Operations in
Obstetrics and Gynecology
Text and Atlas

Video Contents*

*The videos are available on www.emedicine360.com.

Operations in Obstetrics and Gynecology Text and Atlas

Editor

B Ramesh

MBBS MD DGO FCPS Diploma in Gyne Endoscopy (Atlanta, USA) PhD in Urogynecology

Gyne Laparosurgeon, IVF Specialist and Urogynecologist
Medical Director and Chief Laparoscopic Surgeon
Altius Hospitals Pvt Ltd
Bengaluru, Karnataka, India

JAYPEE

JAYPEE BROTHERS MEDICAL PUBLISHERS

The Health Sciences Publisher

New Delhi | London

Jaypee Brothers Medical Publishers (P) Ltd.

Headquarters
Jaypee Brothers Medical Publishers (P) Ltd
4838/24, Ansari Road, Daryaganj
New Delhi 110 002, India
Phone: +91-11-43574357
Fax: +91-11-43574314
Email: jaypee@jaypeebrothers.com

Overseas Office
J.P. Medical Ltd
83 Victoria Street, London
SW1H 0HW (UK)
Phone: +44 20 3170 8910
Fax: +44 (0)20 3008 6180
Email: info@jpmedpub.com

Website: www.jaypeebrothers.com
Website: www.jaypeedigital.com

Operations in Obstetrics and Gynecology: Text and Atlas

First Edition: **2020**

ISBN: 978-93-89776-72-0

Printed at Replika Press Pvt. Ltd.

Dedication

This book is dedicated to my Parents, Shri Bettaiah and Smt Bhadramma and to all my great teachers. My wife, my children Shreyas and Shrusti, fellowship students past and present, and all my endoscopic colleagues from whom I learnt various techniques and to all my patients from whom I learnt the clinical art of Gynecology and techniques of all types of Surgeries.

Contributors

Abdul Basith
MBBS MD Fellowship in Minimal Access Surgery Diploma in Minimal Access Surgery, Post Doctoral Fellowship in Reproductive Medicine
Infertility Specialist
Chennai, Tamil Nadu, India

Aditi Rai MBBS DNB (Obs & Gyn)
Fellow in Minimally Invasive Surgery
Altius Hospitals Pvt Ltd
Bengaluru, Karnataka, India

Apoorva Pallam Reddy
MBBS MS DNB (Obs & Gyn)
Reproductive Endocrinologist (Infertility)
Gynecologist, Laparoscopic Surgeon (Obs & Gyn)
Infertility Specialist
Medical Director
Phoenix Specialty Clinic
Bengaluru, Karnataka, India

B Ramesh
MBBS MD DGO FCPS Diploma in Gyne Endoscopy (Atlanta, USA) PhD in Urogynecology
Gyne Laparosurgeon
IVF Specialist and Urogynecologist
Medical Director and
Chief Laparoscopic Surgeon
Altius Hospitals Pvt Ltd
Bengaluru, Karnataka, India

Bhuvana S MS (Obs & Gyn)
Associate Professor
Department of Obstetrics and Gynecology
Sri Ramachandra Institute of
Higher Education and Research
Chennai, Tamil Nadu, India

Chandramouli MS
MBBS MS (General Surgery) FRCS
Consultant GI and Laparoscopic Surgeon
Fortis Hospital
Bengaluru, Karnataka, India

Dhivya B MS DNB FMIS (Gyne) PGDMLE
Consultant Gynecologist
Rainbow Hospital
Bengaluru, Karnataka, India

Dipak Limbachiya MBBS MD DGO
Director
Eva Women's Hospital and Endoscopy Center
Ahmedabad, Gujarat, India

Divyesh V Shukla
MBBS MD Diploma in Advance Gynecological Endoscopic Surgeries
Director
Isha Hospital
Vadodara, Gujarat, India

G Hemasree MS (Obs & Gyn)
Fellow in Minimally Invasive Surgery
Altius Hospitals Pvt Ltd
Bengaluru, Karnataka, India

GN Vasantha Lakshmi MD
Associate Professor
Department of Obstetrics and Gynecology
Sri Ramachandra Institute of
Higher Education and Research
Chennai, Tamil Nadu, India

Isha Rani MBBS DNB
Fellow in Minimally Invasive Surgery
Altius Hospital Pvt Ltd
Bengaluru, Karnataka, India

Jay Mehta MBBS DNB (Obs & Gyn)
Director
Shree IVF Clinic
Mumbai, Maharashtra, India

Jaya V MD (Obs & Gyn)
Professor
Department of Obstetrics and Gynecology
Sri Ramachandra Institute of
Higher Education and Research
Chennai, Tamil Nadu, India

Jnaneswari TL MBBS MD DNB FIGE
Consultant Obstetrician & Gynecology and Laparoscopic Surgeon
BL Hospital
Bengaluru, Karnataka, India

Kavya Rashmi Rao MBBS MS FMIS
Endoscopy Consultant
Gynecologist Lap Surgeon
Mangaluru, Karnataka, India

Kiruthiga T MS
Assistant Professor
Department of Obstetrics and Gynecology
Sri Ramachandra Institute of
Higher Education and Research
Chennai, Tamil Nadu, India

KS Rajeswari MD
Professor
Department of Obstetrics and Gynecology
Sri Ramachandra Institute of
Higher Education and Research
Chennai, Tamil Nadu, India

Madhuri V MD
Consultant
Altius Hospitals Pvt Ltd
Bengaluru, Karnataka, India

Mala Raj MD
Obstetrician and Gynecologist
Laparoscopy and Infertility Specialist
Aesthetic Gynecologist
Managing Director
Firm Hospitals
Chennai, Tamil Nadu, India

Meenakshi Sundaram
MBBS MD
Consultant Gynecologist
Laparoscopic and Robotic Surgeon
Apollo Hospitals
Chennai, Tamil Nadu, India

Mehul V Sukhadiya MBBS DGO
Consultant
Sumiran Women's Hospital
Ahmedabad, Gujarat, India

MG Dhanalakshmi MD
Professor
Department of Obstetrics and Gynecology
Sri Ramachandra Institute of
Higher Education and Research
Chennai, Tamil Nadu, India

Minal Kumbhalwar MBBS DGO DNB
Fellow in Minimally Invasive Surgery
Altius Hospitals Pvt Ltd
Bengaluru, Karnataka, India

N Palaniappan MD
Professor
Department of Obstetrics and Gynecology
Sri Ramachandra Institute of
Higher Education and Research
Chennai, Tamil Nadu, India

Onimi Syamala MD
Associate Professor
Department of Obstetrics and Gynecology
Sri Ramachandra Institute of
Higher Education and Research
Chennai, Tamil Nadu, India

Pooja Sharma
Consultant
Altius Hospitals Pvt Ltd
Bengaluru, Karnataka, India

Praveen Rathod
MD MCh (Gyn Oncology) International Fellowship in Gyn Oncology/Clinical Visits at RPCI, MSKCC (New York, USA, La Fe Hospital, Valencia, Spain)
Senior Consultant Gynecological Oncology
Laparoscopic Surgery and Associate Professor
Kidwai Cancer Institute/Corporate Hospitals
Bengaluru, Karnataka, India

Preet Agarwal MS (Obs & Gyn)
Associate Professor
Department of Obstetrics and Gynecology
Sri Ramachandra Institute of
Higher Education and Research
Chennai, Tamil Nadu, India

Prijy TP MBBS MS DGO
Consultant Obstetrician and Gynecologist
Malankara Medical Mission Hospital
Thrissur, Kerala, India

Priyanka HK MS (Obs & Gyn) FMIS DMAS
Bengaluru, Karnataka, India

Punitha Rangaraj MBBS DGO
Gynecologist
Laparoscopic Surgeon (Obs & Gyn) Infertility Specialist
Belle Vue's Cambridge Hospital
Bengaluru, Karnataka, India

R Niranjana Radhakrishnan MBBS DNB
Fellow in MIS
Altius Hospitals Pvt Ltd
Bengaluru, Karnataka, India

Rachana Ghanti MBBS MS (Obs & Gyn) FMIS
Senior Resident
Department of Obstetrics and Gynecology
Karnataka Institute of Medical Sciences
Hubballi, Karnataka, India

Ravindranath Nirwani MD
Embryologist
Altius Hospitals Pvt Ltd
Bengaluru, Karnataka, India

Rubina Pandit
MBBS MD (PGIMER) Fellowship in Reproductive Medicine (FIRM-RGUHS)
Consultant
Altius Hospitals Pvt Ltd
Bengaluru, Karnataka, India

Sandip Datta Roy MD
Gynecologist and Laparoscopic Surgeon
Altius Hospitals Pvt Ltd
Bengaluru, Karnataka, India

Shabana Nawaz Ansari MD
Embryologist
Altius Hospitals Pvt Ltd
Bengaluru, Karnataka, India

Shailesh Puntambekar MD
Oncosurgeon
Galaxy Hospital
Pune, Maharashtra, India

Shashikala T MBBS DGO FRM
Laparoscopic Surgeon
Obstetrician and Gynecologist
Milann IVF
Bengaluru, Karnataka, India

Sheila K Pillai MD
Associate Professor
Department of Obstetrics and Gynecology
Sri Ramachandra Institute of
Higher Education and Research
Chennai, Tamil Nadu, India

Shilpi D Shukla MD
Director
Isha Hospital
Vadodara, Gujarat, India

Shruthi Prashanth MS
Assistant Professor
Department of Obstetrics and Gynecology
Sri Ramachandra Institute of
Higher Education and Research
Chennai, Tamil Nadu, India

Shruti Paliwal MBBS MS FMIS
Assistant Professor
Department of Obstetrics and Gynecology
SAIMS Medical College
Indore, Madhya Pradesh, India

Shubhanjali Sen MBBS MS
Fellow in Minimal Invasive Surgery
Altius Hospitals Pvt Ltd
Bengaluru, Karnataka, India

Shwetha Kamath MBBS MS FMIS
Consultant
Altius Hospitals Pvt Ltd
Bengaluru, Karnataka, India

Shwetha Shah MBBS MS DNB
Fellow in Minimal Invasive Surgery
Altius Hospitals Pvt Ltd
Bengaluru, Karnataka, India

Sirisha PNSRS MS
Associate Professor
Department of Obstetrics and Gynecology
Sri Ramachandra Institute of
Higher Education and Research
Chennai, Tamil Nadu, India

Sowmya MS MBBS MS DNB FIMS
Assistant Professor
Department of Obstetrics and Gynecology
Rajarajeshwari Medical College
Bengaluru, Karnataka, India

Supriya Raina MD FIMS
Consultant
Mamatha Medical College
Hyderabad, Telangana, India

Sushila Saini
MBBS MS DGES (Germany) FAMS (USA) FICMCH
Obstetrician and Gynecologist
Doorben Hospital
Jaipur, Rajasthan, India

Swetha Gulabi MS
Assistant Professor
Department of Obstetrics and Gynecology
Sri Ramachandra Institute of
Higher Education and Research
Chennai, Tamil Nadu, India

Tanvi Desai MBBS DNB
Fellow in Minimally Invasive Gynecologist
Altius Hospitals Pvt Ltd
Bengaluru, Karnataka, India

Usha Rani G MD
Professor
Department of Obstetrics and Gynecology
Sri Ramachandra Institute of
Higher Education and Research
Chennai, Tamil Nadu, India

Usha Vishwanath MD
Professor
Department of Obstetrics and Gynecology
Sri Ramachandra Institute of
Higher education and Research
Chennai, Tamil Nadu, India

Preface

Obstetrics and Gynecology is ever expanding with many subspecialties and being a surgical branch, there are innumerable surgeries in each subspecialty. I realized that there is no comprehensive book for all these surgeries. The idea of this book is to bring all the surgeries in one book so that it can serve as a ready reckoner for any gynecologic surgeon and this book is for of practical guide rather than theoretical so that just by looking at the real surgical pictures one can copy the steps during surgery.

The vast majority of chapters are from laparoscopic section because today most of the gyne surgeries are done laparoscopically. There are special chapters on practical aspects of ART, Single Port Surgeries, Uterine Transplant, all in Recent Advances. The clinician should apply their theory knowledge while operating as it is not possible to provide entire information in surgical text. There are many chapters on vaginal surgeries combining the traditional techniques and repairs. There is a good section on Hysteroscopy and a chapter on stem cell injection. It is demonstrated hysteroscopically, which will be useful to ART specialists. Important topics of obstetrics are covered in that section and reader can find any number of books already in the market on obstetric operations. I hope this book will be useful to one and all.

B Ramesh

Acknowledgments

I am grateful to all my teachers who taught the basic steps of gynecology. This book is a culmination of the hard work of many individuals, who has contributed. Especially I am thankful to my parents and family members; my wife Dr Shobha, two beloved children, my son Shreyas and my daughter Shrusti. All of them gave constant support and for allowing me to pursue my dreams.

I am also grateful to all my colleagues and other gynecologists who gave constant encouragement and support, which created a lot of curiosity in doing this book.

I thank especially Mr Shiju, who is an invaluable part of our operating team and our contributor; Dr Punitha Rangaraj, Dr Divyesh V Shukla, Dr Meenakshi Sundaram, Dr Abdul Basith, Dr Jay Mehta, Dr Praveen Rathod, Dr Shashikala T, Dr Jnaneshwari, Dr Apoorva Pallam Reddy, Dr Mala Raj, Dr Mehul Sukhadiya, Dr Sushila Saini, Dr Rachana Ghanti, Dr Shwetha Kamath, Dr Dhivya, Dr Kavya Rashmi Rao, Dr Sowmya MS, Dr Priyanka HK, Dr Supriya Raina, Dr Shruti Paliwal, Dr Prijy, Dr Tanvi, Dr Shubhanjali Sen, Dr Shwetha Shah, Dr Niranjana Radhakrishnan, Dr Aditi Rai, Dr Isha Rani, Dr Minal Kumbhalwar, Dr Garlapati Hema, Dr Rubina Pandit, Mr Ravindranath Nirwani, Ms Shabana Nawaz Ansari, Mrs Hemalata Malini for helping me from time to time for successfully completing this project.

Our special thanks to all the obstetricians and gynecologists of Sri Ramachandra Institute of Higher Education and Research, Chennai, Tamil Nadu, India, Dr Usha Rani G, Dr Jaya V, Dr Usha Vishwanath, Dr N Palaniappan, Dr KS Rajeswari, Dr MG Dhanalakshmi, Dr Onimi Syamala, Dr Sheila K Pillai, Dr GN Vasantha Lakshmi, Dr Preet Agarwal, Dr Bhuvana S, Dr Sirisha PNSRS, Dr Shruthi Prashanth, Dr Kiruthiga T, and Dr Swetha Gulabi, for supporting as a part of publishing this book.

I am thankful to Shri Jitendar P Vij (Group Chairman), Mr Ankit Vij (Managing Director), Mr Venugopal and other staff of M/s Jaypee Brothers Medical Publishers (P) Ltd, New Delhi, India, for their support in publishing this atlas textbook.

Contents

SECTION 1 GYNECOLOGY

SECTION 2 HYSTEROSCOPY

SECTION 3 OBSTETRICS

SECTION 4 IN VITRO FERTILIZATION AND ASSISTED REPRODUCTIVE TECHNIQUE

SECTION 5 SINGLE-PORT SURGERIES IN GYNECOLOGY

1 SECTION

Gynecology

CHAPTER

1

Laparoscopy Instruments

Shruti Paliwal, G Hemasree, B Ramesh

CREATION OF PNEUMOPERITONEUM

VERESS NEEDLE (FIGS. 1 TO 4)

Invented by physician Veres for pleural fluid aspiration.

Sterilized by formalin vapor or glutaraldehyde.

Identification: Available in 4 sizes of length 70, 100, 120 and 200 mm. Particularly for obese patients 120 mm and for thinner patients with scaphoid shape of abdomen 70 mm has to be used. Outer needle of gauge 16 and has sharp end. Its other end is cylindrical. There is another needle inside this needle, which has blunt end and subterminal opening. Other end has luer hub and its lumen is closed by means of 2-way valve. There is spring between two needles, which allows withdrawal of inner needle into outer needle.

Indications: Needle is used for induction of pneumoperitoneum prior to insertion of trocar and sleeve for laparoscopy.

Method of use: Needle is held by cylindrical part of outer needle like pen. Hold the Veress needle like pen at an angle of 45° pointing towards anus to avoid injury to vena cava or aorta. Through a small incision in inferior part of umbilicus, it is passed into abdominal wall and peritoneal cavity while abdominal wall is elevated away from posterior abdominal wall. When the inner blunt needle encounters resistance of abdominal wall, it recedes into outer needle, so sharp point is the advancing point and penetrates abdominal wall with ease. Once peritoneum is pierced, inner needle projects out again, thereby preventing injury to intraperitoneal structures.

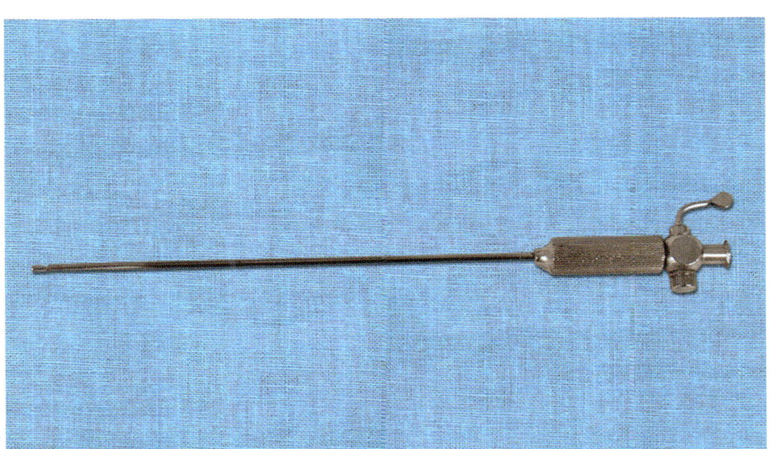

Fig. 1: Veress needle.

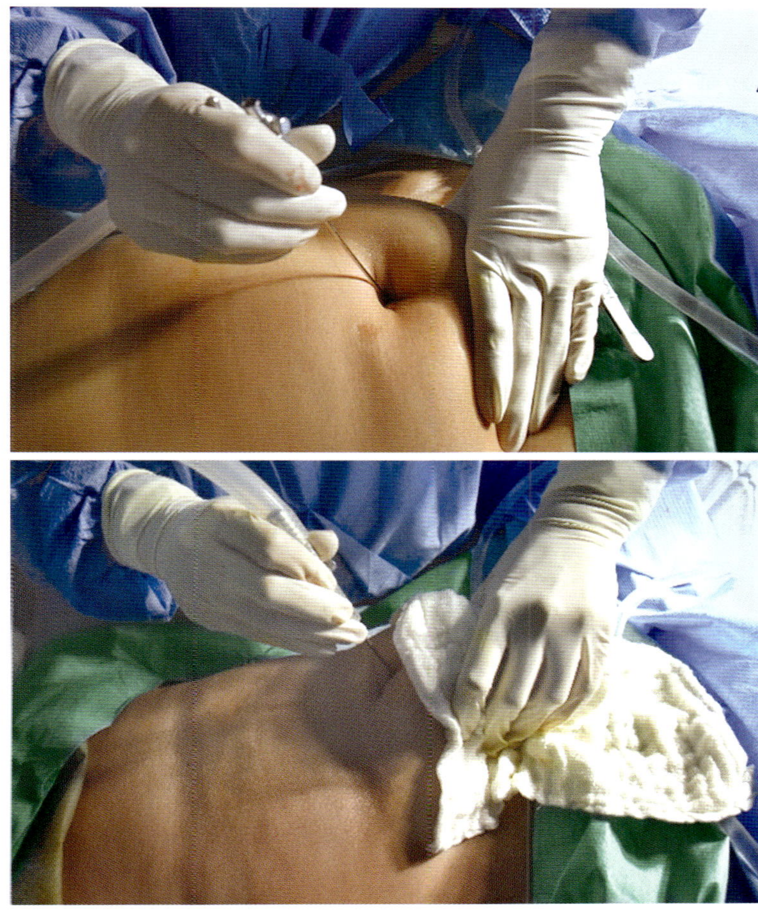

Fig. 2: Insertion of Veress needle.

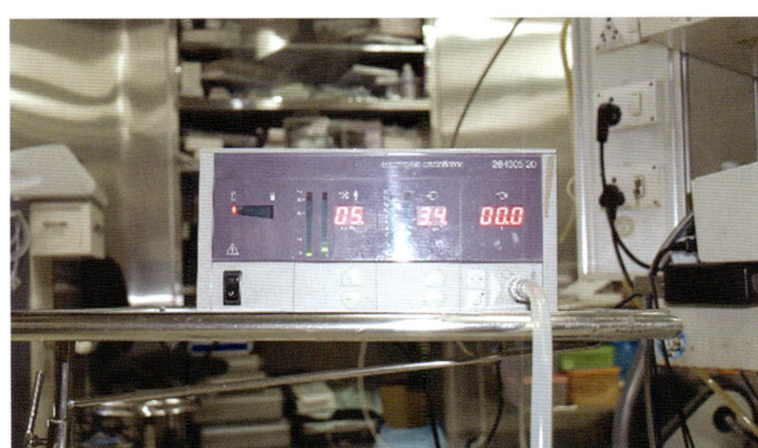

Fig. 3: Veress needle intraperitoneal.

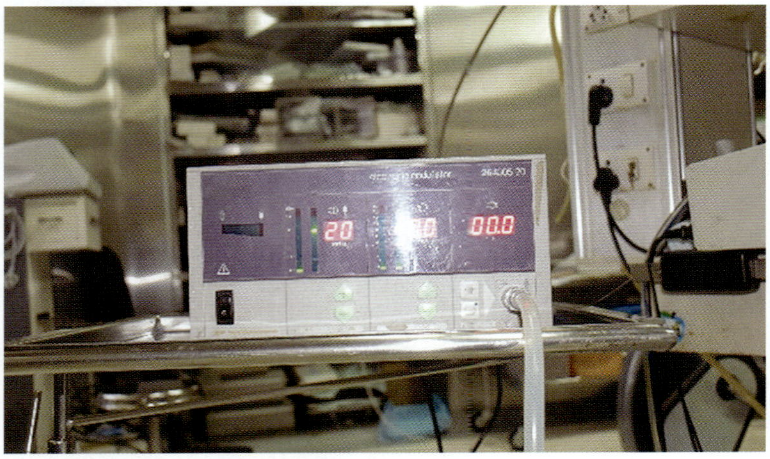

Fig. 4: Veress needle extraperitoneal.

Entry of needle into peritoneal cavity is confirmed by:

- Drop test, whereby a saline drop placed over needle hub gets sucked inside needle because of intra-abdominal pressure is less than atmospheric pressure (plunger test)
- Saline can be freely injected into needle and cannot be reaspirated.
- Movement of tip of needle is free.

Alternate sites for introduction of Veress needle are:

- Supraumbilical, infraumbilical, within umbilicus—superior crease, inferior crease, transumbilical
- Lateral rectus border at either the left subcostal margin or McBurney's point
- Midway between pubic symphysis and umbilicus
- Posterior fornix transvaginally
- Palmer's point (2 cm below the left costal margin).

INSUFFLATORS (FIGS. 5 AND 6)

The electronic CO_2 insufflator is a general-purpose insufflation unit for use in laparoscopic examination and operations. It is a basic prerequisite for surgical laparoscopy, as it offers the option for reducing operating time to minimum. CO_2 is the preferred gas because it does not support combustion, is very soluble and decreases risk of gas embolism and is cheap. Ideal insufflators deliver rapid, accurate flow rates of CO_2 gas up to 15 L/min. In actual measurement, the true amount delivered at end of tube is 60–70% of capable flow rate of insufflator. Some insufflators have heating capability to warm the gas, thus decreasing the intra-abdominal hypothermic effect of cold CO_2 gas and decreased fogging of distal lens of laparoscope. The insufflator compensates for changes in intra-abdominal pressure. The insufflator activates and delivers automatically when intra-abdominal pressure falls below preset pressure. To avoid complications as subcutaneous emphysema, intra-abdominal pressure should not exceed 16 mm Hg.

The basic information that should be supplied by readout of insufflator is:

- Insufflation pressure
- Intra-abdominal pressure
- Insufflation volume per minute
- Total amount of gas used.

TROCAR SLEEVE AND TROCAR (FIGS. 7 AND 8)

Identification: Trocar sleeve is made of metal or nonconductive material as fiberglass or Teflon®. Trocar is made of metal. Size of a

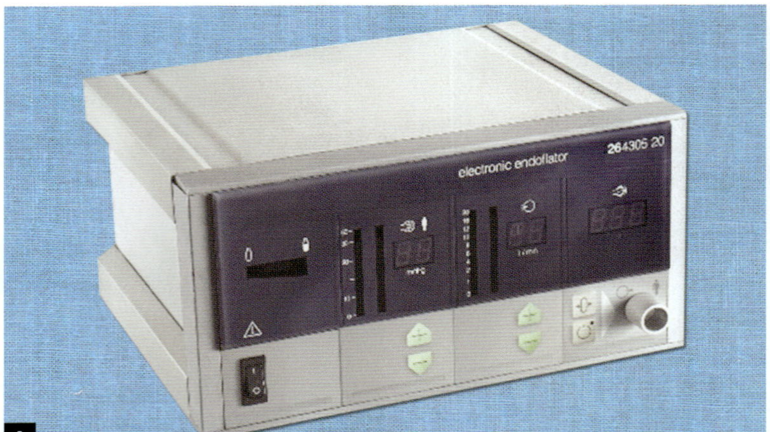

A

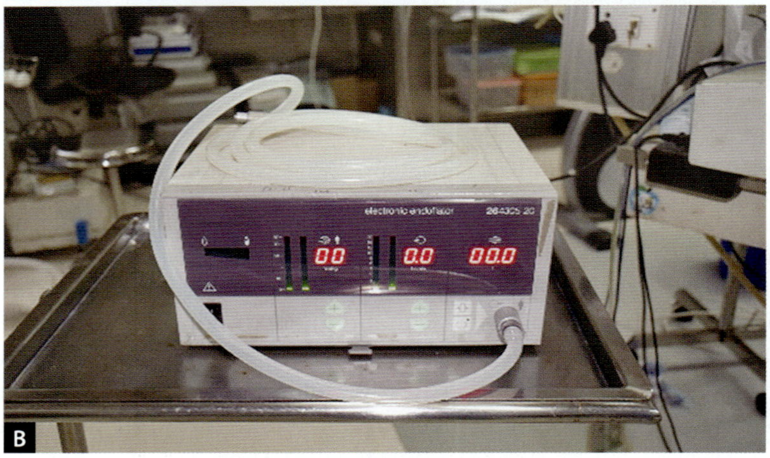

B

Figs. 5A and B: Insufflator.

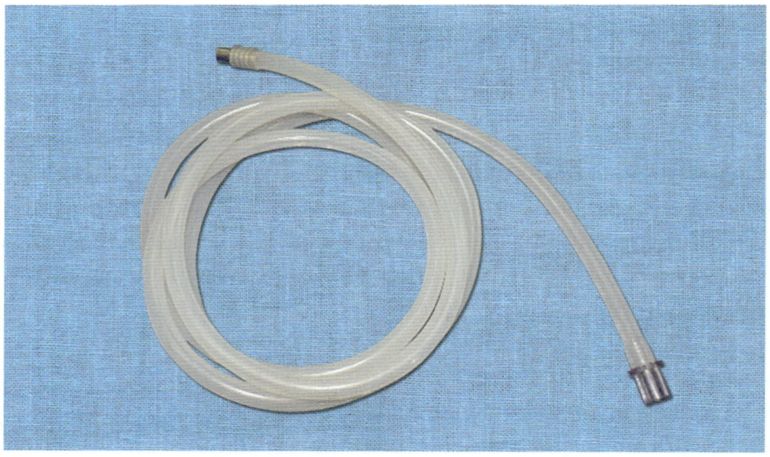

Fig. 6: Insufflator tube.

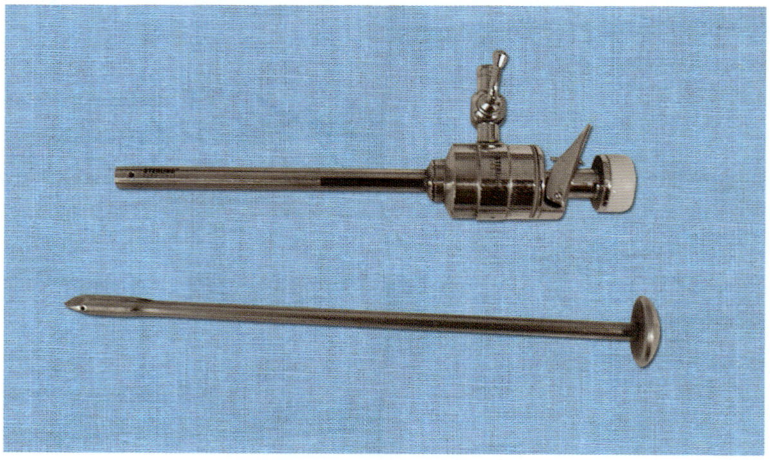

Fig. 7: Trocar sleeve and trocar.

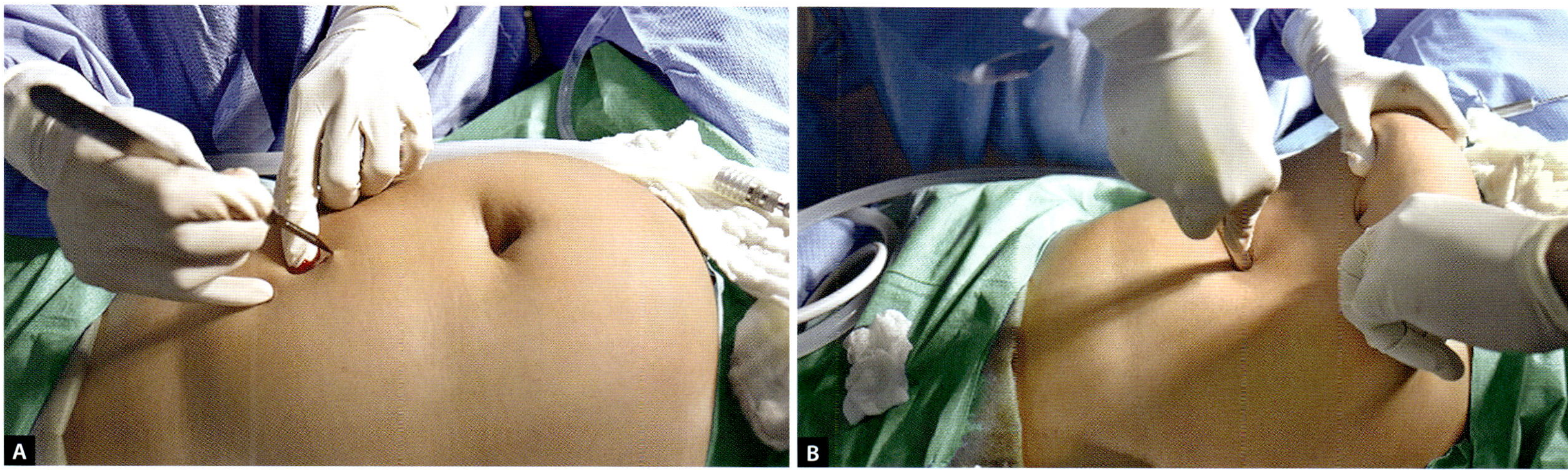

Figs. 8A and B: Insertion of primary trocar.

trocar sleeve depends on size of laparoscope, larger for operative laparoscope. Tip of trocar may be conical or pyramidal. Pyramidal penetrates abdominal wall more easily. Each trocar sleeve has valve, which may be a trumpet valve or flipper valve. Trumpet valve has plunger on side of trocar sleeve which must be pressed before trocar or laparoscope is inserted. It opens automatically on pressure of trocar or laparoscope and closes on removal of latter by spring action. Trumpet valves are mostly found in telescope trocars. Telescope is protected from contamination by tissue and blood particles during insertion by pressing on trumpet valve. Flipper is attached to trocar sleeve with hinge, kept in place by magnetic action. It opens under pressure of tip of trocar and closes on removal of same by magnetic action. Trocar sleeve often has inlet for gas, with 2-way valve. Sleeve has perforations near distal end for flow of gas. Trocar is hollow and cavity communicates with 2–3 openings projecting beyond sleeve. Gas escapes through this opening at the time of exsufflation of peritoneum. EndoTip is used for complicated cases with increased suspicion of adhesion to avoid bowel injury.

In general, trocar with different sizes is used in surgical endoscopy. The standard sizes are 5.5, 11, 12, 15 and 22 mm.

Sterilized by formalin vapor or glutaraldehyde.

Port is best inserted by Hasson's open technique. Benefits include less postoperative pain, less blood loss, faster recovery time, less infections, less need of medications, fewer complications and better cosmetic results.

Trocar and trocar sleeve are used for insertion of laparoscope or the second puncture instrument into peritoneal cavity.

Method of insertion: Trocar is pushed completely into cannula and held with broad end resting against thenar eminence, index finger extending along length and medial three fingers cradling the instrument. Thumb holds the sleeve on other side. Instrument is passed subcutaneously till distal edge of trocar sleeve disappears under skin edge. Then direction changed toward pelvis and passed toward the left and after penetrating rectus sheath toward right to trace zigzag course. During insertion of trocar sleeve, abdominal wall is held away from posterior abdominal wall to avoid accidental injury to retroperitoneal vessels. During insertion, trocar with pyramidal tip is thrust inside without any rotatory movements as cutting edges would churn up tissues. Conical tip can be inserted with rotatory movements also. Sharp pyramidal trocar tips can be positioned relatively easily. Sharp edges can sometimes damage smaller blood vessels and other organs. By using spherical, blunt trocar tips, the blood vessels are pushed aside and protected. However, greater pressure has to be exerted during insertion of blunt trocar. Better protection to prevent trocar slipping out of intraperitoneal space is provided by sheaths with screw threading. However, they caused increased trauma to both abdominal wall and peritoneum. During removal of trocar and sleeve, trocar is pushed in all the way, otherwise omentum and bowel are dragged into sleeve along with trocar and sleeve.

Trocar Sleeve Adaptor (Fig. 9)

It is a small trocar sleeve with rim that fits over the proximal end of large-sized trocar sleeve and a tubular portion that passes into larger-sized trocar sleeve. The opening in proximal broad end is smaller, so instrument with smaller external diameter fits in without permitting leakage of gas of pneumoperitoneum.

Indication: It is used to convert a large-sized trocar sleeve into smaller-sized trocar sleeve, so instrument with smaller external diameter fits in.

LAPAROSCOPE (FIG. 10)

There are two types of telescope, rigid and flexible. Rigid scopes are based on Hopkins rod-lens system. Rigid rod lens provides good resolution and better depth perception.

Three important structural differences in telescope available in market:

- 6–18 rod-lens system telescope are available.
- 0–120° telescopes are available.
- 1.5–15 mm telescope are available.

Laparoscope has an objective, an eyepiece, a light-conducting system connecting the two, a fiber optic bundle for transmission of light from light source to peritoneal cavity and an operative instrument channel if it is an operative laparoscope. The objective, eyepiece and light-conducting image relay system constitutes telescope.

The telescope may have either long glass rods and air lens in between, or long air columns with glass lenses at end. Better telescope have coherent fiber optic bundle instead of long glass rod for transmission of light. System with glass rod or fiber optic bundle is known as Hopkins system. The fiber optic bundle for transmission of light is not coherent; it runs parallel to image-relay system.

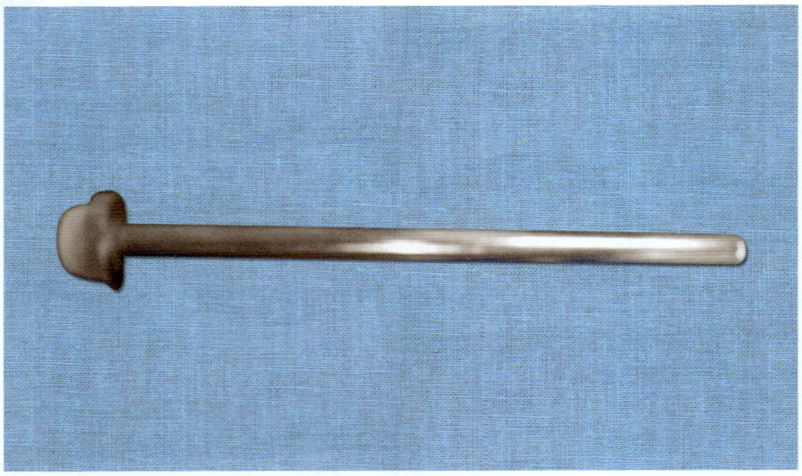

Fig. 9: Trocar sleeve adaptor.

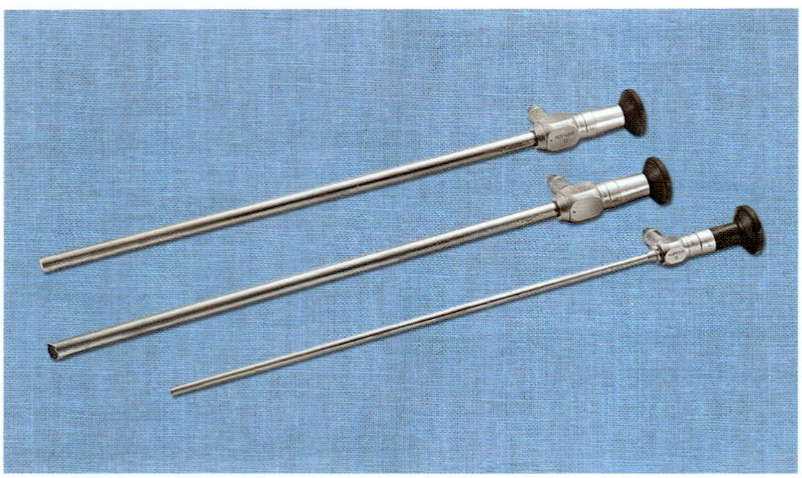

Fig. 10: Laparoscope.

At the proximal end, it can be connected to fiber optic cable that transmits light to the bundle from light source. Fiber optic bundle has more than 200,000 fibers, each fiber 0.05 mm in diameter. Each fiber has outer cladding of low refractive index class fused to it optically by drawing through a furnace together. Light transmission occurs by total internal reflection. It is cold light as heat is dissipated and only light is transmitted.

Hopkins system is better because it transmits light 2.25 times faster, giving a wider viewing angle, increasing the clear aperture of tube and greatly enhancing image quality.

The various telescopes and their application range are described below:

- *0° straightforward telescope:* It has greatest application range because it facilitates orientation and conveys an impression of the area inspected. Direction of view corresponds to natural approach and usual perspective. It is usually preferred in gynecological interventions.
- *30° forward-oblique telescope:* It is used in majority of cases in gynecology, as it gives a better overview and offers better image resolution. It can be rotated to enlarge the field of vision. Use of 30° telescope is advantageous during dissection in Douglas pouch, especially in cases with severe endometriosis, dissection of UV fold, anterior wall lower segment fibroid, and broad ligament fibroid.

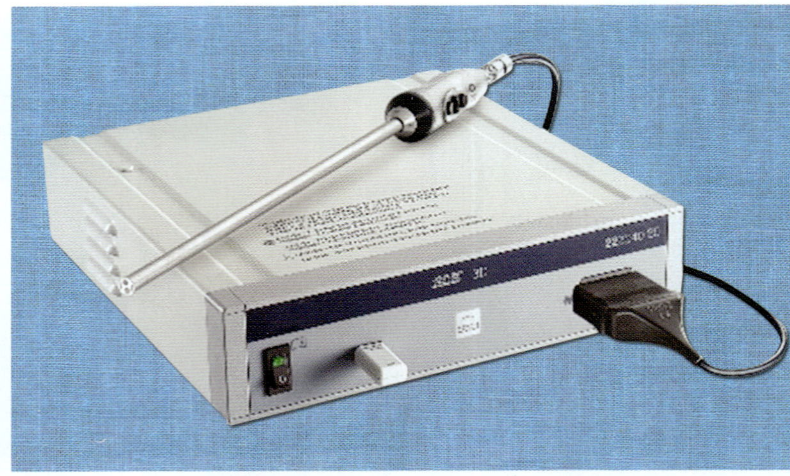

Fig. 11: 3D laparoscope with camera unit.

- 45° telescope.
- *Three-dimensional (3D) laparoscope:* It has improved the depth perception, especially in difficult cases like large size uterus, dense adhesions as in previous cesarean section, endometriosis. Advent of 3D has reduced the operating time significantly.

Angle of vision of laparoscope varies from 130° to 180° and field of vision 60° to 75°. Magnification achieved is product of linear magnification of objective and visual magnification of eyepiece. Zoom effect is achieved at a lesser distance, while magnification is less than 1 at greater distance **(Fig. 11)**.

Configuration available for viewing extension in operative laparoscope is oblique, parallel offset or perpendicular. With oblique and perpendicular types, the number of prisms is reduced so the clarity and brightness of image is better. Oblique type is more convenient for use.

The diameter of diagnostic laparoscope varies between 5 mm and 10 mm and that of operative laparoscope varies between 9 mm and 12 mm. Operative laparoscope carries an operating channel 3–5 mm in diameter, its lightening capacity and image quality are inferior and field of vision is lesser. Operative telescopes are generally 0° straightforward telescope. A 30° telescope gives more space internally and externally. Flexible telescope gives a variable angle of view and is better. If internally flexible scope is not available then an externally flexible scope is used. It removes assistant's hand from surgeon's field. Olympus flexible telescope has secondary flexion capability by which it can be positioned near operating area and locked.

Additional devices can be connected to laparoscope, such as CO_2 laser, for laparoscopic sterilization, tissue fragment or biopsy specimens can be extracted through telescope trocar with aid of grasping forceps, introduced through telescope's instrument channel.

A Veress optical needle with insufflation can be used in some difficult cases in order to perform mini laparoscopy.

Laparoscope is sterilized by exposure to formalin vapors or immersion in glutaraldehyde. It has to be cleaned with normal saline before use.

Laparoscopic Video Monitor (Fig. 12)

Surgical monitors are different from television at home. Monitors last for long time, so it is a high-end product with at least 600 lines

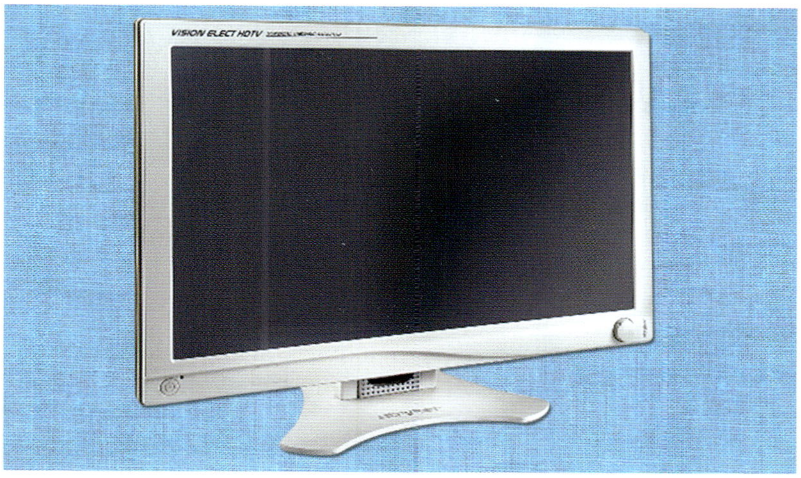

Fig. 12: Laparoscopic video monitor.

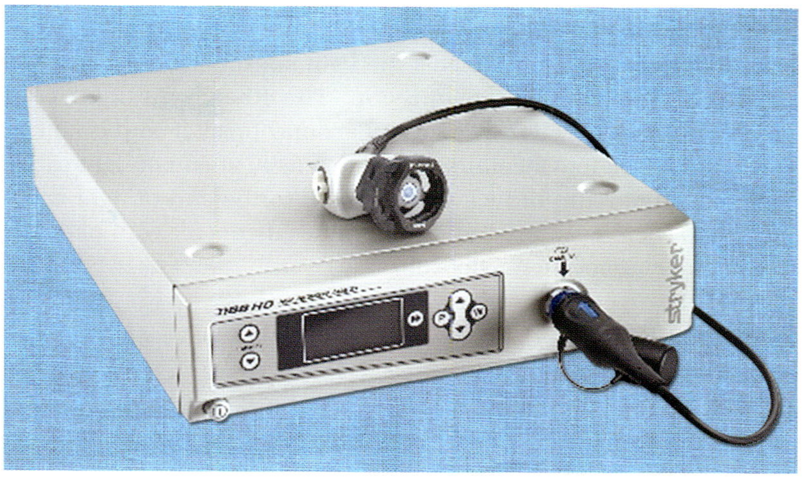

Fig. 13: Full high-definition camera.

resolution. Size of screen varies from 8 inches to 21 inches. The closer the surgeon is to monitor, smaller the monitor should be to get better picture.

In modern practice, additional recording components as digital capture and photo printers are appended. The best pictures come from the fewest devices that the video signal has to pass through. Arranging the components in distributed configuration gives best image quality.

The basic principle of image reproduction is horizontal beam scanning on face of picture tube. Plate is coated internally with a fluorescent substance containing phosphor. This generates electron when struck by beam from the electron gun. As the beam sweeps horizontally and back it covers all the picture elements before reaching original position. This occurs repetitively and rapidly. The method is called horizontal linear scanning. The final image depends upon the number of lines of resolution, scanning lines, pixels and dot pitch. Horizontal resolution is the number of vertical lines that can be seen and vice versa. Pixels denote the number of picture elements and responsible for picture resolution. The more the number of pixels, the better the resolution.

Camera And Light Source (Fig. 13)

First medical camera was introduced by Circon™ Corporation in 1972. 2-chip, 3-chip and high-definition (HD) cameras are available. They are attached to eyepiece of laparoscope at one end and display monitor at other end. Endoscopic findings can be seen on monitor. Improves ease of surgery as well as coordination of assistants who can view the surgery.

The number of pixels determines the resolution. The average chip contains 250,000–380,000 pixels. Cameras are classified according to number of chips. They differ in the way they relay information to the monitor. Color separation is used to create a colored video image from original black and white. In single-chip camera, color separation is achieved by adding a stripe filter that covers the whole chip. Each stripe accepts one of the complimentary colors and each pixel is assigned to one stripe.

In single-chip camera, three primary colors are sensed by single chip. In 3-chip cameras, there are three charge-coupled devices (CCDs) chips for separate capture and processing of three primary colors. In 3-chip cameras, color separation is achieved with prism system that overlies the chips. Each chip receives one of the three primary colors. This system gives a higher resolution and better image quality.

Another type of camera is a combination of scope and camera built together with camera chip integrated at distal end of scope so there are no optical lenses.

High-definition camera and monitor have twice the number of scanning lines than conventional video making image more clear.

Within the head of camera is a CCD that sees an image taken by telescope. The head of camera is attached to ocular of the telescope, and the controller, which is located on trolley along with monitor. The camera head consists of an objective lens that focuses the image of the object on the chip. The CCD then converts optical image into an electrical signal sent through camera cable to camera control unit (CCU) unit. The chip has light-sensitive photoreceptor that generates pixels by transforming incoming photons into electronic charges. Electronic charges are then transferred from the pixels to storage element on chip.

Video Camera Unit (Fig. 14)

Within camera is a CCD that sees the optical image through lens and converts it into electrical image. The image is sent through cables to CCU to monitor input. The monitor converts the electrical image to original optical image seen by human eye.

Light Source (Fig. 15)

Good laparoscopic light source should emit light as much as possible near natural sun light. Two types of light source commonly used are:

- Xenon
- Halogen.

Xenon has a more natural color spectrum and smaller spot size than halogen. Yellow light of halogen bulb is compensated for in the video camera by white balancing. A 250-W halogen or xenon light source provides excellent light intensity. The temperature of 6000 K obtained from xenon provides true white light that enhances visualization to permit recognition of pathological changes. Halogen light field is used in medical field since 20 years but the spectral temperature of these lights is 3200 kelvin which makes it too different and too low from natural sunlight.

Light Cable (Fig. 16)

A fluid light cable that connects the light source with laparoscope provides optimal light transmission. The fiber optic light cord should be handled with care, since fibers may break if cord is kinked or dropped. Due to concentrated light intensity at end of light cable, a significant amount of heat is produced, so the end of light cable should not be placed on drapes, nor allowed contact with patient's skin in order to prevent possible burns.

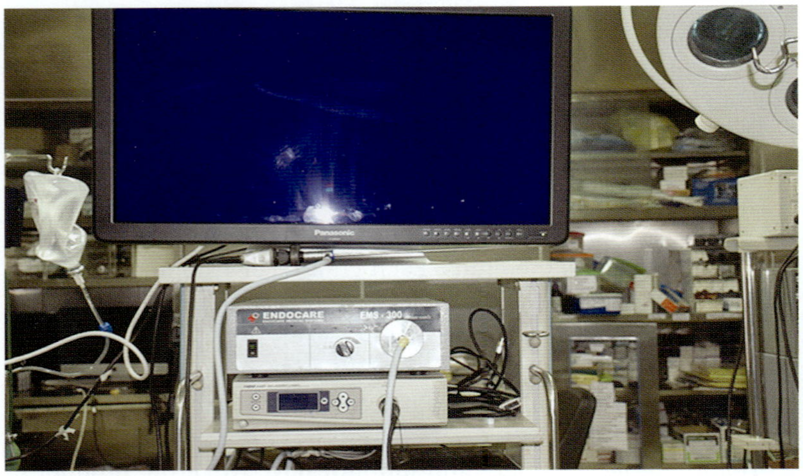

Fig. 14: Video camera unit.

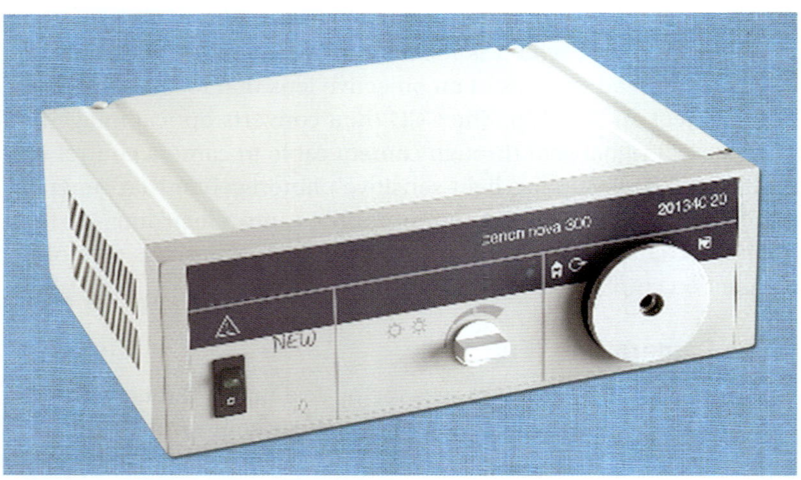

Fig. 15: Xenon light source.

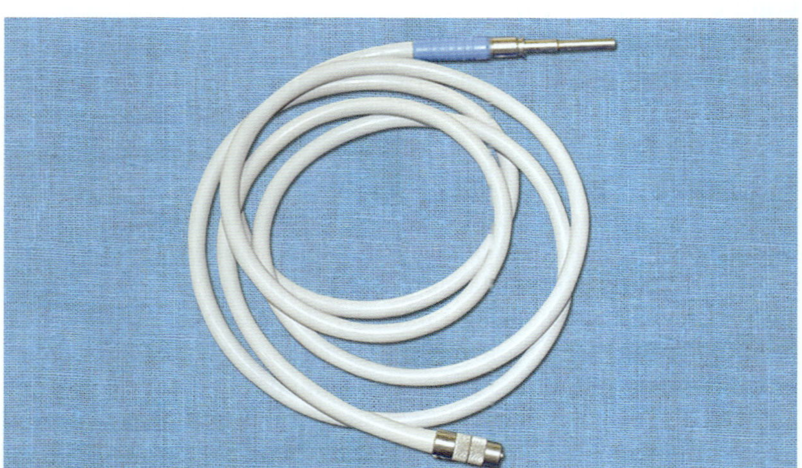

Fig. 16: Light cable.

HAND INSTRUMENTS

GRASPING FORCEPS (FIGS. 17 AND 18)

Identification: They are available in sizes 3–10 mm. The jaws can be blunt or toothed.

Atraumatic grasping forceps have jaws that are flat, long, and oval with fenestrae. They have transverse serrations on inside.

Sterilized by formalin vapor or glutaraldehyde.

Indications:

- To hold the round ligament for manipulation (atraumatic).
- To hold the utero-ovarian ligament to steady the ovary during follicular aspiration (atraumatic).

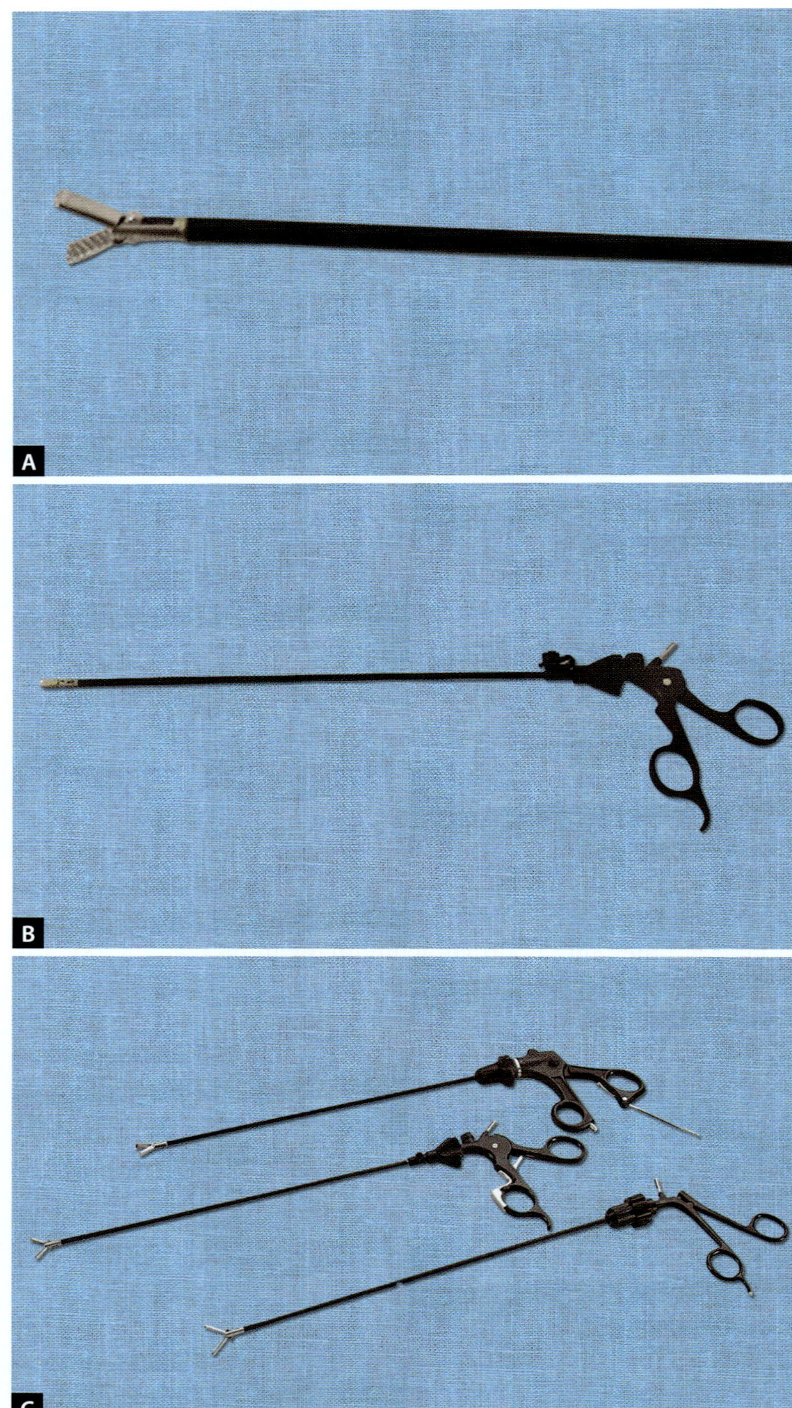

A B C

Figs. 17A to C: Toothed grasper.

- Atraumatic forceps are used to hold Fallopian tube or ureter.
- To hold the UV fold during bladder separation.

Method of use: Instrument is passed into peritoneal cavity through second puncture cannula. Approximation of handle closes the jaws of instrument and structure grasped is securely held.

Toothed Grasper

Uses

- In surgical endoscopy, in case of endoscopic cyst extirpation, they help to fix the ovary capsule properly and remove cystic bag (toothed grasping forceps).
- To hold the myoma during myomectomy.

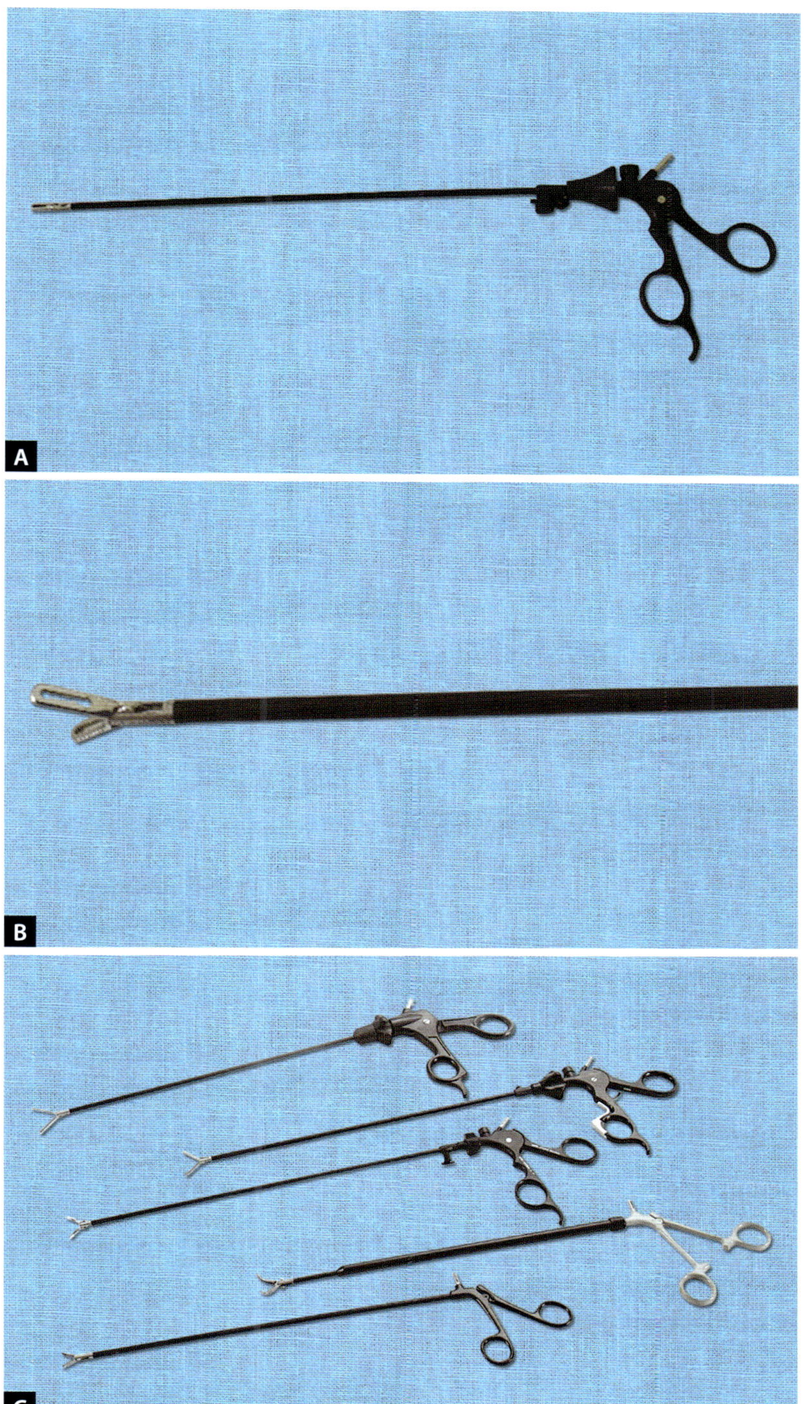

Figs. 18A to C: Nontoothed grasper.

- It can be used as a blunt probe with jaws closed.
- Can give traction with jaws closed.
- It can also serve as needle holder and used to tie suture.

SCISSORS (FIGS. 19 TO 21)

Sterilized by exposure to formalin vapor or glutaraldehyde.

Identification: They can be curved, straight or hooked. Some have an electrical adaptor so they can be combined with unipolar or bipolar electrocoagulation

Indications:

- Used for cutting adhesions or tissues laparoscopically.
- They can divide coagulated tissue and open fallopian tube for salpingostomy.
- Hook scissors are suitable for transecting ligature fibers and for tissue transection.

Method of use: Scissors are passed through second puncture cannula inserted. Hooked scissors have overlapping tips and can cause damage even when closed. Tissue to be divided is hooked on lower blade of scissors and cut. If there is bleeding, it is controlled by electrocoagulation.

Types of scissors:

- *Straight scissors:* Widely used for mechanical dissection in laparoscopic surgery, divide desiccated tissue. They give controlled depth of cutting because it has only one moving jaw.

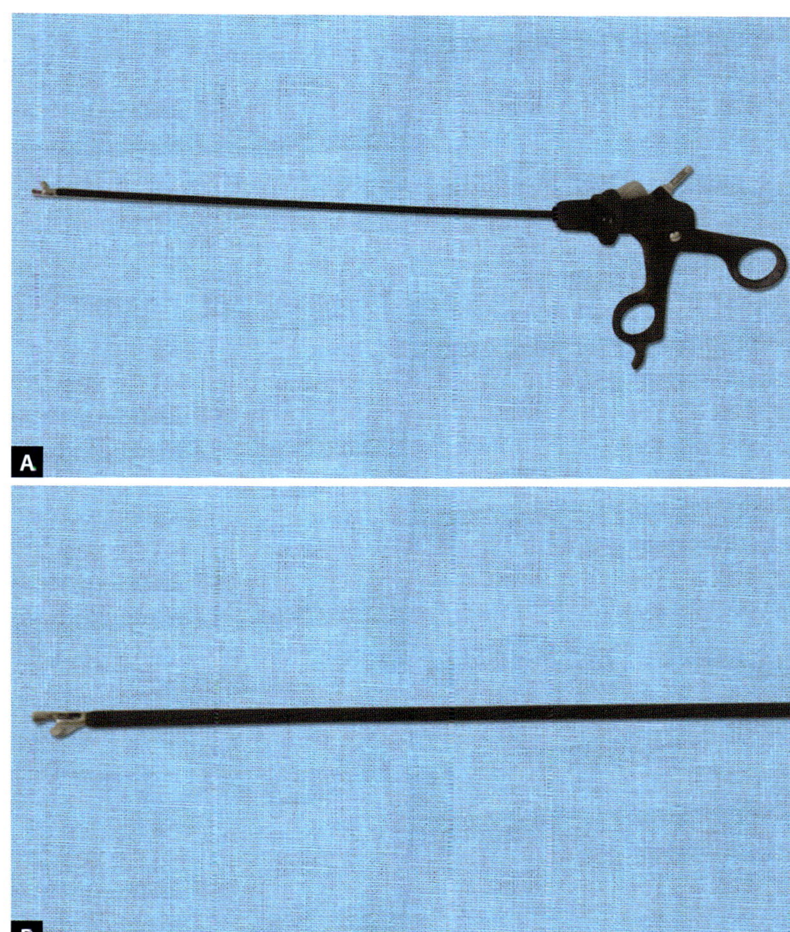

Figs. 19A and B: Hook scissors.

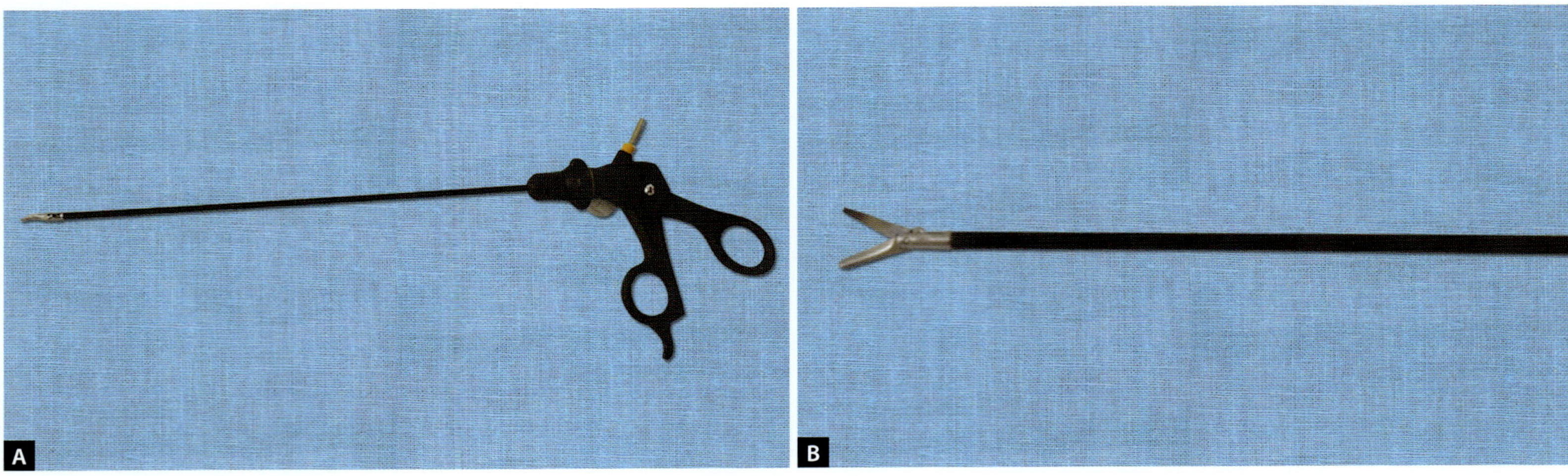

Figs. 20A and B: Curved scissors.

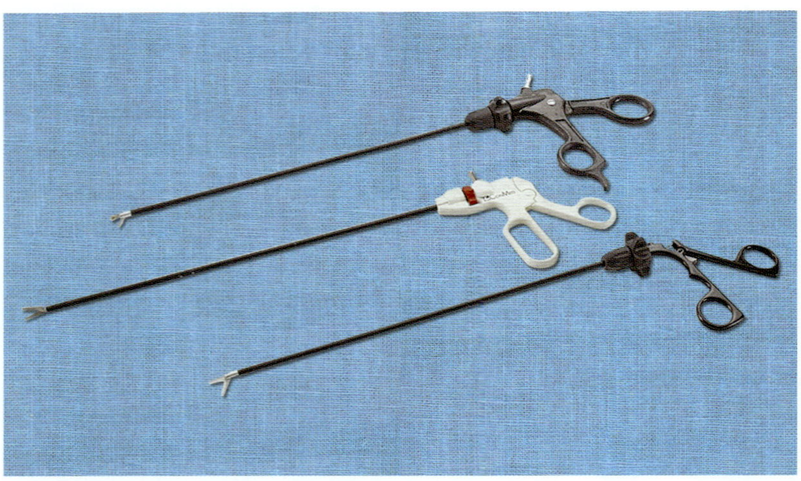

Fig. 21: Hook, straight and curved scissors.

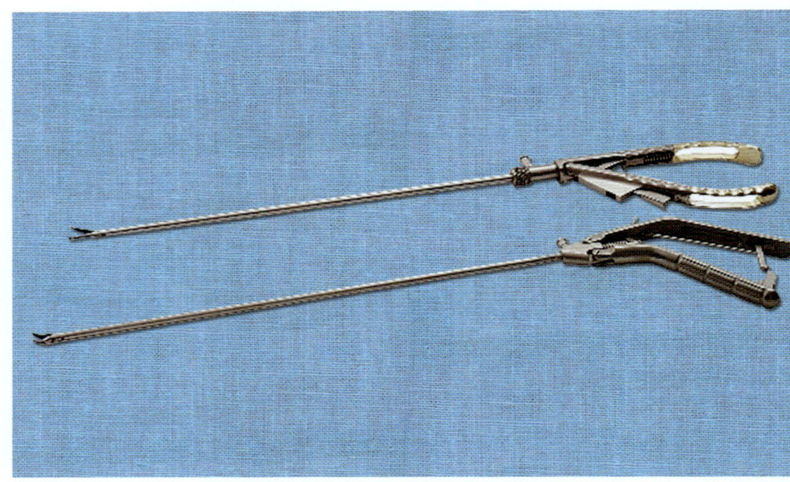

Fig. 22: Needle holder.

- *Curved scissors:* Most widely used in laparoscopic surgeries. They are mounted on curved handle, which is either fixed or retractable. The curvature of blade of these scissors abolishes angle of laparoscopic instrument manipulation. The serrated edges prevent the tissue to slip out of blade. Useful in cutting a slippery tissue or ligature.
- *Hook scissors:* The sharp edge of both the blades is in shape of flattened C. Blades can be partially closed trapping the tissue in the hollow of blade without dividing it and allowing it to be slightly retracted. Advantage of these scissors is that they encircle the structure before cutting it. Tissue is held between jaws and there is no chance of slipping. Especially useful for cutting secured duct or artery in laparoscopic surgery or in tough tissue transection. They have overlapping tips and can cause damage even when closed.
- *Microtip scissors:* They are very fine scissors, either straight or angled, used to partially transect the cystic duct. Advantage is that they can partially cut the duct for facilitating cannulation.

Complications: Injury to adjacent structures, bleeding and complications of electrocoagulation.

NEEDLE HOLDER (FIG. 22)

Needle holder should grasp the needle rock solid hard to prevent rotation. They are available with different type of jaws as curved jaws, flat jaws, or platypus jaws. They are used for laparoscopic knotting and suturing.

CLAW FORCEPS AND TENACULUM (FIGS. 23 TO 25)

It is a 10-mm grasper that requires a 10–11 mm sleeve and is used during myomectomy to remove large pieces of tissue such as suction of tube and ovary or an ectopic pregnancy.

A tenaculum has 10 mm × 35 cm long instrument with single-tooth jaws, fixed shaft and a ratchet handle.

Uses of tenaculum are:

- To steady the uterus during hysterectomy
- To remove the myoma during myomectomy.

MYOMA SCREW (FIG. 26)

The 5-mm and 10-mm myoma screws allow the surgeon to maneuver the myoma and apply traction with improved visibility and access. It can also be used to fix and retract big size uterus at the time of laparoscopic hysterectomy.

ASPIRATION NEEDLE (FIG. 27)

Sterilized by formalin vapor or glutaraldehyde.

Identification: It is 33.5 cm long and has luer hub. Its distal end is thinner than rest of needle being of gauge 21. It is sharp with an

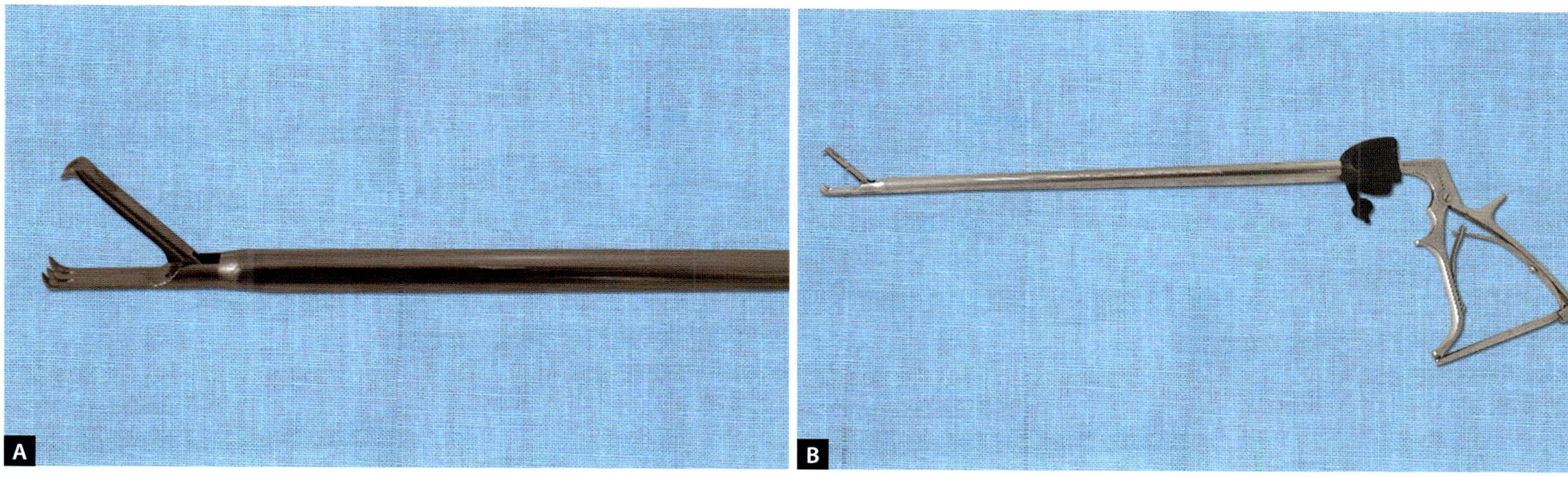

Figs. 23A and B: Claw forceps.

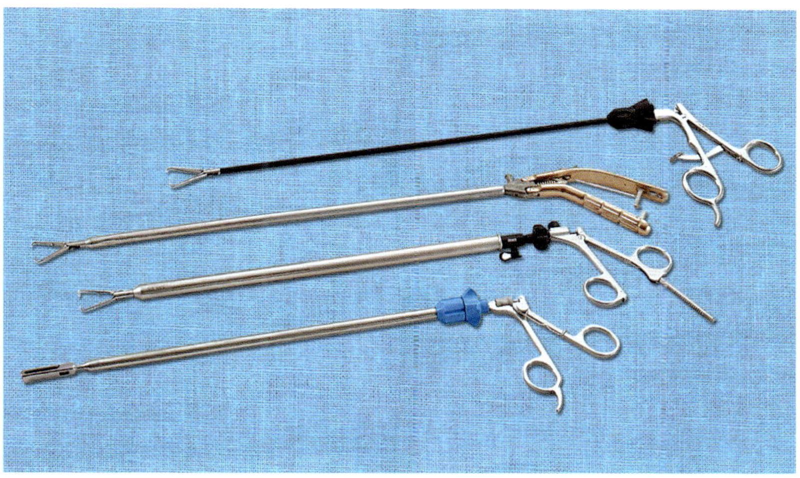

Fig. 24: Claw forceps and tenaculum.

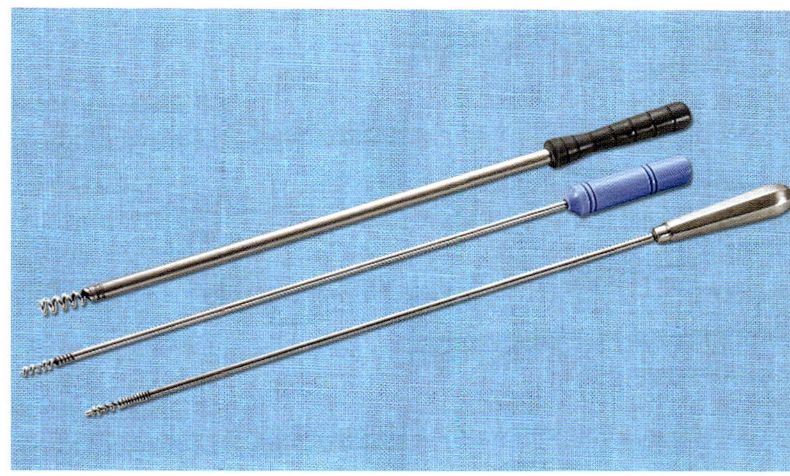

Fig. 26: Myoma screws.

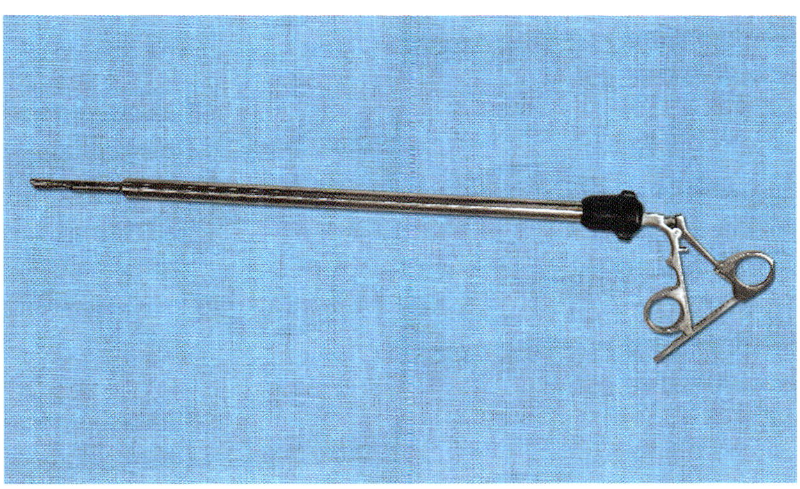

Fig. 25: Tenaculum.

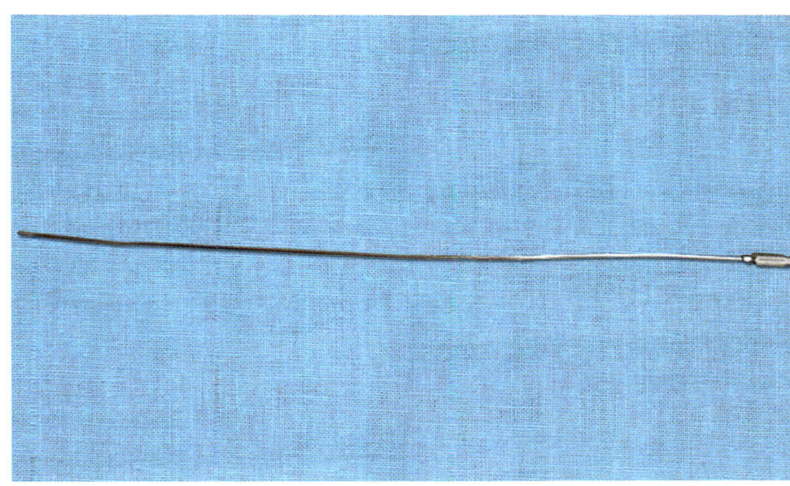

Fig. 27: Aspiration needle.

obliquely cut bevel. When used with a 28-cm probe tip without fenestrations, close-chambered ovarian cyst aspiration can be done.

Indications:

It is used for aspiration of following:

- Ovarian cyst
- Free fluid in the pouch of Douglas
- Free blood in the pouch of Douglas.

It can also be used to inject dilute vasopressin into base of fibroids before myomectomy or into mesosalpinx of tube before salpingostomy for tubal pregnancy. They may also be used for drilling polycystic ovary.

Method of use: It is passed through second puncture cannula suprapubically. Ovarian cyst punctured in avascular area and contents aspirated with syringe attached to needle at other end. Free fluid or blood is aspirated so underlying structure is visualized and analysis of fluid gives clue about presence of fluid When the suction is started and the probe tip is placed on tissue, suction retraction of that tissue results. The needle is inserted into the cyst and leakage of contents is avoided. The 2-cm exposed portion of the needle is etched with 0.5 cm marking to accurately gauge tissue penetration. When a 60-mL syringe is attached to the needle, fluid from aspirated cyst is sent for cytology.

OVARIAN DRILLING NEEDLE (FIG. 28)

Identification: It is a 40-cm long metallic needle with insulation on surface except on terminal 1.5 cm. Diameter of needle is 5 mm, while that of terminal bare part is 1 mm. It has sharp tip for follicular penetration.

Method of use: A monopolar electrocoagulation cable is connected to proximal end. In variant model, terminal portion is hidden within needle and projects on pressing trigger, which activates passage of electric current through tip of needle.

Indication: It is used for ovarian drilling in polycystic ovarian disease resistant to induction of ovulation with drugs.

INJECTION NEEDLE (FIG. 29)

It is used for infiltration of normal saline or vasopressin. A 16- or 22-gauge calibrated aspiration-irrigation needle can be used to aspirate and inject fluids.

Its uses are:

- In linear salpingostomy, injection of diluted vasopressin into mesosalpinx for unruptured midampullary tubal ectopic pregnancy
- Injection of pitressin before myomectomy to reduce blood loss in myomectomy
- During ovarian cystectomy
- Ovarian cyst aspiration.

CLIP APPLICATOR (FIG. 30)

Laparoscopic clip applicator is used through 5–11 mm sleeves for approximation of peritoneal surfaces or hemostasis of medium-sized vessels and application of clips for laparoscopic tubal sterilization.

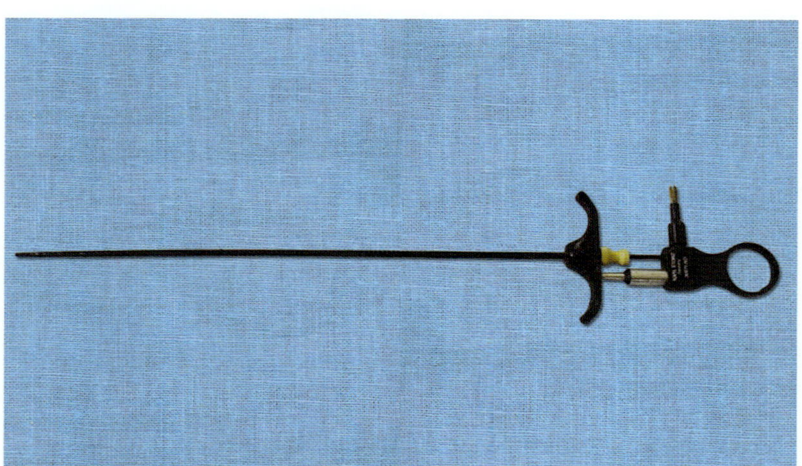

Fig. 28: Ovarian drilling needle.

RING APPLICATOR (FIG. 31)

Yoon and associates introduced the silastic band in 1974. Small silastic band is applied to tube by use of 8-mm applicator and may be used through single puncture 12-mm operating laparoscope. Bands are loaded through plastic-loading device. Applicator is then passed through the channel and grasping hooks deployed from end

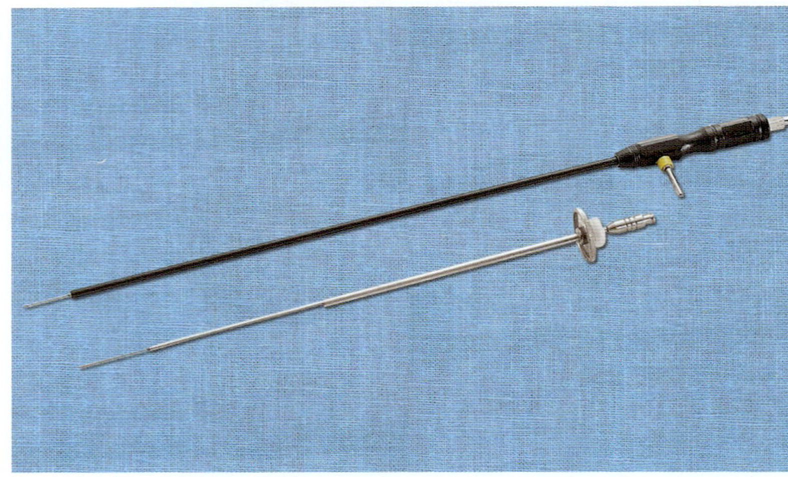

Fig. 29: Injection needles.

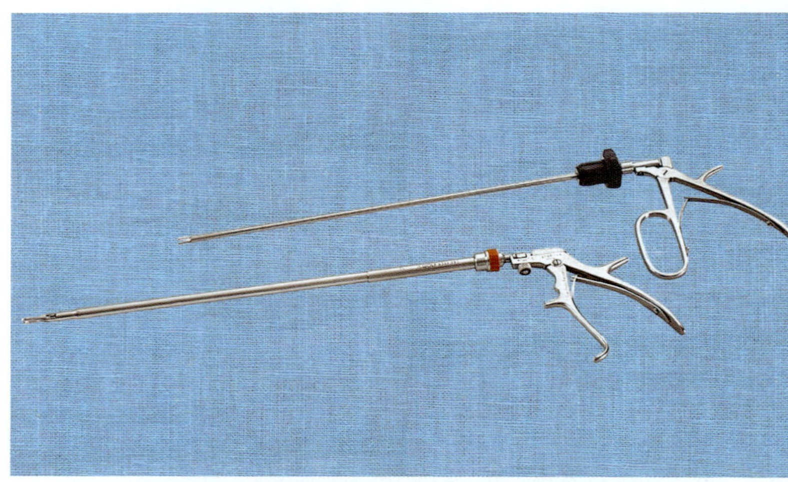

Fig. 30: Clip applicators.

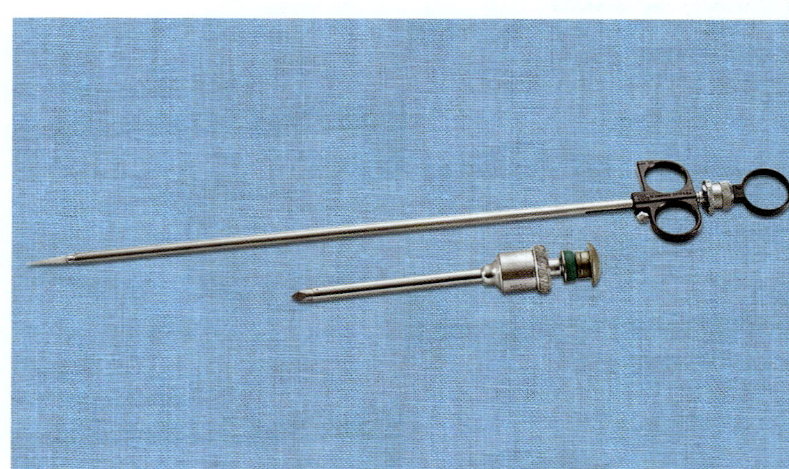

Fig. 31: Ring applicators.

of applicator. Tube is grasped at 3 cm from cornua of uterus in isthmic area. Tube is drawn into inner cylinder of applicator by grasping hooks and silastic band applied by moving outer cylinder forward.

SUCTION AND IRRIGATION TUBE (FIGS. 32A AND B)

Identification: Tube measures 36–43 cm in length and 5 mm in external diameter. Its terminal 1 cm long portion has multiple lateral holes. There is a 2-way stopcock at proximal end.

Method of use: Tube from container of irrigation tube is connected to one outlet, and the tube connected to source of suction is attached to other outlet. 2-way stopcock is operated with single hand control to switch between suction and irrigation. 10 mm suction tube should be used if blood loss is more than 1500 mL of hemoperitoneum or if there are blood clots in abdominal cavity.

Indications:
- Used to irrigate tissues with ringer's lactate during laparoscopic surgery. The fluid and blood collected in peritoneal cavity is removed by suction.
- Sometimes effective irrigation is used for adhesiolysis (hydrodissection).
- Helps with division of tissue planes and space lavage, blunt dissection and smoke and fluid evacuation.

Suction irrigation system has the following characteristics:
- Trumpet valve is designed ergonomically and versatile so that electrosurgical accessories, laser and handheld instruments can be inserted through probe.
- Trumpet valve is easy to use and provides constant control of fluid or suction including valve regulation, rather than on/off mechanism.
- Internal valve diameter is large enough to allow blood and tissue to pass easily through the canister and provide irrigation flow.
- Probe tips are smooth, strong and nonreflective so they can be used for blunt dissection and serve as backstop for CO_2 laser.
- Irrigation pump provides precise and variable irrigation pressures.

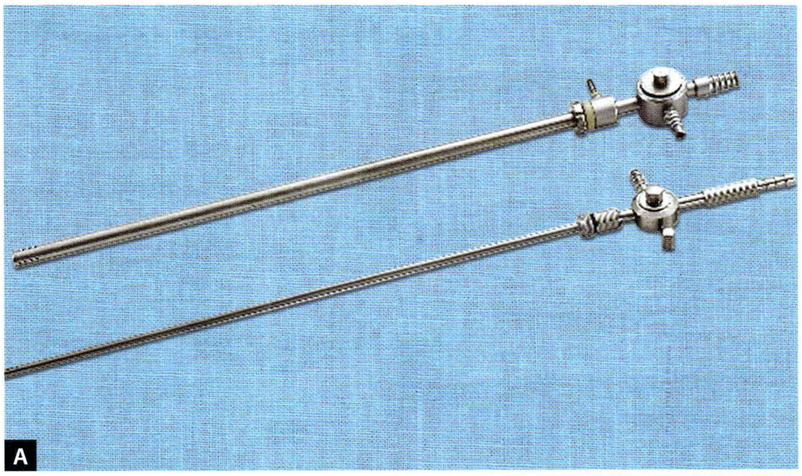
A

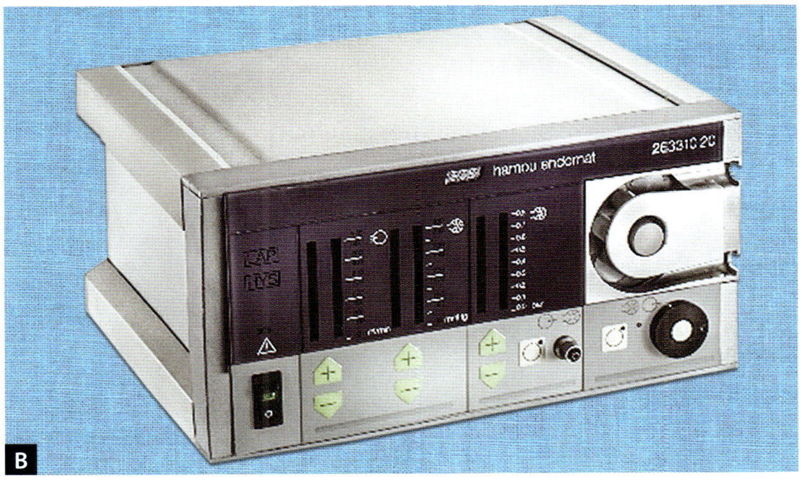
B

Figs. 32A and B: Suction and irrigation system.

PORT CLOSURE NEEDLE (FIG. 33)

It has a pointed tip and single action serrated jaw. It supports smooth introduction through muscle, fascia, and peritoneal layers in simple, single-handed method. It is especially useful when large trocars are used post dilation of port site for organ extraction.

ELECTROMECHANICAL MORCELLATOR (FIGS. 34A TO D)

In the past, laparoscopic surgeons faced the difficult problem of extraction of tissue, often obliged to perform, suprapubic minilaparotomy or transvaginal extraction. The first substantial improvement was development of manual morcellator. Much force and time was required depending on consistency of tissue.

In collaboration with Storz, Steiner developed electromechanical morcellator, consisting of motor driven cutting tube. It is possible with aid of morcellator to extract even large amount of tissues from abdomen, using 11-mm trocar in short period of time. With 12 mm and 15 mm trocar, large quantities of tissue can be extracted within few minutes.

Method of use: Instrument has a motor driven tube with a distal cutting edge. It is inserted into peritoneal cavity through trocar sleeve The motor works at 100–240 VAC, 50–60 Hz electric current. A footswitch permits clockwise, counterclockwise and oscillating rotations.

Clawed forceps are passed into abdomen through the cutting tube and the tissue to be morcellated is grasped. Traction is made on the forceps so tissue presses against cylindrical cutting edge, and cylindrical block of tissue is cut off. Larger masses are broken down into small pieces, which can be removed through trocar sleeve.

Indications: It is used to morcellate tissue for its removal from peritoneal cavity after laparoscopic resection.
- Laparoscopic hysterectomy
- Laparoscopic myomectomy
- Laparoscopic tumor removal.

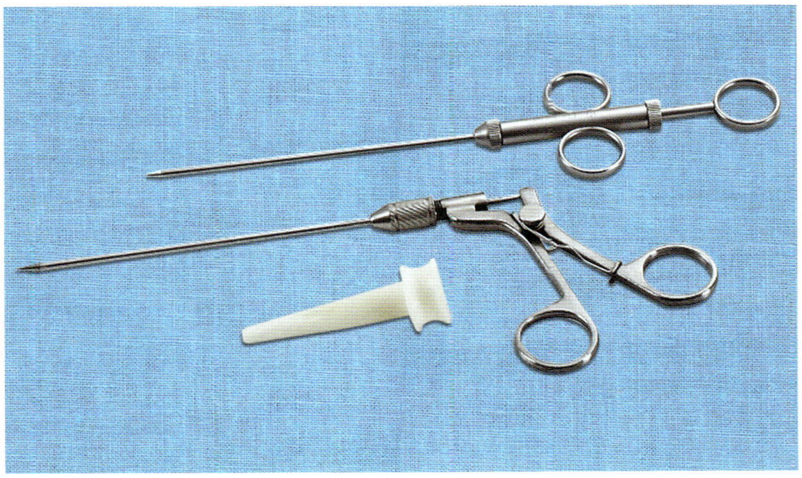

Fig. 33: Port closure needles.

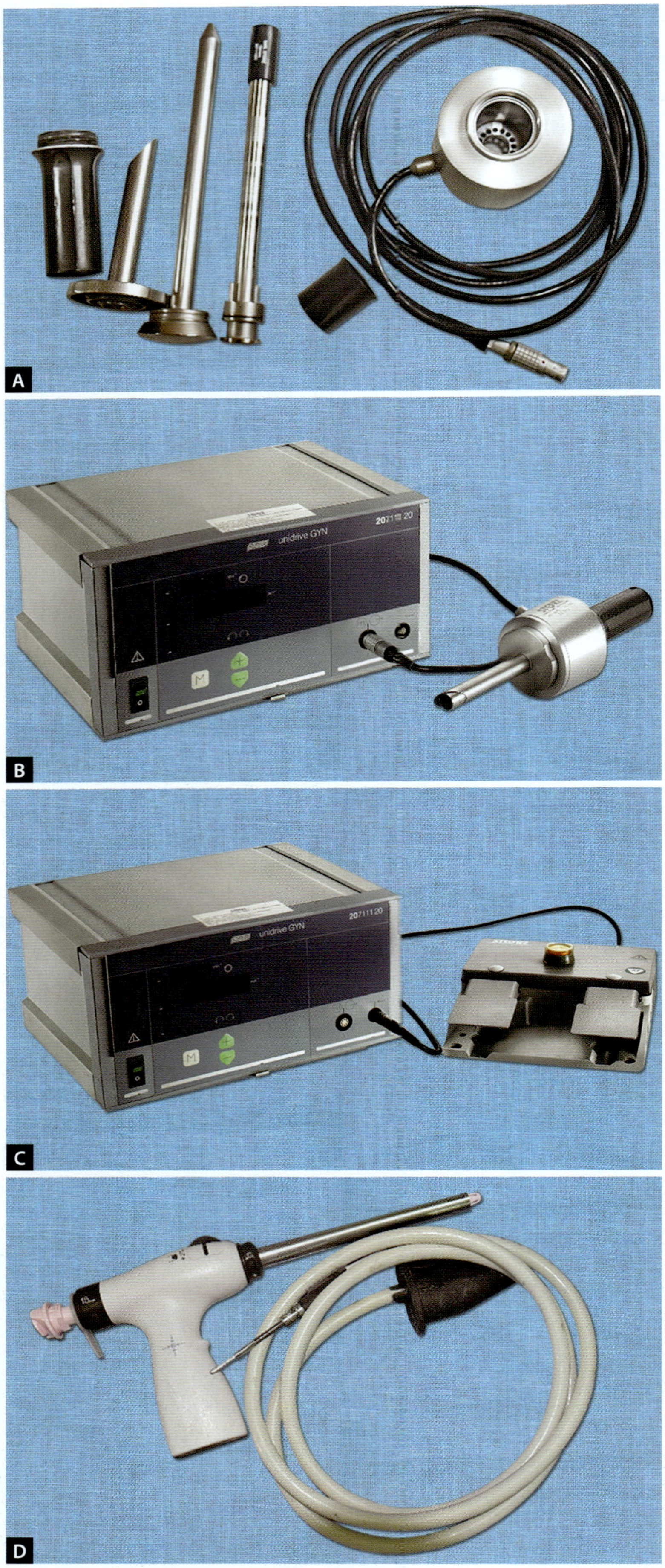

Figs. 34A to D: Electromechanical morcellator.

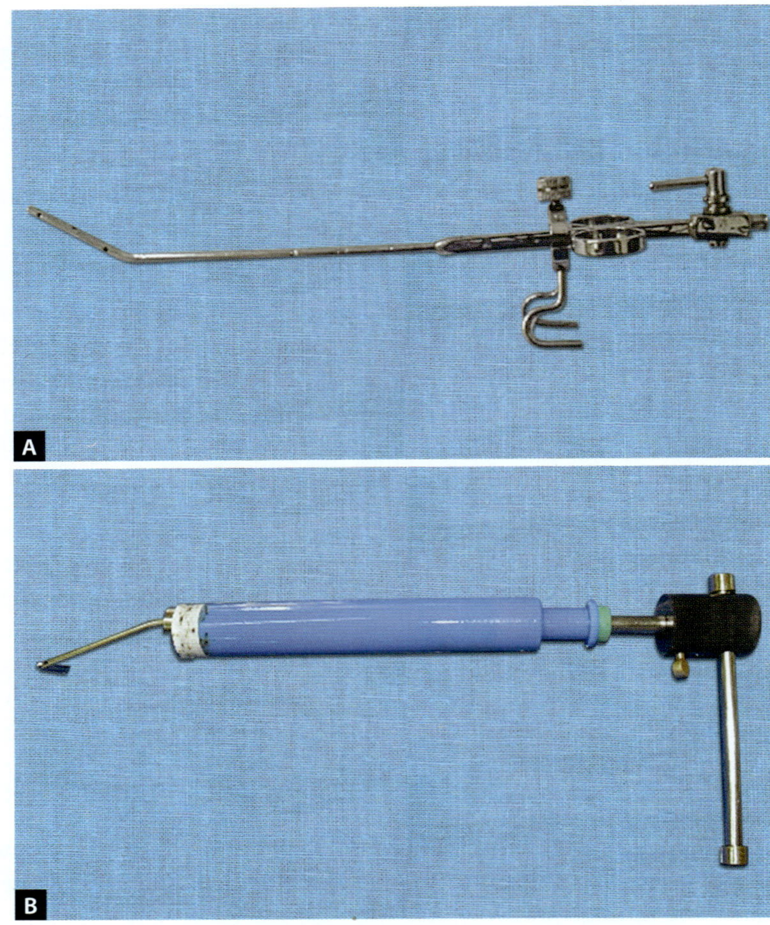

Figs. 35A and B: Uterine manipulators.

UTERINE MANIPULATOR (FIGS. 35A AND B)

Laparoscopic surgery is expedited by use of good uterine manipulator. It is capable of anteverting and positioning the uterus as needed thereby improving access to uterus, fallopian tube, ovary, and posterior and anterior cul-de-sac. It is often used with a tenaculum attached to anterior lip. Uterine manipulators are available in reusable and disposable models. Some manipulators are inserted in fixed position and allow limited uterine mobility, whereas others are hinged and allow the uterus to be moved anteriorly, posteriorly and laterally. They are very essential for mobilization of uterus, identification of vaginal fornices and sealing of vagina during hysterectomy.

A properly designed uterine manipulator should have:

- An intrauterine component or obturator
- A method for fixation of device to uterus
- A channel for chromopertubation
- Prevent escape of pneumoperitoneum during culdotomy.

Commercially available manipulators are:

- Reusable:
    - Semm vacuum cannula
    - Hulka uterine elevator
    - Pelosi uterine manipulator
    - Valtchev uterine mobilizer
- *Partially disposable:* Rumi® uterine manipulator
- *Completely disposable:* Vcare®.

CHAPTER

2

Open Surgery Instruments

Shruti Paliwal, G Hemasree, B Ramesh

SIM'S SPECULUM (FIGS. 1 AND 2)

- Because of shape also called duck-bill speculum.
- It was developed by J Marion Sims out of pewter spoon.
- Most commonly used speculum in obstetrics and gynecology.
- Sterilized by boiling or autoclaving.

Identification: Manufactured out of plastic or stainless steel. Speculum has handle in center and blades at right angle to handle. A trough runs along the instrument to allow free flow of secretions and blood to outside. Bladed are rounded at ends so are atraumatic. A double-blade speculum has two bladed of different sizes, so available in sizes: 25 and 31 mm, 31 and 36 mm, and 36 and 42 mm.

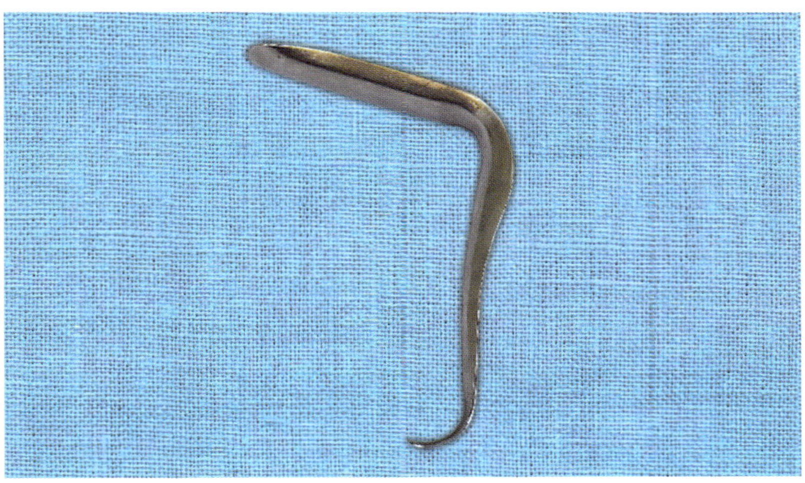

Fig. 1: Sim's single-bladed speculum.

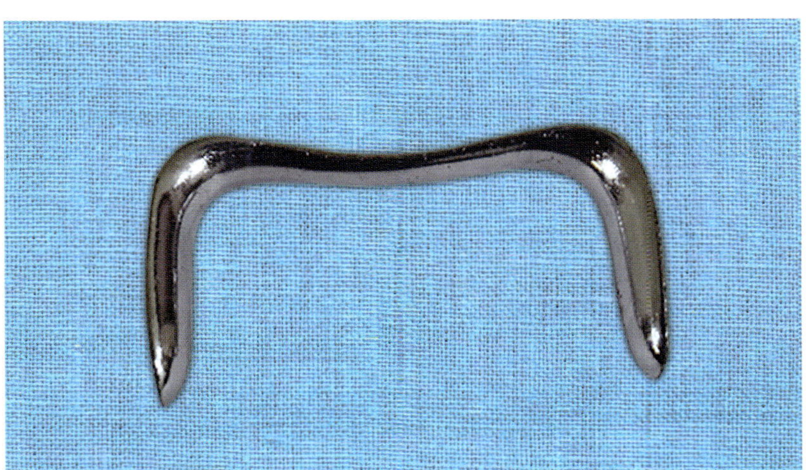

Fig. 2: Sim's double-bladed speculum.

Indications:

- *Visual examination of cervix and vagina for diagnosing:*
  - Leukorrhea
  - Vaginal wall prolapse: Cystocele, urethrocele, enterocele, rectocele, posthysterectomy vault prolapse
  - Uterine prolapse
  - Cervical erosion, chronic cervicitis
  - Cervical carcinoma
  - Cervical polyp
  - Ectropion, cervical tear
  - Vesicovaginal fistula (VVF), rectovaginal fistula (RVF)
  - Stress urinary incontinence (SUI)
  - Vaginal wall cysts
  - Congenital malformations, e.g. transverse vaginal septum, longitudinal vaginal septum, uterus pseudodidelphys.
- Examination for obstetric trauma as cervical tear, vaginal tear.
- *Carrying out operative procedures such as:*
  - Collecting exfoliative cytological smear for genital tract malignancy or hormonal vaginal cytology
  - Cervical biopsy
  - Endometrial biopsy
  - Insertion or removal of intrauterine contraceptive device (IUCD)
  - Polypectomy
  - Dilatation and curettage, dilatation and suction evacuation, blunt curettage for inevitable abortion
  - Tubal patency tests
  - Hysteroscopy
  - Colposcopy, colpomicroscopy
- Colpopuncture, colpotomy
- Insertion of radium into uterine cavity
- Repair of obstetric trauma to cervix or vagina
- Packing uterine cavity and vagina for uncontrolled PPH.

Method of use: The instrument can be inserted in lithotomy, dorsal or Sim's lateral position. Blades are lubricated with antiseptic solution or jelly. Labia minora are held apart and blade is inserted in between transverse axis and long axis of labia. Once in vagina, it is rotated by 90° so as to retract the posterior wall of vagina. Often it has to be used with Sim's anterior vaginal wall retractor. Posterior vaginal wall is examined when speculum is withdrawn.

Drawbacks:
- An assistant is required to hold the speculum during any operative procedure.
- It moves with any movement of assistant, it is not satisfactory for colposcopy and colpomicroscopy.

JACKSON'S SPECULUM (FIG. 3)

It is similar to single-ended Sim's speculum except for shape of blade, which is flatter and less rounded end. It can be used instead of Sim's speculum.

CUSCO'S SPECULUM (FIG. 4)

Sterilized by boiling or autoclaving.

Identification: It has two blades connected by hinge so they open close around a transverse axis. Blades are concave inside with rounded ends. Both blades have handle at right angle and nut and screw to fix distance between the blades. Available in sizes: 75 × 32 mm, 85 × 35 mm, and 95 × 37 mm; for virgins, 70 × 20 mm is available.

Indications:
- Inspection of vagina and cervix as Sim's speculum for ulcer, abnormal discharge, cyst, polyp, growth, bleeding.
- Procedures of cervix and uterine cavity as Sim's speculum. Suitable for short procedures as cytological smear, cervical biopsy, insertion or removal of IUCD, cervical cautery.
- Because it stretches the anterior and posterior vaginal wall, it fixes cervix in center, so suitable for procedures like colposcopy and colpomicroscopy.
- To take cervical and vaginal swab to exclude infections.
- To allow introduction of uterine sound.
- *Obstetric indications:* To diagnose PROM in cases with history of watery vaginal discharge and also to exclude cord prolapse, to exclude local causes of APH.

Method of use: Patient should lie in dorsal or semilithotomy position and separate labia and clean the introitus by antiseptic solution starting from above and going toward perineum. Lubricated blades are inserted between labia minora, transverse axis of blade in long axis of labia. Once in vagina rotated through 90° and opened till cervix visualized satisfactorily. Blades fixed in position with butterfly screw.

Advantages:
- It can be used without assistant
- Self-retaining.

Drawbacks:
- Speculum covers the anterior and posterior vaginal wall, so cannot be used for procedure on these structures.
- Blade occupies space and decreases maneuverability so instrument is not very useful for procedures like dilation and curettage (D&C).

SOONAWALA'S SPECULUM (FIG. 5)

Sterilized by boiling or autoclaving.

Identification: It has two blades at ends directed in opposite directions making speculum Z-shaped. One blade is 6 cm long and other 11.5 cm long. Former has flat surface and square end. The other is round ended much smaller than width of blade at base. Upper surface has raised edges so blood gets collected and drained through longitudinal groove in handle. Weight in center of handle makes speculum self-retaining.

Indications: It was originally designed for vaginal sterilization operations. Not done in current practice.

Now used for:
- Vaginal hysterectomy
- Anterior colporrhaphy
- Kelly's operation for urinary stress incontinence
- Vesicovaginal fistula repair
- Schauta's radical vaginal hysterectomy

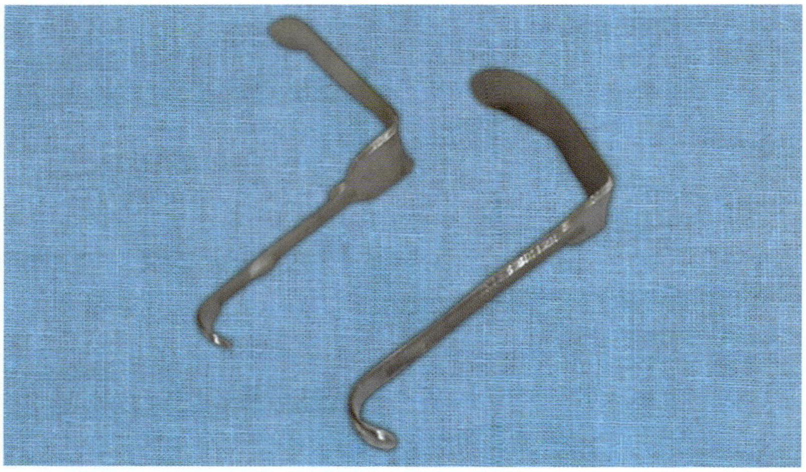

Fig. 3: Jackson's speculum.

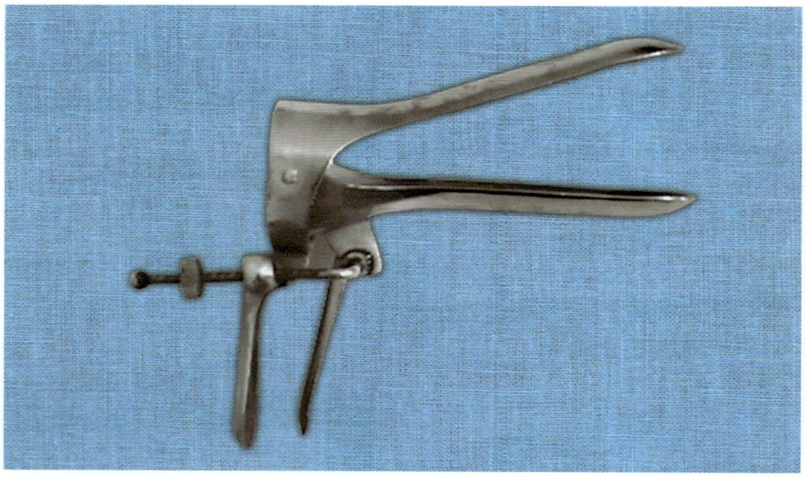

Fig. 4: Cusco's speculum.

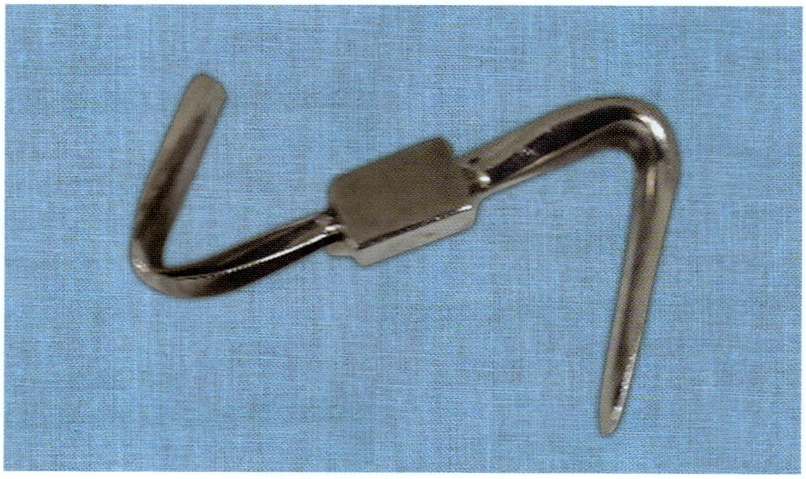

Fig. 5: Soonawala's speculum.

DEAVER'S RETRACTOR (FIG. 6)

Sterilized by boiling or autoclaving.

Identification: Long strip of metal which is bent on both the edges. Blade is thin. Available in three sizes: (1) small, (2) medium, and (3) large.

Indications:
- Used to retract liver in upper abdominal surgeries.
- Useful for retraction of sides of incision and intraperitoneal structures during surgeries on posterior abdominal wall, e.g. ligation of internal iliac artery, Shirodkar's sling operation, etc.

Advantages: Its length and curvature make it an ideal instrument for retraction when working at depth.

Drawbacks: Not good for retraction of sides of abdominal incision because it is narrow and does not retract the sides as well as a broad retractor.

DELEE'S UNIVERSAL RETRACTOR (FIG. 7)

Sterilized by boiling or autoclaving.

Identification: It has a curved blade with greater depth than Doyen's retractor. It has sturdy handle.

Indications: Retraction of anterior abdominal wall for abdominal operations as:
- Cesarean section
- Ruptured ectopic gestation
- Obstetric hysterectomies
- *Abdominal hysterectomies:* Total with bilateral salpingo-oophorectomy or radical
- Ovarian cystectomy, oophorectomy, wedge resection
- *Prolapse repairs:* Purandare's cervicopexy, Shirodkar's sling operation, Khanna's sling operation, Moschcowitz operation, etc.
- *Stress urinary incontinence repair:* Marshall–Marchetti–Krantz operation.

Retractor is used after peritoneum is opened. Broad retracting surface achieves good retraction. Solid blade compresses cut edges of abdominal wall and reduces blood loss.

MORRIS RETRACTOR (FIGS. 8A AND B)

Sterilized by boiling or autoclaving.

Identification: Handle of retractor is straight or curved. Handle has grooves for firm grip. It may be single-ended or double-ended. It has a single blade 5.65 cm deep and 3.75 cm wide.

Indications: Retraction of anterior abdominal wall for abdominal operations as:
- Cesarean section
- Ruptured ectopic gestation
- Obstetric hysterectomies
- *Abdominal hysterectomies:* Total with bilateral salpingo-oophorectomy or radical
- Ovarian cystectomy, oophorectomy, wedge resection

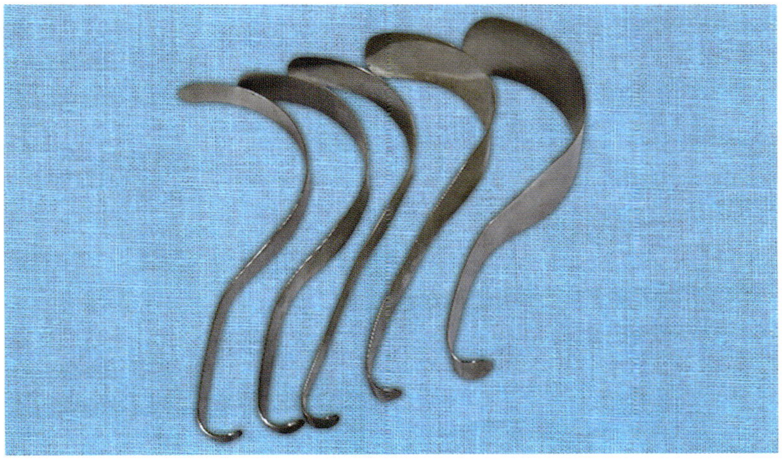

Fig. 6: Deaver's retractor.

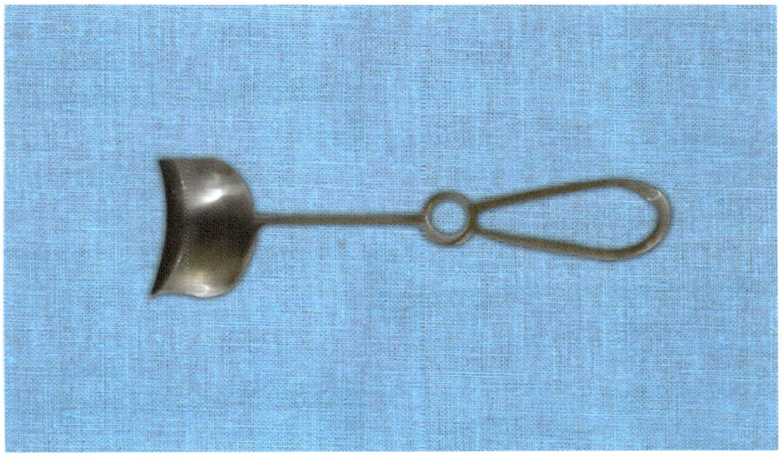

Fig. 7: Delee's universal retractor.

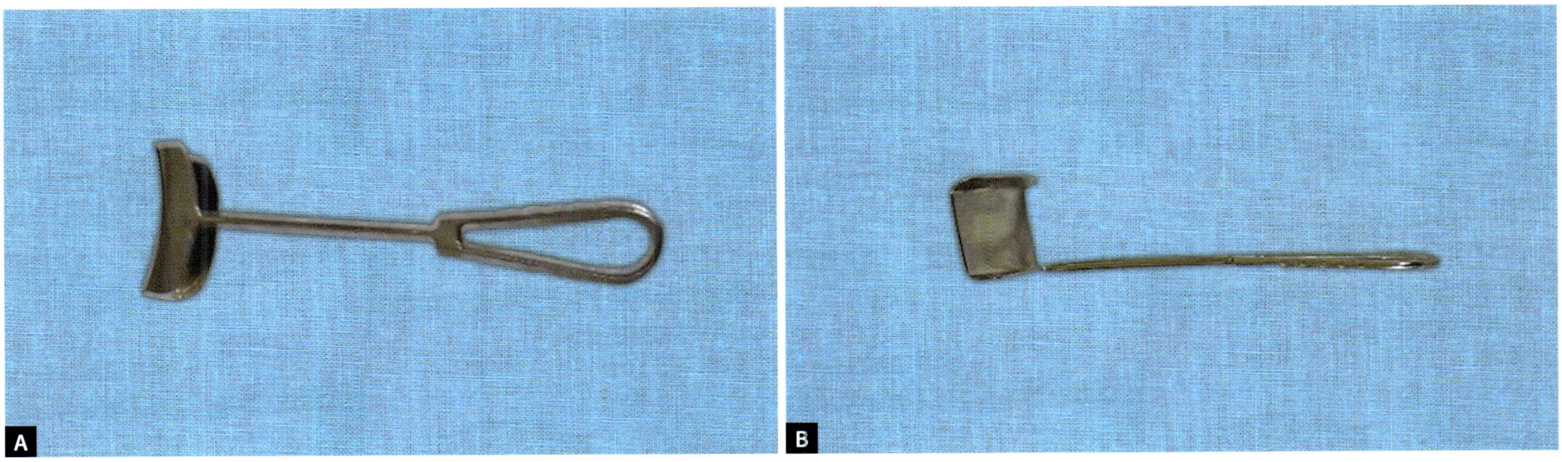

Figs. 8A and B: Morris retractor.

- *Prolapse repairs:* Purandare's cervicopexy, Shirodkar's sling operation, Khanna's sling operation, Moschcowitz operation, etc.
- *Stress urinary incontinence repair:* Marshall–Marchetti–Krantz operation.

Retractor is used after peritoneum is opened. Broad retracting surface achieves good retraction. Solid blade compresses cut edges of abdominal wall and reduces blood loss.

LANDON'S RETRACTOR (FIG. 9)

Identification: It has an L-shaped blade which is 2 cm wide and 8.75 cm long. Handle has fenestra in center for thumb.

Indication:
- It is used to retract the bladder away from cervix during vaginal hysterectomy
- On cystocele and cervix to expose enterocele
- It may be used to retract the lateral and anterior vaginal wall during vaginal operations
- To retract the posterior colpotomy opening for tubal ligation.

Method of use: It is inserted into anterior peritoneal pouch after uterovesical fold of peritoneum is cut.

Advantages: Being narrow and flat, blade occupies very little space, hence ideal for vaginal surgeries where space is less.

LANGENBECK RETRACTOR (FIGS. 10A AND B)

Identification: Blade of retractor is bent at right angle on itself. Distal edge of blade is curved. Handle of instrument is stout.

Uses: Best suited for retraction of bladder away from cervix and vagina during abdominal hysterectomy, especially Wertheim's operation.

SIM'S ANTERIOR VAGINAL WALL RETRACTOR (FIG. 11)

Sterilized by boiling or autoclaving.

Identification: It is a long instrument with spoon-shaped ends, which has transverse serrations on either surface (transverse serrations provide friction against rugous vaginal mucosa and aid efficient retraction). Loops make an angle of 15° with shaft and angled in opposite direction.

Indications:
- Retraction of anterior vaginal wall to visualize cervix with Sim's speculum.
- Blunt curettage when cervix widely open and uterine cavity large as after second-trimester abortion or after delivery of viable baby and bits of placenta are retained.

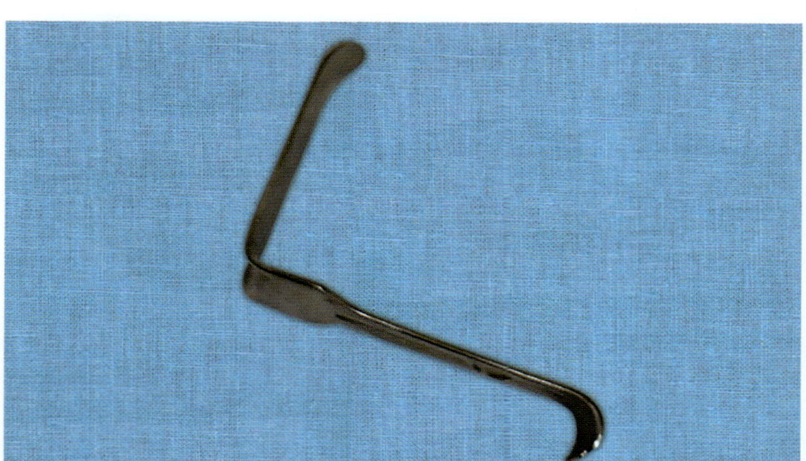

Fig. 9: Landon's retractor.

SPONGE HOLDING FORCEPS (FIG. 12)

Sterilized by boiling or autoclaving.

Identification: It is 22.5 cm long, has ring-shaped ends with transverse serrations on inner surface for better grip. Ratchet lock is present on handle locks the blades.

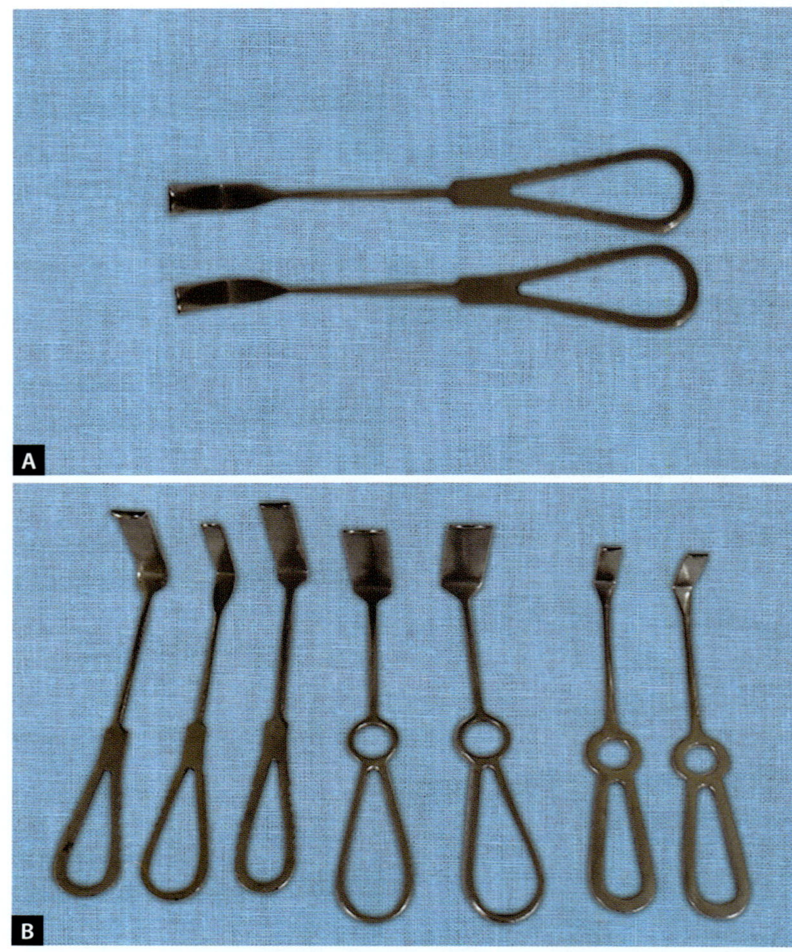

Figs. 10A and B: Langenbeck retractors.

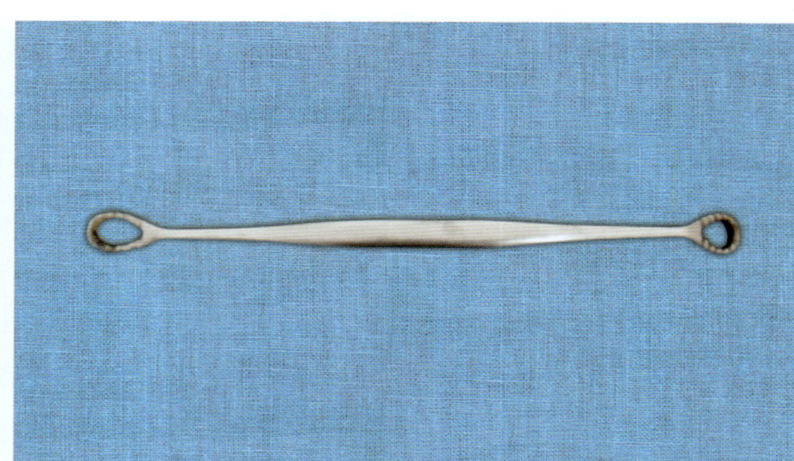

Fig. 11: Sim's anterior vaginal wall retractor.

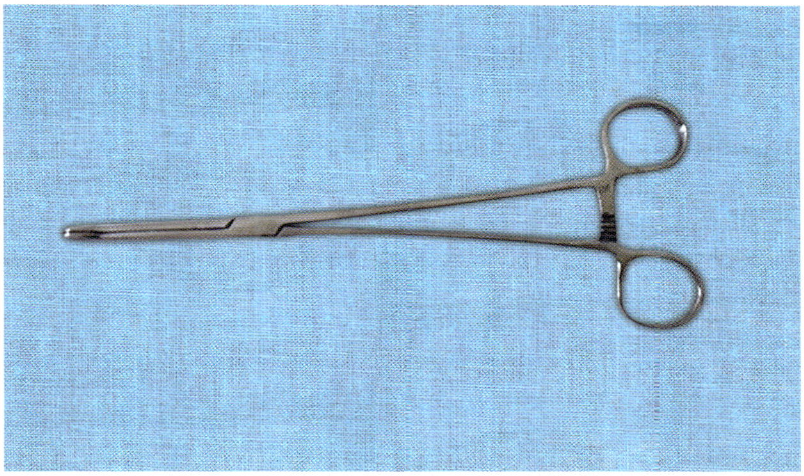

Fig. 12: Sponge holding forceps.

Indications:
- Preparation of vagina, vulva, and abdominal wall for application of detergent and antiseptics.
- To hold sponge to swab blood from distance during surgery.
- To press an oozing area with swab for hemostasis.
- For blunt dissection, e.g. separation of bladder from anterior surface of cervix.
- As temporary nontraumatic clamp over ovarian vessels in infundibulopelvic ligament during conservative surgery like myomectomy, metroplasty, conservative surgery on Fallopian tube for tubal ectopic gestation.
- To hold bowel or omentum away from field of operation by pressure of swab during vaginal surgeries like vaginal hysterectomy.
- To hold the cervix during pregnancy for:
  - Insertion of Foley's extra-amniotically in second-trimester pregnancy termination using ethacridine lactate.
  - Cervical cerclage.
  - Diagnosis of cervical tear after instrumental vaginal delivery, breech extraction, internal podalic version, etc.
  - Repair of cervical tear.
  - To hold and steady the cervix during check curettage for second trimester incomplete abortion.
- To hold cut edges of lower segment during cesarean section for hemostasis and facilitate suturing.
- As substitute for ovum forceps.

TEALES VULSELLUM (FIGS. 13A AND B)

Sterilized by boiling or autoclaving.

Identification: It is a 28 cm long instrument with blades curved on side in gentle manner. The tip of blade has two in three teeth to give good grip to hold structure.

Indications:
- *To hold and steady the cervix:*
  - To differentiate between cystocele and descent of bladder with uterine prolapse.
  - To diagnose enterocele by Telinde's test (posterior lip of cervix is held steady at the normal level of cervix and patient asked to cough. If the highest level of posterior fornix descends below the level of posterior lip of cervix then enterocele is present).
  - To diagnose stress urinary incontinence in presence of massive prolapse of uterus with large cystocele. Huge cystocele can mask urinary stress incontinence by creating posterior urethrovesical angle. So, prolapse held reduced while the patient coughs so diagnosis of stress urinary incontinence can be made.
  - Operations on cervix as cervical biopsy, trachelorrhaphy, amputation, electrocauterization, cryocauterization, endocervical curettage, rapid cervical dilatation, insertion of laminaria tent for cervical dilatation.
  - Operations on uterine cavity, e.g. endometrial curettage, polypectomy, insertion of IUCD, insertion of radium into uterine cavity, endometrial aspiration, first trimester pregnancy termination by dilatation and suction evacuation, hydrotubation, hysterosalpingography, tubal insufflation for tubal patency testing.
  - Vaginal hysterectomy.
  - Anterior colporrhaphy.
  - Colpopuncture.
  - Colpotomy.
  - Culdoscopy.
  - To sound uterine cavity.
- To assess the degree of uterine descent, if the prolapse has been reduced with tampon or pessary and does not descend on straining even after removal of pessary or tampon.
- To hold the uterine fundus during abdominal hysterectomy.
- To hold the uterine fundus down during vaginal hysterectomy after peritoneal pouches have been opened and uterine fundus has been delivered.
- To hold a leiomyomatous polyp and twist it during vaginal myomectomy.

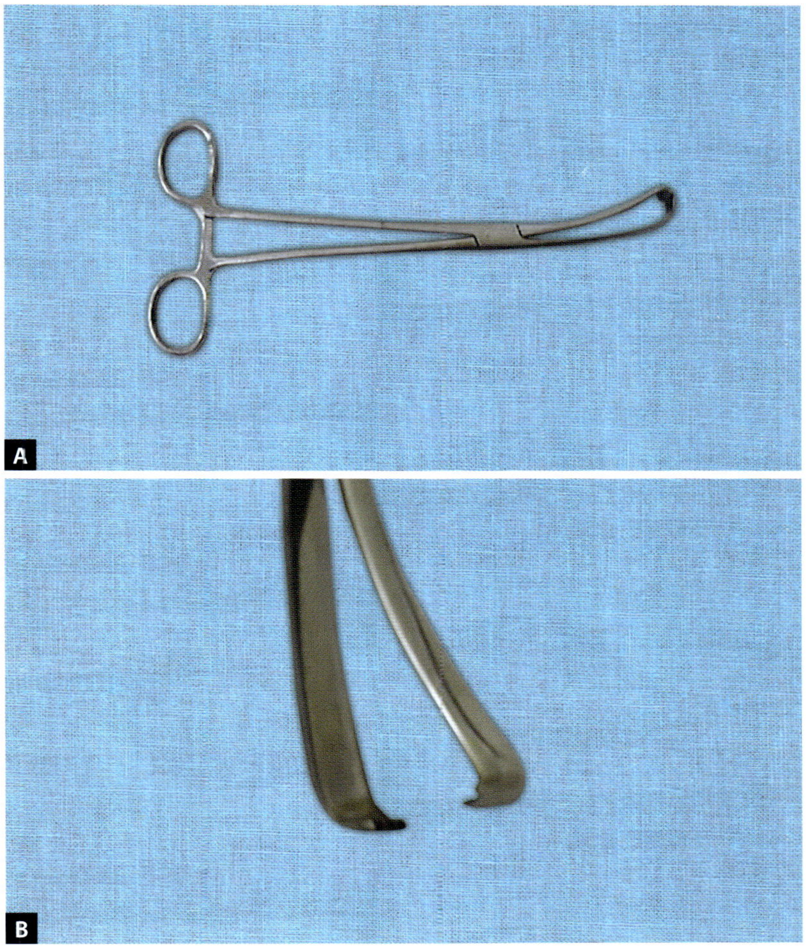

Figs. 13A and B: Teales vulsellum.

- To draw the cervix up through opened anterior vaginal fornix during abdominal hysterectomy.
- To correct a mobile retroversion.
- A stouter vulsellum, known as Schroeder's bulldog vulsellum, is used in situations in which structure held is later removed, e.g. hysterectomy, myomectomy, holding and giving traction on fetal head after craniotomy.

TENACULUM (FIG. 14)

Sterilized by boiling or autoclaving.

Identification: Straight or curved 20 cm long instrument, similar to vulsellum except there is single tooth at the end of each blade.

Advantages of tenaculum over vulsellum:
- Grip more secure because the bite is deeper.
- Suitable for small cervix because two teeth grip a smaller area.

Indication: Same as vulsellum.

Drawbacks: Teeth of vulsellum take a deeper bite into cervix; risk of cervical tissue getting torn is more.

Varieties of tenaculum:
- *Barrett's tenaculum:* 18 cm long and straight
- *Pozzi's tenaculum:* 25 cm long and straight
- *Skene's tenaculum:* 24 cm long and curved
- *Duplay's tenaculum:* 25 cm long and curved.

In general, curved and longer tenaculum is preferred over short and straight.

SIMPSON'S UTERINE SOUND (FIG. 15)

Sterilized by boiling or autoclaving.

Identification: It is a 30 cm long instrument of which 5 cm length is of handle. Rest of instrument graduated in inches or centimeter. It is bent at an angle of 150° at distance of 2.5 inches from tip, i.e. at distance of normal uterocervical length. Sound is olive tipped.

Indications:
- To measure uterocervical length
- To confirm ante- or retroversion of uterus determined first by bimanual examination.
- To measure length of cervical canal and to diagnose elongation of cervix.
- Prior to any procedure on the uterine cavity as D&C.
- To diagnose and differentiate a polyp lying in cervical canal.
- To differentiate between uterine polyp and chronic inversion of uterus: sound can pass by side of pedicle of polyp but arrested by chronic inversion.
- To determine relation of pelvic mass to uterus.
- *Diagnosis of missing IUCD:* Anteroposterior (AP) and lateral view X-ray are taken with sound in uterine cavity.
- Diagnosis of congenital malformations of uterus as bicornuate uterus.
- *Diagnosis of incompetent os:* Passage of sound through internal os without resistance or pain is diagnostic of incompetent os (Shirodkar's test).
- *Diagnosis of cervical stenosis:* Failure of sound to pass through cervix is due to cervical stenosis if not due to other conditions as cochleate uterus, hypertrophy of plicae palmatae, etc.
- *Test the mobility of urethra in stress urinary incontinence:* Sound is passed up to the bladder neck and attempt made to move urethra away from back of pubis. Displacement of urethra away from pubis in region of bladder neck produces incontinence similar to that caused by stress.
- In stress urinary incontinence to identify a point on either side of urethra-vesical junction, so that elevation of point by sound results in control of urinary incontinence. It is a modification of Bonney's test to eliminate the possibility that control of stress urinary incontinence achieved by direct compression of urethra by fingers.
- *Diagnosis of vesicular mole:* Passage of uterine sound for distance at least 10 cm without resistance or rupture of membranes is diagnostic of vesicular mole (Acosta-Sison's test) test is false positive in presence of fetal death or maceration or conducting test prior to 12 weeks of pregnancy, i.e. before fusion of decidua capsularis and parietalis.
- To find direction of cervical canal in first trimester pregnancy termination by dilatation and suction evacuation.
- To find direction of cervical canal and its length prior to insertion of laminaria tents.
- To prevent stenosis of cervical canal after cryo- or electrocauterization of cervix.
- Correction of mobile retroversion of uterus.
- To manipulate the uterus during laparoscopy or minilaparotomy.

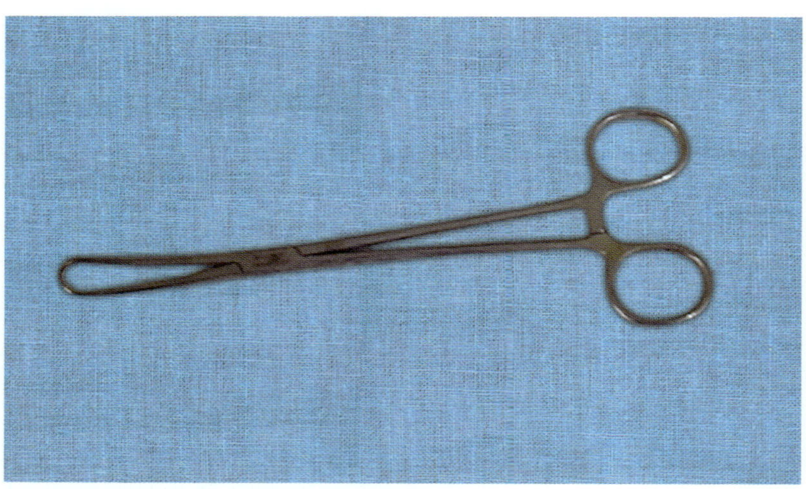

Fig. 14: Tenaculum.

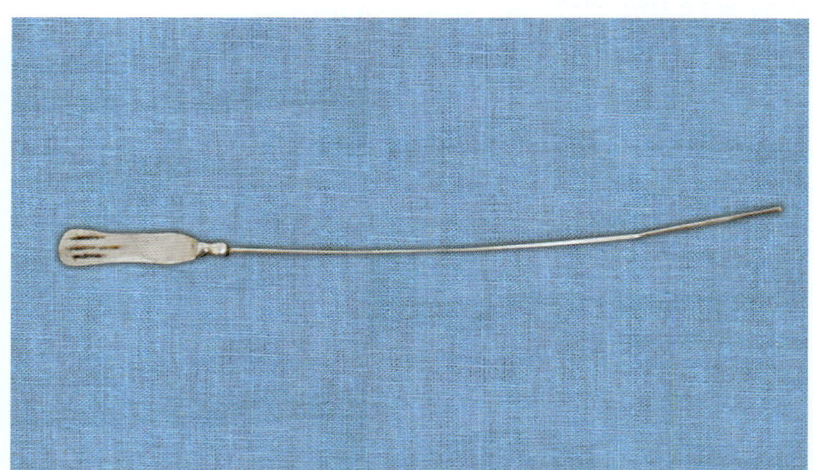

Fig. 15: Uterine sound.

Contraindications: Pregnancy or suspected pregnancy is contraindication to uterine sounding. Because it may rupture membrane resulting in termination of pregnancy or because the uterus is so soft that it can result in termination of pregnancy.

Method of use: Once cervix is exposed and held with vulsellum, sound is passed into cervical canal, sound is dipped in antiseptic solution, held like a pen and passed into cervical canal. When it encounters resistance at level of internal os, length of cervical canal is measured. Subtraction of length of portio vaginalis from it gives length of supravaginal cervix. Sound is passed further till passage is arrested by uterine fundus, thereby it gives total uterocervical length. Angulation of sound is for easy passage in anteverted or retroverted position. For passage into anteverted uterus, sound almost held vertically with angle held toward patient and for retroverted uterus, it is held so that handle lies below level of tip of sound, the angle facing floor.

Drawbacks: Sound can create false passage in cervix if passed with force in presence of resistance.

HEGAR'S DILATOR (FIGS. 16A AND B)

Sterilized by boiling or autoclaving.

Identification: It may be single-ended or double-ended. It is a solid rod, curved near tip and somewhat tapering toward tip. Curve is shallow and dilating portion is within terminal 1.5 cm of dilator. There is a difference of 3 mm in diameter near the tip and maximum dilating portion and is numbered from 3/6 to 23/26 where the numerator is the diameter at tip and denominator is the maximum diameter.

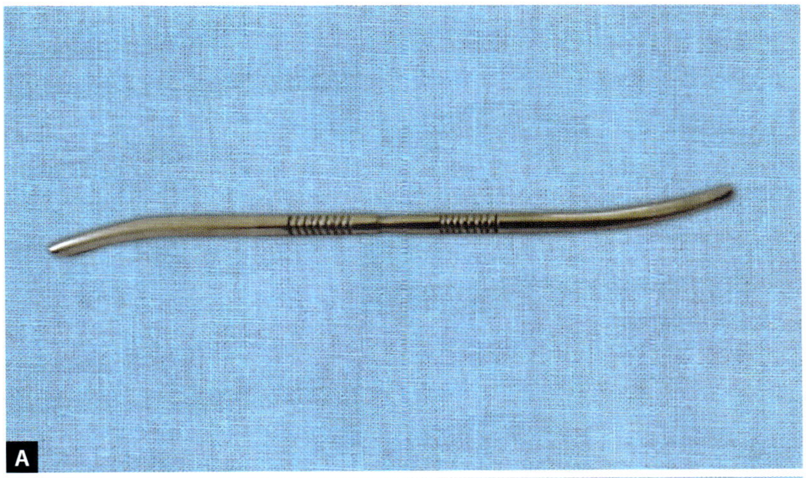

A

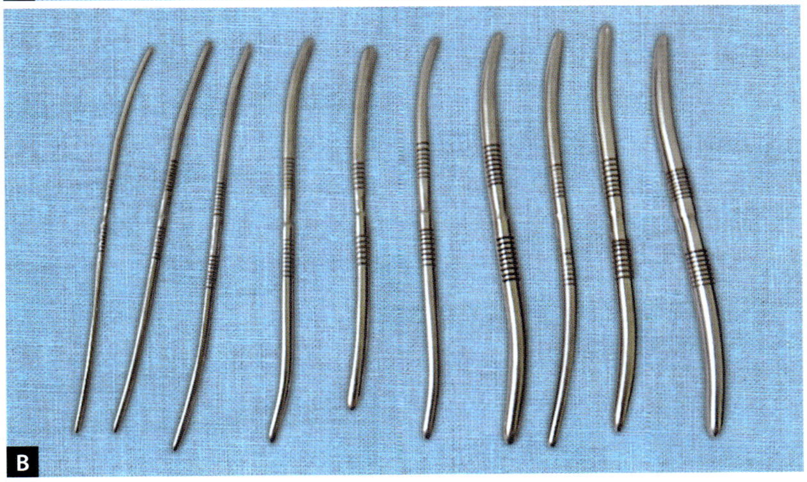

B

Fig. 16A and B: Hegar's dilator.

Indications:

- Prior to endometrial curettage.
- Prior to suction aspiration for first trimester pregnancy termination.
- Prior to suction evacuation of vesicular mole.
- Removal of endometrial polyp, placental polyp, leiomyomatous polyp.
- Removal of intrauterine impacted IUCD by curettage when other measures have failed.
- Hysteroscopy.
- Amputation of cervix, Fothergill's operation, following cervical conization, etc. to aid insertion of Sturmdorf's suture and to prevent cervical stenosis.
- As treatment of cervical stenosis.
- To drain uterine fluid contents, e.g. pyometra, hematometra, hydrometra, etc. when secondary to cervical stenosis.
- Application of intrauterine source of radiation, e.g. radium.
- Primary dysmenorrhea, when all therapies have failed.
- Retrograde dilatation of cervix when found to be closed at time of hysterotomy or elective LSCS.
- *Diagnosis of incompetent os:* Passage of size no 8 Hegar dilator through internal os in nonpregnant state without resistance or causation of pain is said to be diagnostic of incompetent os.
- *Shirodkar's test of incompetent os:* When a size 8 dilator which has been passed through internal os in a nonpregnant woman is withdrawn, there is distinct snap as it passes out of internal os, if os is not incompetent. Absence of snap suggests cervical incompetence.
- It may be used for uterine manipulation during laparoscopy or minilaparotomy.
- Rare cases of pinhole os in labor which fail to dilate even after 100% effacement of cervix: passage of dilator through os results in rapid dilatation of cervix.
- Urethral dilatation.

Method of use: Procedure is carried out under general anesthesia or paracervical block. Cervix is exposed and anterior lip held with vulsellum. Uterine cavity is sounded. Smallest diameter is held like pen and lubricated tip passed into cervical canal. Penetration beyond internal os by widest diameter is avoided by little finger jutting against perineum. Dilator held for 2–3 seconds and then removed so that next dilator is passed. Hegar's dilator has a rapid increase from diameter at tip to maximum diameter.

Complications:

- Cervical tears, dilatation beyond 9 mm results in irreversible damage to cervix.
- *Hemorrhage:* From injury to descending cervical artery, cervical perforation, etc.
- Cervical perforation, uterine perforation.
- Infection.
- Incompetent os, from excessive dilatation of cervix.

HAYWOOD SMITH'S OVUM FORCEPS (FIG. 17)

Sterilized by boiling or autoclaving.

Identification: Spoon shaped, blunt and fenestrated ends which come in contact when forceps is closed. It achieves a good grip on structures held without nipping it at base. There is no catch on the handle, so instrument has no crushing action.

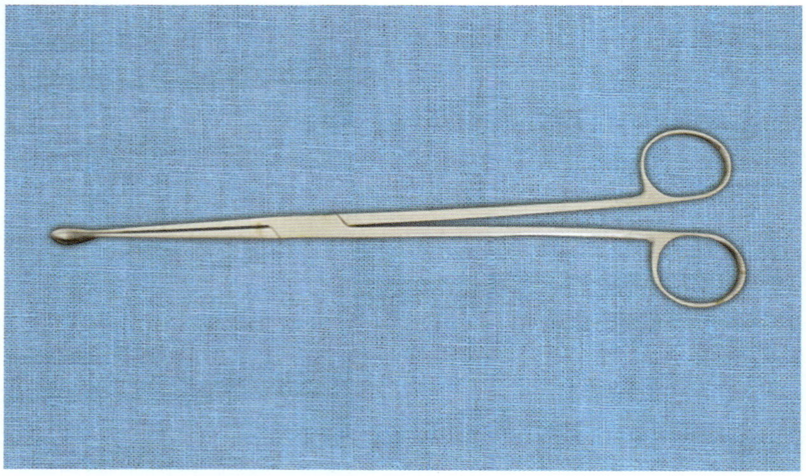

Fig. 17: Haywood smith's ovum forceps.

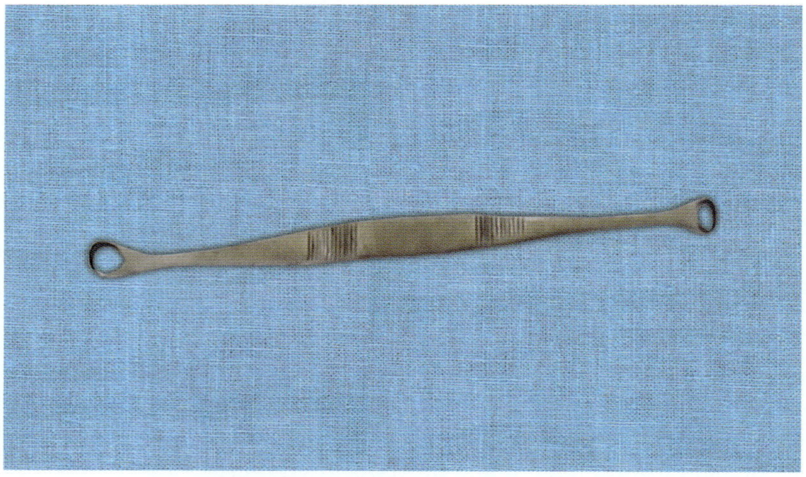

Fig. 18: Blake's uterine curette.

Indications:
- First trimester pregnancy termination, to remove retained products of conception after rapid dilatation of cervix
- Completion of first trimester pregnancy termination
- Removal of bits of membrane and placenta after second trimester pregnancy termination
- Removal of pedunculated cervical or uterine polyps
- Removal of foreign body from vagina
- Manipulation of an enlarged uterus, e.g. after second-trimester abortion for laparoscopic sterilization or minilaparotomy.

Method of use: Procedure can be carried out under general anesthesia or paracervical block and sedation. With the patient in position, cervix is exposed, held with a vulsellum and dilated sufficiently to permit passage of ovum forceps. Ovum forceps held with thumb and ring finger of right hand and two fingers along the length of instrument. Jaws are opened inside uterine cavity; products of conception are grasped and forceps are withdrawn.

Complications:
- Uterine perforation.
- Injury to intra-abdominal structures like small bowel, colon, omentum, etc. secondary to uterine perforation if the latter is undiagnosed and evacuation continued
- Intrauterine infection.
- Incomplete abortion.

BLAKE'S UTERINE CURETTE (FIG. 18)

Sterilized by boiling or autoclaving.

Identification: Central shaft with one small oval loop at each end. Loops are set at an angle to shaft, so tip of loop is directed away from direction of shaft and in opposite direction and curettes endometrium easily. The size of loop varies from 2 × 3 mm to 6 × 10 mm. Edge of the loop is either sharp or blunt.

Indications: For curetting the endometrium, sharp curette used in nonpregnant state.
- Dysfunctional uterine bleeding not responding to hormonal therapy.
- Diagnosis of endometrial tuberculosis.
- Diagnosis of endometrial carcinoma by fractional curettage.
- *Infertility:* To know the hormonal pattern of endometrium.
- Along with Fothergill's operation.
- Prior to myomectomy, to rule out submucosal polyp, endometrial hyperplasia or carcinoma.
- Diagnosis of uterine choriocarcinoma.
- Diagnosis of extension of cervical carcinoma to endometrium.
- Membranous dysmenorrhea.

Blunt curettage is used for curettage in obstetrics because chances of perforation are less than sharp curette. Indications of blunt curette are:
- Check curettage for incomplete abortion
- Postpartum hemorrhage due to retained products of conception
- After evacuation of vesicular mole
- Septic abortion
- Following dilatation and suction evacuation for first trimester-abortion to confirm completeness of procedure
- Following dilatation and evacuation of uterine contents with ovum forceps for first trimester pregnancy termination.

Method of use: Under general anesthesia, sedation or paracervical block after dilatation of cervix to 6–10 mm, curette introduced into uterine cavity and curettage done till grating sensation perceived.

Complications:
- Uterine perforation
- Intrauterine infection
- Intrauterine synechiae.

ALLIS FORCEPS (FIG. 19)

Sterilized by boiling or autoclaving.

Identification: It is available in two sizes, 12 cm and 17 cm in length. Blades are curved inward and have 4 in 5 or 5 in 6 fine teeth. Ratchet lock is present in handles.

Indications:
- *To hold the cut edges of vagina in following situations:*
    - *Abdominal hysterectomy:* After cutting across vagina and removing specimen.
    - *Vaginal hysterectomy:* During closure of vault of vagina.
    - Anterior colporrhaphy, posterior colpoperineorrhaphy, for dissection of vaginal mucosal flaps from underlying bladder and rectum.
    - Excision of vaginal wall cyst.

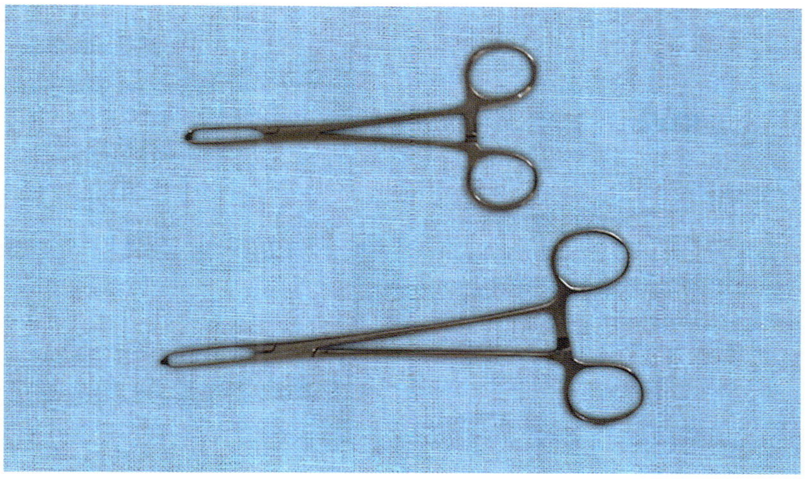

Fig. 19: Allis forceps.

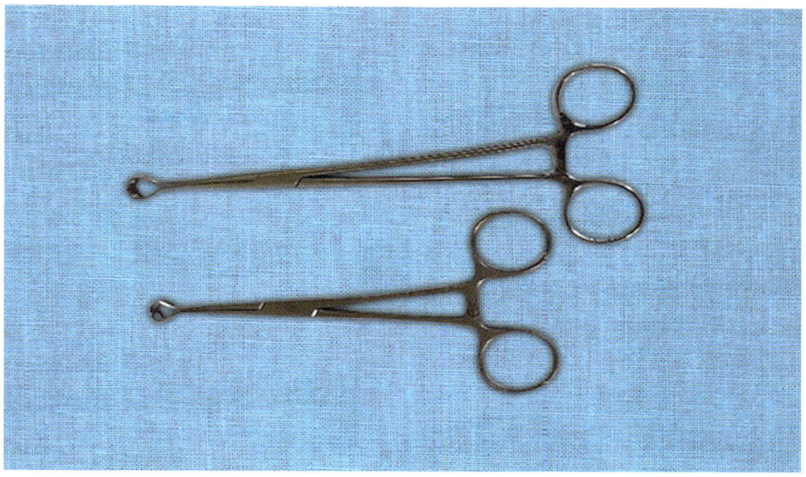

Fig. 20: Babcock's forceps.

- Enterocele repair.
- *Abdominoperineal radical hysterectomy:* For dissection of vaginal cuff.

- *To hold the cervix in following situations:*
  - As a vulsellum
  - *Abdominal hysterectomy:* To draw the cervix up after opening vault of vagina.
- *To hold the uterine fundus in:*
  - *Vaginal hysterectomy:* To draw it down after ligating the uterine vessels and dividing them
  - *Vaginal hysterectomy:* Bisection technique
  - *Abdominal hysterectomy:* To give traction and to manipulate the position of uterus.
- *Myomectomy:* To hold the leiomyoma being enucleated.
- *Metroplasty:* To hold the cut edges of uterus during suturing.
- *Cesarean section:* To hold the cut edges of lower segment for hemostasis and to aid their suturing.
- To hold the edges of rectus sheath during dissection as well as suturing.

BABCOCK'S FORCEPS (FIG. 20)

Sterilized by boiling or autoclaving.

Identification: It has fenestrated triangular blades and grooved jaws. It is available in different sizes which differ in length 12 cm and 17 cm respectively. It is a nontraumatic instrument.

Indications:

- *To hold ureter in:*
  - Wertheim's operation to dissect ureter
  - Ovarian tumor, broad ligament tumor to isolate and safeguard ureter
  - Ureteric reimplantation into sigmoid colon, ileal conduit, urinary bladder, etc.
- *To hold bladder for:*
  - Repair of accidental injury to bladder during gynecological or obstetric operations
  - Vesicovaginal fistula repair
  - Cystostomy.
- *To hold fallopian tube in:*
  - Tubal ligation
  - Tuboplasty
  - Salpingectomy for tubal ectopic gestation.
- *To hold ovary for:*
  - Ovarian cystectomy
  - Wedge resection
  - Endometriosis surgery.
- Dissection of vascular sheaths, ligation of the anterior division of internal iliac artery
- *To hold bowel in:*
  - Rectovaginal fistula repair
  - *Third-degree perineal tear repair:* To hold mucosal edges
  - Repair of bowel injury
  - *Appendicectomy:* To hold appendix and cecum.

KOCHER'S CLAMP (FIG. 21)

Sterilized by boiling or autoclaving.

Identification: It is 20.5 cm long. Tip of blades have one in two teeth. It has transverse serrations on blades. Blades may be curved on flat or straight. Blades can be tightened by Rachet lock on handles.

Indications:

- *Hysterectomy:* To clamp the uterosacral ligaments, uterine blood vessels and the corneal structures or the infundibulopelvic ligaments in vaginal hysterectomy.
- Oophorectomy for ovarian cysts or tumors.
- Removal of pedunculated leiomyomatous polyps.
- Salpingectomy for tubal ectopic gestation.
- Cesarean hysterectomy.
- Clamping the umbilical cord of newborn.
- Artificial low rupture of membranes.
- To hold uterus during abdominal hysterectomy by applying clamp on each side of uterus.

Method of use: Clamp applied with curve facing structure to be removed, so ligature can be passed around clamped to pedicle easily.

Drawbacks:

- Due to absence of longitudinal groove, occlusion of vessels in pedicle is incomplete.
- Not as effective as clamps with longitudinal grooves to prevent slipping of pedicles.

BONNER'S MYOMECTOMY CLAMP (FIG. 22)

Sterilized by boiling or autoclaving. Rubber cap over blades are to be removed for sterilization by chemical methods because heat damages them.

Identification: It is a long clamp 24 cm long made of stainless steel and distal end of blade is covered with rubber tubing to prevent trauma to uterine vessels. There are two pairs of finger grips proximal and distal with a Ratchet lock on handle adjacent to proximal finger grips. The blades are at an angle of 120° with the handles. There are two overlapping transverse bars attached to blade one each. It divides the space between blades into approximately equal parts. Blades are covered with rubber caps distal to site of transverse bars. These caps avoid trauma to uterine vessels.

Indications:
- Myomectomy
- Metroplasty
- Hysterotomy.

Method of use: Instrument is used in these operations to achieve compression of uterine blood vessels to reduce intraoperative blood loss. Distal finger grips are used during application of instrument because blades can be opened wider with finger in distal finger grips rather than in proximal finger grips. For tightening the lock as well as releasing it, proximal grips are used because they offer greater degree of mechanical advantage than distal ones. Instrument is applied with angle downward, so blades go into pelvis over tubes while handle remains horizontal between patient's thighs. Space between the blades distal to transverse bars includes uterus just above cervix and both the round ligaments. The transverse bar prevents the round ligament from slipping. The round ligament holds the uterine fundus down. If uterus is allowed to slip upward, the uterine arteries are not compressed and blood loss during surgery is not controlled. After myomectomy both the clamps are removed. To control blood supply through ovarian vessels a sponge holding forceps is applied over each infundibulopelvic ligament during operation.

Clamp cannot be applied in presence of cervical leiomyoma. In that case cervical leiomyoma is first enucleated and then clamp is applied. The clamp has to be released for 10 minutes after every 20 minutes of application because otherwise the uterine tissue suffers from anoxia, and also histamine and other substances accumulate in uterine circulation and when they enter general circulation cause hypotension and vasodilatation. Clamp is released after closure of myoma bed. Hemostasis has to be confirmed after releasing the clamp.

Complications:
- Myomectomy clamp can injure uterine blood vessels.
- Shock syndrome following release of clamp since clamping may cause crush syndrome effect.

DOYEN'S MYOMA SCREW (FIG. 23)

Sterilized by boiling or autoclaving.

Identification: Sharp pointed hook with handle of different sizes made of stainless steel. It has coarse threaded screw with pointed tip.

Use:
- It is used to hold the leiomyoma during abdominal or vaginal myomectomy.
- To fix the uterine fundus while performing hysterectomy with fibroid uterus.

STRAIGHT LONG CLAMP FORCEPS (FIG. 24)

Identification: Straight long forceps made of stainless steel. The blades are serrated and can be tightened by Ratchet lock on handle.

Indications:
- Hysterectomy
- Ovariotomy
- Salpingectomy.

PLACENTAL CURETTE (FIG. 25)

Sterilized by boiling or autoclaving

Identification: It has wide looped end for curetting and handle at other end. The edges of loop are blunt.

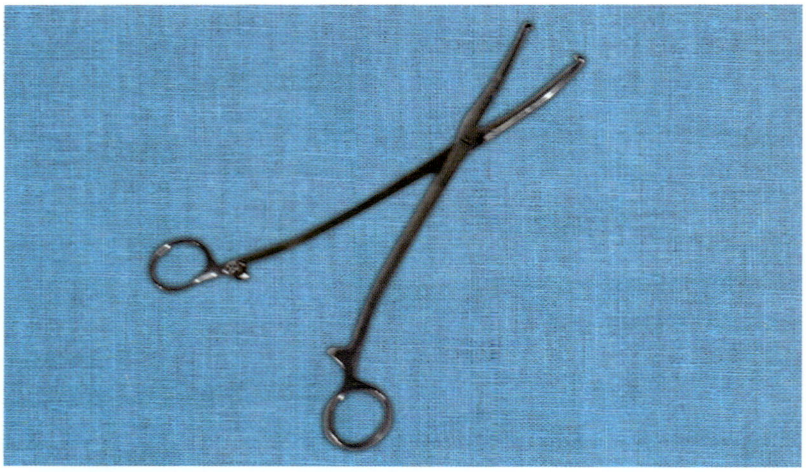

Fig. 21: Kocher's clamp.

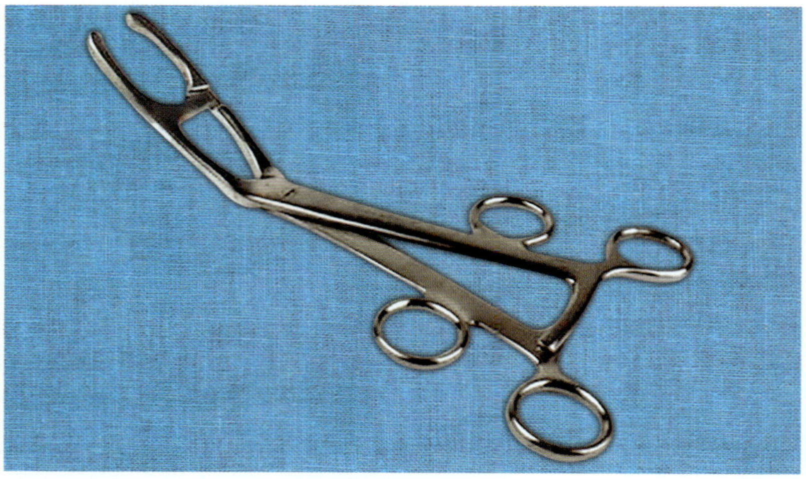

Fig. 22: Bonner's myomectomy clamp.

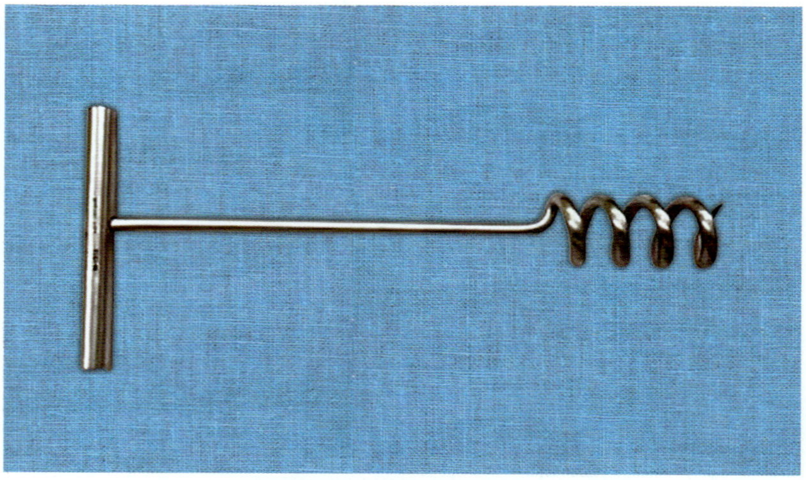

Fig. 23: Myoma screw.

Indications:
- Check curettage or incomplete abortion and retention of placenta in second trimester.
- Retained segments or bits of placenta after delivery of viable fetus.

Method of use: Procedure is carried out under general anesthesia or sedation. With patient in lithotomy position, the cervix is exposed with vaginal speculum and held with sponge holding forceps. Cervical canal is sounded and not the uterine cavity for fear of perforation. After dipping placental curette in antiseptic solution placental curette is inserted in uterine cavity. Uterine cavity is systematically curetted until grating sensation perceived due to scraping of curette against fibrous tissue in basalis.

Complications:
- Uterine perforation
- Intrauterine infection
- Intrauterine synechiae.

GELLHORN'S CERVICAL BIOPSY FORCEPS (FIG. 26)

Sterilized by boiling or autoclaving.

Identification: It is a 22.5 cm long with cup-shaped ends. Edges of cup are cutting and inside of cup has tiny pin that fits into corresponding depression. Pin holds cervical biopsy specimen in place. Handle of instrument are long so as to offer mechanical advantage so biopsy can be taken from firm cervical tissue with application of moderate force. Handles are also bent downward so that they do not obstruct field of vision. There is no catch in handles.

Indications: For taking cervical biopsy—
- Cervical lesion, suspected to be carcinomatous
- Suspicion of cervical carcinoma from Papanicolaou smear
- Abnormal colposcopy findings
- Evaluate the response of radiotherapy for cervical carcinoma
- Diagnosis of persistent cervical carcinoma after radiotherapy
- Diagnosis of recurrence of cervical carcinoma
- Suspected secondaries in cervix
- Differential diagnosis of cervical ulcer
- Diagnosis of DES-associated cervical lesions.

SHIRODKAR FORCEPS (FIG. 27)

Sterilized by boiling or autoclaving.

Identification: It has two finger grips with cross bar connecting the two together. There is a single blade, which is curved on flat and has eye near the tip. There is no joint as with other round ligament forceps, so the problem of joint getting trapped in tissue is avoided.

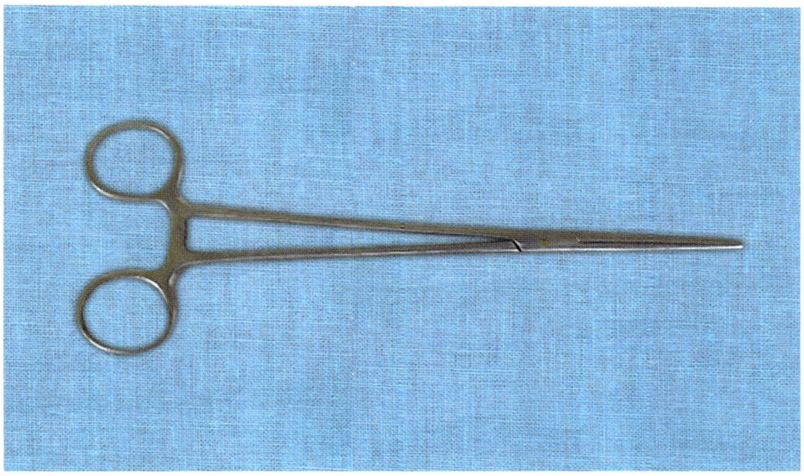

Fig. 24: Long clamp forceps.

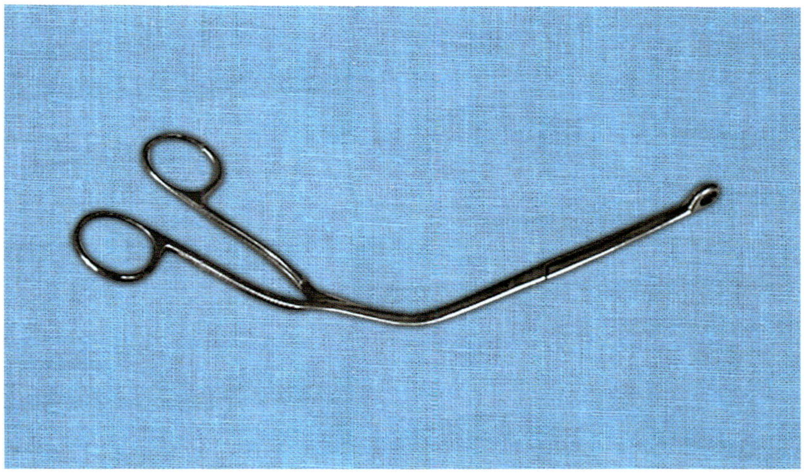

Fig. 26: Gellhorn's cervical biopsy forceps.

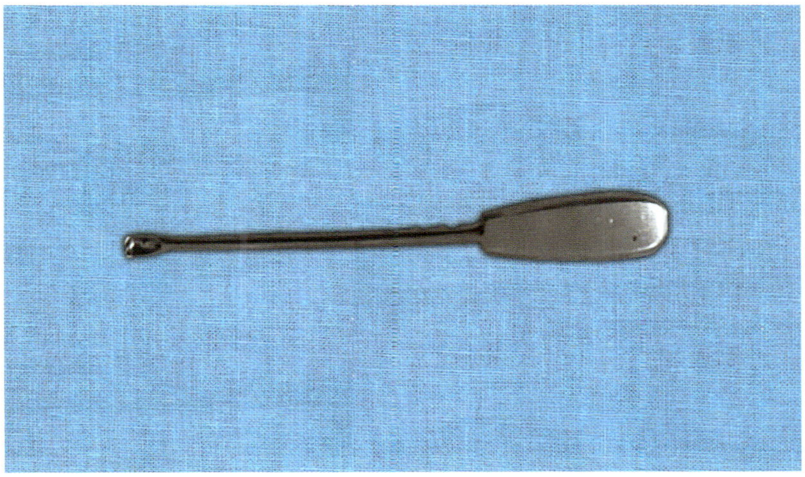

Fig. 25: Placental curette.

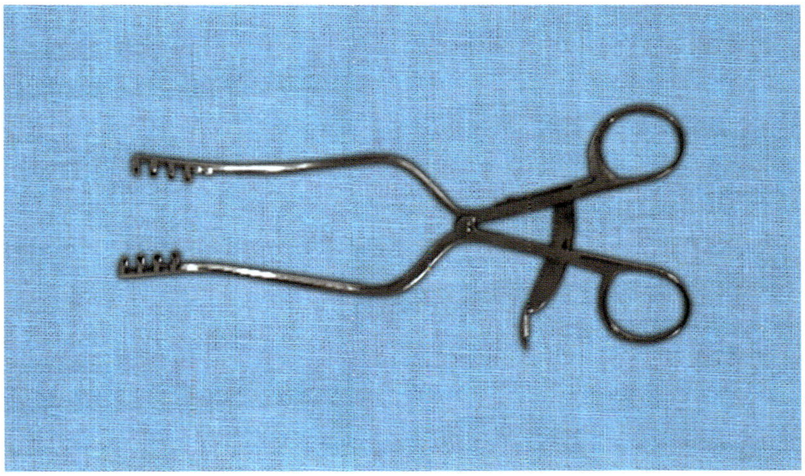

Fig. 27: Shirodkar forceps.

Indications:
- Ventrosuspension by modified Gilliam's operation
- Purandare's cervicopexy—forceps blade is passed starting lateral to rectus abdominis into the broad ligament to emerge in uterovesical space, the strip of rectus sheath or Mersilene tape sutured to its tip through eye. It can be passed by exactly reverse route and rectus sheath strip or Mersilene tape may be drawn back sutured to its tip through eye.

ARTERY FORCEPS (FIG. 28)

Artery forceps are available as straight or curved. Smallest are known as mosquito forceps and they range through to 5 inch Crile's forceps and 7 inch long fine forceps.

Uses: It helps in grasping the tissues, sutures, prosthetic material, vessels, and bleeders; and securing hemostatic by allowing ligation. As they vary in size, they can be used on fine, delicate to larger vascular pedicles and helps in securing the hemostasis.

DISSECTING FORCEPS (FIG. 29)

Forceps are handheld, hinged instrument used for grasping and holding objects. Mechanically forceps employ principle of the lever to grasp and apply pressure. Surgical forceps are made of high-grade carbon steel. Held between thumb and two or three fingers of one hand, with top resting on first dorsal interosseous muscle. Spring tension at one end holds the grasping end apart until pressure is applied. Forceps can be toothed or nontoothed.

Uses: It is used during dissection of vaginal wall and fascia and suturing of tough structures like skin, rectus sheath, and vaginal wall.

BANDAGE SCISSORS (FIG. 30)

They are angled tip scissors with blunt tip on bottom blade, which help in cutting bandages without gouging the skin. They were invented by Henry A Kimmel.

Uses: It is used in anterior colporrhaphy operation to dissect the vaginal flaps from bladder.

NEEDLE HOLDER (FIG. 31)

They can be straight or curved. The handle of the needle holder is long while blades are short. The serrations on inner aspect of blade prevents slipping and turning of needle. The straight holder is used for surface while curved ones are used for depth.

AYRE'S SPATULA (FIG. 32)

Identification: Made of wood, plastic or stainless steel. Instrument is 15–17 cm long. Its one end is broad and has two projections, one projecting beyond other.

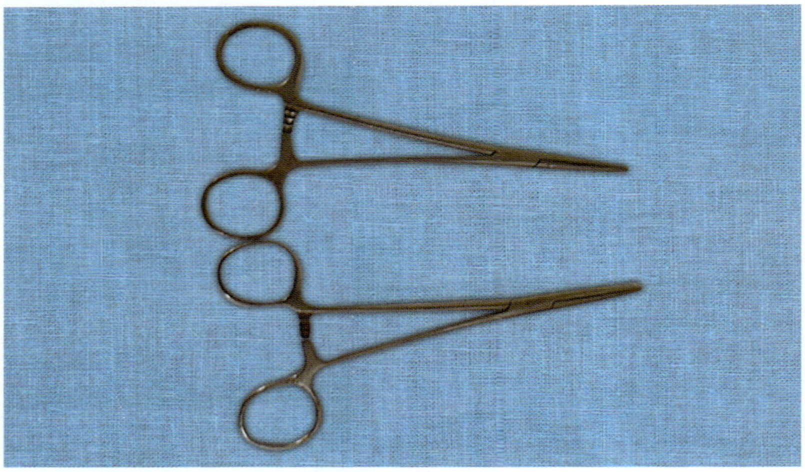

Fig. 28: Artery forceps.

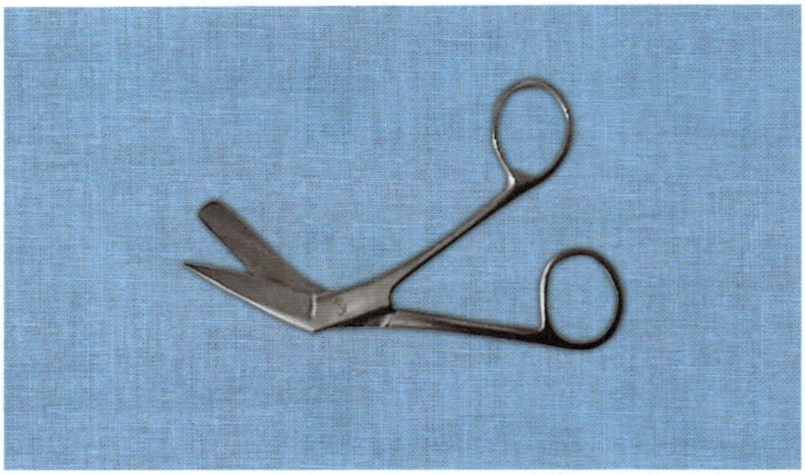

Fig. 30: Bandage scissors.

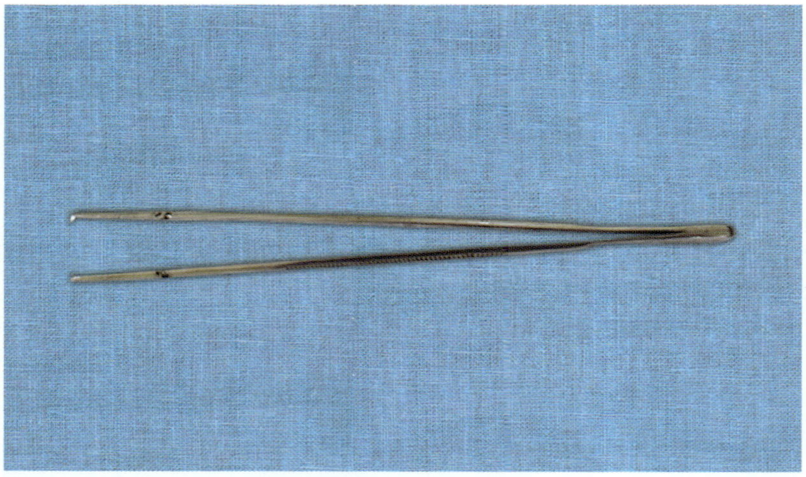

Fig. 29: Dissecting forceps.

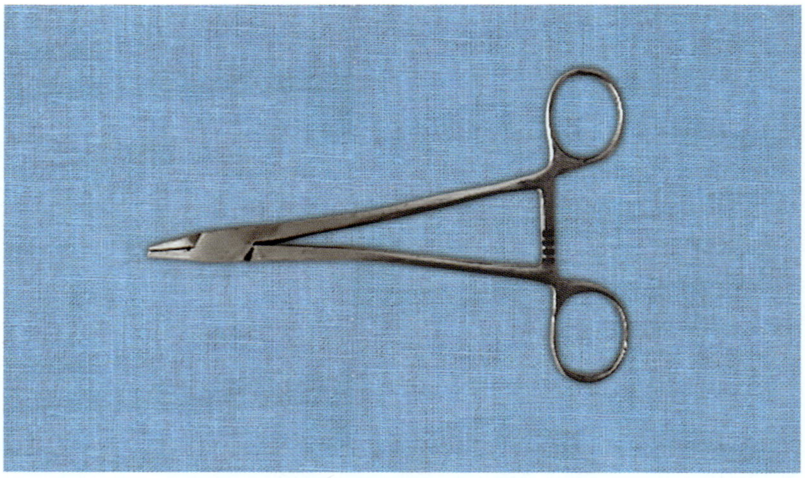

Fig. 31: Needle holder.

Sterilization: Wooden spatula is sterilized by dry heat in hot air oven. Plastic spatula sterilized by immersion in antiseptic solution like cetrimide or Hibitane. Stainless steel spatula sterilized by boiling or autoclaving.

Indications: Used for collecting exfoliative cytological smear from cervix, posterior vaginal fornix, upper one-third of lateral vaginal wall or buccal mucosa as outlined below

- *Cytological screening for cervical carcinoma:* Smear from cervix and posterior fornix.
- *Screening for upper genital tract malignancy:* From posterior fornix in high-risk cases. Incidence of missing diagnosis is high for upper genital tract malignancy.
- *Follow-up of treated case of cervical carcinoma:* From vault of vagina if radical hysterectomy has been done and from cervix after radiotherapy.
- Diagnosis of persistent or recurrent cervical carcinoma.
- *Hormonal cytology:* From upper one-third of lateral vaginal wall.
- Follow-up of cases of CIN treated with CO_2 laser surgery, cryosurgery, electrocauterization, conization or 5-fluorouracil chemosurgery.
- Evaluation of lower genital tract in female offspring of women exposed to DES during pregnancy from cervix and vagina.
- Buccal smear for evaluation of Barr bodies from buccal mucosa.
- Graham's test for predicting response of cervical carcinoma to radiotherapy.

Method of use: No anesthesia required. Prior to taking cervicovaginal smear patient has to avoid sexual relations or vaginal douche for 24 hours. Vaginal examination should not be carried out prior to taking smear. Patient is kept in lithotomy position, cervix is exposed with vaginal speculum. Broad end of spatula is used to make smear from portio vaginalis. Longer end of spatula is inserted into external os while shorter end comes in contact with portio vaginalis. Instrument is rotated through 360° to pick exfoliated cells from portio vaginalis. Smear is made on clean glass slide and smear fixed with equal amount of ether and absolute alcohol. Long and narrow end is inserted into cervical canal and rotated through 360° to pick cells from cervical canal and is fixed as above. Broad end of another Ayre's spatula is used to obtain material for smear from posterior fornix. Broad end can also be used to obtain material from lateral vaginal wall or buccal mucosa. It is known as abrasion cytology. It is better than impression cytology in which smear is obtained by direct contact between slide and surface. Wooden spatula is best because its surface is rough and cells stick on surface more than on plastic or stainless steel. Smear should not be obtained if patient has bleeding per vaginam or has vaginitis.

COPLIN JAR (FIG. 33)

It is a glass jar with glass lid. Inside is square on cross section. There are ridges on opposite walls, so that glass slide fits between ridges without touching one another. Fixative fluid is filled in jar and slides are placed in jar for fixation. Plastic jars are also available with similar design but with secure lid. They can be transported without the fixative spilling out.

LEECH WILKINSON'S CANNULA (FIG. 34)

Sterilized by boiling or autoclaving.

Identification: It is 28 cm long with fixed spiral cone at one end and Luer-Lok mount at other end. A long metal stylet with cannula is supplied for cleaning it.

Indications:

- Hysterosalpingography
- Chromopertubation during laparoscopy
- Hydrotubation

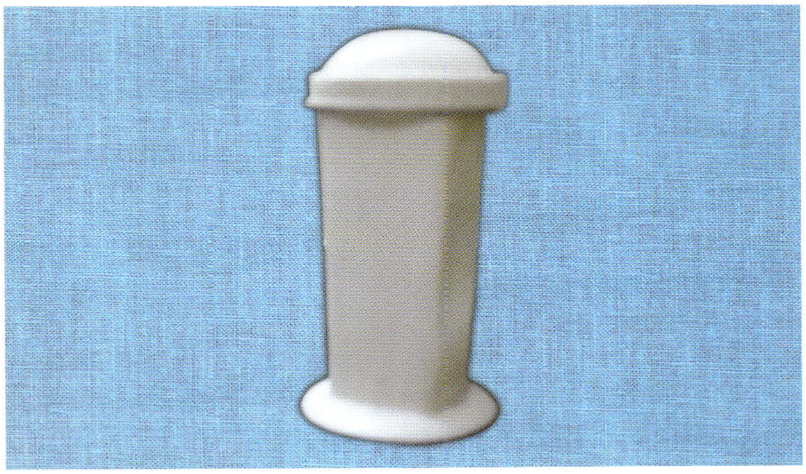

Fig. 33: Coplin jar.

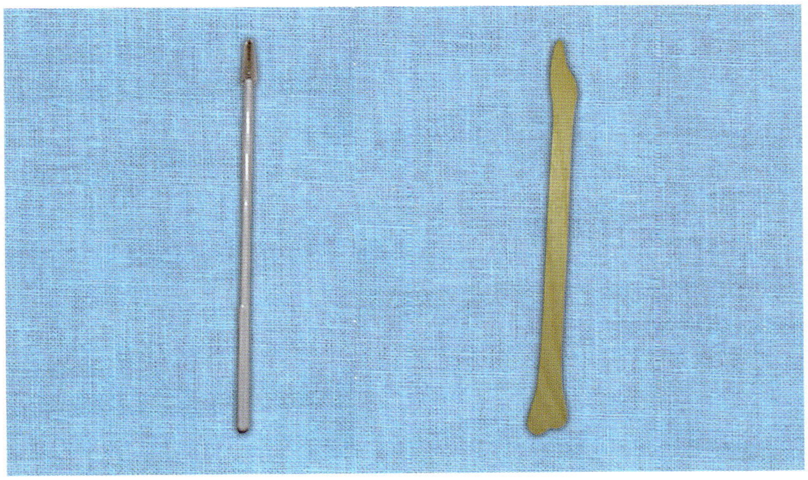

Fig. 32: Ayre's spatula and endocervical brush.

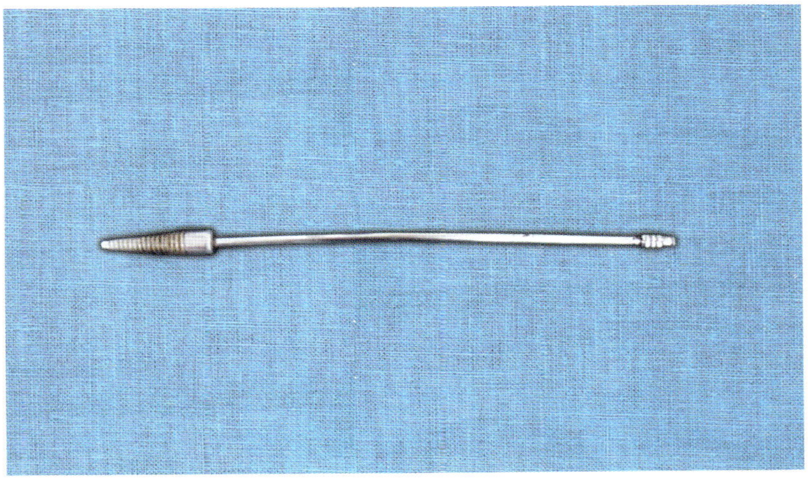

Fig. 34: Leech Wilkinson's cannula

- Rubin's test
- Kymography
- Hysterosalpingography (HSG).

Method of use: It does not require anesthesia. Patient is kept in lithotomy position, cervix is exposed with vaginal speculum and anterior lip held with vulsellum. Cannula is put at external os and rotated clockwise so that it advances in cervical canal and cannula gets fixed in cervix. Syringe is applied on the other end for injection. Spiral cone achieves airtight fit and prevents leak of dye into vagina, especially suited for multiparous cervix, which is usually patulous. For hysterosalpingography 60% sodium iothalamate or 60% methylglucamine diatrizoate is used. Dye is injected under fluoroscopic control or with aid of image intensifier. First plate is taken with filling of uterine cavity, second with delineation of Fallopian tube when peritoneal spill is just occurring and third 15–20 minutes later to show pattern of peritoneal spill.

During chromopertubation, dilute methylene blue is injected and peritoneal spill visualized by laparoscopy.

In Rubin's test, air is injected through cannula and abdomen auscultated at suprapubic areas for sound made by air escaping through Fallopian tube into peritoneal cavity. When the air injection system is connected to kymograph and a graph is plotted of intrauterine pressure on injection of air, it is called kymography. Rubin's test is not done in modern gynecology because it cannot diagnose unilateral tubal blockage or extensive peritubal adhesions if tubes are patent. It can be false positive in presence of large hydrosalpinx. Kymography is also not done because better procedures are available.

Laparoscopy with chromopertubation remains the gold standard.

Complications:
- Uterine perforation, cervical perforation
- Endometrial dislocation
- Bleeding
- Endometritis, pelvic peritonitis
- Venous or lymphatic intravasation.

Contraindications to tubal patency testing and hysterosalpingography:
- Suspected ectopic gestation
- Intrauterine gestation
- Pelvic infection
- Immediate pre- and postmenstrually and during menstruation
- Sensitivity to contrast medium.

CHAPTER

3

Sterilization of Laparoscopic Instruments

Shruti Paliwal, G Hemasree, B Ramesh

INTRODUCTION

Sterilization is the process by which complete destruction of microbes can be attained. It can be achieved by physical, chemical, and physicochemical methods.

Disinfection is the process by which most microorganisms can be eliminated on objects (excluding bacterial spores). It can be achieved by physical or chemical methods.

Types of disinfection **(*Table 1*)**:

- High level: All the microbes are eliminated, sparing spores.
- Intermediate level: Some viruses, spores, and fungi are indestructible.
- Low level: Fungi, viruses, spores, and mycobacteria are spared.

Decontamination is a process of removal of all pathogenic microorganisms from inanimate objects to make them safe to handle/use/discard.

For laparoscopic instruments, ideally, sterilization or at least high level disinfection (HLD) should be used.

SPAULDING CLASSIFICATION OF MEDICAL DEVICES

- *Critical:* Objects which enter normally sterile tissue or the vascular system or through which blood flows should be sterile.
- *Semicritical:* Objects which have contact with mucous membranes or skin that is not intact require a high level disinfection (HLD) which eliminates all microorganisms but high levels of bacterial spores.
- *Noncritical:* Objects which have contact with intact skin require low level disinfection (or nongermicidal detergent).

CLEANING AND STERILIZATION

Steps include:

- Dismantling
- Decontamination
- Cleaning and rinsing
- Drying
- Sterilization
- Storage.

Dismantling

Laparoscopic instruments should be having a design, which allows easy dismantling. Instruments, which cannot be easily dismantled and reassembled, tend to harbor blood or debris within the shafts and poses a risk to safety of patients in whom they are used **(Fig. 1)**.

Decontamination

It is a method by which the bioburden on the reusable medical devices is decreased. The process begins with cleaning the visible blood and body fluids off the instrument in the theater. Container with 0.5% chlorine disinfectant solution is used to soak in all soiled or contaminated instruments for 10 minutes. Instruments designed with an external internal seal that does not totally occlude the internal space, or no gasket should be placed in vertical position in enzymatic cleaning and rinsing solution, instead of standard horizontal position so that air trapped within instrument is allowed to escape and replace with solution **(Fig. 2)**.

Cleaning

Autoclavable instruments require specialized cleaning prior to sterilization. Instrumental surfaces should be free of any residual

Table 1: Types of disinfections.

	Type	*Vegetative*	*TB bacilli*	*Spores*
1	Low level disinfection	+	–	–
2	Intermediate level disinfection	+	+	–
3	High level disinfection	+	+	+
4	Sterilization	+	+	+

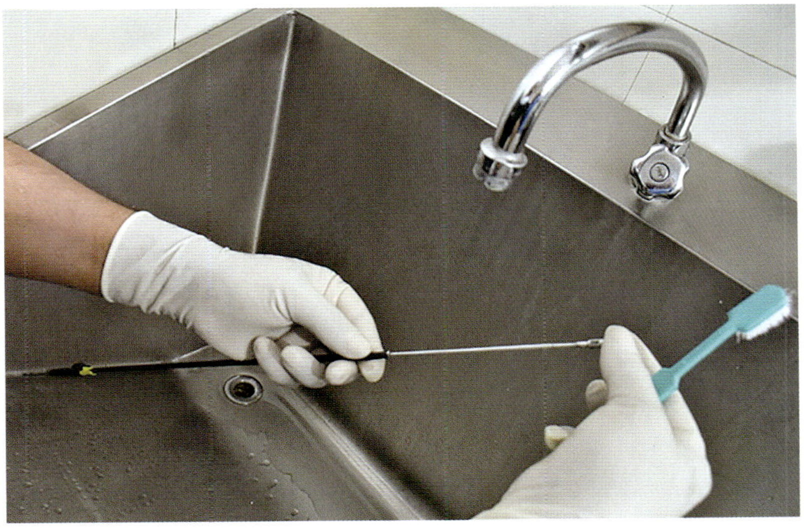

Fig. 1: Dismantling of instrument.

proteinaceous material or organic residues and it is particularly important when instrument has several small moving parts and crevices. The accumulation of residues may lead to corrosive damage and pathogenic colonization. Cleaning of laparoscopic instruments is best carried using soft brushes that allow the inner surface of instrument to be cleaned thoroughly.

Substances harmful for instruments: Saline, bleaching powder, iodine-based preparation, abrasive cleaners, laundry detergents, surgeon's hand scrub, and soap **(Figs. 3A and B)**.

Rinsing

Running water is best used for rinsing of laparoscopic instruments, so that all particulate matter as well as residue of chemicals used for contamination and cleaning are completely cleared from them. Jet of water is better than rinsing in stagnant water **(Figs. 4A to C)**.

Sterilization

Rigid laparoscopic instruments need to be sterile as per Centers for Disease Control and Prevention (CDC) recommendation or if that is not feasible they be high level disinfected. Steam and ethylene oxide are the sterilization processes available.

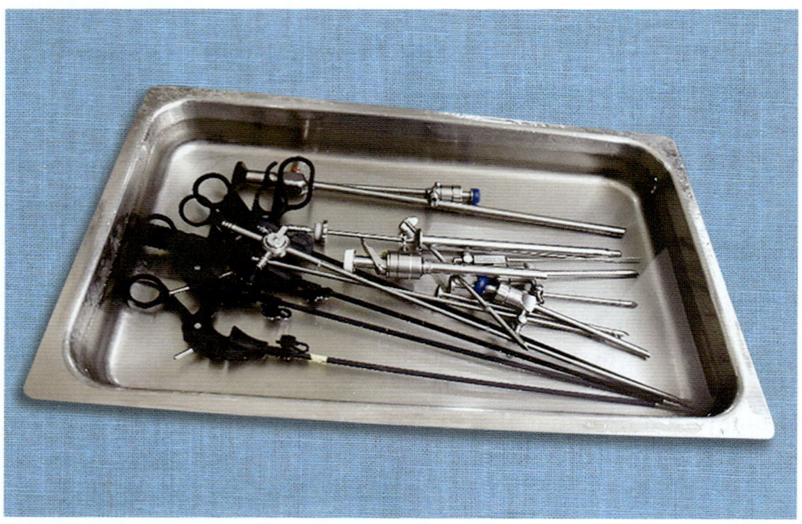

Fig. 2: Instruments soaked in disinfectant for decontamination.

Steam Sterilization

Steam sterilization in an autoclave is one of the most common types of sterilization in hospitals. It is effective, cheap, and nontoxic. Autoclaving at 121°C for 45–60 minutes is suitable for all reusable metal instruments. Before sterilization, all instruments that are insulated, all silicone tubing, and all cords should be doubly wrapped in cloth to prevent contact with hot metallic container. They are then placed in autoclave. Laparoscope may be sterilized by flash or vacuum steam sterilization. Flash sterilization is carried out at 135°C at 30 psi pressure for 4 minutes. This method requires postvacuum and dry cycles. In order to prevent water condensation on lens, the instruments should rest on a sterilizer rack for 45 minutes **(Figs. 5A and B)**.

Low Temperature Steam and Formaldehyde Sterilization

This is a suitable method of sterilization for all kind of heat-sensitive instruments since the temperature used is 55–80°C. It is used for long, narrow, dead end lumen instruments 2 mm and 1–5 meter in length. Cycle takes 5–6 hours depending on temperature used.

Gas Sterilization

Sterilization using ethylene oxide is feasible for all disposable instruments, insulated hand instruments, and all tubings used for gas, suction, and irrigation. It acts by alkylating N position of guanine in DNA directly **(Figs. 6A and B)**. Endoscopic instruments may be sterilized with either cold or warm ethylene oxide gas. With cold gas, temperature is set at 85°C and instruments are exposed for 4 hours 30 minutes followed by aeration for 12 hours. Warm gas sterilization takes place at 145°C for 2 hour 30 minutes, followed by 8 hour aeration. The advantages of ethylene oxide are that items are not damaged, it permeates porous material, and it is noncorrosive to optics. Main disadvantages are its cost, toxicity, need for aeration, and being longer process and risk of inhalation injury and contact injury. It is carcinogenic and mutagenic. Its efficacy is monitored with B subtilis spores.

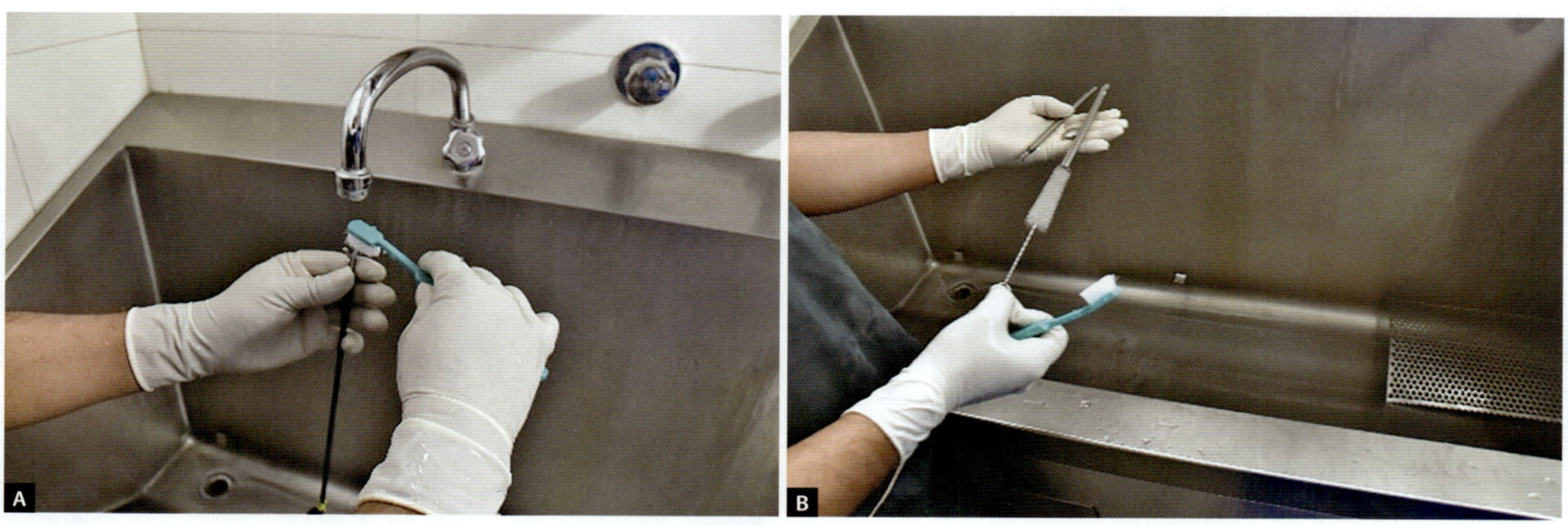

Figs. 3A and B: Cleaning of instruments.

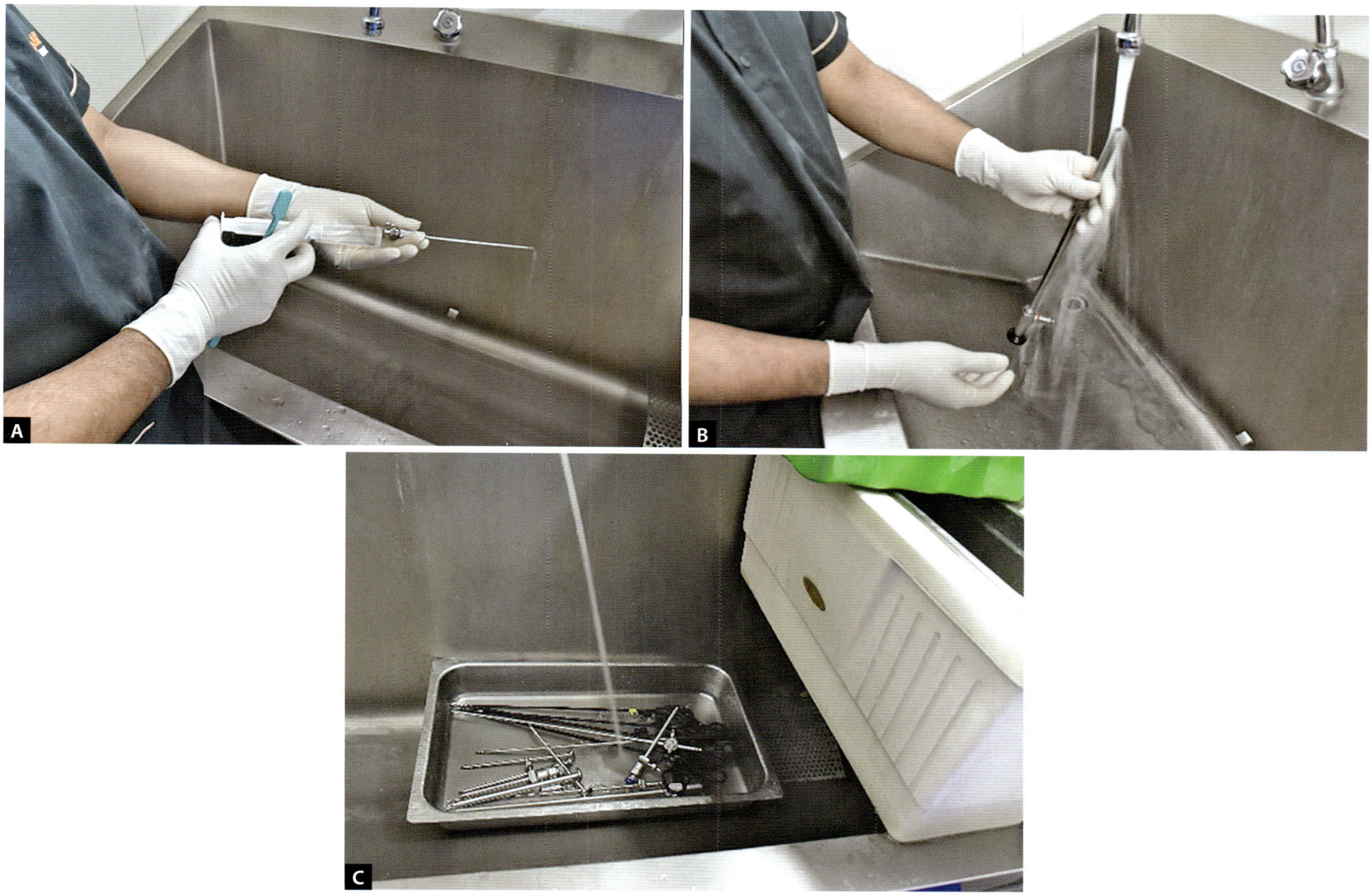

Figs. 4A to C: Rinsing of instruments.

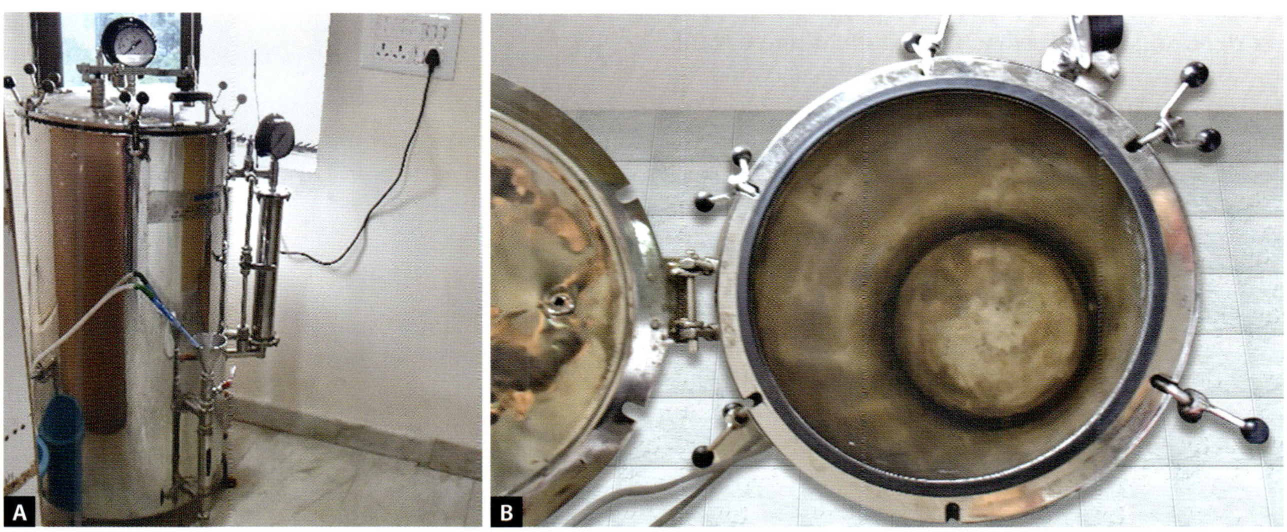

Figs. 5A and B: Autoclave.

HIGH LEVEL DISINFECTION

High level disinfection is used for instrument processing when sterilization is not feasible or available. It eliminates bacteria, fungi, viruses, parasites but does not kill all bacterial endospores which cause diseases such as tetanus, gas gangrene, and atypical mycobacterial infection. It is suitable for items that will come in contact with intact mucus membranes or damaged skin.

Methods of disinfection:

- Low temperature steam—73°C × 20 min
- Boiling water—100°C × 5 min

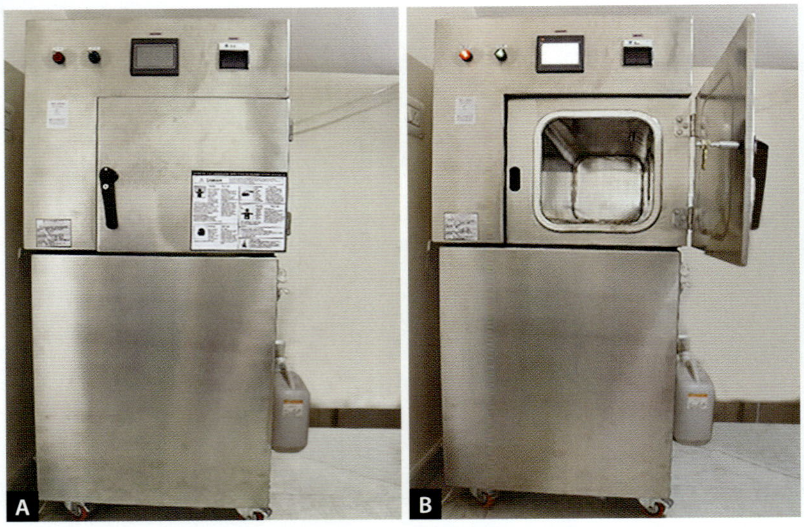

Figs. 6A and B: Ethylene oxide sterilizer.

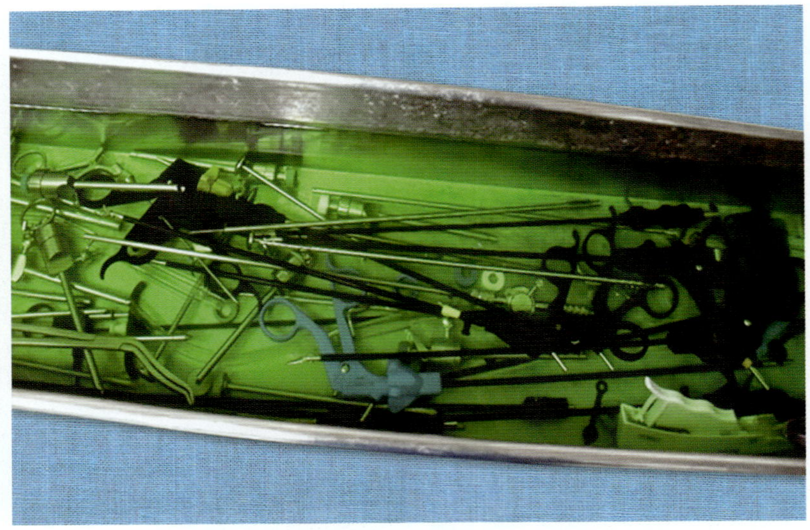

Fig. 7: Disinfection in glutaraldehyde solution.

- Formaldehyde—air tight chamber at 50°C
- Glutaraldehyde 2%—effective against most bacteria, virus including hepatitis B and C/HIV. Cidex solution (2.4% alkaline glutaraldehyde) provides HLD in 20–45 minutes
- Ortho-phthalaldehyde 0.55% (OPA) 12 minutes soak time at room temperature.

Advantages of glutaraldehyde are—good biocidal activity, noncorrosive to optics, and is active in presence of proteins. It destroys microorganisms by alkylation of amino acids. 2.4% alkaline glutaraldehyde solution is called as Cidex. It is efficient in bactericidal, fungicidal, and virucidal activity but slow in mycobactericidal activity. It destroys 99.8% of mycobacterial tuberculosis in 45 minutes at 25°C.

It irritates the skin, eyes, and respiratory tract at concentration of 0.3 ppm. Duration for which the commercially available solution can be used varies between 14 and 30 days. Its potency should be tested daily with manufacturer's test strip. Efficiency of glutaraldehyde is determined by various factors including organic load, contact time and use pattern, concentration, physical configuration of instruments, pH, and temperature.

Occupational Safety and Health Administration's (OSHA) established maximum allowable exposure limit for glutaraldehyde is 0.2 ppm. Fiber optic light cord and telescope need to be soaked in 2% glutaraldehyde for at least 10 minutes and should not exceed 20 minutes. Endocamera may be disinfected by 10 minutes submersion in 2% glutaraldehyde. Care should be taken to leave the plug end of the cord outside solution. Alternately sterile drape over camera and cord can be used. Soakage of other metallic instruments including trochars and hand instruments is recommended for 60 minutes to avoid infection with atypical mycobacterial infection.

Cidex plus, a high level disinfectant, is a 3.4% glutaraldehyde solution (20 minutes at 25°C) **(Fig. 7)**.

Cidex OPA (ortho-phthalaldehyde) requires no activation or mixing. It destroys *Mycobacterium tuberculosis* in 12 minutes at 20°C.

Formaldehyde, glutaraldehyde from phenolic derivatives, hypochlorites, iodophors, phenolics, and quaternary ammonium compounds are unpopular and condemned. Formaldehyde is potentially carcinogenic and extremely irritating to skin, eyes, nose, and respiratory tract. Its efficacy is inadequate and therefore routine use of formaldehyde for sterilizing instruments and other items is not recommended.

Peracetic acid: It acts by denaturing protein and destroys cell membrane. Its byproducts acetic acid, water, and oxygen are nontoxic. Maximum reuse period is 14 days. It is effective in presence of organic material and at low temperature. It has additional tuberculocidal activity.

Ortho-phthalaldehyde solution is an agent that is glutaraldehyde-free agent that provides fast and effective way to HLD. Contact time required with OPA is 12 minutes and is enough to destroy all bacteria, fungi as well as mycobacterial spores. It acts by interacting with amino acid, protein, and microorganisms. Advantages of OPA are—more stability, effective over a 14 day use cycle, and less irritant to eyes. Disadvantage is it stains proteins gray.

Hydrogen peroxide: It has bactericidal, virucidal, sporicidal, and fungicidal properties. It produces hydroxyl-free radicals that can attack membrane lipids, DNA, and other essential cell components. Accelerated hydrogen peroxide (0.5%) kills viruses in 1 minute and mycobacteria and fungi in 5 minutes.

Perasafe: It is 0.08% peracetic acid plus 1% hydrogen peroxide. It acts by denaturing protein and destroys cell membrane. It effectively inactivates mycobacteria resistant to glutaraldehyde. Soak time is 10 minutes **(Table 2)**.

PLASMA STERILIZER

Plasma is the fourth state of matter (solid, liquid, gas, and plasma). It is generated when a gas is heated to an appropriate temperature or exposed to a strong electromagnetic field. Plasma is an ionized gas having some special properties, which are not seen in any other state of matter. It sterilizes by a process called oxidation. All microorganisms are deactivated in a chemical reaction generated by it. Free radicals, which are highly unstable, are generated when hydrogen peroxide is subjected to extreme heat. These free radicles combine with the microorganisms in the load—thus effectively destroying the components of their cells, such as enzymes, nucleic acids, and DNA.

HYDROGEN PEROXIDE PLASMA IN THE STERILIZER

Liquid hydrogen peroxide is placed into the sterilizer and heated up in a vaporizer in order to turn it into gas. Later, the hydrogen peroxide

Table 2: Methods of high level disinfection.

	Autoclave/flash autoclave	*Cidex*	*Perasafe*	*Ethylene oxide*	*Gas plasma*	*Formalin chamber*	*Sterile sleeve*
Camera	X	++	++		+++	+	++
Light cable	+	++	++		+++	+	++
Telescope	+++	++	++		+++	X	X
Tubings/diathermy	X	+	+	+++	+++	+	X
Harmonic scalpel cable	X	++	++		+++	+	++
Heat sensitive hand instruments	x	++	++	+++	+++	X	X
Heat-resistant hand instruments	+++	++	++	+++	+++	X	X
Trocars	+++	++	++	+	+++	X	X

gas is subjected to higher temperatures and plasma is generated. The plasma is dispersed inside the sterilizer chamber in order to oxidize all microorganisms on the load **(Fig. 8)**.

Applications

Common applications for hydrogen peroxide plasma sterilizers include sterilizing the following:

- Doppler, laser probes, ophthalmic lenses, defibrillator paddles, thermometers, harmonic cables, and nonhollow loads, such as electrocautery instruments
- Fiber optic light cables, hollow loads, such as laryngoscopes and their blades, shaver handpieces, and surgical power drills
- Endoscopes, such as rigid and flexible endoscopes.

Hydrogen peroxide plasma has the serious advantage of safety—both for the environment (including the sterilizer operator) and the contents of load. The importance of this safety cannot be overstated. And because hydrogen peroxide does not produce toxic fumes, there are no long aeration/degassing times in the cycle. At the end of the cycle, the plasma is "cracked" into the nontoxic byproducts of water and oxygen, which safely evaporate into the air.

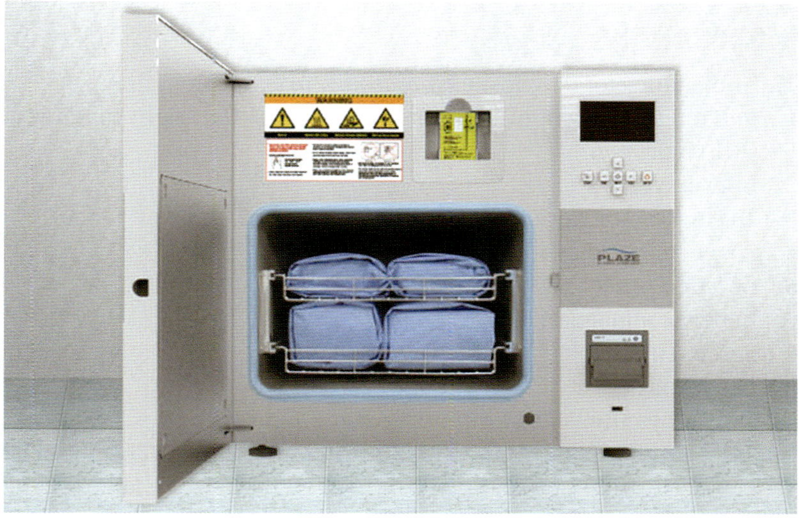

Fig. 8: Plasma sterilizer.

Advantages of Hydrogen Peroxide Plasma

By using hydrogen peroxide plasma as a method of low temperature sterilization, one benefits from:

- No residual chemicals
- Safe handling
- Environmental safety
- Short duration of aeration time.

Disadvantages of Hydrogen Peroxide Plasma

- Liquids, powders, and strong absorbers cannot be sterilized.
- Specific synthetic packaging of the load is needed.
- Smaller sterilization chamber compared to an ethylene oxide sterilizer.

CHAPTER

4

Diagnostic Laparoscopy

B Ramesh, G Hemasree

INDICATIONS

The indications for diagnostic laparoscopy in gynecology are:

1. Pelvic pain, pelvic inflammatory disease (PID), right iliac fossa (RIF) pain, etc.
2. Infertility
3. To confirm the findings of other investigations
4. Suspected pelvic tuberculosis
5. As a part of second look laparoscopy
6. In pelvic malignancies
7. Foreign body
8. Pelvic masses.

Nowadays the role of only diagnostic laparoscopy is limited as imaging modalities are advanced and confirmatory. The modern gynecologist should be ready to continue with operative laparoscopy whenever he does diagnostic laparoscopy. So that both diagnosis and therapy is completed in one sitting under anesthesia.

INSTRUMENTATION

Earlier diagnostic laparoscopy was done with 10 mm telescope and light source without video camera. The surgeon was visualizing the pelvic organs through the eye piece of the telescope. Now with advanced laparoscopic equipment all diagnostic are performed by attaching video camera to the telescope and pelvic organs are seen on the monitor with magnification. So that even small lesions can be picked up easily and disease identified perfectly.

Instrument Required

- Veress needle
- 5 mm trocars
- 5 mm telescope
- Entire videoscope and monitor
- Light source and insulator.

TECHNIQUE

Abdomen, pelvis and perineum are cleaned, scrubbed and draped, bladder emptied, small incision taken at the umbilicus, veress inserted intraperitoneally CO_2 insuflation is done with CO_2 insuflator **(Fig. 1)**. The pressure can go up to 18 mm to prevent primary trocar injuries. The Veress needle is taken out. The incision is slightly enlarged and 5 mm trocar inserted **(Fig. 2)** through the umbilicus or supra umbilicus **(Figs. 3 and 4)**. The 5 mm **(Fig. 5)** telescope connected to videoscope is inserted into the peritoneal cavity to get the clear picture on the monitor **(Fig. 6)**. The surgeon now inspects the whole abdomen and pelvis thoroughly. Another 5 mm trocar is inserted on the flank as same side of the surgeon under vision **(Fig. 7)**. Now 5 mm gasper or any instrument is used to manipulate the pelvic organs, if the patient is infertile chromopertubation is performed and wash is given. If any other pathology is seen ex-endometriosis surgeon proceeds with operative laparoscopy.

CO_2 is evacuated at the end of the procedure and trocars are removed. Band-aid has been put. No sutures required for 5-mm ports.

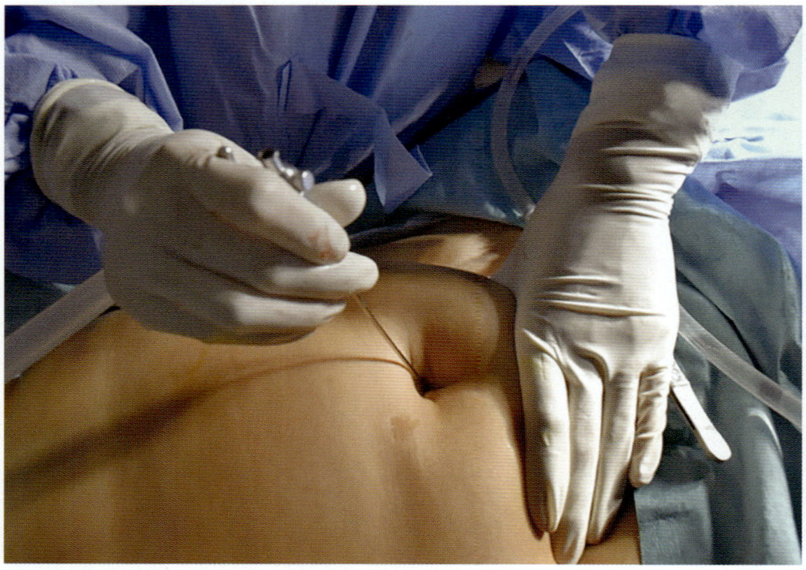

Fig. 1: Veress insertion through umbilicus.

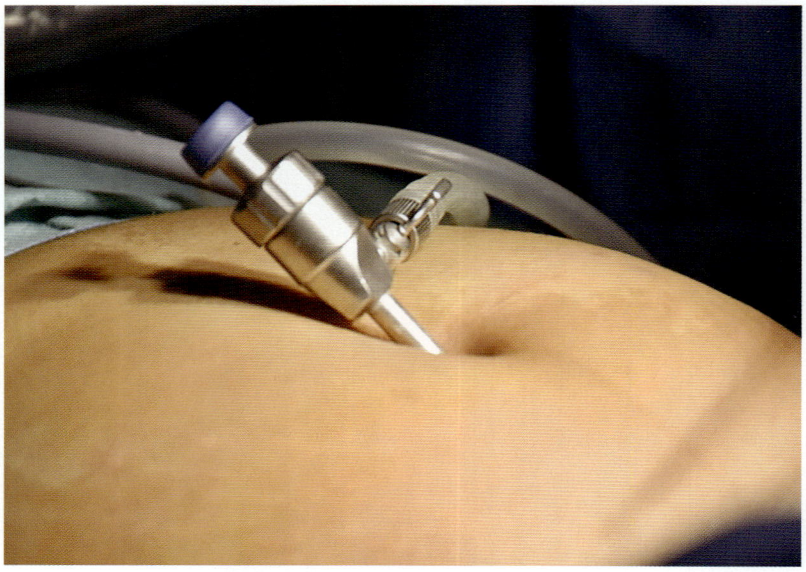

Fig. 2: Trocar placed through umbilicus.

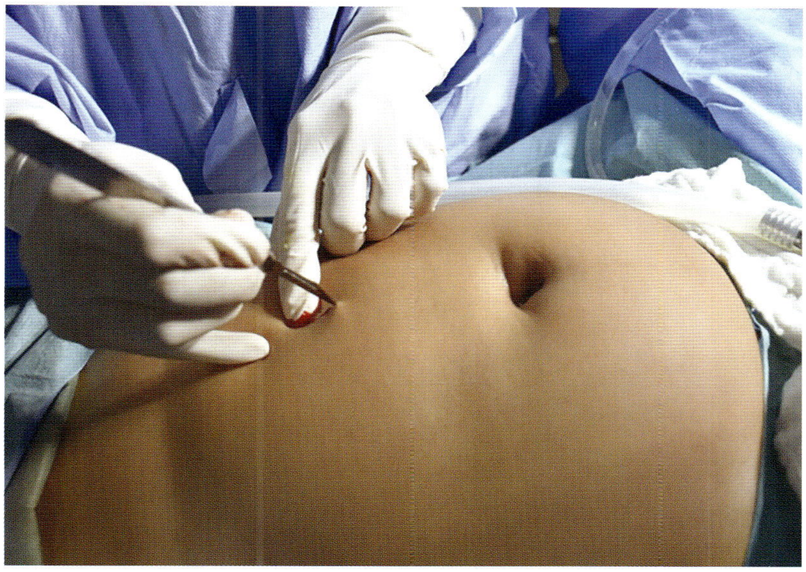

Fig. 3: Incision for supraumbilical trocar.

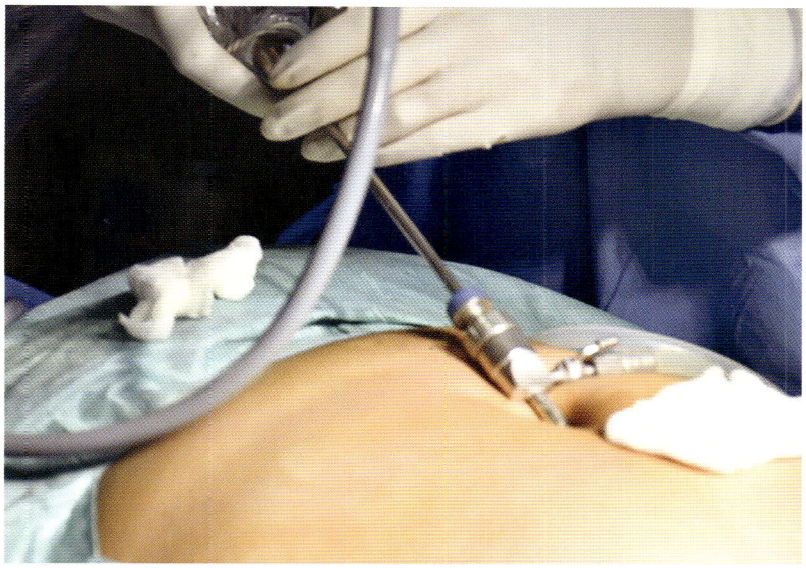

Fig. 5: Telescope inserted.

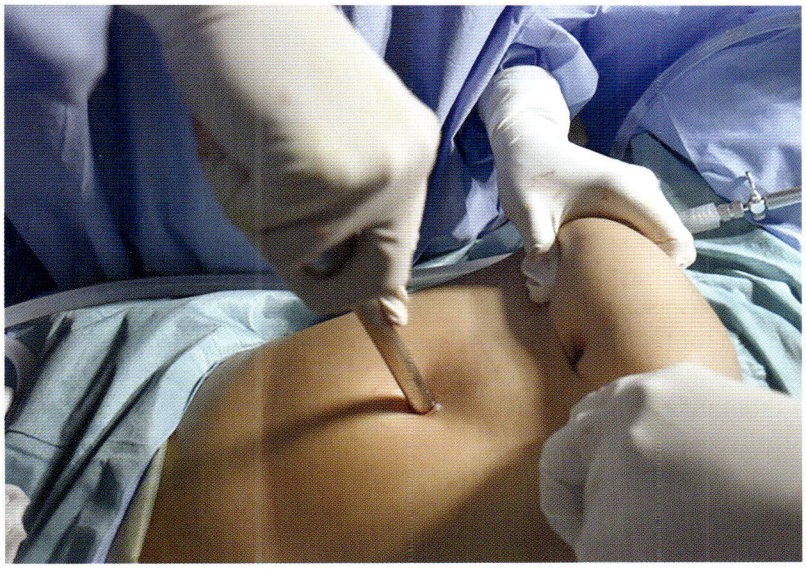

Fig. 4: Supraumbilical trocar placement.

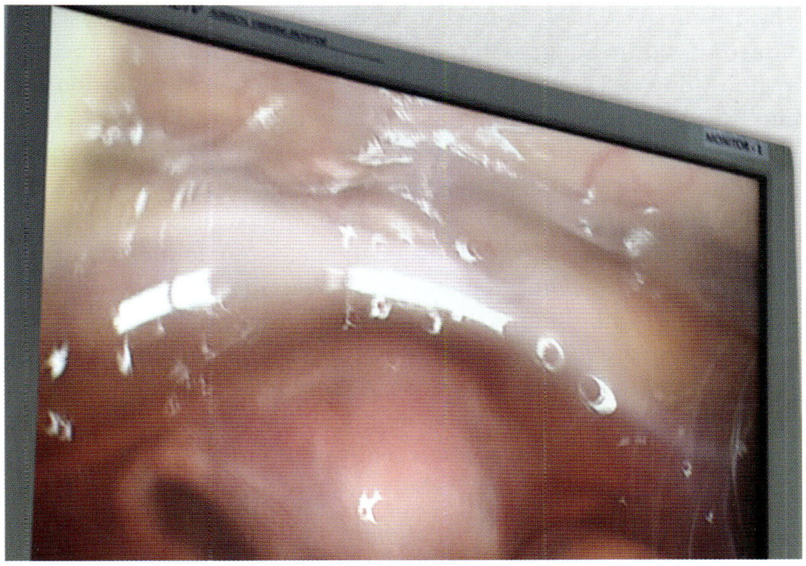

Fig. 6: Picture on the monitor.

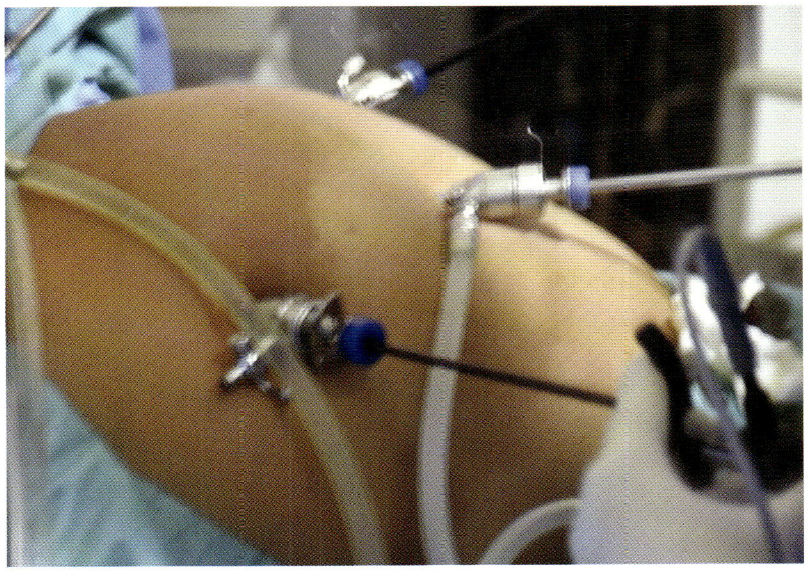

Fig. 7: Insertion of secondary ports.

CHAPTER

5

Laparoscopic Pelvic Anatomy: An Overview

Sandip Datta Roy, Isha Rani

"I did then what I knew how to do. Now that I know better, I do better."—**Maya Angelou**

INTRODUCTION

An excellent knowledge of pelvic anatomy is essential for the safe and successful performance of any gynecological and pelvic surgery. This is more so when it comes to laparoscopic pelvic surgery as the surgeon needs to adapt to the alterations in the appearance of normal anatomy due to the effects of pneumoperitoneum, patient positioning and the use of uterine manipulators. Anterior abdominal structures appear as superior and posterior structures as inferior on the surgical monitor. These limitations are compounded by the loss of depth of field, fixed visual axis, magnification and projection of three-dimensional fields as two-dimensional images. Anatomic orientation of pelvic structures on the monitor may be more challenging when laparoscopes with different angles of view are used. Without proper knowledge of the different structures encountered during dissection, laparoscopy can become hazardous. A thorough description of all the anatomic data of the pelvis is beyond the scope of this chapter. Here, the discussion shall mainly focus on important anatomic structures and understanding of their relationships to ensure a safe pelvic approach during laparoscopy.

THE UMBILICUS, PERITONEAL FOLDS AND POSTERIOR PERITONEUM

The umbilicus is an important anatomic landmark on the anterior abdominal wall as it is primarily concerned with creation of pneumoperitoneum using the Veress needle and the entry of primary trocar in most gynecological endoscopic surgeries. It is located at the level of L3-L4 vertebra, although its location varies with patient's weight, condition of abdominal musculature and, patient's position on the operating table, etc. The aortic bifurcation is located at the level of L4-L5 in 80% of cases.[1] The most dangerous situation is observed in thin patients when the umbilicus is perpendicular to the aortic bifurcation or, in 50% of cases, perpendicular to the left common iliac vein which crosses the sacral promontory near the midline. In thin patients, the umbilicus lies 1–2 cm above the anterior surface of aorta. The umbilicus tends to descend in aged and obese patients and its relation to the aorta is often altered **(Fig. 1)**. The summits of iliac crest are palpable even in obese individual. Aortic bifurcation lies within 1.25 cm above or below the line drawn between the iliac crests in 80% of the individual. Before inserting the Veress needle or direct trocar entry, it is very important to be aware of the position of the umbilicus in relation to the aortic bifurcation because of the risk of major vascular and visceral injury.

There are five peritoneal folds or ligaments on anterior abdominal wall, which has connection with important retroperitoneal landmarks. The *median umbilical ligament* extends from the bladder apex to the umbilicus and encloses the obliterated urachus. Lateral to the median umbilical ligament, on either side, are the *medial umbilical ligaments,* which represent the obliterated umbilical arteries and extend up to the umbilicus **(Fig. 2)**. Further lateral runs the *lateral umbilical folds* formed by the peritoneum overlying the inferior epigastric artery **(Fig. 3)**. These vessels are located between the parietal peritoneum and the fascia transversalis. Before ancillary trocar placement, it is important to identify the inferior epigastric vessels to avoid injuring them. Their location can be confirmed easily under the peritoneum in thin patients by transillumination but not in obese patients. Injury to these vessels during secondary trocar placement can result in significant bleeding and abdominal wall hematoma. Approximately 5 cm above the symphysis pubis, the distance between the inferior epigastric vessels and the midline is 5–6 cm. The mean distance between the medial umbilical ligaments and the inferior epigastric vessels is 2 cm. These distances are significantly greater on the right side than on the left. The lateral trocar should preferably be placed approximately 8 cm lateral to the midline to avoid injuring the inferior epigastric vessels **(Fig. 4)**.

Several important anatomical structures can be identified through the posterior parietal peritoneum. The ureter can be found entering the pelvis over or just below the bifurcation of the common iliac artery **(Fig. 5)**. The internal iliac artery (IIA) runs parallel and just posterior to the ureter. The external iliac artery is seen little lateral and anterior to the IIA on the medial edge of the psoas muscle **(Fig. 5)**. The external iliac vein can be seen posterior and medial to the external iliac artery **(Fig. 6)**. Tracing the internal and external iliac arteries superiorly leads to the point of bifurcation of the common iliac arteries at the pelvic brim overlying the sacroiliac joint **(Fig. 7)**. Tracing the right common iliac artery upward leads to the bifurcation of the aorta, overlying the fourth lumbar vertebra **(Fig. 8)**. The left common iliac artery may be difficult to identify because of the overlying sigmoid mesentery. The left common iliac vein is located posterior and medial to the artery in the presacral space **(Fig. 9)**.

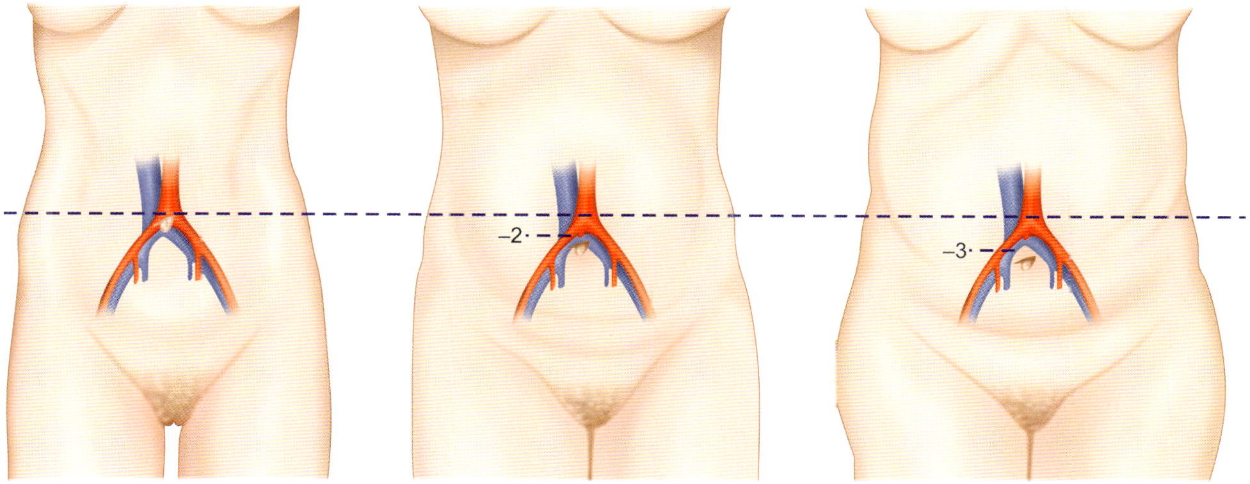

Fig. 1: Position of umbilicus and aortic bifurcation in relation to body weight.

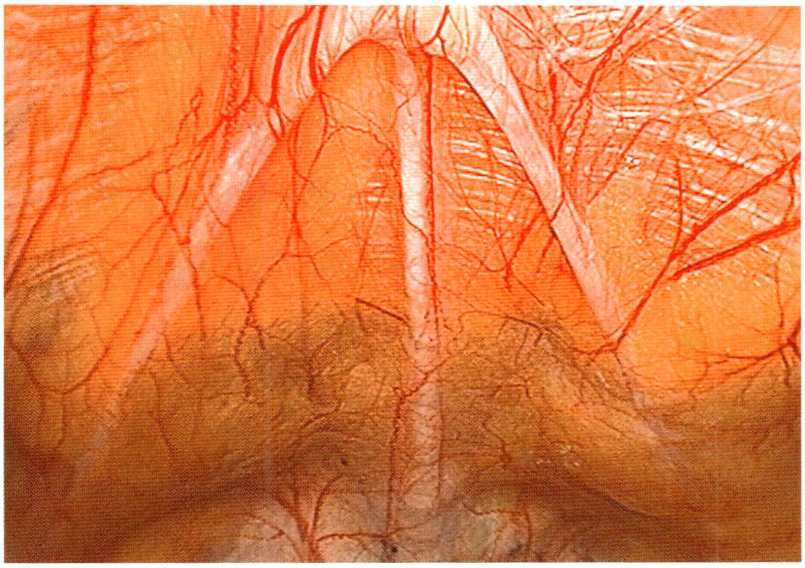

Fig. 2: Medial and mecian umbilical folds.

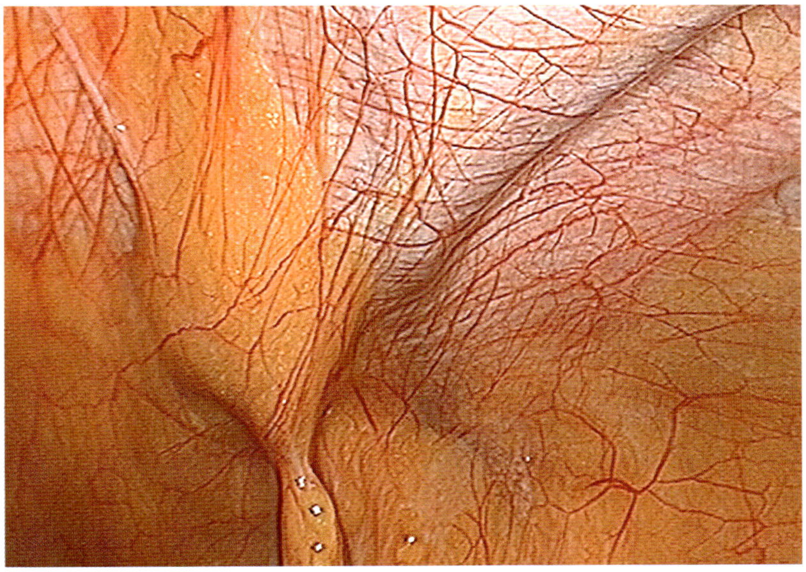

Fig. 3: Lateral umbilical fold (inferior epigastric artery).

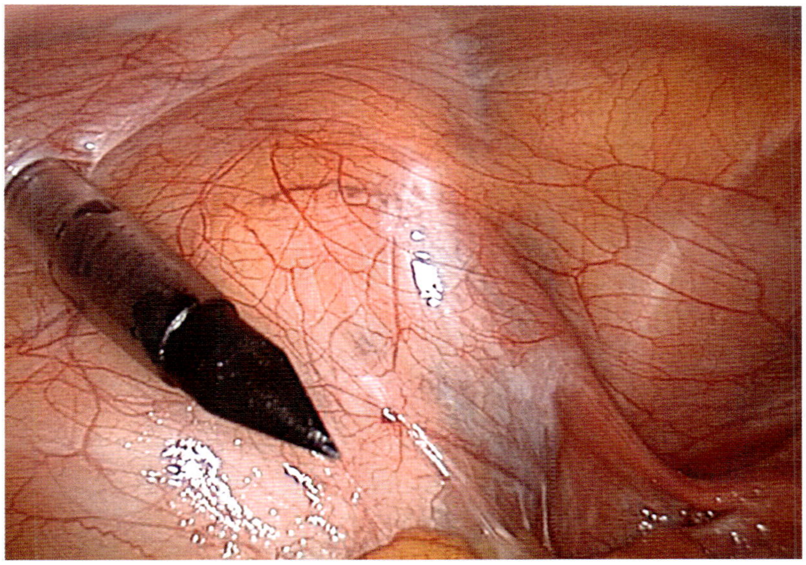

Fig. 4: Trocar placement lateral to the inferior epigastric vessels.

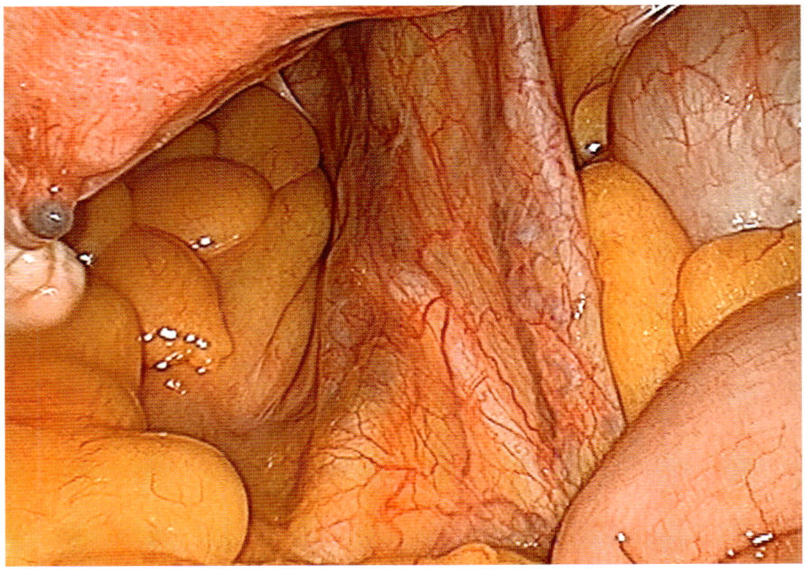

Fig. 5: Ureter entering the pelvis.

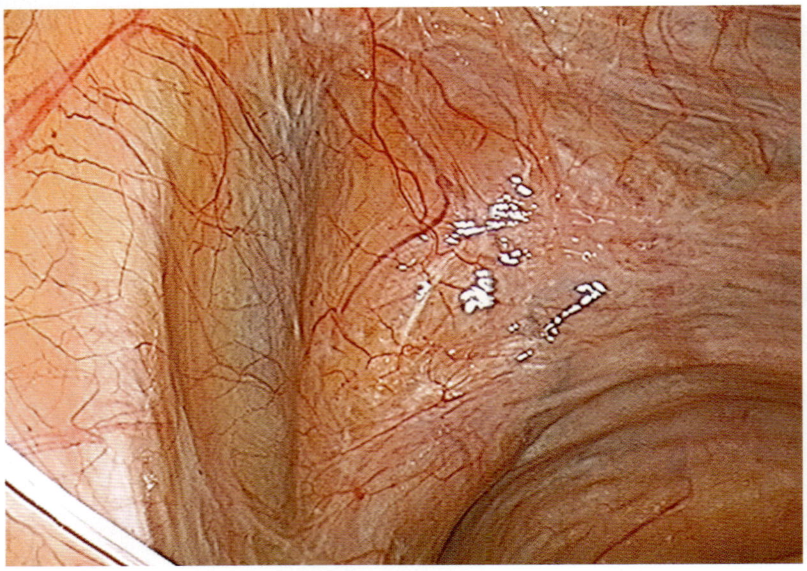

Fig. 6: External iliac artery and vein (left side).

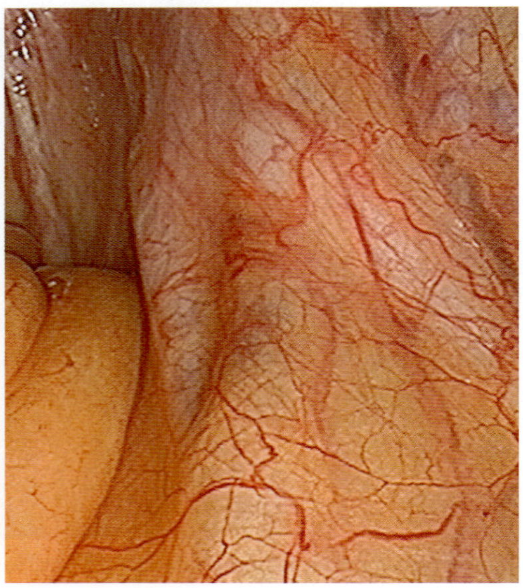

Fig. 7: Bifurcation of common iliac arteries.

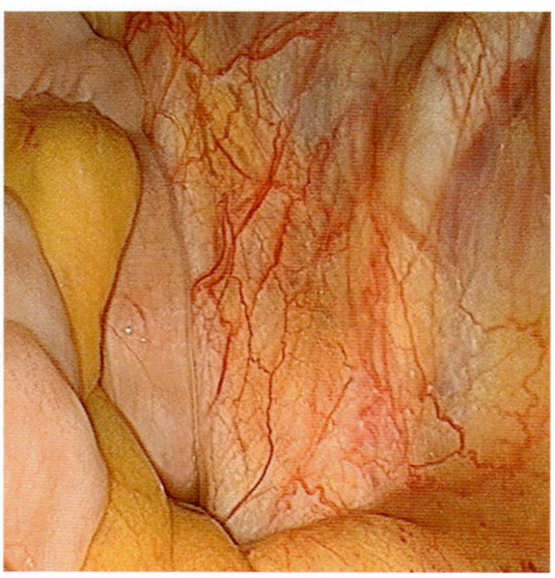

Fig. 8: Aortic bifurcation.

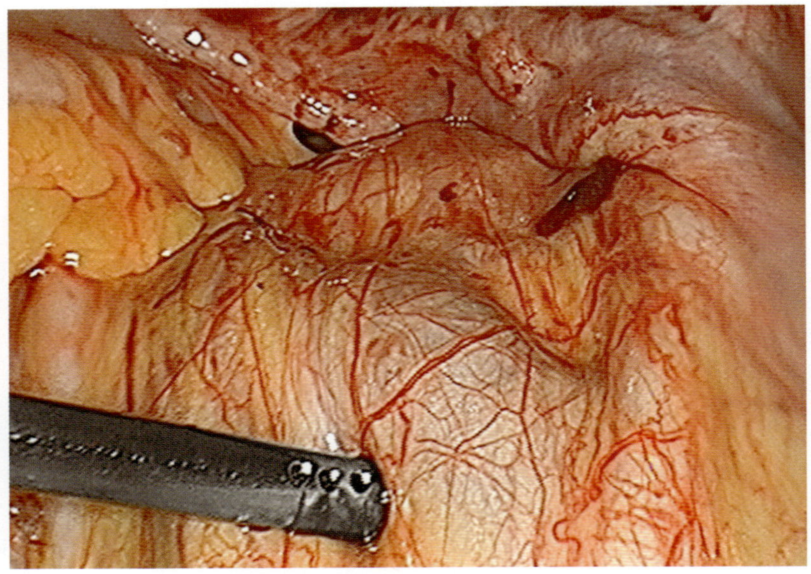

Fig. 9: Left common iliac vein in the midline. Also seen are bilateral ureters entering the pelvis.

STRUCTURES AT THE PELVIC BRIM

Several important structures enter the pelvic cavity at the pelvic brim. Superficially, from lateral to medial, one can find the infundibulopelvic ligaments with the ovarian vessels, the ureter, the bifurcation of the common iliac artery, and the common iliac vein **(Fig. 10)**. Deeper dissection exposes the medial edge of the psoas muscle, the obturator nerve and the fascia overlying the capsule of the sacroiliac joint.

PELVIC SIDEWALL

Pelvic sidewall is entered by opening a triangular peritoneal reflection bounded anteriorly by the round ligament, posteriorly by the infundibulopelvic ligament and laterally by the external iliac vessels **(Fig. 11)**. From superficial to deep, three surgical layers can be dissected based in pelvic side wall. The first layer consists of the parietal peritoneum with the ureter in its fascial sheath. The second layer is a vascular layer composed of the internal iliac vessels and their visceral anterior branches like the uterine, superior vesical and inferior vesical, vaginal, and the middle rectal arteries. The third layer, from anterior to posterior, consists of the psoas muscle with the external iliac artery along its medial border, external iliac vein medial and posterior to the artery and, the obturator internus muscle with the obturator nerve and vessels coursing toward the obturator canal.

BROAD LIGAMENT, ROUND AND OVARIAN LIGAMENTS

The broad ligament consists of a double-layer fold of peritoneum extending from the uterus to the lateral walls of the pelvis. The Fallopian tube is attached in its upper free margin and the ovarian mesentery (*mesovarium*) is attached to the upper part of its posterior leaf. The ovarian vessels and nerves enter into the mesovarium through the infundibulopelvic ligament. The *infundibulopelvic ligament* is the part of broad ligament, which lies between the lateral end of the Fallopian tube and the pelvic wall. It crosses the external iliac vessels approximately 2 cm in front of the ureter **(Figs. 12A and B)**.

The *mesosalpinx* extends between the Fallopian tube and the level of attachment of the ovary to the broad ligament. It contains the infratubal, infraovarian, and tubal branches of ovarian vessels and the infratubal nerve plexus **(Fig. 13)**.

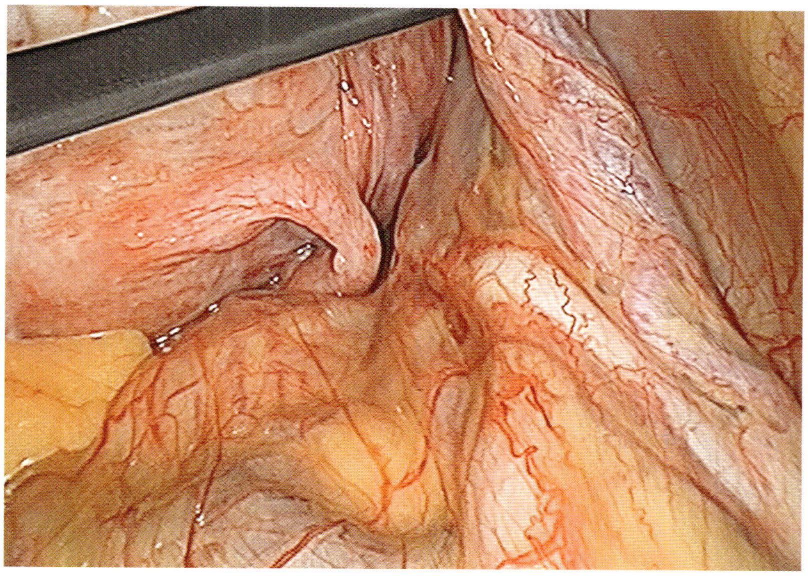

Fig. 10: Structures on the right pelvic brim: Infundibulopelvic (IP) ligament with ovarian vessels, ureter and common iliac artery bifurcation are seen.

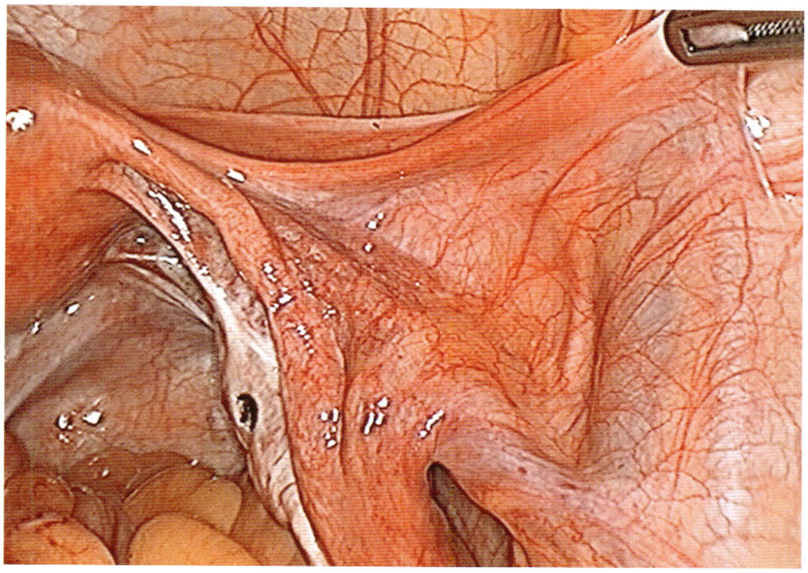

Fig. 11: Triangular peritoneal reflection to enter the pelvic side wall.

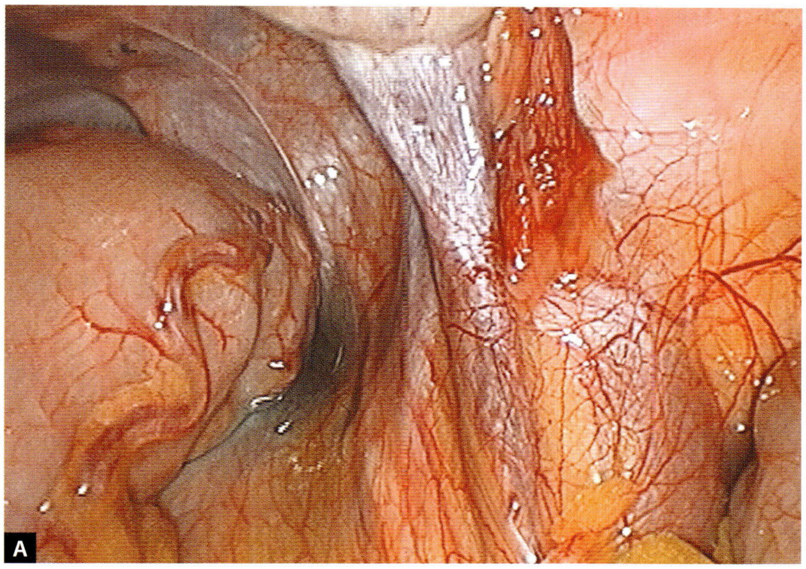

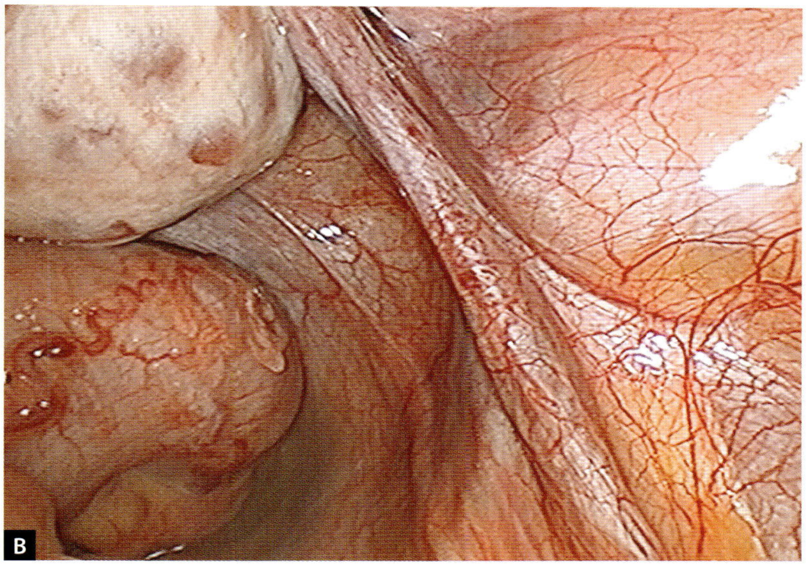

Figs. 12A and B: (A) Infundibulopelvic ligament. Ureter is closely related to this ligament; (B) Infundibulopelvic ligament.

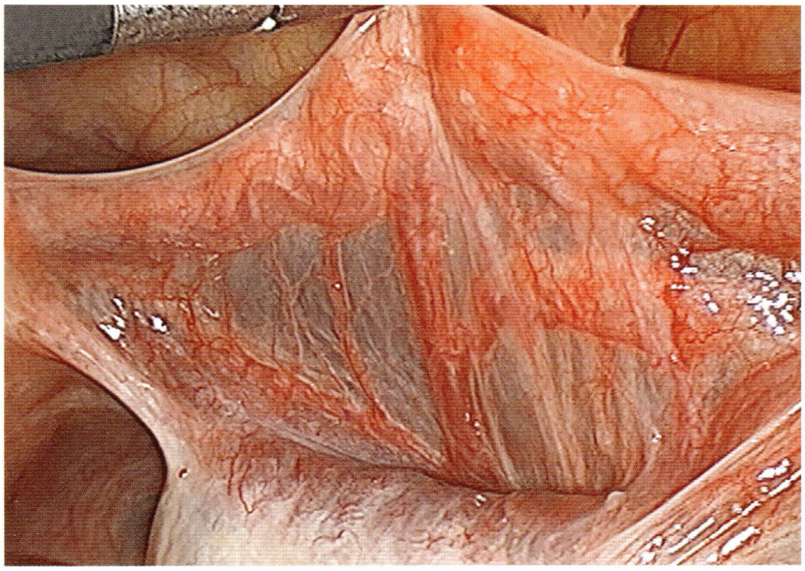

Fig. 13: Mesosalpinx with tubal branches of ovarian artery. Also seen in the ovarian ligament.

The *ovarian fossa* is between the mesovarium anteriorly, the peritoneal fold of the ureter posteriorly and the iliac vessels on the lateral side. The ovaries often become fixed to its fossa in pelvic endometriosis and adnexal infection. An attempt to release such fixed ovaries can occasionally injure the underlying ureter, which may become too intimate to the ovaries due to adhesions.

Anteroposteriorly, the base of the broad ligament is broader than its upper part. The anterior leaf turns toward the uterovesical pouch and the posterior leaf continues downward to a lower level up to the uterosacral ligaments. It contains loose areolar tissue and fat, cardinal ligaments the terminal part of the ureter and the paracervical nerve and the lymphatic plexuses. The upper portion of the cardinal ligament is penetrated by the ureter as it travels into the tunnel of Wertheim just beneath the uterine artery, 1.5–2 cm lateral to the isthmus of the uterus, just lateral to the uterosacral ligament. This is one of the most common sites of ureteric injury in gynecologic procedures as in total laparoscopic hysterectomy. The base of the broad ligament delineates two important spaces: anteriorly the paravesical space and posteriorly the pararectal space. The extent of lateral dissection and excision of the cardinal ligaments determine the class of radical hysterectomy. The round ligament is a fibromuscular cord extending from the uterine cornu to the deep inguinal ring through which it enters the inguinal canal.

PELVIC CELLULAR TISSUES, FASCIA AND LIGAMENTS

All the spaces in pelvis between organs, muscles, and vessels are filled with loose areolar tissues and fat. This cellular tissue can be of two forms: the slack zone, which can be easily dissected (avascular spaces) and the dense zone (fascia and ligaments) which needs to be cut for dissection. In certain areas, the connective tissue is condensed to form fascial ligaments, which contain variable portions of collagen, elastin, and smooth muscles and support the pelvic organs. Some of these structures are described here.

Cardinal or Mackenrodt's Ligament

The cardinal ligament or transverse cervical ligament (Mackenrodt's) is extend from the lateral aspect of supravaginal cervix and upper vagina to the side wall of pelvis. It has a vascular and a nervous part. From above to downward, the superficial uterine vein, the uterine artery, the deep uterine veins, and the middle rectal artery constitute the *vascular part* of the parametrium. In the inferior third of the parametrium, the pelvic splanchnic nerves can be dissected (*nervous part*) of the parametrium. These nerves provide parasympathetic innervation to the bladder and rectum. The cardinal ligaments provide support to the uterus, cervix, and the upper vagina and they are closely related to the uterine artery and the ureter and hence important anatomical structure in hysterectomy.

Uterosacral Ligament

These are paired fibromuscular firm bands, which extend from the posterolateral aspect of the cervix and vaginal fornix to the lateral edge of the second, third, and fourth sacral vertebra. They are the main support of the uterus and hold the cervix posteriorly above the levator plate. Several nerve fibers from the uterus and cervix travel through them. These ligaments are closely related to the ureter. Failure to attach the vaginal vault to the uterosacral ligaments after hysterectomy results in vault prolapse. The inferior hypogastric plexus is located here at the arrival of the hypogastric nerve.

VESICOUTERINE/VESICOCERVICAL LIGAMENTS

The vesicouterine ligaments extend from posterior and lateral aspect of the bladder to the uterine isthmus and the cervix where it fuses with anterior cervicovaginal fascia.

Here two veins, the so-called vesicocervicals veins[2] sketch the outline of the ureter and travel below to drain into the deep uterine veins. Meticulous dissection of this area is important to avoid bleeding near ureter during radical hysterectomy.

PUBOCERVICAL AND RECTOVAGINAL FASCIA

The pubocervical fascia is the part of endopelvic fascia that continues down the anterior vaginal wall beneath the base of the bladder **(Fig. 14)**. Superiorly, it is attached to the endopelvic fascial ring around the supravaginal cervix. Distally, it splits round the urethra and turns forward to be inserted into the body of the pubis and into the upper layer of the urogenital diaphragm. Laterally, the fascia is attached to the arcus tendineus fascia pelvis (fascial white line). At the level of the ischial spine, the uterosacral-cardinal ligament complex fuses with the upper level of the pubocervical fascia to stabilize the pericervical ring. The base of the bladder rests upon the pubocervical fascial platform **(Figs. 15A and B)**. Lateral tear of pubocervical fascia from arcus tendineus fasciae pelvis (ATFP) results in cystocele due to paravaginal defect. Laparoscopic paravaginal repair involves reapproximating the pubocervical fascia to ATFP.

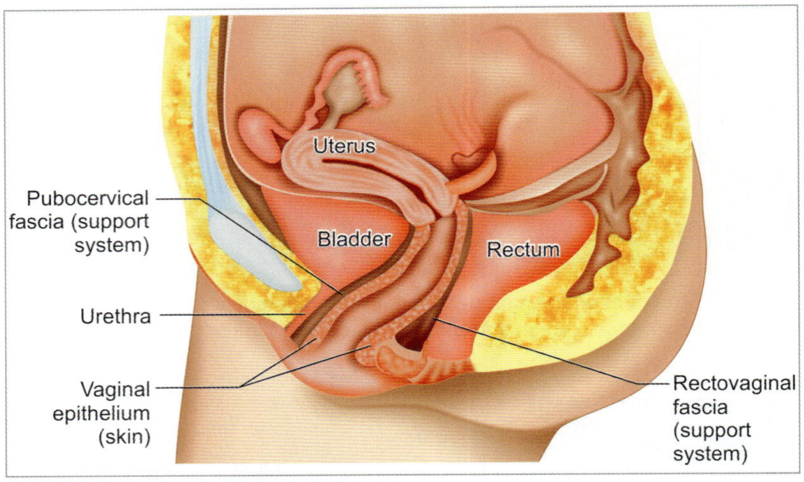

Fig. 14: Pubocervical fascia.

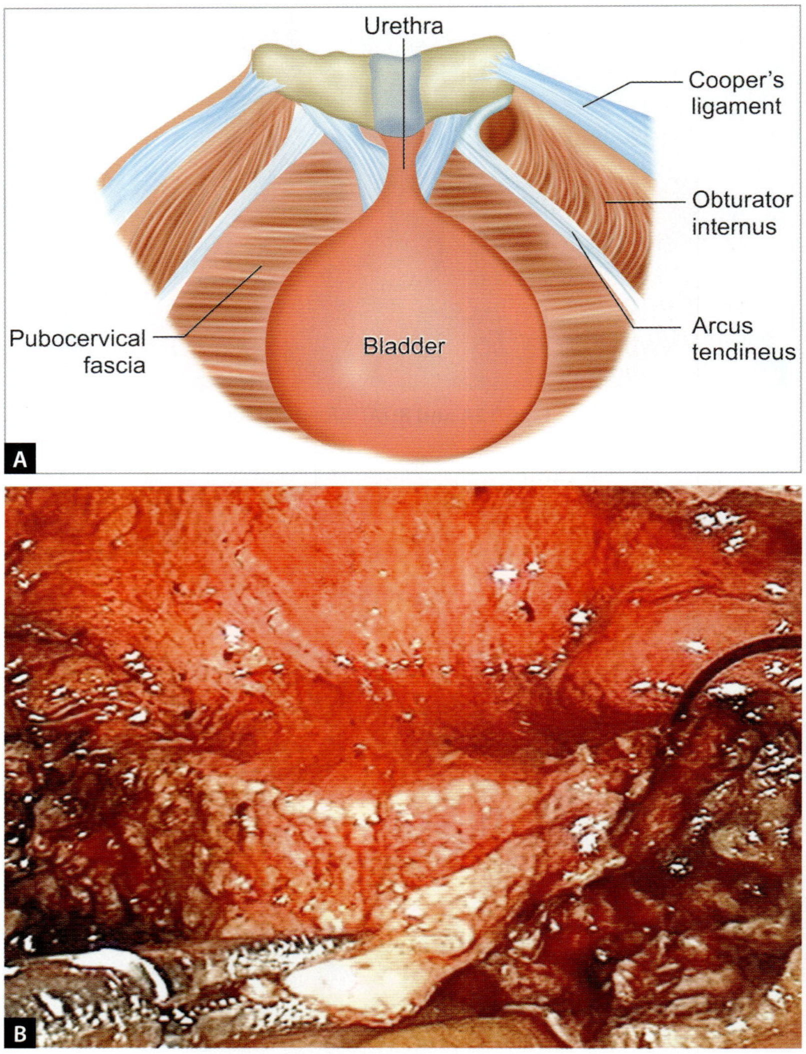

Figs. 15A and B: (A) Pubocervical fascia (PCF) supporting the bladder base; (B) Pubocervical fascia between bladder and vaginal mucosa.

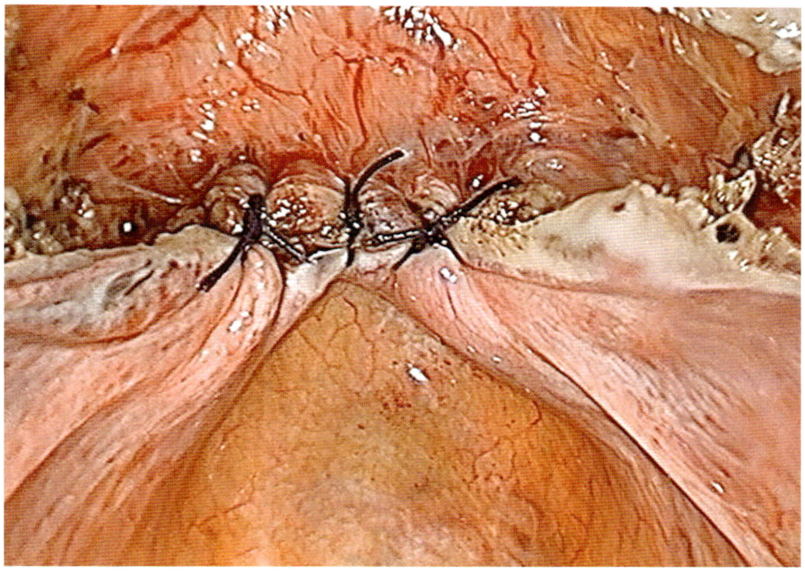

Fig. 16: Incorporation of pubocervical fascia (PCF), rectovaginal fascia (RVF), and uterosacral ligament (USL) in vault.

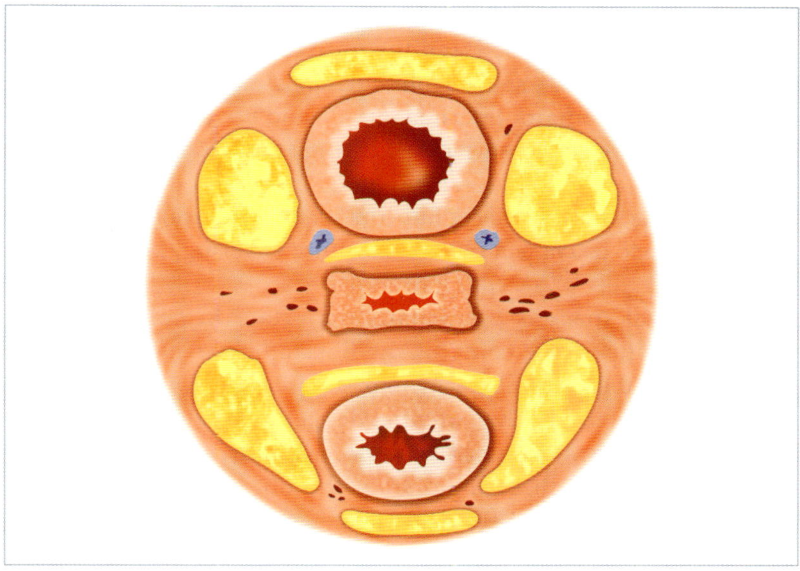

Fig. 17: Different avascular spaces in pelvis.

The rectovaginal fascia or septum (some refer to it as Denonvilliers' fascia) is a sheet of strong connective-type tissue between the rectum and vagina. This layer is immediately beneath the vaginal mucosa and firmly adherent to it. Its principal attachments are peripheral: it merges superiorly with the uterosacral/cardinal ligament complex and the cul-de-sac peritoneum, fuses laterally with the fascia over the levator ani muscle, and merges distally into the perineal body. This layer acts as a supporting structure for the posterior vaginal wall and prevents the rectum from bulging anteriorly into the vagina. Rectoceles represent an isolated defect in this fascia that allows the rectum to protrude anteriorly into vagina. The defects are usually isolated breaks that can be repaired directly with excellent and predictable results.[3] Deeply infiltrating rectovaginal endometriosis can also involve this septum.

The vaginal vault after hysterectomy is formed by the approximation of the pubocervical fascia to the rectovaginal fascia. An enterocele and vault prolapse may result if the pubocervical fascia separates from the rectovaginal fascia in the midline.[4-7] A full thickness closure of the vaginal apex incorporating the pubocervical and the rectovaginal fascia rather than taking only the vaginal mucosa and, reattaching the vaginal vault to the uterosacral ligaments at the time of hysterectomy are the primary steps in preventing future vault prolapse **(Fig. 16)**.

AVASCULAR SPACES OF PELVIS

There are eight different avascular spaces in the pelvis separated by three pairs of different ligaments **(Fig. 17)**. These are: retropubic space, paravesical space (paired), pararectal space (paired), vesicovaginal space, rectovaginal space, and presacral space.

Retropubic Space (Space of Retzius)

The retropubic space is a potential avascular space located between the back of the pubic bone and the anterior wall of the bladder. It is bounded anteriorly by the fascia transversalis, which inserts on the posterior surface of the symphysis pubis. The floor is formed by the urethra, the pubourethral ligament, and the urethrovesical junction. The inferior limit is of the space which is represented by the pubic symphysis and the superior pubic ramus with the pectineal ligament

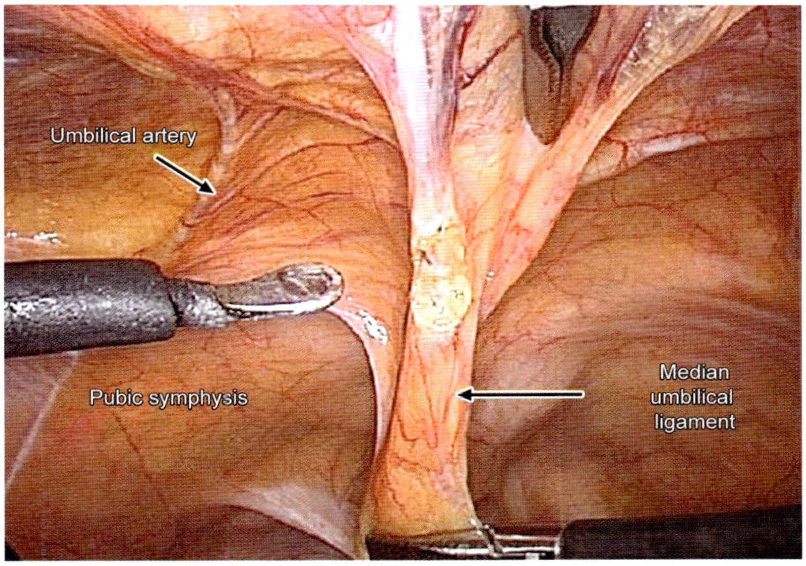

Fig. 18: Entry into retropubic space.

(Cooper's ligament). Laterally, the obliterated umbilical artery separates the retropubic space from the paravesical space. Entry into the space begins by making an incision on peritoneum 3 cm above the dome of the bladder between the obliterated umbilical arteries **(Fig. 18)**. This space is completely avascular and dissected with simple divergent traction. Remaining in contact with the aponeurosis (transversalis fascia) dissection is continued until the fatty tissues anterior to the Cooper's ligament indicate that the superior boundary of the space of Retzius is reached.

Paravesical Space

The paravesical spaces are located anterior to the base of the broad ligament on both sides. It is contiguous medially with the retropubic space, the point of separation being the obliterated umbilical ligament. The development of the paravesical space is initiated with the identification of the obliterated umbilical artery, which is retracted medially, exposing a virtual space whose lateral limit is marked by the external iliac vessels. The dissection is continued deep through the loose areolar tissue of the paravesical space until the obturator internus muscle is reached and the glistening endopelvic fascia is seen at the bottom. The space is bounded medially by the bladder and laterally by the obturator internus muscle and the pelvic diaphragm. The posterior border is represented by the endopelvic fascial sheath around the internal iliac vessels. The floor is formed by the pubocervical fascia, which inserts into the ATFP, the fascial white line. The endopelvic fascia is a fibrous structure covering the levator ani muscles.

Paravesical space is particularly important in pelvic lymphadenectomy. This space contains the obturator nerves and vessels, obturator and the external iliac lymph nodes and is therefore affected by lymphadenectomy. The potential danger at this level is from the internal hypogastric veins and the occasionally present accessory obturator vein, which emerges from the obturator vein near the foramen and ends on the undersurface of the external iliac vein, 1 or 2 cm from the femoral opening. Accessory obturator vein can be avulsed if excessive ventral traction is applied on external iliac vein. Accessory obturator artery arises from the inferior epigastric artery and run across the pectineal ligament on its way to anastomose with the obturator artery in the obturator canal. These aberrant vessels are present in about 25–40% of patients and may be injured during retropubic colposuspension and radical hysterectomy.

The development of the paravesical space enables exposure of the anterior face of the parametrium, which comprises connective and adipose tissue.[8] The vesicohypogastric fascia extends from the superior vesical artery to the lateral edge of the bladder and vesicouterine ligament. In the Piver III level of radicality, this fascia should be sectioned to preserve the superior vesical artery.

Pararectal Space

These are triangular spaces located lateral to the rectum and posterior to the base of the broad ligament, which represents its anterior border. The medial border is represented by the ureter and the lateral border by the internal iliac artery. This virtual space can be developed by dissecting into the loose areolar tissue posterior to the origin of the uterine artery and lateral to the ureter. The dissection continues deep until reaching the plane of the levator ani muscle, which is covered by the endopelvic fascia.

The pelvic ureter and mesoureter can be separated easily from the lateral leaf of the broad ligament until the crossing of the uterine artery by means of soft traction-countertraction movements. The space created between the broad ligament and the mesoureter is named Okabayashi's cranial pararectal chamber.[9] The hypogastric nerve, which originates in the superior hypogastric plexus is found in this space and provides sympathetic innervation to the bladder. Correct dissection is important to prevent injury to the vesical and rectal nerve plexuses in radical surgery.

Vesicovaginal Space

The vesicovaginal space is a potential avascular space limited superiorly by the uterovesical fold of peritoneum. Inferiorly, it extends up to the junction of the proximal one-third and the distal two-thirds of the vagina. Laterally, it is bordered by the vesicocervical ligaments or the bladder pillars. These structures pass just lateral to lower uterine segment and the cervix and course along the anterolateral surface of the upper one-third of vagina to enter the bladder. Entry to this space is initiated by incising the uterovesical fold of peritoneum.

Rectovaginal Space

The rectovaginal (RV) space is located between the rectum and the vagina. Its boundaries are as follows: anteriorly by the posterior vaginal wall, posteriorly by the anterior rectal wall, laterally by the iliococcygeus muscles of levator ani, inferiorly by the perineal body and superiorly by the cul-de-sac peritoneum. The rectovaginal space is entered by incising the peritoneum between the uterosacral ligaments.

Presacral Space

The location of the presacral or the retrorectal space is between the rectum anteriorly and the sacrum posteriorly. The space is bounded anteriorly by the rectum and posteriorly by the sacrum, anterior longitudinal ligament, and the sacral promontory. The lateral boundaries are formed by the ureter and common iliac artery, and also the inferior mesenteric artery on the left side traversing through the sigmoid mesentery. Inferiorly the space terminates at the level of the levator muscles. This space contains the middle sacral vessels, superior hypogastric plexus and lymphatic tissues invested in loose areolar tissues between the bifurcations of aorta.

PARA-AORTIC AREA

Para-aortic area is an anatomical region that extends from the renal vessels to the bifurcation of the common iliac vessels and practically very important in lymphadenectomy for various genital malignancies. This region can be divided into upper and lower para-aortic areas with reference to the origin of the inferior mesenteric artery (an unpaired retroperitoneal artery on the left side emerging from the aorta 2–5 cm proximal to its bifurcation).

PELVIC LYMPH NODES

Pelvic lymph nodes are generally arranged in groups or chains and follow the course of larger pelvic vessels. There are three important groups of pelvic lymph nodes: the external iliac, hypogastric, and the obturator lymph nodes **(Fig. 19)**.

The obturator nodes are found in the *obturator fossa*, which is bounded medially by the internal iliac artery; laterally by the external iliac vein, obturator internus muscle and its fascia; and anteriorly by the obturator vessels and nerve.

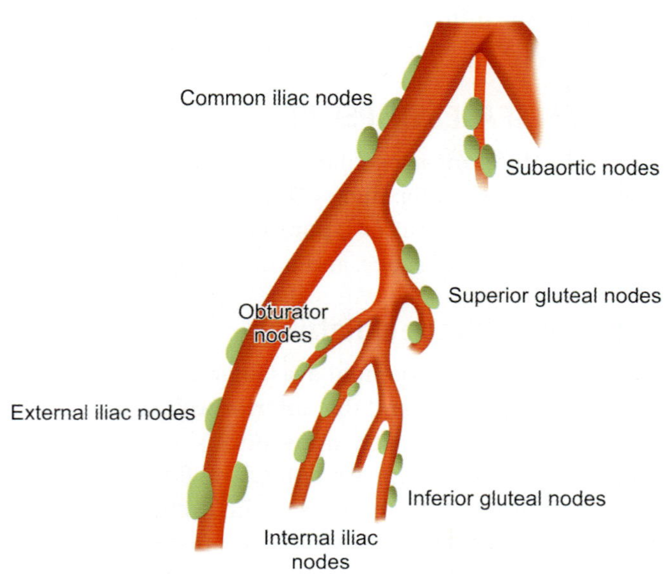

Fig. 19: Pelvic lymph nodes.

VASCULAR RELATIONSHIPS

Vascular supplies of the pelvic organs are derived mainly from the iliac vessels although the adnexa and rectum is mainly supplied from the branches of abdominal aorta. It is not possible here to discuss in detail about the course of all the vessels and the same can be found in any anatomy textbook. However, it is important to know the dangerous anatomic areas, and carefully identify important landmarks and relationships before proceeding with dissection near any vessel. The large vessels like aorta, vena cava, iliac vessels, and their branches and the mesenteric arteries can result in catastrophic outcome when injured and hence their anatomy and relationship should be thoroughly understood. The abdominal aorta bifurcates on the left side of the L4-L5 lumbar vertebra in 80% of cases into right and left common iliac arteries. In 50% of nonobese patients, the point of bifurcation is cephalad to umbilicus. However, this percentage decreases to 30% or less in obese patients.[10]

The *common iliac arteries* run along the medial border of the psoas muscle. The common iliac arteries bifurcate just opposite to the sacroiliac articulation into external and internal iliac arteries. The ureter lies anterior to this bifurcation. The common iliac veins run posteromedial to the arteries.

The *middle sacral artery* arises from the posterior aspect of abdominal aorta, just proximal to its bifurcation **(Figs. 20A and B)**. It descends in the midline in front of the fourth and fifth lumbar vertebrae.

The *external iliac arteries* run along the medial border of psoas muscle downward toward the thigh and become the femoral artery after passing under the inguinal ligament. The IIA gives rise to the principal visceral arteries of pelvis. It divides into anterior and posterior divisions approximately 3–4 cm after its origin. The ureter runs down anterior to this vessel. The posterior division passes through the greater sciatic foramen and gives rise to iliolumbar artery, the lateral sacral artery and the superior gluteal artery. These parietal branches supply the muscles of the buttock.

The branches of the anterior division are: superior vesical, inferior vesical, middle rectal, uterine, vaginal, inferior gluteal, and the internal pudendal artery (terminal branch of IIA).

The uterine artery arises as the first prominent branch from the anterior division of internal iliac artery **(Fig. 21)**. It runs forward and medially in the base of the broad ligament, crossing above and almost at right angles to the ureter and reaches the uterus at the level of the internal os. The uterine artery has three segments: (1) *the parietal segment* descends forward from its origin against the pelvic wall as far as the level of ischial spine. It is related to the ureter medially, and the umbilical and the obturator arteries anteriorly; (2) *the parametrial segment* runs transversely under the parametrium and crosses the ureter anteriorly. Here it gives off a descending cervical branch to supply the lower cervix; and (3) *the mesometrial segment* is more coiled and tortuous and ascends upward alongside the lateral wall of the body of uterus in the mesometrium. It is accompanied by the uterine venous plexus, lymphatic vessels, and sometimes the parauterine lymph nodes. It ends by anastomosing with the ovarian artery near the uterine cornual area, forming a continuous arterial arch **(Fig. 22)**.

The *vaginal artery* runs behind the uterine artery. It is usually a separate branch (or branches) of the IIA but may arise from the first part of uterine artery. It runs anteriorly and medially in the lower part of broad ligament to reach the vaginal fornix. It anastomoses with the azygos branches of the circular artery of cervix in the vaginal wall.

The *obturator artery* proceeds forward, toward the obturator foramen. It is situated against the obturator internus fascia and is bordered by the obturator nerve above and the obturator vein below.

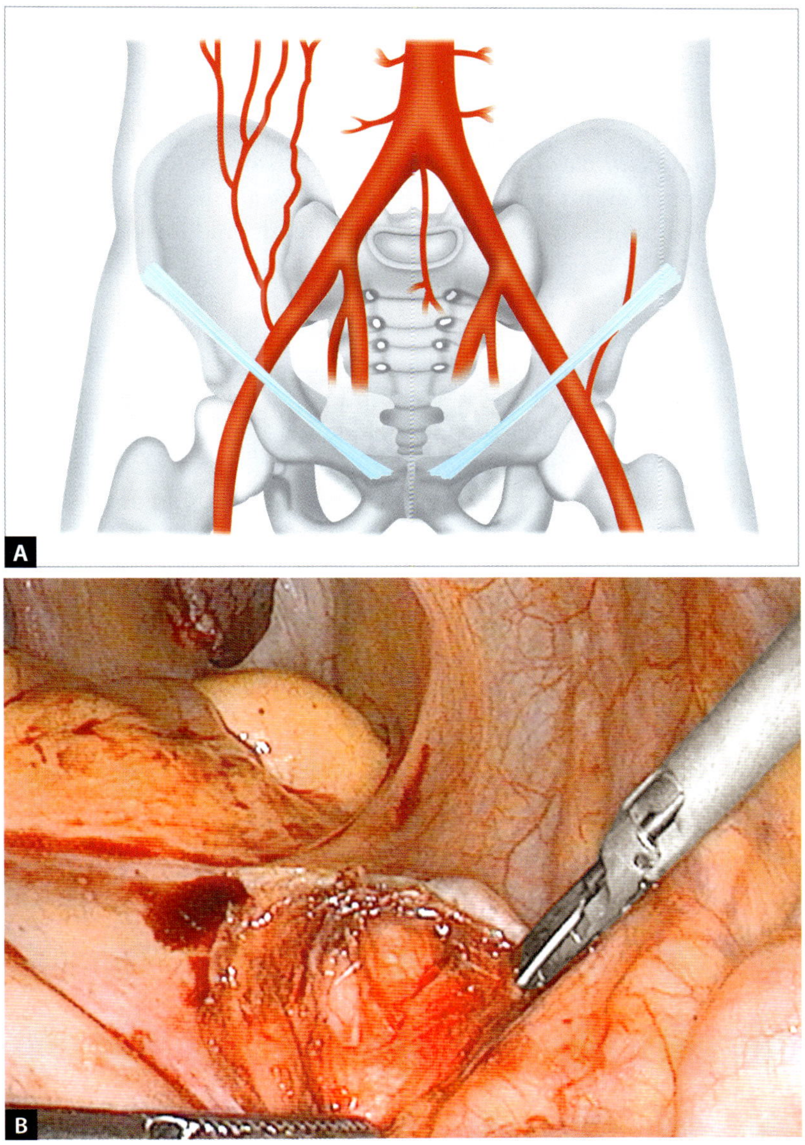

Figs. 20A and B: (A) Middle sacral artery; (B) Middle sacral vessels seen over sacral promontory.

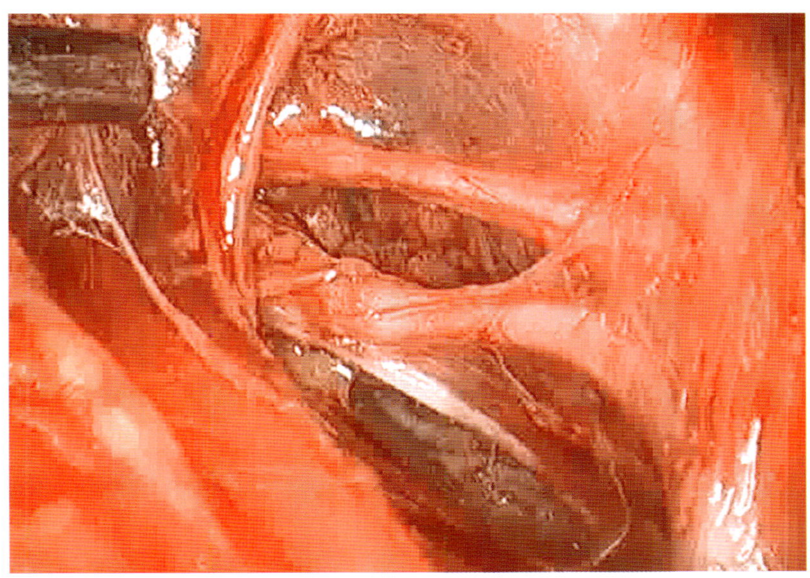

Fig. 21: Origin of uterine artery from internal iliac artery. Also seen is the superior vesical artery.

Its distal part is opposite the obturator lymph nodes. The *middle rectal artery* descends medially toward the lateral aspect of the rectum.

The *internal pudendal artery* is the terminal branch of the internal iliac artery and accompanies the pudendal nerve. It leaves the pelvis through the greater sciatic foramen, passes around the ischial spine and penetrates the ischiorectal fossa through the lesser sciatic notch. In its course to the perineum, it lies with the pudendal nerve within the Alcock's canal, a fascial tunnel over the obturator internus muscle. It ends in two branches: the deep and the dorsal artery of clitoris.

The *ovarian artery* emerges from the ventral aspect of abdominal aorta at the level of L2 vertebra (just below the origin of the renal vessels) and descends downward and laterally in the retroperitoneum and crosses the upper ureter. It runs further down to reach the pelvic brim and enters the infundibulopelvic ligament. Here it divides to give multiple branches to ovary. Either the main artery or a branch travels toward the cornu of the uterus lying below and parallel to the Fallopian tube and makes an end-to-end anastomosis with the terminal part of the uterine artery forming a continuous arterial arch in the mesosalpinx. Vessels from this arch supply the tube and round ligament.

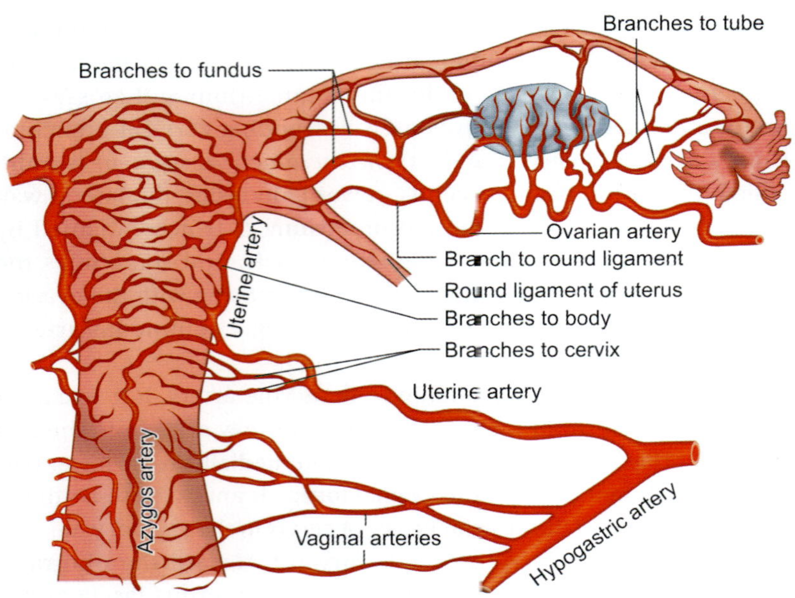

Fig. 22: Course and branches of uterine artery.

There is an efficient anastomotic arterial system in the pelvis between the systemic and pelvic arteries which compensates for all obstruction, even the internal iliac. The iliolumbar, lateral sacral and the middle rectal arteries anastomose with the lumbar, middle sacral, and the superior rectal arteries, respectively. The lumbar arteries arise from the aorta and the superior rectal arteries arise from the inferior mesenteric arteries. The ideal point for IIA ligation is immediately below the last branch of its posterior division.

VENOUS DRAINAGE

The pelvic veins are primarily drained by the internal iliac veins and secondarily by the external iliac, common iliac, superior rectal and ovarian veins. The tributary veins from the pelvic organs follow the arteries and drain the pelvic venous plexus.

NERVOUS ELEMENTS

The pelvis is innervated by both the somatic and autonomic nervous systems. The autonomic nerves include both *sympathetic* (adrenergic) and *parasympathetic* (cholinergic) fibers and provide the primary innervation for genital, urinary, and gastrointestinal visceral structures and blood vessels. Those supplying the important organs and are likely to get injured during pelvic laparoscopic procedures will be discussed here.

Somatic Innervation

The *lumbosacral plexus* and its branches provide motor and sensory somatic innervations to the lower abdominal wall, the pelvic and urogenital diaphragms, the perineum, and the hip and lower extremity **(Fig. 23)**.

The pudendal nerve is the main somatic supply to the pelvic organs. It is formed by the S2, S3, and S4 roots of the sacral plexus and is both motor and sensory in function and is primarily responsible for the innervation of the perineum and the viscera. The nerves important in pelvic laparoscopy include the genitofemoral and the obturator nerves. The genitofemoral nerve emerges from L1 and L2 spinal segments and crosses the psoas muscle to extend in its sheath

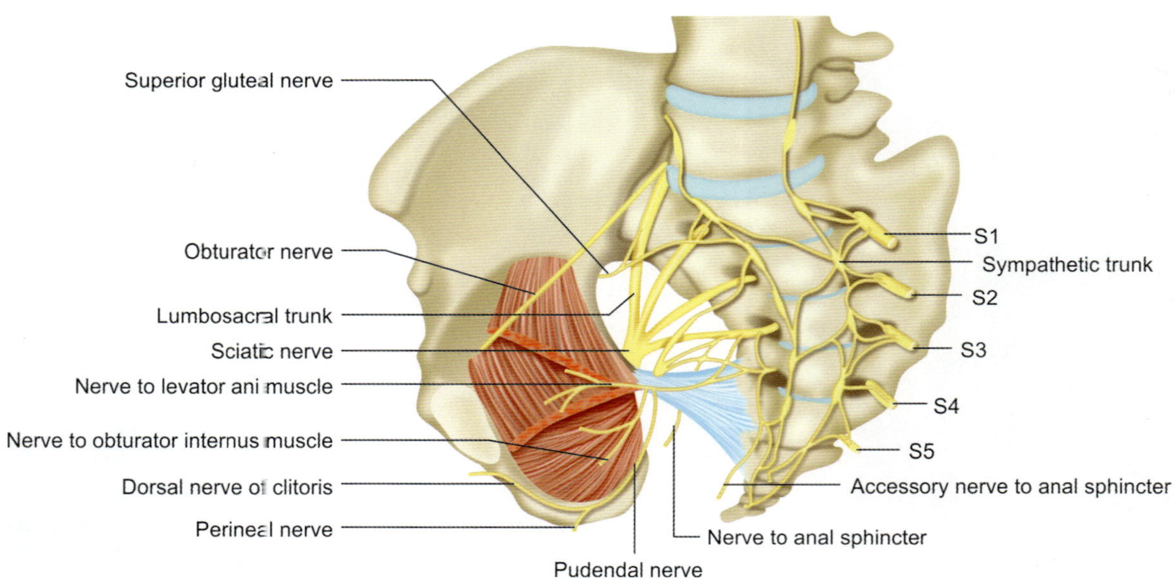

Fig. 23: Lumbosacral plexus.

behind the ureter and the peritoneum. It is very rarely injured in laparoscopy.

The obturator nerve (L2, L3, and L4) provides motor supply to adductor muscles of thigh and sensory supply to medial thigh and leg, hip and knee joints. It emerges in the pelvis between the external and internal iliac veins and extends against the lateral pelvic wall opposite to the ovarian fossa, before entering the obturator foramen. It can be affected at this level by deep infiltrating endometriosis or adnexal infection, leading to obturator neuralgia on the superomedial side of the thigh and the knee. Surgical injury to these nerves can occur during pelvic lymphadenectomy and paravaginal repair, but the functional consequences are often minor.

Autonomic Innervation

Pelvic visceral innervation arises from the autonomic nervous system. The two most important components are the superior and the inferior hypogastric plexus. The ovaries and the distal part of the Fallopian tubes and broad ligament are innervated by the *ovarian plexus*, a network of nerve fibers accompanying the ovarian vessels and derived from the aortic and renal plexuses.

The inferior hypogastric plexus on both sides divides into three important visceral plexuses representing distribution of innervation to corresponding viscera **(Fig. 24)**:

1. *Vesical plexus:* Course along the vesical vessels and innervates the bladder and urethra (external urethral sphincter is supplied by branches of pudendal nerve).
2. *Uterovaginal plexus (Lee-Frankenhauser's ganglion):* Innervates the uterus, vagina, clitoris, and the vestibular bulbs. *Middle rectal plexus:* Course along the middle rectal vessels and innervates the rectum.

AFFERENT INNERVATION

Afferent or sensory fibers from the pelvic viscera and blood vessels follow the same pathways to provide sensory input to the central nervous system. They are also involved in reflex arcs needed for bladder, bowel, and genital tract function.

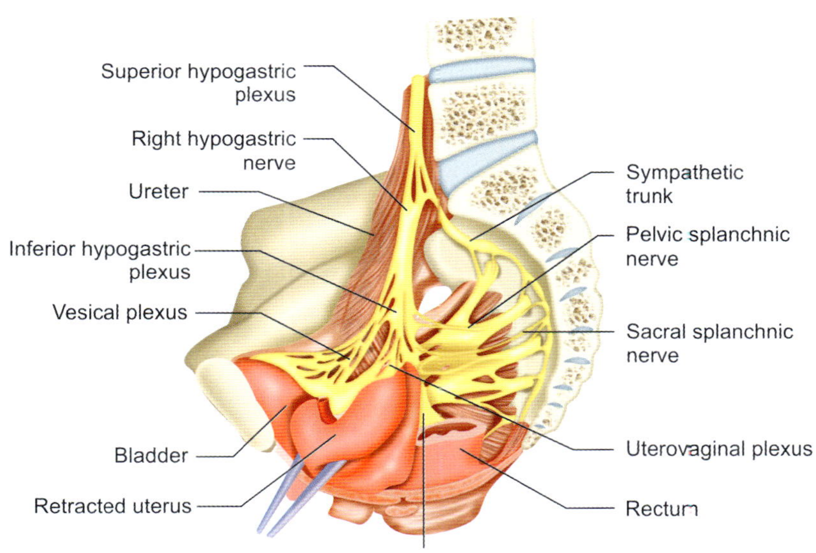

Fig. 24: Pelvic-visceral-nerve-plexuses.

THE URETER

The lumbar ureter runs anterior to the psoas muscle and lateral to the tip of the transverse process of the lumbar vertebrae. It lies medial to the ovarian vessels and is encountered in gynecology only by specialists who perform para-aortic lymphadenectomy. It enters the pelvic cavity over the bifurcation of common iliac artery. In a thin patient, it is easy to identify under the peritoneum by its characteristic peristaltic movement. The right ureter crosses the right external iliac artery anteriorly just distal to its origin. The left ureter crosses in front of the bifurcation of the common iliac artery. Both the ureters are closely related to the infundibulopelvic ligaments and therefore vulnerable to thermal injury when this ligament is desiccated for hemostasis **(Fig. 25A)**.

With reference to the broad ligament, the course of pelvic ureter can be described as retroligamentary, intraligamentary, and retrovesical ureter.

The retroligamentary ureter runs forward and medially, along the posteromedial aspect of the uterine artery, approaching almost up to the uterosacral ligament origin. However, this course may be modified in case of adhesions due to endometriosis, previous surgery or pelvic infection and it can come in contact with the ovaries or the uterosacral ligaments and thus more vulnerable to injury during dissection. The distance of the ureter from the uterosacral ligament, and the infundibulopelvic ligament is small, but significantly more on the left side. It is located about 1–3 cm from the uterosacral ligament and the infundibulopelvic ligament.

The intraligamentary ureter courses beneath the uterine vessels (*water under the bridge*) and the cardinal ligaments of the uterus from back to front to enter into the bladder. Here it lies just beneath the uterine artery, approximately 1.5–2 cm lateral to the isthmus and 10 mm from the lateral vaginal fornix **(Fig. 25B)**. At this point, it travels medially and anteriorly to pass on the anterolateral aspect of the upper third of the vagina to enter into the trigon of bladder (retrovesical ureter).

Ureter receives its blood supply from multiple feeding vessels along its course. Above the pelvic brim, the blood supply comes mainly from the medial side whereas below the pelvic brim, it receives supply mainly from the lateral side. Upper segment is supplied mainly by branches from renal and ovarian arteries. The middle segment receives branches from aortic and common iliac arteries. The pelvic ureter is supplied by branches from uterine, vaginal, middle rectal, and inferior vesical arteries **(Fig. 25C)**. Longitudinal arteries and veins run through the adventitia and provide vital circulation along the course of the ureter. Injury to the adventitia during dissection can compromise the ureteral blood supply and result in tissue sloughing and fistula formation.

Ureter is particularly vulnerable to injury at four areas: (a) the pelvic brim where the ureter passes over the IIA and beneath the infundibulopelvic ligament, (b) the ovarian fossa, (c) lateral to the cervix where the ureter passes under the uterine arteries, and (d) lateral to the vaginal fornix.

URINARY BLADDER

Surgical Anatomy and Relations (Figs. 26A to C)

The bladder is a hollow muscular pelvic organ with a capacity of 300–600 mL. Its size, position, and relations vary according to the volume of urine. It has one superior surface (top), two inferolateral surfaces (sides), and a posterior surface (base or back). Bladder neck is the inferior most part of the bladder that gives origin of the urethra and relatively fixed. The superior surface is triangular and covered by peritoneum of uterovesical peritoneum. The base is related with the supravaginal cervix and the anterior fornix.

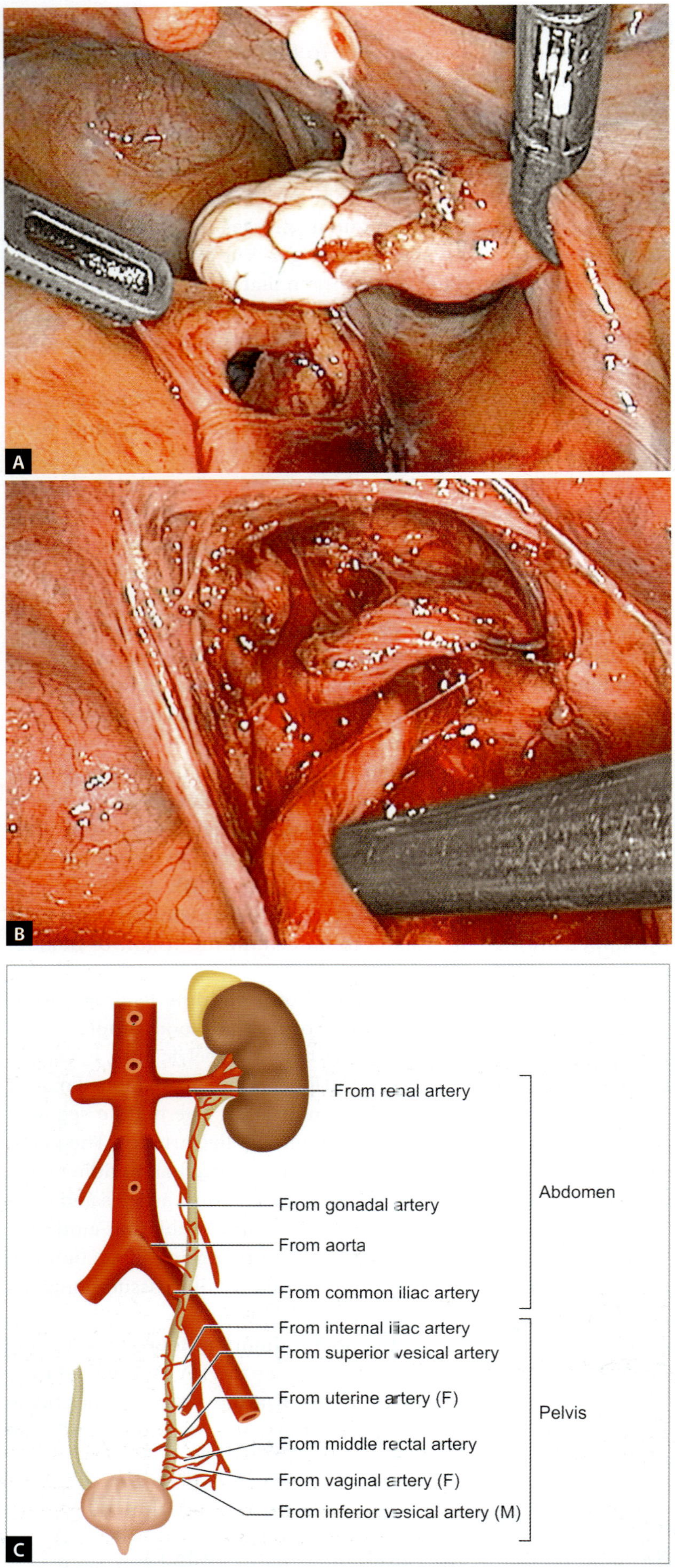

Figs. 25A to C: (A) Ureter in relation to infundibulopelvic ligament; (B) Ureter beneath the uterine artery; (C) Blood supply of ureter.

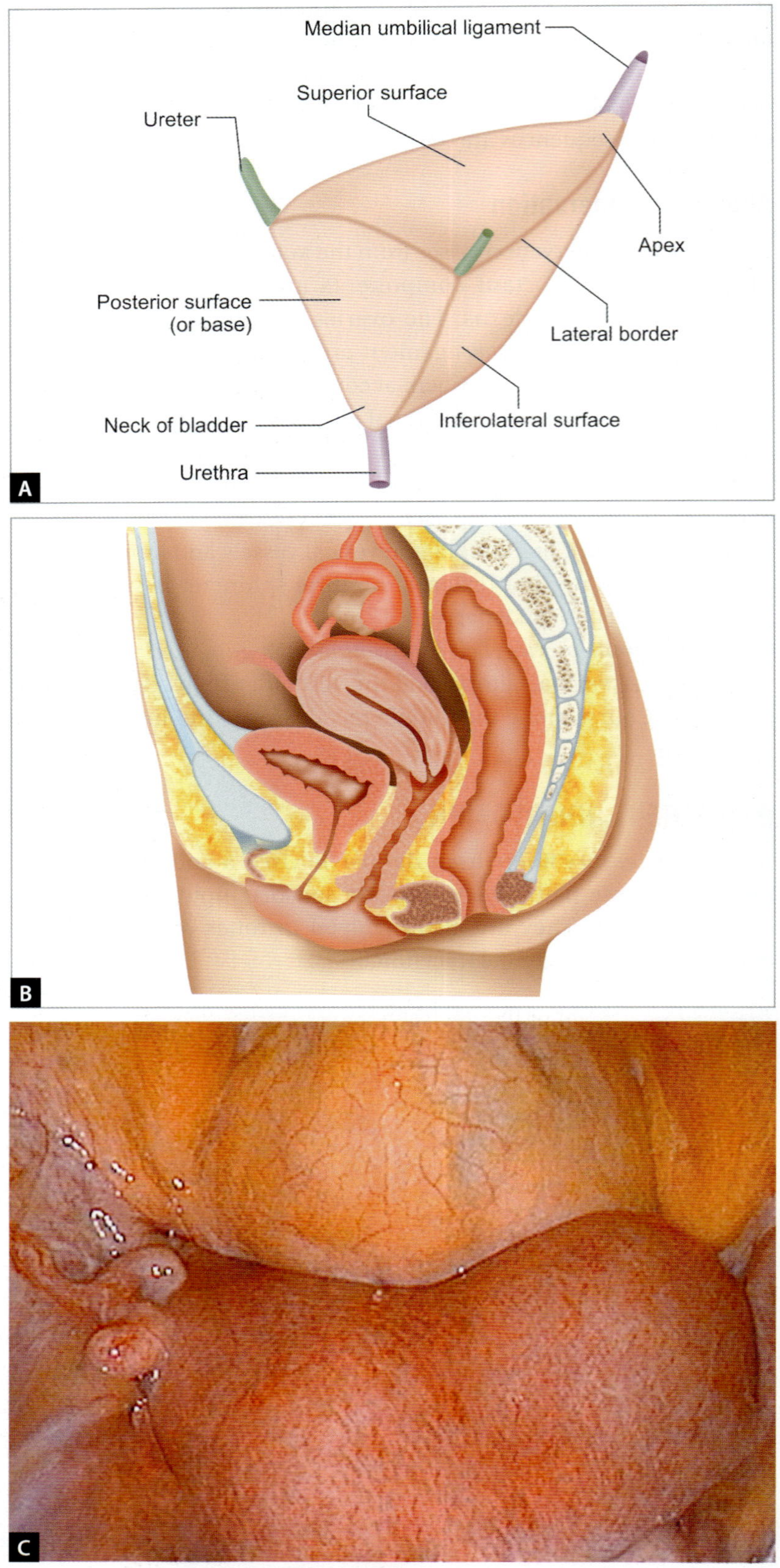

Figs. 26A to C: (A) 3D view of bladder with surfaces and opening of ureter and urethra; (B) Relation of uterus with bladder and rectum; (C) Laparoscopic view of full bladder in relation to the uterus.

The bladder is bordered *anteriorly* by the retropubic space, rectus abdominis muscles, and pubic symphysis; *inferiorly* by the levator ani muscles and obturator internus muscles; *posteriorly* by the lower uterine segment, cervix, and vagina; and *superiorly* by the anteverted uterus. The bladder neck rests on the superior layer of the urogenital diaphragm.

The arterial blood supply is mainly contributed by the IIA through the superior, middle, and inferior vesical arteries. In addition, the vaginal arteries supply the bladder neck. The venous drainage from the bladder is via the hypogastric vein. The nerve supply includes the hypogastric sympathetic plexus and the pelvic splanchnic nerves, which accompany the vessels. The bladder wall is composed of three muscle layers: outer longitudinal, middle circular, and inner longitudinal. These muscle layers converge on the base to form the trigone, a triangular area marked by the ureteric orifices, and the internal urethral meatus. Between the ureteral orifices lies the interureteric ridge (Mercier's), which also demarcates the roof of the trigone. The bladder mucosa is lined by transitional epithelium.[11] Bladder endometriosis, adhesion due to previous cesarean section, lower segment myoma, pelvic inflammatory disease PID, a distended bladder, etc. can predispose the bladder to injury during laparoscopic hysterectomy and other procedures like laparoscopic bladder neck suspension, vault prolapse repair, etc.

SIGMOID AND RECTUM

The most important parts of bowel in gynecological laparoscopy are the sigmoid colon and the rectum. The sigmoid colon extends from the pelvic brim to the third sacral segment. Posteriorly it is related to the left external iliac vessels, left piriformis muscle and the left sacral plexus. The rectum extends from the third sacral segment to below the tip of the coccyx. It is separated from the vagina by the rectovaginal septum and from uterus by small intestinal coils. Several pathological conditions may affect sigmoid and rectum and make it prone to injury during dissection. Severe endometriosis may involve the rectosigmoid and the rectovaginal septum. Laparoscopic mobilization of lower colon with shaving and disk excision may be required in severe rectal and rectovaginal endometriosis. Rectal injury is a potential risk under such circumstances, and, if any doubt exists, a diagnostic test by air or dye injection in the rectum may be necessary.

CONCLUSION

Pelvic anatomy forms the basis of advanced laparoscopic gynecological procedures. Although the basic facts of anatomy do not change with time, our understanding of specific anatomic relationships and the development of new clinical and surgical correlations continue to evolve. Alteration in normal pelvic anatomy due to various disease conditions, congenital variation and intraoperative complications may make normal anatomy look unfamiliar. Special emphasis must be given to the anatomy of pelvic vessels, bowel, and the urinary system as their injury can be disastrous. Surgical anatomy should preferably be reviewed before every difficult pelvic procedure. Every devoted pelvic surgeon should remain a passionate student of anatomy regardless of his/her skill and experience.

REFERENCES

1. Nezhat F, Brill AI, Nezhat CH, et al. Laparoscopic appraisal of the anatomic relationship of the umbilicus to the aortic bifurcation. J Am Assoc Gynecol Laparosc. 1998;5:135-40.
2. Fujii S, Takamura K, Matsumura N, et al. Precise anatomy of the vesico-uterine ligament for radical hysterectomy. Gynecol Oncol. 2007;104(1):186-91.
3. Richardson AC. The rectovaginal septum revisited: its relationship to rectocele and its importance in rectocele repair. Clin Obstet Gynecol. 1993;36(4):976-83.
4. Richardson AC. The anatomic defects in rectocele and enterocele. J Pelvic Surg. 1995;1:214-21.
5. Ross JW. Apical vault repair, the cornerstone of pelvic vault reconstruction. Int Urogynecol J Pelvic Floor Dysfunct. 1997;8(3):146-52.
6. DeLancey JO. Anatomy and biomechanics of genital prolapse. Clin Obstet Gynecol. 1993;36(4):897-909.
7. Richardson AC, Lyon JB, Williams NL. New look at pelvic relaxation. Am J Obstet Gynecol. 1976;126(5):568-73.
8. Jimenez AM, Colomer AT. An update of anatomical references in total laparoscopic radical hysterectomy: from surgical anatomy to anatomical surgery. J Minim Invasive Gynecol. 2008;15(1):4-10.
9. Yabuki Y, Asamoto A, Hoshiba T, et al. Dissection of the cardinal ligament in radical hysterectomy for cervical cancer with emphasis on the lateral ligament. Am J Obstet Gynecol. 1991;164(1 Pt 1):7-14.
10. Hurd WW, Bude RO, De Lancey JO, et al. The relationship of the umbilicus to the aortic bifurcation: implications for laparoscopic technique. Obstet Gynecol. 1992;80(1):48-51.
11. Bent AE, Cundiff GW. Cystourethroscopy. In: Baggish MS, Karram MM, (Eds). Atlas of Pelvic Anatomy and Gynecologic Surgery. Philadelphia: WB Saunders. 2001:721-46.

CHAPTER

6

Suture Materials

Shruti Paliwal, G Hemasree, B Ramesh

INTRODUCTION

Characteristics of ideal suture material are as follows:

- Its use should be possible in any operation, only variable being diameter as determined by tensile strength.
- It should allow easy and comfortable handling.
- Tissue reaction stimulated should be minimal and should not be favorable for bacterial growth.
- The breaking strength should be high in small caliber.
- The knot should hold securely without fraying or cutting.
- Material should not shrink in tissues.
- It should have uniform physical properties.
- Material should be nonelectrolytic, noncapillary, nonallergic, and noncarcinogenic.
- It should be sterile.
- It should be absorbed with minimal tissue reaction.

CATGUT SUTURE (FIG. 1)

Processed ribbon of sheep or beef intestinal submucosa are spun into strands of varying sizes ranging from 7-0 to 3. Raw material is collagen. It is absorbed through cellular and tissue proteases. Plain catgut is untreated and digested relatively quickly by body enzymes. It resists absorption for about 7 days. It is useful for tissues, which heal rapidly, e.g., ligating blood vessels and suturing subcutaneous fatty tissue.

Advantage of plane catgut: Ease of handling.

Disadvantage of plane catgut: Most rapid loss of tensile strength and knot strength.

When treated with 20% chromium salt solution in water with five parts of glycerin for 1–96 hours, it becomes chromic catgut. Chromic catgut resists body enzymes and prolongs the absorption time to 4–6 weeks. The chromicizing process either bathes each ribbon before spinning into strands (true chromicizing) or applies the solution to the finished strand (surface chromicizing). The concentration of chromium salt and duration of chromicizing process are precisely controlled to distribute chromatin uniformly. The treatment alters the color of catgut from yellowish tan shade of plain catgut to darker shade of brown.

Advantages of chromic catgut: Less irritating and cause less tissue reaction. It is easy to handle and knot is more secure.

Disadvantage of chromic catgut: Variability of absorption in infected field and rapid decrease in tensile strength.

POLYGLACTIN 910 SUTURE (FIG. 2)

It is a copolymer of lactide and glycolide. Copolymer is extruded and braided into strands varying in sizes from 9-0 to 3. It may be dyed violet or left undyed. Monofilament sutures are available in sizes 10-0 and 9-0. A controlled combination of lactide and glycolide results in structure maintaining 55% of original strength for 14 days and 20% of tensile strength for 21 days. Absorption process is minimal till the 40th day and completed by 60–90 days. It is absorbed by process of

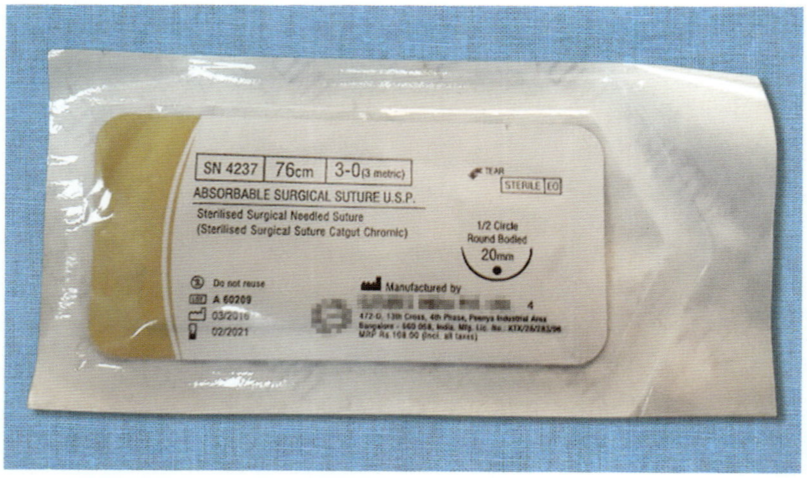

Fig. 1: Catgut suture.

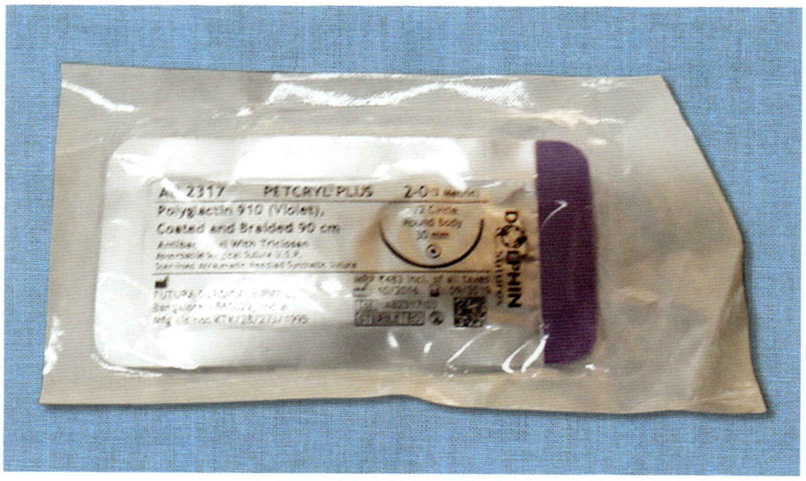

Fig. 2: Polyglycolic acid 910 suture.

slow hydrolysis. It is not affected by infection because its degradation is by hydrolysis and not inflammatory cell enzymatic degradation.

Advantages: Excellent tensile strength, longer tensile half-life, and low tissue reactivity.

Disadvantage: Tendency to gather tissue. It cannot be used when extended approximation of tissues under stress is required. Now coated polyglactin 910 suture is available, varying in sizes from 8-0 to 2. The coating is of equal parts of polyglactin 370 and calcium stearate. The coating produces smoothness, allows adjustable knot tension for precise knot placement, and causes less tissue drag than uncoated polyglactin 910 suture.

POLYGLYCOLIC ACID SUTURE (FIG. 3)

It is synthetic, absorbable, and braided suture. It is a homopolymer of glycolic acid. Filaments are dyed green to enhance visibility in tissues. The filaments are uniform in size and tensile strength but are smaller in diameter than polyglactin 910 suture. The suture sizes vary from 8-0 to 2 dyed green and from 7-0 to 2 natural beige. The tensile strength at 14 days' postimplantation is about 55% original value and at 21 days 20% original value. Tissue reaction is minimal. A microscopic layer of fibrous connective tissue grows over and into the suture material. Absorption from tissue is minimal at 7–15 days, significant at 30 days, and maximum after 60–90 days.

Advantages:
- The rate of absorption of polyglycolic acid suture is slower than that of polyglactin 910 suture.
- Suture is not affected by infection.

Disadvantage: It is an inferior knot security. A 2 + 1 + 1 + 1 knot configuration is secure.

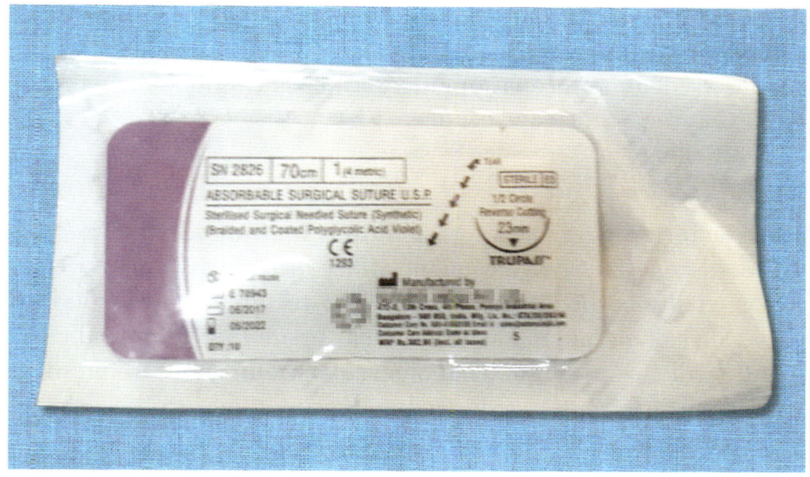

Fig. 3: Polyglycolic acid suture.

POLYDIOXANONE (FIG. 4)

Polydioxanone (PDS) is a synthetic, monofilament, and absorbable suture material. It is prepared from polyester polydioxanone. It is colored by adding D&C Blue No. 6 and D&C Violet No. 2 during polymerization. It is also available undyed in natural clear form. At 14 days after implantation, 70% tensile strength retained; at 28 days, 50% is retained; and at 56 days, 14% is retained. Absorption is minimal till the 90th day and is complete within 6 months.

Disadvantages: Less knot security. Vaginal mucosal suture causes localized irritation, if left for more than 10 days, and should be removed as indicated. Subcuticular suture may cause erythema and reaction during absorption.

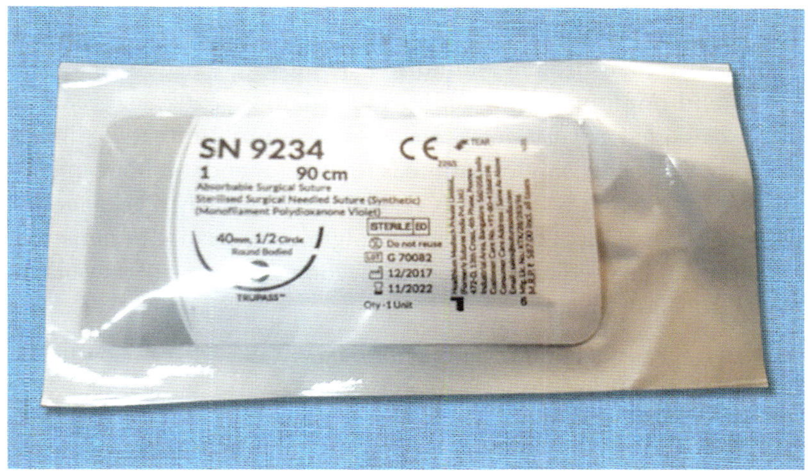

Fig. 4: Polydioxanone suture.

POLIGLECAPRONE 25 (FIG. 5)

It is a monofilament, synthetic and absorbable suture material. It is a copolymer of 75% glycolide and 25% caprolactone. It is available in natural undyed golden color and in dyed violet color.

Advantages: It is supple, pliable, and compliant. It is virtually memory free when dispensed. Its smooth surface ensures that it gently glides with minimum effort. It is relatively inert and well tolerated in tissue from initial placement until absorption is complete. It has a high initial tensile strength that is double that of chromic catgut when placed in tissue.

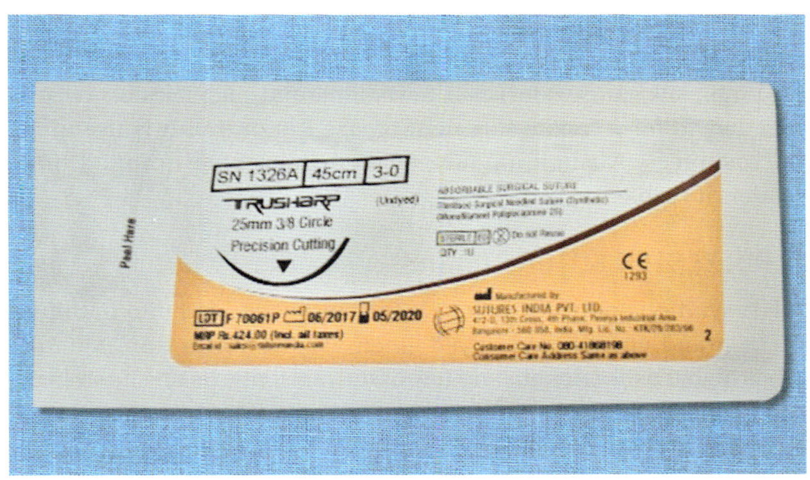

Fig. 5: Poliglecaprone 25.

At 7 days postimplantation, approximately 50–60% of tensile strength remains. At 14 days, 20–30% of tensile strength remains with wound support continuing up to 21 days. At 7 days postimplantation, approximately 60% of original tensile strength remains. At 14 days, approximately 30% strength remains, with wound support continuing up to 28 days. It is broken down by hydrolysis. The time required for complete absorption of material is 90–120 days postimplantation.

It is used for bowel anastomosis, peritoneal closure, subcutaneous closure, and subcuticular closure.

BARBED SUTURE (FIG. 6)

Self-anchoring with no knots required for wound closure. It is prepared from size 0 polydioxanone, which reabsorbs within 26 weeks. It has axially barbed segments directed in opposite direction on either sites of midpoint. Each suture has premium cutting and taper point needle with NuCoat technology. It is useful for gastrointestinal wound closure. It is useful in laparoscopic surgery because of elimination of knot tying.

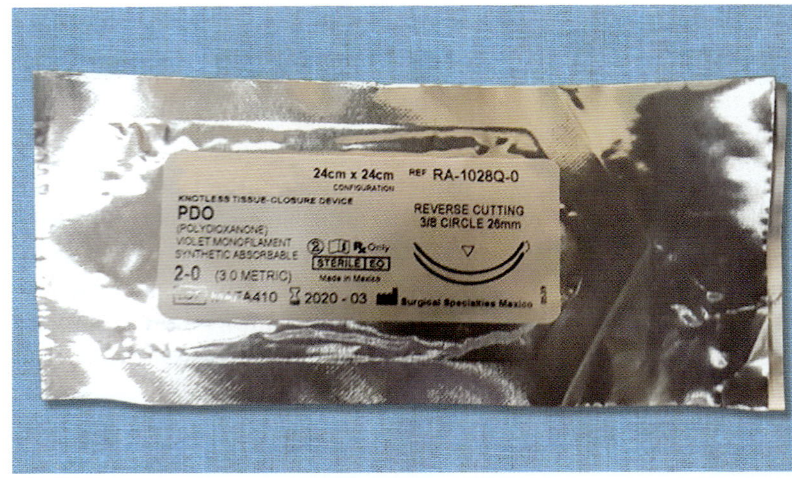

Fig. 6: Barbed suture.

SURGICAL SILK (FIG. 7)

The raw material is a protein thread, a continuous fiber spun by silkworm larva in making its cocoon. It is cream or orange in raw state. The fibers are braided together to form suture strand. Although it is classed as nonabsorbable, found to lose most of tensile strength in 1 year and not found in tissue for more than 2 years. So, it can be better classified as very slowly absorbable suture. Untreated silk has capillary action. So, surgical suture is treated to render it noncapillary and serum proof. It is dyed with vegetable dye, usually black, and for enhancing visibility. Loses tensile strength on exposure to moisture. It should not be used in presence of infection. Surgical silk is available in size from 9-0 to 5.

Advantage: Ease of handling and knot security. A 2 + 1 knot configuration is secure.

Disadvantage: Low tensile strength and tendency to form urinary stones.

Twisted silk fibers, encased in nonabsorbable coating of tanned gelatin or other protein, are called dermal suture. The coating prevents ingrowth of tissue cells, which could interfere with suture removal after the use for skin closure. Dermal suture is used for suturing skin in areas of tension.

Virgin silk suture consists of several natural silk filaments twisted together to form fragile fragment of size 8-0 or 9-0. It is useful for microsurgery. A small amount of methylene blue dropped on it renders it visible.

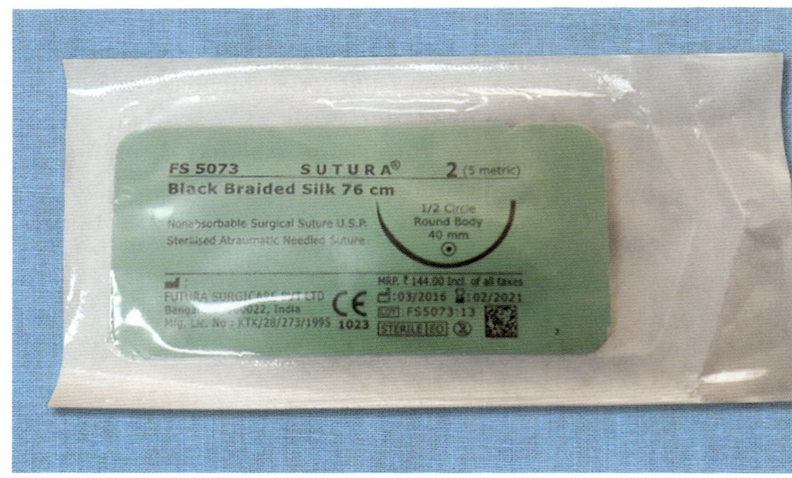

Fig. 7: Surgical silk.

POLYESTER SUTURE (FIG. 8)

It is a synthetic polymer. Its fibers are closely braided into multifilament strand. It is white or dyed green. Its size varies from 6-0 to 5. It has high tensile strength and low tissue reactivity. Its tensile strength is retained in tissues for long periods. Its knots are secure. Polyester is stiff and harder to handle. It has sawing or tearing effect when passed through tissues.

Braided polyester suture may be coated with polybutilate, which serves as a surgical lubricant. Polybutilate is polyester material, which adheres strongly to braided polyester strand. Coated polyester suture exhibits less tissue reaction than uncoated one. Its passage through tissue is smoother and makes handling easier. It is white or dyed green. Its range varies from 7-0 to 5.

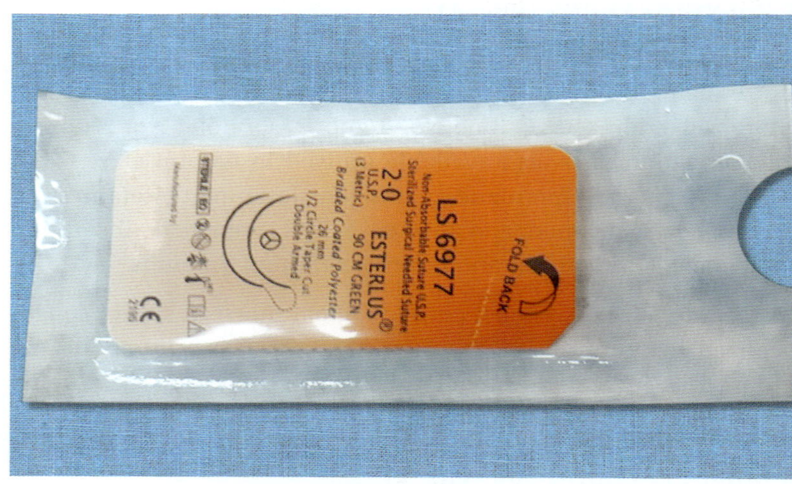

Fig. 8: Polyester suture.

NYLON (POLYAMIDE) (FIG. 9)

It is a synthetic polyamide polymer and can be monofilament or multifilament. Monofilament nylon has greater tensile strength, remarkably smooth infection rate is less, excellent knot security, no tissue adherence, infection resistant, and minimal tissue trauma. They are available in black color. They are available in size from 2 to 10-0.

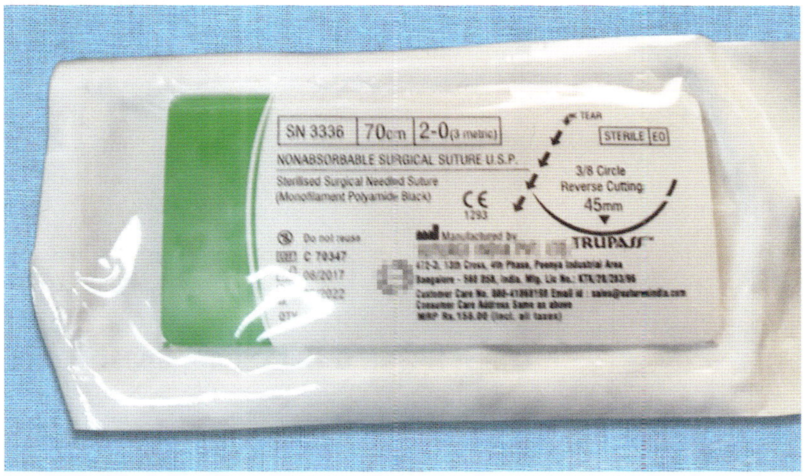

Fig. 9: Nylon suture.

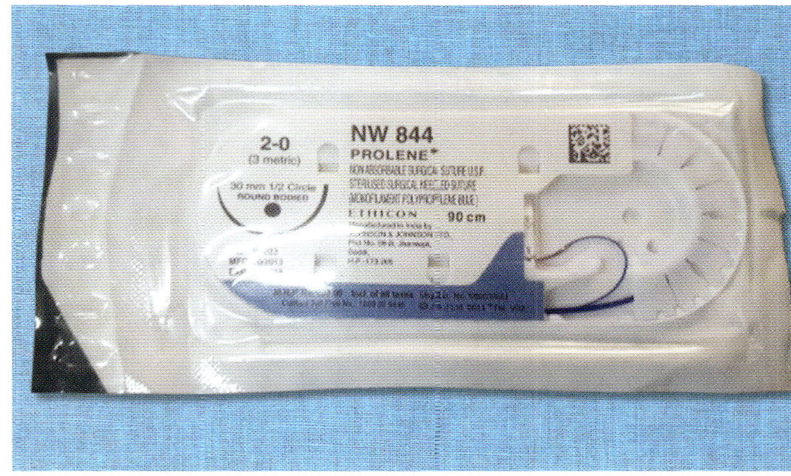

Fig. 10: Prolene suture.

Table 1: Characters of different suture materials.

Suture	*Composition*	*Color*	*Absorption*	*Breaking strength*	*Tissue reaction*	*Uses*	*Caveats*
Braided synthetic vicryl (ethicon), polysorb, and dexon (synthetic)	Copolymer of glycolide and lactide (vicryl and polysorb) or homopolymer of glycolic acid (dexon)	Undyed (white) or dyed (violet or green)	++	+++	+–	Interrupted deep dermal closure, oral mucosa, and vessel ligation	Interrupted than running suture
Braided synthetic vicryl rapide (ethicon)	Copolymer of glycolide and lactide	Undyed (white) or dyed (violet or green)	++++	+++	+–	Interrupted deep dermal closure, oral mucosa, and vessel ligation	Use an interrupted than running suture. Can be substituted plain gut due to absorption
Monofilament synthetic PDS III and monocryl (ethicon), maxicon, biosyn, and caprosyn	Various polymers	Undyed (clear) or dyed (violet)	+ PDS III and maxicon ++ monocryl and biosyn +++ caprosyn	+ Caprosyn ++ monocryl and biosyn +++ maxicon	++	Subcuticular closure and fascia	Causes less tissue reaction
Plain gut	Serosa of beef intestine or submucosa of sheep intestine	Light tan	++++	+	++++	Eyelid close to lip margin (where suture removal would be difficult)	Uses five ties
Chromic gut	Same as above but treated with chromic salts to delay absorption	Brown	+++	+	+++	Oral and nasal mucosa	When it is used inside mouth, it is used within 1–2 weeks
Fast-absorbing gut	Plain gut treated with heat to facilitate more rapid absorption	Light tan	++++	+	++++eyelid close to lid margin	Facial wounds under low tension	Maintain strength 7 days and is completely absorbed within 2 weeks

(PDS: polydioxanone)

PROLENE (POLYPROPYLENE) (FIG. 10)

It is a synthetic polymerized propylene, monofilament, generally blue color and has high tensile strength.

Advantages: It has least tissue reaction. It is unaffected by tissue reaction and can be used during infection. They are extremely durable and long lasting.

Disadvantages: Fragility, high plasticity, high expense, and difficulty of use.

It is available in size from 10-0 to 2. A 2 + 1 + 1 + 1 + 1 + 1 + 1 knot configuration is secure.

CHAPTER 7

Colposcopy

Tanvi Desai, G Hemasree, Shashikala T

WHAT IS COLPOSCOPY?

Colposcopy was discovered by Hans Hinselmann of Germany in 1924.

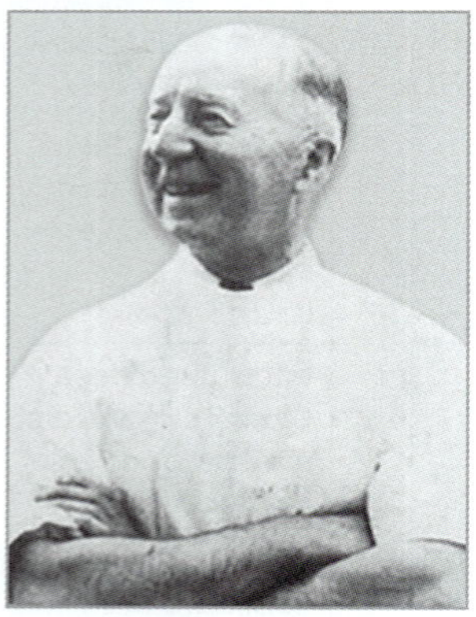

Hans Hinselmann

Colposcopy (kol-POS-kuh-pee) is a procedure to closely examine the cervix, vagina, and vulva for signs of disease. During colposcopy, a special instrument called a colposcope is used. A colposcope can greatly enlarge the normal view. This examination allows the healthcare provider to visualize problems that cannot be seen by the naked eye alone. A colposcope is a low-power, stereoscopic, and binocular field microscope with a powerful light source used for magnified visual examination of the uterine cervix to help in the diagnosis of cervical neoplasia.

ANATOMY OF CERVIX

The female reproductive system is made up of vulva, vagina, uterus, fallopian tubes, and ovaries **(Fig. 1)**. The cervix is the lower, narrow part of a women's uterus. It connects the main body of uterus to the vagina **(Fig. 2)**.

STRUCTURE

The cervix is about 2 cm (1 inch) long. It is made up mostly of connective tissue and muscle. It is divided into two main parts:

1. The endocervix is the inner part of the cervix lining the canal leading into the uterus.
2. The ectocervix, or exocervix, is the outer part of the cervix. It is rounded, lip-like, and sticks out into the vagina.

The endocervical canal is the passageway from the uterus to the vagina.

The two main types of cells in the cervix are:

1. Columnar cells line the endocervical canal. They are glandular cells that make mucus.
2. Squamous cells line the ectocervix and vagina. They are flat and thin like the scales on a fish.

The squamous cells join the columnar cells in an area of the cervix called the *squamocolumnar junction*. This is also called the *transformation zone* because the tall columnar cells are constantly being changed into flat squamous cells, especially during puberty and childbearing years. Precancerous changes of the cervix and most cervical cancers start in the transformation zone **(Figs. 3A and B)**.

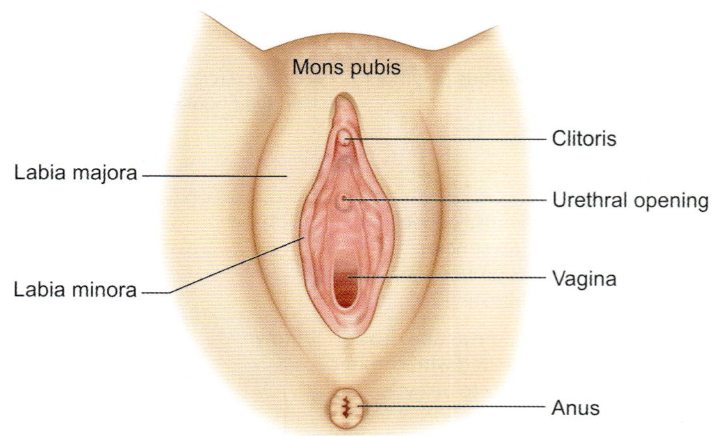

Fig. 1: Female reproductive system.

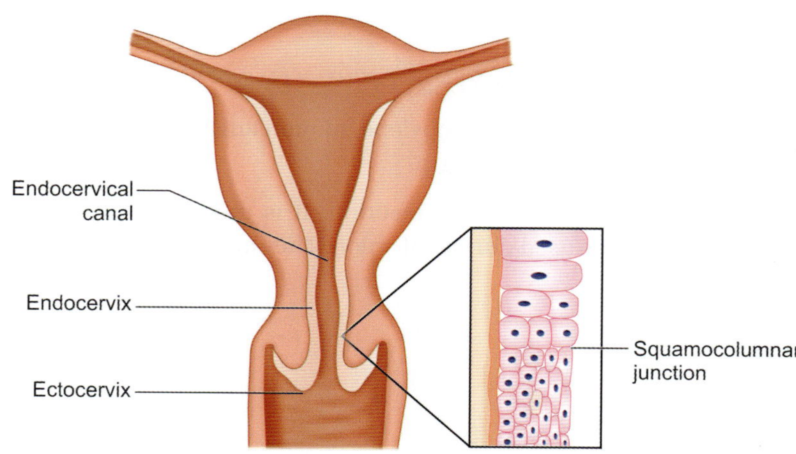

Fig. 2: The cervix.

Physiological changes in the cervix:

- From birth until puberty, the endocervical epithelium is composed of columnar cells and the ectocervical epithelium of native squamous cells. The interface between the two is termed the original squamocolumnar junction **(Fig. 4)**.
- During puberty and at the first pregnancy, the cervix increases in volume in response to hormonal changes. The endocervical epithelium everts onto the ectocervix (portio vaginalis) exposing it to the acidic pH of the vagina. This provides a stimulus for metaplastic change of the columnar epithelium **(Fig. 5)**.
- *The process of metaplasia is a patchy one:* It starts initially in the crypts and at the tips of the endocervical villae, which gradually fuse. Eventually, the whole of the everted endocervical epithelium may be replaced by squamous epithelium. The squamocolumnar junction undergoes eversion after puberty and pregnancy and recedes into the endocervical canal at the menopause **(Fig. 6)**.
- Immature metaplasia develops as a transformation zone between the squamocolumnar junction and the ectocervix from basally situated reserve cells **(Figs. 7 to 10)**.

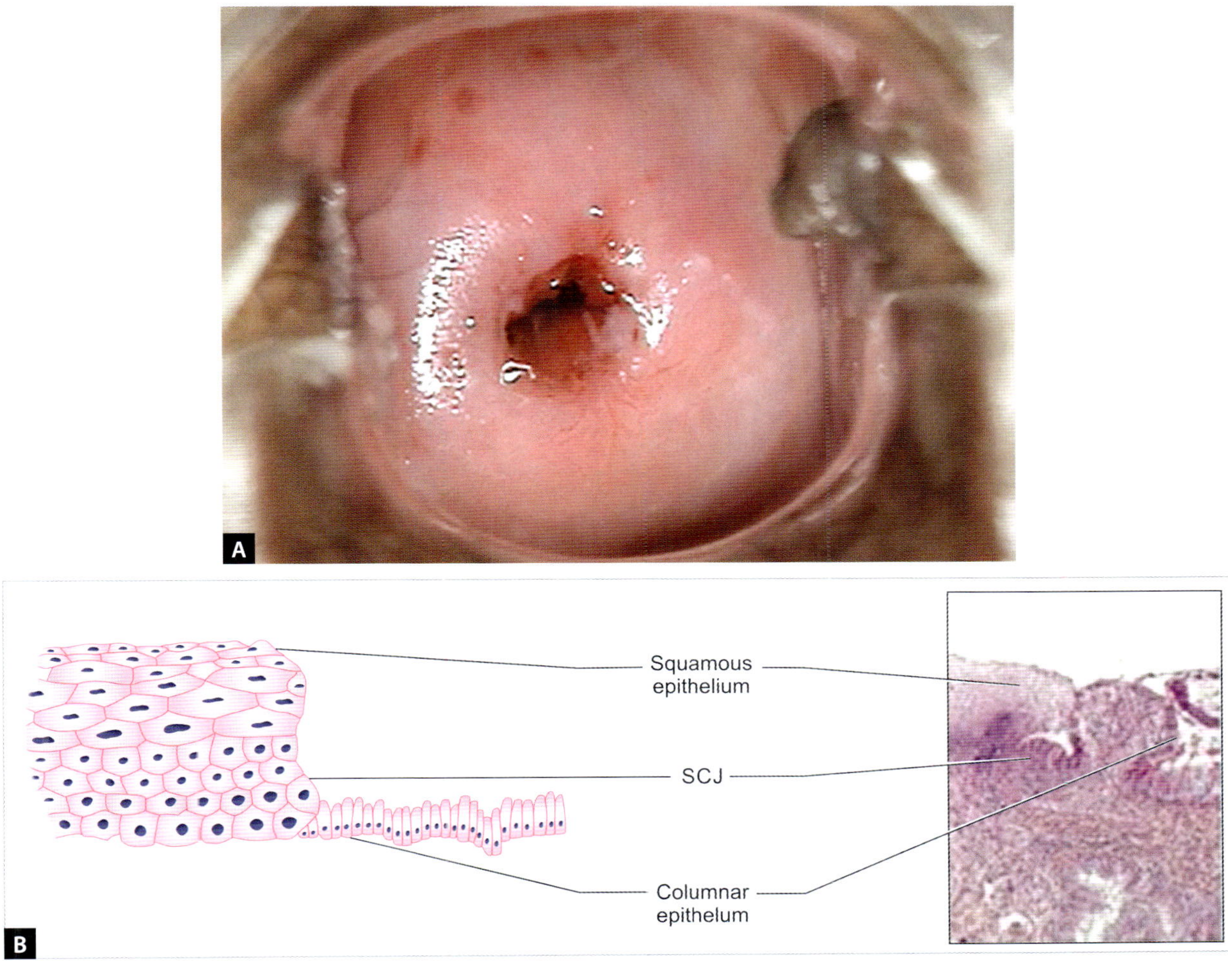

Figs. 3A and B: (A) Squamocolumnar junction (SCJ) and (B) Squamocolumnar junction (×10).

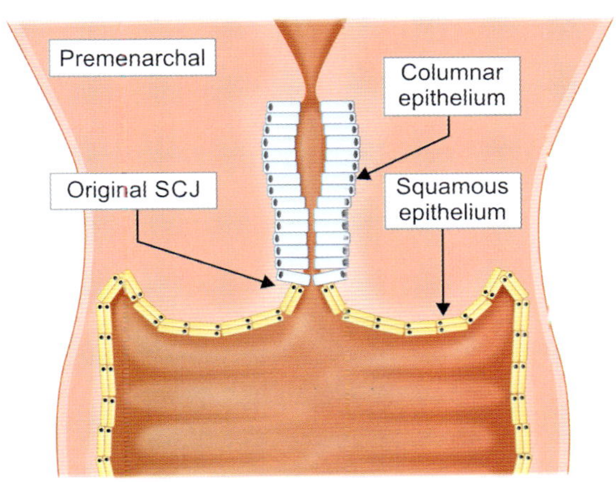

Fig. 4: Premenarchal squamocloumnar junction [original squamoco umnar junction (SCJ)].

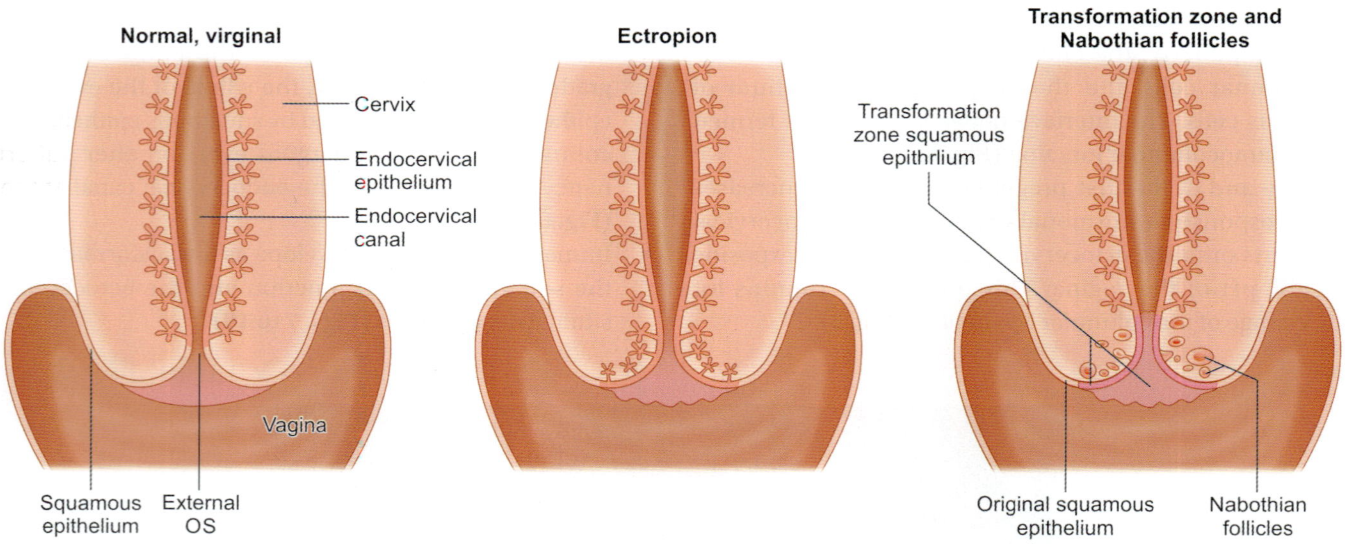

Fig. 5: Puberty changes.

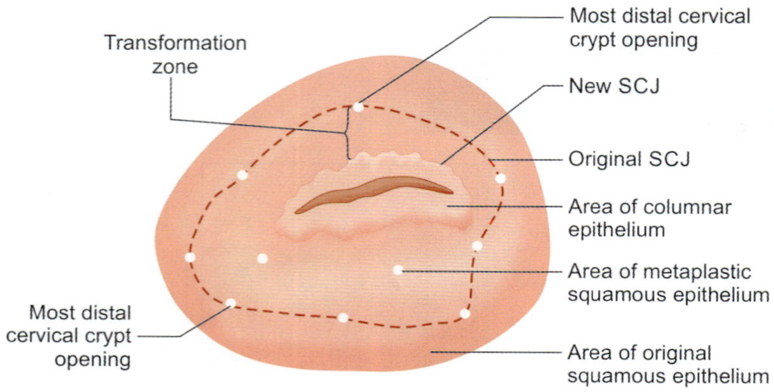

Fig. 6: A method of identifying outer and inner borders of the transformation zone. (SCJ: squamocolumnar junction)

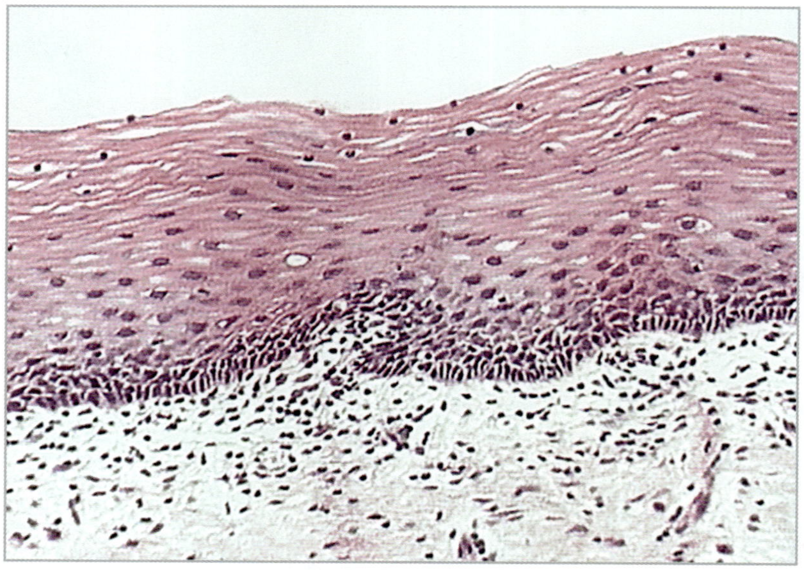

Fig. 8: Nabothian follicles.

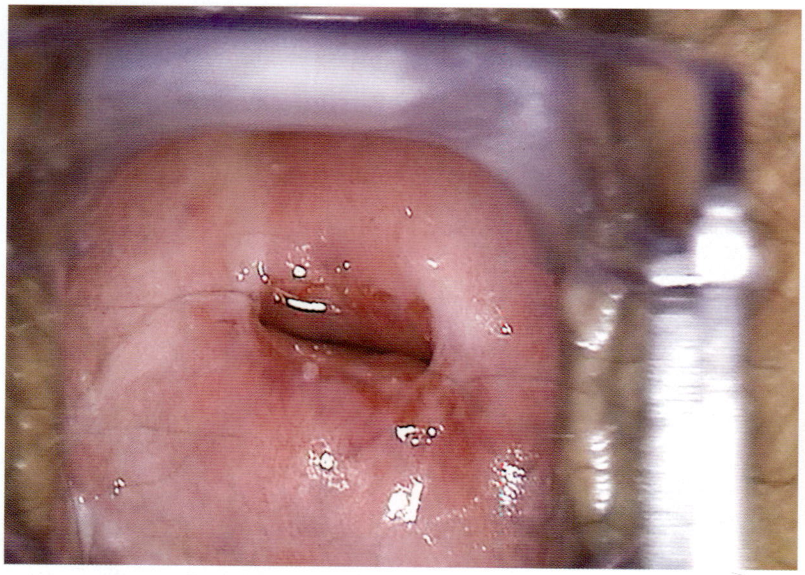

Fig. 7: Mature and immature metaplastic cells are shown in the transformation zone.

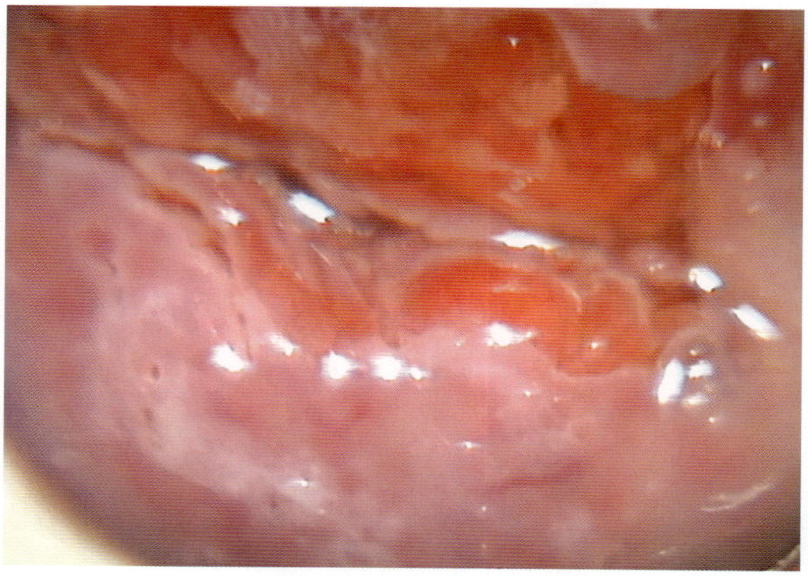

Fig. 9: Gland opening.

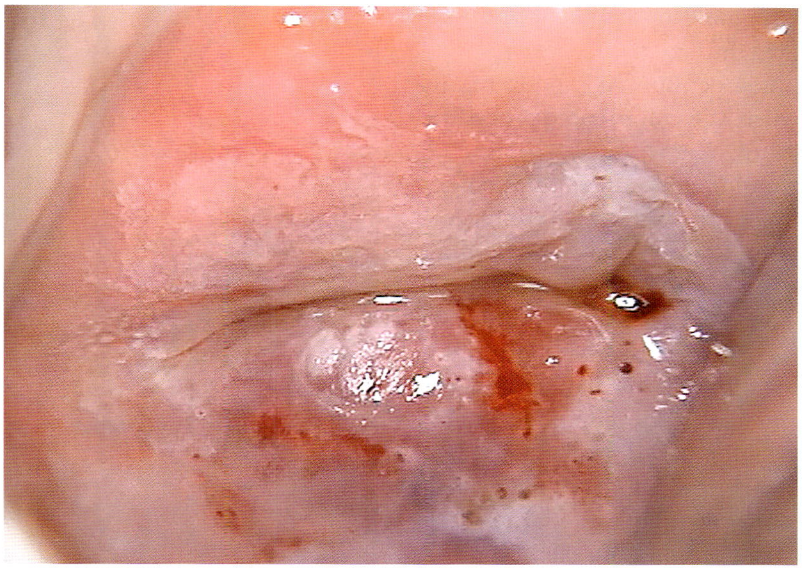

Fig. 10: Columnar epithelium surrounded by metaplastic squamous epithelium.

FINE REGULAR PATTERN OF MOSAIC VESSEL (FIGS. 11 AND 12)

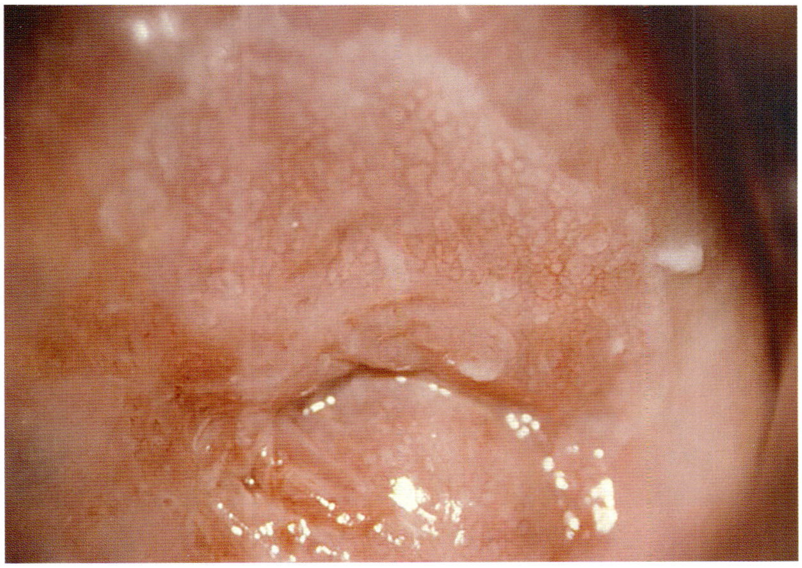

Fig. 11: Dilated capillaries terminating on the surface.

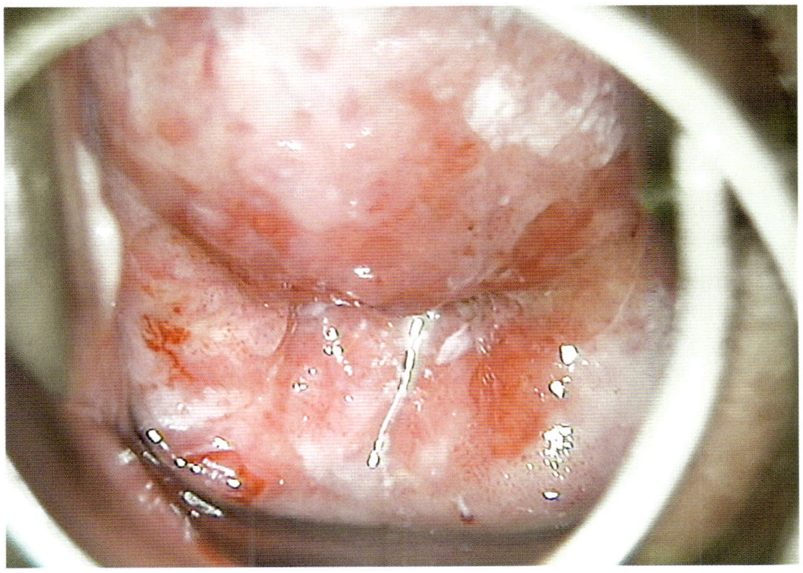

Fig. 12: Appears on end on view as a collection of dots.

WHAT ARE THE INDICATIONS FOR COLPOSCOPY?

- The most common indication of referral for colposcopy is positive screening tests [e.g. positive cytology, positive on visual inspection with acetic acid (VIA), etc.]
- Cervical intraepithelial neoplasia (CIN) 2 or CIN 3 on cytology
- Suspicious looking cervix
- Invasive carcinoma on cytology
- Persisting low-grade abnormalities (CIN 1) on cytology for more than 12–18 months
- CIN 1 on cytology
- Persistently unsatisfactory quality on cytology
- Infection with human papillomavirus (HPV)
- Acetopositivity on VIA
- Acetpositivity on visual inspection with acetic acid with magnification (VIAM)
- Positive on visual inspection with Lugol's iodine (VILI).

PROCEDURE

Colposcopy is done in a doctor's office **(Fig. 13)**.

Magnification can be changed by changing the power of an eye piece.

The procedure is best done when a woman is not having her menses. This gives the healthcare provider a better view of the cervix. For at least 24 hours before the test, one should not:

- Douche
- Use tampons
- Use vaginal medications
- Have intercourse.

It is important to explain the examination procedure and reassure the woman before colposcopy. This will ensure that the woman relaxes during the procedure.

Written informed consent should be obtained from the woman before the colposcopic examination.

Relevant medical and reproductive history should be obtained before the procedure.

A strict adherence to the essential steps involved in colposcopic examination ensures that common errors are avoided.

As with a pelvic examination, the patient is given lithotomy position. A *speculum* is used to hold apart the vaginal walls so that the inside of the vagina and the cervix can be seen. The colposcope is placed just outside the introitus. The vagina is cleaned using normal saline and cotton swab before visualizing through the colposcope.

It is important to visualize the squamocolumnar junction in its entire circumference **(Fig. 14)**, otherwise, the colposcopic procedure is termed "unsatisfactory" **(Fig. 15)**.

One should identify the transformation zone during the colposcopic procedure. The proximal limit of the transformation zone is defined by the squamocolumnar junction, while the distal limit of the transformation zone is identified by finding the most distal crypt openings or Nabothian follicles in the lips of the cervix and by drawing an imaginary line connecting these landmarks. This is followed by application of 3–5% dilute acetic acid and Lugol's iodine solution successively to examine the cervical epithelium. It is difficult to study the vascular pattern of the cervix after acetic acid/Lugol's iodine **(Fig. 16)**. Hence, physiological saline is applied first before acetic acid/Lugol's iodine to study the subepithelial vascular pattern in detail **(Fig. 17)**. It is essential to obtain directed biopsies, under colposcopic control, from abnormal/suspicious areas identified.

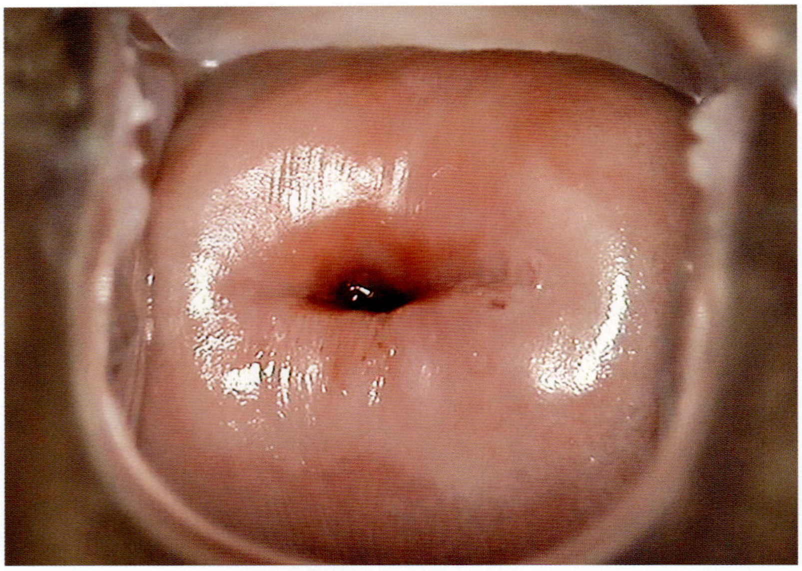

Fig. 15: Unsatisfactory colposcopy.

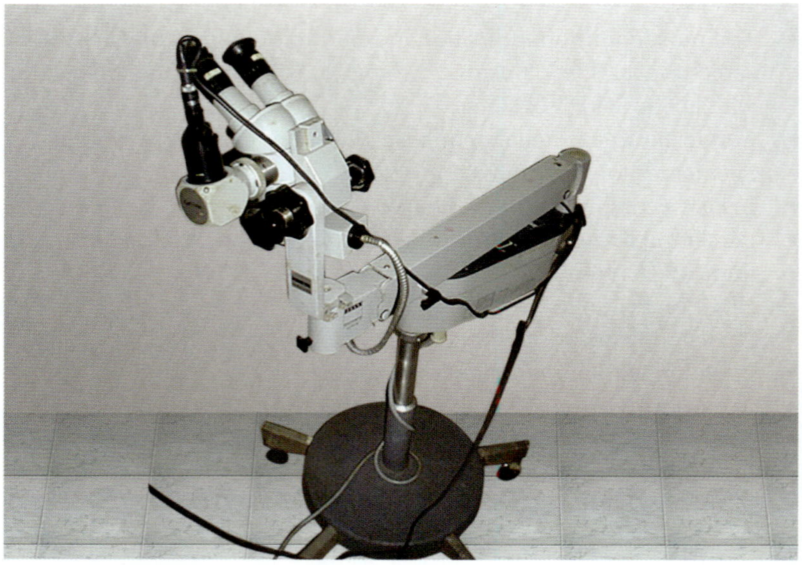

Fig. 13: Colposcope: Single objective lens with fixed focal distance.

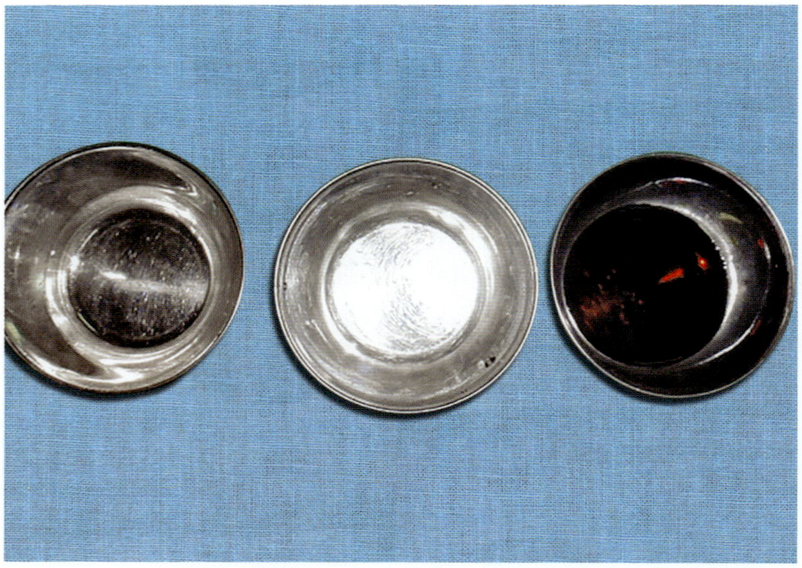

Fig. 16: Normal saline/acetic acid/Lugol's iodine.

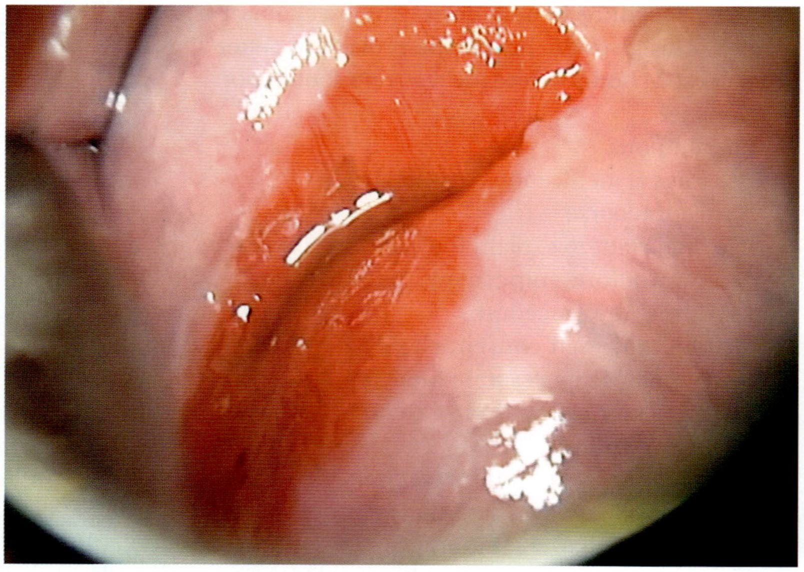

Fig. 14: Satisfactory colposcopy.

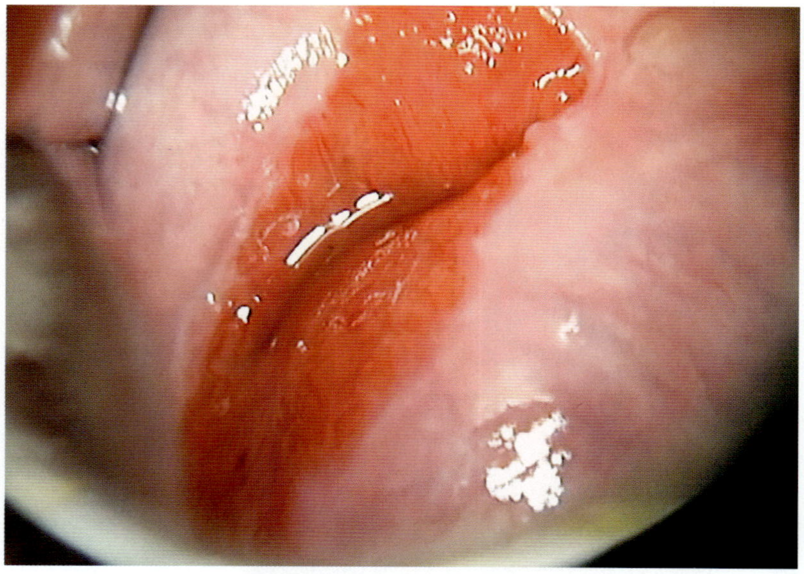

Fig. 17: Normal colposcopic appearance.

Acetic Acid Test

About 3–5% acetic acid is usually applied with a cotton swab. It helps in coagulating and clearing the mucus. Acetic acid causes swelling of the epithelial tissue, columnar, and any abnormal squamous epithelial areas in particular. It causes a reversible coagulation or precipitation of the nuclear proteins and cytokeratins. Thus, the effect of acetic acid depends upon the amount of nuclear proteins and cytokeratins present in the epithelium. When acetic acid is applied to normal squamous epithelium, little coagulation occurs in the superficial cell layer, as this is sparsely nucleated. Areas of CIN undergo maximal coagulation due to their higher content of nuclear protein and prevent light from passing through the epithelium. As a result, the subepithelial vessel pattern is obliterated and difficult to see and the epithelium appears white. This reaction is termed acetowhitening, and produces a noticeable effect compared with the normal pinkish color of the surrounding normal squamous epithelium of the cervix, an effect that is commonly visible to the naked eye.

The acetowhite appearance **(Fig. 18)** can also be seen in certain other conditions where nuclear protein is increased like immature squamous metaplasia, congenital transformation zone, in healing and regenerating epithelium (associated with inflammation), leukoplakia (hyperkeratosis), and condyloma. Acetowhitening associated with CIN and invasive cancer quickly appear and persist for more than 1 minute **(Fig. 19)**. The acetic acid effect reverses much more slowly in high-grade CIN lesions and in early preclinical invasive cancer than in low-grade lesions, immature metaplasia, and subclinical HPV changes. It may last for 2–4 minutes in the case of high-grade lesions and invasive cancer.

Schiller's (Lugol's) Iodine Test (Figs. 20 and 21)

The principle behind the iodine test is that original and newly formed mature squamous metaplastic epithelium is glycogenated, whereas CIN and invasive cancer contain little or no glycogen. Columnar epithelium does not contain glycogen. Immature squamous metaplastic epithelium usually lacks glycogen or, occasionally, may be partially glycogenated. Iodine is glycophilic and hence the application

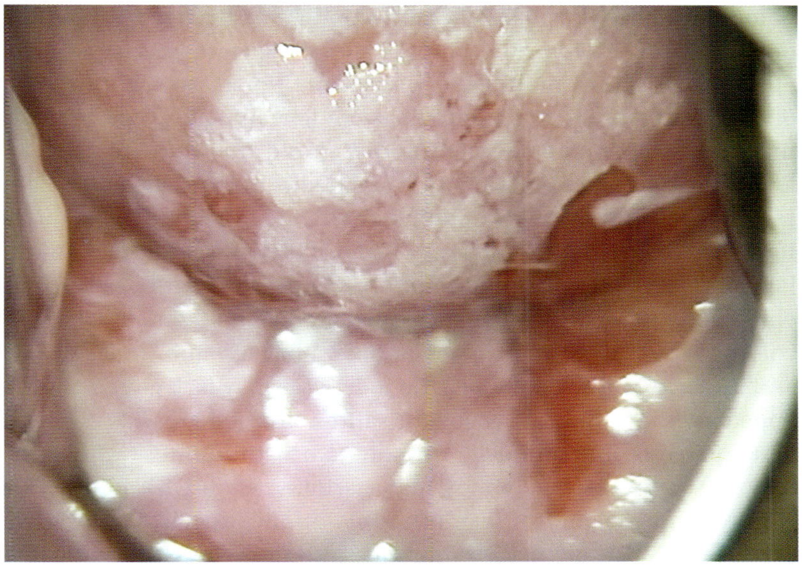

Fig. 19: Acetowhite positive.

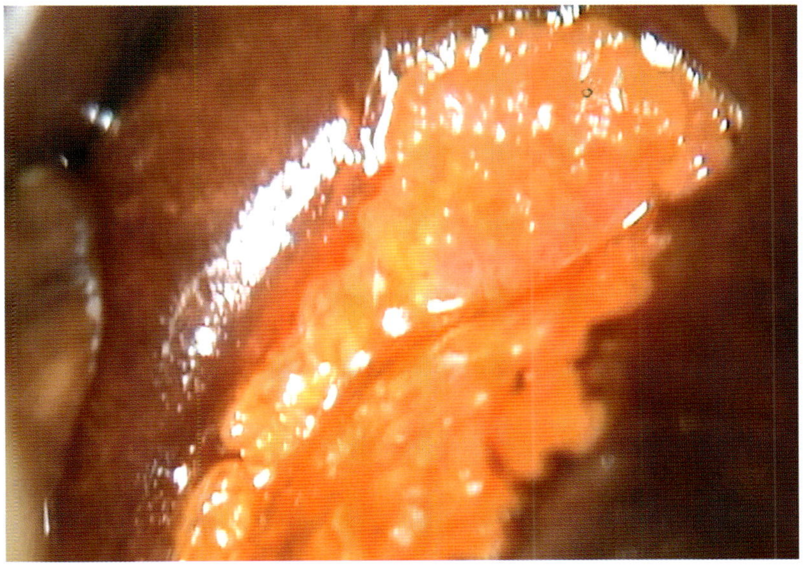

Fig. 20: Lugol's iodine appearance.

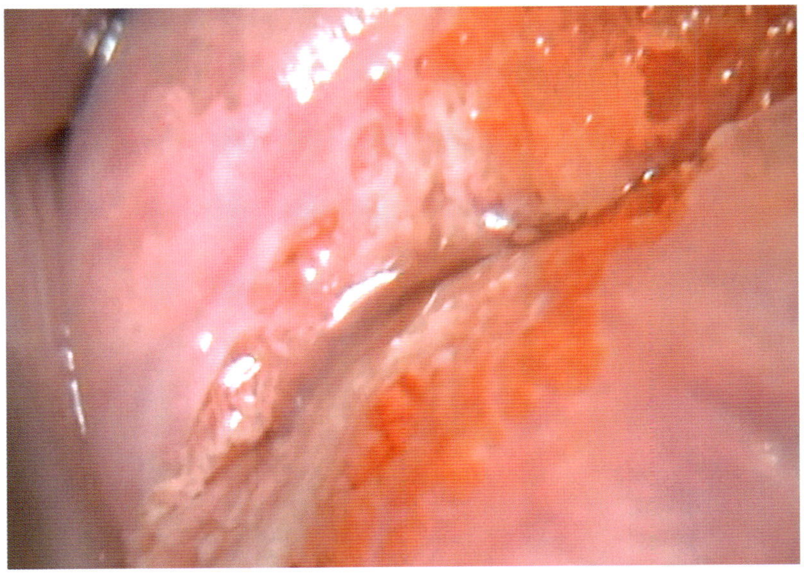

Fig. 18: Acetowhite appearance.

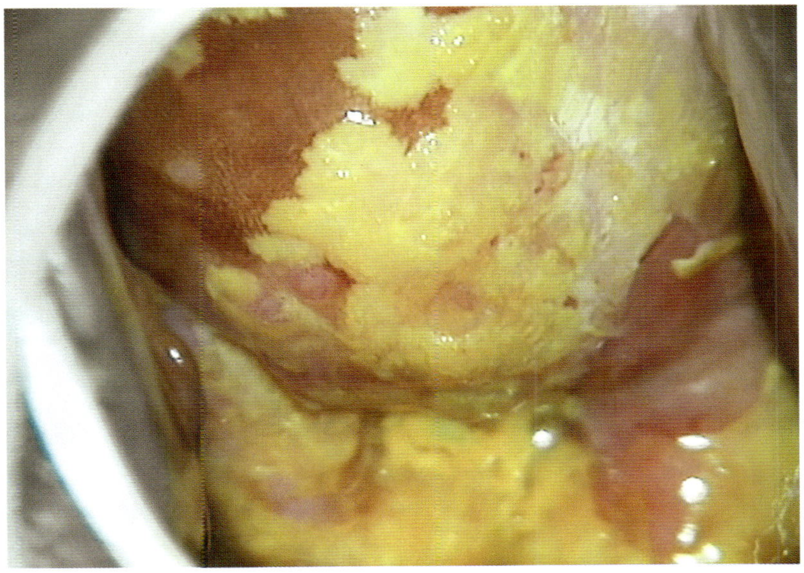

Fig. 21: Iodine negative appearance.

of iodine solution results in uptake of iodine in glycogen-containing epithelium. Therefore, the normal glycogen-containing squamous epithelium stains mahogany brown or black after application of iodine. Columnar epithelium does not take up iodine and remains unstained, but may look slightly discolored due to a thin film of iodine solution; areas of immature squamous metaplastic epithelium may remain unstained with iodine or may be only partially stained. If there is shedding (or erosion) of superficial and intermediate cell layers associated with inflammatory conditions of the squamous epithelium, these areas do not stain with iodine and remain distinctly colorless in a surrounding black or brown background. Areas of CIN and invasive cancer do not take up iodine (as they lack glycogen) and appear as thick mustard yellow or saffron-colored areas. Areas with leukoplakia (hyperkeratosis) do not stain with iodine. Condyloma may not, or occasionally may only partially, stain with iodine. We recommend the routine use of iodine application in colposcopic practice as this may help in identifying lesions overlooked during examination with saline and acetic acid and will help in delineating the anatomical extent of abnormal areas much more clearly, thereby facilitating treatment.

WHEN IS CERVICAL BIOPSY PERFORMED?

The main objective of colposcopy is to differentiate lesions that are insignificant and not requiring biopsy and those that are suspicious and requiring biopsy.

During colposcopy, the healthcare provider may see abnormal areas. A biopsy of these areas may be done. During a biopsy, a small piece of tissue is removed from the cervix. The sample is removed with a special device.

Cells also may be taken from the canal of the cervix. A special device is used to collect the cells. This is called endocervical curettage (ECC).

Once an abnormal transformation zone is detected, the area is evaluated and compared with other areas of the cervix. If any other abnormal zones are present, the colposcopist should then decide from where a biopsy or biopsies should be taken. It is essential to obtain one or more directed punch biopsies from areas colposcopically identified as abnormal and/or doubtful. Biopsy should be obtained from the area of the lesion with worst features and closest to the squamocolumnar junction. Biopsy always should be done under colposcopic control by firmly applying the biopsy instrument, with the jaws wide open, to the cervical surface to be sampled.

After the biopsy has been obtained, it is advisable to indicate the site of the target area which has been biopsied, on the diagram of cervix in the reporting form. It is important to place the freshly obtained biopsy specimen in a labeled bottle containing 10% formalin.

The biopsy site(s) may be cauterized with Monsel's paste or with a silver nitrate stick immediately after the procedure to control any bleeding.

WHAT IS LARGE LOOP EXCISION OF THE TRANSFORMATION ZONE?

It is also called loop electrosurgical excision procedure (LEEP), this is the most common way of removing cervical tissue for examination and treating precancerous changes of the cervix. The abnormal tissue is removed using a thin wire loop that is heated electrically. Sometimes the doctor can remove all visible abnormal cells **(Fig. 22)**.

A large loop excision of the transformation zone (LLETZ) is usually done under a local anesthetic in the doctor's office or, sometimes, under a general anesthetic in hospital. It takes about 10 minutes. Sometimes, it is done at the same time as a colposcopy, but this is uncommon. The tissue sample will be sent to a laboratory for examination under a microscope. The results will be available in about a week.

WHAT IS CONE BIOPSY?

This procedure is similar to an LLETZ and is used when there are abnormal glandular cells in the cervix or when early-stage cancer is suspected. In some cases, it is also used to treat very small, early-stage cancers. A surgical knife (scalpel) is used to remove a cone-shaped piece of tissue from the cervix. The cone biopsy is usually done under a general anesthetic and involves a day or overnight stay in the hospital. Results are usually available in a week **(Fig. 23)**.

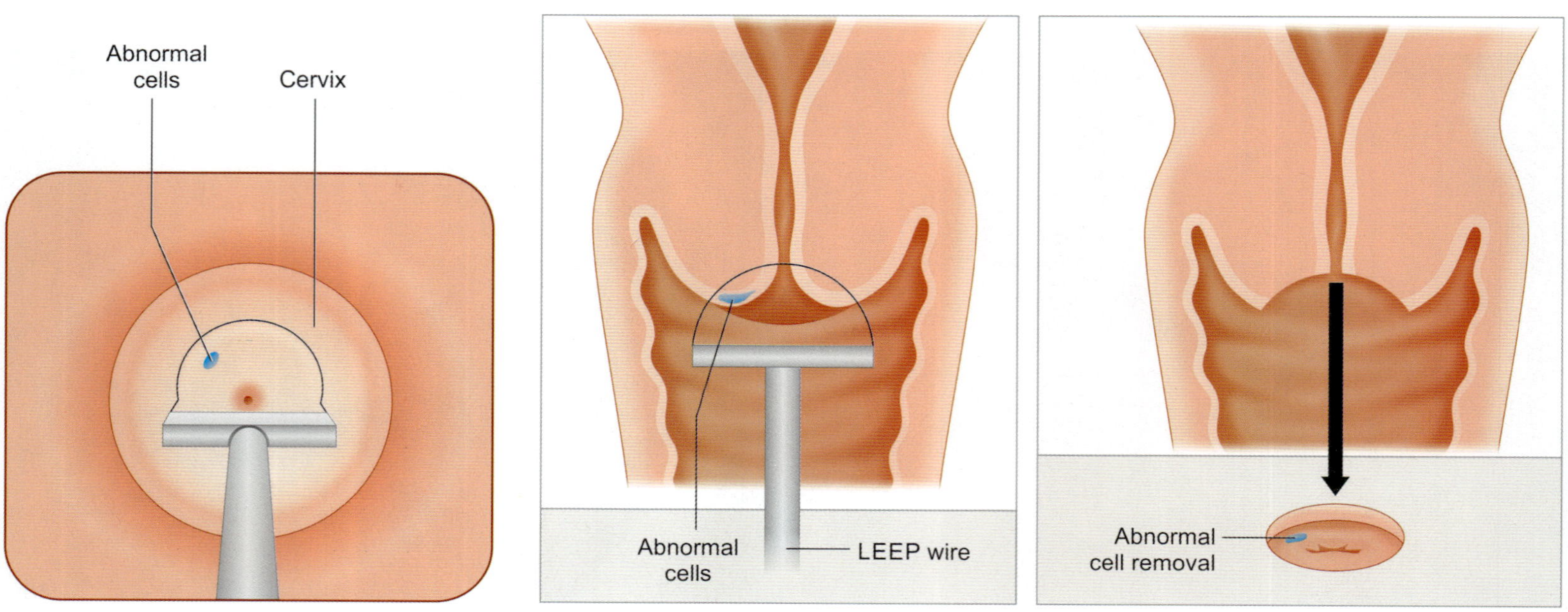

Fig. 22: Loop excision.

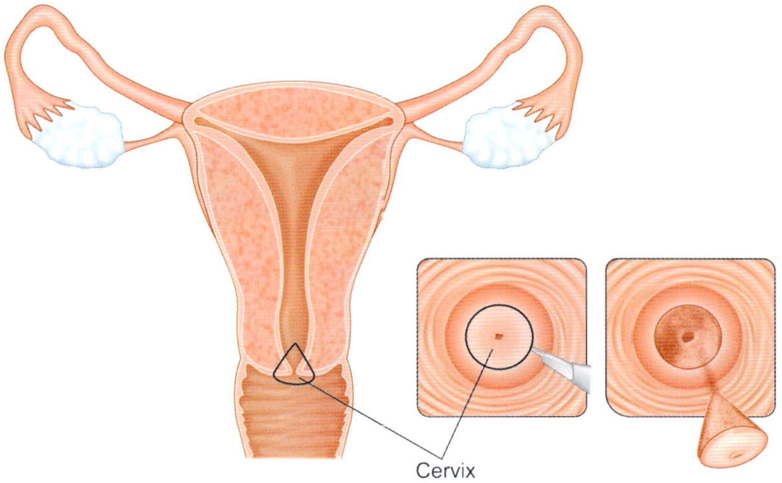

Fig. 23: Cone biopsy.

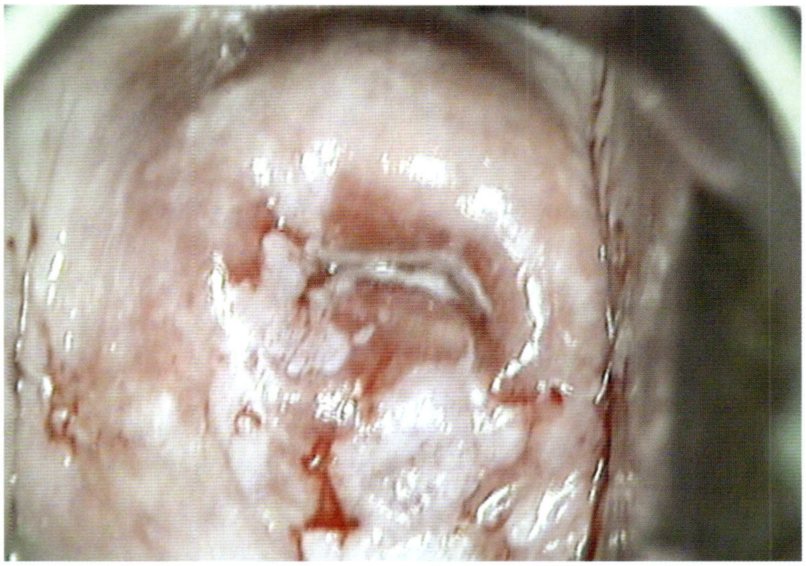

Fig. 26: Dense AWA—CIN II CIN III, invasive Ca.

Abnormal Colposcopic Findings (Figs. 24 to 36)

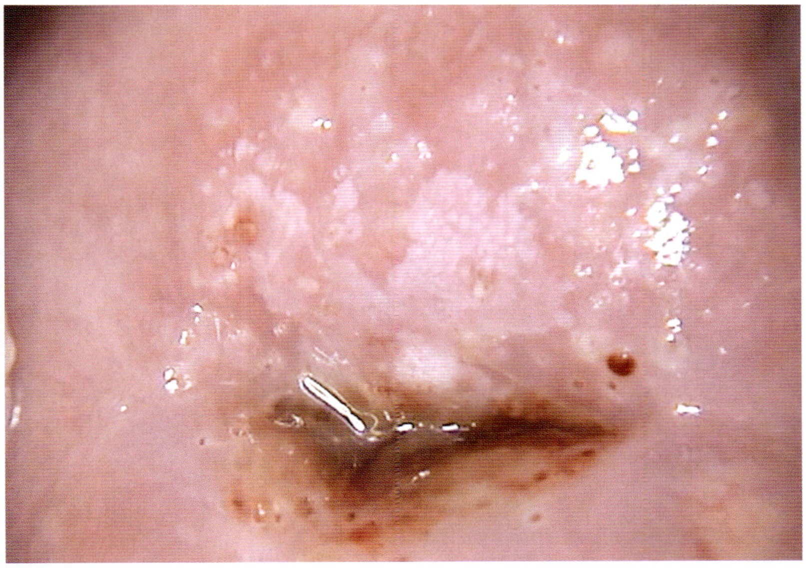

Fig. 24: Mild degree of acetowhite area (AWA)—immature metaplasia and CIN I.

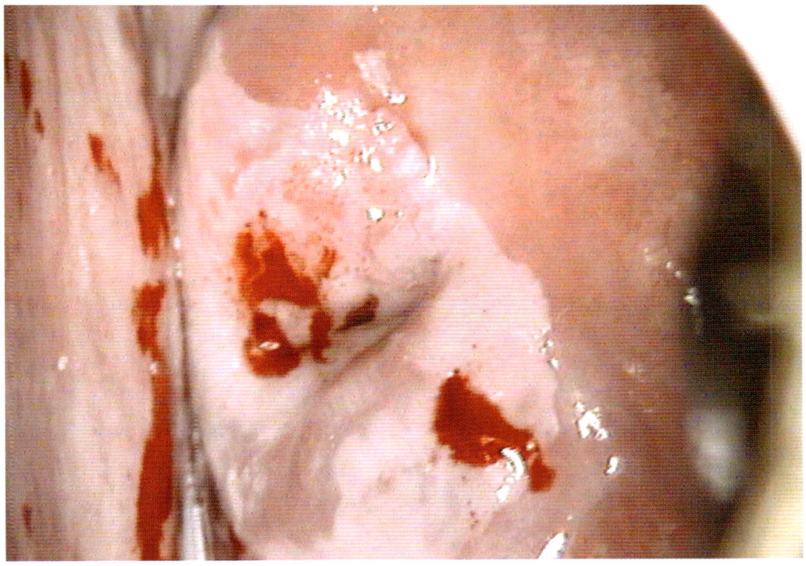

Fig. 27: Coarse punctations—high-grade lesion and invasive Ca.

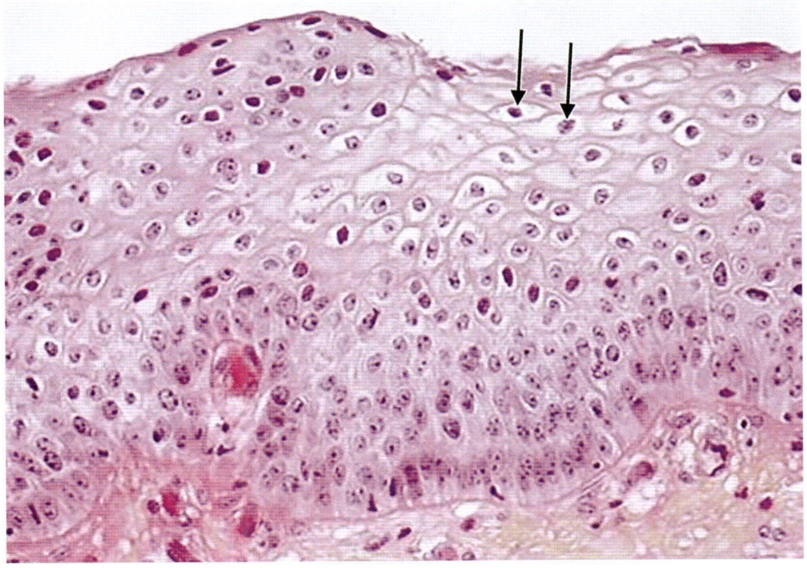

Fig. 25: *Histology of CIN 1:* Dysplastic cells are confined to lower third of epithelium. Koilocytes indicated by arrows are observed in upper layers of epithelium.

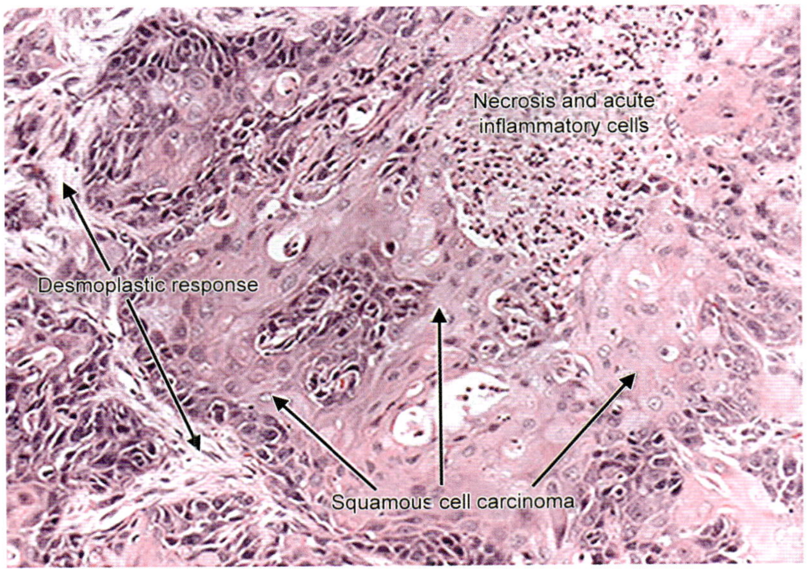

Fig. 28: Histology of Invasive Ca cervix—squamous cell carcinoma.

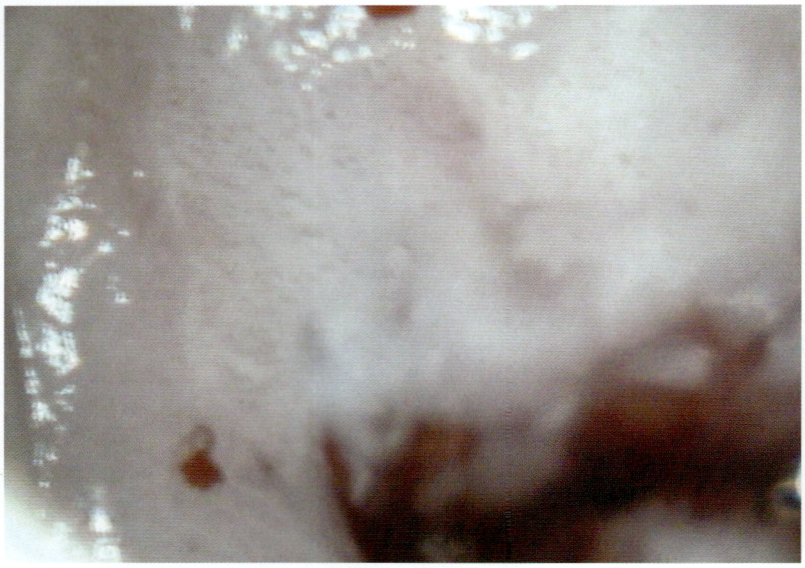

Fig. 29: Fine punctations—metaplasia, inflammation, and low-grade lesion.

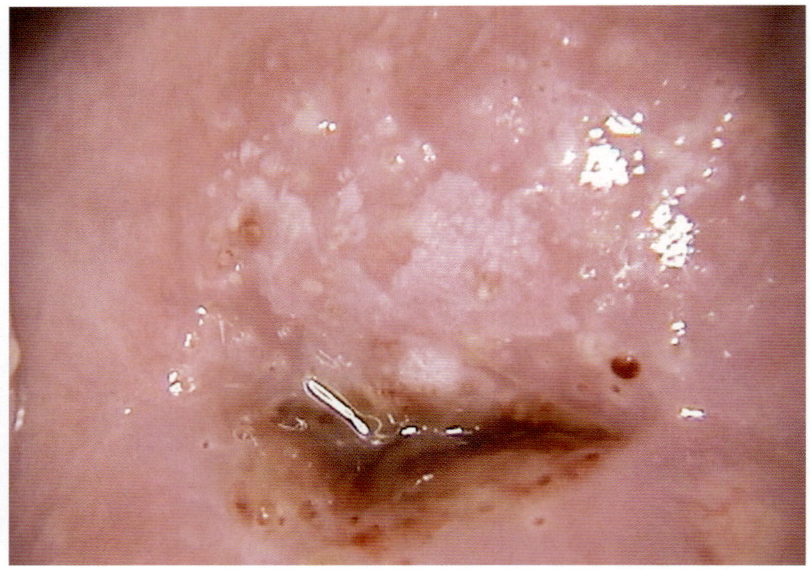

Fig. 30: Fine mosaic—metaplasia, inflammation, and low-grade lesion.

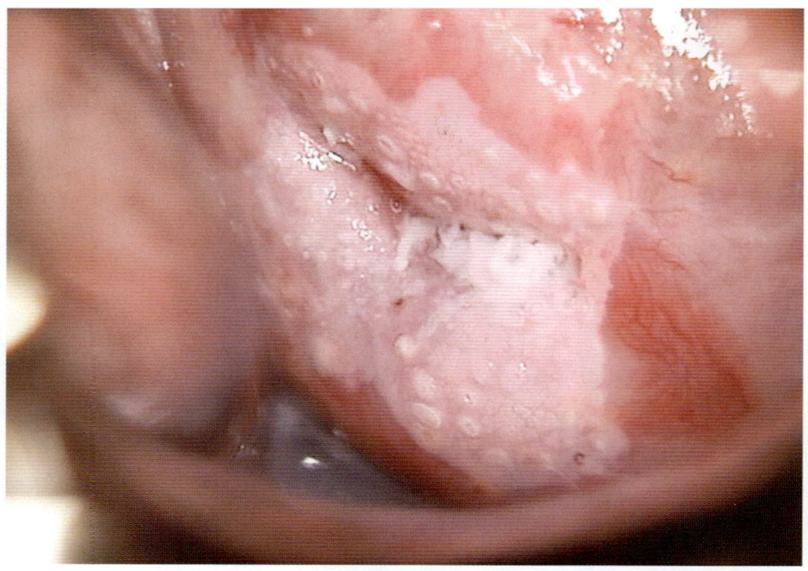

Fig. 31: Coarse mosaic—high-grade lesion and invasive Ca.

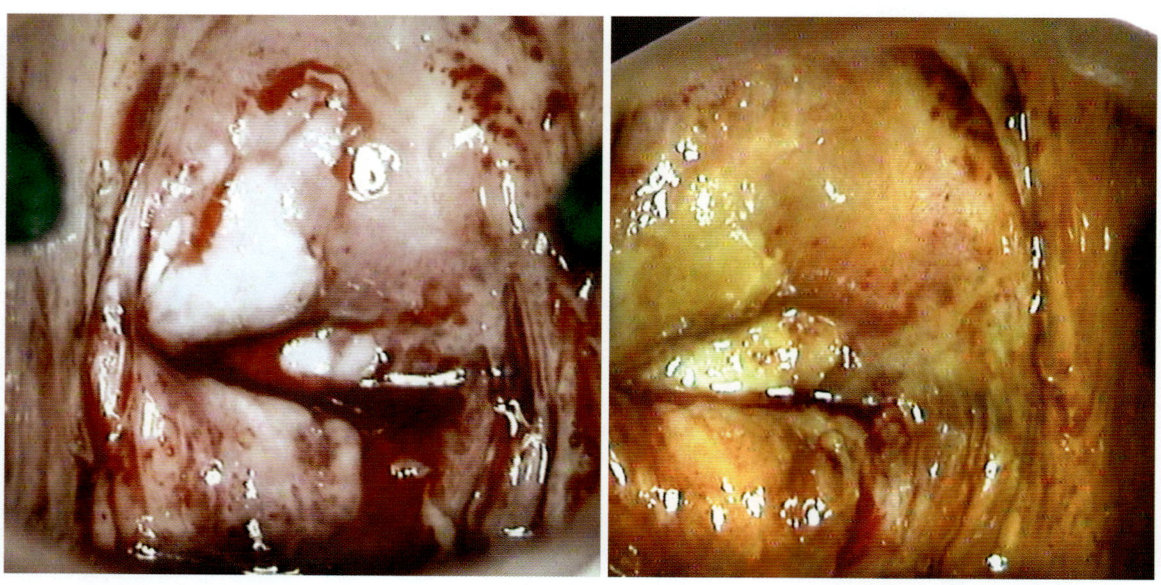

Fig. 32: Dense AWA, irregular surface, distinct margin, iodine negative, coarse punctations and coarse mosaic highly suggestive of high-grade squamous intraepithelial lesion (HSIL) and Ca.

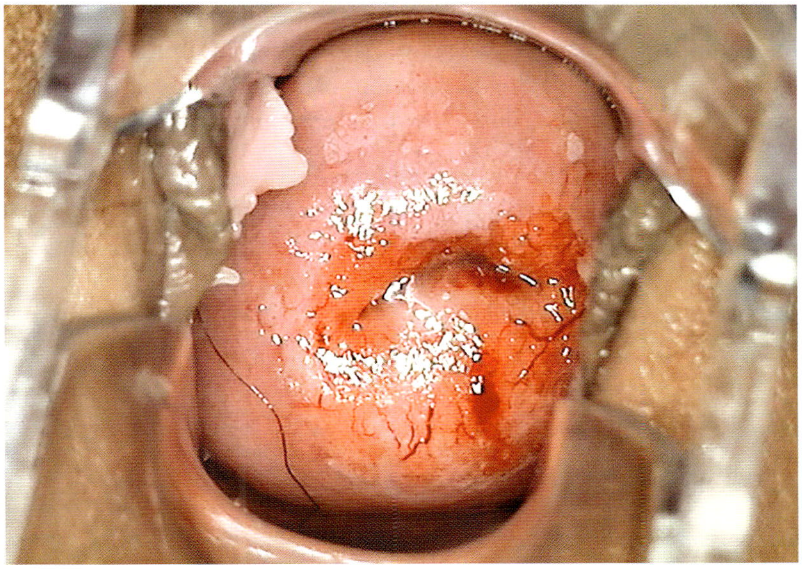

Fig. 33: Nonsuspicious vascular pattern—regular course and branching, terminal loops have normal intercapillary distance, diffusely distributed, and present in poorly circumscribed areas.

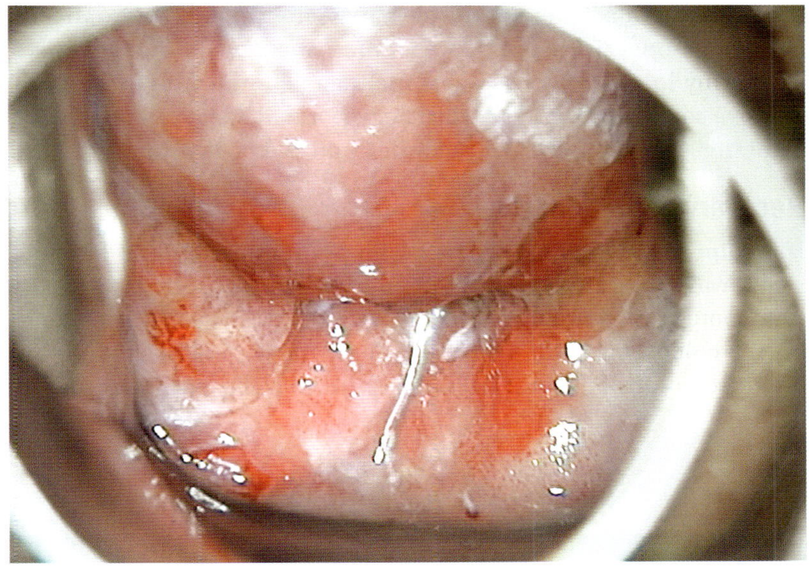

Fig. 36: Atypical vessels—haphazard shape, great variation in caliber, abrupt changes in direction with acute angle and increased intercapillary distance.

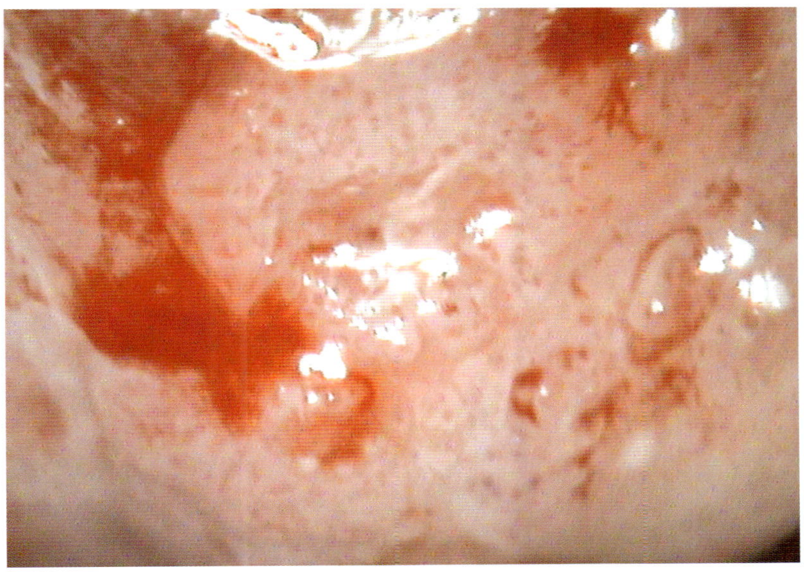

Fig. 34: Suspicious vascular pattern—haphazard branching, great variation in caliber. Increased intercapillary distance, corkscrew, and comma-shaped vessels.

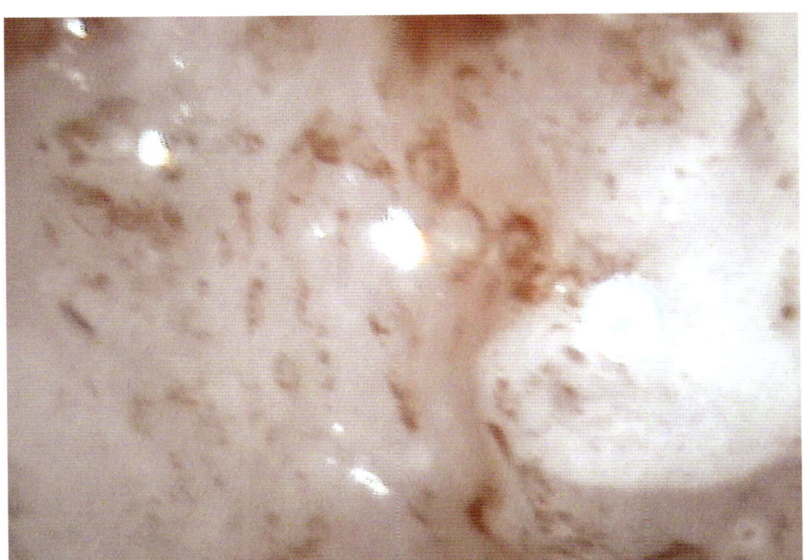

Fig. 35: Abnormal vessel suspicious of malignancy—abnormal vessels are present in a sharply circumscribed dense AWA areas.

If the woman is pregnant: The effects of pregnancy on the cervix are edema, an increase in the area of the epithelium, enlargement and opening of the os, and eversion. As the pregnancy progresses, these changes are exaggerated, so that an inadequate examination at the beginning of pregnancy may become adequate by a later stage due to eversion. Certain difficulties in examination, however, become more pronounced as pregnancy progresses: the vaginal walls tend to be redundant and collapse, obscuring the view; cervical mucus is increased; increased vascularity leads to easily induced bleeding; the blood vessel pattern in cervical pseudodecidual tissue tends to mimic invasive cancer; and CIN tends to appear as a more severe grade than it actually is (due to increased size, increased edema, and vasculature pattern). Thus, considerable experience is required for colposcopy in pregnancy.

The steps in the colposcopic procedure for a pregnant woman are similar to those for a nonpregnant woman, but extra care must be taken not to injure any tissues when a digital examination or speculum insertion is performed. If a repeat cytology smear is needed, this may be performed using a spatula, by applying gentle pressure to avoid bleeding. Some may prefer to obtain a cytology sample at the end of the colposcopic procedure, in order to avoid inducing bleeding that may obscure the colposcopic field, but this may result in a poor hypocellular sample, as cells might have been washed away during the different steps of the colposcopic procedure.

As the pregnancy progresses, cervical biopsy is associated with an increased probability and degree of bleeding, which may often be difficult to control. The risk of biopsy should always be weighed against the risk of missing an early invasive cancer. All lesions suspicious of invasive cancer must be biopsied or wedge excised. Sharp biopsy forceps should be used, as they will produce less tearing of tissue. Biopsy should always be carried out under colposcopic vision to control depth. The prompt application of Monsel's paste or silver nitrate to the biopsy site, immediate bed rest for 15–30 minutes, and the use of a tampon or other hemostatic packing to put pressure on the biopsy site are helpful to minimize bleeding. Some women may need an injection of pitressin into the cervix or suturing for hemostasis. To avoid a large amount of tissue slough, due to the effect of Monsel's paste, hemostatic packs should not be left in place for more than a few hours after the paste has been applied. Alternatively, cervical biopsy in a pregnant woman may be performed with diathermy loop. If colposcopy is inadequate and cytology suggests invasive cancer, a conization must be performed, ideally in the second trimester. Noninvasive lesions may be evaluated postpartum.

Recovery after Colposcopy

If a colposcopy is done without a biopsy, patient should feel fine right away. She can do the routine things normally. She may have a little spotting for a couple of days.

If a colposcopy with a biopsy is done, the patient may have pain and discomfort for 1 or 2 days. Over-the-counter pain medications can be helpful. She may have some vaginal bleeding. Patient also may have a dark discharge for a few days. This may occur from medication used to help stop bleeding at the biopsy site. While the cervix heals, do not have intercourse, do not use tampons, and do not douche.

Report to the healthcare provider right away if has any of the following problems are present:

- Heavy vaginal bleeding (using more than one sanitary pad per hour)
- Severe lower abdominal pain
- Fever
- Chills.

CASE STUDIES (FIGS. 37 TO 50)

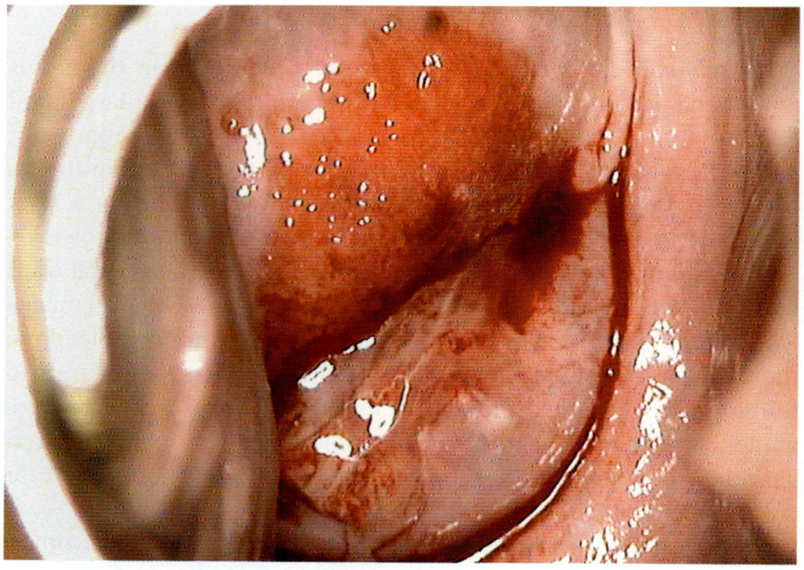

Fig. 37: A 38-year-old female, history of (H/O) white discharge per vagina (WDPV) on and off. Pap not done: Satisfactory colposcopy subjective of (s/o) cervical ectopy.

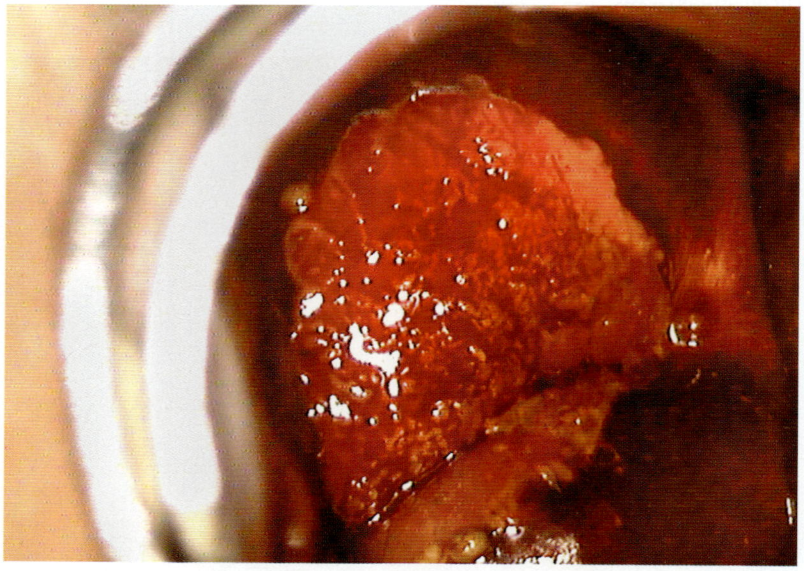

Fig. 39: No iodine negative area. Pap taken. Human papillomavirus (HPV) test advised.

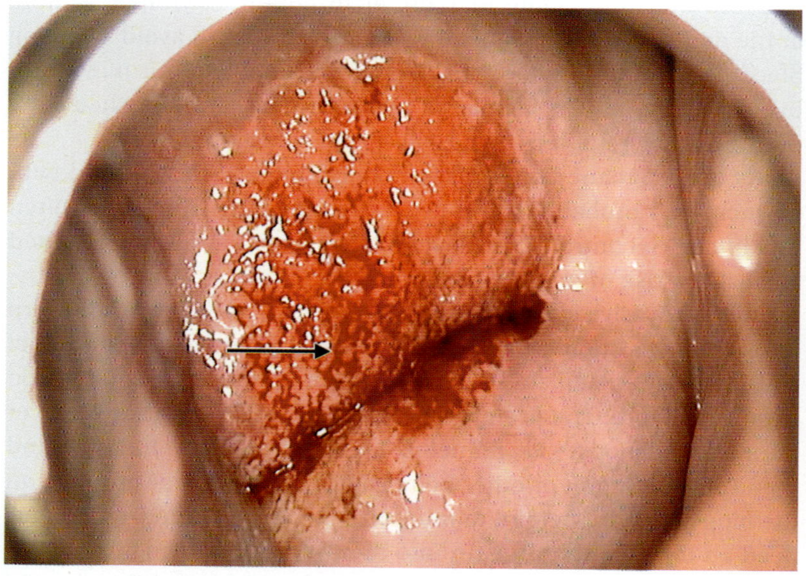

Fig. 38: Grade 1 AWA at 6 o'clock, and no abnormal vessel.

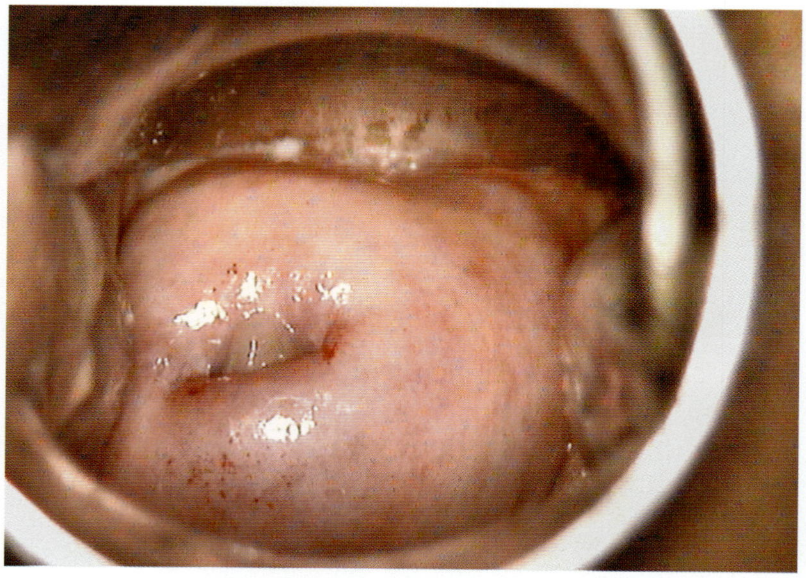

Fig. 40: A 62-year-old female with history of vulval itching (unsatisfactory colposcopy)

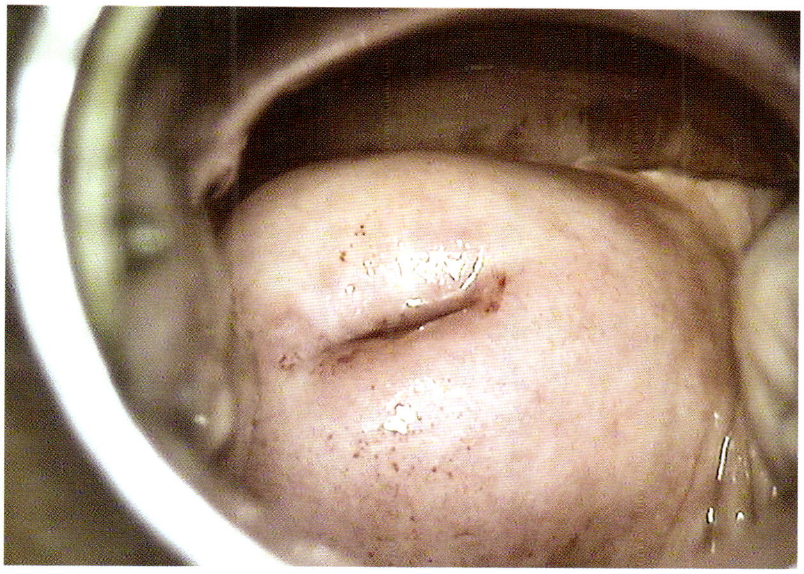

Fig. 41: Postmenopausal cervix, green filter.

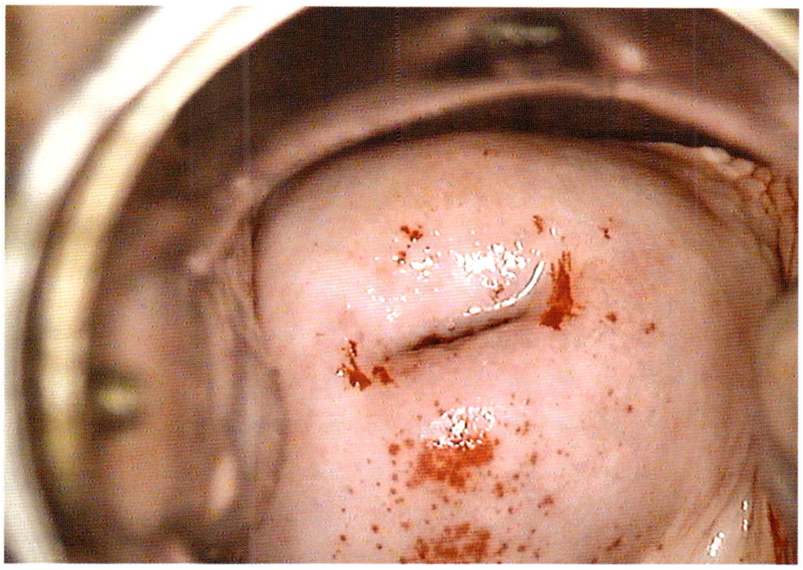

Fig. 42: Subepithelial hemorrhage seen after acetic acid mimicking punctation.

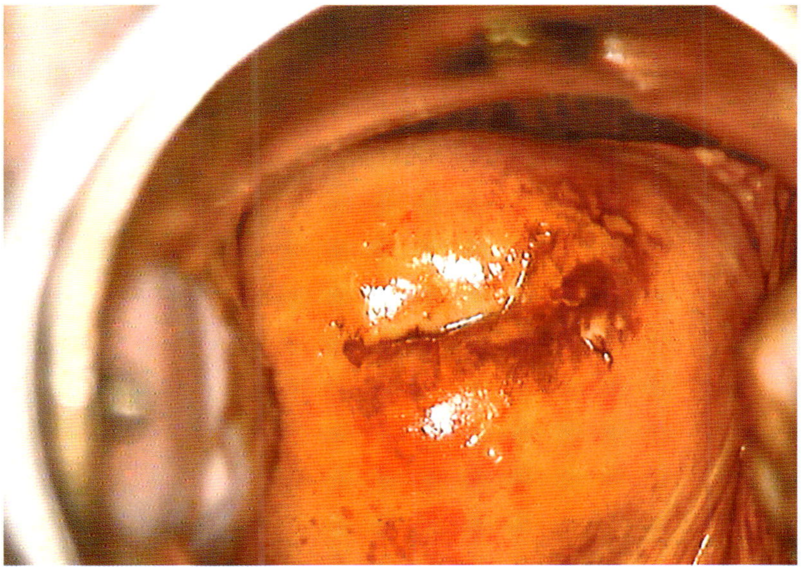

Fig. 43: Postmenopausal women, iodine negative.

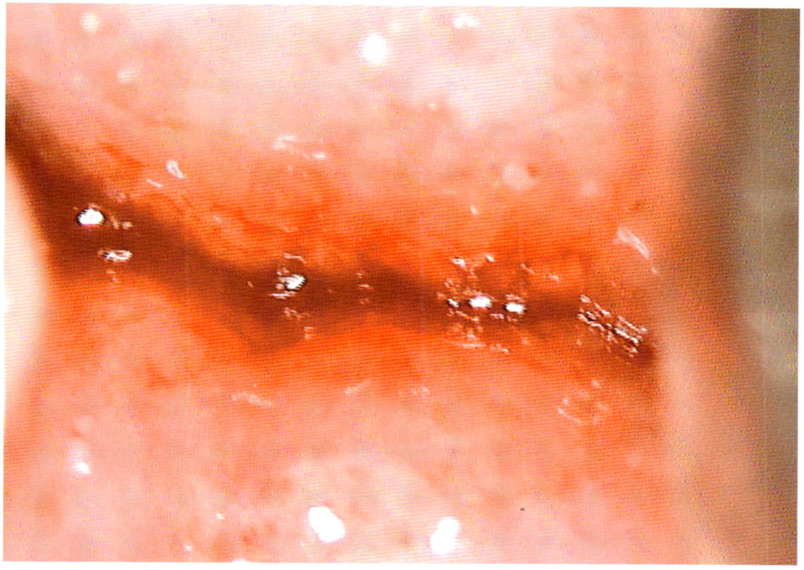

Fig. 44: A 50-year-old: P2L1. Satisfactory colposcopy.

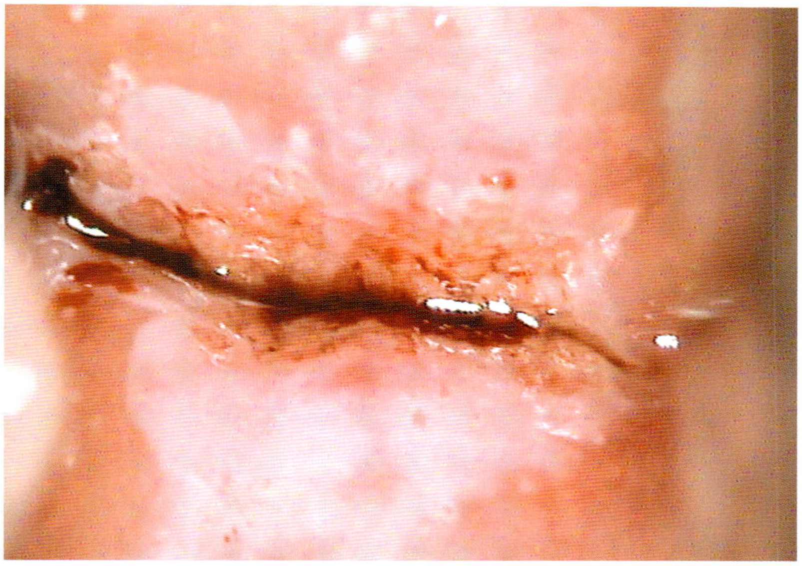

Fig. 45: Grade 1–2 AWA at anterior and posterior lips of cervix.

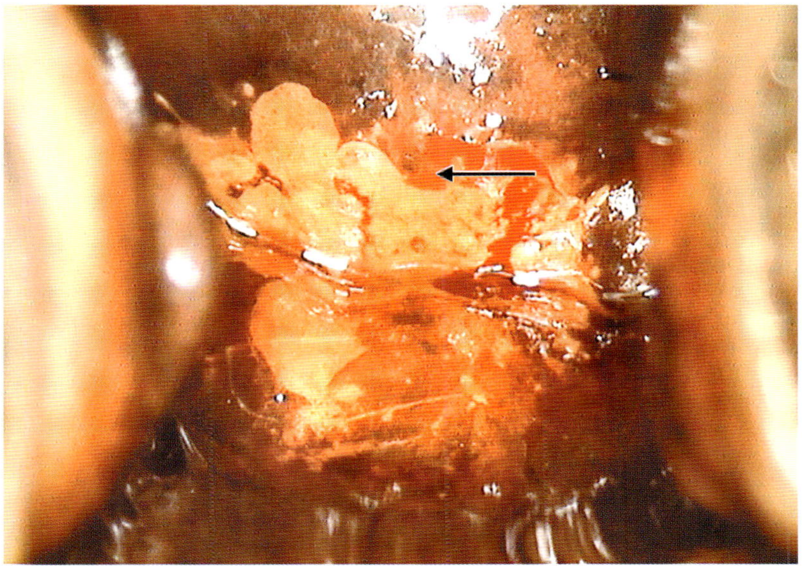

Fig. 46: Mustard yellow area.

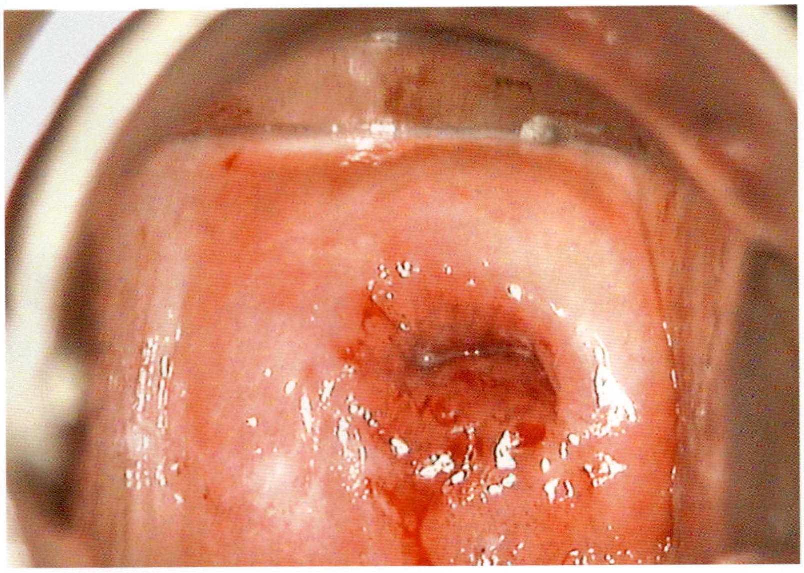

Fig. 47: A 57-year-old: Pap smear—unsatisfactory and blood stained, biopsy cervical intraepithelial neoplasia 3, unsatisfactory colposcopy, fine+ coarse punctation at 6'o clock position and atypical vessels.

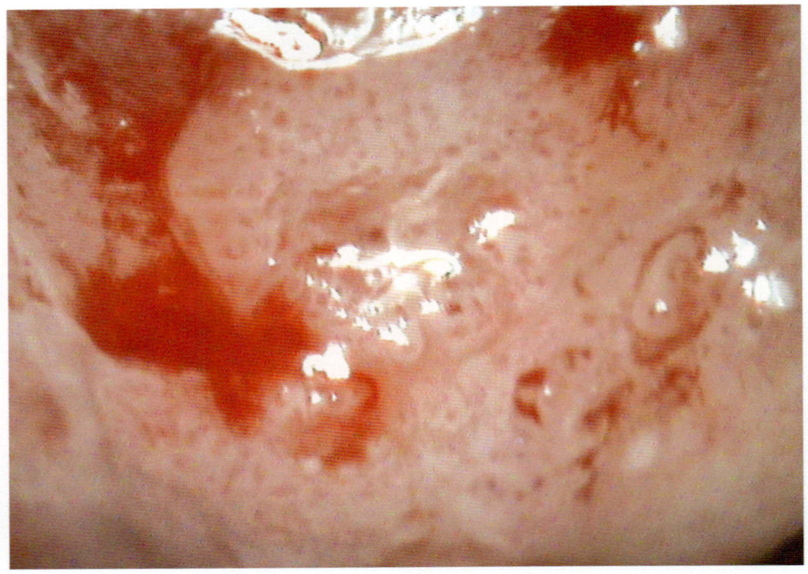

Fig. 49: Comma-shaped abnormal blood vessels.

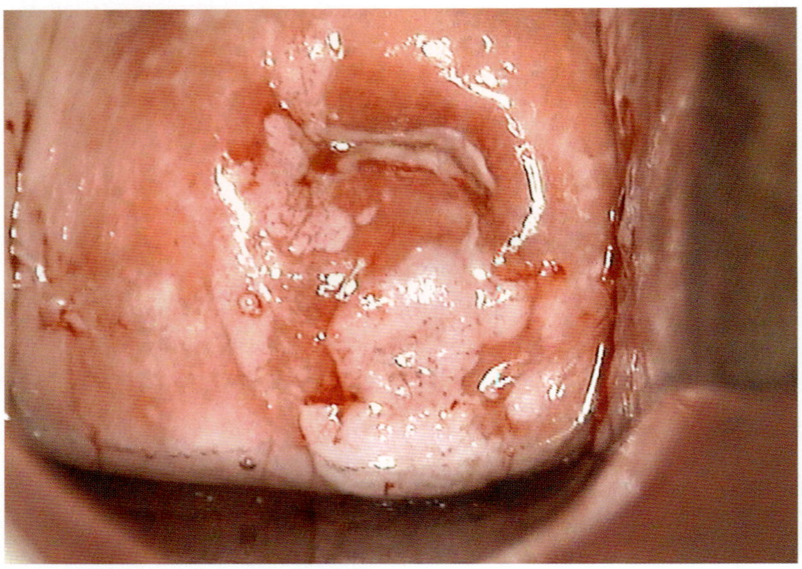

Fig. 48: Dense AWA at 5 to 8 o' clock position, grade I to II AWA at external os.

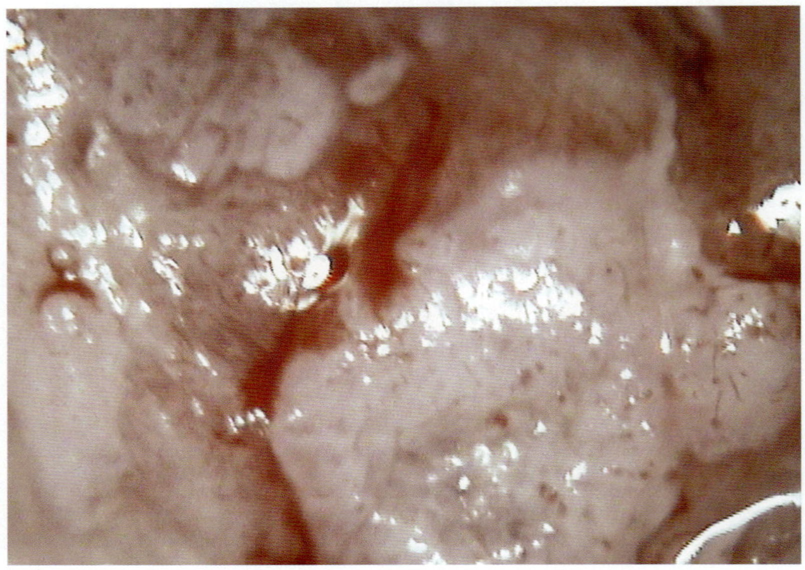

Fig. 50: Comma-shaped abnormal blood vessels in dense AWA.

SUGGESTED READING

1. Canadian Cancer Society. The cervix. [online] Available from: http://www.cancer.ca/en/cancer-information/cancer-type/cervical/cervical-cancer/the-cervix/?region=on#ixzz5QlNygLun. [Last accessed December, 2019].
2. https://www.eurocytology.eu/en/course/934
3. Mayo Clinic. Colposcopy. [online] Available from: https://www.mayoclinic.org/tests-procedures/colposcopy/about/pac-20385036. [Last accessed December, 2019].
4. World Health Organization. An introduction to colposcopy: indications for colposcopy, instrumentation, principles and documentation of results. In: Sellors JW, Sankaranarayanan R, (Eds). Colposcopy and Treatment of Cervical Intraepithelial Neoplasia: A Beginners' Manual. [online] Available from: screening.iarc.fr/colpochap.php?chap=4. [Last accessed December, 2019].
5. The American College of Obstetricians and Gynecologists. Colposcopy. [online] Available from: https://www.acog.org/Patients/FAQs/Colposcopy. [Last accessed December, 2019].
6. World Health Organization. The colposcopic examination step-by-step. In: Sellors JW, Sankaranarayanan R (Eds). Colposcopy and Treatment of Cervical Intraepithelial Neoplasia: A Beginners' Manual. [online] Available from: screening.iarc.fr/colpochap.php?chap=5. [Last accessed December, 2019].

CHAPTER

8

Principles of Electrosurgery

Jnaneshwari TL, Isha Rani

INTRODUCTION

Electrosurgery is an integral part of all surgeries. Laparoscopy with all its advantages depends a lot on electrosurgical instruments to increase the efficacy and the ease of the operating technique. The dependency on the use of electrosurgery has led to lot of research and continuing advancements and improvements in technology to help in making the surgical procedures easy and definitely safer.

BRIEF HISTORY OF EVOLUTION OF ELECTROSURGERY

The uses of heat are known to humans since ancient times. Anecdotes suggesting the use of heated stones for achieving hemostasis and antisepsis are well known. After the discovery of electricity and its uses, the quest for improvisations and its applications in various fields began.

In 1881, Morton found out that a current at 100 Hz frequency can pass through a human without causing burns, the research expanded. In the late 19th century and early 20th century, the use of current or diathermy to treat carcinomatous tumors, vascular lesions, and hemorrhoids became common.[1]

In 1920s, Mr William Bovie, an electrophysicist, designed the first electrosurgical unit (ESU) that delivered current, which could cut and coagulate the targeted tissues, helping surgeons perform complicated surgeries by reducing blood loss and operating times.[2]

This heralded new research and improvements in ESUs in delivery of the current, making them more efficient, compact, affordable, and safe.

PHYSIOLOGY OF ELECTROSURGICAL UNITS

Properties of Electricity

Current is defined as the flow of electrons during a period of time and is measured in amperes and needs the following parameters to flow:

- *Circuit* is the pathway needed for the uninterrupted flow of electrons.
- *Voltage* is the force that pushes the current through the path with resistance and is measured in volts.
- Resistance is the obstacle to the flow of current in the circuit and is measured in ohms (impedance = resistance).

The original source of these electrons is the earth (ground). A complete circuit is needed for the flow of the current and any break in the path will result in stoppage of the flow. To complete the circuit, the electrons must return to ground, i.e. to the source. Hence, all the circuits must be grounded and any grounded object can complete the circuit, thus allowing the electrons to flow to ground and become a path.

Types of Current

Direct current: The current flows in one direction through a circuit.

Alternating current (AC): When AC flows through a circuit, the movement of electrons reverses direction at regular intervals, expressed as cycles per second. This is the type of current used by the ESU.

Any current when it passes through the human body can cause burns and excessive neuromuscular stimulation. Standard appliances used in houses use current at 60 Hz and can cause electrical accidents. But when the frequency of current exceeds 100 Hz, the neuromuscular junctions cannot recognize the passage of current and this prevents burns and electrocution.

The main job of the ESU is to pick the current from the wall socket, amplify it to more than 200 Hz (200,000 cycles/min) and render it to the instrument which touches the tissue and causes the desired effect.

Principles of Electrosurgery in the Operating Theater

With this brief introduction, to facilitate the use of current in surgery, we need a source that produces current, a machine that makes the current safe for use during surgery, a path for the flow of the current and a path for the return of the current into the ground.

- The electrosurgical generator is the source of electron flow and voltage.
- The circuit is composed of a generator, active electrode, patient, and patient return electrode.
- Pathways to ground are numerous including OR table, stirrups, staff members, and equipment
- Patient's tissue provides impedance and heat is produced as electrons overcome the impedance.

The completion of the circuit is essential for the flow of the current. There is a point of entry of the current and exit of the current from the patient's body. The point of entry is called the *active electrode* and the point of return from the body is called *passive electrode.*

The two most common types of electrosurgical circuits, which are usually used in the operating room, are as follows:

1. Bipolar circuit
2. Monopolar circuit.

Bipolar Circuit (Figs. 1A and B)

- Active output and patient return functions are both accomplished at the site of surgery.
- Current path is confined to tissue grasped between forceps tines.
- Patient return electrode need not be applied for bipolar only procedures.

Monopolar Circuit (Figs. 2A and B)

Monopolar is the most commonly used electrosurgical modality. This is due to its versatility and clinical effectiveness.

- The active electrode is in the wound.
- The patient return electrode is attached somewhere else on the patient.
- The current must flow through the patient to the patient return electrode.

TISSUE EFFECTS OF ELECTROSURGERY

When current is applied to the tissue, it gets heated up and the subsequent results are due to the temperature rise, which causes various effects at the cellular level to bring about the desired effects.

The effects on the tissue depends on final temperature and kinetics of temperature increase are as follows:

- <40°C—reversible thermal damage
- 45°C—necrosis
- 80°C—coagulation of proteins
- 100°C—desiccation
- >100°C—carbonization (formation of eschar/charring; **Fig. 3**).

The other factors that affect the electrosurgical technique include:

- *Tissue character:* Fluid filled (wet) tissues improve better conduction.
- *Tip of the electrode:* A sharp tip will definitely get a better effect with low current settings as the delivery point has more concentration of the energy.
- Time of activation of the electrode.
- The waveform used.
- The power settings in the generator.
- Tissue impedance.
- The formation of eschar—prevents passage of current.

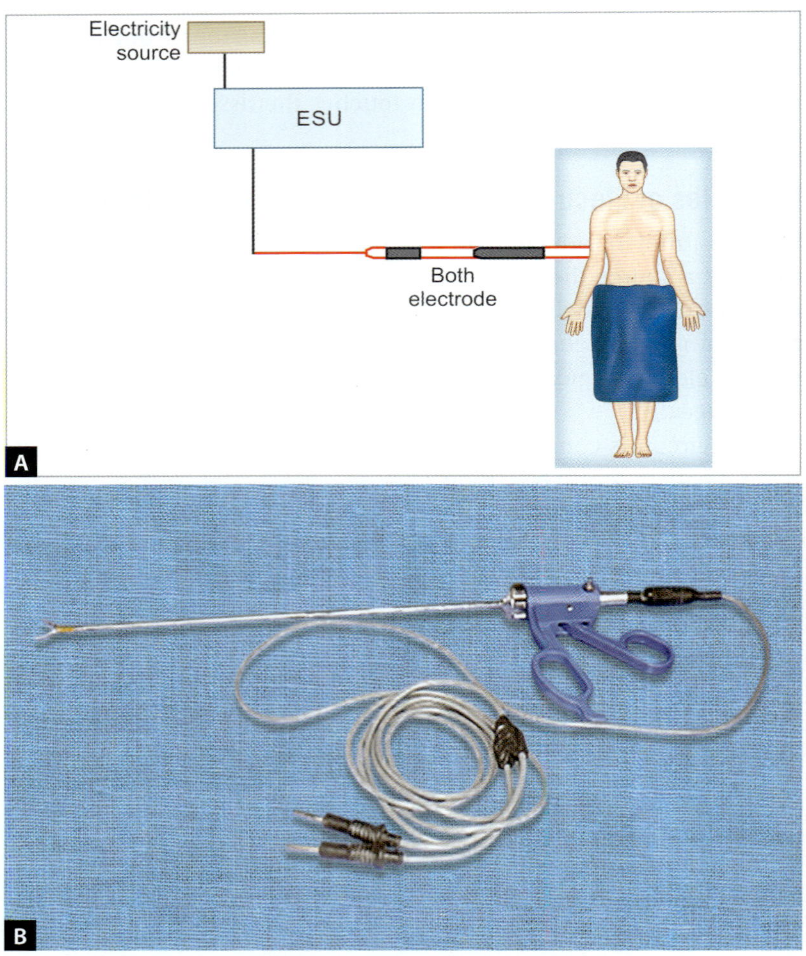

Figs. 1A and B: Bipolar circuit.

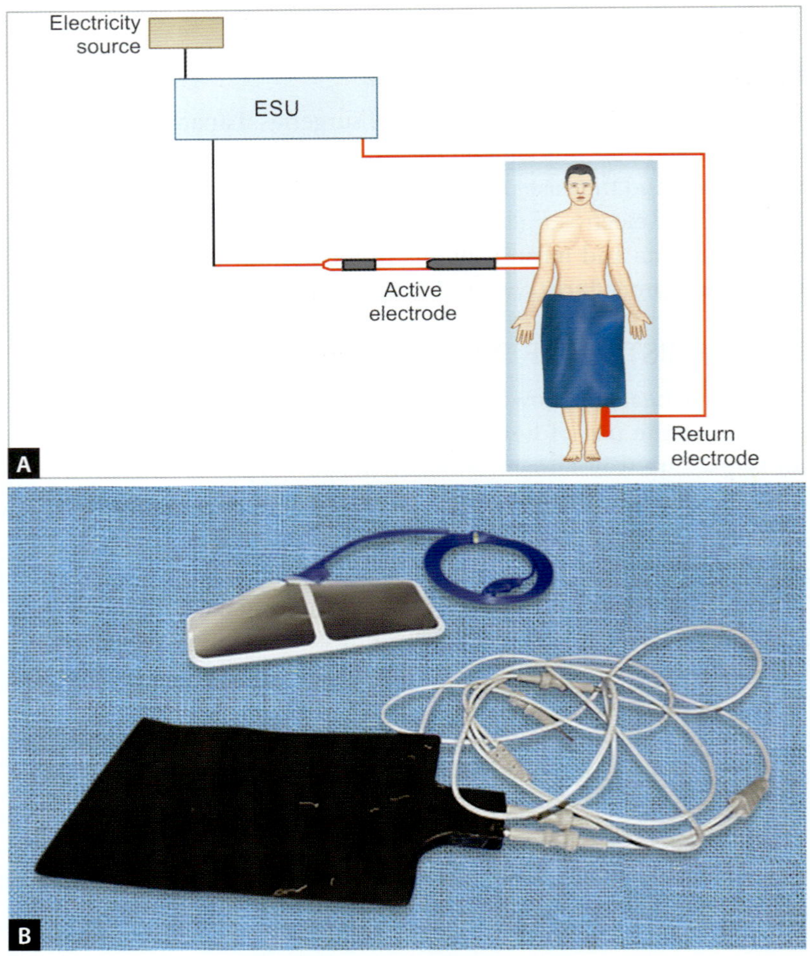

Figs. 2A and B: Monopolar circuit.

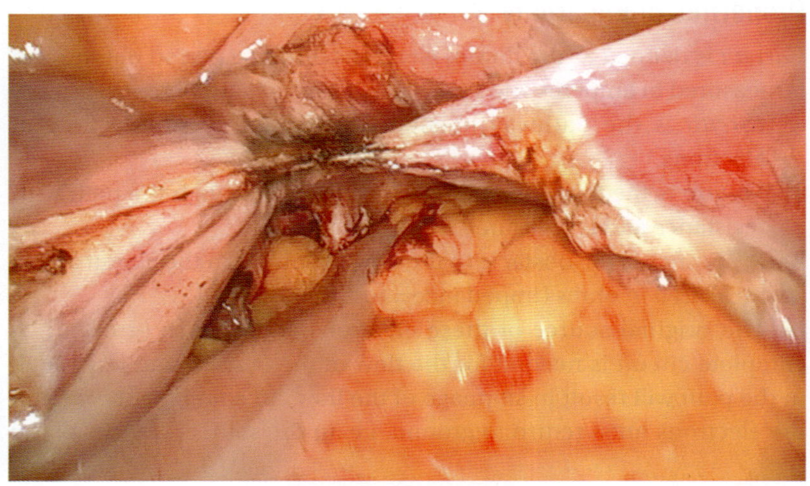

Fig. 3: Eschar/charring.

Basically, two wave forms of current are used, the *cut* and the *coagulation* **(Fig. 4)**.

Cut: This is a continuous waveform with low voltage—the current is delivered at a constant setting whenever the electrode is activated. This produces high heat in a short time and causes desiccation by vaporizing the water content of the cells. This is achieved by keeping the activated electrode a little away from the targeted tissue, so that an arc of electrons passes through the intervening gas and cuts. If the electrode touches the tissue, a coagulum is formed as heat gets directly dispersed to the tissue, rather than a sharp cut.

Coagulation: This is an intermittent wave of current delivered at a high voltage. During the activation of the electrode, only 6% of the time the current gets delivered at a high voltage. Thus, while using this waveform, we use high-voltage current and keep the electrode under activation for longer duration to get the desired effect. This causes a slow delivery of the heat leading to coagulation of proteins forming a coagulum.

The surgeon must know this while using the coagulation waveform as higher voltage is used for longer duration to bring about the desired effect. This definitely will lead to more heat generated, spread of this heat to surrounding tissues (lateral spread; **Fig. 5**), and causing unintended damage to them, leading to complications.

Fulguration uses a spray of current causing a spark in air between the electrode and tissue without touching, causing heat and necrosis.

Desiccation causes deep necrosis due to contact with the tissue.[3]

There are various modifications attempted by the generators in delivering the current by varying the on-off time in the waveform leading to blend waveforms **(Figs. 6A and B)**.

A "blended current" is not a mixture of both cutting and coagulation current, but rather a modification of the duty cycle.

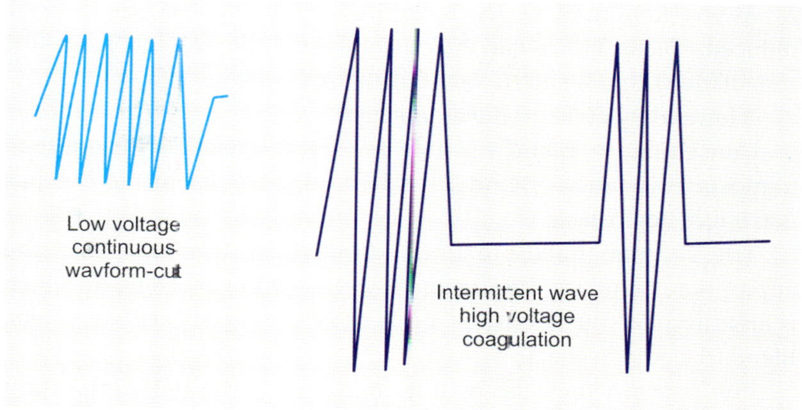

Fig. 4: Monopolar current waves.

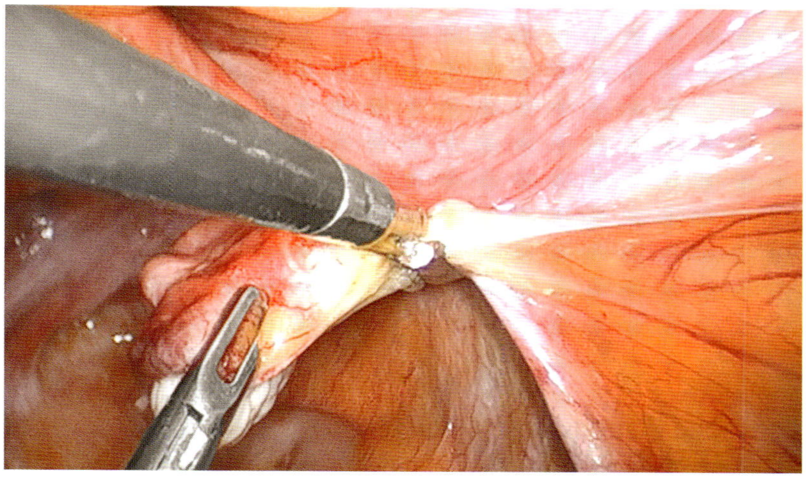

Fig. 5: Lateral spread in bipolar.

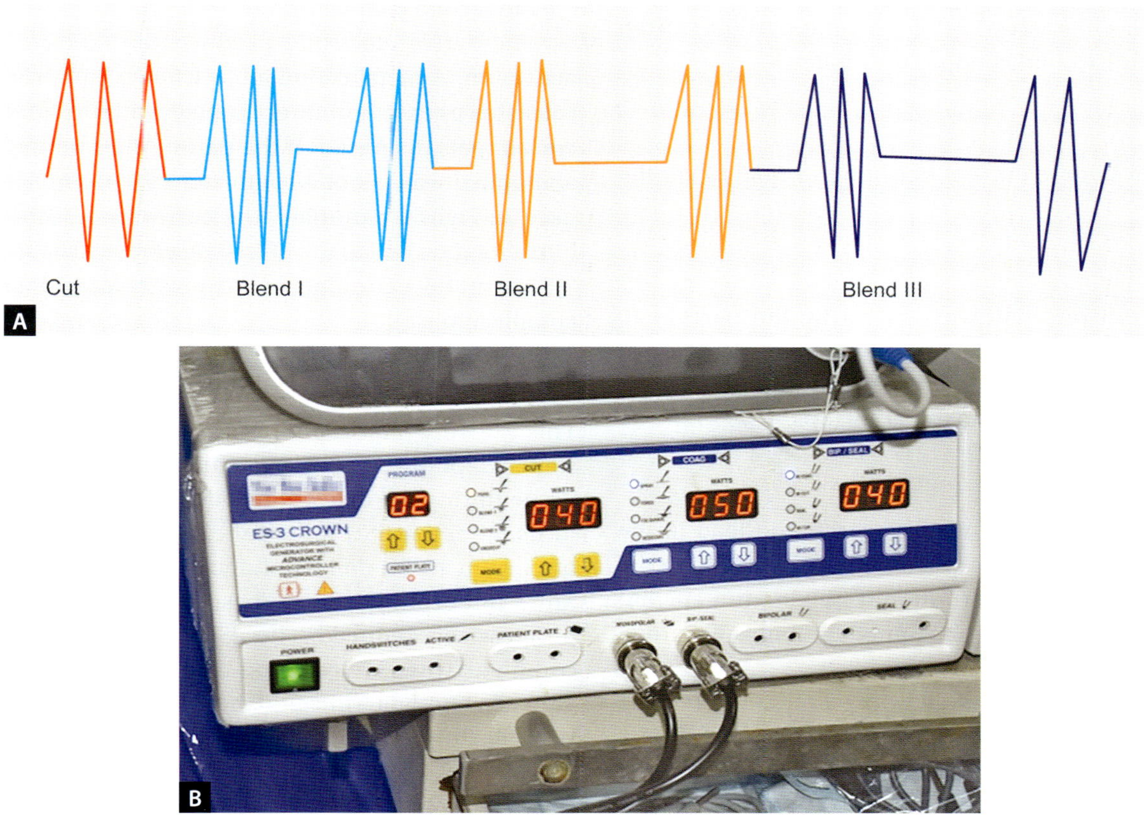

Figs. 6A and B: ESU demonstrating blend waveforms.

As you go from Blend I to Blend III, the duty cycle is progressively reduced—Blend I (80% cut, 20% coagulation), Blend II (60% cut, 40% coagulation), and Blend III (50% cut, 50% coagulation).[3]

A lower duty cycle produces less heat.

Consequently, Blend I is able to vaporize tissue with minimal hemostasis, whereas Blend III is less effective at cutting but has maximum hemostasis

The surgeon needs to understand these modes to use the appropriate blend for the surgery. If you need to cut the tissue which is less vascular you can use Blend 1, but if the tissue is very vascular, Blend III would be ideal.

The rate at which the heat is produced is the most important variable that determines the tissue effect. High heat causes vaporization, while low or slow heat causes formation of a coagulum.

This constant change in tissue characteristics, while doing a surgery needs continuous change in the current dynamics to perform the procedure with precision and minimal lateral tissue damage. This calls for the presence of trained and educated personnel in the operation theater (OT) during the procedure making it dependent.

The newer ESUs have automatic programs, which sense the tissues changing characteristics, and modulate the current flow and output accordingly (Enseal and LigaSure). This eliminates the need for changing the controls on the ESUs and produces only necessary output that is necessary to achieve the desired effect on the tissue or seal a vessel.

EVOLUTION OF ELECTROSURGICAL UNITS

Grounded Electrosurgical Units

Initially, the concept was that ground was the source of all the current and the returning of the electrons to the ground, completing the circuit. But the problems started when the current started returning to the ground through more than one paths. Wherever a conductor was in contact with the patient and the ground, like the metal OT table, stirrups or even the anesthesiologist, the current started seeking alternate pathways. Complications are as follows:

Current Division

Due to multiple pathways, more current became essential to get the job done.

Alternate Site Burns

As there were more than one pathways taken by the current to return to the ground, wherever the current exited from the body at a higher concentration, it resulted in alternate site burns such as ECG (electrocardiogram) electrodes and metal stirrups.

Isolated Electrosurgical Units

The above complications prompted more research and lead to the emergence of isolated ESUs. The system attempted at abolishing the other conductive pathways of the current and making the current compulsorily return to the ground through only the return electrode and not through any other path.

This eliminated the problems of current division and alternate site burns. But the problem of *return electrode burns* remained. If the concentration of the current at the return site was high and concentrated at a small point, deep burns happened.

To prevent *return electrode burns*, systems with *return electrode monitoring* started. The units are made in such a way, that if the return electrode is not applied properly, the circuit gets automatically interrupted.

The return electrode burns can be prevented even by proper application of the return plate.

The active electrode that delivers the current to the tissues usually has a sharp tip at which a high concentration of the current produces the desired effect. The return electrode or the return plate, as it is usually known, is not necessarily a passive electrode, it collects the same amount of current over a larger surface area, which lets the heat get dissipated over a relatively large area and thus does not cause burns at the place of return.

The ideal place of application of the return plate:

- Must not have fat
- Must not be over bony prominences, raw areas, hairy areas, and scar tissue
- Must have a good adhesive and good conductive gel
- Must be placed near the site of surgery—to reduce the distance taken by the current in the patient's body before returning.

Other than return electrode burns, the other complications that can occur in monopolar circuit are as follows:

- *Direct coupling:* If the active electrode by mistake touches another instrument, which is not insulated, it becomes a conductor and if it is resting on the bowel or any other tissue, burns happen.[4]
- *Insulation failure:* Prolonged use of the instrument, over a period of time leads to breaks in the insulation of instrument which leads to current leakage. If such an instrument touches the tissue along the path, it causes burns.[5]
- *Capacitative coupling:* A capacitor creates an electrostatic field between the two conductors and, as a result, a current in one conductor can, through the electrostatic field, induce a current in the second conductor.

The active electrode produces an electric field at the site of activation. A metal cannula has its own electrical field, but does not cause burns as it is in direct contact with the abdominal wall and the current gets dispersed. If the part of the cannula in contact with the abdominal wall is not a conductor of current, like plastic, which was used in Hybrid cannulae, the current does not get dispersed, and burns happen due to the persisting electrical fields.[6]

All metal cannulae or all plastic cannulae do not have this complication.

VESSEL SEALING TECHNOLOGY

This is a very important innovation in bipolar circuit. There is constant adaptation of the current according to the resistance of the tissue during the activation cycle. When the sealer grasps the tissue in its jaws, the ESU judges the tissues and decides on the amount of current to be delivered according to the tissue characteristics. More importantly, as the tissue gets coagulated, the current gets progressively reduced. The ESU also gives a beep when the seal is complete, when we can stop the activation. The seal so established has been found to withstand the rise in the systolic pressures, making it very effective. This technology enables us to seal vessels at a single go. The other most important advantage is very minimal lateral spread of 1 mm, almost comparable to that of ultrasonic scalpel.[7]

- *Enseal:* It uses tissue impedance technology and can cut after the seal is complete **(Fig. 7)**.
- *LigaSure:* It uses the above the technology—fuses collagen and elastin of the vessel walls **(Figs. 8A and B)**.
- *Thunderbeat:* It combines this technology with ultrasonic energy.

Complications happen with the use of electrosurgery, and one of the most important one is due to the *lateral spread* of the generated heat.

Eschar formation: Occurs due to impedence of heat

Monopolar systems have the maximum spread of up to 2 cm at times, if the current of higher voltage for longer times is used.

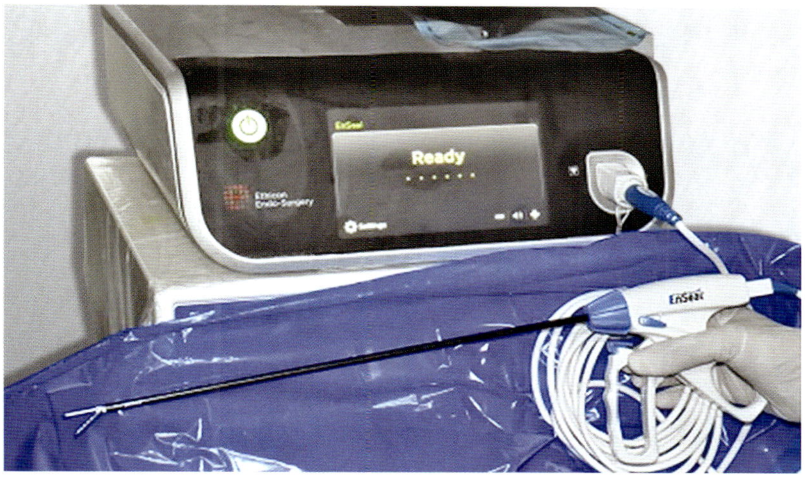

Fig. 7: Enseal tissue sealer.

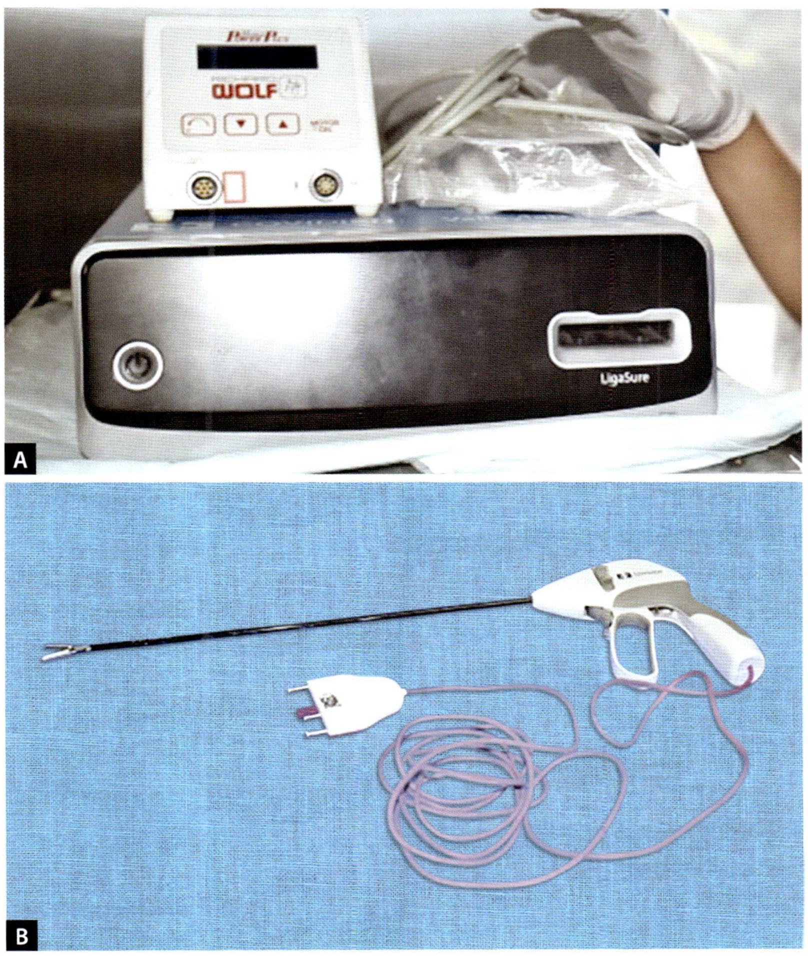

Figs. 8A and B: LigaSure vessel sealer system.

Bipolar systems are relatively safer, with electricity being delivered to only the tissue grasped in the jaws, but can still be up to 1 cm.

Ultrasonic scalpel and tissue impedance systems have the least lateral spread of 1 mm.

SMOKE IN OPERATION THEATER

The burning of tissues releases toxic gases containing benzene-like gases, which are precancerous. It is usually more when monopolar instruments are in use. It is better to suction out the fumes to clear the vision, rather than venting it out from a port, as we will be inhaling it once it leaves the body cavity and enters into the OT atmosphere. Special smoke evacuators have been designed to remove the gases and can be connected to a port vent. There are some filters that are available, which filter out the toxic substances, before releasing it to the OT atmosphere.

We, in this era of minimally invasive surgery, are very lucky, when all the above complications have led to the design of a composite ESU with all the safety mechanisms, leading to the delivery of precise modulating current, eliminating return burns, and mishaps due to coupling.

But still, what we use is electricity which can always cause complication. We are becoming more and more dependent on the energy sources. *We must be aware of all the mechanics and consciously be careful to avoid complications.*

Some tips to avoid complications are as follows:

- Buy an ESU with return electrode monitor (REM) to avoid return burns.
- Use all metal or all plastic cannulae.
- Regularly inspect the insulation of all the instruments to look for "blow holes."
- Use low-voltage waveforms.
- Use brief intermittent activation, instead of continuously keeping on. This gives some time for the surrounding tissues to cool off.
- Apply return plate well.
- Never activate in open circuit.
- Never activate unless the instrument and its whole path is under vision.
- Never activate when some other conductor is nearby which can cause coupling.
- Wet tissues increase the depth of the penetration of the current and constant irrigation while sealing a vessel, improves depth penetration and cools the surrounding tissues, reducing lateral spread.
- Do not activate the current until eschar is formed—it is not necessary to char the tissue to form a seal and it gets stuck to the jaws of the instrument, which leads to avulsion of the adherent tissue and bleeding.
- In case of a bleed from the vessel, do not panic, clear the field by suctioning, irrigate the area for identifying the bleeder, grasp it, if possible, lift it from the surrounding tissues without much traction, and coagulate it. Never blindly reach in the field and activate the current; other tissues may get held and get coagulated. Put an extra port, if necessary for retraction and exposure of the bleeding vessel.
- Use bipolar circuit whenever feasible.
- Never use a new instrument or ESU when you are operating in a new set up or in a difficult case.

- Do not anchor the electrical cords with metal clips.
- Use smoke evacuators to prevent inhalation of toxic precancerous gases.
- Use ESUs which judge tissue impedance and seal big vessels when dealing with vessels beyond 5–7 mm.
- Use vasopressin in dilution, wherever and whenever feasible, which prevents bleeding from small oozers and eliminate the need of coagulation, especially ovarian cystectomy, myomectomy, etc.

Other alternate sources of heat have been developed to overcome the problems due to electric current and have been met with various levels of success. The most successful one is the harmonic scalpel which uses ultrasonic waves to produce heat. The detailed discussion is out of the purview of this chapter, but is a very useful equipment which dissects, coagulates, and cuts with very minimal lateral spread. But large vessels continue to pose a challenge. It is a very useful equipment to have in your armamentarium, especially in dealing with dense adhesions doing oncosurgery.

Radiofrequency ablators and argon beam lasers are other modalities that are being tried for safe implementation.

ELECTROSURGERY IN HYSTEROSCOPY (FIGS. 9 TO 11)

Both monopolar and bipolar circuits are available.

Monopolar energy usage needs glycine as the nonelectrolyte distention medium to prevent ionization, and hence a little unsafe due to distention medium complications. Underwater cutting modality must be available in the ESU for it to work. Current settings are usually above 100 W. The advantage is faster and easier accomplishment of the procedure.

Bipolar electrode uses normal saline as distention medium and is relatively safer. The intended procedure takes more time due to the lesser diameter of the loop.

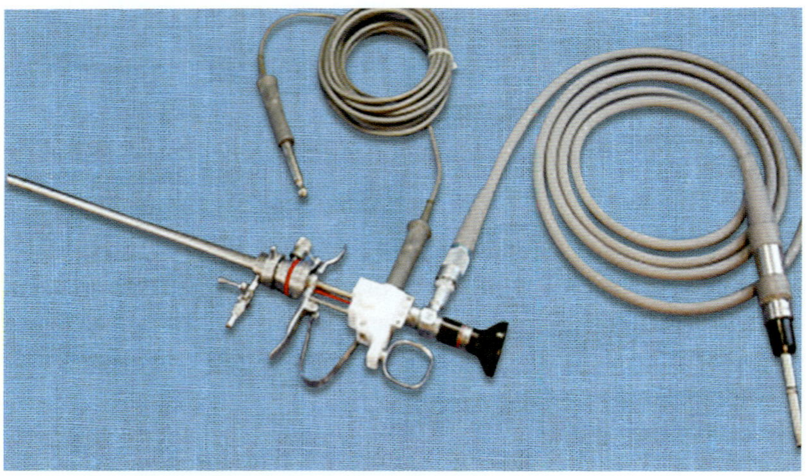

Fig. 9: Resectoscope with electrosurgical connection.

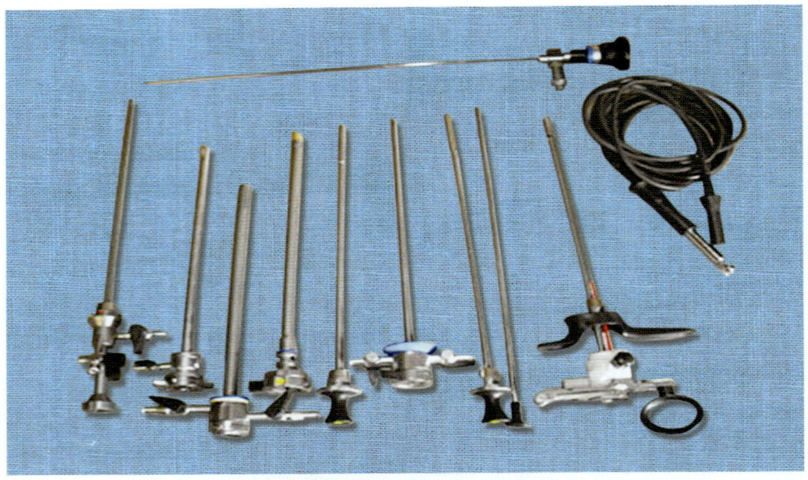

Fig. 10: Parts of resectoscope.

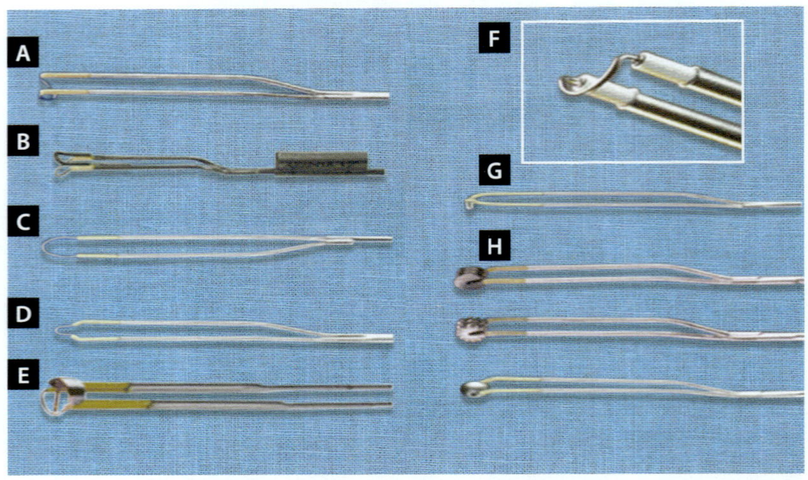

Figs. 11A to H: Different electrodes used in resectoscope.

REFERENCES

1. Glover JL, Bendick PJ, Link WJ. The use of thermal knives in surgery: electrosurgery, lasers, plasma scalpel. Curr Probl Surg. 1978;15(1):1-78.
2. O'Connor JL, Bloom DA. William T. Bovie and electrosurgery. Science Direct Surgery. 1996;119(4):390-6.
3. Wang K, Advincula AP. Current thoughts in electrosurgery. Int J Gynaecol Obstet. 2007;97:245-50.
4. Covidien. Valleylab. Principles of electrosurgery. 1999. pp. 1-23.
5. Vancaillie TG. Active electrode monitoring. How to prevent unintentional thermal injury associated with monopolar electrosurgery at laparoscopy. Surg Endosc. 1998;12(8):1009-12.
6. Odell RC. Electrosurgery: biophysics, safety and efficacy. In: Mann WJ T, Stovall G, (Eds). Mann/Stovall Gynecologic Surgery. New York: Churchill Livingstone; 1996. pp. 55-67.
7. Camran Nezhat, Michael Lewis, Louise P. King. Prevention and management of laparoscopic surgical complications, 3rd edition, Laparoscopic Vessel Sealing Devices.

CHAPTER

9

Lasers in Gynecology

Apoorva Pallam Reddy, Isha Rani

A BRIEF HISTORY OF LASERS IN GYNECOLOGY

With regards to precision tissue removal, laser beams are probably the only upgrade that surgeons have had since the scalpel was invented around 400 BC. The comparison is hardly fair however, as lasers do a lot more than just divide tissue and can be used to treat and cure a number of conditions as well. What is interesting to note, is that while it was none other than Albert Einstein himself who discovered the key mechanisms and concepts behind laser technology back in 1917, it would be almost half a century before "coherent" light would see the light of day. In fact, it was not until May 16th 1960 that the first working laser was developed by Theodore Maiman, using a synthetic ruby as the lasing medium. The first carbon dioxide laser was developed 3 years later in 1963 by Dr C Kumar N Patel from Baramati, India.

Now while carbon dioxide lasers are quite a staple in gynecology today, it took over a decade from initial development to first application in gynecology. This major gap in the timeline was mostly because appropriating depth of penetration was a lot harder than anyone had anticipated at the time. While there were developments like Dr Kaplan increasing wattage and adding an articulated delivery system and Dr Bellina expanding applications by using it to treat infertility, it was not until 1978 that the next breakthrough occurred. This was Anderson and Hartley emphasizing the actual mechanics for the depth of cervical involvement in 1978, following which further refinement proved the CO_2 laser to be a safe, practical and efficacious alternative to treat a number of gynecological conditions **(Fig. 1)**.

DIFFERENT TYPES OF LASERS

Lasers are named according to the medium or "lasing material" that is being activated to produce the beams, so if the medium is a ruby, it is a ruby laser, if the medium is CO_2, it is a CO_2 laser and so on.

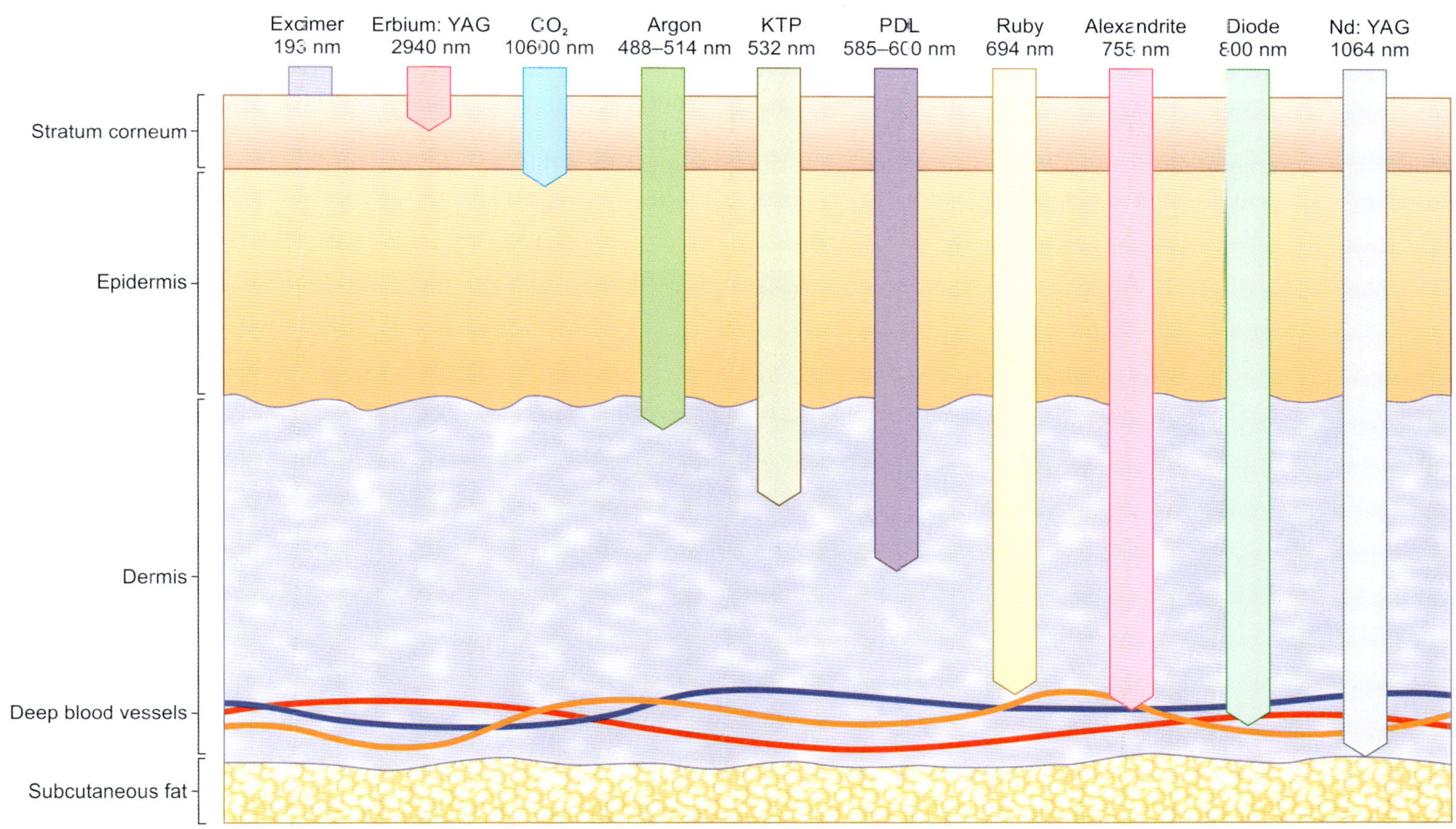

Fig. 1: Depth of penetration by various lasers. In normally epidermis, absorption is usual in the range of 200–10,000 nm and for dermis in the range of 280–1,300. (KTP: potassium titanyl phosphate; Nd:YAG: neodymium:yttrium-aluminum-garnet; PDL: pulsed dye laser)

To make things a bit easier, lasers are also divided into the types of lasing material employed, thereby giving us four subgroups which are: (1) solid state, (2) gas, (3) dye, and (4) semiconductor. The ones we are already familiar with are pretty easy to place; ruby, neodymium:yttrium-aluminum-garnet (Nd:YAG), and KTP (potassium titanyl phosphate) are solid state lasers, while CO_2 and argon are obviously gases. Since only solid state and gas lasers are relevant to gynecology, they are the only two we are going to focus on for now. An interesting observation is due to the specific wavelengths that different mediums emit, each laser produces different colored beams based on the medium. The first laser that used a ruby as medium emitted a pink light.

Solid state lasers are named for employing a lasing material distributed in a solid matrix. What this means is the medium is often a minority ion that makes up about 1% of the solid state host. A good example is the neodymium:yttrium-aluminum-garnet (Nd:YAG) laser, made by doping the medium (Nd) into the host (YAG). Rare earth elements are the most common "dopants", while glass or crystalline materials are the most common hosts. Gas lasers on the other hand, use either a gas or a mixture of gases, confined within a glass tube. Gas lasers are used in applications that require laser light with very high beam quality and long coherence lengths. The most popular example here is the helium–neon laser that uses a mixture of helium and neon (HeNe) and emits a visible red color. Another interesting fact about the color spectrum is both the CO_2 and Nd:YAG lasers emit light that is invisible to the human eye.

MECHANISM OF ACTION (FIGS. 2A AND B)

Now with regards to gynecology in particular, laser action can be broken down into tissue cutting, coagulation and vaporization, or if you really want to get technical: excision, incision, ablation, vaporization and coagulation. The concept behind all the different actions are constant however and works on the principles of targeting chromophores in your skin to promote coagulation. If you are wondering what chromophores are, they are what gives our skin its color and that part of our skin that gets targeted by the lasers. Lucky for us, our chromophores are made mostly of water, while the CO_2 laser has an unusually high absorption by water in our skin. What this means is a minimal amount of radiant exposure is needed for vaporization and neocollagenesis or tissue remodeling, is often achieved with just residual dermal heating.

While it may be difficult to imagine how vaporizing cells in our body can be constructive, what you have to remember is we are strategically promoting collagen production through a wound healing process. Collagen is what we need to remodel connective tissue so it remains firm, while also maintaining elasticity. In fact, the laser action is just the tip of the iceberg when you look at the big picture and a lot of the heavy lifting is actually done by our own bodies. The physiological and functional recovery of the vaginal mucosa can be broken down into three stages, the first is an early thermal effect where you shrink collagen and elastic fibers. This is followed immediately by proliferation, where you have new collagen fibers and epithelial cells and then remodeling that typically occurs 20–40 days after the procedure. Remodeling includes formation of mature collagen fibers, new blood vessels, lubrication and vaginal pH and fauna normalization.

Now while it is important to note that most of the recovery work is done naturally by our bodies, this would never be possible without the mechanism of a laser. This is because unlike the surgical blade that requires a surgeon to press down on the tissue or exert mechanical action, the power density of the focused laser beam already comes with its own mechanical force packed in it. This greatly reduces the margin of error and reduces surrounding tissue damage to almost negligible. This is the reason why laser procedures are so precise, come with almost no downtime whatsoever and do not require you to be hospitalized before or after the procedure. Considering hospital room charges are normally the biggest part of the bill and the fact that zero downtime means you can keep working, comparing lasers and steel blades really does seem a bit unfair **(Fig. 3)**.

APPLICATIONS OF LASERS IN GYNECOLOGY

Here we can breakdown the clinical applications of lasers in gynecology into surgical and nonsurgical procedures. Surgical here refers to minimally invasive surgeries like fiber optic laser laparoscopy, where the surgeon is basically using a laser as a replacement for his scalpel. This means an incision still has to be made to insert

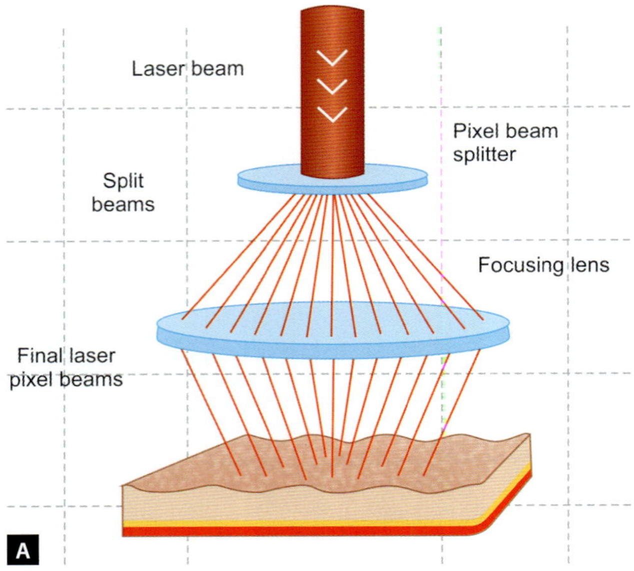

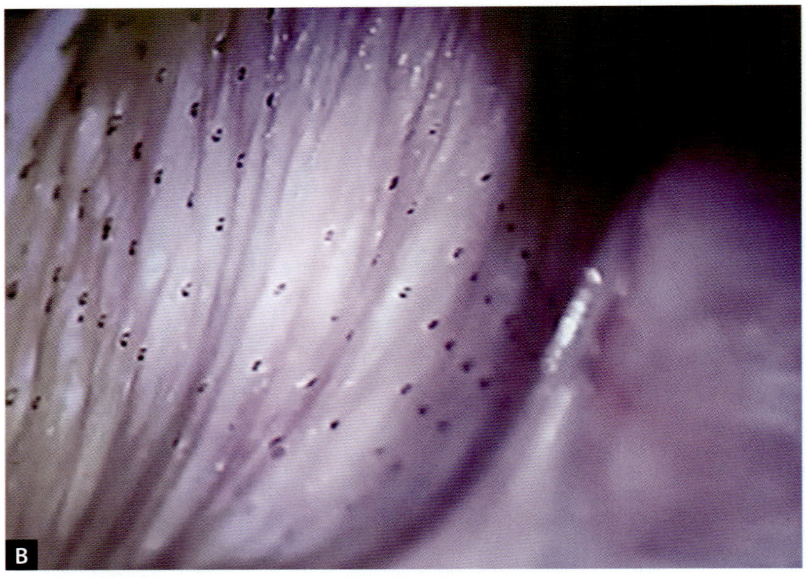

Figs. 2A and B: Mechanism of laser.

the laser and sutures will definitely be required to close that up. Nonsurgical applications however, are procedures where no incisions are made and no sutures are required whatsoever. These are procedures where ablation and vaporization are used strictly to get desired esthetic effects and are typically done without anesthesia of any sort.

While a lot of the applications of lasers in gynecology are surgical and involve removing fibroids and life-threatening tumors, the good news is there are a number of conditions that are dealt with nonsurgically as well. These include treatments for stress urinary incontinence (SUI), vulvodynia, vulvar vestibulitis syndrome, and genitourinary syndrome of menopause (GSM) among others. While some of these conditions cause localized pain and discomfort, almost all of them cause some level of psychological trauma, sexual dysfunction and generally a lower quality of life. Dealing with these issues without going under the knife would probably be impossible in the past, but today thanks to the laser technology, a "surgery-free" cure is very much a possibility.

In addition to being used to help cure gynecological conditions, lasers are also being used for pure esthetic and quality of life improvements as well. These esthetic procedures are noninvasive, involve zero downtime and also help cure conditions like dryness, vaginal laxity, and urinary incontinence **(Figs. 4A and B)**. Vaginal rejuvenation **(Figs. 5A to C)**is one of the most popular esthetic procedures and is often referred to as vaginoplasty. More recently, vaginoplasty procedures have also been marketed as "designer vagina" procedures, inferring patients can customize their procedures (and results) considerably. Other popular esthetic procedures include bleaching, nonsurgical vaginal tightening, wart removal, and treatment for dryness.

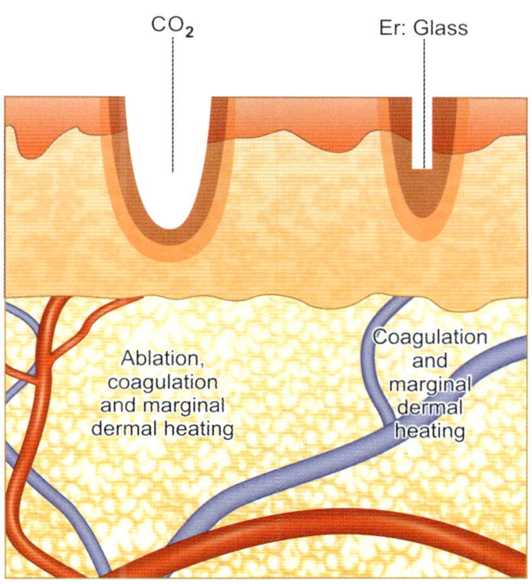

Fig. 3: Mechanism of laser effect.

PREPROCEDURE CHECKLIST

Not unlike regular surgery where you have a bunch of tests to make sure you are fit and healthy and not allergic to any of the medication, laser procedures have some considerations as well. One absolute must is having a detailed discussion if the desired results are indeed achievable. A negative pregnancy test and Pap smear are also prerequisites to the procedure, among other things. Those include making sure you are not on any medication that causes photosensitivity, you do not have any active vaginal or urinary tract infections, you are not undergoing chronic corticosteroid therapy and you do not have herpes or any oncological pathologies. It is also advisable to not smoke as much as possible before and after the procedure as smoking slows down the wound healing process substantially.

Caution to be Exercised during the Procedure

Safety needs to be the number one priority while handling lasers, for both patients and staff alike. It is important that all personnel present in the treatment area wear appropriate protection, which is OD > 7 for the CO_2 wavelength. Headpieces need to be lubricated without covering the laser's energy window. The lubrication has to be oil based and not water based to make sure it does not affect the efficacy of laser. The probe covers should be single-use, hygienic, lubricated and of the right size. The treatment area also needs to be periodically cleansed with gauze to remove any excessive mucus. Saline, Betadine or any water-based solutions should not be used to clean the vaginal area. Additionally, always ensure that the laser safety shutter is in the closed position, an appropriate alert appears on screen if it is not so, pay attention to alerts, as well as the laser temperature indicator.

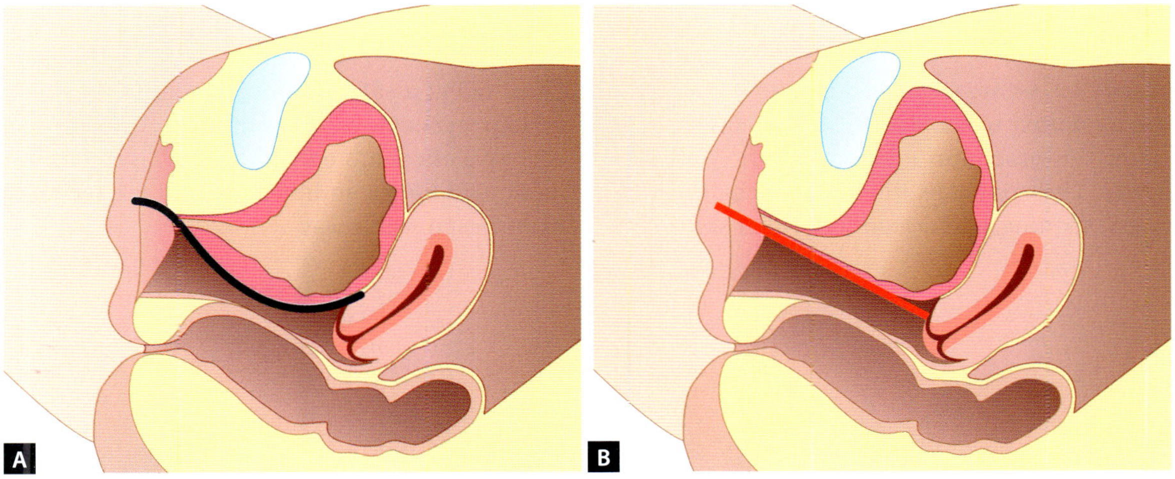

Figs. 4A and B: Vaginal canal (A) before and (B) after laser for stress urinary incontinence (SUI).

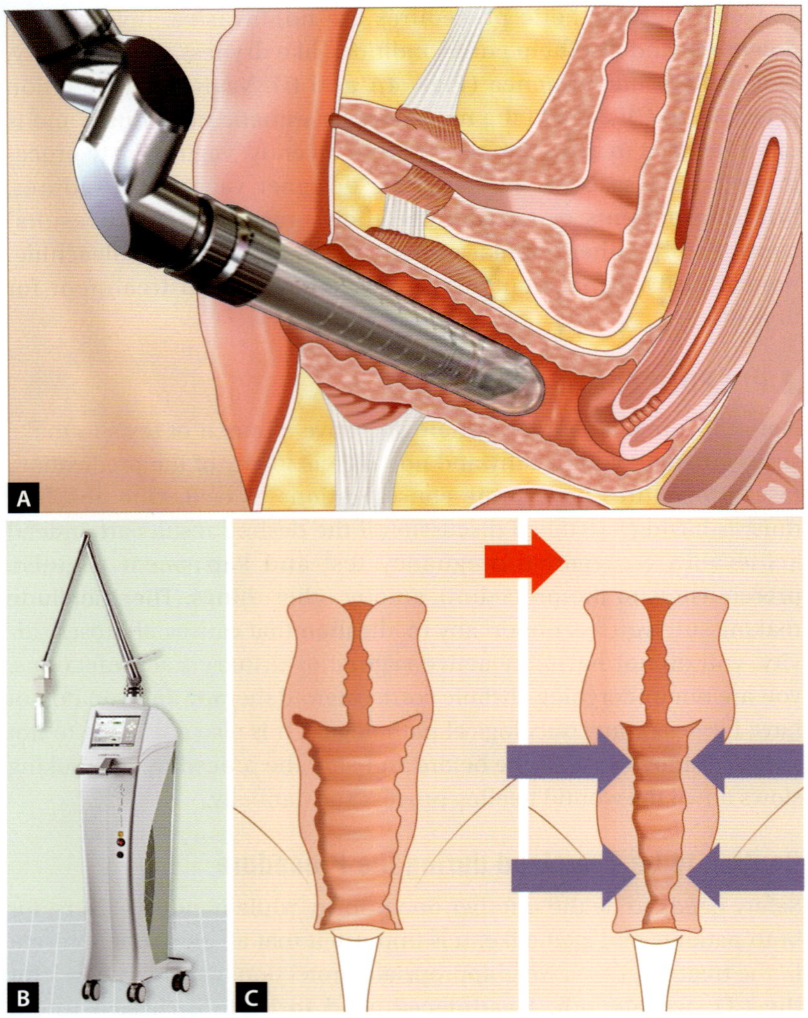

Figs. 4A to C: Steps of laser use for vaginal rejuvenation.

POSTPROCEDURE CARE

The wound healing process is completely natural and no special medication or treatment is required. A couple of things that need to be avoided for 3 days postprocedure however, are sexual intercourse and tampons, following which no extra care or precautions are necessary. While results may be visible immediately after the procedure, it is best to assess results after the wound-healing process is complete, which is typically a 3–6-month period. Follow-up maintenance sessions are also advisable to further enhance results.

SIDE EFFECTS

Most of the energy-based devices are safe when operated by trained professional. There are a number of short-term side effects that can occur immediately after the procedure, depending on your skin type and sensitivity levels. These include, itching, redness, swelling, inflammation, tenderness, spotting, and discomfort. Other short-term reactions may include burning upon urination, mild vaginal bleeding, pink or brown vaginal discharge, and a mild-to-profuse watery vaginal discharge. A major concern for patients and clinician alike is the carcinogenic potential of energy-based devices. It should be kept in mind that most energy based do not work at the level of epithelium and work at connective tissue level. Even CO_2 gas lasers are nonionizing and do not carry any longer term carcinogenic risk.

COST OF PROCEDURE

The cost of the machines ranges from 35 lacs to 50 lacs depending on the specifications. Apart from the machine cost, most devices have a disposable probe cover or handle piece that is used for individual patient. The procedure cost for 3–4 sessions can be determined keeping these factors in mind. In Western countries the cost can range from 3000$ to 4000$ for four sessions. In India, the cost ranges from 600$ to 1000$ for four sessions.

RESEARCH AVAILABLE

The evidence supporting the role of energy-based devices for gynecological conditions is on the rise.

There are a number of clinical studies that prove the effectiveness of CO_2 lasers in gynecology, one of which is the evaluation of CO_2 laser therapy on vulvovaginal atrophy in oncological patients. The study was conducted by Dr Isabella Pagano and colleagues on 33 postmenopausal patients with vaginal atrophy or SUI. Each patient underwent three vaginal CO_2 laser treatment sessions in 1 month intervals. Ninety percent of the patients were satisfied with the procedure and reported significant improvements in their quality of life as well as reduction in frequency and severity of SUI symptoms. Additionally, no adverse events were reported throughout the study and post-histology treatment samples showed significant restoration of epithelial and subepithelial structures.

Another study worth mentioning is the one conducted by Dr Ksenija S Martinec from Slovenia on the treatment of urinary incontinence with the CO_2 laser. What is interesting about this study is not only it is on a rather large study group of 94 patients, but it also includes extensive documentation recorded over a 9-month follow-up period. While the results indicate over 25% of the patients reported complete resolutions, 82% of patients said it had improved their quality of life. Additionally, with regards to urine leakage, the original 35% that reported leakage at least once a day, postprocedure were reporting an average of 1–3 episodes a week.

CONCLUSION

Laser offers a safe, noninvasive and effective means for managing various gynecological conditions. Any new technology introduced is always encountered with a lot of skepticism. Embracing advancement with better understanding of the technology helps us using it in the best possible way.

CHAPTER

10

Laparoscopic Suturing

Mala Raj, Minal Kumbhalwar

INTRODUCTION

Laparoscopic suturing has evolved a long way, ever since Kurt Semm in 1970 reported using endoloops for mobile pedicles. Reich and Clarke introduced technique to use curved needle and knot pushes for placing extracorporeal knots. However, complex surgeries like myomectomy, pelvic floor surgeries and tubal recanalization required prolonged suturing which was difficult with extracorporeal suture technique, also need of expertise in intracorporeal suturing was felt. To be skilled in laparoscopic endosuturing one needs to adapt to the laparoscopic procedures and get training for adequate depth perception, constant practice, hand-eye coordination, direct tactile sensation, and patience too. The concept of ipsilateral suturing pioneered by Dr Charles H Koh is a boon to laparoscopy.

For successful intracorporeal suturing, it is mandatory to have the right set of instruments like two laparoscopic needle holders of which one could be toothed, so that it could be utilized to suture with left hand as well and also to grasp the tissues while suturing. The choice of needle holder is again important. There are two types of needle holder. One is self-righting holder with fixed lock mechanism, but only limitation is that we cannot grasp the suture with this holder because it will damage suture material and also we cannot take bites in any direction. The second type of needle holder is the articulating jaw needle holder. The main advantage of this is that it helps in angling the needle according to stitch and for manipulating the suture. Ideally while holding the needle holder, it should be held at an angle greater than 90° and the insertion angle on to the target tissues should be 80–100°. The needle should be held at the junction of anterior two-thirds and posterior one-third from tip of the needle to get the ideal smiley position. Adjusting the needle to get this position could be challenging in the initial days. The needle can be repositioned by holding it to and fro in between the needle holder and grasper.

Another method for repositioning the needle is to place the needle on some solid tissue, and to release the grip, which is followed by moving the needle holder until correct alignment is reached. Third method of holding the needle is by hanging the needle by needle holder vertically at right angle to patient's body with the concavity facing toward the pelvis.

The right needle holder can easily grasp the needle at the junction of anterior two-thirds and posterior one-third and the needle is turned horizontally in such a way that the concavity of the needle faces anterior abdominal wall in the "smiley position **(Fig. 32)**" or "half-moon position" and convexity of the needle facing down. This type of suturing is called *vertical zone suturing* **(Fig. 13)**, which means the needle passes from below upward with the needle holder in horizontal direction and the needle in the vertical alignment passing across tissues from below upward. Once correct alignment is achieved, suturing can be started. The needle should be held perpendicular to the shaft of the instrument and the needle should be perpendicular to the suture line. The entrance and exit bite has to be very carefully planned. The site and amount of tissue to be taken is determined based on the function of the organ and reconstruction goal. The assisting grasper should be 60–90° and 6–7 inches apart to avoid a "chopstick effect".[1] Once a good bite is taken, the first knot is made which is a "surgeon's square knot". With the right hand needle holder, a "C-loop" is form and the left hand needle holder enters it from down and two throws put and free tail end of the sutures is grasped. After securely tied, another throw is made which is reinforced by pulling in opposite direction. The direction of pull is important to tighten the knot, and then the sutures are cut.

For continuous suturing, the bites on the tissues are taken in a similar manner and needle is regrasped as it appears from the upper end without dropping it and putting repeated bites. This saves quite a lot of time and energy. The continuous suture is closed by holding the needle with the right holder in smiley position and the left needle holder comes from below end and two throws are taken grasping free end and surgeon knot is secured. This is reinforced by putting one more throw.

Once suturing is complete, the needle along with remaining suture removed out of the abdomen by removing lower accessory 5 mm trocar under vision, to avoid dragging on soft tissue. Basically, intracorporeal suturing is of two types—(1) ipsilateral suturing and (2) contralateral suturing. Ipsilateral suturing is better than contralateral as it is more accurate, ergonomically less tedious and quite physiological. Ipsilateral suturing is surgical technique where the hands operate in normal resting position allowing surgeon to be at ease and precision.

For effective and comfortable suturing, proper port placement is mandatory. The lower accessory port is placed 1–2 cm above anterior superior iliac spine and the second accessory port is placed on the midclavicular line 4–6 cm from the first accessory port to avoid chopstick effect inside the abdomen.

INTRODUCTION OF NEEDLE INTO THE PERITONEAL CAVITY

Introduction of needle inside the peritoneal cavity can be done by either Reich technique or by Backloading technique.

In Reich technique, the suture is held in the left lower needle holder about 2 cm from needle hub, and inserted into the peritoneal cavity. In Backloading technique, remove the left lower 5 mm trocar and backload the needle on a 5 mm valve less trocar which is held on a needle holder. Then introduce the needle holder along with the trocar into the peritoneal cavity and pull the suture inside.

SUTURE MATERIAL

The length of suture material and type of suture material determines good suturing. Length of suture to be taken depends on the length of the incision. It is difficult to suture with too long or too short suture materials. For a single stitch, thread should be approximately 14 cm long. A good rule of thumb for running suture is to allow 14 cm for the first stitch and about 2–3 cm for each additional stitch. A suture incision ratio of 9:1 is best for long suture line and 10:1 for short suture line.[2] However, the most import aspect in suturing is choosing the ideal suture material. The choice of suture material is based on the following criteria like:

- Duration needed for the sutured tissue requiring exogenous support.
- Characteristics and biochemical properties of the suture materials.

Types of Suture Material

Sutures can be smooth braided (twisted) or barbed based on the strand's surface texture. Smooth sutures are monofilament strands with a surface that is directionally and topographically uniform. Braided sutures combine thinner suture filaments together to create a multifilament strand that is directionally uniform but topographically varied in a weaved configuration. Barbed sutures are smooth monofilament strands that is directionally uniform but topographically in a weaved configuration.

From a production perspective, there are two methods of barbed suture manufacturing. The first method involves cutting into the shaft of a strand of smooth suture with a blade of some fashion.[3] The second method involves press-forming or compound profile punching in which suture elements protrude from an intact core and serve as the barbs by which tissue holding is achieved.[4,5] Regardless of the difference in design or production, barbed sutures are designed to easily pass through tissues in one direction and provide resistance to backward migration. Barbed sutures do not require knots to anchor the tissues. Elimination of knots has many potential advantages, ensuring adequate wound closure strength, less foreign body reaction and inflammation.

Strength of Wound

Vakil et al. in 2017 tested the hypothesis that wound closure using No. 2 barbed polydioxanone suture would have equivalent closure integrity to No. 1 polyglactin 910 interrupted sutures in arthrotomy closures on cadaveric knees.[6] In support of their hypothesis, they found that after 2,000 flexion cycles, the interrupted suture or continuous barbed suture did not had a single failure. In the same trial, they also sought to determine if cutting the barbed suture line would lead to failure than interrupted suture closures. To test this, the integrity of the wounds was further observed after cutting sequential throws stitches and continuing cyclical testing.

It was observed that while smooth and barbed sutures closures serviced first throw cutting, the barbed suture fared much better when multiple cuts were made. Once wound closed with interrupted suture sustained three cuts, they all failed, while the barbed sutures sustained up to seven cuts. So, it was concluded that wounds closed with barbed sutures are at least as strong as those closed with interrupted sutures and are likely better to maintain tissue tension even when portion of suture line fail.

Inflammation and Wound Healing

Given the topographic variation in the surface that is created by the barbs, there is theoretical concern for increased adhesion formation induced by the adherence of nontarget tissues to the exposed barbs as well as increase in inflammation. Similar to that seen with braided sutures as compared with smooth sutures.

Einarsson et al. studied the adhesion formation and investigated the effect of barbed sutures versus smooth suture on formation of adhesion after closure of ovine myometrium.[7] In this animal study, a 5 cm myometrial defect was made in each horn of a bicornuate uterus of sheep. One horn was then closed with 2-0 polyglactin 910 and another horn with barbed polydioxanone with each sheep acting as her own control. Three months later, the animals were sacrificed; autopsy was performed to grossly analyze adhesion formation. It was found that adhesion formation was not different between the two groups. The majority of the animals that formed adhesions did so at both horns. However, more studies are clearly needed before any final conclusion regarding inflammation and wound healing can be made.

Efficiency of Sutures

Another important characteristic of any suture material is the efficiency. Efficiency is important to minimize procedure times, affecting with infections and blood loss. In various in vivo studies, closure times with barbed sutures were found significantly faster. A randomized controlled study by Ting et al. demonstrated 32% faster. Closure times when using barbed suture (average 9.3 minutes) compared with closures using knotted suture (average 13.6 minutes), during primary total hip and knee arthroplasties.[8]

FOREIGN BODIES EFFECT ON WOUND HEALING

The presence of any foreign body like suture material produces inflammatory tissue responses, which would reduce cellular mechanism against infection, interfere with the proliferative phase of wound healing and weaken the strength of the wound due to excessive scar tissue formation.[9] Generally, some inflammatory response is physiologically necessary after surgical trauma. However, in optimum circumstances without the presence of foreign bodies or infection, these reactions subside within a week. However, some degree of an inflammatory reaction will persist as long as the foreign body remains within the tissue. So, the degree of inflammatory response and subsequent integrity of the scar ultimately depends on the chemical nature and physical characteristics of the suture materials used.

TENSION ON SUTURE LINE IN WOUND HEALING

Tension on suture line influences wound healing. Both loose reapproximation and excessive tension can reduce wound strength. While loose reapproximation may not allow the wound to appropriately interact to create (fibroblast, bridging) excessive tension can cause localized hypoxia, edema and necrosis. These effects both reduce fibroblast proliferation and yield excessive tissue overlap both of which lead to reduced strength in wound healing.[10]

Wound tension within a suture loop is affected by several factors like type and volume (bite) of tissue including the suture size, diameter, and the amount of force applied while knotting. It is found that tissues with lower collagen content appear more susceptible to injury due to suture tension than collagenized tissues.[11]

KNOTS ON WOUND HEALING

The surgical knots are now simply considered as necessary evil, which is only used to anchor smooth sutures and produces a lot of untoward effects, thereby weakening the wound. First, the knot is the weakest portion of any suture line and the second weakest point is the portion immediately adjacent to the knot. This is because the knot causes stretching of the molecular bond, which reduces the tensile strength.[12] The tensile strength of the suture has been reported to be reduced from 35% to 95% depending on the suture material used[13] and suture breakage occurred immediately adjacent to the knot 74% of the time.[14] Empirically, the knot creates an uneven distribution of tension across the wound with higher tension burden placed on the knots, where the suture line is at its weakest. Secondly, knot volume is directly related to grade of inflammatory reaction and it produces the highest density of foreign body reaction.[15] So, eliminating the knot size or eliminating knots altogether should be beneficial as long as the wound holding strength of suture line is not compromised.

CLINICAL APPLICATION OF LAPAROSCOPIC SUTURING

Suturing in Myomectomy (Figs. 1 to 11 and 26, 27, 33, 34)

Laparoscopic suturing of myoma is as good as laparotomy suturing in experienced hands with advance suturing skills. However, the key factor during laparoscopic suturing is to avoid dead space and avoid energy sources on the uterus, to maintain the integrity of the scar. The myometrial vascularity after laparoscopic myomectomy using continuous and interrupted sutures was analyzed using contrast-enhanced magnetic reasonable imaging. It was concluded that after 3 months of surgery, a vascularity index in continuous sutures group was higher than of single interrupted sutures group stating that continuous suturing leads to a poorer vascular recovery of the myometrium.[16]

In our center, if the dead space is more, we suture in three layers. Initial layer in figure of eight interrupted, second layer is continuous without locking and third layer is for the serosa, which is baseball stitch. The main advantage of "Baseball" **(Figs. 8A and B, 9, 25, 28)** suture technique is it avoids exposing the raw area and thereby prevents adhesion formation.

Suturing in Total Laparoscopic Hysterectomy (Figs. 14 to 16)

Suturing the vault in total laparoscopic hysterectomy (TLH), one needs to pay attention to suturing of vaginal angles. Monofilament delayed absorbable suture is used to suture the vaginal angles which involves the uterosacral angle and compresses the smaller vessels medial to the uterine pedicle to increase perfect hemostasis. This is usually done as an extracorporeal stitch and can be used to give traction as well or continuous intracorporeal stitch. The vaginal cuff is sutured in a transverse manner, starting at the distal angle, incorporating the vaginal mucosa, pubocervical as well as rectovaginal fascia. Suturing can be continuous running suture or interrupted "figure of eight" sutures or barbed suture. To prevent necrosis suture locking **(Figs. 29, 30, 37)** should be avoided and the sutures need to be placed approximately 1 cm apart.

Suturing the Bladder

Bladder heals very well when sutured laparoscopically, if care is taken while suturing by avoiding necrosis of the tissues. We use Vicryl 3-0 curved, round body needle or barbed sutures to suture the bladder. One needs to identify the trigone and ureteric orifices before starting the suture.

Suturing the Bowel

Repair of bowel is done with Vicryl 3-0 on a small curved needle. It is sutured in two layers. The most important aspect is tension-free suture line. The second layer reinforces the first layer and as it is sutured in continuous pattern, it is closed at the end by putting a square knot. After repair of large intestine, an underwater check for tight closure is done by introducing air through a Foley catheter inserted in the rectum. If air bubbles appear from the suture site, more reinforcing sutures are needed.

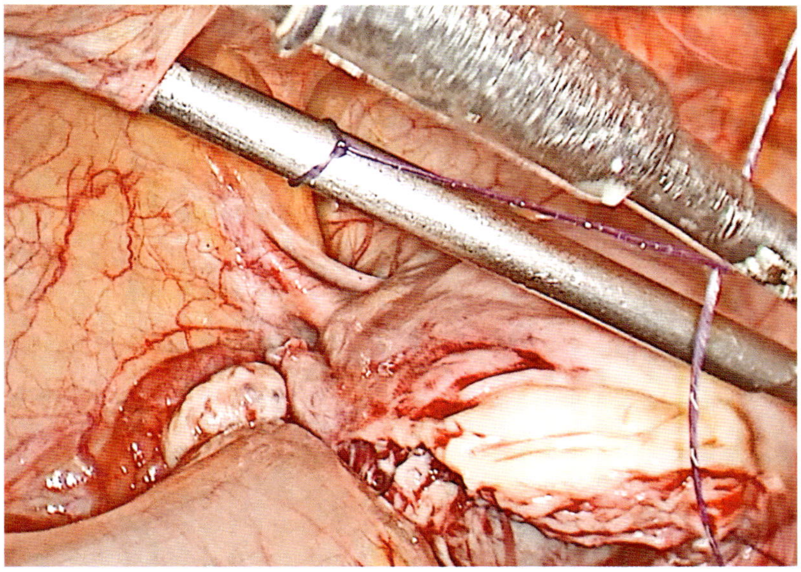

Fig. 1: Loop of barbed suture drawn inside.

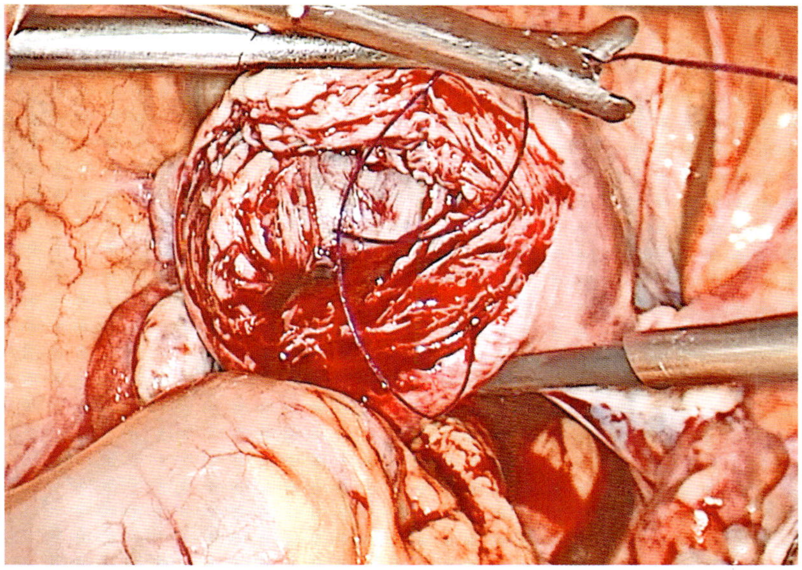

Fig. 2: Loop of barbed suture.

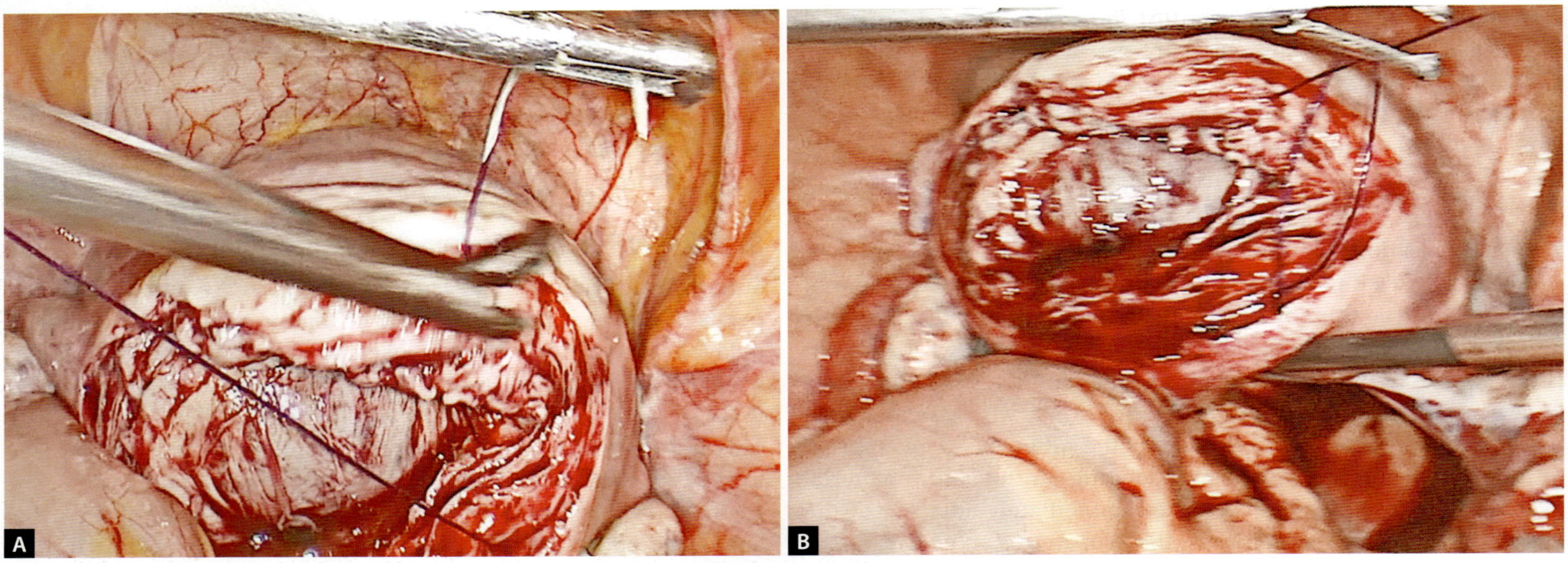

Figs. 3A and B: Suturing the upper flap.

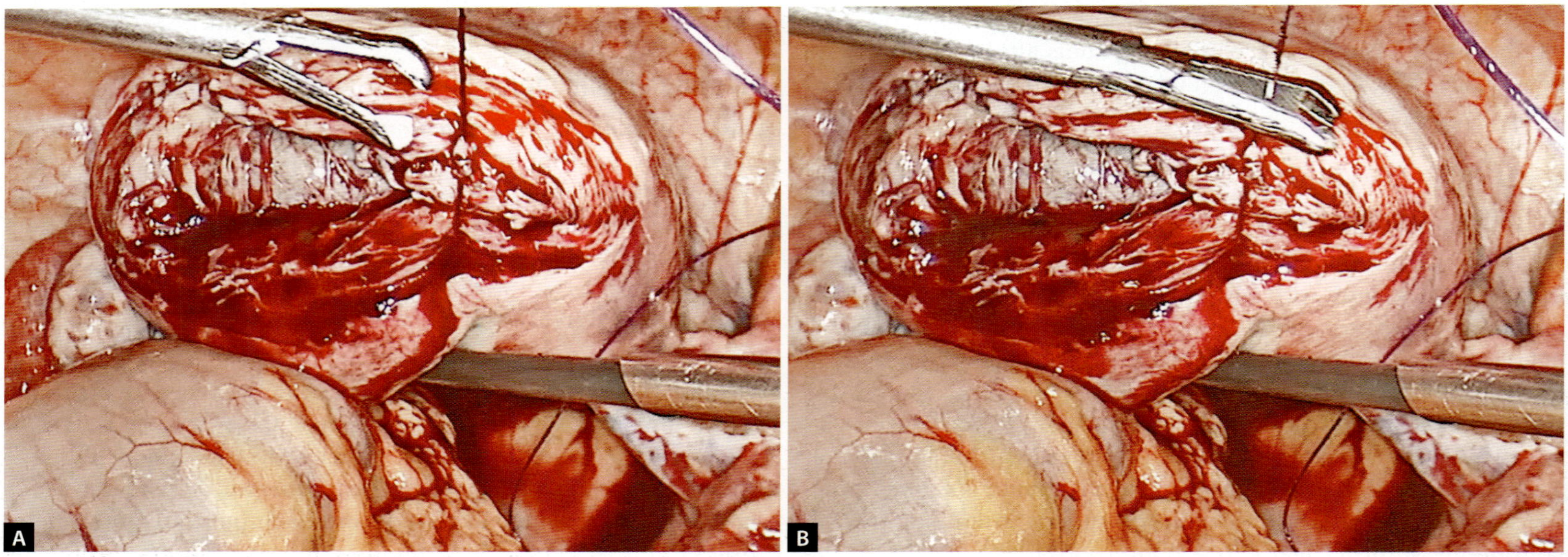

Figs. 4A and B: Tightening the upper flap suture.

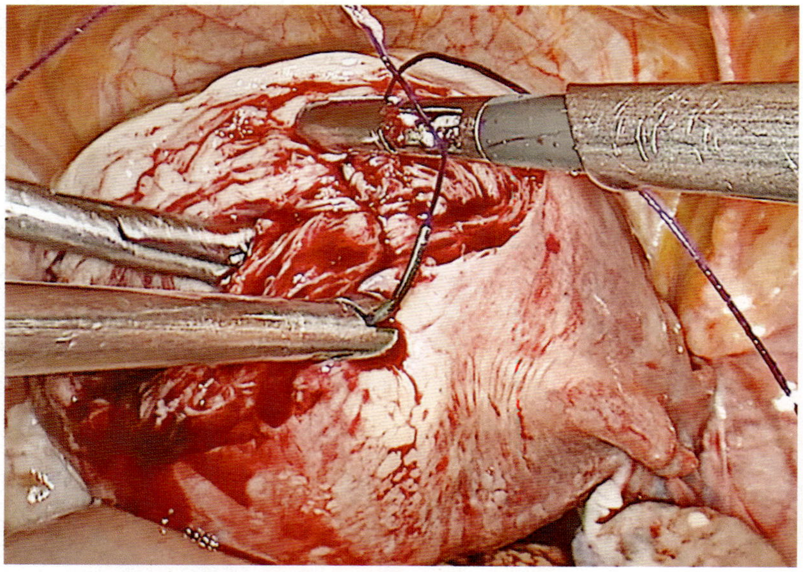

Fig. 5: Stitch on the lower flap with barbed suture.

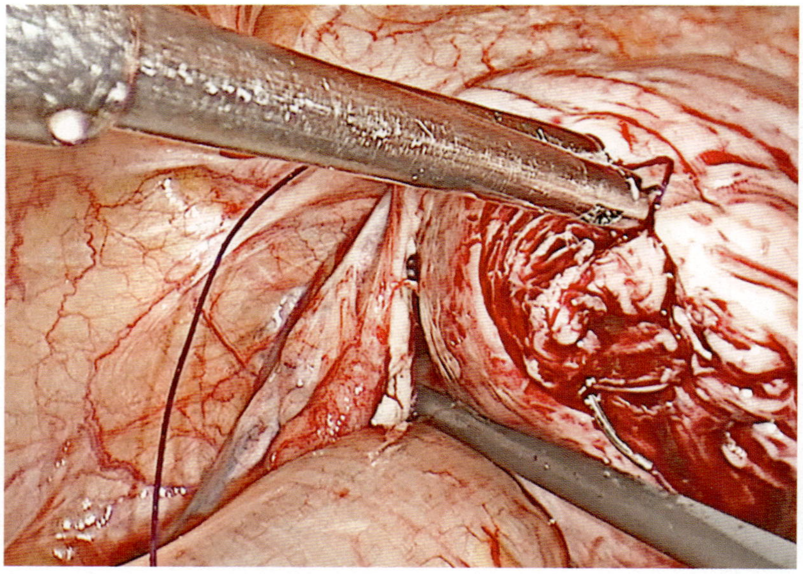

Fig. 6: Stitch on the lower flap.

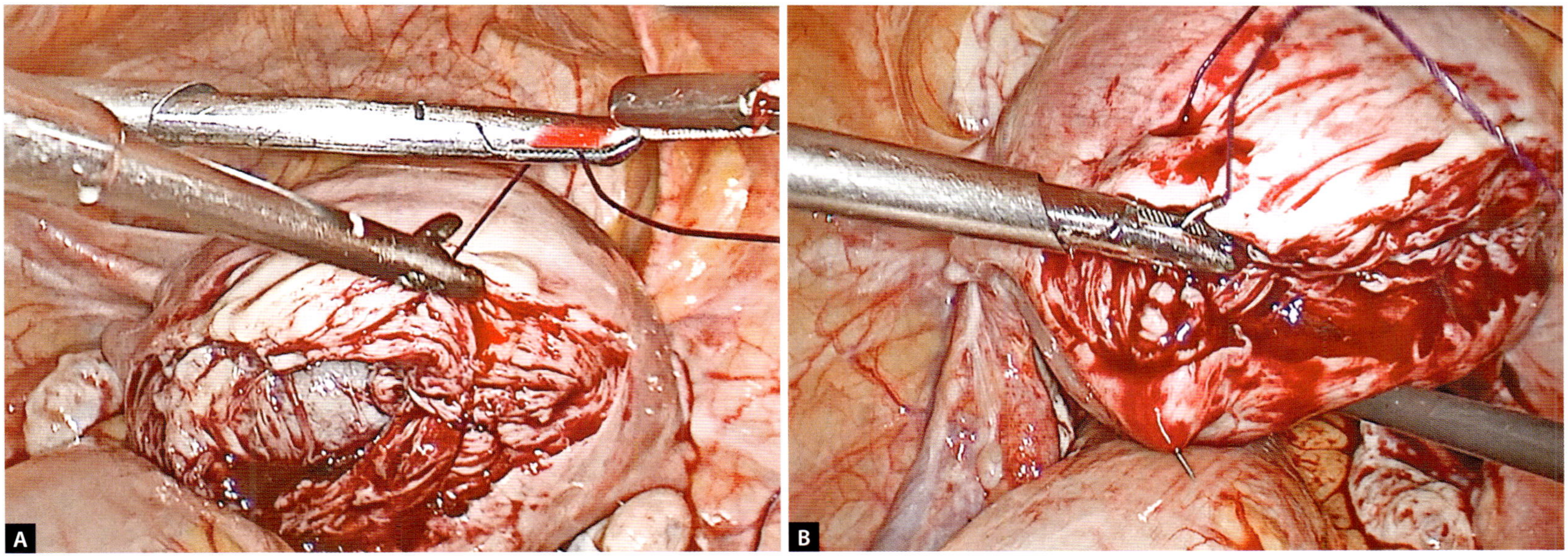

Figs. 7A and B: Stitch on the upper flap.

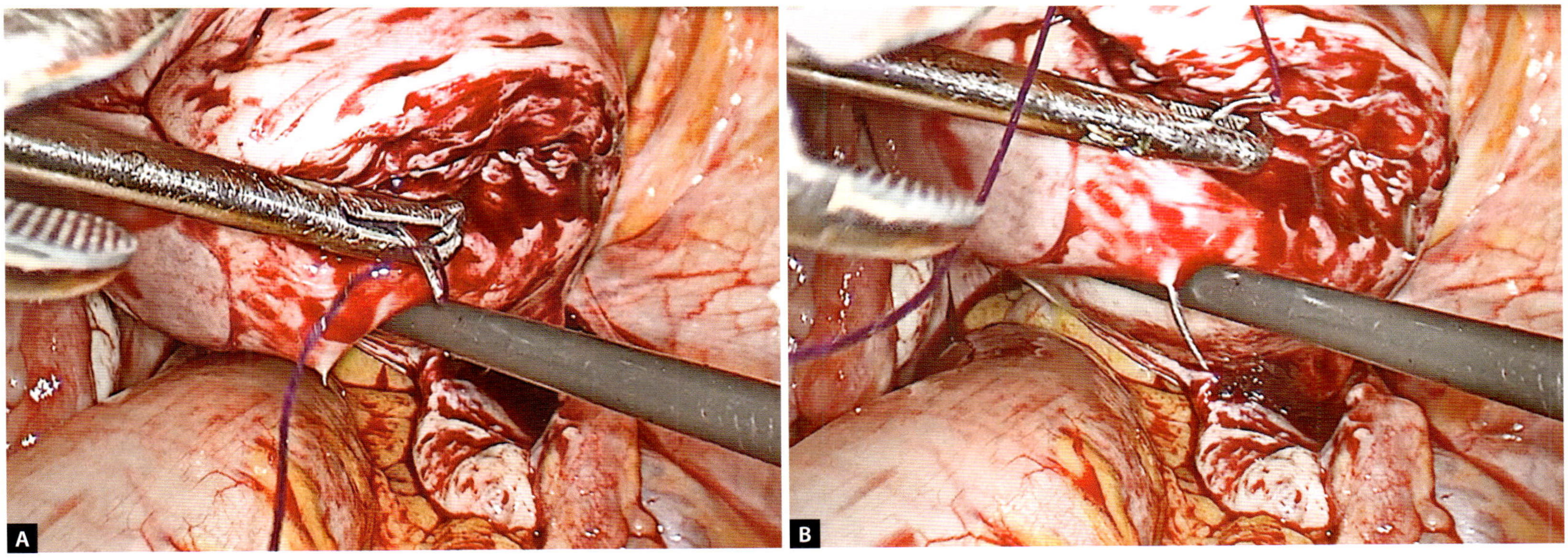

Figs. 8A and B: Baseball stitch of the lower flap

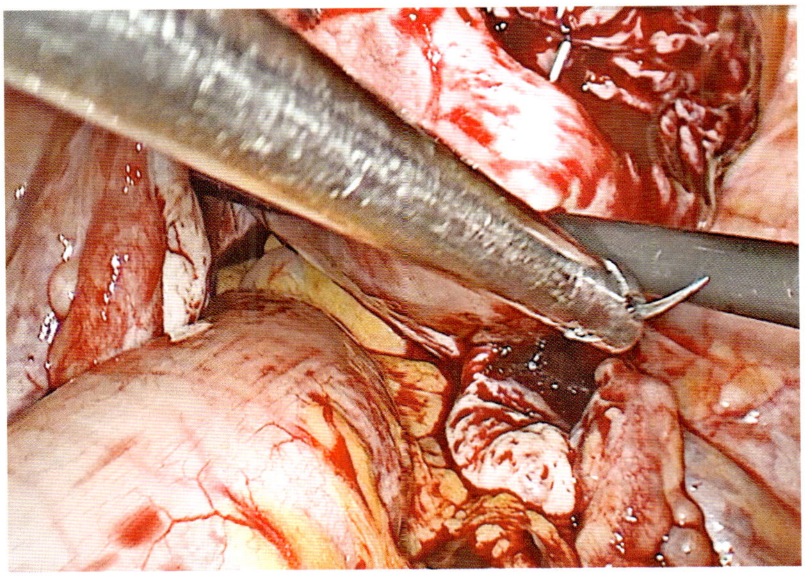

Fig. 9: Baseball stitch of the upper flap.

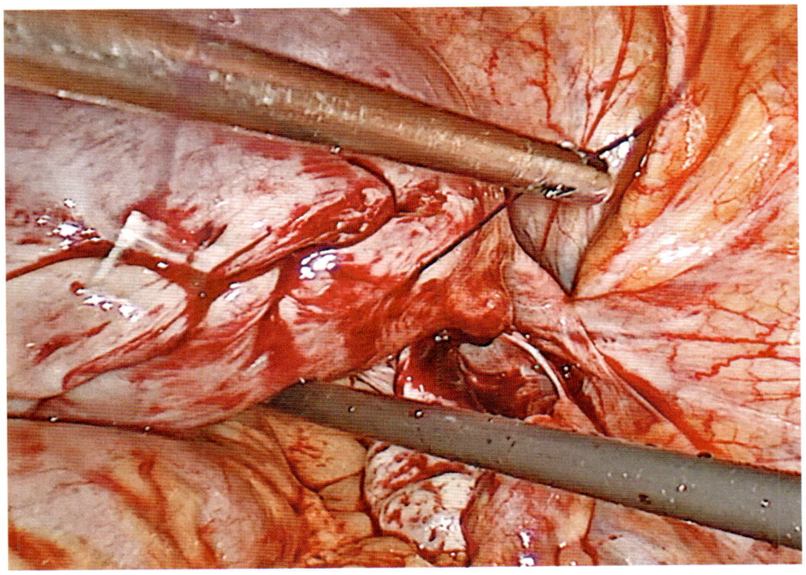

Fig. 10: Delivering the needle in the lower flap.

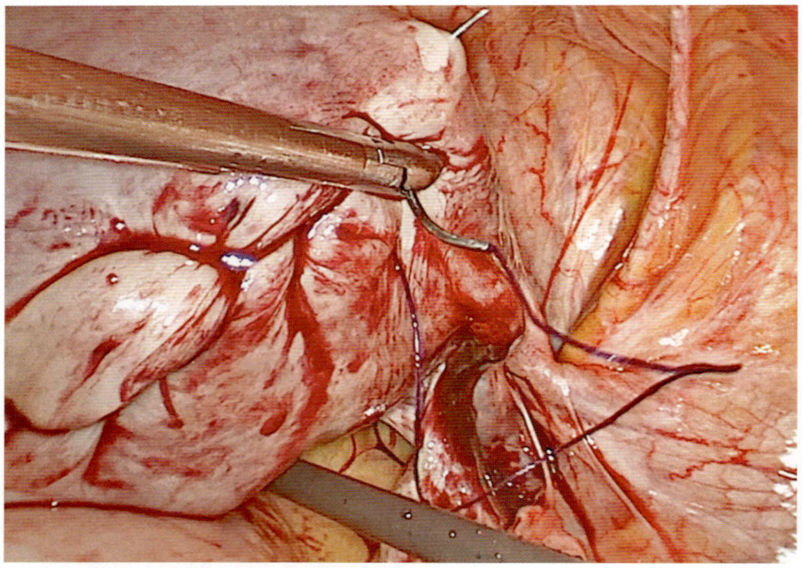

Fig. 11: Baseball stitches.

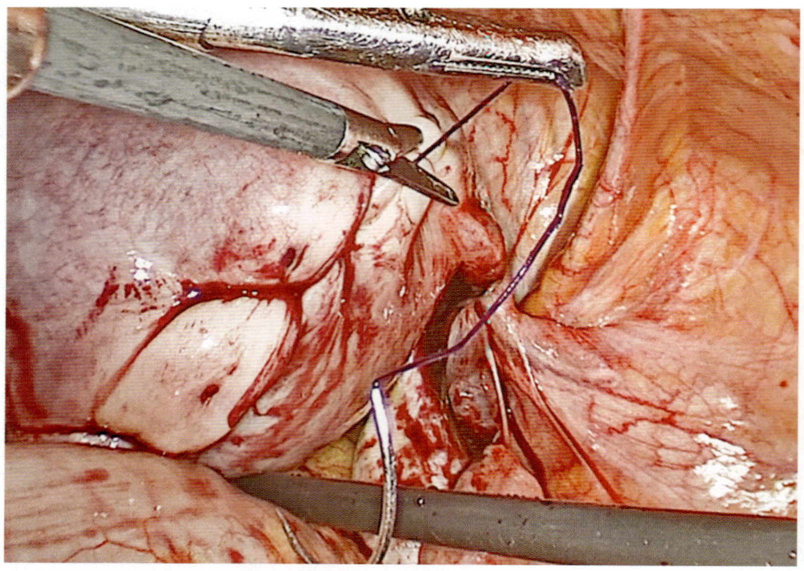

Fig. 12: Completion of the baseball stitch.

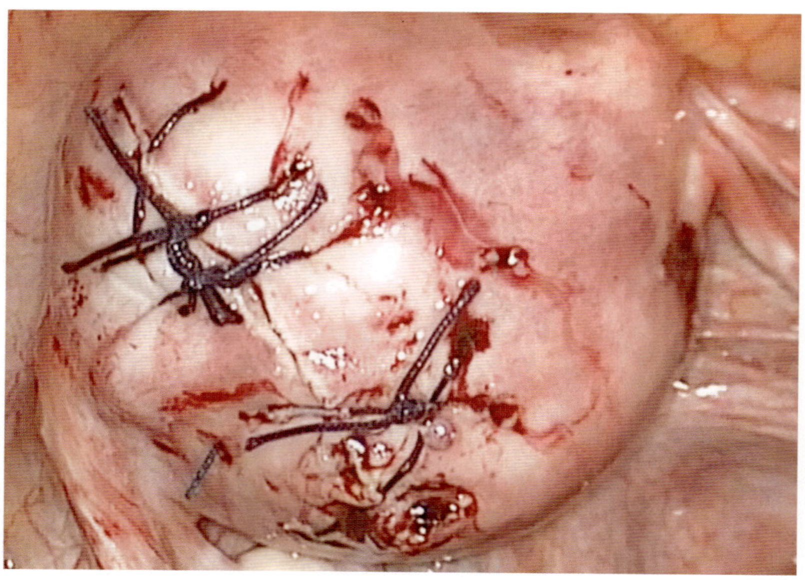

Fig. 13: Vertical suturing.

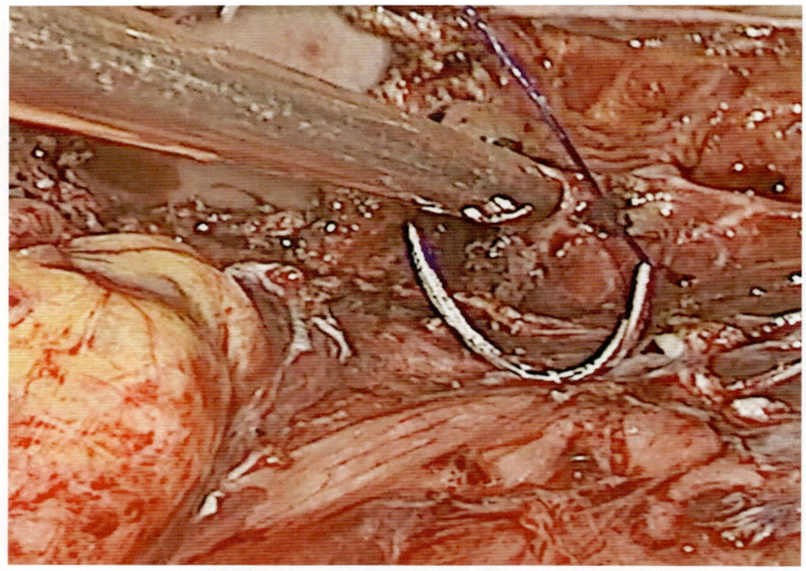

Fig. 14: Suturing the vault in total laparoscopic hysterectomy (TLH).

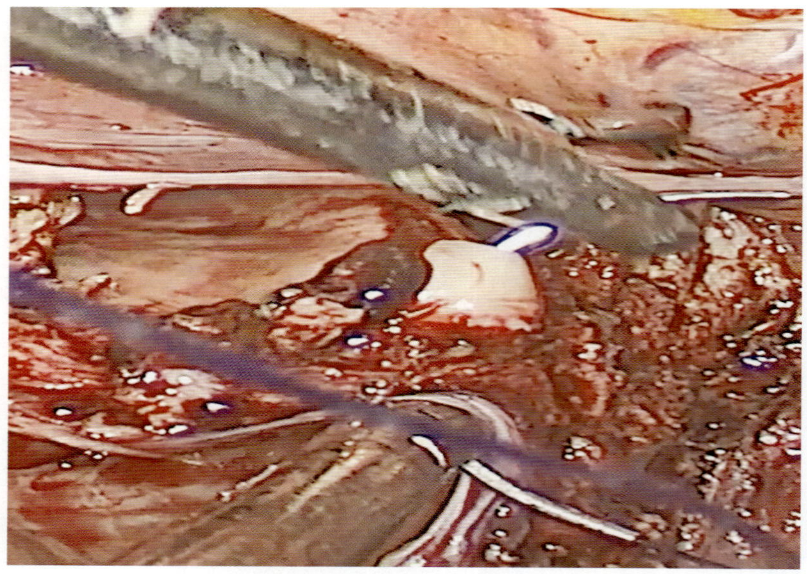

Fig. 15: Bite in the lower flap.

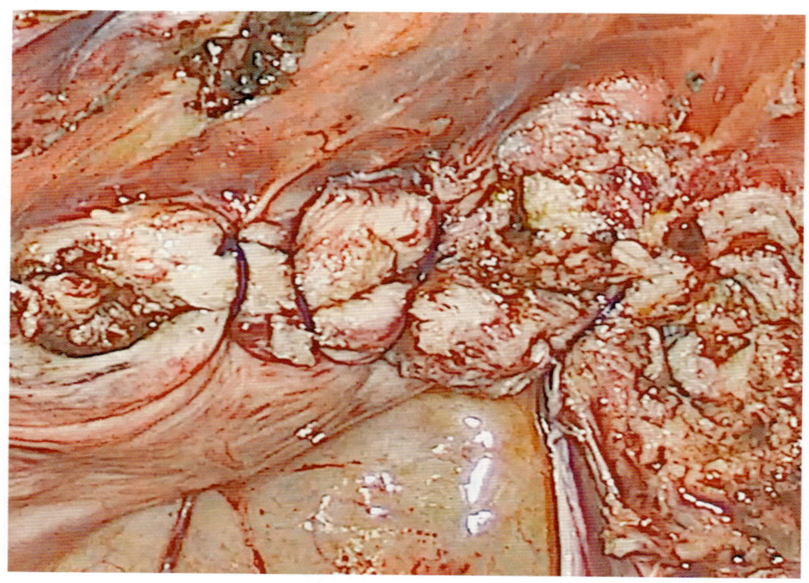

Fig. 16: Suturing of the vault.

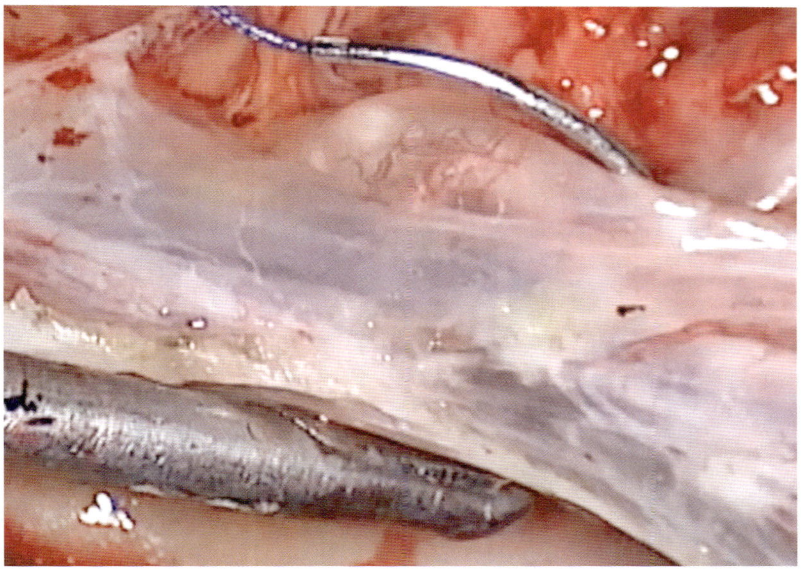

Fig. 17: Suturing of uterine artery.

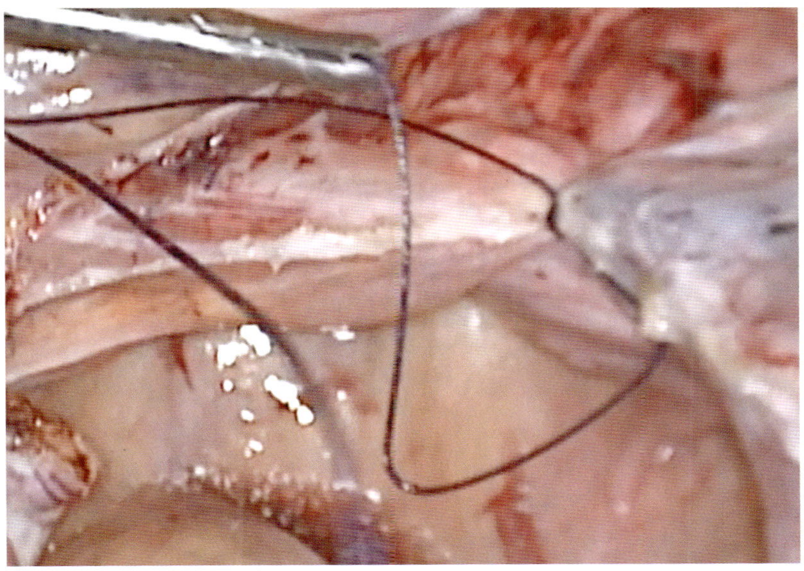

Fig. 18: Uterine artery ligated.

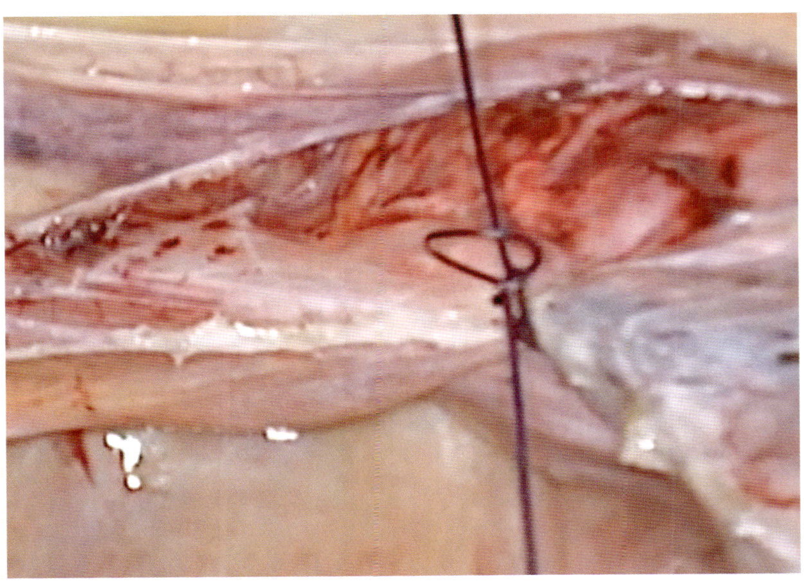

Fig. 19: Knot n the uterine artery.

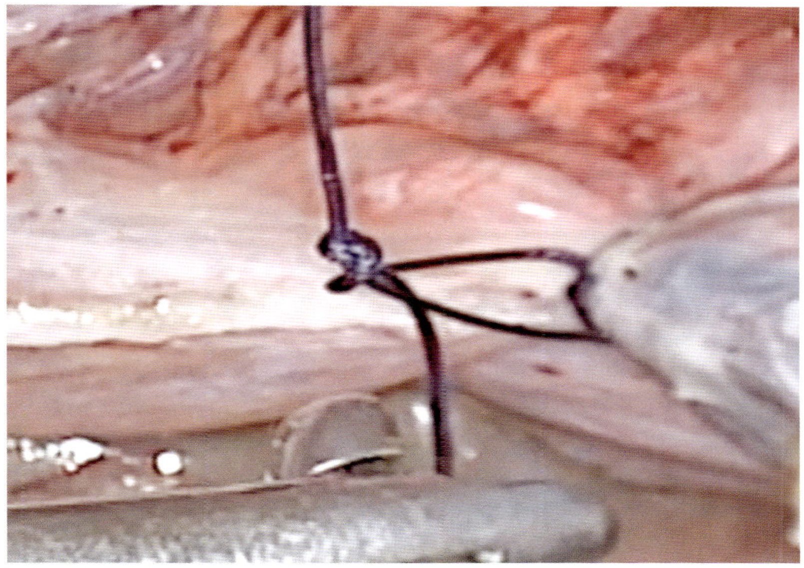

Fig. 20: Tightening of knct in uterine artery.

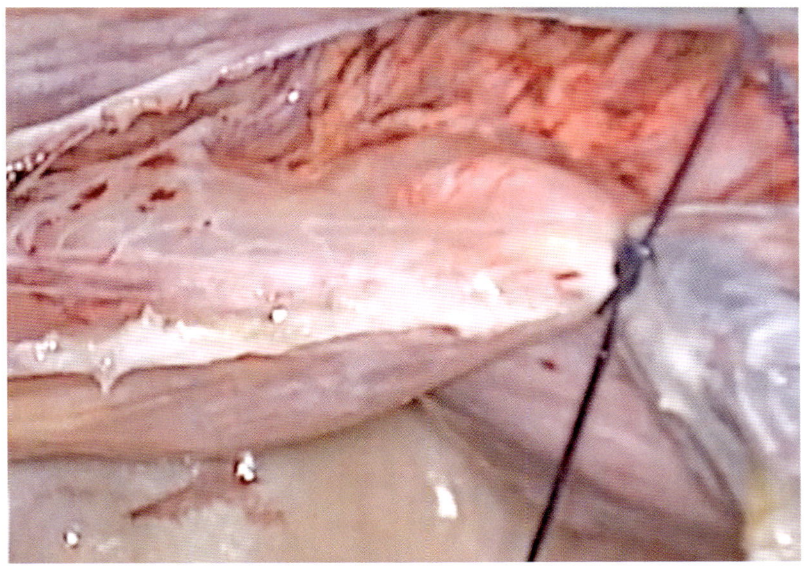

Fig. 21: Squaring the krot in uterine artery.

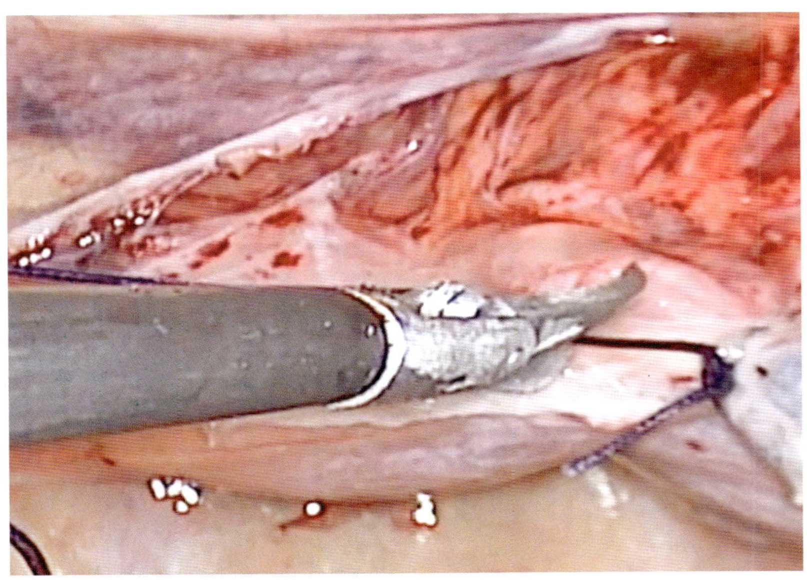

Fig. 22: Completion of uterine artery ligation.

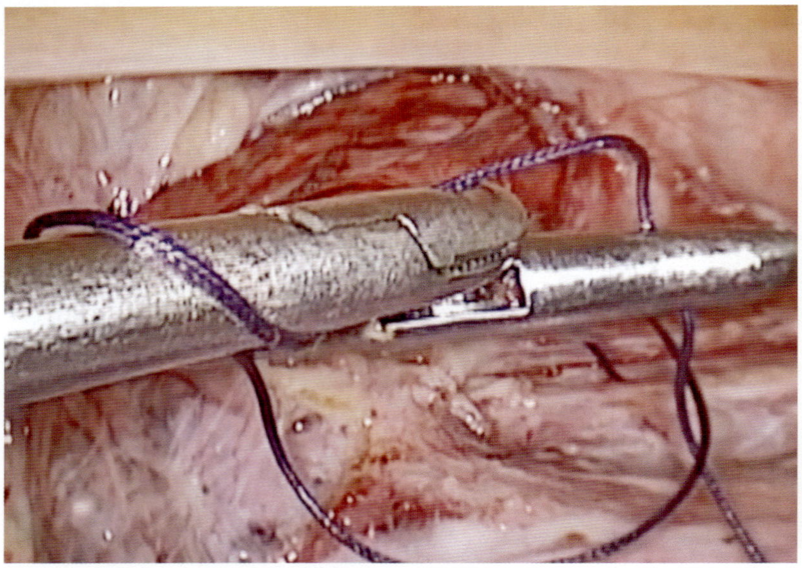

Fig. 23: Throwing of the knot.

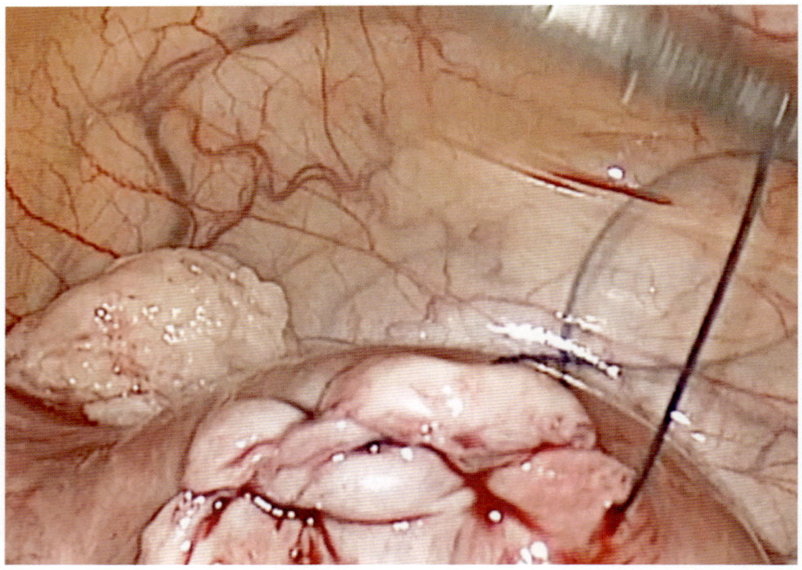

Fig. 25: Baseball suturing.

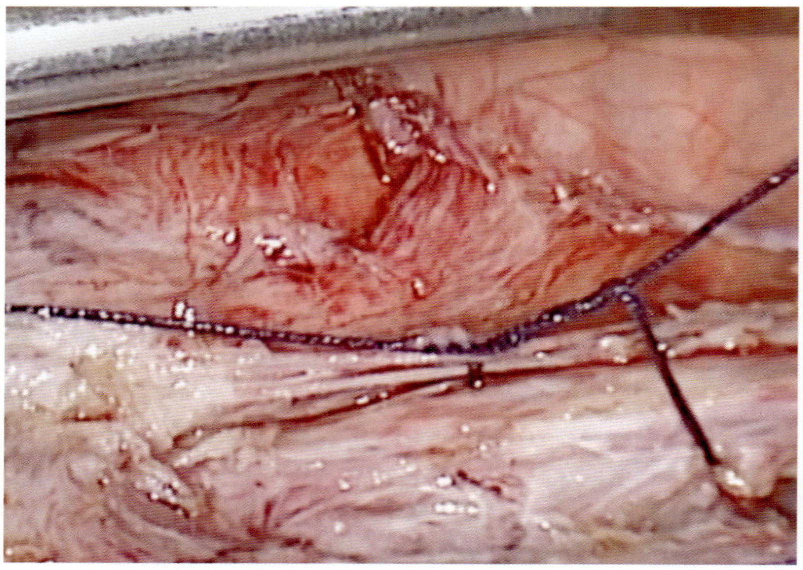

Fig. 24: Squaring the knot.

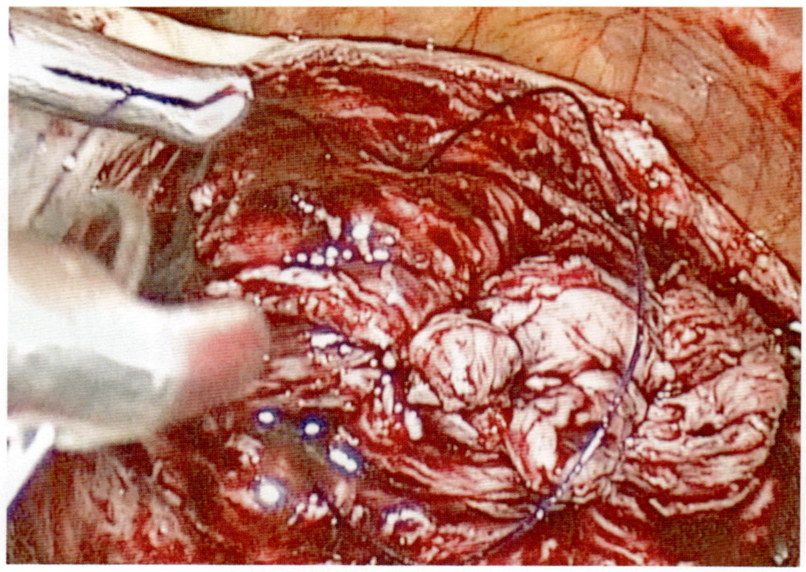

Fig. 26: Suturing of myometrium in layers.

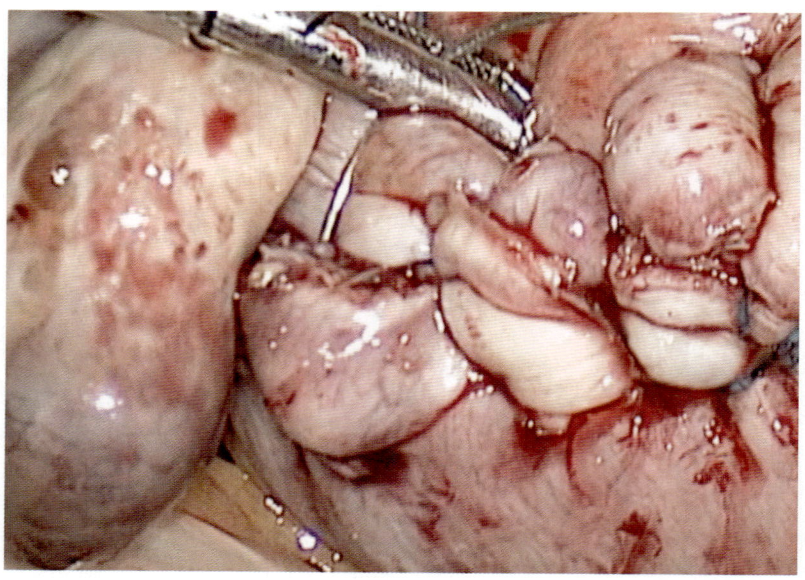

Fig. 27: Suturing in layers.

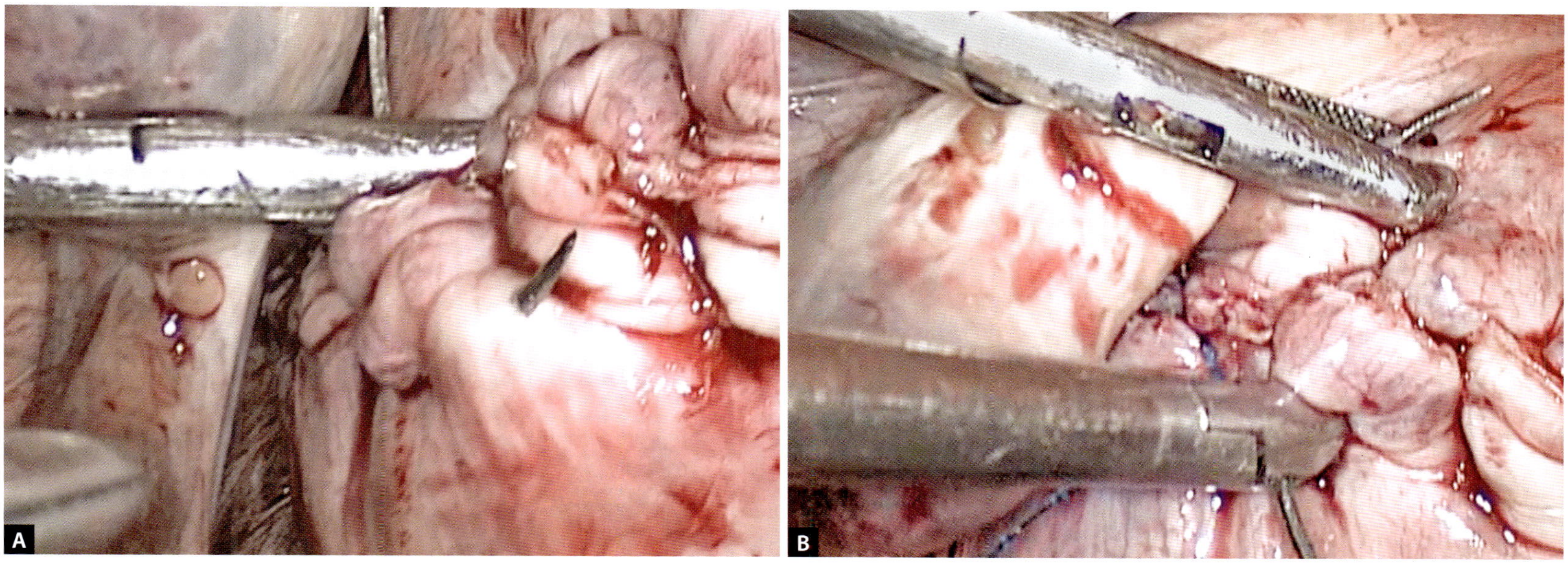

Figs. 28A and B: Baseball stitch of serosa.

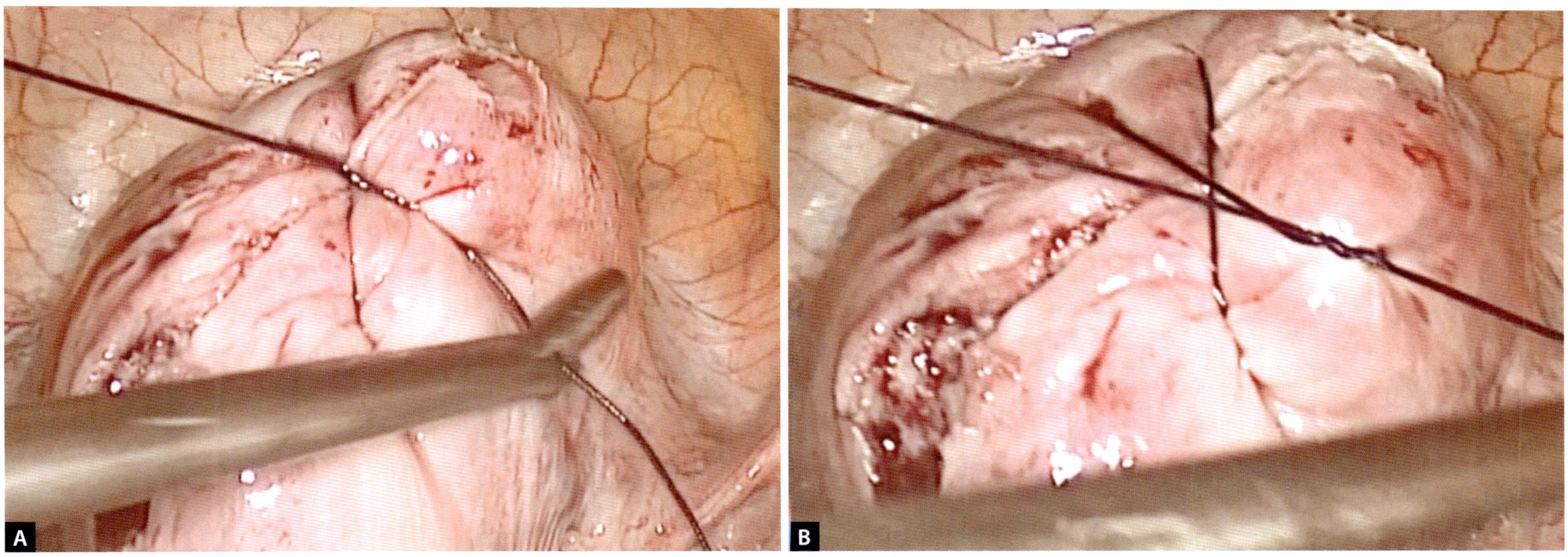

Figs. 29A and B: Figure-of-eight suturing.

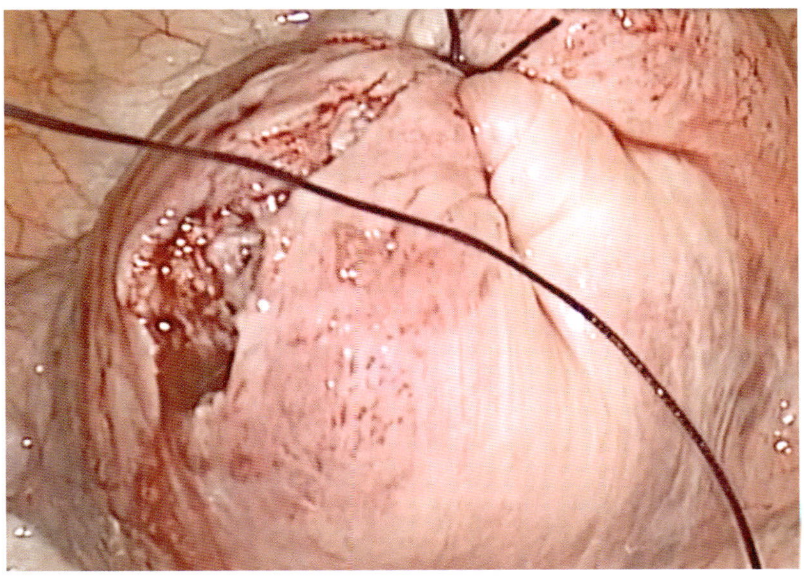

Fig. 30: Completion of figure-of-eight suturing.

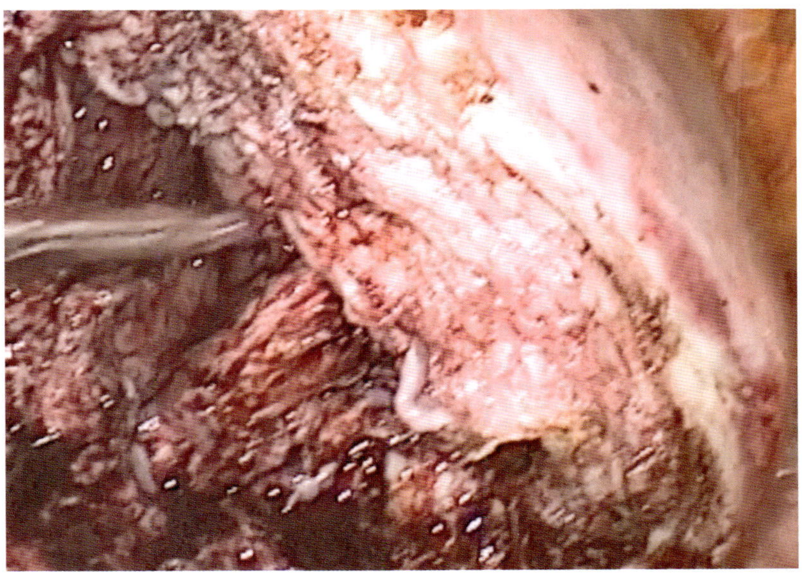

Fig. 31: Submucous myoma fibroid position removed laparoscopically.

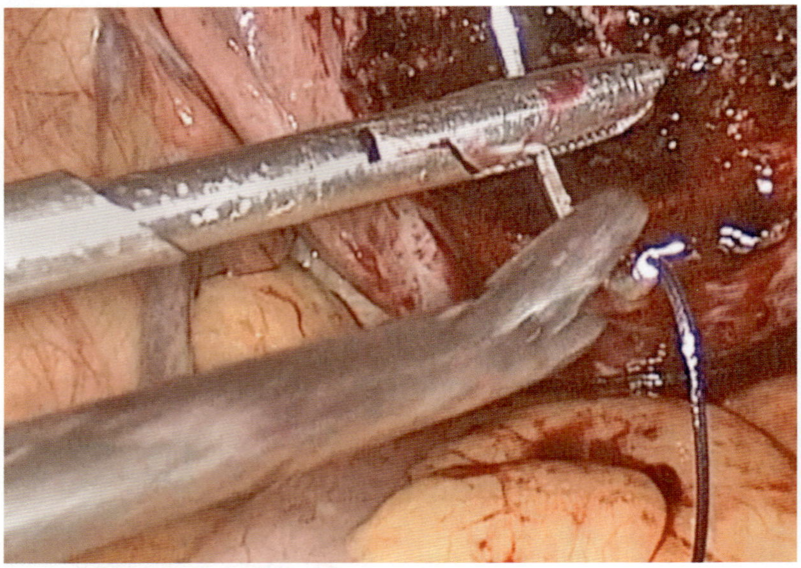

Fig. 32: Holding the needle in smiley.

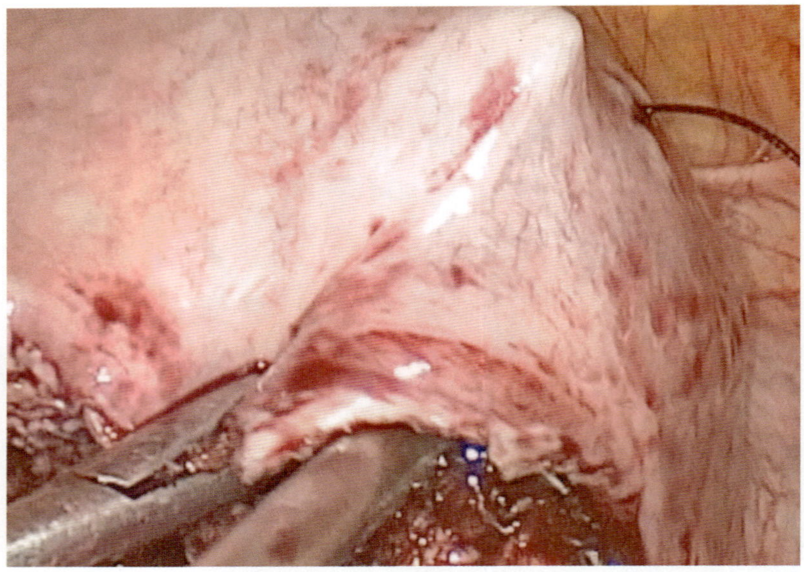

Fig. 34: Thick bite in upper flap.

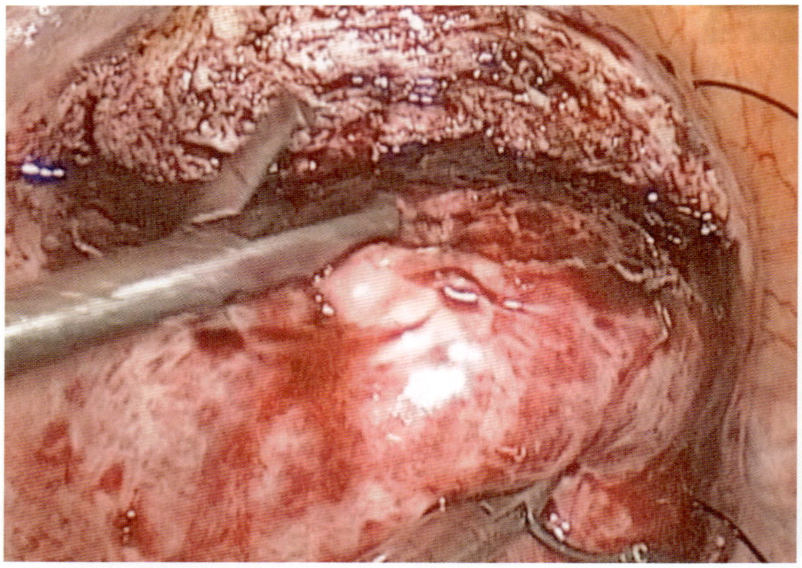

Fig. 33: Thick bite in the lower flap.

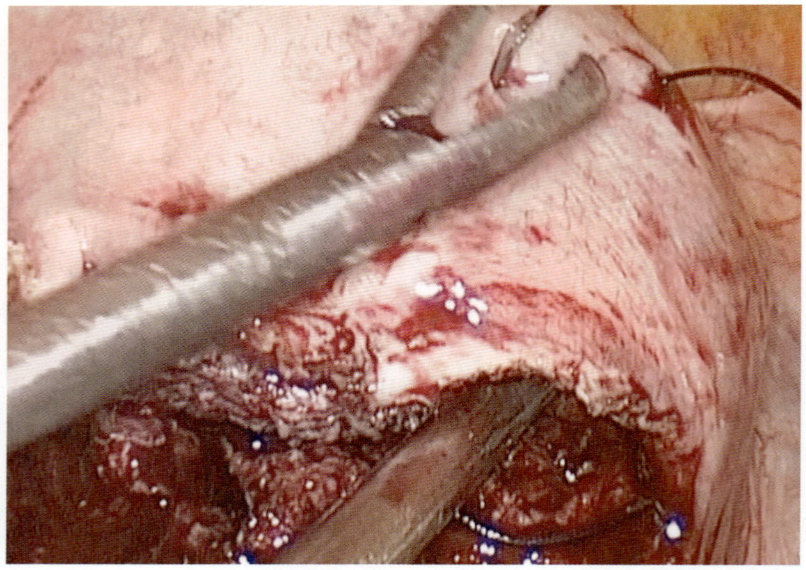

Fig. 35: Delivering of the needle.

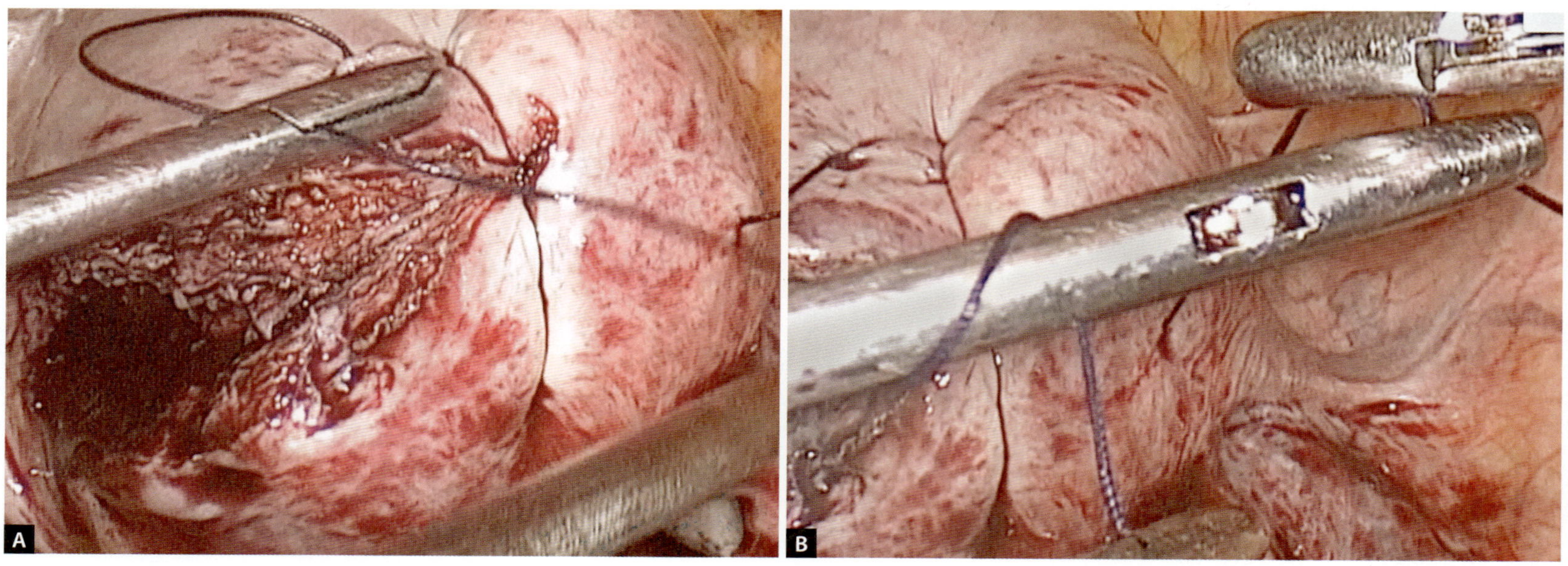

Figs. 36A and B: Throwing the knots.

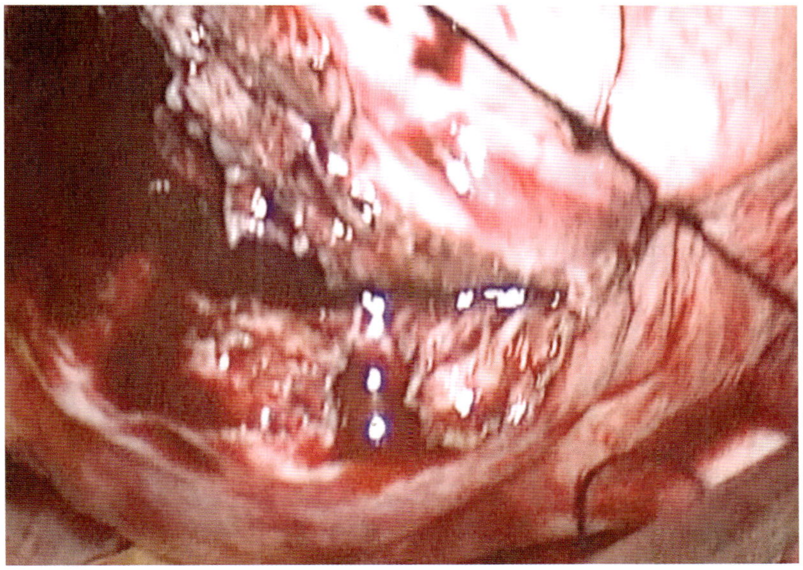

Fig. 37: Figure-of-eight.

CONCLUSION

Although the skills necessary to properly perform intra- or extra-corporeal knot tying for laparoscopic surgery requires patience, it is a challenging skill that most surgeons need to expertise to perform advanced laparoscopic procedures.

REFERENCES

1. Nathanson LK, Nathanson PD, Cuschieri A. Safety of vessel ligation in laparoscopic surgery. Endoscopy. 1991;23:206-9.
2. Desai PJ, Moran ME, Calvano CJ, et al. Running suturing: the ideal length facilities this task. J Endoural. 2000;14:191-4.
3. Genova P, Williams RC, Jewett W. Method for variable-angle cutting of a suture to create tissue retainers of a desired shape and size. US Patent; 2011. pp. 8, 015,678.
4. Maiorino N, Buchter MS, Primavera M, et al. Method of forming barbs on a suture. US Patent. 2012; pp. 8, 161, 618.
5. Lindh D, Nawrocki JG, Collen JP. Tissue holding devices and methods for making the same. US Patent; pp. 7, 850, 894.
6. Vakil JJ, O'Reilly MP, Sutter EG, et al. Knee arthrotomy repair with a continuous barbed suture: a biomechanical study. J Arthroplasty. 2011;26(5): 710-3.
7. Einarsson JI, Vonnahme KA, Sandberg EM, et al. Barbed compared with stranded suture: effects on cellular composition and proliferation of the healing wound in the ovine uterus. Acta Obstet Gynecol Scand. 2012;91:613-9.
8. Ting NT, Moric MM, Della Valle CJ, et al. Use of knotless suture for closure of total hip and knee arthroplasties: a prospective, randomized clinical trial. J Arthroplasty. 2012;27:1783-8.
9. Witte MB, Barbul A. Role of nitric oxide in wound repair. Am J Surg. 2002;183:406-12.
10. Stone IK, von Fraunhofer JA, Masterson BJ. The biomechanical effects of tight suture closure upon fascia. Surg Gynecol Obstet. 1986;163:448-52.
11. Klink CD, Binnebosel M, Alizai HP, et al. Tension of knotted surgical sutures shows tissue specific rapid loss in a rodent model. BMC Surg. 2011;11:36.
12. Greenberg JA, Goldman RH. Barbed suture: a review of the technology and clinical uses in obstetrics and gynecology. Rev Obstet Gynecol. 2013;6:107-15.
13. Chu CC, von Fraunhofer JA, Greisler HP. Wound Closure Biomaterials and Devices, 1st edition. Boca Raton, FL: CRC Press; 1997. pp. 68-122.
14. Marturello DM, McFadden MS, Bennett RA, et al. Knot security and tensile strength of suture materials. Vet Surg. 2014;43:73-9.
15. Van Rijssel EJ, Brand R, Admiraal C, et al. Tissue reaction and surgical knots: the effect of suture size, knot configuration, and knot volume. Obstet Gynecol. 1989;74:64-8.
16. Fujimoto A, Morimoto C, Hosokawa Y, et al. Suturing method as a factor for uterine vascularity after laparoscopic myomectomy. Eur J Obstet Gynecol Reprod Biol. 2017;211:146-9.

CHAPTER

11

Permanent Female Sterilization

Sowmya MS, Aditi Rai, B Ramesh

INTRODUCTION

Female sterilization is the surgical procedure used to end a woman's ability to become pregnant. The procedure involves ligation, with or without resection or blocking of both the Fallopian tubes, so that the egg and the sperm do not meet. Rarely hysterectomy is also performed for the same purpose if other valid grounds are present. No nonsurgical method of female sterilization has been found to be effective and safe as yet.

USAGE

Female sterilization or tubal ligation is the most accepted method of contraception in India. Currently, the female sterilization accounts for 85% whereas male sterilization accounts for 10–15% of all sterilizations in India in spite that males sterilization is much easier than its counterpart. The most popular method used in female sterilization in India is the laparoscopic tubal occlusion. Over 85.3% of all persons who have adopted this method of contraception availed this service from government facilities.

Sterilization is a permanent method and offers many advantages over other methods—it is a single step procedure, provides the most effective method against pregnancy, the less chances of risk if done in accordance to accepted medical standards, it is cost-effective. It has been estimated that each procedure averts 1.5–2.5 births per woman.

GUIDELINES FOR STERILIZATION

Sterilization services are provided free of charge in Government institutions. There are several criteria:

- The age of the husband should be in between 25 years and 50 years of age.
- The age of the wife should be in between 20 years and 45 years of age.
- The couple must have at least two living children at the time of operation.
- If the couple has three or more number of children, the age of the husband or the wife can be relaxed at the discretion of the operating surgeon.
- It is sufficient if the acceptor declares having the consent of his/her spouse to undergo sterilization without outside pressure.

SELECTION OF CASES

Cases for contraception are selected nowadays on the basis of World Health Organization (WHO) medical eligibility criteria **(Table 1)**.

Table 1: World Health Organization (WHO) medical eligibility criteria.

Category C WHO: Extra caution	
Young age	Hypothyroidism
Obesity: More than 90 kg body weight	Mild cirrhosis
Hypertension: Adequately controlled BP or raised BP (systolic 140–159 mm Hg) or diastolic (90–99 mm Hg)	Schistosomiasis with fibrosis of the liver
History of ischemic heart disease	Liver tumors
History of cardiovascular heart disease Uterine fibroids	Thalassemia
Past pelvic inflammatory disease (PID) without subsequent pregnancy	Sickle cell disease
Diabetes without vascular disease	Diaphragmatic hernia (laparoscopy may be dangerous)
Kidney disease	Depressive disorders
Severe nutritional deficiencies	Previous abdominal or pelvic surgeries
Category D WHO: Delay the procedure (condition must be treated and resolved before the procedure)	
Pregnancy	Unexplained vaginal bleeding before evaluation
Postpartum (7 to <42 days)	Malignant gestational trophoblastic disease
Severe preeclampsia/eclampsia	Cervical or endometrial or ovarian cancers (as treatment makes a woman sterile)
Prolonged rupture of membranes (24 h or more)	PID
Puerperal sepsis	Sexually transmitted infection
Severe antepartum or postpartum hemorrhage	Current gallbladder disease
Severe trauma to the genital tract at the time of delivery	Active viral hepatitis
Postabortion sepsis	Severe postabortion hemorrhage
Acute hematometra	Sterilization concurrent with emergency abdominal surgery or any infectious condition
Current deep venous thrombosis (DVT) or pulmonary embolism	Current ischemic heart disease
Category S WHO: Special precaution/refer client (refer client to center with facilities for general anesthesia and other medical support where an experienced surgeon or staff can perform the procedure)	
Postpartum or postabortion uterine rupture or perforation	Severe cirrhosis
Multiple risk factors for arterial cardio-vascular diseases (old age, smoking, diabetes mellitus and hypertension	Diabetes with nephropathy/retinopathy or neuropathy

Contd...

Contd...

Category S WHO: Special precaution/refer client (refer client to center with facilities for general anesthesia and other medical support where an experienced surgeon or staff can perform the procedure)	
Endometriosis	Coagulation disorders
AIDS (use of condom required poststerilization)	Chronic asthma, bronchitis
Known pelvic tuberculosis	Fixed uterus due to previous surgery or infection
Hyperthyroidism	Abdominal wall or umbilical hernia (hernia repair should be done concurrently)

COUNSELING

Prior to the procedure proper counseling is required as to remove any misconceptions from the patient's mind. Some of the following points need to be explained:

- The procedure should be considered as permanent as reversal of tubal ligation is difficult and chances of ectopic pregnancy are increased.
- Possible failure of operation is possible even though the chances are remote.
- All alternative methods of contraception must be considered before going for tubal ligation such as intrauterine devices (IUDs), vasectomy, etc. each of them has their own pros and cons.
- Complications such as bleeding and infection can happen, though they are rare.
- Menstrual disturbances, postsurgery, are not due to the surgery. They mostly affect those who were already using oral contraceptives (OCs) up to the time of surgery and had menstrual irregularities.
- Some women put on more weight postsurgery due to the rest they get and more nourishment as they stop having children every few years.

Types of tubal ligation depending on the timing of the operation:

- *Cesarean ligation*—when tubal ligation is combined with cesarean section.
- *Puerperal ligation*—when done early in the puerperium for those who desire sterilization after the delivery of the baby. Advantages are:
  - Technically easy as uterus is large
  - Postoperative and postpartum periods convalesce, so no extra hospital stay required. Optimum time is after 6 hours.
- *Interval ligation*—done in nonpregnant women or 6 weeks after normal delivery. Should be done within 7–10 days of onset of menstruation. When done in the later part of the cycle or lactational amenorrhea, vacuum aspiration or dilatation and curettage needs to be done to avoid failure of procedure.
- *Postabortal ligation* or sterilization.
- *Gynecological ligation*—in cases of genital prolapsed when family is complete and a vaginal plastic repair is being performed, unless the patient is more than 40 years and she requires a vaginal hysterectomy.

Tubal ligation may be done by an open method (minilaparotomy), vaginally or laparoscopically.

Minilaparotomy

Tubal ligation is done by means of minilaparotomy method.

For minilaparotomy, local anesthesia in the form of 0.5% lignocaine with epinephrine 1:200,000 (safe dose 100 mL), preceded by an intramuscular injection of meperidine 100 mg and promethazine hydrochloride 50 mg given 30–40 min before the procedure, is quite sufficient.

During a preoperative counseling and health checkup, the patients are selected carefully. Those with fatty abdomen, retroverted uterus, and restricted mobility due to previous surgery or infection are not suitable for minilaparotomy.

This procedure is usually meant for interval tubal ligation but may be utilized in a modified way for puerperal and postabortal sterilization, as in this case uterine elevation is not always required. The operation is performed in an outpatient procedure and the patients are advised to come with an empty stomach.

Procedure: The patient is placed in semilithotomy position or in a Trendelenburg position. She voids urine before coming to the operating table, and the preoperative medications are given. After cleaning the abdominal and perineal parts, sterile drapings are applied.

A preliminary vaginal examination is done to note the mobility, size and shape of the uterus and for the presence of any adnexal masses. The cervix is cleaned with 5% povidone-iodine solution after introducing speculum and the anterior lip of cervix is held with a tenaculum or atraumatic forceps, and the uterine elevator is introduced. Various instruments are used to elevate the uterus such as the Rubin's insufflations cannula with rubber stop, pair of ring forceps with gauze pad.

The abdomen is opened using a transverse incision of about 3 cm wide. In a puerperal tubal ligation, this incision is taken 2 cm below the fundus and in interval tubal ligation it is taken about 2.5 cm above the pubic symphysis. In cases of obese patients, a larger incision may be taken depending on the experience of the surgeon. The incidence of ventral hernia is lesser with a transverse incision than a vertical one, though some doctors still prefer a vertical incision. The abdomen is opened in the usual way.

After retracting the incision to one side using retractors, the pelvic organs are explore and if required any adhesions are separated, the Fallopian tubes are identified on each side and brought out of the abdomen using atraumatic forceps like Babcock forceps and Allis forceps by manipulation with the fingers. The confirmation of the structure must be done by identifying the fimbrial end as the round ligament may sometimes be mistaken for the Fallopian tube.

After elevating the uterus by the assistant, the tubal ligation is carried out by one of the ways described below. Tubal ligation is mostly performed by Pomeroy's method with or without modifications, or by Parkland's method. The tubes may also be occluded by Hulka-Clemens clips.

The major complications following minilaparotomy procedure are bladder injury, bleeding, uterine perforation or tubal injury which was encountered in less than 2% (IFRP study).

The patient is kept in the side room or overnight and given analgesics for postoperative pain. She is asked to follow-up after 5–7 days for stitch removal. She can resume sexual and other activities after the pain has abated.

Advantages of minilaparotomy:

- It is a safe, effective, and convenient method of tubal ligation.
- It can be done by junior doctors.
- Does not require special training.

- Can be used for mass sterilization for population control.
- The complications are minor.
- It can be performed soon after childbirth, abortion or for interval sterilization.

Disadvantages of minilaparotomy over laparoscopy:
- Higher chances of wound and pelvic infections.
- Longer convalescence period.
- Longer duration and severity of postoperative pain.
- Larger incisional scar than that needed for laparoscopy.

Pomeroy Technique

After bringing out the Fallopian tubes outside the incision, about 4 cm lateral to the fundus the tube is clamped. Avoiding the blood vessels by observation against light, the mesosalpinx is pierced using a round bodied needle with chromic catgut No. 0. The base of the loop is tied, neither too tight nor with fine suture so as to not cut through, producing stump hemorrhage. Particularly in puerperal sterilization when the tubes are friable, congested and edematous. The base of the loop is tied so as to keep at least 2 cm of the loop above the tie **(Fig. 1)**. The loop is then cut with the stump not too close to the base. The stumps are then cleaned with a gauze to confirm that the tubes are cut completely (by noting the sprouting of the tubal mucosa) and also that perfect hemostasis has been achieved.

The opposite tube is ligated in the same way.

The abdominal wall is closed in layers the usual way. Skin is closed.

Catgut stitches are used in the Pomeroy technique to ligate the loop of the tube and so the tubal cut ends remain widely apart after the absorption of the catgut, reducing the risk of failure. More failure has been noted after the use of silk sutures.

The Pomeroy technique is the most simple and safe procedure of tubal ligation and is also used in minilaparotomy and vaginal sterilization. However, it has got a failure rate of 1 in 300–400 operations. Though recent modifications have reduced the failure rate.

Irving Technique

This technique was developed to counteract the failure rates due to the conventional Pomeroy's method. In this technique, the Fallopian tube is doubly ligated with chromic catgut about 2.5 cm lateral to the uterine cornua and then severed, the sutures kept long. The medial end of the tube is dissected from the mesosalpinx. A tunnel is made near the posterior surface of the uterus near the cornua in an avascular area. Both the ligatures attached to the medial stump are threaded with a needle and passed through the tunnel and brought out of the uterine wall 1 cm away from the first suture and tied together **(Fig. 2)**.

This technique is particularly useful for tubal ligation during cesarean section, as the retraction of the uterus further compresses the Fallopian tube ends occluding it.

The Irving technique requires considerable exposure, larger incision, and more time, and is more hemorrhagic. But this technique has a low failure rate, less than 1 in 1,000 cases.

Oxford Technique

A similar procedure that can be applied in the interval situation is the Oxford technique as described by Williams. As in the Irving procedure, the oviduct is divided and a segment of the isthmus is removed. The proximal end of the oviduct is passed under the round ligament and tied in this location. The distal tube is then tied on the opposite side of the round ligament.

Uchida Technique

In this technique, saline with epinephrine is injected into the mesosalpinx, which enables separation of the muscular tube from the mesosalpinx. The mesosalpinx is then cut and the loop of Fallopian tube is brought out. The tube is ligated at two places enough to remove 5 cm of the tube. The medial end is then buried into the mesosalpinx and the mesosalpinx is then closed. The lateral end is left outside **(Fig. 3)**.

Although no failure cases have been noted with this technique, it is not very popular but can be done during a minilaparotomy.

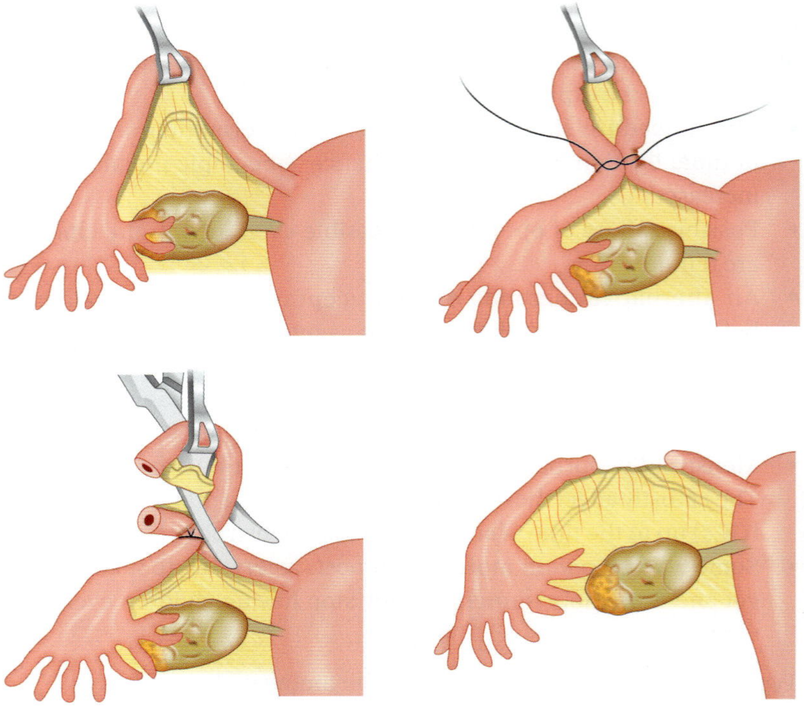

Fig. 1: Pomeroy's method.

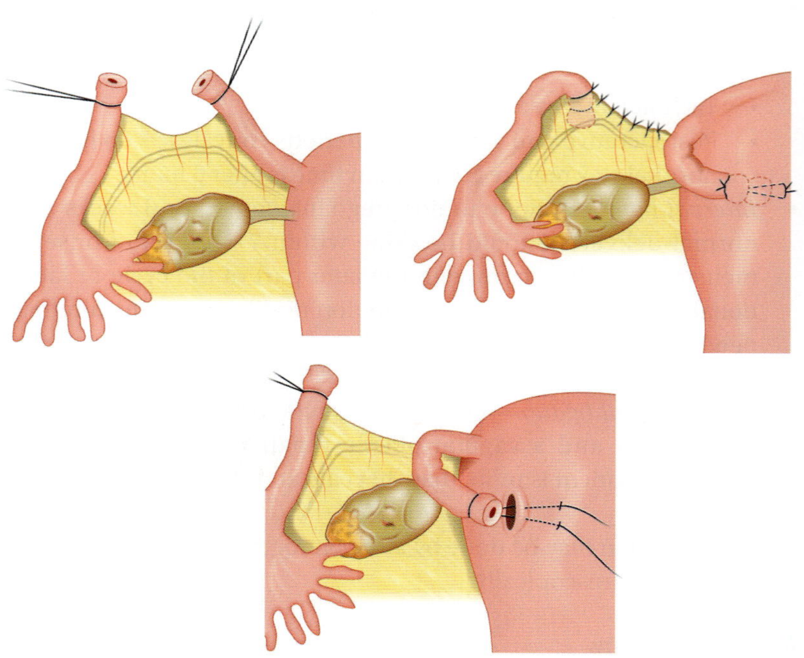

Fig. 2: Irving method.

Fimbriectomy (Kroener's Techniaue)

The fimbrial end in this technique is doubly ligated with silk or catgut sutures **(Fig. 4)**. This technique can be used in vaginal tubal ligation also. Although, this technique has a low failure rate, it is not very popular. Also the success of reversal of female sterilization is also very poor. It is considered in patients who have had precious tubal ligation failure.

Madlener's Technique

A loop of tube in the middle one-third is crushed at its base and ligated with silk or catgut. Although it is a simple procedure, it has a high failure rate (0.3–2%) hence abandoned **(Figs. 5A and B)**.

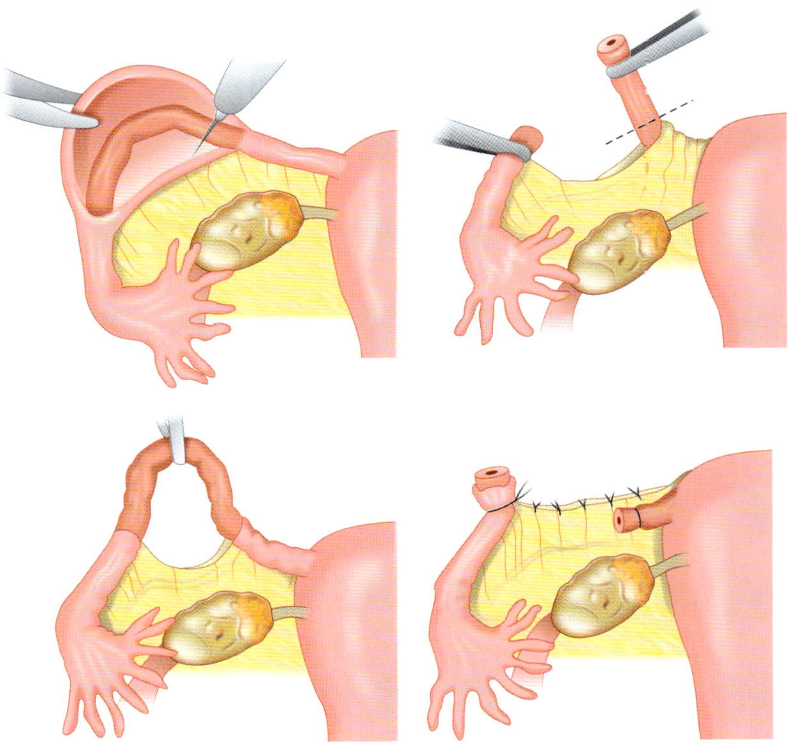

Fig. 3: Uchica technique.

Aldridge's Technique

In Aldridge procedure, Fallopian tube remains intact **(Figs. 6A and B)**. The fimbrial end is drawn into a pocket beneath the peritoneum of the broad ligament and buried fimbrial end just beneath the peritoneum, which is secured by nonabsorbable suture material.

Parkland Technique

In this technique, a window is created in the mesosalpinx in an avascular area, using an artery forceps so as to separate the tube from the mesosalpinx for about 2.5 cm. About 2 cm of the tube is excised and the free ends are ligated. The tubes are replaced inside the abdomen after confirmation of hemostasis. The failure rate of this method is 1 in 400.

Various other procedures such as cornual resection, salpingectomy, and simple ligation and modifications of other techniques such as Pomeroy's have been advocated. But they only involve unnecessary extra steps and no improvement in the failure rate. Hence, mostly only Pomeroy's and Parkland's method are used, rest are all abandoned.

Vaginal Tubal Ligation

Tubal ligation by vaginal approach also called as colpotomy. Tubal ligation is done in nonpregnant cases. Some surgeons perform vaginal tubal ligation with safety following first trimester abortions. Some surgeons are against postabortal vaginal tubal ligation because of more complications of bleeding, infection and a higher failure rate. Hence, it is mostly performed as an interval tubal ligation.

Contraindications to vaginal tubal ligation are endometriosis, infection, previous surgeries producing lessened mobility of the uterus or producing masses, obesity, recent second trimester abortions, and vaginal infection. However, the procedure can be carried out after waiting for 2–4 weeks following abortion and after cure of infection.

It is usually done under general or regional anesthesia as local and intravenous analgesia fails more often causing difficulties. The procedure can be done in an outpatient setting and can be advised rest for about 4–6 hours or overnight.

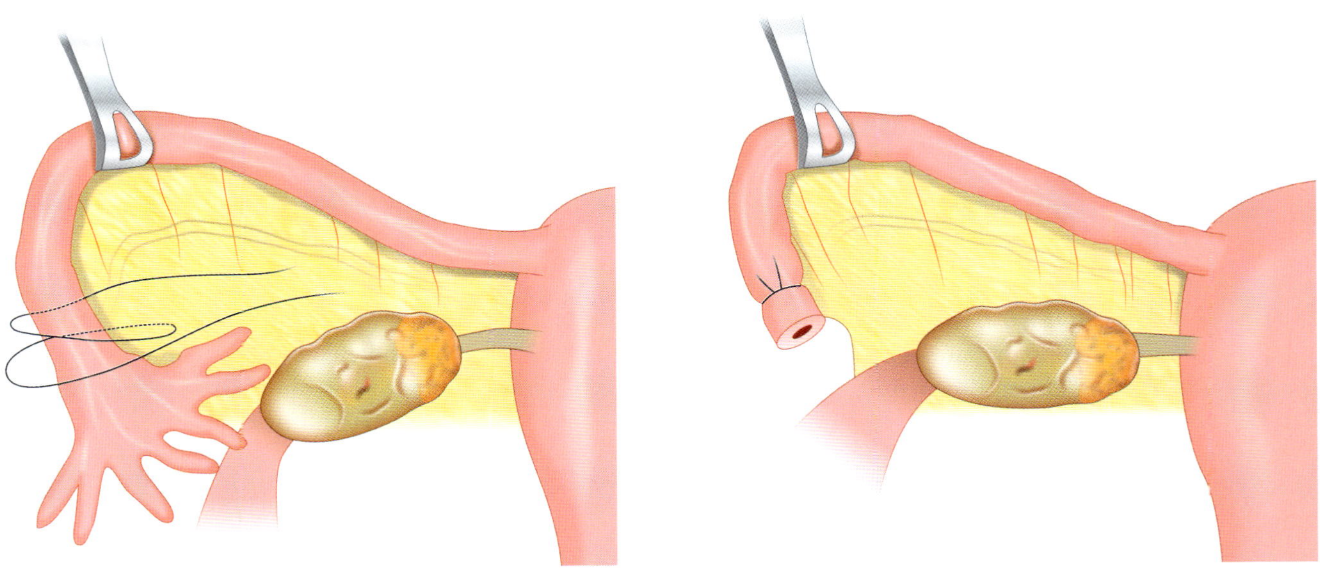

Fig. 4: Kroener's technique.

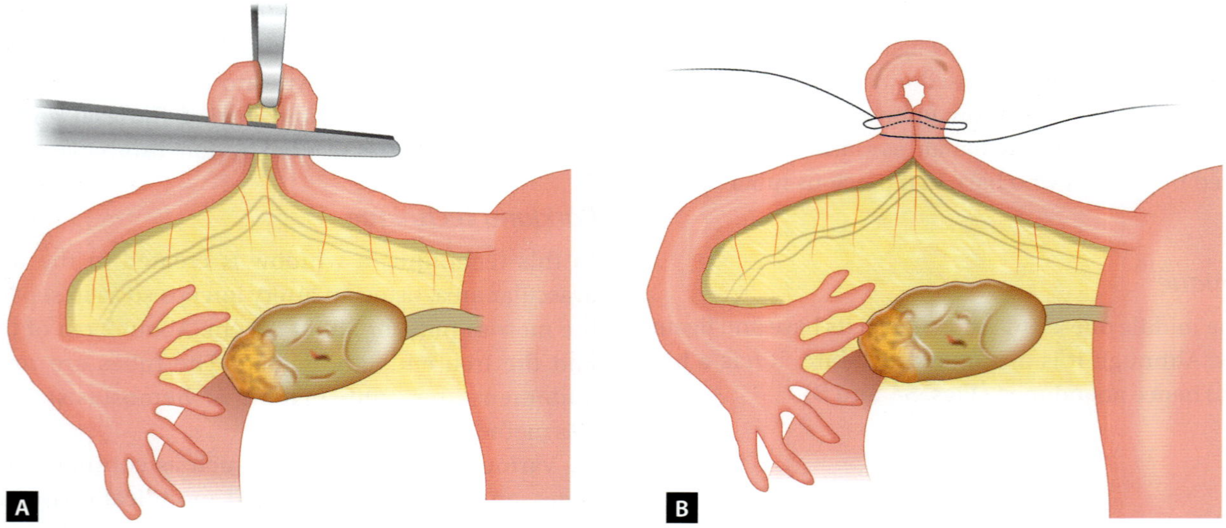

Figs. 5A and B: Madlener's technique.

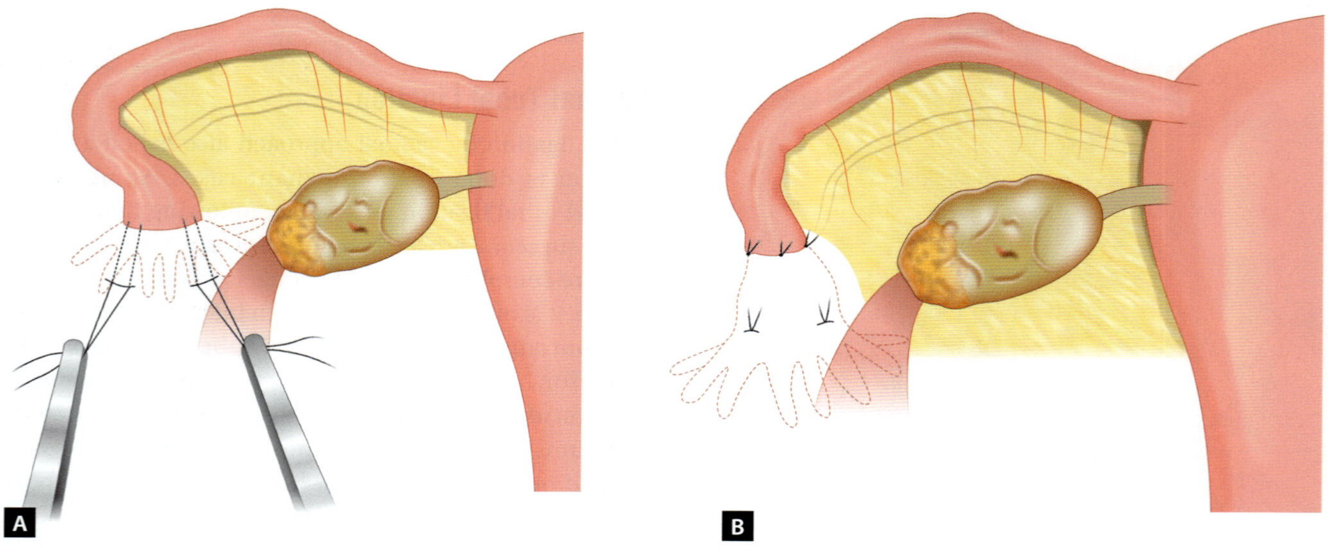

Figs. 6A and B: Aldridge technique.

In cases of vaginal prolapse during vaginal plastic repair, tubal ligation is done mostly by anterior colpotomy, otherwise done through posterior colpotomy.

Procedure: After general anesthesia, the patient is in semilithotomy position with head down; parts are cleaned with antiseptic solution and covered with sterile dressings. After a preliminary vaginal examination, the posterior lip of the cervix is held with the vulsellum. An Allis forceps is applied to the posterior fornix and the posterior vaginal vault and peritoneum is opened by means of a scalpel and scissors. If there is too much oozing from the cut vaginal mucosa, hemostasis is secured with a continuous locked suture. The uterus is pushed to one side using a Deaver's retractor or right angled anterior vaginal retractor, and the tube is bought down by a curved atraumatic forceps or Babcock's forceps. There may be difficulty in bringing the tubes down due to adhesions. Manipulations with sponge holding forceps or fingers or pulling down the ovarian ligament by means of a forceps may be needed at times.

Tubal ligation is done mostly by Pomeroy's method or by fimbriectomy or occlusion using Hulka-Clemens clip of silicone bands. The opposite tube is ligated by the same way and the colpotomy wound is closed with one layer of catgut stitches.

On discharge, the patients are given prophylactic antibiotics and are advised to resume ordinary work after pain relief. Abstinence is advised for 3 weeks at least as it may result in rupture of the vault with severe hemorrhage.

Advantages of vaginal ligation:
- It can be performed as an outpatient procedure.
- No abdominal scar is left.
- No special instruments required.
- Minimal postoperative pain.

Major drawbacks:
- Technically more difficult, requires training.
- Chances of failure.
- General anesthesia is required in most cases.
- Intraperitoneal contamination and infection is more frequent.
- Laparotomy is needed to complete the operation or deal with complications in at least 2–3% cases.
- Sexual intercourse is delayed.

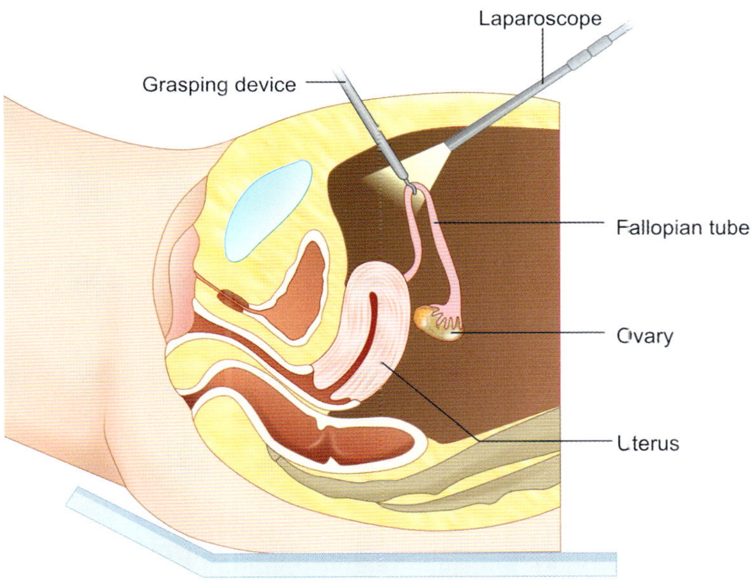

Fig. 7: Positioning for diagnostic laparoscopy. A secondary port at the suprapubic area for grasper to grasp fallopian tubes.

Laparoscopic Sterilization

Female sterilization with the use of an operating laparoscope is becoming more and more popular because it has been found to be safe, simple and an effective procedure that can be performed through one or two very small incisions or holes in the abdomen, mostly under sedation and local anesthesia on an outpatient basis. However, this procedure needs some special instruments and special training **(Fig. 7)**.

The use of laparoscope for female sterilization is widely being used since the 1970s.

Instruments

A gynecological minor set is required along with the following special instruments:

- *Laparoscopes:* Modern laparoscopies are thin metal tubes of 5–10 mm diameter with inbuilt lenses and prisms so as to give direct vision of the operating field; they have a fiber optic light bundle system to transmit cold light from an external source directly into the abdomen. There are two main types: (1) Straight type, with a built-in operating system used for applying clips on the Fallopian tubes. (2) Angled type, in which the view finder is set off from the main part and has a special sheath for introducing the operating system for fulguration or the use of silastic bands.
- *Lighting system:* A fiber optic external light source of sufficient power is used to provide intra-abdominal illumination through the laparoscope.
- *Gas insufflation apparatus:* This is used to produce controlled pneumoperitoneum of appropriate pressure and volume.
- *Veress needle:* This is a narrow needle with a spring-loaded obturator to cover the cutting edge of the needle upon entering the abdomen; it is used to introduce gas or air for pneumoperitoneum. This is safer than the Tuohy needle, which is also used for this purpose.
- *Trocars:* One or two steel trocars with pyramid-shaped points are used to puncture the abdominal wall; they have trocar sleeves through which laparoscopes are introduced. The flapper valve model is better because it allows laparoscopes to be introduced or withdrawn without escape of gas.
- *Intrauterine devices:* A combined sound and tenaculum or a Rubin's insufflation cannula is inserted into the uterus and manipulated by the assistant during the procedure.

The instruments are most effectively sterilized by soaking for at least 10 minutes in a solution containing 10% formaldehyde and glutaraldehyde (Cidex).

Anesthesia

Usually local anesthesia with slight sedation is used and more safe than general anesthesia which may be preferred by some surgeons and anesthetists.

Preoperative Preparations

Apart from the basic routine investigations such as hemoglobin, total and differential WBC count and ordinary urine analysis, the patient is required to starve for 6–8 hours before the operation.

Surgical Procedure

The patient is placed in the dorsal lithotomy position. Bladder should be emptied by urinary catheter.

The uterine manipulator is inserted to mobilize the uterus. Pneumoperitoneum is created by Veress needle with the help of CO_2 gas. First, after putting trocar site we should rule out omentum or small bowel injury. Next, the uterus, ovaries, and Fallopian tubes are viewed by anteverting or retroverting the uterus with the manipulator.

The Fallopian tubes are identified through the fimbrial end and which is differentiating them from the round ligament. They are then grasped and ligated by the various methods using clips or rings or by electrocoagulation techniques as discussed here.

All laparoscopic sterilization techniques should avoid medial segment of the Fallopian tube (2 cm) near the uterus. Direct pressure for prolonged time on this segment may increase the risk of tuboperitoneal fistula formation. The presence of a fistula increases the risk of pregnancy.

This procedure may be carried out through a single incision or a double incision in which the laparoscope is inserted through the primary port and the grasper through the other port.

Once both the tubes are ligated, the port sites are closed and patient is given rest till the postoperative pain fades away.

Contraindications

There are a few contraindications such as a large abdominal mass (uterine or ovarian tumor) needing laparotomy, decompensated heart disease, severe respiratory dysfunction, hiatus hernia and a history of abdominal surgery (especially the bowel).

Relative contraindications are gross obesity with thick abdominal wall and pelvic adhesions due to previous pelvic surgery or infections.

Methods of Tubal Occlusion

Laparoscopic tubal occlusion is done by electrocoagulation or nonelectrical methods using silastic bands or spring loaded clips (Hulka–Clemens). The electrocoagulation methods cause less pain but may produce serious gastrointestinal burns, burns of other organs, vessels and abdominal wall. Unipolar coagulation causes a greater extent or burns hence now almost given up.

Bipolar electrocoagulation technique: To reduce the chance of burns due to unithermal electrocoagulation, bipolar electrocoagulation was introduced. In this technique, the current flowing from the electrotherm machine enters and leaved the body through the same instrument. The forceps grasps the mobile midportion of the tube, and a current is passed for about 10 seconds from the bipolar generator. The fulguration involves only a small portion of the tube and some part of the mesosalpinx. Some surgeons cut the fulgurated part of the tube, but as it produces more complications, it is discouraged.

Clips: Two types of clips are mostly used, the spring loaded clip (Hulka–Clemens clip) and the silicone titanium clip (Filshie clip). The current model of Hulka–Clemens clip consists of two plastic jaws with interlocking teeth. The jaws are held together by together by a stainless steel spring which is pushed forward to lock the clip in place over the tube. A clip is placed at the isthmus about 2–3 cm away from the uterus **(Fig. 8)**.

The *Filshie clip* is made with titanium with the inner surface lined by silicone. When the clip is applied over the tube, the upper jaw latches under a hook in the lower jaw. The latest models have hinged jaws that open and close easily, allowing easy removal and repositioning when needed. The clips are more suitable in young women who may need reversal and in postabortal cases when the tubes are edematous. The clips cause least damage to the tubes (about 1 cm) **(Fig. 9)**.

Falope rings: This was introduced by Yoon in 1974. At present in India, this silastic band is most popular. It is used in laparoscopic tubal ligation. The Falope ring is made up of a silicone rubber with 5% barium sulfate having an outer diameter of 3.6 mm and inner diameter of 1.0 mm and thickness of 2.2 mm. The specially equipped laparoscope is loaded with the two Falope rings and is inserted in the standard fashion. After identifying one of the Fallopian tubes, the tongs of the band applicator are extended and the tube grasped about 3 cm from the uterus, choosing a thin portion of the tube. The tube is then brought into the applicator and the band is pushed over the knuckle of the tube. The tongs are then released and the tube is dropped. The other tube is occluded by the same way. If a double-incision technique is used, the band applicator is inserted through the second trocar **(Fig. 10)**.

The clips cause least damage (1 cm), Falope rings (3 cm), and with the Pomeroy method (3–4 cm). Hence, chances of reversal are best with clips and postoperative pain is most with the band technique.

Advantages of Laparoscopic Sterilization

- Very effective method of contraception as compared to long-term temporary methods.
- Cost effective.
- Does not need long-term motivation.
- Reversal possible.
- Very low complication rate.
- Limited restriction of activity postoperatively, can be done as an outpatient procedure.

Disadvantages

- Steep learning curve.
- Rate of complication is low but if complications occur, they can be dangerous.
- Postoperative shoulder and chest pain due to insufflations of abdomen with gas.
- Equipment is costly and difficult to maintain.

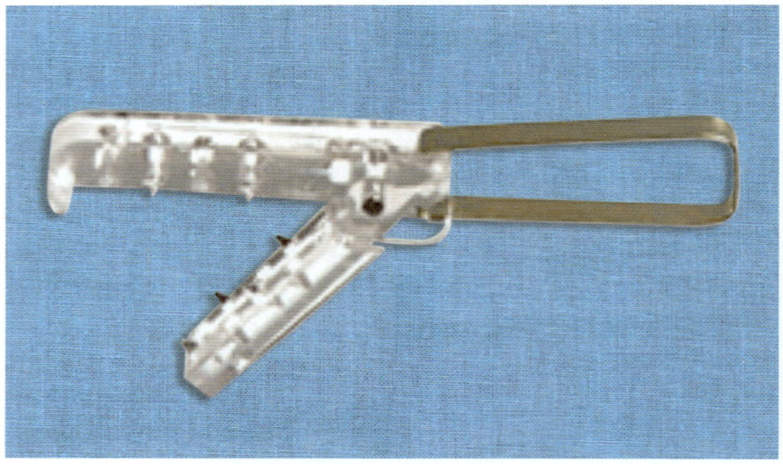

Fig. 8: Hulka–Clemens clip.

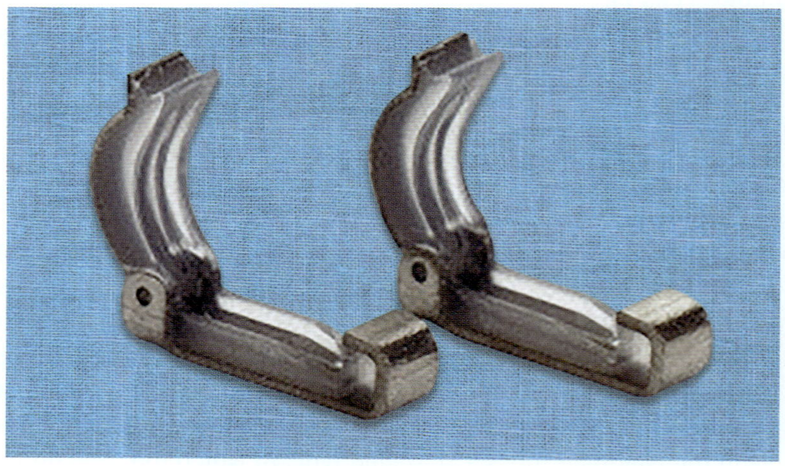

Fig. 9: Filshie clip.

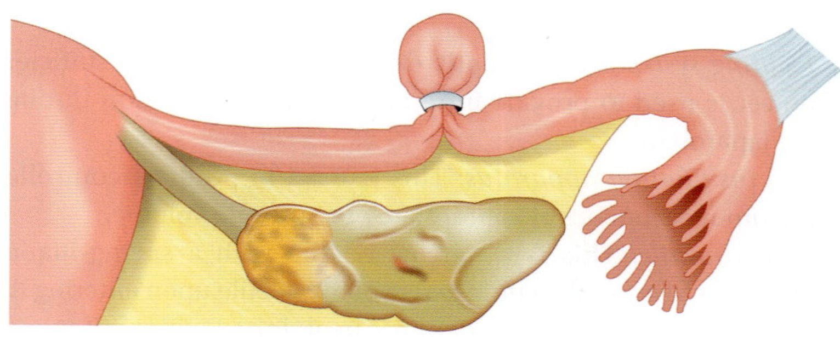

Fig. 10: Falope ring.

Complications

Actual complications are rare but if they happen—wound sepsis, abdominal wound hematoma, surgical emphysema, and uterine injury are the minor complications.

Serious and more dangerous complication include anesthetic hazards, injury to intestines, large vessels, burns of gastrointestinal tract and other pelvic organs, mediastinal emphysema, cardiorespiratory embarrassment and even death.

Failure Rates

Typical failure rate following female sterilization by laparoscopic sterilization in India are reported as 0.2–1.3%. Failure rates can be higher when performed by inexperienced surgeons and in camp setup.

Failure rate has also been the highest when spring clips were used or when coagulation procedures were followed, rather than when silicone bands were used.

Long-term Risks (Real or Suspected)

- Chances of ectopic pregnancy
- Regret following sterilization
- *Post-tubal sterilization syndrome*: Abnormal menstrual bleeding, dysmenorrheal and premenstrual distress. But various studies done have shown no association between these symptoms and tubal ligation.

OTHER METHODS OF FEMALE STERILIZATION

- *Essure:* It is a microcoil (formerly called STOP) developed lately, which is a spring-like device. This is introduced using a hysteroscope inserted through the vagina into the uterus then the Fallopian tubes. In 3 months' time, a scar tissue grows into the device and plugs the Fallopian tube. It is an outpatient procedure and done under local anesthesia. It is successful in 90–95%. The placement is confirmed by USG or X-ray after 3 months; hence till then another form of contraception needs to be used. It is not very popular and yet to be FDA approved **(Figs. 11A to C)**.
- *Hysterectomy:* It is used as sterilization method only in special cases such as mentally ill patients who cannot take care of themselves and require hysterectomy for other pathologies also.
- Substances like Quinacrine were widely used in the past, as it is a sclerosing agent; however since it is a blind procedure and has harmful side effects, it is not routinely used now. Also it has high failure rates.

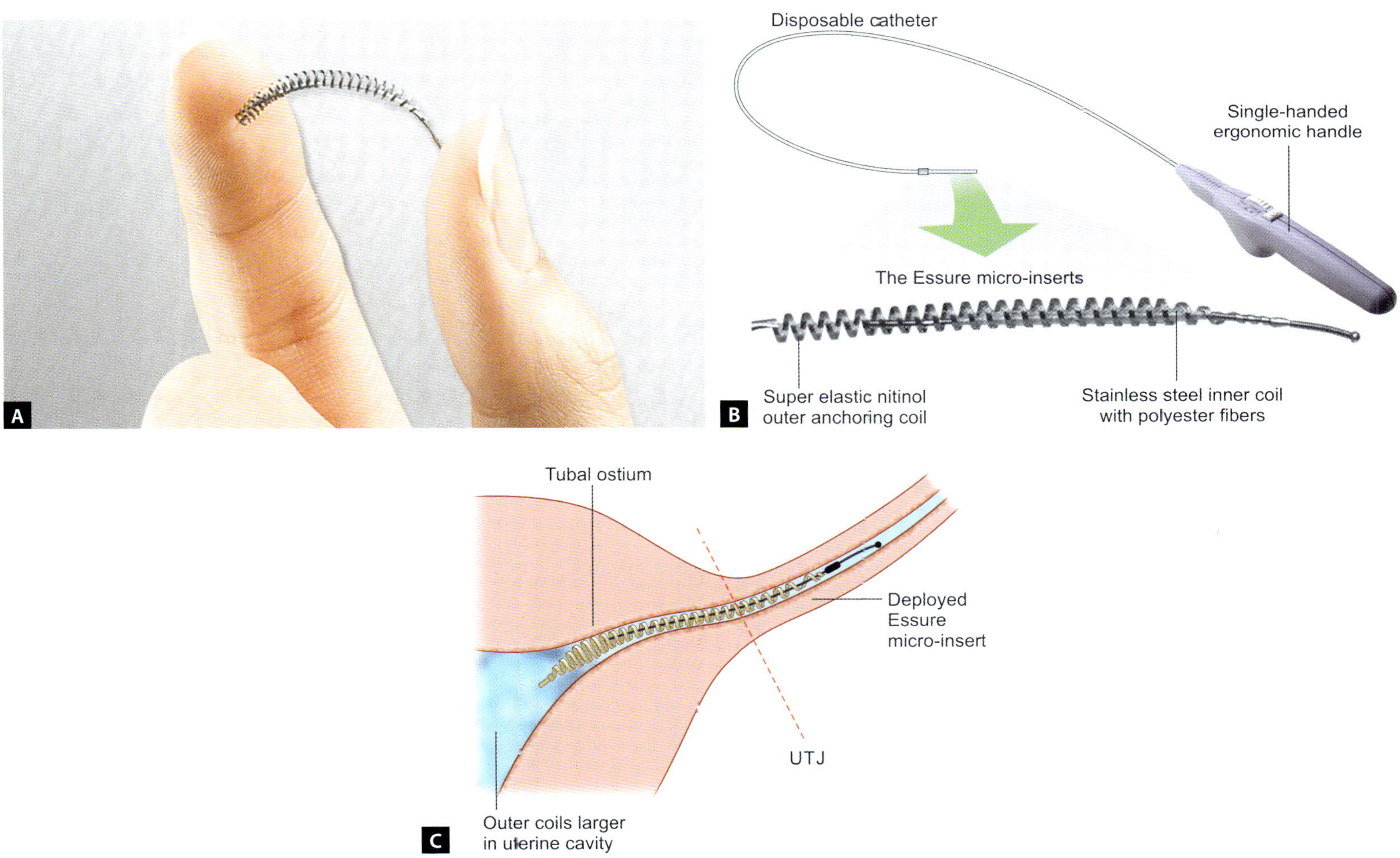

Figs. 11A to C: Essure coil placement hysteroscopically.

LAPAROSCOPIC BILATERAL TUBAL LIGATION (FIGS. 12 TO 31)

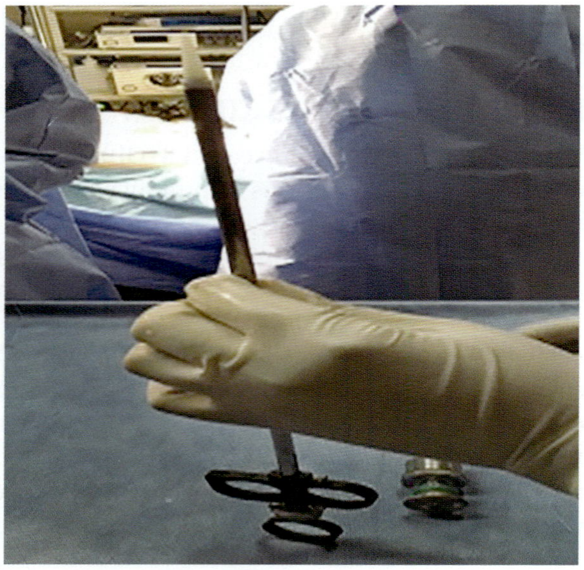

Fig. 12: Ring applicator.

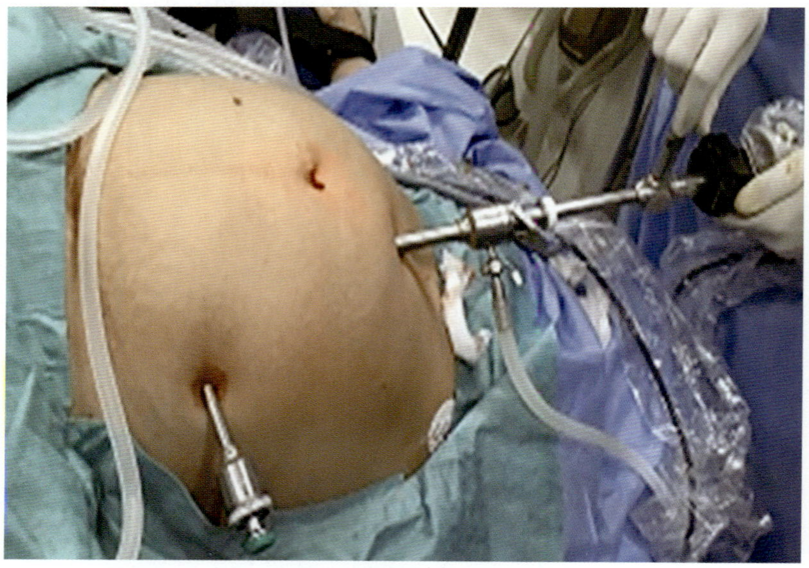

Fig. 13: Placement of trocars.

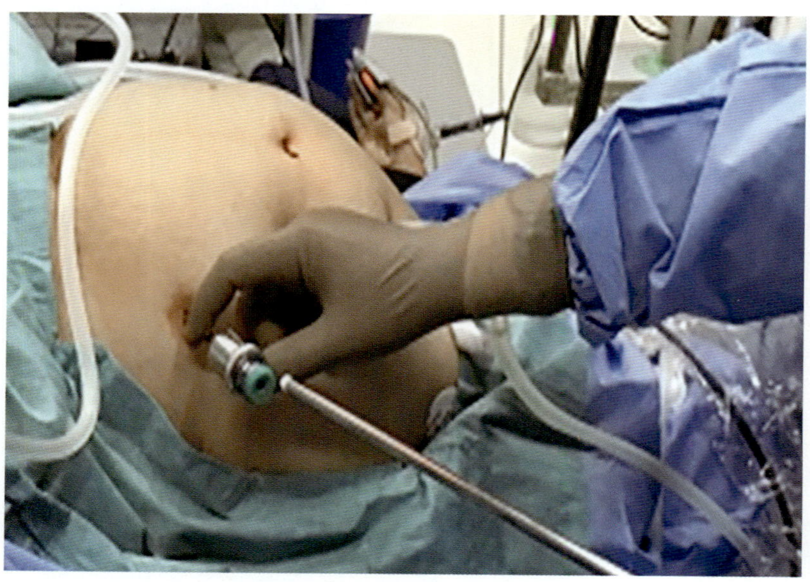

Fig. 14: Introduction of ring applicator.

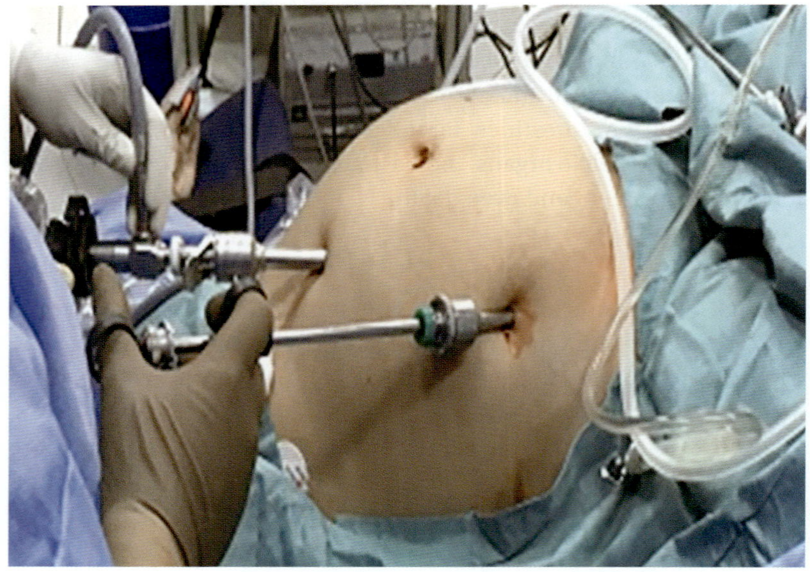

Fig. 15: 7-mm trocar as left lateral secondary port.

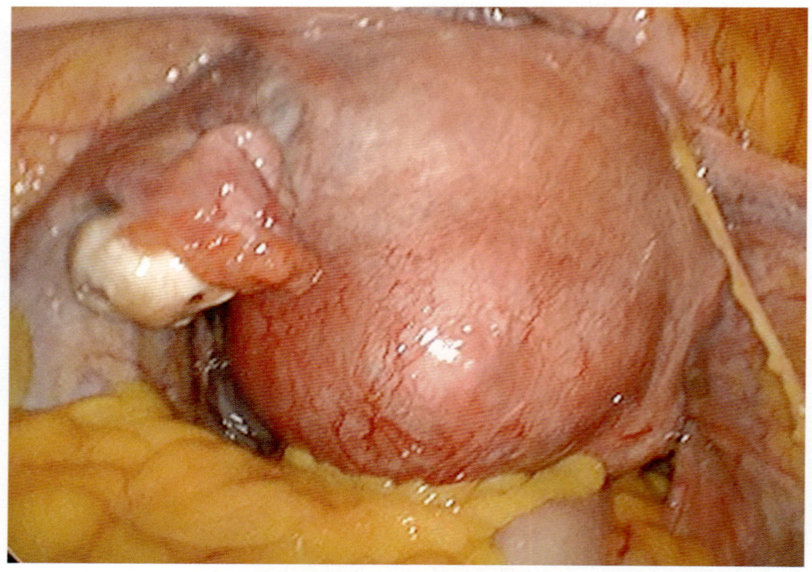

Fig. 16: Tubal ligation in patient with previous three lower segment cesarean section.

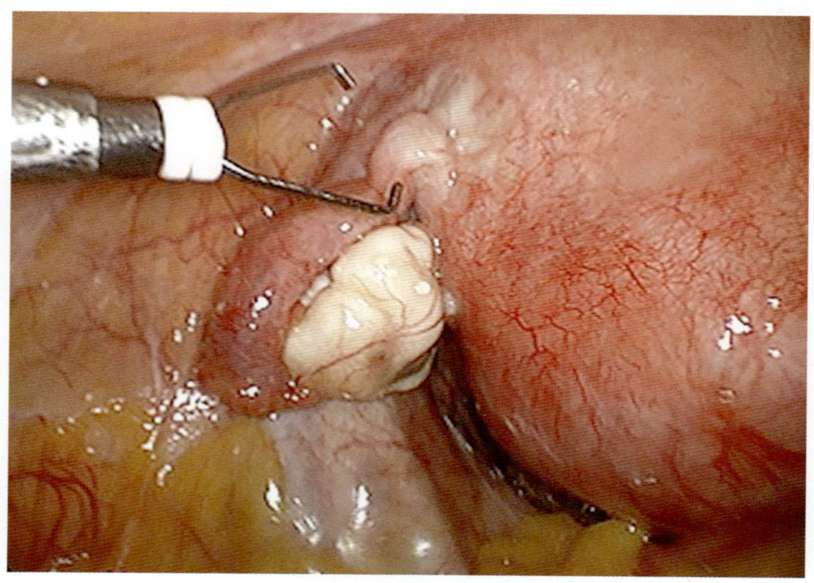

Fig. 17: Opening the prongs.

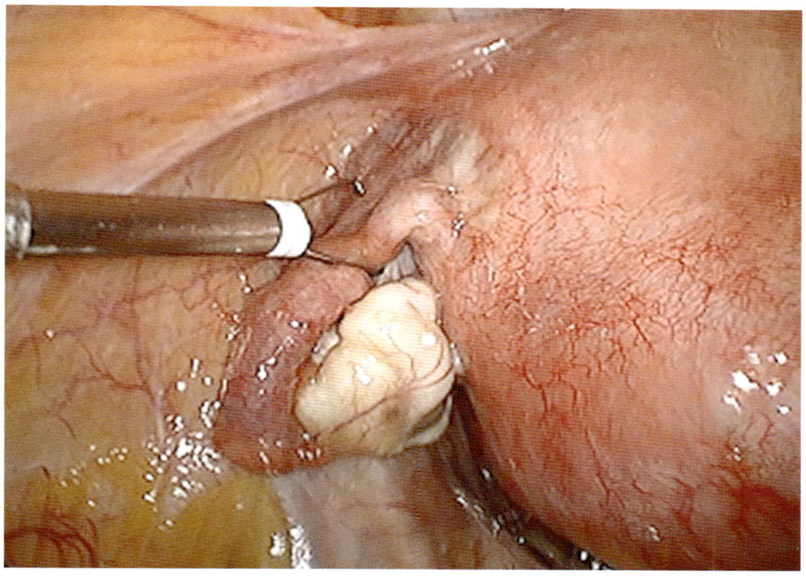

Fig. 18: Hold the fallopian tubes near isthmic portion.

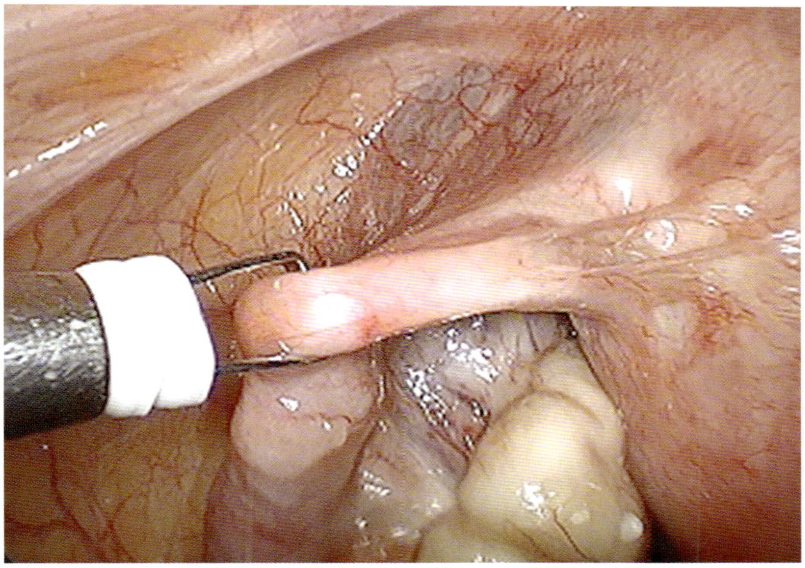

Fig. 19: Pull the prongs into applicator along with fallopian tube.

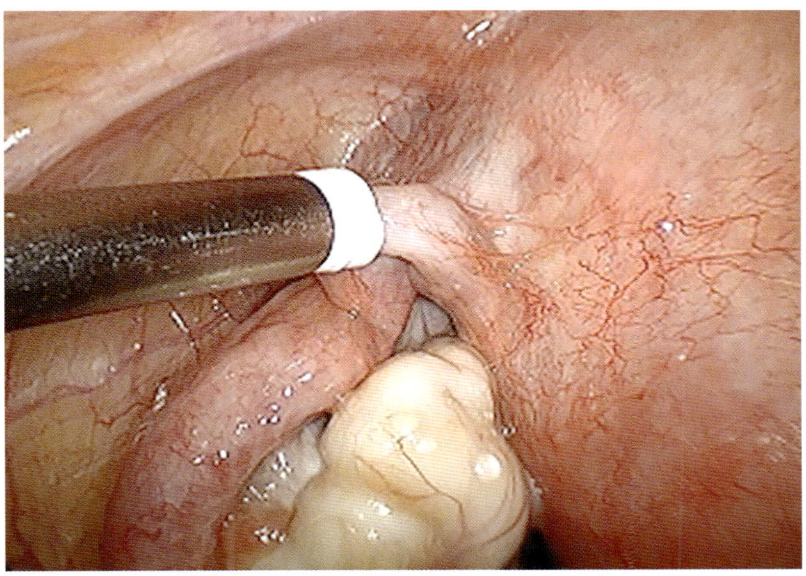

Fig. 20: Applicator should encircle tube.

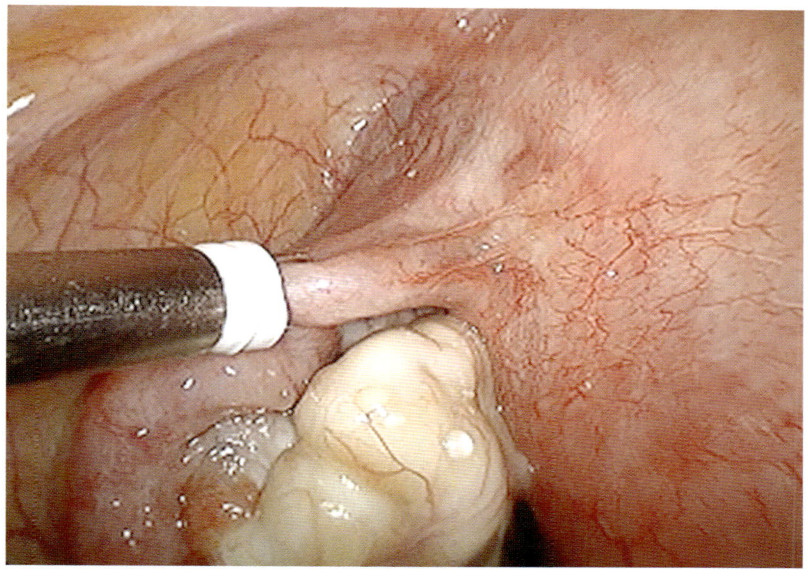

Fig. 21: 1.5–2-cm tube is pulled in.

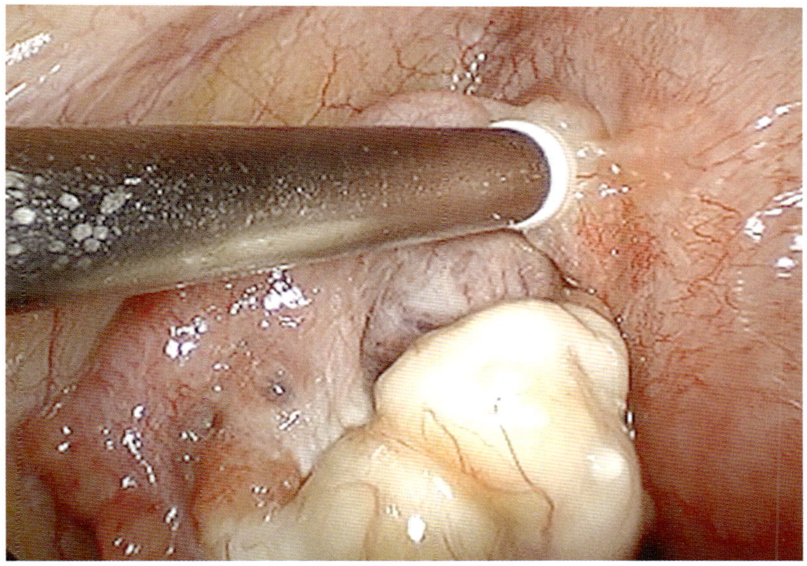

Fig. 22: Large sheath will push the tube toward fallopian tube (left).

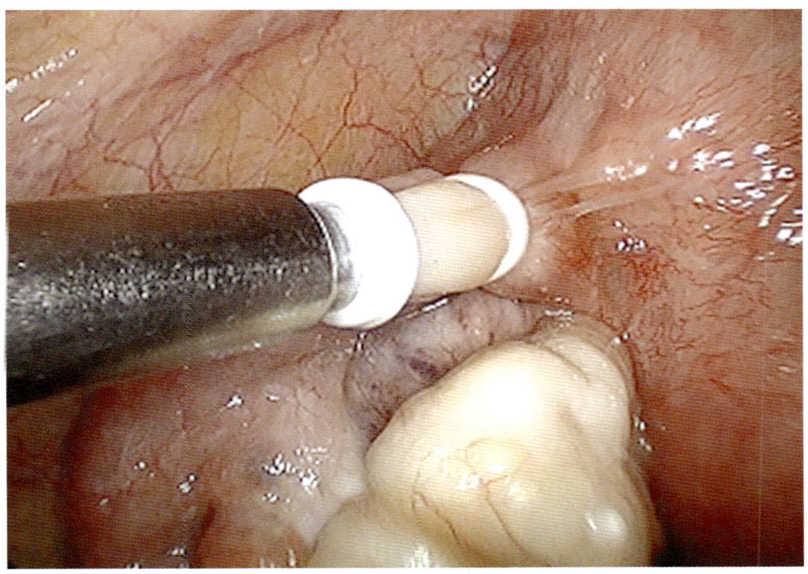

Fig. 23: Falope ring over loop of tube grasped by prongs.

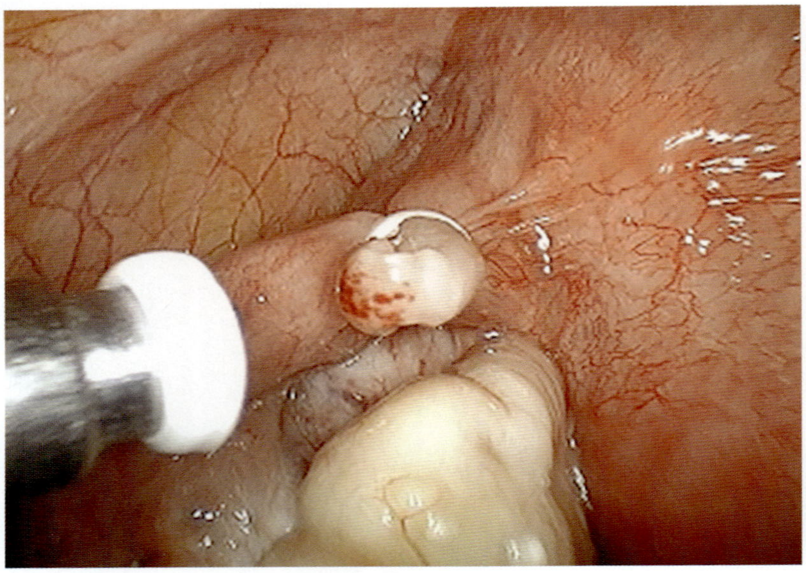

Fig. 24: Left side tubal ligation.

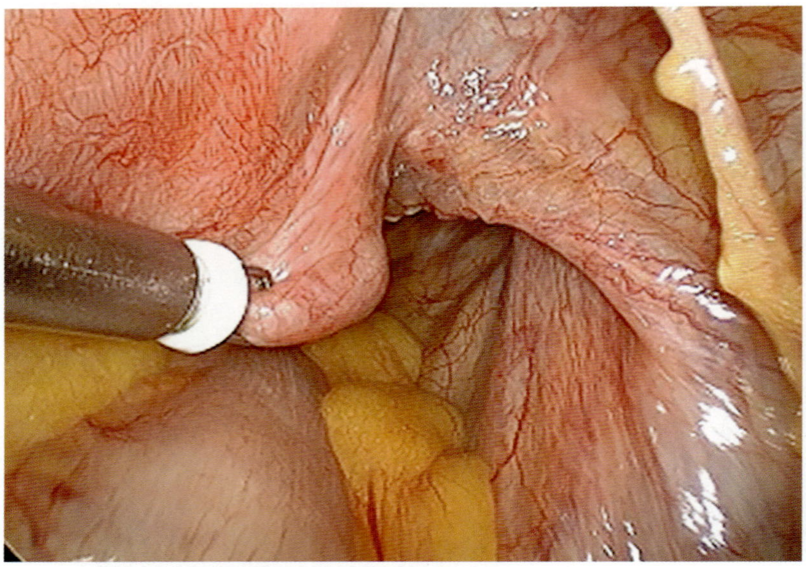

Fig. 25: Introduction of applicator.

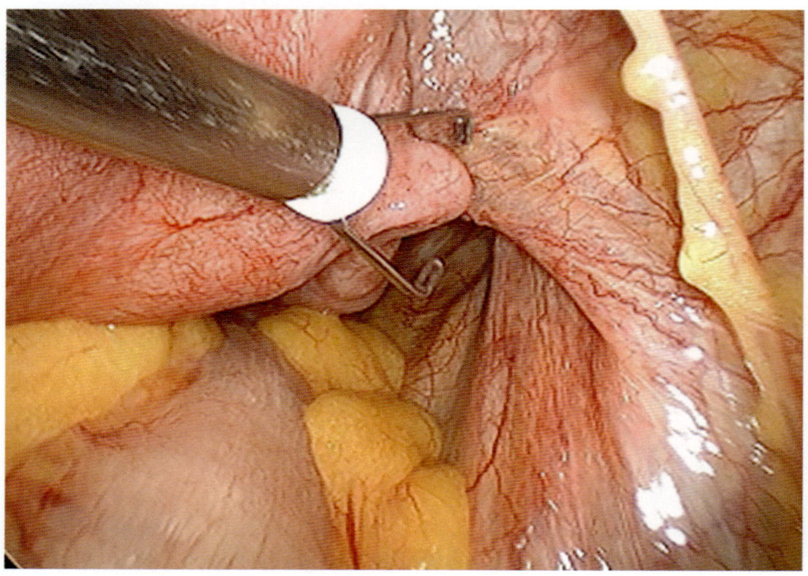

Fig. 26: Opening prongs of applicator.

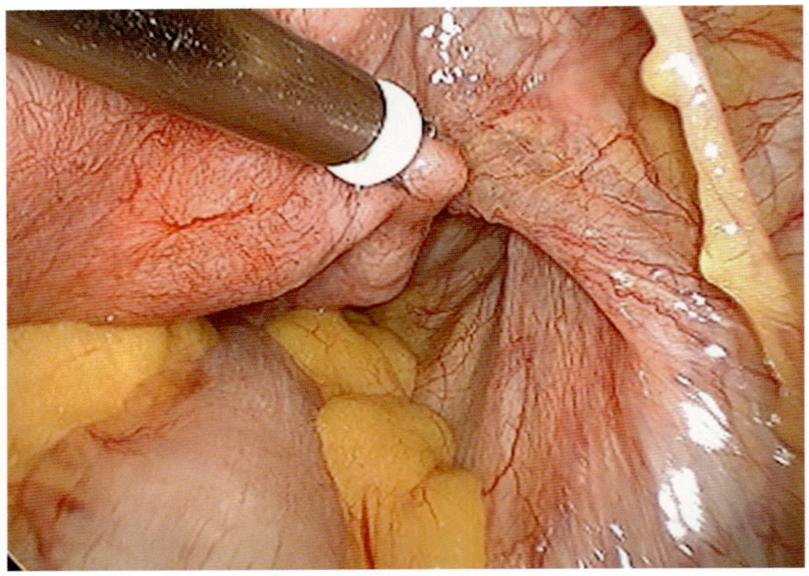

Fig. 27: Pull the prongs into applicator.

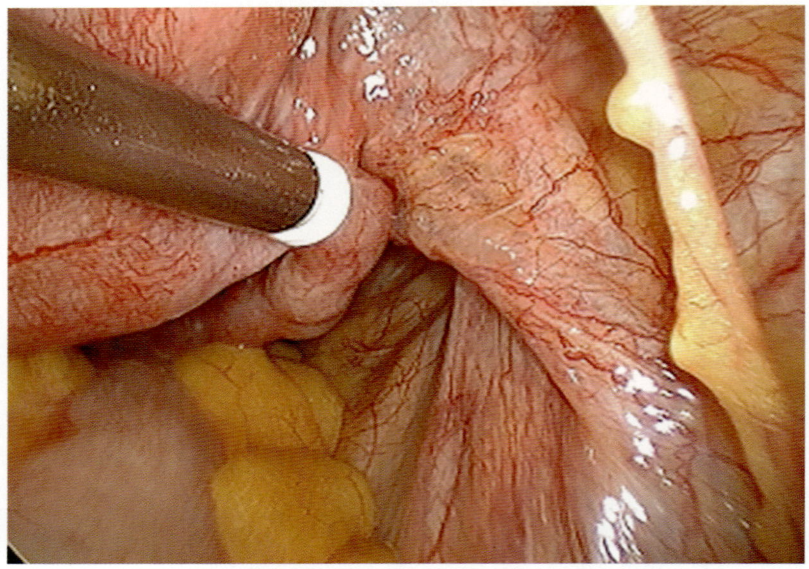

Fig. 28: Large sheath will push the tube toward uterus fallopian tube (right).

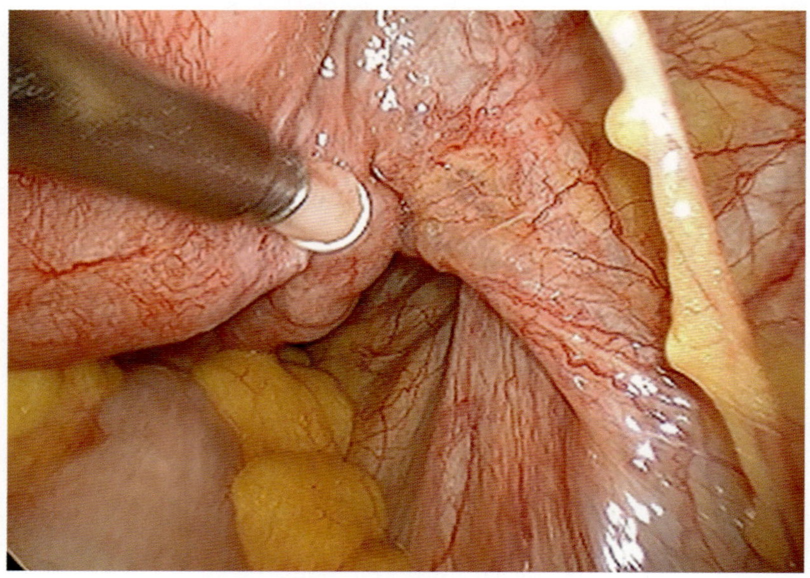

Fig. 29: 1.5–2 cm tube is pulled in aplicator.

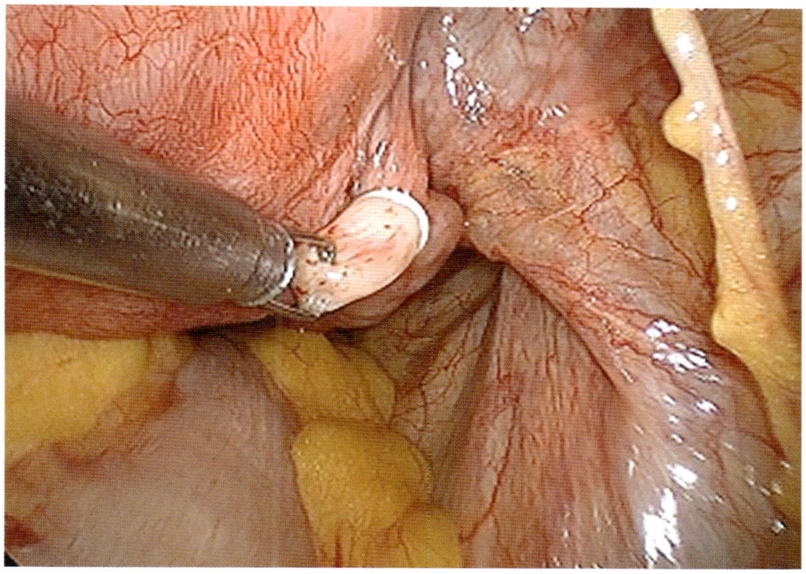

Fig. 30: Falope ring over loop cf tube grasped by prongs.

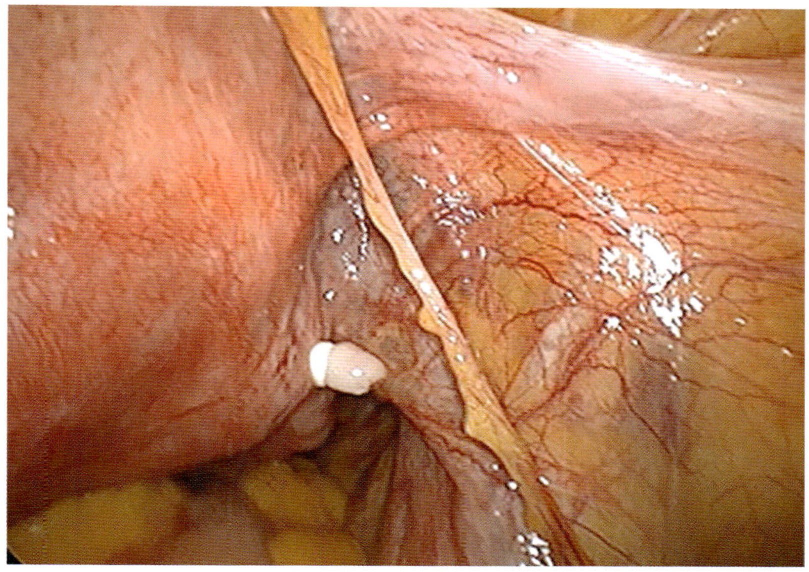

Fig. 31: Right-sided tubal ligation.

BILATERAL TUBAL LIGATION IN BICORNUATE UTERUS (FIGS. 32 TO 38)

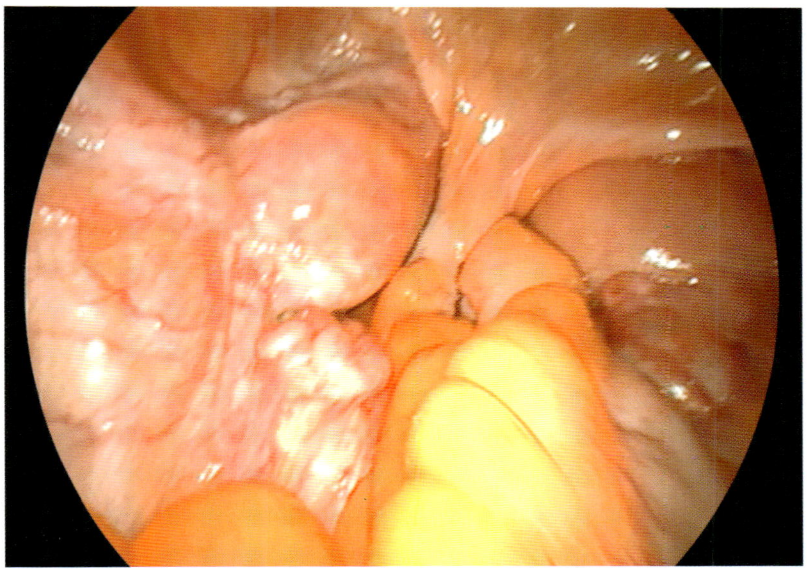

Fig. 32: Bicornuate uterus.

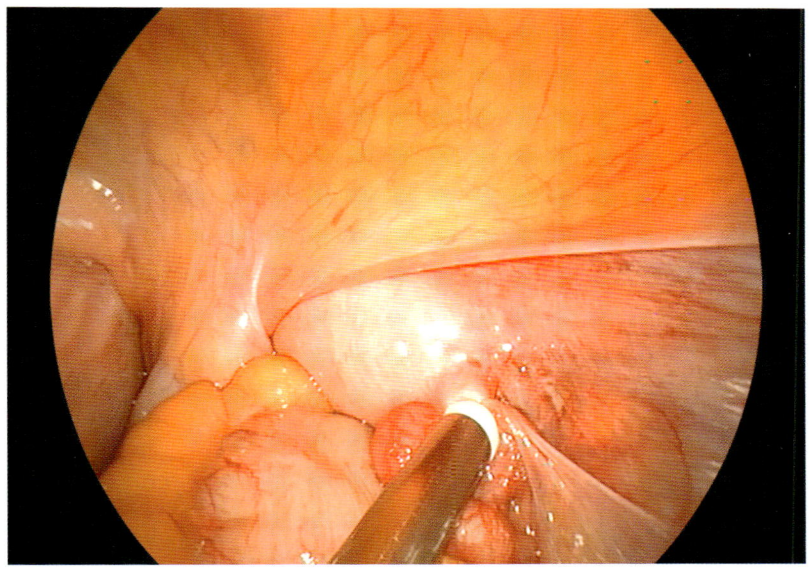

Fig. 34: Pull the prongs nto applicator.

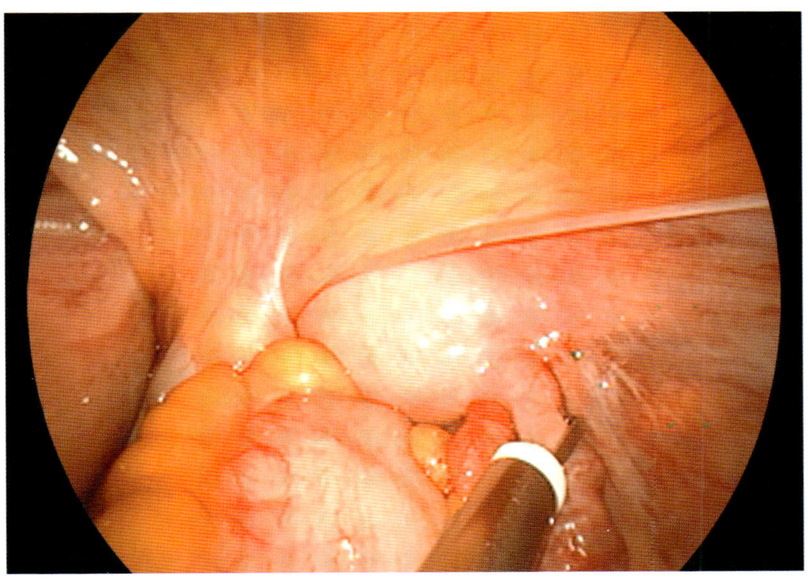

Fig. 33: Opening prongs of applicator.

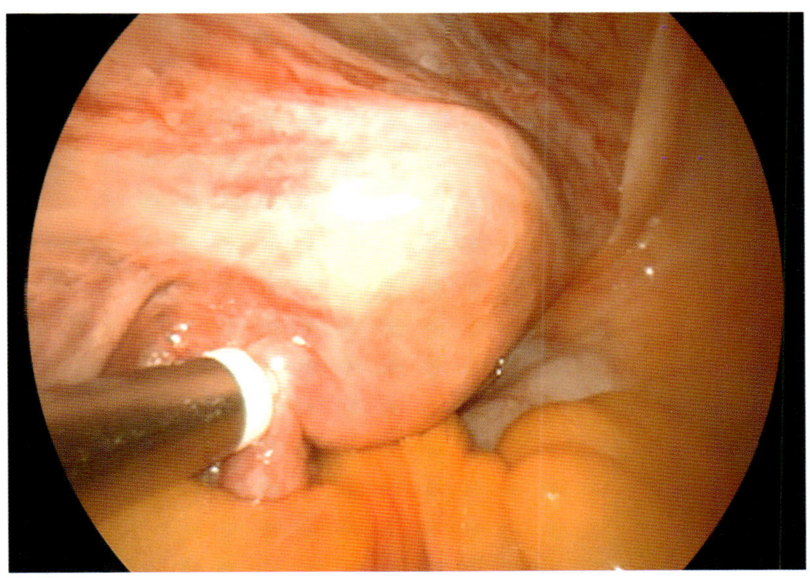

Fig. 35: 1.5–2 cm tube is pulled in.

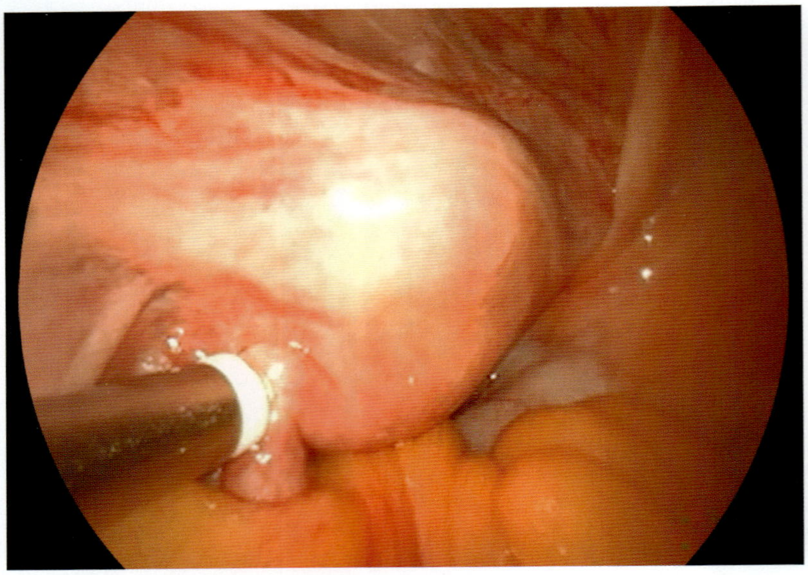

Fig. 36: Falope ring over loop of tube grasped by prongs.

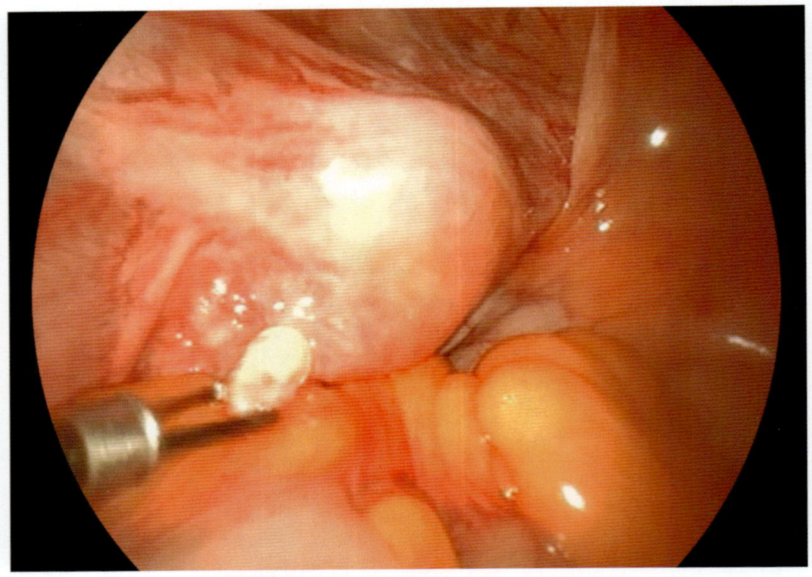

Fig. 37: Right-sided tubal ligation done.

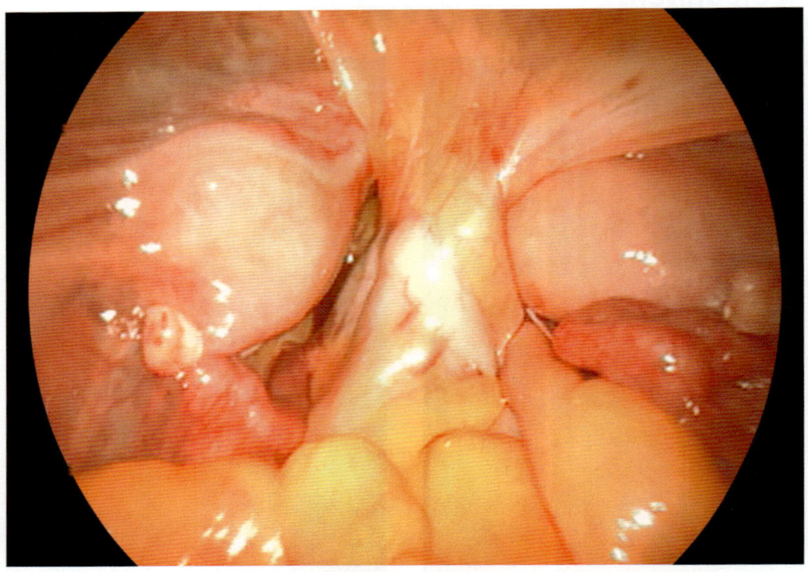

Fig. 38: Bilateral tubal ligation of bicornuate uterus.

CHAPTER

12

Salpingostomy

Sowmya MS, Isha Rani, B Ramesh

INTRODUCTION

Increase in the diagnosis of ectopic pregnancy is seen in the recent past due to the advent of sensitive human chorionic gonadotropin (hCG) assays and widespread use of transvaginal sonography. With technical advancement, even the treatment options have increased.

As a result, ectopic pregnancy is identified early, and medical or surgical therapy can be given promptly. Surgical treatment can be performed, either radical or conservative. It can be performed both by laparotomy and by laparoscopy, laparoscopic approach being the gold standard. Other modality of treatment of ectopic pregnancy being expectant management and medical management using methotrexate and other drugs.

Mode of treatment is decided on various parameters, one of them being level of hCG. Methotrexate (MTX) is the drug of choice for medical management. MTX suspension under laparoscopic guidance was a common mode used until 1993 (Fujishita et al., 1995).[1] However, MTX therapy has some disadvantages such as inadequate decline of hCG concentration after MTX injection, and the requirement for additional MTX injection or surgical interventions. Women with ectopic pregnancy tend to reject MTX therapy because of its side effects and uncertainty of treatment.

Bruhat et al. described a method for conservative laparoscopic surgery in ectopic pregnancy for the first time.[2] Since then, due to the technical developments, today the technique includes both radical treatment and various conservative pharmacological management strategies.[3] In women who wish to preserve future fertility, conservative surgery by linear salpingotomy is the gold standard for the management. Laparoscopic conservative surgery has been reported to have advantages in terms of efficacy, safety, cost, and subsequent reproductive outcome in comparison with laparotomic surgery.[4-6]

SURGICAL PROCEDURE

The laparoscopic procedure was performed as described by Pouly and Tulandi and Saleh.[3,7] Briefly described, usually two operating trocars (5 mm) at lateral suprapubic site are used, but in the cases of salpingotomy with suturing, a 5-mm suprapubic ancillary port is added. In patients with hemoperitoneum, aspiration of blood and washing is done for better visibility. Either regular suction pump with normal saline is used or single roller pump is used for suction and irrigation of fluids. Evaluation of the tubal site for operation and measurement of the lengthwise and crosswise extension of swelling tubes was done using a 5-mm probe.

In order to prevent hemorrhage, vasopressin (20 U in 200 mL of normal saline) is injected to the mesosalpinx. An incision is made over the antimesenteric border of the fallopian tube, at the point of maximum bulge unipolar electrocautery, the argon laser, or CO_2 laser may be used. If bleeding persists, it should be controlled by pressure or micropinpoint cautery. Use of energy sources should be as minimal as possible. The irrigation and suction tube (5 mm) is then introduced through the salpingotomy incision, and all clots and trophoblastic tissues are aspirated. In most cases, aspiration removed the product of conception entirely. In some cases, hydrodissection (saline solution was injected under high pressure) or grasping forceps, is attempted to separate the trophoblast from the tubal wall. Surgical specimens were generally withdrawn through the 10-mm trocar sleeve after grasping the tissue with claw forceps and passing through the operating channel of the laparoscope. All the clots and products of conception should be removed and contralateral fallopian tube should be inspected. If any bleeding or oozing of blood from inside the lumen or tubal wall happens, or there is complete tubal damage, salpingotomy should be switched to salpingectomy.

Incision is either closed two layers or is left open and employed a running locked suture for hemostasis.[5] Semm described a laparoscopic method of reapproximation with an ethicon endosuture system using the extracorporeal knot.[3] Bruhat et al. preferred to leave the tubal incision open.[2] Reich et al. initially used Klepinger bipolar forceps to pinch the cut ends together; however, they later abandoned this technique in favor of Bruhat's method.[9] Nelson et al. compared primary and secondary closure of ampullary salpingotomy in a rabbit and found no statistically significant difference in subsequent pregnancy rate, nidation indices, or percentage of adhesions. Studies have shown no significant difference between tubal suturing and keeping the salpingostomy open in the number of subsequent intrauterine pregnancies and repeat ectopic pregnancies. Based on these data, it seems reasonable to speculate that primary closure of the tubal wall is unnecessary.[10]

Contraindications

There are no absolute contraindications to salpingostomy. However, in certain conditions, caution has to be exercised.

The relative contraindications to be considered are as follows:

- *Interstitial pregnancy*, as the incision can be followed by an acute hemorrhage which may be difficult to control.

- *Massive bleeding with tubal rupture.* It can be impossible to stop the bleeding without salpingectomy.
  As already explained earlier, there is a risk for persistent trophoblastic disease, risk is further increased in the following situations, hence making them relative contraindications:
- Hematosalpinx of size >4 cm
- High hCG level (>10,000 IU)
- Ectopic pregnancy with a living fetus.

POSTOPERATIVE WORK-UP

Postoperative complications are rare, but persistent trophoblast can occur after conservative treatment.

The persistence of trophoblast is infrequent after salpingectomy (0.2%) as a whole segment of fallopian tube is removed. If milking of fallopian tube, trans abdominal or trans trocar extraction of specimen is done, there is risk of persistence of trophoblast as during extraction a part may drop down and get implanted in peritoneum. So, in order to ensure complete resolution monitoring of hCG level is done weekly till it is negative. This level must be <2% of the initial level.

After salpingotomy, this risk is greater. The incidence differs largely from one series to another. In the Epidemiological Register for Ectopic Pregnancy in Auvergne (EREPA), the risk was <5%,[11,12] but some series have reported risks at over 20%. These failures occur for two different reasons. Poor operative technique explains largely the failures in the high-frequency series. This is the reason why we have underlined some of the technical aspects, such as the place of salpingostomy, the size of the aspiration device, and the danger of "milking", However, even with a perfect technique, a risk exists, related to deep infiltrating trophoblast in cases of active pregnancy. Hagström et al.[13] demonstrated that a rapid kinetics of the hCG, a high hCG level and a high progesterone level are predictive of this risk of failure.

The early detection of a failure also forms part of the treatment; the drop in hCG must be monitored. In 1992, a monitoring algorithm was published that still holds good.[14] The relative hCG level must be measured on the second postoperative day and later if necessary. If it is still over 35% on the second day, failure is extremely probable and subsequent treatment must be applied.

In case persistent trophoblastic disease is suspected, MTX injection should be an option rather than a second laparoscopy, as it reduces hCG levels in >95% cases.

STEPS OF SALPINGOSTOMY (FIGS. 1 TO 13)

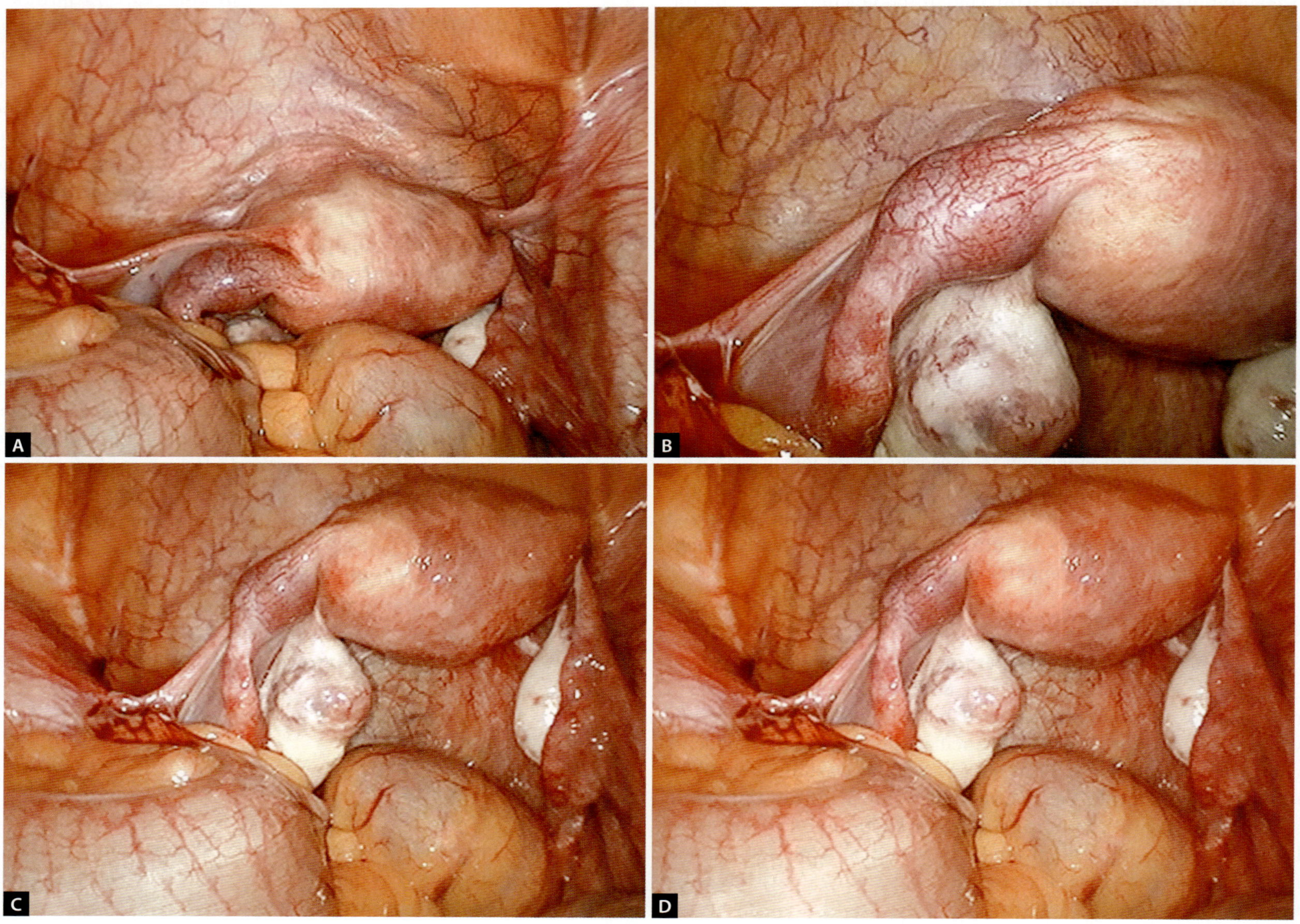

Figs. 1A to D: Panoramic view of left-sided unruptured ectopic gestation.

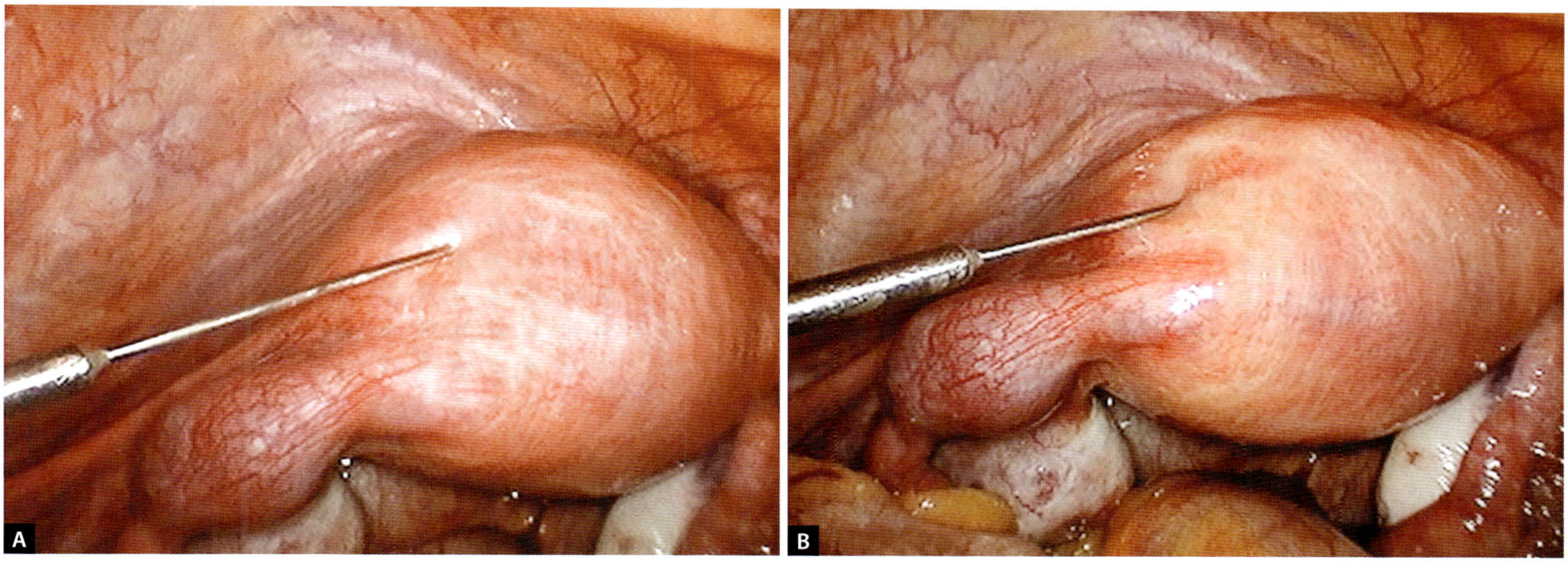

Figs. 2A and B: Injection of diluted vasopressin into uterine wall.

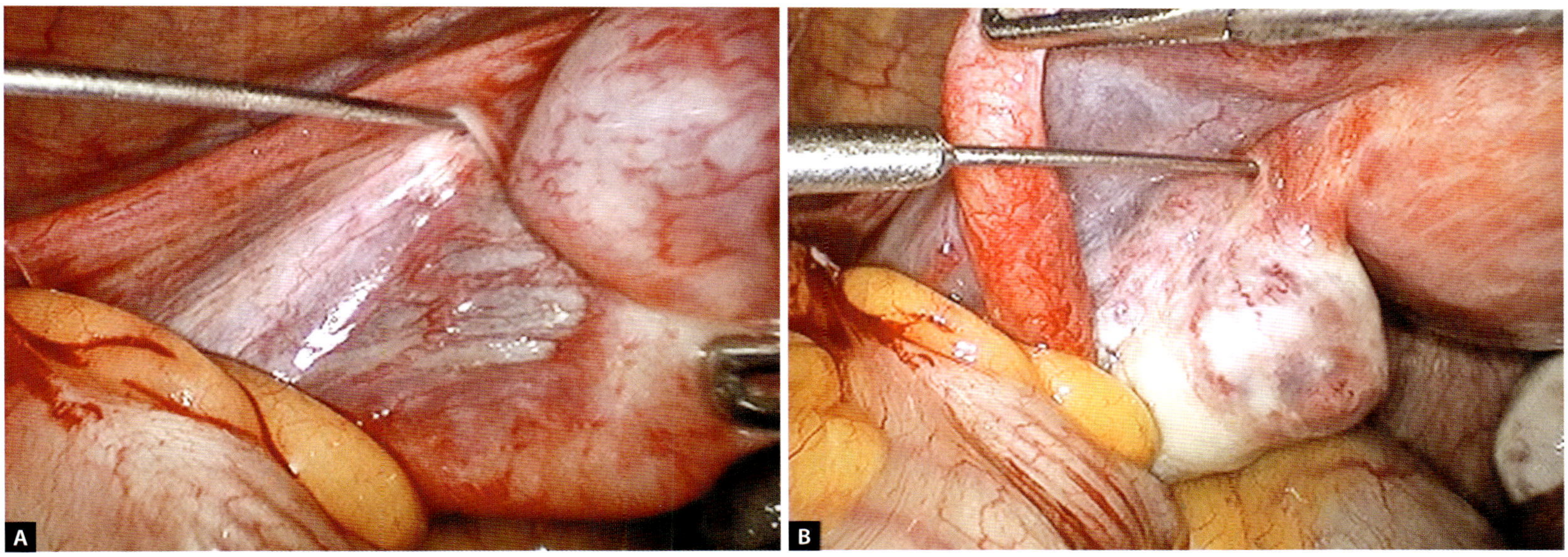

Figs. 3A and B: Injection of diluted vasopressin into mesosalpinx.

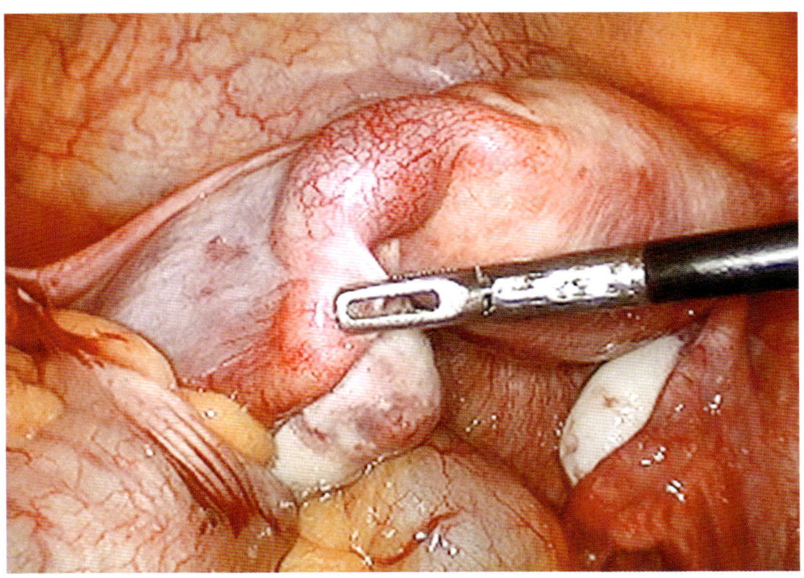

Fig. 4: Mesosalpinx after injection vasopressin.

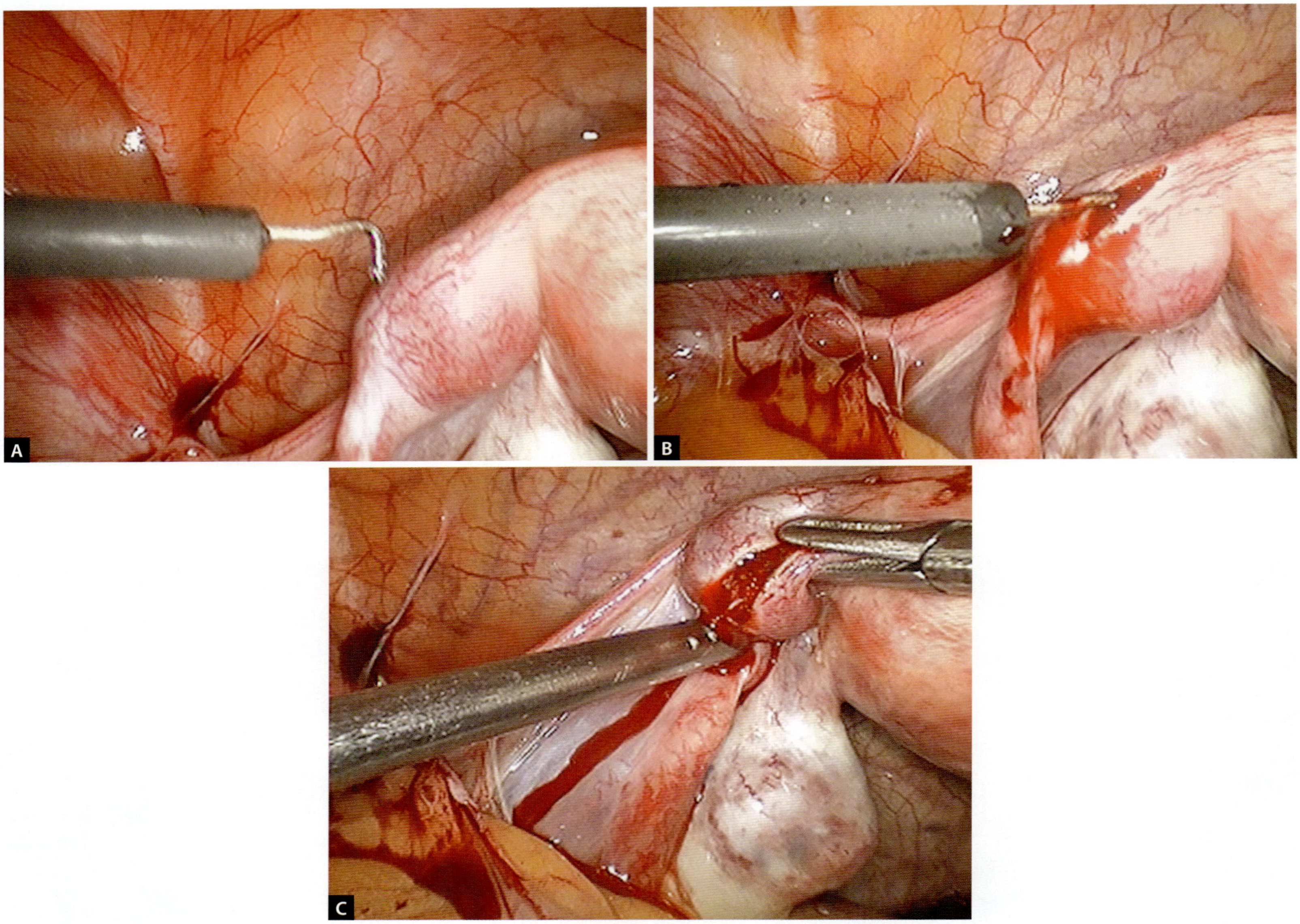

Figs. 5A to C: Incision taken over ectopic sac with monopolar needle.

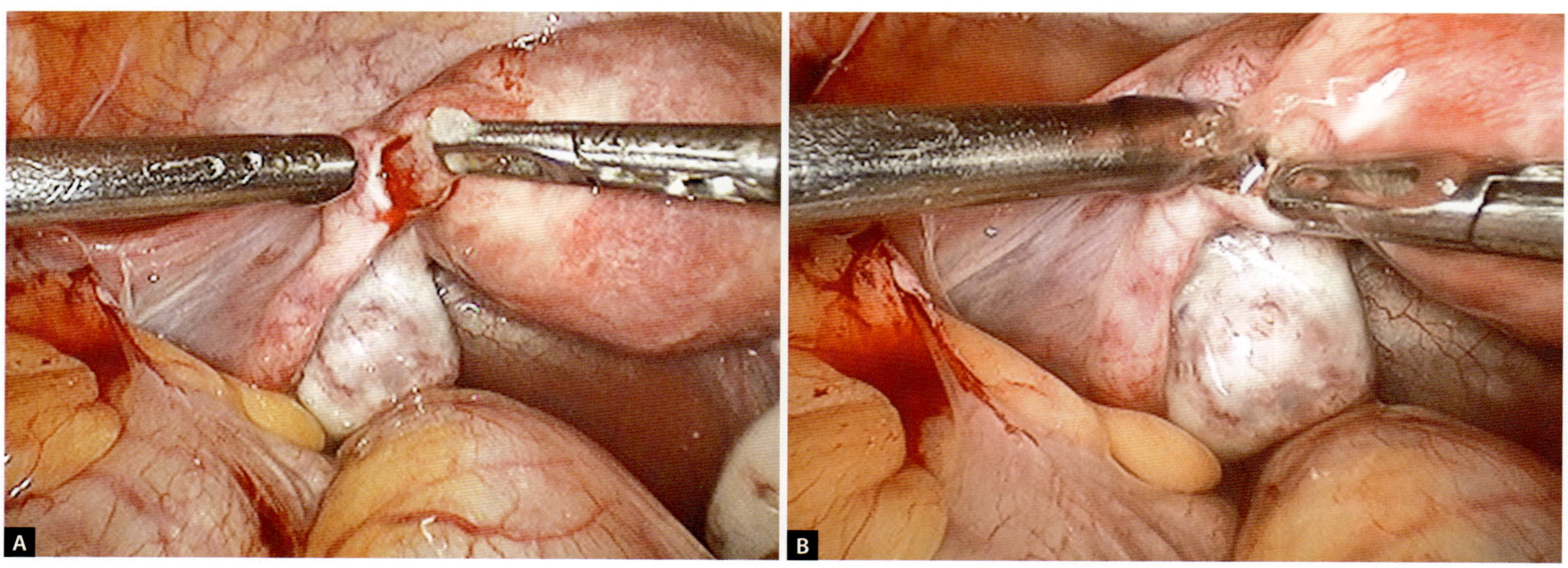

Figs. 6A and B: Removal of ectopic sac with grasper and suction cannula.

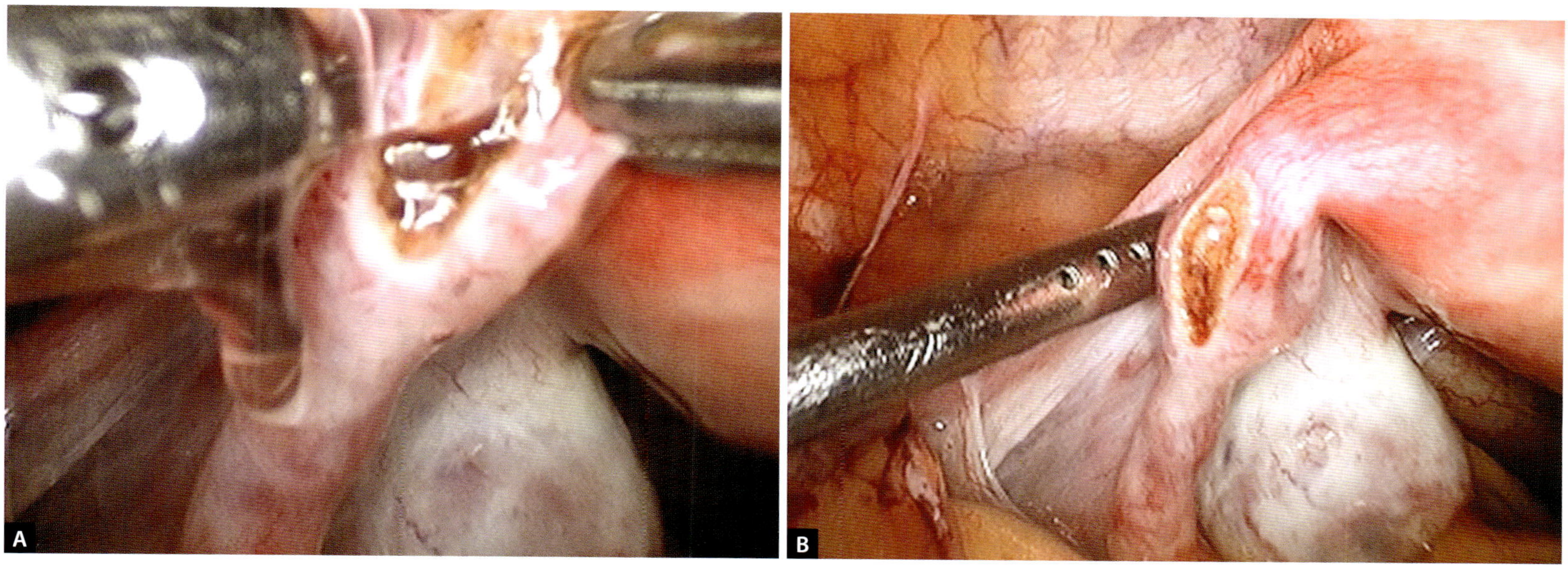

Figs. 7A and B: Irrigation of tube at the site of ectopic.

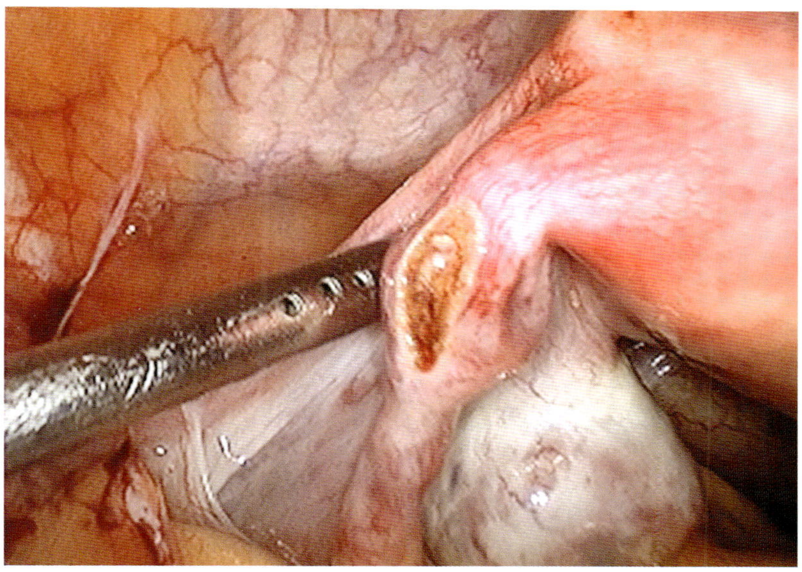

Fig. 8: Postsalpingostomy status of tube.

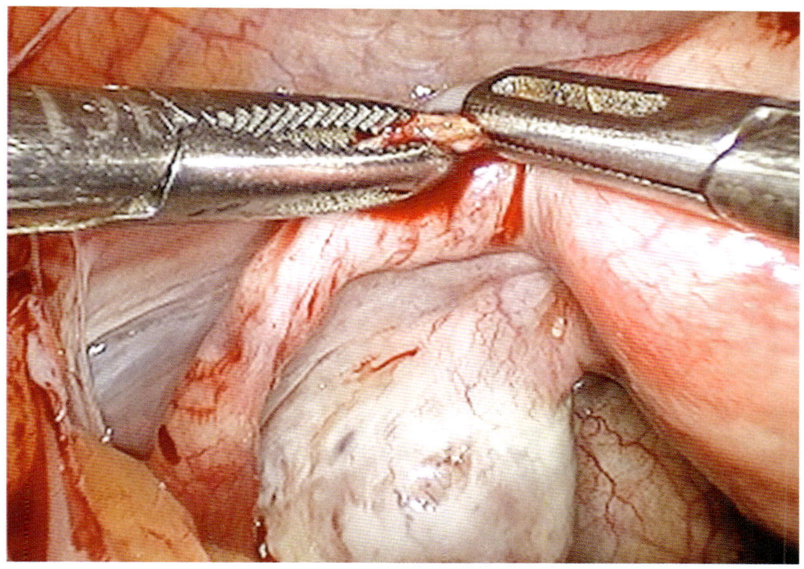

Fig. 10: Compression continued.

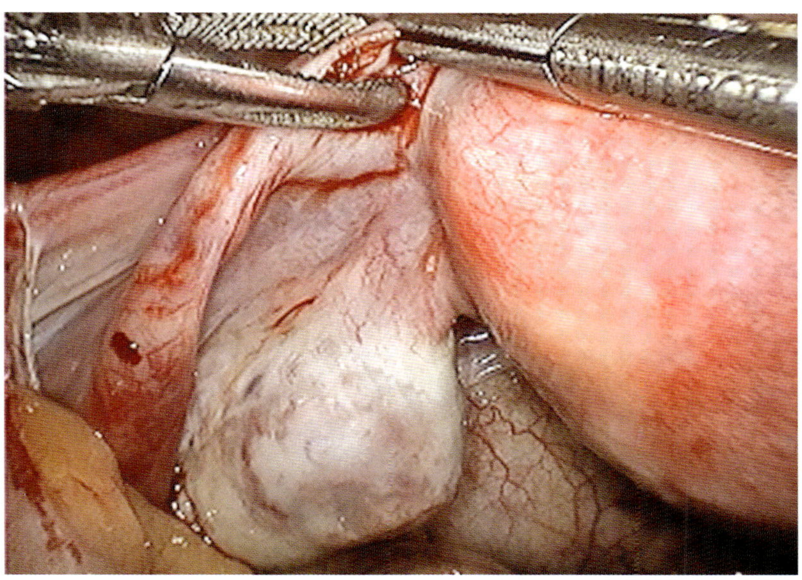

Fig. 9: Mechanical compression of salpingostomy site with plain graspers.

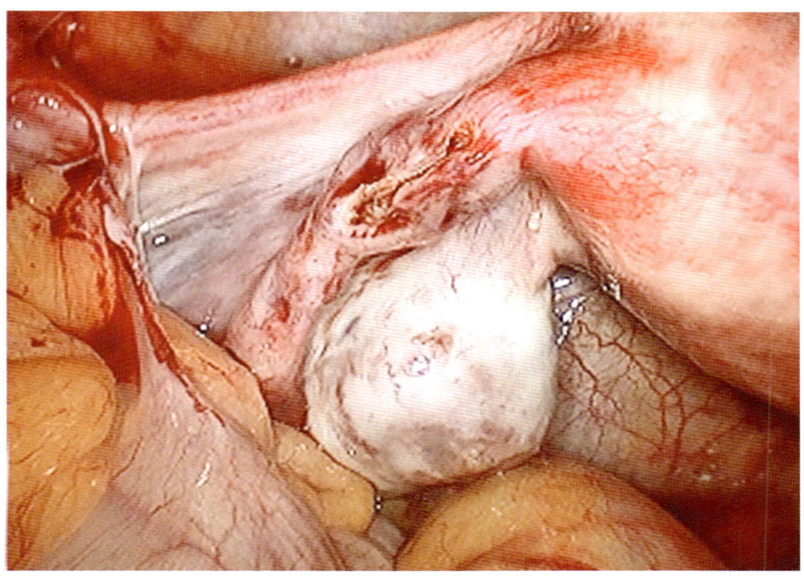

Fig. 11: Release of compression.

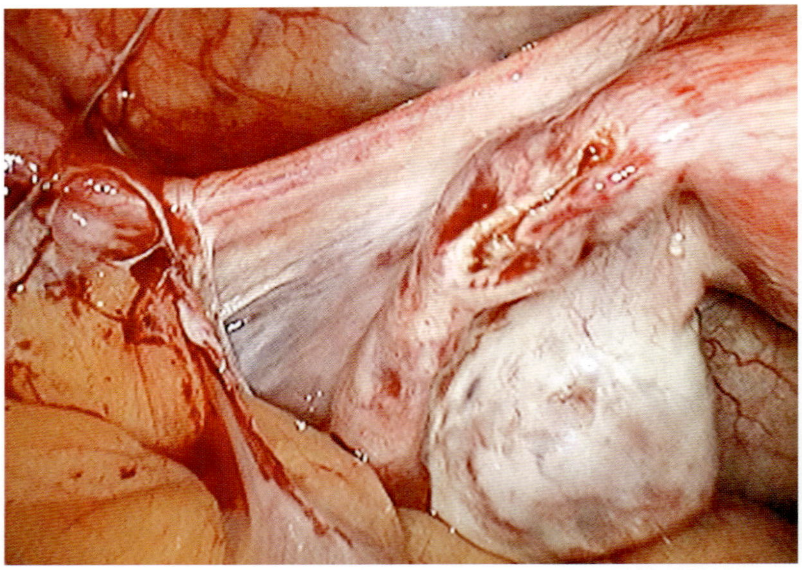

Fig. 12: After mechanical compression postsalpingectomy status hemostasis achieved.

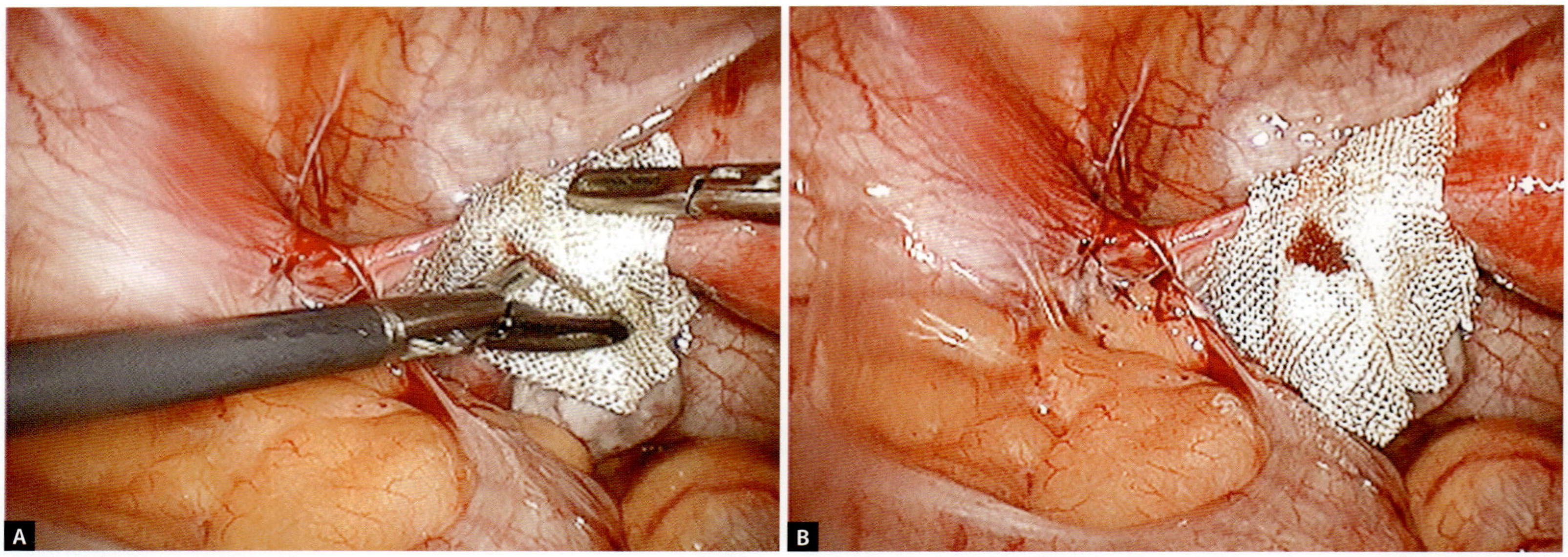

Figs. 13A and B: Placement of interceed over salpingostomy site.

SALPINGOSTOMY WITH SUTURING (FIGS. 14 TO 20)

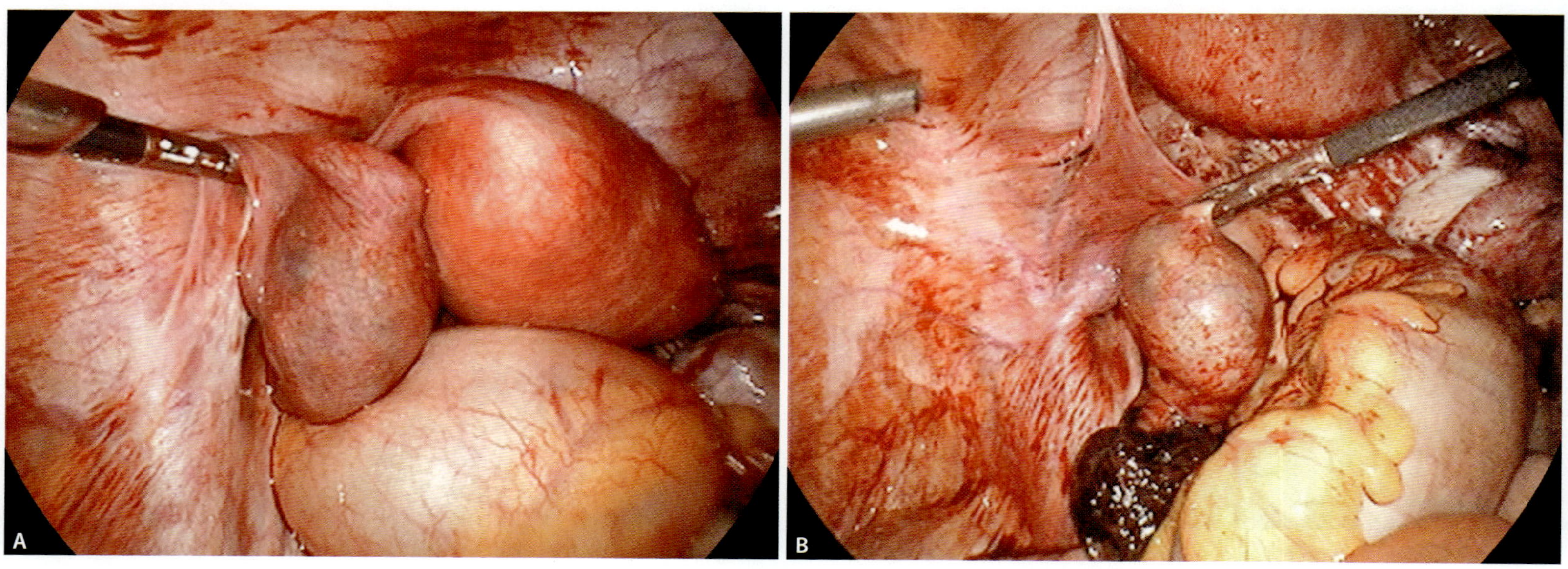

Figs. 14A and B: Panoramic view of left sided unruptured tubal ectopic.

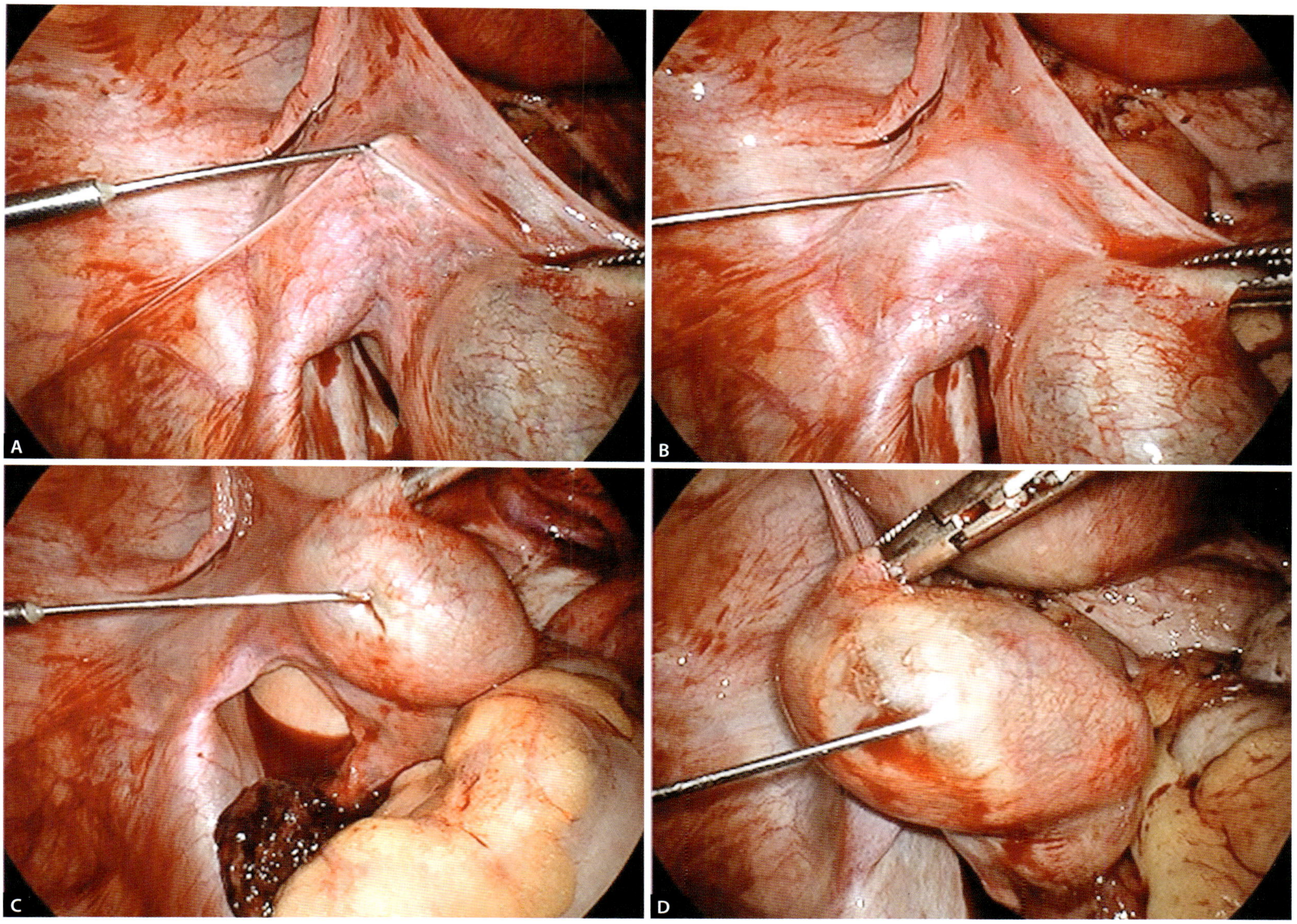

Figs. 15A to D: Injection of diluted vasopressin into mesosalpinx and ectopic sac.

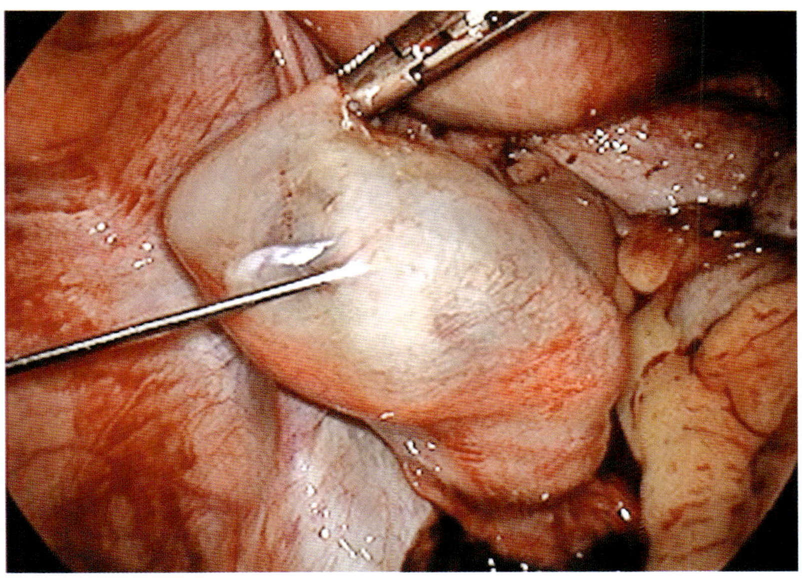

Fig. 16: Blanching of tubes seen after vasopressin injection.

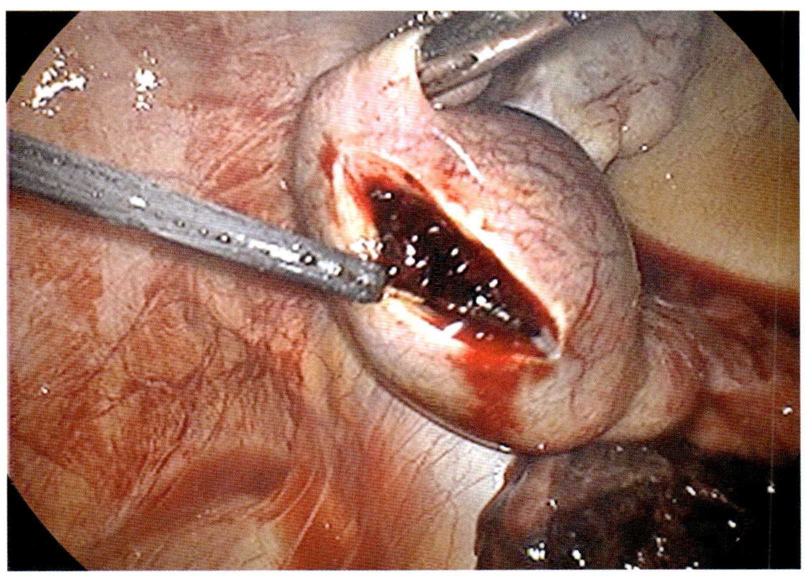

Fig. 17: Incision of ectopic sac with monopolar.

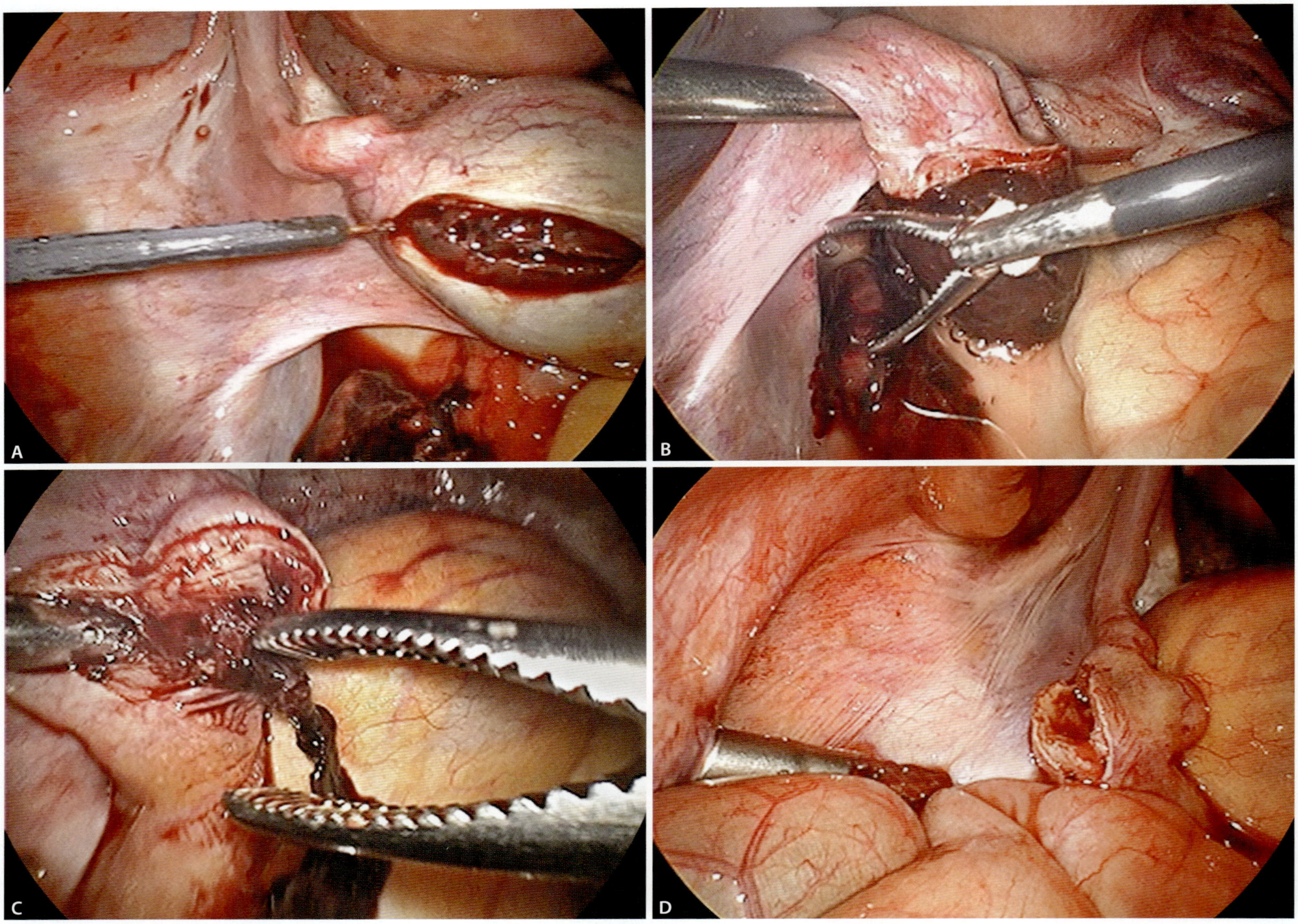

Figs. 18A to D: Removal of gestational sac with plain graspers.

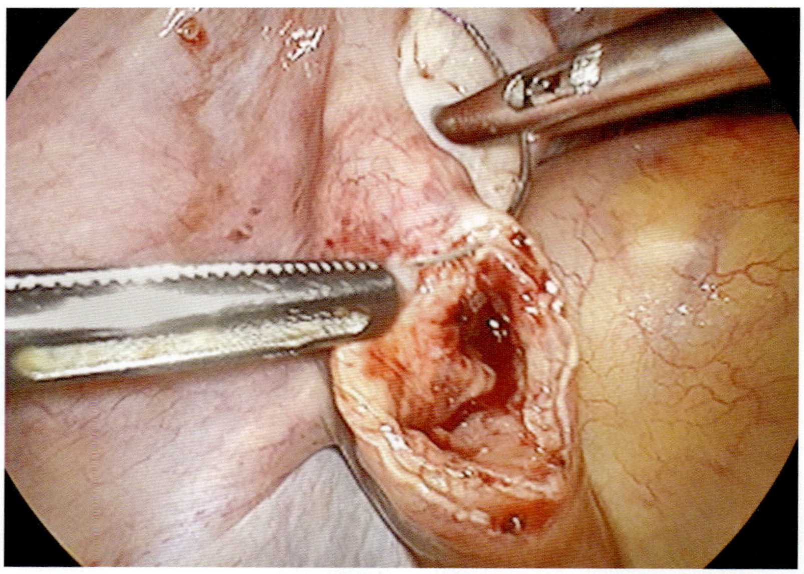

Fig. 19: Fallopian tube after retrieval of sac.

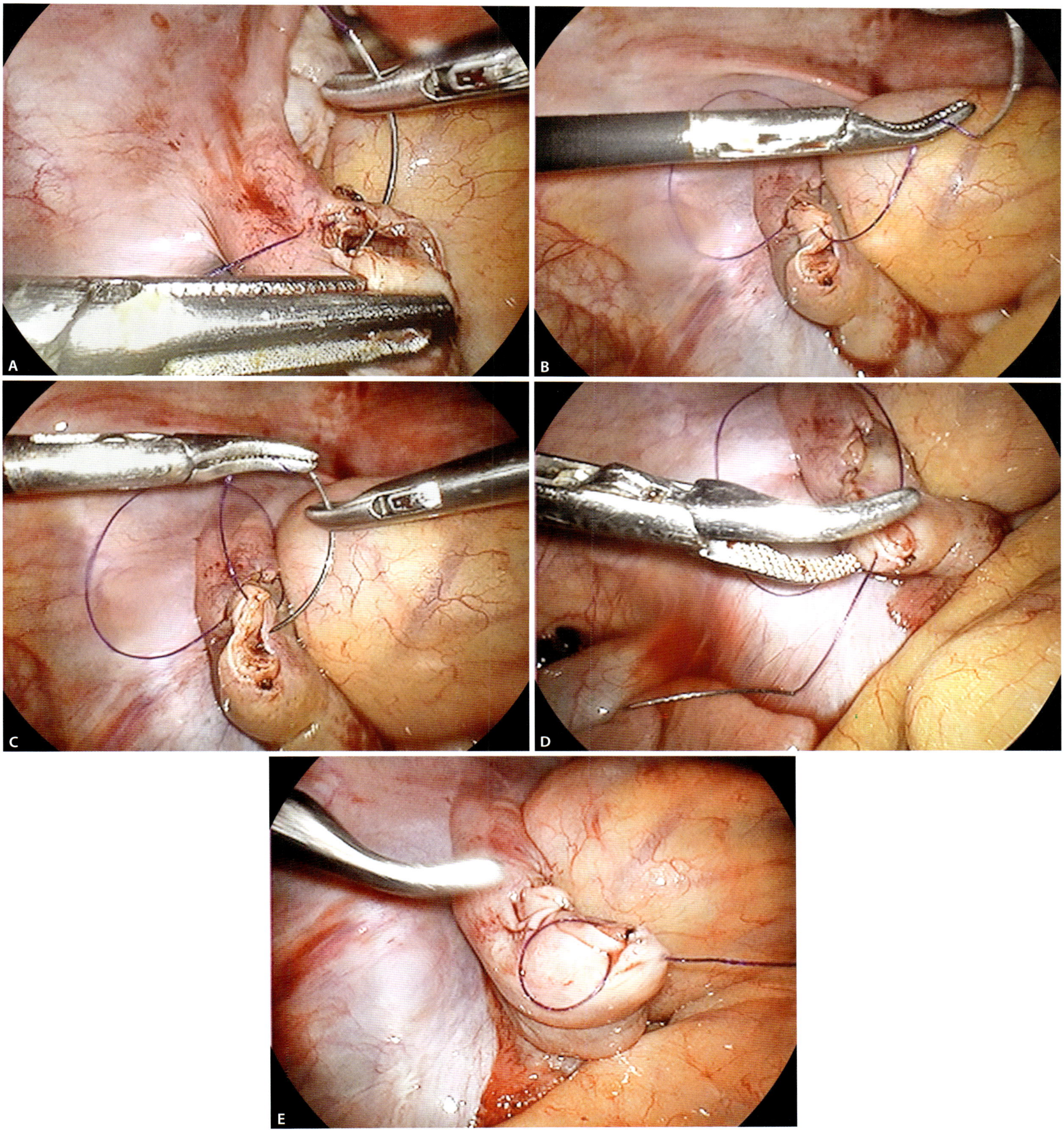

Figs. 20A to E: Using No. 3-0 quilled barbed suture, muscularis and mucosa sutured in continuous fashion.

REFERENCES

1. Chen C, Wang P, Chiu L, Liu W. The Treatment of Ectopic Pregnancy with Laparoscopy-Assisted Local Injection of Chemotherapeutic Agents. 2014;(October 2011).
2. Bruhat MA, Manhes H, Mage G, et al. Treatment of ectopic pregnancy by means of laparoscopy. Fertil Steril. 1980;33:411-4.
3. Pouly JL, Mahnes H, Mage G, et al. Conservative laparoscopic treatment of 321 ectopic pregnancies. Fertil Steril. 1986;46:1093-7.
4. DeCherney AH, Diamond MP. Laparoscopic salpingostomy for ectopic pregnancy. Obstet Gynecol. 1987;70:948-50.
5. DeCherney AH, Kase N. The conservative surgical management of unruputured ectopic pregnancy. Obstet Gynecol. 1979;54:451-5.
6. DeCherney AH, Romero R, Naftolin F. Surgical management of unruptured ectopic pregnancy. Fertil Steril. 1981;35:21-4.
7. Tulandi T, Saleh A. Surgical management of ectopic pregnancy. Clin Obstet Gynecol. 1999;42:31-8.
8. Semm K. Advances in pelviscopic surgery. Curr Probl Obstet Gynecol. 1982;5:20-5.
9. Reich H, Freifeld ML, McGlynn F, et al. Laparoscopic treatment of tubal pregnancy. Obstet Gynecol. 1987;6:275-9.
10. Nelson LM, Margara RA, Winston RMK. Primary and secondary closure to amupullary salpingotomy compared in the rabbit. Fertil Steril. 1986;45:292-5.
11. Bouyer J, Fernandez H, Coste J, et al. Fertility after ectopic pregnancy: 10-year results in the Auvergne Registry. J Gynecol Obstet Biol Reprod (Paris). 2003;32:431-8.
12. Seifer DB, Gutmann JN, Doyle MB, et al. Persistent ectopic pregnancy following laparoscopic linear salpingostomy. Obstet Gynecol. 1990;76:1121-5.
13. Hagström HG, Hahlin M, Bennegarg-Eden B, et al. Prediction of persistent ectopic pregnancy after laparoscopic salpingostomy. Obstet Gynecol. 1994;84:798-802.
14. Pouly JL, Chapron C, Wattiez A, et al. The drop in the level of hCG after conservative laparoscopic treatment of ectopic pregnancy. J Gynecol Surg. 1992;7:211-7.

CHAPTER 13

Dermoid Cyst

Priyanka HK, Minal Kumbhalwar, B Ramesh

INTRODUCTION

Ovarian dermoid cyst and mature cystic ovarian teratoma are interchangeable terms often used to refer the most common ovarian neoplasms. These are slow-growing tumors, which contain elements from multiple germ cell layers and these are best assessed with ultrasound.

Dermoid cyst and teratomas have similar imaging appearances, but the fundamental histological difference is that a dermoid is composed only of dermal and epidermal elements; however, teratomas have mesodermal as well as endodermal elements.

EPIDEMIOLOGY

Mature cystic teratomas account for ~15% (range 10–20%) of all ovarian neoplasms. They tend to occur mainly in young women, typically around the age of 30 years and also they are the most common ovarian neoplasm in patients below 20 years.

CLINICAL PRESENTATION

Uncomplicated ovarian dermoid tends to be asymptomatic and are often incidentally discovered. However, they are more prone for ovarian torsion, and patient may present with acute pelvic pain.

PATHOLOGY

Mature cystic teratomas are encapsulated neoplasms with mature organ or tissue components. They are composed of well-differentiated entities from at least two out of three germ cell layers (i.e., ectoderm, mesoderm, and endoderm). They contain developmentally mature skin, which is complete with hair follicles and sweat glands. Sometimes clumps of long hair, pockets of sebum, blood, fat, bone, nails, teeth, eyes, cartilage, and thyroid tissue are also found. Typically, their diameter ranges below 10 cm, but rarely can be more than 15 cm. Organ structures like teeth and bone fragments may be present in ~30% of cases **(Figs. 1A to D)**.

LOCATION

They can be bilateral in 10–15% of cases **(Figs. 2A and B)**.

VARIANTS

Struma ovarii tumor: Contains thyroid elements, which are separately classified as specialized teratomas of the ovaries.

RADIOGRAPHIC FEATURES

X-ray

May show calcific and tooth components with the pelvis.

Pelvic Ultrasound

Ultrasound is the preferred imaging modality of choice. Typically, an ovarian dermoid appears as cystic adnexal mass with few mural elements. Most of the lesions are unilocular.

The spectrum of sonographic features includes:

- Diffusely or partially echogenic mass with posterior attenuation due to sebaceous material and hair inside the cyst cavity **(Figs. 3A and B)**
- An echogenic interface at the edge of mass which obscures deep structures: The tip of the iceberg sign
- Echogenic, shadowing calcific or dental (tooth) components
- Mural hyperechoic Rokitansky nodule: Dermoid plug
- The presence of fluid–fluid levels
- Multiple thin, echogenic bands caused by the hair in the cyst cavity: The dot dash pattern
- *Color Doppler:* No internal vascularity. Presence of internal vascularity requires workup to exclude malignancy
- Appearance of intracystic floating balls is rare but is considered characteristic.

Computed Tomography

Computed tomography (CT) has high sensitivity in the diagnosis of cystic teratomas although not routinely recommended due to its ionizing radiation.

Typically, CT images demonstrate fat (areas with very low Hounsfield values), fat-fluid level, calcification (sometimes dentiform), Rokitansky protuberance, and tufts of hair **(Figs. 4A and B)**. The presence of above features is diagnostic of ovarian cystic teratomas in 98% cases. If the size exceeds 10 cm or soft tissue plugs and cauliflower appearance with irregular borders are seen, malignant transformation should be suspected always.

When ruptured, the characteristic hypoattenuating fatty fluid can be found as anti-dependent pockets, particularly below the right hemidiaphragm, a pathognomonic finding. The spilled cyst content also leads to a chemical peritonitis and it causes stranding of the mesentery and peritoneal thickening, which mimics peritoneal carcinomatosis.

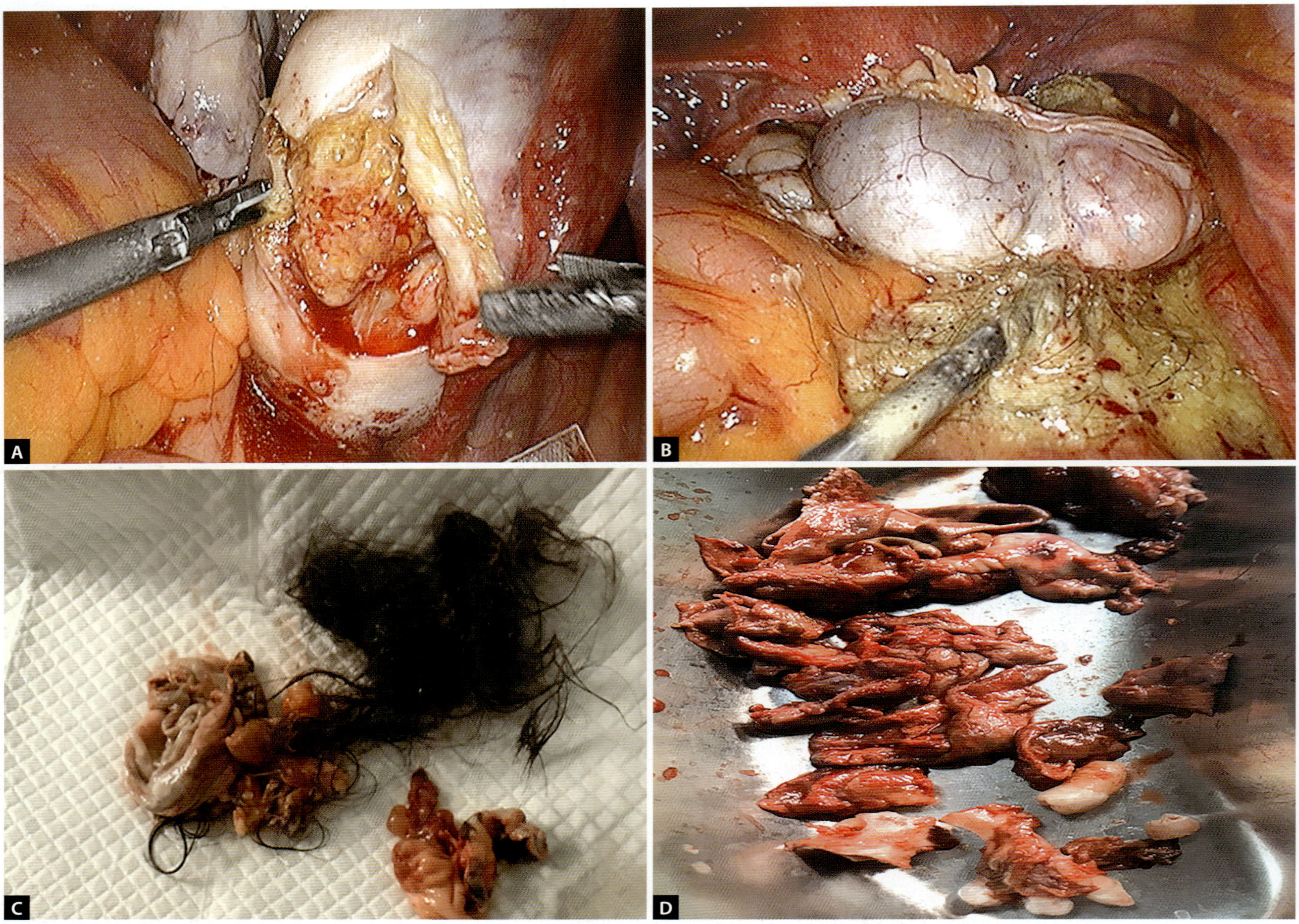

Figs. 1A to D: Dermoid cyst.

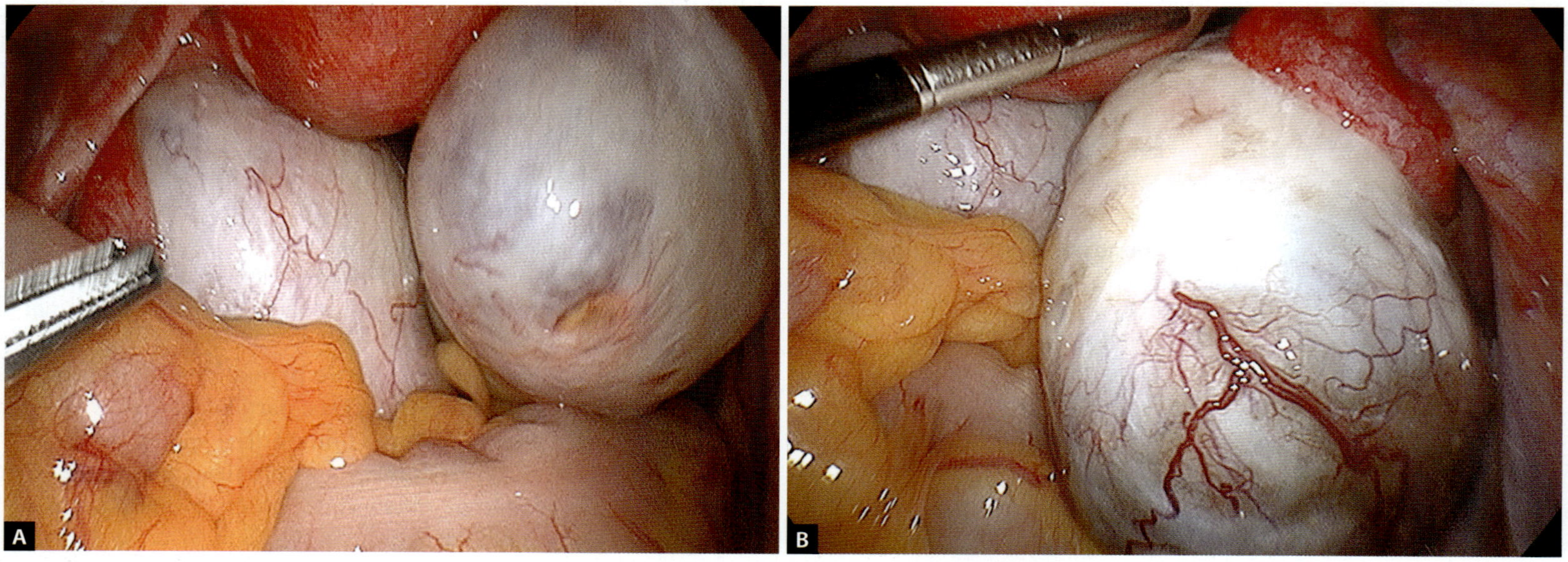

Figs. 2A and B: Bilateral coexistence of dermoid cyst.

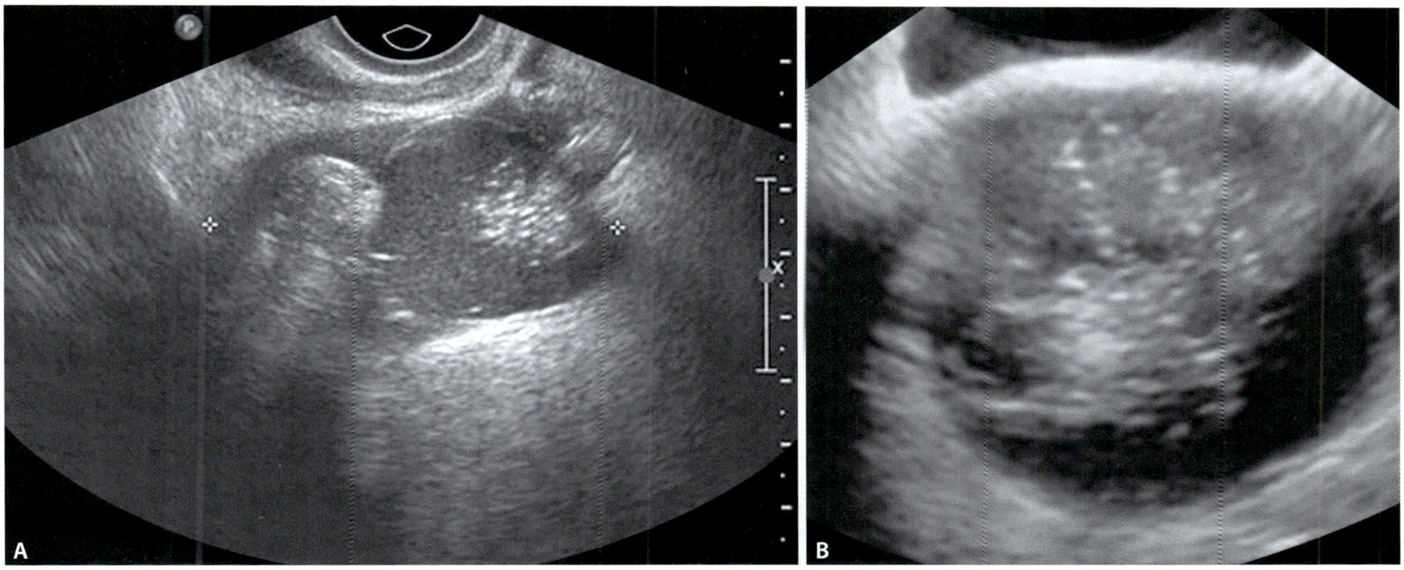

Figs. 3A and B: The mass exhibits posterior enhancement, low-level echogenicity of part of the content, focal areas of high echogenicity some of which also cause shadowing. One area exhibits the clustered punctate high amplitude echo pattern typical created by "hair in fat".

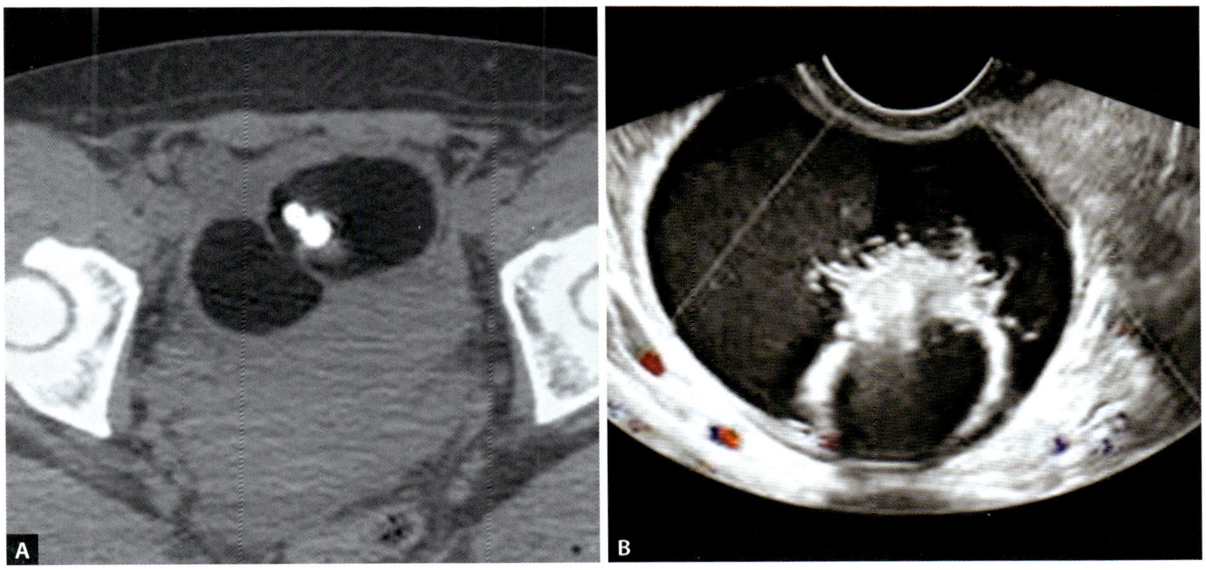

Figs. 4A and B: CT-scan pictures of dermoid.

Pelvic Magnetic Resonance Imaging

Magnetic resonance imaging (MRI) evaluation is usually reserved for difficult cases but it is exquisitely sensitive to fat components. Both fat suppression techniques and chemical shift artefact can be used to confirm the presence of fat **(Figs. 5A to D)**.

Also, enhancement can identify solid invasive components, and hence can be used to accurately stage locally malignant variants.

TREATMENT PROGNOSIS

Mature ovarian teratomas are slow growing (1–2 mm per year) and, therefore, few offer nonsurgical management. Larger lesions are usually surgically removed. Treatment options include cystectomy or salpingo-oophorectomy depending on age of the patient. Ovarian cystectomy is performed in benign conditions of the ovary in which in toto removal of cyst is possible and when it is desirable to leave a functional ovary in place. This is particularly true for women of reproductive age group. Laparoscopic cystectomy indications include serous, mucous, dermoid and endometriotic cysts. Although various modalities of removal of dermoid cysts are available, laparoscopy being superior to laparotomy is always preferred.

PREOPERATIVE EVALUATION

Routine preoperative investigations include complete blood count, bleeding time, clotting time, renal function tests, viral markers, thyroid function tests, electrocardiography (ECG), and urinalysis. However, tests like liver function tests, serum electrolytes, prothrombin time and international normalized ratio (PT-INR), activated partial thromboplastin time (aPTT), chest radiography, 2D-echocardiography, CT, MRI and contrast MRI should be done whenever indicated. Preanesthetic fitness is obtained. Preanesthetic assessment is an essential step prior to surgery in an attempt to decrease the morbidity related to anesthesia and surgery. Patient is advised for admission in the evening one day prior to surgery. Appropriate informed consent is obtained from the patient after detailed explanation of the planned operation, its potential risks and benefits, the possibility of laparotomy, hysterectomy, blood transfusion and

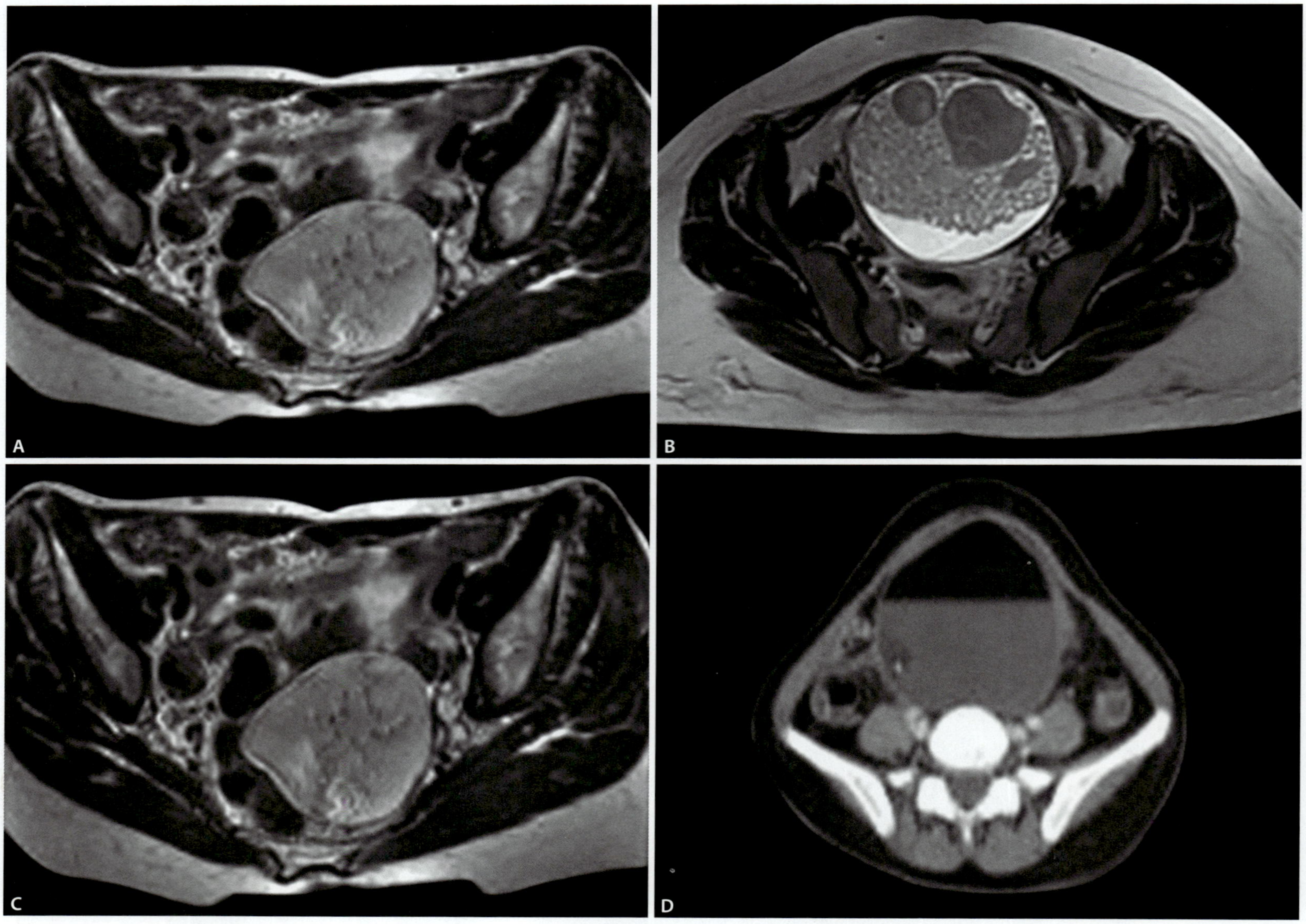

Figs. 5A to D: MRI showing dermoid.

therapeutic alternatives. Aspirin and warfarin need to be stopped 5 days prior to surgery. 24 hours before surgery patients are advised to have light food. An oral mechanical bowel preparation like Dulcolax® tablets are administered. Patient is kept nil per oral 8 hours prior to surgery.

SURGICAL EQUIPMENT

Routine laparoscopic equipment essential for performing laparoscopic cystectomy includes:

- A laparoscopic tower with a high-flow CO_2 insufflator, camera and a light source
- An operating table with leg stirrups
- Vasopressin injection needle
- 2 laparoscopic toothed graspers for grasping and manipulating the cyst
- Laparoscopic plain grasper to manipulate adnexal structures and bowel
- Suction irrigator is required for clearing out fluid, blood and clots
- Uterine sound for uterine manipulation
- Harmonic scalpel, monopolar electricity generator, bipolar electricity generator and bipolar forceps
- Laparoscopic scissors.

TECHNIQUE OF LAPAROSCOPIC OVARIAN CYSTECTOMY

In our center, the surgical technique followed for laparoscopic ovarian cystectomy is described next. Patients should be placed on the operating table in the dorsal lithotomy position. A thorough examination under anesthesia is performed. The bladder should be emptied with a catheter. The abdomen, perineum, and vagina are surgically prepared. Povidone-iodine is applied to the abdominal area and vagina extending from the nipple line up to the inner thighs and draping is done. The use of a nasogastric tube prior to the establishment of the pneumoperitoneum is recommended in cases where adhesions are expedited. Prophylactic antibiotics are administered approximately 1 hour before procedure. The umbilical area is the most common site for Veress needle insertion. CO_2 is commonly preferred gas for most laparoscopic procedures. Veress needle is checked for patency prior to insertion. A stab incision is made either at the umbilicus or at Palmer's point in flat position. The Veress needle is inserted at a 45° angle (90° if obese) at the midline and directed toward the uterine fundus. Initial intra-abdominal insufflation pressure should not exceed 10 mm Hg, and it is the most reliable parameter for monitoring insufflation and proper needle placement. If the needle is properly placed, the peritoneal cavity is insufflated with 3–6 L of CO_2. After insufflating about 1.5–2 L of CO_2, intra-abdominal pressures will begin to rise. Insufflation should be continued until the pressure reaches at least up to 18–20 mm Hg. Insertion of the Veress needle through the subcostal space in the left midclavicular line (Palmer's point) is safer alternative where adhesions are contemplated. The left upper quadrant is easily accessible and is usually free of intra-abdominal adhesions. Few surgeons suggest using Hasson's technique of open entry or an optical Veress in such cases. Once adequate pneumoperitoneum is achieved, sensorcaine infiltration is done at the site of primary port placement. A 5-mm skin incision is made 3–4 cm above the umbilicus or higher, depending on the size of the uterus and the primary port is placed with 45–60° angulation. The periumbilical area is inspected and adhesion of anterior abdominal wall to underlying omentum and bowel are evaluated. Trendelenburg position is adopted. The abdominal wall is transilluminated by the laparoscope at the site of the secondary trocar placement laterally in order to visualize and avoid injury to deep epigastric blood vessels. The secondary 5 mm trocars usually two in number are placed on the left and right lateral walls, 8–10 cm lateral to the umbilicus, lateral to the inferior epigastric vessels, under vision in a similar manner. In a bigger cyst, all the ports are placed higher, depending on the size. If necessary, a third suprapubic midline port can be placed. The placement of secondary trocar under vision is noted in **Figures 6 and 7**.

The step-by-step approach is described below **(Figs. 8A to T)**:

1. The utero-ovarian ligament is grasped with an atraumatic forceps introduced from the side of tumor, so that ovaries are exposed adequately **(Fig. 8A)**.
2. *Step 1:* Injecting diluted vasopressin using cyst aspiration needle in between ovarian cortex and cyst wall to create a tissue plane and to reduce blood loss from the ovarian bed **(Figs. 8B-F)**.
3. *Step 2:* Making an incision in the ovarian cortex overlying the cyst.
4. *Step 3:* Separation of the cyst wall from the surrounding ovarian cortex. The ovarian cyst is held with atraumatic forceps and the ovarian cortex is grasped with another forceps which is placed close to cyst. By traction and countertraction, the dissection is carried out with ease and cyst is removed **(Figs. 8G-L)**.
5. *Step 4:* Dissection should be done till the hilus to ensure total removal of cyst wall.
6. *Step 5:* The interior surface of ovarian cortex is rinsed thoroughly. Hemostasis is achieved with thorough saline wash, if not bipolar forceps can be used sparingly.

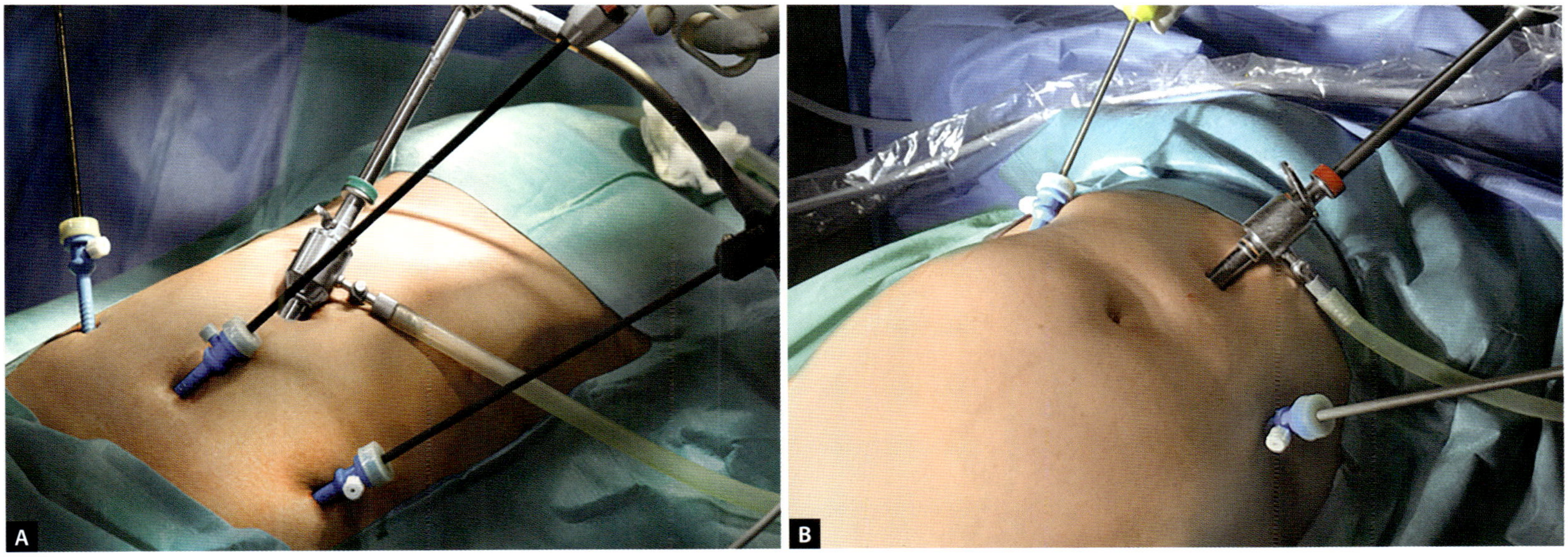

Figs. 6A and B: Primary and secondary trocars placement.

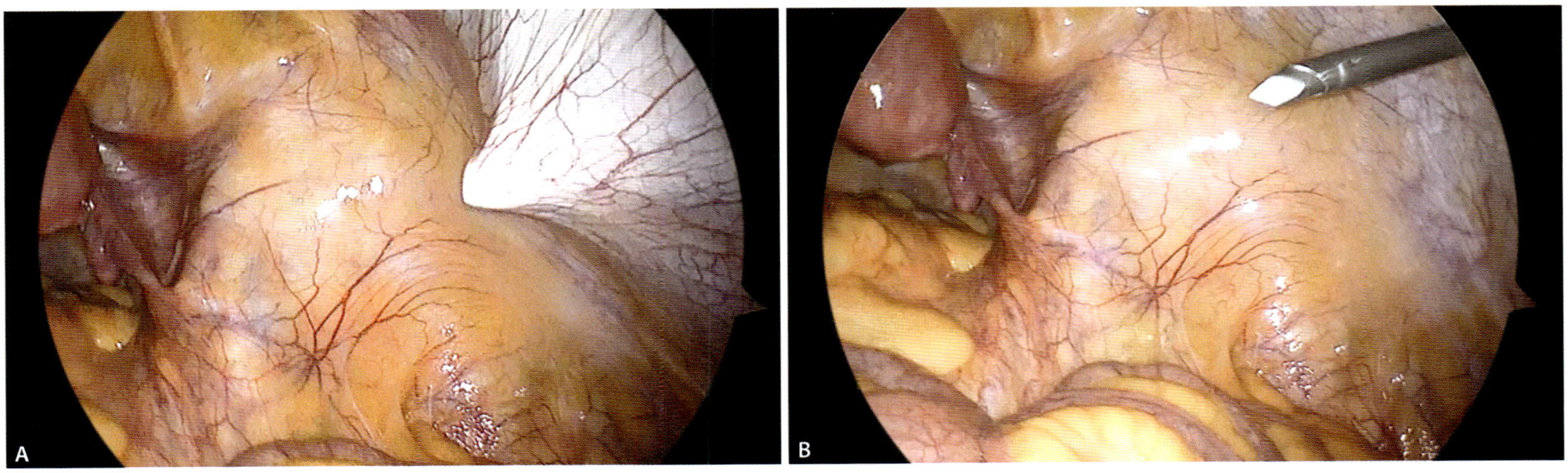

Figs. 7A and B: Secondary trocar insertion under laparoscopic vision.

Ovarian Reconstruction

It has been shown that approximation of ovarian surface for ovarian reconstruction by keeping the ovarian tissue apposed to each other with bowel grasper for 5 min without using sutures **(Figs. 9A to D)** was associated with shorter operating times, better morphological ovarian reconstruction and good pregnancy outcome.

Whereas in cases of large cysts, approximation does not occur spontaneously, so closure can be done using the following methods.

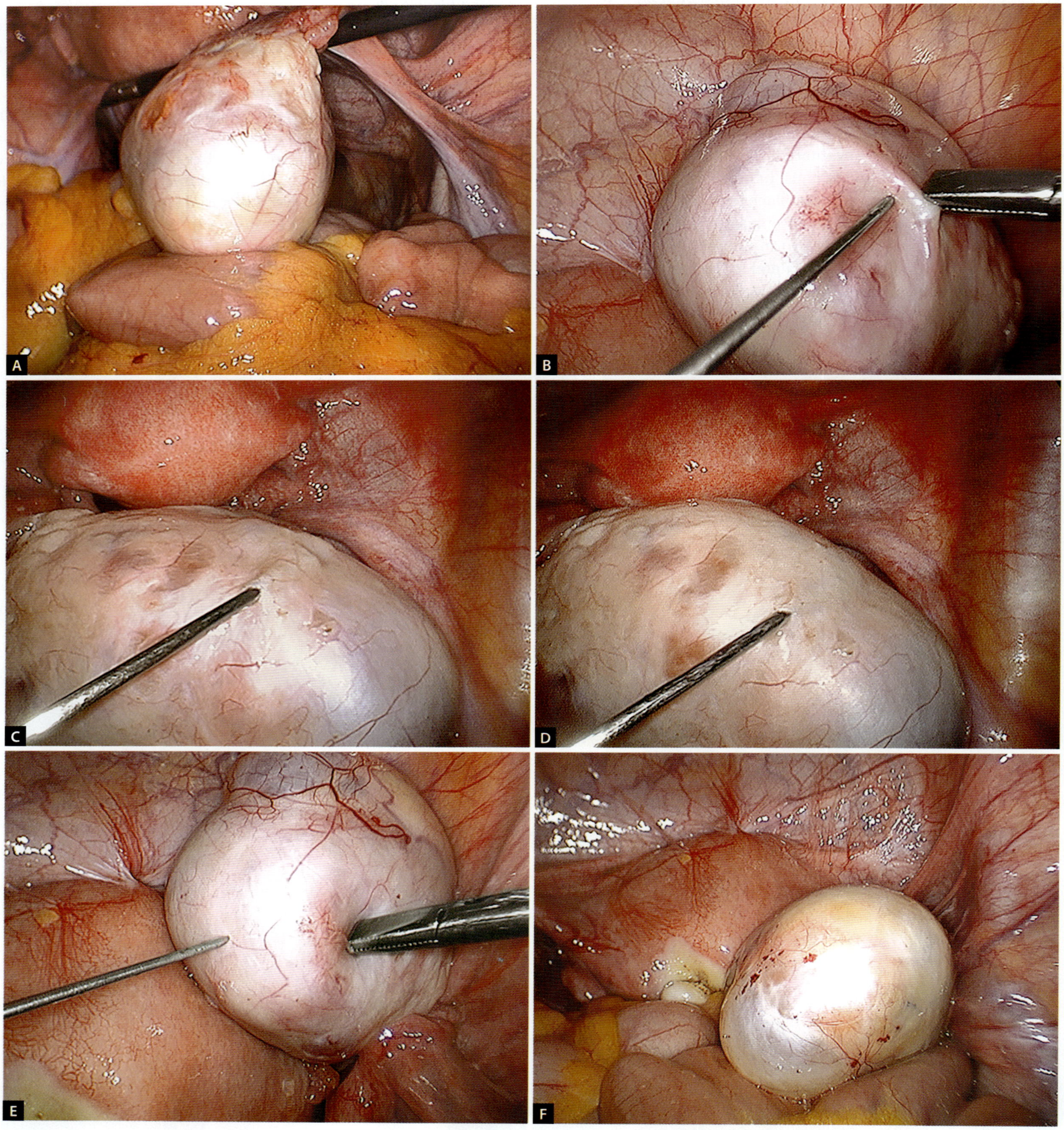

Figs. 8A to F: (A) Utero-ovarian ligament is grasped with an atraumatic forceps; (B to F) Injection of diluted vasopressin.

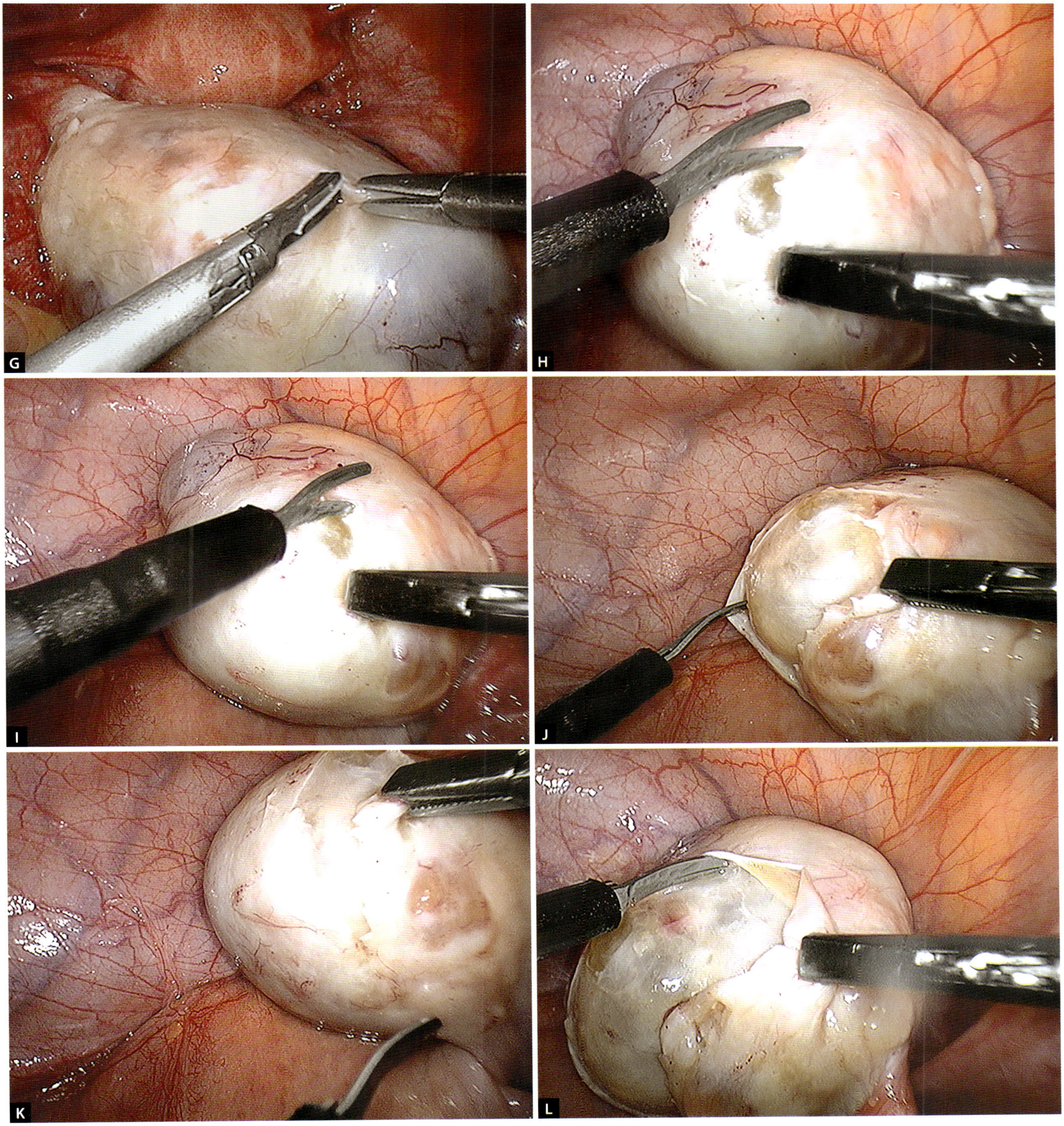

Figs. 8G to L: (G) Incision made with harmonic; (H to L) Incision extenced with scissors.

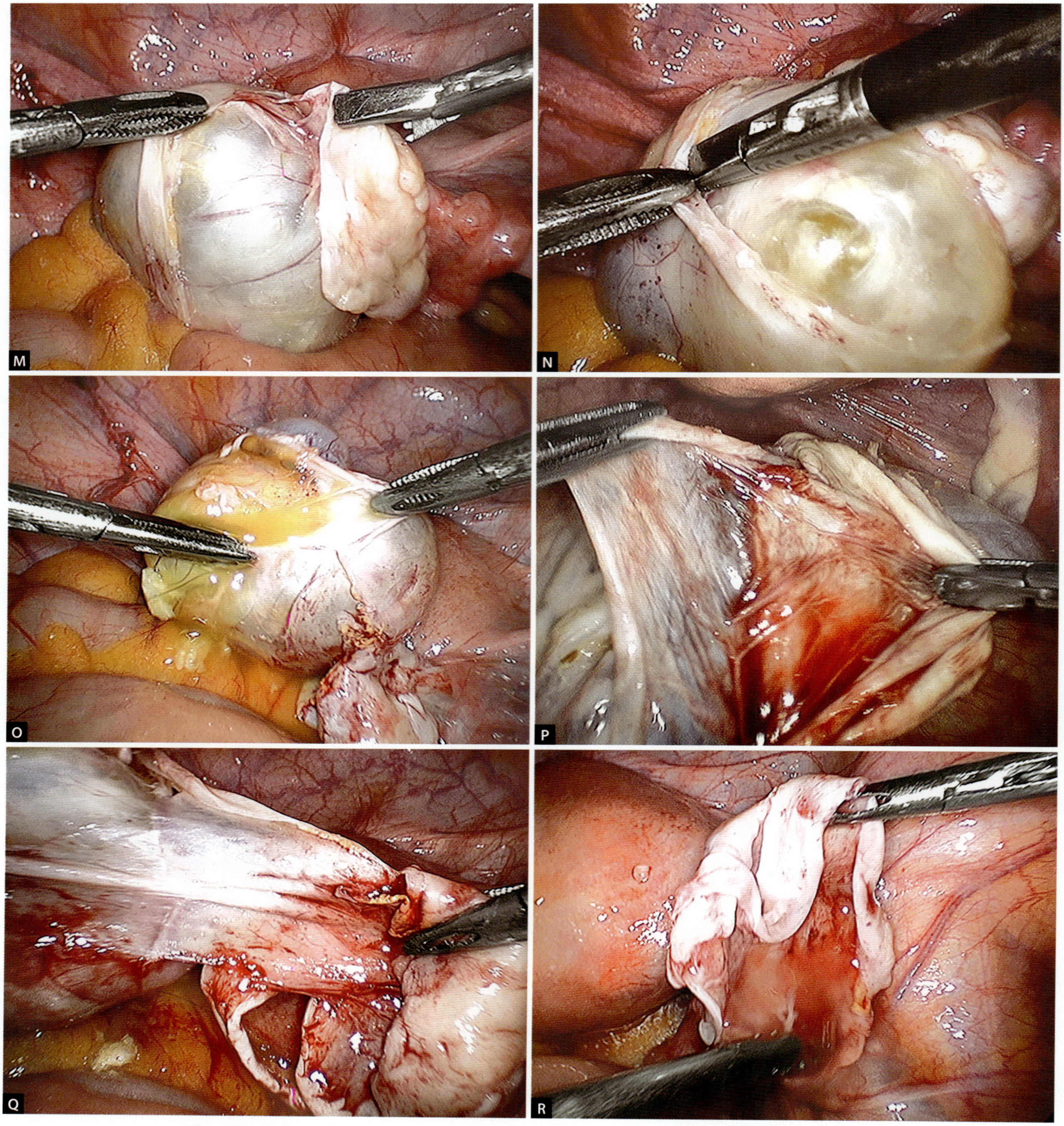

Figs. 8M to R: Cyst wall separated from ovarian cortex using graspers. Q-ovarian cortex following cystectomy.

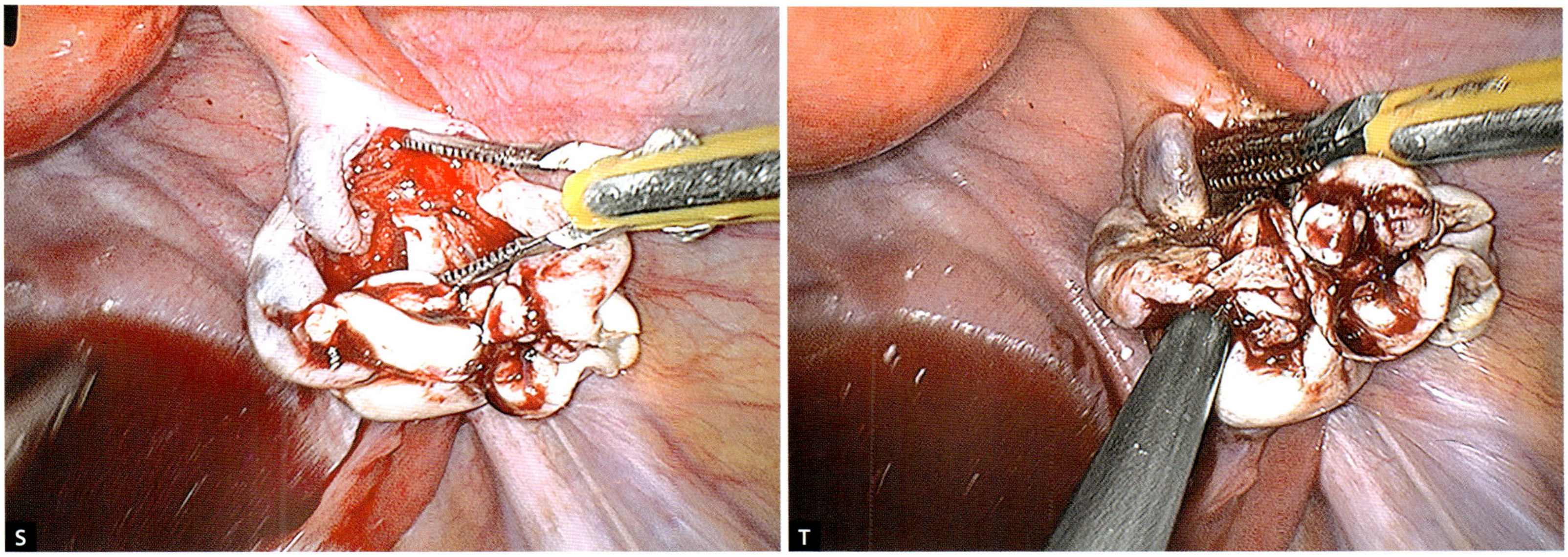

Figs. 8S and T: Fulguration of ovarian hilus.

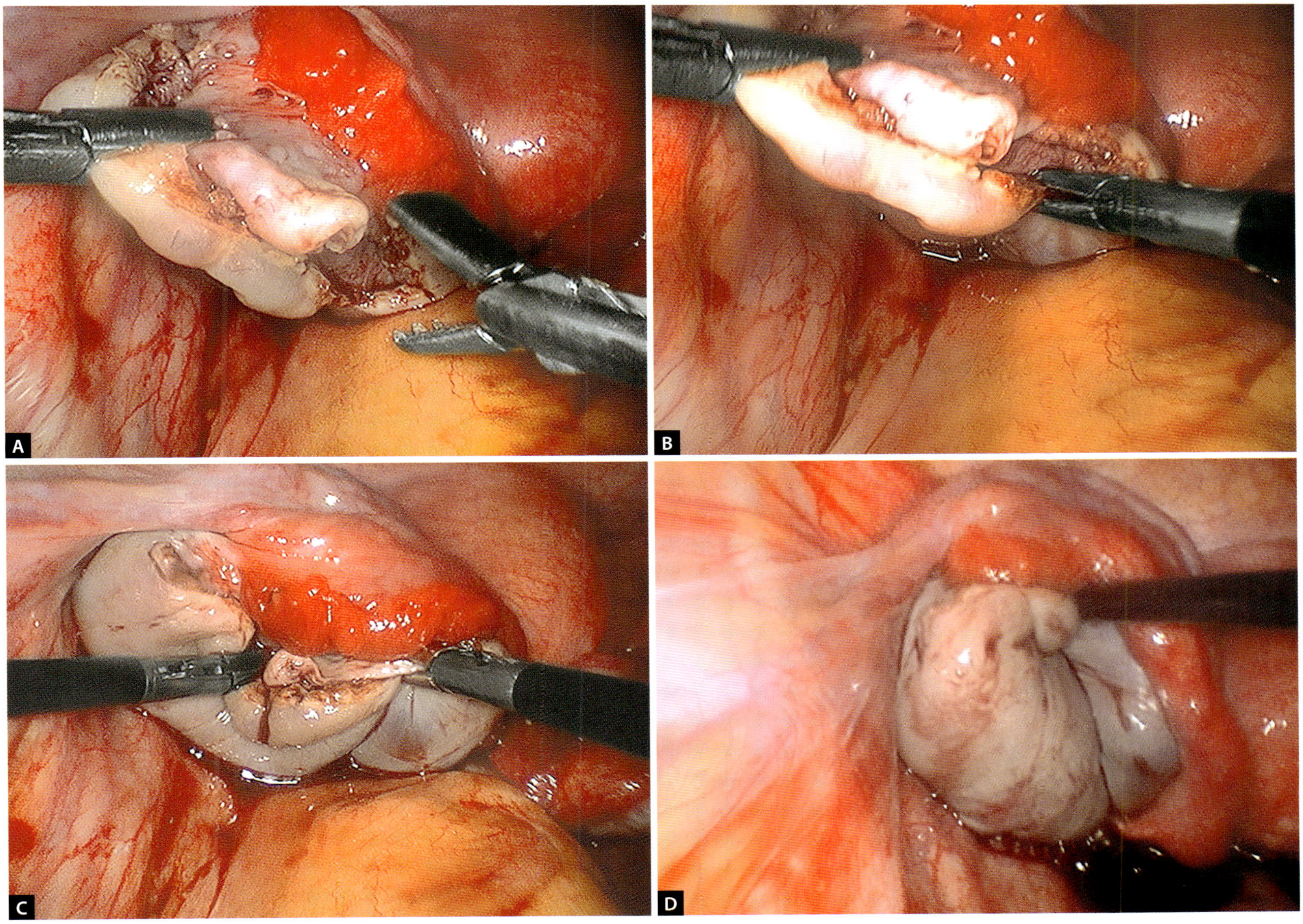

Figs. 9A to D: Ovarian reconstruction.

- *Suturing:* Two lower abdominal accessory ports are necessary through which laparoscopic needle holder and graspers are introduced to manipulate the needle, suture, and tissue involved. The suture material used is 6-0 polydioxanone **(Figs. 10A to G)**.
- Clips can also be used for closing the ovarian cortex. The clip is made of titanium, an inert, nonreactive metal and can vary from medium to large size. Three or four clips are applied using the 10-mm clip applicator, which is usually sufficient to achieve ovarian closure.
- Fibrin sealant

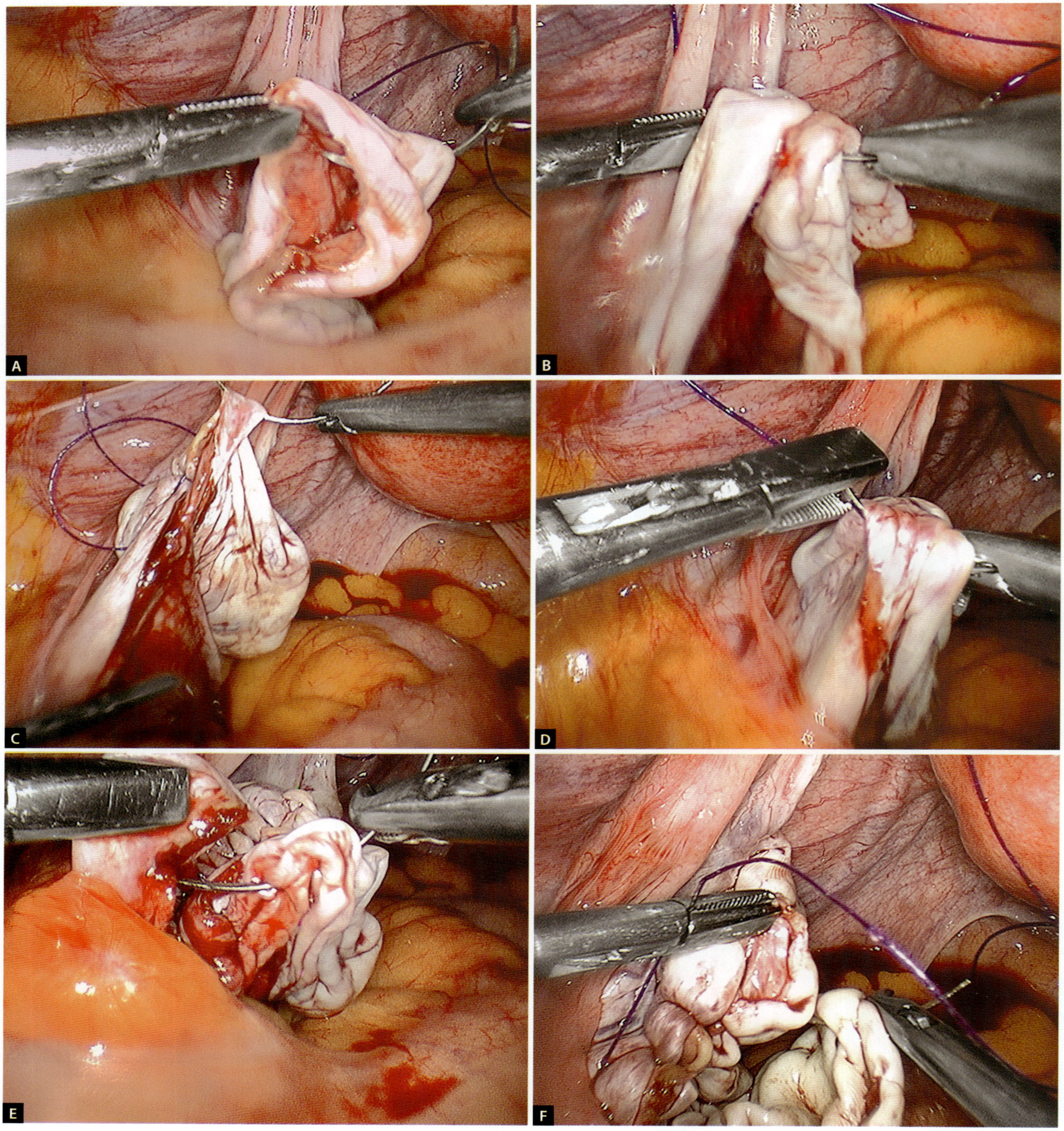

Figs. 10A to F: Different steps of ovarian reconstruction.

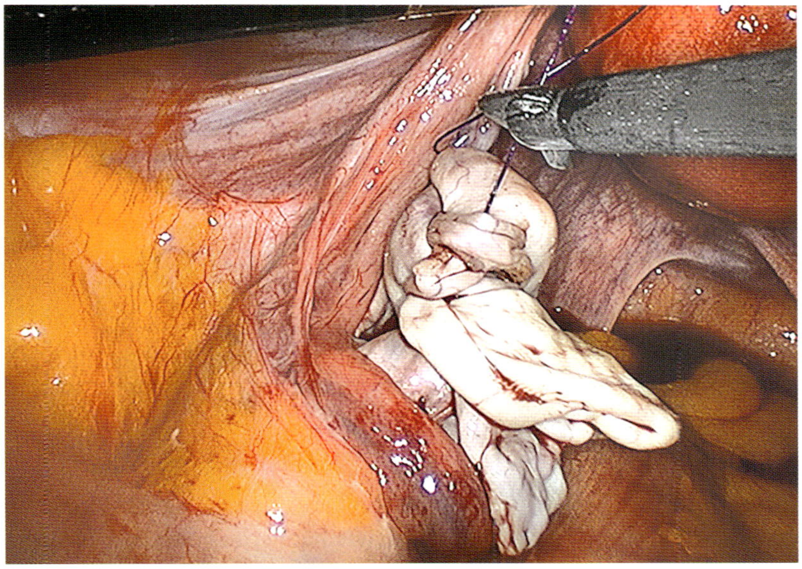

Fig. 10G: Ovarian reconstruction by suturing.

COMPLICATIONS

It mainly includes:

- Ovarian torsion: seen in 3–16% of ovarian teratomas, considered as the most common complication
- Rupture in 1–4%
- Malignant transformation in 1–2%, usually into squamous cell carcinoma (adults) and rarely into endodermal sinus tumors (pediatrics)
- Superimposed infection in 1%
- Autoimmune hemolytic anemia in less than 1%
- Paraneoplastic anti-N-methyl-D-aspartate receptor (anti-NMDA receptor) associated limbic encephalitis (rare).

DIFFERENTIAL DIAGNOSIS

General differential imaging considerations include:

- Hemorrhagic ovarian cyst
- *Endometrioma:* High T1 signal that do not suppress with fat saturation T2 shading
- Pedunculated lipoleiomyoma of the uterus
- Immature teratoma
- *Ovarian serous or mucinous cystadenoma/cystadenocarcinoma:* This is usually a serious consideration if typical features of mature teratoma are absent (i.e., fat is absent) and usually it occurs in older age group than dermoid cysts.

Accompanying Video: Laparoscopic dermoid cyst.

CHAPTER

14

Serous Cystadenoma

Priyanka HK, Minal Kumbhalwar, B Ramesh

INTRODUCTION

Ovarian serous cystadenomas are benign type of ovarian epithelial tumor at the nonmalignant end of the spectrum of ovarian serous tumors **(Fig. 1)**.

EPIDEMIOLOGY

Serous cystadenomas account for ~60% of serous tumors of ovaries. They are the most common ovarian epithelial neoplasm. The peak incidence ranges between fourth to fifth decades of life.

CLINICAL PRESENTATION

Generally, serous cystadenomas are asymptomatic but if symptoms are present, they usually occur due to pressure effect with displacement of adjacent organs, e.g. bowel loops, adnexal torsion.

ETIOLOGY

Serous cystadenomas are derived from ovarian epithelial inclusions, which itself is derivative of Fallopian tube epithelium.

LOCATION

They are bilateral in ~15% of cases.

MACROSCOPIC APPEARANCE (FIGS. 2A TO D)

Serous cystadenomas are usually unilocular (or at times multilocular) cysts filled with clear watery fluid. Their average diameter ranges between 10 cm, but may be extremely large. The cyst lining is flat or may have small papillary projections.

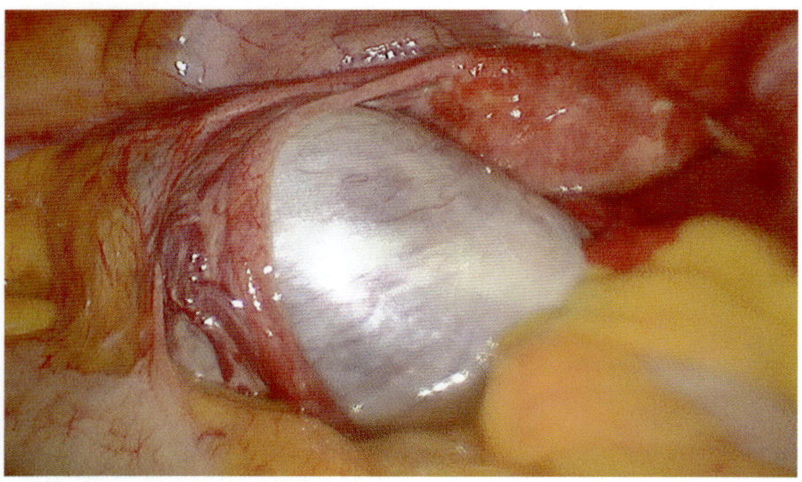

Fig. 1: A left ovarian serous cystadenoma.

MICROSCOPIC APPEARANCE

Composed of a solitary layer of benign epithelium which resembles mucosa of Fallopian tube and it may form papillary structures. Psammomatous calcification can also be a feature as like other serous tumors.

Ultrasound (Figs. 3A and B)

- Usually appears as a unilocular cystic/anechoic adnexal mass
- Papillary projections are absent:
  - If there is any wall irregularity, it is thin, with an acute angle with the cyst wall and has a regular surface
- Some lesions may contain sonographically detectable septations
- On color Doppler imaging, no flow is detected
- When compared to malignant neoplasms they have higher resistive and pulsatility indices on pulsed Doppler.

Computed Tomography

Typically seen as a unilocular (or multilocular) cystic mass with homogeneous computed tomography (CT) attenuation, with a thin regular wall or septum, and usually no endocystic or exocystic vegetation. Cysts can be enough large in size sometimes can be seen filling most of the lower pelvis with extension into the upper abdomen.

Magnetic Resonance Imaging

The typical magnetic resonance imaging (MRI) image of serous cystadenoma is a unilocular thin-walled adnexal cyst. MRI sometimes shows a beak sign which suggests an ovarian origin.

Signal characteristics within the cyst are usually homogeneous.

- T1: Cyst content shows hypointense signal in uncomplicated cases
- T2: Cyst content is of fluid (hyperintense) signal.

T1 C + (Gd): Cyst wall may show enhancement sometimes after contrast administration.

TREATMENT AND PROGNOSIS

They are benign lesions with a good prognosis. However, ovarian cystadenocarcinoma is thought to occur from ovarian cystadenoma evoluting into borderline serous tumors and invasive carcinoma. Surgical options include resection or oophorectomy. Cystadenomas do not recur following oophorectomy.

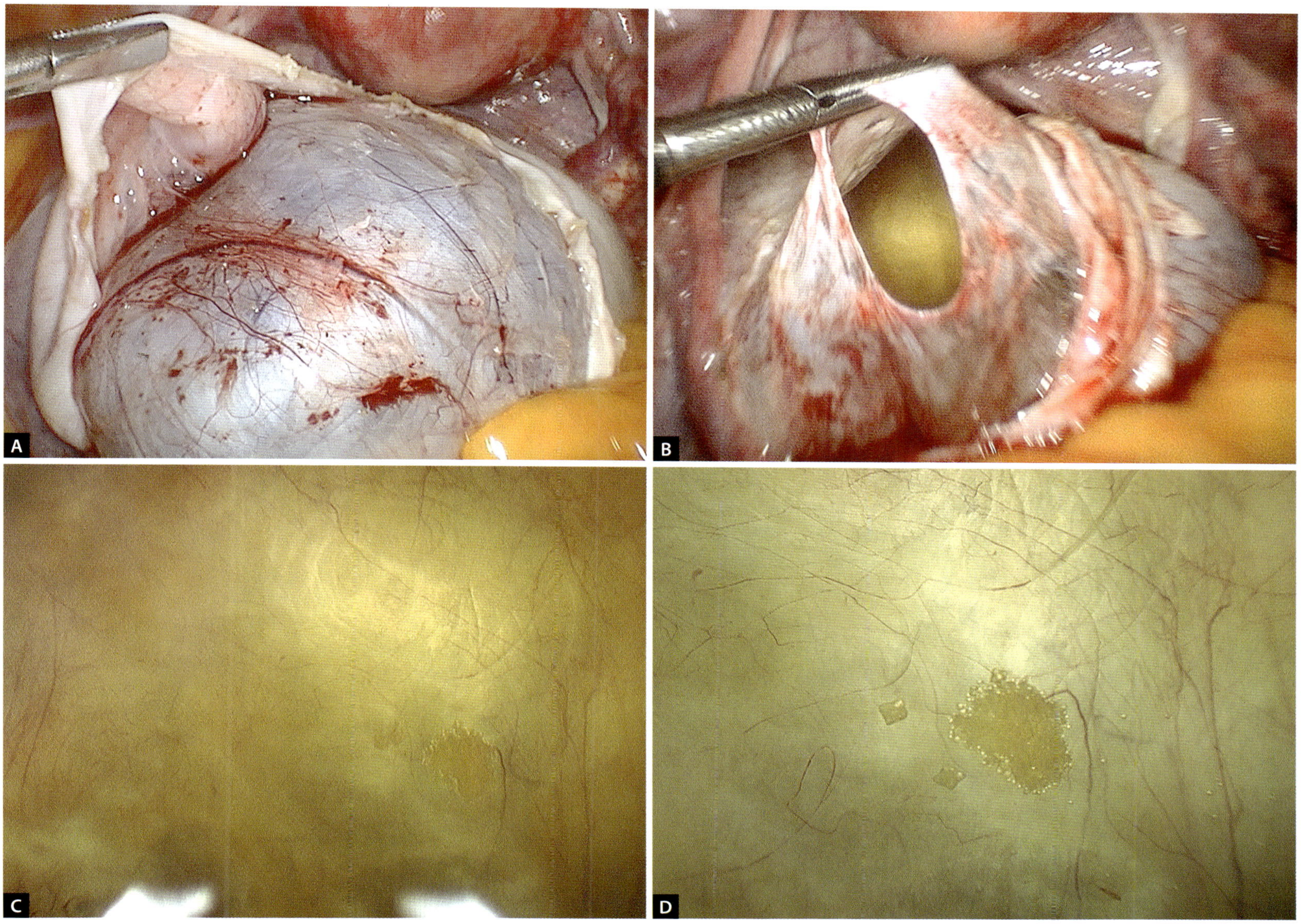

Figs. 2A to D: (A and B) Left unilocular serous cyst with clear watery fluid; (C and D) Cystoscopy—visualization of interior of cyst presents clear watery fluid.

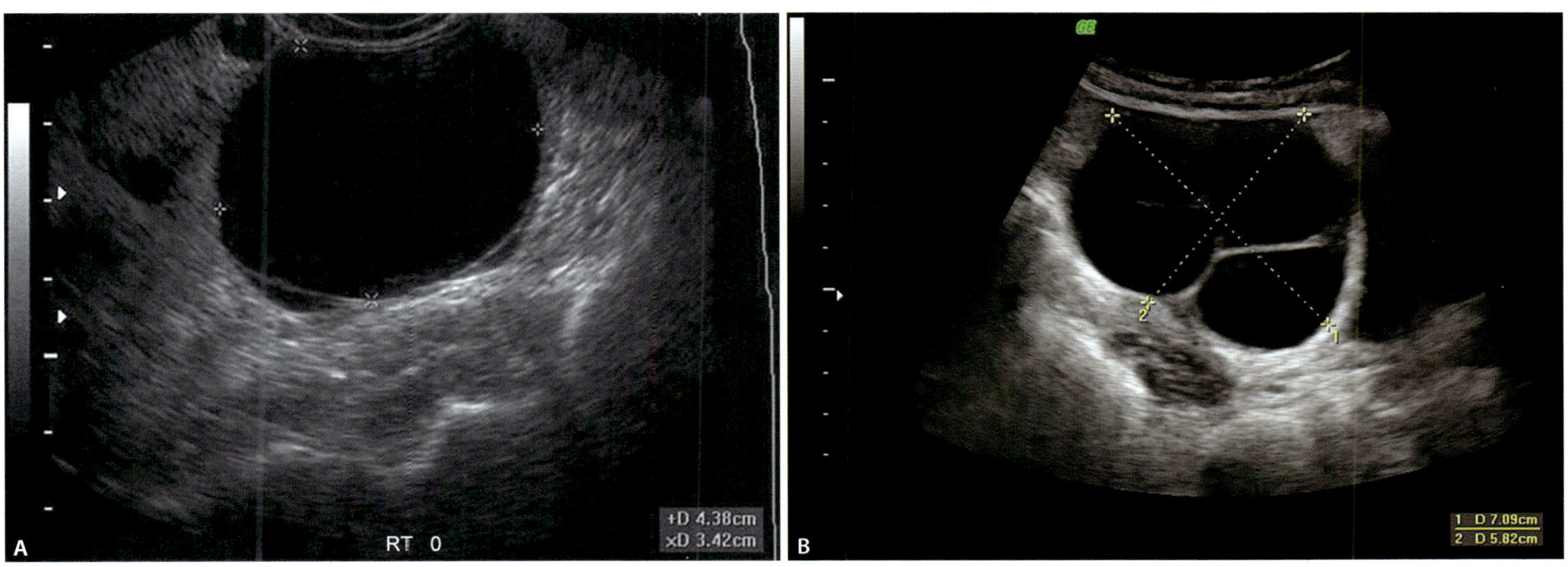

Figs. 3A and B: Ultrasound features of serous cystadenoma.

OVARIAN MUCINOUS CYSTADENOMA

Epidemiology

Ovarian mucinous cystadenoma is a benign tumor arising from the surface epithelium of the ovary. Of all ovarian tumors, mucinous tumors comprise 15%. They are typically seen between the third and the fifth decades.

Clinical Presentation

- It tends to be huge in size.
- Mucinous cystadenomas usually are large, multiloculated cystic mass with mucus-containing fluid.
- The average size at presentation is 18 cm, and they can become extremely large so as to fill the entire abdominopelvic cavity, occasionally can present with ureteral obstruction or abdominal compartment syndrome.
- About 80% of mucinous tumors are benign, 10% are borderline, and 10% are malignant. Borderline tumors, also known as tumors of low malignant potential (LMP tumors), can be more common than invasive primary mucinous ovarian carcinomas, and it comprises up to 67% of mucinous neoplasms that are not categorized strictly as benign.

Location

Mucinous cystadenomas are termed depending upon organ/location:
- Ovary—ovarian mucinous cystadenoma
- Pancreas—pancreatic mucinous cystadenoma
- Liver—mucinous cystadenoma of the liver
- Vermiform appendix—appendiceal mucinous cystadenoma
- Peritoneum—peritoneal mucinous cystadenoma.

Bilateral: These are bilateral in 5–10% of cases.

Diagnosis

Mucinous tumors are evaluated using ultrasound, CT scan, or MRI. Findings on imaging studies are nonspecific.

Ultrasound shows large multiloculated cystic lesion in the adnexa.

Some of the locules are anechoic while few of them contain uniform low-level echoes, consistent with proteinaceous content, such as mucin or hemorrhage. The septations are usually thin and avascular. There are no solid components **(Figs. 4A and B)**.

In spite of absent vascularity and absent solid components, the size and the multiloculated aspect of this lesion makes it suspicious for a cystic neoplasm and warrants further evaluation.

The contrast-enhanced CT shows similar features. The locules are of different attenuation, consistent with varying protein content.

There is no evidence of ascites or peritoneal deposits and also no lymphadenopathy.

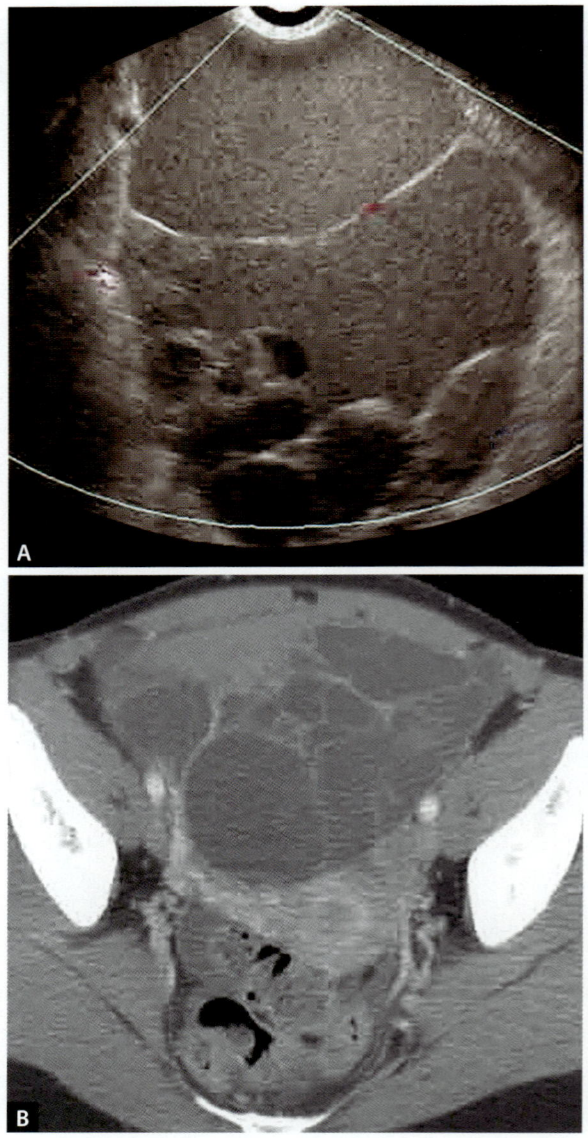

Figs. 4A and B: Ultrasound and MRI features of ovarian mucinous cystadenoma.

Pathology

Macroscopic Appearance (Fig. 5)

It is a multilocular cyst with smooth outer and inner surfaces.

These tumors are usually multiseptated, cystic masses with thin walls.

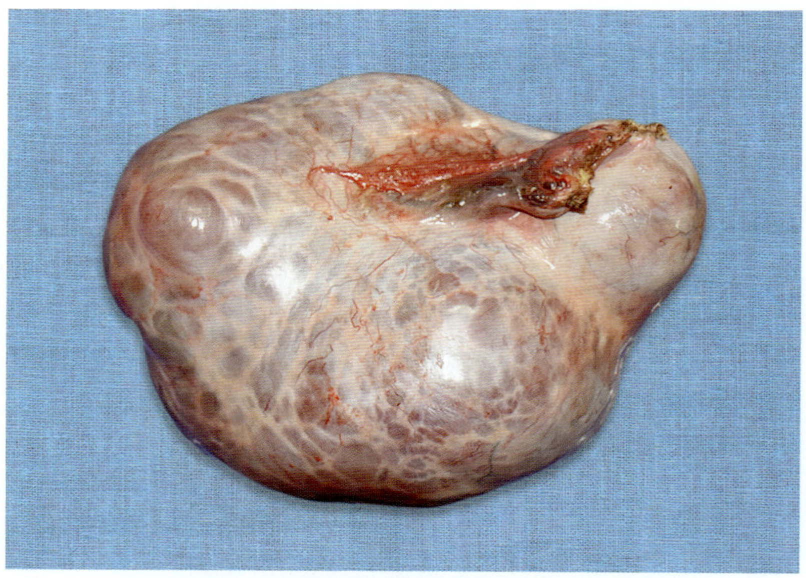

Fig. 5: Multiloculated cyst.

Microscopic Appearance

They also contain varying amounts of solid tissue comprising of proliferating stromal tissue, papillae, or malignant tumor cells **(Fig. 6)**.

Treatment

Exploratory laparotomy with removal of the involved adnexa is done for large mucinous tumors of the ovary. If the patient is postmenopausal, a total hysterectomy with bilateral salpingo-oophorectomy is the preferred option regardless of the histology. However, many patients are premenopausal and mucinous tumors being unilateral most of the time, whether benign, borderline, or invasive primary ovarian cancers, it allows fertility preservation with conservation of contralateral ovary and the uterus in early stage disease.

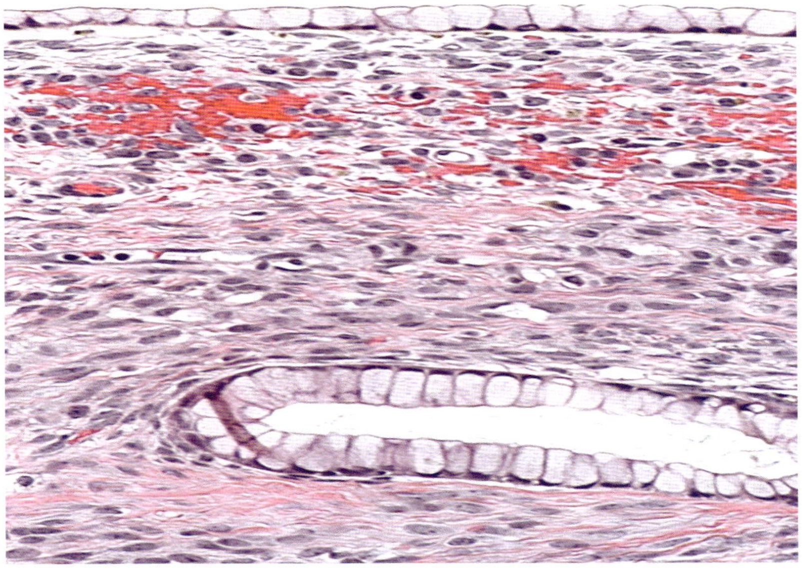

Fig. 6: Microscopic appearance.

LAP-ASSISTED OOPHORECTOMY (FIGS. 7 TO 9)

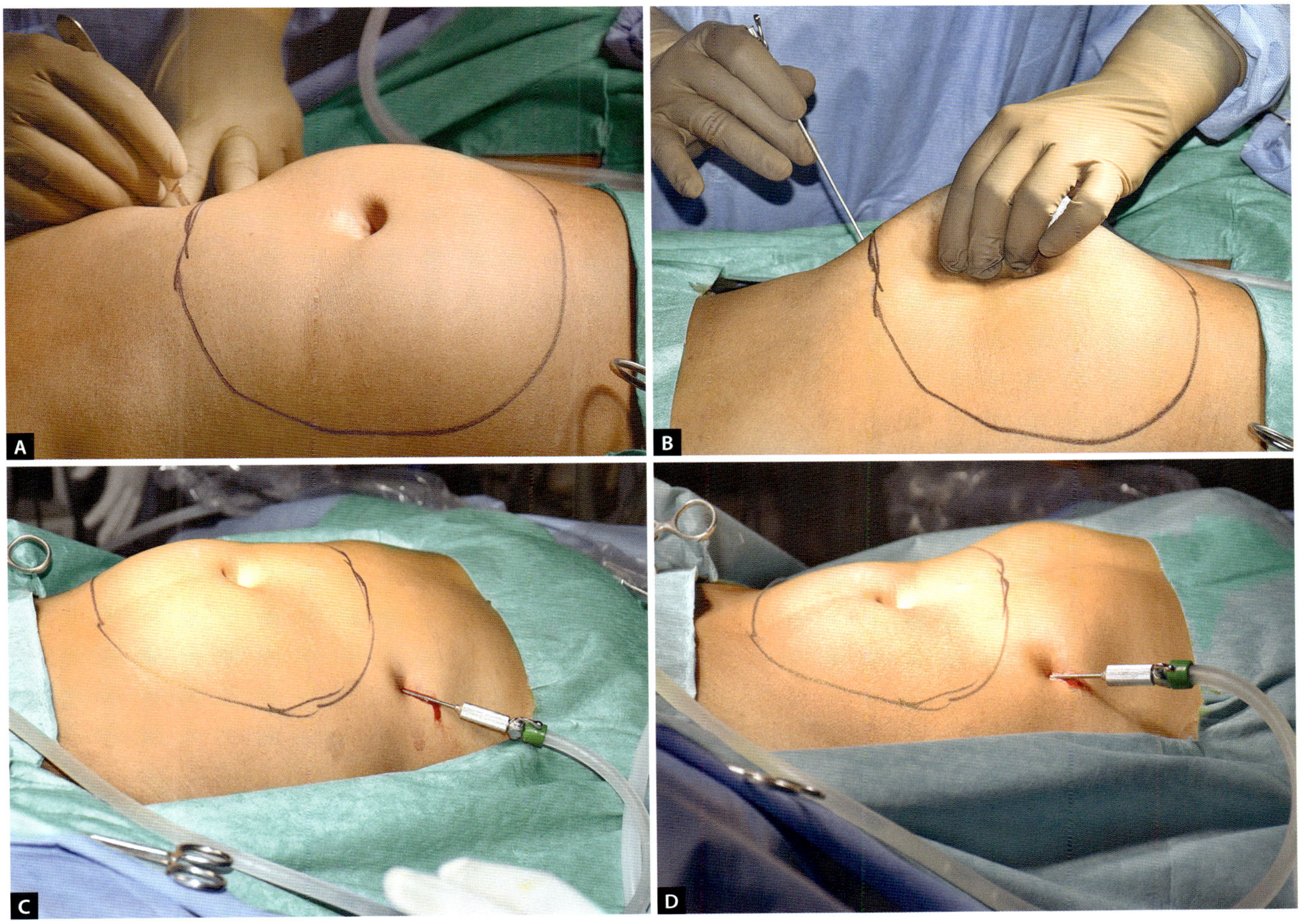

Figs. 7A to D: Laparoscopic part.

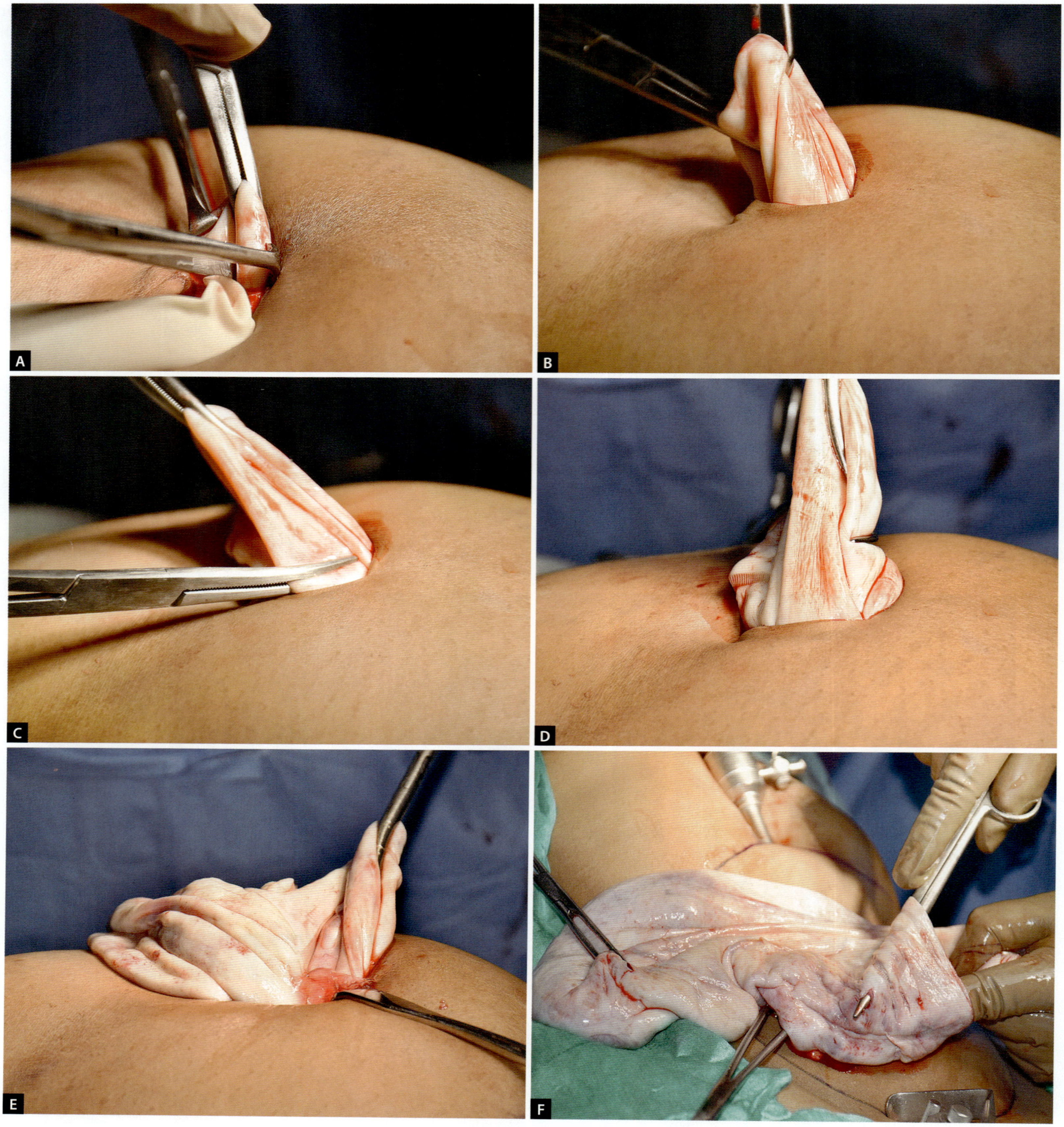

Figs. 8A to F: Cyst brought out through the umbilicus.

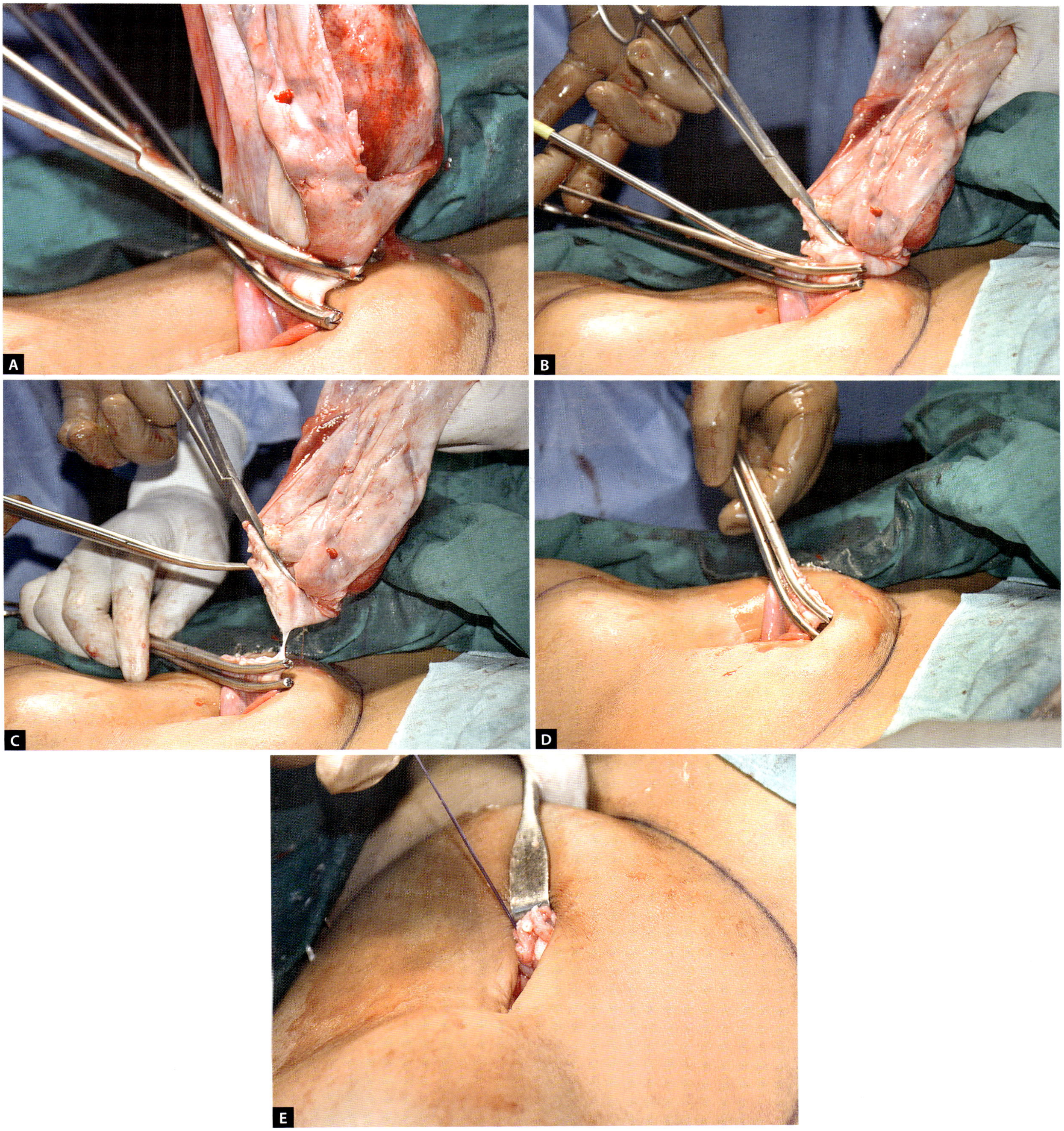

Fig. 9A to E: (A to D) Oophorectomy done by clamping and ligation; (E) Closure.

Laparotomy for Huge Cyst (Figs. 10A to I)

Step 1: Midline vertical incision made and abdomen opened in layers

Step 2: Cyst brought out of the abdomen

Step 3: Biclamp applied to infundibulopelvic ligament, cauterized, and cut

Step 4: Pedicle visualized for hemostasis

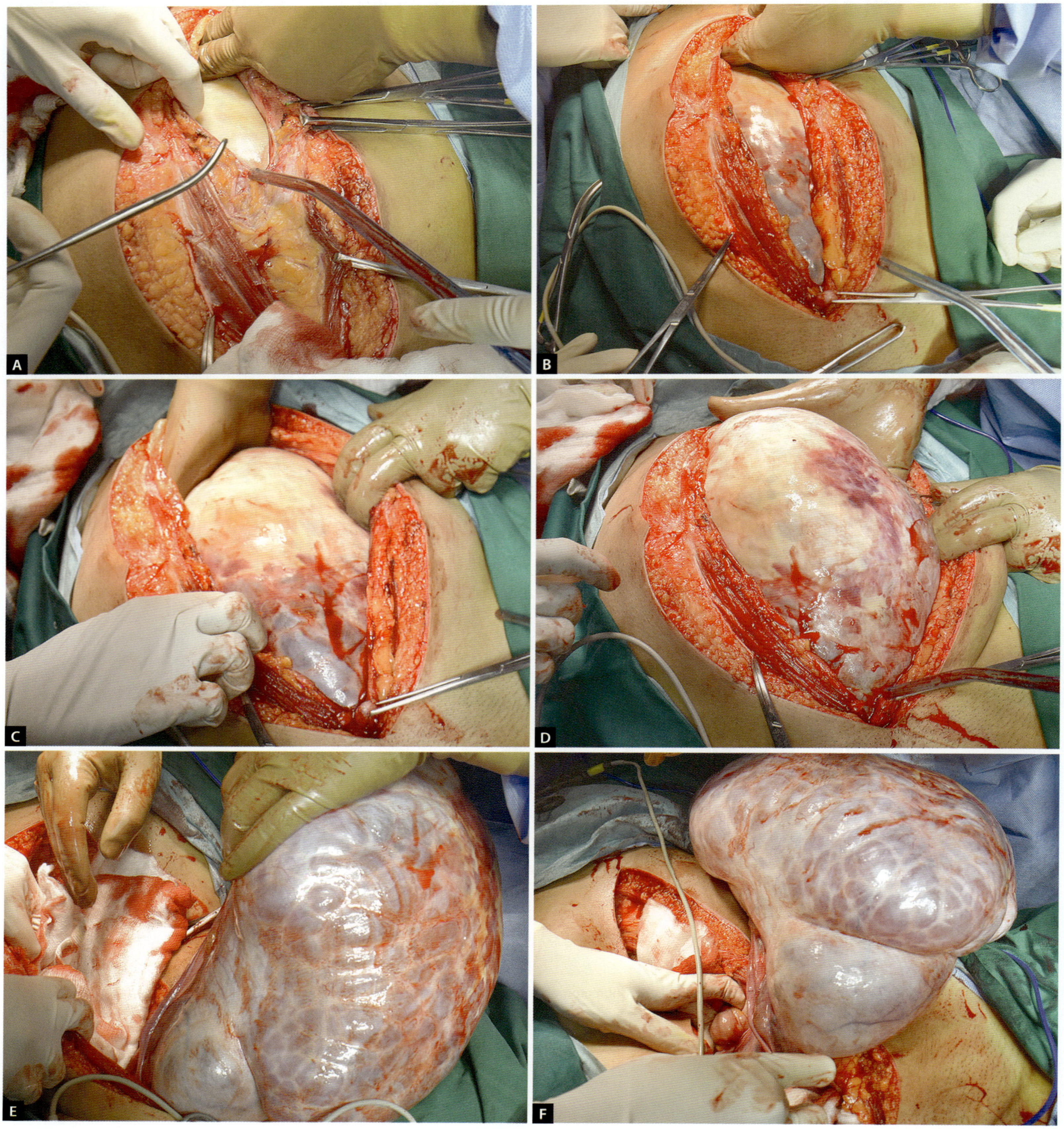

Figs. 10A to F

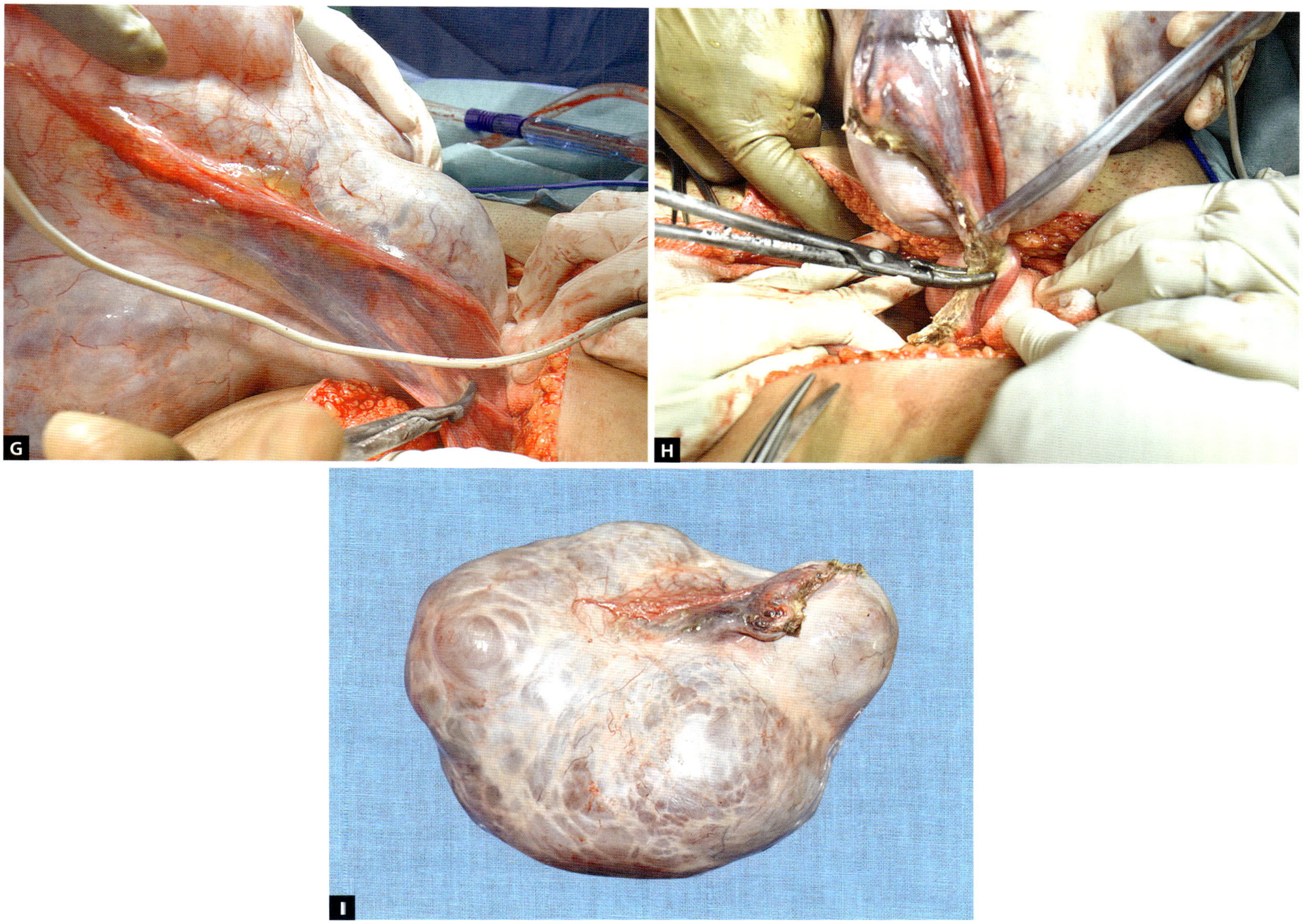

Figs. 10G to I

Figs. 10A and I: Specimen

CHAPTER 15

Bartholin's Gland Surgery

Prijy TP, Isha Rani, B Ramesh

INTRODUCTION

The Bartholin's glands are essential organs of female reproductive system. The function of Bartholin's gland is to secrete mucus to maintain lubrication of vagina and vulva. The Bartholin's glands can easily get infected and may form abscess prone to infections and abscess formation. In such scenario, presentation will be vulvar pain and dyspareunia. Other complications are formation of Bartholin's cyst and rarely, malignancy.

While deciding management for pathological conditions of Bartholin's gland, goal should be to preserve the gland and its function as much as possible. Generally, office-based procedures such as insertion of a Word catheter for a duct cyst or gland abscess, and marsupialization of a cyst are carried out. Broad-spectrum antibiotic is treatment of choice in presence of cellulitis. In perimenopausal and menopausal women presenting with Bartholin's gland mass where adenocarcinoma is suspected, excisional biopsy is done.

ANATOMY

The Bartholin's glands, also known as greater vestibular glands, are pea-sized glands bilaterally located at the posterior region of the vaginal opening **(Fig. 1)**. The glands were first described in the 17th century by the Danish anatomist, Casper Bartholin.[1] The glands are homologous to the male bulbourethral or Cowper's glands.[2] The glands have an oval shape and are located posterior to vestibular bulbs and lateral to the bulbocavernosus muscle in the deep perineal pouch, located between deep and superficial fascia of the urogenital diaphragm. Bartholin's gland opens at 4 and 8 o'clock position via a duct of width approximately 2.5 cm and drains mucus into the vaginal vestibule.[3,4]

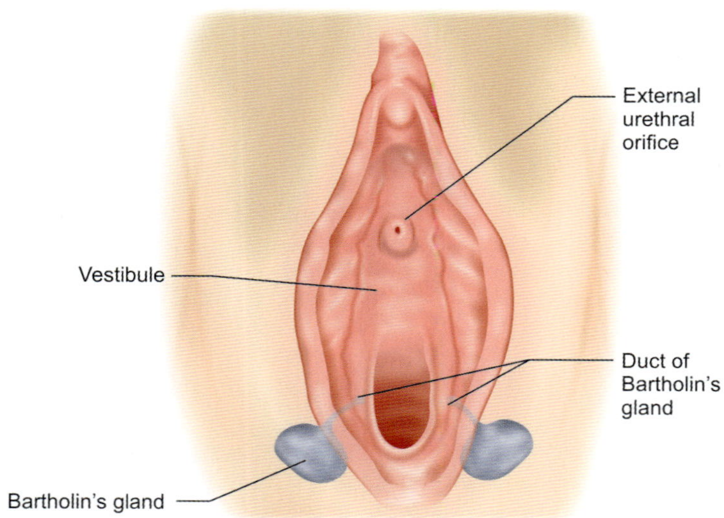

Fig. 1: Bartholin's cyst.

Embryologically, the Bartholin's glands originate from the urogenital sinus, hence supplied by external pudendal artery and vein. The gland derives its nerve supply from pudendal nerve. The lymphatic vessels drain into superficial inguinal and pelvic nodes.[1]

A diagnosis of Bartholin's cyst is made on clinical appearance, but the distinction between cyst of the duct and cyst of the gland can only be made on histopathology. The duct is lined by transitional epithelium, whereas the lining of the gland acinus is a single layer of columnar or cubical epithelium.

EPIDEMIOLOGY

Bartholin's duct cysts are most common cystic growths in the vulva,[5] occurring in labia majora. 2% of women develop a Bartholin's duct cyst or gland abscess at some time in life.[6] Abscesses are three times more common than cysts.

The size of Bartholin's gland increases during sexual activity and stabilizes/shrinks in women with reduced sexual activity. As cyst develops due to accumulation of Bartholin's gland secretions resulting from obstruction, occurrence of Bartholin's duct cyst and gland abscess is seen during the reproductive years, especially between 20 years and 29 years of age. Almost all cases are seen between 20 years and 50 years, 72% occurring before 30 years of age and 10% in women more than 40 years of age.[1]

Bartholin's cysts and abscesses are exceedingly rare before puberty and in postmenopausal women. In postmenopausal women if Bartholin's cyst is seen, there should be a high suspicion of malignancy and should be deemed malignant until proved otherwise. Due to reduced frequency of sexual activity and reduced secretory response, cyst formation due to collection of secretion is less likely and excisional biopsy is required.

ETIOLOGY

Bartholin's cysts are due to occlusion of the main duct which opens into the vestibule, arising in the duct system of the Bartholin's gland.[1] Ductal obstruction occurs secondary to mucus, trauma, or from infection and edema. If incomplete treatment is provided, there is an increased risk of recurrence, due to scarring and stenosis of duct opening.

A Bartholin's abscess more commonly results from polymicrobial nongonorrheal infection of the cyst fluid rather than primary infection of the gland or duct. Rarely, Bartholin's cyst or abscess occurs after episiotomy, trauma, or vulvovaginal surgery.

Bartholin's gland adenocarcinoma is a rare type of gynecological malignancy. It forms 2–7% of all vulvar malignancies. The incidence is highest in postmenopausal age group, highest being in women of age >60 years.

CLINICAL PRESENTATION AND SYMPTOMS

If Bartholin's duct cyst is small and not inflamed, it will be incidentally found during regular gynecological examination or patient may appreciate as a small swelling in the genital region **(Fig. 2)**. Bartholin's gland cyst is painless but painful if abscess is formed **(Fig. 3)**. Abscess might be associated with cellulitis and lymphangitis. Larger cysts and abscess tend to cause intense vulvar pain, dyspareunia, and swelling such that the patient experiences difficulty in walking, sitting, and engaging in sexual intercourse (dyspareunia). During examination, an abscess presents as a tender mass in the lower vestibular region surrounded by erythema and edema. When the abscess grows large enough to extend to the upper labia, it may result in rupture and spontaneously drain. The patient may experience a sudden relief of pain after a discharge that suggests spontaneous rupture. Cysts can present in the form of inguinal hernia.

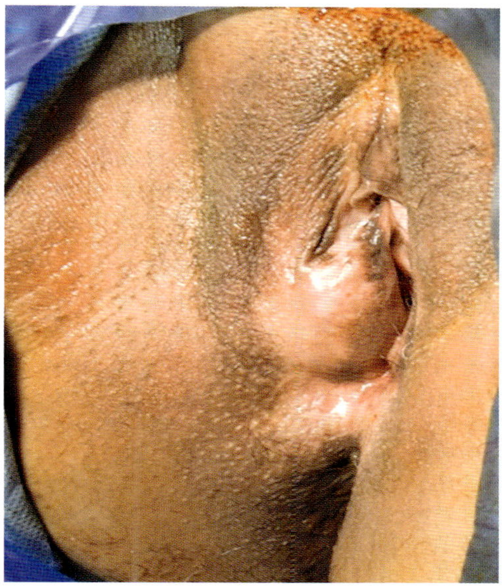

Fig. 2: Bartholin's duct cysts.

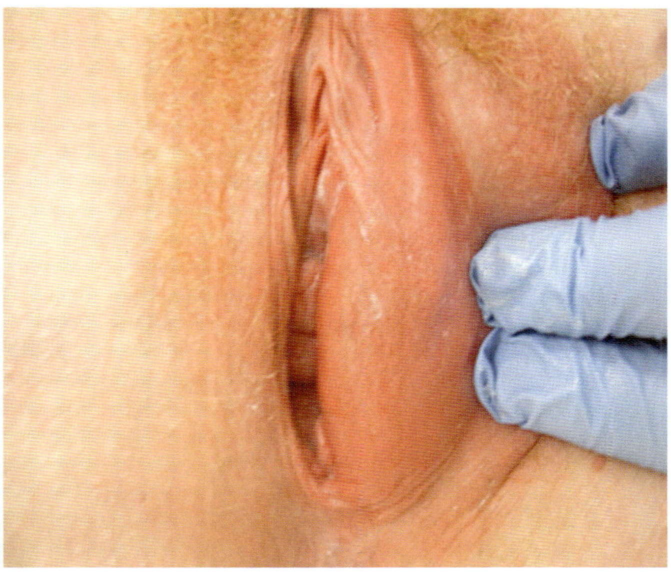

Fig. 3: Swelling of bartholin's gland.

In a neonate, Bartholin's duct cyst is associated with hydroureteronephrosis and contralateral renal cyst may present with urinary retention.[7] Bartholin's gland adenocarcinoma presents as painless mass vulvar region. Mass fixated to the underlying tissue is suspicious of malignancy. First detection of sentinel node may lead to suspicion of adenocarcinoma of Bartholin's gland.[8]

Bartholin's duct cysts and gland abscesses must be differentiated from other vulvar masses such as epidermal inclusion cyst, Skene's duct cyst, hidradenoma papilliferum, and lipoma. As Bartholin's glands usually shrink during menopause, a vulvar growth in a postmenopausal woman should be evaluated for malignancy, especially if the mass is irregular, nodular, and persistently indurated.

The diagnosis of Bartholin's cysts and abscesses is clinical and readily made on visual inspection of the vulva. Further investigations are not required to make the diagnosis.

TREATMENT OPTIONS[9]

Asymptomatic Cyst

First Conservative Management

A small, quiescent, and asymptomatic cyst can be managed with sitz baths or warm compresses to aid drainage.

Symptomatic Cyst

- First marsupialization adjunct broad-spectrum antibiotics
- First Word catheter drainage adjunct broad-spectrum antibiotics
- Second surgical excision
- Third silver nitrate cauterization
- Third alcohol sclerotherapy.

Bartholin's Abscess

First conservative management ± incision and drainage plus broad-spectrum antibiotics after resolution of infection/inflammation adjunct marsupialization or catheter insertion.

If spontaneous rupture of abscess occurs, conservative management with regular sitz bath and analgesics is advised.

Small unruptured abscesses can also be treated with local application of warm, wet dressings, or regular sitz baths to promote spontaneous drainage or development to a stage suitable for incision and drainage.

Incision and drainage may be required if spontaneous drainage does not occur. Packing the cavity may reduce the risk of recurrence. Abscess may recur after incision and drainage recurs in up to 15% of patients.

Adjunct Broad-spectrum Antibiotics

- *Primary options—trimethoprim/sulfamethoxazole:* 160/800 mg orally twice daily for 7 days.
- *Secondary options—amoxicillin/clavulanate:* 875 mg orally twice daily for 7 days, clindamycin: 300 mg orally four times daily for 7 days, cefixime: 400 mg orally once daily for 7 days, and clindamycin: 300 mg orally four times daily for 7 days.

Word Catheter

Word catheter[10] is commonly used to treat Bartholin's duct cysts and gland abscesses. It is made from No. 10 French Foley's catheter with 1-inch long stem. The balloon tip at the word catheter can be inflated with 3ml of saline **(Fig. 4)**. After sterile preparation and the administration of a local anesthetic, the wall of the cyst or abscess is grasped with a small forceps, and using No. 11 blade, a 5-mm (stab) incision is made into the cyst or abscess. The cyst wall should be grasped before the incision is made to prevent it from collapsing, as otherwise can lead to a false tract formation. The incision should be within the introitus external to the hymenal ring in the area of the duct orifice. Care should be taken regarding the size of the incision as too large incision will cause the Word catheter to fall off.

After making the incision, the Word catheter is inserted and the balloon tip is inflated with 2–3 mL of saline solution injected through the hub of the catheter **(Figs. 5A to C)**. The inflated balloon allows the catheter to remain within the cavity of the cyst or abscess. The free end of the catheter can be placed in the vagina to allow drainage of the secretions. Word catheter is placed for 4–6 weeks, to allow epithelization. Sitz baths taken 2–3 times daily may aid patient comfort and healing during the immediate postoperative period. Coitus may be resumed after catheter insertion. Unless, there is an evidence of cellulitis, antibiotic therapy is not necessary. If cellulitis is present, cultures are sent, but empirical broad-spectrum antibiotics are started and then are changed as per the culture report. If a Bartholin's cyst or abscess is too deep, Word catheter placement is impractical and other options must be considered.

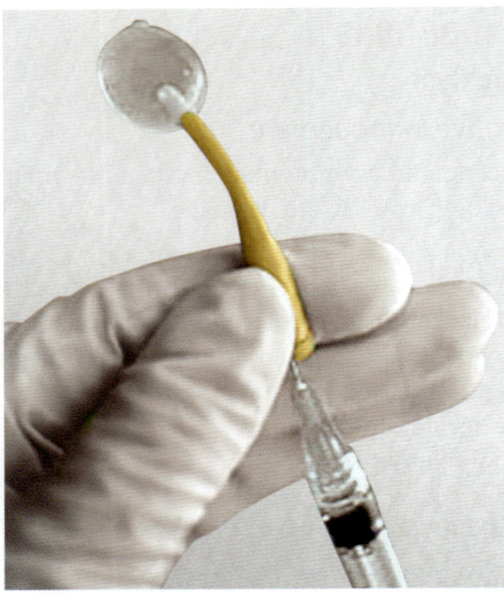

Fig. 4: Balloon tip of the word catheter being inflated.

Marsupialization

An alternative to Word catheter placement is marsupialization of a Bartholin's cyst **(Figs. 6A and B)**.[10] A new mucocutaneous junction is created between the wall of the cyst and the skin of the labia, and to place it in anatomically normal position. By doing so, this allows for patency of the gland to be maintained so that secretory function is not lost. However, if infection is present accompanied by marked inflammation and necrosis, sutures will pull through the friable tissue and marsupialization will not be possible. It can be performed under pudendal nerve block or local anesthetic.

Marsupialization can be performed in the office setting or, if the cyst is deeply seated, in an outpatient surgical suite. It is performed under local anesthesia and under all aseptic precaution. The cyst wall is held with two small hemostats and a vertical incision of about 1.5–3 cm depending on the size of the cyst is made in the vestibule over the center of the cyst and outside the hymenal ring.

After the cyst is vertically excised, the cavity drains spontaneously; it is then irrigated with saline solution. Loculations if present are broken with artery forceps. The cyst wall is everted and approximated to the edge of the vestibular mucosa with interrupted 2-0 absorbable suture. Daily sitz baths should begin on the first postoperative day. Approximately 5–15% of Bartholin's duct cysts recur after marsupialization. Complications, which may occur with the procedure, are dyspareunia, hematoma, and infection.

Excision

Surgical excision may be necessary in recurrent cases. Excision is not an office-based procedure.

Excision of the Bartholin's gland should be considered in patients who do not respond to conservative attempts[10] to create a

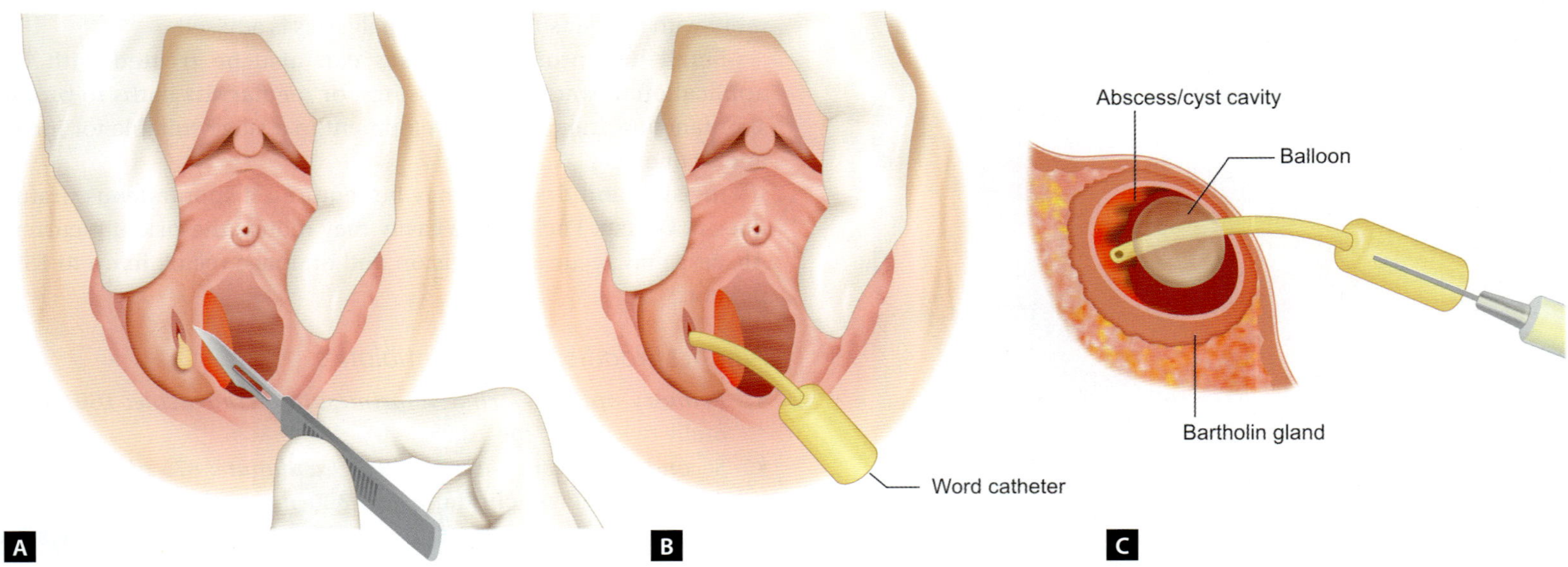

Figs. 5A to C: Incision catheter inserted in to the cyst bulb inflated.

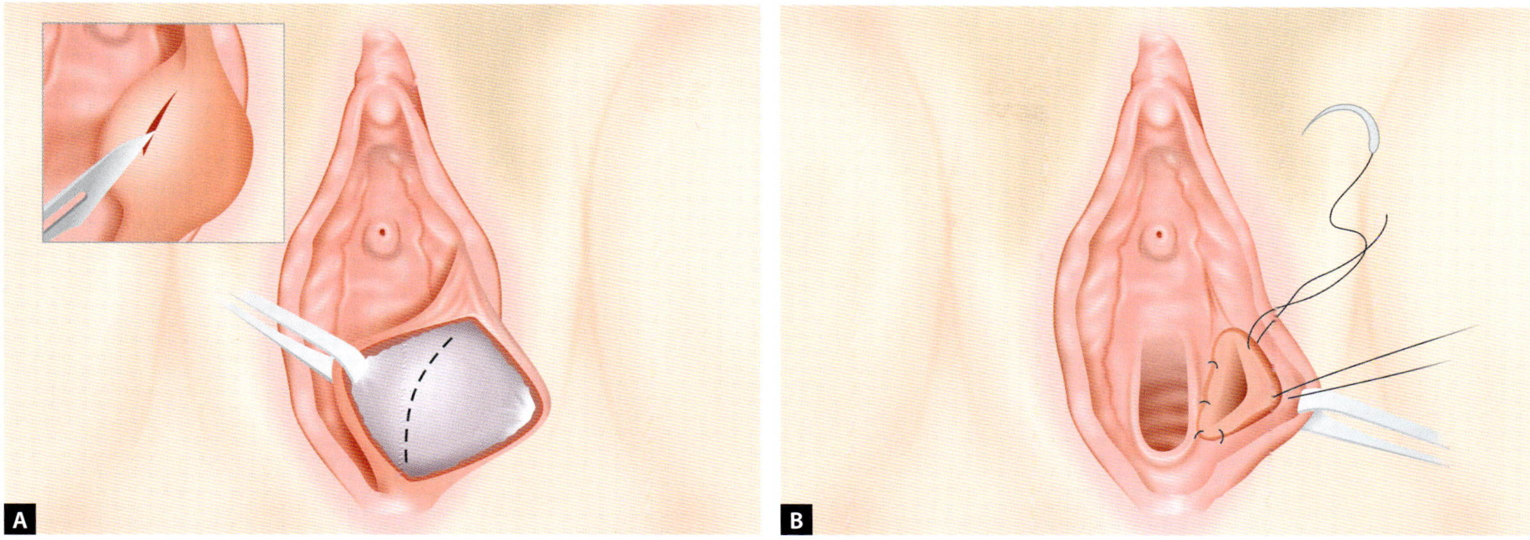

Figs. 6A and B: Marsupialization of Bartholin's duct cyst. (A) A vertical incision is made over the center of the cyst to dissect it free of mucosa; (B) The cyst wall is everted and approximated to the edge of the vestibular mucosa with interrupted sutures.

drainage tract. The procedure should be performed after treating an active infection. If multiple attempts have been made to drain a cyst or an abscess, adhesions may form, making excision difficult leading to increased postoperative scarring and chronic pain in the area. Some surgeons recommend excision of the Bartholin's gland in patients >40 years of age to exclude adenocarcinoma when cysts or abscesses occurs.

Excision of the Bartholin's gland has been called the "bloodiest little operation in gynecology".[11] It is indicated for persistent and recurrent Bartholin's gland abscess and cyst. The key to successful excision is hemostatic control of the copious blood supply to the gland.

The purpose of the operation is to remove the entire Bartholin's gland.

Physiologic Changes

Bilateral removal of Bartholin's gland eliminates the secretion of fluid from the gland that is useful as a vaginal lubricant. In the well-estrogenized vagina, however, this is generally not a clinical problem.

Points of Caution

Meticulous hemostasis is essential. The branches of the pudendal artery are frequently lacerated during the excision of the Bartholin's gland. They must be carefully identified, clamped, and tied, or postoperative vulvar hematoma will result.

The labia are retracted laterally with several Allis clamps. For resection of the Bartholin's gland, it is preferable to make the incision over the vaginal mucosa, directly over the meatus of the gland, rather than incision in the skin of the labia **(Fig. 7)**.

The vaginal mucosa is retracted medially and the skin of the introitus is retracted laterally to expose the wall of the gland. Its meatus may be seen if not distorted by an old infection and scarring.

A small Metzenbaum scissors is used to lyze the filmy adhesions between the wall of the abscess or cyst and the overlying vaginal mucosa and subcutaneous tissue of the labia majora **(Figs. 8A to G)**. Either forceps or an Allis clamp is placed on the wall of the cyst. The wall is retracted to allow adequate dissection and identification of the blood supply to the gland from branches of the pudendal artery.

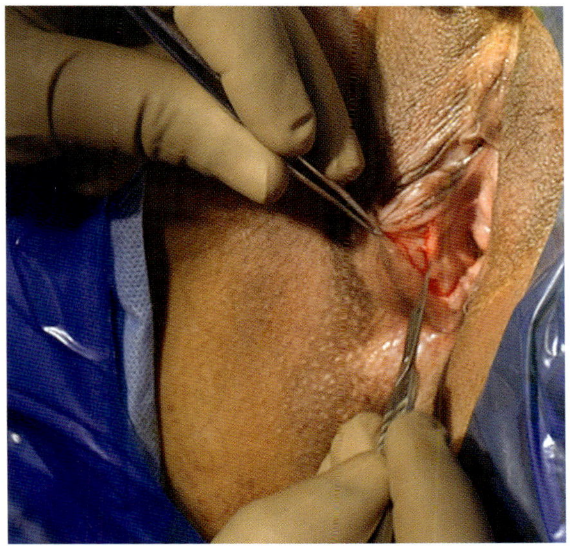

Fig. 7: Incision over the vaginal mucosa.

The bed of the gland **(Fig. 9)** should be closed with interrupted 3-0 absorbable suture to eliminate dead space **(Figs. 9 to 12)**.

Other Treatment Modalities

Other methods of treating Bartholin's gland cyst and abscess include silver nitrate gland ablation, laser, needle aspiration with or without alcohol sclerotherapy, and gland excision.

Due to the disadvantage of recurrence, scarring, persistent drainage, and hemorrhage associated with commonly used treatments, CO_2 laser serves as an advantageous method of avoiding such results. Incision on the cyst is made with CO_2 laser and the wall is vaporized from the inside. In reported cases, the cysts healed with no scar formation and minimal incidence of recurrence.

Silver nitrate topical: Silver nitrate is a simple, cost-effective germicide and a chemical sclerosing agent. Its use has been described in the outpatient treatment of both cysts and abscesses. Benefits of silver nitrate application include less incidence of early and late morbidity, low recurrence rate, and avoiding sutures. A prospective randomized controlled trial found that using silver nitrate and marsupialization

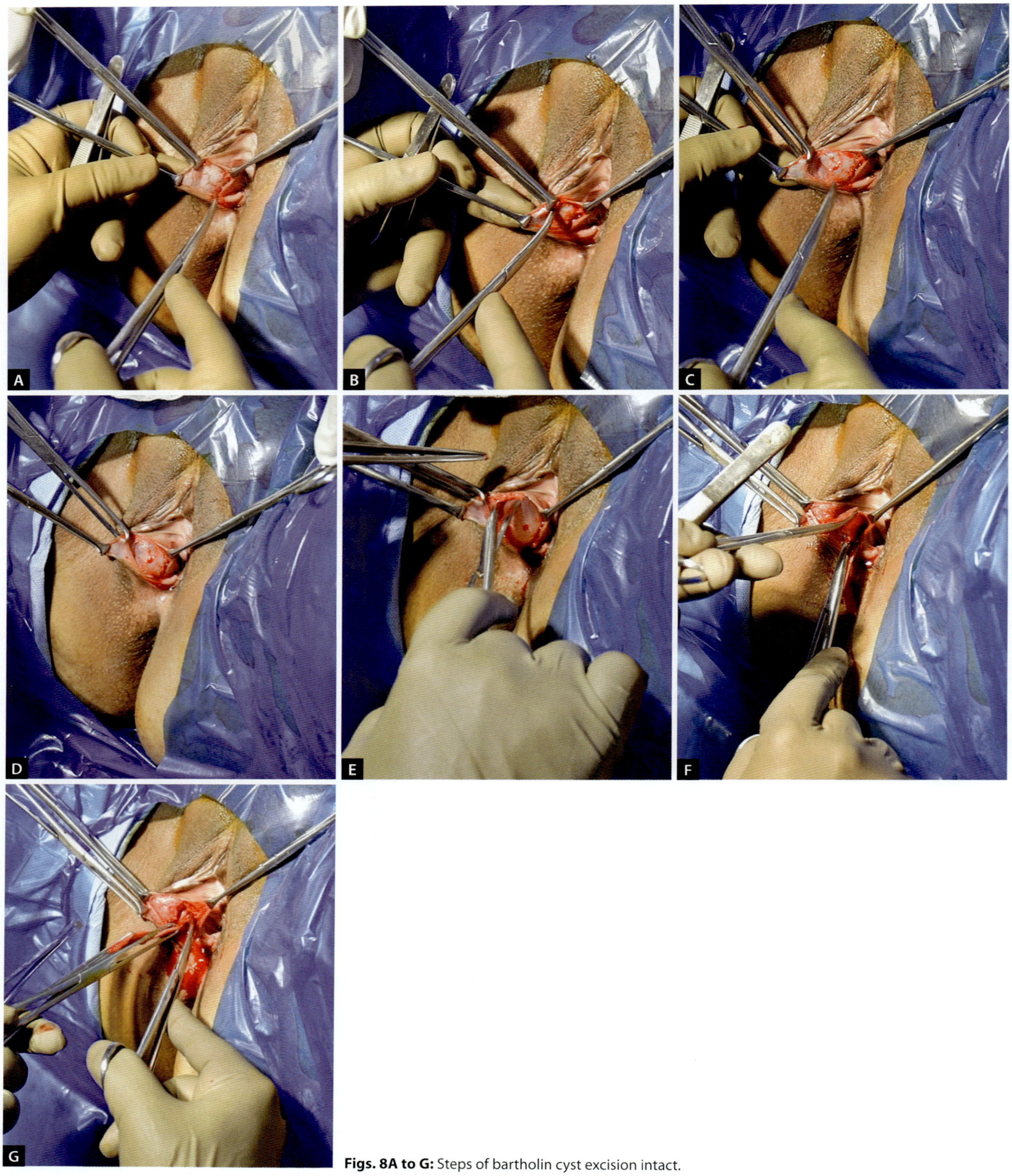

Figs. 8A to G: Steps of bartholin cyst excision intact.

were equally effective, with less scar formation noted with the use of silver nitrate. Complications include chemical burns of the labial or surrounding mucosa, labial edema, hemorrhagic or purulent discharge, and cyst recurrence.

Alcohol sclerotherapy is compared with aspiration; instillation of alcohol for sclerotherapy reduced treatment time with a low recurrence rate. Complete evacuation of the injected alcohol is essential to avoid necrosis of the cyst wall. Compared with silver nitrate, alcohol sclerotherapy was as effective, with fewer complications and a faster healing time. There were no recurrences at 24-month follow-up.

Treatment of Bartholin's adenocarcinomas[12] can be either surgical, i.e. vulvectomy or radiotherapy. Hyperbaric oxygen[13] therapy may be used following radical vulvectomy to promote wound healing. Primary adenoid cystic carcinoma is a rare malignancy of Bartholin's cancer. Depending on the stage of adenocarcinoma, lymphadenectomy is planned.[14]

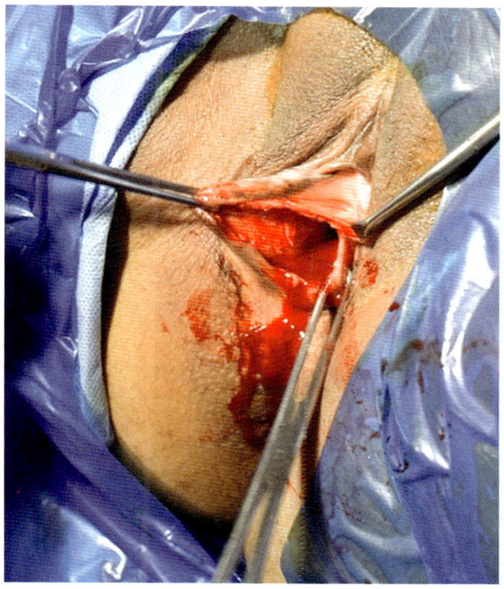

Fig. 9: Bed of the gland.

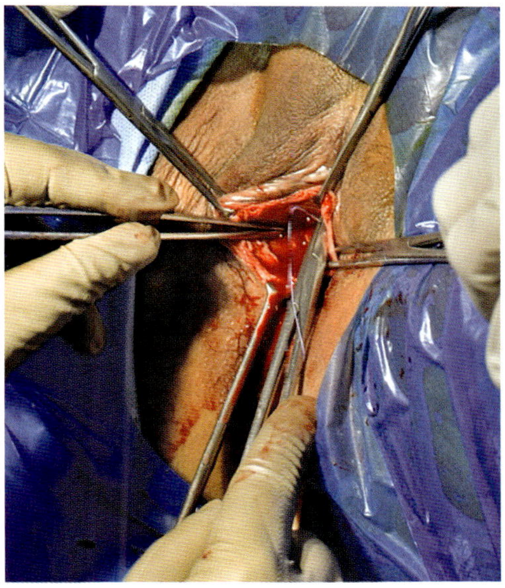

Fig. 10: Obliteration of bed.

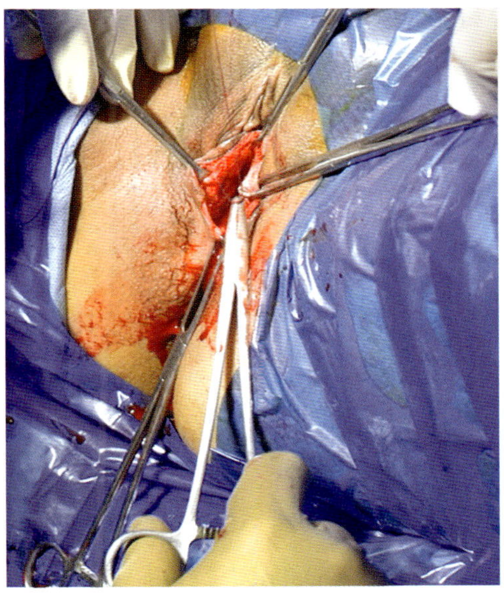

Fig. 11: Suturing continued.

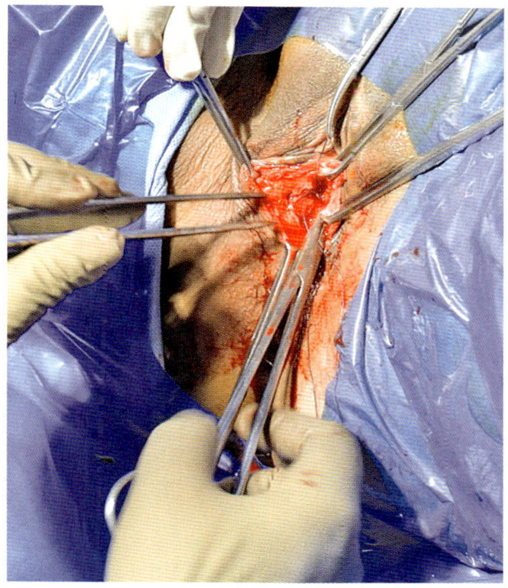

Fig. 12: Closure.

CONCLUSION

The Bartholin's glands form a crucial part of the female reproductive system by causing vaginal lubrication. Cyst forms due to blockage of the gland ducts that may lead to abscess formation. Asymptomatic small cysts can be left untreated, large cysts and abscess require proper treatment. Appropriate management should be chosen, healing depends on level of infection, treatment method, and patient's condition.

REFERENCES

1. Lee MY, Dalpiaza A, Schwamb R, et al. Clinical pathology of Bartholin's gland: A review of literature. Curr Urol. 2015;8(1):22-5.
2. Stenchever MA, Droegemueller W, Herbst AL, et al. Comprehensive Gynecology, 4th edition. St. Louis: Mosby; 2001. pp. 482-486, 645-646.
3. Hill DA, Lense JJ. Office management of Bartholin gland cysts and abscesses. Am Fam Physician. 1998;57(7):1611-6.
4. Govan AD, Hodge C, Callander R. Gynaecology Illustrated, 3rd edition. New York: Churchill Livingstone; 1985. pp. 19, 195-196.
5. Kaufman RH. Benign Diseases of the Vulva and Vagina, 4th edition. St Louis: Mosby; 1994. pp. 168-248.
6. Aghajanian A, Bernstein L, Grimes DA. Bartholin's duct abscess and cyst: a case-control study. South Med J. 1994;87(1):26-9.
7. Cevik M, Savas M, Guldur ME, et al. Urinary retention as the presentation of Bartholin's duct cyst in a neonate. J Pediatr Adolesc Gynecol. 2012;25(3): e65-7.
8. Balepa L, Baeyens L, Nemec E, et al. First detection of sentinel node in adenocarcinoma of Bartholin's gland. J Gynecol Obstetbiol Reprod (Paris). 2004;33:649-51.
9. BMJ best practice - bartholin cyst, march 2018.
10. Omole F, Simmons BJ, Hacker Y, Management of Bartholin's duct cyst and gland abscess. Am Fam Physician. 2003;68(1):135-140.
11. Wheeless CR, Roenneburg ML, Parker JE. Atlas of Pelvic Surgery. Baltimore: M. Roenneburg & C. Wheeless; 2007.
12. Duun S. Adenoid cystic carcinoma of Bartholin's gland—a review of the literature and report of a patient. Acta Obstet Gynecol Scand. 1995;74(1): 78-80.
13. Reedy MB, Capen CV, Baker DP, et al. Hyperbaric oxygen therapy following radical vulvectomy: an adjunctive therapy to improve wound healing. Gynecol Oncol. 1994;53(1):13-6.
14. Hsu ST, Wang RC, Lu CH, et al. Report of two cases of adenoidcystic carcinoma of Bartholin's gland and review of literature. Taiwan J Obstet Gynecol. 2013;52(1):113-6.

CHAPTER

16

Uterovaginal Prolapse

Kavya Rashmi Rao, Isha Rani, B Ramesh

INTRODUCTION

In the past century due to increase in the life expectancy in developed country, there is increased need for clinicians having experience in disorders of the elderly.

Pelvic organ prolapse (POP) is protrusion of pelvic organs and adjoining vaginal segment into or through the vagina, due to reduced strength of their normal attachment. POP most often is accompanied with urinary incontinence, are commonly seen to affect many females. It is a common and costly affliction of older women and quite distressing.

In this era as there is increased incidence of POP, it is more important than ever to continue researches and study to understand pathophysiology and risk factors associated, and device measures to prevent it.

Furthermore, continued efforts are needed to understand factors that result in long-lasting and site-specific repair of POP in patients undergoing surgery.

HISTORY

Uterine prolapse was first mentioned in the Kahun Papyri in 2000 BC. Hippocrates described numerous nonsurgical treatments for this condition. In 98 CE, first description of removal prolapsed uterus was by Soranus of Rome when it turned black. The first successful vaginal hysterectomy for the cure of uterine prolapse as described by Willouby, was self-performed by a peasant woman named Faith Raworth in1670.

Starting from century, there has been many modifications and advancement in the surgical procedure.

RISK FACTORS

Factors increasing the chances of uterine prolapse include:

- Increasing number of pregnancies and normal delivery
- Increased age/postmenopausal status
- Obesity
- Previous history of pelvic surgeries
- Chronic constipation or frequent straining during bowel movements
- Family history of weakness in connective tissue
- Chronic cough with chronic airway disease
- Hispanic or white.

INDICATIONS

- To attain relief from symptoms
- Restoration of the normal anatomy and function of the pelvic structures
- Prevention of recurrence of prolapse
- Repair of other associated defects in pelvis
- Cystocele, if association with bladder outlet obstruction
- Surgery is offered to all symptomatic patients.

CONTRAINDICATIONS

Cystocele repair is contraindicated in following conditions:

- Local vaginal diseases, vaginitis, and neoplasms
- Medically unfit for surgery
- Not willing for major surgery
- Early disease with asymptomatic cystoceles.

PATHOPHYSIOLOGY

Pelvic organ prolapse results from weakness of structures supporting the pelvic organs either due to break in the connective tissue or neuromuscular dysfunction or both.

Vaginal canal is supported mainly by endopelvic fascia, which envelops the vagina and condenses at the apex, forming the triradiate ligament complex (Mackenrodt's, uterosacral, and pubocervical ligament). The first line of support is endopelvic connective tissue, is intimately associated with pelvic diaphragm. Levator ani and coccygeus muscles forms major component.

These muscles forms diaphragm through which the urethra, vagina, and rectum, hence supporting these structures **(Fig. 1)**. Muscular support provides basal tonicity and support of the pelvic structures; when contracted as in the setting of increased abdominal pressure, the rectum, vagina, and urethra are pulled anteriorly toward the pubis.

CLASSIFICATION OF PROLAPSE

- Anterior vaginal wall:
  - Upper two-thirds—cystocele **(Fig. 2)**
  - Lower one-third—urethrocele
- Posterior vaginal wall:
  - Upper one-third—enterocele
  - Lower two-thirds—rectocele
- Uterine descent
- Decent of cervix to vagina (I degree)
- Decent of cervix up to the introitus (II degree)
- Decent of cervix outside the introitus (III degree).

DEFINITIONS

The pelvic supports disorders includes rectoceles and cystoceles, enteroceles, and uterine prolapse. These terminologies signify displacement of the rectum, bladder, small intestines, and uterus,

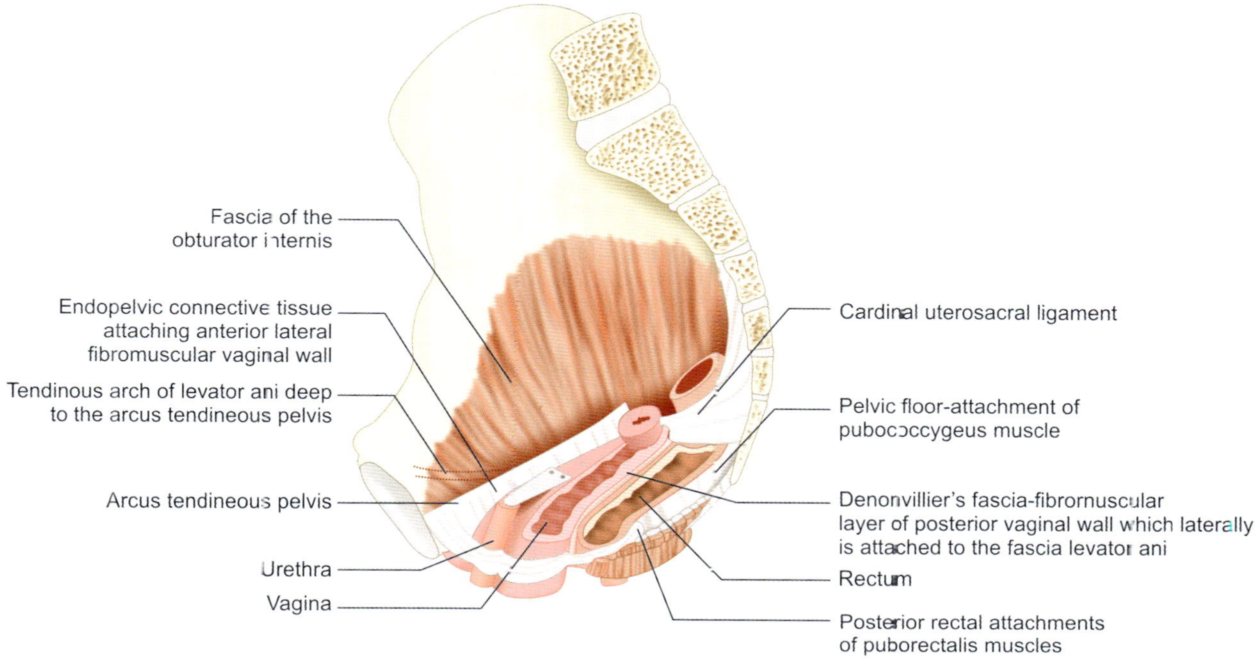

Fig. 1: Anatomy of the pelvic floor.

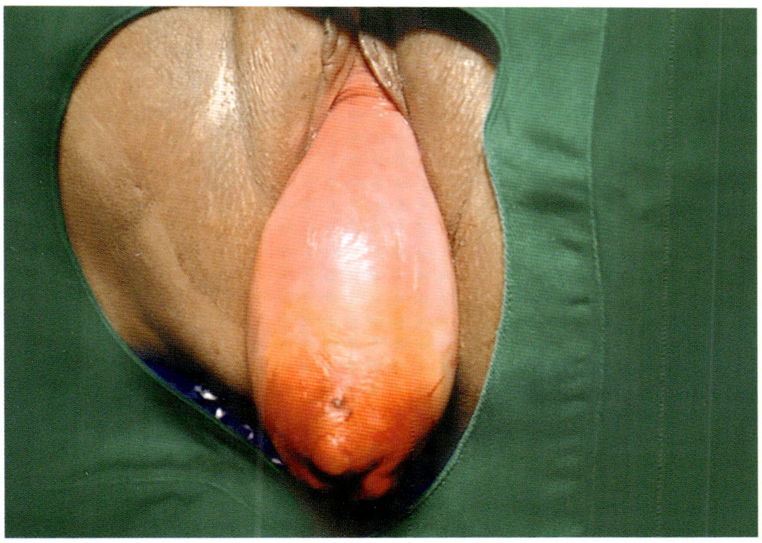

Fig. 2: Prolapse.

respectively which resulted from failure of the endopelvic connective tissue and muscular support (levator ani), or both.

Rectocele

Protrusion of the rectum through posterior vaginal wall resulting from weakness in the muscular wall of the rectum and the paravaginal musculoconnective tissue, which holds the rectum in place posteriorly.

Enterocele

It is defined as herniation of the peritoneum and small bowel. It is the only true hernia among the pelvic support disorders. Most enteroceles occur between the uterosacral ligaments and the rectovaginal space, but they may also occur primarily apically, especially in the setting of a previous hysterectomy, so special steps should be performed during surgery to prevent occurrence of enterocele.

Cystocele

It is defined as herniation of the urinary bladder through anterior vaginal wall. Cystoceles usually occur due to pubocervical musculoconnective tissue weakness, midline or detachment from its lateral or superior connecting points.

Uterine Prolapse

Uterine prolapse is generally results from weakness of cardinal or uterosacral ligament which forms the apical support, causing downward displacement of the cervix and uterus toward the introitus.

Procidentia

It is defined as complete prolapse of the uterus and vagina, and total vaginal vault prolapse, which can occur after hysterectomy, represent eversion of the entire vagina.

These terms are just for description and terms are somewhat inaccurate and misleading as they do not focus on the specific defects. These terminologies focus on the organ descending with the respective vaginal wall like bladder, rectum, small bowel, or uterus and does not give any idea about the defect. Specific defect support issues will be discussed in the setting of the surgical management section.

PELVIC ORGAN PROLAPSE QUANTIFICATION SYSTEM

In literature may systems have been described for staging of prolapse. Typically it is graded on a scale of 0–3 or 0–4, with the grade increasing with the severity of prolapse. Currently the International Continence Society has approved terminology Pelvic Organ Prolapse Quantification system, or POP-Q for grading the POP.

This standardized quantification system facilitates communication between physicians in practice and research and enables following the progression of the conditions more accurately.

In this system, we get to know about the site specific defects and it also helps in the follow-up. The system identifies nine locations in the

Table 1: Stages of pelvic organ prolapse.

Stage 0	No prolapse is demonstrated. Points Aa, Ap, Ba, Bp are all at -3 cm, and point C is between total vaginal length (TVL) and -(TVL -2 cm).
Stage I	The most distal portion of the prolapse is >1 cm above the level of the hymen.
Stage II	The most distal portion of the prolapse is <1 cm proximal or distal to the plane of the hymen.
Stage III	The most distal portion of the prolapse is <1 cm below the plane of the hymen but no further than 2 cm less than the total vaginal length.
Stage IV	Complete to nearly complete eversion of the vagina. The most distal portion of the prolapse protrudes to > + (TVI -2) cm.

vagina in centimeters relative to the hymen, which are used to assign stage (from 0 to IV) of prolapse at its most advanced site **(Table 1)**.

Although probably more detailed than necessary for clinical practice, but gynecologists should be familiar with POP–Q system because it is provides uniformity for describing research result in the published studies. Its two most important advantages over previous grading systems are:

1. It is standardized technique with quantitative measurements at straining relative to a constant reference point (i.e. the hymen), and
2. Its ability to assess prolapse at multiple vaginal sites.

Female pelvic organ prolapse (POP–Q classification): The diagram shows the anatomic position of the POP–Q sites, six sites involving the anterior (Aa, Ba), middle (C, D), and posterior (Ap, Bp) compartments along with genital hiatus (GH), perineal body (PB), and total vaginal length (TVL).

There are six points along the vagina (two points on the anterior, middle, and posterior compartments) measured taking hymen as the reference point of 0. Positions of six points are measured in centimeters, proximal to hymen is assigned as negative and distal to hymen is a positive number. Other three measurements are not assigned negative or positive.

The measurement of GH is taken from the middle of the external urethral meatus to the posterior midline hymen. The PB is taken from the posterior margin of the GH to the midanal opening. The TVL is greatest depth of the vagina measured in centimeters. It is measured after reducing the prolapse to normal. All measurements except the TVL are measured during maximal straining.

On anterior vaginal wall Aa and Ba points are located, Ba point moving depending on the amount of anterior compartment prolapse. Point Aa represents a point on the anterior vagina 3 cm proximal to the external urethral meatus, corresponding to the bladder neck. Taking this definition, position of Aa ranges from –3 to +3. Point Ba is the most distal or dependent point of any portion of the anterior vaginal wall from point Aa to just anterior to the vaginal cuff or anterior lip of the cervix. Position of this point depends on the nature of the defect.

The middle compartment consists of points C and D. C represents the most dependent edge of the cervix or in patients post hysterectomy position of vaginal cuff. D represents location of the posterior fornix; and is not considered in patient following hysterectomy. This point corresponds to the level of the attachment of the uterosacral ligament to the posterior cervix. It is intended to differentiate suspensory failure from cervical elongation.

The posterior compartment is measured similarly to the anterior compartment. The corresponding terms are Ap and Bp. The nine

Table 2: Possible ranges of the six site-specific pelvic organ prolapse quantitative examination measurements.

Points	*Description*	*Range*
Aa	Anterior wall 3 cm from hymen	-3 cm to + 3 cm
Ba	Most dependent portion of rest of anterior wall	- 3 cm to + TVL
C	Cervix or vaginal cuff	± TVL
D	Posterior fornix (if no prior hysterectomy)	± TVL or omitted
Ap	Posterior wall 3 cm from hymen	-3 cm to +3 cm
Bp	Most dependent portion of rest of posterior wall	-3 cm to + TVL

(TVL: total vaginal length)
(*Source*: Bump RC, Mattiasson A, Bo K, et al. The standardization of terminology of female pelvic organ prolapse and pelvic floor dysfunction. Am J Obstet Gynecol. 1996;175:11-12.)

measurements can be recorded as a simple line of numbers (i.e. –3, –3, –8, –10, –3, –3, 11, 4, and 3 for points Aa, Ba, C, D, Ap, Bp, total vagina length, GH, and PB). The six vaginal sites have possible ranges that depend on the total vaginal length. After collection of the site-specific measurements, stages are assigned according to the most dependent portion of the prolapse **(Table 2)**.

The POP–Q examination might appear confusing initially, proper demonstration using devices (i.e. a marked ring forceps or marked cotton-tip applicator) is necessary for those unfamiliar with the staging system. The POP–Q examination is a standardized tool for assessments of postoperative outcome accurately and to ensure uniform, reliable, and site-specific descriptions of POP.

EVALUATION

Although as many as 50% of women older than age 50 have some degree of POP, fewer than 20% seek treatment. This may be due to a number of reasons:

- Asymptomatic
- Feeling embarrassment
- Misconceptions and taboos regarding surgery and other treatment options.

Pelvic organ prolapse though not life-threatening have an impact on psychological well-being and overall quality of life by causing significant restriction of activities.

SYMPTOMS

Pelvic organ prolapse often is accompanied by symptoms of voiding dysfunction, including:

- Urinary incontinence,
- Obstructive voiding symptoms,
- Urinary urgency and frequency
- Urinary retention and upper renal compromise with resultant pain or anuria.

Other symptoms often associated with POP include:

- Pelvic pain,
- Problems in defecation (e.g. constipation, diarrhea, tenesmus, and fecal incontinence),
- Back and flank pain,
- Pelvic discomfort,
- Dyspareunia.

An informed choice regarding the treatment modality is made after taking into consideration degree of prolapse and severity of symptoms, general condition of patient, and effect on the activity of patient.

PHYSICAL EXAMINATION

For systematic evaluation of the patient it is important to divide the pelvis into three compartments and examine them separately to assign defects to specific compartment. To evaluate apical compartment, Graves speculum or Baden retractor is used.

Sims univalve speculum is used to examine anterior and posterior compartment, speculum is placed posteriorly while examining anterior compartment and placed anteriorly while examining posterior compartment.

Rectovaginal examination is used to differentiate between dissecting apical enterocoele and posterior wall defect. Sometimes both defects can coexist. If an anterior lateral detachment defect is suspected, an open ring forceps (or a Baden retractor) may be placed in the vagina at a 45° angle posteriorly cephalad to hold the lateral fornices adjacent to the pelvic sidewall.

During the evaluation of each compartment, in order to ascertain full extent of prolapse, patients are asked to perform Valsalva. If description of patient's symptoms is not consistent with the findings while performing Valsalva, patient is examined while straining in standing position with empty bladder.

BLADDER EVALUATION

Patients with prolapse commonly presents with urinary symptoms. It is necessary to evaluate bladder and urethral function in all patients irrespective of symptoms.

Cases of severe POP and procidentia are associated with urethral kinking, which can mask minor degree of stress urinary incontinence (SUI). So, examination should be done after reducing the prolapse that mimics bladder and ureteral function after correction.

Minimal required tests performed before the surgery are: (1) a clean catch or catheterized urine sample to test for routine and culture sensitivity, (2) ultrasound for a postvoid residual (PVR) volume, and (3) assessment of bladder sensation, which can be performed as a part of office cystometrics.

Although there is no consensus on what constitutes an abnormal PVR volume, provided the patient has voided 150 mL or more, a PVR less than or equal to 100 mL is acceptable. Reduction stress testing at the time of simple office cystometrics can be performed with the use of a pessary, large cotton swab, ring forceps, or using speculum—posterior blade.

Care should be taken that urethra should not be overly straightened (with a resultant false-positive test result) or obstructed (with a resultant false-negative test result), or that tension is not placed on the puborectalis muscles by excessive posterior retraction. These risks can be minimized by orienting the vaginal apex toward the sacrum.

IMAGING

Diagnostic imaging is not necessary for management in women with POP. However, if clinically indicated, tests that may be performed include fluoroscopic evaluation of bladder function, ultrasound of the pelvis, and defecography for patients in whom intussusception or rectal mucosal prolapse are suspected. Magnetic resonance imaging (MRI) is increasingly being used for the evaluation of pelvic pathology such as mullerian anomalies and pelvic pain; however, generalized use in women with prolapse is not currently clinically indicated and is used primarily for research purposes.

Role of Magnetic Resonance Imaging

As the technology advances and high quality surface coils and rapid T2-weighted imaging techniques are made available as an imaging modality, the importance of cystourethrography, ultrasonography, and defecography may be reduced for the evaluation of these women. The pelvic floor defects are diagnosed quickly and accurately when MR images are used and hence help in treatment planning. Complete imaging of female pelvis is done in less than 15 minutes if a standardized MR imaging protocol is carried out.

Patient Evaluation and Selection

Pelvic floor damaged is diagnosed by physical examination. Examination is done at rest and at stain to locate several anatomic landmarks and the degree of pelvic descent.

In order to determine the type of surgery performed, site of defect is determined by physical examination and correlating it with the symptoms. Depending on the defects, site-specific corrective surgery is planned. If only cystocele is present it is treated with retropubic (Burch) colposuspension, in this procedure lateral aspect of the bladder is suspended from the pelvic side walls. Paravaginal fascial repair is added if detachment of fascia from the tendinous arch is suspected. When hysterectomy is planned for uterine prolapse uterosacral suspension is done with or without mesh to provide extra support to the tissues. In presence of enterocoele approximation of rectovaginal fascia is done and posterior colporrhaphy is done for rectocele.

Majority of patients are diagnosed based on physical examination and basic urodynamic studies. There is no need of MRI in such patients. In women following delivery pelvic floor weakness is always present but no evaluation in the form of imaging is needed if they do not have any symptoms.

Magnetic resonance imaging may form an important preoperative tool in patients having symptoms involving multiple compartments and will require complex repair and in women presenting with recurrence following a repair. Despite surgeon's best efforts recurrence of symptoms occurs in 10–30% of patients, and is mainly because of pelvic floor defects which were not recognized earlier, in such conditions MRI can be helpful in identifying subtle defects.

Magnetic Resonance Imaging Evaluation of Pelvic Floor Weakness

Imaging Protocol

Best position to evaluate pelvic floor defects is in standing but however MRI evaluation is done in supine position. There is no requirement of oral or intravenous contrast agents, and the protocol takes approximately 15 minutes to complete. A specialist radiologist who is well versed with signs of pelvic descent is required.

After voiding, patient is positioned in supine position and multicoil is wrapped low around the pelvis. First midline sagittal section is obtained by taking the image identifying pubic symphysis, urethra, vagina, rectum, and coccyx.

Next, 10-mm-thick sagittal images of the midline are taken with a rapid half-Fourier T2-weighted imaging sequence, such as single-shot fast spin echo (SSFSE; GE Medical Systems, Milwaukee, WI) or half-Fourier acquisition single-shot turbo spin echo (HASTE; Siemens, Iselin, NJ), and a 30-cm field of view. These images are obtained while the patient is at rest and during the Valsalva maneuver. Coaching prior to imaging may be required for many patients to achieve maximal pelvic strain. Next, 5-mm-thick axial T2-weighted images of the pelvic floor centered on the puborectal muscle are obtained with a 20-cm field of view and a standard high-resolution sequence such as fast spin echo. Coronal images are optional.

Image Interpretation

For the interpretation of the sagittal MR images the pubococcygeal line is drawn, either electronically or by using a wax pencil. This line extends from the inferior border of the pubic symphysis to the last joint of the coccyx and represents the level of the pelvic floor. The distance from the pubococcygeal line to the bladder neck, cervix, and anorectal junction should be measured on images obtained when the patient was at rest and at maximal pelvic strain. The bladder neck is easily identified in all women because of the high T2 signal of urine. The cervix and anorectal junction can be harder to identify; however, a reasonable estimate of their locations is usually possible. In healthy women, there is minimal movement of the pelvic organs, even with maximal strain. In a symptomatic patient, organ descent of greater than 1 cm below the pubococcygeal line indicates pelvic floor laxity, and surgical intervention is indicated if organ descent greater than 2 cm.

The next measurements to be made are the H line and the M line. These lines, which were initially described by Comiter et al., are not used by all surgeons but may be helpful for confirming pelvic floor laxity. The H line is the anteroposterior width of the levator hiatus and is drawn from the inferior aspect of the pubic symphysis to the posterior wall of the rectum at the level of the anorectal junction. The M line is the vertical descent of the levator hiatus and is drawn as a perpendicular line dropped from the pubococcygeal line to the most posterior aspect of the H line. Both of these lines become elongated during the Valsalva maneuver in the patient with pelvic floor laxity. The posterior urethrovesical angle is extremely variable among continent and incontinent women and is of little value in the identification of significant pelvic floor weakness.

At last, the angle formed at the levator plate with the pubococcygeal line is measured. In women without prolapse, the levator plate will be parallel to the pubococcygeal line at rest as well as during pelvic strain. Loss of posterior muscular support is identified by increased caudal inclination. Descent of the small bowel more than 2 cm between the vagina and rectum is indicative of enterocele. Anterior bulging of the rectum is evidence of an anterior rectocele. Sphincter tears and rectal ulcers are not identified by MRI.

On the axial and coronal images, thinning and tears of puborectal and iliococcygeal muscles should be looked for. The width of the levator hiatus is not a reliable marker for pelvic floor laxity; it rarely exceeds 4.5 cm in women with intact pelvic floors. Paravaginal fascial tears can be identified if there is displacement of posterior wall of the vaginal fornix. On axial images, the anterior external urethral sphincter and thin fascial condensations that support the upper portion of the urethra (sometimes called the lateral pubovesical ligaments) can also be seen **(Fig. 3)**.

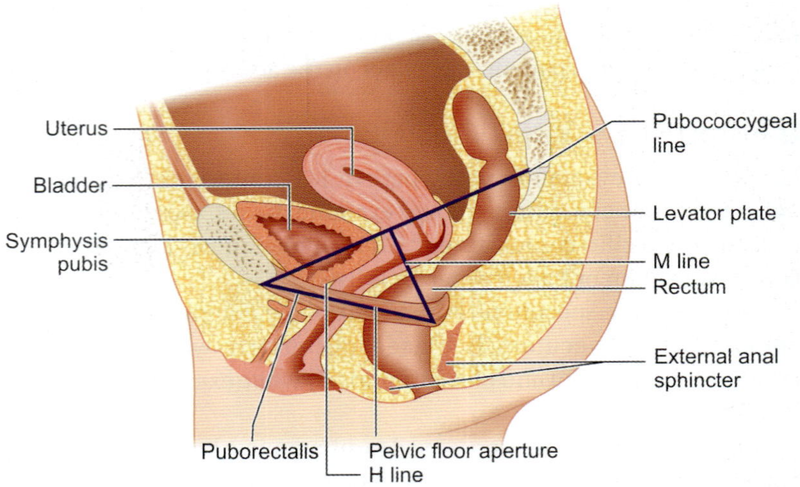

Fig. 3: Drawing of the sagittal midline view of the female pelvis shows bony landmarks and the puborectal muscle, also called the levator sling. The pubococcygeal, H, and M lines and the levator plate are delineated in red.

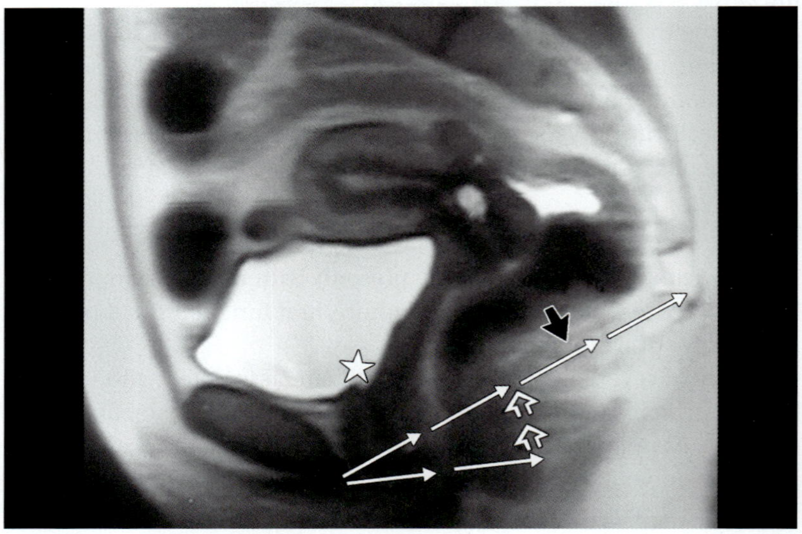

Fig. 4: Pelvic MR images of a 46-year-old healthy, continent volunteer. (a, b) Sagittal T2-weighted images (2,200/96 [repetition time ms/echo time ms]) of the subject at rest (a) and during pelvic strain (b) show minimal (<1 cm) inferior movement of the pelvic viscera. The bladder neck is marked with a star. The levator plate (black arrows) remains parallel with the pubococcygeal line (upper line of white solid arrows). The H (lower line of white solid arrows) and M (open arrows) lines are less than 5 cm and 2 cm in length, respectively, indicating an intact levator hiatus. (c) Axial T2-weighted image (4,200/12) shows the normal butterfly shape of the vagina. The puborectal sling is intact (arrows). The anterior external urethral sphincter and lateral pubovesical ligaments (arrowheads) support the upper portions of the urethra and are part of the extrinsic continence mechanism.

Normal Appearance of the Pelvic Floor

In healthy, continent women, MR images do not demonstrate much of descent of pelvic organs even on maximal downward pelvic strain **(Figs. 4 and 5)**. Normal location of bladder neck, vaginal fornices, and anorectal junction is at or above the pubococcygeal line. Sagittal images are also taken; with strain urethra is seen slightly anterior to the bladder. Cutoff for H line and M line is 5 cm and 2 cm, respectively. On axial images, the entirety of the levator sling should be of similar thickness and homogeneous low signal intensity. The right aspect of the puborectal muscle may appear slightly thinner than the left, a finding that is caused by chemical shift artifact in most cases. On coronal images, the iliococcygeal muscle should be intact and

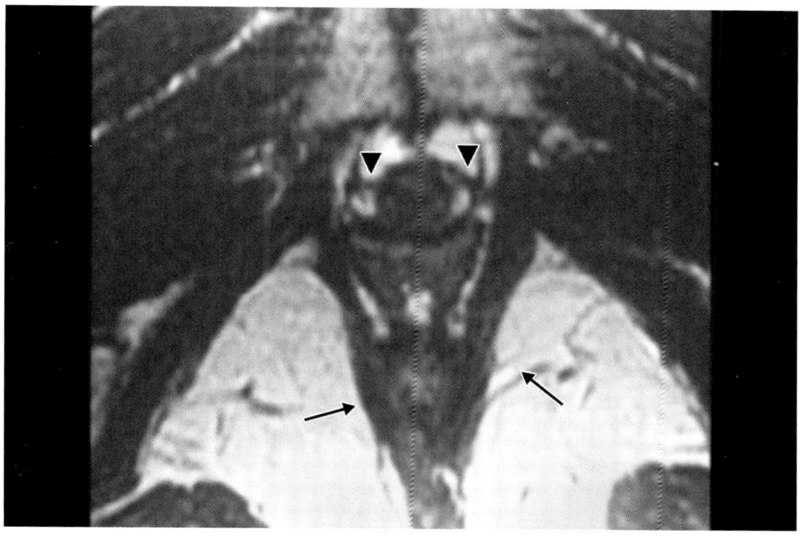

Fig. 5: Pelvic MR images of a 46-year-old healthy, continent volunteer. (a and b) Sagittal T2-weighted images (2,200/96 [repetition time msec/echo time msec]) of the subject at rest (a) and during pelvic strain (b) show minimal (<1 cm) inferior movement of the pelvic viscera. The bladder neck is marked with a star. The levator plate (black arrows) remains parallel with the pubococcygeal line (upper line of white solid arrows). The H (lower line of white solid arrows) and M (open arrows) lines are less than 5 cm and 2 cm in length, respectively, indicating an intact levator hiatus. (c) Axial T2-weighted image (4,200/12) shows the normal butterfly shape of the vagina. The puborectal sling is intact (arrows). The anterior external urethral sphincter and lateral pubovesical ligaments (arrowheads) support the upper portions of the urethra and are part of the extrinsic continence mechanism.

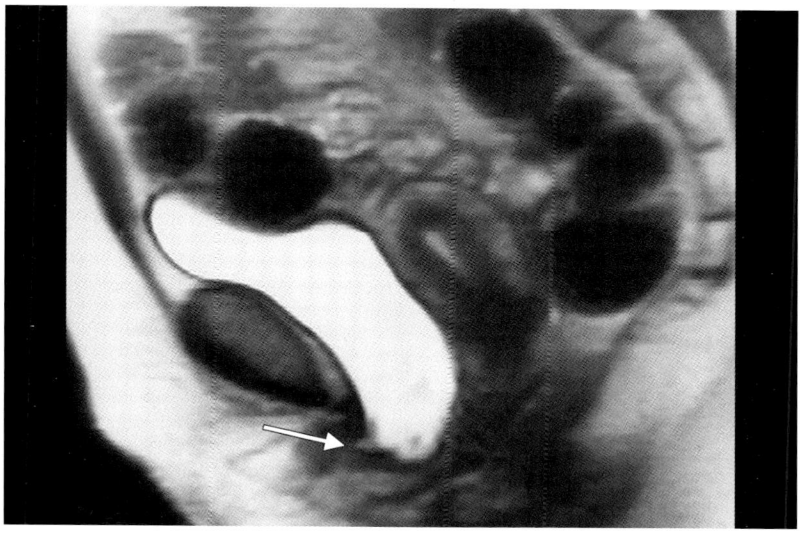

Fig. 6: Stress incontinence and incomplete bladder emptying in a 55-year-old woman. (a) Sagittal T2-weighted image (2,200/96) of the patient at rest shows the pelvic organs and floor, which have a normal appearance. (b) Sagittal T2-weighted image (2,200/96) of the patient during pelvic strain demonstrates development of a cystocele and rotation of the urethra into the horizontal plane (arrow), indicating damage to the internal sphincter.

convex upwards. With age there is thinning of levator ani muscle that does not denote tears. The adequate lateral fascial support is indicated by H shape of vagina.

Cystocele and Stress Incontinence

Posterior aspect of the bladder descent below the pubococcygeal line and bulge to the anterior vaginal wall due to stretching or tearing of the pubocervical fascia and levator ani muscle. MR images obtained during strain show the change in position of the bladder and the resulting cystocele. The H line exceeds 5 cm and the M line 2 cm fascial defects may be midline, lateral, or both. Beaking of the bladder neck at rest and at pelvic strain is a common finding and should not be considered as indication of incontinence.

Woman with moderate pelvic floor laxity on physical examination. The H line (from the pubic symphysis to the posterior wall of the rectum) and the M line (from the posterior aspect of the H line to the pubococcygeal line) are delineated by dots. (a and b) Sagittal T2-weighted images (2,200/96) of the patient at rest (a) and during pelvic strain (b) show significant descent of the bladder below the pubococcygeal line, forming a cystocele (white arrow). A large fibroid (black arrow) likely prevents descent of the uterus. On the strain image, the H and M lines are elongated and the levator plate is almost vertical (arrowheads), indicating loss of anterior and posterior support. (c) Axial T2-weighted image (4,200/112) shows intact pubovesical ligaments (arrows) and mild widening of the levator hiatus (distance between asterisks).

For uncomplicated stress incontinence, a retropubic urethropexy is offered to the patient. Loss of intrinsic urethral sphincter integrity and anterior fascial supports of the bladder neck leads to rotation of the bladder and urethra anteriorly and superiorly. In severe cases, due to apposition of the urethra and anterior bladder wall symptoms of stress incontinence gets masked **(Fig. 6)**. It is important to identify this urethral hypermobility because it usually requires a pubovaginal sling procedure for adequate repair.

Uterine or Vaginal Vault Prolapse

Due to muscle damage and stretching or tearing of uterosacral ligament leads to descent of the vaginal fornices and uterus below pubococcygeal line. Diagnosis is made by sagittal MR images obtained during pelvic strain, the H and M lines appear elongated. On axial images, there is loss of H shape of vagina and cervix is at the level of pubic symphysis along with posterior displacement of the fornix on the affected side. Sometimes puborectal muscles are seen to be avulsed from its insertion on the pubic rami, it is associated with severe grade. If coronal image is taken, iliococcygeal muscle is seen as flat or convex downward.

In uterine or vaginal vault prolapse uterosacral suspension provides support and in severe cases sacrocolpopexy with mesh can be done **(Fig. 7)**.

Rectocele, Sigmoidocele, and Enterocele

Loss of posterior muscular support will appear as caudal inclination of the levator plate. Angulation of greater than 10° is indicates significant posterior weakness. Rectocoele is determined by obtaining sagittal MR images obtained during pelvic strain, which shows anterior bulging of rectum. Tearing of rectovaginal fascia is suspected if there is descent of small bowel loops more than 2 cm into the rectovaginal space. Many physicians believe that small bowel loops resting on the sigmoid colon or rectum give patients the feeling of incomplete evacuation and lead to repetitive and unproductive straining. On axial images, loops of sigmoid or small bowel can be seen insinuated between the rectum and vagina.

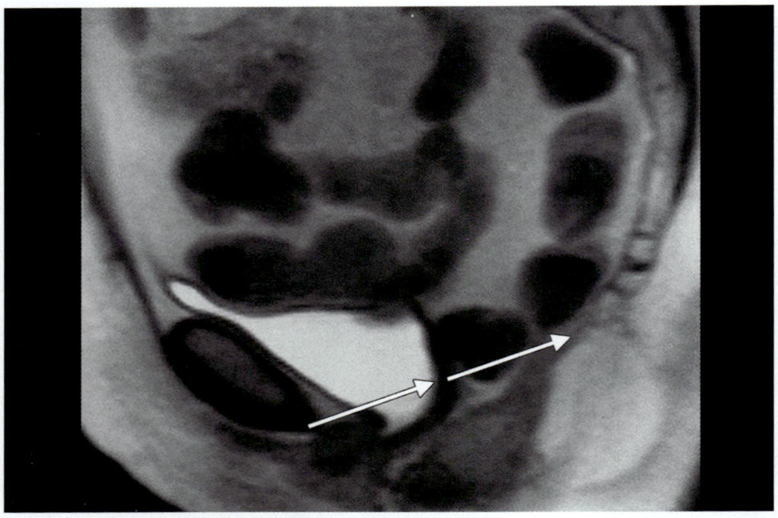

Fig. 7: Firm, painful mass lateral to the left wall of the vagina in a 62-year-old woman. (a) Sagittal T2-weighted image (2,200/96) of the patient during pelvic strain shows only minimal descent of the pelvic organs below the pubococcygeal line (arrows). (b) Axial T2-weighted image (4,400/112) of the patient at rest shows detachment of the right aspect of the puborectal muscle from the parasymphyseal area and deformation of the right vaginal fornix (arrow). (c) Coronal T2-weighted image shows mild convex downward deformity of the iliococcygeal muscle (arrow). The intact, left aspect of the levator ani muscle was in spasm and responded well to biofeedback therapy.

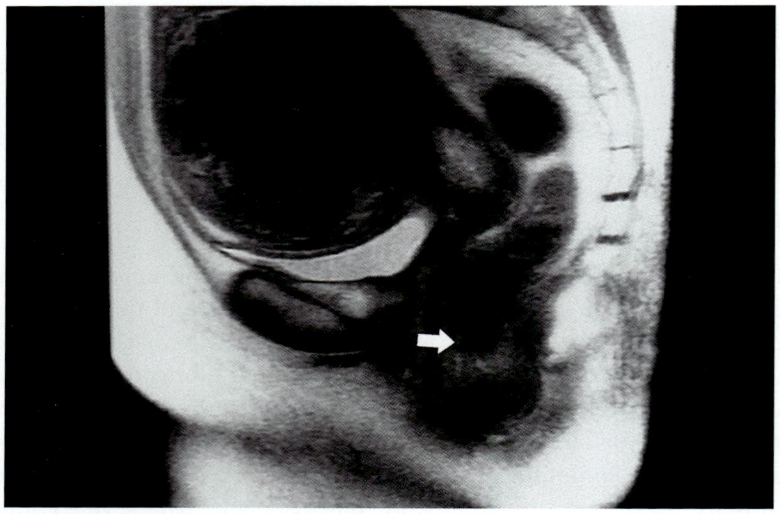

Fig. 8: Incomplete bowel evacuation and posterior pressure in a 63-year-old woman. Sagittal T2-weighted images (2,200/96) of the patient at rest (a) and during pelvic strain (b) show descent and anterior bulging of the rectum consistent with a rectocele (white arrows). The levator plate is nearly vertical (black arrow). The large uterine fibroid likely prevents descent of the middle and anterior compartments.

Enterocoele is treated by culdoplasty. Posterior colporrhaphy is required for adequate repair of fascial defects adjacent of sigmoid and rectum **(Fig. 8)**.

Reporting Magnetic Resonance Imaging Findings

While reporting the image details of location demonstrating laxity and number of compartments involved along with measure of descent of bladder, vagina, and rectum. In the presence of severe damage to all the three compartments, the term global pelvic wall weakness is used. The damage to the pelvic floor may be so severe that all three compartments are involved. This is called global pelvic floor weakness. The presence or absence of enterocele and rectocele should be noted. In presence of muscle tears and inferred fascial tears their location should also be specified.

Other measurements such as H line, M line, and angle of the levator plate can be reported as if desired by the radiologist or requested by referring surgeon. The measurements reported are useful for comparisons in patients presenting with recurrence of symptoms. These measurements may be useful for quantification of descent and for comparison with future images in patients who return for evaluation of recurrent symptoms.

Postoperative Imaging

In the postoperative period it can be used in patient with persistent and recurrent symptoms though not clinically necessary. Use of clips and metallic artifacts in reparative procedure is not a problem. Many women have been imaged successfully less than 2 months after the initial surgical procedure.

Advanced Imaging Techniques

For preoperative evaluation in symptomatic patient with pelvic floor weakness MRI protocol described above is all that is required. The use of open-configuration MRI technique has been described by several authors. This technique maximizes the evidence of all weakness, however it rarely helps in identifying new defects or changes the therapeutic approach. Using 3D imaging determine levator ani volume helps to select the treatment plan either conservative or surgical. It still remains a research technique.

SURGICAL MANAGEMENT

Aims

- The primary aims of surgery are to *relieve symptoms*, which may be caused by prolapse, and, in most cases, to restore vaginal anatomy so that sexual function may be maintained or improved without significant adverse effects or complications.
- Occasionally, when sexual function is not desired, *obliterative or constrictive surgery* is more appropriate and also may relieve symptoms.

There is no steadfast rule as to when surgery is indicated. Many patients with more advanced prolapse have few or no symptoms, whereas some with lesser degrees of prolapse have what they term severe symptoms. This is confounded by the observation that many of the "symptoms" may not be specifically related to the anatomic defect or may be worsened by anxiety. In general, surgery should be offered to patients who have tried conservative therapy and were not satisfied with the results or who do not desire conservative therapy.

The prolapse should be symptomatic or should be greater than or equal to stage II with apparent progression. All patients should be given the alternative of trying conservative treatments when applicable.

Approaches to surgery include vaginal, abdominal, and laparoscopy or a combination of approaches **(Fig. 9)**.

Depending on the extent and location of prolapse, surgery may involve a combination of repairs directed to the anterior vagina, vaginal apex, posterior vagina, and perineum. Concomitant surgery may be planned for urinary or fecal incontinence. The surgical route is chosen based on the type and severity of prolapse, the surgeon's training and experience, the patient's preference, and the expected or desired surgical outcome.

Procedures for prolapse can be broadly categorized into three groups: (1) restorative, which use the patient's endogenous support structures; (2) compensatory, which attempt to replace deficient

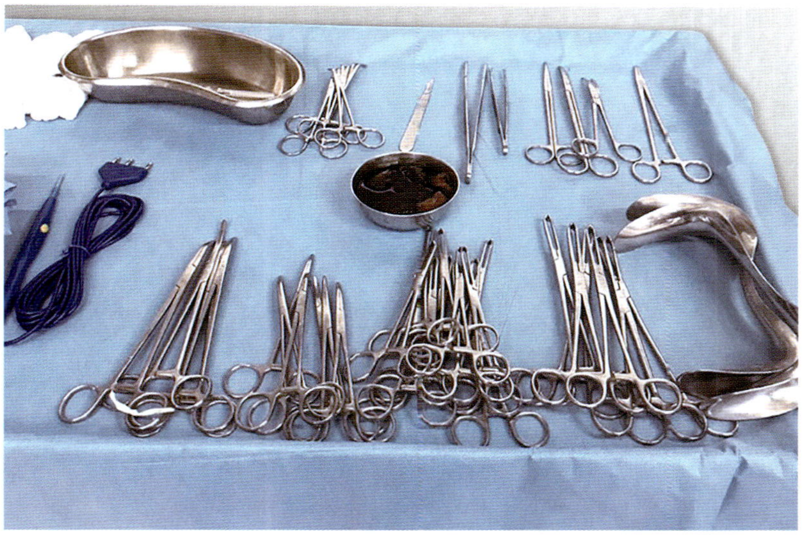

Fig. 9: Surgical equipment for vaginal hysterectomy + cystocele rectocele repair.

support with permanent graft material; and (3) obliterative, which close or partially close the vagina.

Preoperative Evaluation

Routine preoperative tests include a complete blood count, bleeding time, clotting time, renal function tests, evaluation of thyroid status, viral markers, electrocardiography (ECG), and urinalysis. However, tests like liver function tests, serum electrolytes, prothrombin time and international normalized ratio (PT-INR), activated partial thromboplastin time (aPTT), chest radiography, 2D echocardiography, CT, MRI, and contrast MRI should be done as indicated. Preanesthetic fitness is obtained. Preanesthetic assessment is an essential step prior to anesthesia in an attempt to decrease the morbidity related to anesthesia and surgery. Patient is advised for admission the evening before the surgery. Appropriate informed consent is taken from the patient after explaining the planned operation thoroughly along with its benefits and risks, including possibility of laparotomy and therapeutic alternatives. Aspirin and warfarin are to be stopped 5 days prior to surgery. All patients are advised to eat lightly for 24 hours before surgery. An oral mechanical bowel preparation like Coloprep or Peglac is administered. Patient is kept nil per oral 8 hours prior to surgery and blood is kept reserved.

Non-decent Vaginal Hysterectomy with Bilateral Salpingo-oophorectomy: Abnormal Uterine Bleeding (Normal Sized Uterus)

Procedure

A circular incision is taken over the cervix below bladder sulcus, and vaginal mucosa dissected off the cervix all around. The pouch of Douglas is identified posteriorly and peritoneum incised. The bladder is now pushed upwards until the uterovesical peritoneum is visible, and is similarly incised. The uterus is now free in the front and behind. Next, the pedicles containing Mackenrodt's and uterosacral ligaments are clamped on either side close to the cervix, cut on the uterine side and the pedicles transfixed. Next, the uterine vessels are identified, BiClamp applied, and cauterized and cut. The upper portion of the broad ligament holding the uterus contains round and ovarian ligaments and the fallopian tube are clamped and cauterized with BiClamp and cut. These are similarly dealt with on both sides, and the uterus removed. The peritoneal cavity is closed with a purse-string suture, using Vicryl 2-0.

Cervicovaginal epithelium incised posteriorly and extended anteriorly uterosacral and cardinal ligament and base of surgical bladder pillar clamped and ligated BiClamp used to clamp the uterine on either side cauterized and cut **(Figs. 10 and 11)**.

Vaginal Hysterectomy with Anterior Colporrhaphy: Third Degree Uterine Prolapse with Cystocele

Saline of 200 mL infiltrated into the pubocervical fascia and a circular incision is taken over the cervix below bladder sulcus. Vaginal mucosa dissected off the cervix all around. The pouch of Douglas is identified posteriorly and peritoneum incised. The bladder is now pushed upwards until the uterovesical peritoneum is visible, and is similarly incised. The uterus is now free in the front and behind. The pedicles containing Mackenrodt's and uterosacral ligaments are clamped on either side close to the cervix, cut on uterine side and pedicles are transfixed. Next, the uterine vessels are identified, using BiClamp cauterized and cut. The upper limit of the broad ligament holding uterus contains round and ovarian ligaments and the fallopian tube are clamped and cauterized with BiClamp and cut. These are similarly dealt with on both sides, and the uterus removed, following which ovarian ligament clamped and ovary with the cyst delivered out

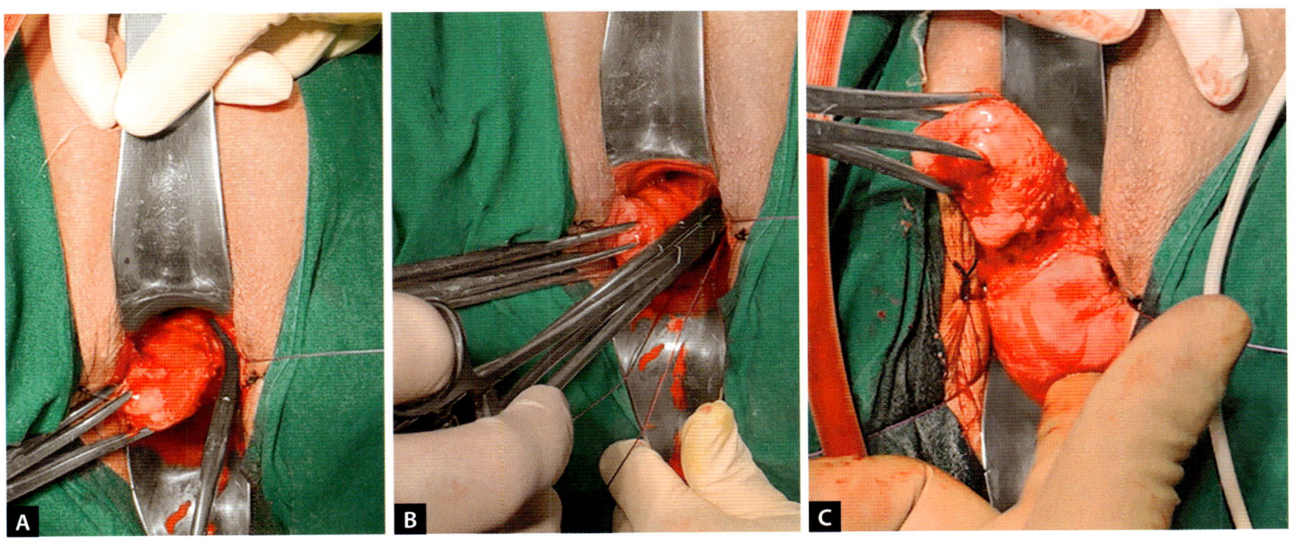

Figs. 10A to C: Uterine artery clmaped, cut and ligated.

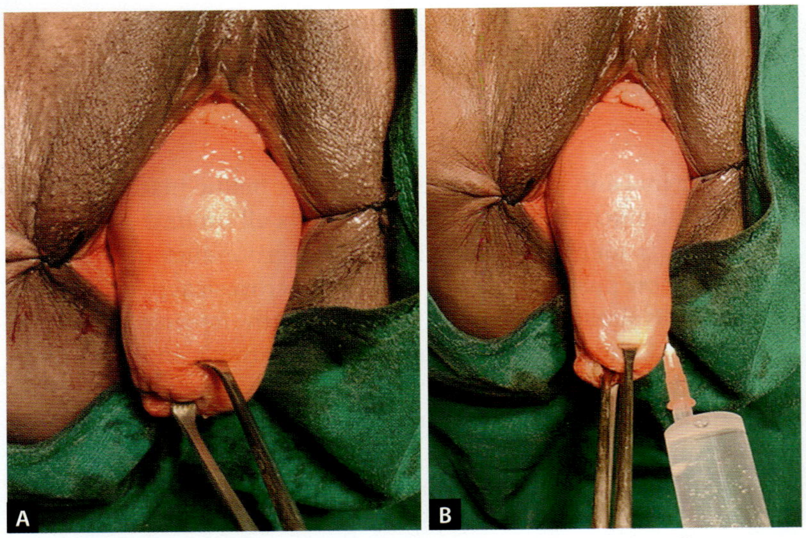

Figs. 11A and B: 200 mL of saline infiltrated into anterior vaginal wall.

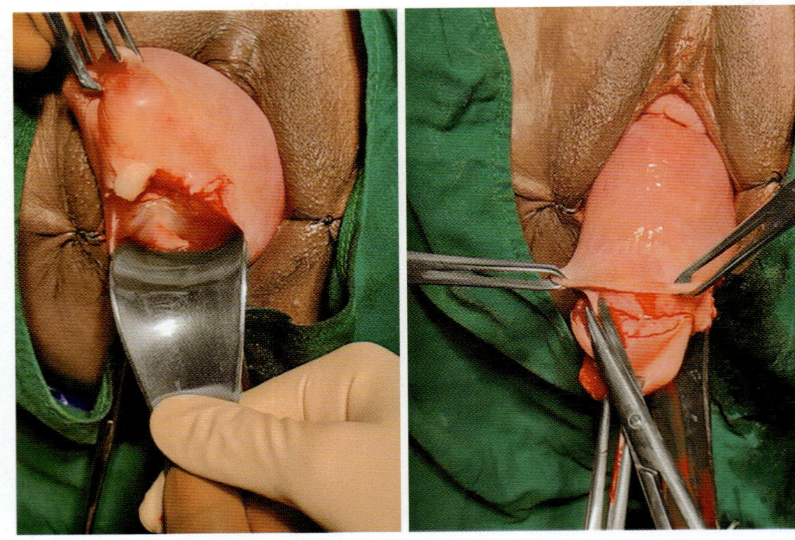

Figs. 13A and B: Sims speculum inserted into the posterior cul-de-sac.

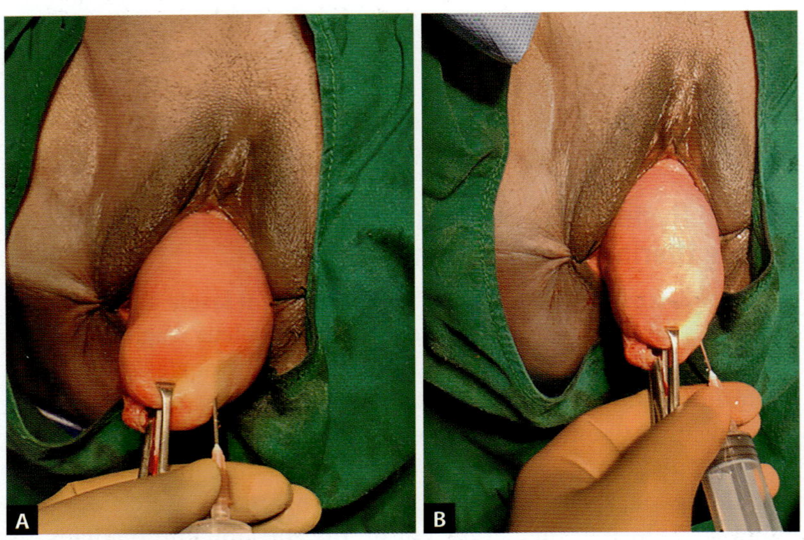

Figs. 12A and B: al fascia and opened posterior cul-de-sac.

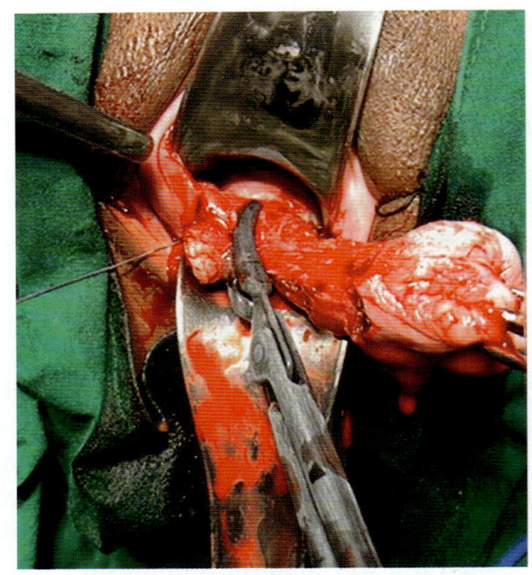

Fig. 14: Uterosacral and cardinal ligament with base of surgical bladder pillar clamped using BiClamp cauterized and cut.

by suctioning the fluid and ovariotomy done **(Fig. 11)**. Salpingo-oophorectomy done on the other side too. Paravaginal defect corrected by taking lateral suture from vaginal mucosa to arcus tendineus fasciae pelvis (ATFP) on either side followed by peritoneal cavity is closed with a purse-string suture, using Vicryl 2-0 and anterior colporrhaphy done **(Figs. 12 and 13)**.

BiClamp used to clamp the uterine either side cauterized and cut. BiClamp used to clamp tubo-ovarian round ligament cauterized and cut close to the fundus **(Fig. 14)**.

Ovarian cyst held with Babcock's forceps and delivered out gently. Other side normal ovarian ligament clamped using BiClamp cauterized and cut.

Paravaginal defect repaired—laterally vaginal epithelium sutured to the arcus tendineus fasciae pelvis (white line).

Cystocele/Anterior Wall Prolapse (Flowchart 1)

Anterior vaginal wall prolapse (AWP) which constitutes cystocele and urethrocele is the most common form of female POP. 81% of females undergoing surgery for POP undergo the anterior vaginal wall repair. It has highest recurrence rate AWP carries the highest risk for recurrence, with reported recurrence rate being15–30%.

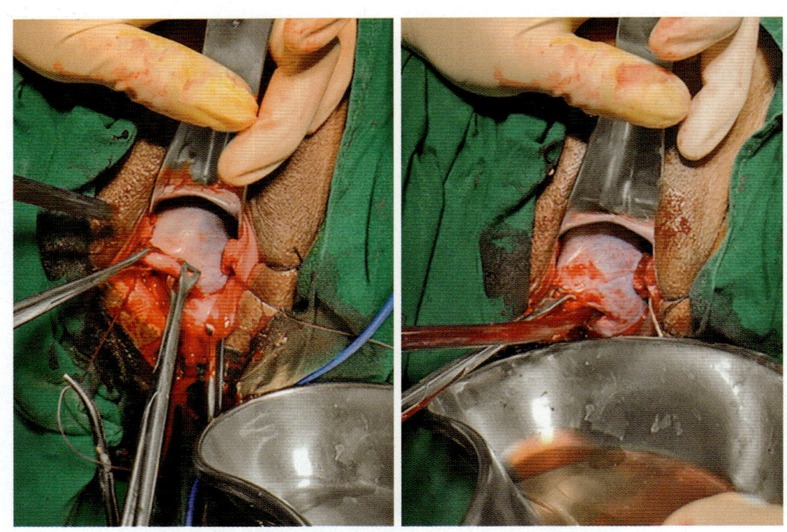

Fig.15: Ovarian cyst punctures and fluid suctioned out.

The vaginal wall is supported by many fascia and ligaments. DeLancey had divided vaginal support into three levels:

1. *Level 1*: The cardinal-uterosacral ligament complex also known as triradiate ligament, which functions as suspensory "leashes" supporting cervix and upper vagina.

Flowchart 1: Diagnosis and management of cystocele.

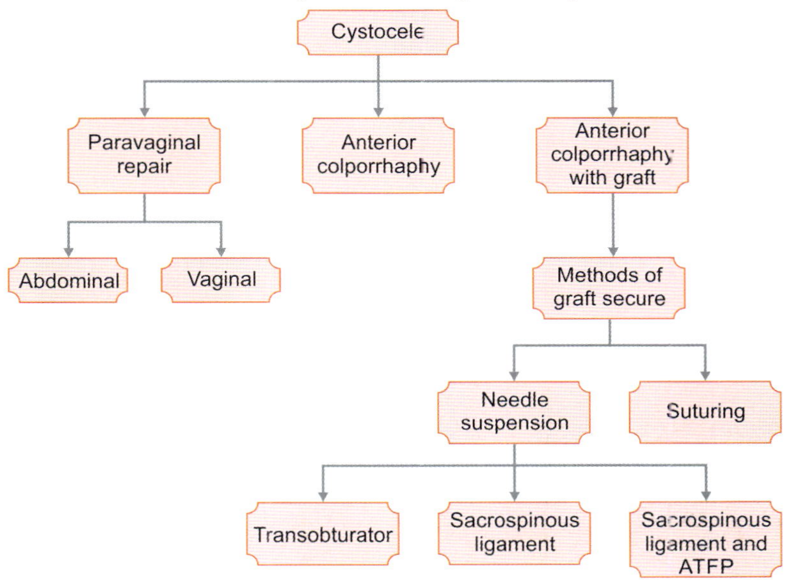

2. *Level 2*: The lateral connections of the vagina to the ATFP, or "white line", it supports the middle portion of the vagina.
3. *Level 3*: Lower vagina is supported by fascial connections to the perineal membrane anteriorly and the PB posteriorly.

Disruption of one or more of these support structure precipitate POP-cystocele. Site of fascial detachment determines the type of cystocele, midline defect of the pericervical fascia causes central cystocele (1%), detachment of pericervical fascia from ATFP, lateral cystocele (80–85%), detachment of uterosacral ligament or the pericervical ring, and apical cystocele (15%).

Combination of defects can coexists, common being lateral with central cystocele. Surgical repair should take into consideration all the existing defects.

Procedure: Anterior Colporrhaphy

There are three basic techniques for cystocele repair:

1. Anterior colporrhaphy
2. Paravaginal repair
3. Anterior colporrhaphy with graft.

Patients having advanced cystocele (stage III and beyond), restoration of anatomy and function usually requires more than one repair: concomitant posterior, apical, and enterocele repairs are usually required.

Anterior Colporrhaphy

Procedure: In anterior colporrhaphy the main step is plication of the pubocervical fascia with the aims of repairing the midline fascial defects and strengthening of the stretched out fascia.

Patient is positioned in lithotomy and 16 French Foley catheter is inserted into the bladder for continuous drainage. Appropriate exposure of the vaginal mucosa is necessary ad is made sure by using labial retractors and weighted vaginal speculum. The incision is taken at a point proximal to bladder neck which is extended proximally to 2 cm from the vaginal apex. Vaginal wall is held with 2 Allis clamp and hydrodissection is done by injecting saline submucously, this step also ensures hemostasis.

After hydrodissection, a longitudinal incision is taken on the anterior vaginal wall with a No. 5 blade. Using Metzenbaum scissors and blunt dissection with 4 × 4 wet gauze piece vaginal epithelium is separated from the pubocervical fascia.

Dissection is continued laterally till vaginal sulci and proximally till vaginal cuff (if the patient is posthysterectomy). Hemostasis is maintained by using both the electrocautery and hemostatic sutures. Ascia is then approximated from side-to-side using interrupted sutures.

Excessive plication of the fascia should be avoided, as doing so may cause urethral kinking and obstruction. Usually, one layer of plication is sufficient, though more than one layer may be required in patients with advanced (stage III and IV) cystoceles. In order to minimize the risk of recurrence, fascia should be reattached to the supported vaginal apex. If cystocele is coexistent with apical prolapse, apical suspension sutures are taken.

At the end, redundant vaginal flap excised and vaginal skin is sutured back.

Vaginal Approach

Vaginal paravaginal repair is done to repair lateral vaginal wall defects. In this vaginal mucosa is sutured to arcus tendineus fasciae pelvis using 2-0 polyglactin sutures **(Figs. 16 to 21)**.

Huge Cystocele Repair with Vaginal Mesh

In order to provide extra support to the weakened tissue biologic or synthetic graft **(Figs. 22 to 26)** may be used. It is sutured to cardinal-uterosacral ligament complex proximally, the endopelvic fascia distally, and the obturator fascia laterally. The procedure is started in similar manner as anterior colporrhaphy (see above). Graft is trimmed to trapezoid shape, size of which should be similar to anterior vaginal wall. Two sutures (2-0 polyglactin) are taken through the cardinal ligaments proximally and two sutures through the pericervical fascia close to the pubic bones, each side. The graft is secured to these sutures then lateral sutures (3-0 polyglactin) are used to secure the graft to the obturator fascia.

After the graft arms are passed, tension is adjusted, the graft arms are cut flush with the skin, and the skin punctures are glued. The vaginal skin is trimmed as required, the wound is thoroughly irrigated, and the vaginal incision is closed.

Rectocele Repair: Colpoperineorrhaphy

Up to one-third or one-half of women undergoing surgery for prolapse will involve the posterior vaginal wall. Rectoceles are one type of posterior compartment prolapse that consists of the rectum protruding into the vagina. Other conditions that impact the posterior wall include enteroceles, sigmoidoceles, intussusception, and rectal prolapse. Posterior vaginal wall prolapse can present just as an asymptomatic bulge or with symptoms such as constipation, pelvic pressure, and problems in defecation including obstructed defecation, splinting.

Anatomy

An understanding of pelvic anatomy and location of weakness in the anatomy of the posterior vaginal wall is paramount to successful repair of rectoceles **(Fig. 27)**. DeLancey originally divided the vaginal axis into three levels of support for the posterior vaginal wall. At the apex, cardinal-uterosacral complex suspends the vagina. The middle of the vagina is supported by the endopelvic fascia and the levator ani. Level three support, at the most caudal portion of the vagina, is represented by the PB and perineal membrane. Identification of the

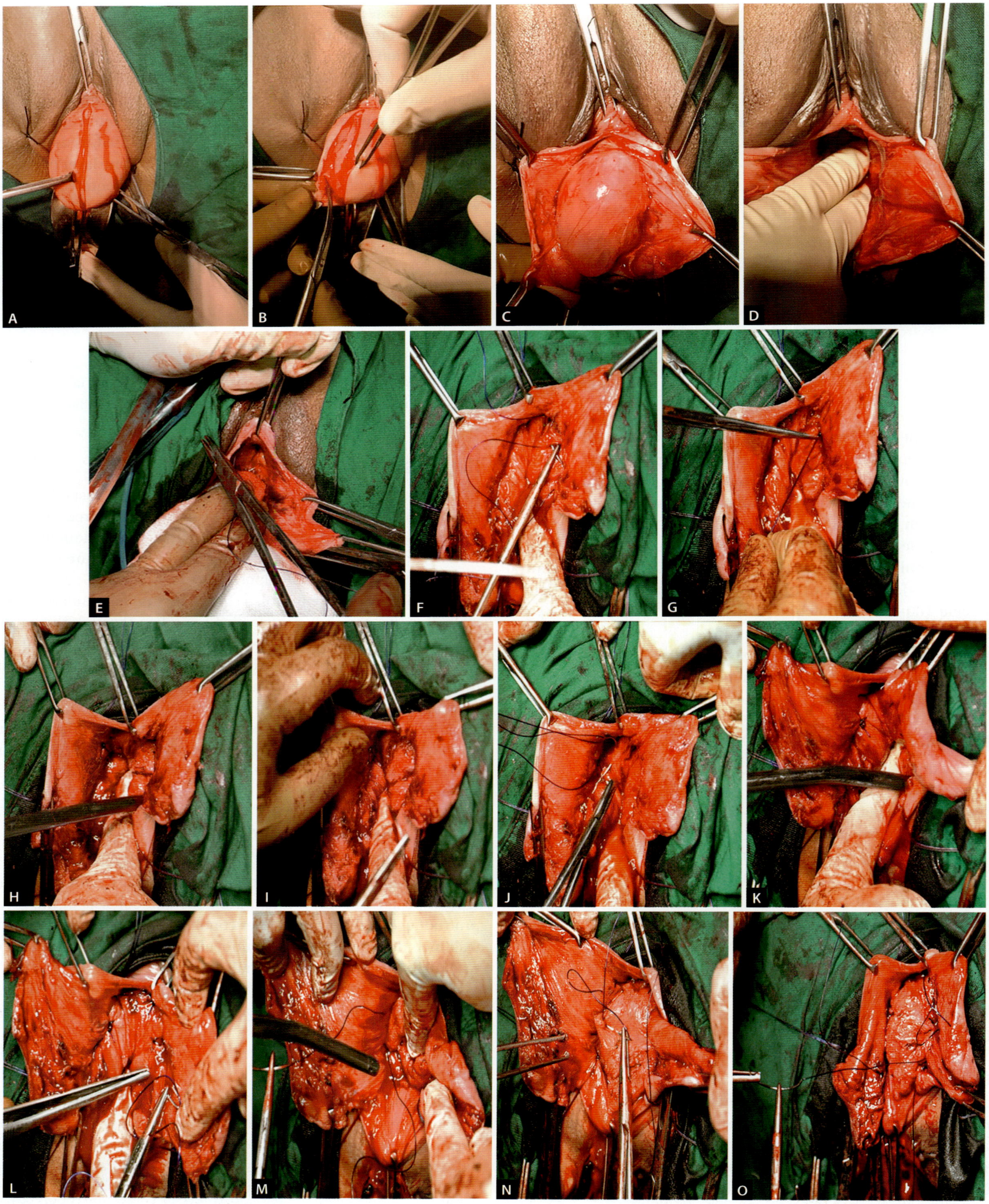

Figs. 16A to O: (A and B) Saline infiltrating into the vesicovaginal fascia and cystocele separating underlying mucosa; (C) Longitudinal incision taken over the vaginal epithelium, separating vaginal mucosa and submucosal layer from fibromuscular layer (D) Cystocele separated off the underlying mucosa and pushed inside; (E) Paravaginal defect repaired—laterally vaginal epithelium sutured to the arcus tendineus fasciae pelvis (white line); (F to O) Triple plication—suture taken on paravaginal epithelium to pubocervical mucosa and then paravaginal epithelium multiple areas.

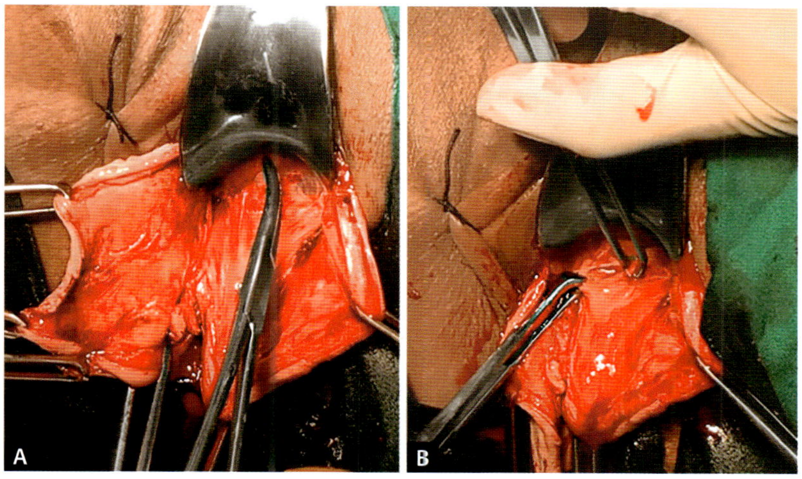

Figs. 17A and B: Peritoneal tissues over the bladder held and buttressing of the vesicovaginal fascia done with interrupted Vicryl 2-0 sutures.

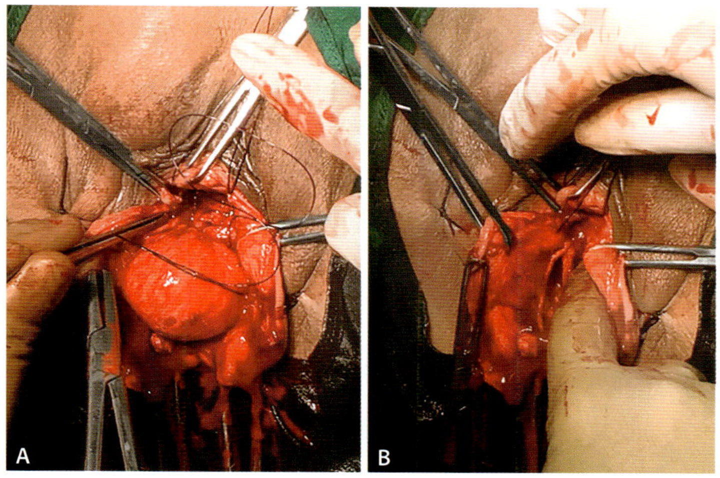

Figs. 19A and B: Buttressing suturing done.

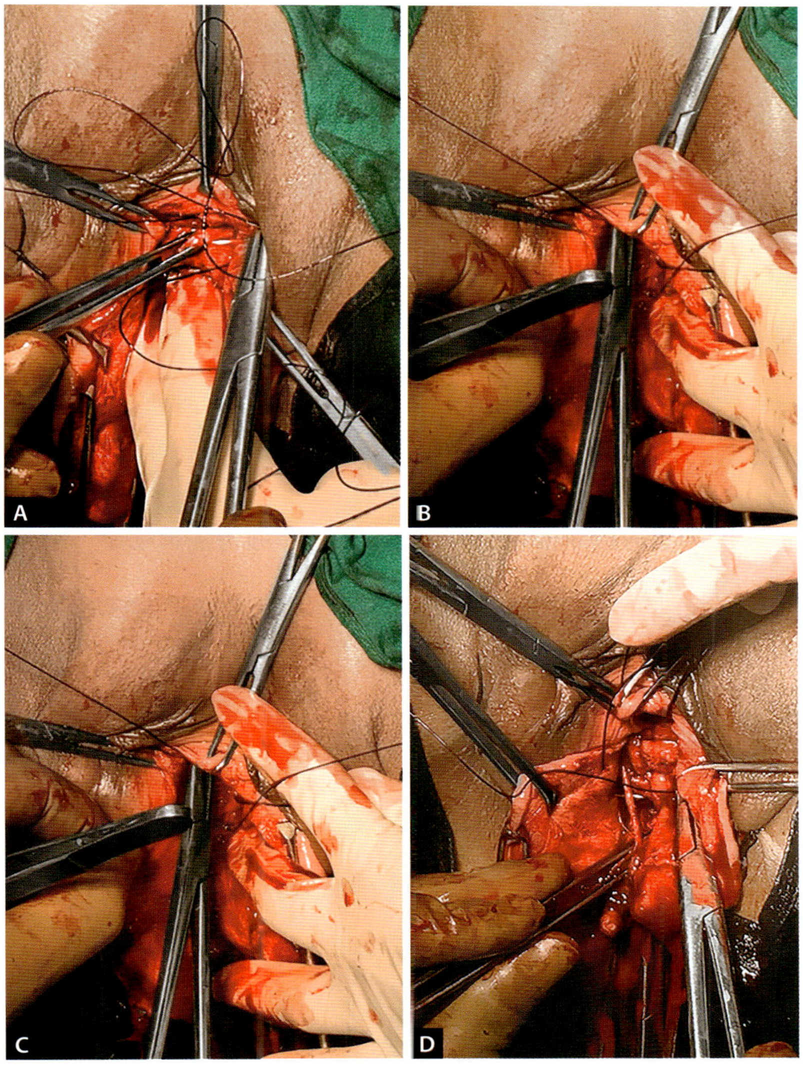

Figs. 18A to D: Buttressing of vesicovaginal fascia done with interrupted sutures.

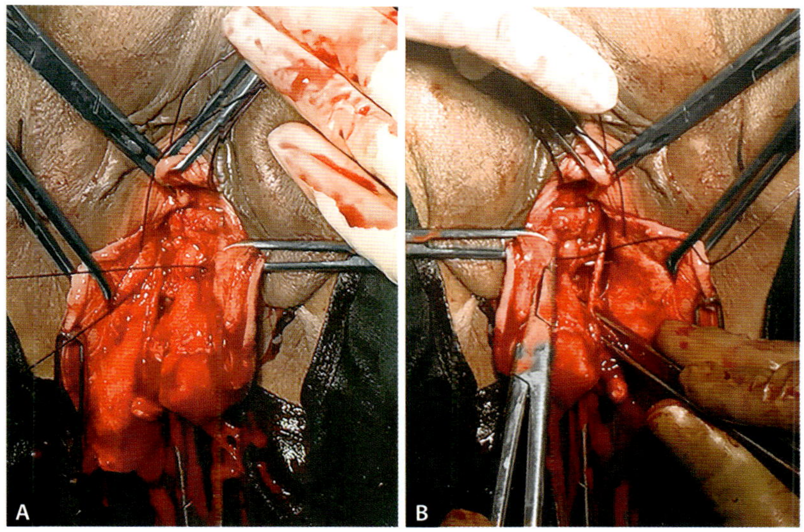

Figs. 20A and B: Excess vaginal tissue excised.

breakdown in each level of support as well as addressing each level of support with repair will help in surgical planning and prevent the need for reoperation.

The integrity of posterior vaginal wall is maintained by rectovaginal septum. It runs downward and gets integrated into the PB distally. This tissue forms anterior surface of the rectovaginal space and is thinnest along the midline. The rectovaginal septum is made of dense fibromuscular elastic tissue. During childbirth due to distension there might be tearing of these fibers leading to posterior wall prolapse. Separation of the rectovaginal septum transversely causes the uppermost type of rectocele.

Procedure: Posterior Colporrhaphy

Before starting the procedure it is important to first assess the degree of rectocoele and GH to plan the incision. Most often perineorrhaphy is performed along with rectocoele repair, in such cases incision is made will likely incorporate portions of the PB. It is important to not extend the incision beyond the desired GH, for there is risk of constricting vaginal introitus, which results in dyspareunia.

Allis clamp is placed on the vaginal epithelium at the most proximal and distal aspect the rectocele. If perineorrhaphy is also planned, two additional Allis clamps are placed mucocutaneous junction of the widened introitus at the desired level of closure. Placing the Allis clamp assists to delineate the borders for the incision as well as acts as countertraction aiding during dissection. 200 mL saline is injected below the vaginal epithelium to aid hydrodissection.

Incision is made using electrocautery or sharp dissection between the two clamps. If perineorrhaphy is also done, incision is taken on the skin in the shape of an inverted isosceles from the perineum. In case of deficient perineum, defined as PB less than 2 cm, the triangular

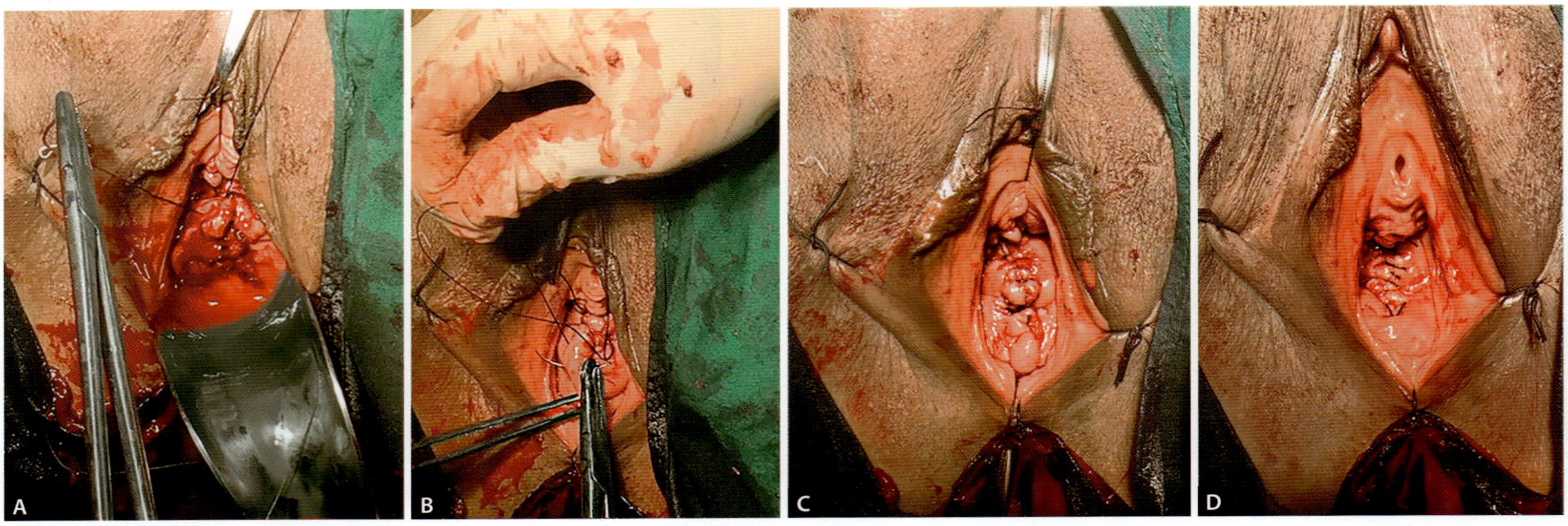

Figs. 21A to D: Vaginal mucosa sutured using Vicryl 1-0.

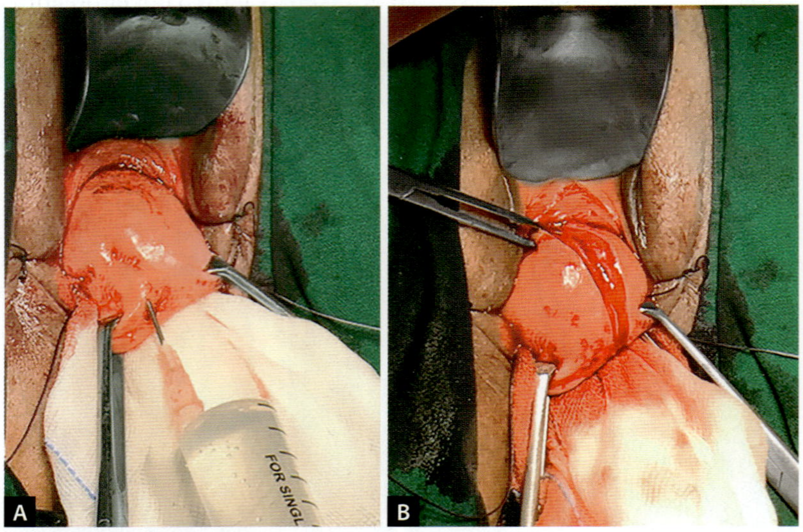

Figs. 22A and B: Saline injected into vaginal epithelium and vertical incision taken.

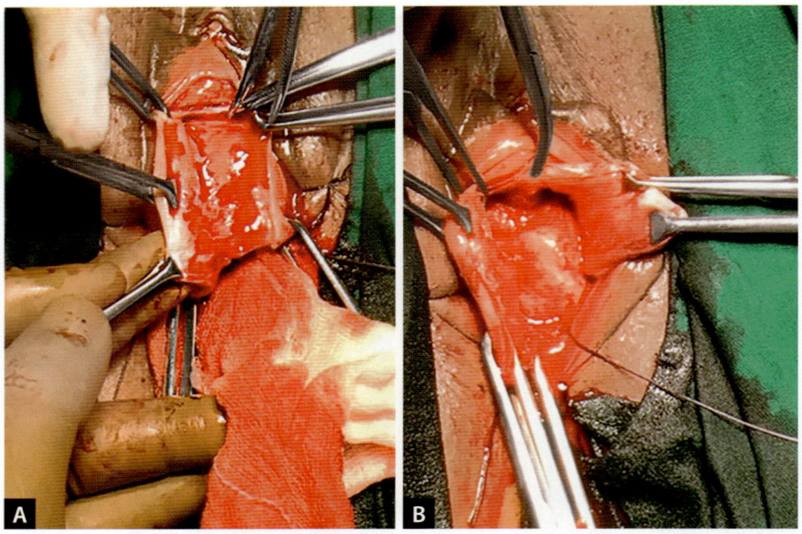

Figs. 23A and B: Bladder is separated from underlying mucosa.

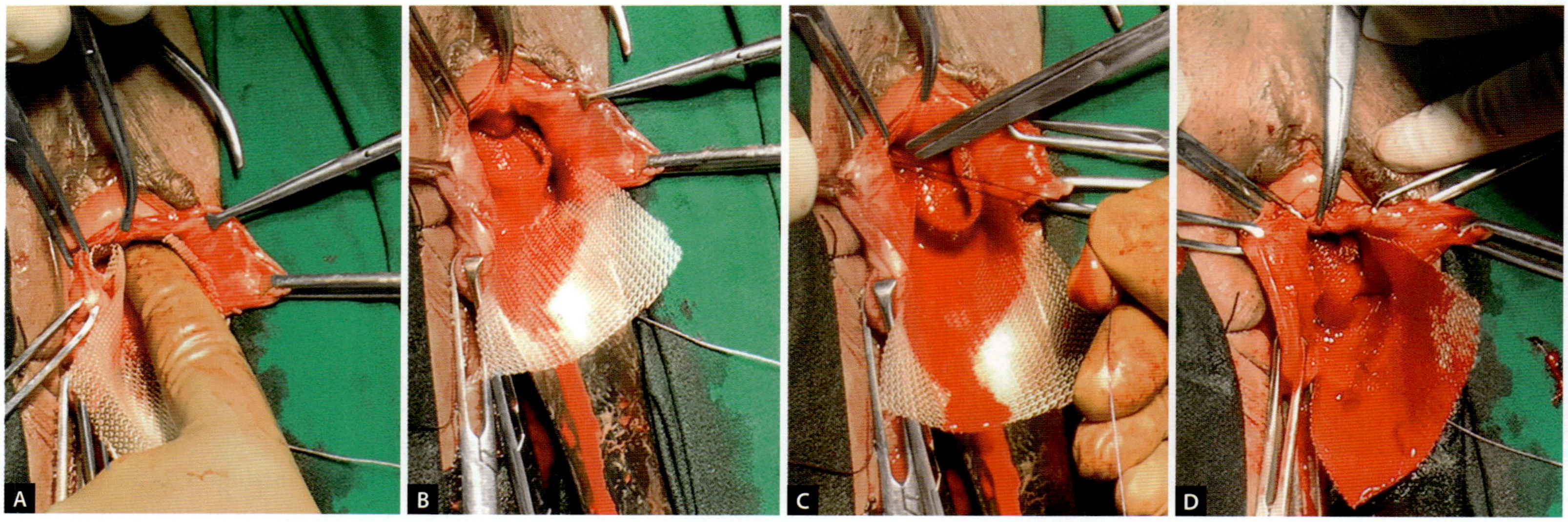

Figs. 24A to D: Polypropylene mesh placed between vaginal mucosa and bladder and fixed all over using Vicryl 2-0.

incision may not be possible. This is done to prevent redundant skin after the repair.

While creating tension on the vaginal wall, vaginal epithelium is dissected off the underlying tissue with sharp dissection. Nondominant index finger is then placed in the rectum to determine the thickness of the tissue being dissected. In most cases, the dissection should continue only to the point slightly above the defect and should always be carried out to the sidewalls.

After mobilizing the vaginal epithelium off the underlying rectocoele, rectovaginal septum is then plicated in the midline

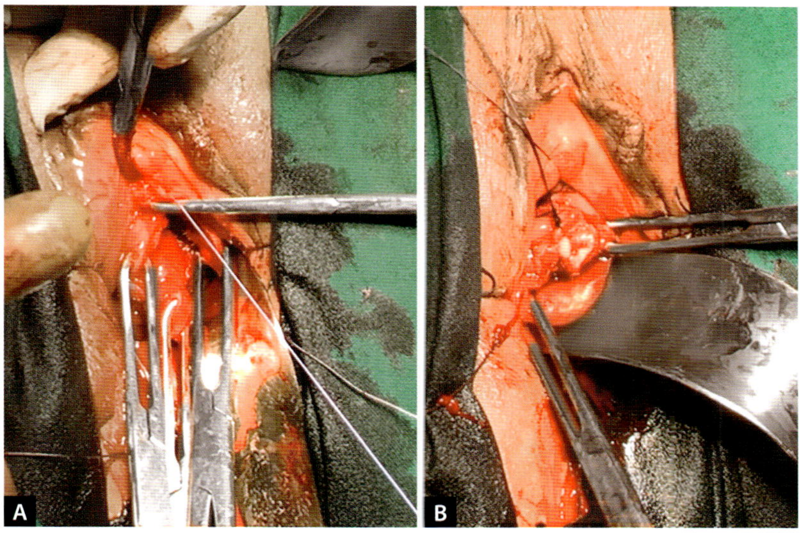

Figs. 25A and B: Vaginal mucosa sutured over the mesh.

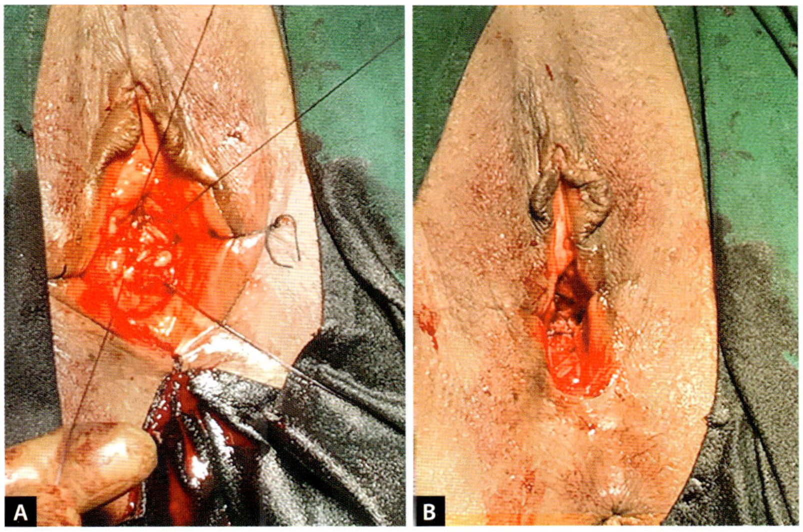

Figs. 26A and B: Skin closed using Vicryl 1-0.

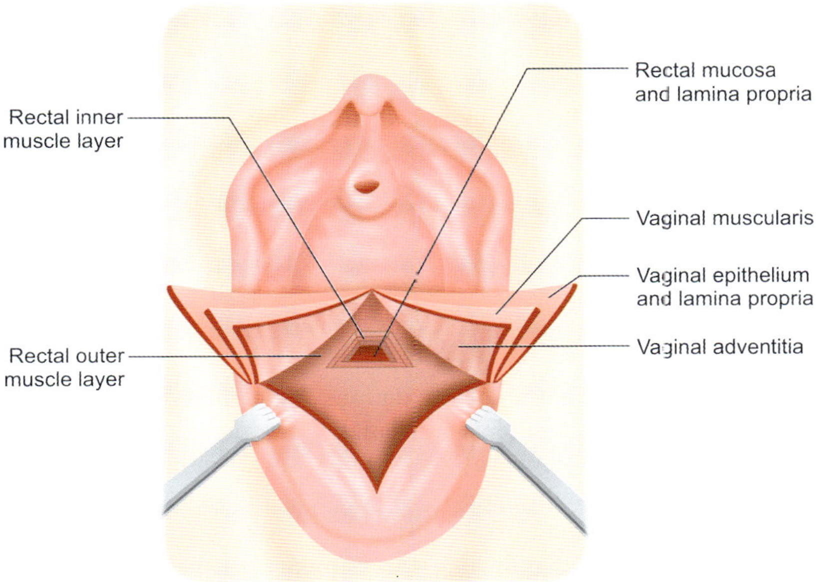

Fig. 27: In presence of normal support, the vagina is pulled posteriorly towards the sacrum by uterosacral ligaments and to a lesser degree cephalad by cardinal ligaments, resulting in an almost horizontal orientation in the proximal two-thirds.

using 2-0 absorbable interrupted sutures. Care should be taken to avoid rectal mucosa while taking the sutures, and to make sure that vagina was not overly constricted. At this point the rectocele will be fully reduced and a perineorrhaphy can be performed, which is discussed here.

Excess tissue is excised and vaginal epithelium is closed. Prior to closure care is taken as to not overly trim the vaginal epithelium as it may lead to scarring and contracture. Reattachment of rectovaginal connective tissue to PB is done only if separation is observed.

Perineorrhaphy

Perineorrhaphy is performed along with posterior compartment repair in patients in whom separation of the perineal muscles is detected. Free ends of the bulbocavernosus and transverse perineal group of muscle is plicated and is reattached to the rectovaginal septum with 2-0 absorbable suture. Perineorrhaphy should be performed with any posterior repair where there is separation of the perineal muscles. While finishing this step care should be taken to allow 3 finger breadths space at genital hiatal to allow adequate sexual function. Denonvilliers' fascia is mobilized from the vaginal epithelium and reattached to perineal body.

COMPLICATIONS

Complications of cystocele repair and rectocele repair may occur either intraoperative or postoperatively.

Intraoperative Complications

Bleeding

Excessive vaginal bleeding is defined as amount of bleeding causing the need for blood transfusion. It is reported that blood transfusion rate for prolapse surgeries (including cystocele repair) was 3 out of 519 patients. Bleeding is more common in patients in those where vaginal reconstructive surgery is also performed alongside especially sacrospinous fixation or hysterectomy. Increased body mass index is also found as associated factor causing increased bleeding.

If bleeding occurs, using good exposure with appropriate retractors and the use of headlights bleeding point is localized and measures are taken to stop the bleeding. Measures taken to stop bleeding could be packing, electrocauterization, suture ligation, and embolization by interventional radiology are treatment options. Lost blood should be replaced with packed cells. In the postoperative period continuous monitoring of vitals sign and periodic check of blood parameters are done.

Injury to Bladder, Ureter, or Urethra

Injury to the urinary tract varies from 4% to 11%, bladder injury being the most common. Uncommon forms of urinary tract injuries are also seen in vaginal reconstructive surgery and these are ureteral obstruction (when the ureters are tied or kinked), urethral traumas, and suture transfixation to the bladder. Kwon et al. reported that after anterior colporrhaphy the incidence of ureteral obstruction is 2%.

To treat and prevent long-term consequences of urinary tract injury, cystoscopy is performed intraoperatively during most vaginal surgical procedure. A 70° lens is used with a full bladder and 1 ampule of indigotindisulfonate and furosemide 10 mg injected intravenous. Bladder is inspected with special attention to anterolateral bladder walls, ureteral orifices, and urethra. If the trocars are in place on moving their exact sites of bladder perforation can be confirmed.

Primary repair of intraoperative cystotomy gives the best outcome so it is imperative to not miss the injury caused. Cystotomy caused by the passed trocars is managed by removal of the trocars and repositioning after complete emptying of the bladder. The trocars should "hug" the bone as they are passed. Ureteral obstruction, as diagnosed by failure to see free fluid efflux, should be managed by revising the sutures. Urethral trauma is managed by urethrorrhaphy, and avoiding synthetic slings and long catheter drainage of at least 1 week's duration.

Nerve Injury

Common reasons for nerve injury is improper positioning or direct nerve trauma. Sciatic nerve injury is suspected if patient complains of pain at the buttock and back of the thigh radiating downward, with or without foot drop. This usually occurs after prolonged use of free-hanging stirrups. It can also occur during sacrospinous ligament fixation and removing sutures usually solves the problem.

In femoral nerve injury patient presents with inability to flex the hip or extend the knee associated with pain or paresthesia at the anteromedial aspect of the thigh and leg. It usually occurs due to prolonged compression while using abdominal retractors or hyperabduction of the hips. Other common nerve injuries after pelvic procedure include peroneal, iliohypogastric, ilioinguinal, obturator, and pudendal nerve injuries.

Intraoperative nerve injury is avoided by taking care of patient. Patient should be properly positioned using well-padded stirrups, pressure points, overlay stretch should be avoided, and retractor blades should be always placed under direct vision. Furthermore, knowledge of the neuroanatomy of the female pelvis is important to avoid and to recognize common sites of nerve involvement.

Bowel Injury

Bowel injury is rarely encountered during repair of POP. It is generally encountered during rectocoele repair. Small bowel can be injured during enterocele repair or sacrospinous fixation procedure. Bowel preparation should be done before all procedures as in cases bowel injury primary repair is facilitated.

Other Complications

As in any other surgical procedure anesthesia-related complications are possibility. Other complications accompanying cystocele repair includes deep venous thrombosis (DVT), and pulmonary embolism (PE).

Postoperative Complications

Infection

Vaginal surgeries are clean-contaminated procedure and carry a risk of postoperative infection. Risk of postoperative infection further increases in advanced patient age, prolonged surgeries, excessive intraoperative bleed or immunocompromised patient. Preoperative antibiotic prophylaxis and appropriate intraoperative field preparation is required to decrease the risk of postoperative infection.

Graft-related Complications

Presence of mesh can cause erosion of the mucosa and ultimately leading to extrusion of mesh into part of urinary tract of vagina it is in contact with. It is initially managed by local estrogen application. Drake et al. in a study reported that rate of mesh extrusion was 10.9% after dermal allograft and 13 weeks of local estrogen therapy was 100% successful in treating the extrusion. In case local estrogen does not have effect, mesh excision is required either partial or complete. Other mesh-related complications include dyspareunia, pelvic or vaginal pain, vaginal narrowing, vaginal bleeding, and discharge.

De Novo Voiding Symptoms

In women undergoing anterior colporrhaphy, 10% develop voiding symptoms. The reason being dissection related nerve injury and plication resulting in bladder outlet obstruction or both.

Sexual Dysfunction

A study reported that 18% women complained of dyspareunia resulting in deteriorated sexual function after undergoing anterior colporrhaphy with posterior colpoperineorrhaphy. A study from Taiwan concluded that though mesh repair for severe cystocele was safe and effective, it had effects on sexual activity and voiding. A prospective study conducted in Germany concluded that in patients with symptomatic POP surgical correction using mesh implants caused improved sexual function.

Recurrence

A study by Eilber et al. addressed the role of combining apical support with cystocele that reviewed public use file data on a 5% random national sample of female Medicare beneficiaries. They found that out of women who had surgery for POP in 1999, after 10 years cumulative reoperation rates were highest in women who had isolated anterior repair (20.2%) and it exceeded those who had concomitant apical support procedure (11.6%, $p < 0.01$).

Rectocele Repair Complications

One of the common complications of rectocele repair intraoperatively is fecal contamination. In order to prevent this, an adhesive drape is placed on the perineum over anus. Other method would be to put a purse-string suture to close the anus, but may cause ballooning of ballooning of distal rectum and prevent rectal examination during the surgery. Bowel preparation is not recommended as it may risk of contamination, surgeon can evacuate the rectal vault as needed prior to starting surgery.

Postoperative dyspareunia occurs in patients undergoing levator plication. It is generally not recommended as part of a posterior vaginal prolapse repair for patients who are sexually active. Vaginal epithelium should not be trimmed excessively as it leads to tissue scarring and contracture along the incision, increasing risk of dyspareunia.

VAGINAL VAULT PROLAPSE

International continence society defines vaginal vault prolapse as downward displacement of vaginal cuff below a point 2 cm less than total vaginal length. A bulge is seen in upper vagina or outside vagina. is bulge of upper vagina into or outside vagina. In 72% of patient there may be coexistent pelvic floor defect (cystocele, rectocoele or enterocoele). Before planning the management it is necessary to assess the defects of the various vaginal compartments as due to associated urinary, anorectal, and coital dysfunction there is negative impact on the quality of life of these women.

In order to minimize the risk of posthysterectomy vault prolapse, a clear understanding of the supporting mechanisms for the uterus and the vagina is necessary to strategize and decide on the corrective procedure taking into consideration all the weak supports.

SACROSPINOUS COLPOPEXY

The sacrospinous ligament originates from the ischial spine, runs along the lateral aspect of the sacrum, and attaches medially with the sacrotuberous ligament **(Figs. 28A and B)**. Sedera was the first person to use the sacrospinous ligament as a secure point of attachment in patients with vaginal vault and uterine prolapse as early as 1958. Richter popularized the procedure in Europe in 1968, and Randall and Nichols introduced the technique in the USA in 1971.

Indications

It has become one of the favored methods for restoring vaginal support in women with following conditions:

- Vault prolapse,
- Massive eversion of the vagina, and
- Procidentia (complete uterine prolapse).

Defects in apical vaginal support should be recognized by examination and addressed when undertaking surgery for prolapse. The upper third of the vagina (level I) is supported by vertical fibers of the paracolpium (continuation of cardinal ligament) attaching it to the pelvic wall. The uterosacral and sacrospinous ligament suspension restores vaginal support (level I). The age-specific incidence increased with advancing age and thus better surgical techniques are required. In cases with marked uterovaginal prolapse and vault prolapse transvaginal sacrospinous ligament fixation technique is used. Possible complications were injury to the pudendal nerve, internal pudendal artery and vein, ureter, and rectum. In order to avoid injury to rectum direct visualization and adequate exposure of sacrospinous ligament coccygeus muscle complex is necessary by adequate dissection of pararectal space. By placing fixation suture minimally 1.5 cm medial to the ischial spine injury to the pudendal nerve and the internal pudendal vessels is avoided. Vaginal prolapse results from weakness of pelvic floor due to childbirth and postmenopausal atrophy. In the pelvis upper vagina is suspended by cardinal uterosacral ligament complex (caudal part), it attaches cervix and upper vagina to the pelvic wall at greater sciatic foramen. On being damaged, the cervix, upper vagina prolapses downward away from the greater sciatic foramen, and fall below the normal position at the level of the ischial spine. During performing hysterectomy it is necessary to reconstruct the suspensory apparatus, if not done there is increased risk of vault prolapse. The exact incidence of vaginal vault prolapse following hysterectomy is not commonly reported but is estimated approximately 0.5% of patients. Various surgical methods are described for vaginal prolapse correction and prevention of recurrence. Advantages of sacrospinous fixation includes vaginal approach hence avoiding complication of laparotomy, faster recovery, shorter hospital stay, and maintenance of sexual potency. Studies has proven that a simple procedure as sacrospinous fixation should be done routinely with massive uterovaginal and vault prolapse avoids recurrence on follow-up.

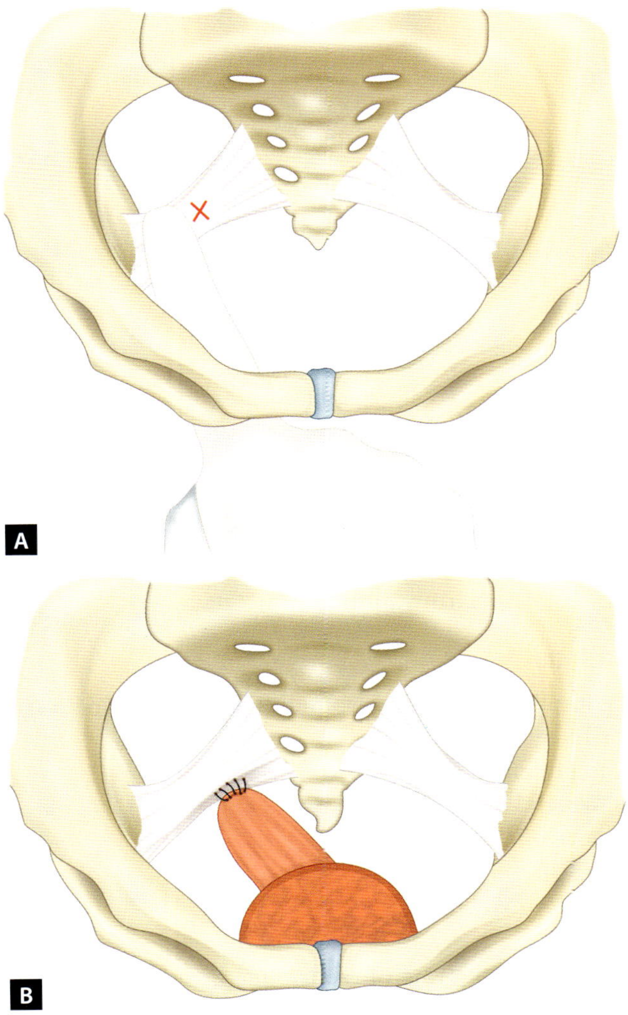

Figs. 28A and B: (A) Sacrospinous ligament fixation for proper suture location (X), at a point two finger breadths medical to the ischial spine (right index finger); (B) The upper vaginal is secured to the sacrospinous ligament, restoring vaginal wall support, and correcting prolapse.

Symptoms and Signs

When there is total prolapse of the vagina it often interferes with bladder, bowel, and sexual function. There may not be correlation between extent of prolapse and symptoms. Often patient have occult stress incontinence that is SUI is not evident when patient presents but becomes evident after corrective surgery. Therefore, examination should be done for SUI after correction of prolapse. Also during the surgery, measures are taken to ensure that the intravesical pressure does not exceed the intraurethral pressure, other than in the act of micturition.

After correction of the defect rectal function improves, for good sexual function adequate length of the vagina should be maintained along with introital dimensions.

Procedure

Patients are positioned in lithotomy and choice of anesthesia is general anesthesia **(Figs. 29 and 30)**. Vaginal hysterectomy is done as an initial step in patients of marked uterovaginal prolapse. For sacrospinous fixation, a longitudinal incision is taken on posterior vaginal wall and rectovaginal space is exposed. Lateral dissection of epithelium is done to open pararectal space on the right side. The suspension is preferred on the patient's right for ease of retraction of rectum and right handed surgeon prefer to pass suture forehanded. A window is created by blunt finger dissection between ischial spine and rectovaginal space. If correctly identified, the plane will usually develop without any difficulty. Dissection is done until ischial spines are reached. Sacrospinous ligament is palpated and ischial spine is used as a guide or landmark,

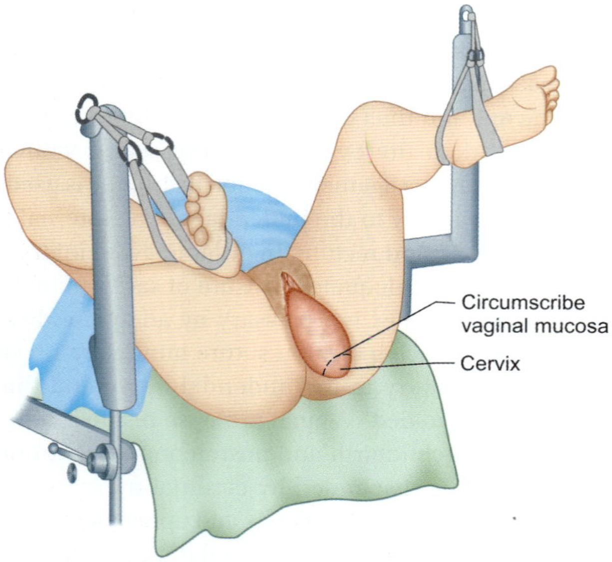

Fig. 29: After placing the patient in lithotomy position, painting, and draping is done in usual manner.

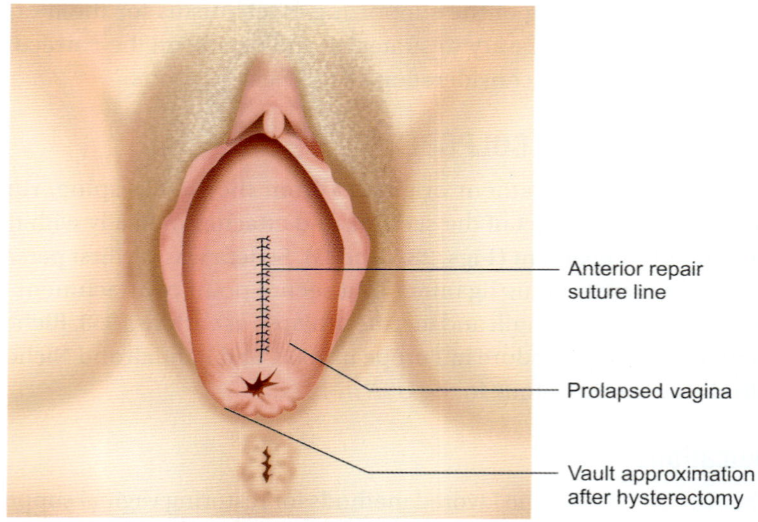

Fig. 31: A perineal view of complete prolapse of the vagina following the vaginal hysterectomy and anterior repair is shown.

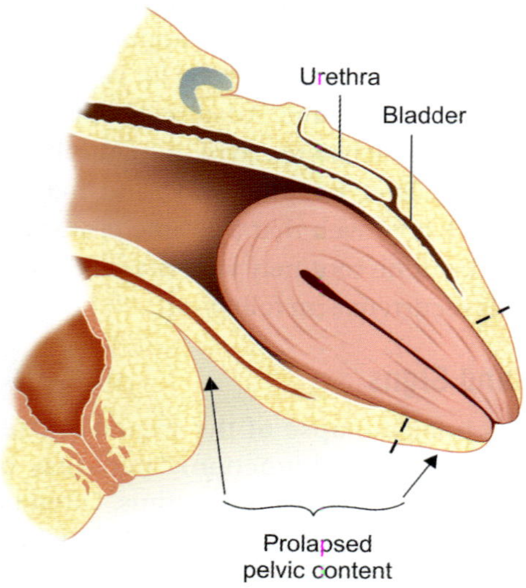

Fig. 30: In the presence of uterus, a circumferential incision is taken at the junction of cervix and vagina, as is done during vaginal hysterectomy.

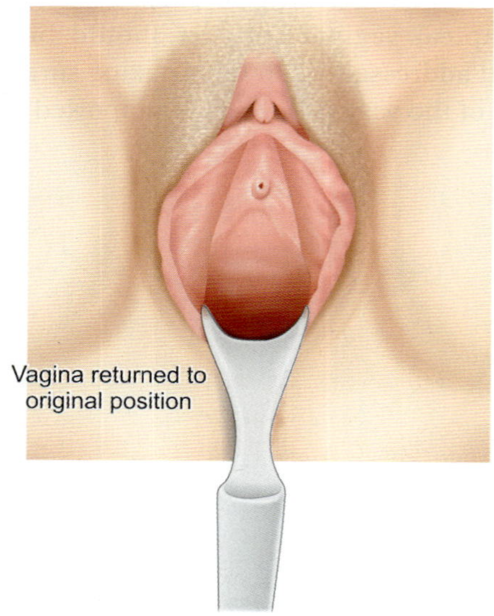

Fig. 32: Prolapsed vagina is returned to its original position.

this ligament passes from the ischial spine to the lower part of the sacrum. Now, three narrow malleable retractors are used to retract the peritoneum and rectum, to visualize clearly sacrospinous ligament. The upper border of the ligament will now be clearly defined. In all cases, a delayed absorbable suture 0 monofilament polydioxanone, 1.5 m (loop) on 40 mm half-circle, a heavy round body needle is used for this procedure. With a 12 inch long needle holder, the suture is placed through the sacrospinous ligament coccygeus muscle complex starting from the superior border in an upside down direction, it should be 2 cm medial to the ischial spine, so that neurovascular bundle is not injured. When this suture is retrieved it is in the form of a loop, it is then divided to form two sutures. Two suture pairs thus established are established with one pass. After enterocele closure and anterior colporrhaphy (if indicated), sacrospinous sutures are placed through the full thickness of vaginal muscularis at the point of new vaginal apex. Vaginal cuff is now sutured and closed. The sutures of sacrospinous ligament are now tied. This tying of sutures brings the sacrospinous ligament in contact with the vaginal epithelium directly **(Figs. 31 to 48)**. When healing occurs, vaginal epithelium is fused with the sacrospinous ligament and vault remains suspended up nicely thereafter. Postoperatively women were given broad-spectrum antibiotic for 5 days.

Complications

Potential complications of sacrospinous ligament fixation include:

- Hemorrhage
- Injury to pudendal nerve
- Injury to rectal or bladder
- Recurrence of AWP
- De novo SUI.

Outcomes

Follow-up showed that rate of recurrence or persistence of anterior vaginal wall was 20% after 1 year of surgery. After this procedure the anterior segment of vaginal wall is placed under undue tension due to alteration of the vaginal axis in the posterolateral direction will predispose for prolapse at the site opposite the repair.

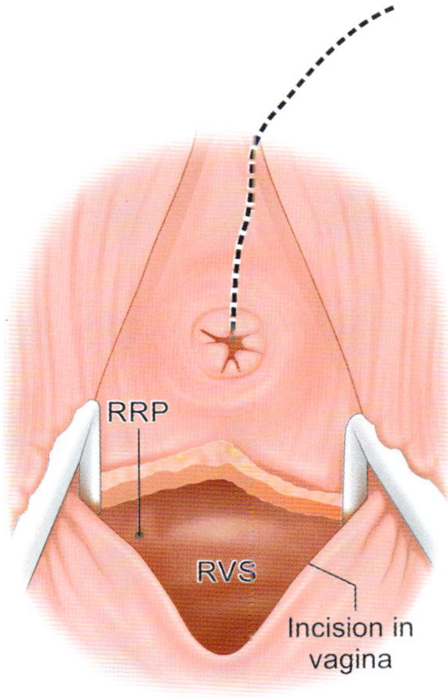

Fig. 33: Following anterior repair, posterior vaginal mucosa is opened as done during posterior repair. Through the posterior vaginal mucosa, a finger is inserted through the incision, and the rectovaginal space (RVS) is dissected. Identification of rectal pillars is done and then bluntly perforated either with finger or with long Kelly clamp.

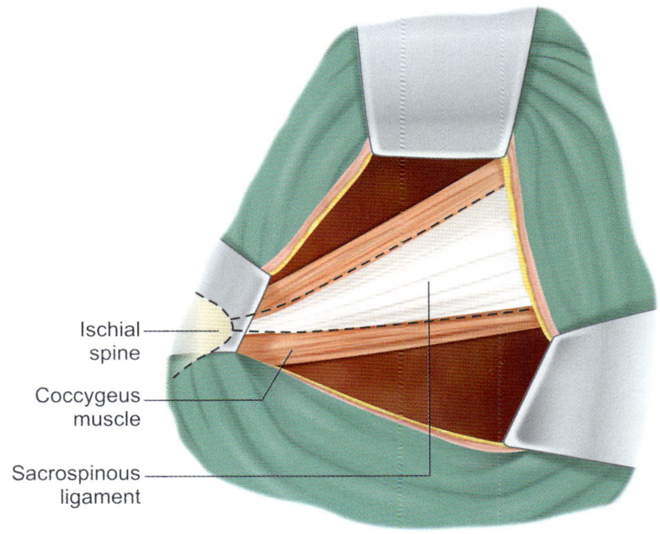

Fig. 35: Long thin retractors are used to displace rectum to left and cardinal ligament along with ureter is displaced anteriorly. To displace side walls of the pelvis a narrow right angle retractor is used to displace the side walls of the pelvis and perineum. In order to visualize sacrospinous ligament directly by removing areolar tissue after exposing the superior surface of pelvic diaphragm and dissecting sacrospinous ligament using a sponge dissector.

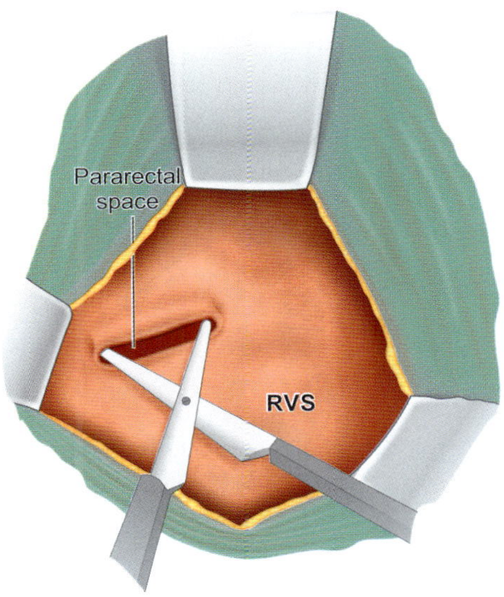

Fig. 34: In order to enter the pararectal space rectovaginal space is exposed. A narrow Deaver retractor may be used for that purpose; however, Breisky–Navratil retractors are more effective owing to its curve corresponding to pelvic curve. Adequate retraction of cardinal ligament, vagina, and rectum is required for better exposure and prevention of injuries. Some surgeons use bright fiber optic head lampcan for illumination of pararectal space.

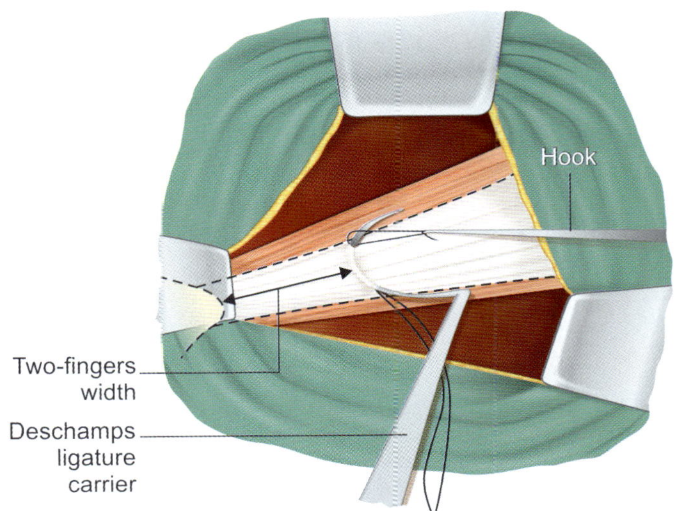

Fig. 36: The Deschamps ligature carrier is loaded with 0 monofilament nylon suture then it is directly inserted into the ligament. Skin hook is used to hold the suture and Deschamps carrier is removed. Sutures should be placed approximately two fingers width from the ischial spine to prevent the risk of nerve entrapment.

ILIOCOCCYGEAL FIXATION

Inmon was the first one to describe iliococcygeal fixation, in this technique vaginal apex is everted and secured to the iliococcygeal fascia bilaterally, just below the ischial spine. This technique was successfully performed in 3 women with atrophied uterosacral ligaments.

Technique

Midline incision taken on the posterior vaginal wall and opened in the same manner as done while performing posterior colporrhaphy. Rectovaginal space is created by blunt dissection bilaterally, dissection is done laterally in the direction of levator muscles and posteriorly in the direction of ischial spines. Rectum is depressed down and medially using the nondominant hand, and a single stitch is placed into iliococcygeus and fascia at point 1 and 2 caudal to ischial spine using 0 polyglycolic suture. Both ends of the suture is passed through posterior vaginal apex of the same side and held with artery forceps. Same is done on the other side.

Vaginal epithelium is usually not excised in order to maintain good vaginal length and circumference (**Fig. 49**). On complition of posterior colporhapy posterior vaginal wall is closed and both iliococcygeal fixation sutures are tied in place.

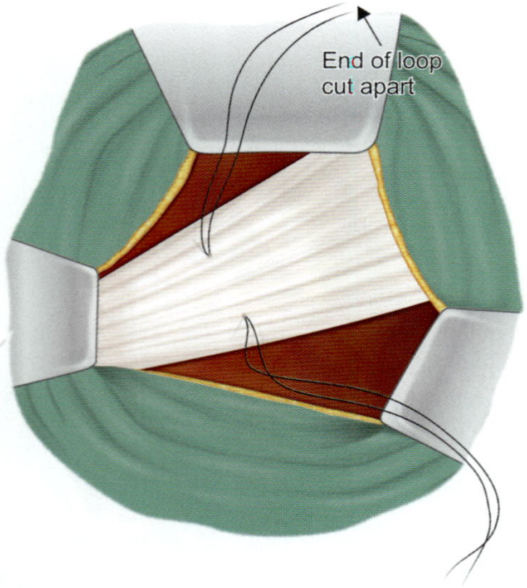

Fig. 37: For second suture Deschamps ligature carrier is used and after loading is passed through sacrospinous ligament.

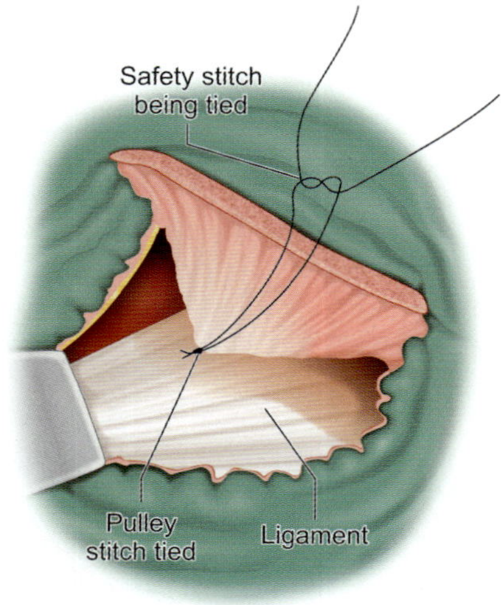

Fig. 39: The pulley stitch is tied and the ends of the suture is cut. The safety stitch is then tied.

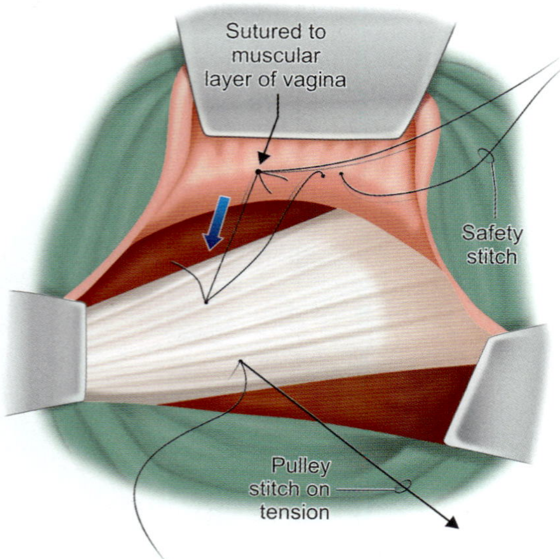

Fig. 38: The first suture is taken through the sacrospinous ligament is then placed through the muscular layer of the vagina. In a similar manner, the second suture is placed. The opposite end of the suture in the sacrospinous ligament is left free and held on a small artery forceps. Traction applied on this suture will draw the vaginal vault directly to the ligament, where a square knot will promptly affix it to the sacrospinous ligament.

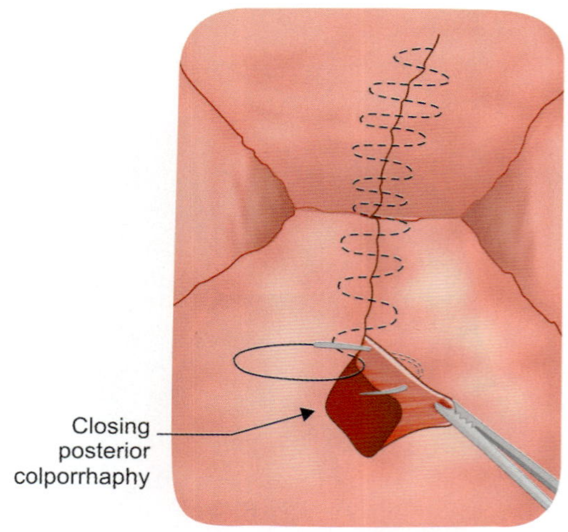

Fig. 40: A posterior colporrhaphy is done in the routine manner, and the vaginal mucosa closed.

Complications

Shull and colleagues studied 42 women who underwent iliococcygeus suspension and along with repair of coexisting pelvic support defects. Out of 42 women, 2 (5%) presented with recurrence of cuff prolapse on follow-up, of which 1 required surgery (she had recurrence of an inguinal hernia that had been repaired at the original surgery). Another patient, with history of five pelvic surgeries in the past, presented with cuff prolapse grade 2. On follow-up 6 patients presented with weakness at other sites, out of which 1 required surgery. 95% of women faced no persistence or recurrence of cuff prolapse on 6 weeks to 5 years follow-up. Meeks and colleagues also applied the Inmon technique in 110 women presenting with posthysterectomy vault prolapse or total uterine procidentia. In both studies, the most common complications reported was hemorrhage (1.2%), others being bladder/rectal perforation (1.2%), and recurrent vault prolapse (8%).

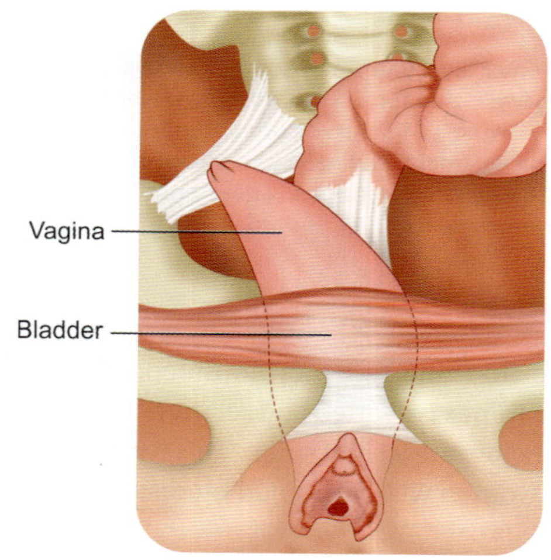

Fig. 41: On completion of the procedure the apex of the vagina is suspended from the sacrospinous ligament approximately 2 cm away from the ischial spine as shown. An indwelling catheter is left in situ for minimum of 4 days. Thereafter, management of bladder function is similar to that following surgery for urinary incontinence. No vaginal packs or drains are used.

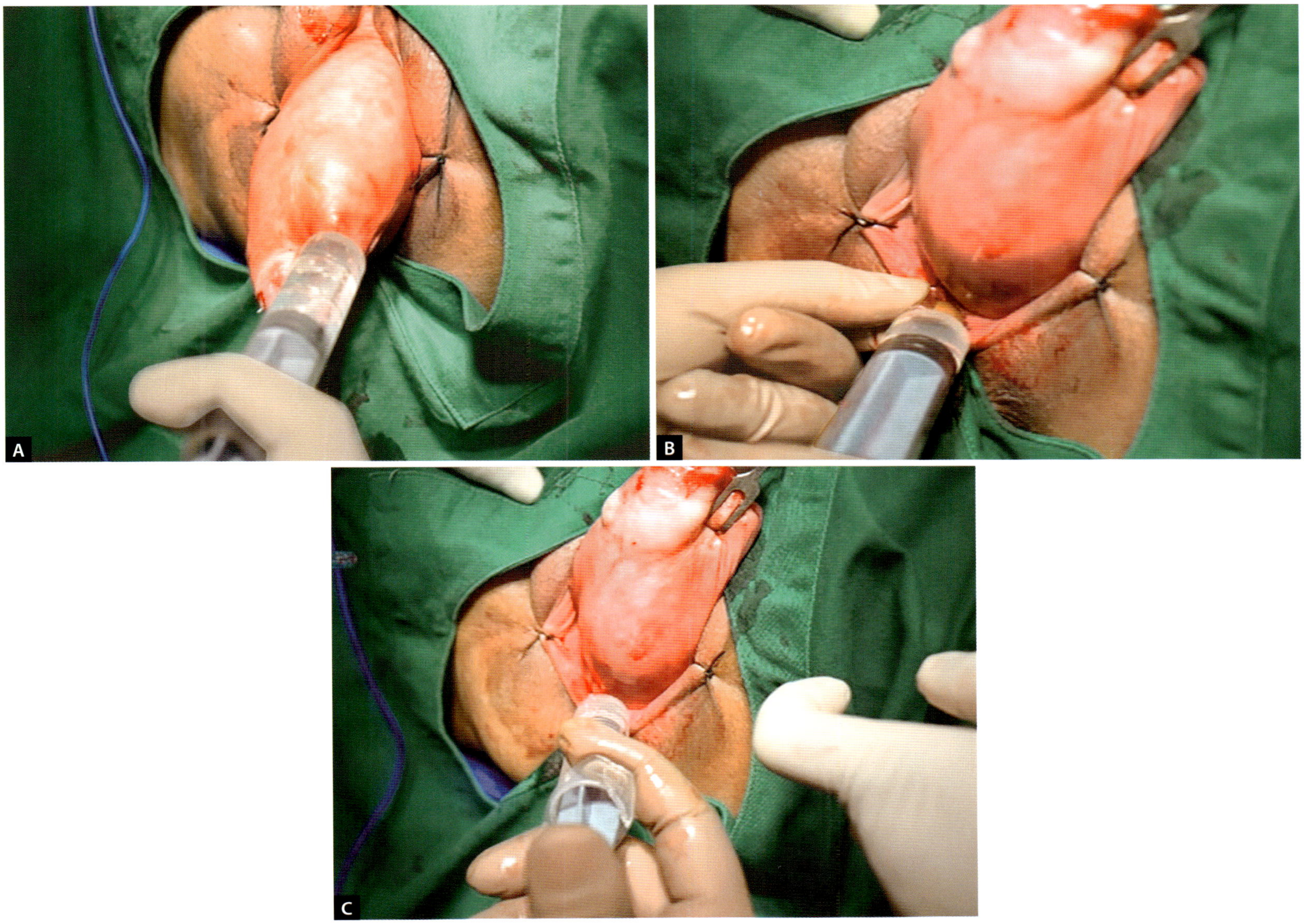

Fig. 42A to C: (A) Procidentia. (B and C) Incision taken in the rectovaginal space. 200 mL saline infiltrating the vag nal epithelium.

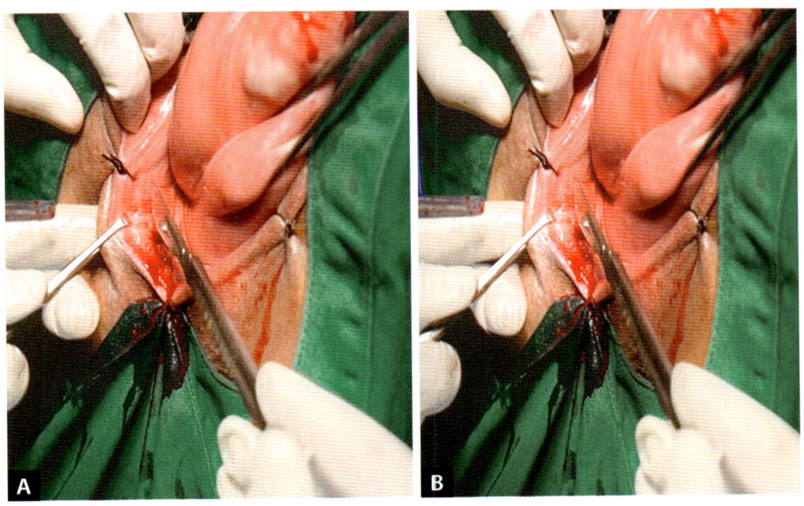

Figs. 43A and B: Blunt dissection done over rectovaginal space.

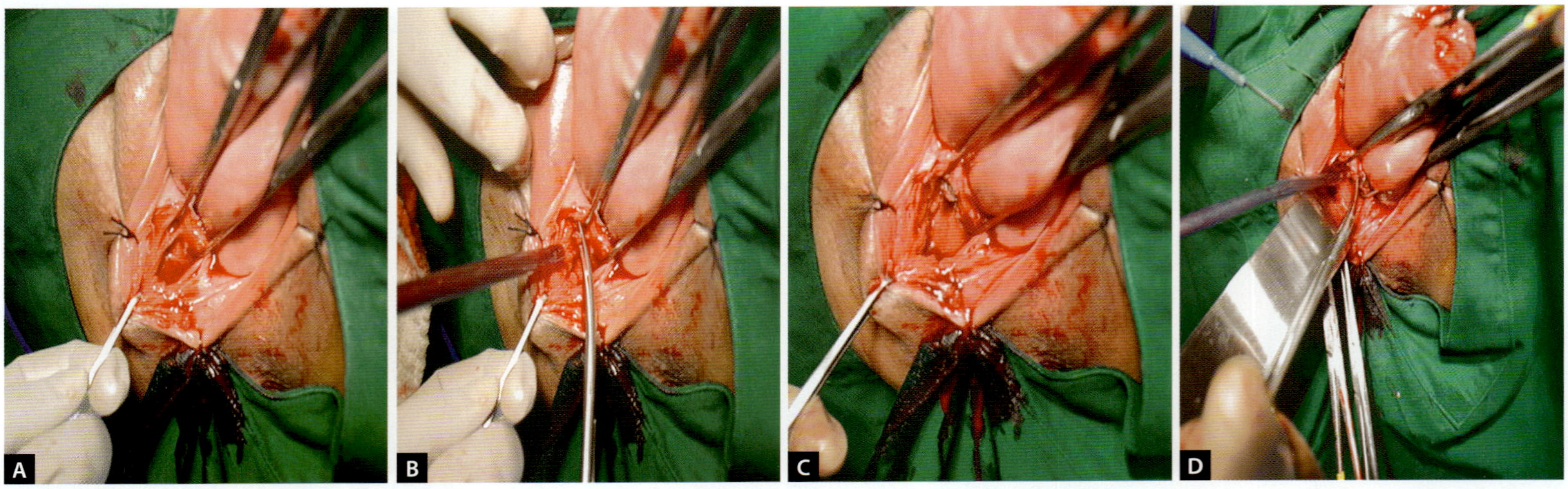

Figs. 44A to D: Space dissected till ischial spines and sacrospinous ligament felt.

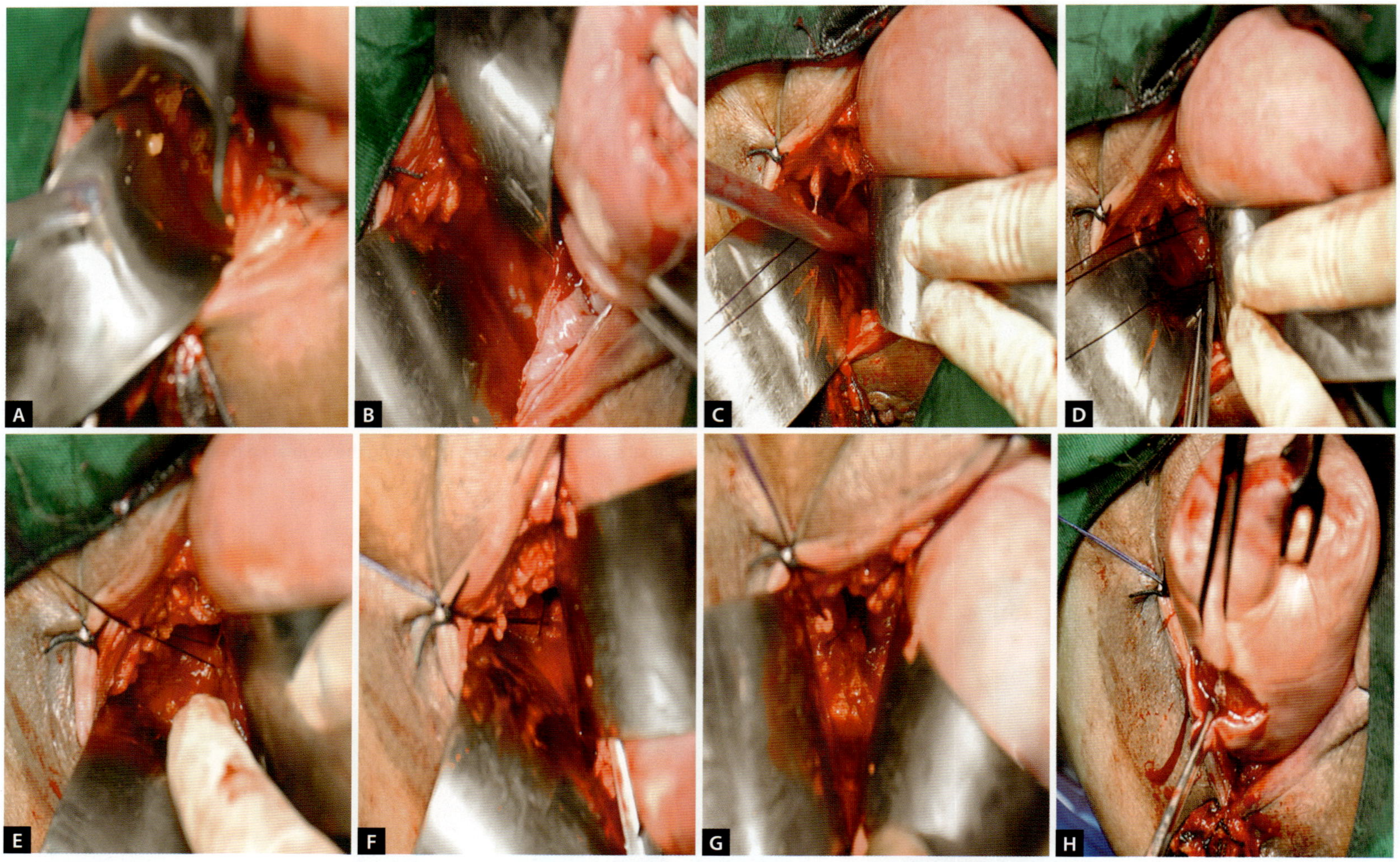

Figs. 45A to H: (A to F) Polydioxanone (PDS) No. 2 suture taken through the sacrospinous ligament 1.25 cm medial to the ischial spines; (G and H) Triple plication of pubocervical fascia to vaginal epithelium done.

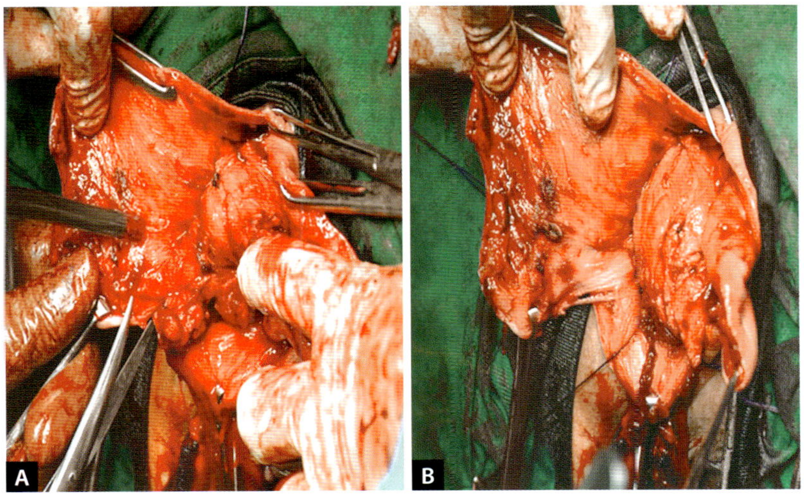

Figs. 46A and B: Following cystocele repair, suture through sacrospinous ligament is brought out via vaginal apex and knot placed.

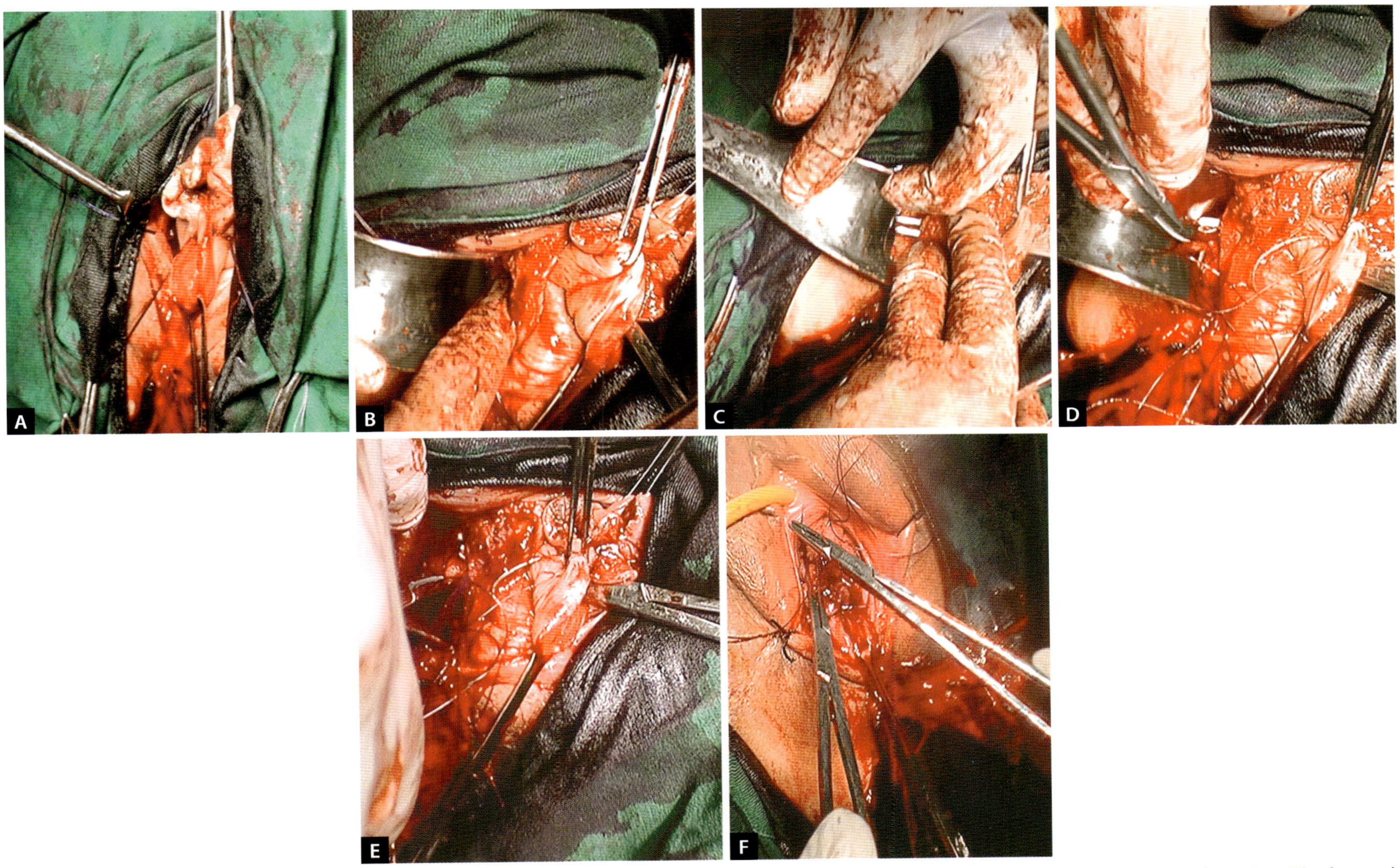

Figs. 47A to F: The end of the suture which was taken through the sacrospinous ligament is placed in the muscular layer, similarly the second stitch is taken. The free end of the suture material is left free and held with hemostat. Traction on the suture will pull vault towards the sacrospinous ligament, and a square knot is placed to promptly fix it to the ligament.

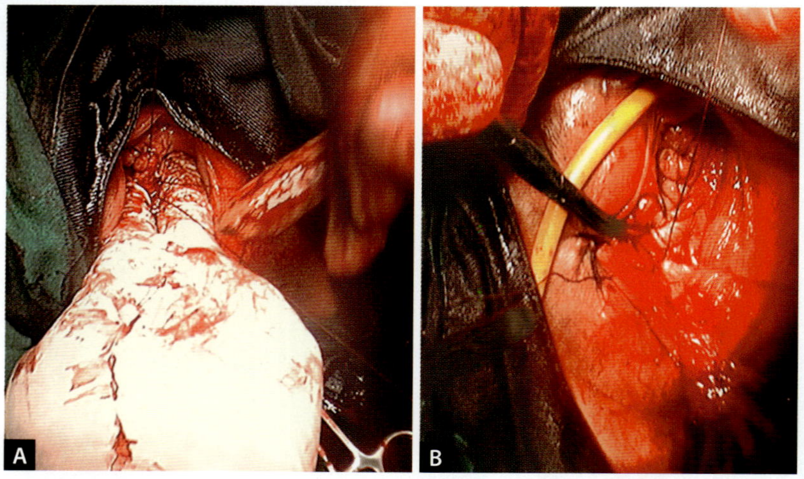

Figs. 48A and B: The pulley stitch is tied and the ends of sutures are cut. At last safety stitch is tied.

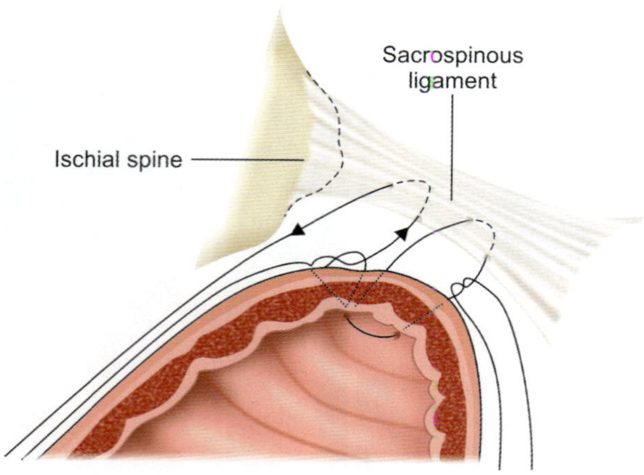

Fig. 49: Pulley stitches.

Benefits

In comparison with sacrospinous ligament fixation, iliococcygeus fixation is easier to perform technically and anterior vaginal wall is under less tension.

SUGGESTED READING

1. Baden WF, Walker T. Genesis of the vaginal profile. Clin Obstet Gynecol. 1972;15:1048-54.
2. Beck RP. Pelvic relaxation prolapse. In: Kase NG, Weingold AB (Eds). Principles and Practice of Clinical Gynecology. New York, NY: John Wiley & Sons; 1983. pp. 677-85.
3. Blaivas JG, Appell FA, Fantl JA, et al. Standards of efficacy for evaluation of treatment outcome in urinary incontinence: recommendations of the urodynamic society. Neurourol Urodyn. 1997;16:145-7.
4. Brown JS, Waetjen LE, Subak LL, et al. Pelvic organ prolapse surgery in the United States, 1997. Am J Obstet Gynecol. 2002;186(4):712-6.
5. Bump RC, Mattiasson A, Bo K, et al. The standardization of terminology of female pelvic organ prolapse and pelvic floor dysfunction. Am J Obstet Gynecol. 1996;175:10-17.
6. Comiter CV, Vasavada SP, Barbaric ZL, et al. Grading pelvic prolapse and pelvic floor relaxation using dynamic magnetic resonance imaging. Urology. 1999;3:454-7.
7. Fielding JR, Griffiths DJ, Versi E, et al. MR imaging of pelvic floor continence mechanisms in the supine and sitting positions. AJR Am J Roentgenol. 1998;171:1607-10.
8. Fielding JR, Versi E, Mulkern RV, et al. MR imaging of the female pelvic floor in the supine and upright positions. J Magn Reson Imaging. 1996;6:961-3.
9. Goodrich MA, Webb MH, King BF, et al. Magnetic resonance imaging of pelvic floor relaxation: dynamic analysis and evaluation of patients before and after surgical repair. Obstet Gynecol. 1993;82:883-91.
10. Gufler H, Laubengerger J, DeGregorio G, et al. Pelvic floor descent: dynamic MR imaging using a half-Fourier RARE sequence. J Magn Reson Imaging. 1999;9:378-83.
11. Harris TA, Bent AD. Genital prolapse with and without urinary incontinence. J Reprod Med. 1990;35:792-8.
12. Healy JC, Halligan S, Reznek RH, et al. Patterns of prolapse in women with symptoms of pelvic floor weakness: assessment with MR imaging. Radiology. 1997;203:77-81.
13. Hoyte L, Schierlitz L, Zou K, et al. Two- and 3-dimensional MRI comparison of levator ani structure, volume, and integrity in women with stress incontinence and prolapse. Am J Obstet Gynecol. 2001;185:11-9.
14. Kelvin FM, Maglinte DDT, Hale DS, et al. Female pelvic organ prolapse: a comparison of triphasic dynamic MR imaging and triphasic fluoroscopic cystocolpoproctography. AJR Am J Roentgenol. 2000;174:81-8.
15. Klutke C, Golomb J, Barbaric Z, et al. The anatomy of stress incontinence: magnetic resonance imaging of the female bladder neck and urethra. J Urol. 1990;143:563-6.
16. Law PA, Danin JC, Lamb GM, et al. Dynamic imaging of the pelvic floor using an open-configuration magnetic resonance scanner. J Magn Reson Imaging. 2001;13(6):923-9.
17. Leinemann A, Anthuber C, Baron A, et al. Dynamic MR colpocystorecto-graphy assessing pelvic-floor descent. Eur Radiol. 1997;7:1309-17.
18. Molander U, Milsom I, Ekelund P, et al. An epidemiological study of urinary incontinence and related urogenital symptoms in elderly women. Maturitas. 1990;12:51-60.
19. Norton P, Baker J, Sharp H, et al. Genitourinary prolapse: relationship with joint mobility. Neuro Urodyn. 1990;9:321-2.
20. Nygaard IK, Kreder KJ. Complications of colposuspension. Int Urogynecol J. 1994;5:353-60.
21. Olsen AL, Smith VJ, Bergstrom JO, et al. Epidemiology of surgically managed pelvic organ prolapse and urinary incontinence. Obstet Gynecol. 1997;89(4):501-6.
22. Ozasa H, Mori T, Togashi K. Study of uterine prolapse by magnetic resonance imaging: topographical changes involving the levator ani muscle and the vagina. Gynecol Obstet Invest. 1992;24:43-8.
23. Pelsang RD, Bonney WW. Voiding cystourethrography in female stress incontinence. AJR Am J Roentgenol. 1996;166:561-5.
24. Richardson AC, Edmonds PB, Williams NL. Treatment of stress urinary incontinence due to paravaginal fascial defect. Obstet Gynecol. 1981;57:357-62.
25. Richardson AC, Lyon JB, Williams NL. A new look at pelvic relaxation. Am J Obstet Gynecol. 1976;126:568-73.
26. Rush CB, Entman SS. Pelvic organ prolapse and stress urinary incontinence. Med Clin North Am. 1995;79:1473-9.
27. Samuelsson EC, Arne Victor FT, Tibblin G, et al. Signs of genital prolapse in a Swedish population of women 20 to 59 years of age and possible related factors. Am J Obstet Gynecol. 1999;180:299-305.
28. Schoenenberger AW, Debatin JF, Guldenschuh I, et al. Dynamic MR defecography with a superconducting, open-configuration MR system. Radiology. 1998;206:641-6.
29. Shull BL, Baden WF. A six-year experience with paravaginal defect repair for stress urinary incontinence. Am J Obstet Gynecol. 1989;160:1432-40.
30. Silva WA, Kleeman S, Segal J, et al. Effects of a full bladder and patient positioning on pelvic organ prolapse assessment. Obstet Gynecol. 2004;104:37-41.
31. Smith AR, Hosker GL, Warrell DW. The role of partial denervation of the pelvic floor in the aetiology of genitourinary prolapse and stress inconti-nence of urine. A neurophysiological study. Br J Obstet Gynaecol. 1989;96(1):24-8.
32. Tan IL, Stoker J, Zwamborn AW, et al. Female pelvic floor: endovaginal MR imaging of normal anatomy. Radiology. 1998;206:777-83.
33. Tapp A, Cardozo L. The effect of epidural anesthesia on postpartum voiding. Neurourol Urodyn. 1987;6:235-9.
34. Tunn R, Paris S, Fischer W, et al. Static magnetic resonance imaging of the pelvic floor muscle morphology in women with stress urinary incontinence and pelvic prolapse. Neurourol Urodyn. 1998;17:579-89.
35. Unterweger M, Marincek B, Gottstein-Aalame N, et al. Ultrafast MR imaging of the pelvic floor. AJR Am J Roentgenol. 2001;176:959-63.
36. Wall LL, Versi E, Norton P, et al. Evaluating the outcome of surgery for pelvic organ prolapse. Am J Obstet Gynecol. 1998;178:877-88.
37. Yang A, Mostwin JL, Rosenshein NB, et al. Pelvic floor descent in women: dynamic evaluation with fast MR imaging and cinematic display. Radiology. 1991;179:25-33.

CHAPTER

17

Total Laparoscopic Hysterectomy

Dhivya B, Minal Kumbhalwar, B Ramesh

INTRODUCTION

Hysterectomy is one of the commonly performed gynecological surgeries worldwide, second only to cesarean section. In 1813, Conrad Langenbeck performed the first planned vaginal hysterectomy followed by Abdominal Hysterectomy by Clay and Koeberle in 1863. American Congress of Obstetricians and Gynecologists (ACOG) committee opinion (2009)[1] states that vaginal hysterectomy should be the approach of choice whenever feasible, for benign causes, in uterus less than 12 weeks taking into account the higher morbidity associated with abdominal approach. Contraindications to vaginal hysterectomy include presence of severe endometriosis, adnexal masses, previous pelvic surgeries, and malignancy. The ideal approach to hysterectomy in such cases would be one which includes the advantages of vaginal hysterectomy like avoiding a large incision, with added advantage of a panoramic view of the entire pelvis and easy manipulation, all of which is feasible in laparoscopic hysterectomy. The role of the laparoscope in assisting vaginal hysterectomy has been described by Semm[2,3]since 1984. Newer innovations in technology lead to first laparoscopic hysterectomy by Harry Reich[4] in 1989. In 1992, Nezhat et al.[5] reported that laparoscopically assisted vaginal hysterectomy (LAVH) could replace most abdominal hysterectomies for benign lesions. The extent of dissection laparoscopically and vaginally depends on the gynecologist's expertise, experience, and preference. Despite consensus statements by both the ACOG and the American Association of Gynecologic Laparoscopists (AAGL) stating that laparoscopic hysterectomy should be the standard of care; even now more than 50% of hysterectomies are done as open procedures for benign etiologies. Slow acceptance of minimally invasive laparoscopic hysterectomy amongst practicing Gynecologists (OB/GYNs), specifically conventional laparoscopic hysterectomy, has been attributed to long learning curves and insufficient laparoscopic training in OB/GYN residencies.[6]

SURGICAL ANATOMY (FIG. 1)

The uterus is a pear-shaped, inverted, muscular organ of the female reproductive system, situated between the rectum and bladder. This *muscular* organ having expansion capability for accommodating growing fetus, is attached laterally to the Fallopian tubes and distally to vagina.

The *uterus* is composed of three parts:

1. *Fundus:* Uterine top above entry site of the Fallopian tubes
2. *Body:* Site of blastocyst implantation
3. *Cervix:* Lower portion of uterus between internal and external os.

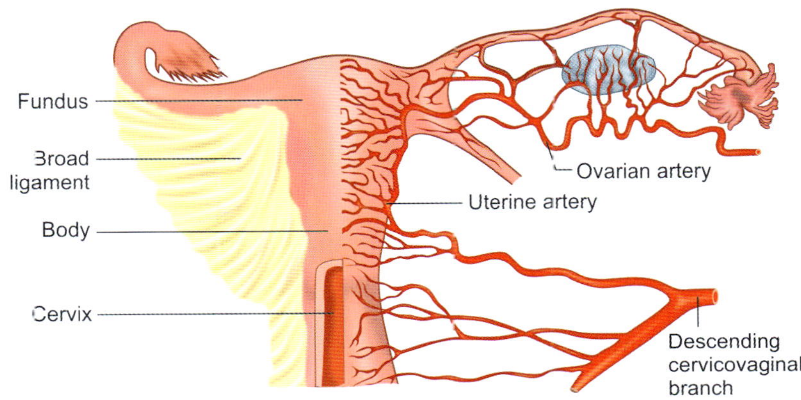

Fig. 1: Anatomy of uterus.

With respect to vagina, the uterus is anteverted and anteflexed with respect to the cervix. The uterus mainly fundus and body are made up of three layers:

1. *Perimetrium:* A double membrane, covering the uterine muscle which is in continuation with peritoneum of abdomen.
2. *Myometrium:* Thickened smooth muscle.
3. *Endometrium:* The mucous membrane lining the uterine cavity internally having two parts—(1) the deep layer *stratum basalis* and (2) superficially *stratum functionalis (hormone sensitive layer that cyclically sheds and regenerates)*.

Uterus supports mainly divided into primary and secondary supports:

- *Primary supports further includes muscular supports and ligamentous support:*
  - Muscular support consists of pelvic diaphragm, perineal body, and urogenital diaphragm
  - Ligamentous support includes:
    - Mackenrodt ligament, i.e. transverse cervical or cardinal ligament
    - Uterosacral ligament
    - Round ligament
    - Pubocervical ligament
    - Uterine axis.
- *Secondary supports includes:*
  - Broad ligament
  - Uterovesical fold of peritoneum
  - Rectovaginal fold of peritoneum.

The *uterine artery* is the main blood supply for uterus. Venous drainage is through broad ligament plexus which flows into *uterine veins*. Lymphatic supply is through the *iliac, aortic, sacral,* and *inguinal lymph nodes*. Sympathetic nerve supply for uterus is from the *uterovaginal plexus* which consists of *anterior* and *intermediate* portion of *inferior hypogastric plexus*. Parasympathetic nervous supply is from the *splanchnic nerves (S2-S4)*. The cervix receives nerve supply by *uterovaginal plexus* via *inferior* fibers. The afferent fibers via *inferior hypogastric plexus* enter the spinal cord through *T10-T12* and *L1* fibers.

A good knowledge of regional anatomy is necessary to reduce damage to bowel and ureter. The uterine artery crosses above the ureter 1 cm on lateral aspect of the internal os (water under the bridge). During hysterectomy, one should be cautious enough while clamping uterine arteries for not to include ureter.

DEFINITIONS

A review of the literature suggests multiple definitions of a laparoscopic hysterectomy. According to Donnez et al.,[7] there are five types of laparoscopic hysterectomy as given in **Table 1**.

Type 1 laparoscopic hysterectomy is performed in suspected cases of pelvic adhesions or mild pelvic endometriosis to assess the feasibility of performing a vaginal hysterectomy. Type 2, namely laparoscopy-assisted vaginal hysterectomy (LAVH) involves initial steps like adhesiolysis, excision of endometriosis being done laparoscopically followed by vaginal hysterectomy. Type 3, laparoscopic hysterectomy comprises bilateral ligation of the uterine arteries laparoscopically. Type 4, complete laparoscopic hysterectomy is one in which laparoscopic dissection is done and uterus is freed from its attachments with peritoneal cavity and vaginal closure is done laparoscopically or vaginally. Type 5 involves laparoscopic closure of the vault. Additional terms include laparoscopic supracervical and laparoscopic radical hysterectomy. Laparoscopic supracervical hysterectomy (LSH) is a technique where the upper uterus is completely detached from the cervix and then retrieved, while the cervix, uterosacral ligaments, and cardinal ligaments are left behind. Laparoscopic radical hysterectomy done for early endometrial and cervical cancers, involves removal of the uterus, supporting ligaments, upper vagina together with pelvic, and para-aortic lymph nodes, as necessary.

INDICATIONS

The number of hysterectomies has been on the rise in the previous three decades. According to the VALUE trial, three-quarters of hysterectomy were performed through the abdominal route, while the rest were done vaginally.[8,9] Vaginal hysterectomy, previously done predominantly for pelvic organ prolapse, has recently found a resurgence due to reduced hospital stay, better patient comfort, and early return to normal life in comparison to abdominal hysterectomy. Though abdominal hysterectomy has increased risks of febrile and postoperative morbidity and a longer postoperative hospitalization and convalescence period, this route is preferred due to the ease and convenience offered by the large incision, especially in larger and bulky uterus, pelvic inflammatory disease, endometriosis, previous surgeries, and narrow vagina.[10] However, the route selected depends on the pelvic pathology, previous surgeries and most importantly, the surgeon's expertise.[11] In cases where adhesions are suspected, laparoscopy can reveal whether a vaginal approach is appropriate. Of late, laparoscopy has been adopted to such an extent that it can be considered as a replacement to abdominal hysterectomy. Indications for laparoscopic hysterectomy include:

- Abnormal uterine bleeding
- Leiomyomas
- Adenomyosis
- Endometriosis
- Uterine prolapse
- Ovarian tumors
- Adnexal masses
- Pelvic inflammatory disease
- Failure of transcervical resection of the endometrium (TCRE)
- Gynecologic malignancies—laparoscopic hysterectomy can also be performed in early endometrial cancer stage 1.[12-15]

Table 1: Types of laparoscopic hysterectomy.

Type	*Procedure*
1	Diagnostic laparoscopy followed by vaginal hysterectomy
2	Laparoscopy-assisted vaginal hysterectomy
3	Laparoscopic hysterectomy
4	Complete laparoscopic hysterectomy
5	Laparoscopic closure of the vagina

CONTRAINDICATIONS

There are very few contraindications to laparoscopic hysterectomy, which are the same as for any other operative laparoscopic procedures. With advances in anesthesia and laparoscopic innovations, most of the patients can undergo laparoscopic hysterectomy safely.

Absolute Contraindications

- Severe cardiac problems
- Pulmonary disease.

These patients may not tolerate an adequate pneumoperitoneum and deep Trendelenburg position for satisfactory vision and maneuverability.

Relative Contraindications

- Multiple previous major surgeries
- Morbid obesity
- Severe, chronically ill patients
- Malignancy.

In patients with multiple previous surgeries with adhesions, introduction of Veress through Palmer's point, primary port insertion under vision or Hasson's open entry technique might be required. However, in cases with extensive adhesions, it would be a wiser decision to convert to laparotomy as and when required. In morbid obesity,[16] problems encountered are difficulty in Veress needle insertion, restricted mobility of laparoscopic instruments, and fat deposition in omentum obscuring the operative field. The reposition of panniculus is required for ease of instrumentation. Depending on pannus mobility, it can be taped or weighted on the lower part of body. Longer instruments with extra accessory ports facilitate the bowel manipulation for better visualization. Though malignancy is considered a contraindication, especially in cases where rupture and spillage of cyst are to be avoided, magnified view of pelvic anatomy with laparoscopy by experts provides an excellent opportunity for performing radical hysterectomy with lymphadenectomy.

INSTRUMENTS (FIGS. 2A TO F)

Routinely equipment essential for performing laparoscopic hysterectomy successfully includes:

- A laparoscopic tower with camera, light source, and high-flow CO_2 insufflator **(Fig. 2A)**.
- An operating table with leg stirrups.
- Two laparoscopic graspers (toothed and nontoothed) with longer jaws for holding and manipulating the adnexal structures, uterus, and bowel **(Fig. 2B)**.
- Suction aspirator and irrigator are required to clear out the blood, clots, and smoke.
- Vasopressin injection needle.
- Simple uterine manipulator with vaginal tube **(Fig. 2C)** is used for manipulating the uterus which is capable of extreme anteversion, retroversion, and movement in 45° arc toward right and left side.
- Monopolar electricity generator, bipolar electricity generator **(Fig. 2D)** and bipolar forceps, harmonic generator **(Fig. 2E)** and harmonic scalpel[17] **(Fig. 2F)**, or LigaSure vessel sealing instrument[18]

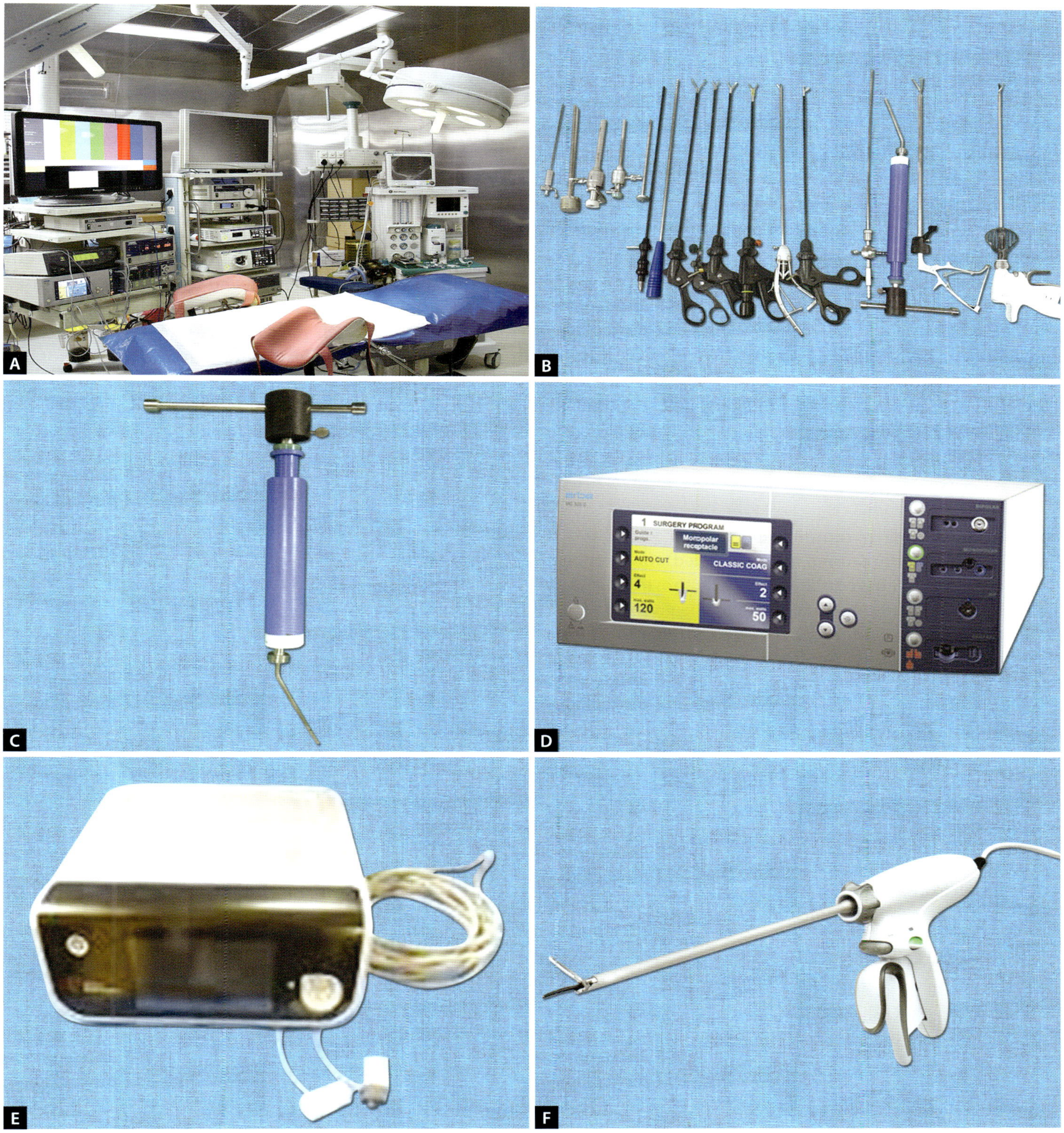

Figs. 2A to F: (A) Laparoscopic tower and OR setup; (B) Instruments used in total laparoscopic hysterectomy; (C) Simple uterine manipulator; (D) Electrosurgical generator with vaginal tube; (E and F) Harmonic generator with handle.

- Laparoscopic scissors.
- Laparoscopic myoma screw for manipulation of bulky and large uterus.
- A needle holder and hooked scissors are used for suturing the vault and cutting the suture, respectively.

PREOPERATIVE EVALUATION

Routine preoperative investigations include a complete blood count, bleeding time, clotting time, renal function tests, serum electrolytes, evaluation of thyroid status, viral markers, Pap smear, electrocardiography (ECG), and urinalysis. However, tests like prothrombin time and international normalized ratio (PT-INR), activated partial thromboplastin time (aPTT), tumor markers, endometrial biopsy, liver function tests, chest radiography, 2D-echocardiography, computed tomography (CT), magnetic resonance imaging (MRI), and urodynamic studies should be done, as indicated. Preanesthetic fitness is obtained. Preanesthetic assessment is an essential step prior to anesthesia in an attempt to decrease the morbidity and mortality related to anesthesia and surgery. Patient is advised for admission the evening before the surgery. Appropriate written, informed, and verbal consent is obtained from patient after detailed explanation of proposed surgery, its benefits, risks, and complications, the possibility of converting to laparotomy, and medical/therapeutic alternatives for surgery. Aspirin and warfarin are to be stopped 5 days prior to surgery. All patients are advised to eat lightly for 24 hours before surgery. Oral laxative tablets (bisacodyl) are given the night before. If adhesions or difficult surgery is contemplated, an oral mechanical bowel preparation like Coloprep or Peglec is administered. Patient is kept nil per oral 8 hours prior to surgery.

ANESTHESIA

Laparoscopic hysterectomy is routinely performed with general anesthesia. Laparoscopic operations are performed after tracheal intubation under controlled ventilation; hence short as well as intermediate-acting neuromuscular blockers must be given based on surgery duration. However, in non-obese patients, general anesthesia can be safely performed without intubation with ProSeal laryngeal mask airway. Extreme care has to be taken for patients with higher airway pressures (>30 cm H_2O) or when possibilities of extreme head-down tilt is expected.

POSITION (FIG. 3)

Providing appropriate position to patient is a crucial component of laparoscopic gynecological procedures. Accurate patient positioning for laparoscopic surgery decreases the risk of grievous nerve injury in both upper and lower extremities.[19] The patient is provided dorsolithotomy position with the buttocks reaching up to the table end with arms tucked securely to the patient's side, providing adequate area on both side of the patient's head and shoulders for operating and preventing brachial plexus injury. For patients with huge breast mass, towels are placed behind the scapula, i.e. shoulder blades for elevating the head above the chest level facilitating intubation and airway access during surgery. After proper insertion of manipulator and Foley's catheter, the position is changed to low lithotomy position for the rest of the surgery. The bladder is drained prior to ancillary trocar placement for decreasing chances of any potential injury. Shoulder braces are placed on the acromion process to prevent nerve injury during steep Trendelenburg position. Mild degree of Trendelenburg is useful during placement of the uterine manipulator. Proper positioning and boot stirrups decrease neuronal injury, specifically when laparoscopic procedures prolong for more than 2 hours. External pressure over the legs should be avoided. Important components of accurate lithotomy positioning **(Fig. 3)** are—(1) hip flexion of 60–170°; (2) knee flexion of 90–120°; (3) hip abduction of 90° or less, and (4) minimal external hip rotation. If electrosurgery is to be used during the procedure, a return plate for monopolar instruments must be appropriately placed under the patient's thigh, and full contact surface of plate with thigh should be assured.

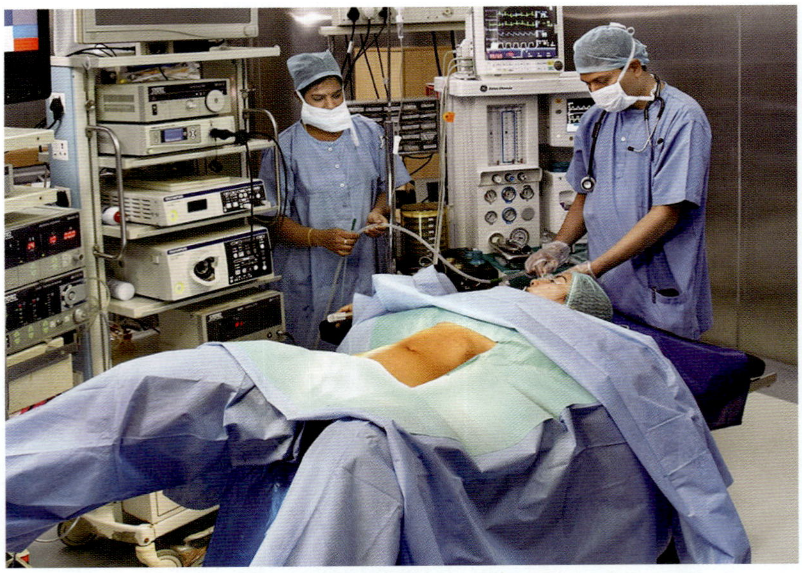

Fig. 3: Positioning of patient.

SURGICAL TECHNIQUE

Port Placement (Figs. 4A to D)

Povidone-iodine is applied over the operating field of abdomen and vagina starting from nipple line up till inner thighs and proper draping is done. The nasogastric tube is inserted before creating pneumoperitoneum in cases where adhesions are expedited. Prophylactic antibiotics are administered approximately 1 hour prior to the procedure. The most preferred site for Veress needle insertion is umbilicus. CO_2 is most commonly used gas for most laparoscopic hysterectomy. Veress needle is checked for patency prior to insertion. A stab incision is made either at the umbilicus or at Palmer's point in flat position. The Veress needle is introduced at a 45° angle (90° if obese) in the midline and directing toward uterine fundus or pelvis. Initially intra-abdominal insufflation pressure should not be more than 10 mm Hg and it acts as reliable indicator for monitoring insufflation and accurate needle insertion. After proper needle placement, 3–6 L of CO_2 is insufflated inside the peritoneal cavity. After 1.5–2 L of CO_2 insufflation, intra-abdominal pressures will start increasing. Insufflation has to be continued till the pressure reaches up to 18–20 mm Hg. Insertion of the Veress needle through the Palmer's point, i.e. subcostal space in the left sided midclavicular line is safest alternative in cases where adhesions are contemplated.[20] The left upper quadrant is usually free of intra-abdominal adhesions and also easily accessible. Some also suggest using Hasson's technique of open entry[21] or an optical Veress in such cases.

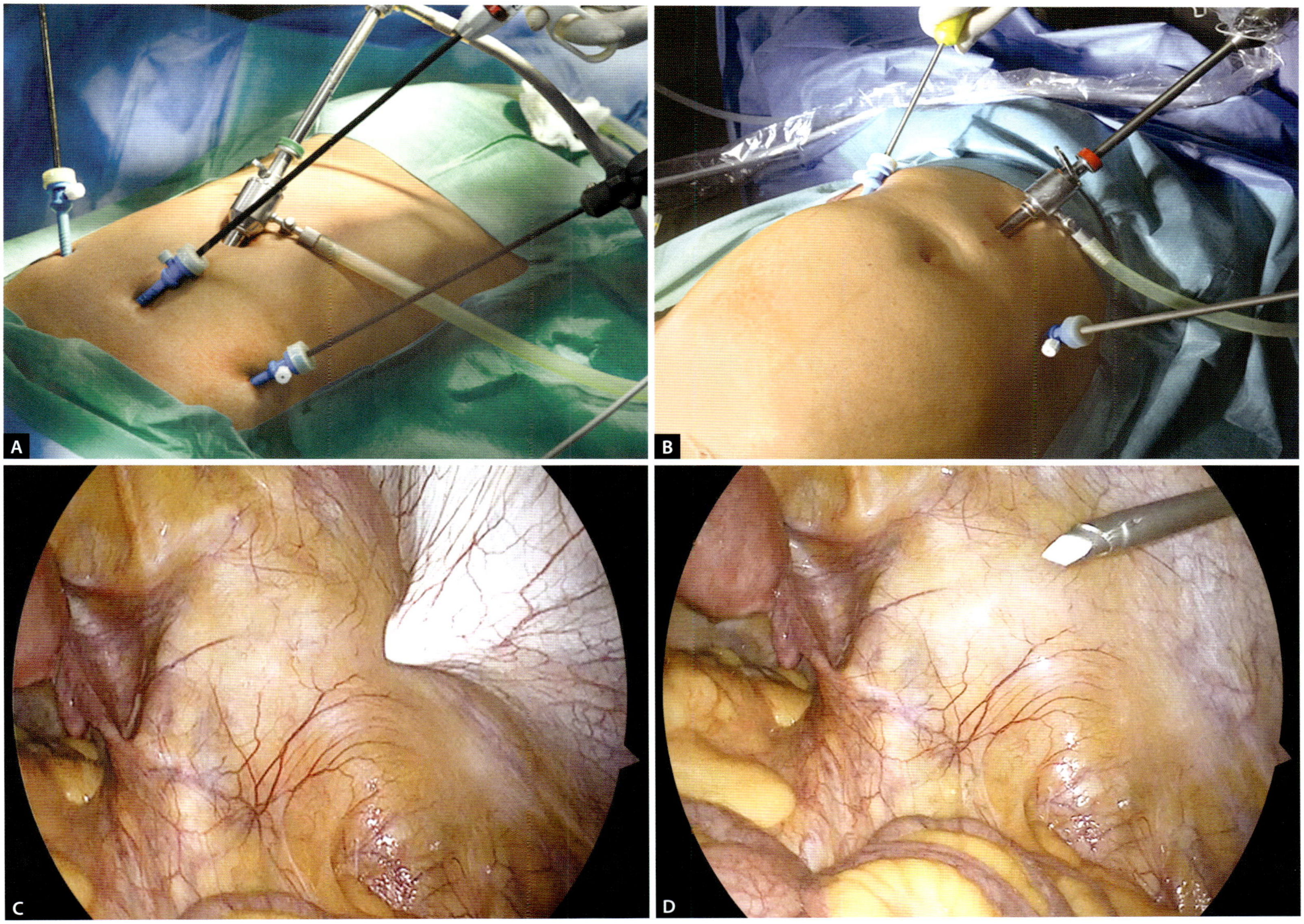

Figs. 4A to D: (A) Ports in normal sized uterus; (B) Ports in big uterus (20 weeks size); (C and D) Ancillary port placement under vision.

Once adequate pneumoperitoneum is achieved, sensorcaine infiltration is done at the site of primary port placement. Considering uterine size, 5-mm skin incision is made 3–4 cm above the umbilicus or even higher up and primary port is placed with angulation of 45–60°. The periumbilical area is inspected for any underlying omental or bowel adhesions with the anterior abdominal wall. Trendelenburg position is adopted. At the site of secondary trocar placement, laparoscopic transillumination of the abdominal wall is done to avoid injury to deep epigastric blood vessels. The secondary 5-mm trocars usually two in number are placed on the left and right lateral walls, approximately 8–10 cm on lateral side of the umbilicus, lateral to the inferior epigastric vessels, under vision in a similar manner **(Fig. 4A)**. In a bigger uterus, all the ports are placed higher **(Fig. 4B)**, depending on the uterine size. If necessary, a third suprapubic midline port can be placed **(Fig. 4A)**. The placement of secondary trocar under vision is noted in **Figures 4C and D**.

The step-by-step approach for total laparoscopic hysterectomy (TLH) is described here:

Upper Pedicles (Figs. 5A to G)

Abdomen is inspected for presence of omental or bowel adhesions. If present, adhesiolysis is done with bipolar and scissors or harmonic.[17]

Diluted injection vasopressin 10–20 units in 100 mL normal saline is infiltrated into the uterus till blanching occurs, as this procedure reduces the blood loss.[22] This is followed by coagulation of the round ligament, proximal part of the uterine tube, mesosalpinx, and the ovarian ligament with bipolar introduced from the ipsilateral side. Three adjacent areas are coagulated followed by cutting with laparoscopic scissors in the mid part. The uterus is mobilized to the right side to provide tension on left uterine-ovarian ligament with a uterine manipulator to facilitate the process. To avoid back bleeding, medial part (upper lateral uterine border) is desiccated with bipolar. The remaining part of the broad ligament adjoining the uterus is taken down up to the Mackenrodt's ligament in similar fashion. The same procedure is repeated on the opposite side.

To prevent ovarian cancers, bilateral tubes are cauterized and cut with harmonic[17] as illustrated in **Figures 6A and B**.

Development of Bladder Flap (Figs. 7A to C)

The upper junction of the uterovesical peritoneal fold (white line) is the area where the peritoneum is very loosely adhered to the cervix and hence it can be easily separated. Dissection in false tissue plane provokes unnecessary bleeding. The uterus is retroverted and pushed cephalad to aid dissection. The peritoneum of the vesicouterine space is then grasped and elevated with forceps, while harmonic[17] or scissors are used to dissect the vesicouterine space **(Figs. 7A to C)**. Hydrodissection[23] also separates broad ligament leaves by distending the vesicouterine space and making out the bladder tendinous attachments clear in this area. The middle loose connective tissue band is the vesicocervical ligament while the lateral bands on sides of the cervix are pubocervical ligament, i.e. bladder pillars. These pillars contain blood vessels and hence proper desiccation is necessary, these are coagulated with bipolar or harmonic.[17] Coagulation followed by sharp dissection is used to divide peritoneum down

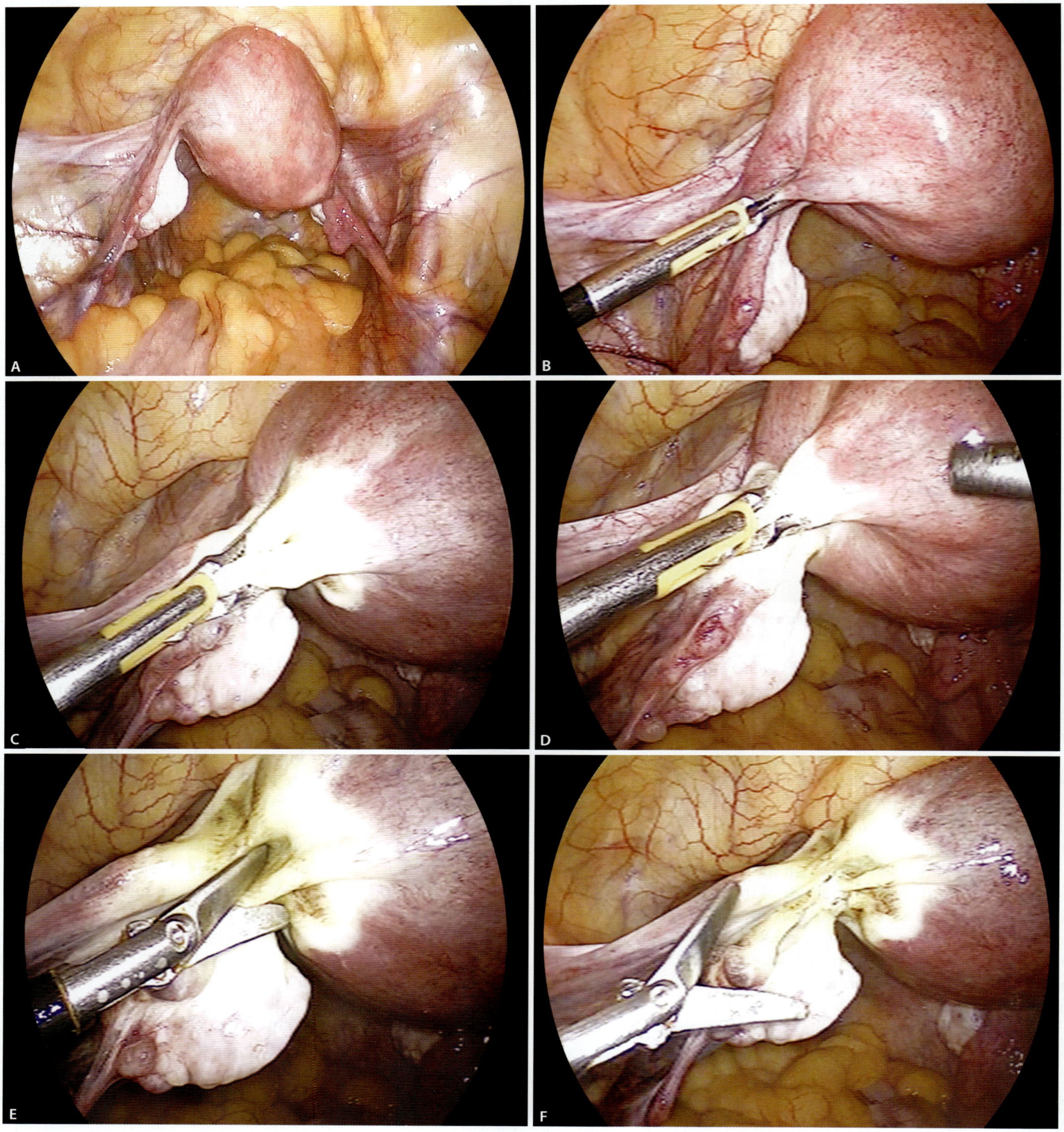

Figs. 5A to F

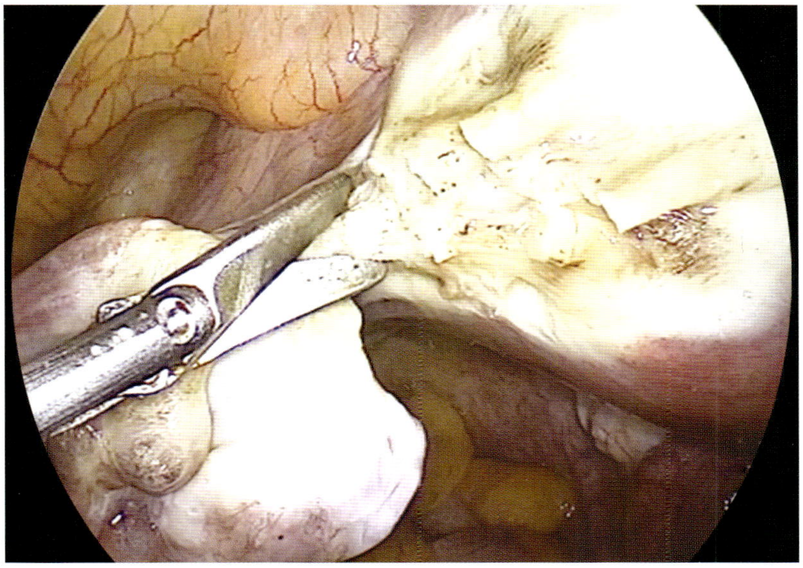

Fig. 5G

Figs. 5A to G: (A) Laparoscopic appearance of uterus; (B to D) Coagulation of left upper pedicle with bipolar forceps; (E to G) Cutting of the upper pedicle with scissors illustrated.

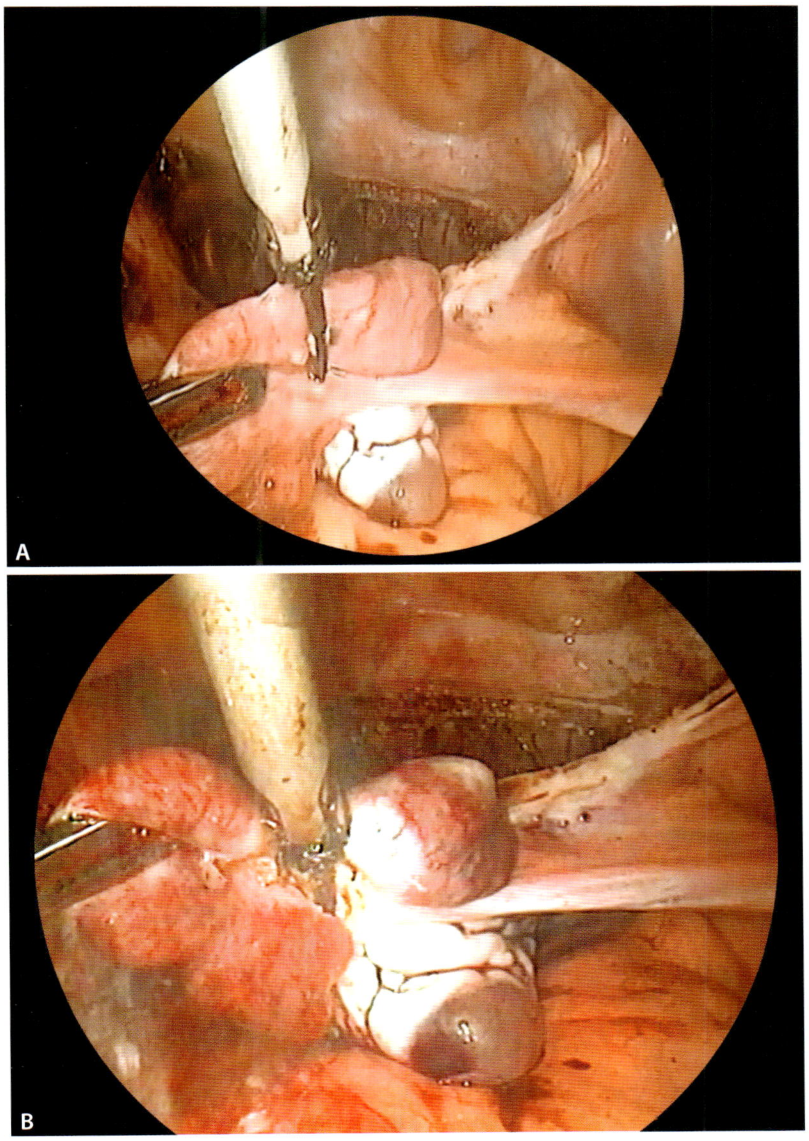

Figs. 6A and B: Right salpingectomy with harmonic demonstrated.

to the uterosacral ligaments. The bladder is dissected from uterus by blunt probe dissection pushing downward along the vesicocervical plane till the anterior pouch is exposed adequately **(Figs. 7B and C)**. Lateral bladder dissection helps to push the ureters away from the cervix.

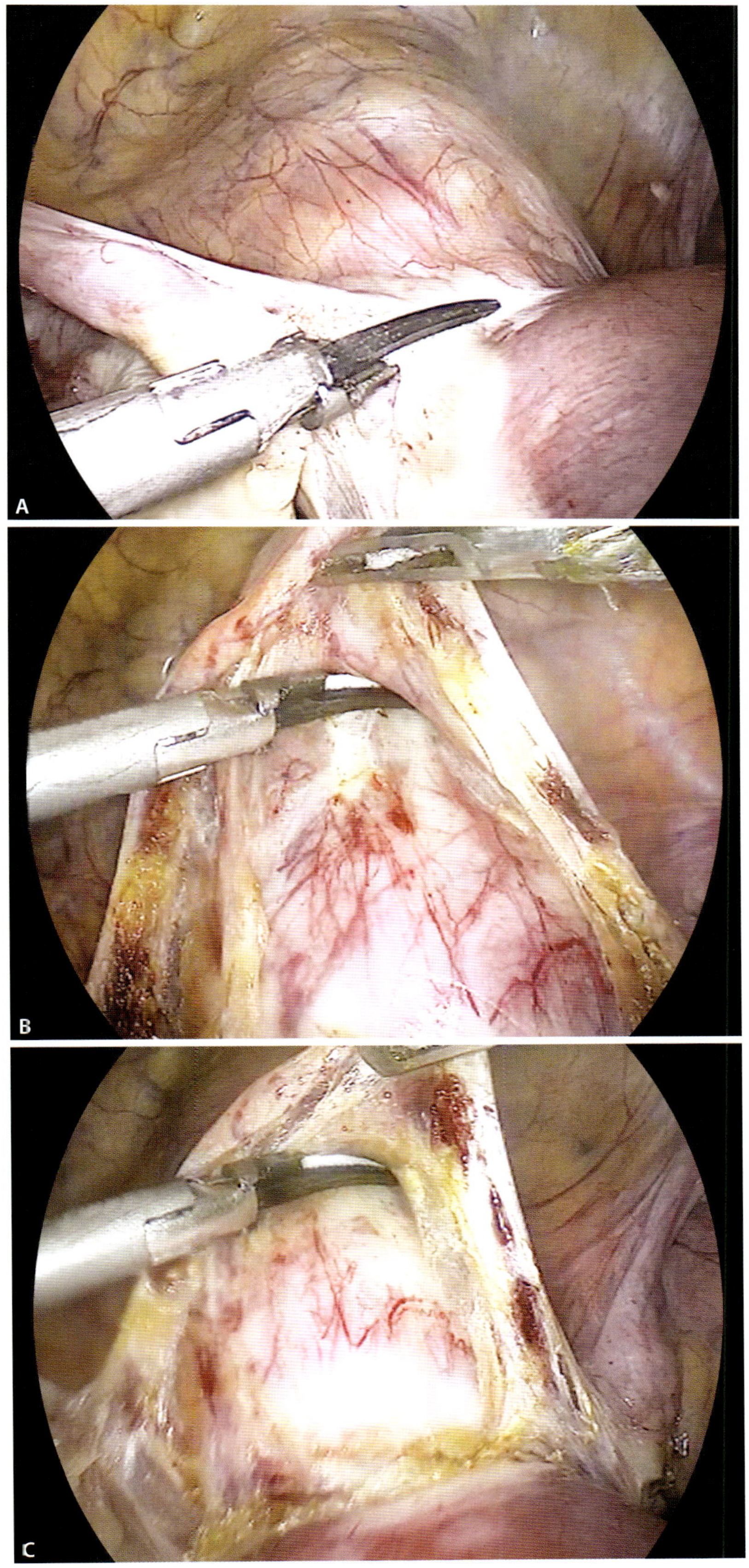

Figs. 7A to C: Bladder dissection.

UTERINE ARTERIES (FIGS. 8A TO G)

This is the most crucial step of this surgery. The broad ligament peritoneum on both sides anteriorly and posteriorly is opened downward mainly toward the cervix after skeletonization of the uterine arteries. With proper dissection, the uterine vessels are visualized at ureteric canal as it crosses above the ureter. Detailed knowledge of the anatomy and ureteric course is required to prevent injury. After the bladder is dissected from the anterior cervix, the uterine vessels are identified, desiccated with bipolar, as recommended by Canis et al.,[24] and cut with laparoscopic scissors to free uterus lateral border.

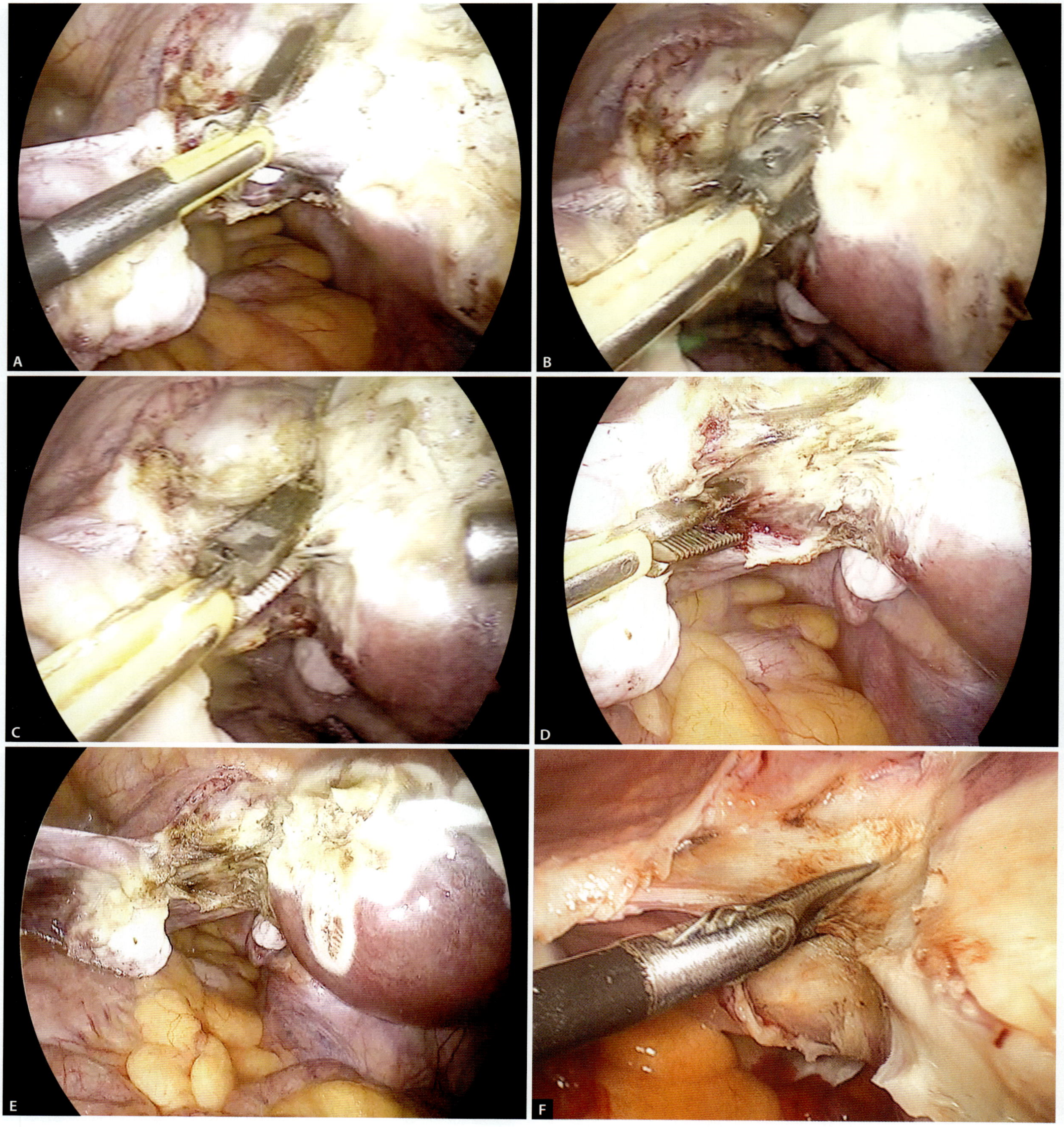

Figs. 8A to F

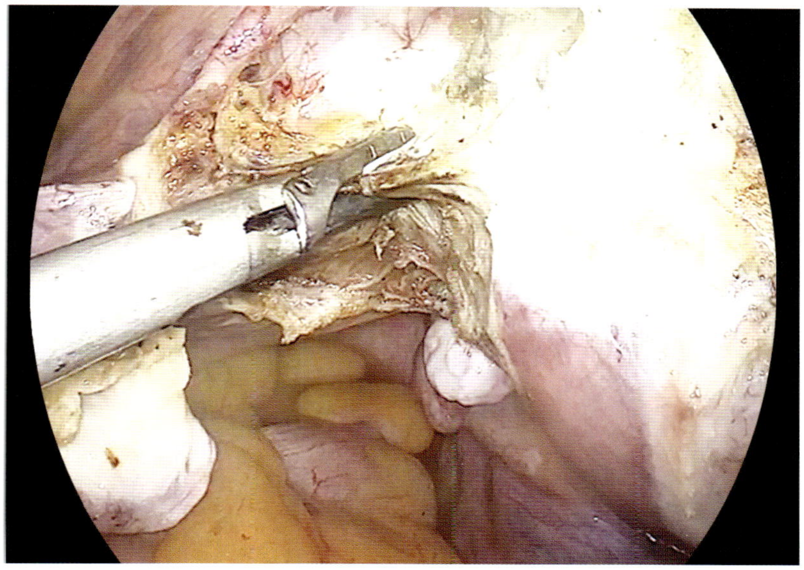

Fig. 8G

Figs. 8A to G: (A) Coagulation of uterine artery pedicle; (B) Wetting tissues with irrigator with bipolar; (C) Enhanced coagulation after wetting; (D) Repeated coagulation of uterine artery; (E) Appearance after repeated coagulation; (F) Cutting of uterine artery with scissors; (G) Cutting of uterine artery with harmonic illustrated.

EnSeal[25] or Harmonic[17] can also be used for combination coagulation and cutting. As the uterine vessels are grasped, ureteric position and safety should be judiciously checked Some gynecologists prefer suture ligation[26] of the vascular bundle. It is preferable to perform repeated coagulation of uterine artery pedicles with bipolar, so as to prevent bleeding at ligation of the vessels.

CARDINAL LIGAMENTS

At the level of the cardinal ligaments, the ureter and descending branches of uterine artery are near to each other and to cervix. Therefore, Mackenrodt's ligament dissection must be precisely done avoid in bleeding and ureteral injury. The shorter distance between the cervix and the ureter puts the ureter at greater risk of injury. By contralateral retraction of the uterus, the cardinal ligament is dissected to identify tissue planes, vessels, and the ureter. Once the ureter falls on lateral aspect, the cardinal ligament tissue closest to the cervix is coagulated and transected. The harmonic scalpel[17] or LigaSure[18] may be used as an alternative.

Colpotomy (Figs. 9A to F)

The rim of the vaginal tube used along with simple uterine manipulator can be easily visualized and palpated. A transverse incision with harmonic[17] or monopolar hook is made between the bladder and vagina and continued circumferentially and colpotomy is completed. The vagina is separated above uterosacral ligament insertion to the paracervical ring preserving the anatomical arch made by the uterosacral ligaments bilaterally and thereby preventing vaginal prolapse later. In most cases, extrafascial hysterectomy is performed, where the uterus is removed along with its fascial layer. In cases where bladder is adherent to cervix, the outer endopelvic fascia is dissected and finally, is left attached to the bladder (intrafascial), as shown in **Figure 10**. The uterus is removed by morcellation vaginally or laparoscopically. Vaginal morcellation is more advantageous than laparoscopic morcellation as it is simpler, easier, and faster and no sophisticated equipment or extra port is required. Postoperatively, there is reduced risk of injury to major organs and no risk of spillage.[27] The gas escapes rapidly outside peritoneal cavity at the time of morcellation. A mop placed inside a surgical glove is inserted in vagina to give temporary seal to maintain the pneumoperitoneum.

Adnexectomy (Figs. 11A to C)

When adnexectomy is required, the adnexa are freed first. The infundibulopelvic ligament (the suspensory ligament of the ovary) is identified and adequately exposed by applying traction from opposite side to the adnexa with a grasping forceps. Bipolar forceps compress and desiccate the vessels, which are then cut with scissors closer to desiccation ensuring that pedicle remains compressed. Harmonic[17] can serve both the purposes of coagulation and cutting. We recommend removal of the tubes and ovaries after hysterectomy to aid in obtaining adequate area for maneuvering the adnexa.

CLOSURE OF THE VAGINAL VAULT (FIGS. 12A TO M)

Vaginal vault is irrigated after specimen retrieval **(Fig. 12A)** and inspected for any active bleeding **(Figs. 12B and C)**. Bipolar should be judiciously used at the vaginal cuff to avoid tissue necrosis and subsequent wound breakdown, if the sutures are placed in nonviable tissue. To facilitate apical vaginal suspension, the vault angles are sutured to same sided uterosacral ligaments at the level of the ischial spine, incorporating the cardinal ligament at the corner and the lateral part of the anterior vaginal fornix. Adequate care has to be taken to incorporate full thickness of vagina and not to include the ureters. The vaginal cuff is closed laparoscopically using bidirectional quill barbed suture No. 1 continuous **(Figs. 12D to I)** or a Vicryl No. 1 continuous or intermittent suture.[27,28] Vault closure can also be done vaginally with Vicry 1-0 or 2-0 suture. Any existing cystocele or rectocele is repaired. Laparoscopic vault closure is always superior to vaginal vault closure as it is done under direct vision and there are lesser chances of vault complications postoperatively.[27] The pneumoperitoneum is restored again to inspect the abdomen and pelvis. Irrigation and suction are performed. The pedicles are examined. To ensure hemostasis, 300 mL Ringer's lactate is instilled into the pelvis which neutralizes pneumoperitoneal pressure and

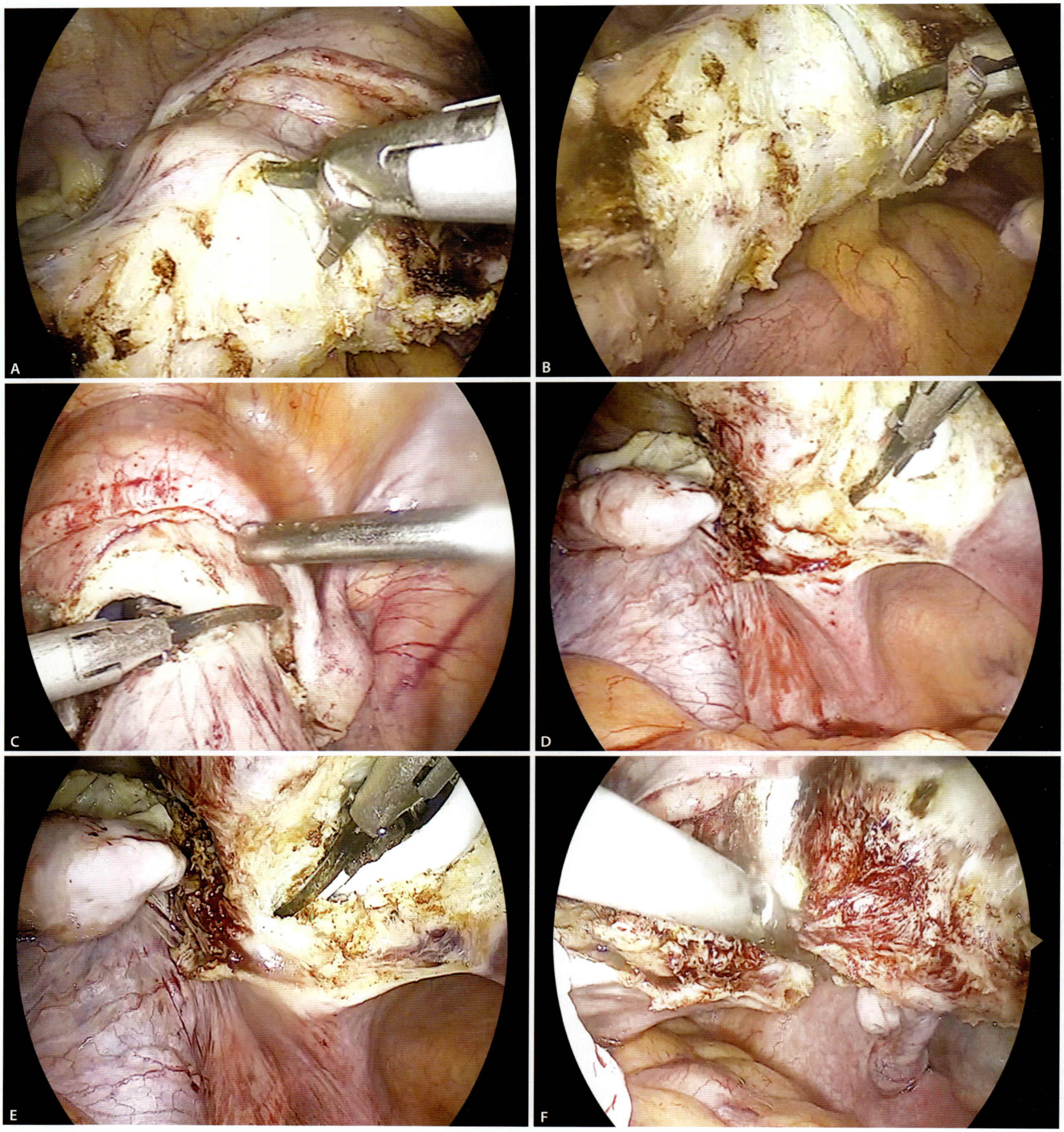

Figs. 9A to F: Colpotomy illustrated.

hence allows visualization of minute bleeders. The vault is checked by inserting laparoscope underwater to visualize for bleeding in reverse Trendelenburg position.[29] The trickle of blood which is observed as "red smoke" sign helps to identify bleeding. At last step, the fluid should be clear in the pelvis and visualizing ureters should confirm peristalsis and anatomic integrity. At the end of the procedure, bladder integrity is observed by filling the bladder with 100–150 mL of blue solution (5–10 mL methylene blue in 100 mL normal saline)

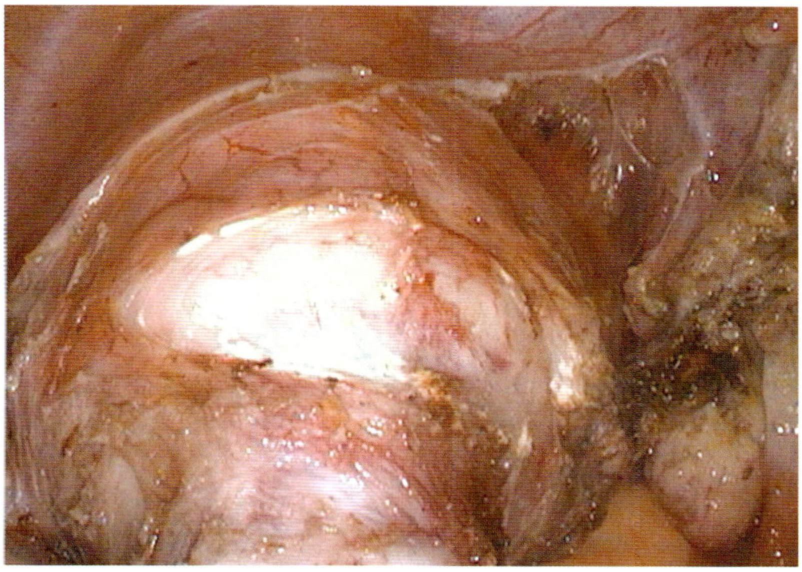

Fig. 10: Intrafascial hysterectomy—pubocervical fascia dissection.

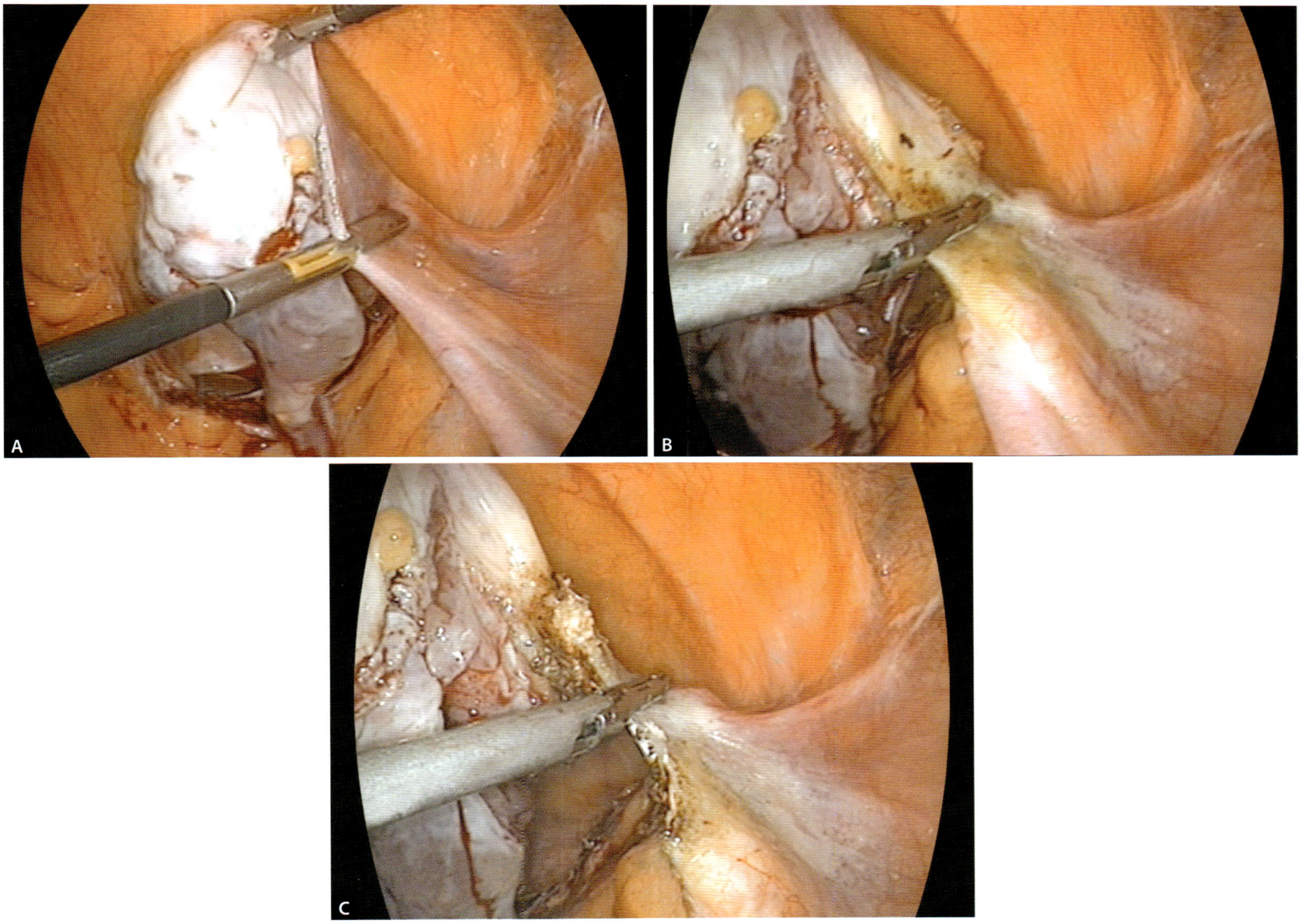

Figs. 11A to C: (A) Coagulation of IP ligament with bipolar; (B) Cutting of IP ligament with harmonic; (C) Demonstration of salpingo-oophorectomy.

and inspecting for leakage laparoscopically. To reduce postoperative pain, 20 mL of 0.25% bupivacaine is infiltrated intraperitoneally over the vaginal vault and pelvic sidewalls up to the paracolic gutters and subdiaphragmatically using the endoscopic applicator.[30] After satisfactory observation, pneumoperitoneum is released, trocars are removed. For preventing incisional hernia, omental, and bowel strangulation after trocar removal of more than 5-mm size, the fascial defect has to be repaired using delayed absorbable sutures. Instillation of 20 mL of 0.25% bupivacaine into laparoscopic port sites is done before closure.[31] Subsequently, the port sites are closed with Monocryl 3-0 subcuticular sutures.

POSTOPERATIVE CARE

Close monitoring of vitals along with strict vigil on input and urine output is recommended in the immediate postoperative period. Adequate analgesia should be administered. Oral antibiotics are advised in most cases; however, intravenous antibiotic can be

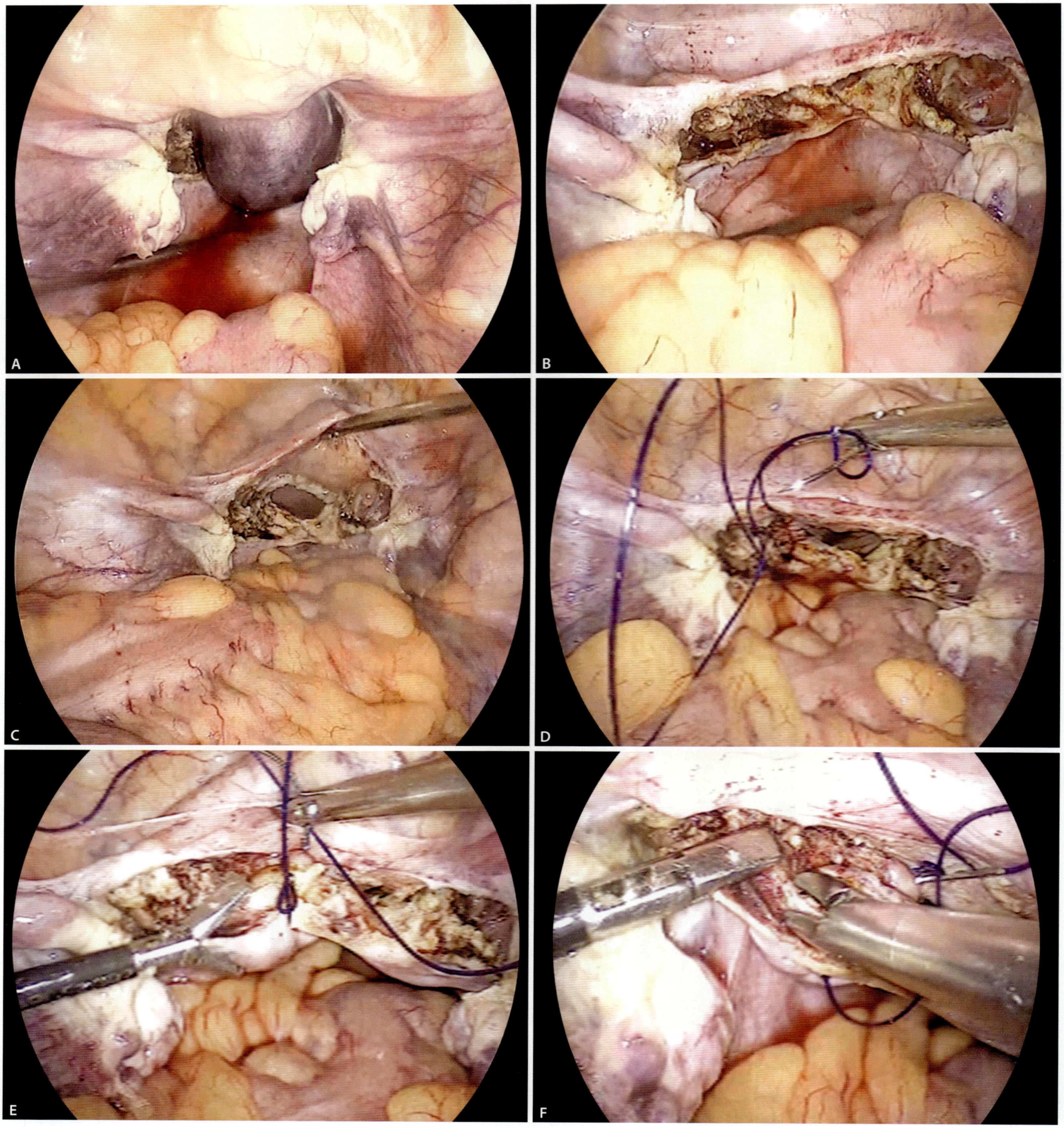

Figs. 12A to F

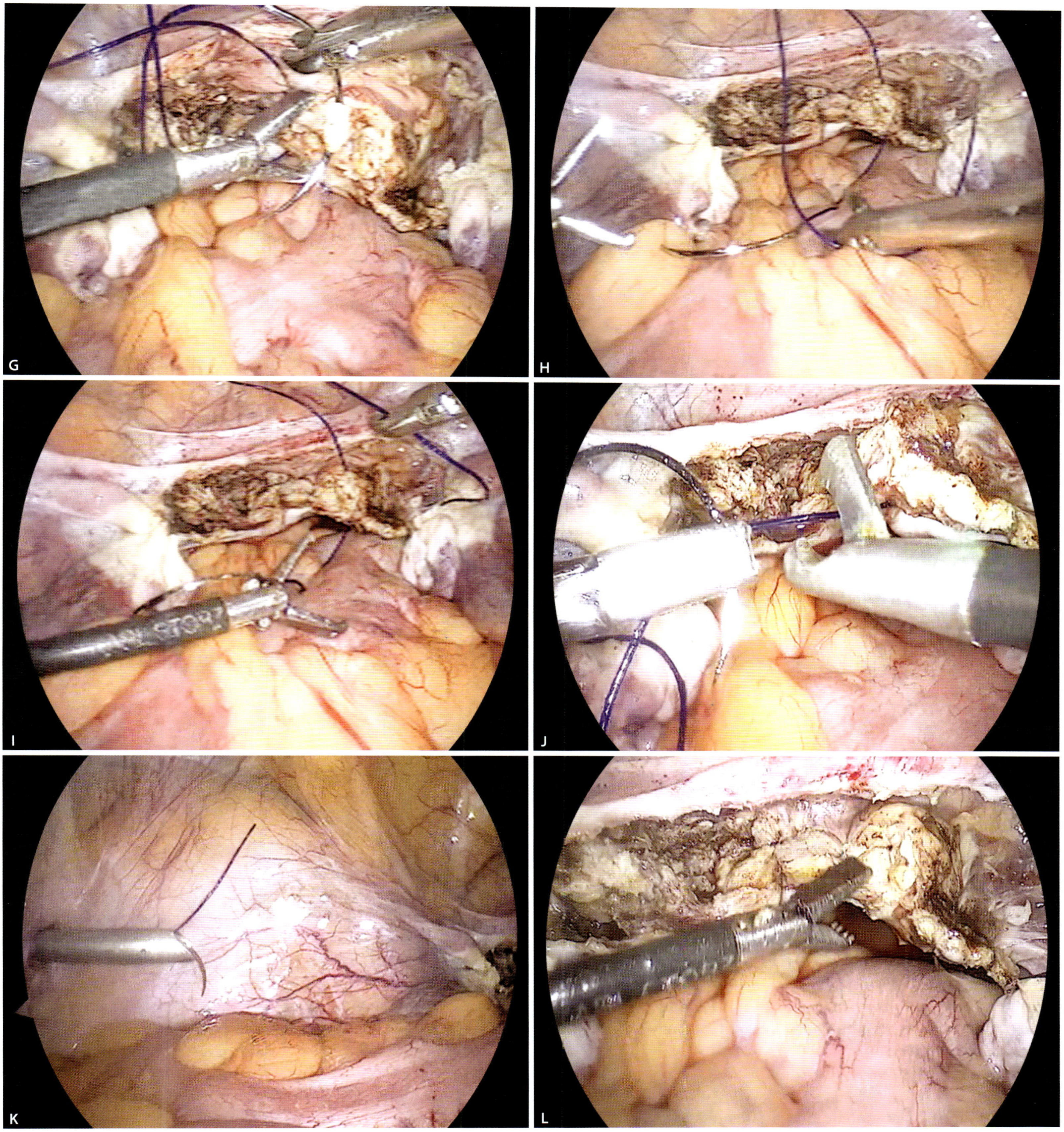

Figs. 12G to L

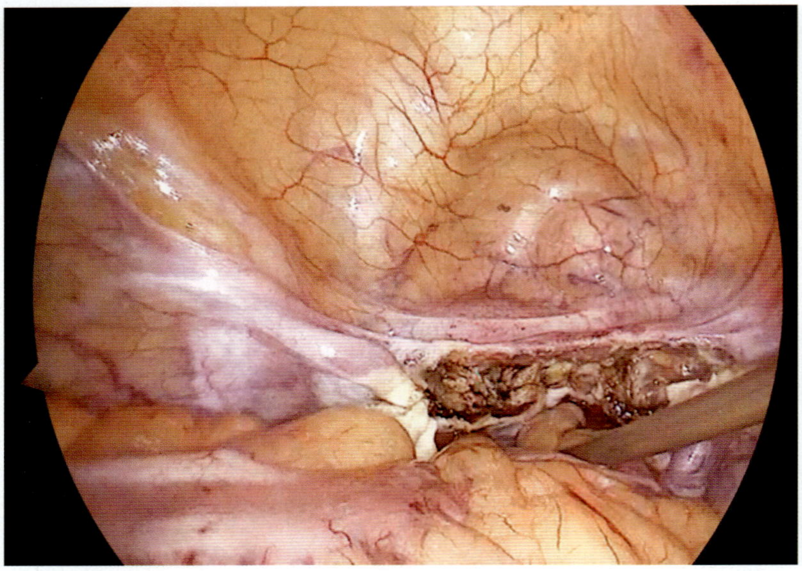

Fig. 12M

Figs. 12A to M: (A) Specimen retrieval; (B) Laparoscopic appearance of vault; (C) Laparoscopic appearance of vault after suction; (D to I) Vault suturing demonstrated; (J) Suture being cut; (K) Suture retrieval demonstrated; (L to M) Appearance of vault after suturing.

administered, if necessary. Graded compression stockings and low molecular weight heparin are administered in patients prone to deep vein thrombosis (DVT). Patients are initially allowed clear liquids, once bowel sounds resume. If tolerated, the diet is shifted to "soft diet" for 2–3 days, which is then followed by regular diet with ample intake of fluids. Medications taken preoperatively (stopped temporarily) are usually resumed once patient crosses the immediate postoperative period. Although minimally invasive, hysterectomy is considered a major surgery and patients are observed for at least 24 hours postoperatively. Once patient voids without discomfort, tolerates a regular diet, and ambulates wall, she can be discharged.

COMPLICATIONS

While laparoscopic surgery has become a boon in the abdominal and pelvic surgeries, it brings with it all risks and complications also. This includes anesthesia-related complications as well as surgery-related complications. The surgery related-complications include:

- Febrile morbidity (0.6%)
- Hemorrhage (0.1%)
- Urinary tract injuries (2.7%)—bladder—1.5%, Ureter—1.2%
- Bowel injuries (0.4%)
- Vascular injuries (1.2%)
- Conversion to laparotomy (0.3%)
- Deep venous thrombosis and related complications
- Pulmonary complications
- Incisional hernia (0.02%)
- Mortality.

The incidence of complications associated with laparoscopic surgeries varies considerably between reports, depending on the expertise of doctor and the complexity of surgery involved. Postoperative recovery after laparoscopic surgery should provide progressive improvement and patient should feel better each day **(Box 1)**. Delay in improvement or worsening postoperative status should alert the gynecologist. Since unrecognized injury can occur, vigilant attention and early diagnosis of complications are an absolute requirement for the laparoscopic surgeon.

Box 1: Complications in total laparoscopic hysterectomy.

- Hemorrhage (0.1%)
- Febrile morbidity (0.6%)
- Bladder and ureteric injury (2.7%)
- Bowel injuries (0.4%)
- Vascular injuries (1.2%)
- Conversion of surgery to laparotomy (0.3%)

Vascular injuries are generally life-threatening event and are auspicious within first 24 hours of procedure. They are the most common causes of trocar injuries related mortality reported. Ureteric injury manifests usually within the first 48–72 hours postoperatively, but may present later with fever, flank pain, peritonitis, leukocytosis, hematuria, and abdominal distention. Bowel injuries are inseparable part of laparoscopic procedure. Symptoms may appear days to weeks after the initial surgery, leading to delayed complications. The patient may present with symptoms such as malaise, nausea fever, abdominal tenderness, and leukocytosis. In suspicious cases, routine blood tests, X-rays, ultrasonography (USG) abdomen, as well as CT imaging of pelvis, and abdomen may be needed. To evaluate for ureteral injury, IV contrast should be given. To evaluate for intestinal injury, erect X-ray abdomen, oral and rectal contrast should be given. When there is doubt, it is better not to hesitate and perform a second-look laparoscopy than overlooking a possible complication.

ADVANTAGES

The advantages of laparoscopic hysterectomy are well-documented—fewer postoperative infections and pain, shorter hospitalization, faster recovery, and rapid normalization of routine day-to-day activities. A Cochrane meta-analysis comparing TLH with total abdominal hysterectomy (TAH) showed decreased trend in morbidity—specifically decreased perioperative complications, lesser blood loss, and shorter duration of hospital stay.[27,32] Laparoscopy enables the surgeon to have enhanced visualization, minimizes blood loss, and magnifies the operative field.

LIMITATIONS

The disadvantages of laparoscopy mentioned include more operative time, fixed visual angles, conversion of a 3D to 2D image, steep and long learning curve, and associated increased costs. Multiple studies have proved that operative time is similar and in many times reduced, especially for patients with a high body mass index. With the advent of 3D-laparoscopy, some of the above problems can be overcome. *New England Journal of Medicine*[33] states that laparoscopic hysterectomy is less expensive than other approaches, if reusable instruments are used. Once the surgical technique is mastered, many concomitant procedures can be performed, which shows the efficacy of the minimally invasive approach for different surgical operations in gynecology, without any need for conversion to laparotomy or a second surgery.[27]

Vaginal hysterectomy is a signature of every trained gynecologist. However, whenever the vaginal route is contraindicated, laparoscopy should be the route of choice to avoid the disadvantages of a laparotomy due to the more favorable adverse effect profile with no change in the technique of operative reconstructive surgery. Detailed anatomical knowledge of pelvic floor is mandatory before performing TLH. Multiple RCTs have shown that with increasing experience, the rate of complications and operating time can be minimized. Hence, the younger generation of gynecologists should practice the laparoscopic approach to hysterectomy.

REFERENCES

1. ACOG Committee Opinion No. 444. Choosing the route of hysterectomy for benign disease. Obstet Gynecol. 2009;114:1156-8.
2. Semm K. Operationslehref¨urendoskopische Abdominalchirugie–operative Pelviskopie. Stuttgart, Germany: Schattauer; 1984.
3. Semm K, Friedrich ER. Operative Manual for Endoscopic Abdominal Surgery. Chicago: Year Book Medical Publishers; 1987.
4. Reich H. New techniques in advanced laparoscopic surgery. Clin Obstet Gynecol. 1989;3:655-81.
5. Nezhat C, Nezhat F, Gordon S, et al. Laparoscopic versus abdominal hysterectomy. J Reprod Med. 1992;37:247.
6. Jacoby VL, Autry A, Jacobson G, et al. Nationwide use of laparoscopic hysterectomy compared with abdominal and vaginal approaches. Obstet Gynecol. 2009;114:1041-8.
7. Donnez J, Nisolle M, Squifflet J, et al. Laparoscopy-assisted vaginal hysterectomy and laparoscopic hysterectomy in benign diseases. In: Donnez J, Nisolle M (Eds). An Atlas of Operative Laparoscopy and Hysteroscopy. Carnforth, UK: Parthenon Publishing; 2001. pp. 251-60.
8. Bachmann GA. Hysterectomy: a critical review. J Reprod Med. 1990;35: 839-62.
9. Dicker RC, Scally MJ, Greenspan JR, et al. Hysterectomy among women of reproductive age. JAMA. 1982;248:323-7.
10. White SC, Wartel LJ, Wade ME. Comparison of abdominal and vaginal hysterectomy: a review of 600 operations. Obstet Gynecol.1971;37:530-7.
11. Lee NC, Dicker RC, Rubin GL, et al. Confirmation of the preoperative diagnoses for hysterectomy. Am J Obstet Gynecol. 1984;150:283-7.
12. Mage G, Wattiez A, Chapron C, et al. Hystérectomie per-coelioscopique: resultatsd'uneserie de 44 cas. J Gynecol Obstet Biol Reprod (Paris). 1992;21:436-44.
13. Querleu D, Leblanc E, Castelain G. Laparoscopic pelvic lymphadenectomy in the staging of early carcinoma of the cervix. Am J Obstet Gynecol. 1991;164:579-81.
14. Reich H, McGlynn F, Wickie W. Laparoscopic management of stage 1 ovarian cancer: A case report. J Reprod Med. 1990;35:601-4.
15. Donnez J, Nisolle M, Anaf V. Place de l'endoscopiedans le cancer de l'endomètre. In: Dubuisson JB, Chapron CH, Bouquet de Jolinière J (Eds). Coelioscopieet Cancerologieen Gynecologie. Paris: Arnette; 1993. pp. 77-82.
16. Lamvu G, Zolncun D, Boggess J, et al. Obesity: physiologic changes and challenges during laparoscopy. Am J Obstetr gynecol. 2004;191(2):669-74.
17. Winter ML, Mendelsohn SA. Total laparoscopic hysterectomy using the harmonic scalpel. JSLS. 1999;3(3):185-6.
18. Greenberg JA. LigaSure Advance™ instrument. Rev Obstetr Gynecol. 2009;2(2):132-3.
19. Barnett JC, Hurd WW, Rogers RM, et al. Laparoscopic positioning and nerve injuries. J Minim Invasive Gynecol. 2007;14(5):664-72.
20. Reich H, Levie M, McGlynn F, et al. Establishment of pneumoperitoneum through the left ninth intercostal space. Gynaecol Endosc. 1995;4:141-3.
21. Hasson HM. Open laparoscopy: a report of 150 cases. J Reprod Med. 1974;12:234-8.
22. Ghomi A, Makhlouf F, Kasturi S, et al. Intramyometrial injection of vasopressin in laparoscopic supracervical hysterectomy. J Minim Invasive Gynecol. 2008;15(2):197-201.
23. Kobayashi E, Iwamiya T, Isobe M, et al. A novel technique for the management of the vesicouterine ligament during radical hysterectomy. Gynecol Oncol. 2009;115(1):56-9.
24. Canis M, Mage G, Wattiez A, et al. Vaginally assisted laparoscopic radical hysterectomy. J Gynecol Surg. 1992;8:103-5.
25. Rothmund R, Kraemer B, Brucker S, et al. Laparoscopic supracervical hysterectomy using EnSeal vs standard bipolar coagulation technique: randomized controlled trial. J Minim Invasive Gynecol. 2013;20(5):661-6.
26. Reich H. New laparoscopic techniques. In: Sutton C, Diamond M (Eds). Endoscopic Surgery for Gynaecologists. London, UK: WB Saunders; 1993. pp. 28-39.
27. Bettaiah R, Reddy CA. Laparoscopic hysterectomies: our 10 Years experience in a single laparoscopic center. J Obstetr Gynecol India. 2016;66(4):274-81.
28. Medina BC, Giraldo CH, Riaño G, et al. Barbed suture for vaginal cuff closure in laparoscopic hysterectomy. JSLS. 2014;18(1):83-8.
29. Nezhat C, Nezhat F, Burrell M. Laparoscopically assisted hysterectomy for the management of a borderline ovarian tumor: a case report. J Laparoendosc Surg. 1992;2:167-9.
30. Rivard C, Vogel RI, Teoh D. Effect of intraperitoneal bupivacaine on postoperative pain in the gynecologic oncology patient. J Minim Invasive Gynecol. 2015;22(7):1260-5.
31. Dath D, Park AE. Randomized, controlled trial of bupivacaine injection to decrease pain after laparoscopic cholecystectomy. Can J Surg. 1999; 42(4):284-8.
32. Aarts JW, Nieboer TE, Johnson N, et al. Surgical approach to hysterectomy for benign gynaecological disease. The Cochrane Library. 2015;(8): CD003677.
33. J. Hart J, Chatzipapas IK, Magos A. The cost of a hysterectomy in a UK hospital. J Obstetr Gynaecol. 1999;19(5):522-5.

Accompanying Video: Total laparoscopic hysterectomy.

CHAPTER

18

Vesicovaginal Fistula

B Ramesh, Jay Mehta, Aditi Rai, Mehul V Sukhadiya

INTRODUCTION

Vesicovaginal fistula (VVF) can be repaired either vaginally or abdominally nowadays. Laparoscopic repair is slowly replacing the abdominal method because of its high success rates and minimally invasive in nature.

Generally, infratrigonal fistulas are repaired vaginally because the approach is easier vaginally.

Supratrigonal fistulas and complicated fistulas are repaired abdominally or laparoscopically.

VAGINAL REPAIR (FIGS. 1 TO 9)

Commonly done vaginal method is Latzko method or layer method.

Principles of Repair

- Repair should be done on noninfected and noninflamed tissues
- Tissues are approximated without tension
- Microsurgical principles are applied.

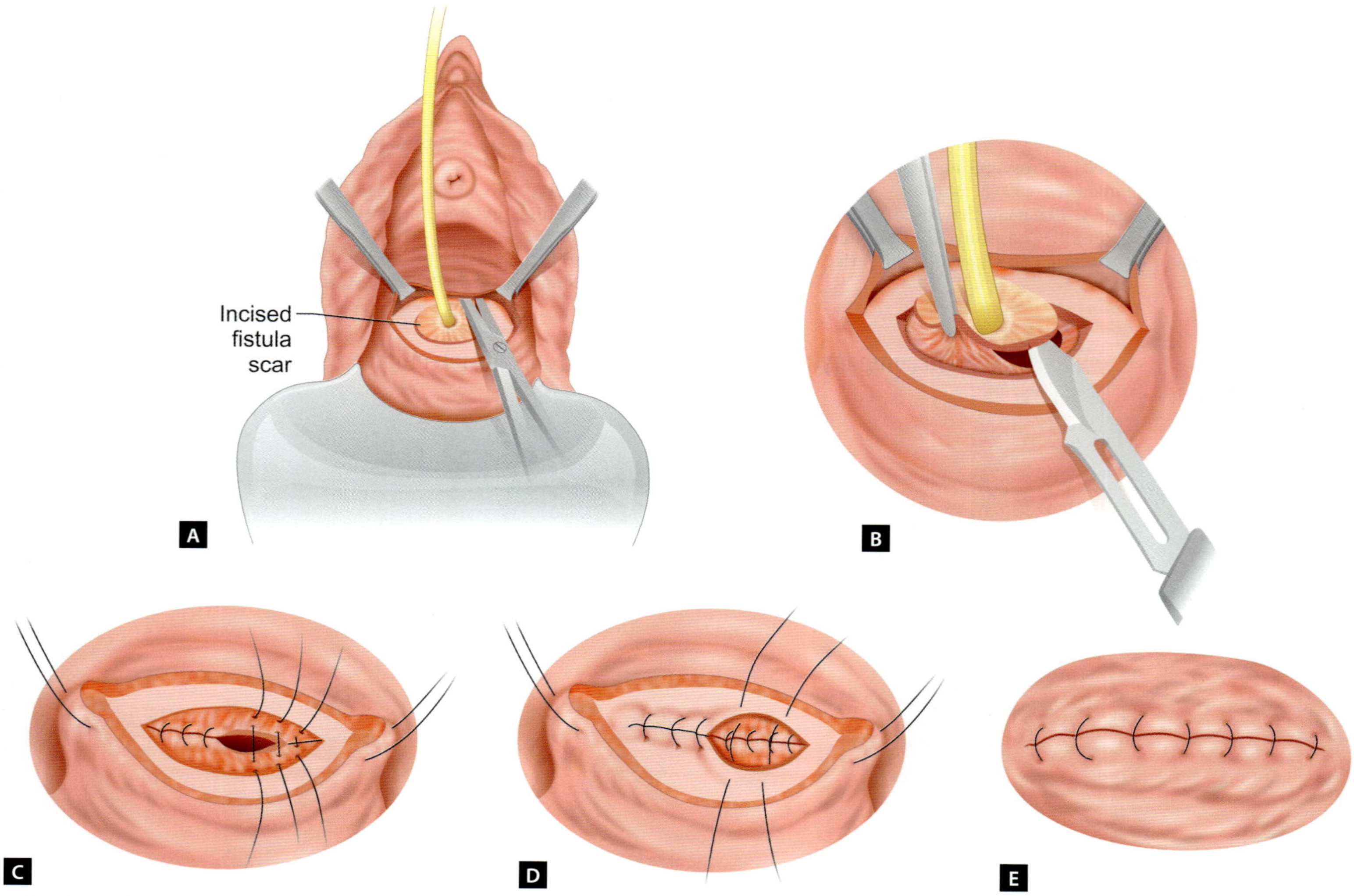

Figs. 1A to E: Traditional vesicovaginal fistula repair. (A) Initial incision of a circumferential collar around the fistulous opening. The vaginal epithelium is sharply dissected radially from the collar; (B) The fistula is excised sharply, making sure that the healthy tissue is left to be reapproximated. Excessive trimming, increasing the loss of tissue, should be avoided; (C) Interrupted fine, delayed absorbable suture on a small tapered needle is used, extramucosally if possible, to close the first layer. Stitches are placed approximately 0.5 cm apart with sufficient purchase of tissue to securely close the defect; (D) The second layer imbricates over the first with suture being placed in a staggered fashion into the bladder muscularis so as not to overlap the sutures of these layers; (E) The vaginal epithelium is closed with interrupted delayed absorbable suture after ensuring proper hemostasis in the vesicovaginal space.

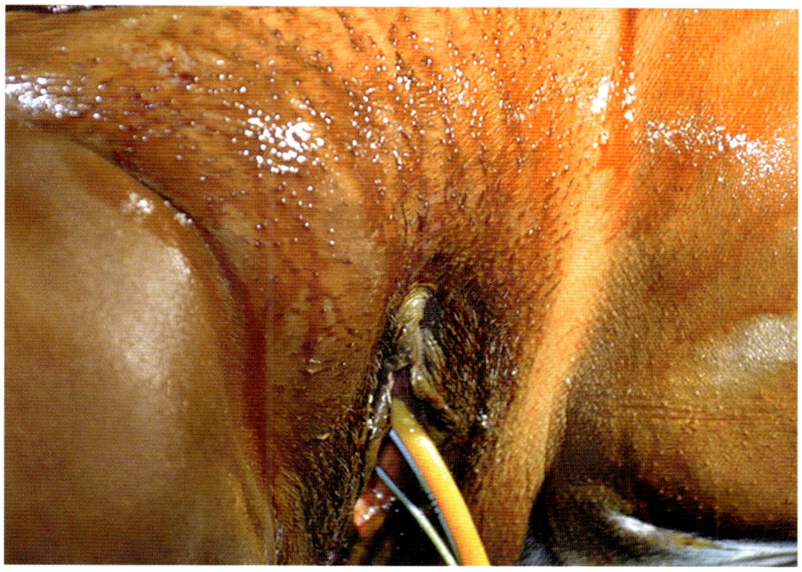

Fig. 2: Fistula with ureteric stents inserted.

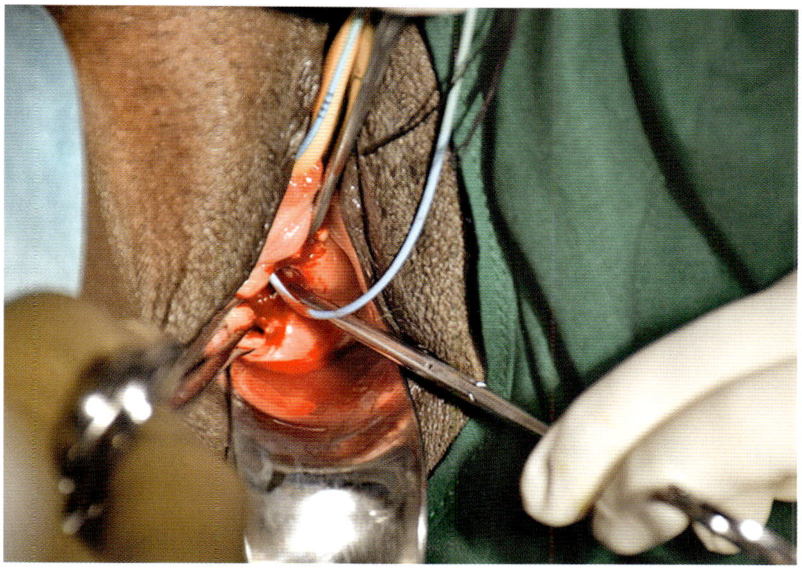

Fig. 4: Vagina incised around the fistula.

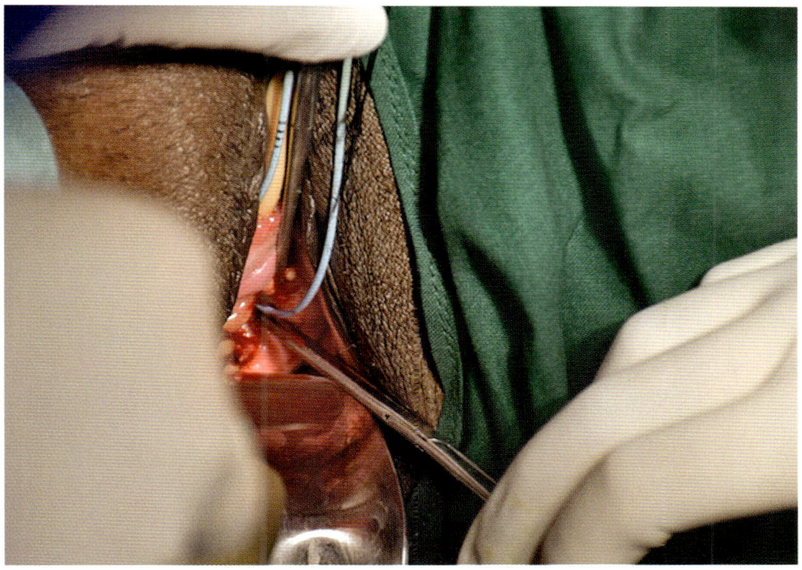

Fig. 3: Fistula with stent inserted into the fistula through cystoscopy for identification.

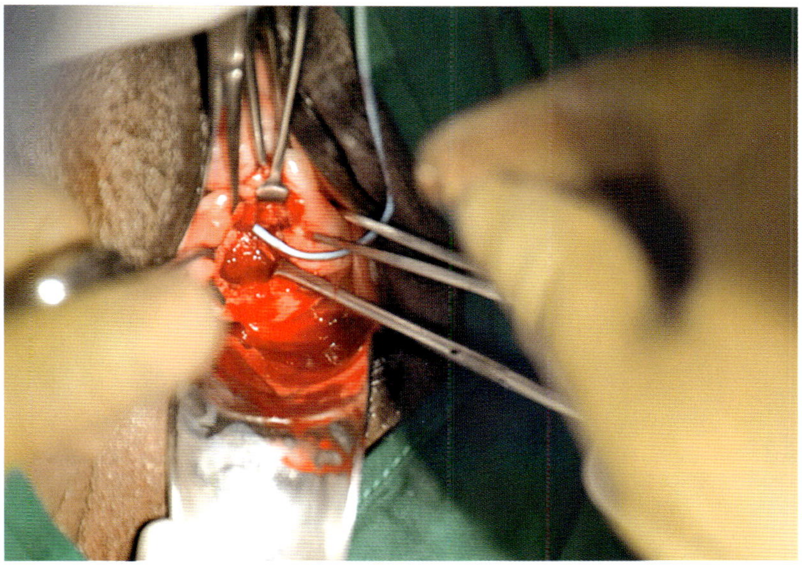

Fig. 5: Vaginal epithelium excised and fistula exposed further.

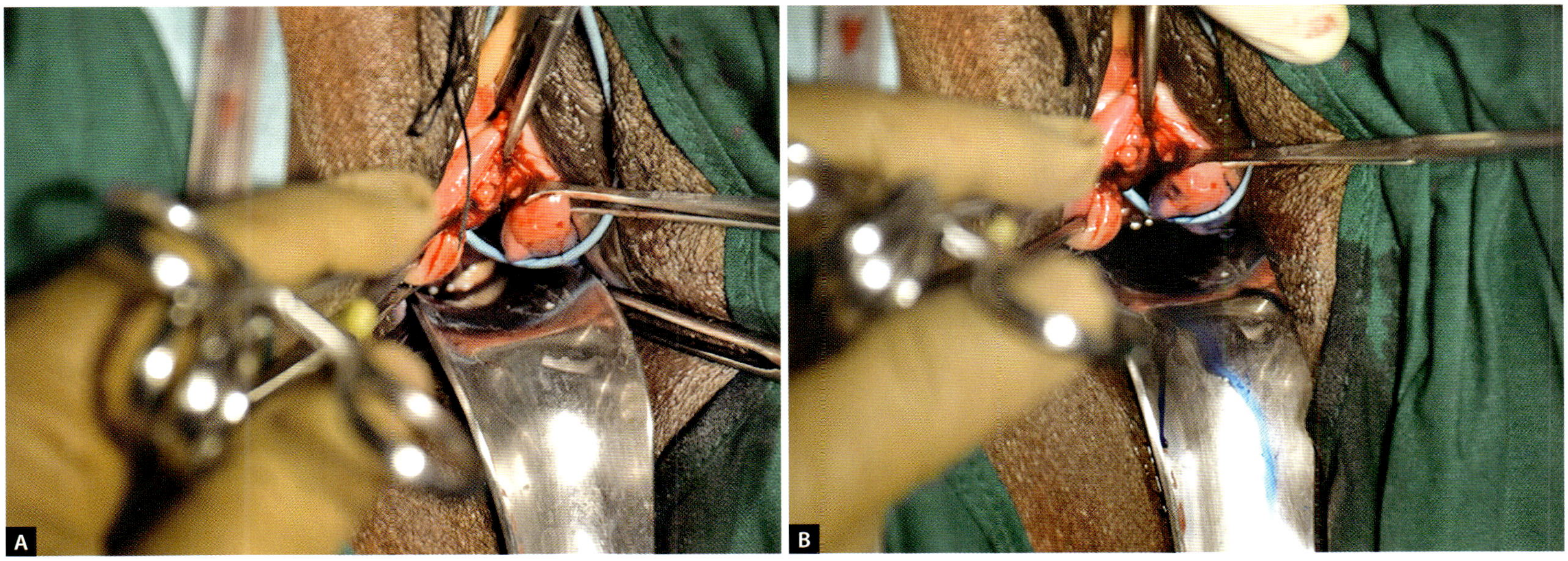

Figs. 6A and B

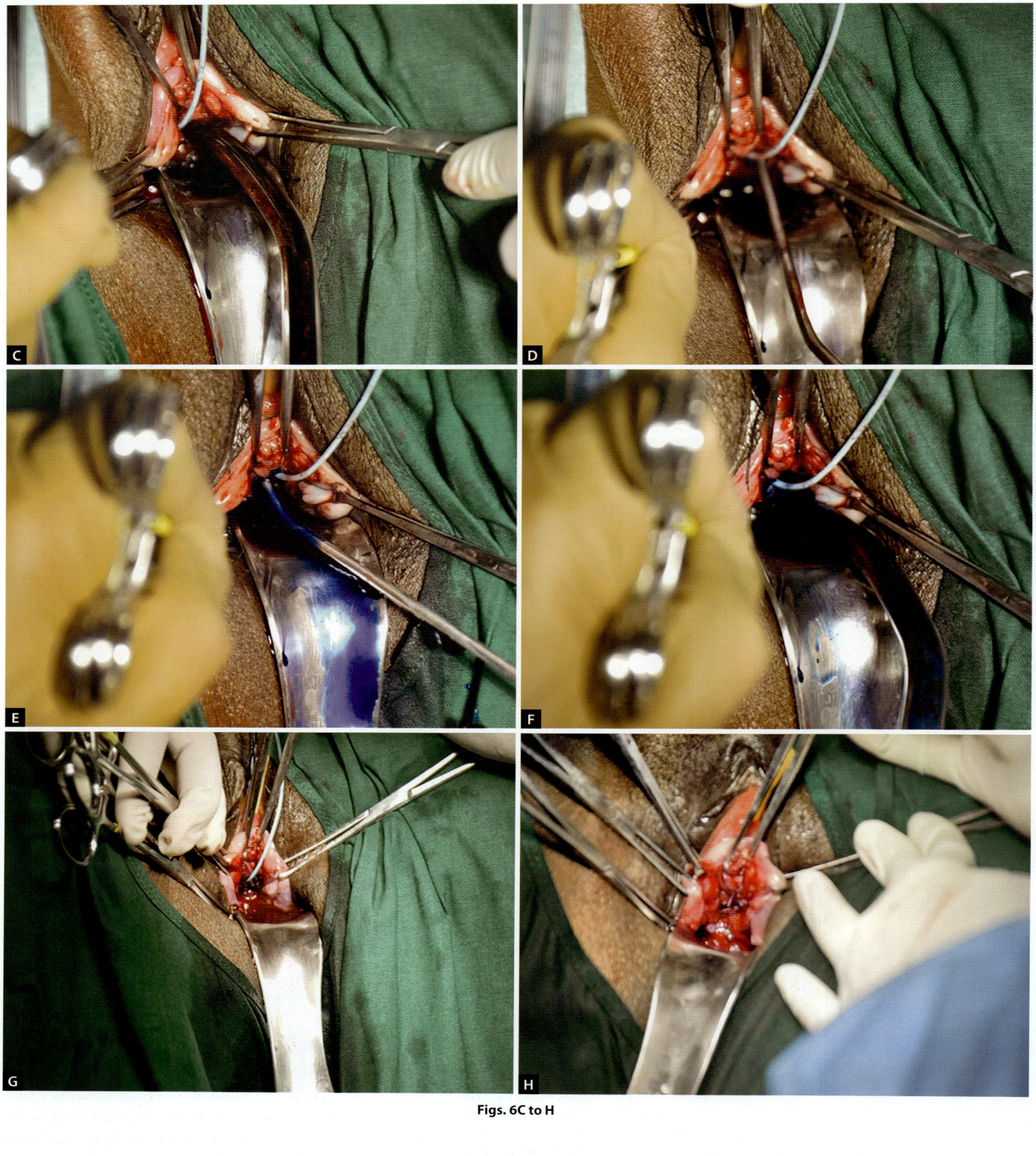

Figs. 6C to H

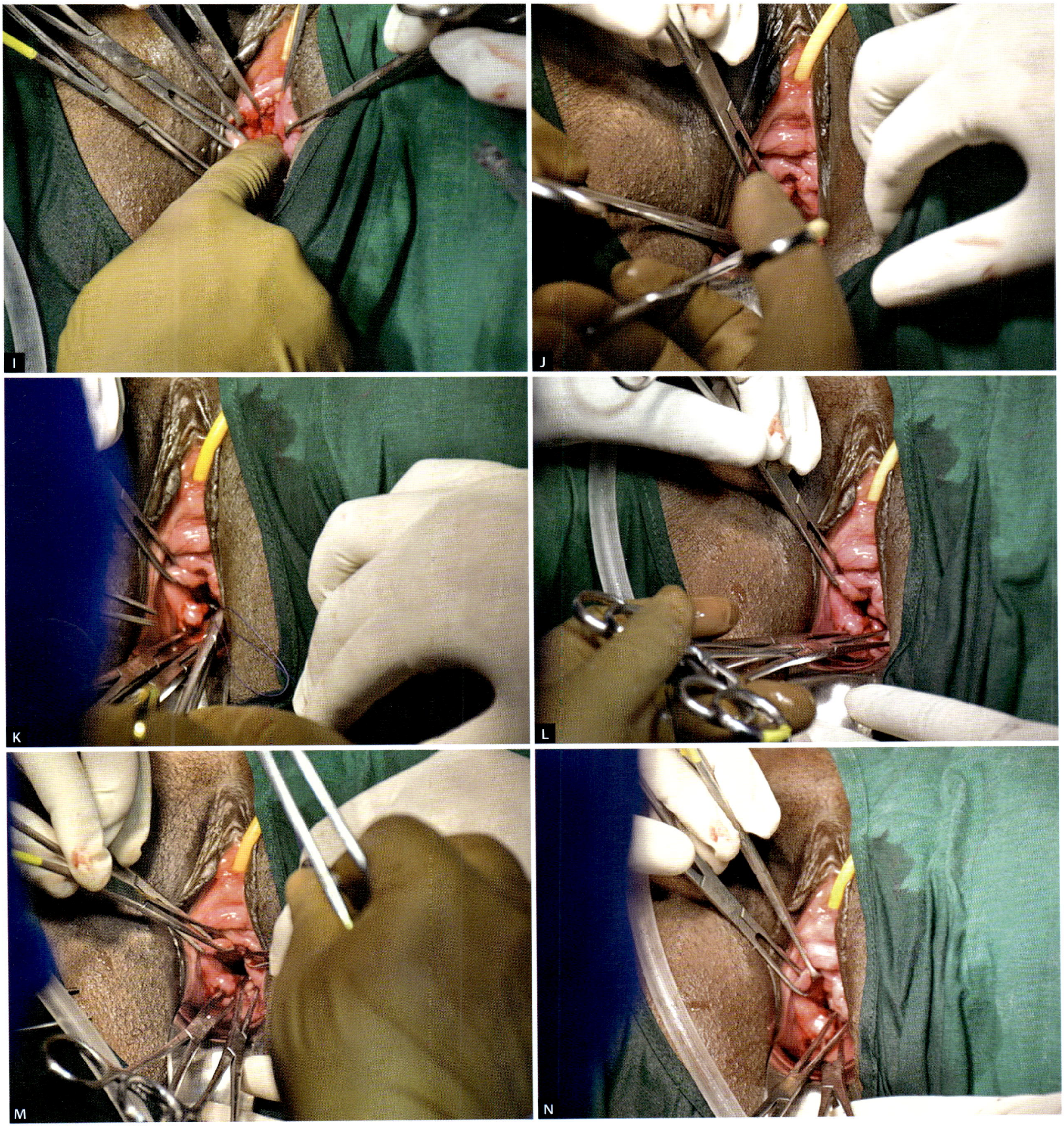

Figs. 6I to N

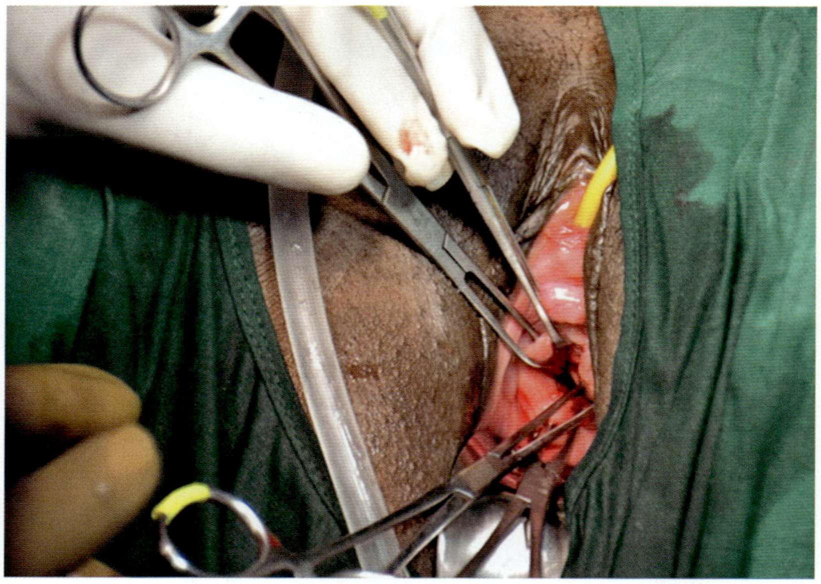

Fig. 6O

Figs. 6A to O: Bladder mucosa identified.

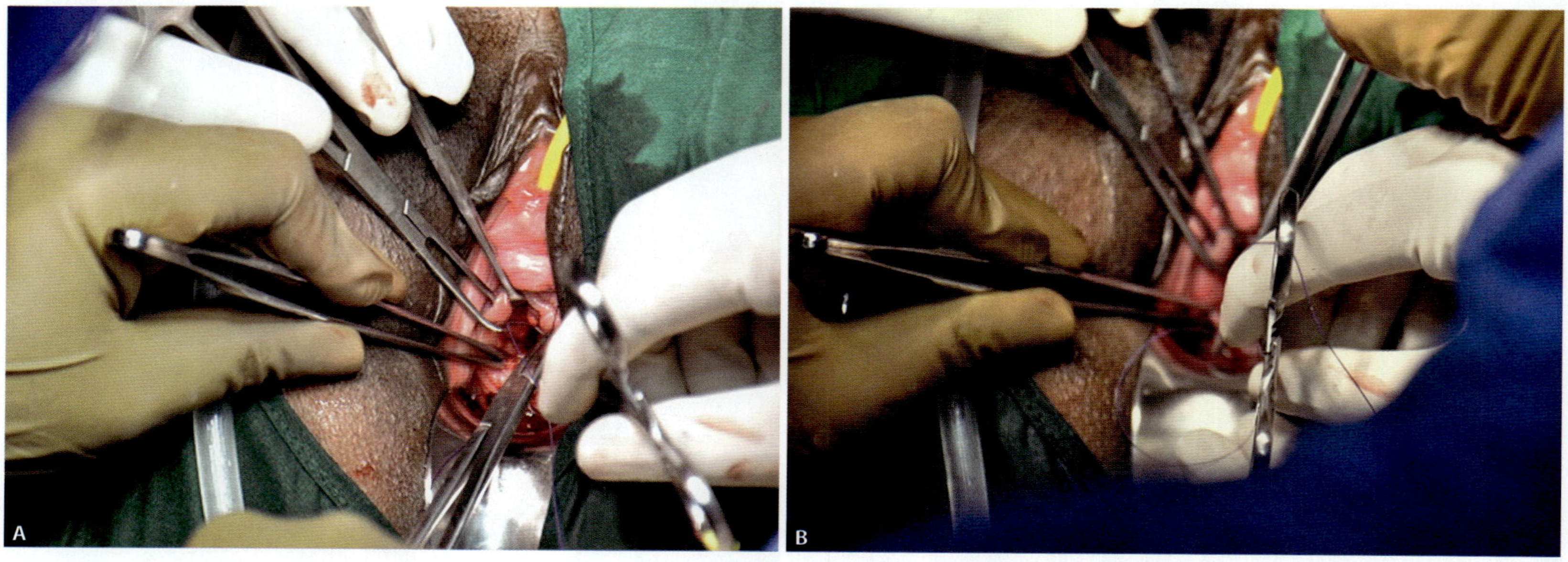

Figs. 7A and B: Using 3-0 Vicryl bladder mucosa sutured.

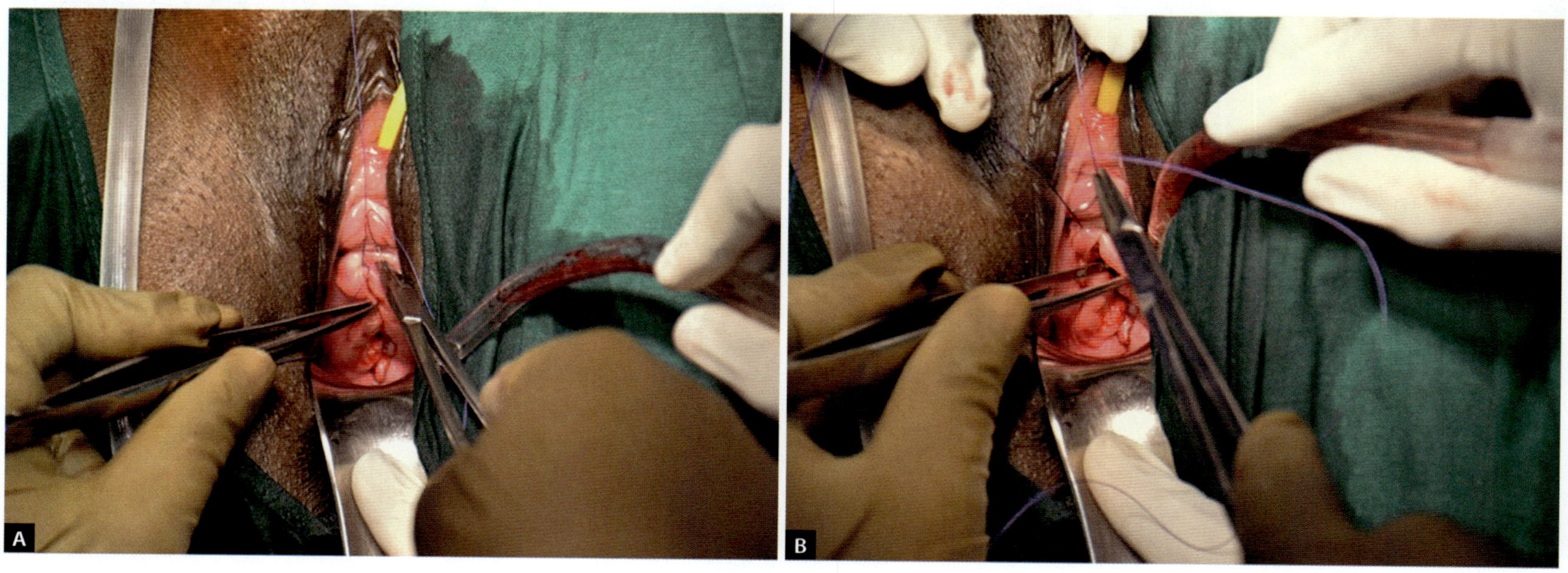

Figs. 8A and B

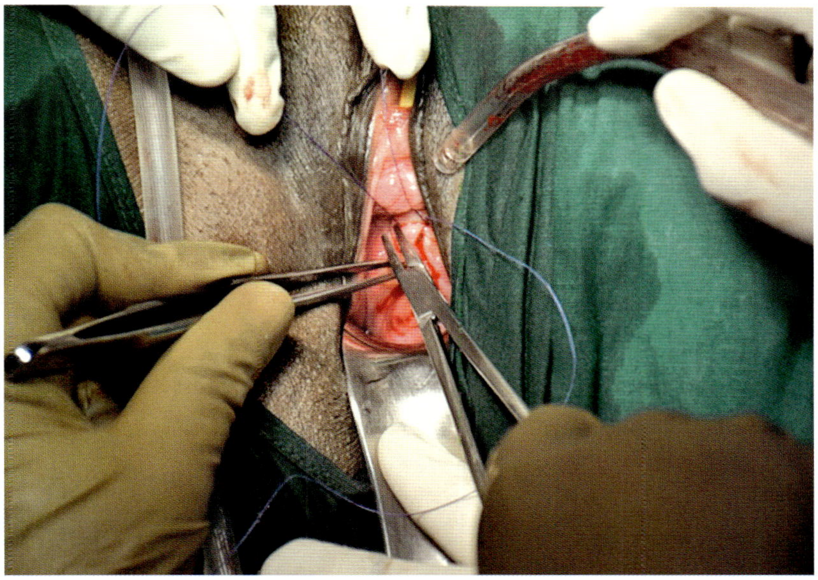

Fig. 8C

Figs. 8A to C: Second layer of seromuscular closed with 3-0 continuous suture.

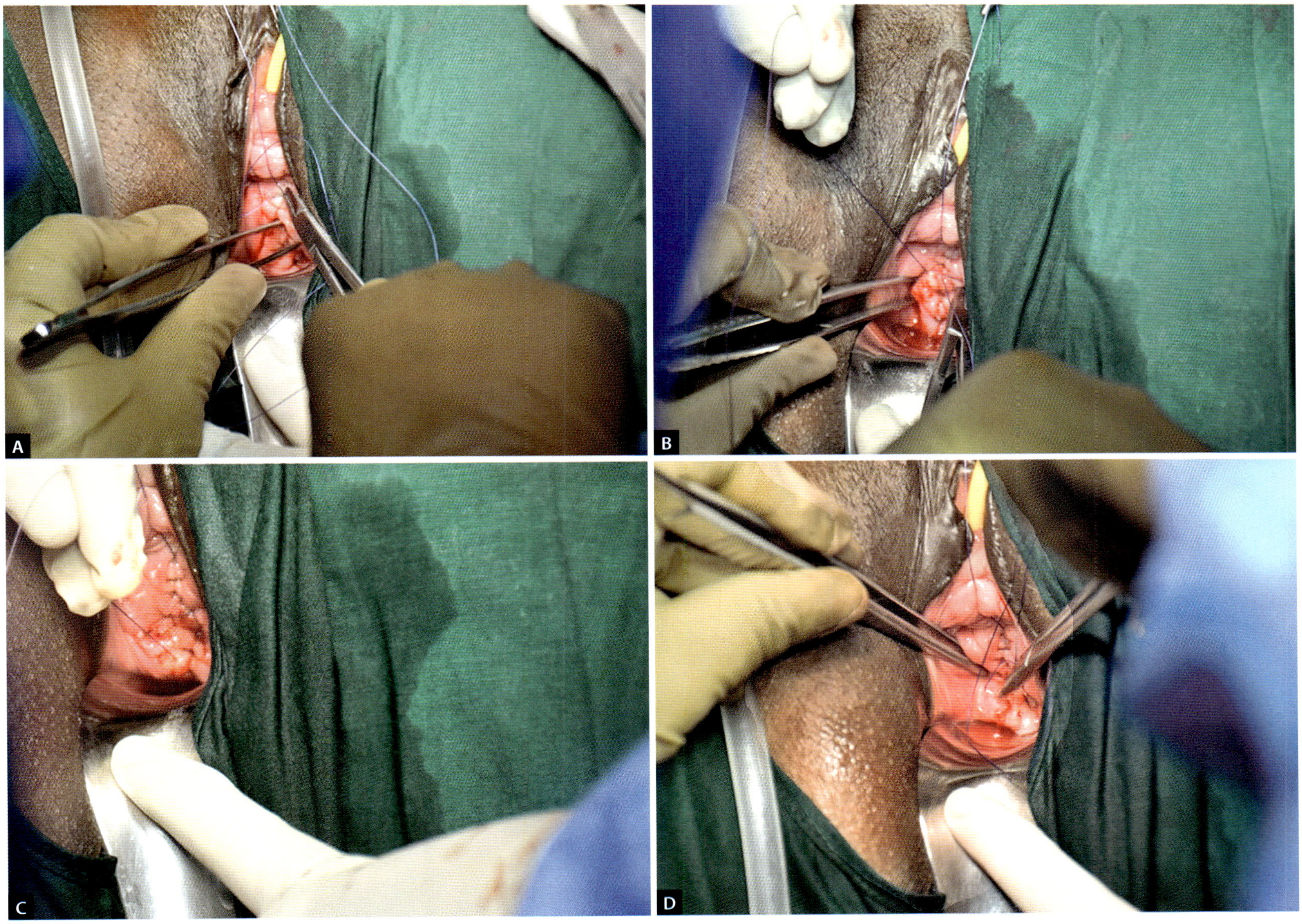

Figs. 9A to D

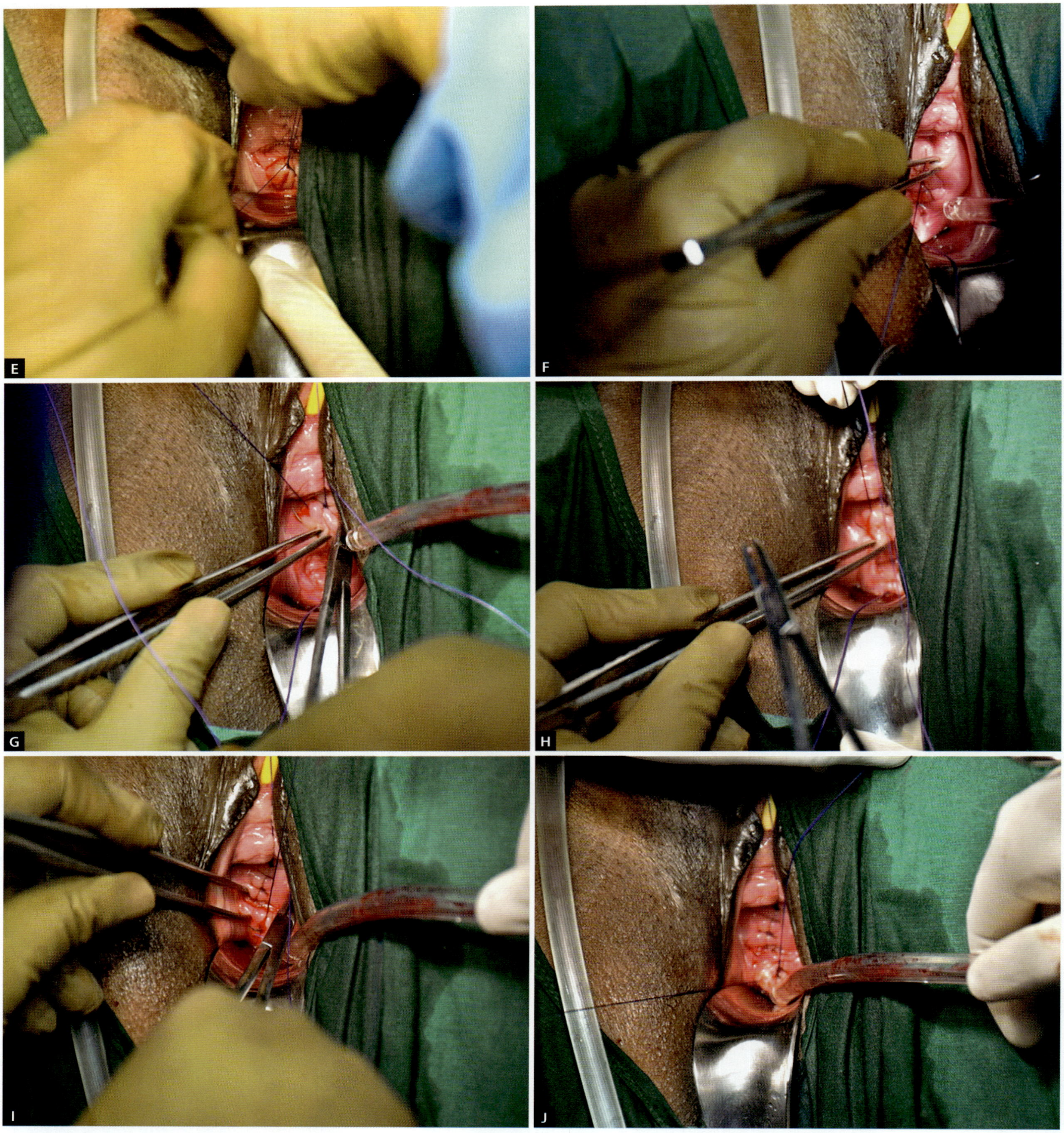

Figs. 9E to J

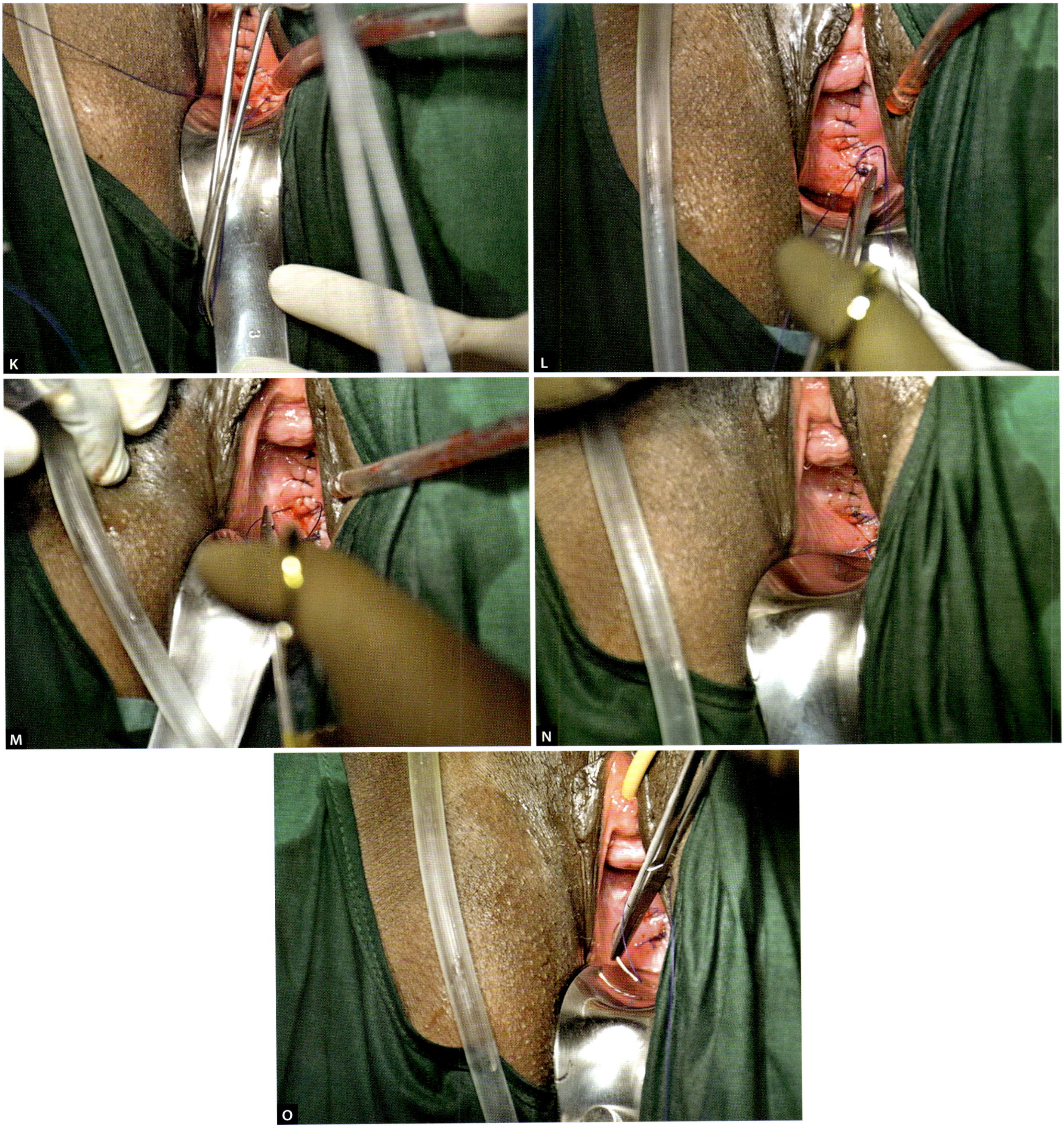

Figs. 9K to O

Figs. 9A to O: Vaginal epithelium closed with 3-0 Vicryl.

Timing of Repair

If the fistula occurs within few days of the surgery or insult, it can be repaired immediately before inflammatory reaction sets in.

If the wound and fistula is not clean and healthy delay of 4–8 weeks is recommend.

Steps

The fistula is exposed vaginally, a circumferential and incision taken around the fistula, the vaginal epithelium and fibrous tissues are excised with sharp dissection. The fistulous tract is not excised.

First ,the bladder mucosa is closed with 3-0 Vicryl with interrupted sutures. Next, the fibromuscular layer is closed with either interrupted or continuous 3-0 Vicryl.

It may be necessary to put the third layer. Methylene blue injected with bladder and water tightness confirmed.

- Insert 18 Fr Foley catheter for 14 days for continuous drainage.

LAPAROSCOPIC METHOD (FIGS. 10 TO 20)

Laparoscopy offers excellent vision and magnification of the fistula, 3D gives the depth also and the success rates are higher.

There are two methods of laparoscopy for VVF repair:
1. Transvesical method
2. O'Conner's method.

Commonly done is O'Conner's method. The bladder is filled with saline and catheter passed through fistula for identification. Bladder is bivalved with harmonic or monopolar hook the same incision is extended to include the fistula. Now the bladder mucosa is separated from the fistula with sharp dissection the separated vagina and fibrous tissues are excised. The proximity of the fistula to the ureteric orifices is examined if necessary. Bilateral ureteric stents are placed. Now using 2-0 Vicryl or barbed sutures the bladder mucosa is sutured continuously from the apex till the bladder is completely closed. Omental graft is mobilized and placed between the bladder and vagina, so that it acts

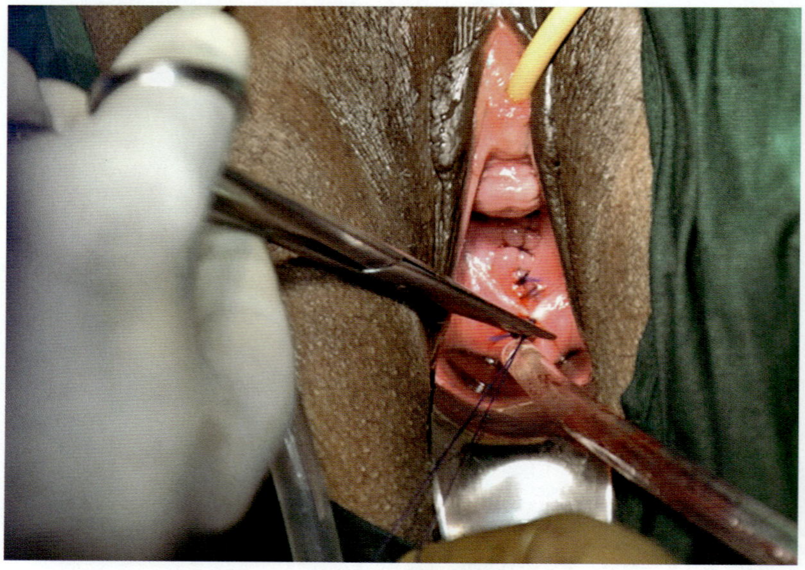

Fig. 10: Final picture.

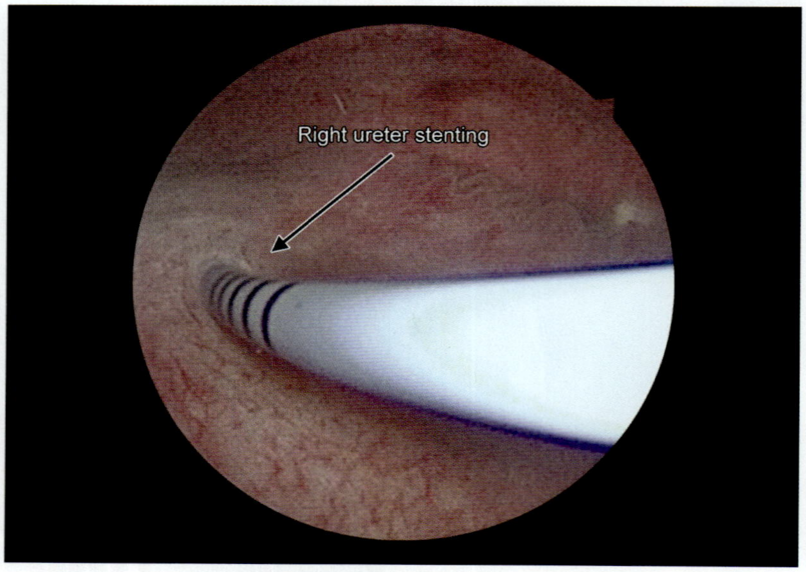

Fig. 12: Right ureter stenting.
Courtesy: Dr Jay Mehta.

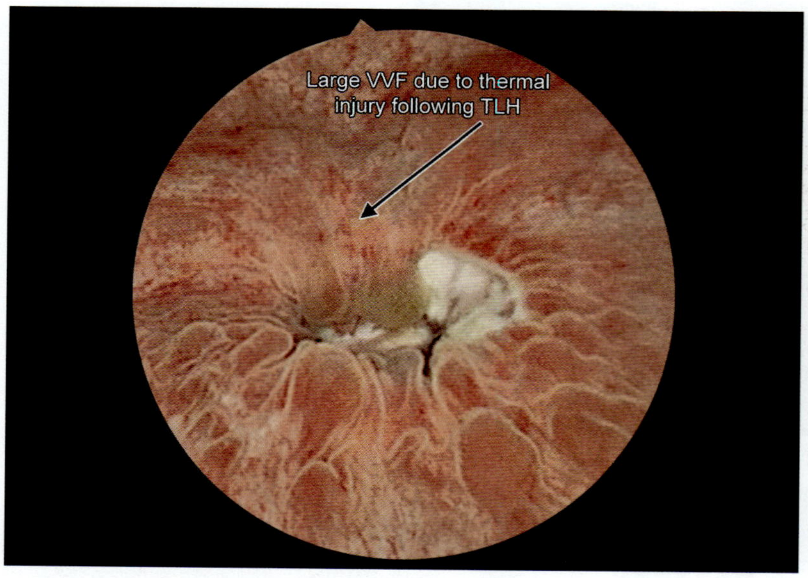

Fig. 11: Cystoscopic appearance of large fistula caused by thermal burn.
(TLH: total laparoscopic hysterectomy; VVF: vesicovaginal fistula)
Courtesy: Dr Jay Mehta.

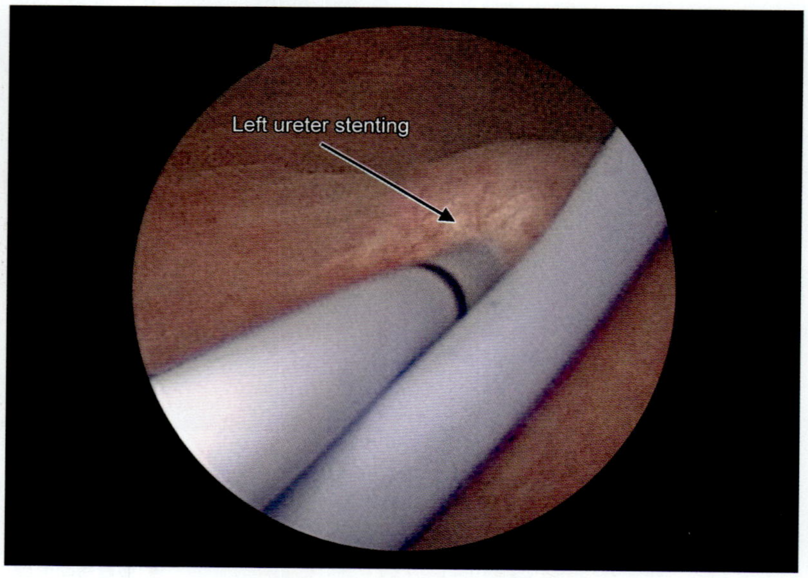

Fig. 13: Left ureter stenting.
Courtesy: Dr Jay Mehta.

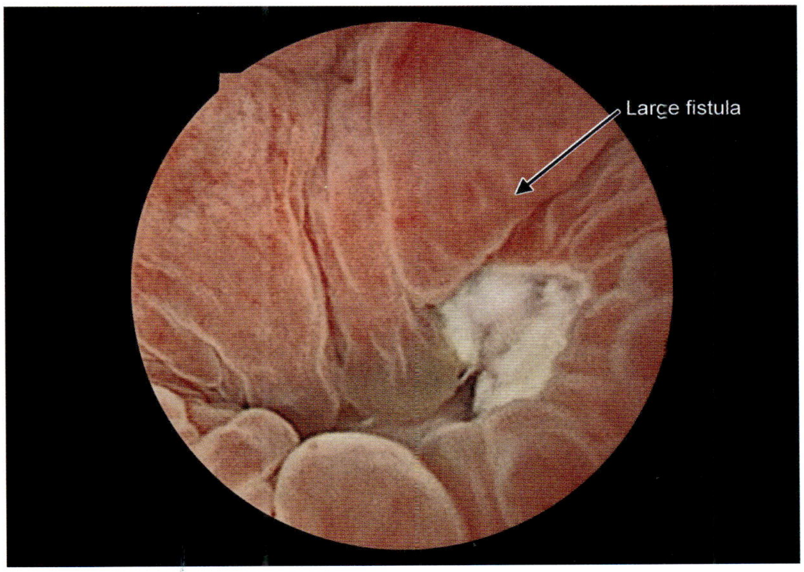

Fig. 14: Large fistula.
Courtesy: Dr Jay Mehta.

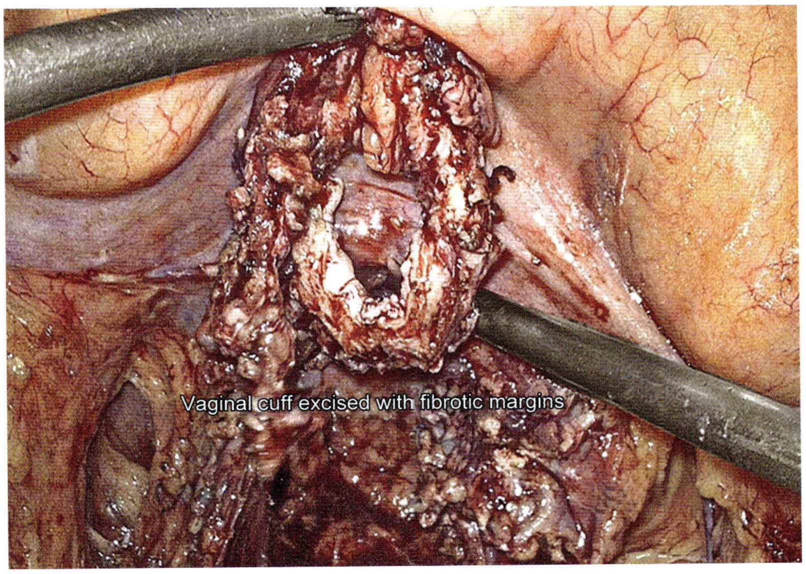

Fig. 15: Vaginal cuff excised with fibrotic margins.
Courtesy: Dr Jay Mehta.

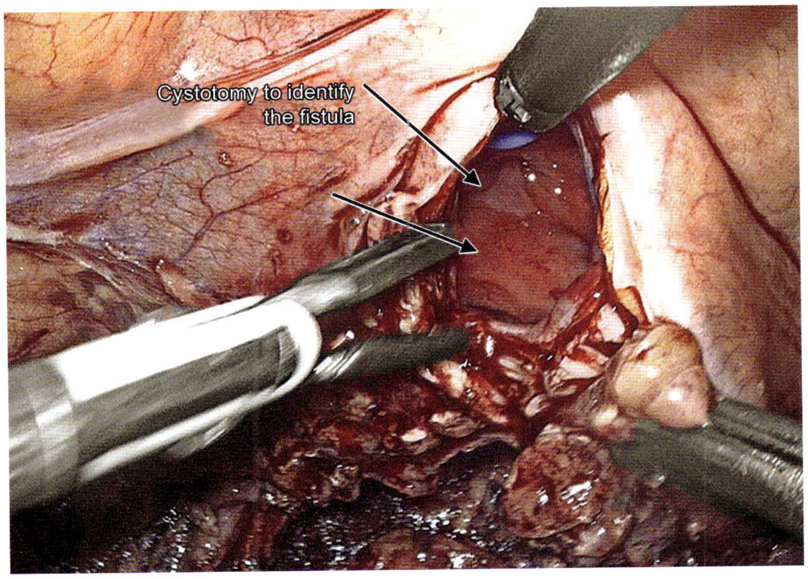

Fig. 16: Cystotomy to identify the fistula.
Courtesy: Dr Jay Mehta.

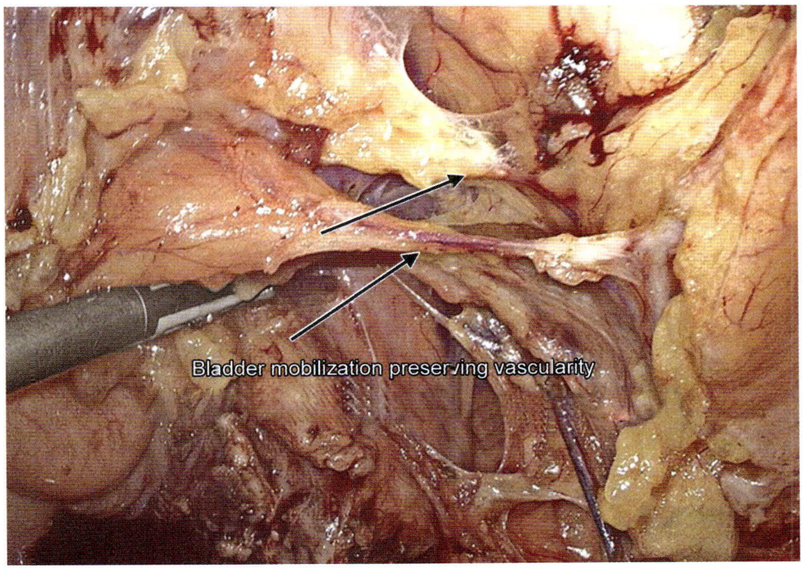

Fig. 17: Bladder mobilization preserving vascularity.
Courtesy: Dr Jay Mehta.

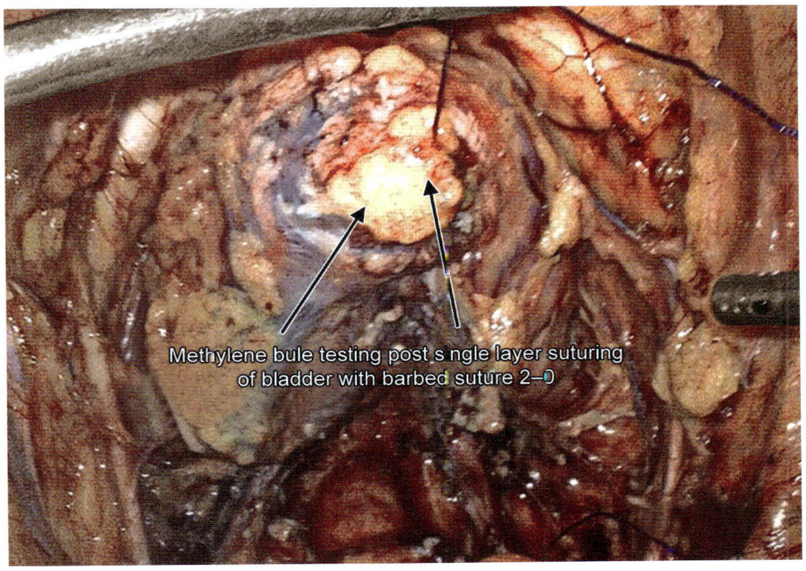

Fig. 18: Methylene blue testing post single layer suturing of bladder with barbed suture 2-0.
Courtesy: Dr Jay Mehta.

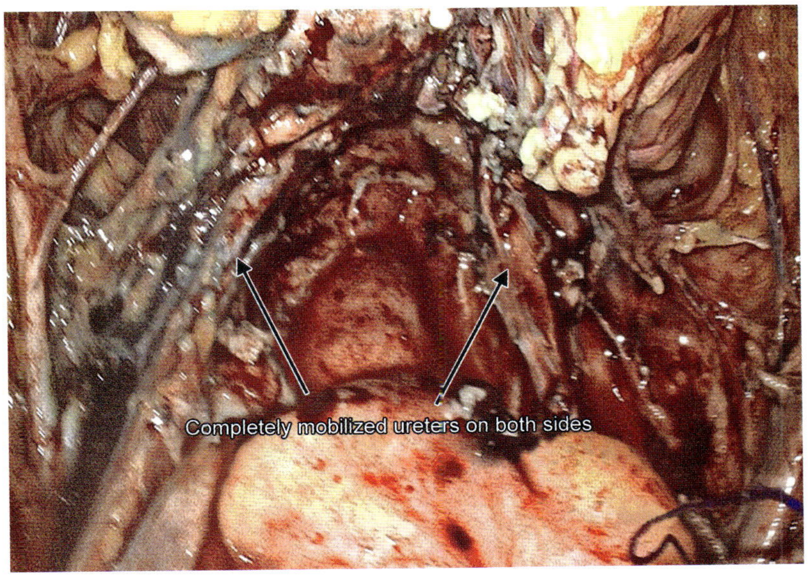

Fig. 19: Completely mobilized ureters on both sides.
Courtesy: Dr Jay Mehta.

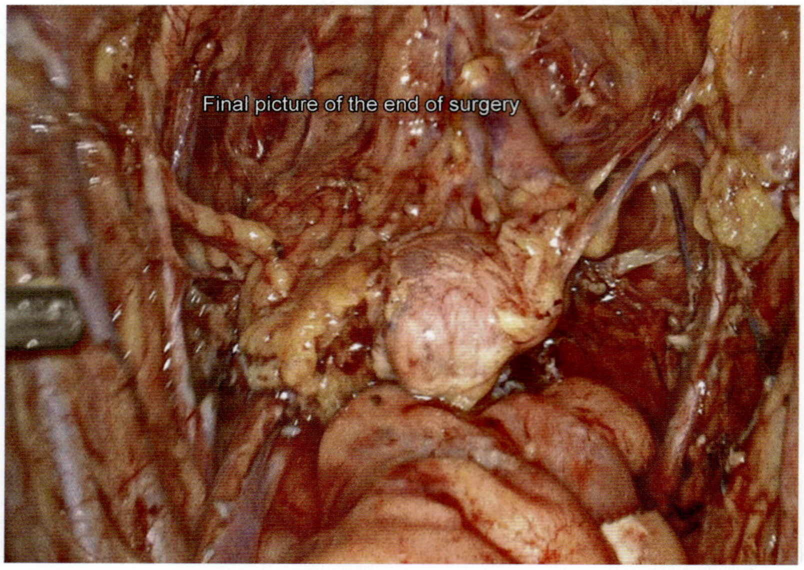

Fig. 20: Final picture of the end of surgery.
Courtesy: Dr Jay Mehta.

a interposition tissue and also it gives blood supply to the area so that healing is better. Once the bladder is completely closed, methylene blue is injected and tested for water tightness if necessary additional in tempted sutures are put.

An 18 Fr Foley catheter is inserted into the bladder for continuous drainage for 3 weeks.

With O'Connor's method success rates could be 90–100%, if done properly.

CHAPTER

19

Leiomyoma Uterus

Rachana Ghanti, Aditi Rai, B Ramesh

INTRODUCTION

Uterine fibroids, most common pelvic tumor in women, also known as *uterine leiomyoma, myoma, fibromyoma, fibroleiomyoma*, are benign smooth muscle tumors of the uterus. They are estimated to be present in a high percentage of all women of reproductive age and may be discovered incidentally during routine annual examination. Asymptomatic fibroids may be present in 40–50% of women older than 35 years of age.[1] Using ultrasonography screening, other authors have estimated a cumulative incidence by age 50 of greater than 80% in African-American women and nearly 70% in white women.[2]

Leiomyomas may occur singly but often are multiple. They may be subserosal, intramural, or submucosal in location within the uterus or located in the cervix, in the broad ligament, or on a pedicle. Most fibroids start in the muscular wall of the uterus. With further growth, some lesions may develop toward the outside of the uterus or toward the internal cavity. Secondary changes may develop within fibroids hemorrhage, necrosis, calcification, and cystic degenerations.

If the uterus contains too many to count, it is referred to as *diffuse uterine leiomyomatosis*.

Laparoscopic myomectomy was described for the first time as early as 1970s when it was exclusively restricted for subserosal myomas. Surgical science has seen a tremendous shift from open to minimal access surgery and with the recent advances in video endoscopic imaging technology and energy devices coupled with improved skill acquisition of the surgeons, laparoscopic myomectomy is being now preferred at most good centers worldwide. It is not any longer restricted to moderate <9 cm myoma or less than 5–7 myomas. Size, number, and location are no longer a restriction in experienced hands, although the technique has its learning curve.

Debatable issues about excessive blood loss, long time involved in surgery, and the strength of the obstetric scar are of lesser concern with the evolving trends showing results equal to if not better than the open approach.

However, the recent evolving concern is of morcellation and the upcoming contained bag morcellation is being advocated to combat this debate.

Although different studies reveal different criteria, it is generally considered that the laparoscopic approach is not feasible if there are three myomas of a diameter of about 8 cm each or a uterus of about 16 weeks with a 12-cm myoma. Nezhat recommends up to 15 cm in diameter.

SURGICAL ANATOMY

Classification of Fibroids

We can classify leiomyomas on the basis of their origin, location, symptoms they cause and the ease of removal/resection **(Table 1 and Figs. 1 to 13)**.

Classification of leiomyomas based on their location in the uterine wall:

- Subserosal
- Intramural
- Submucous

Submucous fibroids cause menorrhagia, dysmenorrhea, and infertility and need to be treated.

Table 1: Classification of leiomyoma based on their location.

Uterine	*Extrauterine*		*Unusual variants*
Fundus	Cervical		Diffuse leiomyomatosis
Body	Peritoneal		Lipoleiomyomatosis
Cornual	Broad ligament		Leiomyosarcoma
	True	Pseudo	
Lower segment	Parasitic fibroid		
Lateral wall			

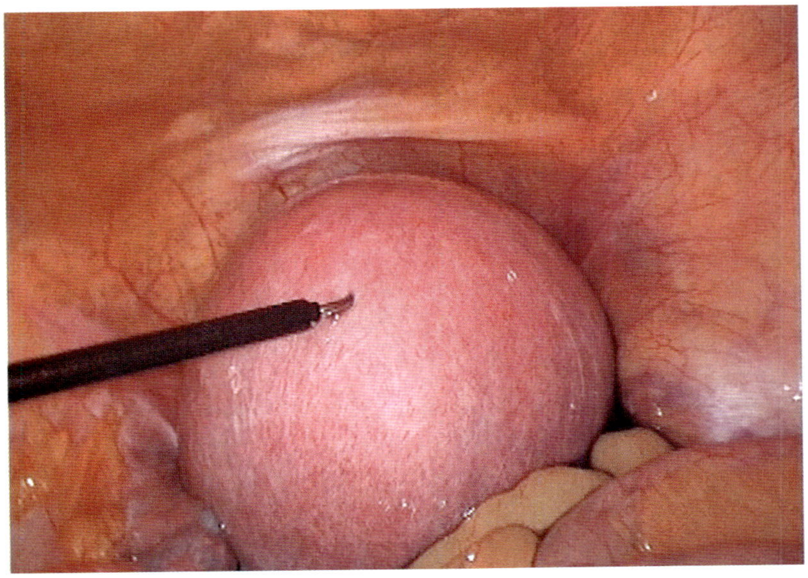

Fig. 1: Fundal fibroid.

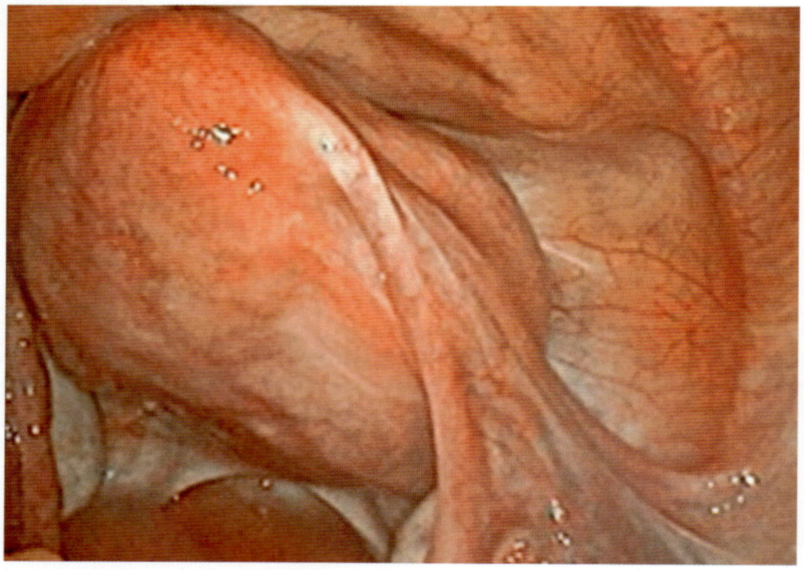

Fig. 2: Lower segment.

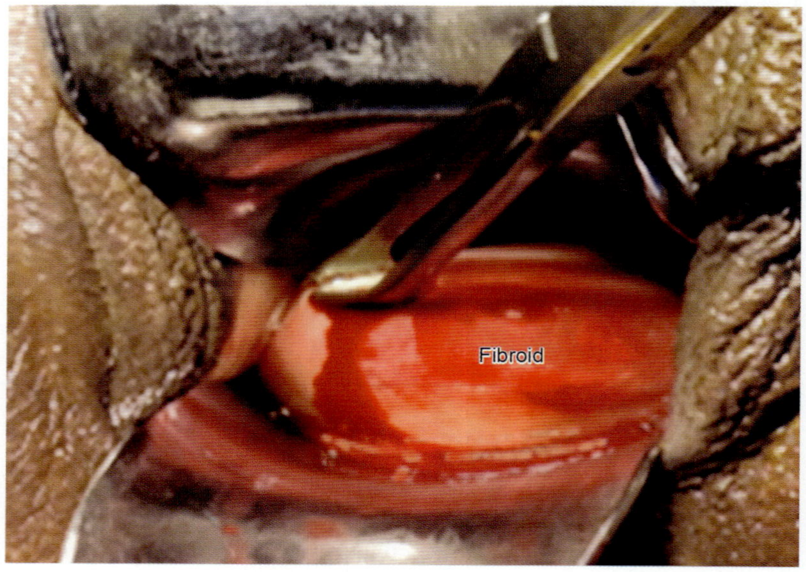

Fig. 4: Cervical fibroid.

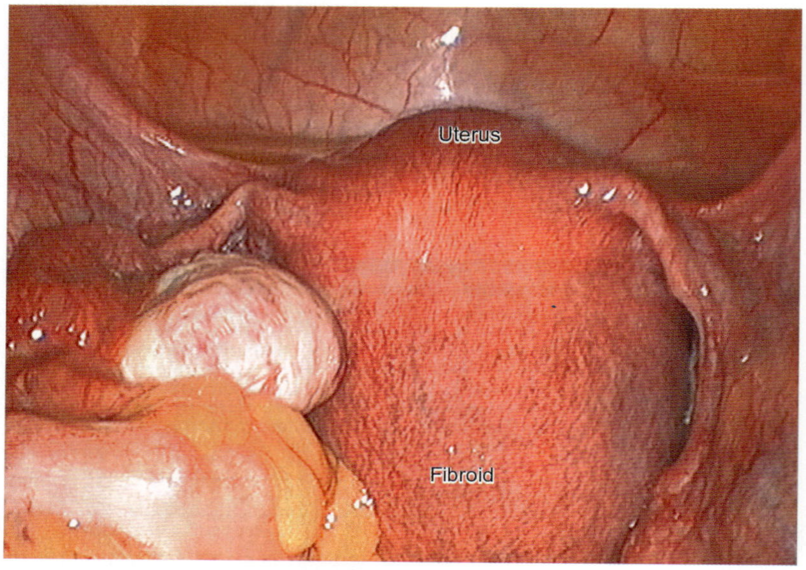

Fig 3: Posterior wall fibroid.

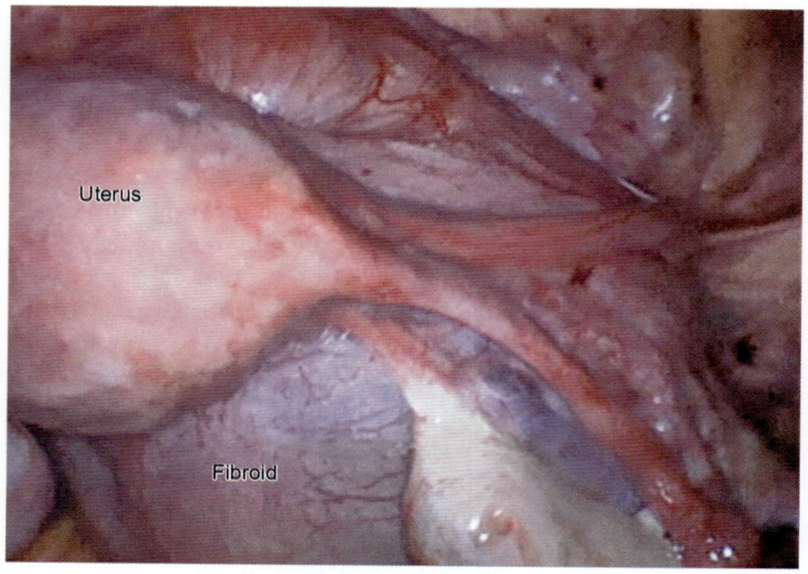

Fig. 5: Pseudobroad ligament.

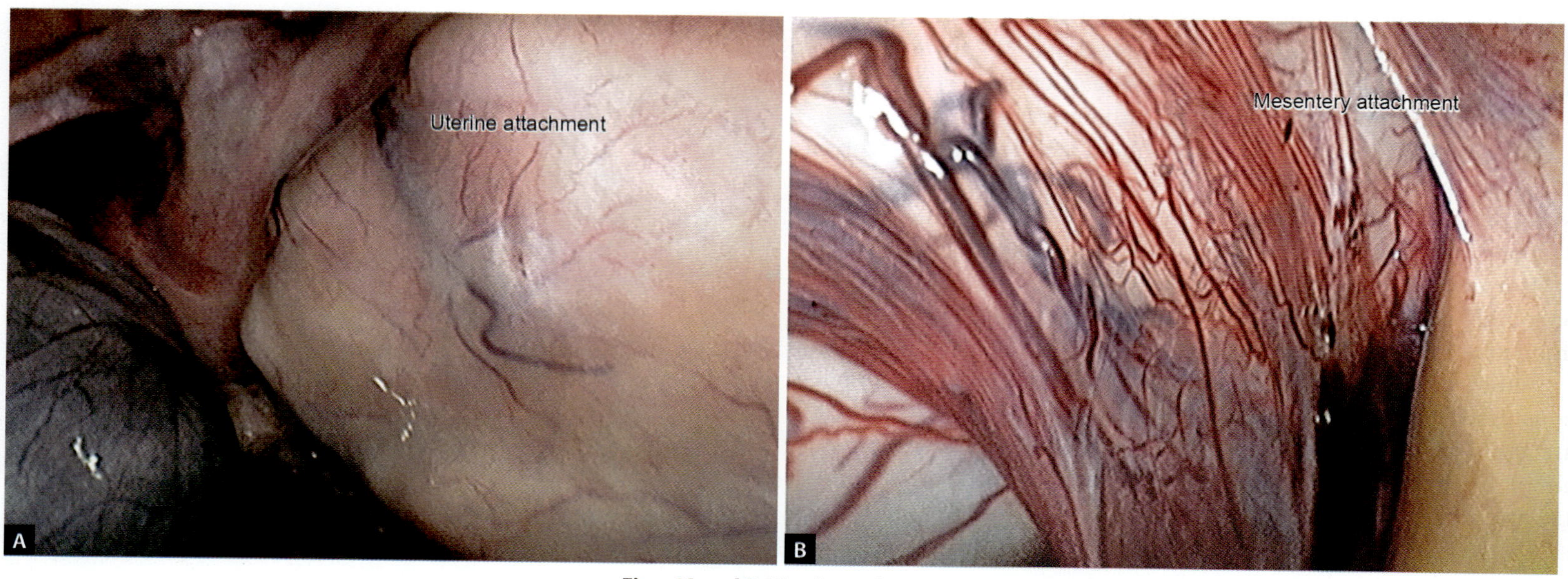

Figs. 6A and B: Wandering fibroid.

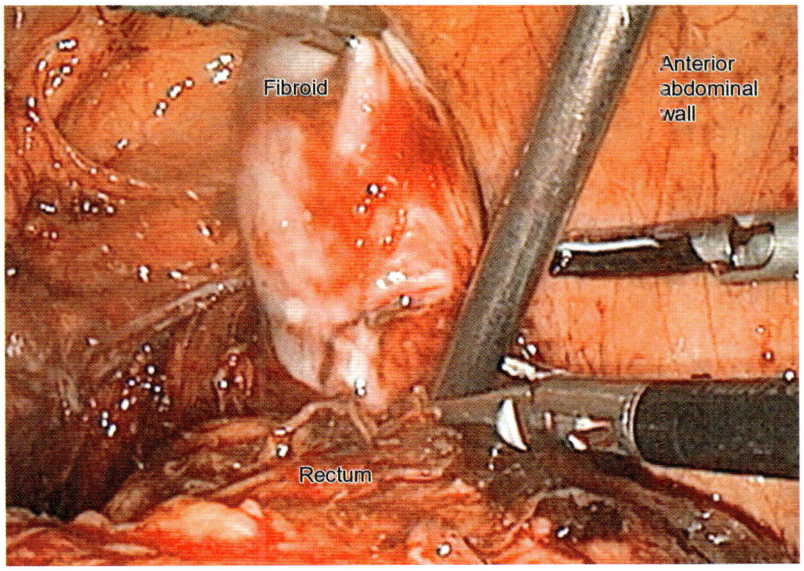

Fig. 7: Parasitic fibroid in the pelvic floor.

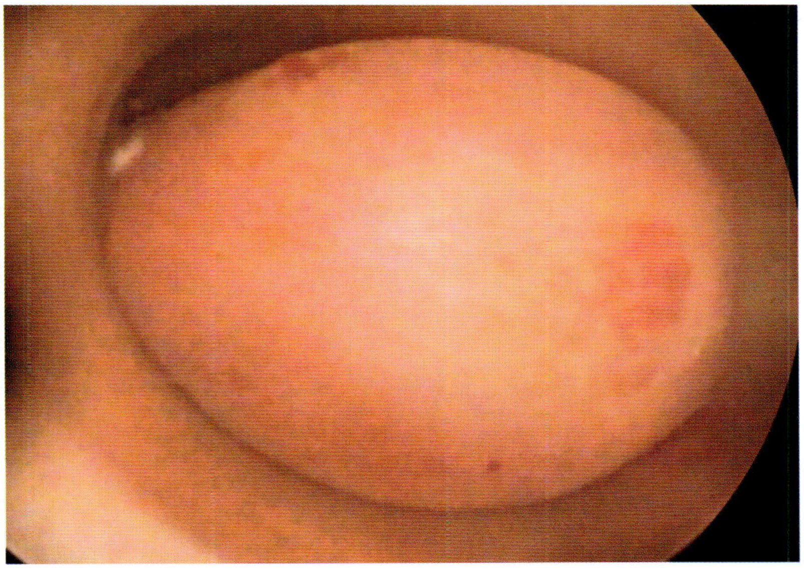

Fig. 10: Submucous fibroid.

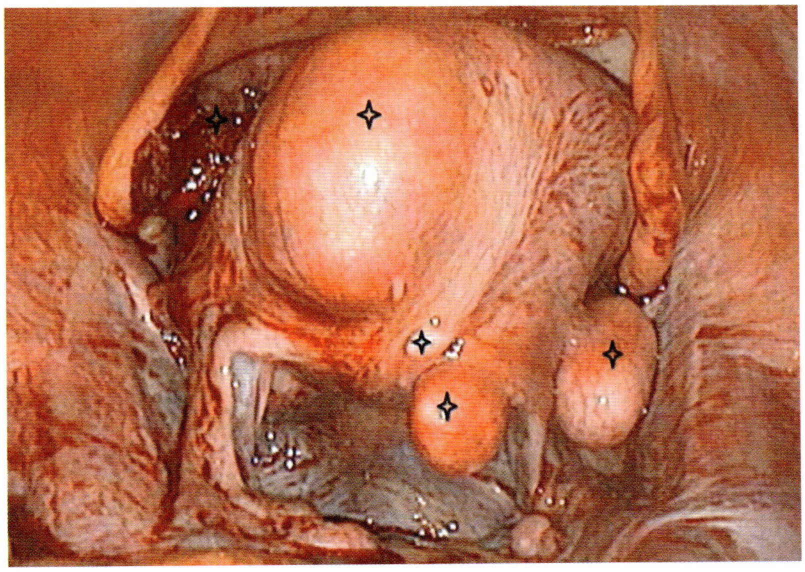

Fig. 8: Diffuse leiomyomatosis.

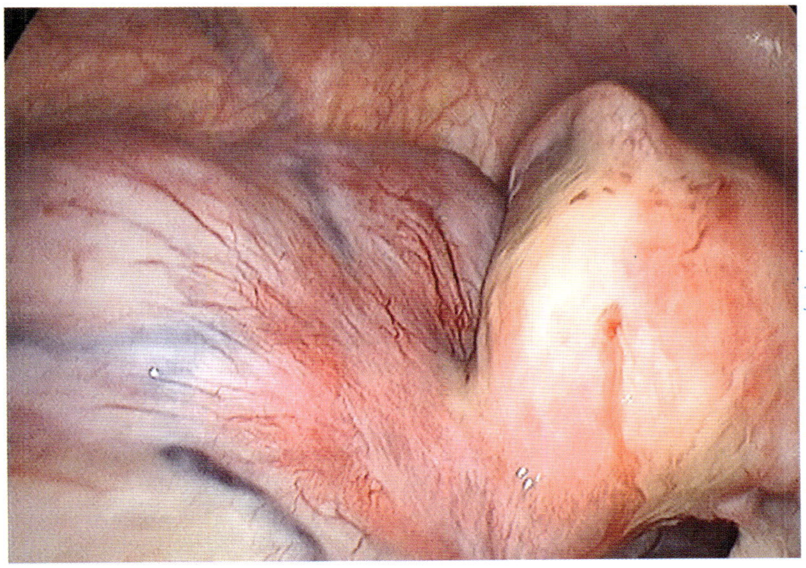

Fig. 11: Subserous fibroid.

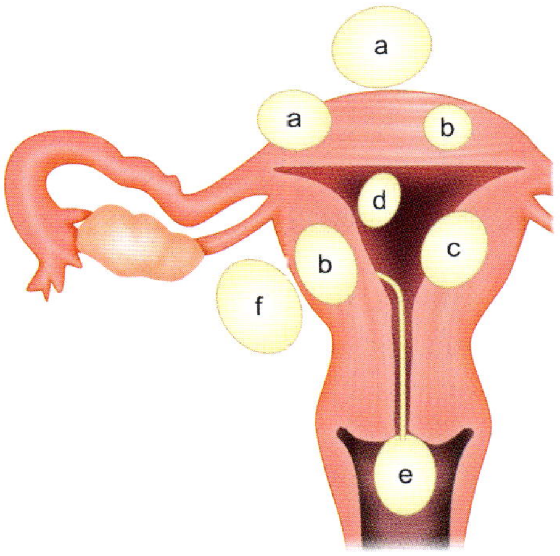

Fig. 9: Schematic drawing of various types of uterine fibroids. a: subserosal fibroids; b: intramural fibroids; c: submucosal fibroid; d: pedunculated submucosal fibroid; e: pedunculated cervical fibroid; and f: fibroid of the broad ligament.

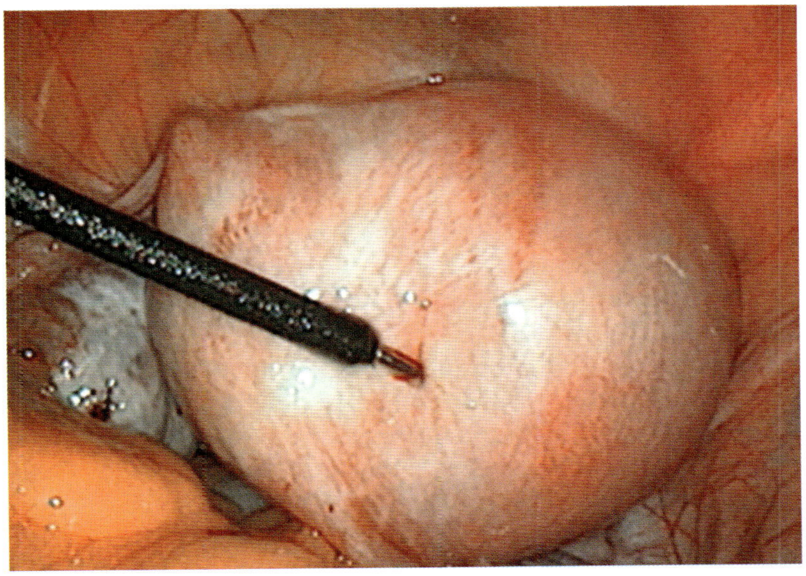

Fig. 12: Intramural fibroid.

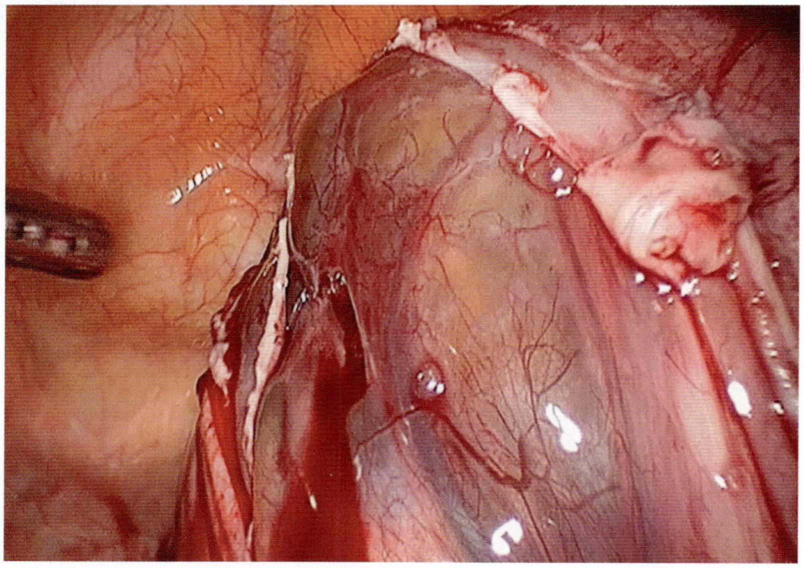

Fig. 13: Cystic degeneration with loss of plane.

Table 2: Classification of leiomyoma based on complications to the leiomyoma.

Uncomplicated	*Complicated*
	Degeneration
	Torsion
	Hemorrhage
	Malignant transformations

Intramural fibroids can be left alone if they are asymptomatic until they are more than 4–5 cm.

Subserous fibroids are usually asymptomatic and rarely cause any complications.

Classification of leiomyomas based on the symptoms ***(Table 2)****:*
- *Symptomatic*—menorrhagia, adjacent organ compression
- *Asymptomatic*

Classification of submucous fibroids has been proposed on the basis of feasibility of hysteroscopic resection of the same. This scoring system gives a fair idea about the possibility of complete hysteroscopic resection, necessity of multiple settings, need of laparoscopic assistance, and the probability of increased incidence of complications. This enables the operating team to formulate the approach strategy and helps in discussing the various options with the patient and preparing them for the outcome.

European Society for Gynaecological Endoscopy (ESGE): Classification of submucous myomas:
- *Type 0:* Pedunculated myoma within endometrial cavity.
- *Type I:* <50% myometrial extension (sessile), <90° angle of myoma surface to uterine wall.
- *Type II:* >50% myometrial extension (sessile), >90° angle of myoma surface to uterine wall.

Source: Modified from Wamsteker K, Emanuel MH, de Kruif JH. Transcervical hysteroscopic resection of submucous fibroids for abnormal uterine bleeding: results regarding the degree of intramural extension. Obstet Gynecol. 1993;82:736-40.

Myometrial extension is important when evaluating women for resectoscopic surgery. Thus, an ESGE type 2 leiomyoma that reaches the serosa is considered to be a type 2–5 lesion and therefore is not a candidate for resectoscopic surgery.

INDICATIONS

Surgery for uterine leiomyomata is complex and it is depend upon their medical comorbidities, surgical history, clinical scenario, and patient preference.

This procedure is considered when patient either has a *desire for future fertility or feels strongly about retaining their uterus*. The criteria are directed at relieving symptoms or improving quality of life by decreasing the patient's concerns. No indications exist for removing asymptomatic fibroids.

Excessive uterine bleeding:
- Heavy menstrual bleeding which changes the lifestyle of the person.
- Uterine bleeding leads to cause anemia.

Pelvic discomfort caused by myomata: Acute and severe.

Chronic lower abdominal pain or low back or pelvic pressure with evidence of sizeable leiomyoma on imaging studies.

Leiomyomata those are palpable abdominally: A definite risk exists for myoma recurrence after myomectomy and, with it, the need for a repeat surgical procedure in the future. If the patient no longer desires to retain her fertility or her uterus, hysterectomy is the usual procedure of choice.

PREOPERATIVE EVALUATION AND TREATMENT

If medical management failed and her symptoms are sufficiently severe, then surgery is the main option.[3] In women who complain of menorrhagia, the hematocrit is used to assess the degree of anemia. For anemic patients, preoperative gonadotropin-releasing hormone agonists (GnRH agonists) treatment will reduce the size of myoma, restoration of hematocrit value and decrease chance for blood transfusion. While some studies show a decrease in intraoperative blood loss after a course of GnRH agonist therapy.[4] After taking GnRH agonist, surgeons will get difficulty during procedure[5] because of loss of cleavage plane due to hydropic degeneration of myoma. Saline infusion sonography determines endometrial distortion by submucous fibroids. Periodic pelvic ultrasound examinations help monitor the growth rate of asymptomatic myomas. The presence of large broad ligament myoma needs for an intravenous urography to rule out ureteral obstruction. Patients are counseled regarding the risk of intra- and postoperative bleeding, adjacent organ injury, need for blood transfusion, and required laparotomy and rarely hysterectomy.

TYPES OF MYOMECTOMY

- *Total laparoscopic myomectomy*
- *Laparoscopically-assisted myomectomy:* Laparoscopically assisted myomectomy (LAM) is a safe alternative to laparoscopic myomectomy (LM). It is less difficult and requires less time to complete the decision to perform LAM. LAM may be superior to LM in the situation where myoma size is more than 8 cm, many myomas requiring extensive morcellation, and a deep, large, intramural myoma that requires uterine repair in multiple layers.

  Three major objectives of LAM are reduction of blood loss, prevention of postoperative adhesions, and maintenance of myometrial integrity. LAM, with "open" morcellation and conventional suturing, reduces the duration of the operation and the need for more extensive laparoscopic experience.

- *Single-incision laparoscopic surgery (SILS)—myomectomy*
- *Robotic myomectomy and robotically-assisted myomectomy:* Robotic surgery has more advantage over straight laparoscopy such as shorter learning curves, a three-dimensional vision system, wristed instrumentation, and ergonomic positioning.[6] Because of its inherent advantages and principles similar to open surgery, robotic technology has the potential to facilitate utilization of a less invasive approach to the surgical management of myomas, thereby increasing this option for patients.
- *Myolysis:* Laparoscopic myolysis or leiomyoma coagulation can be used as an alternative to laparoscopic myomectomy for the treatment of small intramural or subserosal leiomyomas. The procedure was developed in Germany in 1986 and was first performed in the United States by Goldfarb in 1990.[7,8] Myolysis is designed to destroy the blood supply and subsequently cause stromal death of symptomatic myomas in order to achieve a decrease in their size.
- *High-intensity focused ultrasound (HIFU)*
- *Uterine artery embolization:* It involves the catheterization of both uterine arteries and the instillation of microparticles [polyvinyl alcohol (PVA)] to cause occlusion of blood supply to the myomas and subsequently leading to devascularization and infarction. Embolization did result in significant improvements in patient symptomatology.

MANAGEMENT OF FIBROIDS: LAPAROSCOPIC MYOMECTOMY

Surgical Equipment (Figs. 14 and 15)

- Gas insufflators
- Light source
- Video camera unit
- Suction irrigation device
- Monitor and documentation system
- Telescopes **(Figs. 15A and B)**:
  0°—10 mm, 30°—10 mm
  4 mm—30° standard hysteroscope
- *Trocars:* One 10 mm, two to three 5 mm
- *Operating instruments* ***(Figs. 15A and B)***—atraumatic and traumatic graspers:
  - Dissecting and hook scissors
  - Injection needle
  - *Myoma screw:* 5 mm and 10 mm
  - Needle holder
  - Port closure needle
- Energy sources—harmonic scalpel:
  - Bipolar forceps
  - Monopolar hook
- Morcellator **(Figs. 16A and B)**
- Suture materials

Steps of Surgery (Figs. 17 to 20)

- Ports placement
- Vasopressin injection **(Figs. 20A and B)**
- Uterine incision
- Enucleation
- Uterine repair
- Extraction of myoma
- Port closure

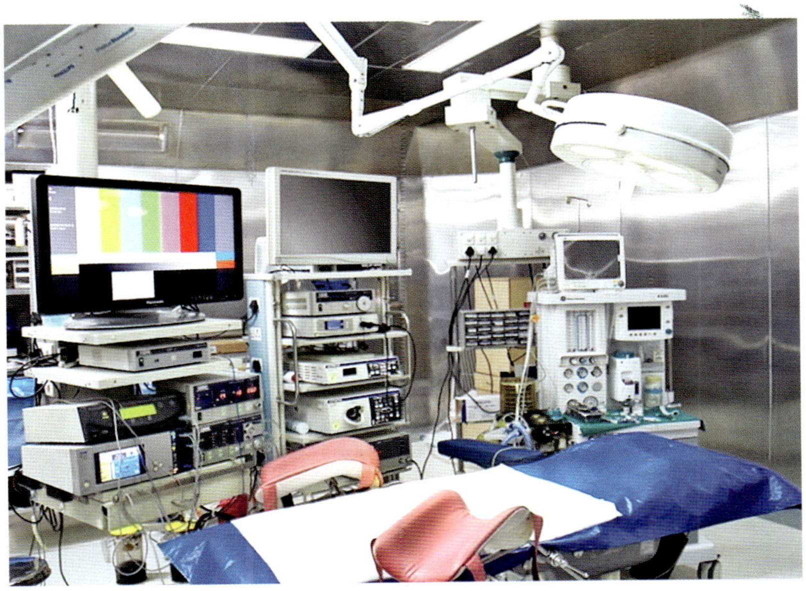

Fig. 14: Operation room (OR) setup.

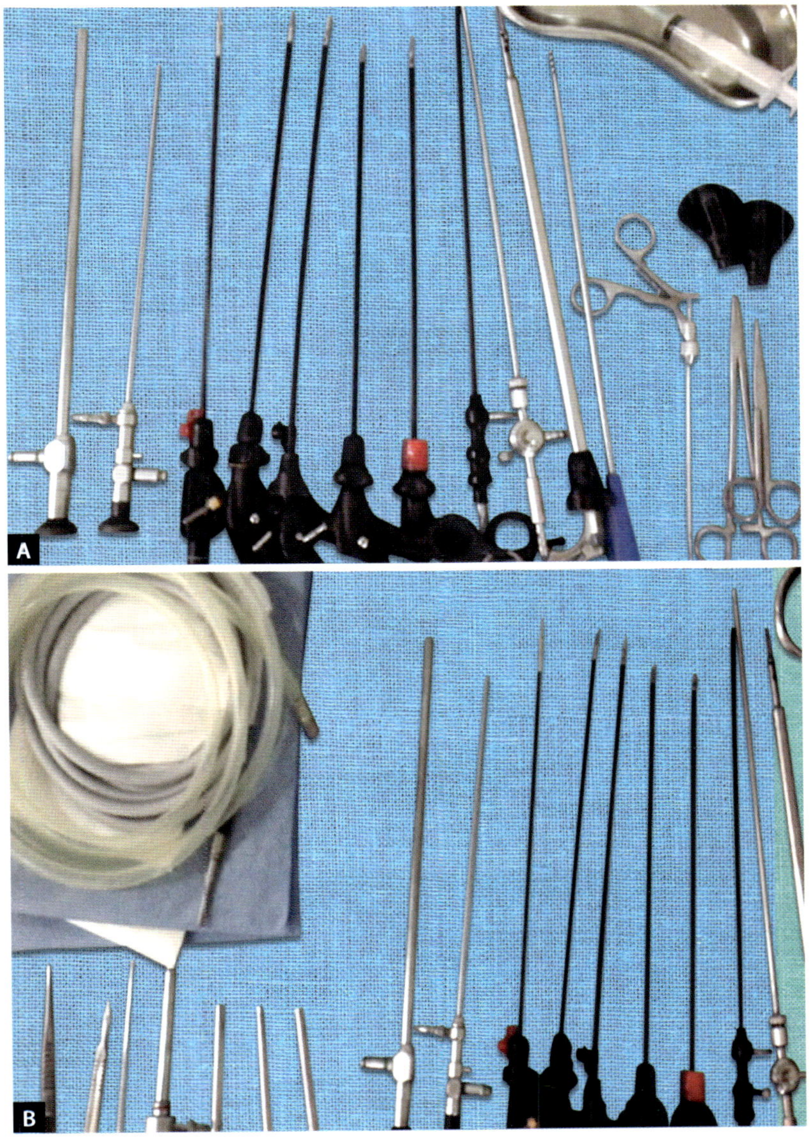

Figs. 15A and B: (A) Instruments—telescopes, graspers, scissors, suction irrigation cannula, myoma screw, claw forceps, port closure needle, and dilute vasopressin; and (B) Instruments—light cable, insufflations tube, trocars, and Veress.

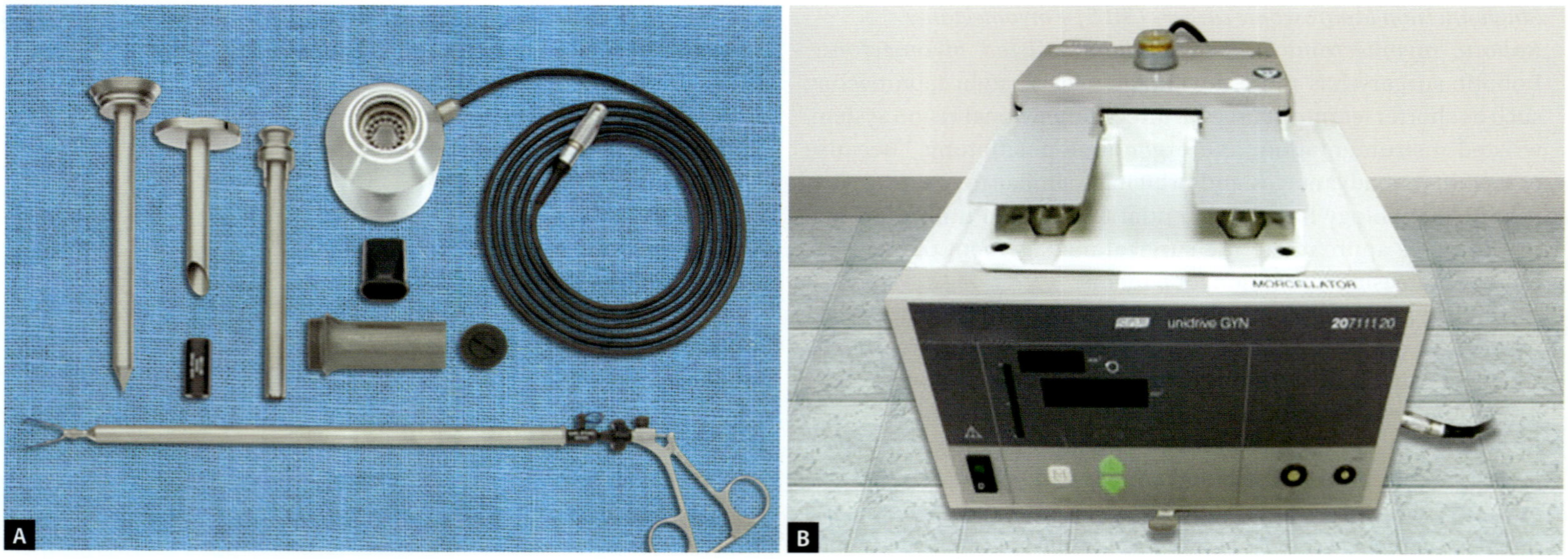

Figs. 16A and B: (A) Rotocut morcellator (conventional); and (B) Motor unit (Karl Storz unidrive).

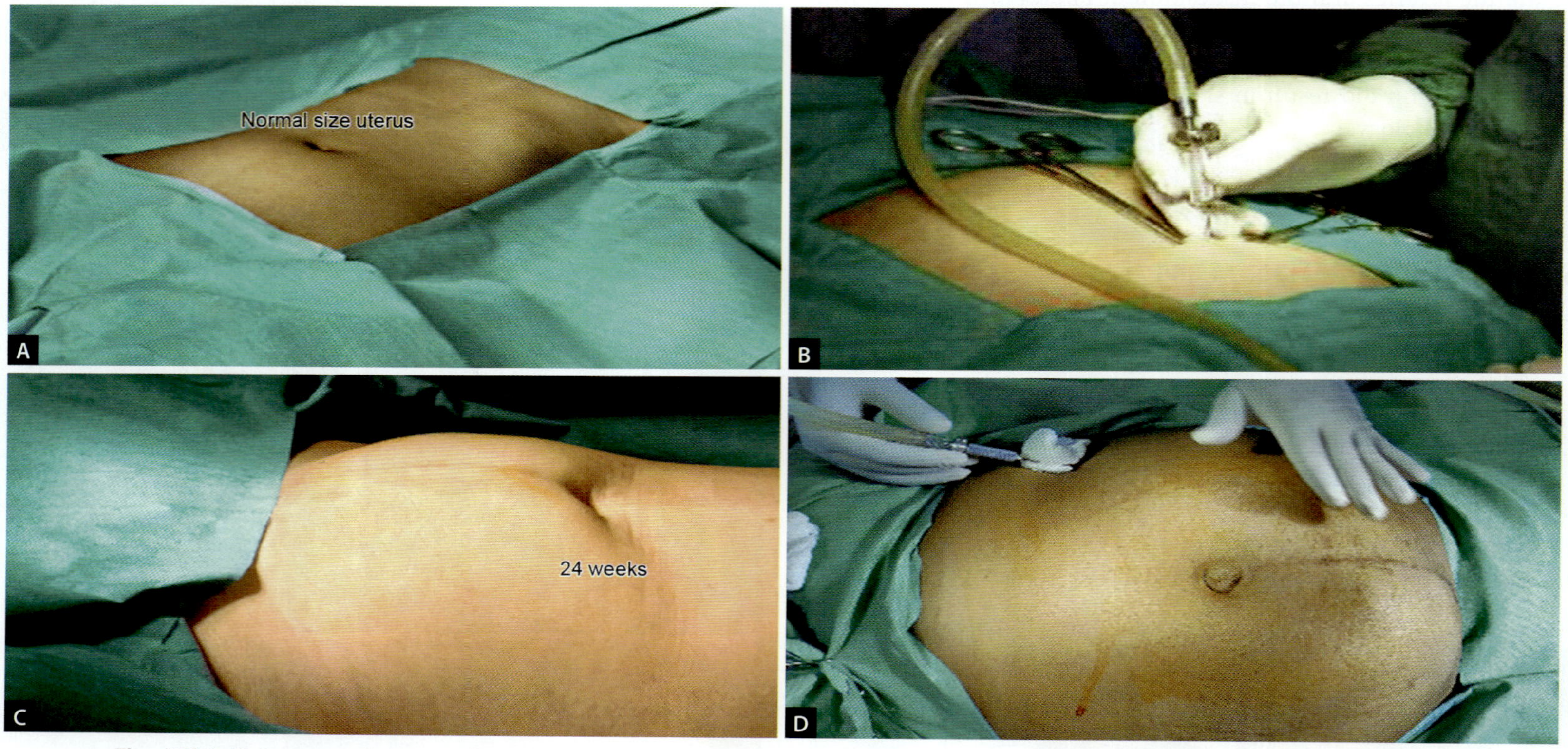

Figs. 17A to D: Pneumoperitoneum—Veress insertion. (A) Normal size uterus; (B) Intraumbilical Veress placement; (C) 24 weeks size fibroid uterus; (D) Veress through Palmer's point.

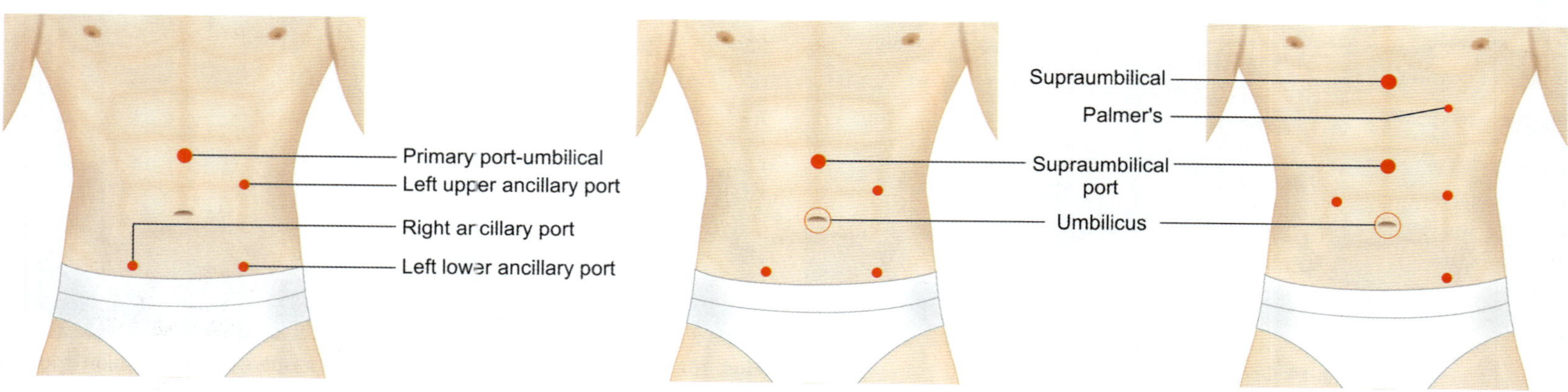

Fig. 18: Schematic diagram showing various primary and ancillary ports.

Abdominal Entry and Port Placement

Each surgeon has his own entry protocol. We generally use the Veress needle through umbilicus **(Fig. 17B)** or Palmer's point **(Fig. 17D)** and insufflate to a pneumoperitoneum of about 18 mm Hg. If myoma or pathology is small (size < 8–10 cm), an umbilical or supraumbilical trocar 5 mm or 10 mm **(Fig. 18)** is put or else a primary trocar (5 mm) is taken at left upper quadrant which actually visualizes the fibroid and overall size of uterus and then accordingly a supraumbilical entry above the umbilicus is chosen and a 10-mm trocar is introduced under direct vision of a 5-mm optical trocar **(Figs. 19A to D)**.

A total of three 5-mm working ports are taken which may be chosen as per the style of suturing preferred by the surgeon. We generally choose two left ports lateral to inferior epigastric vessels and one lower right port for assistant. Many surgeons use a third suprapubic port.

Incision and Enucleation

Refer to **Figures 21A to D**.

Enucleation of Myoma

Refer to **Figures 22A to D**.

Suturing of Myoma Bed

Refer to **Figures 23A to D**.

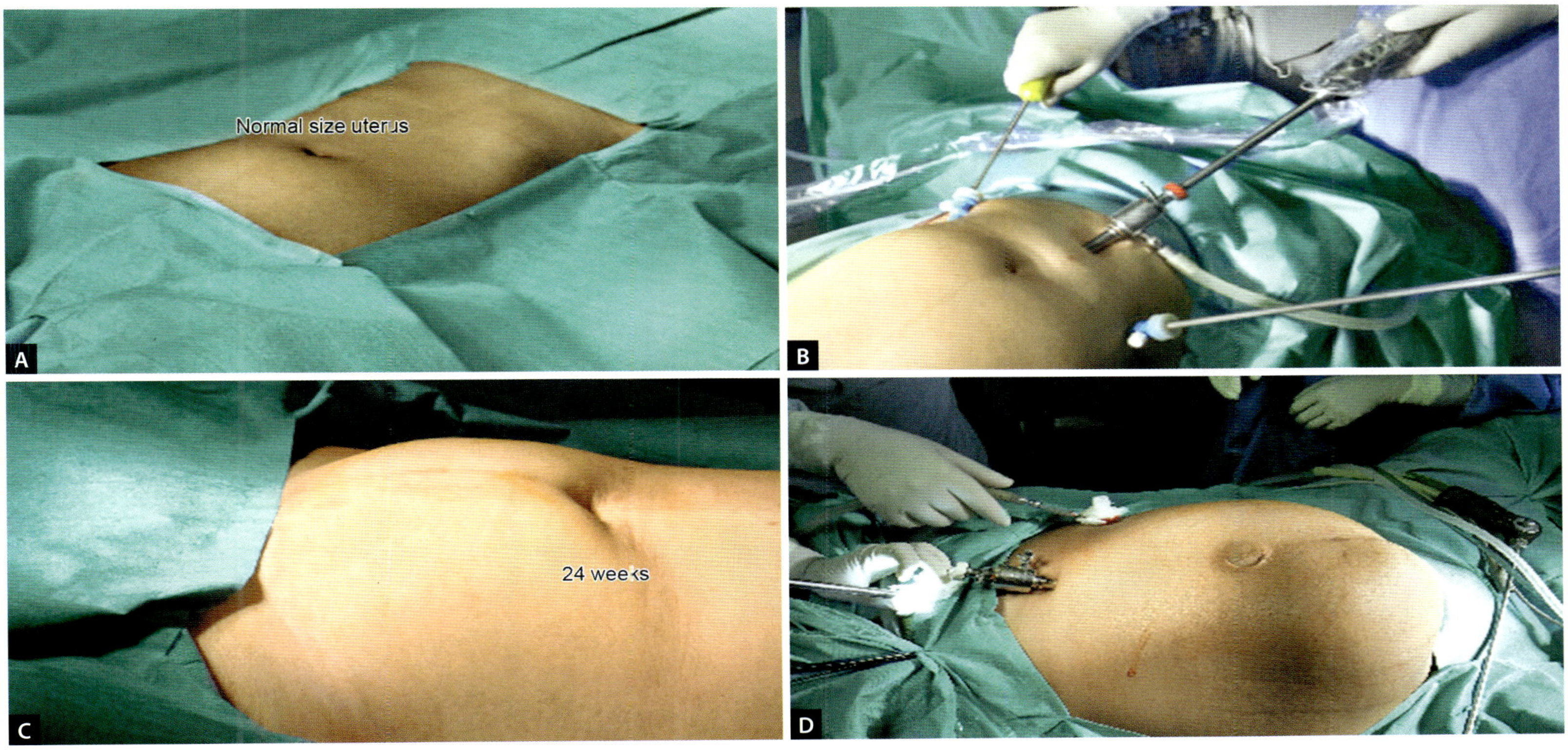

Figs. 19A to D: Port placement. (A and B) Primary and secondary port placement in normal size uterus; and (C and D) Primary port placement in a 24 weeks size uterus. Note higher placement of trocar just below xiphisternum (provides proper panoramic view for performing surgery).

Injection of Vasopressin

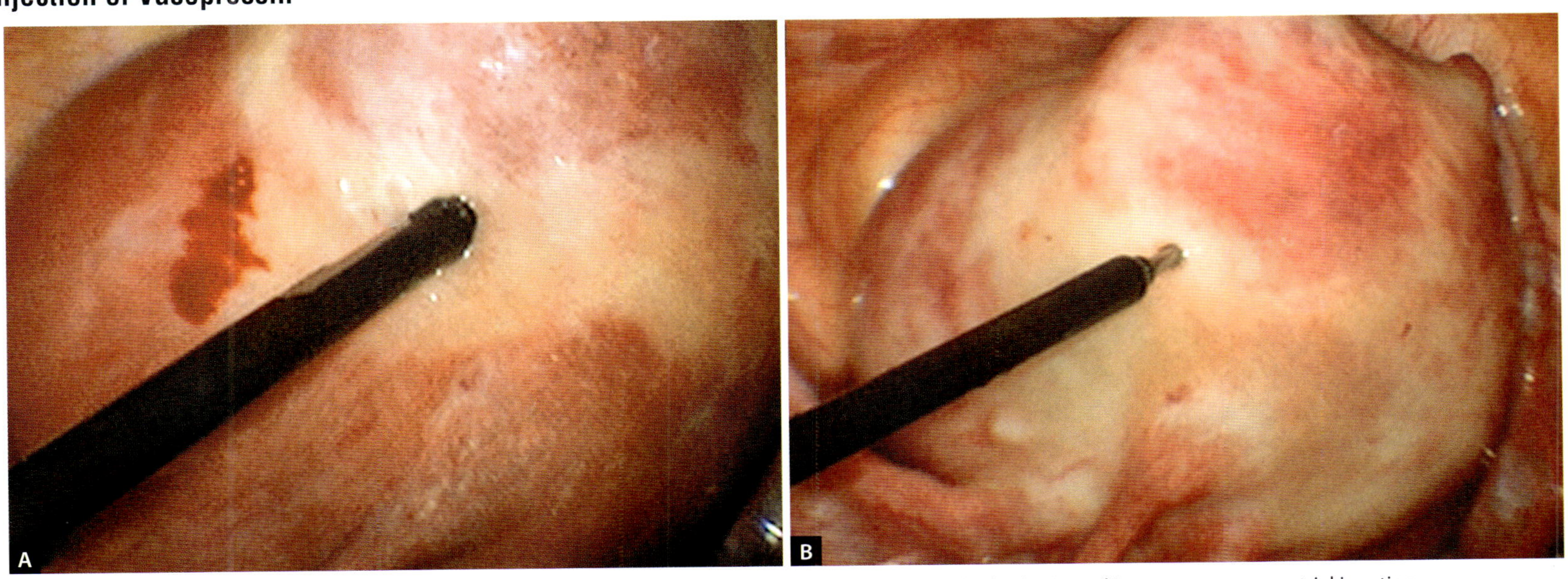

Figs. 20A and B: Vasopressin injection. (A) Diluted vasopressin (20 U in 200 mL of normal saline) injected into myoma myometrial junction; (B) Note the blanching seen after injection.

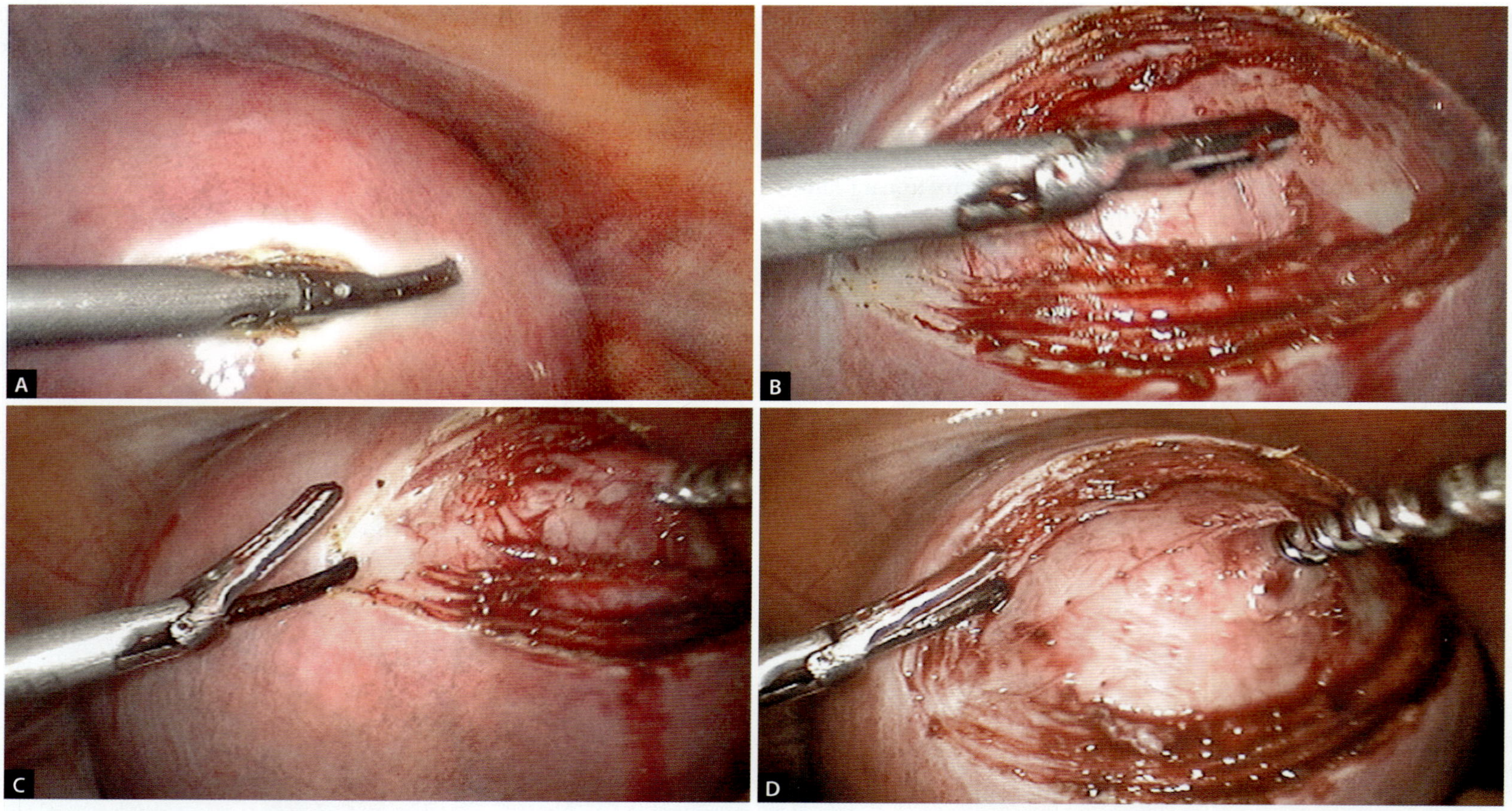

Figs. 21A to D: Sequential images of incision and enucleation. (A) Incision over myoma using harmonic in an oblique fashion; (B) Myoma screw used to stabilize the uterus while incising with harmonic; (C) Myometrial layers and pseudocapsule being cut with harmonic. *Note:* Proper plane identification is the key step in enucleation; (D) Enucleation in process using 5 mm myoma screw.

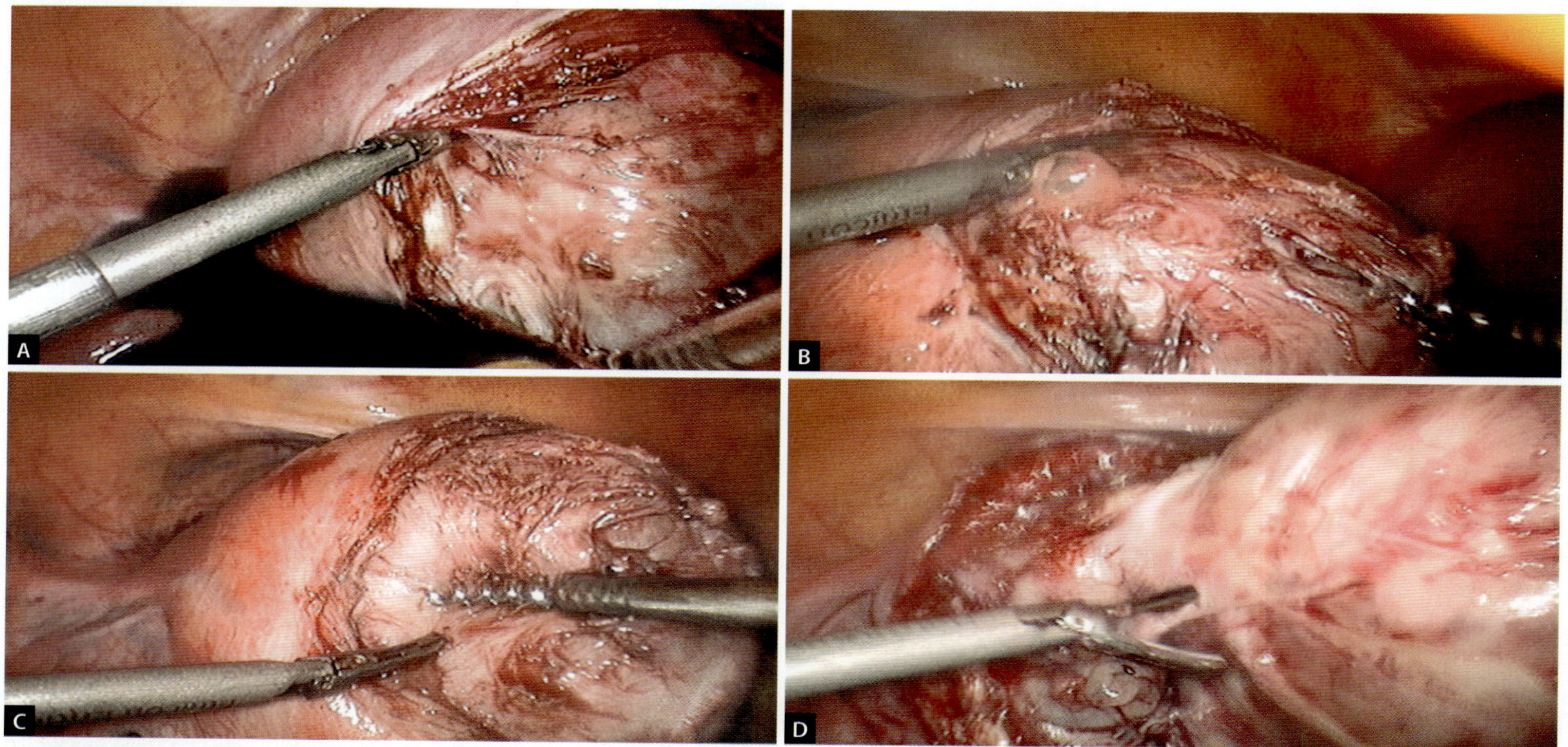

Figs. 22A to D: Continuation of enucleation. (A and B) Traction and countertraction with harmonic and myoma screw, (B) Myoma screw advanced near the margin to aid in enucleation; (C) Harmonic is used to cut through the tissues which hold back the myoma; and (D) Final step of enucleation. Myoma is cut from the bed.

Baseball technique of suturing ***(Figs. 24 and 25)****:* Note the undermining of suture material and approximation of edges. Buried suture line prevents adhesion formation. Bites are taken inside out on both sides of the edges and suture tightened each time.

Suture materials: The author generally either uses standard Vicryl polyglactin no. 1 or 1-0 on a cutting needle (40 mm size) or (50 mm size) in large myomas for standard suturing. The author also finds the use of barbed suture useful.

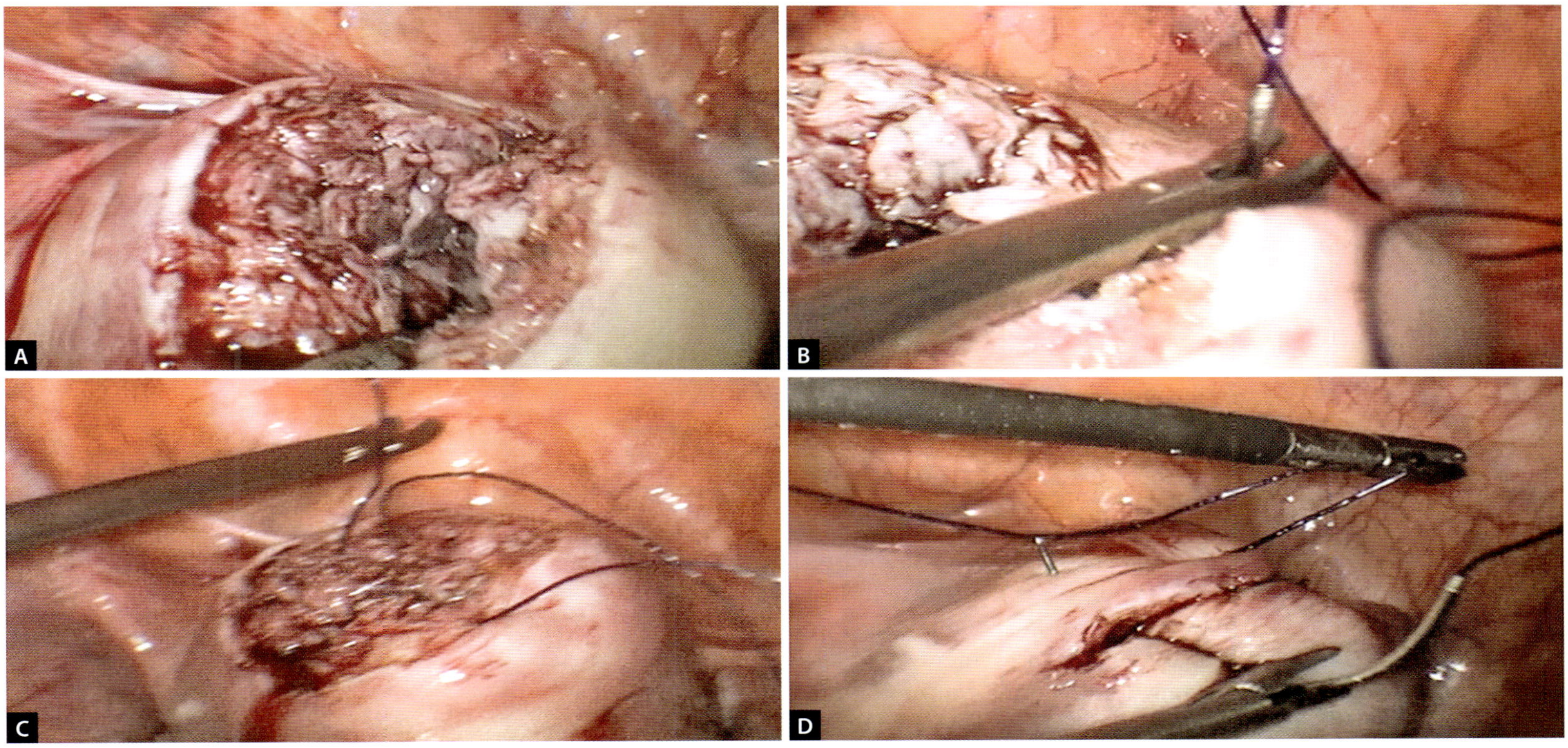

Figs. 23A to D: Suturing—continuous nonlocking with barbed sutures. (A) Myoma bed after complete enucleation; (B) Holding the needle with needle holder. Note the angle at which needle is held; (B and C) First layer sutured using barbed sutures in continuous nonlocking manner; and (D) Second layer suturing in similar manner. Approximation of edges is very important.

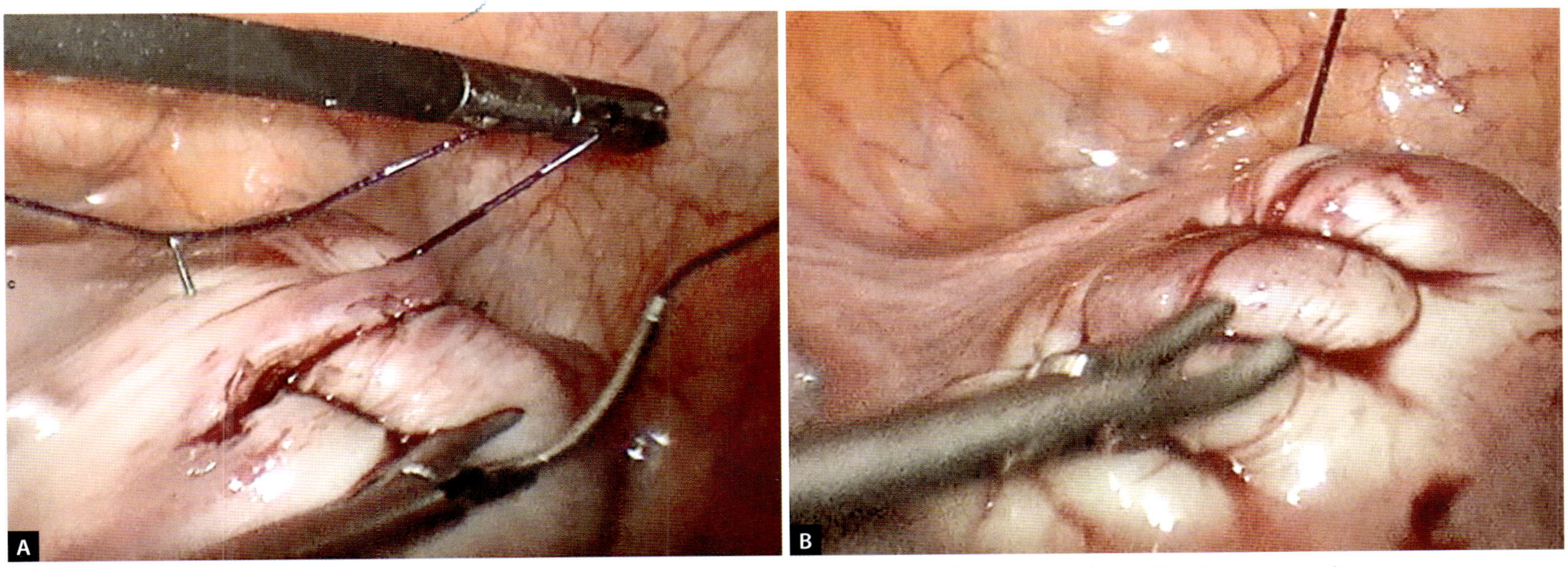

Figs. 24A and B: Final step of suturing. (A) Going beyond the angles of suture line. Note the depth of the bite taken; and (B) Suture line after completing second layer closure. Note the proper approximation of edges and the final bite should go beyond the angle of incision line.

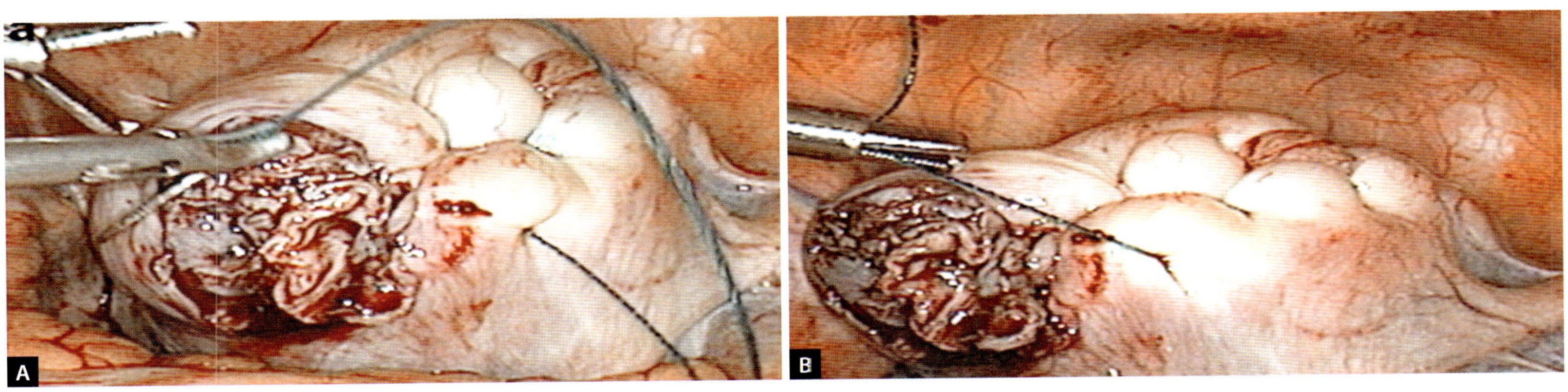

Figs. 25A and B

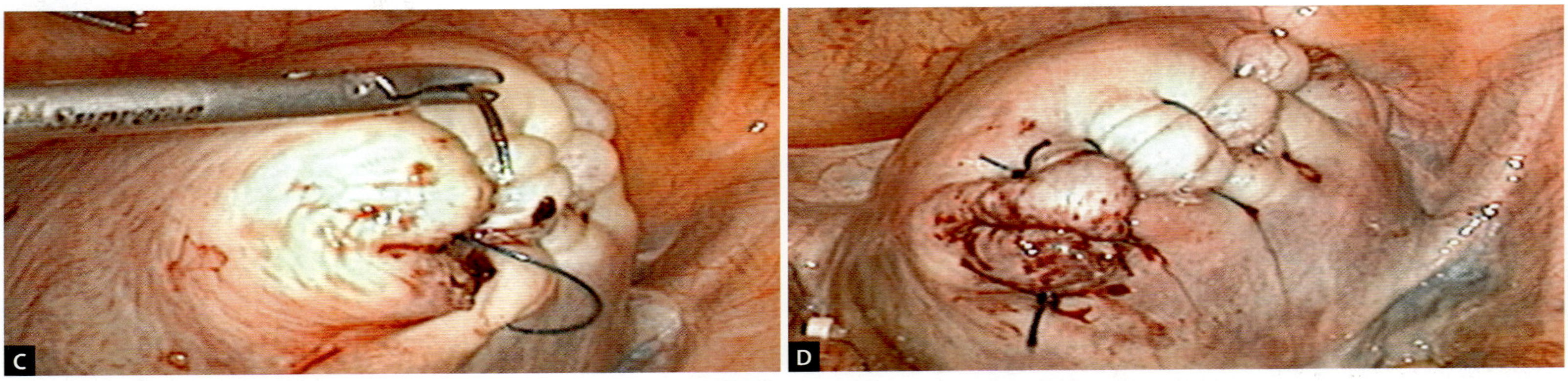

Figs. 25C and D

Figs. 25A to D: Baseball suturing.

Barbed suture **(*Fig. 26*)**: An innovation in suture design.

The bidirectional barb sutures were first introduced in 2007 in United States (Angiotech Pharmaceuticals). The material is polydioxanone, nylon or polypropylene, but it is the suture design that makes it revolutionary. This suture consists of standard suture material with tiny barbs cut into the length of filament **(Fig. 26)** in a helical array set facing in opposite directions from midpoint with a needle at each end. This allows tissues to be reapproximated without need of tying a surgical knot. It has had a profound impact on laparoscopic suturing, especially in laparoscopic myomectomies.

The tension on the suture material is evenly distributed across the length of suture rather than only on the ends at the knot. Unidirectional barbed sutures are also available **(Fig. 27)**.

In minimally invasive surgery, especially laparoscopic myomectomy, the ability to perform suturing quickly and properly is a challenge. In cases where knot tying is difficult, the use of barbed suture can approximate the tissues compactly with less time and with even distribution of tension.[9]

In the author's own experience, the use of barbed suture is very valuable especially when dealing with large myomas, where the suturing time is crucial. Also hemostasis obtained is much better than traditional sutures.[10]

The V-LOC suture by Covidien, introduced in 2009, is a unidirectional barbed suture with a loop at one end for facilitated fixation **(Fig. 28)**. This suture also makes suturing easy and fast.

The Stratafix by Ethicon-Endosurgery is also available.

The adhesion formation with barbed suture in animal studies has not been found to be different in comparison to standard suture materials.[11]

Significantly faster closure time in myomectomy with barbed suture has been seen in several in vivo studies now.[12]

Pregnancy outcomes are also comparable following suturing with barbed suture when compared with standard suture.[13]

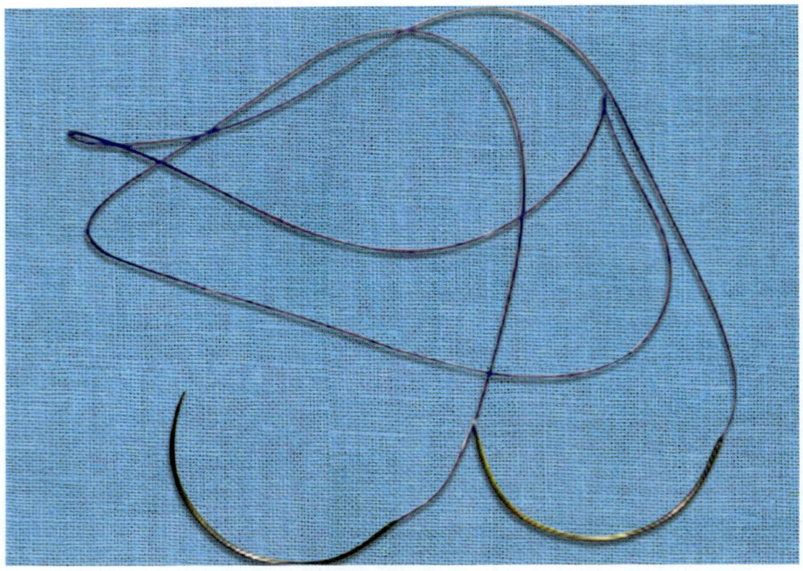

Fig. 26: Bidirectional barb suture.

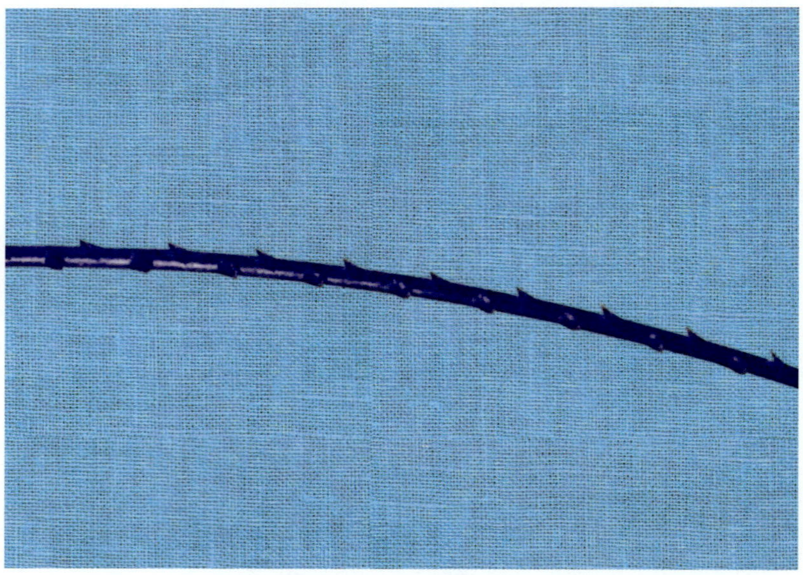

Fig. 27: Unidirectional barb suture loaded on a single needle.

Extraction

Various methods are possible for extraction of myomas:

- Standard electromechanical power morcellation
- Via posterior colpotomy
- Via Endoknife—appropriate for small myoma < 2–4 cm in diameter
- Contained morcellation in isolation bags
- Via minilaparotomy

Standard electromechanical morcellation: This was first introduced in 1993 to improve speed and ease of tissue extraction without the need of laparotomy.

Standard morcellation involves extension of the port size to 12–15 mm and guiding the morcellator under vision **(Figs. 16 and 29)**. It is recommended to activate the blade of the morcellator inside a trocar with an oblique end so that simple traction on the myoma peels it like an "orange" without small fragments. "Swiss cheese" effect should be avoided as this leads to fragmentation.

The technique has potential for vascular and visceral injury and has to be performed under strict visual guidance and control. Concern regarding the power morcellation is further discussed in the upcoming sections below **(Figs. 30A to D)**.

Contained morcellation: 1 in 400 females undergoing surgery of myomas are at risk of having a leiomyosarcoma (American Cancer Society).

5-year survival for leiomyosarcoma is poor as seen from the data:

- Stage I: 60%
- Stage II: 35%
- Stage III: 22%
- Stage IV: 15%

Several studies have reported an increase in recurrence rate and decrease in rate of survival following morcellation which results in upstaging of disease. So, the methods of bag morcellation, minilaparotomy, and colpotomy are proposed to overcome this problem. For larger specimens a minilaparotomy with or without use of self-retaining retractors is advised.

In April 2014, Food and Drug Administration (FDA) issued a warning about power morcellation, concerning morcellation of unsuspected leiomyosarcomas.

According to American Association of Gynecologic Laparoscopists (AAGL) most females with uterine cancer can be diagnosed prior to surgery. 1 in 400 to 1 in 1000 females undergoing myomectomy will have uterine leiomyosarcoma, prognosis of these females is unusually poor and may be worsened in setting of power morcellation.

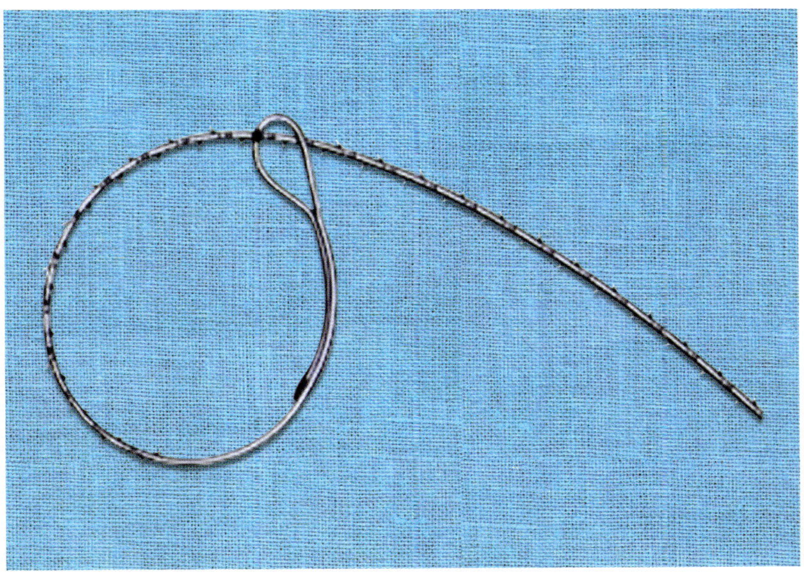

Fig. 28: V-Loc by Covidien.

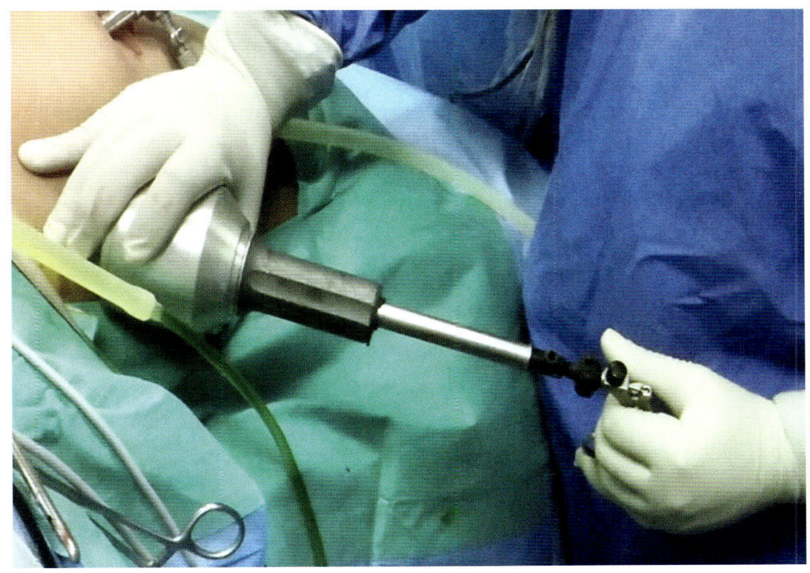

Fig. 29: Outside view of standard morcellator assembled and ready for morcellation.

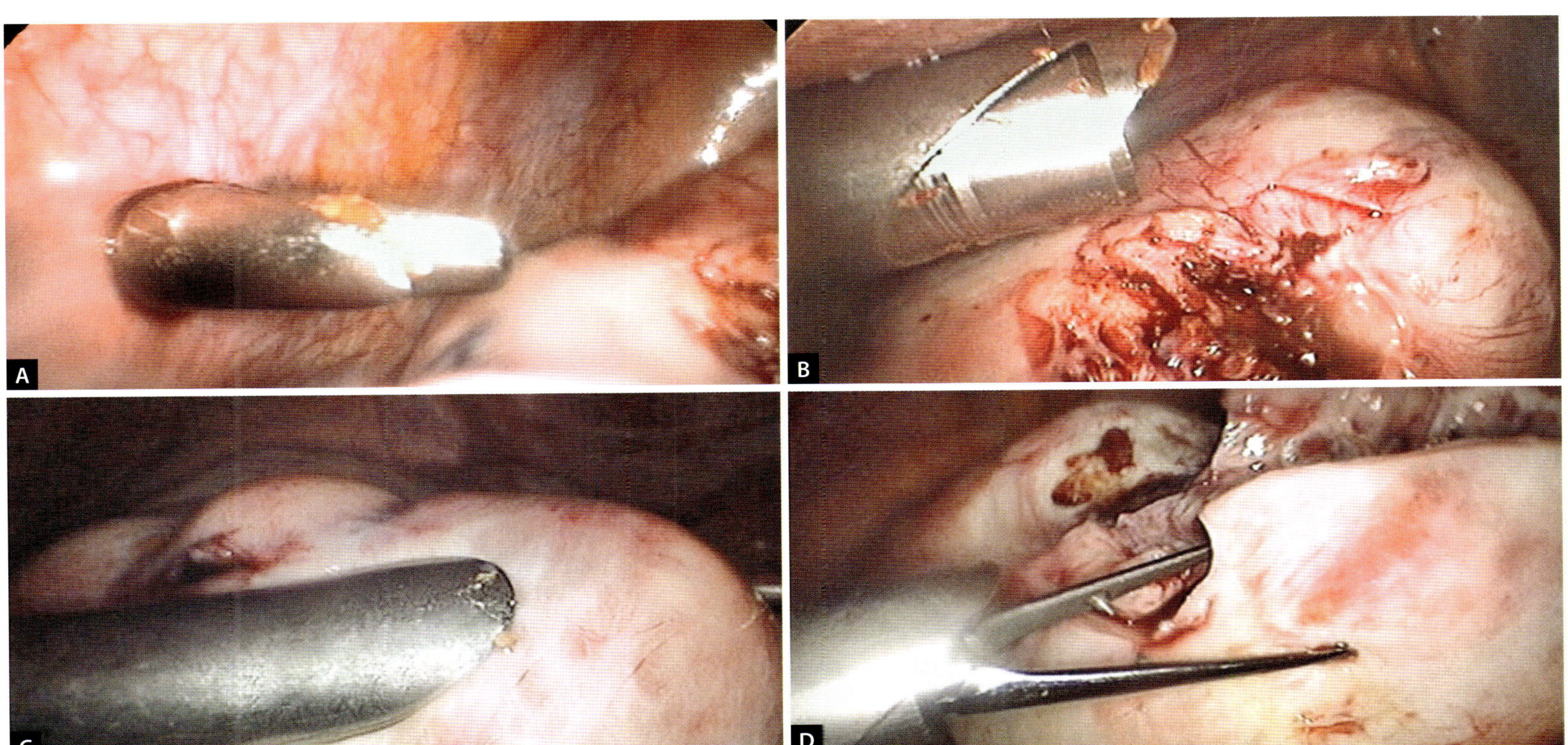

Figs. 30A to D: Laparoscopic view of morcellation. (A) 12 mm trocar inserted; (B) Outer sheath with rotating inner blade; and (C and D) Morcellation in process.

Steps of in-bag morcellation **(Figs. 31A and B)**: In-bag morcellation seems to be a viable alternative to open power morcellation and offers the advantage of no spillage of tissues or fluids during morcellation.[14]

This technique involves the placement of the specimen into a large plastic bag within abdomen, exteriorizing the opening of the bag, insufflating the bag within the peritoneal cavity and then using the power morcellator within the bag to remove the specimen in a contained manner.

A recent study from January 2013 to April 2014 which included 73 patients, concluded this as a feasible technique. Methods of morcellating uterine tissue in a contained manner may provide an option to minimize the risks of open power morcellation while preserving the benefits of minimally invasive surgery (level of evidence II).[15]

In the author's own personal experience, this method, once a couple of cases are performed, is fairly easy to perform and the author has morcellated specimens up to 2.3 kg with relative ease and without spill.

In addition to the risk involved to viscera and vessels, there has been concern for tissue dissemination. Retrospective studies show that disseminated parasitic myomas occur in 0.1–1% of cases with power morcellation.[16,17] The use of contained morcellation is likely to substantially reduce this particular complication.

Description of technique: The isolation bag **(Fig. 32)** is available in various sizes. The average size of large bag may be as big as 50 × 50 cm. The basic steps are illustrated in the following steps:

First step involves folding the bag in an accordion style and the air is compressed out of it **(Fig. 33)**. This folded bag is then placed inside the plastic trocar sleeve which holds the folded bag completely along its length and this trocar is now introduced through the side port being used for the morcellation **(Fig. 34)**.

After being completely pushed in the peritoneal cavity the plastic sleeve is withdrawn **(Fig. 35)** and the bag is spread inside in such manner that it gets unfolded by a coordinated action of the surgeon and his assistant **(Fig. 36)**.

- The closed base of the bag is placed snugly at the pouch of Douglas and the bag is opened wide with the instruments of the surgeon and assistant ports.
- Next, the parked specimen (usually right upper quadrant) is grasped and placed into the bag **(Figs. 37A and B)**.

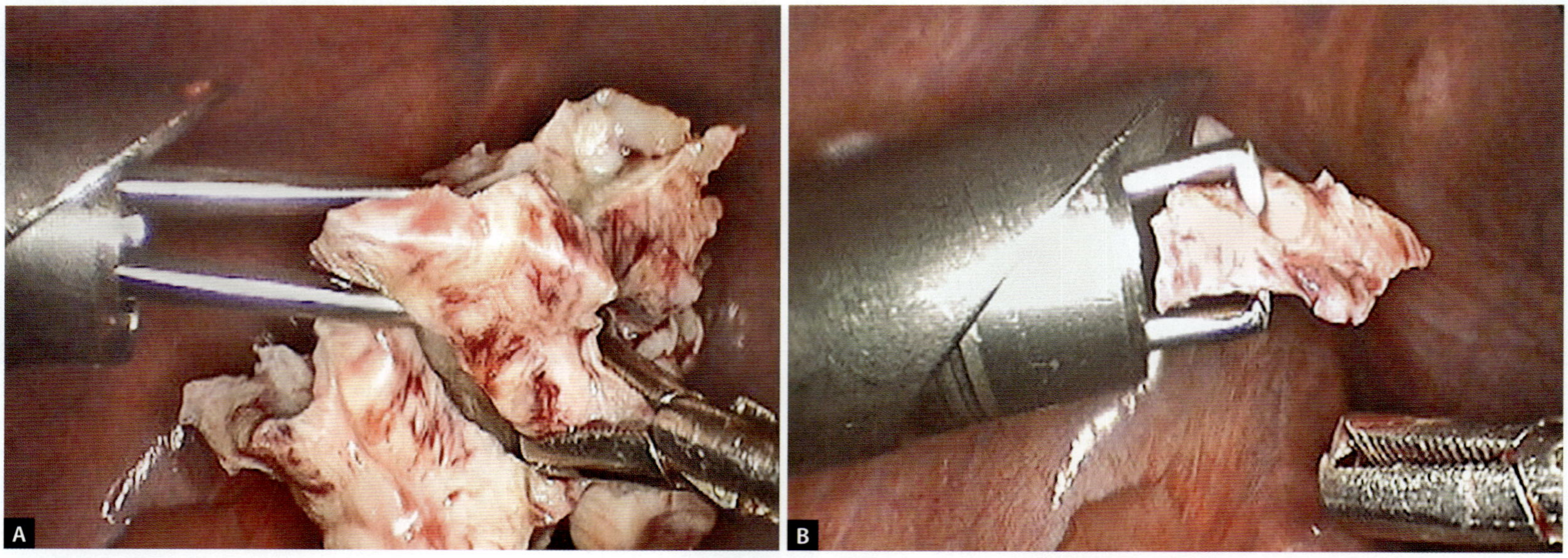

Figs. 31A and B: Final steps of morcellation.

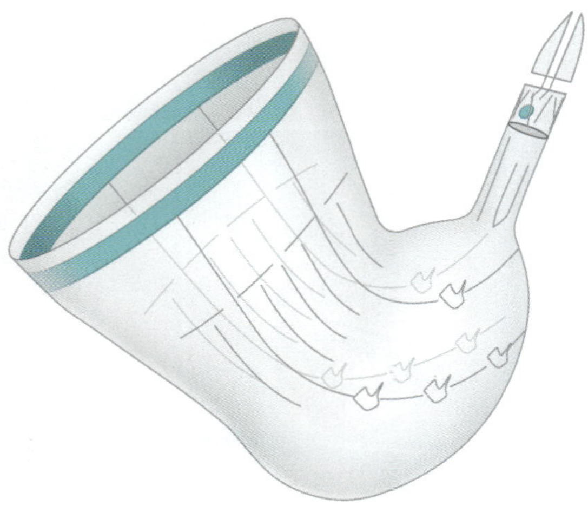

Fig. 32: MorSafe—Endobag.

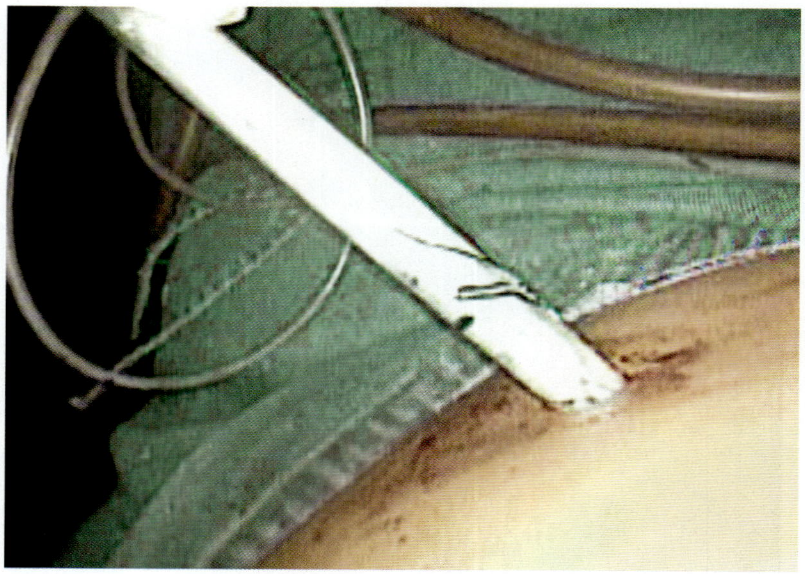

Fig. 33: Rolled bag placed inside sleeve.

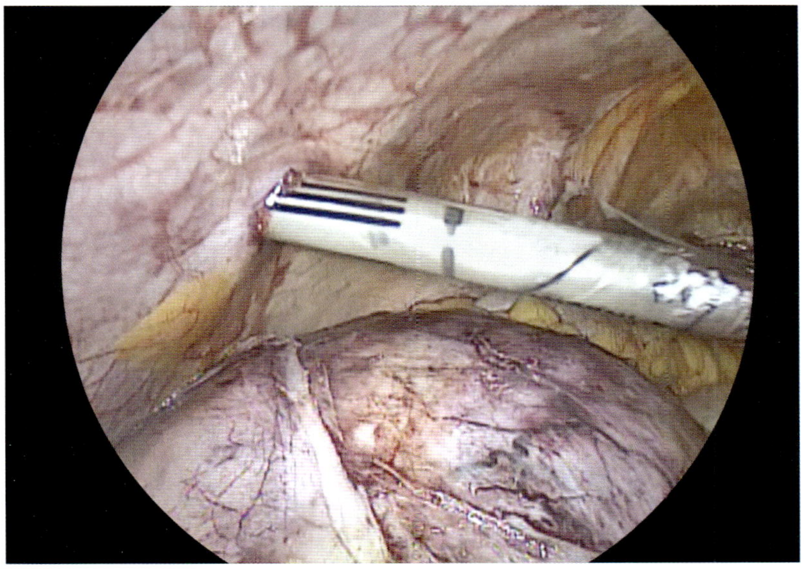

Fig. 34: Inside view of bag in the sleeve.

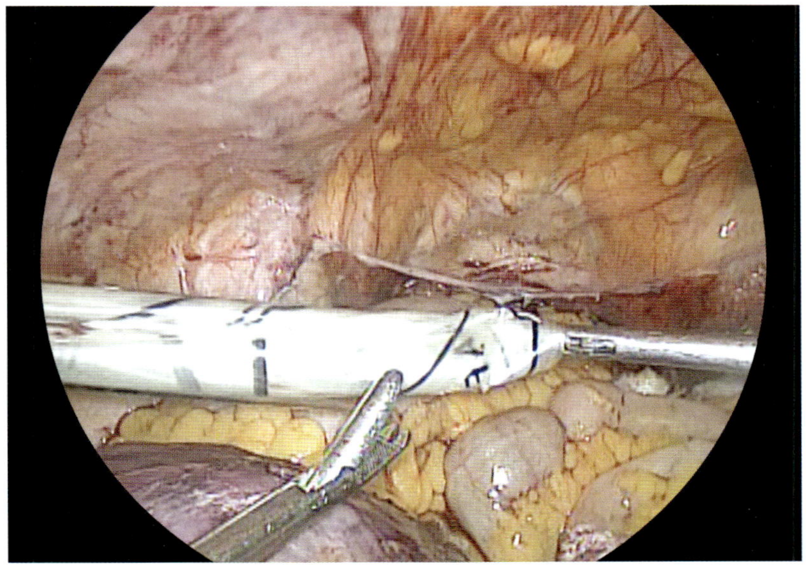

Fig. 35: Sleeve is withdrawn and bag retained in.

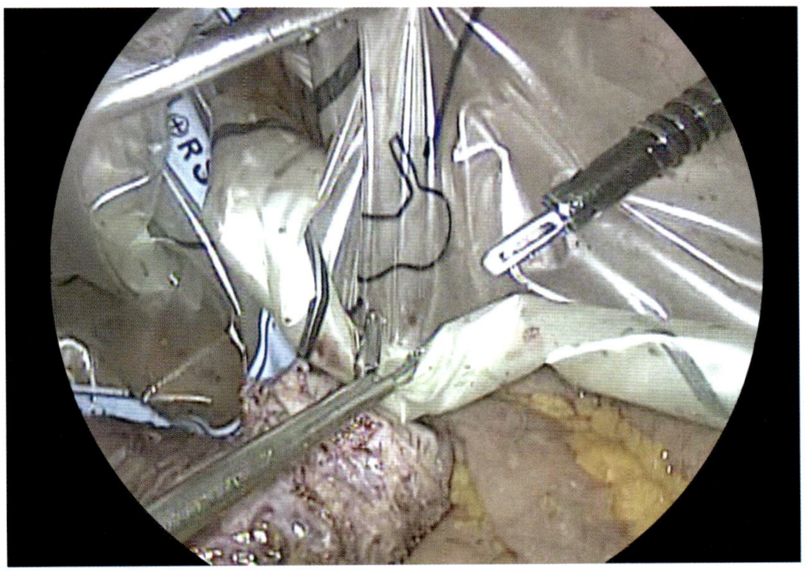

Fig. 36: Unrolling the bag.

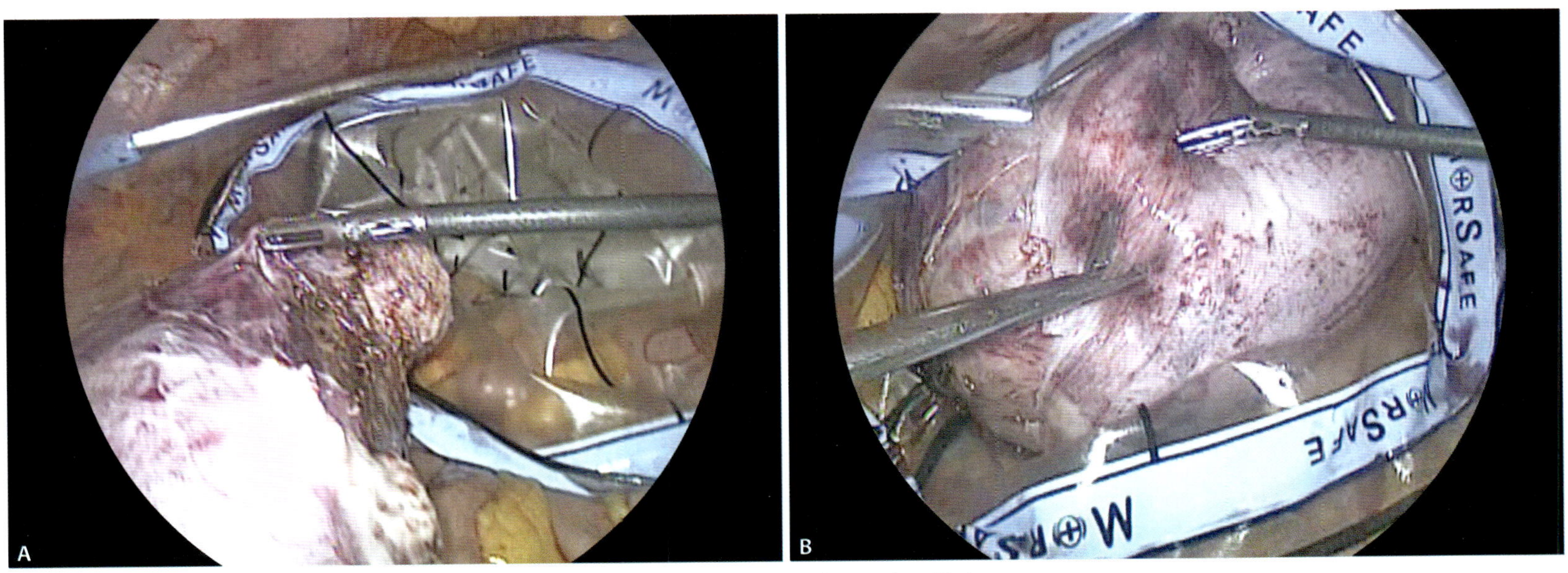

Figs. 37A and B: Specimen being placed in bag.

- Next, the rim of the bag is railroaded out through morcellator port then the morcellator port and the base is resealed so that gas does not leak out **(Fig. 38)**.
- The bag has other additional sleeve which is used for passing the optical trocar with the gas connection. This sleeve is now railroaded out through the optical (11 mm) port **(Fig. 39)**.
- The sleeve is opened with a small nick and the optical trocar with the scope is introduced inside the bag and the pneumoperitoneum created within the bag **(Fig. 40)**.
- Once the bag pneumoperitoneum is established, the morcellator is introduced under the vision and entire specimen is morcellated within bag and railroaded out ensuring no spill and also safety to neighboring viscera and vessels **(Figs. 41 to 44)**.

Via minilaparotomy: This is a safe and effective minimally invasive alternative to laparoscopic myomectomy. Further advantages are that it allows for the freedom to additionally palpate the uterus and also effectively close it in three layers. This makes the technique very important for those surgeons with limited suturing skills **(Figs. 45 and 46)**.

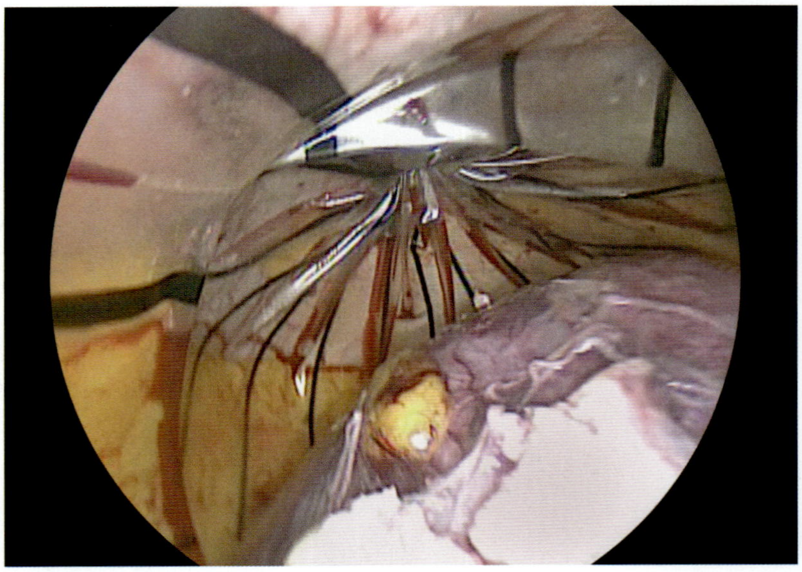

Fig. 40: Establishment of pneumoperitoneum in the bag via the extension end.

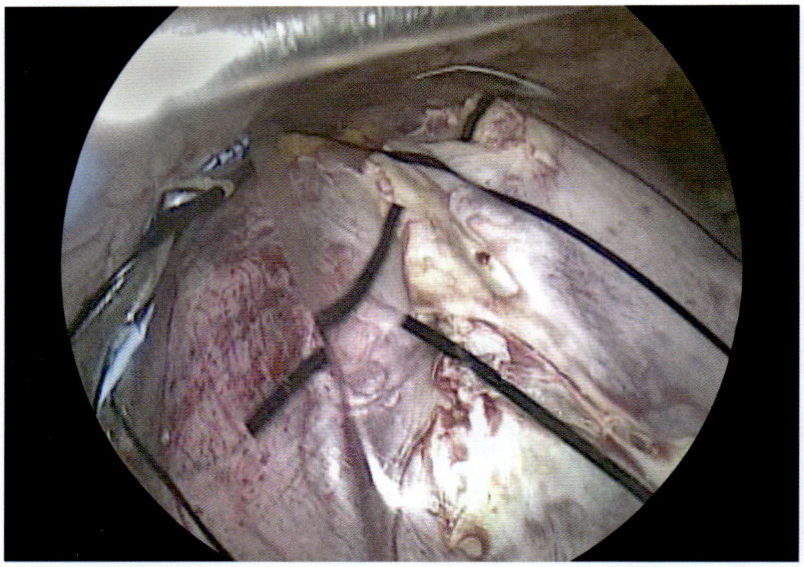

Fig. 38: The bag's edges being taken out of morcellator port (with the specimen inside).

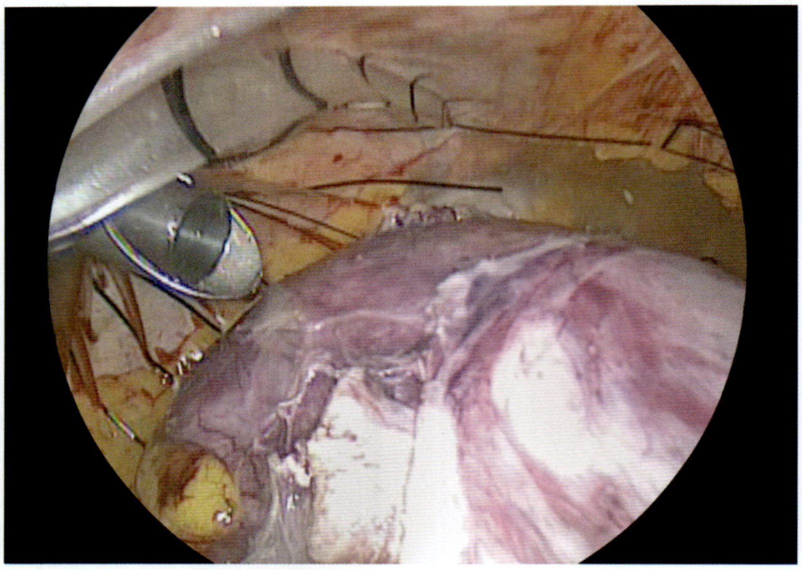

Fig. 41: Morcellator—introduced in bag.

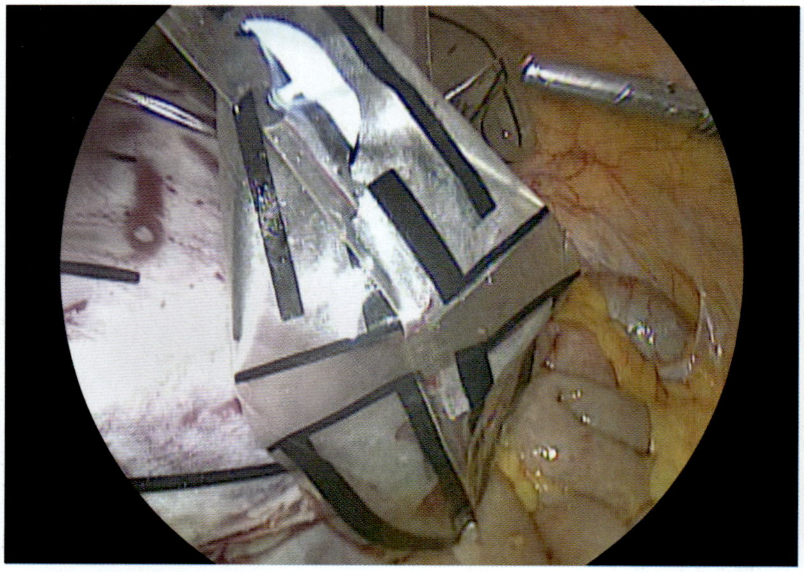

Fig. 39: Identifying tail end and railroading it out of primary port.

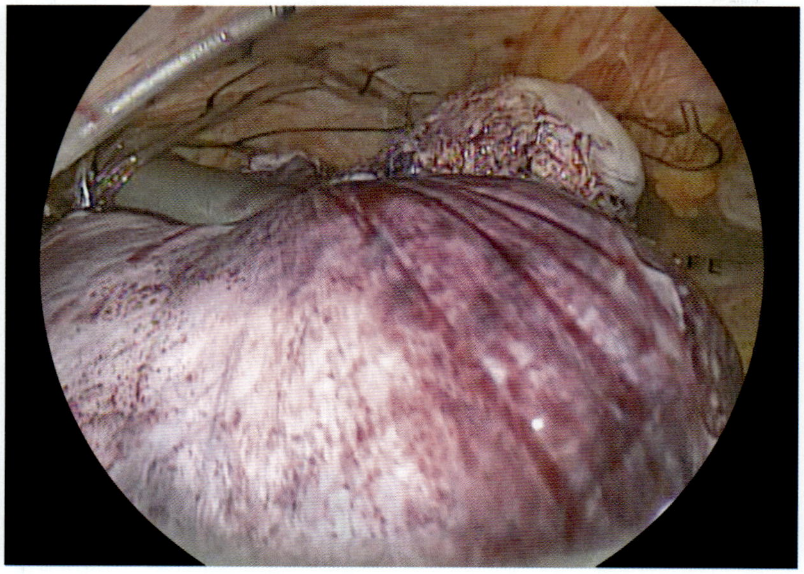

Fig. 42: Morcellation being carried out.

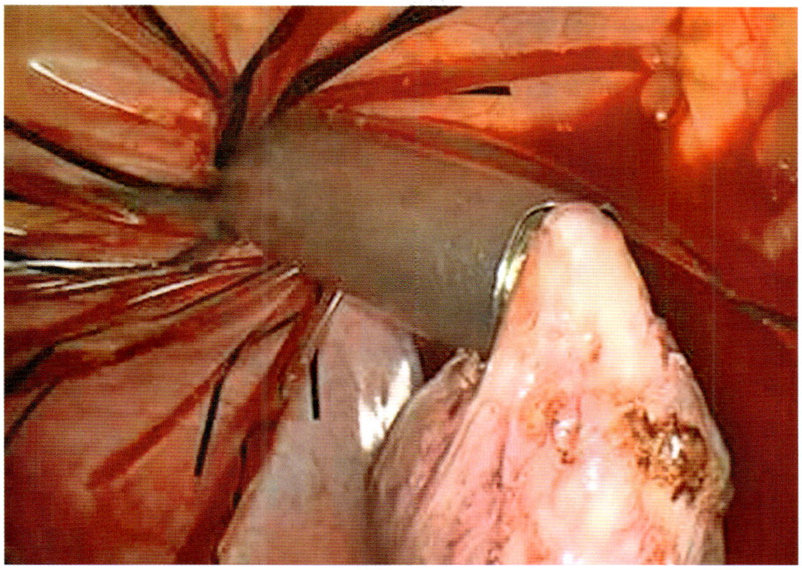

Fig. 43: Morcellation in bag is in progress.

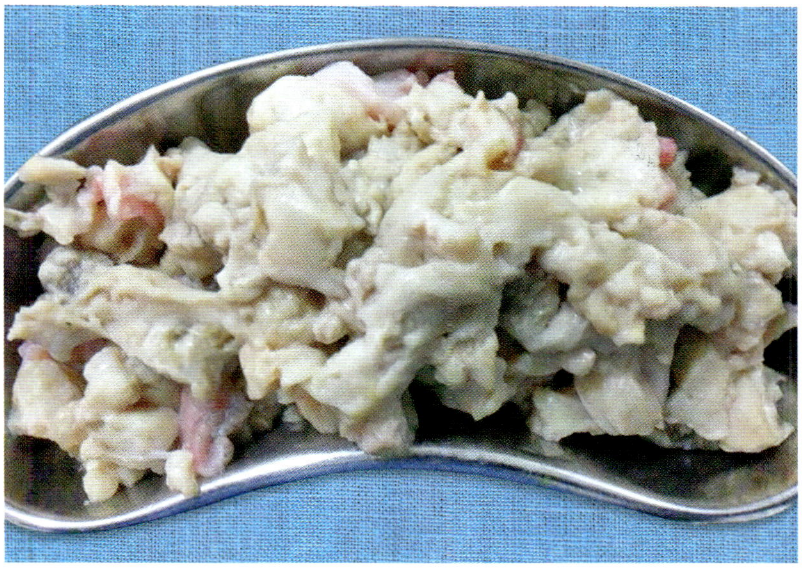

Fig. 45: Myoma strips after complete morcellation.

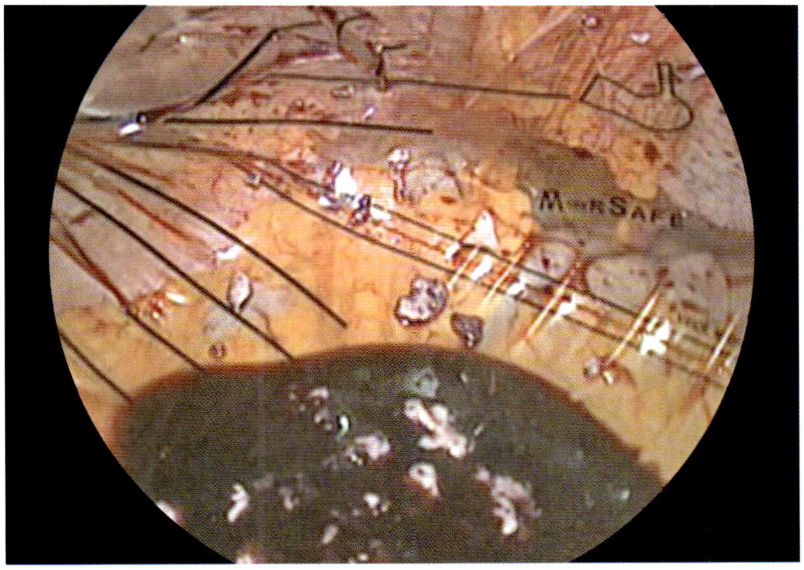

Fig. 44: The entire blood and small fragments of myoma collect at base of bag.

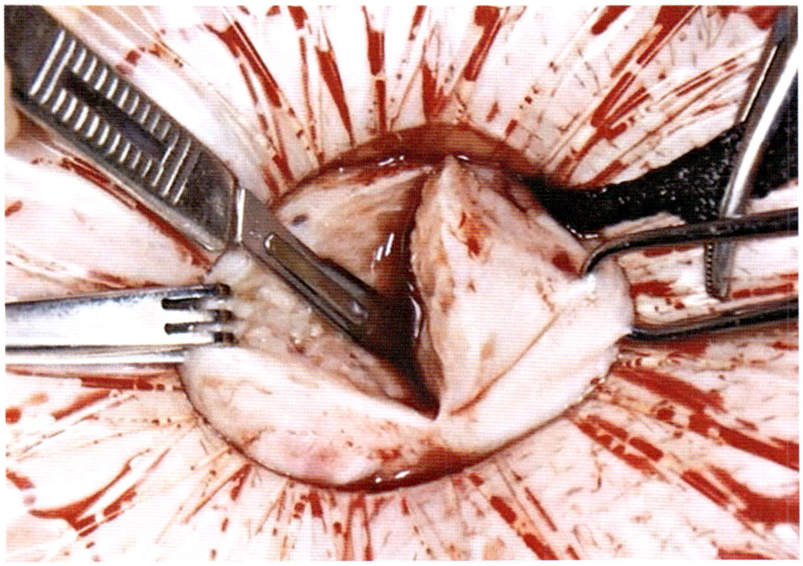

Fig. 46: Myoma morcellation in progress through minilap with ring retractor in place.

- Minilaparotomy incision may vary from 3 to 6 cm suprapubic transverse incision. This is adequately small and also cosmetic.
- The incision is taken 2–3 finger breadths above the symphysis pubis. The skin and subcutaneous tissue are incised horizontally till the level of fascia. Next the finger is used to dissect bluntly in the vertical direction, working up toward the umbilicus and down toward the pubis. The fascia is then opened in midline for about 6 cm. The rectus muscle is then separated at midline and peritoneum grasped and nicked vertically taking care not to injure the urinary bladder **(Figs. 47A1 to B2)**.
- Elastic abdominal retractors are now available which are then introduced **(Figs. 47 and 48A)** (e.g. Mobius retractors). The surgeon and assistant both work in coordinated manner to adjust the top and bottom rings so that they adjust firmly and snugly. Usually 2–3 twists of the retractor will give a round opening of ring size and keep the subcutaneous fat, muscle, peritoneum out of the way. This provides the room for removal by morcellation and also for repair of the hysterotomy. If the situation is found to be more complicated as in broad ligament myoma or inaccessible low posterior wall or cervical myoma, then the retractor is removed and incision is extended to conventional laparotomy.

The rules of myomectomy after this manner are same. The only difference is that contrary to laparoscopic myomectomy wherein multiple incisions are generally required for enucleating different myomas, here we may attempt the removal of multiple myomas through a single strategic incision and proceed as in the open method.

The myomas are morcellated using number 10/11 blade **(Fig. 48B)**. Thereafter, the entire uterus defect can be exteriorized for easy and compact suturing[18]

Posterior colpotomy: Posterior colpotomy allows for the large myomata to be extracted.[19] Some people have suggested that this approach may cause postoperative adhesions in colpotomy site.[20-22] A monopolar hook may be used or even a harmonic scalpel **(Fig. 49)** to create an incision in the posterior vagina **(Figs. 50 and 51)** over a colpotomizer through which the fibroid is extracted. This incision may be closed laparoscopically or vaginally **(Figs. 52 to 54)**. Some authors have also described the opening of the posterior fornix under direct vision by a 10–12 mm trocar introduced vaginally in the posterior fornix under laparoscopic vision.[23]

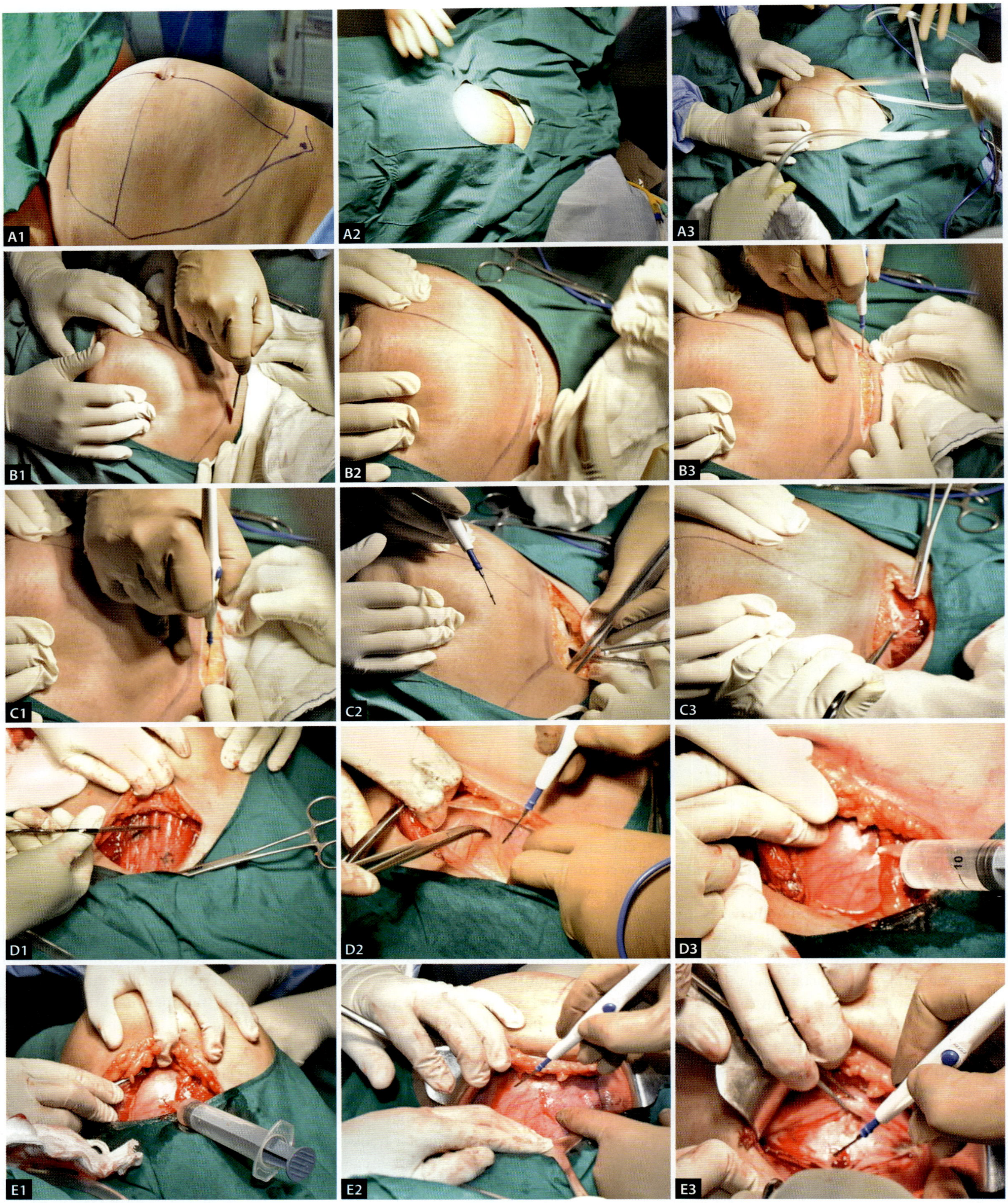

Figs. 47A1 to E3

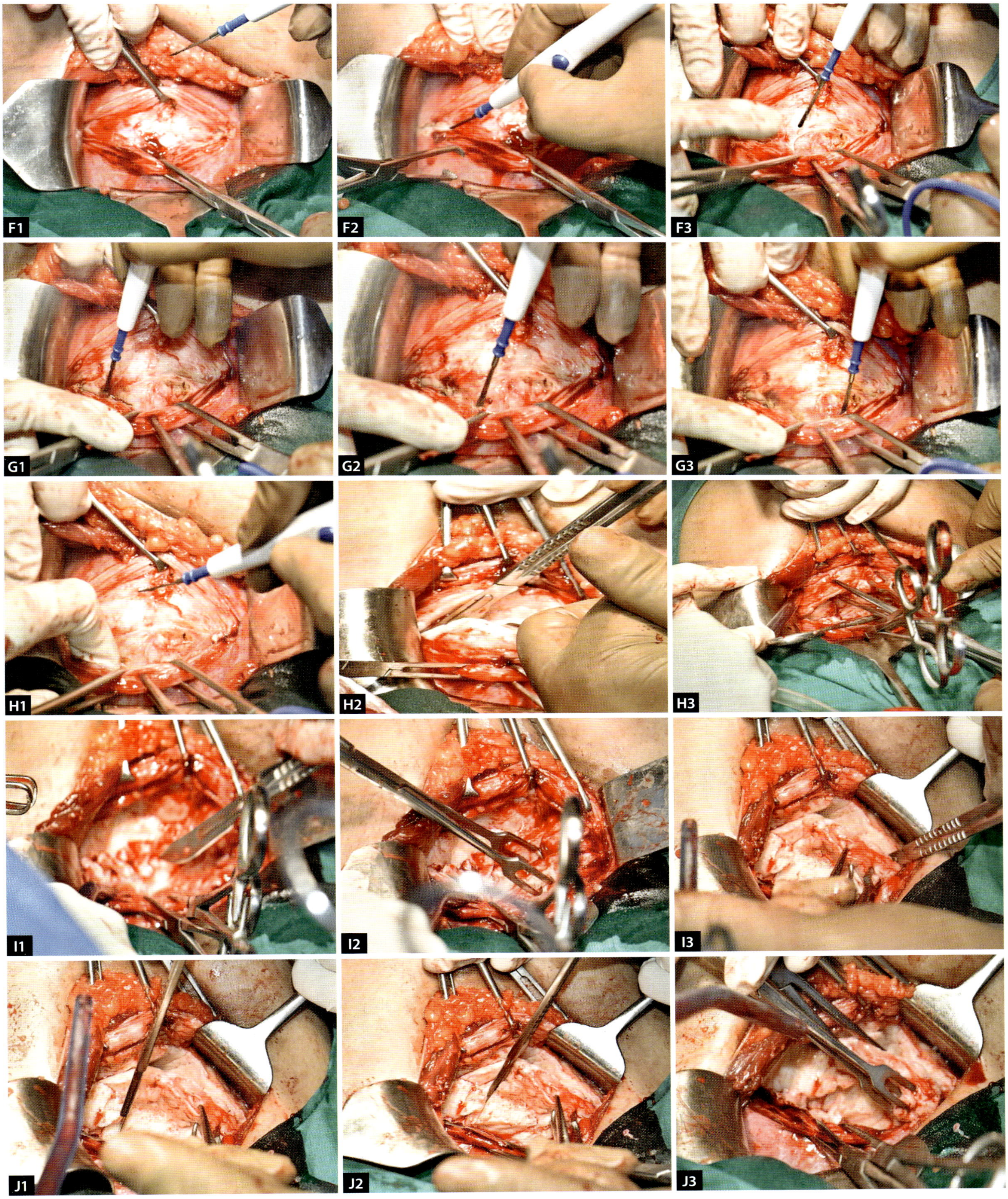

Figs. 47F1 to J3

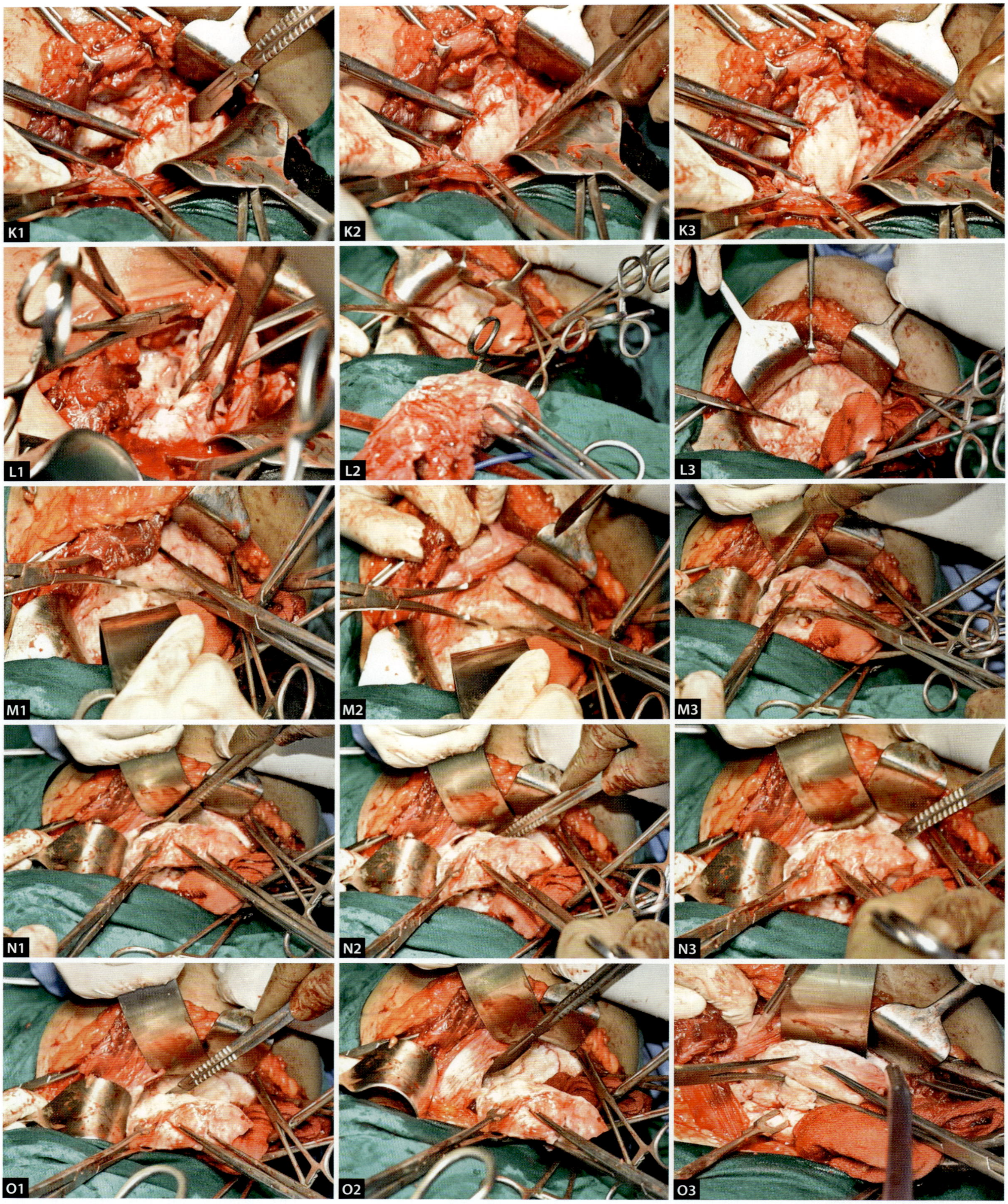

Figs. 47K1 to O3

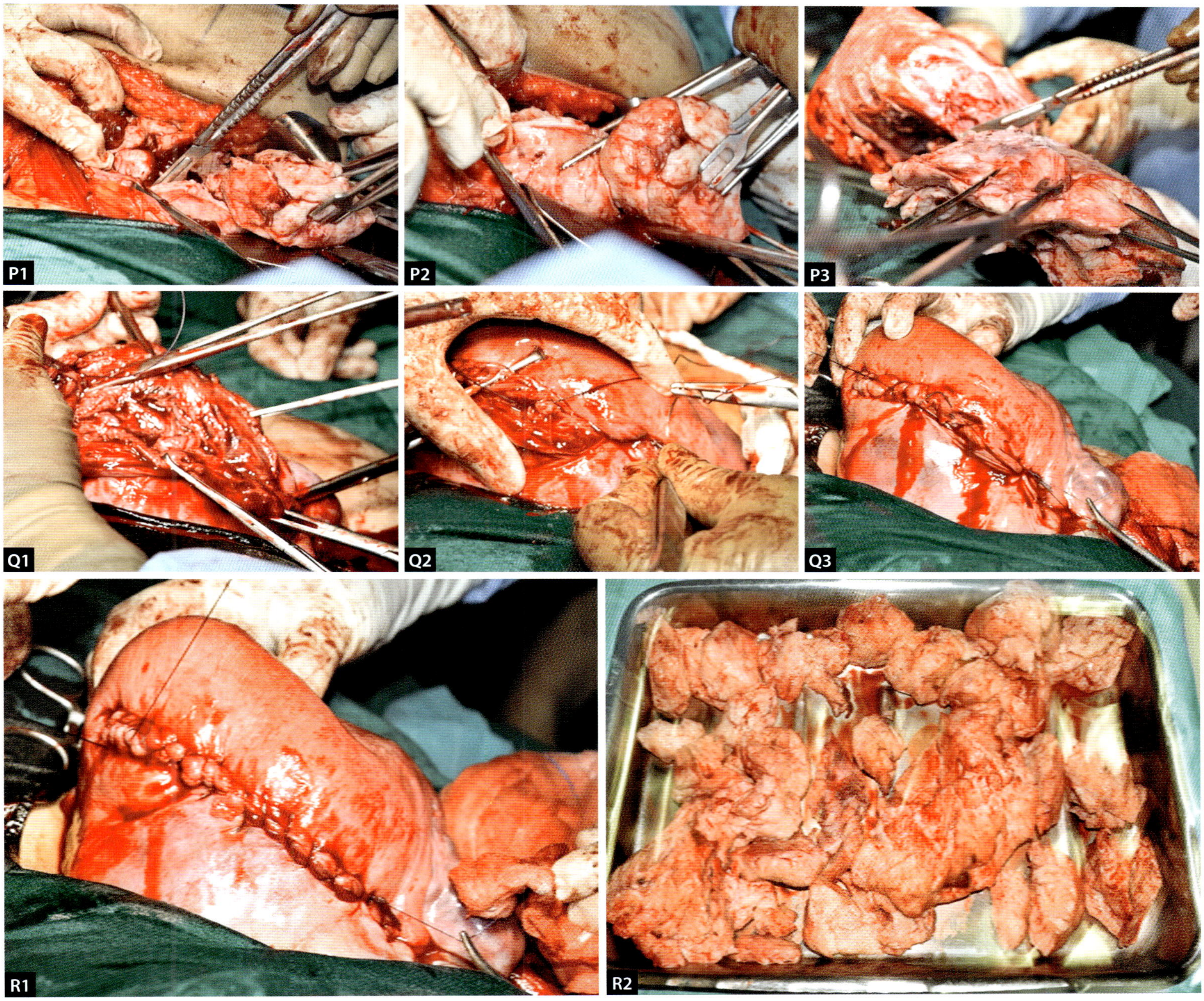

Figs. 47P1 to R2

Figs. 47A1 to R2: Steps of minilaparotomy. (A1 to A3) Planning of skin incision; (B1 to D2) Opening of abdomen in layers; (D3 to E1) Vasopressin infiltration; (E2 to I1) Incision over myoma; (I2 to P3) Laparoscopy-assisted enucleation of myoma; (Q1 to R1) Laparoscopy-assisted myoma bed suturing; and (R2) Morcellated myomectomy specimen.

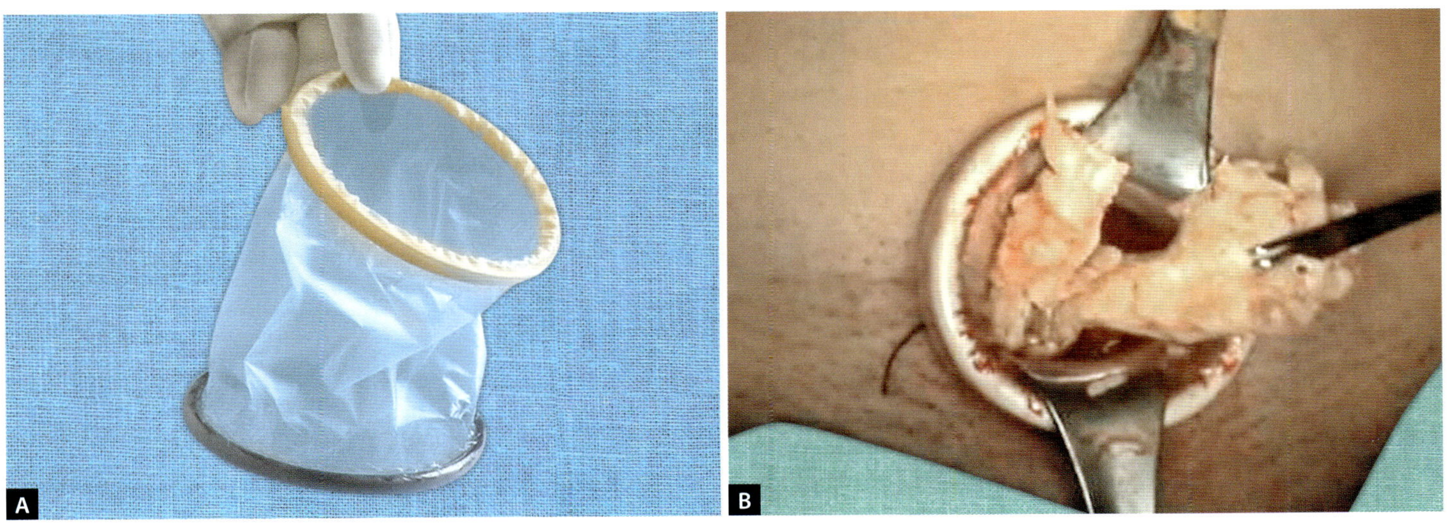

Figs. 48A and B: (A) Mobius retractor for minilap; and (B) Extraction of the myoma strips via minilap.

Colpotomy Retrieval

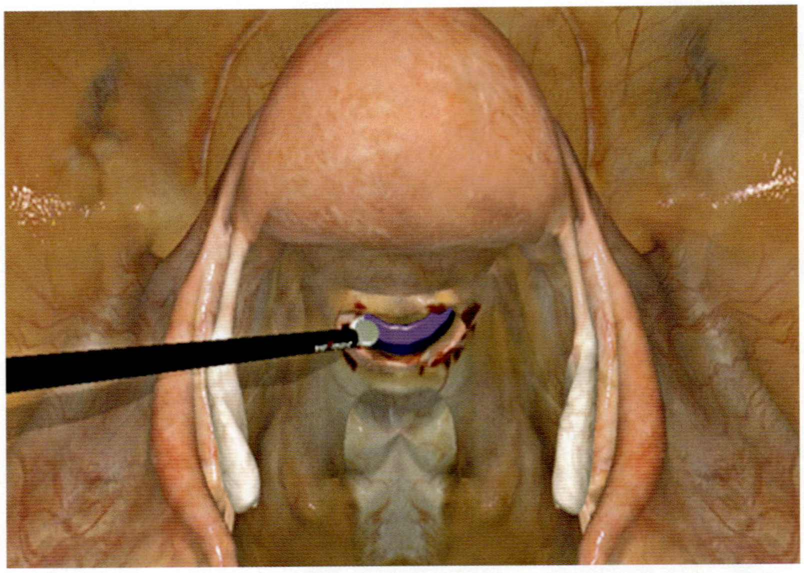

Fig. 49: Site of incision between uterosacral ligaments.

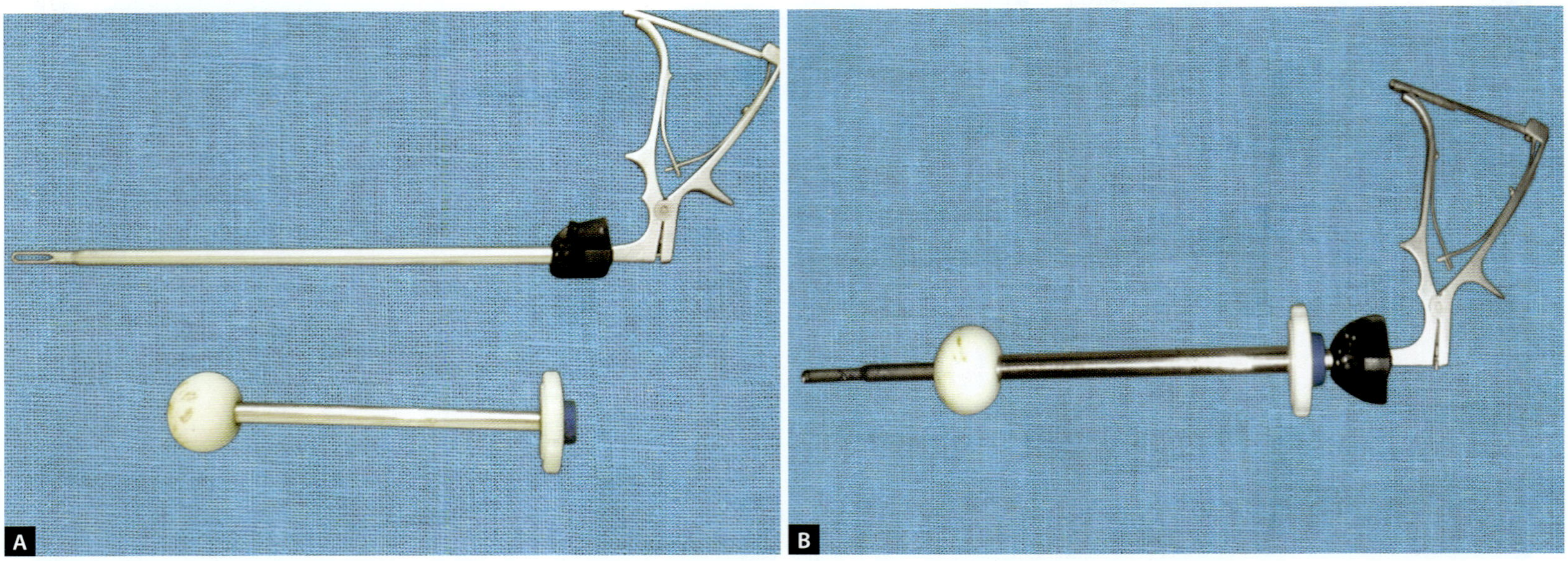

Figs. 50A and B: Vaginal colpotomizer with a claw forceps to catch fibroid in vivo.

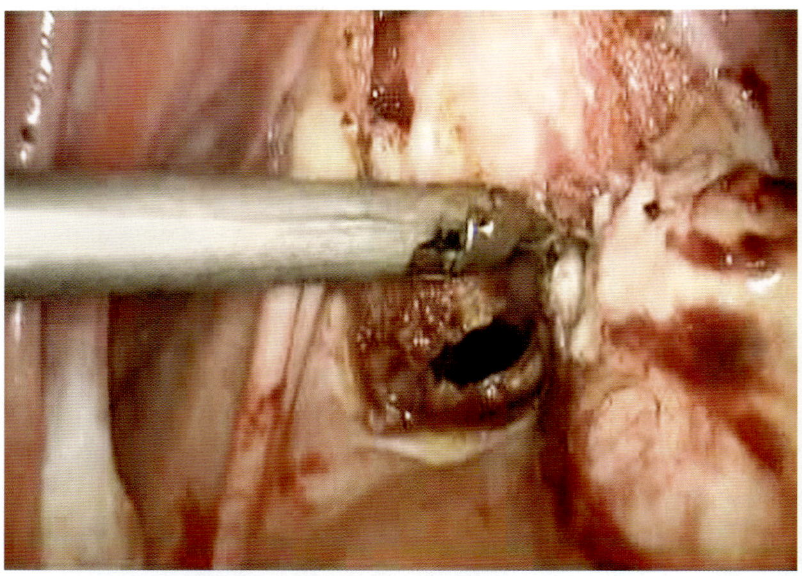

Fig. 51: Incision of colpotomy in laparoscopy.

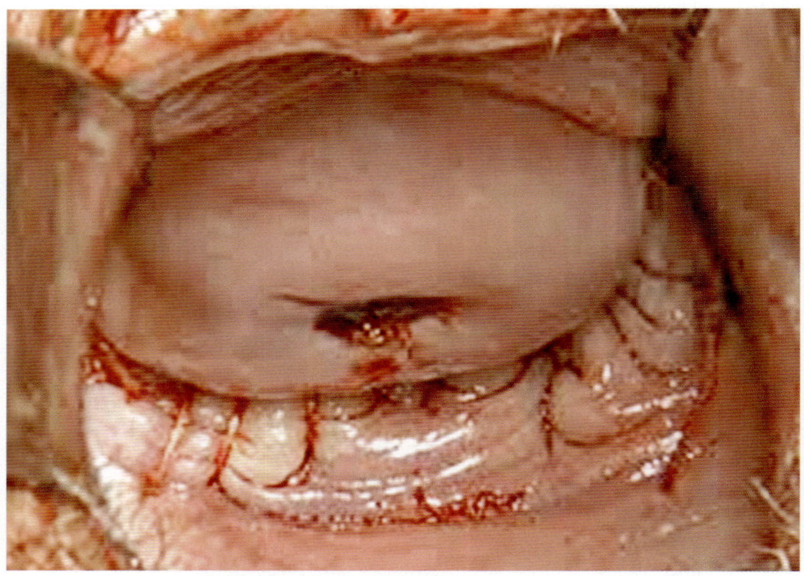

Fig. 52: Closure of colpotomy seen from vaginal view.

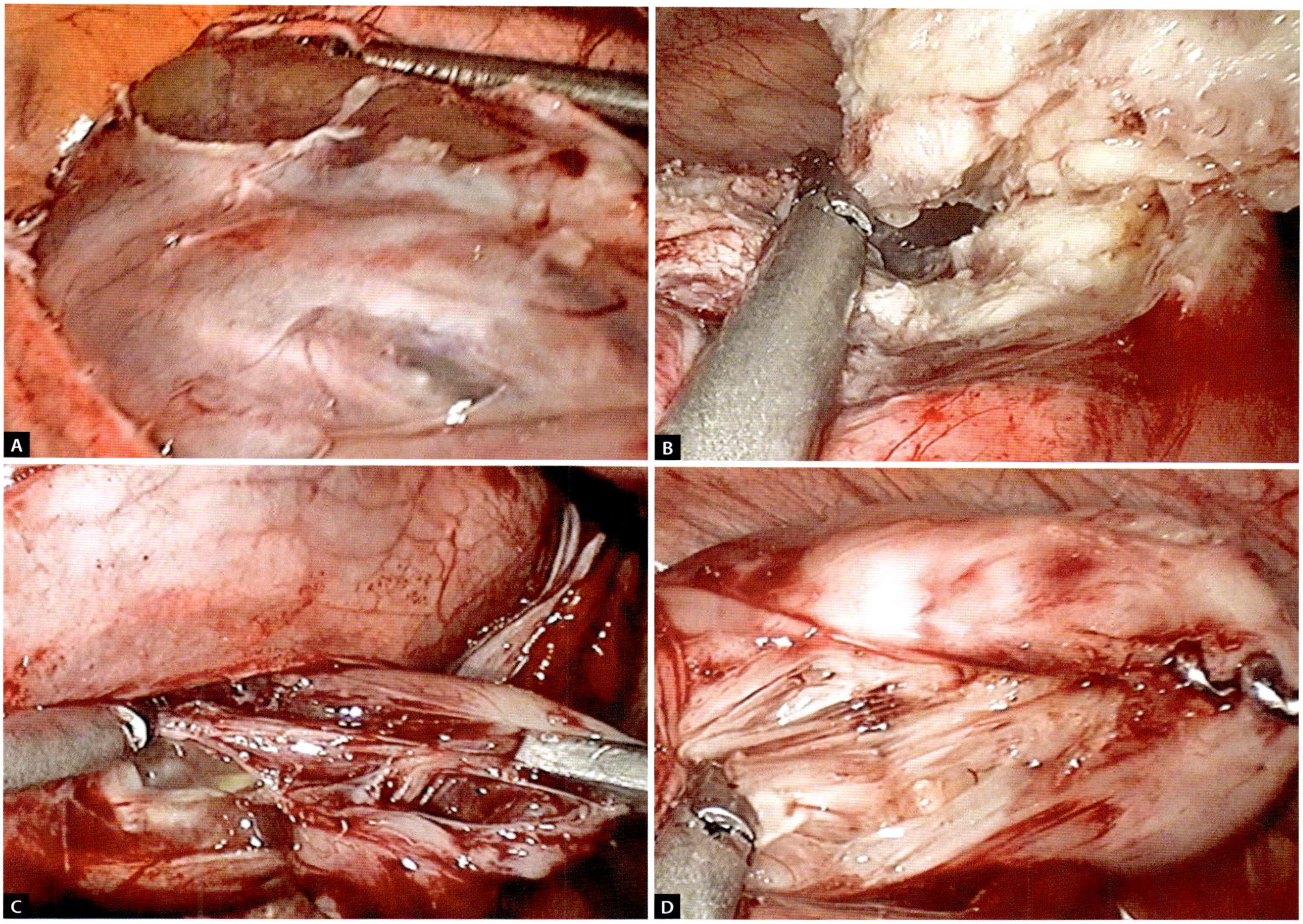

Figs. 53A to D: Difficult myoma excision in case of cystic degeneration of fibroid because of improper plane: piecemeal removal of degenerated fibroid. (A) Cystic degeneration of fibroid; (B and C) Piecemeal removal of fibroid using harmonic and myoma screw; and (D) Note the loss of plane between myoma and uterine myometrium, making enucleation difficult.

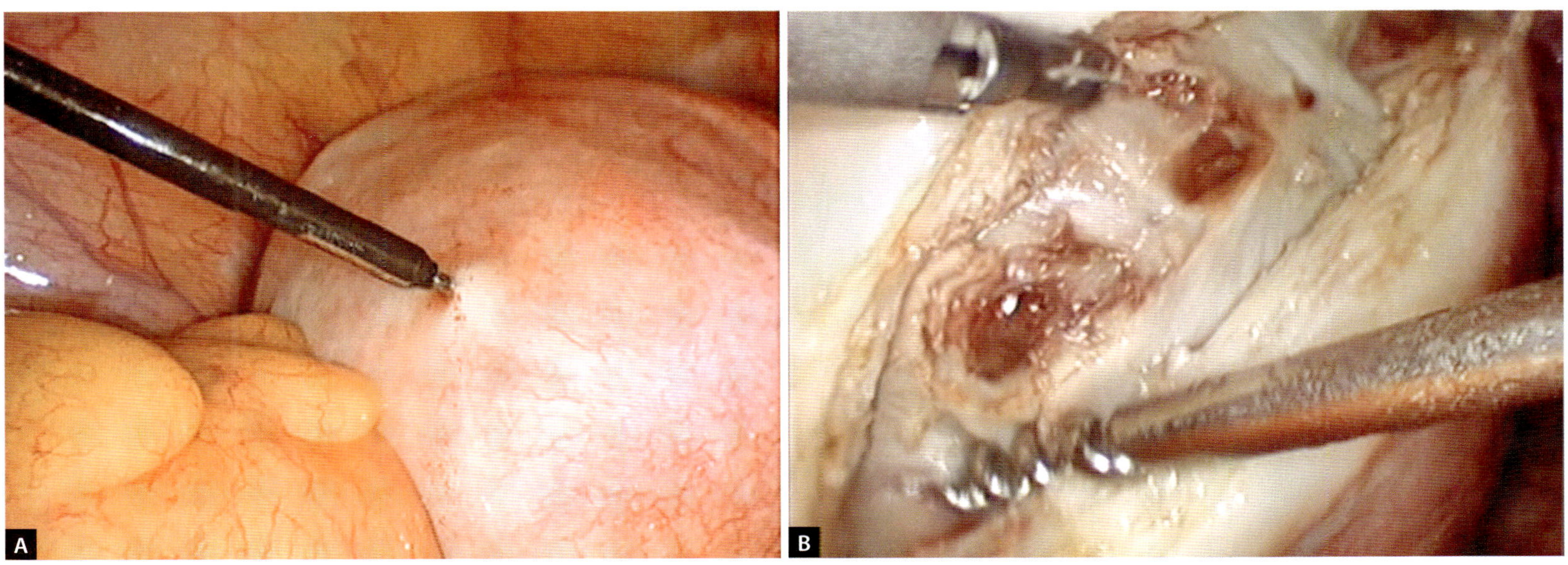

Figs. 54A and B

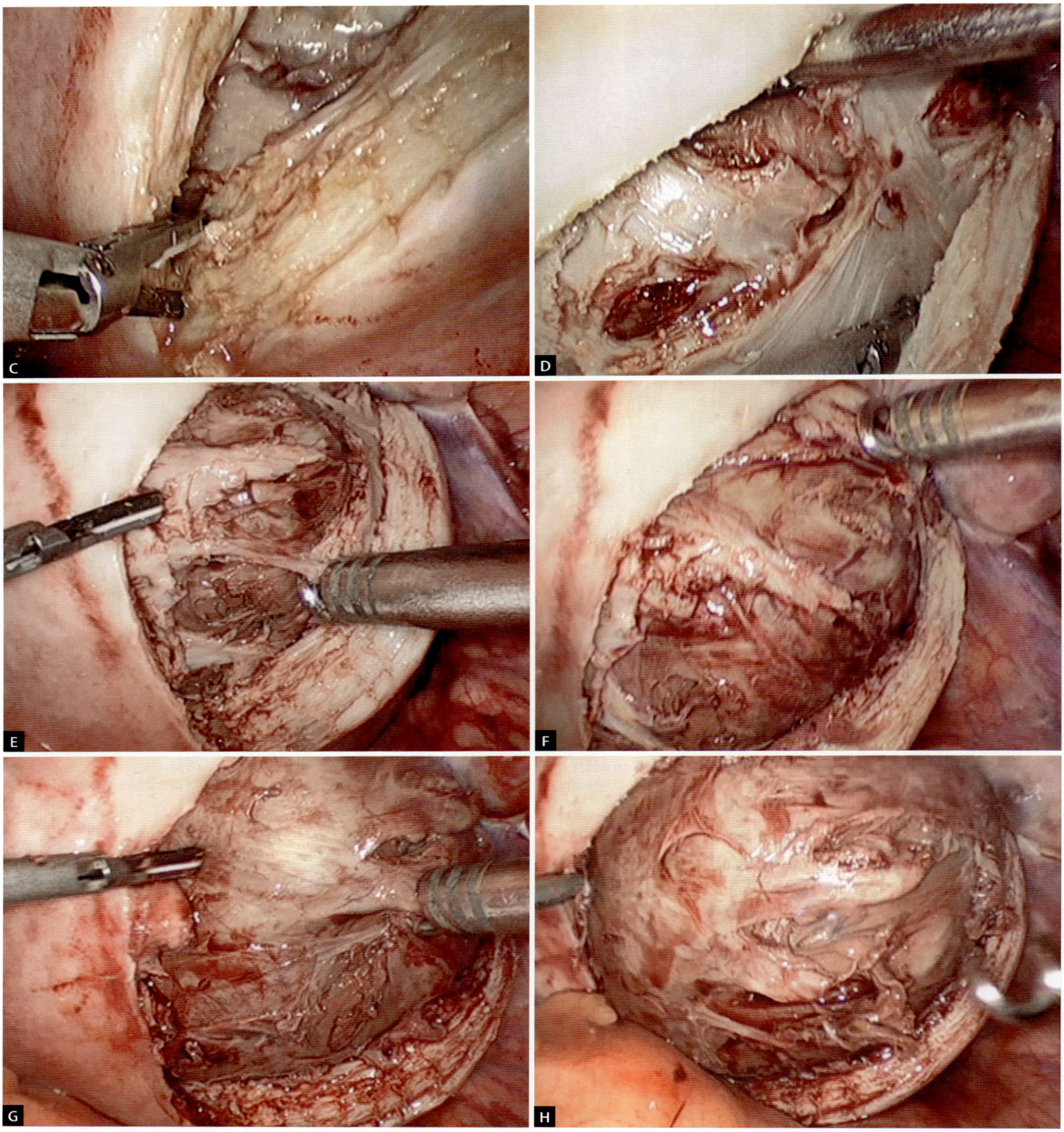

Figs. 54C to H

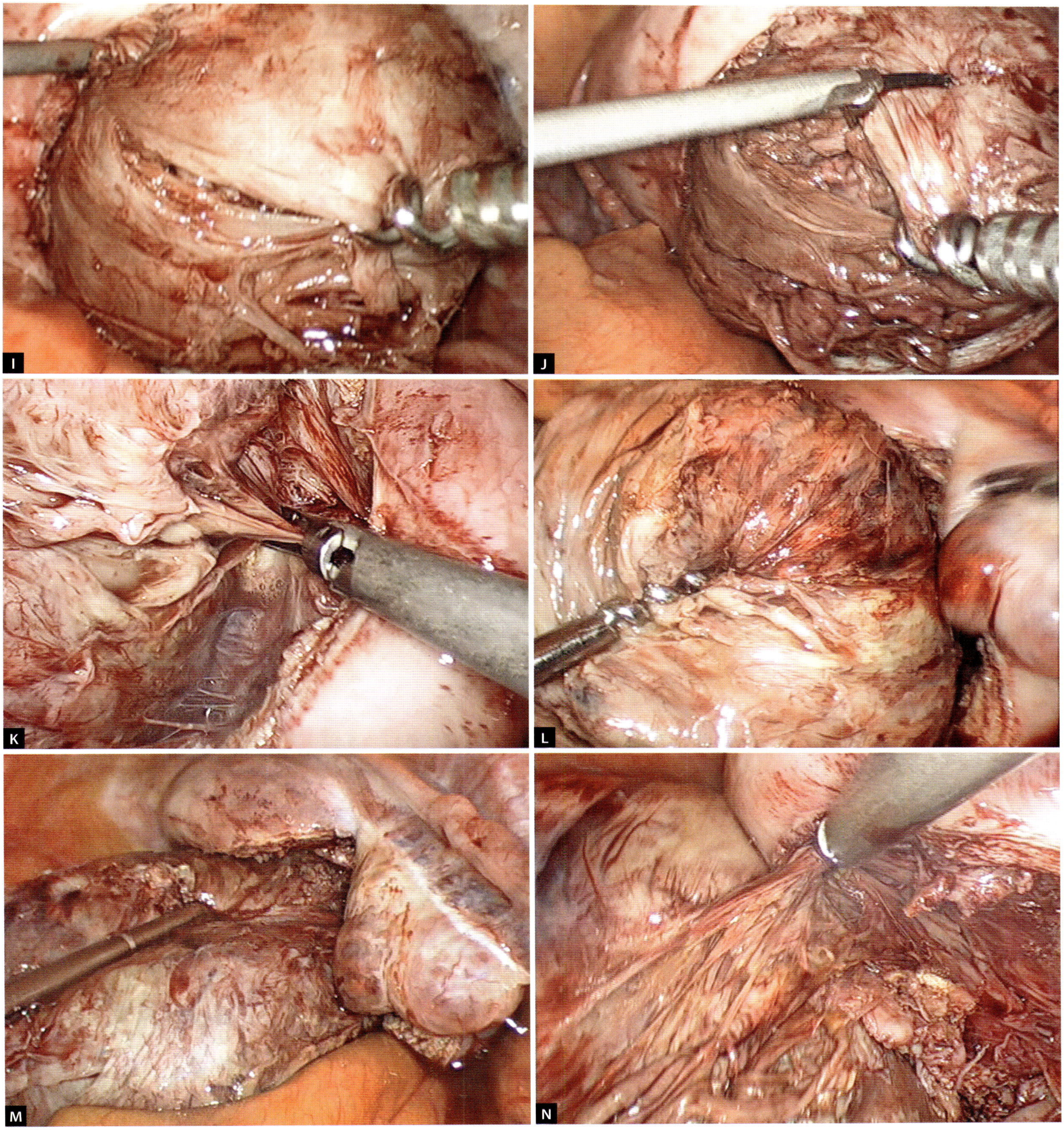

Figs. 54I to N

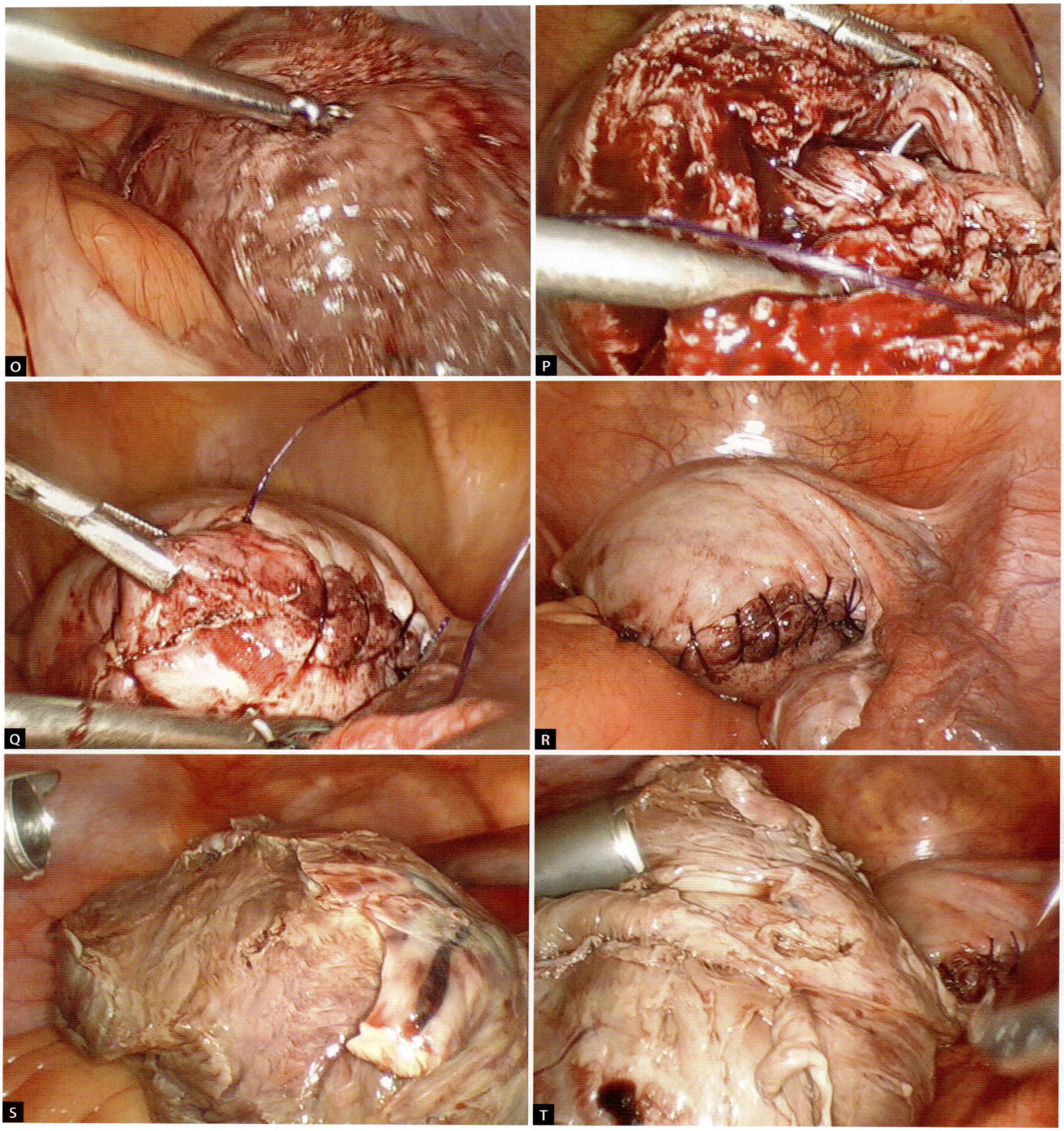

Figs. 54O to T

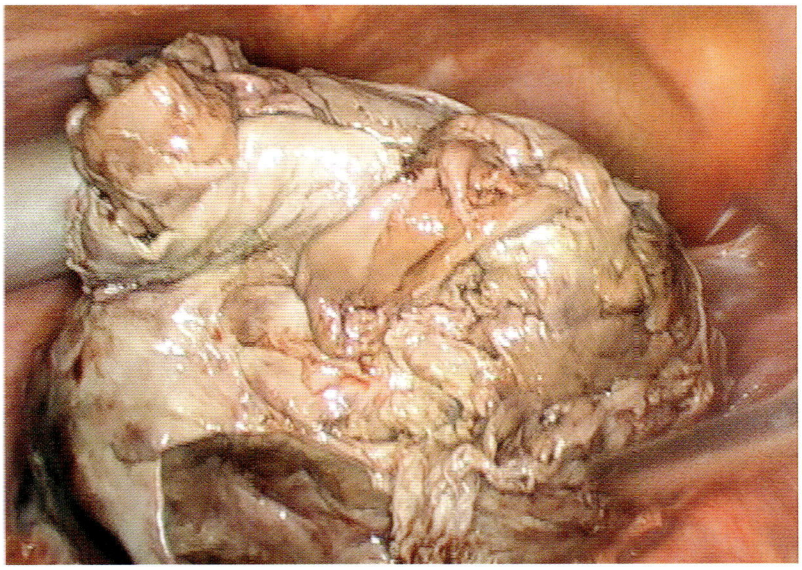

Fig. 54U

Figs. 54A to U: Difficult myomectomy in a case of red degeneration of fibroid.

ROLE OF UTERINE ARTERY LIGATION

This method has been adopted by some surgeons to reduce blood loss and in the author's opinion is of use specially when dealing with multiple and large myomas.

Transitory ligation at level of internal os after reflecting the uterovesical fold is possible. The uterine artery can be ligated at the origin too. The option to permanently leave the suture behind or release the suture remains open.

In a study, which compared uterine artery ligation with a control group with no ligation, it was found that although the mean operative time was larger (107 min vs. 93 min; $p = 0.03$), there was less blood loss (84 mL vs. 137 mL; $p < 0.001$) in the uterine artery ligation group.[24]

Another study in which temporary clipping of uterine artery was done documented a statistically effective less hemoglobin drop in clipped group versus control group.[25]

Transitory clipping of uterine arteries at the origin has been described to decrease intraoperative blood loss. At the end of surgery, the declipping is performed if fertility is desired or may be left occluded if there is no desire for fertility. Also selectively unilateral ligation may be done if largest myoma is lateral, e.g., right artery in right lateral myoma. Bilateral occlusion is done if myoma is vascularized by both arteries.[26]

Also observational comparative studies on uterine artery ligation and its effect have found an improvement in the effectiveness of treatment both on the clinical symptoms and recurrence of the leiomyomas.

Three approaches to UAL are:

1. Lateral approach
2. Anterior approach
3. Posterior approach

Lateral Approach (Figs. 55A to D)

The line of dissection is in the triangle bounded by the round ligament anteriorly, infundibulopelvic ligament medially and pelvic sidewall (external iliac vessels) laterally. The peritoneum opened and paravesical and obturator space developed by a blunt dissection. Start dissecting retrograde on medial aspect of obliterated umbilical artery in the paravesical space and continue till it gets obstructed by uterine artery which traverses from lateral to medial side. Subsequently, distancing differentiating uterine vessels from the ureter, uterine artery is occluded either by coagulation and cutting or clipping or ligating uterine artery just medial to the origin from the hypogastric artery.

Anterior Approach (Fig. 56)

In cases where the large posterior broad ligament fibroid fills the pelvic cavity and lateral pelvic wall, the anterior approach to the uterine artery through the anterior broad ligament makes ligation feasible. In this approach, uterine artery can be occluded at the transverse or the ascending part of uterine artery.

Surgical Method

Careful inspection of the anterior broad ligament over the paravesical area can often reveal pulsation of the uterine artery to assist in mapping its course. This peritoneum is elevated, then incised transversely using monopolar scissors over the avascular window between the limit of the paravesical fat and the round ligament. The potential space between the leaves of the broad ligament is opened using a combination of pneumodissection and blunt dissection, thus enabling access to the base of the broad ligament.

The preferred site of UA ligation is lateral to its crossing over the ureter because it is away from the ureter and is less intimately intertwined with the uterine vein. The UA can be identified more proximally as it branches off the internal iliac artery. Once the artery has been sufficiently skeletonized, including a segment of artery for proximal control of the vessel in case of unexpected bleeding, a single clip can be applied.

Posterior Approach (Figs. 57A to C)

In posterior approach the pelvic parietal peritoneum is incised over 15 mm under the ovarian fossa opposite the uterine artery, whose path runs parallel to the path of the ureter located just below. The ureter, therefore, has to be previously identified by transparency by its crawling movement so that the peritoneal incision is carried

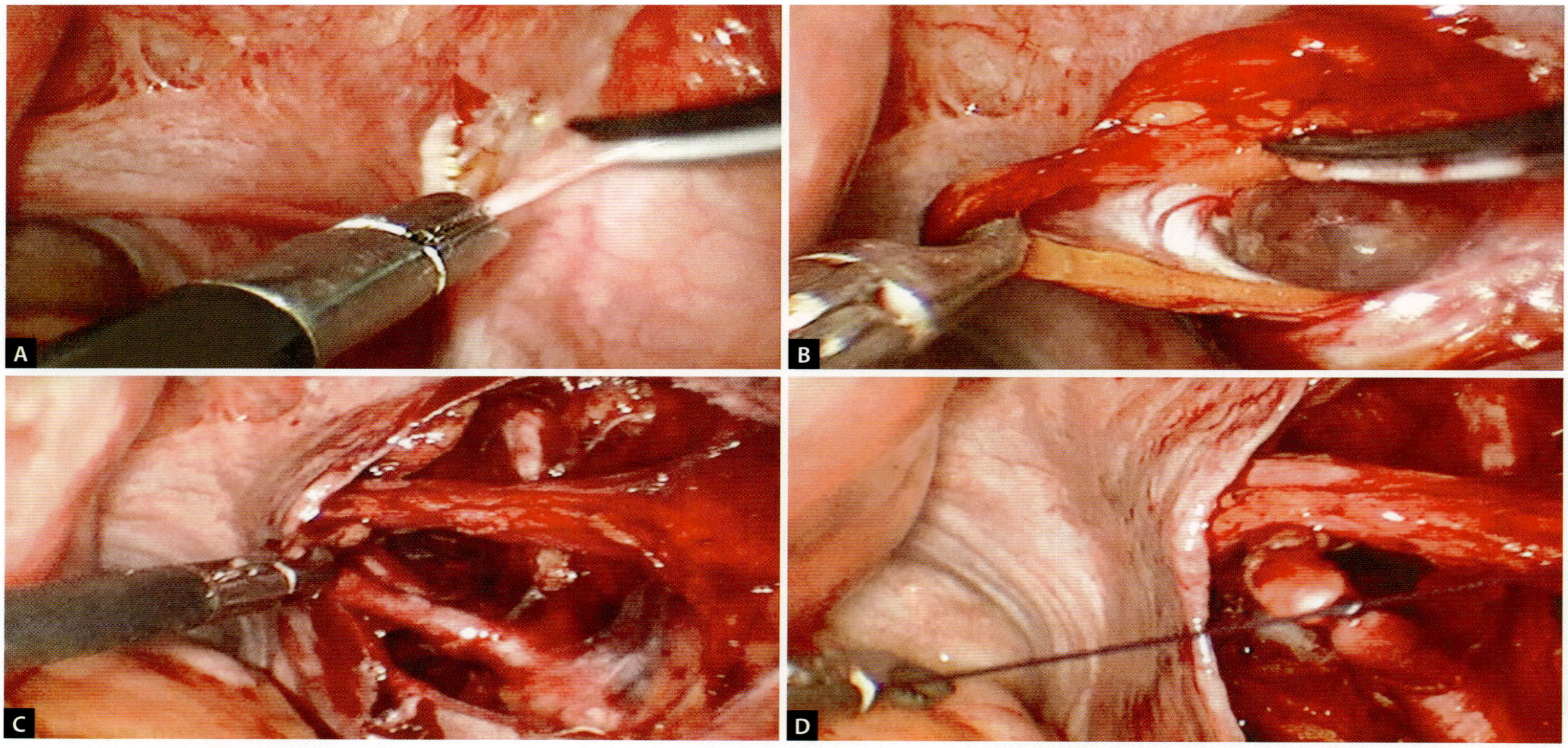

Figs. 55A to D: Uterine artery ligation—lateral approach. (A) Incision of peritoneum in the lateral pelvic wall overlying ureter; (B) Dissection parallel to ureter; (C) Identification of uterine artery; and (D) Ligation of artery using Vicryl no. 1-0.

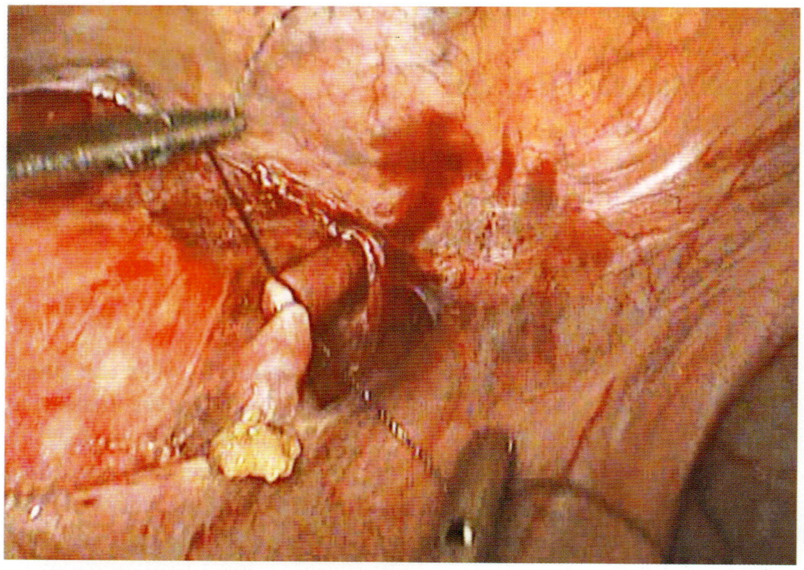

Fig. 56: UAL at internal os level—anterior approach.

out parallel to its path 10 mm above it. Occlusion of the artery can be performed by applying 5-mm or 10-mm vascular clip or by ligation using Vicryl no. 1 or by harmonic scalpel. The technique can be facilitated by temporarily fixing the ovary to the abdominal wall ipsilaterally.

COMPLICATIONS OF LAPAROSCOPIC MYOMECTOMY (TABLE 3 AND FIGS. 58 TO 68)

The main complications that can occur in a laparoscopic myomectomy are:

- *Intraoperative and immediate postoperative:*
  - Hemorrhage and hematoma formation
  - Conversion to laparotomy
  - Hysterectomy (very rare)
  - Morcellator injury
  - Lost needles and myomas
  - Dilutional coagulopathy
  - Minor complications like pyrexia, abdominal pain, vaginitis, metrorrhagia, dysuria, etc.
- *Late:*
  - Recurrence of myomas
  - Scar dehiscence during pregnancy
  - Port site hernia

Other complications generally associated with laparoscopy such as shoulder pain, subcutaneous emphysema, atelectasis, gas embolism, pneumothorax, and rarely diaphragmatic rupture can also occur.

Hemorrhage

Refer to **Figures 58 and 59**.

Morcellator Injuries

The first specimen removal during laparoscopic surgery was done in 1973. Despite this innovation, it took extensive amounts of time to remove even small specimens due to the manual force necessary. In 1993, the Steiner Morcellator revolutionized laparoscopic specimen removal.

In contrast, the electromechanical morcellator makes it easy to remove even relatively large sections of tissue from the abdomen within a short period through the existing incisions.

It is very important to close the bigger port site laparoscopically to avoid incidence of Richter's hernia. A special port closure needle is used and the rest closed laparoscopically. After removing the morcellator, port closure needle enters the abdomen through one end of the 15 mm incisions, carrying no. 1 Vicryl suture along with it.

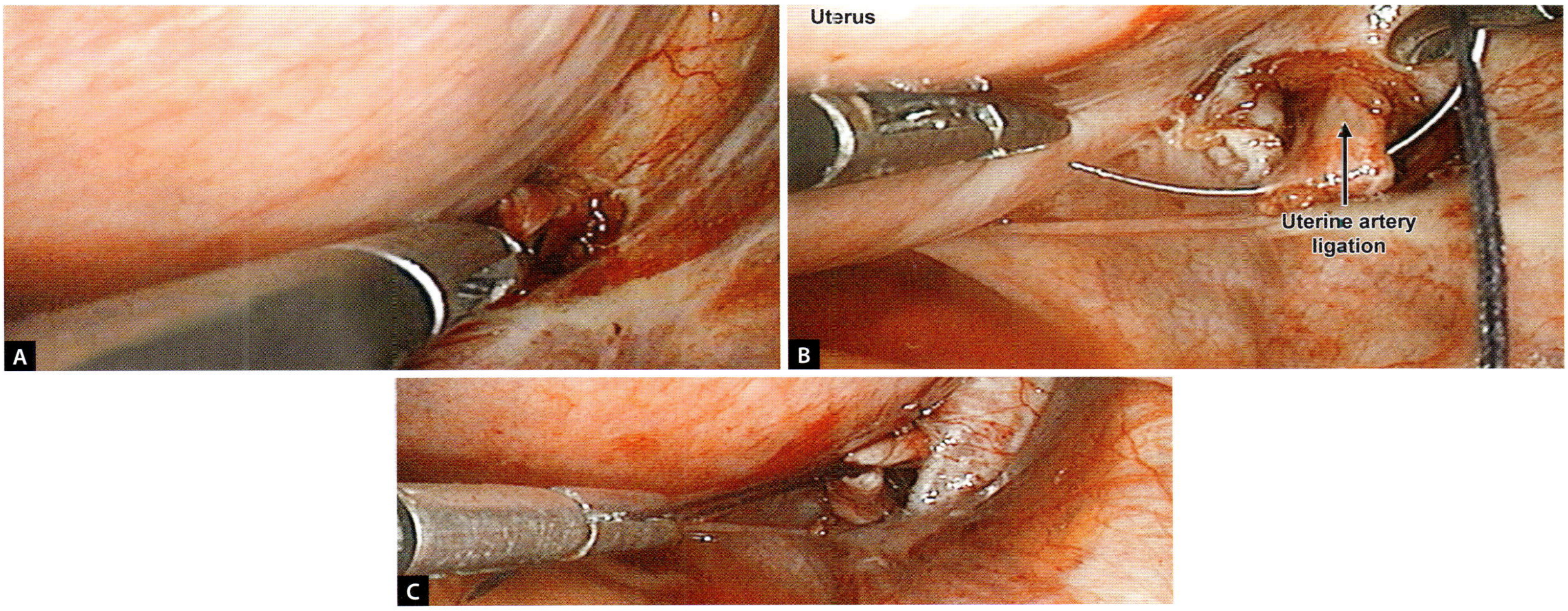

Figs. 57A to C: Uterine artery ligation—posterior approach. (A) Incision of peritoneum under the ovarian fossa; (B) Ligation of uterine artery using Vicryl no. 1; (C) Uterine artery after ligation.

Table 3: Complications of laparoscopic myomectomy in incidence.

Complications	*Incidence*
Hemorrhages requiring blood transfusion	0.14%
Postoperative hematomas	0.48%
Bowel injury	0.04%
Postoperative acute kidney failure	0.04%
Unexpected sarcomas	0.09%
Failure to complete planned surgery/conversion to hysterectomy	0.34%
Spontaneous uterine rupture during pregnancy	0.26%
Recurrence	4–30%

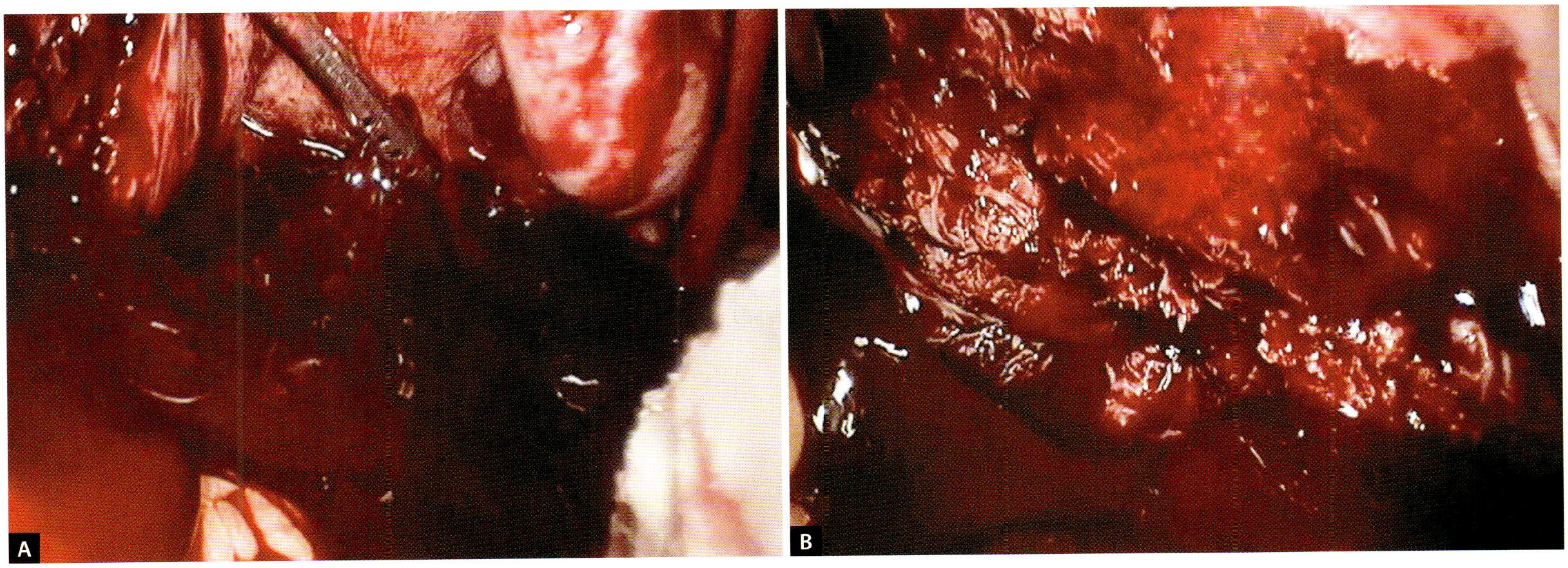

Figs. 58A and B: Intraoperative hemorrhage at myoma bed after large myoma excision.

The suture is released and the needle withdrawn. It is reintroduced from the other end of the incision. The first free end of suture in the peritoneal cavity is grasped and brought out over the abdomen. When the suture is tied the defect in the peritoneum and the rectus sheath gets adequately closed and eliminates the risk of bowel and omental herniation. Care should be exercised during introduction of morcellator. Vital tissue damage can be sustained by inadvertent morcellation beyond the myoma or uterus.

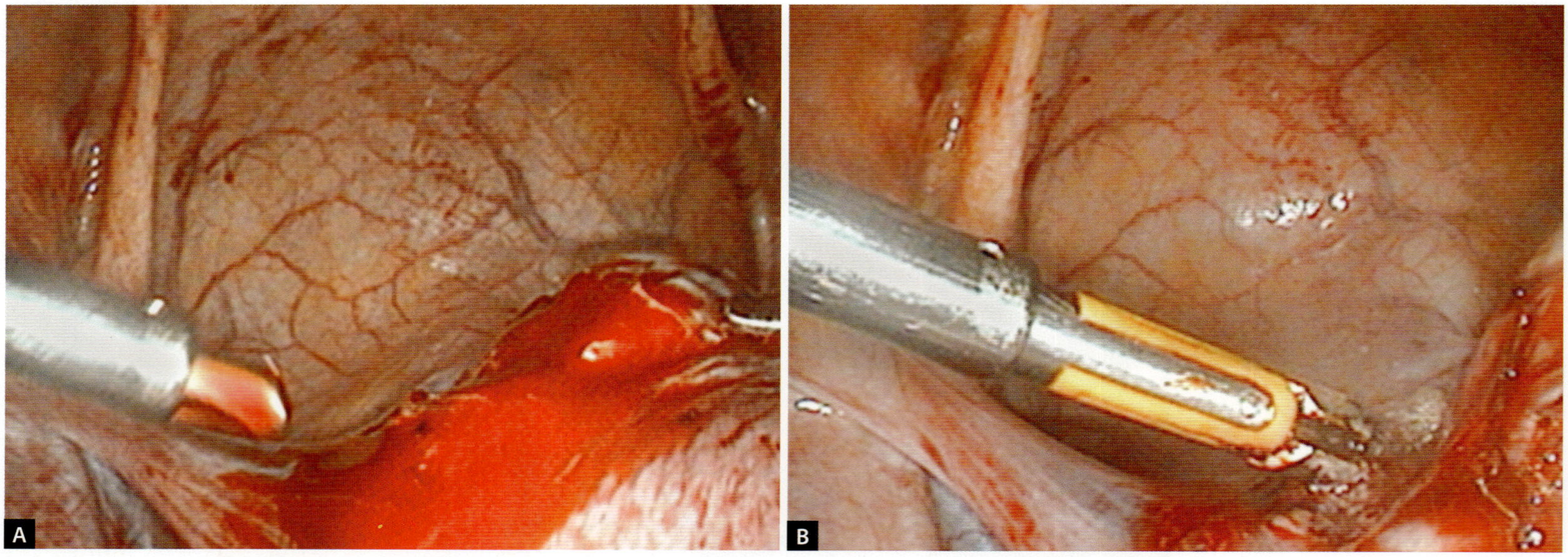

Figs. 59A and B: (A) Active bleeding from feeding vessel of myoma; and (B) Bleeding managed using bipolar energy source.

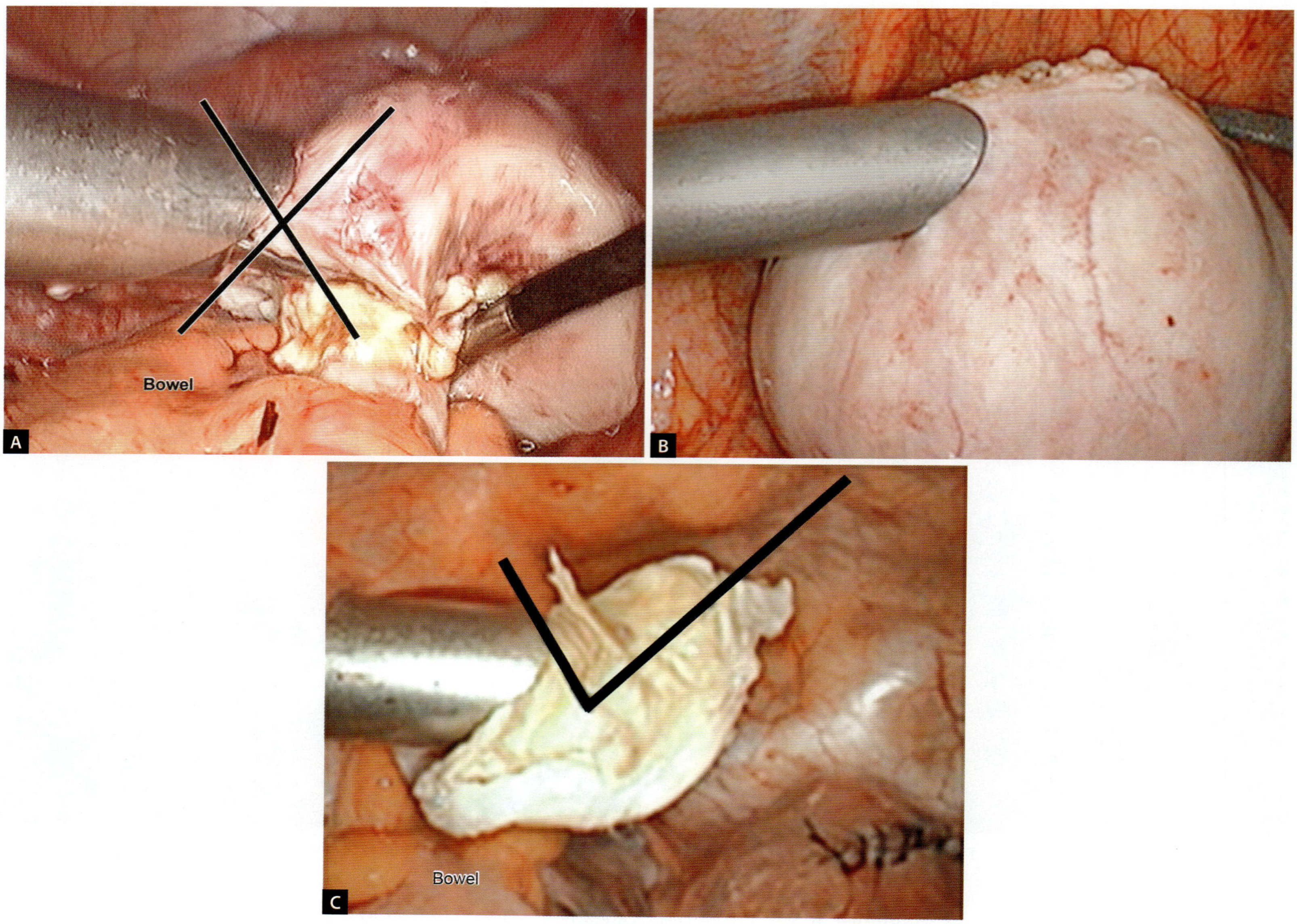

Figs. 60A to C: Panoramic view of morcellation showing wrong and correct method.

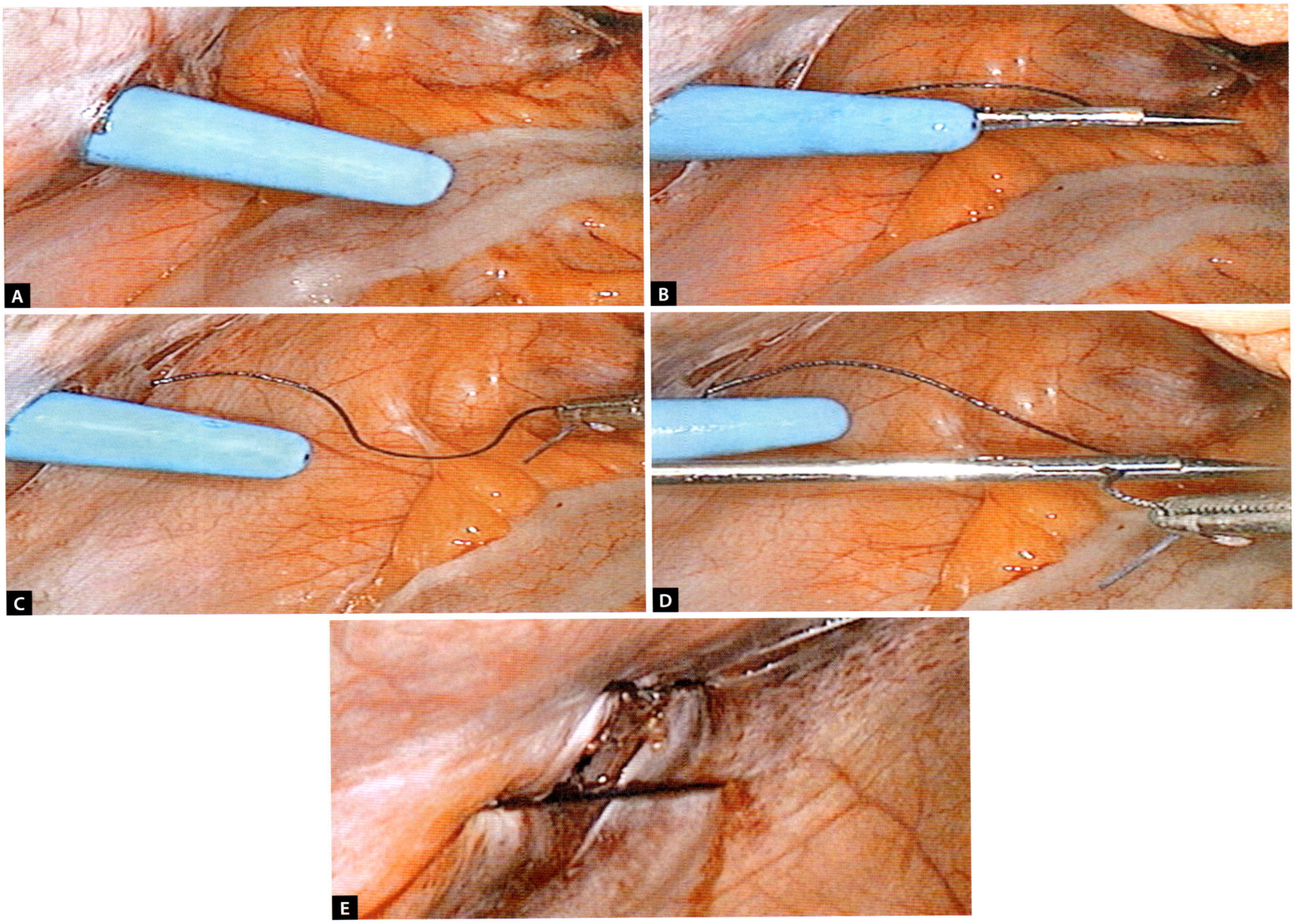

Figs. 61A to E: Step-by-step closure of port site (15 mm morcellator port).

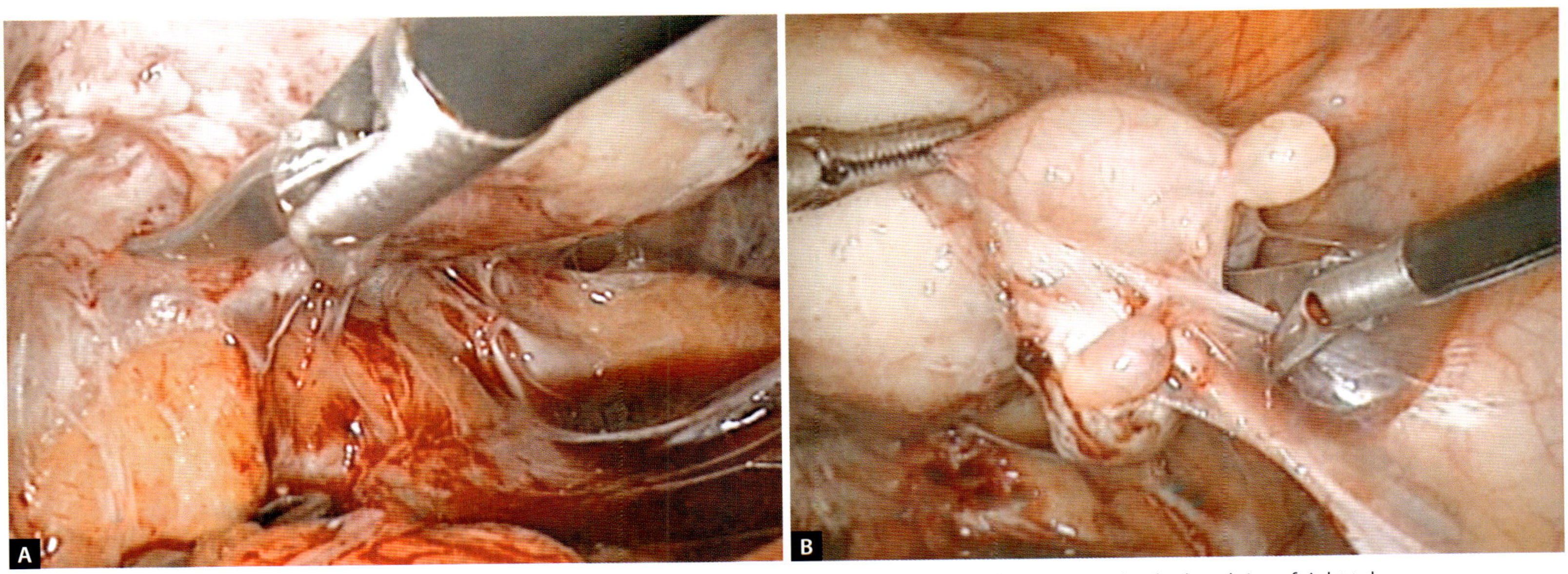

Figs. 62A and B: (A) Postmyomectomy adhesions—released; and (B) Postmyomectomy adhesions causing hydrosalpinx of right tube.

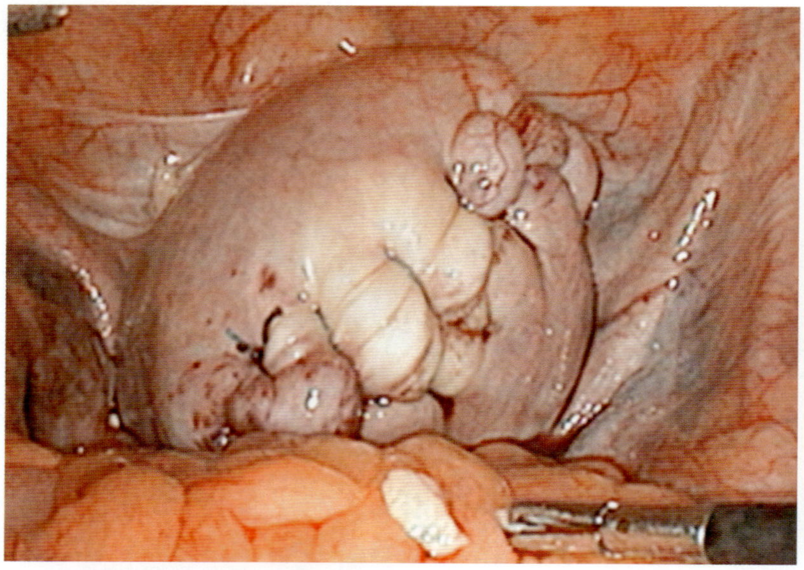

Fig. 63: Removing bits of myoma after morcellation using toothed grasper.

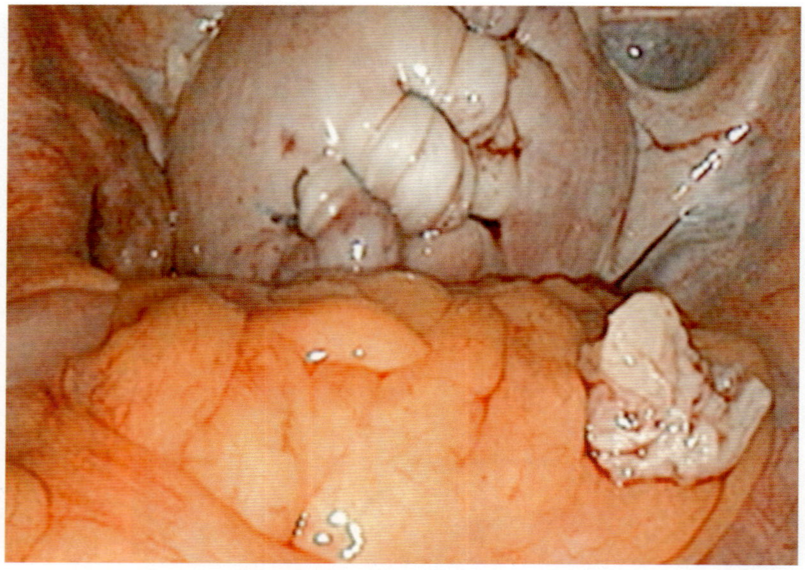

Fig. 64: Morcellation inside the endobag—prevents spillage of fragments in the cavity.

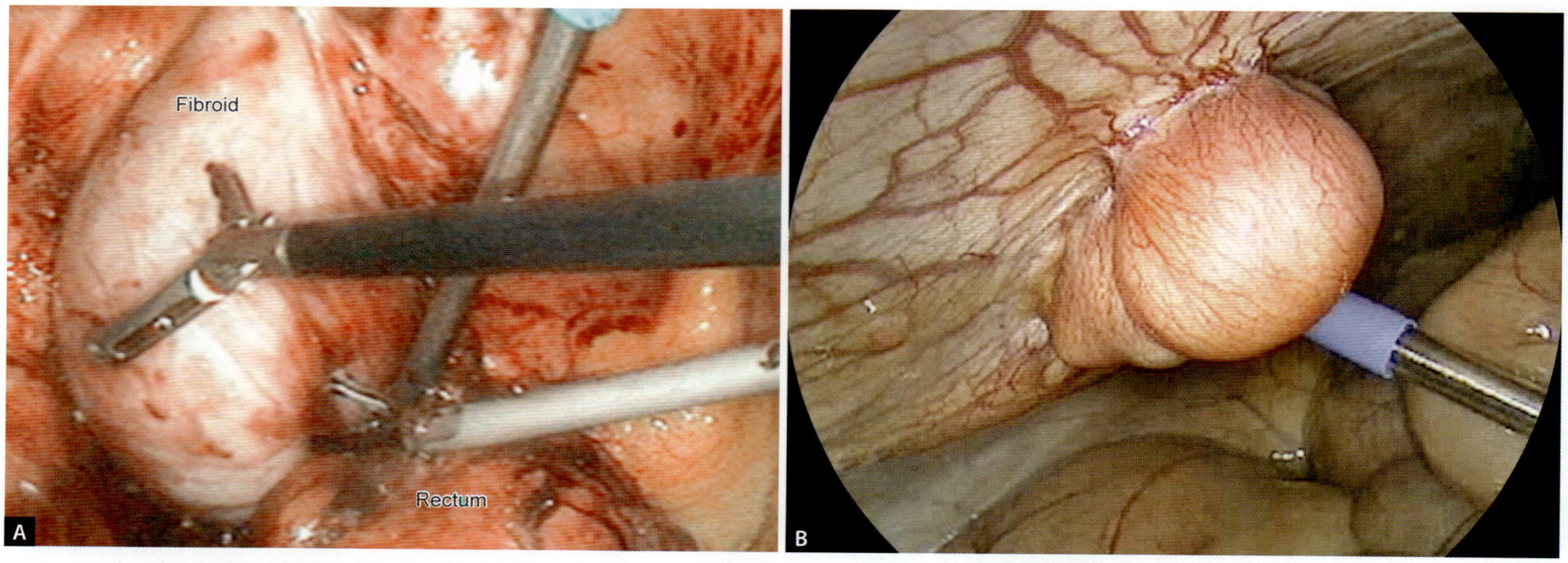

Figs. 65A and B: (A) Parasitic fibroid postmyomectomy seen in the pelvic floor; and (B) Parasitic fibroid seen in the anterior abdominal wall.

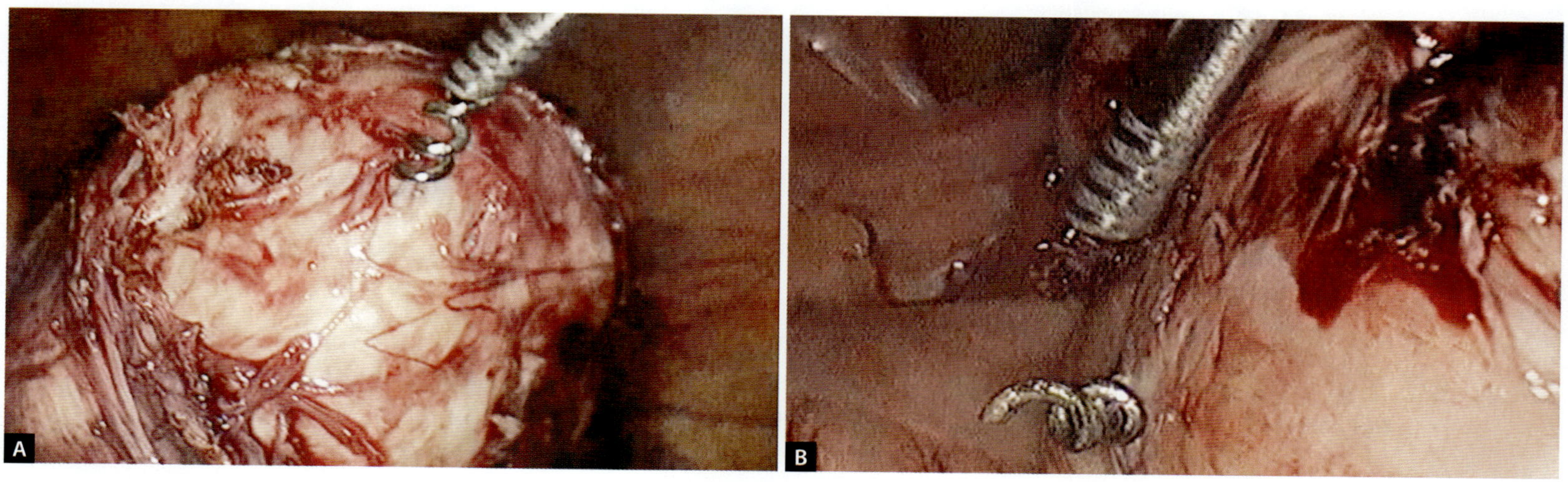

Figs. 66A and B

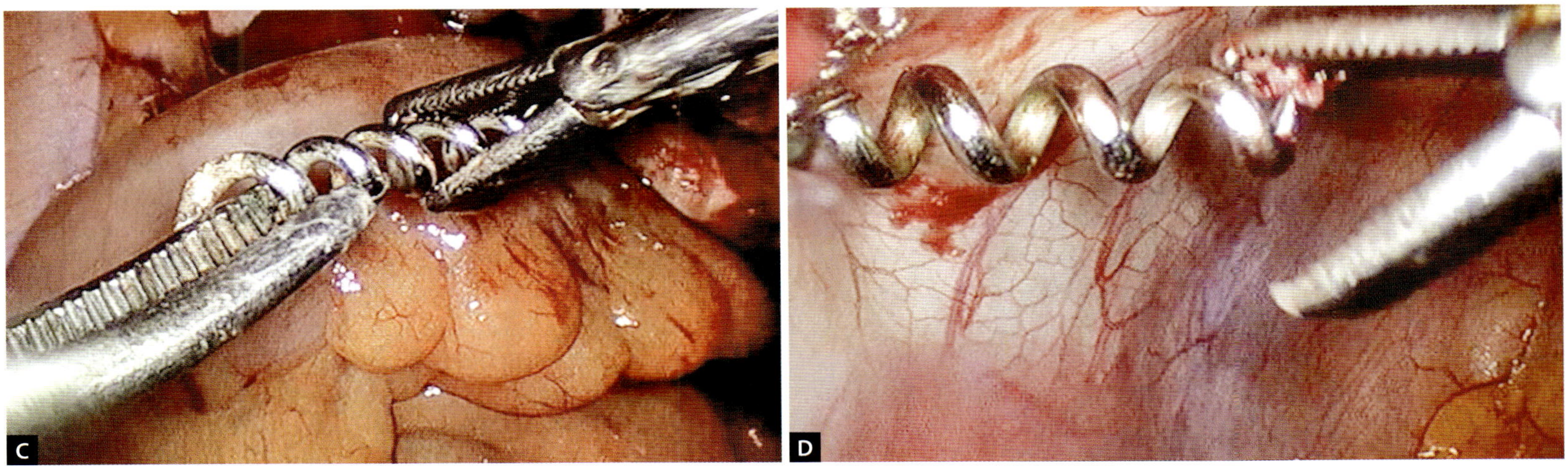

Figs. 66C and D

Figs. 66A to D: Rare case of broken myoma screw. (A) Myoma screw being used for traction of the myoma; (B) Broken screw during traction; (C and D) Retrieval of myoma screw from lateral port.

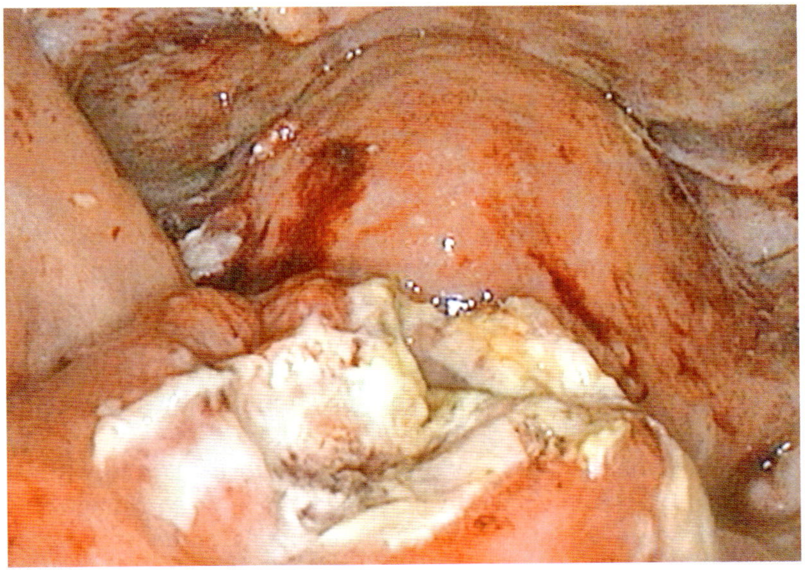

Fig. 67: Evidence of bowel necrosis and localized peritonitis on postoperative day 5.

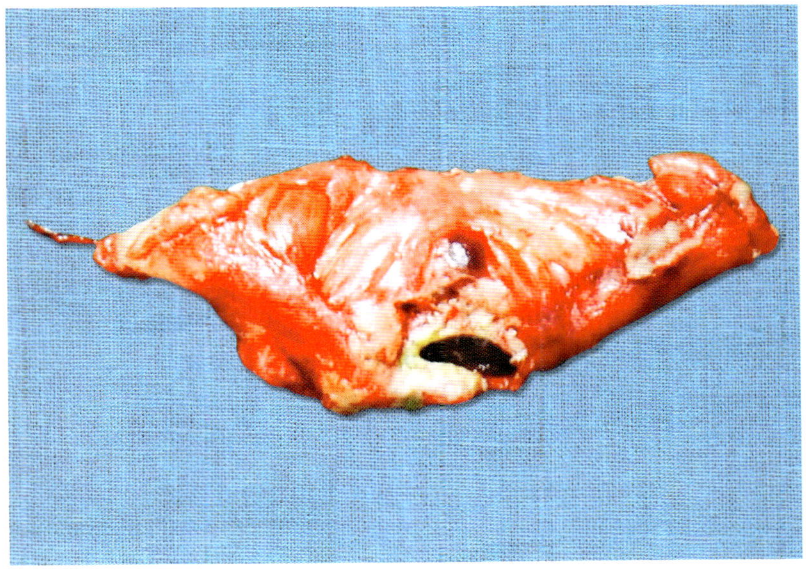

Fig. 68: Specimen of wide segmental bowel resection by minilaparotomy.

Tips to Avoid Morcellator Injuries

- The removing blade should always remain as anterior as possible.
- Excellent pneumoperitoneum should be maintained.
- Adequate panoramic view allows the operator to visualize the blade at all times **(Figs. 60A to C)**.
- The specimen should be completely separated from surrounding structures and vessels.
- Specimen should always be pulled into the morcellator rather than pushing the morcellator into the specimen.
- The individual holding the handpiece should also be responsible for its activation.
- Use of a laparoscopic bag to retain the specimen should not create a false sense of security with vital structures located in such close proximity. If the bag is torn during morcellation, the surgeon should immediately deactivate the morcellator and consider carefully inspecting surrounding viscera for injury.
- It is very important to close the morcellator port site laparoscopically using a port closure needle to avoid incidence of Richter's hernia.

It is ideal if morcellation can be done inside a bag so that pieces of the myoma do not get left out in the abdomen. Also in the rare case of an unsuspected sarcoma, the chance of disseminating it is minimized. The tip of the morcellator should always be visible and the morcellation should be like the peeling of an onion so that you do not create holes in the myoma.

The FDA's current recommendations discourage the use of power morcellators during hysterectomy or myomectomy for fibroids and that if, after carefully weighing the available options, the doctor feels that laparoscopic power morcellation (LPM) is the best option for the patient, then the doctor should inform the patient that the fibroid may contain unexpected cancerous tissue and that lap. Power morcellator may spread the disease significantly worsening their prognosis ***(Figs. 61A to E)****.*

Pelvic Adhesions Postlaparoscopic Myomectomy (Figs. 62A and B)

Incidence

Varies from 18 to 30%.[27]

When the incision on the myoma is posterior, the incidence rises. The incidence also rises when the patient also already had adhesions at initial surgery

Prevention

Use minimum cautery:

- Avoid using posterior incisions and multiple incisions as far as possible.
- The initial incision should be placed such that you can enucleate most of the myomas through it. For this, proper fibroid mapping prior to the procedure by the surgeon will help. Transvaginal sonography (TVS) and hysteroscopy may be used.
- Thorough hemostasis and use of barriers like *interceed* have been shown to prevent adhesions at second-look laparoscopy.
- One must not allow the tissues to become charred.
- Frequent irrigation to keep the tissue moist also helps in preventing adhesions.

Uterine Rupture during Pregnancy

Exact incidence not known. But it is rare.

Cause

The integrity of myometrium compromised badly.

Prevention

Huge myomas especially intramural reaching submucous plane are more likely to give way. There should be good approximation of the tissues with no dead space. When the myoma cavity is deep, it should be closed in layers. There should be no dead space to allow a hematoma to form there when the action of vasopressin wears off. Barbed sutures and baseball suturing technique will help. Preferably do not violate the endometrial cavity if possible during myomectomy.

The risk of uterine rupture in pregnancy postlaparoscopic myomectomy is there when intramural myomas are excised. Studies by Hasson,[21] Roemisch and Nezhat[28] as well as one study by Miller[20] revealed no uterine rupture either pre- or intrapartum, but Miller recommends cesarean section for all postmyomectomy patients.

Recurrence of Myomas

Incidence

Approximately 23–25%.

Cause

Missing small myomas and deep intramural myomas at original surgery. Recurrence risk increases after preoperative GnRH agonist usage.

Prevention

- Thorough mapping of all myomas by transabdominal as well as TVS, if necessary, hysterosonogram, MRI, etc.
- Do not use GnRH agonists prior to laparoscopic myomectomy. It also makes dissection more difficult by shrinking the myomas, thus making them more likely to be missed.

Mean time of recurrence was 42 months with 4.08% of patient requiring repeat surgery.[29]

Lost Needles/Myoma Bits in Peritoneal Cavity

Refer to **Figures 63 to 65**.

CURRENT CONTROVERSY OVER POWER MORCELLATION

Recent media attention on a highly publicized case of disseminated leiomyosarcoma after laparoscopic hysterectomy utilizing power morcellator was the reason behind scrutinizing this procedure. US FDA issued a warning on use of LPMs in a statement on April 17, 2014 saying not to use LPM in suspected or known uterine malignancy. If LPM is performed in women with unsuspected uterine sarcoma, there is a risk that the procedure will spread the cancerous tissue within the abdomen and pelvis, significantly worsening the patient's likelihood of long-term survival. For this reason, and because there is no reliable method for predicting whether a woman with fibroids may have a uterine sarcoma, the FDA discourages the use of LPM during hysterectomy or myomectomy for uterine fibroids. FDA clearly states that usage of LPM should be individualized, after a careful benefit-risk evaluation. If LPM is considered as the best therapeutic option for an individual, the healthcare provider should:

- Inform patients that their fibroid(s) may contain unexpected cancerous tissue and that power morcellation may spread the cancer, significantly worsening their prognosis.
- Be aware that some clinicians and medical institutions now advocate using a specimen "bag" during morcellation in an attempt to contain the uterine tissue and minimize the risk of spread in the abdomen and pelvis.

Responding to the US FDA, AAGL issued a statement on July 11, 2014 stating that the risk of death from abdominal hysterectomy is slightly higher than from laparoscopic hysterectomy with power morcellation including LMS and potential dissemination.[30] Measuring the effectiveness and benefits of LPM, AAGL clearly mentioned that the procedure needs to be improved not abandoned and full benefit of the procedure can be obtained only by preoperative screening and selecting appropriate cases.

On November 24, 2014 US FDA issued a fresh warning against the use of LPMs in the majority of women undergoing myomectomy or hysterectomy for treatment of fibroids. Limiting the patients for whom laparoscopic morcellators are indicated, the strong warning on the risk of spreading unsuspected cancer and the recommendation that doctors share this information directly with their patients, are part of FDA guidance to manufacturers of morcellators.[31] The guidance strongly urges these manufacturers to include this new information in their product labels.

But following the April 2014 FDA safety communication, regarding power morcellation, the cases of minimally invasive myomectomy decreased with consequent increase in hospital stay and the potential complications of open surgery.[32]

In January 2016, a group of 49 physicians led by William H Parker wrote a commentary disagreeing with the US FDA view. While FDA estimated the risk of occult LMS as 1 in 458, this group reanalyzed the data and estimated the risk as 1 in 1,550.[33]

However, a recent cohort study of 34,728 women who underwent hysterectomies for leiomyomas found the incidence of occult uterine sarcoma as 1 of 278 and the incidence of leiomyosarcoma as 1 of 429.[34]

The American College of Obstetricians and Gynecologists (ACOG) issued a recent statement which states "Without question, morcellation of an undiagnosed sarcoma can disseminate malignant tissue. However, by allowing some women to avoid the higher morbidity and mortality associated with open abdominal surgery, morcellation can also save lives". It further states "As a result of the continuing conversation about morcellation, obstetrician-gynecologists are better able to evaluate each individual woman's risk of an undiagnosed sarcoma and to counsel her to receive the right approach for her own unique medical needs".[34]

Leaving needles is rare.

Suturing technique should be good. Do not hold the needle too close to swaging. The needles should be removed from the peritoneal cavity after each sequence of suturing. If you need to suture in another place it can be reintroduced.

Management: If, even after thorough inspection of the peritoneal cavity, one is unable to find the needle, it can be removed using a C-arm.

Small myoma bits are sometimes missed. To prevent this morcellation should preferably be done in endobags. Orange peel method of morcellation should be used. It should be done under vision. When small pieces do fall off they should be picked up and removed immediately before starting another bout of morcellation. Some surgeons prefer to keep a gauze piece below so that the pieces may be later picked off it **(Figs. 66A to D)**.

Role of Transvaginal Sonography

Transvaginal sonography has a very important role to play in laparoscopic myomectomy. The exact sit, size, and number of myomas should be known to the operating surgeon prior to surgery so that all of them get removed. The distance from endometrium, cornu as well as relative position from one another in case of multiple myomas is important. It is ideal if the surgeon himself does this only the day prior to surgery. This is of immense importance since the tactile findings are minimal during laparoscopic surgery. This also helps in planning port selection and incisions.

Intraoperative Ultrasound in Laparoscopic Myomectomy

Use of high frequency ultrasound (10–12 MHz) transducer placed directly on the surface of an organ provides sharper images than might be obtained through the abdominal wall.

In a study done by David Levine et al. laparoscopic ultrasound (LUS) transducer was placed through a 10–12 mm port to map the uterus and then identify the location, type size, and number of myomas to be treated via radiofrequency thermal ablation. Gynecologic surgeon performed the scan.

The transducer was passed over each wall systematically (anterior, right, posterior, left, and fundus). Scanning was done from lower segment up to the fundus. Laparoscopic ultrasound enabled imaging of the entire extent of the myoma in all planes. When a myoma was identified, the surgeon could determine its location and anatomical relationship to the serosa, the myometrium and endometrium. These parameters enabled proper classification of the myoma. LUS could identify more myomas when compared with contrast enhanced MRI. So the conclusion is that LUS should be used at the time of myoma treatment to maximize detection of their number and location and therefore enable treatment of most if not all myomas. Thus, recurrences can be prevented.

Thromboembolism Prevention

American College of Obstetricians and Gynecologists recommends that until more evidence is accumulated patients undergoing laparoscopic surgery should be stratified by risk category and should receive prophylaxis similar to that provided in patients undergoing open surgery.[35]

Early ambulation and/or pneumatic compression stockings may be adequate if the patient is not obese and the surgery does not last more than 30 minutes.

All other patients especially if obese, aged more than 40 years, who have been immobilized recently or have been prescribed estrogens or progestogens recently should receive low-molecular-weight heparin 40 mg administered subcutaneously 12 hours before surgery and once a day postoperatively till discharge.

Bowel Injury

Incidence: 0–0.5%.[36]

Causes: Thermal/trauma by entry technique instruments/instruments of myomectomy procedure.

Prevention: High degree of suspicion, cold scissors for dissection, and avoid electrical energy source for cauterization directly on the bowel rather than suturing using No. 3-0 delayed absorbable suture material are preferred. Previous surgical history should be recorded for difficult surgery and dense adhesions.

Diagnosis: Stormy postoperative period with fever, rising ESR and CRP, evidence of peritonitis such as fever, abdominal distension, absent or sluggish bowel sounds, passage of purulent stools can be diagnosed by CT abdomen/diagnostic laparoscopy.

Management: Timely detection. Wide segmental resection with coverage of broad spectrum antibiotics **(Figs. 67 and 68)**.

Postoperative Course

Two randomized clinical trials have demonstrated that laparoscopic myomectomy has proven advantages compared with the laparotomic approach in terms of the postoperative course. The laparoscopic approach may offer the benefits of less postoperative pain and shorter recovery time in comparison with laparotomy. It also reduces the hospital stay and transient episodes of febrile morbidity.

REFERENCES

1. Marshall LM, Spiegelman D, Barbieri RL, et al. Variation in the incidence of uterine leiomyoma among premenopausal women by age and race. Obstet Gynecol. 1997;90:967-73.
2. Baird DD, Dunson DB, Hill MC, et al. High cumulative incidence of uterine leiomyoma in black and white women: ultrasound evidence. Am J Obstet Gynecol. 2003;188:101-7.
3. Hurst BS. Laparoscopic Myomectomy. In: Ricardo A, Anna Alvarez M (Eds). Practical Manual of Operative Laparoscopy and Hysteroscopy, 2nd edition. New York: Springer; 1997. pp. 163-72.
4. Zullo F, Pellicano M, Dicarlo C, et al. Ultrasonographic prediction of the efficacy of GnRH agonist therapy before laparoscopic myomectomy. J Am Assoc Gynecol Laparosc. 1998;5:361-6.
5. Takahashi K, Kawamura N, Ishiko O, et al. Shrinkage effect of gonadotropin releasing hormone agonist treatment on uterine leiomyomas and t(12;14). Int J Oncol. 2002;20:279-83.
6. Visco AG, Advincula AP. Robotic gynecologic surgery. Obstet Gynecol. 2008;112:1369-84.
7. Gallinat A, Leuken RP. Current trends in the therapy of myomata. In: Leuken RP, Gallinat A (Eds). Endoscopic Surgery in Gynecology. Berlin: Demeter Verlag; 1993. pp. 69-71.
8. Goldfarb HA. Nd:YAG laser laparoscopic coagulation of symptomatic myomas. J Reprod Med. 1992;36:636-8.

9. Greenberg JA, Goldman RH. Barbed suture: A review of technology and clinical uses in obstetrics and gynaecology. Rev Obstet Gynecol. 2013;6: 107-15.
10. Nett M, Avelar R, Sheehan M, et al. Watertight knee arthrotomy closure: Comparison of novel single bi-directional barbed self-retaining suture versus conventional interrupted sutures. J Knee Surg. 2011;24:55-9.
11. Einarrson II, Vonnahme KA, Sandberg EM, et al. Barbed compared with standard suture: effects on cellular composition and proliferation of the healthy wound in the ovine uterus. Acta Obstet Gynecol Scand. 2012;91:613-9.
12. Huang MC, Hseih CH, Su TH, et al. Safety and efficacy of unidirectional barbed sutures in minilaparotomy myomectomy. Taiwan J Obstet Gynecol. 2013;52:53-6.
13. Sandberg EM, Cohen SL, Hill-Lydecker CI, et al. Pregnancy outcomes after laparoscopic myomectomy closure with bidirectional barbed suture. J Minim Invasive Gynecol. 2013;20:492-8.
14. Einarsson JI, Cohen SL, Fuchs N. In-bag morcellation. J Minim Invasive Gynaecol. 2014;21:951-3.
15. Cohen SL, Einarsson JI, Wang KC, et al. Contained power morcellation with an insufflated isolation bag. Obstet Gynaecol. 2014;124:491-7.
16. Ciecaella G, Granese R, Calagna G, et al. Parasitic myomas after endoscopic surgery: an emerging complication in the use of morcellator? Description of four cases. Fertile Steril. 2011;96:e 90-6.
17. Leren V, Langbrekke A, Quigstad E. Parasitic leiomyomas after laparoscopic surgery with morcellator. Acta Obstet Gynecol Scand. 2012;9:1233-6.
18. Glasser MH. Minilaparotomy myomectomy: A minimally invasive alternative for the large fibroid uterus. J Minim Invasive Gynaecol. 2005;12:275-83.
19. Mangeshikar PR. New instrumentation and technique for laparoscopic myomectomy. J Am Assoc Gynecol. 1995;2:S29.
20. Miller CE, Johnston M, Rundell M. Laparoscopic myomectomy in the infertile women. J Am Assoc Gynecol Laparosc. 1996;3:525-32.
21. Hasson HM, Rotman C, Rana N, et al. Laparoscopic myomectomy. Obstet Gynecol. 1992;80:884-8.
22. Clark LE, Gulden Menderes G, Azodi M, et al. A simple approach to specimen retrieval via posterior colpotomy incision. JSLS. 2015;19: e2015.00222.
23. De Grandi P, Chardonnens E, Gerber S. The morcellator knife: a new laparoscopic instrument for supracervical hysterectomy and morcellation. Obstet Gynecol. 2000;95:777-8.
24. Chang WC, Huang PS, Wang PH, et al. Comparison of laparoscopic myomectomy using in situ morcellator with and without Uterine Artery ligation for treatment of symptomatic myomas. J Minim Invasive Gynecol. 2012;19:715-21.
25. Vercellino G, Erdemoglu E, Joe A, et al. Laparoscopic temporary clipping of uterine artery during laparoscopic myomectomy. Arch Gynecol Obstet. 2012;286:1181-6.
26. Dubuisson J, Ramyend L, Streuli I. The role of preventive uterine artery occlusion during laparoscopic myomectomy: A review of literature. Arch Gynecol Obstet. 2015;291:737-4.
27. Dubisson JB, Faucontier A, Chapron C, et al. Second look after laparoscopic myomectomy. Human Reprod. 1998;13:2102-6.
28. Roemisch M, Nezhat FR, Nezhat C. Pregnancy after laparoscopic myomectomy. JMIG. 1996;3:s42.
29. Doridot Y, Dubuisson JB, Chapron C, et al. Recurrence of leiomyomata after laparoscopic myomectomy. J Am Assoc Gynecol Laparosc. 2001;8: 495-500.
30. Brown J. AAGL advancing minimally invasive gynecology worldwide: statement to the FDA on power morcellation. J Minim Invasive Gynecol. 2014;21:970-1.
31. Johnson LA. (2014). FDA strengthens warning on device linked to cancer. [online] Available from https://medicalxpress.com/news/2014-11-fda-device-linked-cancer.html [Last accessed January, 2020].
32. ACOG. (2015). ACOG Statement on FDA Regulation of Morcellation. [online] Available from http://www.acog.org/About-ACOG/News-Room/Statements/2015/ACOG-Statement-on-FDA-Regulation-of-Morcellation [Last accessed on January, 2020].
33. Troy Brown RN. (2015). Leading Physicians Refute FDA Warning on Morcellation. http://www.medscape.com/viewarticle/855654#vp_2 [Last accessed January, 2020].
34. Parker WH, Kaunitz AM, Pritts EA, et al. U.S. Food and Drug Administration's guidance regarding morcellation of leiomyomas: well-intentioned, but is it harmful for women?. Obstet Gynecol. 2016;127:18-22.
35. Cheng Z, Yang W, Dai H, et al. Laparoscopic uterine artery occlusion combined with myomectomy for uterine myomas. J Minim Invasive Gyneacol. 2008;15:346-9.
36. Magrina JF. Complications of laparoscopic surgery. Clin Obstet Gynecol. 2002;45:469-80.

Accompanying Video: Laparoscopic myomectomy.

CHAPTER

20

Ovarian Torsion

Shwetha Shah, Aditi Rai, B Ramesh

INTRODUCTION

Ovarian torsion accounts for about 2–3% of gynecological emergencies. Lower abdominal pain is the common chief complaint, as there are many causes of lower abdominal pain, ovarian torsion should be considered, as missing the diagnosis would lead to loss of ovary and poor outcomes such as infertility. As the clinical features are nonspecific, ultrasound is the mainstay to make preoperative diagnosis.[1,2] The exact incidence is unknown as the diagnosis can be made definitively on surgery.

DEFINITION

Complete or partial rotation of ligamentous supports which includes lymphatics, arteries, and veins due to mechanical obstruction resulting in ischemia and infarction[3] **(Fig. 1)**.

Adnexal torsion is the torsion of the Fallopian tubes and ovaries together. It occurs in 67% of cases of adnexal torsion.[4,5]

NORMAL ANATOMY OF OVARIES (FIG. 2)

The infundibulopelvic and utero-ovarian ligaments suspend the movable ovary, and also contain the arterial, venous, and lymphatic supply to the ovaries.[6] As the ovaries are mobile, they are capable of undergoing twisting by any benign or malignant growth within it.

PATHOPHYSIOLOGY OF TORSION (FIG. 3)

Torsion of ovary causes twisting of suspensory ligaments and vascular pedicles resulting in venous occlusion and congestion and, in severe cases, arterial occlusion and ischemia.

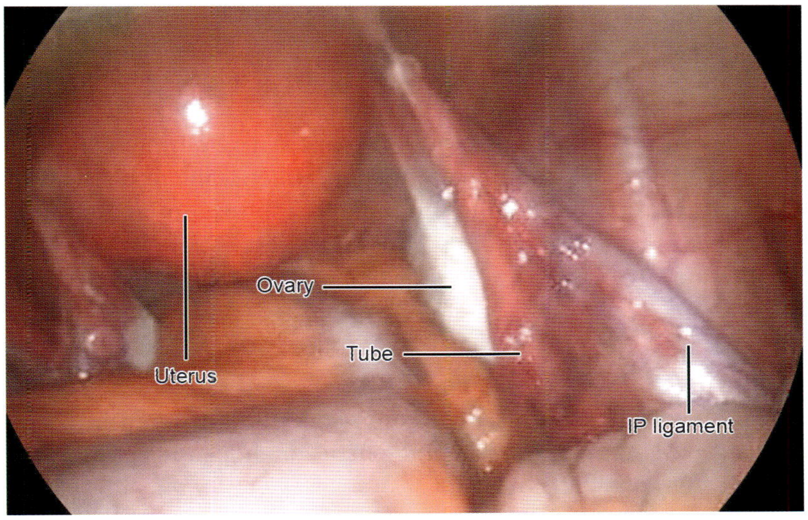

Fig. 2: Normal anatomy of ovaries.

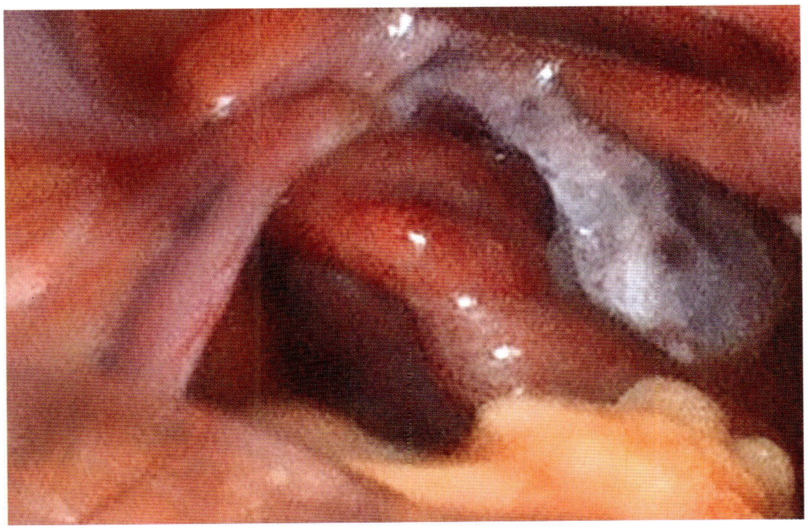

Fig. 1: Torsion of ligaments and vessels.

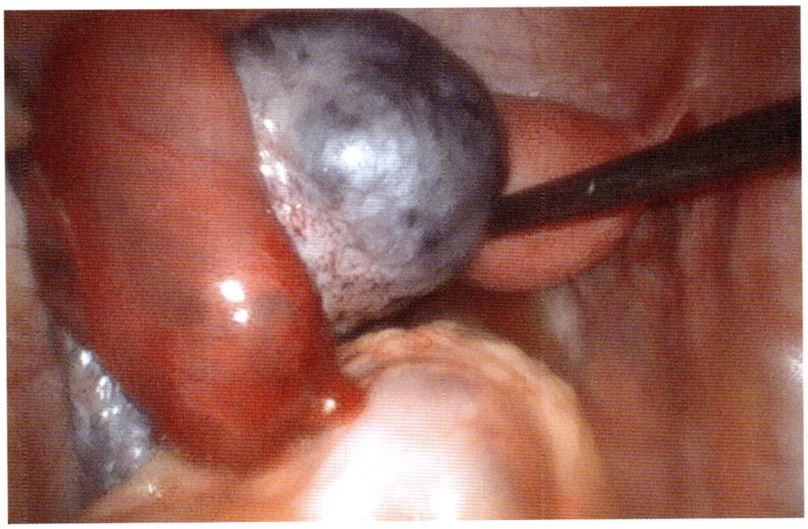

Fig. 3: Pathophysiology of torsion.

Ovarian torsion occurs when the mobile ovary rotates on its supports.

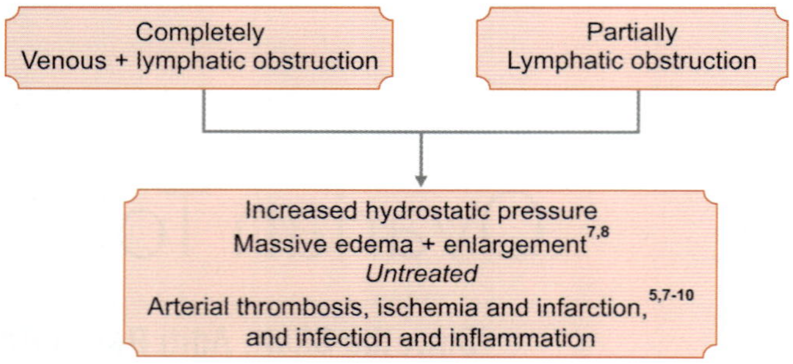

ETIOLOGY

- The most common cause is cysts in the ovaries[11-13] which includes benign cystic teratoma, cystadenoma,[4,14] and hemorrhagic cyst, cysts caused by ovulation-inducing agents.[15]
- Torsion of a normal ovary is more common in adolescents, causes include the following:
  - Markedly mobile fallopian tubes or mesosalpinx
  - Elongated pelvic ligaments
  - Abrupt changes in intra-abdominal pressure.[5,16,17]
- Pelvic inflammatory disease, endometriosis, or malignancies are not associated with torsion commonly as adhesions make the ovaries immobile.[7,8,18]
- Ovarian torsion can be seen after laparoscopic hysterectomy.[19] This is due to less adhesion formation, which is the result of lesser peritoneal trauma and inflammatory response in laparoscopic surgeries.[20,21]
- Torsion involving paratubal or paraovarian cysts has also been found.[22-24]

CLINICAL FEATURES

Most commonly seen in adolescents and young women in child-bearing age groups and less common in postmenopausal age groups.[8]

A history of acute colicky pain in a lower quadrant, with nausea and vomiting should raise the suspicion of torsion. On bimanual examination, a palpable mass is felt with adnexal tenderness.[12,25] These classical symptoms and signs are rarely present, leading to delay in diagnosis and treatment. In some cases, due to repeated episodes of torsion and detorsion, acute pain is interspersed with asymptomatic intervals. The following differentials should be considered while evaluating such a patient.

DIFFERENTIAL DIAGNOSIS

- Appendicitis
- Ruptured ovarian cyst
- Urinary tract infection
- Nephrolithiasis
- Pelvic inflammatory disease
- Uterine leiomyoma
- Diverticulitis
- Bowel obstruction
- Ectopic pregnancy.

DIAGNOSIS

Definitive diagnosis of ovarian torsion requires laparoscopy. There is no serum marker for a diagnosis of adnexal torsion. Some studies have found an association between an increased level of serum interleukin-6[26,27] and ovarian torsion, although further research is needed.[28]

IMAGING FEATURES OF OVARIAN TORSION

Gray-scale Ultrasonography (USG)

As the clinical features are nonspecific, ultrasound is the mainstay to make preoperative diagnosis.[1,2]

The most common finding in ovarian torsion is unilateral ovarian enlargement. The ovarian stroma may be heterogeneous due to hemorrhage and edema. A complex adnexal mass may be found which can be predominantly cystic, solid, or both.[4,7,18]

Color Doppler Imaging

The pathognomonic finding is the absence of arterial flow and the whirlpool sign on color Doppler; however, it may be associated with normal findings[4,29] as the ovaries have dual blood supply by ovarian and ovarian branches of uterine artery.[9] The abnormal arterial flow is almost always accompanied by either decrease or absence of venous flow, which shows that veins are affected earlier in the pathogenesis of torsion.[4] The whirlpool sign is the visualization of coiled circular vessels around the enlarged ovaries. It has been associated with necrotic or infarcted ovaries intraoperatively.[10,30]

MANAGEMENT

The gold standard to treat ovary torsion is surgery, and this is also the only way to confirm the torsion. There are two surgical methods—laparoscopy and laparotomy. A laparoscopic approach has become a popular procedure.

The current recommendations suggest that surgical detorsion and ovarian conservation[30] rather than oophorectomy are the best surgical practices **(Figs. 4A and B)**.

If malignancy is suspected, a salpingo-oophorectomy is warranted. According to many observational studies, detorsion is associated with preserved ovarian function.[31-35] The earlier the approach to torsion, the higher is the chance to preserve function. An animal study showed that necrosis might develop after occlusion of ovarian vessels for 36 hours or longer[36] **(Fig. 5)** After the symptoms have developed, ovarian conservation reportedly decreases with time.[37,38] No evidence suggests that detorsion increases adverse events postoperatively.[39]

Laparoscopy in pregnancy has divided opinion. Nezhat et al. demonstrate the benefits of operative laparoscopy and subsequent successful pregnancy outcomes.[40] Schelling recommends laparoscopy to be avoided in pregnancy due to complicated access, prolonged operating times, and a theoretical risk of fetal acidosis due to an increased abdominal pressure and consequent decrease in uterine perfusion.[41] Pucci and Seed report that no adverse fetal effects due to carbon dioxide pneumoperitoneum have been detected.[42] Taking this into consideration when operating on pregnant women, certain steps are recommended.

These include:
- Monitoring arterial blood gas and carbon dioxide level
- Avoiding pneumoperitoneum pressure >12 mm Hg
- Left lateral position.

Neonates with ovarian torsion often present with irritability and the condition can be treated with laparoscopic surgery.[43-45]

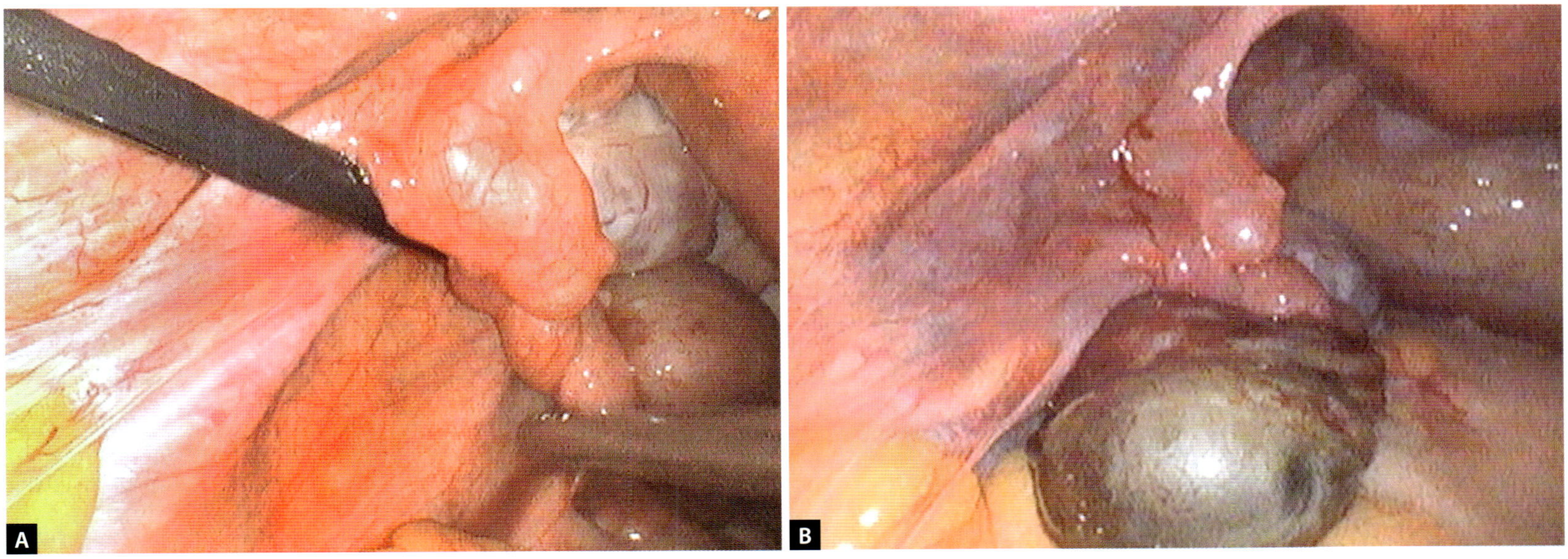

Figs. 4A and B: Lap image of torsed and detorsed ovaries.

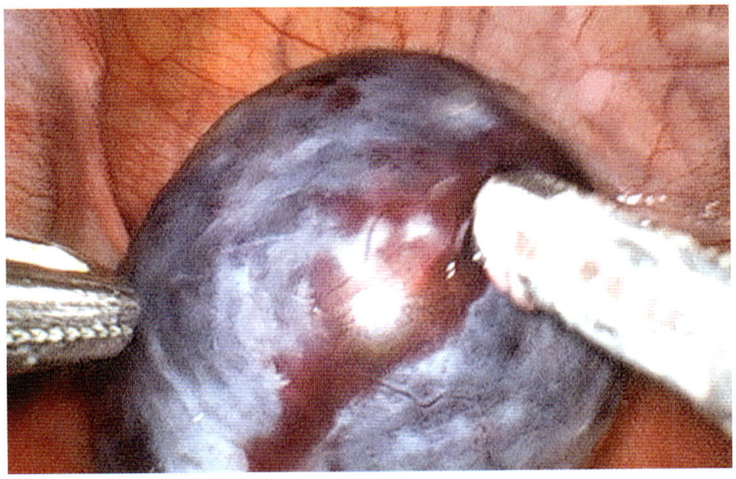

Fig. 5: Lap image of gangrenous ovary.

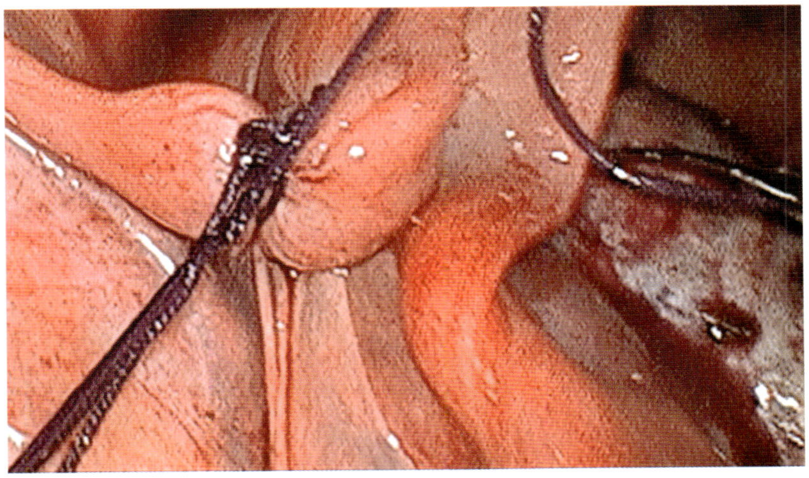

Fig. 7: Lap oophoropexy.

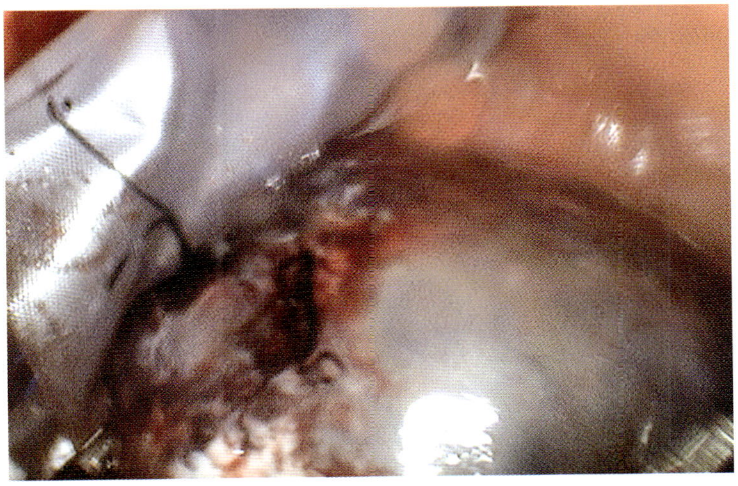

Fig. 6: Lap oophorectomy in a postmenopausal woman and tissue retrieval in endobag.

In postmenopausal women, however, the treatment of choice is bilateral oophorectomy[8] **(Fig. 6)**.

More recently, debate has sparked over the issue of oophoropexy and what the best practice is. Oophoropexy or fixation of the ovary is performed with the goal of decreasing further episodes of torsion, therefore maintaining long-term fertility. However, there is a lack of evidence regarding the long-term outcome of oophoropexy. Theoretical concerns in regard to oophoropexy include concerns regarding the disruption of tubal blood supply or a communication between ovary and fallopian tube.[46] There is also debate over the appropriateness of oophoropexy of the contralateral ovary in cases of children who have lost an ovary due to torsion and necrosis.

Methods of oophoropexy include fixation of the ovary to the:

- Lateral pelvic wall **(Fig. 7)**
- Posterior abdominal wall
- Plication of the utero-ovarian ligaments is another method which can be employed to prevent recurrence.

The preferred technique of oophoropexy is plication of utero-ovarian ligament. A combined approach of fixation of the ovary and shortening of the ligament may be more efficacious in preventing recurrence.[47]

KEY NOTES

- Diagnosis of ovarian torsion is mainly on laparoscopy.
- The most consistent finding is an enlarged ovary, without which the diagnosis is unlikely to be ovarian torsion. Comparison with the asymptomatic contralateral side is typically very helpful.
- Because the majority of cases of adnexal torsion occur in young women, a conservative operation is ideal.

- The most important factor in preservation of ovarian function is early recognition and treatment. Several studies have reported high salvage rates when treatment is initiated within the first 24 hours of the onset of symptoms.

REFERENCES

1. Bharathan R, Ramsawak L, Kelly A. Ovarian torsion: opportunities to improve clinical management. J Obstet Gynaecol. 2012;32(7):683-6.
2. Swenson DW, Lourenco AP, Beaudoin FL, et al. Ovarian torsion. Case-control study comparing the sensitivity and specificity of ultrasonography and computed tomography for diagnosis in the emergency department. Eur J Radiol. 2014;83(4):733-8.
3. Sasaki KJ, Miller CE. Adnexal torsion: review of the literature. J Minim Invasive Gynecol. 2014;21(2):196-202.
4. Albayram F, Hamper UM. Ovarian and adnexal torsion: spectrum of sonographic findings with pathologic correlation. J Ultrasound Med. 2001;20(10):1083-9.
5. Breech LL, Hillard PJ. Adnexal torsion in pediatric and adolescent girls. Curr Opin Obstet Gynecol. 2005;17(5):483-9.
6. Anne A, Dalley A. Grant's Atlas of Anatomy, 13th edition. Philadelphia: Lippincott Williams & Wilkins; 2012.
7. Warner MA, Fleischer AC, Edell SL. Uterine adnexal torsion: sonographic findings. Radiology. 1985;154(3):773-5.
8. Lee AR, Kim KH, Lee BH, et al. Massive edema of the ovary: imaging findings. AJR Am J Roentgenol. 1993;161(2):343-4.
9. Oelsner G, Shashar D. Adnexal torsion. Clin Obstet Gynecol. 2006;49(3):459-63.
10. Rosado WM, Trambert MA, Gosink BB, et al. Adnexal torsion: diagnosis by using Doppler sonography. AJR Am J Roentgenol. 1992;159(6):1251-3.
11. Varras M, Tsikini A, Polyzos D, et al. Uterine adnexal torsion: Pathologic and gray-scale ultrasonographic findings. Clin Exp Obstet Gynecol. 2004;31(1):34-8.
12. Houry D, Abbott JT. Ovarian torsion: a fifteen-year review. Ann Emerg Med. 2001;38(2):156-9.
13. White M, Stella J. Ovarian torsion: 10-year perspective. Emerg Med Australas 2005;17(3):231-7.
14. Lee EJ, Kwon HC, Joo HJ, et al. Diagnosis of ovarian torsion with color Doppler sonography: depiction of twisted vascular pedicle. J Ultrasound Med. 1998;17(2):83-9.
15. Gorkemli H, Camus M, Clasen K. Adnexal torsion after gonadotrophin ovulation induction for IVF or ICSI and its conservative treatment. Arch Gynecol Obstet. 2002;267(1):4-6.
16. Littman ED, Rydfors J, Milki AA. Exercise-induced ovarian torsion in the cycle following gonadotrophin therapy: case report. Hum Reprod. 2003;18(8):1641-2.
17. Mordehai J, Mares AJ, Barki Y, et al. Torsion of uterine adnexa in neonates and children: a report of 20 cases. J Pediatr Surg. 1991;26(10):1195-9.
18. Graif M, Shalev J, Strauss S, et al. Torsion of the ovary: sonographic features. AJR Am J Roentgenol. 1984;143(6):1331-4.
19. Mashiach R, Canis M, Jardon K, et al. Adnexal torsion after laparoscopic hysterectomy: description of seven cases. J Am Assoc Gynecol Laparosc. 2004;11(3):336-9.
20. Gutt CN, Oniu T, Schemmer P. Fewer adhesions induced by laparoscopic surgery? Surg Endosc. 2004;18(6):898-906.
21. Roberston D, Lefebvre G; Clinical Practice Gynaecology Committee. Adhesion prevention in gynaecological surgery. J Obstet Gynaecol Can. 2010;32(6):598-608.
22. Muolokwu E, Sanchez J, Bercaw JL, et al. The incidence and surgical management of paratubal cysts in a pediatric and adolescent population. J Pediatr Surg. 2011;46(11):2161-3.
23. Schrager J, Robles G, Platz T. Isolated fallopian tube torsion: A rare entity in a premenarcheal female. Am Surg. 2012;78(2):118-9.
24. Said MR, Bamigboye V. Twisted paraovarian cyst in a young girl. J Obstet Gynaecol. 2008;28(5):549-50.
25. Gillmer MD. Morris PJ, Wood WC. Ovarian accidents. Section. 36.4. Oxford Textbook of Surgery, 2nd edition. New York, NY: Oxford University Press; 2000.
26. Cohen SB, Wattiez A, Stockheim D, et al. The accuracy of serum interleukin-6 and tumour necrosis factor as markers for ovarian torsion. Hum Reprod. 2001;16(10):2195-7.
27. Daponte A, Pournaras S, Hadjichristodoulou C, et al. Novel serum inflammatory markers in patients with adnexal mass who had surgery for ovarian torsion. Fertil Steril. 2006;85(5):1469-72.
28. Laganà AS, Sofo V, Salmeri FM, et al. Oxidative stress during ovarian torsion in pediatric and adolescent patients: changing the perspective of the disease. Int J Fertil Steril. 2016;9(4):416-23.
29. Peña JE, Ufberg D, Cooney N, et al. Usefulness of Doppler sonography in the diagnosis of ovarian torsion. Fertil Steril. 2000;73(5):1047-50.
30. Vijayaraghavan SB. Sonographic whirlpool sign in ovarian torsion. J Ultrasound Med. 2004;23(12):1643-9.
31. Hubner N, Langer JC, Kives S, et al. Evolution in the management of pediatric and adolescent ovarian torsion as a result of quality improvement measures. J Pediatr Adolesc Gynecol. 2017;30(1):132-7.
32. Harkins G. Ovarian torsion treated with untwisting: second look 36 hours after untwisting. J Minim Invasive Gynecol. 2007;14(3):270.
33. Mashiach S, Bider D, Moran O, et al. Adnexal torsion of hyperstimulated ovaries in pregnancies after gonadotropin therapy. Fertil Steril. 1990;53(1):76-80.
34. Bider D, Mashiach S, Dulitzky M, et al. Clinical, surgical and pathologic findings of adnexal torsion in pregnant and nonpregnant women. Surg Gynecol Obstet. 1991;173(5):363-6.
35. Dolgin SE, Lublin M, Shlasko E. Maximizing ovarian salvage when treating idiopathic adnexal torsion. J Pediatr Surg 2000;35(4):624-6.
36. Taskin O, Birincioglu M, Aydin A, et al. The effects of twisted ischaemic adnexa managed by detorsion on ovarian viability and histology: an ischaemia reperfusion rodent model. Hum Reprod. 1998;13(1O):2823-7.
37. Anders JF, Powell EC. Urgency of evaluation and outcome of acute ovarian torsion in pediatric patients. Arch Pediatr Adolesc Med. 2005;159(6):532-5.
38. Aziz D, Davis V, Allen L, et al. Ovarian torsion in children: is oophorectomy necessary? J Pediatr Surg. 2004;39(5):750-3.
39. Zweizig S, Perron J, Grubb D, et al. Conservative management of adnexal torsion. Am J Obstet Gynecol. 1993;168(6 Pt 1):1791-5.
40. Nezhat FR, Tazuke S, Nezhat CH, et al. Laparoscopy during pregnancy: a literature review. JSLS. 1997;1(1):17-27.
41. Schelling M. Adnextumoren in der Schwangerschaft. In: Schneider H, Husslein P, Schneider KTM, (Eds). Geburtshilfe, Heidelburg: Springer-Verlag; 2000.
42. Pucci RO, Seed R. Case report of laparoscopic cholecystectomy in the third trimester of pregnancy. Am J Obstet Gynecol. 1991;165(2):401-2.
43. Crombleholme TM, Craigo SD, Garmel S, et al. Fetal ovarian cyst decompression to prevent torsion. J Pediatr Surg. 1997;32(10):1447-9.
44. Alrabeeah A, Galliani CA, Giacomantonio M, et al. Neonatal ovarian torsion: report of three cases and review of the literature. Pediatr Pathol. 1988;8(2):143-9.
45. Bryant AE, Laufer MR. Fetal ovarian cysts: incidence, diagnosis and management. J Reprod Med. 2004;49(5):329-37.
46. Fuchs N, Smorgick N, Tovbin Y. Oophoropexy to prevent adnexal torsion: how, when, and for whom? J Minim Invasive Gynecol. 2010;17(2):205-8.
47. Simsek E, Kilicdag E, Kalayci H, et al. Repeated ovariopexy failure in recurrent adnexal torsion: combined approach and review of the literature. Eur J Obstet Gynecol Reprod Biol. 2013;170(2):305-8.

Accompanying Video: Laparoscopic surgery for ovarian torsion.

CHAPTER

21

Imperforate Hymen

B Ramesh, G Hemasree

INTRODUCTION

Imperforate hymen follows failure of inferior end of the vaginal plate to canalize and incidence approximates 1 in 1,000 to 2,000 females (Parazzini, 1990).

After menarche, adolescents with imperforate hymen present with trapped menstrual blood behind the hymen (hematocolpos) which creates a bluish bulge at the introitus with cyclic menstruation. The vaginal canal greatly distends leading to formation of hematometra and hematosalpinx cyclic pain, amenorrhea, abdominal pain, and difficulty with urination or defecation may be the presenting symptoms (Bakos 1999). Retrograde menstruation may lead to development of endometriosis.

Incision and drainage is the treatment for imperforate hymen and hematocolpos **(Figs. 1A to H)**.

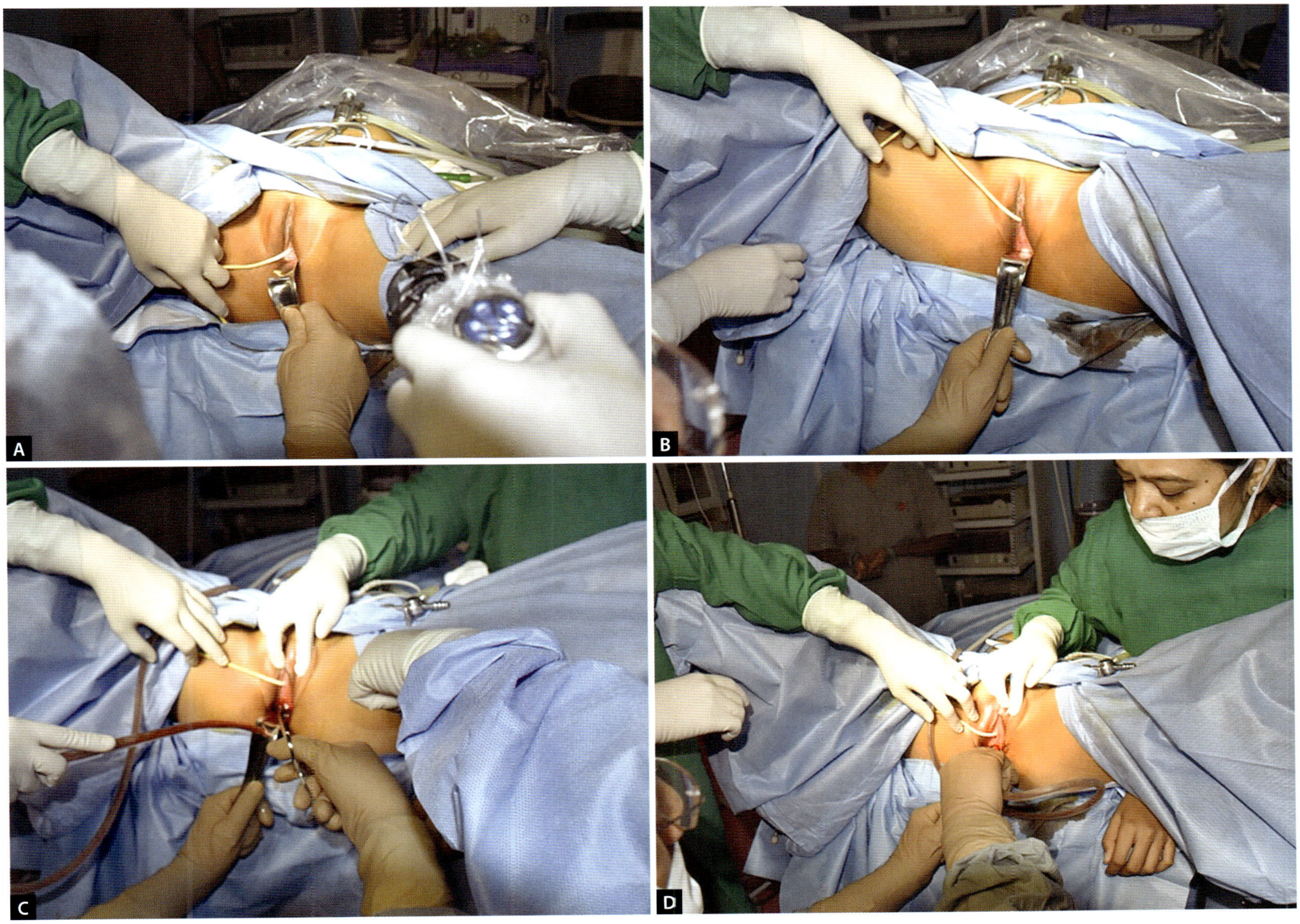

Figs. 1A to D

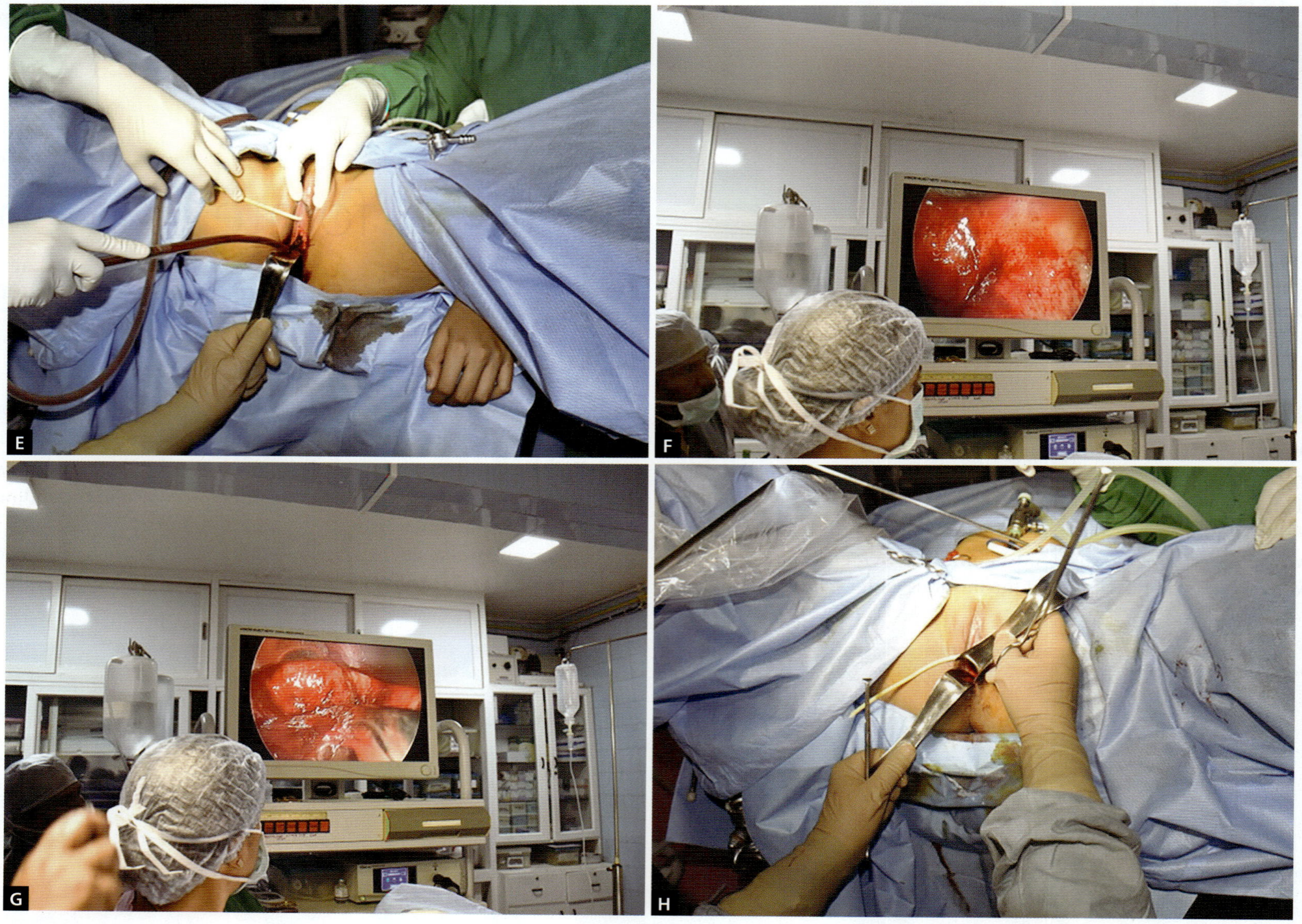

Figs. 1E to H

Figs. 1A to H: (A to E) Drainage of hematocolpos; (F to H) Laparoscopic inspection of the pelvis in the same case.

CHAPTER 22

Surgical Treatment of Endometriosis

Priyanka HK, Minal Kumbhalwar, Isha Rani, B Ramesh

INTRODUCTION

Endometriosis is a condition where tissue similar lining the uterus (the endometrial stroma and glands) is found elsewhere in the body.

An estimated 10% of all women during their reproductive years (from the onset of menstruation to menopause) are affected by endometriosis.

Patients may present with various symptoms majorly including pain, subfertility, or a combination of these problems. The disease may be suspected from pelvic examination or imaging studies. The primary focus of investigation and treatment should be directed at resolution of the presenting symptom(s). However, as endometriosis is a chronic, relapsing disorder, clinicians should develop a long-term plan of management with each patient that is dependent on her symptoms and goals for fertility and quality of life.

ETIOLOGY

Many studies demonstrate that women with endometriosis have an increased volume of peritoneal fluid, as well as increased peritoneal fluid concentrations of prostaglandins, proteases, and cytokines including inflammatory cytokines such as interleukin-1 (IL-1), IL-6, and tumor necrosis factor-α (TNF-α), and angiogenic cytokines, such as IL-8 and vascular endothelial growth factor (VEGF) produced by macrophages. Several studies have also demonstrated elevated concentrations of inflammatory cytokines in the serum of women with endometriosis, implying that endometriosis is outcome of systemic inflammation. It is unknown if inflammation causes, or is result of, endometriosis.

At present, there is no consensus on the origin of endometriosis. Failure of immune mechanisms to destroy the ectopic tissue and abnormal differentiation (metaplasia) of endometriotic tissue have been suggested as underlying mechanisms in a stromal-cell defect associated with increased estrogen and prostaglandin production, along with resistance to progesterone.

Sampson is credited with the theory of retrograde menstruation, where menstrual tissue refluxes through the Fallopian tubes and implants on pelvic structures. This mechanism has been consistently observed in humans and is supported by the anatomic distribution of implants of endometriotic tissue. This theory does not explain the observation that reflux menstruation occurs in most women but the disease in only 5–10% of the female population.

In the coelomic metaplasia theory, endometriotic lesions develop when coelomic mesothelial cells of the peritoneum undergo metaplasia. Another theory postulates the circulation and implantation of ectopic menstrual tissue via the venous or the lymphatic system, or both.

Although none of these theories can completely explain the origin and behavior of this enigmatic disease, our present understanding of the molecular mechanisms of endometriosis forms the basis for much of our therapeutic approach.

Endometriosis diagnosis is based on the women's history, symptoms, and signs; the diagnosis is corroborated by physical examination and imaging techniques, and should be proven by histology of either a directly biopsied vaginal lesion, from a scar, or of tissue collected during laparoscopy. The visual recognition of endometriosis during laparoscopy alone is of limited value as it has a high false-positive rate. On the other hand, diagnosis during laparoscopy is dependent on the ability of the surgeon to recognize peritoneal disease in all its different appearances. If the surgeon performing, the laparoscopy is not familiar with these appearances, endometriosis may be missed and left untreated—your eyes see only what your mind knows. This is especially relevant in deep infiltrating disease, where sometimes endometriosis is hidden beneath the peritoneal surface.

DIAGNOSTIC LAPAROSCOPY

Initially, the surgeon explores the pelvic cavity to assess the extent of disease and identify abnormalities or distortions of the pelvic organs. The location and boundaries of the bladder, ureter, colon, rectum, pelvic gutters, uterosacral ligaments. and major blood vessels are noted. The upper abdominal organs, abdominal walls, liver, and diaphragm should be evaluated for endometriosis or any other condition that may contribute to the patient's symptoms. The omentum and the small bowel are evaluated for disease. A rectovaginal examination is accomplished to evaluate deep and retroperitoneal endometriosis found in the lower pelvis at the rectovaginal septum, uterosacral ligament, lower colon, and pararectal area. In 15% of patients with endometriosis, the appendix is involved and should be examined. The diagnostic laparoscopy is extended to an operative procedure, if the patient has been advised of this possibility.

OPERATIVE LAPAROSCOPY

The operative procedure begins by lysing adhesions between the bowel and the pelvic organs obtaining adequate exposure of pelvic cavity. The ovaries are dissected from the cul-de-sac or pelvic side wall, and the tubes are freed from adhesions to restore the anatomy. If patient has presented with complaints of infertility, chromopertubation is done. Endometrial implants and endometriomas are resected or fulgurated, and if the patient has significant midline pelvic pain, uterosacral nerve ablation or presacral nerve resection is done.

TREATMENT OF MINIMAL TO MODERATE ENDOMETRIOSIS

The best primary treatment of minimal and mild endometriosis in individuals attempting to achieve a pregnancy remains controversial. Surgical treatment is advocated by some. It has been demonstrated that surgical treatment of endometriosis appears superior to other treatment forms, and the laser ablation may provide a higher pregnancy rate than laparoscopic diathermy ablation.

Peritoneal Implants

Superficial peritoneal endometriosis is either vaporized with the laser, coagulated with monopolar or bipolar current, or excised. Implants less than 2 mm are coagulated, vaporized, or excised. When lesions exceed 3 mm, vaporization or excision is needed **(Figs. 1A and B)**.

OVARIAN ENDOMETRIOSIS

The ovaries are most common site for endometriosis. The accepted histologic criterion for the diagnosis of endometriosis is the presence of endometrial glands and stroma.

Endometriotic implants or endometriomas less than 2 cm in diameter are either coagulated, laser ablated, or excised, using scissors, biopsy forceps, lasers, or electrodes. Draining the endometrioma or partially resecting its wall is inadequate because the endometrial tissue lining the cyst can remain functional and may cause recurrence.

Excision of Endometriotic Implants

Refer to **Figures 2A to D**.

Coagulation of Endometriotic Implant Using Bipolar Forceps

Refer to **Figures 3A to D**.

Fulguration of Endometriotic Cyst Wall with Bipolar

Ovarian endometriosis is treated during first-look laparoscopy, if penetration of not more than 3 cm into the ovary and if the cyst diameter is no larger than 3 cm. Small (<1 cm in diameter) endometriotic implants of the ovary are fulgurated or cauterized until follicles containing fluid are encountered or no further pigmented tissue is seen. Large (<3 cm in diameter) endometriomas are treated by excision. A 3–4-mm portion of the top of the cyst, the chocolate-colored material is aspirated and the cyst is completely opened and washed out with irrigation fluid. After washing, the interior wall of the cyst is carefully examined to confirm the diagnosis of an endometrioma and the absence of any intracystic lesions suspected of being malignant (ovarian cystoscopy). At a power setting of 40 W and with continuous mode application, the interior wall of the cyst is then cauterized to destroy the lining of the cyst as it is made up of stroma and is continued until no further pigment is visualized **(Figs. 4A to E)**.

Endometriosis: Cystectomy

The procedure begins with adhesiolysis. Once the cyst is mobilized, the cortex is grasped with forceps introduced through a second trocar. Diluted vasopressin (10 U in 100 mL) of 8–10 mL can be injected between the cortex and cyst wall. The cortex is incised using laser or scissors. The incision must be made on the antimesenteric surface, as far as possible from the ovarian hilus. The incision is extended with scissors, and hydrodissection can be used to separate the cyst wall from the ovarian stroma. If the cyst is opened and spillage occurs, peritoneal irrigation must be performed in order to remove the chocolate-colored fluid. The cyst is decompressed by suction drainage and washed. The cyst wall is then exposed and inspected to confirm the diagnosis of an endometrioma.

After identifying the correct plane of cleavage between the wall of the cyst and the ovarian tissue by applying opposite bimanual traction with two 5-mm grasping forceps, providing strong but nontraumatic traction, the inner lining of the cyst is stripped from the normal ovarian tissue. The bed of the cyst needs to be carefully inspected to detect possible bleeding zones that may require coagulation with bipolar forceps.

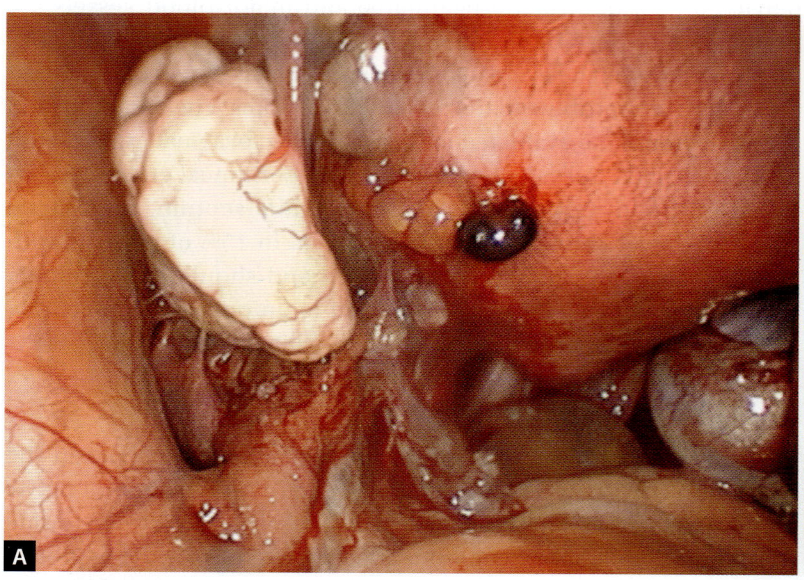

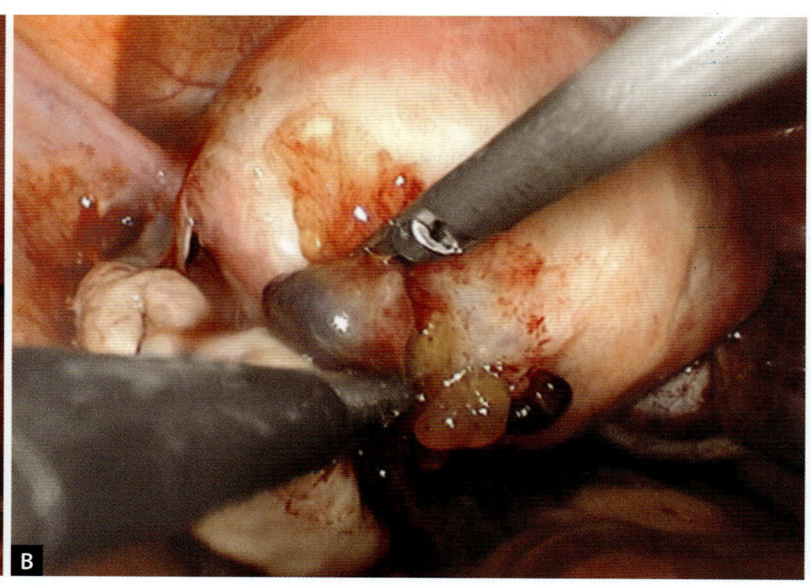

Figs. 1A and B: Peritoneal implants.

The endometrioma is removed through the 10-mm trocar. If the volume exceeds the dimensions of the trocar, an endobag can be used.

The ovary does not usually require suturing **(Figs. 5 to 12)**.

Ovarian Reserve Following Cystectomy

Ovarian reserve is defined as the quantitative and qualitative supply of follicles in the ovaries that can potentially develop into mature

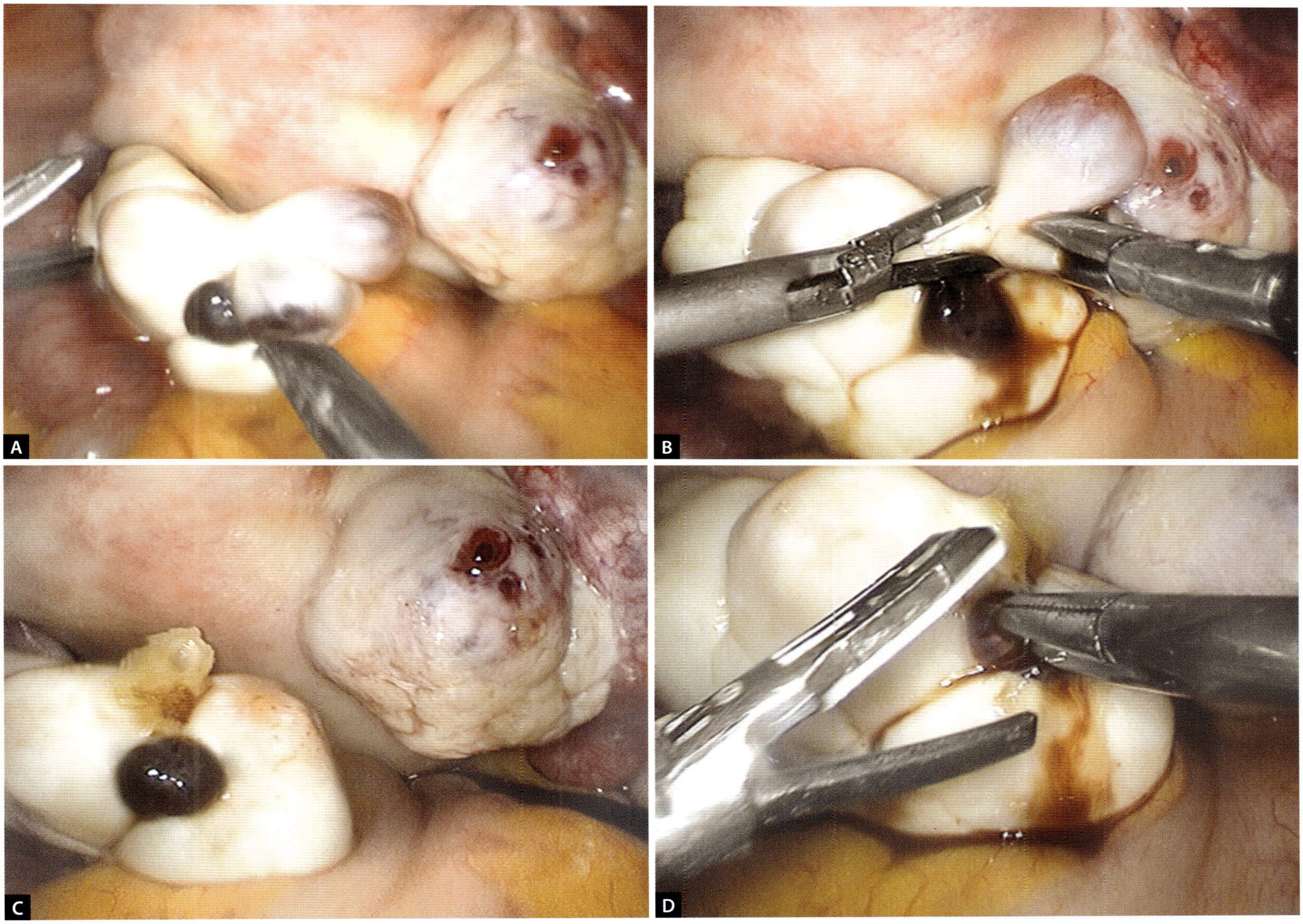

Figs. 2A to D: Excision of endometriotic implants.

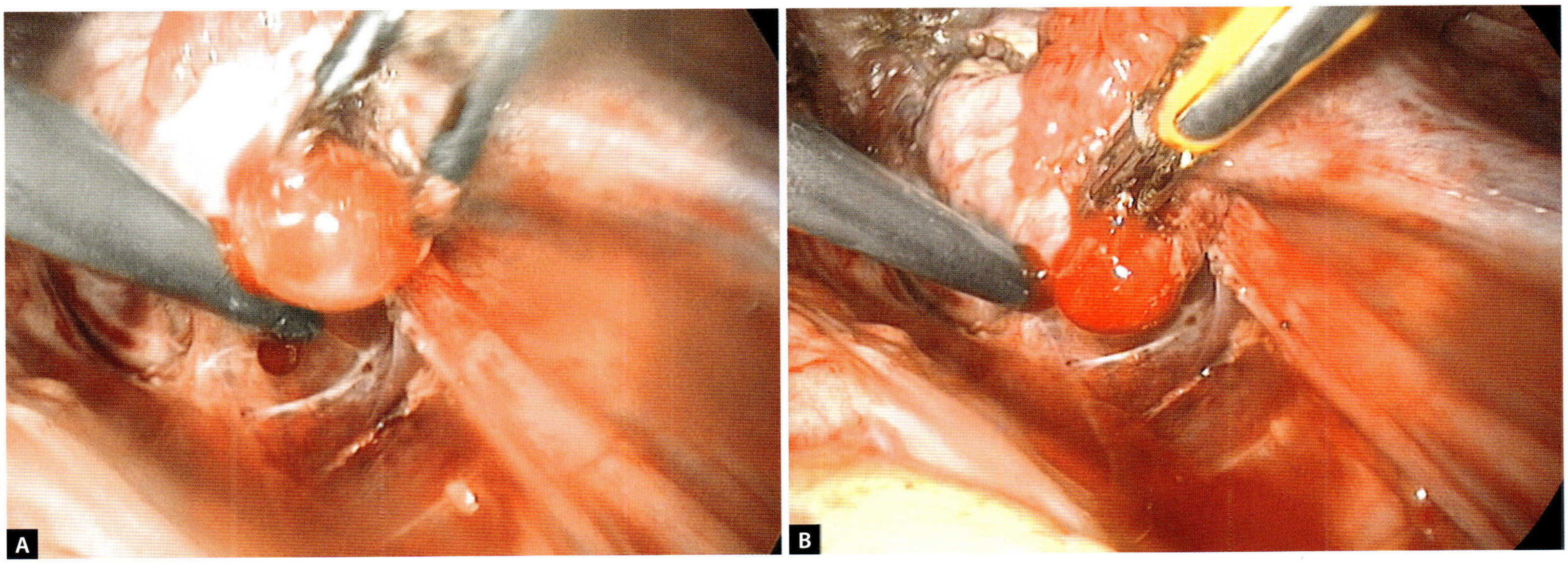

Figs. 3A and B

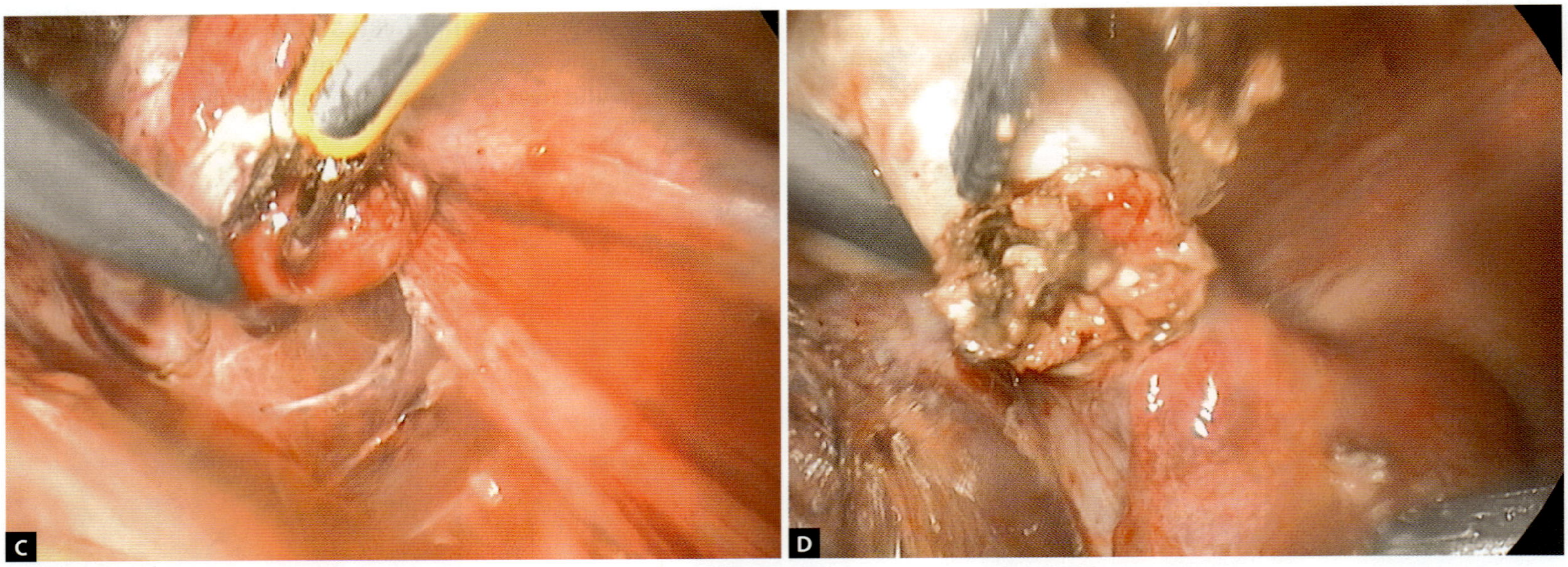

Figs. 3C and D

Figs. 3A to D: Coagulation of endometriotic implant using bipolar forceps.

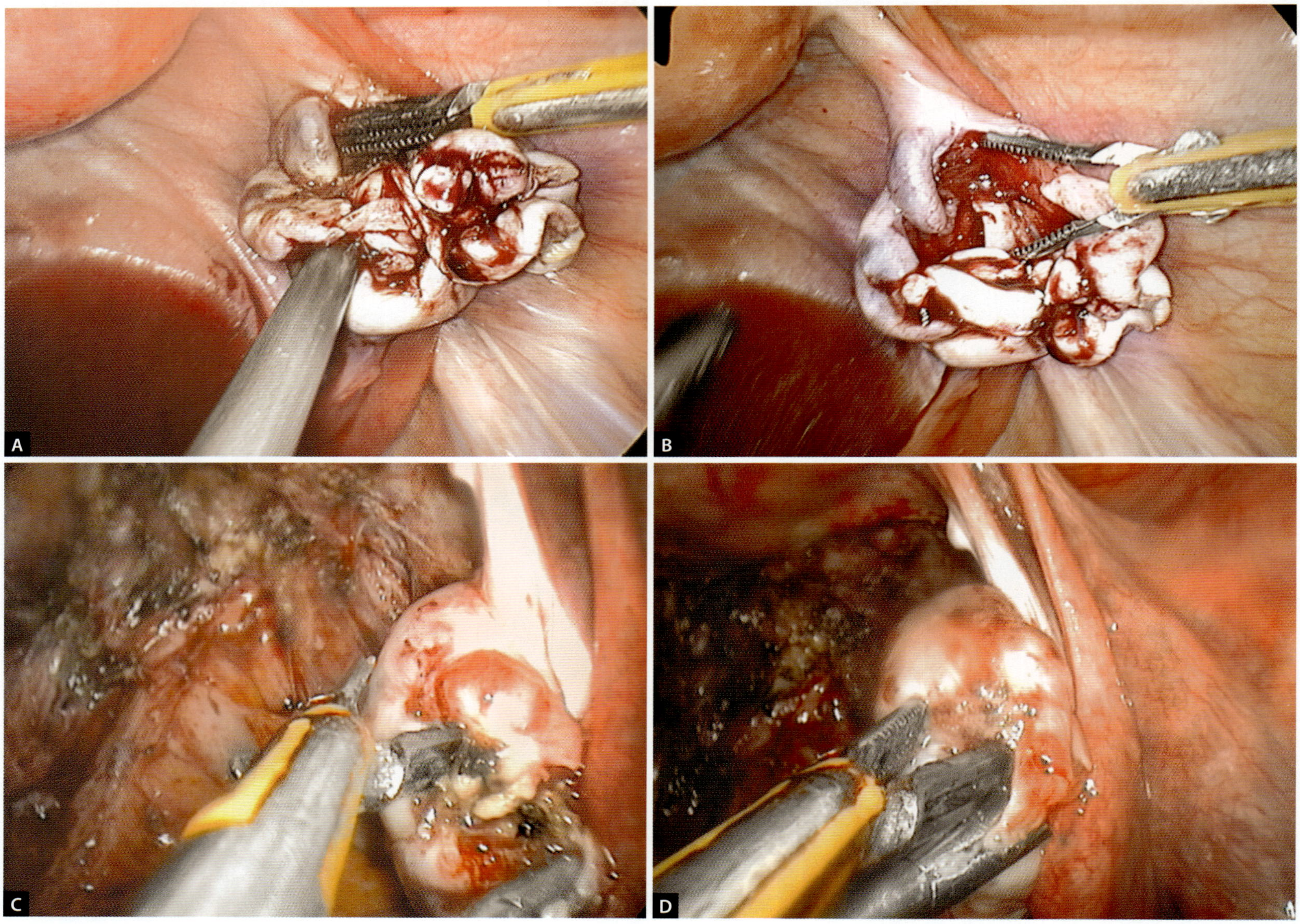

Figs. 4A to D

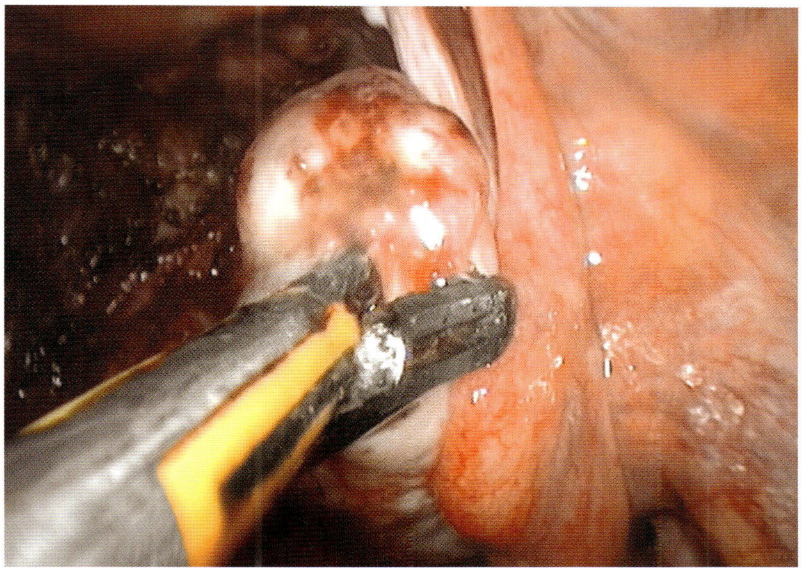

Fig. 4E

Figs. 4Ato E: Fulguration of endometriotic cyst wall with bipolar.

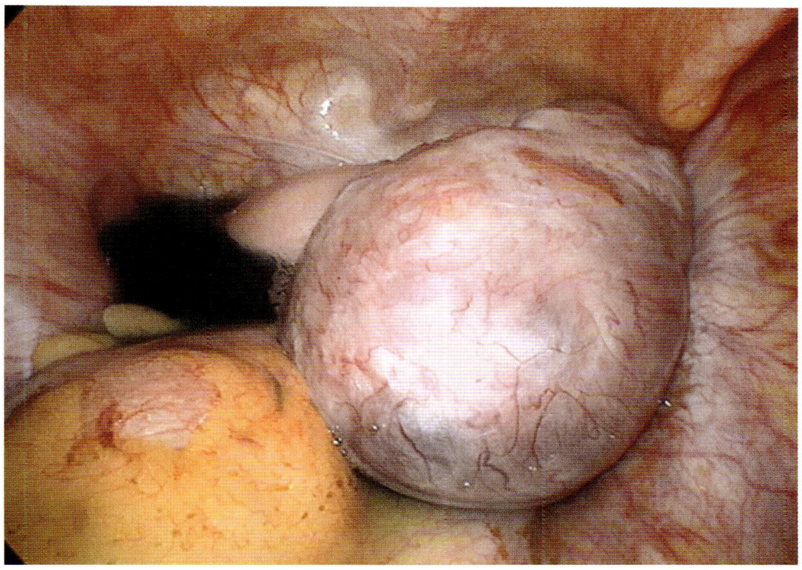

Fig. 5: Right endometriotic cyst.

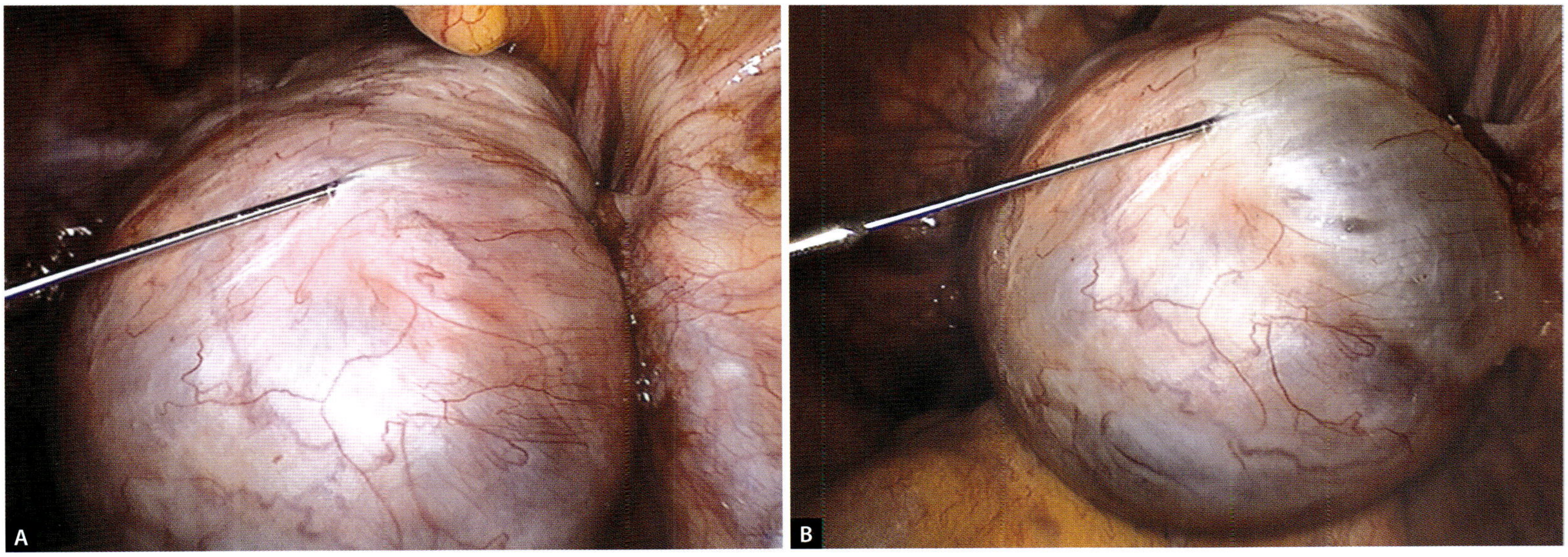

Figs. 6A and B: Injection of diluted vasopressin between ovarian cortex and cyst wall using cyst injection needle.

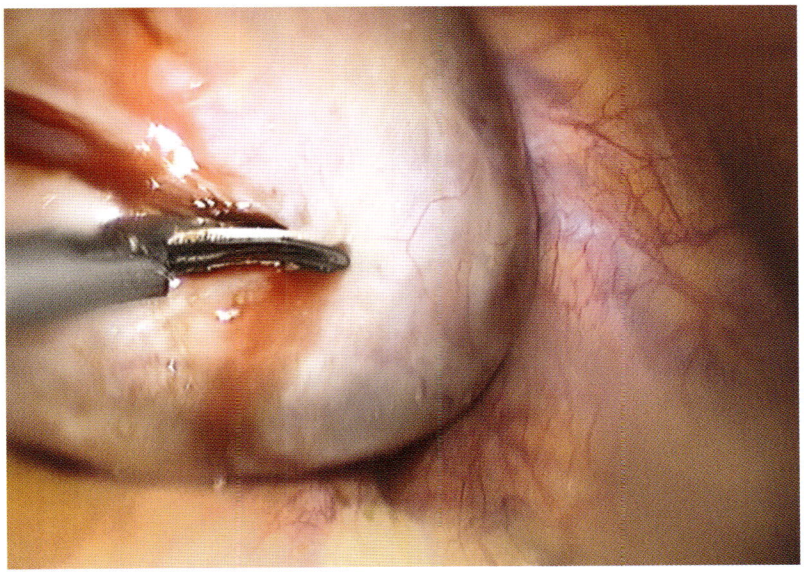

Fig. 7: Incision made over cyst wall using harmonic.

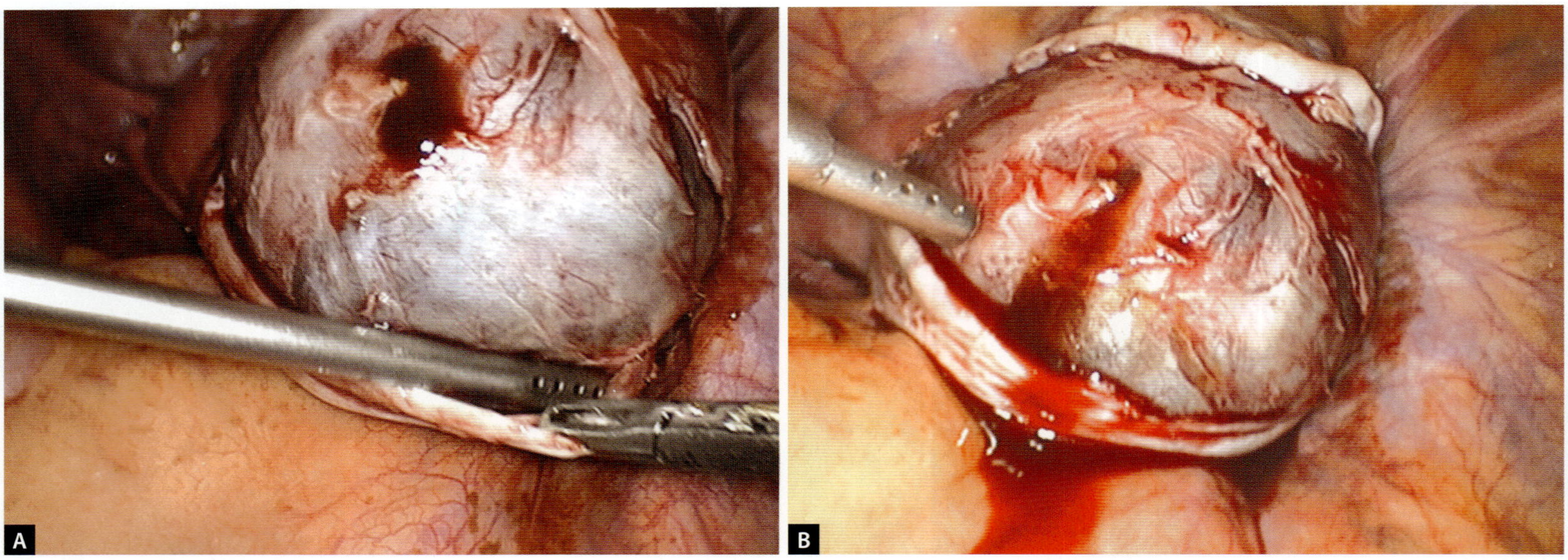

Figs. 8A and B: Cyst wall separated from ovarian cortex by blunt dissection with atraumatic graspers and suction irrigator.

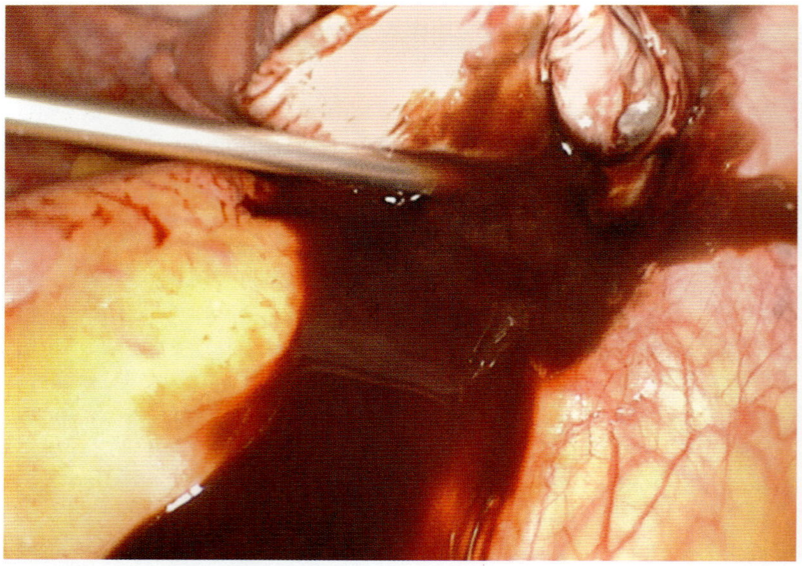

Fig. 9: Cyst ruptured and contents aspirated.

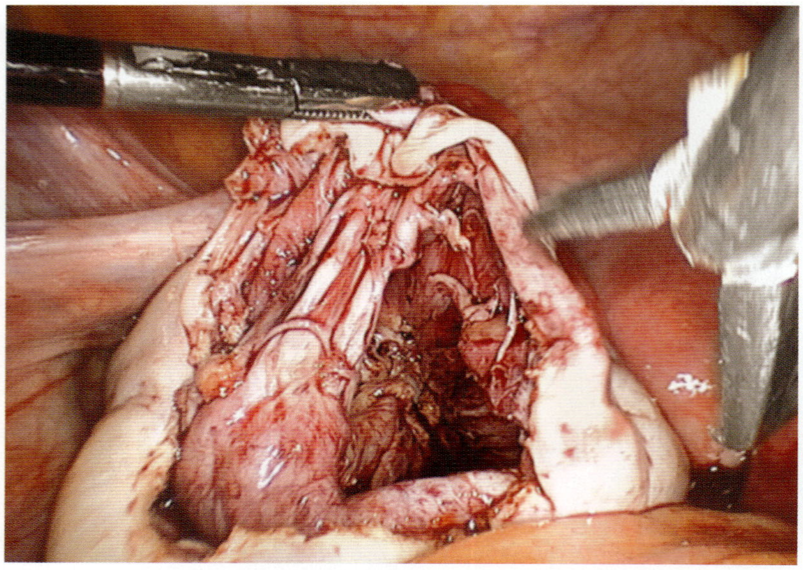

Fig. 10: Cyst wall attached to ovarian cortex at hilum.

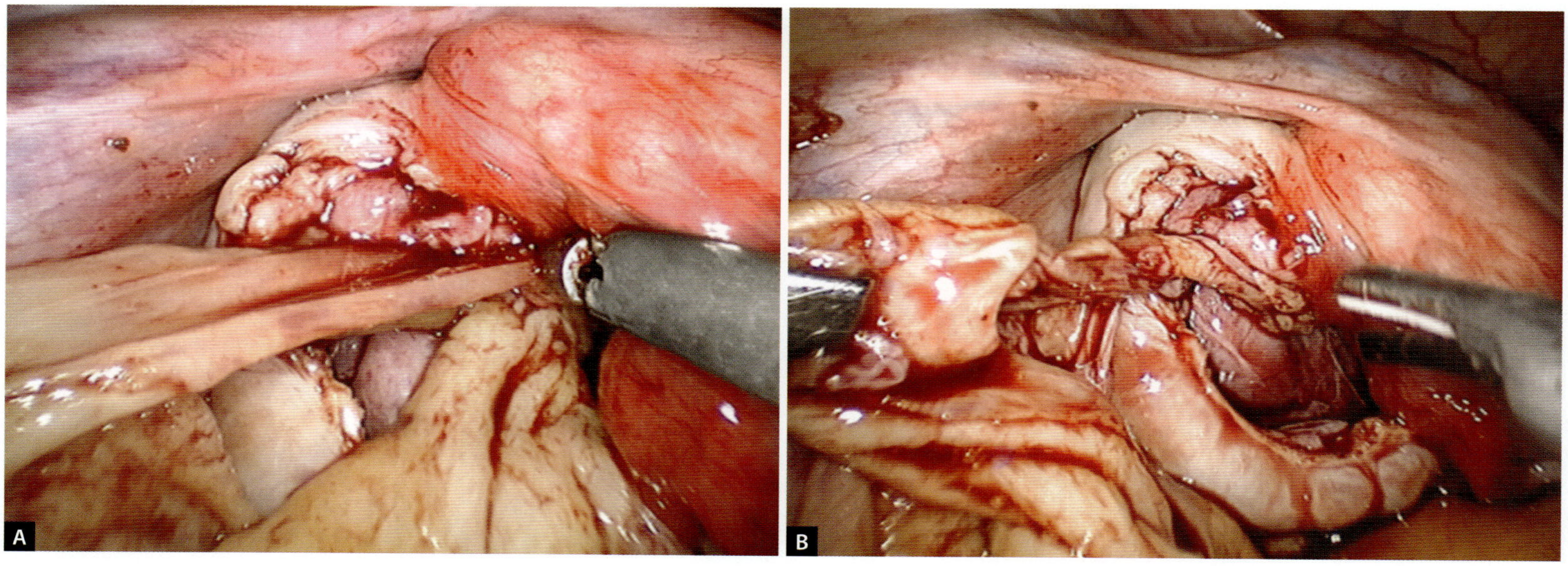

Figs. 11A and B: Cyst wall excised using harmonic.

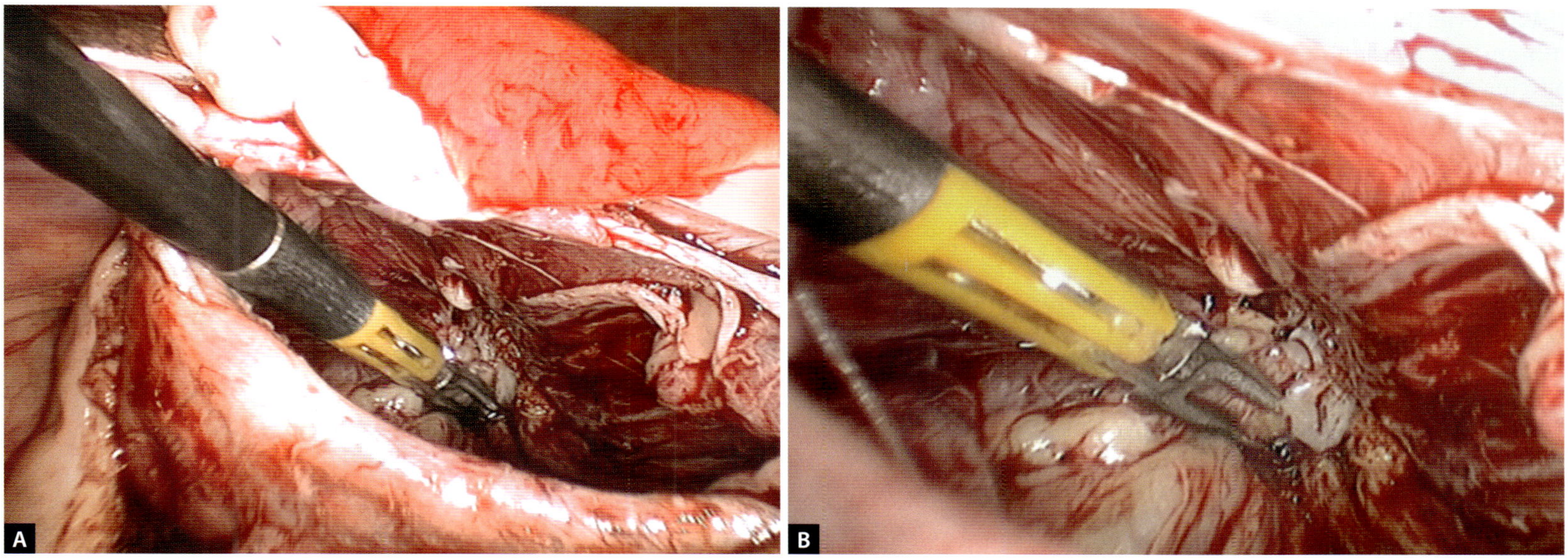

Figs. 12A and B: Coagulation at ovarian hilus using b polar.

follicles that in effect determine a woman's reproductive potential. Benign ovarian cysts form within the ovarian parenchyma and are often removed either using a minimally invasive procedure such as laparoscopy or an open abdominal procedure called the laparotomy. Both, the cyst in itself and the cystectomy, i.e. excision and enucleating of cyst from the ovary can reduce the ovarian reserve.

A study was conducted by Melanie Henes et al. on influences of ovarian cyst removal on ovarian reserve showed that it was dependent on histology, size, and type of operation. According to that study, the size of the cysts had an influence on the ovarian reserve, only larger ovarian cysts with a diameter of 5 cm or more showed a statistically significant reduction in anti-Müllerian hormone (AMH). Their data showed a significant decrease in AMH levels after surgery on the ovaries.

In another study conducted by Chamnan Tanprasertkul et al. AMH changes after laparoscopic ovarian cystectomy for endometrioma compared with the nonovarian conditions concluded that laparoscopic ovarian cystectomy in case of endometrioma had negative impact on the ovarian reserve, measured by serum AMH. This effect was sustained at least 6 months after operation.

Comparison between Cyst Wall Fulguration versus Cystectomy

Endometrioma is one of the frequent adnexal mass seen in the premenopausal population, but there is no validated recommendation for its treatment. Medical therapy is inefficient and cannot be recommended in the management of ovarian endometriomas. While the surgical treatment of choice is laparoscopy, for conservative treatment, the preferred method is controversial. Cystectomy can be destructive for the ovarian parenchyma hence causing loss of follicles, whereas ablation may be incomplete which pose a great risk of recurrence. Draining the endometrioma or partially resecting its wall is inadequate, because the endometrial tissue lining the cyst remains functional and may cause the symptoms to recur. Cystectomy of ovarian endometriomas improves spontaneous pregnancy rates and reduces pain. In addition, it may improve the response to in vitro fertilization (IVF). It has been shown that laparoscopic cystectomy for ovarian endometriomas >4 cm in diameter improves fertility compared to drainage and coagulation. Drawbacks of surgery include postoperative adhesion formation and incomplete removal of the disease.

Var et al. found that there was significant reduction in antral follicle count (AFC) and ovarian volume following laparoscopic endometriotic cystectomy. Said et al. concluded that removal of endometriotic cysts with the stripping technique is associated with direct trauma to the ovarian cortex leading to destruction of the follicles. In a study by Ercan et al., on the 2nd postoperative day a significant increase in the ovarian volume was detected on the operated ovary, which may be the result of edema due stripping procedure. They were followed up for 3 months and they found no significant difference between the operated and nonoperated ovarian volume. AFCs of the operated side were significantly lower on 2nd postoperative day and the decrease persisted 3 months after surgery. In a study by Celik et al., compared preoperative measurements with 6 weeks and 6 months postoperatively, the AFC increased both at week 6 and 6 months postoperatively, but there was a significant decrease in serum AMH levels.

Hart et al. concluded that there is good evidence to suggest that excisional surgery for endometrioma provides for a better outcome than drainage and ablation with regard to the recurrence of the endometrioma, recurrence of pain symptoms, and in women who were previously subfertile, subsequent spontaneous pregnancy. Consequently this approach should be the favored. However in women who may subsequently may undergo fertility treatment insufficient evidence exists to determine the favored surgical approach.

DIRECT TROCAR INSERTION

For large endometriomas, the cyst can be punctured with the 5-mm trocar and aspirated with the suction—irrigator probe. Then high-pressure irrigation at 500–800 mm Hg is used to irrigate the cyst, causing it to expand, and is aspirated several times **(Figs. 13 to 15)**.

Fertility Following Laparoscopic Conservative Surgery

The effect of endometrioma on ovarian reserve is given in following text.

Whatever the hypothesis, endometriomas develop in contiguity with surface ovarian cortex, where there is pooling of primordial follicles that constitute ovarian reserve. The development of endometriotic lesion may initiate marked inflammation in surrounding tissue and the function of ovarian cortex as reservoir of dormant follicles is affected by developing endometriomas. It is possible that

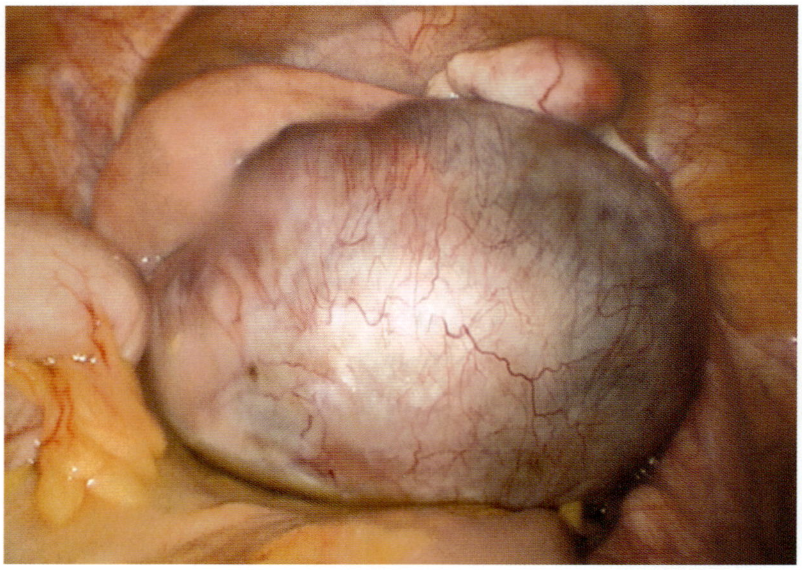

Fig. 13: Left endometriotic cyst 8 × 8 cm.

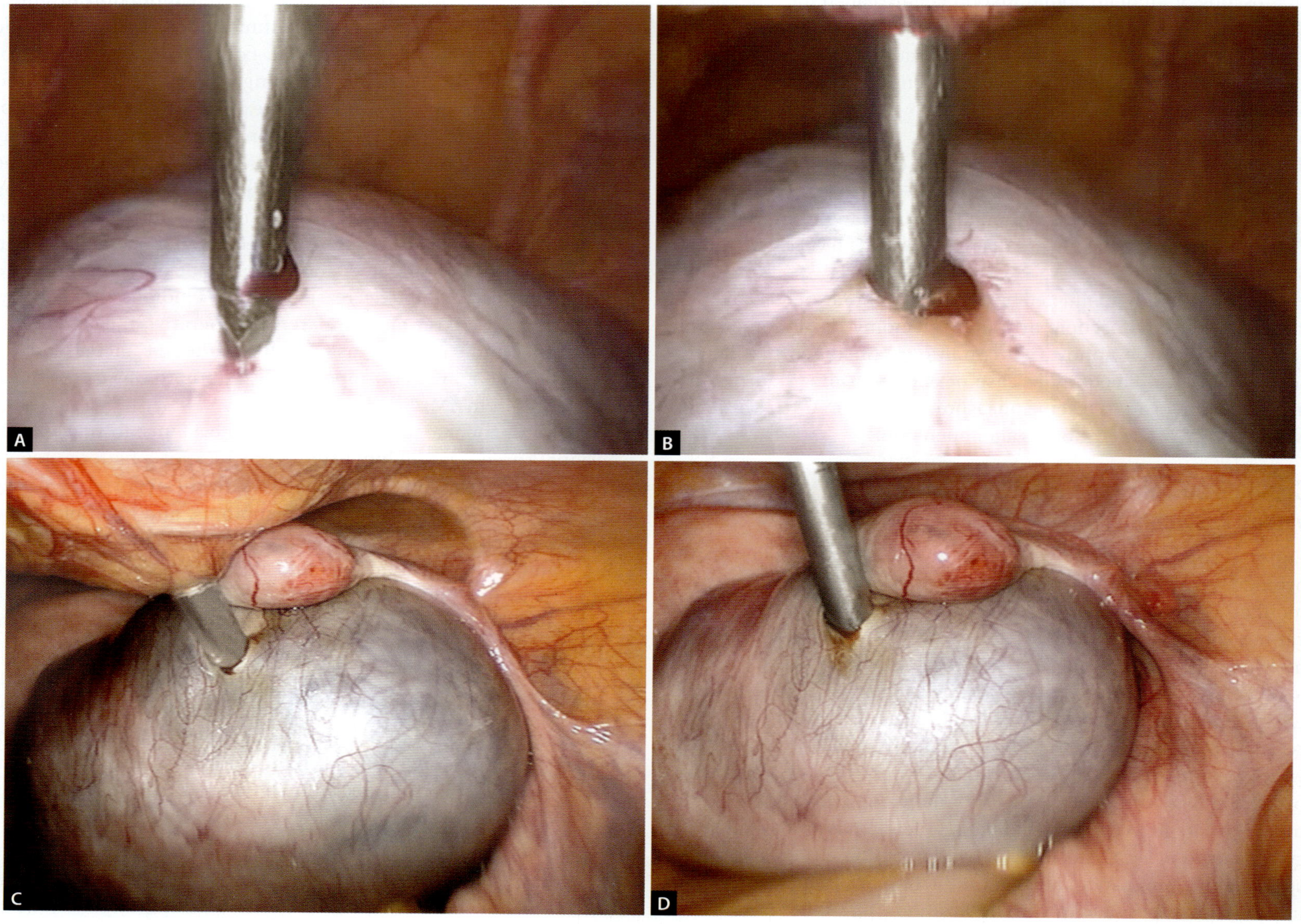

Figs. 14A to D: Cyst punctured with trocar and cannula.

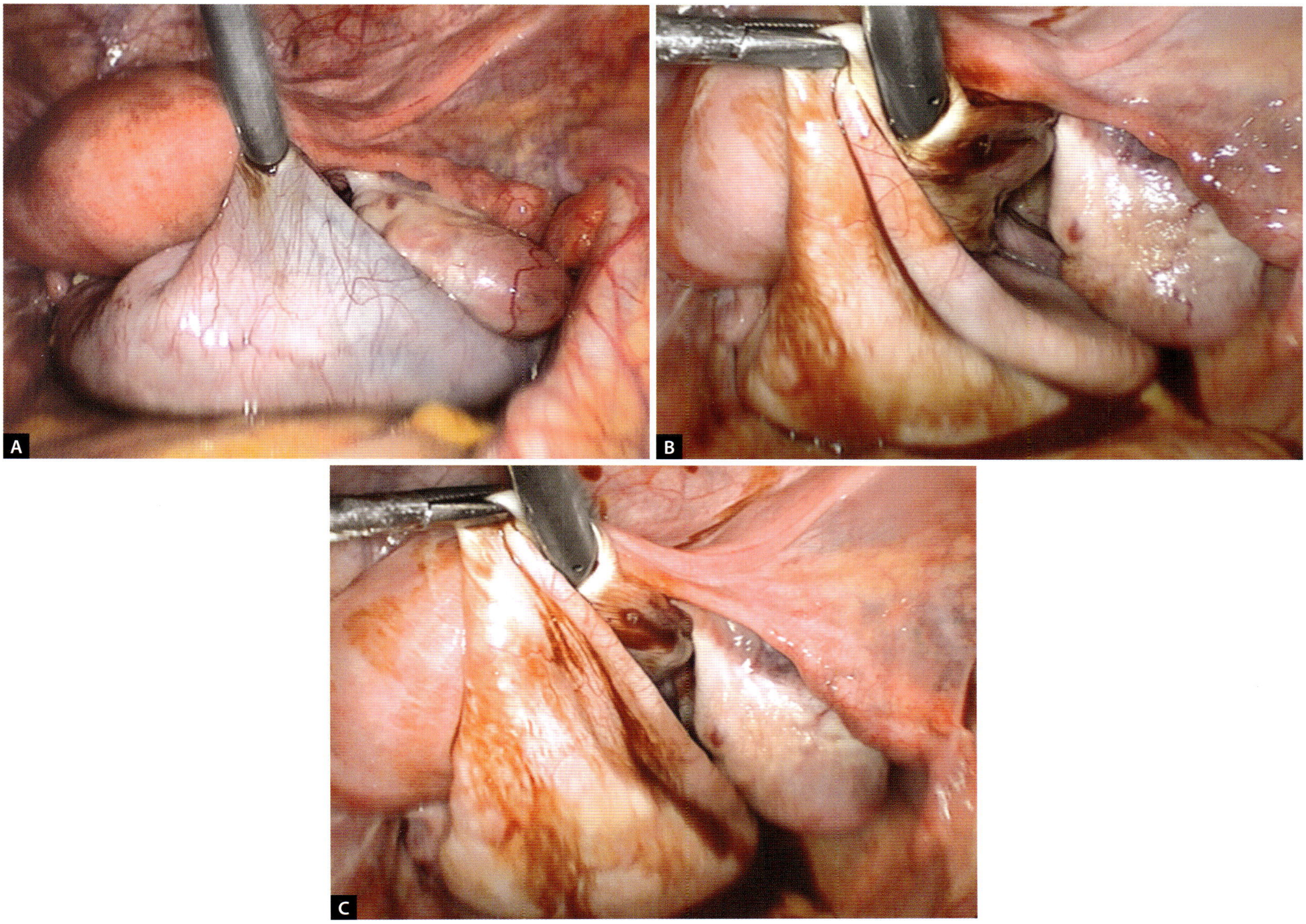

Figs. 15A to C: Contents of cyst aspirated with suction irrigation cannula.

detrimental effects on ovarian reserve by endometriomas may be accentuated by the surgical damage.

Ovarian cortex from ovaries with endometriomas on examination showed decreased follicular density compared to those of contralateral healthy ovaries or nonendometriotic benign ovarian cyst. In addition, ovaries with endometriomas showed significant fibrosis formation in ovarian cortex that is proportional to decrease of follicular density. These results support that the inflammation and transformation of normal cortical structure caused by development of endometriomas may affect physiological functions of adjacent ovarian cortex as follicular reservoir. Accelerated follicular recruitment and, at the same time, increased atresia of early follicles were found in the ovarian cortex derived from ovaries with endometriomas comparing to those of contralateral intact ovaries. These results indicate "burn-out" of ovarian reserve along with the development of endometriomas could be responsible for decreased fecundity in women with endometriosis.

There is controversy regarding the surgical management of endometriomas in women undergoing infertility treatment. While surgical treatment may improve spontaneous pregnancy rates by restoring the pelvic anatomy, it remains controversial as to whether surgical intervention on the ovary itself is beneficial as it may not reverse, the inflammatory and biomolecular changes shown to influence fertilization and implantation. Furthermore, there are concerns regarding the safety of surgical treatments, with reported reduction in the ovarian reserve and the added risk of requiring an oophorectomy though small. In contrast, concerns have been raised about the effect of an endometrioma on oocyte quantity and quality. Owing to this conflict, management should be individualized and based on clinical factors, including pain, size of the cysts, and concerns over potential malignancy.

Consideration should be given to surgical treatment being undertaken by a surgeon with specific expertise in endometriosis and fertility, in order to minimize the impact on the ovarian reserve and provide a holistic assessment regarding future fertility management.

When surgical management is opted, ovarian endometriomas are best managed by performing a cystectomy, as opposed to drainage and coagulation, which is associated with an overall lower recurrence risk and higher spontaneous postoperative pregnancy rate, especially when the size of cyst is 3 cm or more in diameter. Hart et al. summarized two randomized controlled trials (RCTs) which showed beneficial effect of excisional surgery over drainage or ablation of an endometriotic cyst in achieving a spontaneous pregnancy in subfertile women. However, this can lead to a significant reduction in the number of ovarian follicles. Data from observational controlled studies investigating ovarian endometrioma drainage and ablation using energy with minimal thermal spread, such as CO_2 laser or plasma energy, indicated good results.

Surgical Treatment Prior to IVF

Surgical treatment of endometriomas prior to IVF is widely practiced, although its need and effect is debatable. A systematic review (five controlled studies; n = 655) reported similar live birth (OR, 0.9; 95% CI, 0.63–1.28), clinical pregnancy (OR, 0.97; 95% CI, 0.78–1.2) and miscarriage rates (OR, 1.32; 95% CI, 0.66–2.65) following IVF treatment in women with and without surgically treated endometriomas. The number of oocytes retrieved and the cancellation rates were comparable in both the groups, women with a surgically treated endometrioma had a lower AFC and required higher doses of gonadotropins for ovarian stimulation.

Interestingly, women who had undergone surgical management for a unilateral endometrioma had a lower number of oocytes retrieved from the surgically treated ovary (mean difference; 2.59; 95% CI; 4.13–1.05) when compared with the contralateral normal ovary, indicating a reduction in the ovarian reserve following surgical intervention, as has been reported in several other studies.

The potential physiological compensation by the normal ovary for the compromised ovary is seen, in conjunction with the higher follicle stimulating hormone doses required for ovarian stimulation, may account for the similar IVF outcomes noted in women who have undergone surgical treatments for their endometriomas.

A Cochrane review incorporating two small RCTs has reported similar pregnancy rates for surgical (cystectomy or aspiration) and expectant management. There was no differences in pregnancy rates following a cystectomy and aspiration of an endometrioma, while cystectomy is associated with a lower ovarian response following controlled stimulation, with a lower number of mature oocytes retrieved, raising concern about the potential adverse influence of a cystectomy on ovarian reserve. In contrast, a meta-analysis including three controlled studies (including non-RCT studies) reported similar ovarian responses and pregnancy rates following IVF in women with an endometrioma surgically managed with a cystectomy compared to transvaginal aspiration prior to IVF treatment. Based on the available evidence, the ESHRE guideline group concluded that a cystectomy for an endometrioma of size more than 3 cm, prior to undergoing IVF treatment, does not improve pregnancy rates. However, surgery prior to ART can be considered for the management of endometriosis-associated pain, for increasing the accessibility of the follicles and ease during oocyte retrieval procedures, or to ameliorate any concern for malignancy.

ADNEXECTOMY/SALPINGO-OOPHORECTOMY

Refer to **Figures 16 to 20**.

URETEROLYSIS

Ureteral involvement by endometriosis is rare and occurs in about 0.1–0.4% of cases. It most commonly affected part is the distal ureter, less commonly the mid-ureter, and rarely the proximal ureter. Lesions are typically extrinsic, with a smaller fraction of cases involving the lumen of the ureter (i.e. intrinsic). Depending on the extent of ureteral involvement, ureterolysis with or without ureteral resection can be performed safely and effectively with the laparoscopic approach. The ultimate goal is to avoid ureteral obstruction and loss of renal function. While performing ureterolysis, care is taken to preserve the periureteral vascular supply if the ureter is not directly affected by endometriosis, fibrosis, or inflammation.

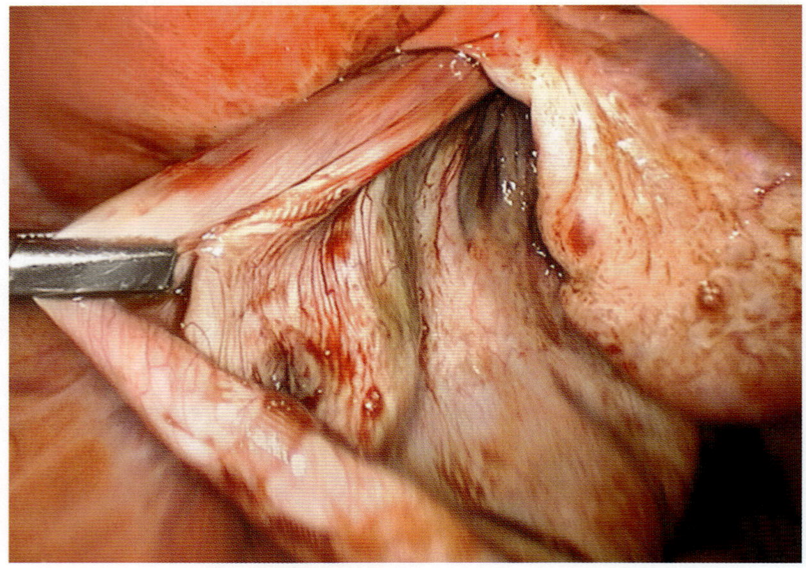

Fig. 16: Ovary held with tooth grasper and traction applied.

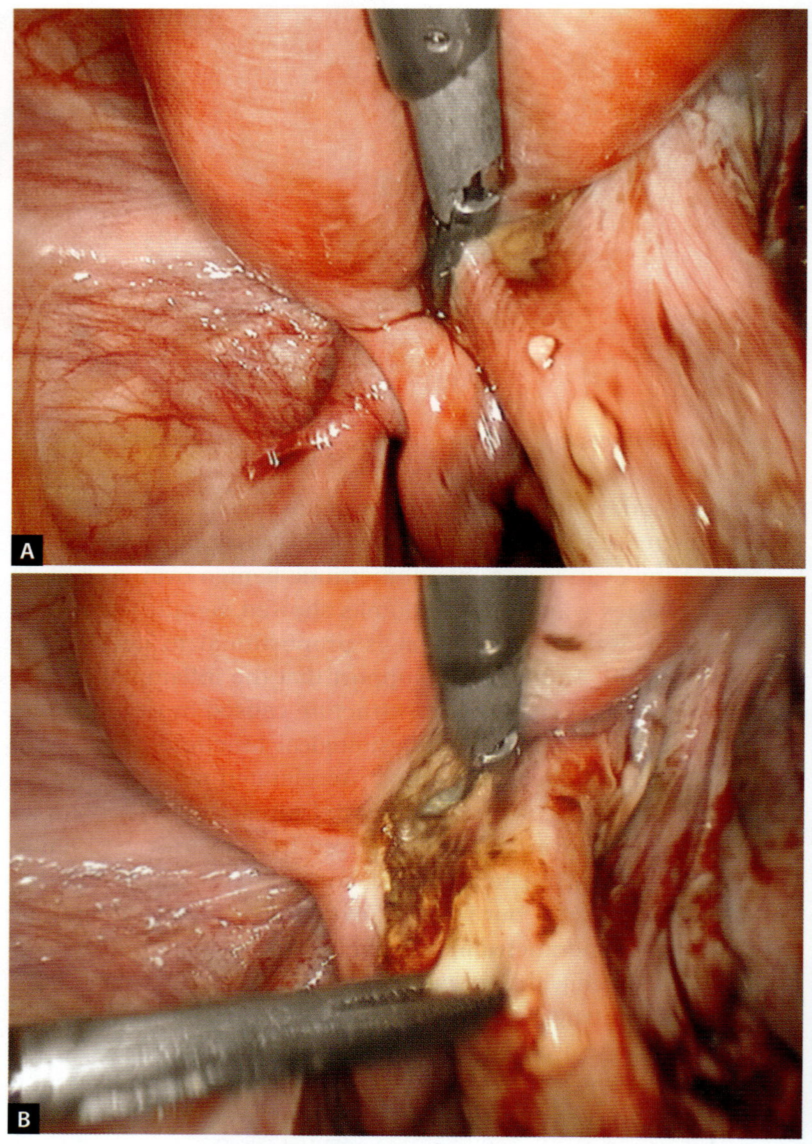

Figs. 17A and B: Ovarian ligament cauterized and cut with harmonic.

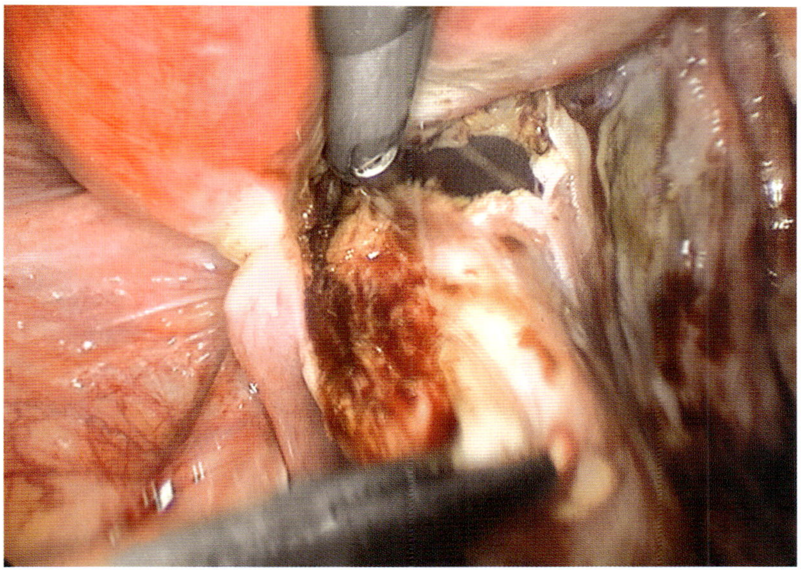

Fig. 18: Incision extended with harmonic while traction is applied with tooth grasper.

The blood supply to the distal ureter typically comes laterally from the iliac artery, whereas the mid- and proximal ureters' blood supply comes medially from the aorta. There is also a fine network of vessels that travel along the length of the ureter. Thus, while performing ureterolysis care should be taken to preserve the periureteral tissue and adventitia of the ureter. In cases in which extrinsic ureteral involvement is minimal, ureterolysis alone may be needed to relief the symptoms.

Steps of Ureterolysis

- Identification of ureter **(Figs. 21A and B)**
- Incision made lateral to ureter over the peritoneum on the lateral pelvic wall triangle **(Figs. 22A to C)**
- Incision extended cephalad up to pelvic brim **(Fig. 23)**
- Loose areolar tissue dissected **(Fig. 24)**
- Incision extended up till uterosacral ligament (USL) **(Fig. 25)**
- Ureter freed by grasping with an atraumatic grasper and surrounding fascia dissected with harmonic **(Figs. 26A and B)**
- Postureterolysis **(Fig. 27)**.

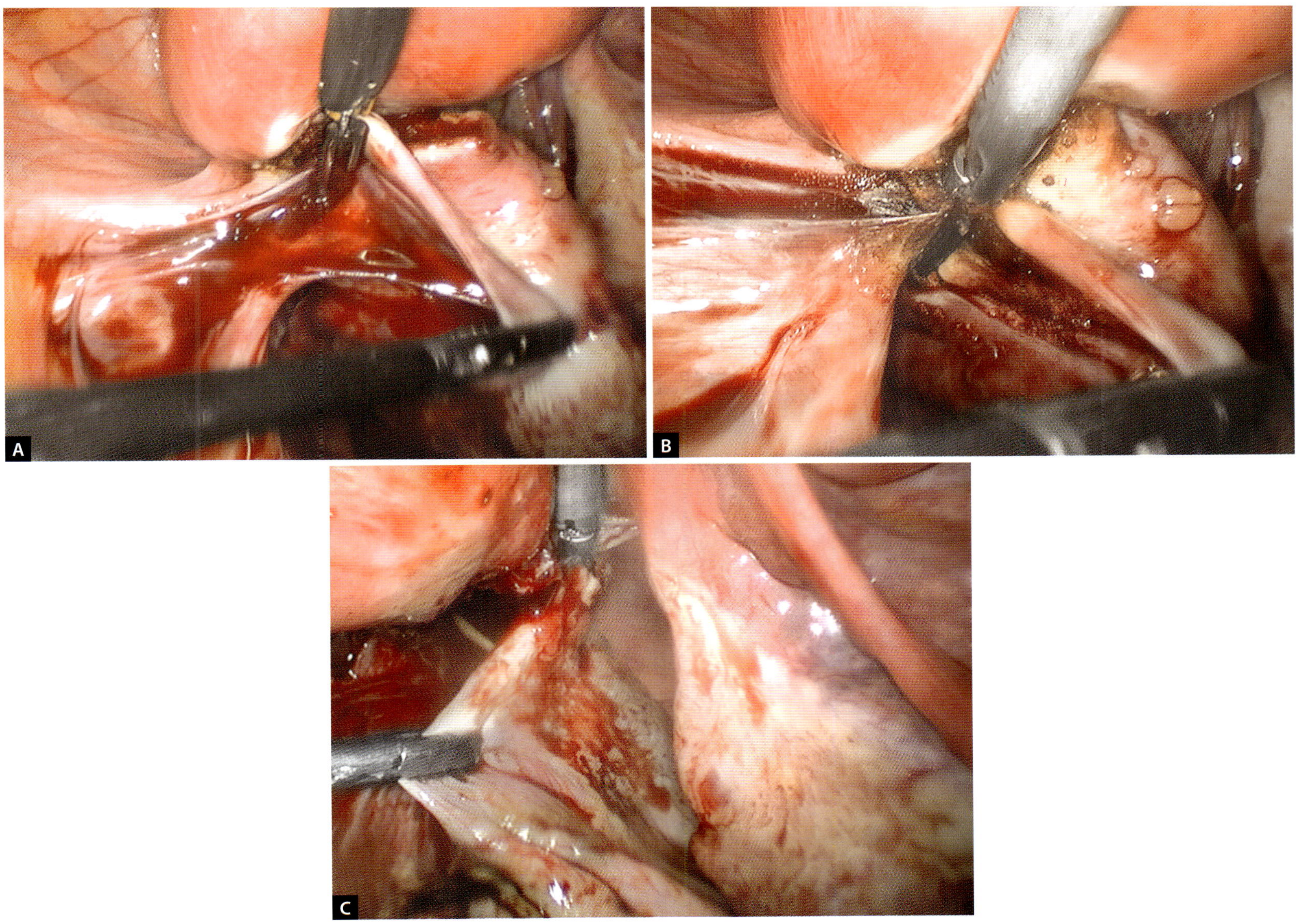

Figs. 19A to C: Infundibulopelvic ligament is cauterized with bipolar and cut with harmonic/scissor.

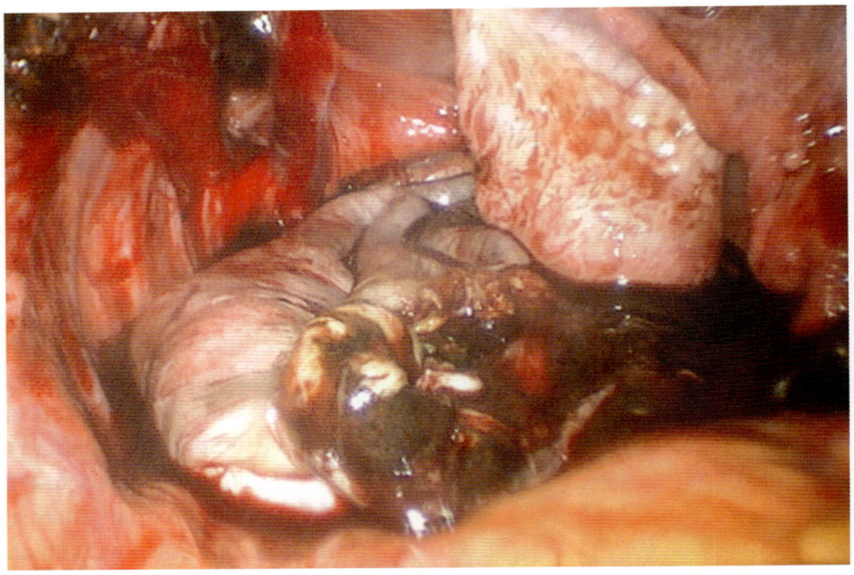

Fig. 20: Specimen of ovary and tube postadnexectomy.

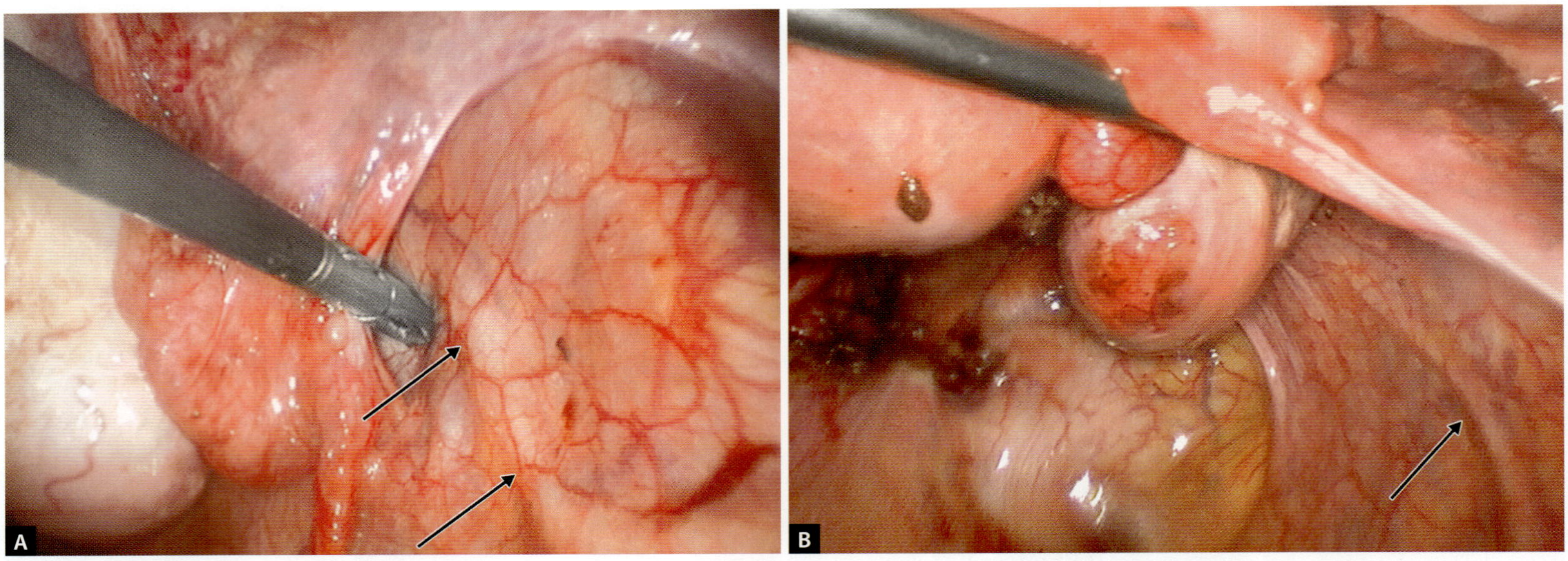

Figs. 21A and B: Identification of ureter.

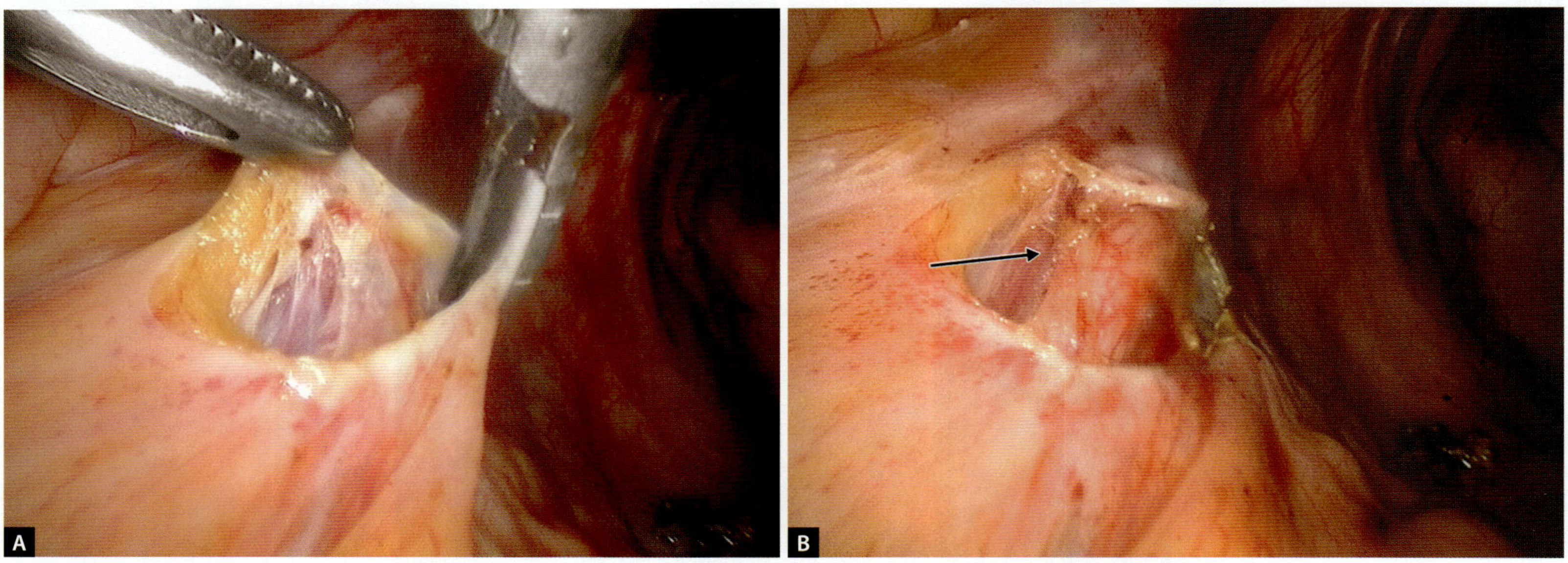

Figs. 22A and B

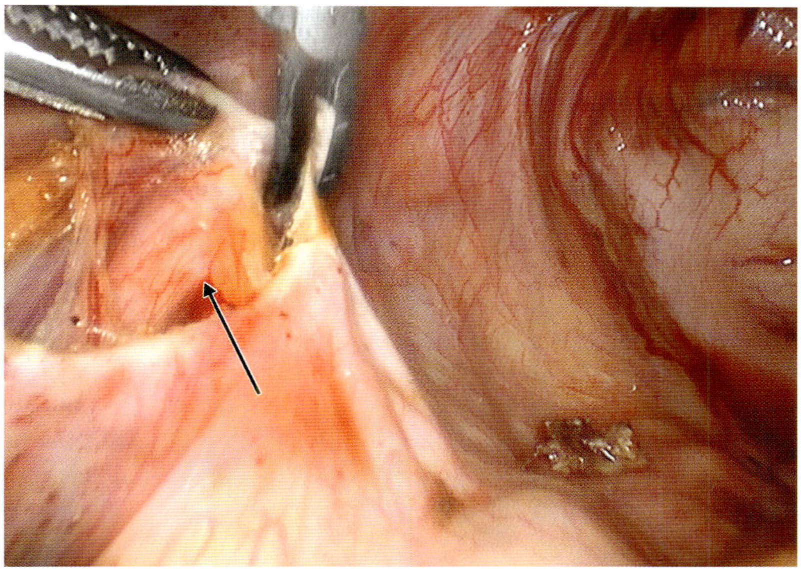

Fig. 22C

Figs. 22A to C: Incision made lateral to ureter over the peritoneum on the lateral pelvic wall triangle.

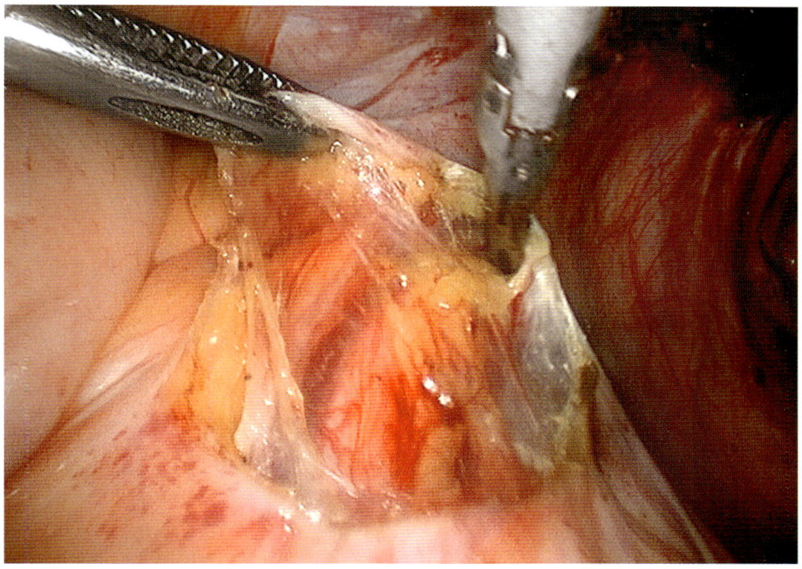

Fig. 24: Loose areolar tissue dissected.

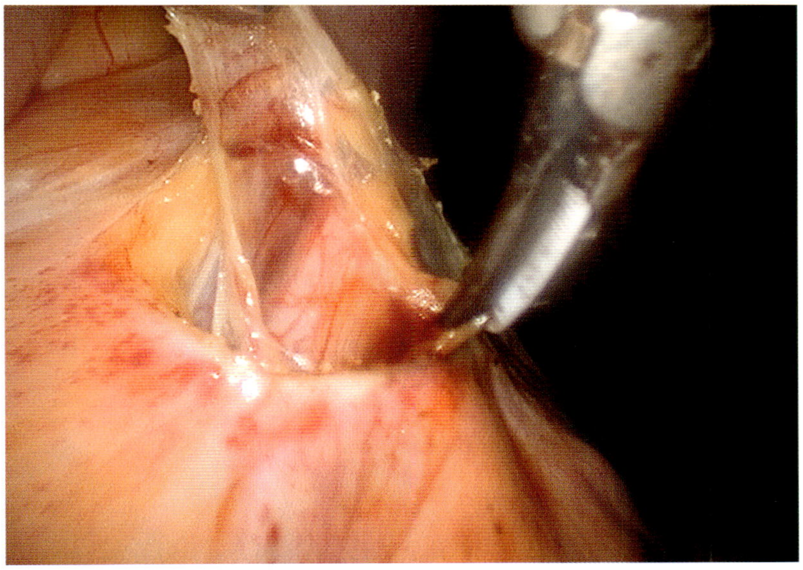

Fig. 23: Incision extended cephalad up to pelvic brim.

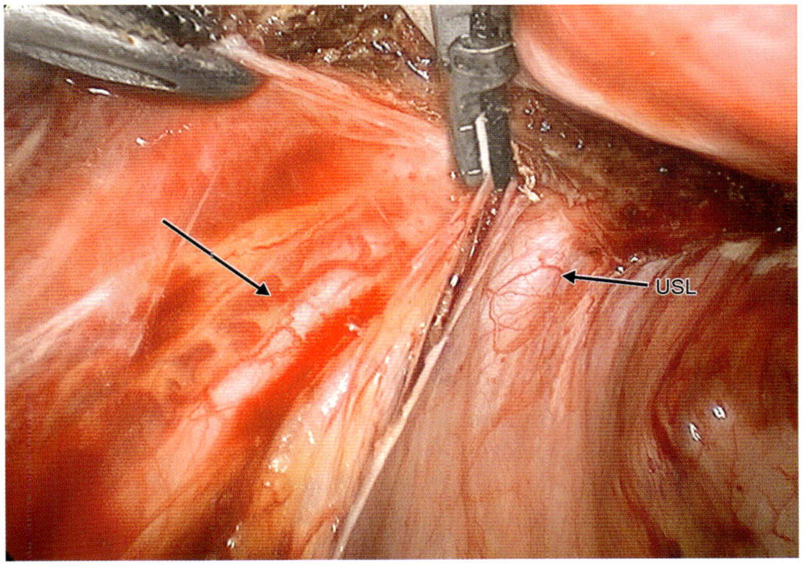

Fig. 25: Incision extended up till uterosacral l gament (USL).

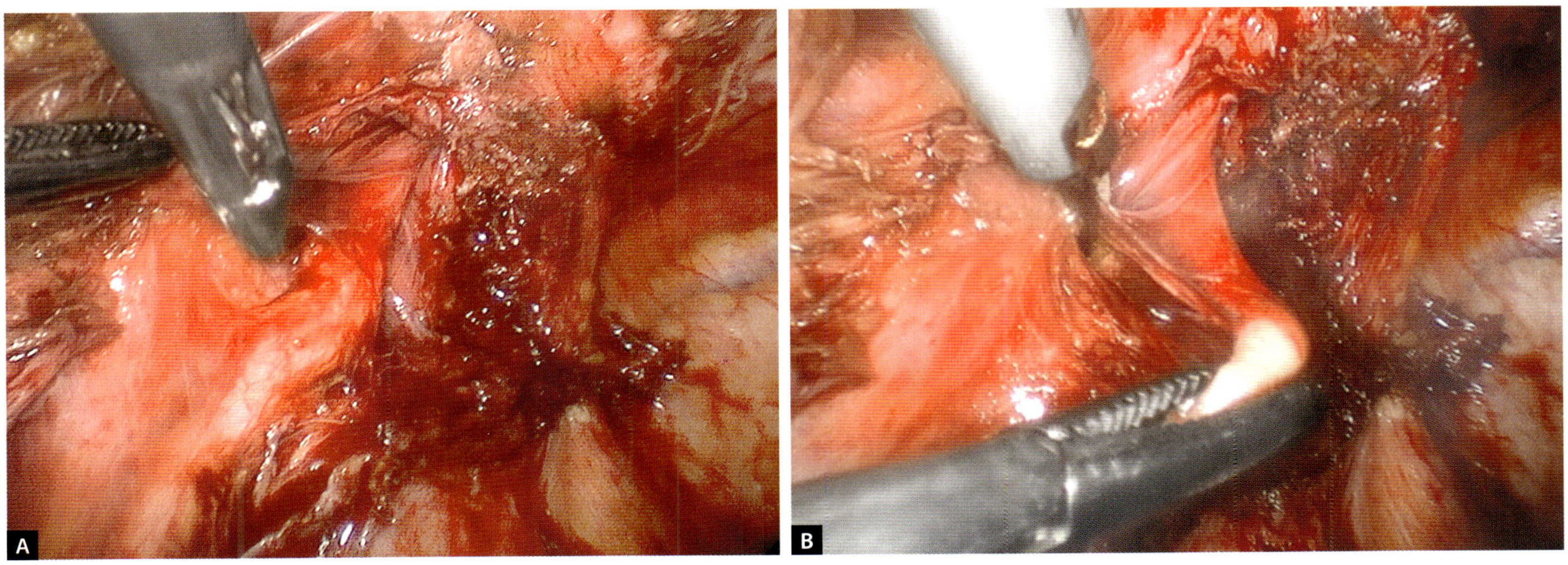

Figs. 26A and B: Ureter freed by grasping with an atraumatic grasper and surrounding fascia dissected with harmonic.

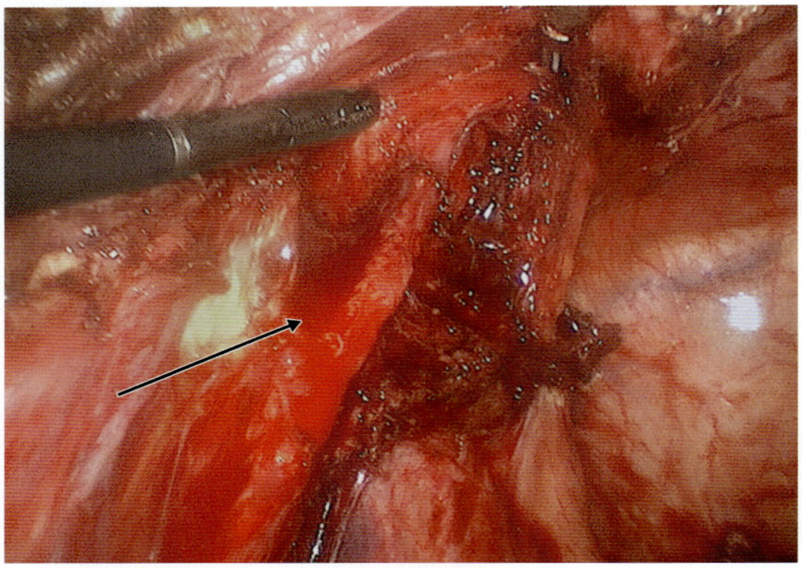

Fig. 27: Postureterolysis.

PRESACRAL NEURECTOMY

A percentage of women with chronic pelvic pain and/or dysmenorrhea does not respond or respond poorly to medical treatment. Surgery may represent the final therapeutic option for these patients. Appropriate patient selection is crucial and increases success rate.

The procedure involves isolating and transecting superior hypogastric nerve plexus (SHP) which is collection of several nerve fibers arising from uterus, cervix, upper vagina, broad ligament, and proximal one-third of Fallopian tube. Pain impulses from the cervix, the body of the uterus, and the proximal Fallopian tube get transmitted through afferent fibers that accompany sympathetic nerves into the spinal cord at the thoracic and lumbar region. The sympathetic nerves that emerge from the uterus pass through the uterosacral ligament along the Mackenrodt's ligament and join the pelvic plexus. Parasympathetic fibers from S1-S4 travel with the nervi erigentes through the pelvic plexuses (Frankenhauser ganglia) which lies lateral to the cervix to reach the bladder, rectum, and uterus. The presacral nerve is a plexus of nerves also known as the superior hypogastric plexus. SHP is continuous with inferior hypogastric nerve plexus.

Within the interiliac trigone, the common iliac artery and ureter lie on the right and the common iliac vein lies on the left. The inferior mesenteric, superior hemorrhoidal, and midsacral arteries are at the center of the prelumbar space. This trigone is defined caudally by the sacral promontory and laterally by the common iliac arteries. The superior edge of the triangle is delineated by the aortic bifurcation. Centrally and to the left, multiple nerve fibers, sometimes in bundles, run caudally from the aortic plexus above and through the interiliac trigone to form the superior hypogastric plexus. These fibers, representing the presacral nerve, are buried in loose areolar tissue. They display no particular patterns and vary among individuals. Both ureters, which lie to the right and left of the trigone, are identified before transection of the nerve bundle continues.

Indications

- Midline pelvic pain
- Failed medical management
- Desires conservative surgery.

Complications

- *Visceral:*
  - Constipation—responds well to medical therapy
  - Urinary urgency—responds minimally to medical therapy.

Vascular Injuries

Bleeding is the most important intraoperative complication of presacral neurectomy.

Injury mostly occurs to the middle sacral vessels, common iliac vein, or vena cava. The middle sacral vessels are present in the midline between the presacral nerve and the periosteum of the sacral promontory. Usually, the nerve is dissected anterior to the vessels and ligation is not necessary. Hemostasis is obtained by ligation or coagulation. However, an inadvertent injury to the common iliac vein or vena cava may require an immediate laparotomy.

Steps of Presacral Neurectomy

- Sigmoid colon is deflected laterally to expose interiliac triangle **(Figs. 28A to C)**
- Grasping and tenting peritoneum over sacral promontory with atraumatic grasper **(Fig. 29)**
- Incision made with harmonic and extended superiorly over aortic bifurcation **(Figs. 30A to C)**
- Left peritoneal edge is lifted, dissected and inferior mesenteric artery (IMA) identified (Note: IMA serves as left lateral border of dissection) **(Figs. 31A to C)**
- Right ureter is identified, which serves as right lateral border of dissection **(Figs. 32A and B)**.
- Superior hypogastric plexus identified, held with grasper and dissected **(Figs. 33A to E)**
- Superior hypogastric plexus (about 2–3 cm length) is transected up till aortic bifurcation **(Figs. 34A and B)**
- Postexcision of SHP **(Fig. 35)**
- Specimen of SHP retrieved through 5-mm lateral port **(Fig. 36)**

DEFINITIVE SURGERY IN ENDOMETRIOSIS

Definitive surgery involves bilateral oophorectomy and may include removal of the uterus and Fallopian tubes and excision of all visible endometriotic nodules and lesions. It should be considered in women who have significant pain and symptoms despite conservative treatment, do not desire future pregnancies and have severe disease, or are undergoing hysterectomy because of associated other pelvic conditions, such as fibroids or menorrhagia.

Laparoscopy is the preferred route for surgical management of endometriosis, irrespective of severity, advantage includes greater visualization through a magnified view and the quicker patient recovery and return to normal activity when compared with laparotomy. Patients with invasive endometriosis, including bowel and bladder involvement, should be referred to those with experience or advanced training in managing these cases through a multidisciplinary approach.

Steps of Total Laparoscopic Hysterectomy in Endometriosis

Our technique for a total laparoscopic hysterectomy (TLH) is described further, since other types of laparoscopic hysterectomy

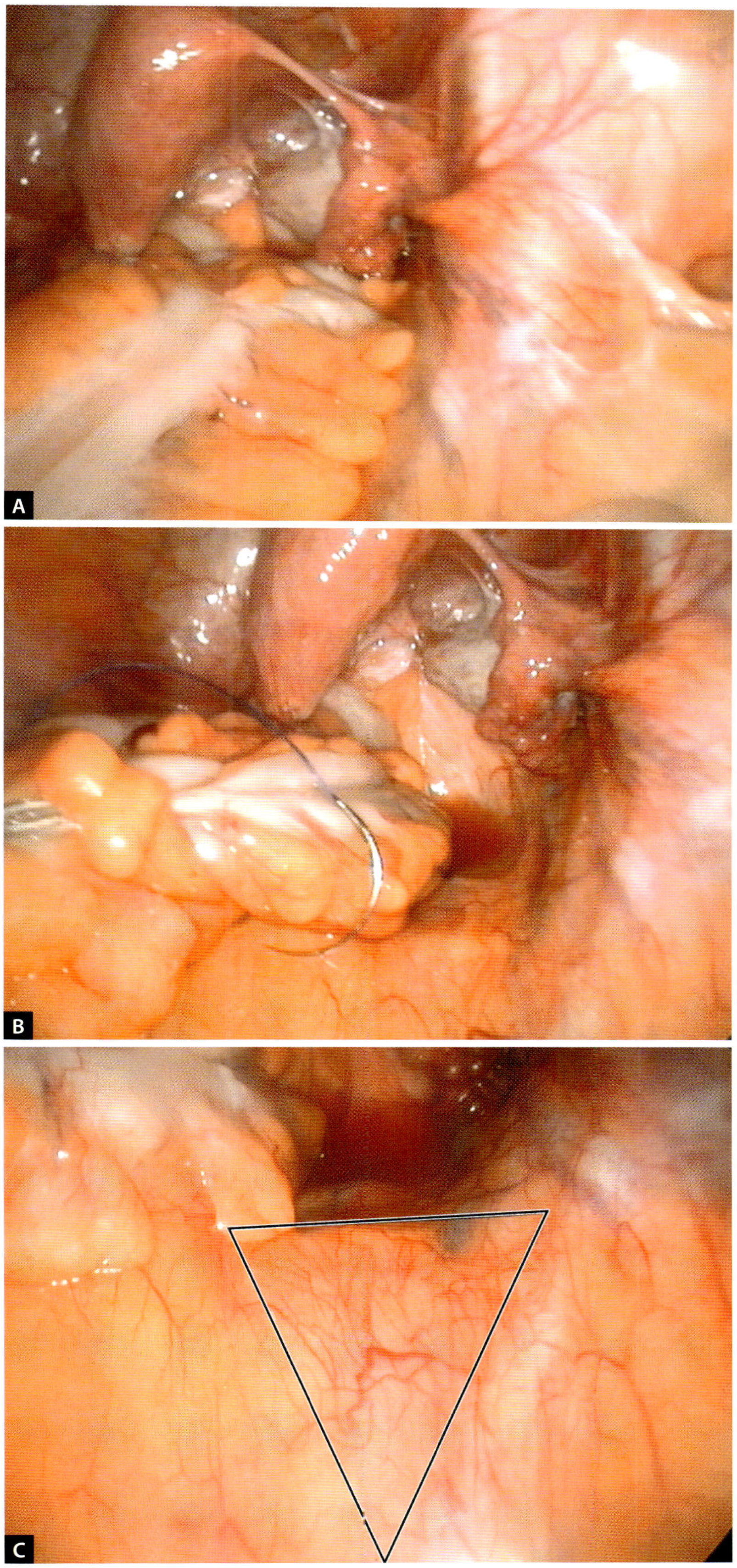

Figs. 28A to C: Sigmoid colon is deflected laterally to expose interiliac triangle.

[e.g. laparoscopic-assisted vaginal hysterectomy (LAVH) or LH] are mere modifications of this more extensive procedure. These steps are designed to prevent complications, which are anticipated during surgery.

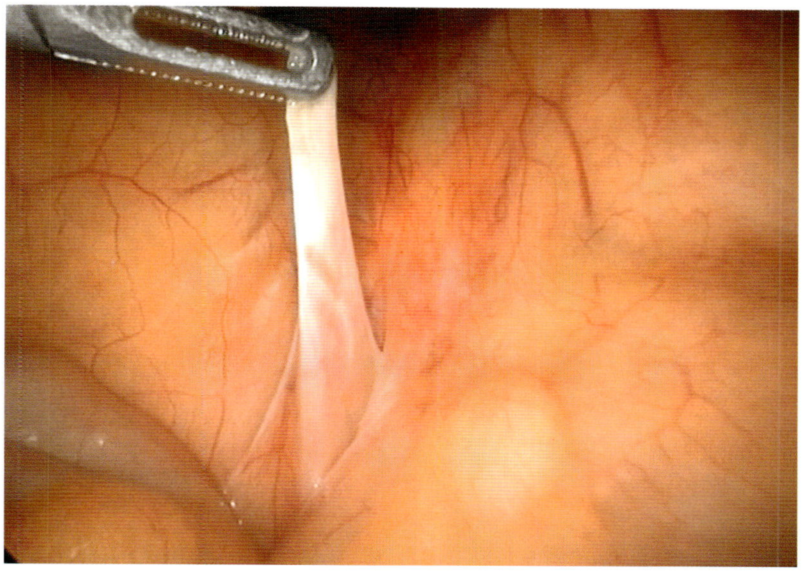

Fig. 29: Grasping and tenting peritoneum over sacral promontory with atraumatic grasper.

Preoperative Preparation

- The patient is optimized medically for preexisting problems
- Patients are encouraged to hydrate with clear liquids
- On the day before surgery. Coloprep containing Picolax and sodium sulfate as active ingredients, divided into two doses, is given to evacuate the bowel
- All laparoscopic procedures are done using general anesthesia with endotracheal intubation, with orogastric tube suction to minimize bowel distension. The patient's arms are tucked at her side (no armboards), and shoulder braces are positioned at the acromioclavicular joint
- We use one dose of a prophylactic antibiotic 1 hour before surgery.

Incisions

Three laparoscopic puncture sites including the umbilicus are used—10-mm supraumbilical, ancillary ports 5 mm right and 5 mm left lower quadrant. Additional ports are planned after inspecting the lesions. Pneumoperitoneum to 20 mm Hg is obtained before primary trocar insertion, and reduced to 12 mm Hg afterward.

Vaginal Manipulator

We use a Sukhadia uterine manipulator which allows for not only anterior and posterior manipulations but also permits lateral manipulations of uterus.

Exploration

Whole abdomen is inspected, and the appendix is identified.

If appendiceal pathology is present, i.e. adhesions or endometriosis, appendectomy is done.

Adhesiolysis

Normal pelvic anatomy should be restored using sharp dissection with harmonic/scissors or blunt dissection using suction/irrigation cannula.

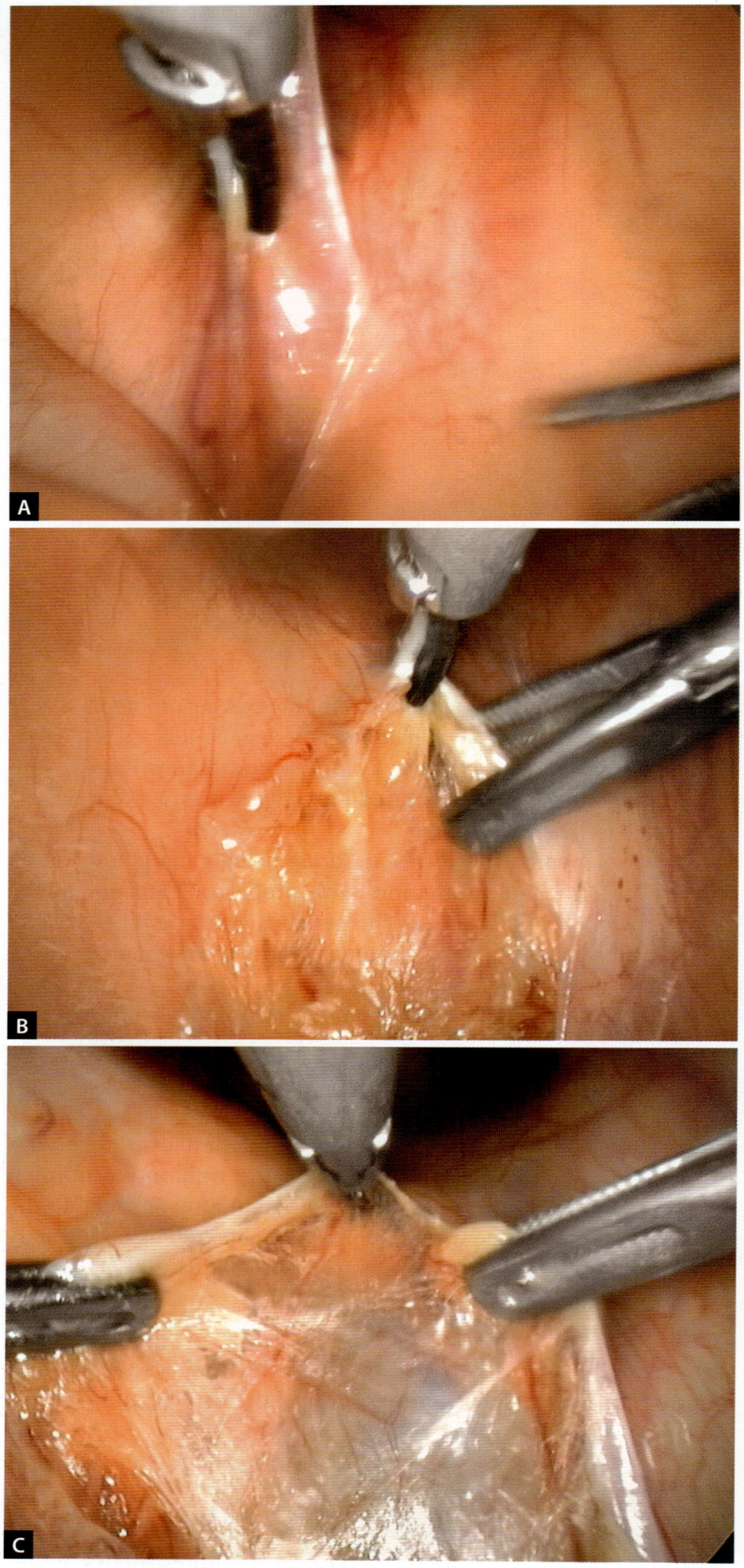

Figs. 30A to C: Incision made with harmonic and extended superiorly over aortic bifurcation.

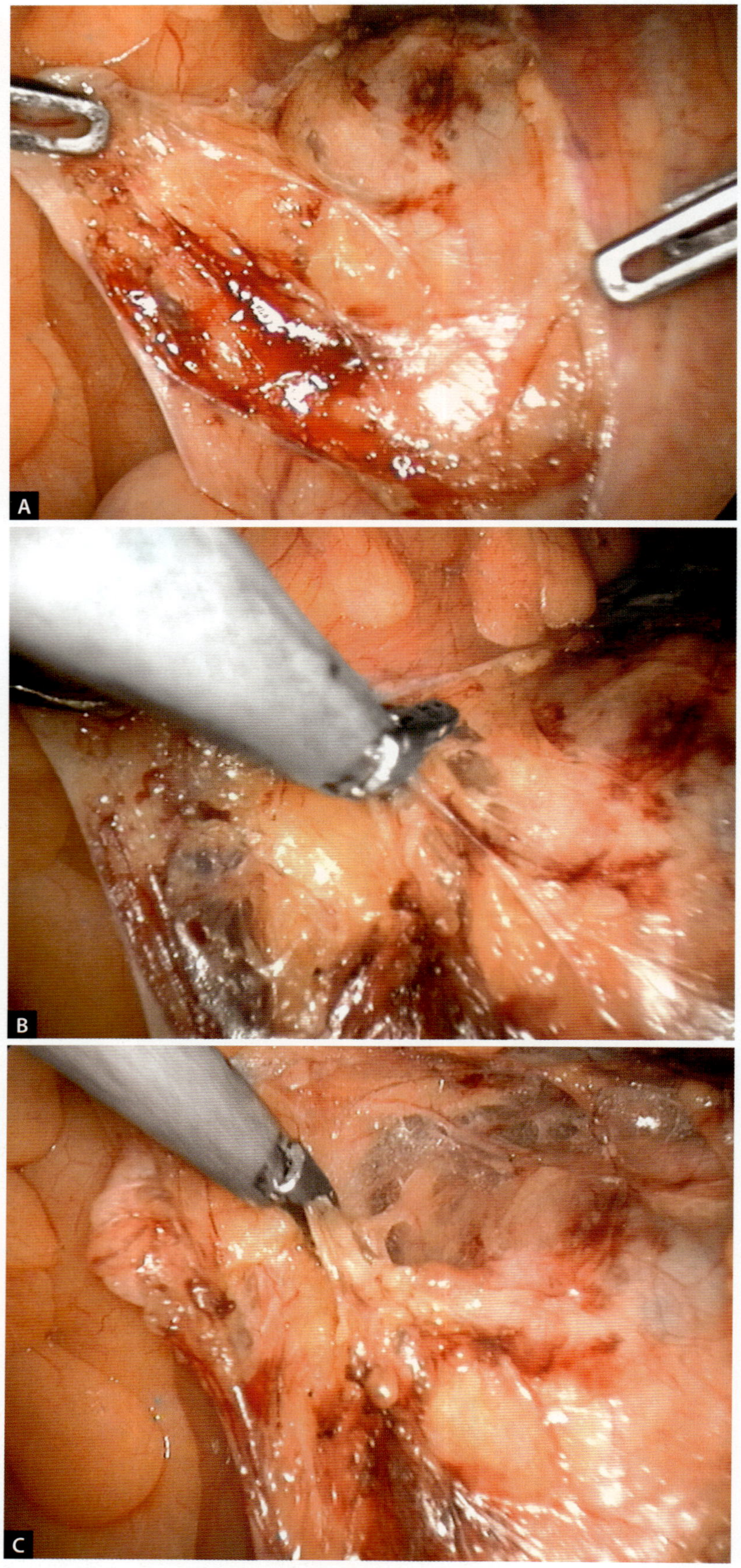

Figs. 31A to C: Left peritoneal edge is lifted, dissected and inferior mesenteric artery (IMA) identified (Note: IMA serves as left lateral border of dissection).

Lysis of bowel adhesions: Bowel adhesions vary in thickness, vascularity, and cohesiveness. Some adhesions can be stretched without tearing the tissue, excised using a laser harmonic scalpel or electrosurgery at the points of attachment to the pelvic organs, and removed. Dense adhesions are excised with scissors or any other cutting instrument (energy source) **(Figs. 37 to 57)**.

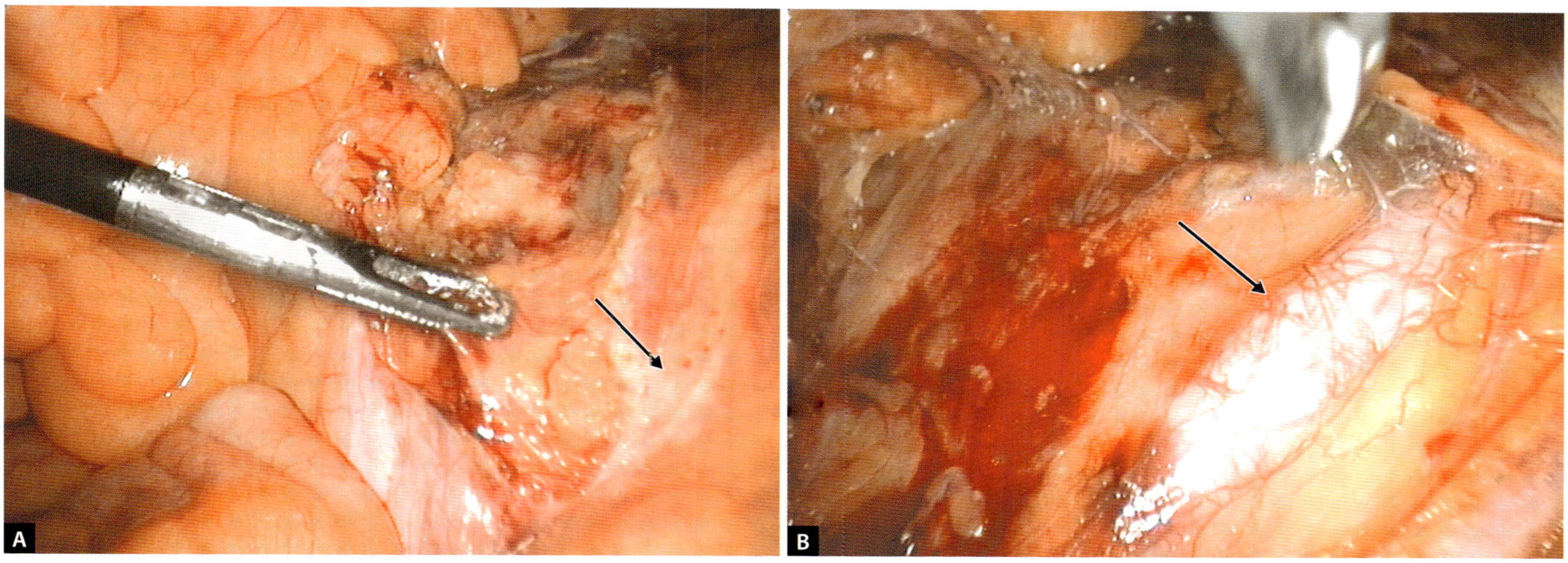

Figs. 32A and B: Right ureter is identified, which serves as right lateral border of dissection.

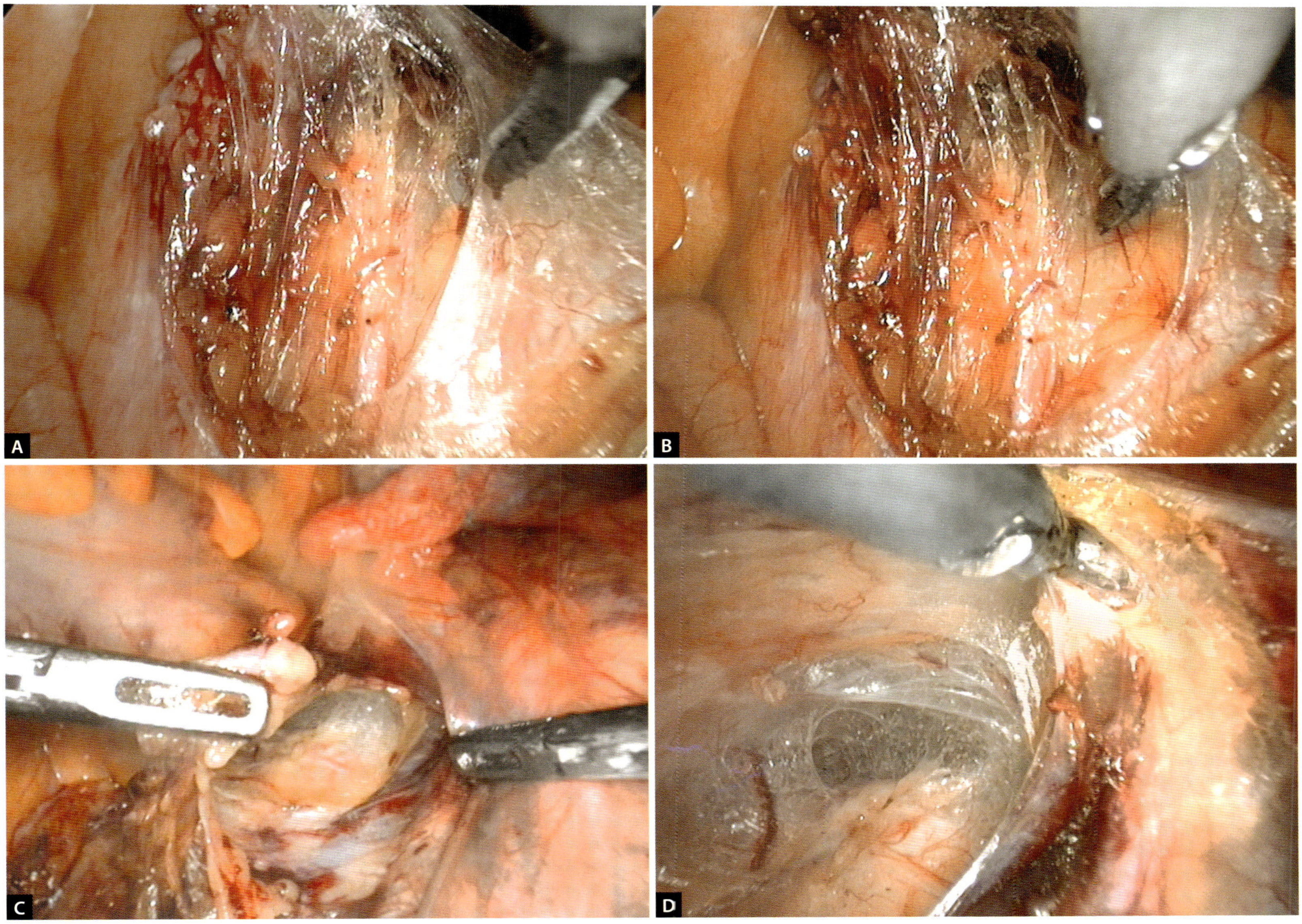

Figs. 33A to D

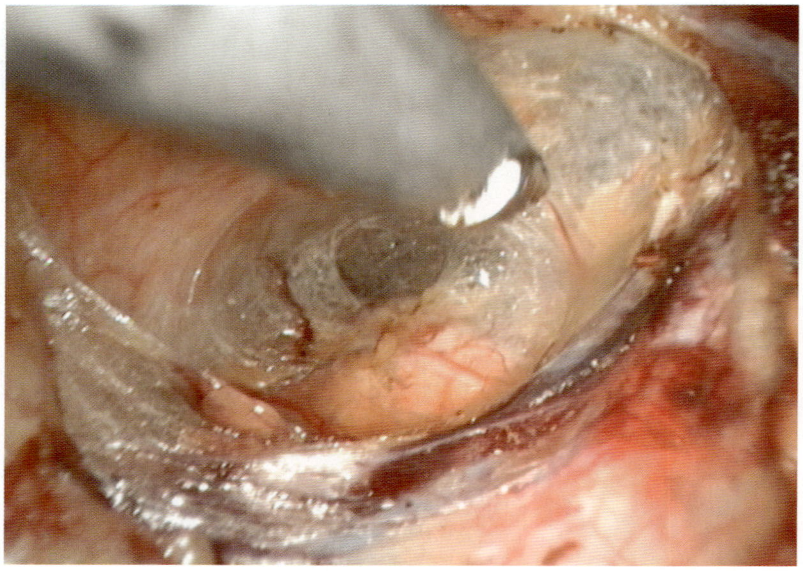

Fig. 33E

Figs. 33A to E:-Superior hypogastric plexus identified, held with grasper and dissected.

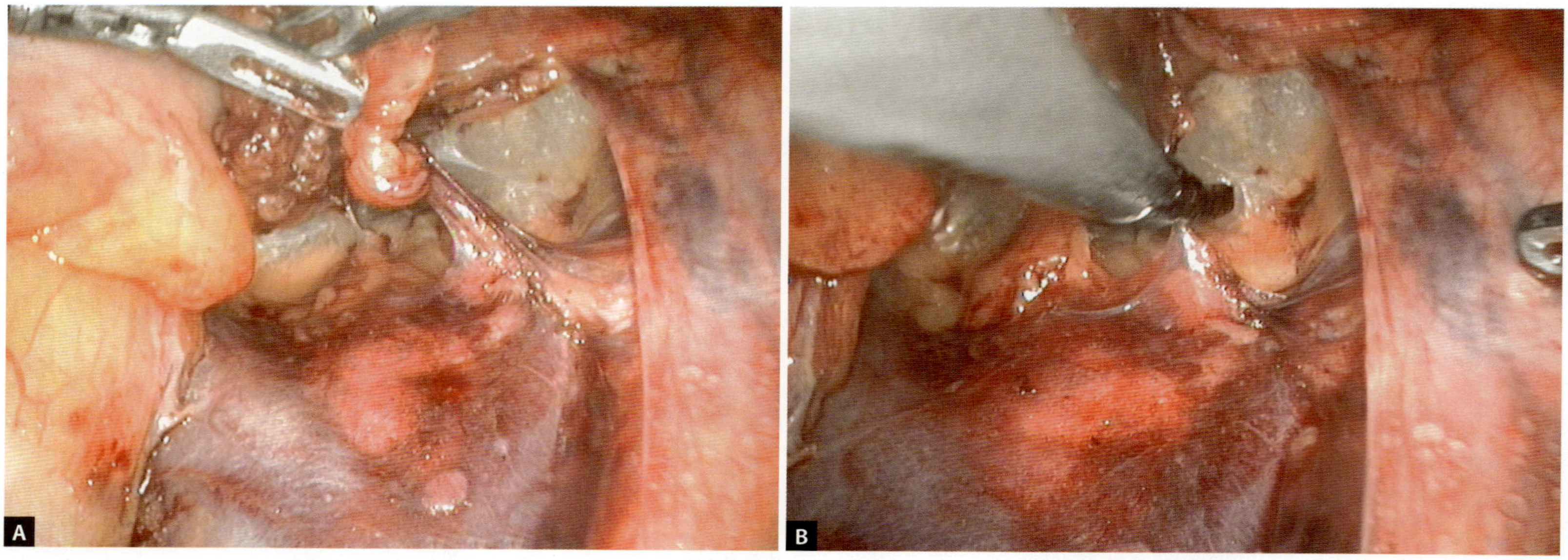

Figs. 34A and B: Superior hypogastric plexus (about 2–3 cm length) is transected up till aortic bifurcation.

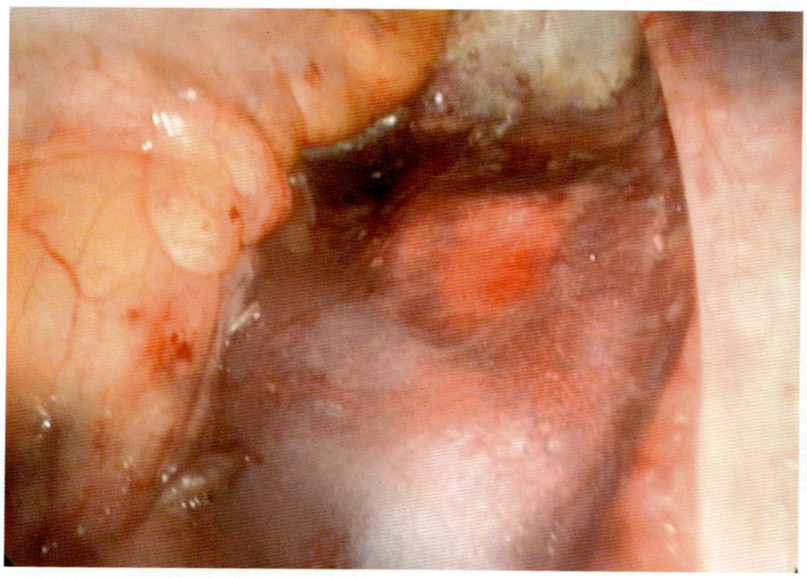

Fig. 35: Postexcision of superior hypogastric plexus.

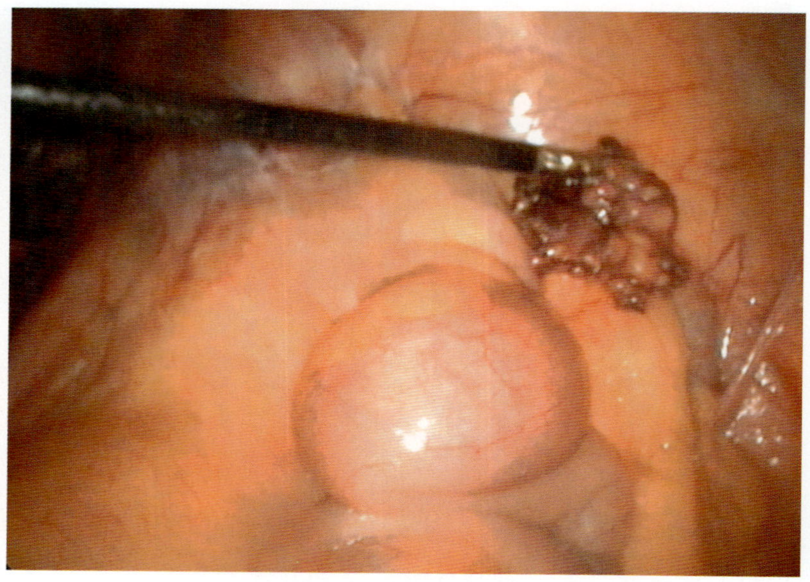

Fig. 36: Specimen of superior hypogastric plexus retrieved through 5-mm lateral port.

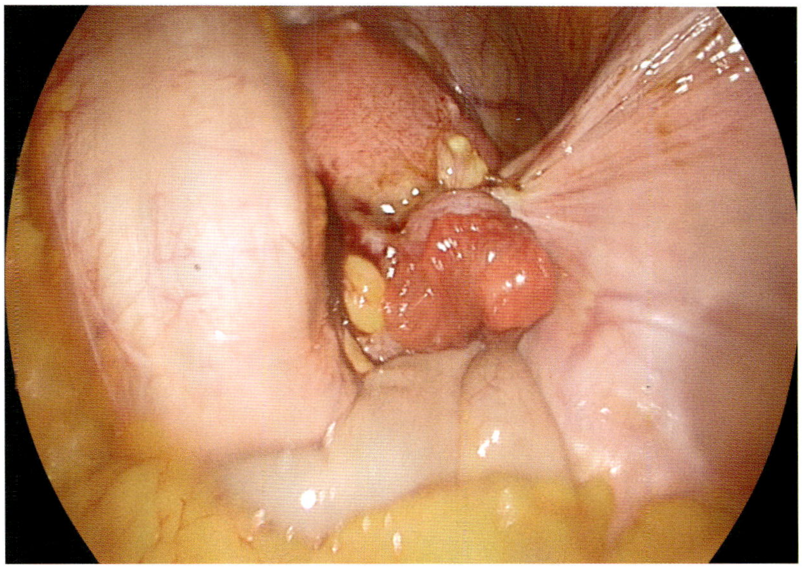

Fig. 37: Grade IV/severe endometriosis.

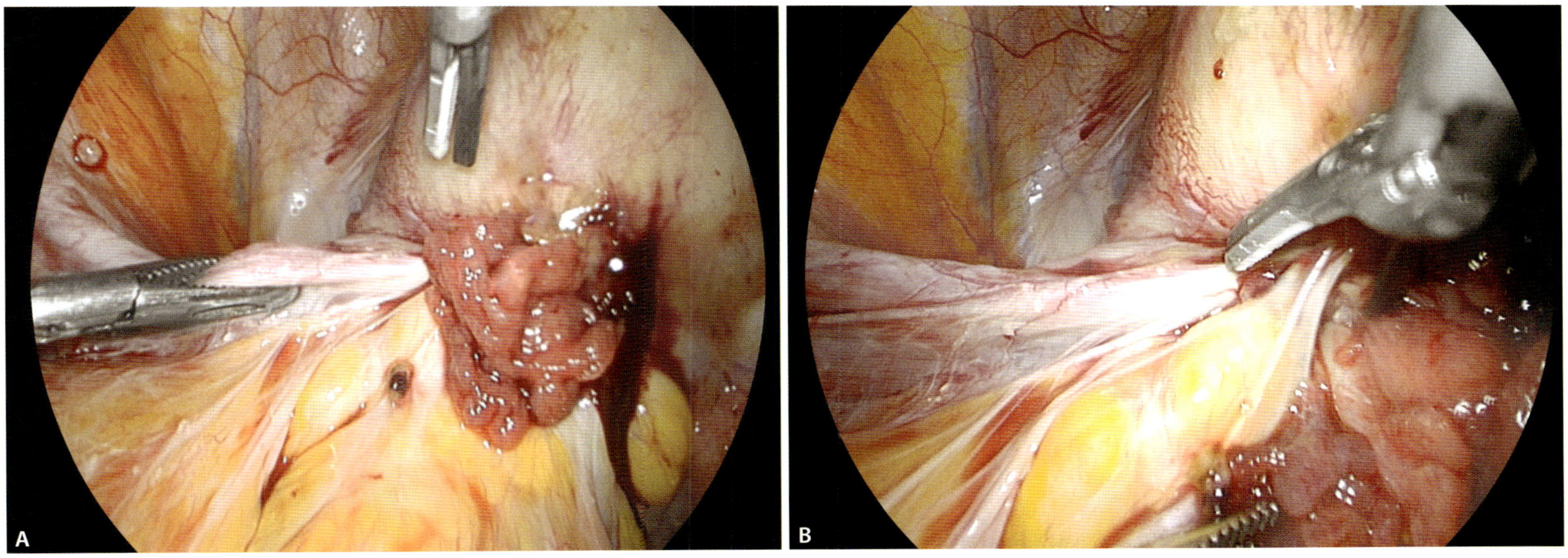

Figs. 38A and B: Lysis of bowel adhesions using an atraumatic grasper and harmonic.

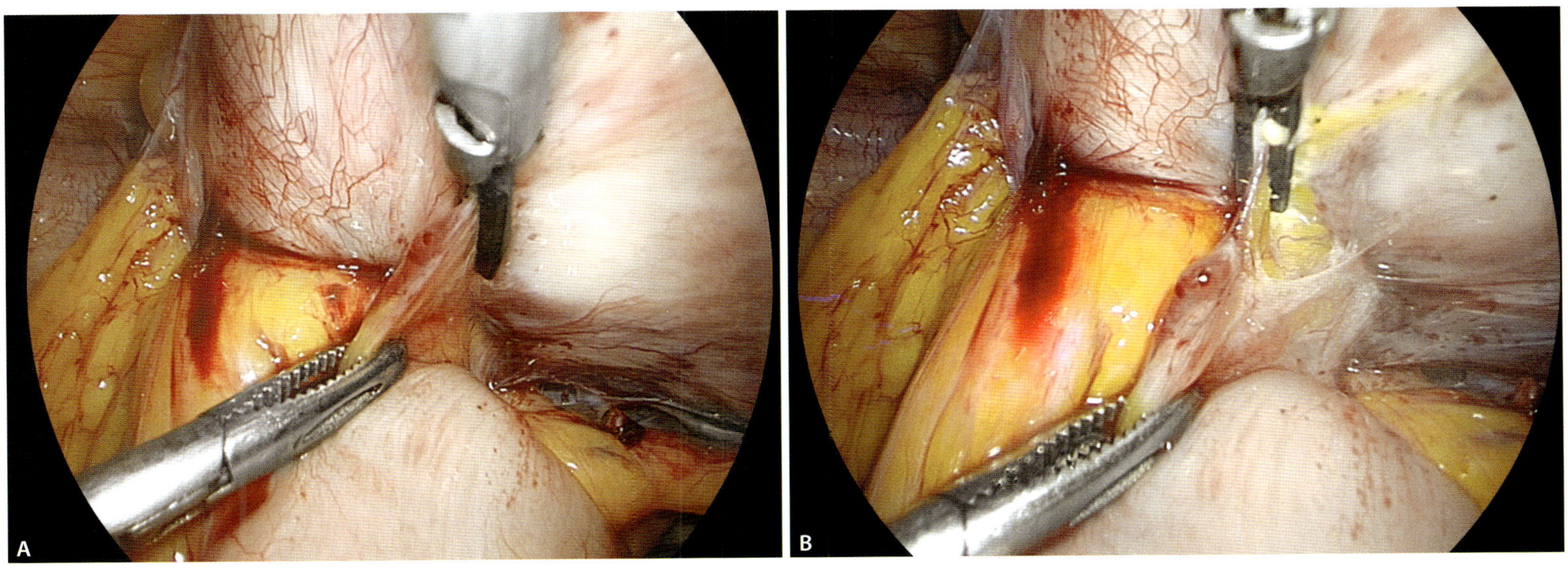

Figs. 39A and B

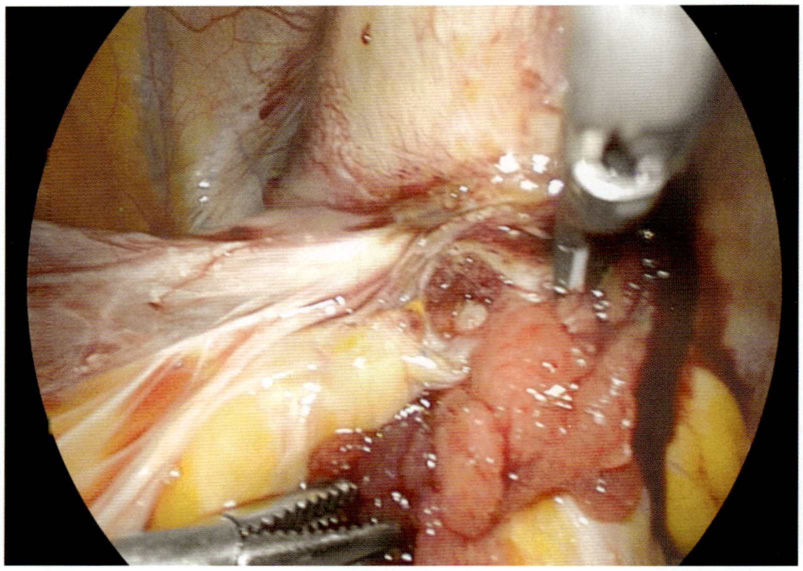

Fig. 39C

Figs. 39A to C: Bowel is held with grasper and cut close to the uterine surface.

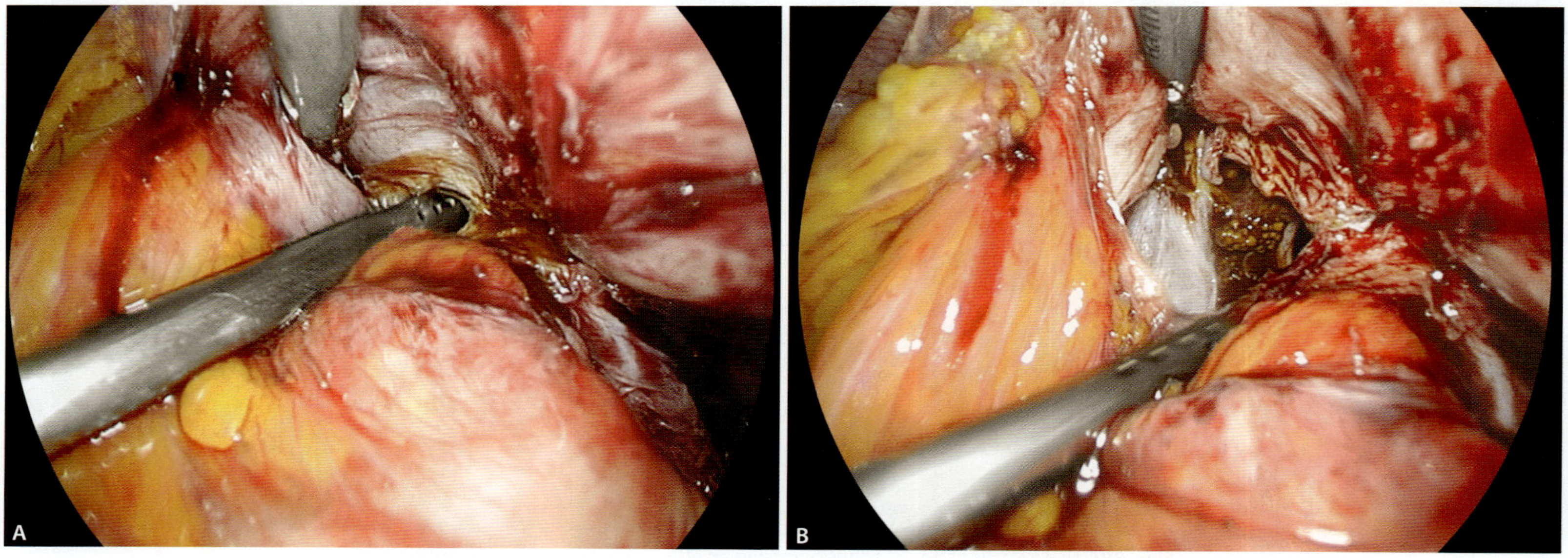

Figs. 40A and B: Adhesiolysis of bowel adhesions using suction/irrigation cannula and hydrodissection.

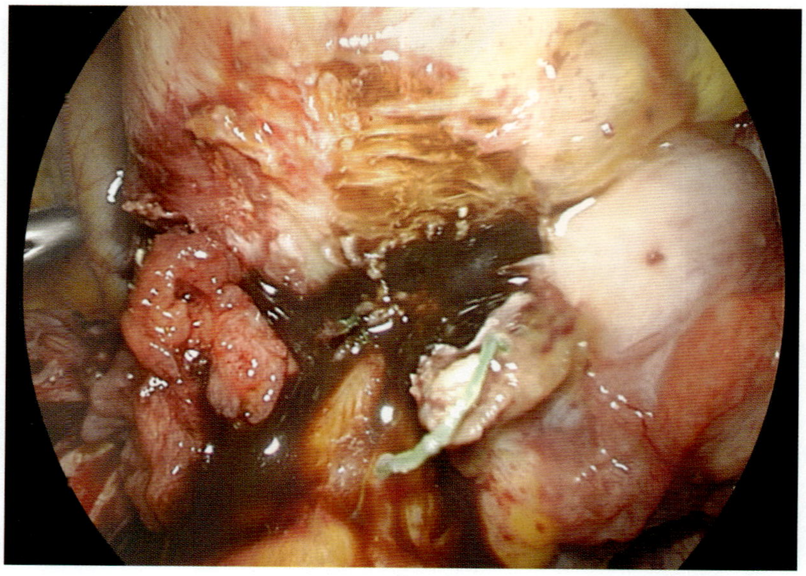

Fig. 41: Spillage of chocolate colored material seen during adhesiolysis.

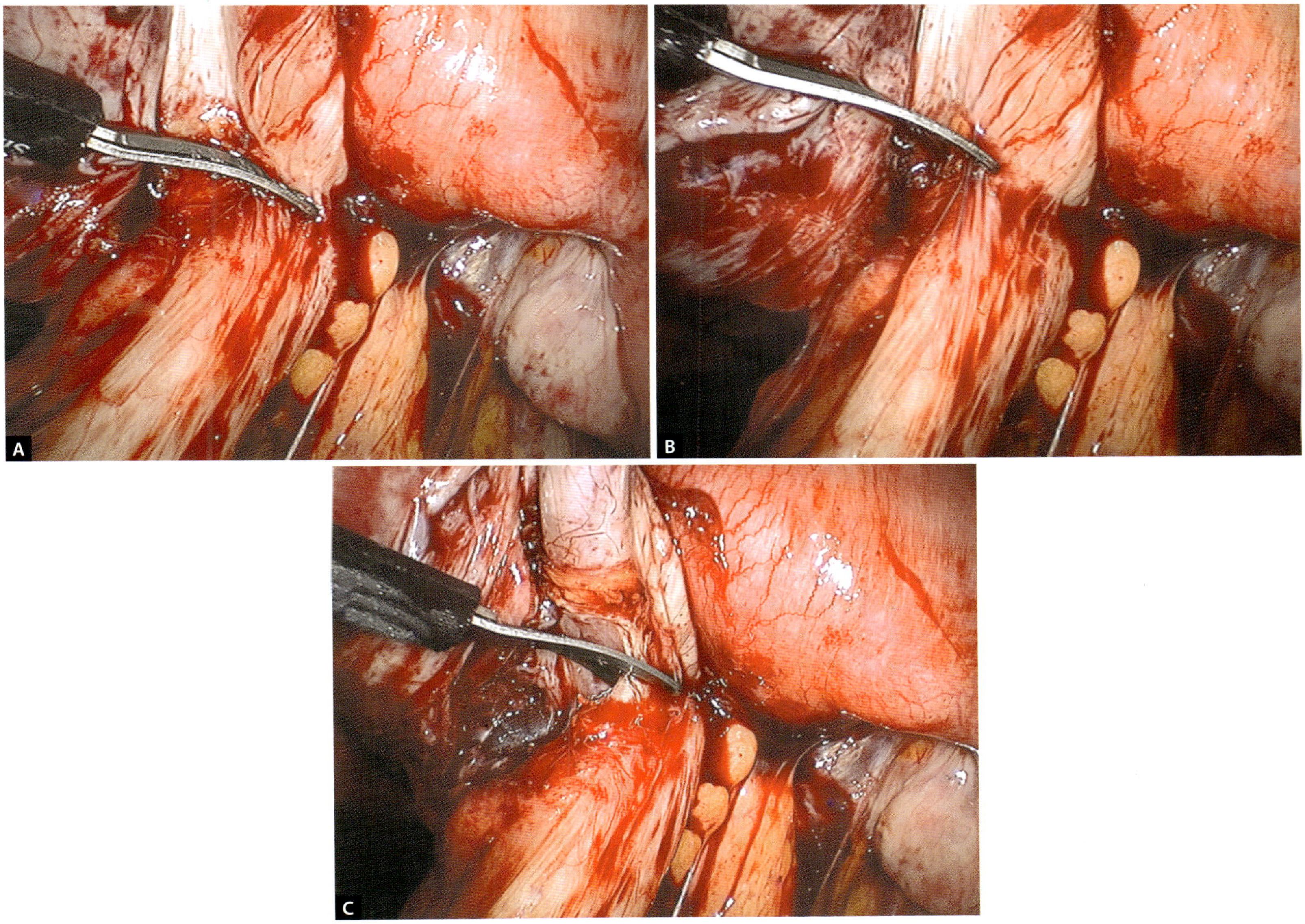

Figs. 42A to C: Lysis of bowel adhesions using cold scissors.

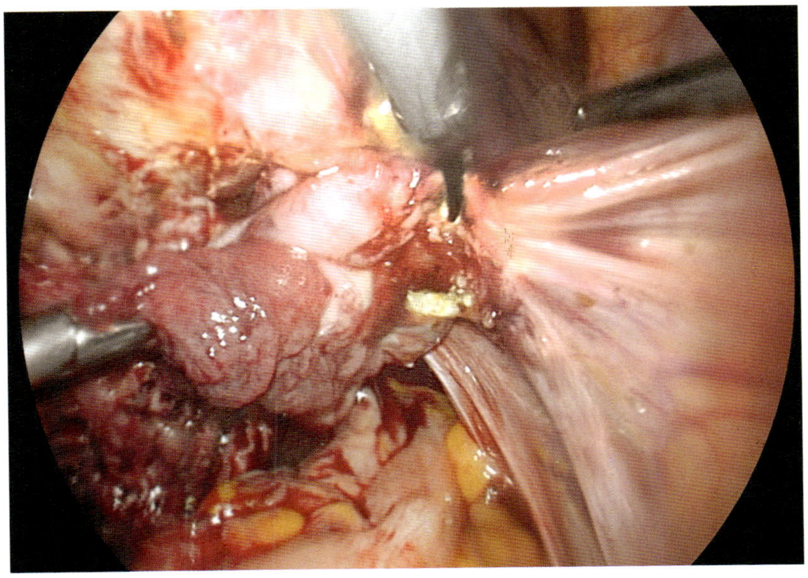

Fig. 43: Bilateral infundibulopelvic ligaments are cauterized and cut using bipolar forceps or harmonic.

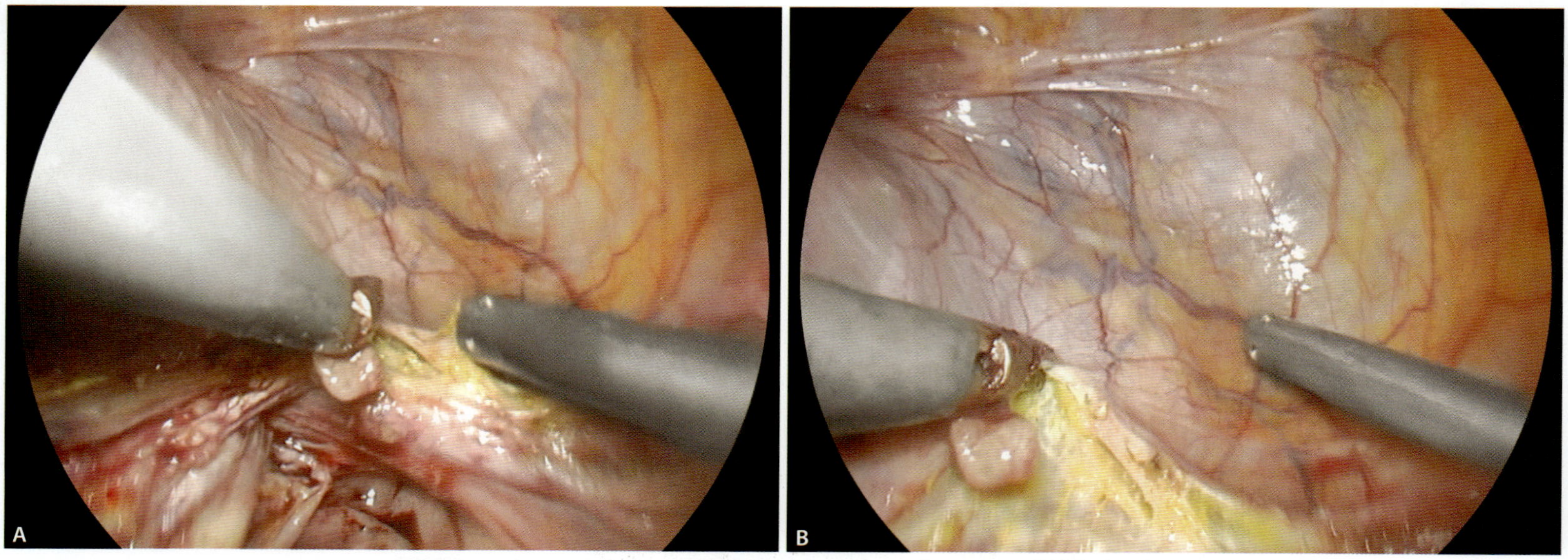

Figs. 44A and B: Uterovesical fold opened through lateral window using harmonic.

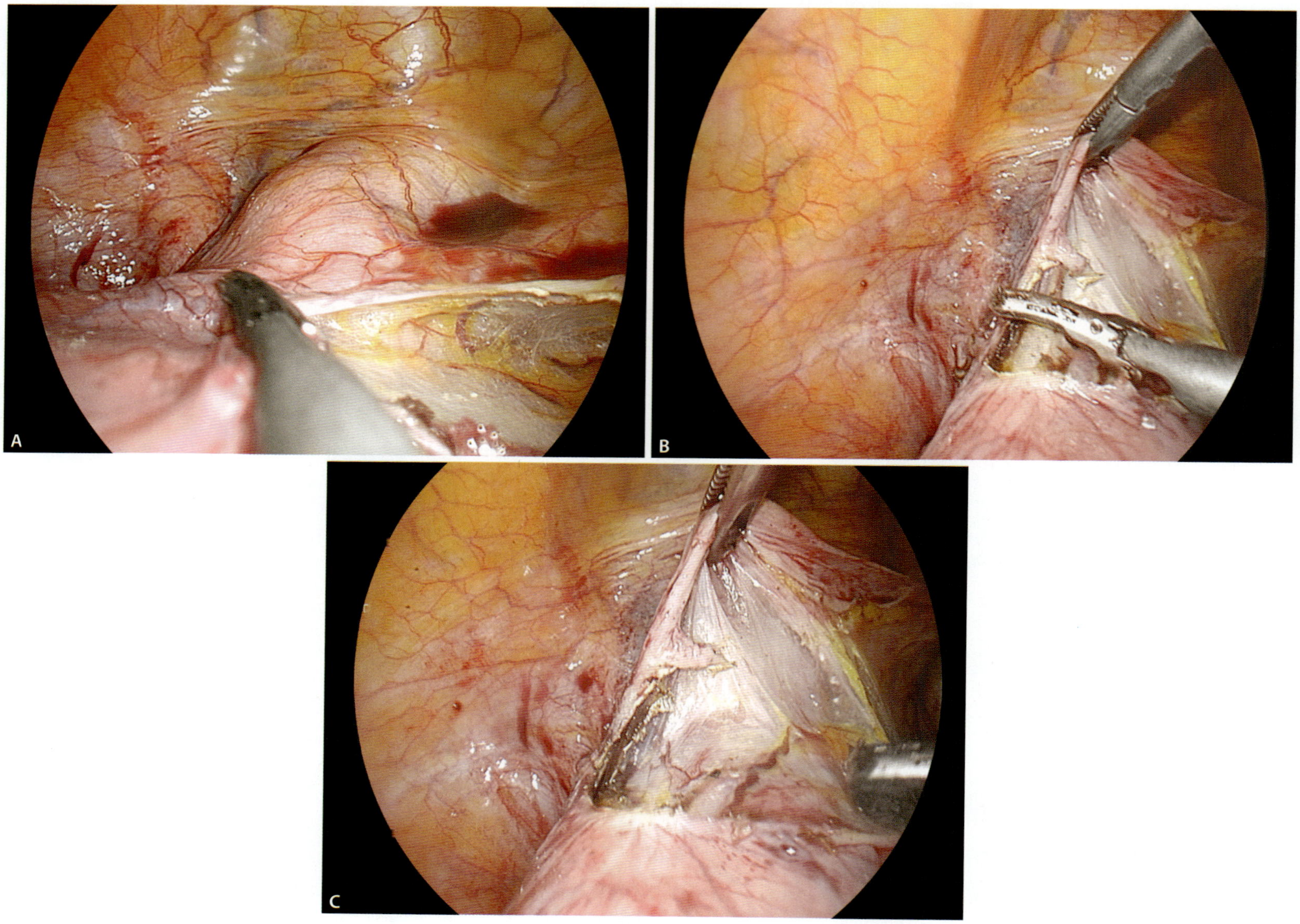

Figs. 45A to C: Incision extended centrally.

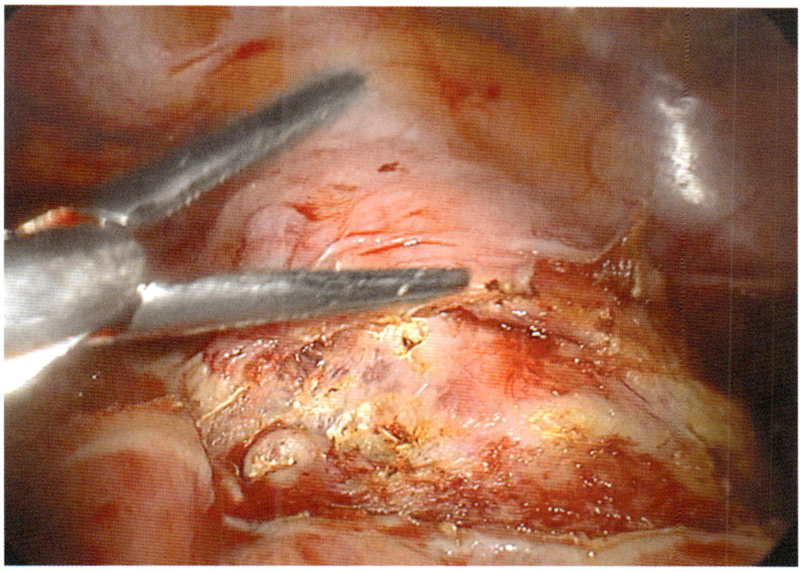

Fig. 46: Incision extended onto the other side.

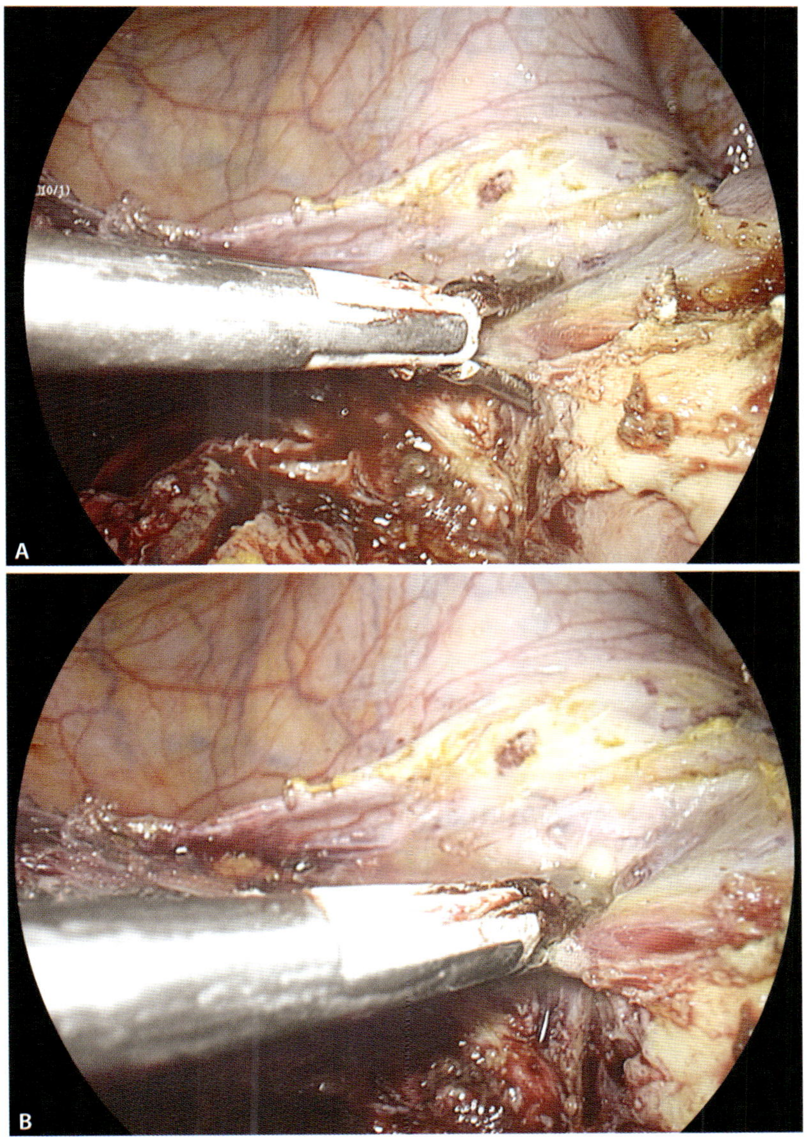

Fig. 47A and B: Bilateral uterine vessels cauterized using bipolar.

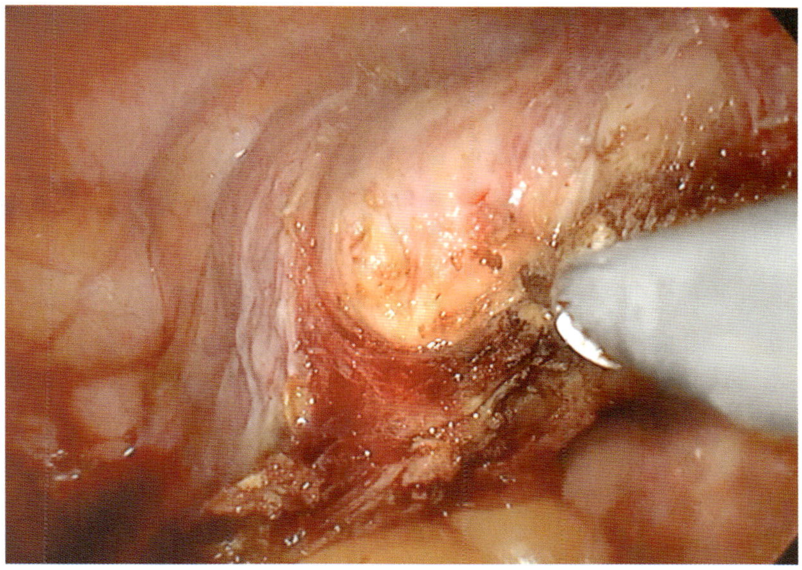

Fig. 48: Uterine vessels cut with harmonic.

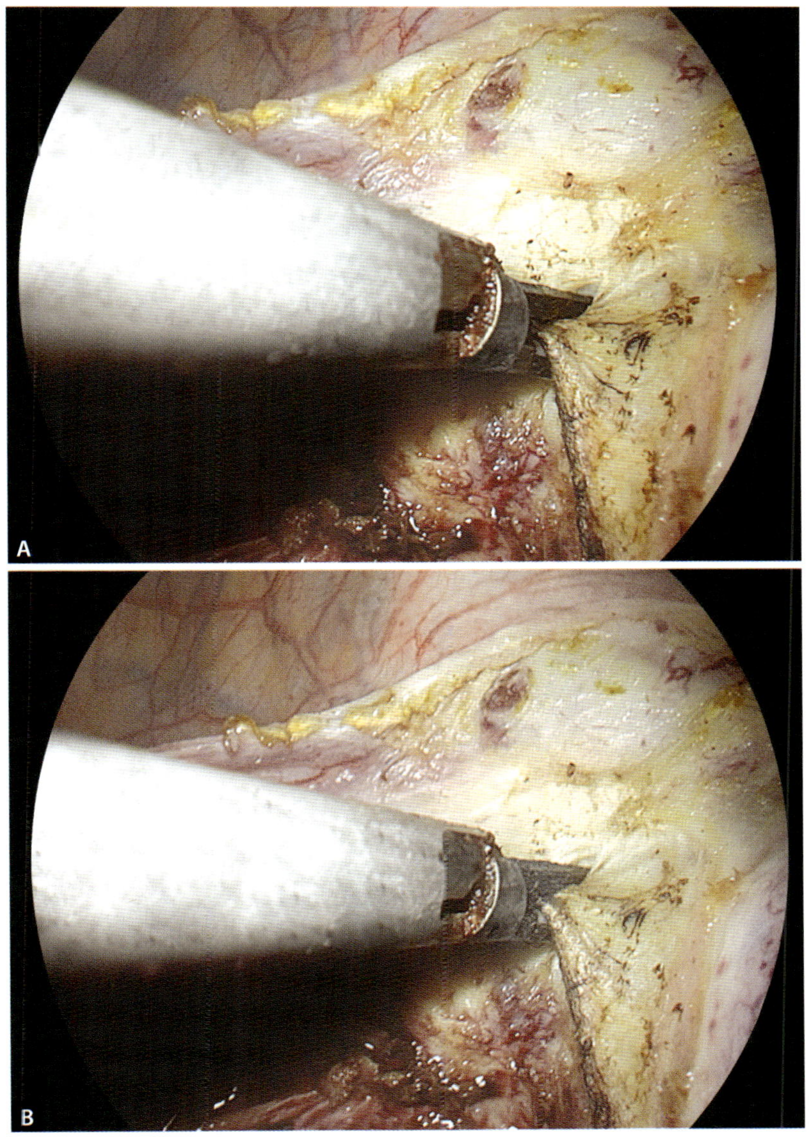

Figs. 49A and B: Bilateral Mackenrodt's cauterized and cut with harmonic.

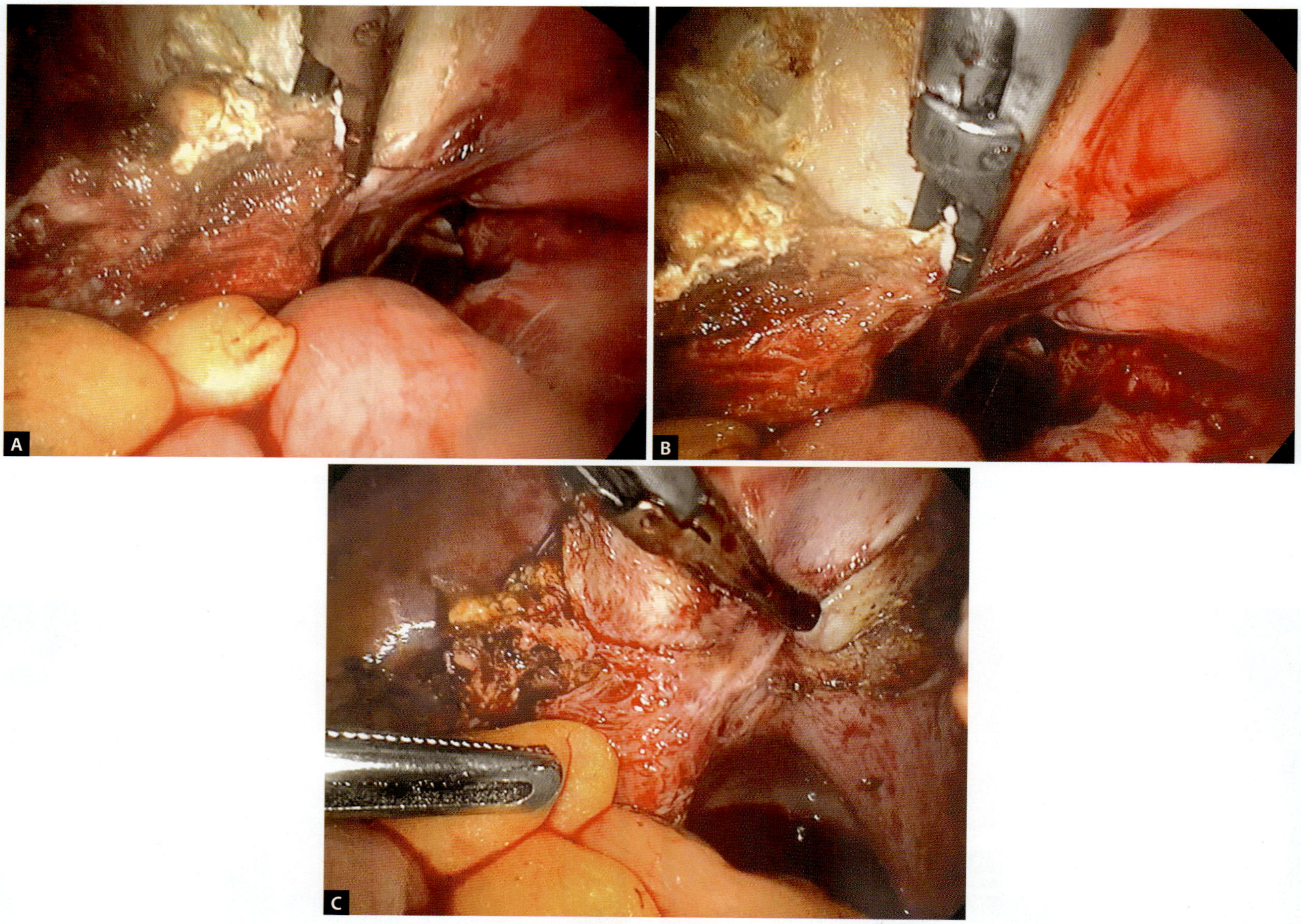

Figs. 50A to C: Bilateral uterosacrals cauterized and cut with harmonic.

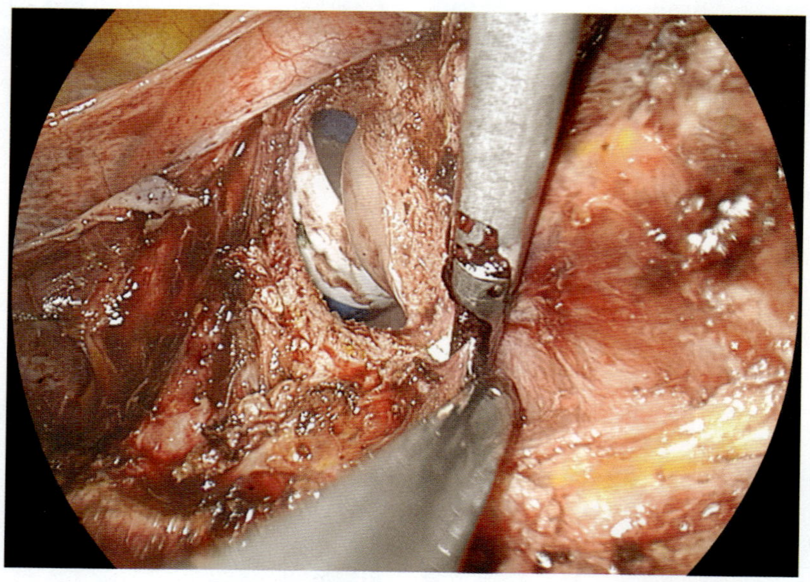

Fig. 51: Vault opened with harmonic.

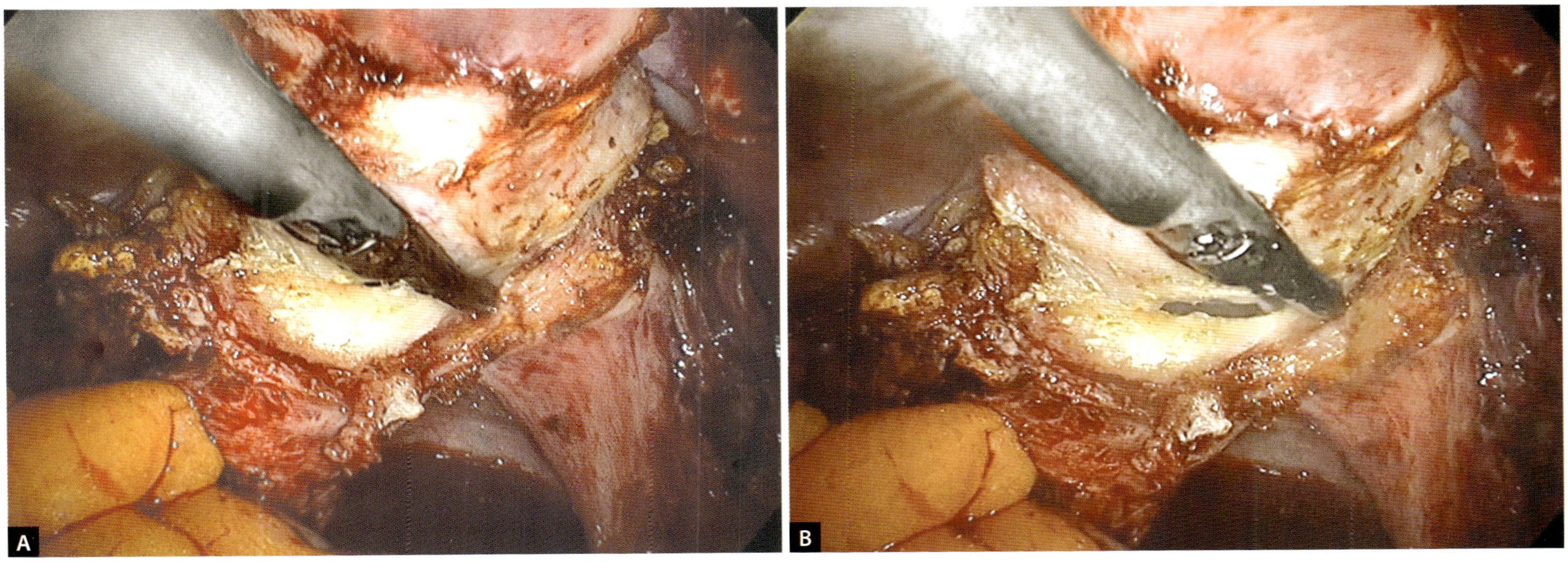

Figs. 52A and B: Vault incision extended posteriorly above arch of uterosacrals.

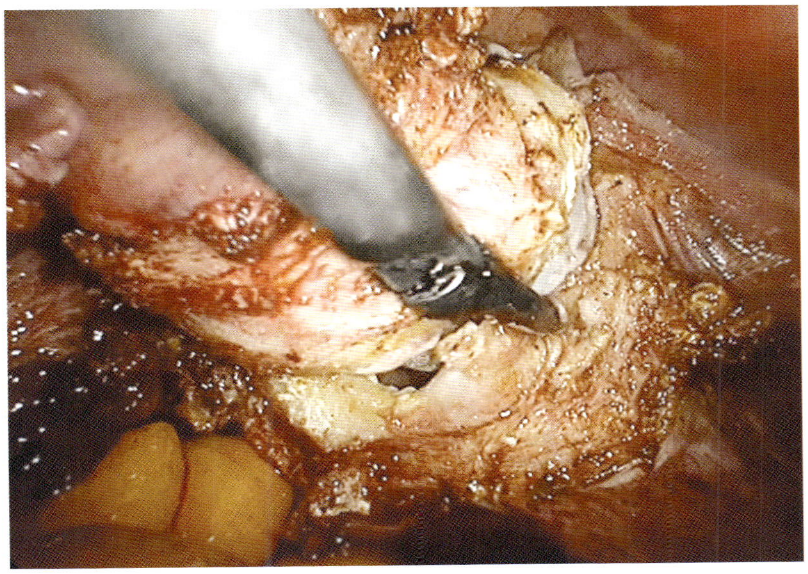

Fig. 53: Incision extended to opposite side.

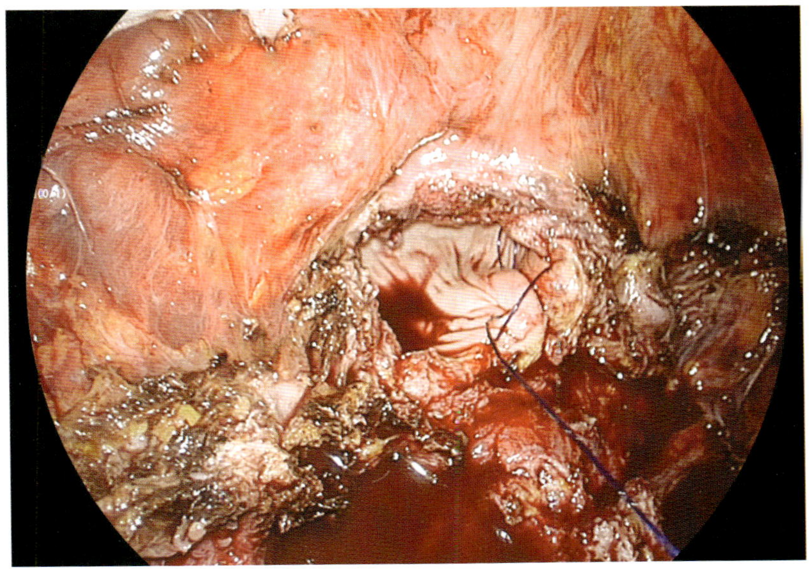

Fig. 54: Vault sutured laparoscopically using barbed sutures starting from right angle.

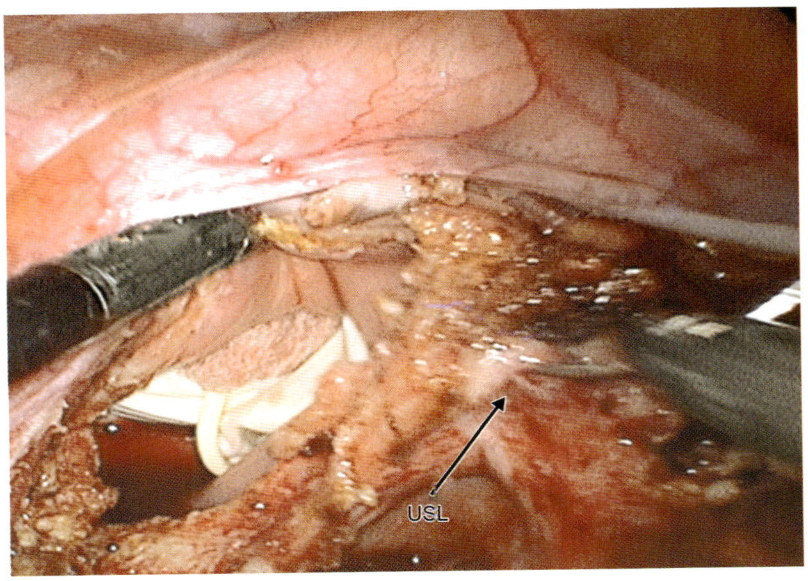

Fig. 55: Inclusion of uterosacral stump with the ipsilateral angle.

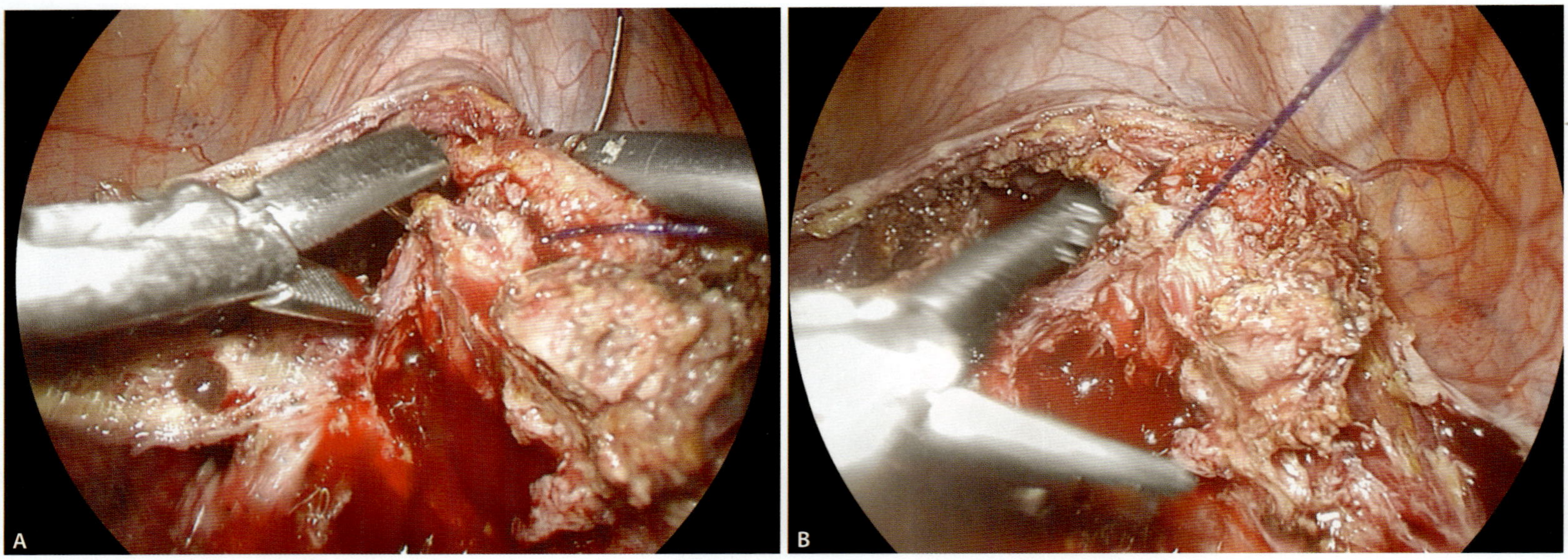

Figs. 56A and B: Approximation of anterior and posterior vaginal walls with barbed sutures.

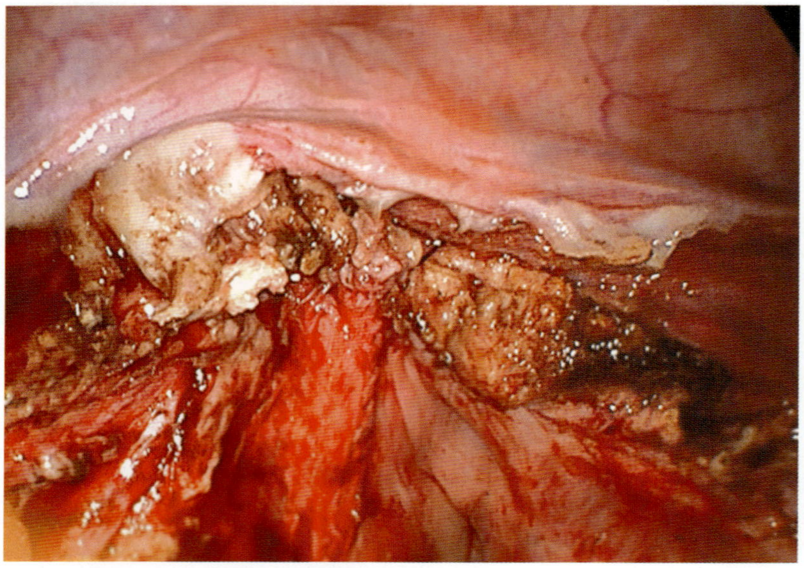

Fig. 57: Appearance of vault postsuturing.

RECTAL SHAVING IN ENDOMETRIOSIS

Rectal shaving is used as treatment for deep endometriosis infiltrating the rectum. In the literature, the terms shaving or partial thickness excision implies removal of endometriotic nodules from the rectal wall without entering the lumen.

In literature, postoperative outcomes of rectal shaving are evaluated through retrospective case series, the investigators emphasized low rates of postoperative complications, which were presumed inferior to those after colorectal segmental resection. In addition, postoperative digestive function related to conservation of mesorectum and overall rectal capacity was better after rectal shaving than after colorectal resection. However, the rate of postoperative recurrences could be higher, especially in women seeking fertility and who have stopped contraceptive pill intake.

Steps

- Incision made posteriorly in between uterosacral ligaments **(Figs. 58A and B)**
- Rectovaginal space created by separating posterior vaginal wall from rectum **(Fig. 59)**
- Rectovaginal fibrotic nodule held with tooth grasper and excised using harmonic **(Figs. 60A to C)**
- Rectovaginal fibrotic nodule **(Fig. 61)**.

SECOND-LOOK LAPAROSCOPY

Second look laparoscopy is performed after first attempt at surgery or course of treatment to determine if patient is disease free. If lesions are seen, further procedures are usually carried out in order to achieve a near complete excision. Also indicated when primary surgery was incomplete due to advanced disease.

When endometrioma is more than 10 cm in size, a first laparoscopy is performed for confirmation of diagnosis of an endometrioma and to open it wide and rinse it. Followed by gonadotropin-releasing hormone (GnRH) for 12 weeks to reduce size of the cyst. After 6–8 weeks of treatment, ultrasound is performed to assess the residual cyst size. If endometrioma is seen and its size is larger than 4 cm, an ultrasound-guided transvaginal puncture of the cyst is performed. GnRH therapy is pursued for one more month. Second-look laparoscopy is then performed to open and rinse the endometrioma and fulgurate its internal wall. Women undergoing the above procedure, showed a greater increase in AMH levels and significant increase in AFC compared to women who underwent a single step procedure.

MEDICAL VERSUS SURGICAL TREATMENT

Treatment for Pain

Pharmacological Treatment

Nonsteroidal anti-inflammatory drugs (NSAIDs) act by inhibiting production of prostaglandins, which are responsible for pain sensation. It is prescribed by many clinicians for endometriosis-related pain due to their high availability and low cost. However, the latest Cochrane analysis identified only two RCTs that compared NSAIDs to placebo for endometriosis-related pain, and only one was considered methodologically reliable. The remaining article showed there was no benefit of NSAIDs over placebo for pain relief. Use of additional analgesia or side effects, but was too small for making any

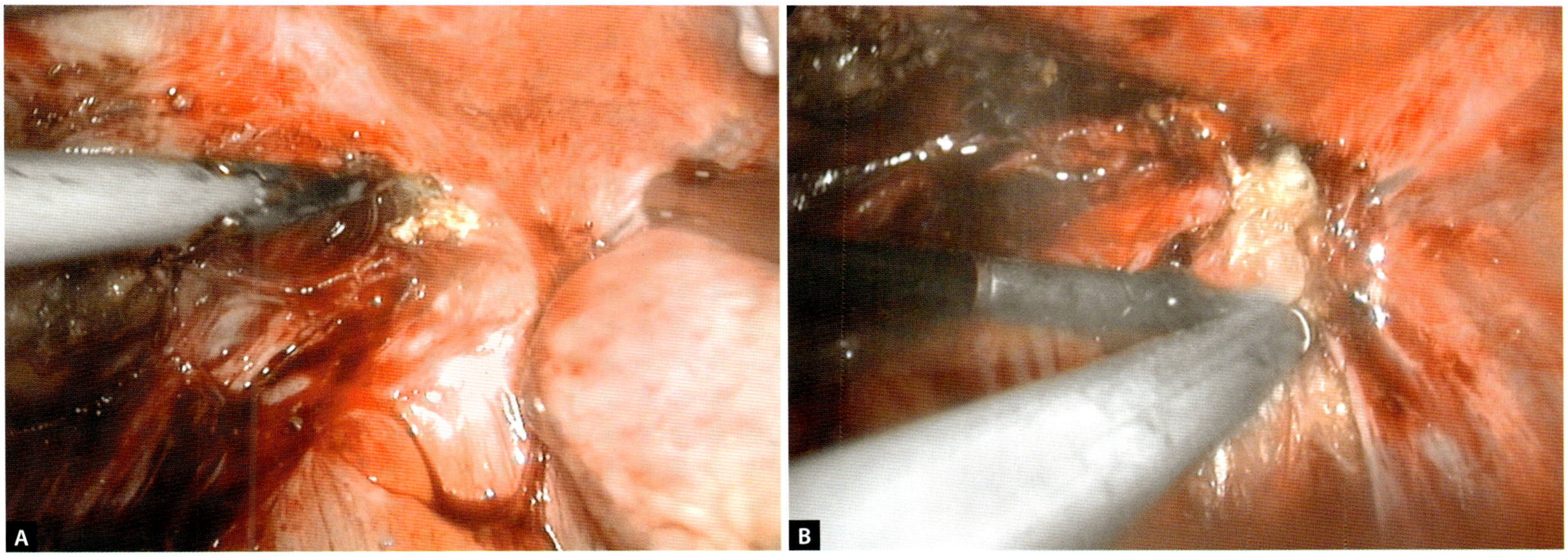

Figs. 58A and B: Incision made posteriorly in between uterosacral ligaments.

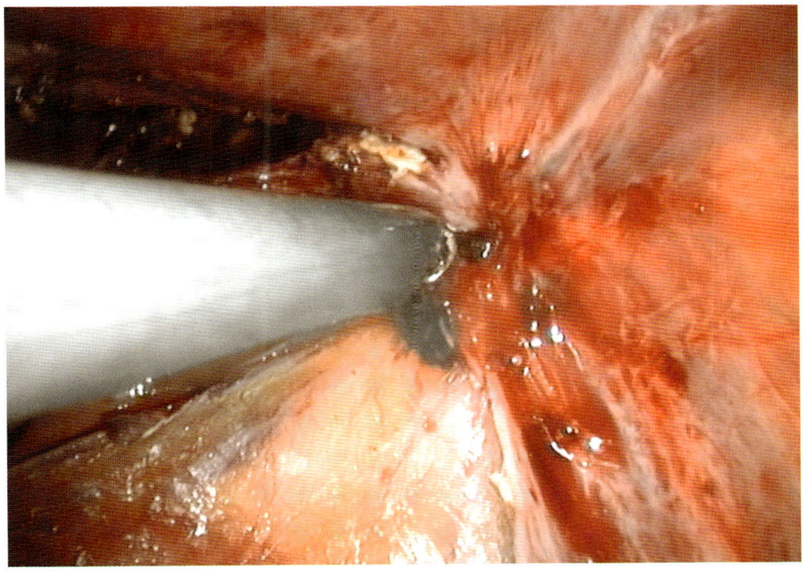

Fig. 59: Rectovaginal space created by separating posterior vaginal wall from rectum.

conclusive recommendation. The next commonly used pharmacological group for pain treatment in endometriosis is hormonal agents, which suppress the influence of sex steroids on endometriosis lesions, such as GnRH agonists and different progestogens. A recent update concluded that all commonly used hormonal agents were effective in endometriosis pain alleviation with no superiority of a specific agent. Preference should consider safety and adverse effect profiles, including possible loss of bone mineral density with long-term use of GnRH agonists. Combined oral contraceptive pills also demonstrated some efficacy in suppressing implants and endometriomas, and effective pain relief in a several studies, but showed high relapse rate after completion of therapy. Modern delivery systems, such as the vaginal ring and the transdermal patch, demonstrated similar results in pain relief, but were associated with reduced patient adherence and bleeding control, disadvantage being it was not cost effective.

Dienogest is a new selective progestin with no androgenic, mineralocorticoid, and glucocorticoid activity. It is shown to be more effective than placebo for reducing endometriosis-associated pelvic pain. In a randomized, multicenter study, dienogest was compared with leuprolide acetate in women with endometriosis. and displayed similar efficacy to leuprolide acetate in treatment of endometriosis symptoms. It also demonstrates specific quality-of-life benefits, such as satisfaction with work productivity and energy level, and better safety profile.

The levonorgestrel intrauterine system, labeled as a contraceptive and a heavy menstrual bleeding treatment, is also seen to be effective in reducing endometriosis lesion severity and the size of rectovaginal lesions. A multicenter RCT demonstrated that the levonorgestrel intrauterine system was as effective as the GnRH analog for the treatment of endometriosis-related pain, with avoidance of hormonal suppression. It also seems, according to recent accumulating data, to reduce the recurrence of symptoms in women undergoing surgical treatment for endometriosis.

Surgical Treatment

Surgical management of endometriotic lesions has the potential for definitive cure hence avoiding the side effects of prolonged medical treatment. A recent update summarized results from noncomparative studies in regard to outcomes of surgery for endometriosis-related pelvic pain. Most studies demonstrated improvement in menstrual and nonmenstrual pain, dyspareunia and life quality postsurgery, but recurrence rate being up to 54% and risk of undergoing repeat surgery, particularly in young women.

The latest Cochrane meta-analysis assessed the efficacy of laparoscopic surgery in treatment of endometriosis-related pelvic pain, as studied in RCTs. The analysis highlighted improved pain outcomes when compared with diagnostic laparoscopy alone, but no conclusions could be drawn in regard to severe endometriosis treatment or specific surgical interventions. Moreover, there were no published RCTs that compared effectiveness of surgery versus medical treatment for pain associated with endometriosis. There is some evidence that, in regard to deep dyspareunia, surgical treatment results in better outcomes and fewer side effects compared with medical treatment. Women that underwent surgeries for excision of deep endometriotic lesions, including vaginal, rectal, or sigmoid resection,

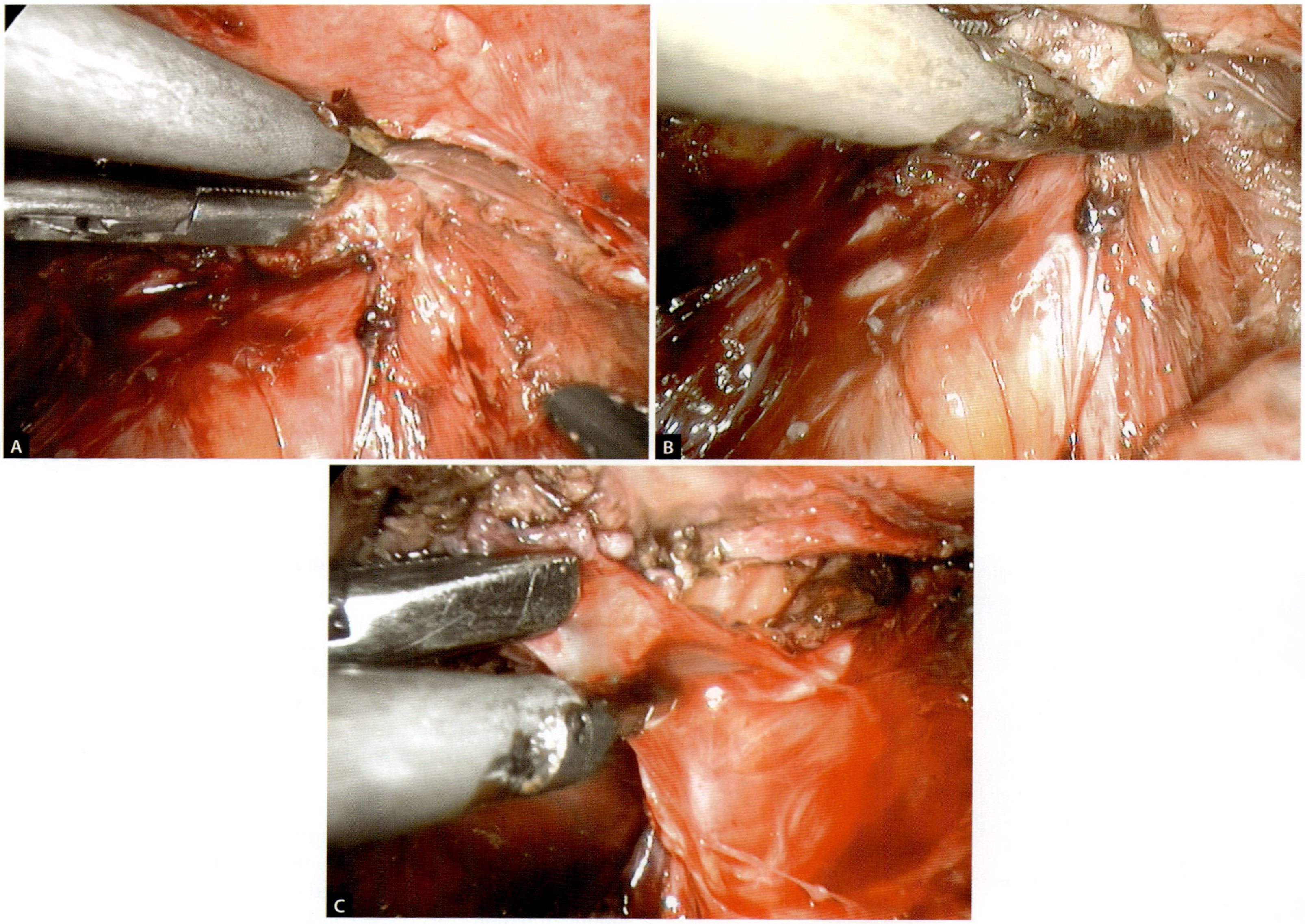

Figs. 60A to C: Rectovaginal fibrotic nodule held with tooth grasper and excised using harmonic.

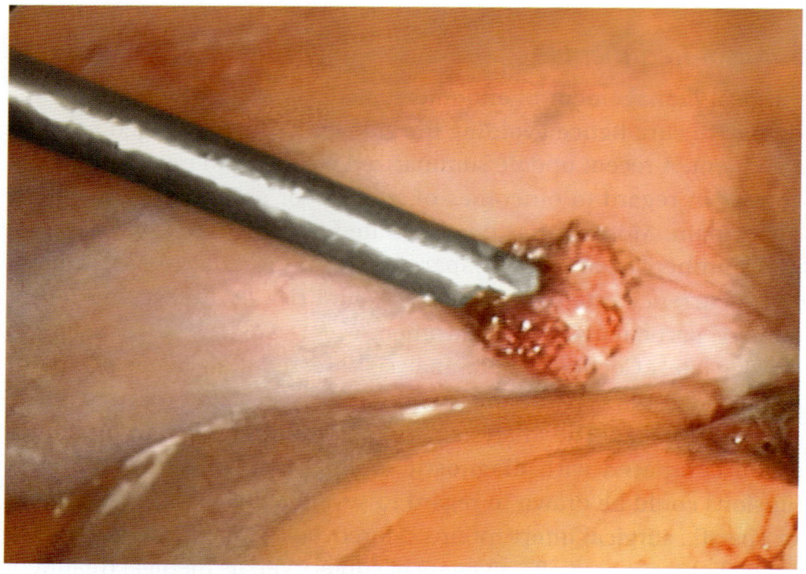

Fig. 61: Rectovaginal fibrotic nodule.

experienced significant improvement in sexual functioning, quality of life and pelvic pain. However, possible complications of extensive surgery must always be thoroughly discussed with the patient preoperatively.

Treatment for Infertility

Pharmacological Treatment

No evidence of improvement in fertility was shown with the use of different ovulation suppression agents or the anti-inflammatory pentoxifylline, in subfertile women having endometriosis who were interested in pregnancy. On the contrary, women with endometriosis who underwent IVF may benefit from prolonged GnRH agonists administration before treatment, as well as from oral contraceptive pills administration for 6–8 weeks prior to treatment with assisted reproductive technologies. IVF outcomes in women with endometriosis seem, overall, similar to outcomes among patients with other indications when controlled for age, despite earlier reports of reduced pregnancy rates when compared with other indications. Superovulation with or without intrauterine insemination increases pregnancy rates in women with mild endometriosis, while IVF should be suggested as first-line treatment for women with more severe disease, particularly if compromised tubal function is present.

Surgical Treatment

A meta-analysis of randomized trials showed an advantage of laparoscopic surgery when compared with diagnostic laparoscopy in the treatment of subfertile women with minimal and mild endometriosis in regard to clinical pregnancy rates Conservative surgery was also suggested as effective for natural conception during the first year after the operation. Surgery for more severe disease lacks conclusive support from randomized trials.

Controversy still exists in regard to the influence of endometriomas on fertility, the response to IVF treatments, and the possibility of diminished ovarian reserve following endometrioma resection.

ROLE OF GnRH

Compared to eutopic endometrium, endometriotic implants are characterized by overproduction of prostaglandins and increased local production of estrogens and cytokines, which synergize the activities of each other, promoting implantation and invasion of ectopic endometrium causing pain associated with endometriosis. In addition, there is aromatase overactivity resulting in increased COX-2 expression, which favors prostaglandin E production, hence, upregulating estrogen synthesis pathways. Interventions that reduce ovarian estrogen production reduce this synergistic process, thereby reducing or eliminating endometriosis-related pain.

Notably, the GnRH analog inhibits cell proliferation and increases apoptosis in eutopic endometrial cell cultures, an effect that appears to be mediated by an increase in the expression of the pro-apoptotic proteins Bax and FasL and a decrease in the expression of the antiapoptotic protein Bcl-2. GnRH analogs bind to receptors in the pituitary they have a longer half-life when compared native GnRH and hence resulting in down-regulation of the pituitary-ovarian axis and hypoestrogenism.

A long-term follow-up study of patients treated with a GnRH—a alone for 6 months revealed a 53% recurrence of disease or symptoms 2 years after completion of treatment.

A combination of surgical treatment and medical therapy (preoperative and postoperative) has been suggested for endometriosis. Surgical treatment followed by medical treatment may prolong pain-free (or reduced-pain) interval compared to surgery alone. In women wishing to preserve their reproductive potential, the rates of recurrent pain symptoms are 44% with surgical management and 53% with medical management.

CHAPTER

23

Total Laparoscopic Hysterectomy in Endometriosis

Shwetha Shah, Aditi Rai, B Ramesh

"In the middle of every difficulty lies opportunity"—**Albert Einstein**

INTRODUCTION

Endometriosis is defined as presence of endometrial glands and stroma outside the uterus, which induces chronic inflammatory reaction. The most common sites of implantation are pelvic viscera and peritoneum. It mainly affects women of reproductive age, but is also seen in adolescents and postmenopausal women.[1] It is found in women of all ethnic and social groups.

Hysterectomy with or without oophorectomy is the approach reserved for patients with advanced endometriosis, recurrence, and severe pain symptoms in whom open surgery is the usual approach. Patients with deep infiltrating endometriosis should be approached by total laparoscopic hysterectomy (TLH) and a more radical surgery is safe and valid than standard hysterectomy to address the deeper lesions.

Severe and deep infiltrating endometriosis should be managed in a multidisciplinary approach as the goal of surgery is complete removal of all the disease as far as possible and to provide a symptom free life to the patient. Hence, such surgeries should be undertaken by an experienced laparoscopic surgeon with thorough knowledge of retroperitoneal anatomy and pelvic radical surgery. The aim of this chapter is to highlight on the challenges that we routinely encounter while performing TLH in cases of endometriosis which in turn will help to reduce complications and patient morbidity.

ROLE OF ENDOSCOPY IN ENDOMETRIOSIS

Laparoscopy has now become the gold standard for diagnosis and excision of all forms of endometriosis. The advantages of operative laparoscopy include faster patient recovery and reduced cost and less adhesion formation.[2]

In a recent prospective study, laparoscopic excision of endometriosis significantly reduced pain and improved quality of life for up to 5 years. The results have been more promising with radical surgery, including extensive excision of deep disease and also removal of portions of bowel and bladder containing significant endometriosis. There may be a continuing role for hysterectomy in the management of endometriosis, but the evidence for concomitant oophorectomy is less convincing.

INDICATIONS FOR TOTAL LAPAROSCOPIC HYSTERECTOMY IN ENDOMETRIOSIS

Women with symptomatic endometriosis who have completed child bearing:

- With failed medical line of management
- When conservative measures have failed
- Rectovaginal endometriosis or nodule
- Recurrent disease

TARGET POPULATION

Patients with endometriosis, including patients with advanced disease undergoing hysterectomy, are much younger as compared to those treated with same procedure for other indications. Uccella S et al. comparing patients with endometriosis treated with TLH with those treated with TLH for other benign indications found a mean age difference of 2 years (42 vs. 44, $p < 0.001$).[3]

Another challenge among these patients is that most of them have undergone previous multiple surgeries in the past either open or laparoscopic for endometriosis[4] and this poses an increased risk dense adhesions involving both the peritoneum and retroperitoneum during subsequent surgery, more so in cases where previous attempts of performing a radical surgery have failed.

ROLE OF OOPHORECTOMY

Bilateral oophorectomy is done for the purpose of the elimination of the estrogen that sustains and stimulates the ectopic endometrium.[5] According to Reich, at least one ovary can be preserved.[6] The decision to perform bilateral oophorectomy at the time of surgery is dependent upon many factors, one of which is the discretion of the operating surgeon and if ovaries are clearly the cause of pelvic pain. Namnoum and colleagues[7] had determined the risk of reoperation and/or recurrence of symptoms after hysterectomy for the treatment of endometriosis. Among 138 women, 39 had a hysterectomy with ovarian preservation and 109 had all ovarian tissue removed. Of those whose ovaries were preserved, 62% had recurrent pain and 31% required intervention.

The authors concluded that the women with ovarian preservation had six times the risk of developing recurrent pain and an eightfold greater risk of reoperation. At present, there is no consensus on this subject.

PREOPERATIVE EVALUATION

Good preoperative evaluation is must for planning surgery and preoperative patient counseling. Most of these patients have pain as the debilitating complain and hence planning of surgery should be done with the aim of adequate pain relief.

A thorough history of especially pain symptoms, physical examination should include a per rectal examination, in patients with complaints of dyspareunia and dyschezia to rule out rectovaginal involvement. A tranvaginal ultrasound can help to identify associated abnormalities like adenomyosis and fibroids. Adnexal evaluation should be done to identify whether the endometrioma is single or multiloculated. A magnetic resonance imaging (MRI) pelvis is indicated in patients with bowel or urinary complaints.

In cases that are at high risk for bowel or urinary involvement, a colorectal and an urologist skilled in advanced laparoscopic surgery should be consulted in advance. A multidisciplinary approach is of prime importance in such cases to avoid complications and medicolegal litigations.

PREOPERATIVE PREPARATION

Patient is optimized medically for pre-existing comorbidities. A detailed well-informed consent is obtained in all cases. Patient is admitted 1 day prior to surgery and allowed liquid diet night before surgery. Patient is kept nil orally for 6 hours. Bowel preparation is done using Coloprep which contains picolax and sodium sulfate as active ingredients. Antibiotic prophylaxis is given 30 minutes prior shifting to OT.

INSTRUMENTS AND EQUIPMENT

Apart from standard instruments, very few special instruments are required as extensive retroperitoneal dissection is expected during the surgery. Uterine manipulators help to improve ergonomics, increase space, and facilitate nodule resection. We use Sukahdia uterine manipulator which facilitates anterior, posterior as well as lateral manipulation of uterus.

A bowel manipulator may be needed in some cases of dense bowel adhesions. A rectal probe may be needed if POD is obliterated. A combination of bipolar electrosurgery and ultrasonic energy is our choice for dissection.

PROCEDURE

Surgery is performed under general anesthesia with nasogastric tube to minimize bowel distension. Arms are placed by the side without arm boards and shoulder braces are positioned at the acromioclavicular joints. Legs are positioned in Allen stirrups. Intermittent pneumatic compression device is used for prevention of deep venous thrombosis in all patients. Low molecular weight heparin is administered prophylactically in all patients 12 hours prior to surgery.

Abdominal Entry and Port Placement

Veress needle is introduced at umbilicus or palmers' point to create pneumoperitoneum. Pneumoperitoneum up to 20 mm Hg is obtained before primary trocar insertion and then subsequently reduced to 12 mm of Hg.

Primary 10-mm-trocar is placed supraumbilically and abdominopelvic inspection is done for omental and bowel adhesions. A steep head low position is given to displace the bowel and help in adequate visualization of pathology. Three to four ancillary secondary 5-mm ports, two on left lower quadrant lateral to inferior epigastric artery, one on lower right side, and one suprapubically depending upon uterine size, are used.

Dilemmas in Defining the Operative Target

While performing TLH in cases of endometriosis, three options should be considered:

1. Excision of large endometriotic lesions first
2. Perform hysterectomy first and then subsequently address the nodule
3. To remove the uterus and disease en block

The first approach is favored as uterine manipulation facilitates dissection of retroperitoneal spaces, which further helps in development of correct surgical planes. Identification of vital structures like ureter, vessels, and nerves becomes easy. Complications can be detected easily and tackled. Vaginal excision and reconstruction is precise. The only unfavorable point is excision of large nodules becomes difficult due to space limitations and altered ergonomics.

PRINCIPLES OF SURGERY

The goal of surgery is complete removal of all endometriotic lesions, which can be achieved by:

- Maximum uterine mobility
- Clear operative field.

Most of these patients have adhesions due to previous surgery and these combined with the adhesions of the disease itself, make mobility and visibility difficult. This further becomes more challenging as most of these adhesions are dense, vascular, firm, and they involve vital adjacent organs like bowel, ureter, and rectum obliterating the pouch of Douglas (POD) to various degrees.

Maneuvers to Enhance Uterine Mobility and Visibility

- Division of round ligaments
- Extensive division of anterior leaf and posterior leaf of broad ligament
- Adhesiolysis
- Decompression of endometriomas.

Anatomical Correction

Endometriosis is associated with gross anatomical distortion in almost all cases, hence before proceeding for hysterectomy, anatomical correction of uterus and adnexa should be done.

This refers to adhesiolysis and decompression of endometriomas, which in turn will safeguard the ureter and bowel during hysterectomy.

Adhesiolysis

Omental adhesions to anterior abdominal wall are released with the help of harmonic Ace **(Fig. 1)**. Sharp dissection close to parietal peritoneum is employed to achieve lysis of bowel adhesions to anterior abdominal wall. Bowel adhesions vary in thickness, vascularity, and cohesiveness. Some adhesions are stretched without

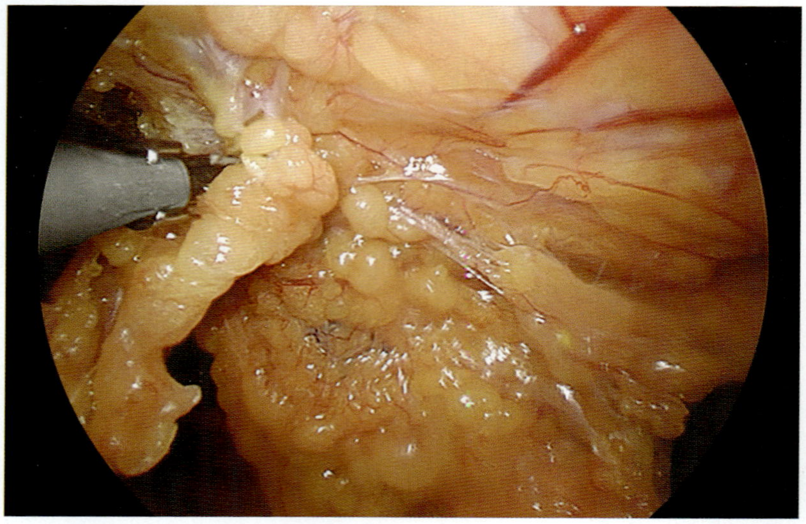

Fig. 1: Dense omental adhesions to anterior abdominal wall released with harmonic.

tearing the tissue. Bowel adhesions to uterus or adnexa are also released by sharp dissection. Dense bowel adhesions should be dissected toward the uterine serosa. Complete rectosigmoid adhesiolysis is not possible because of severity of adhesions and poor accessibility due to enlarged uterus and adnexa **(Figs. 2 to 5)**.

Adnexal adhesions to pelvic side wall are released by combination of blunt and sharp dissection. The dissection is started from normal peritoneum using suction irrigation cannula while maintaining traction with grasper from ipsilateral port **(Fig. 6)**. Identification of uterus to avoid inadvertent injury to them. Adnexal adhesions to rectosigmoid are released with scissors.

Obliteration of POD due to uterosacral scarring and retroflexion of uterus is commonly seen with endometriosis. Use of uterine manipulators will expose the POD and combination of sharp and blunt dissection will allow adherent rectum to fall away.

Ureterolysis

Ureteral involvement occurs in 0.1–0.4% cases. The most common site of affection is distal ureter. The lesions are typically extrinsic and rarely it may involve the lumen of ureter. Depending on the extent of ureteral involvement, ureterolysis with or without ureteral resection can be performed safely and effectively with the laparoscopic approach. The ultimate goal is to avoid ureteral obstruction and loss of renal function.

As the ureter is invariably adhered to the diseased peritoneum of ovarian fossa or involved by the disease process itself, dissection of ureter up to the ureteric tunnel is must when performing TLH. In case of severe endometriosis, fibrosis causes retraction, which leads to medial displacement of ureter from its normal lateral position. Another important aspect is preservation of periureteral vascular supply and adventitia of ureter. Ureteric involvement should be suspected when there is clinical involvement of uterosacrals. While performing ureterolysis, a combined lateral and medial approach is preferred as it is safe and more appropriate **(Figs. 7 to 12)**. When extrinsic ureteric involvement is minimal, management includes ureterolysis alone.[8] The principles for management include—atraumatic handling of ureter with interposition of normal tissue like omentum. When the ureter is directly involved by the disease process, management includes complete resection of the diseased ureter and reimplantation with temporary stenting.

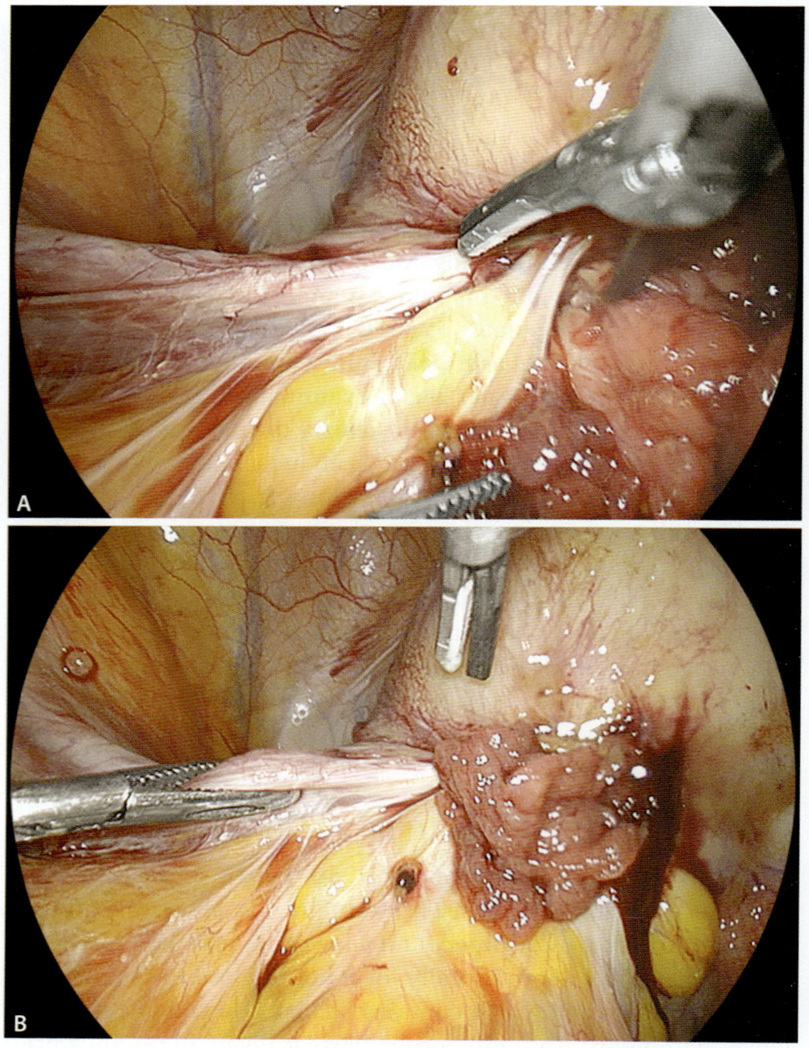

Figs. 2A and B: Lysis of bowel adhesions with atraumatic graspers and harmonic.

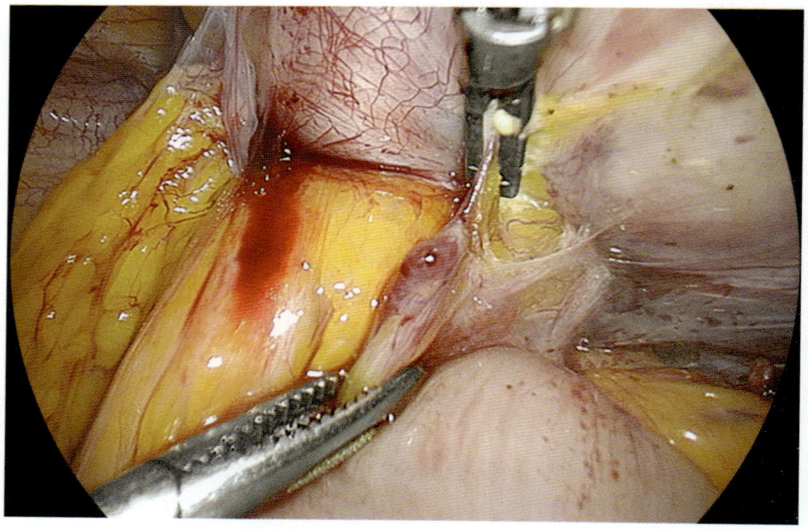

Fig. 3: Bowel is held with grasper and cut close to uterine surface.

Rectal Shaving

It was first described by Donnez and Squiffle.[9] It is reserved in cases of deep endometriosis involving the rectum wall not beyond the muscular layer.[9] It is referred as removal of endometriotic nodules from the rectal wall without opening the lumen and therefore, it does not require suturing of the rectal wall except in cases where the

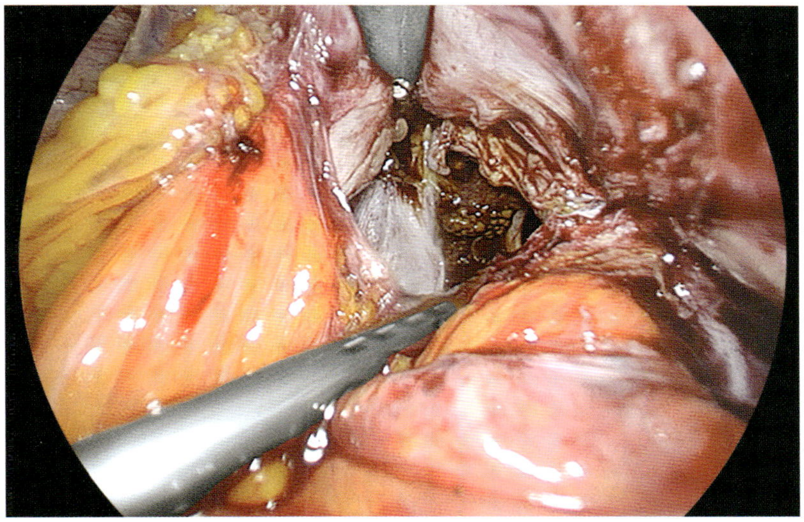

Fig. 4: Adhesiolysis of bowel adhesions using suction/irrigation cannula.

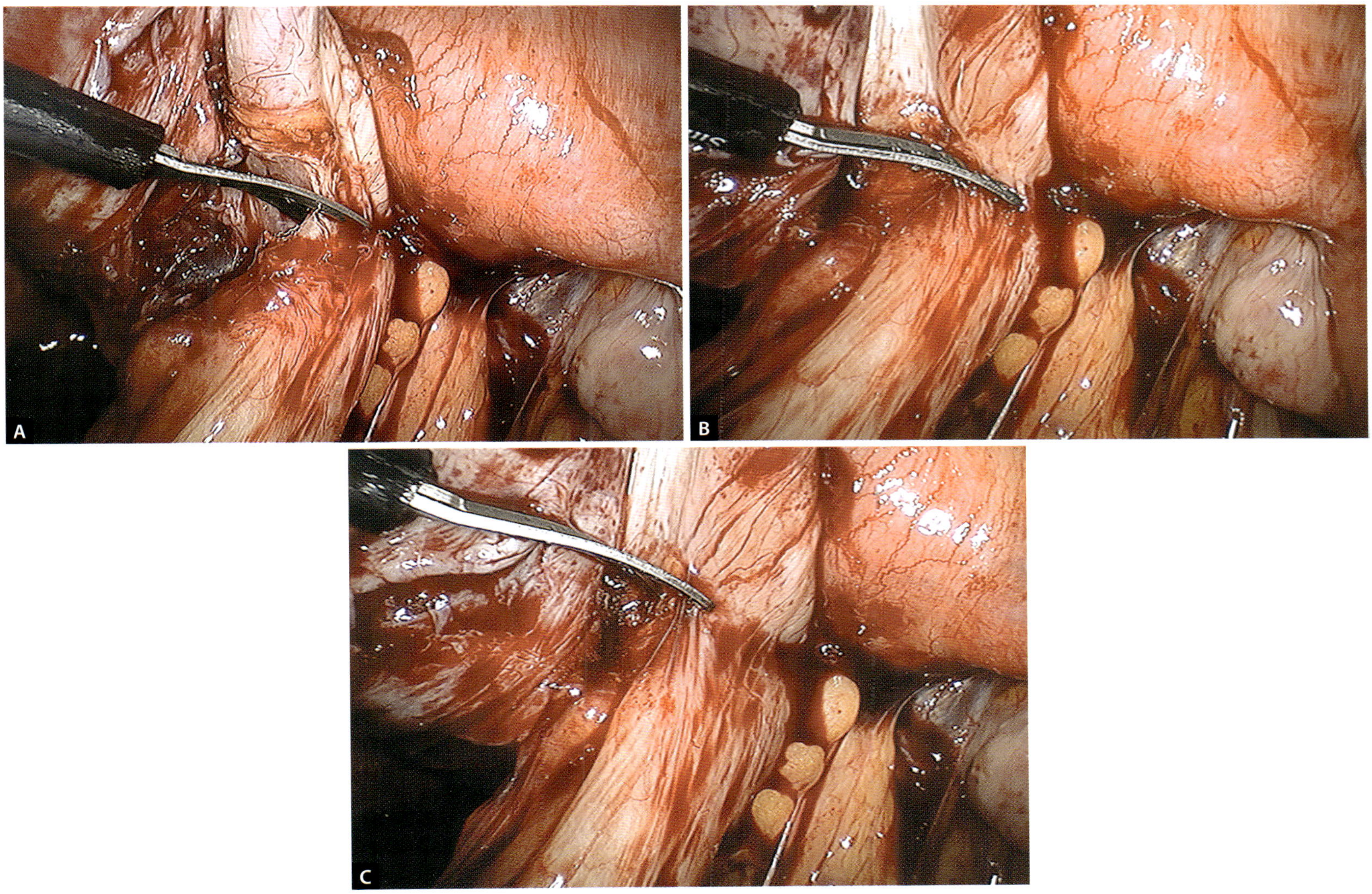

Figs. 5A to C: Lysis of bowel adhesions using cold scissors.

shaved rectal wall is excessively thin. Postoperative outcomes have been analyzed in literature which claim lower complication rates when compared to colorectal resection.[10] In addition, postoperative digestive function related to conservation of mesorectum and overall rectal capacity could be better after rectal shaving than after colorectal resection.[11]

The deep subperitoneal space located between the uterosacral ligaments and the rectum is longitudinally opened to avoid injury of the hypogastric and splanchnic nerves.[12] Dissection is performed in close contact with the lateral wall of the rectum and is directed toward the healthy rectovaginal space located below the endometriotic nodule. Once the lateral wall of the rectum is freed, the rectal shaving

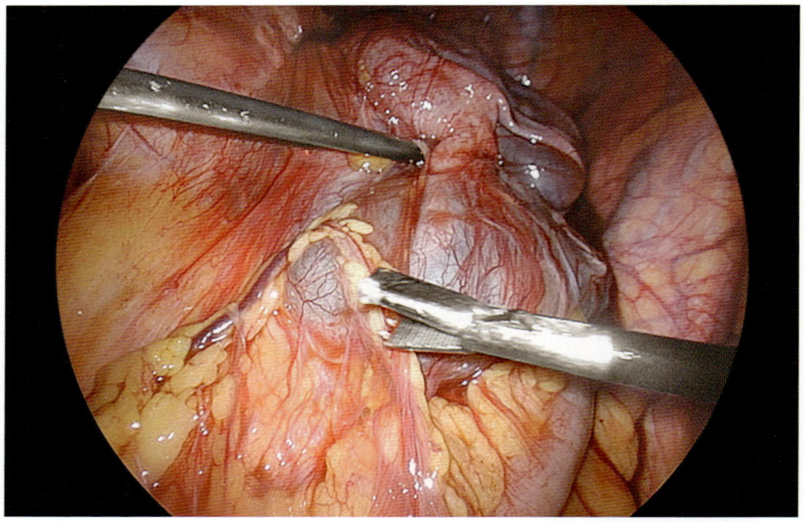

Fig. 6: Adnexal adhesions released with help of suction cannula and graspers.

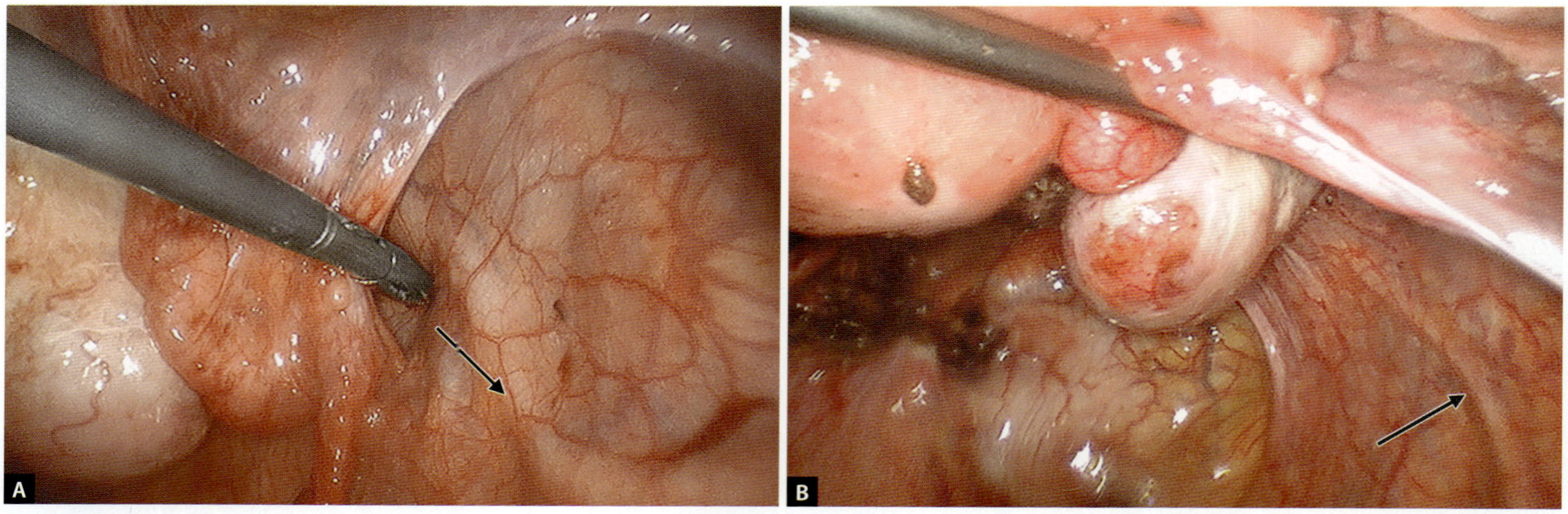

Figs. 7A and B: Identification of ureter.

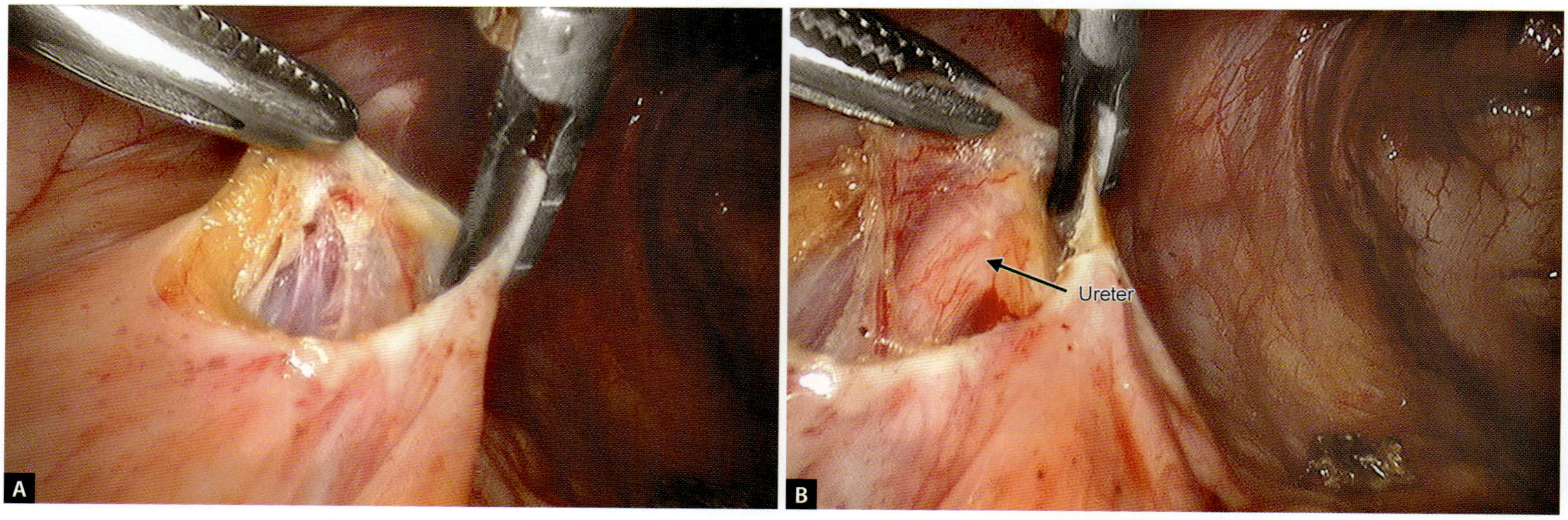

Figs. 8A and B: Incision made lateral to ureter over the peritoneum on the lateral pelvic wall triangle.

is performed as deeply as possible into the thickness of the rectal wall to remove abnormal fibrous lesions involving rectal layer. The deep endometriotic nodule is then treated by resection of vaginal fornix and anterior root of uterosacral ligaments **(Figs. 13 to 16)**.

Development of Retroperitoneal Spaces

The prerequisite for performing a safe TLH in severe endometriosis is mastering retroperitoneal anatomy. The principles of dissection are similar to those of radical hysterectomy but the major hindrance is

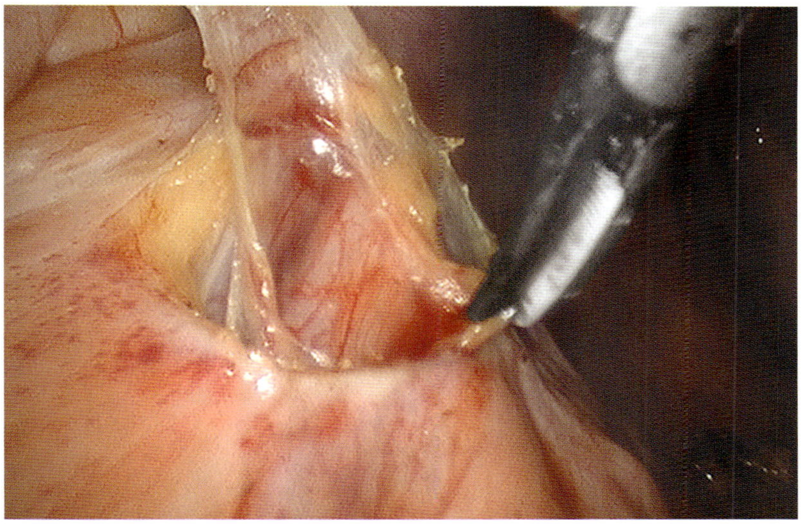

Fig. 9: Incision extended cephalad up to pelvic brim and loose areolar tissue dissected.

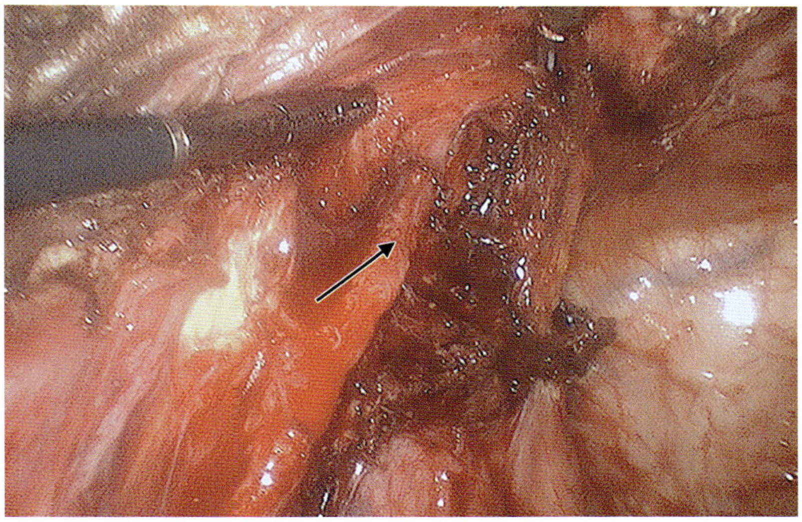

Fig. 12: Postureterolysis.

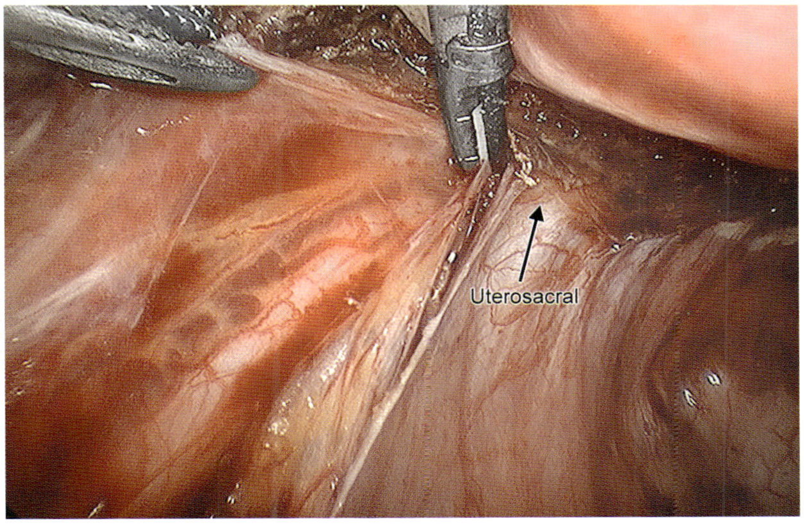

Fig. 10: Incision extended up till the uterosacral ligament (USL).

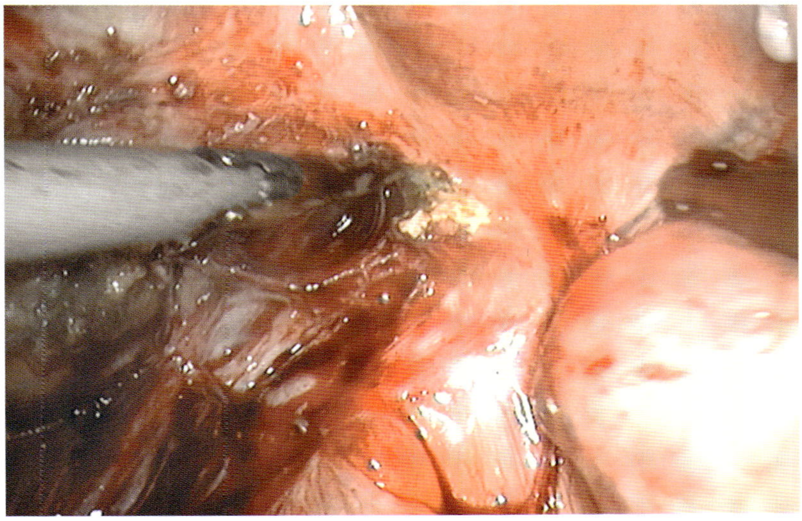

Fig. 13: Incision made posteriorly between two uterosacral ligaments.

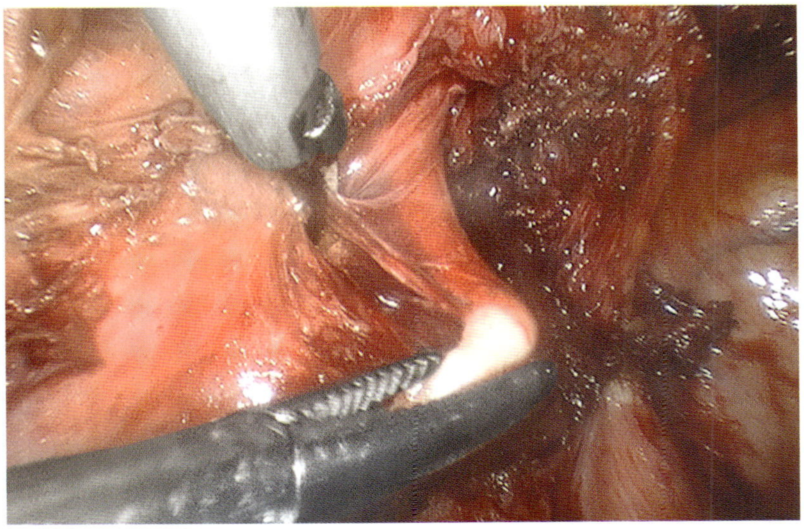

Fig. 11: Ureter grasped with atraumatic grasper and surrounding fascia separated with harmonic.

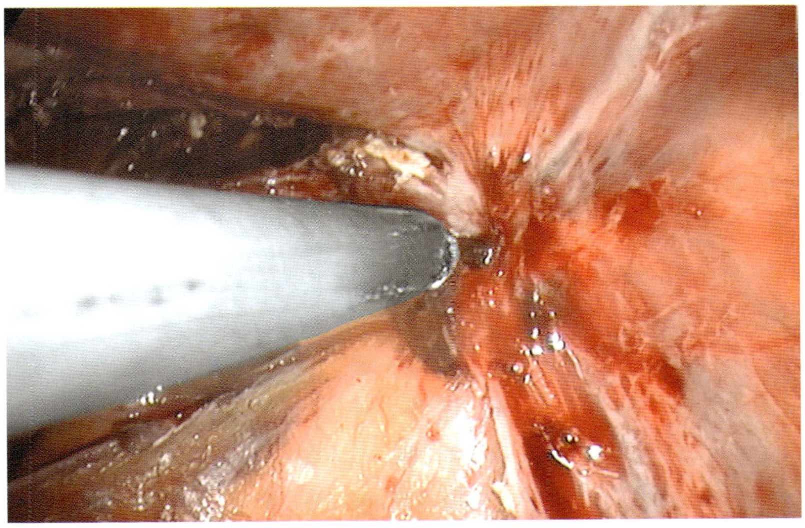

Fig. 14: Rectovaginal space created by separating posterior vaginal wall from rectum.

infiltration of these spaces by the disease process itself. Furthermore, due to previous inadequate surgery, the risk of complication increases. Development of any space may be needed at any point during the surgery, especially when radicle excision of the nodule is planned. Dissection should start from healthy to diseased side with the aim of circumscribing the nodule, following the planes developed by the gas.

Care should be taken to prevent creation of pseudo spaces and also use of irrigation should be minimum.

Adnexectomy

The difficulties encountered include multiple previous ovarian surgeries for endometriomas and also recurrent ovarian disease. The pelvic peritoneum is diseased and distorted and also vital structures like ureters are adhered densely to the ovaries. This poses difficulty in identifying the ureter separately from the infundibulopelvic ligament. Anticipating all these anatomical variations during surgery, a lateral approach should be considered while performing adnexectomy **(Figs. 17 to 21)**.

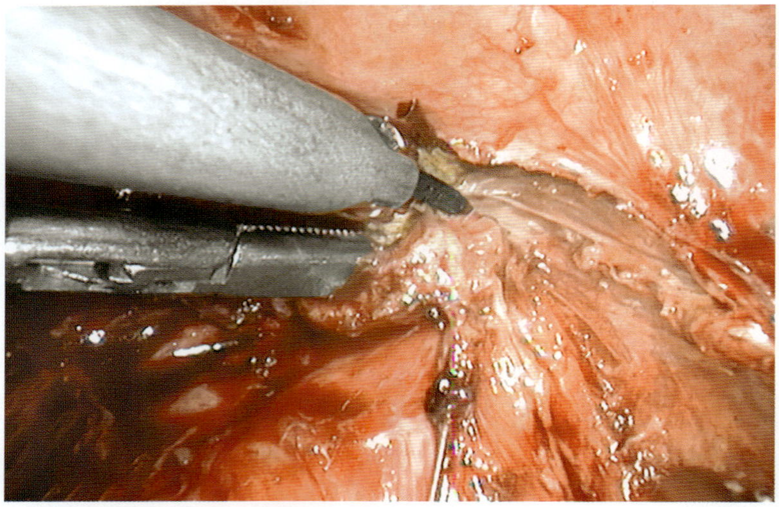

Fig. 15: Rectovaginal fibrotic nodule held with tooth grasper and excised using harmonic.

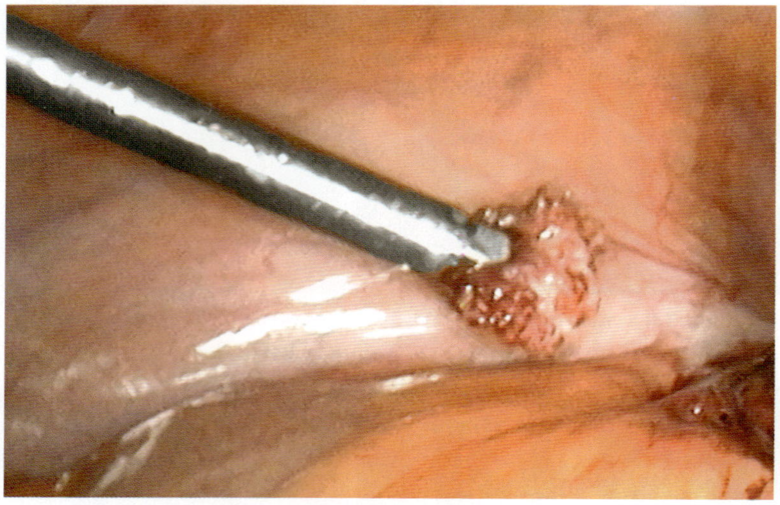

Fig. 16: Rectovaginal fibrotic nodule excised.

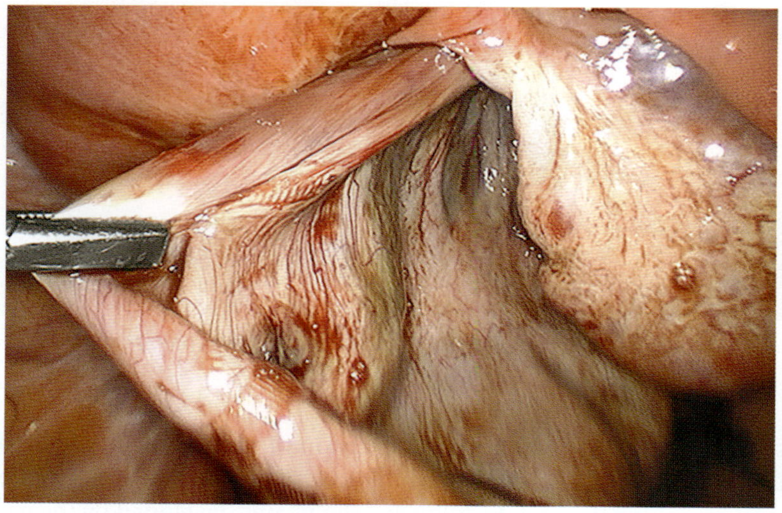

Fig. 17: Ovary held with tooth grasper and traction applied.

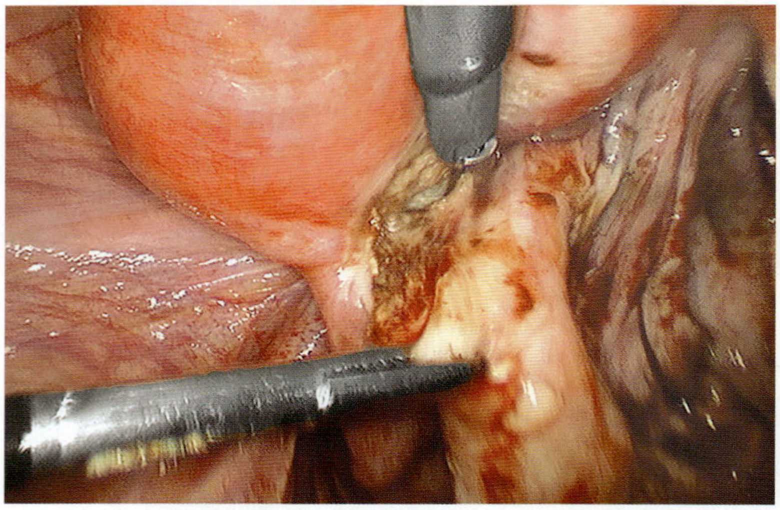

Fig. 18: Ovarian ligament cauterized and cut with harmonic.

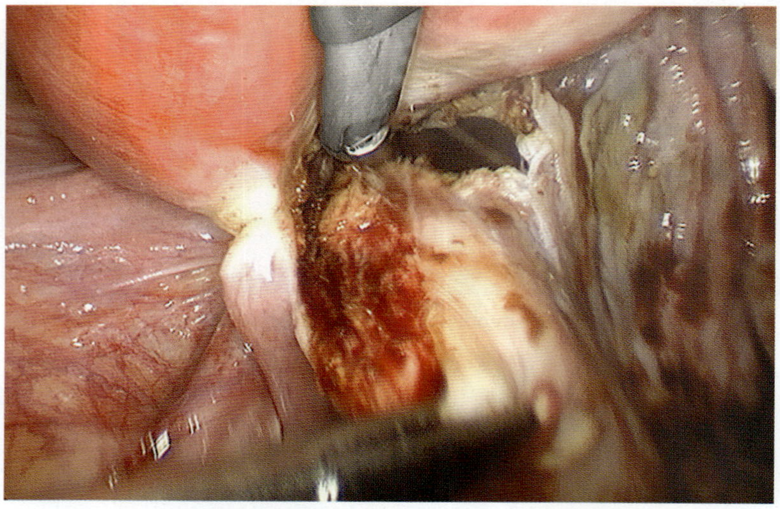

Fig. 19: Incision extended with harmonic while traction is applied with tooth grasper.

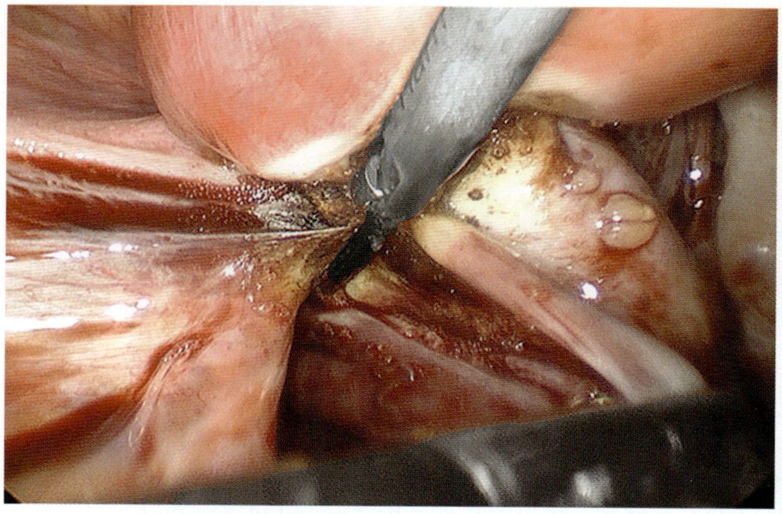

Fig. 20: Infundibulopelvic ligament cauterized with bipolar and cut with harmonic.

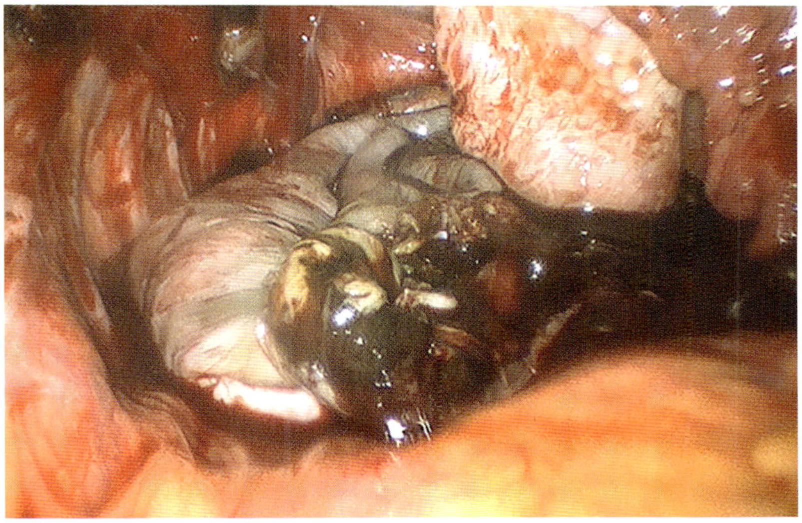

Figs. 21: Specimen of tube and ovary postadnexectomy.

Nerve Sparing Technique

Unlike the TLH procedure for benign indications where a nerve sparing approach is not relevant, it plays an important role while performing TLH in cases of deep infiltrating endometriosis. In deep infiltrating endometriosis, the lesions may extend into areas with dense autonomic innervation, and hence an effort at pelvic nerve sparing should be made, at least an unilateral preservation. This can be aided by the digital zoom function of the laparoscope, which helps in identification of inferior hypogastric plexuses and preservation of the urinary function. A key step in nerve sparing approach is that it helps in correct identification of anatomic structures in the posterior parametrium prior to removal of lesions. The surgeon should take the time to distinguish the cranial structure (uterosacral ligaments), the caudad structure (rectovaginal ligaments), and the lateral caudad structure (lateral rectal ligaments). These structures hold the autonomic nerves, which innervate the pelvic viscera. Damage of only the inferior hypogastric nerve may result in changes in the feeling for bladder filling, whereas damage of the inferior hypogastric plexus leads to bladder dysfunction with urinary retention. A prospective nonrandomized study comparing a non-nerve-sparing technique with a nerve-sparing technique proved that the complete laparoscopic nerve-sparing excision of endometriosis seems to be feasible and offers good results in terms of less bladder morbidity with apparently higher satisfaction than the non-nerve-sparing technique.[13]

COMPLICATIONS

- Intraoperative hemorrhage
- Rectovaginal fistula, bowel fistula, and bladder fistula
- Anastomotic leaks and stenosis, bowel obstruction
- Urinary retention
- Constipation
- Dyschezia
- Dysuria.

CONCLUSION

Surgery is the mainstay for diagnosis and management of endometriosis in cases were family is completed. Laparoscopy with histological confirmation is gold standard approach. Definitive surgery in the form of hysterectomy with or without removal of ovaries and all endometriotic lesions should be performed in all cases whenever feasible for complete cure of disease. Laparoscopic identification of the inferior hypogastric nerve and inferior hypogastric plexus is a feasible procedure for trained laparoscopic surgeons who have a good knowledge not only of the retroperitoneal anatomy, but also of the pelvic neuroanatomy as this qualification could prohibit long-term bladder and voiding dysfunction. Clinicians should refer women with suspected or diagnosed deep endometriosis to a center of excellence that offers multidisciplinary approach.

REFERENCES

1. Eskenazi B, Warner ML. Epidemiology of endometriosis. Obstet Gynecol Clin North Am. 1997;24:235-58.
2. Luciano AA, Lowney J, Jacobs SL. Endoscopic treatment of endometriosis-associated infertility: therapeutic, economic and social benefits. J Reprod Med. 1992;37:573-6.
3. Uccella S, Marconi N, Casarin J, et al. Impact of endometriosis on surgical outcomes and complications of total laparoscopic hysterectomy. Arch Gynecol Obstet. 2016;294(4):771-8.
4. Hidaka T, Nakashima A, Hashimoto Y, et al. Effects of laparoscopic radical surgery for deep endometriosis on endometriosis-related pelvic pain. Minim Invasive Ther Allied Technol. 2012;21(5):355-61.
5. Nezhat F, Nezhat C, Silfen SL. Videolaseroscopy for oophorectomy. Am J Obstet Gynecol. 1991;165:1323-30.
6. Reich H, Secktin T, Reich JM. Laparoscopic hysterectomy for advanced endometriosis and rectosigmoid disease. In: Donnez J (Ed). Atlas of Laparoscopy and Hysteroscopy, 3rd edition. London: Informa UK; 2007. pp. 93-110.
7. Namnoum AB, Hickman TN, Goodman SB, et al. Incidence of symptom recurrence after hysterectomy for endometriosis. Fertil Steril. 1995;64:898-902.
8. Watanabe Y, Ozawa H, Uematsu K, et al. Hydronephrosis due to ureteral endometriosis treated by transperitoneal laparoscopic ureterolysis. Int J Urol. 2004;11:560-2.
9. Donnez J, Squifflet J. Complications, pregnancy and recurrence in a prospective series of 500 patients operated on by the shaving technique for deep rectovaginal endometriotic nodules. Hum Reprod. 2010;25:1949-58.
10. Nezhat C, Nezhat F, Ambroze W, et al. Laparoscopic repair of small bowel and colon: a report of 26 cases. Surg Endosc. 1993;7:88-9.
11. Roman H, Vassilieff M, Tuech JJ, et al. Postoperative digestive function after radical versus conservative surgical philosophy for deep endometriosis infiltrating the rectum. Fertil Steril. 2013;99:1695-704.
12. Kondo W, Bourdel N, Tamburro S, et al. Complications after surgery for deeply infiltrating pelvic endometriosis. BJOG. 2011;118:292-8.
13. Landi S, Ceccaroni M, Perutelli A, et al. Laparoscopic nerve-sparing complete excision of deep endometriosis is it feasible? Hum Reprod. 2006;21(3):774-81.

Accompanying Video: Total laparoscopic hysterectomy in endometriosis.

CHAPTER

24

Scar Endometriosis

B Ramesh, Punitha Rangaraj, Minal Kumbhalwar

INTRODUCTION

Cesarean section scars are the most common site of scar endometriosis. It can also occur at skin, subcutaneous tissues, abdominal wall, trocar sites, pelvic side wall, episiotomy scar, following uterine surgery patients with scar endometriosis may be asymptomatic or present with cyclical pain during menstrual cycle. Ultrasound, CT, and MRI may be used to detect scar endometriosis.

On clinical examination, a nodule is felt which may be tender.

SURGERY

Scar endometriosis is temporarily suppressed and gives relief by medications such as progesterones, gonadotropin-releasing hormone (GnRH), oral contraceptive (OC) pills, etc.

Surgical explorations and en bloc excision with surrounding clear on margins are performed **(Figs. 1 to 3)**.

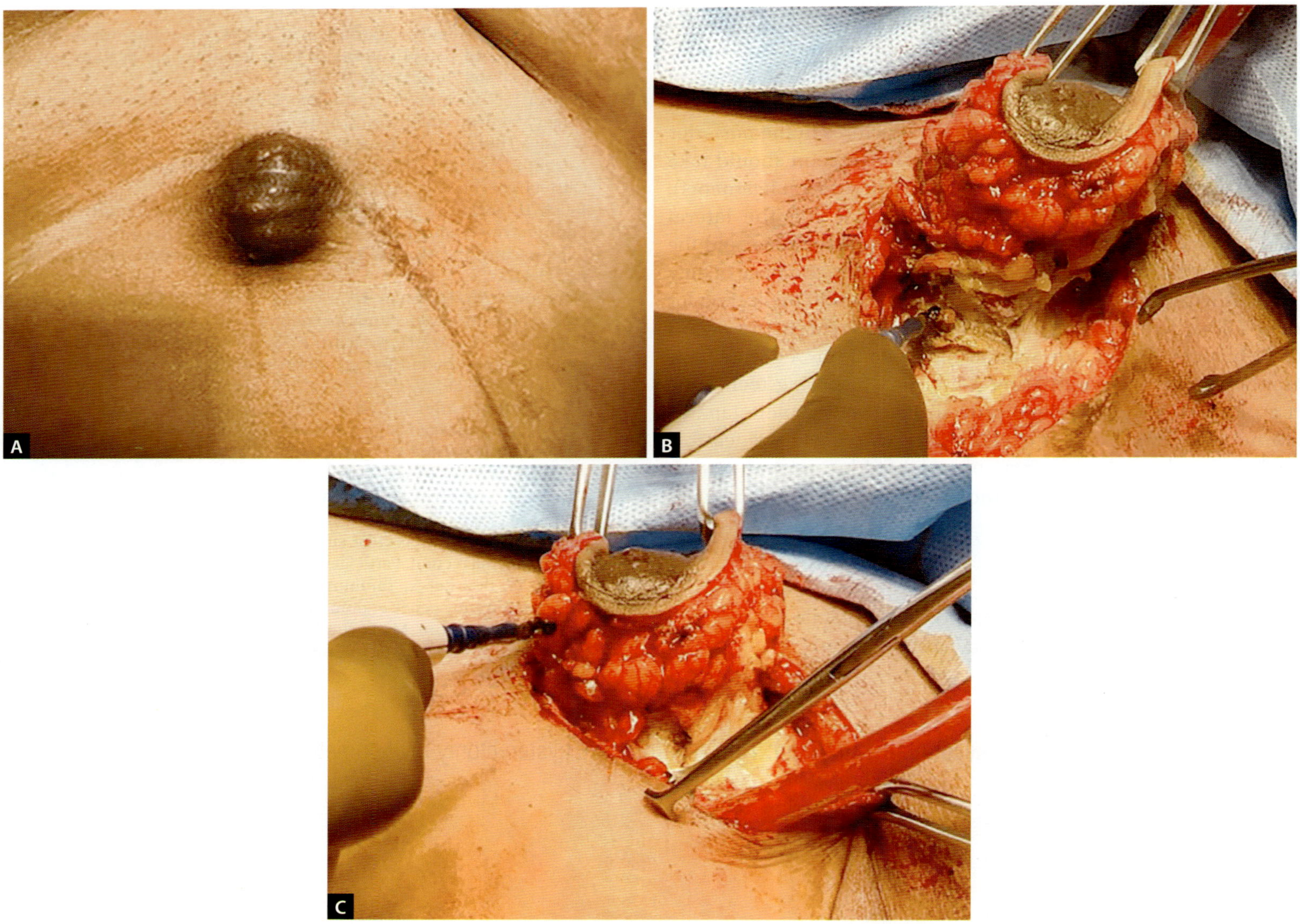

Figs. 1A to C: (A) Clinical photograph showing blackish discoloration nodule in the abdominal wall with previous operated scar; (B) Reddish-white fibrous area along with fascia and subcutaneous fat; (C) Excision of the endometrioma along with subcutaneous tissue.

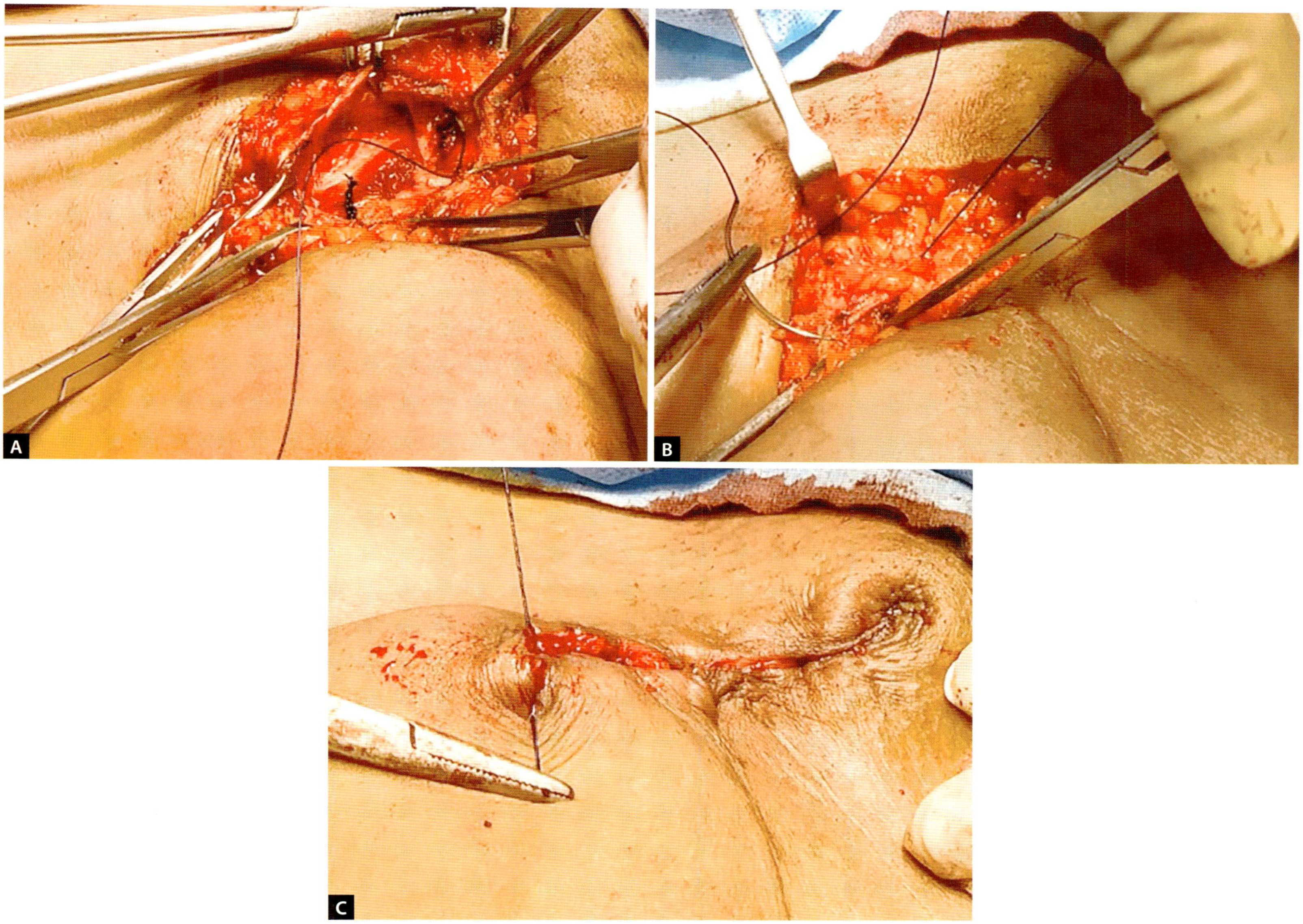

Figs. 2A to C: Suturing back in layers after excision.

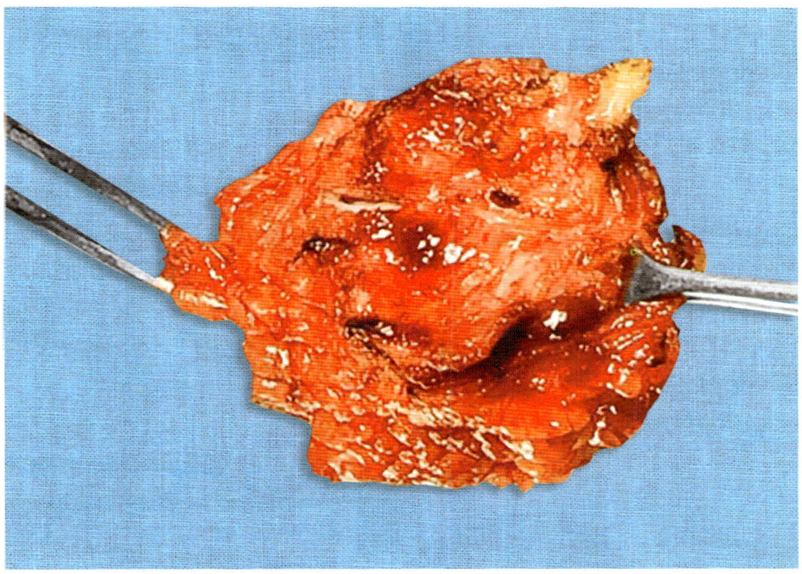

Fig. 3: Gross specimen of recurrent scar endometriosis.

CHAPTER

25

Laparoscopic Adenomyomectomy

Dhivya B, Aditi Rai, B Ramesh

INTRODUCTION

Adenomyosis also known as "endometriosis interna". The most common age group is late reproductive years. Presence of endometrial glands and stroma within the myometrium is defined as uterine adenomyosis and because of the histologic criteria adopted for diagnosis prevalence is extremely variable (14–66%) and the technique used to obtain myometrial samples.[1-5] Adenomyosis can either be diffuse or localized (focal), depending on the extent of myometrial invasion.[6] Young women will have more severe symptoms with mild disease, whereas older patients with enlarged uteri will have minimal symptoms. Moreover, in up to 80% of cases, adenomyotic uteri is associated with other pathology, such as myomas.[7] At the time of diagnosis, up to 35% of women are asymptomatic.[8] Most common symptoms are menorrhagia (50%), 30% and 20% have dysmenorrhea and metrorrhagia, respectively.[9,10] Around 20% of patients experience both menorrhagia and severe dysmenorrhea.[11] Less common symptoms are dyspareunia and chronic pelvic pain.[12] Severity of symptoms may be based on depth of uterine disease.[13] Hysterectomy is the treatment of choice; however, adenomyomectomy as an alternative option for those who have not completed childbearing or want to retain uterus.

SURGICAL ANATOMY

The junctional zone myometrium[14] have a specific characteristic that distinguishes it from other similar junctions in the human body. Pelvic MRI is helpful to diagnose and characterize adenomyosis, and sensitivity is 78–88% and specificity is 67–93%.

Magnetic resonance imaging (MRI), T2-weighted images display three distinct layers in healthy women:[15]

1. The endometrial mucosa shows high intensity signal.
2. Junctional zone myometrium is low intensity signal which is localized just beneath the endometrium.
3. Myometrium.

Gordts et al.[16] proposed a classification for adenomyosis based on MRI:

- Simple hyperplasia of junctional zone (zone thickness ≥8 mm to <12 mm)
- Partial or diffuse adenomyosis (thickness ≥12 mm; high-signal intensity myometrial foci and involvement of the outer myometrium)
- Adenomyoma (myometrial mass with indistinct margins of primarily low-signal intensity).

Two-dimensional (2D) transvaginal sonographic features of adenomyosis are as follows:[17-22]

- Globally or asymmetrically enlarged uterus.
- Round cystic space within the myometrium **(Fig. 2)**
- Radiating pattern appears in myometrial hypoechoic area (fan-shaped shadowing)
- Ill-defined endometrial stripe.

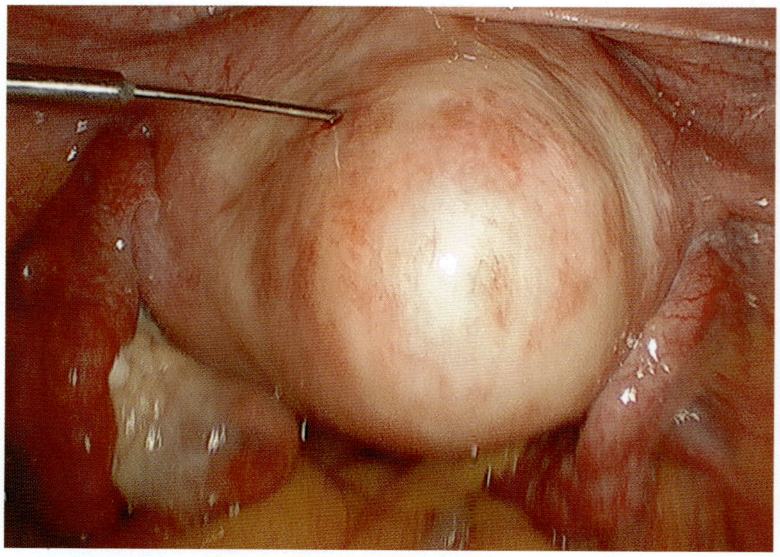

Fig. 1: Laparoscopic appearance of adenomyotic uterus.

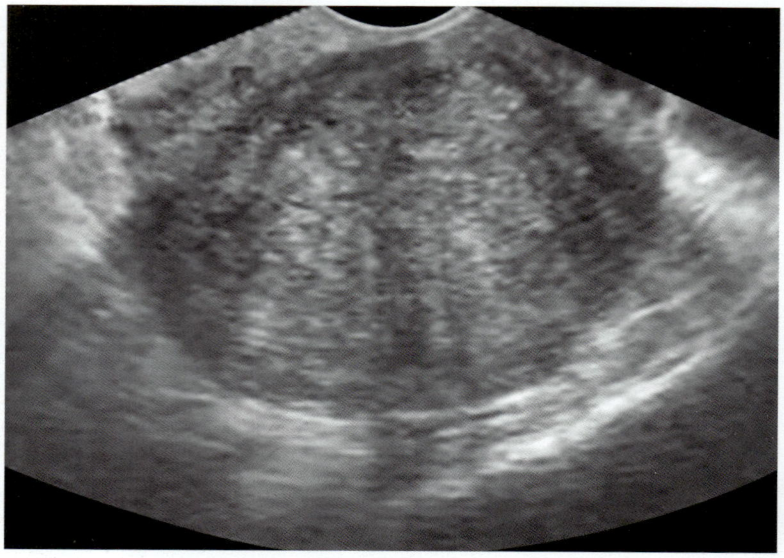

Fig. 2: Ultrasonographic appearance of adenomyosis.

Unlike fibroids, adenomyoma grows inside the myometrium displacing the surrounding myometrium and cause myometrial hypertrophy, adenomyosis infiltrates normal myometrium; hence, there is no capsule separating adenomyosis from myometrium.

The "question mark sign" **(Fig. 3)**—the corpus uterus is bent backward, the fundus facing the posterior pelvic compartment, and the cervix faced towards urinary bladder.[22]

MRI FINDINGS

Ectopic endometrial tissues become brighter on T1-weighted images when menstrual hemorhage occurs. Bright foci are being detected with increasing frequency of using high-resolution technique. These features may manifest as myometrial cysts, myometrial nodules, linear striations, pseudowidening of the endometrium, and poor definition of the endometrial junction. MRI findings **(Figs. 4 and 5)** of extent and location of adenomyosis help in determining the need for adenomyomectomy in patients with focal adenomyosis.

LAPAROSCOPIC ADENOMYOMECTOMY

Though there are various modalities for treating adenomyosis ranging from hormonal preparations, myometrial electrocoagulation to surgery, Grimbizis et al.,[23] in their study, mentioned that first-line approach for focal adenomyosis is laparoscopic excision of adenomyoma; in women who are keen for future pregnancy with diffuse adenomyosis, aggressive excision of the lesion with restoration of the uterine wall gives best results. However, due to advances in laparoscopy, excision and suturing by laparoscopic adenomyomectomy can be achieved with better patient comfort and equally achievable pregnancy rates.[24,25]

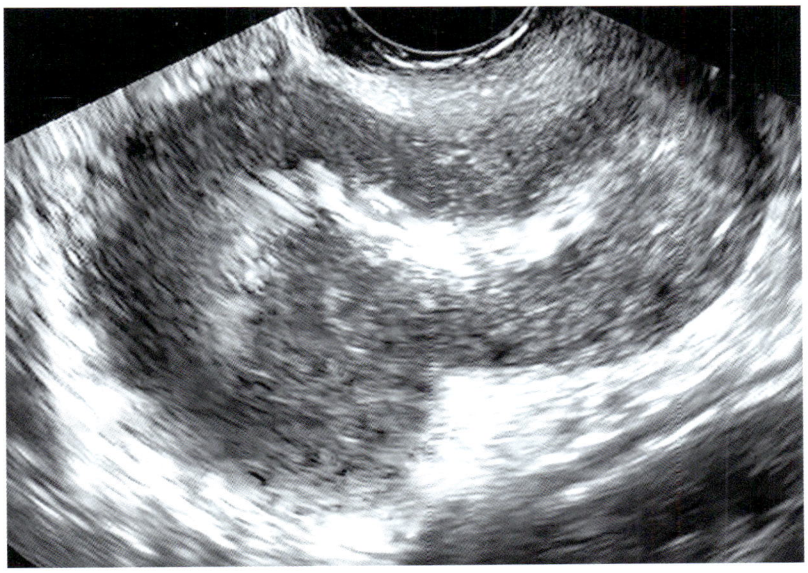

Fig. 3: Question mark sign.

Indications

- Symptomatic adenomyosis
- Focal adenomyosis
- Failure of medical management
- Desire for future pregnancy
- Young patients
- Desire to avoid hysterectomy.

Adenomyosis may be associated with infertility; because of dysregulation of myometrial architecture and function, structural and functional defects of the uterine junctional zone (JZ), disturbed uterine peristalsis and sperm transport and altered endometrial function and receptivity.

Contraindications

- Diffuse adenomyosis
- Age >40 years
- No wish for further conception
- Severe cardiorespiratory illness
- History of previous conservative surgery.

Surgical Equipment

Routine laparoscopic equipment essential for performing laparoscopic adenomyomectomy includes **(Figs. 6A to C)**:

- A laparoscopic tower with a high-flow CO_2 insufflator, camera and a light source
- An operating table with leg stirrups
- Vasopressin injection needle
- *Hysteroscope:* Hysteroscopy is done to rule intrauterine structural pathology
- Myoma screw for fixing the adenomyoma
- Laparoscopic toothed grasper for grasping and manipulating the uterus
- Laparoscopic plain grasper to manipulate adnexal structures and bowel

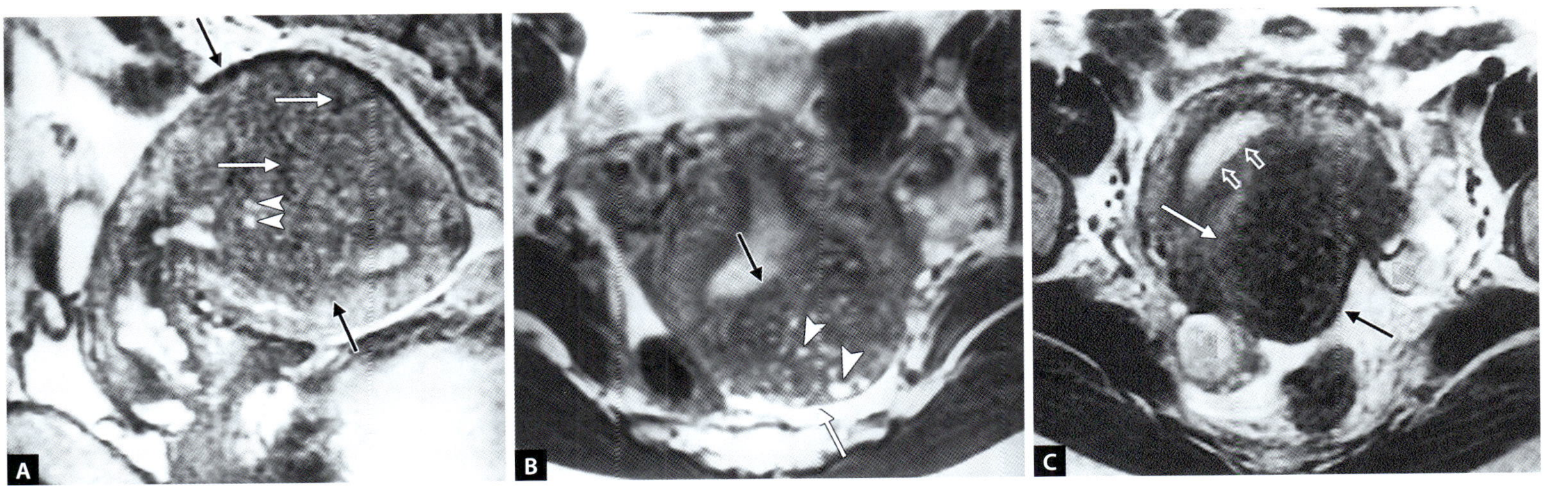

Figs. 4A to C: Magnetic resonance images of focal adenomyosis showing low signal intensities in the myometrium.

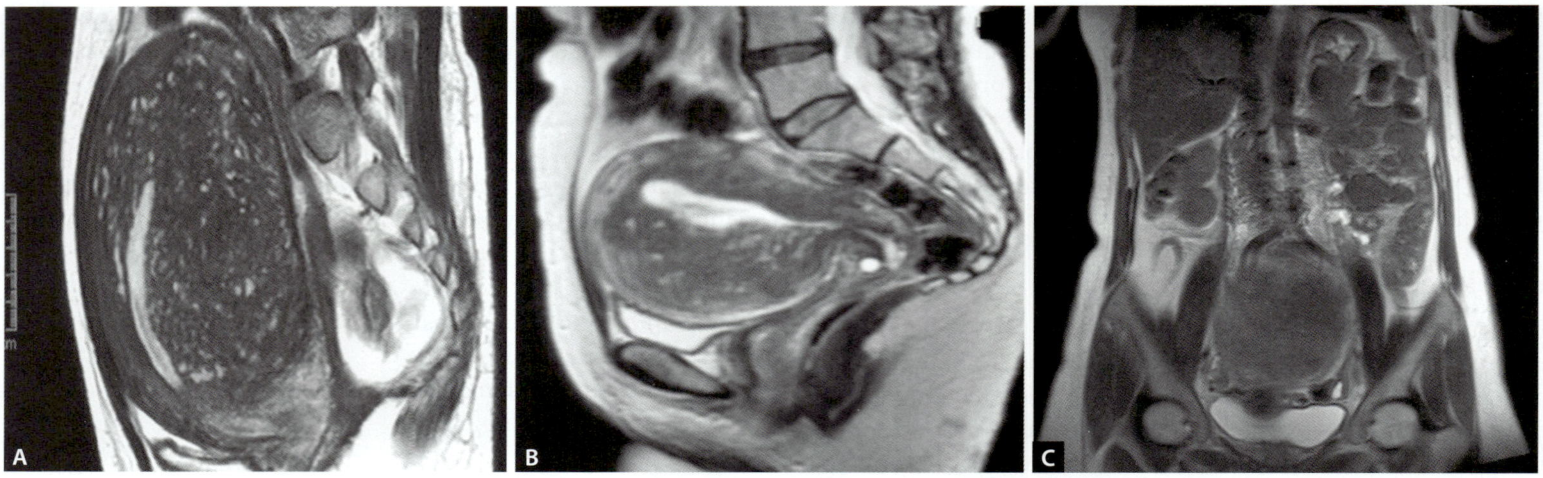

Figs. 5A to C: The MRI findings showing uneven and diffuse adenomyosis.

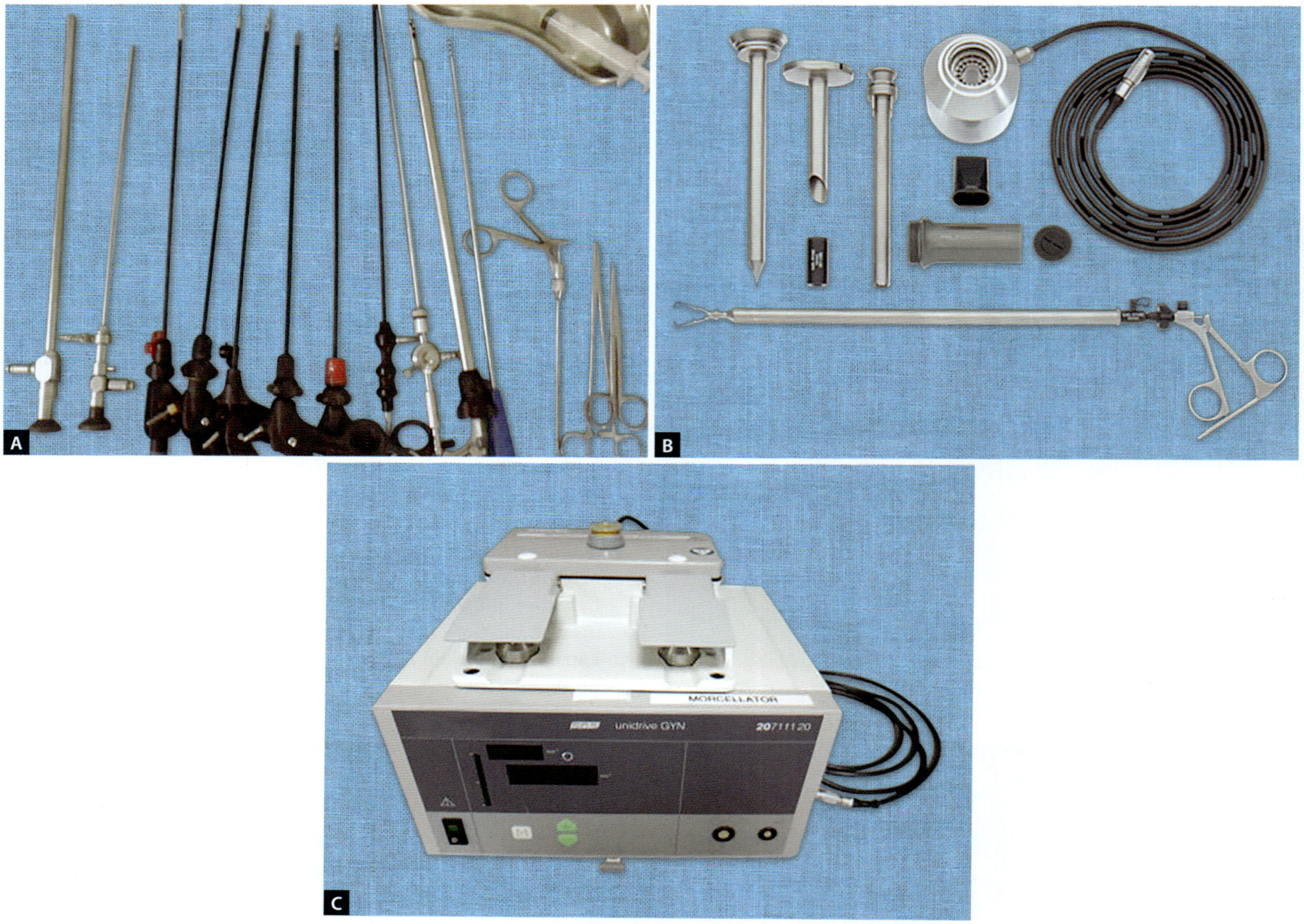

Figs. 6A to C: (A) Instruments for laparoscopic adenomyomectomy; (B and C) Electromechanical morcellator.

- Suction irrigator is essential to clear out the smoke, blood and clots
- Uterine sound for uterine manipulation
- Harmonic scalpel, monopolar electricity generator, bipolar electricity generator and bipolar forceps
- Laparoscopic scissors
- A needle holder and hooked scissors is used for suturing the vault and cutting the suture, respectively
- Morcellator **(Figs. 6B and C)** for specimen retrieval.

Preoperative Evaluation

Routine preoperative tests include a complete blood count, bleeding time, clotting time, renal function tests, evaluation of thyroid status, viral markers, electrocardiography (ECG), and urinalysis. However, tests like liver function tests, serum electrolytes, prothrombin time and international normalized ratio (PT-INR), activated partial thromboplastin time (aPTT), chest radiography, 2D-echocardiography, CT, MRI and contrast MRI should be done as indicated. Preanesthetic fitness is obtained. Preanesthetic assessment is an essential step prior to anesthesia in an attempt to decrease the morbidity related to anesthesia and surgery. Patient is advised for admission at the evening before the surgery. Informed consent should take after a thorough explanation of the planned operation, its potential risks and benefits, the possibility of laparotomy, hysterectomy, blood transfusion and therapeutic alternatives. Aspirin and warfarin are to be stopped 5 days prior to surgery. All patients are advised to eat lightly for 24 hours before surgery. An oral mechanical bowel preparation like Coloprep or Peglec is administered. Patient is kept nil per oral 8 hours prior to surgery and blood is kept reserved.

Surgical Technique (Figs. 7 to 10)

In our center, the surgical technique followed predominantly for laparoscopic adenomyomectomy is described next. The surgical procedure is as follows—infiltrating the uterus with diluted solution of vasopressin (20 units in 200 mL). Once blanching is achieved, excision of adenomyosis after T-shaped incision with subsequent reconstruction of the uterus. Adenomyoma is fixed with myoma screw and excised from surrounding myometrium with harmonic, leaving a myometrial thickness, from the serosa above and the endometrium below, of 1 cm. Care is also taken to avoid damage to the Fallopian tube. After removing adenomyoma, small residual of adenomyoma will be there, since there is no capsule or tissue plane as in myoma. Surgical approximation and suturing the adenomyoma bed can be challenging to the surgeon. We need to preserve good thickness of myometrium while excising the adenomyoma. Three-flap technique or inverted T-shaped incision gives good opportunity to retain good myometrial thickness. The future scar integrity depends on how well the margins are approximated without leaving dead space in the wound. Barbed sutures have brought a revolution

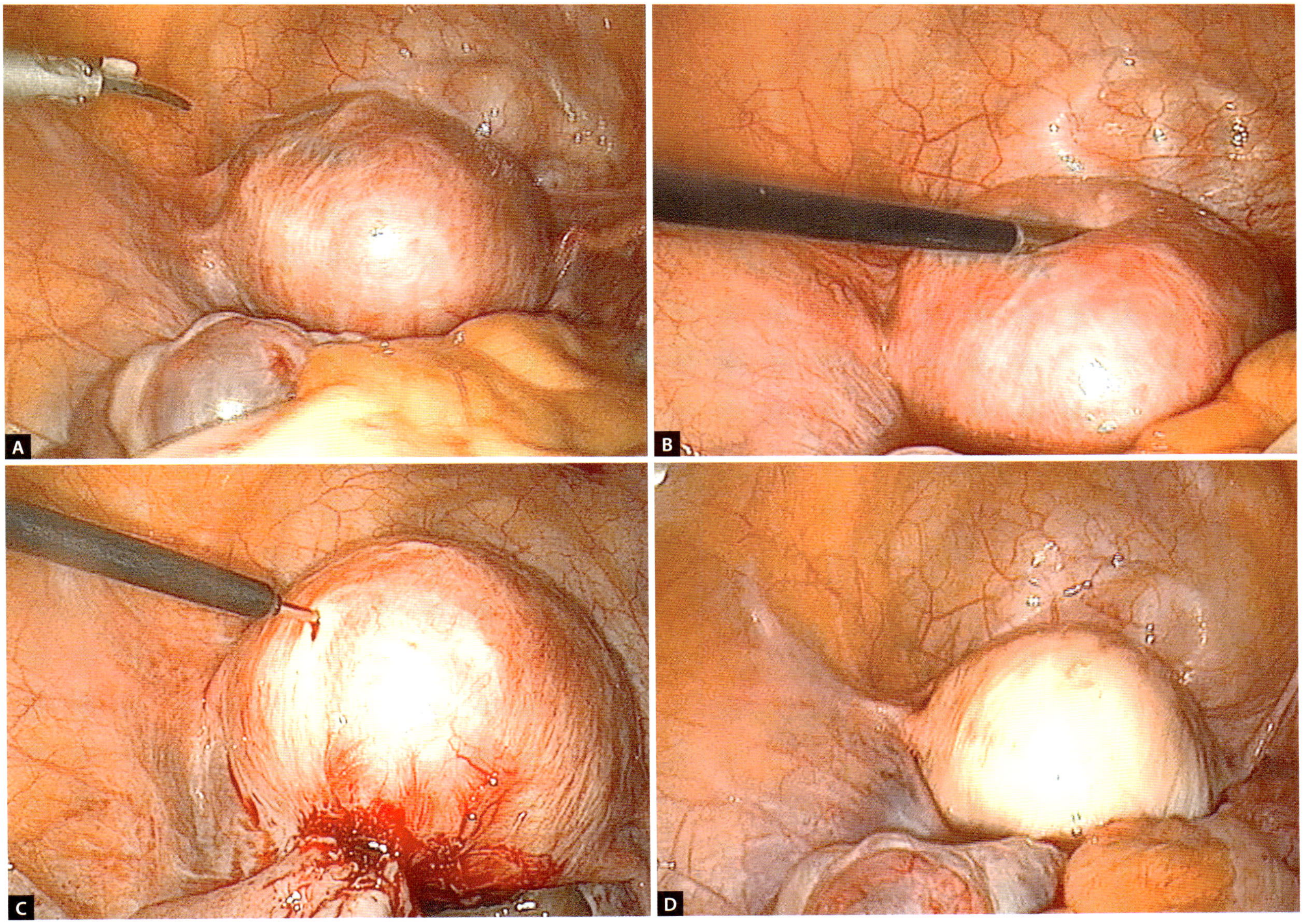

Figs. 7A to D: (A and B) Laparoscopic appearance of bulky and adenomyotic uterus; (C) Vasopressin infiltration; (D) Blanching effect of vasopressin.

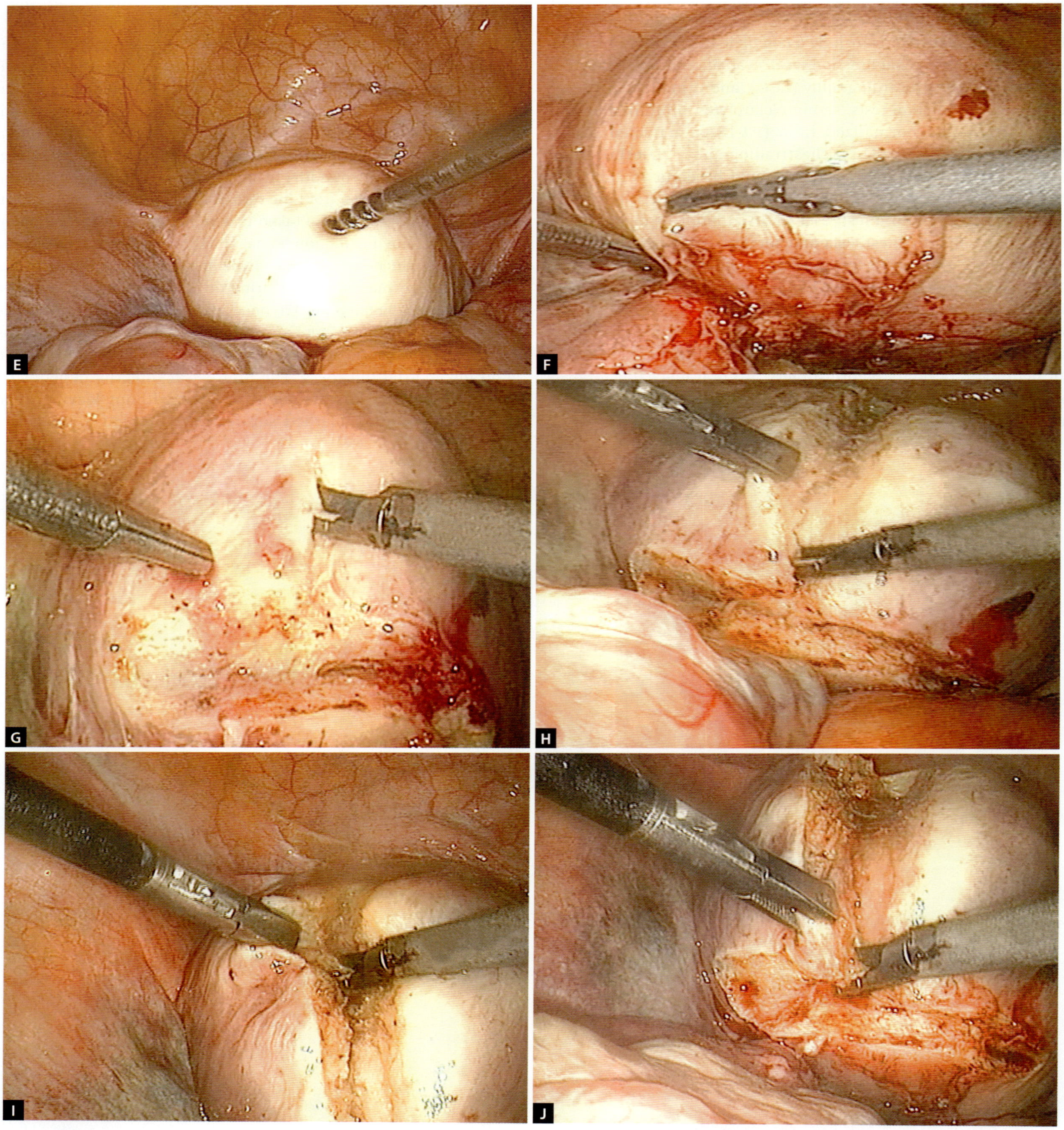

Figs. 7E to J: (E) Fixing the adenomyomatic uterus; (F) Incision made with harmonic; (G) T-shaped incision made; (H) Deepening of T-shaped incision; (I) Deepening of vertical limb; (J) Approaching the adenomyotic area.

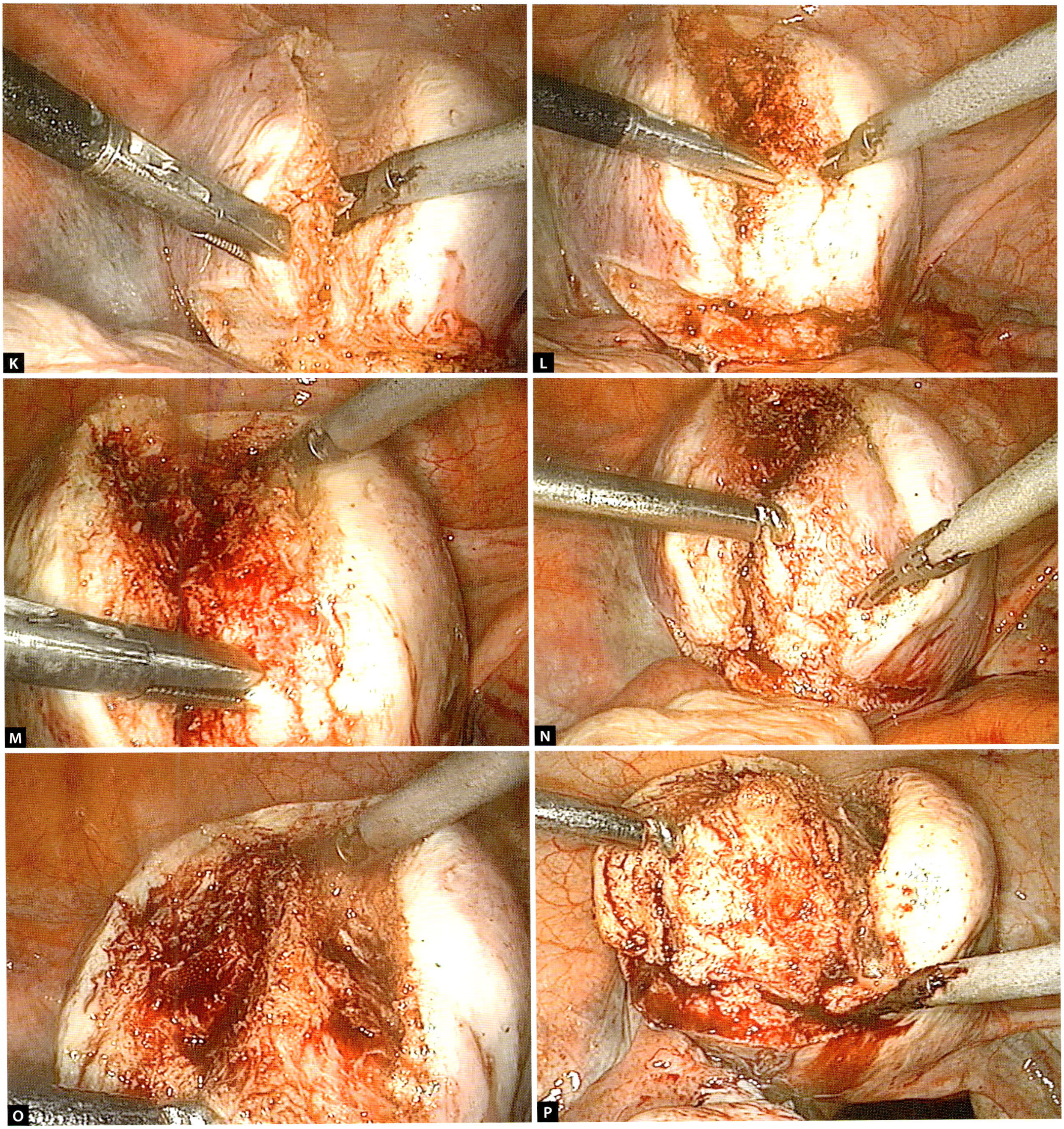

Figs. 7K to P: (K) Further deepening of incision; (L) Dissection of seromuscular layer from adenomyoma; (M) Dissecting the upper portion of adenomyoma; (N) Fixing adenomyoma with myoma screw; (O) Deepening the apex of the incision; (P) Traction with myoma screw.

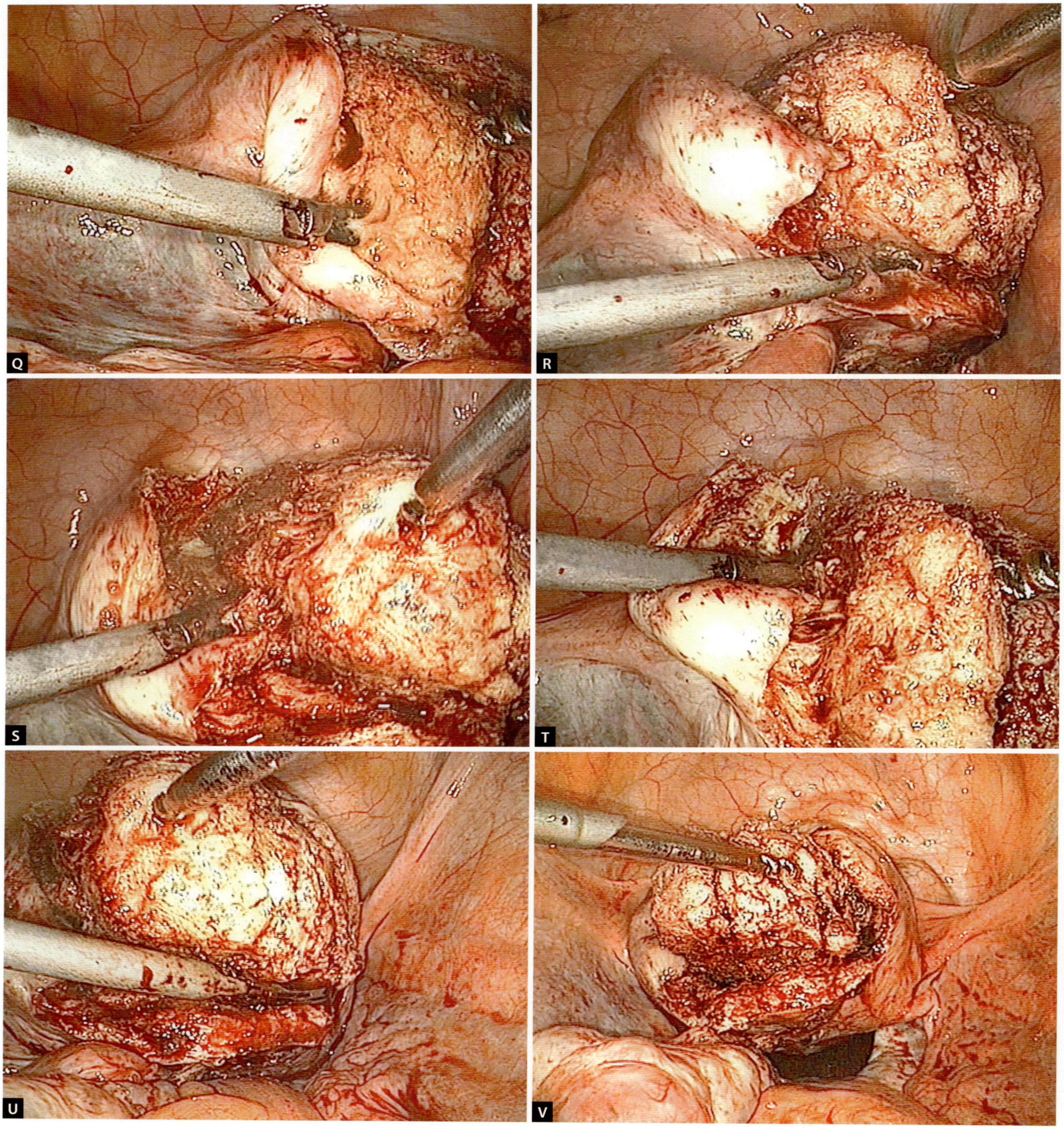

Figs. 7Q to V: (Q and R) Excision to dissect left lobe of adenomyoma; (S) Traction and countertraction to aid in dissection; (T) Separation of seromuscular layer; (U and V) Enucleation of adenomyoma.

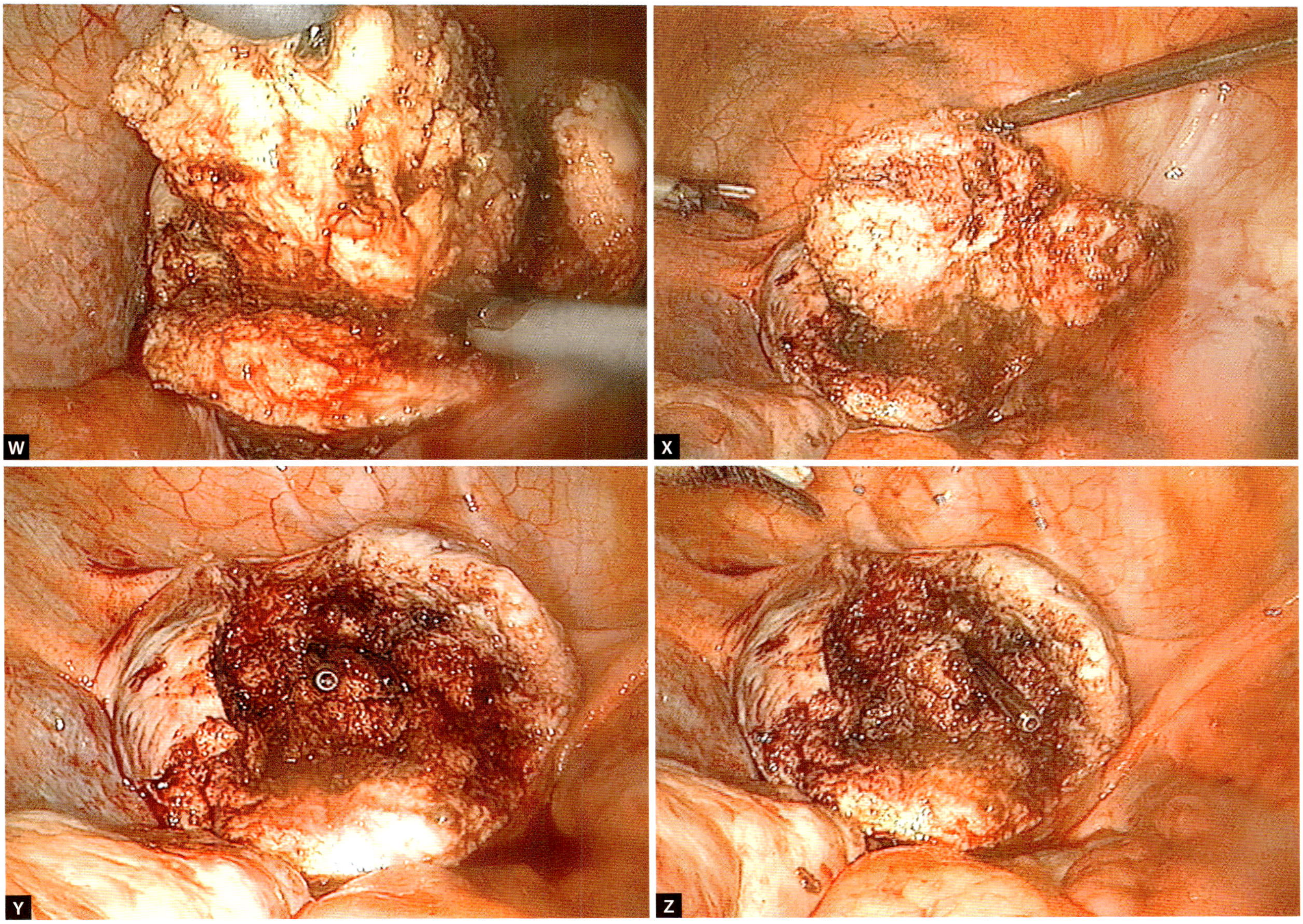

Figs. 7W to Z: (W and X) Enucleation of adenomyoma (continued); (Y) Apperance of adenomyoma bed after excision; (Z) Relation of uterine manipulator (cavity) to adenomyoma.

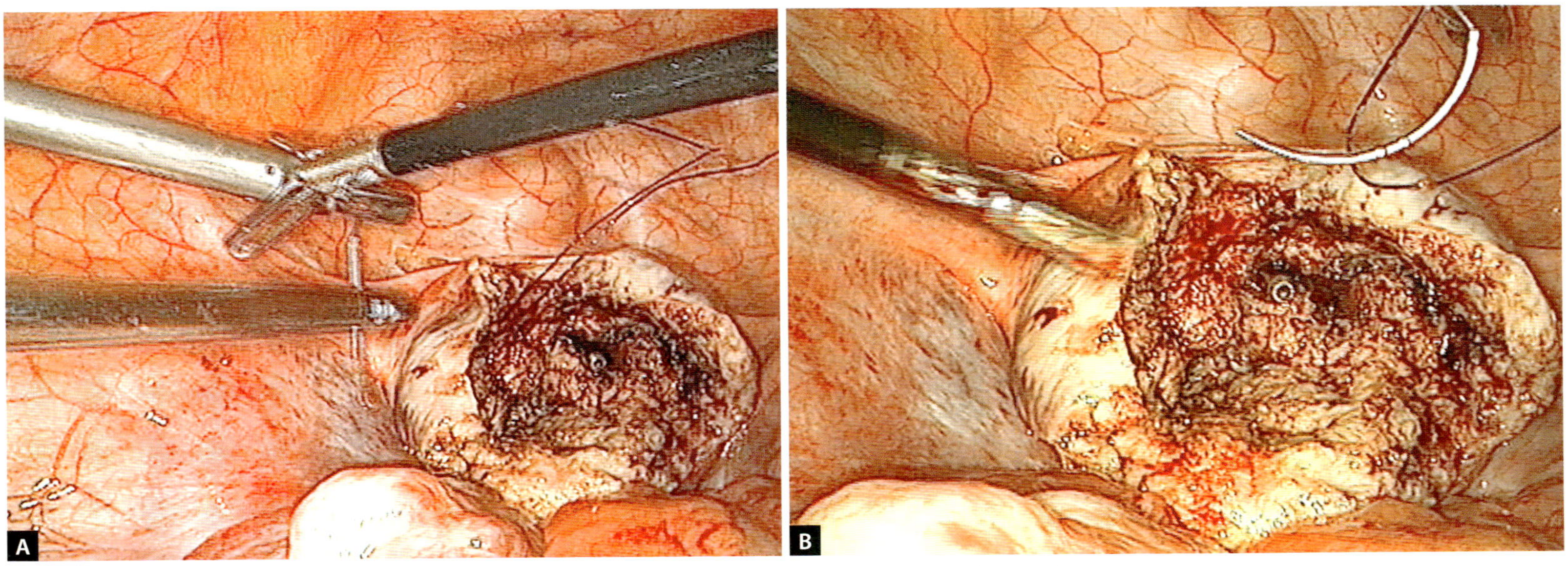

Figs. 8A and B: Suturing the bed of adenomyoma (first layer).

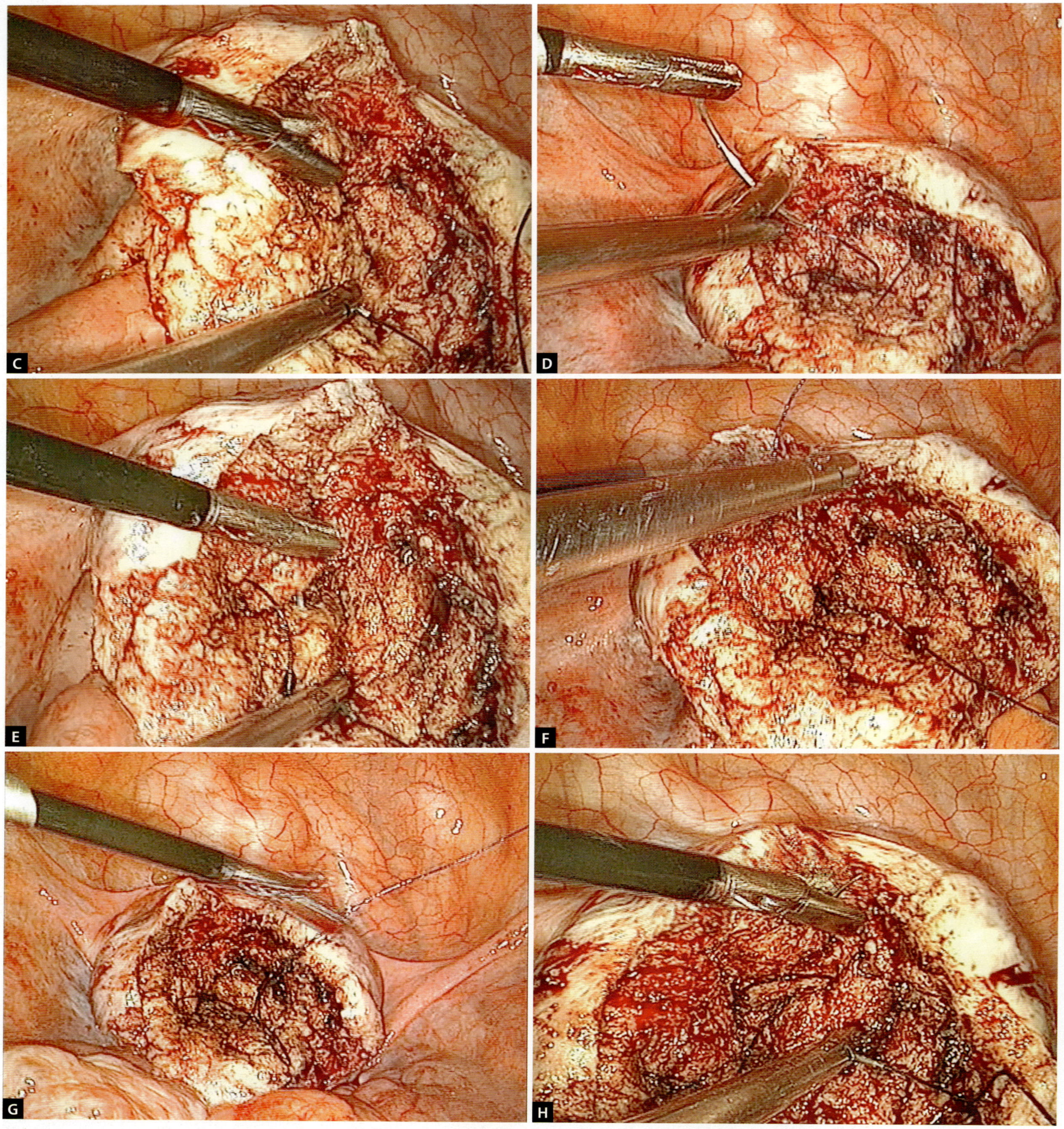

FIGS. 8C to H: (C to H) Suturing the bed of adenomyoma (first layer)

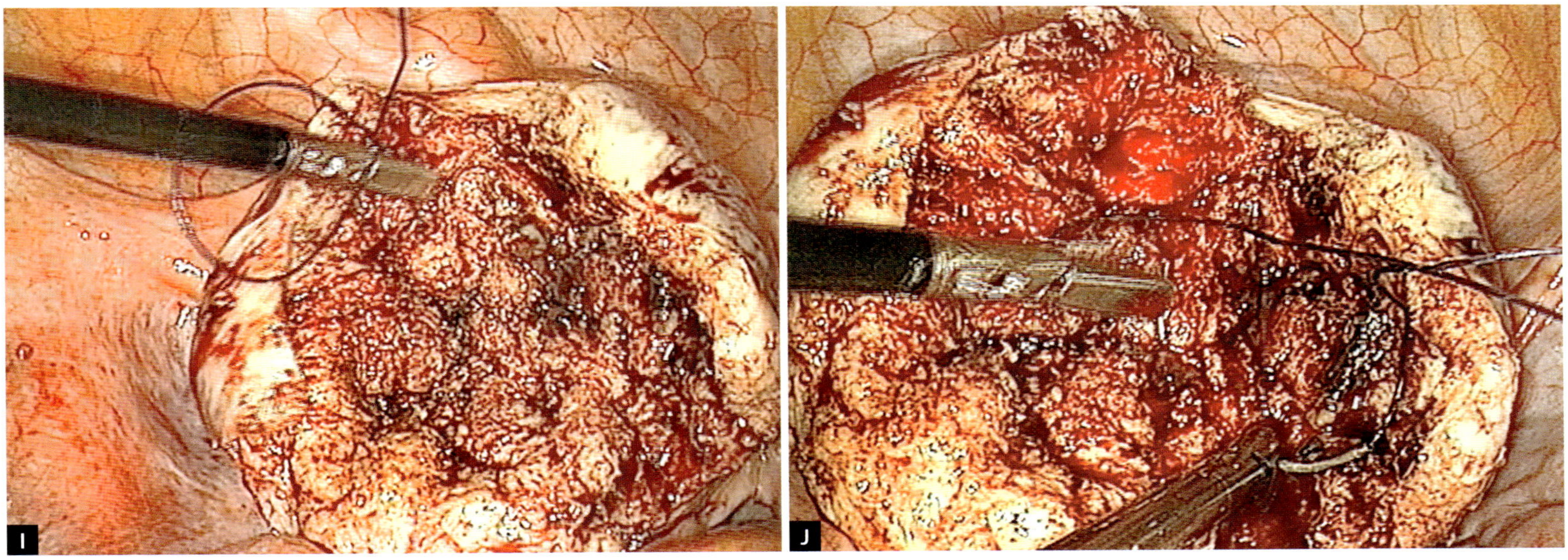

Figs. 8I and J: Suturing the bed of adenomyoma (first layer continued).

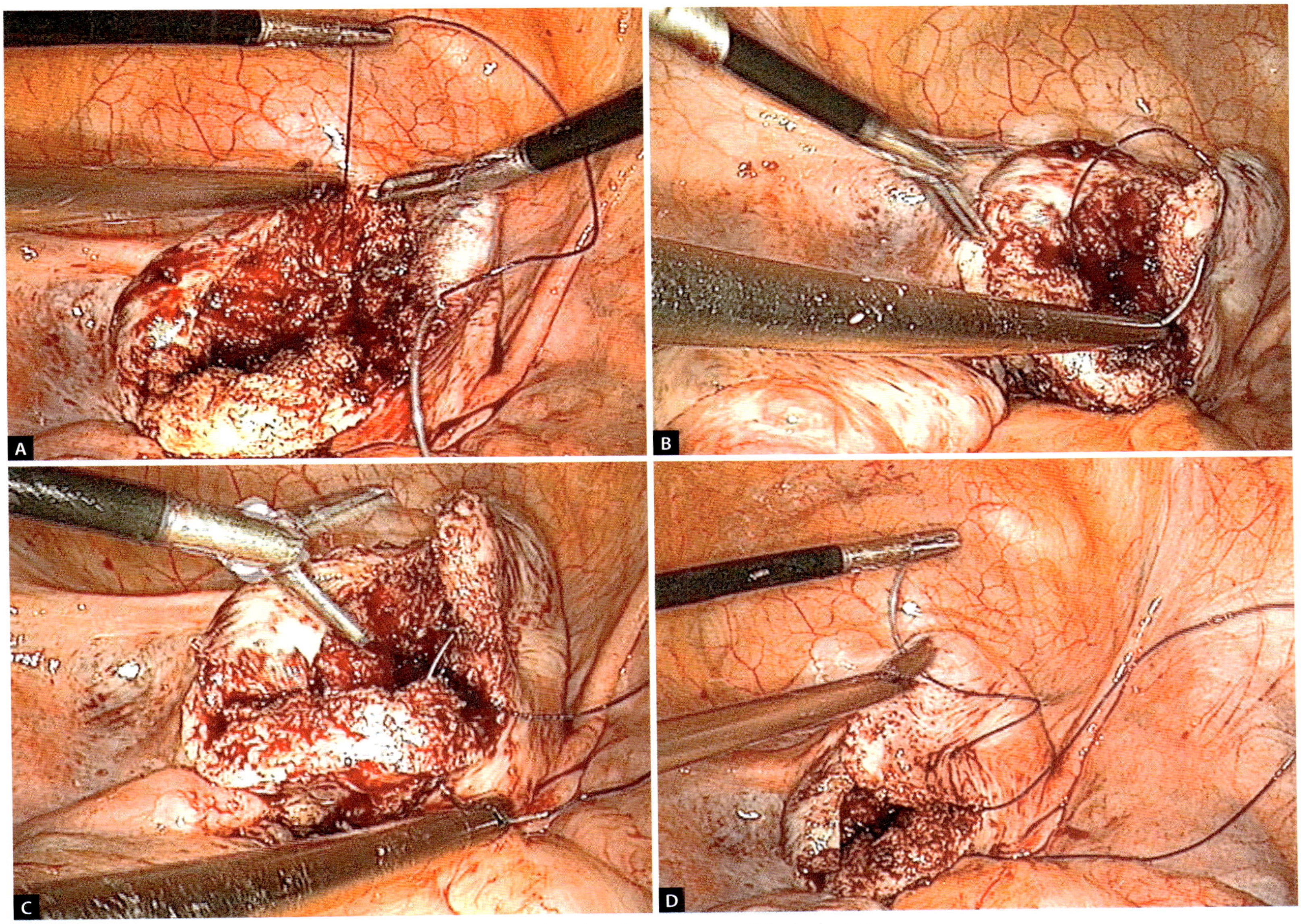

Figs. 9A to D: Suturing of second layer with barbed suture.

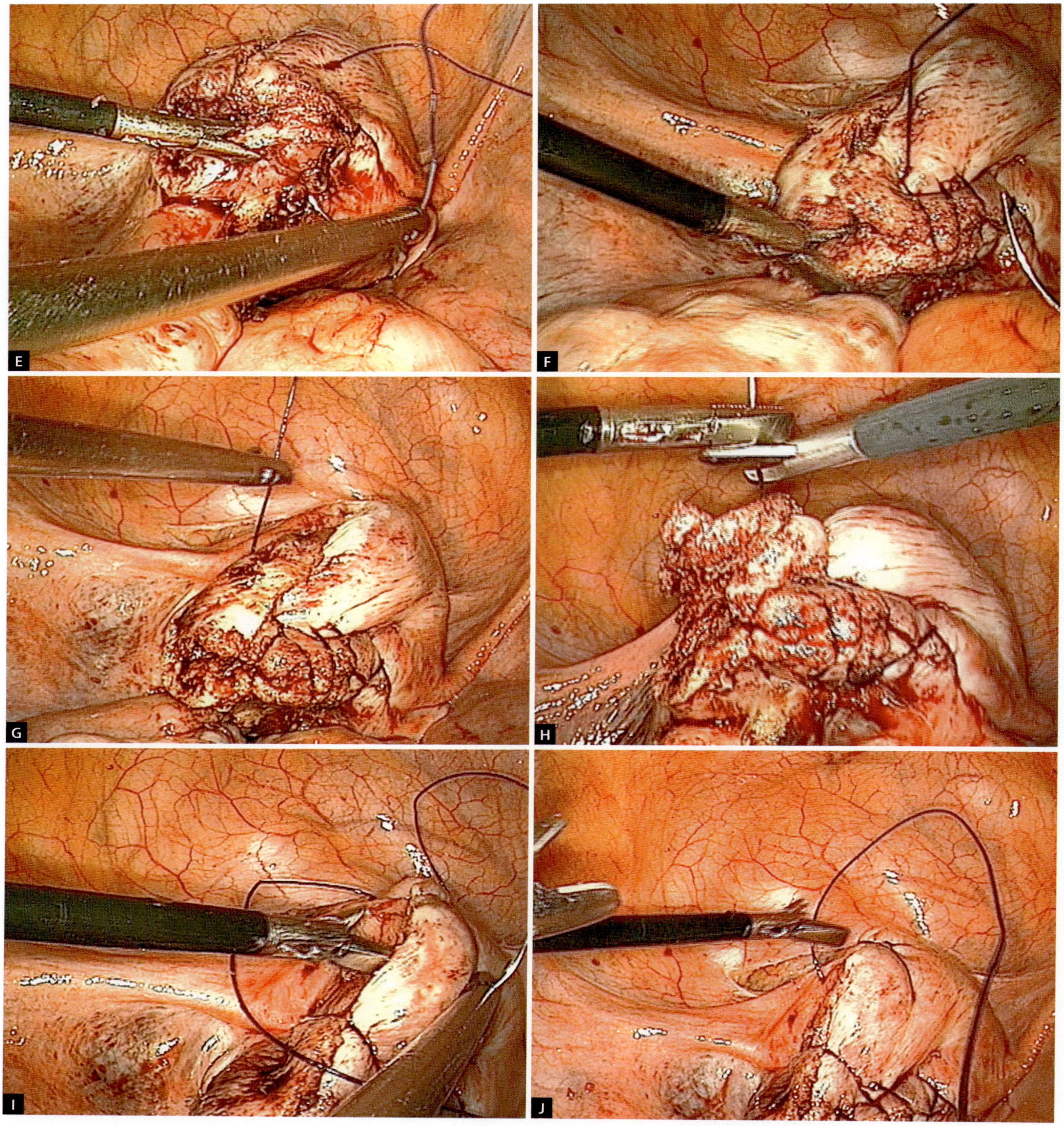

Figs. 9E to J: Suturing of second layer with barbed suture (continued).

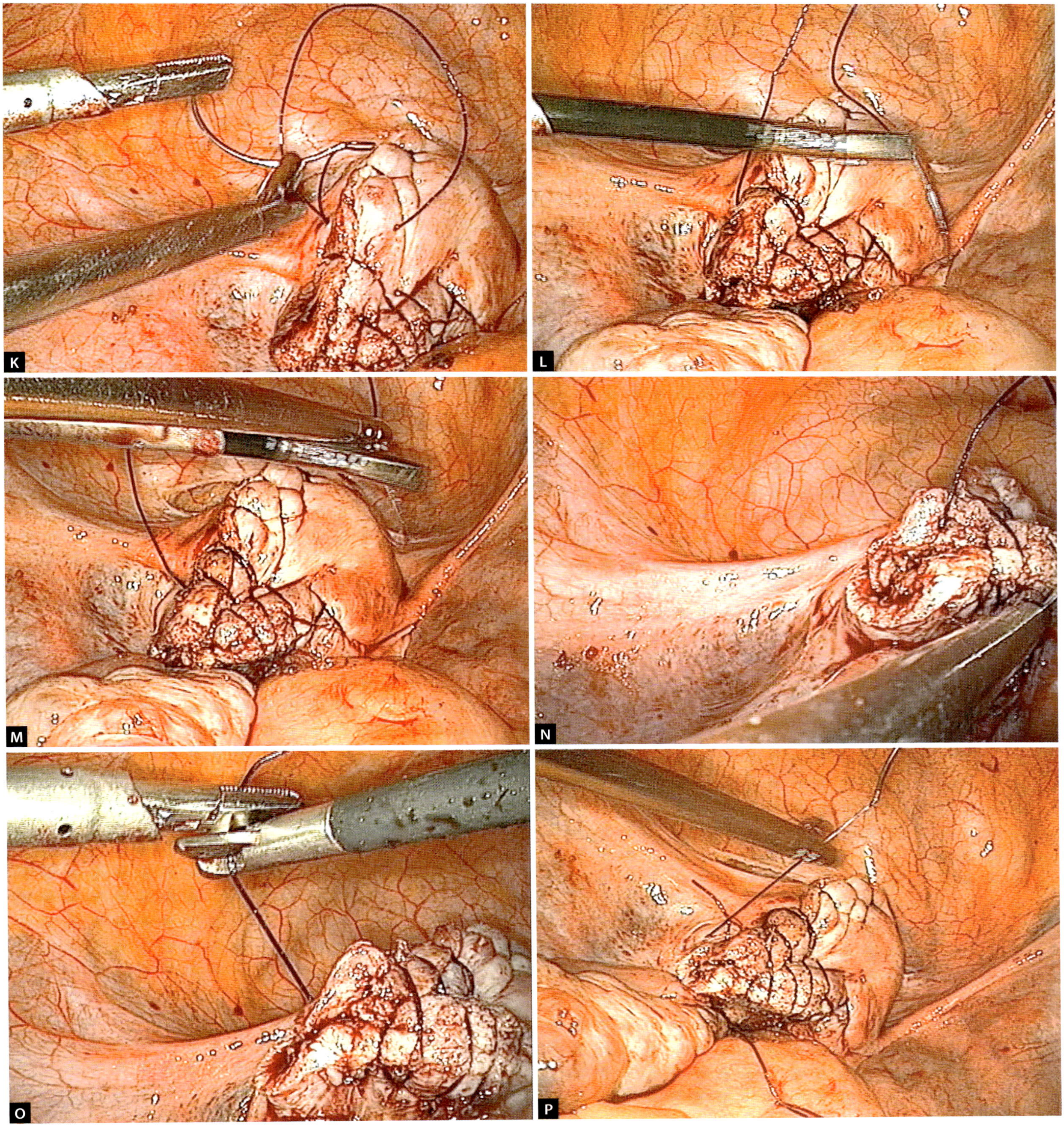

Figs. 9K to P: (K and L) Suturing of second layer with barbed suture (continued); (M to P) Suturing of final layer with barbed suture.

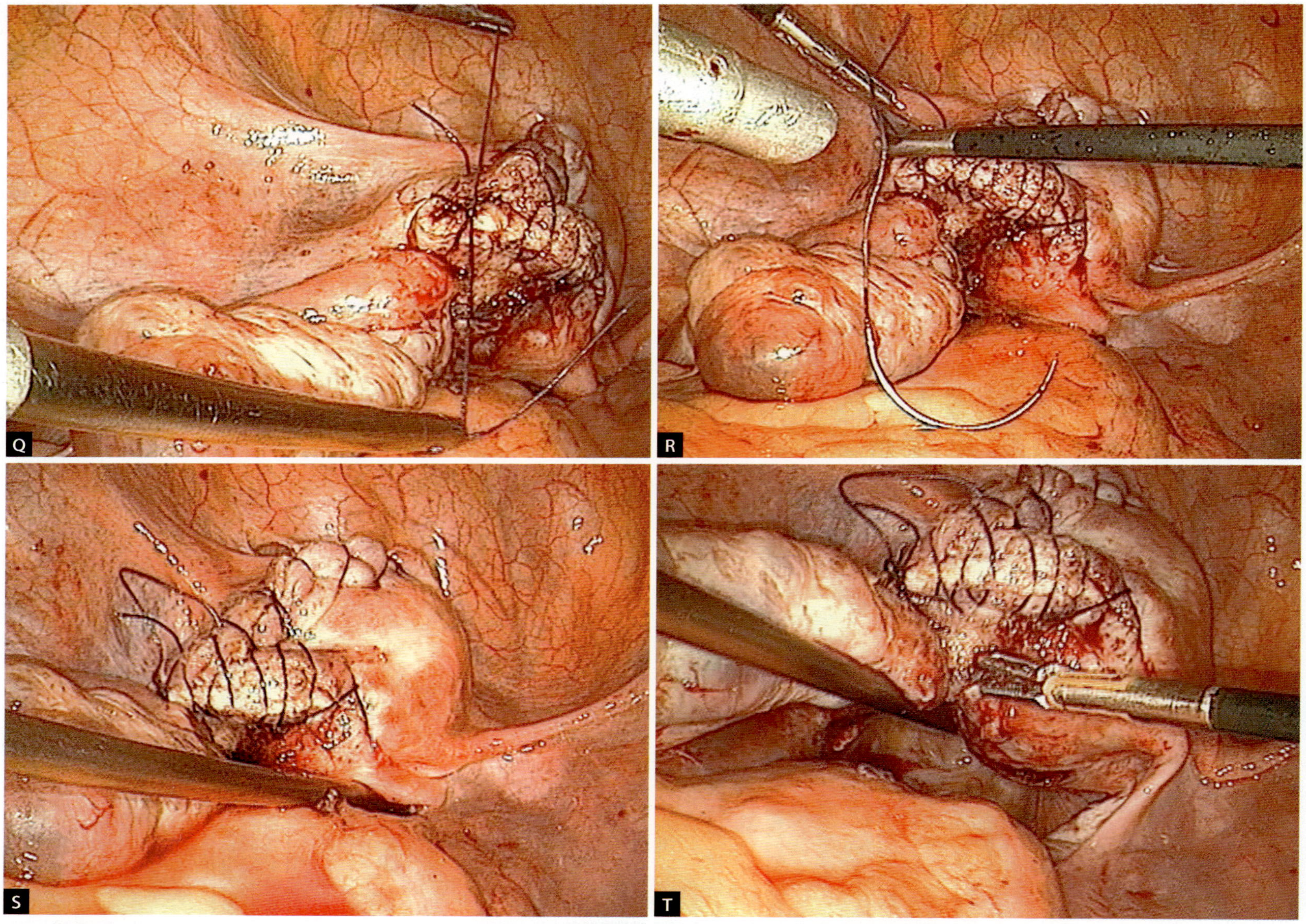

Figs. 9Q to T: (Q) Tying the knot; (R) Suture being cut with hooked scissors; (S) Appearance of the uterus after suturing; (T) Achieving hemostasis.

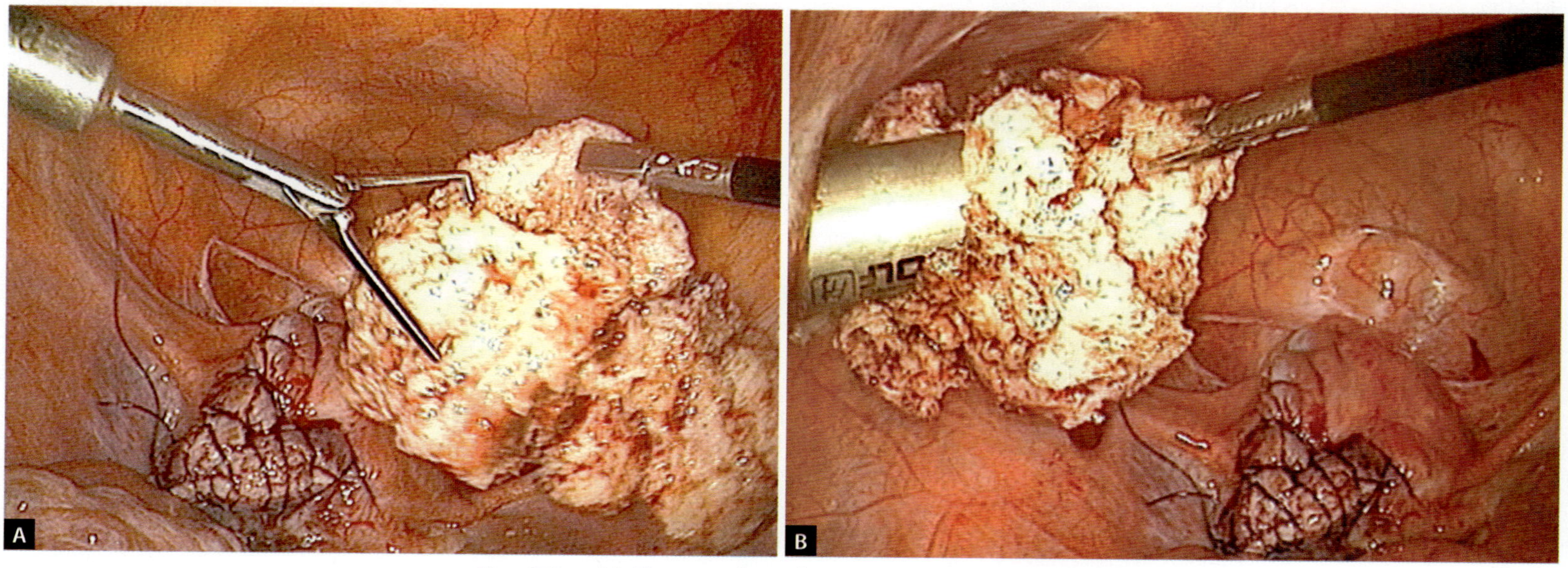

Figs. 10A and B: Electromechanical morcellation of adenomyoma.

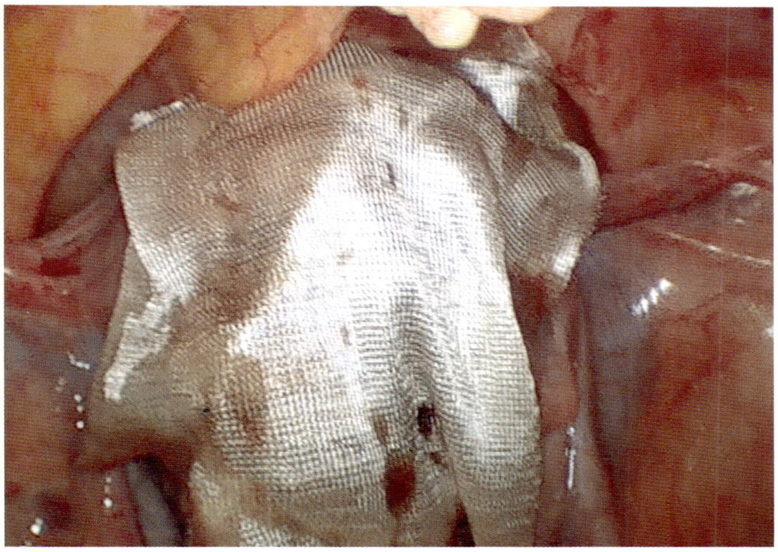

Fig. 10C: Interceed placement.

in laparoscopic suturing. If there is deeper defect, the closure has to be in layers obliterating the dead space with layer-by-layer suturing. There should be fine approximation for the last layer without eversion of the margins. Good hemostasis is the key. Interceed or any anti-adhesive barrier should be placed on the top of the wound to prevent adhesions.

Comparison in Surgical Technique between Adenomyoma and Fibroid

When compared to excision of leiomyoma **(Figs. 11A to N)**, adenomyomectomy poses more difficult as adenomyosis is more of an infiltrative process Due to absence of a definite cleavage plane, excision of adenomyomatous from healthy tissue will be difficult. Suturing of the adenomyoma bed is also more challenging when compared to a fibroid.

While removing adenomyoma, part of the myometrium is removed resulting in a defect, which is difficult to be sutured.

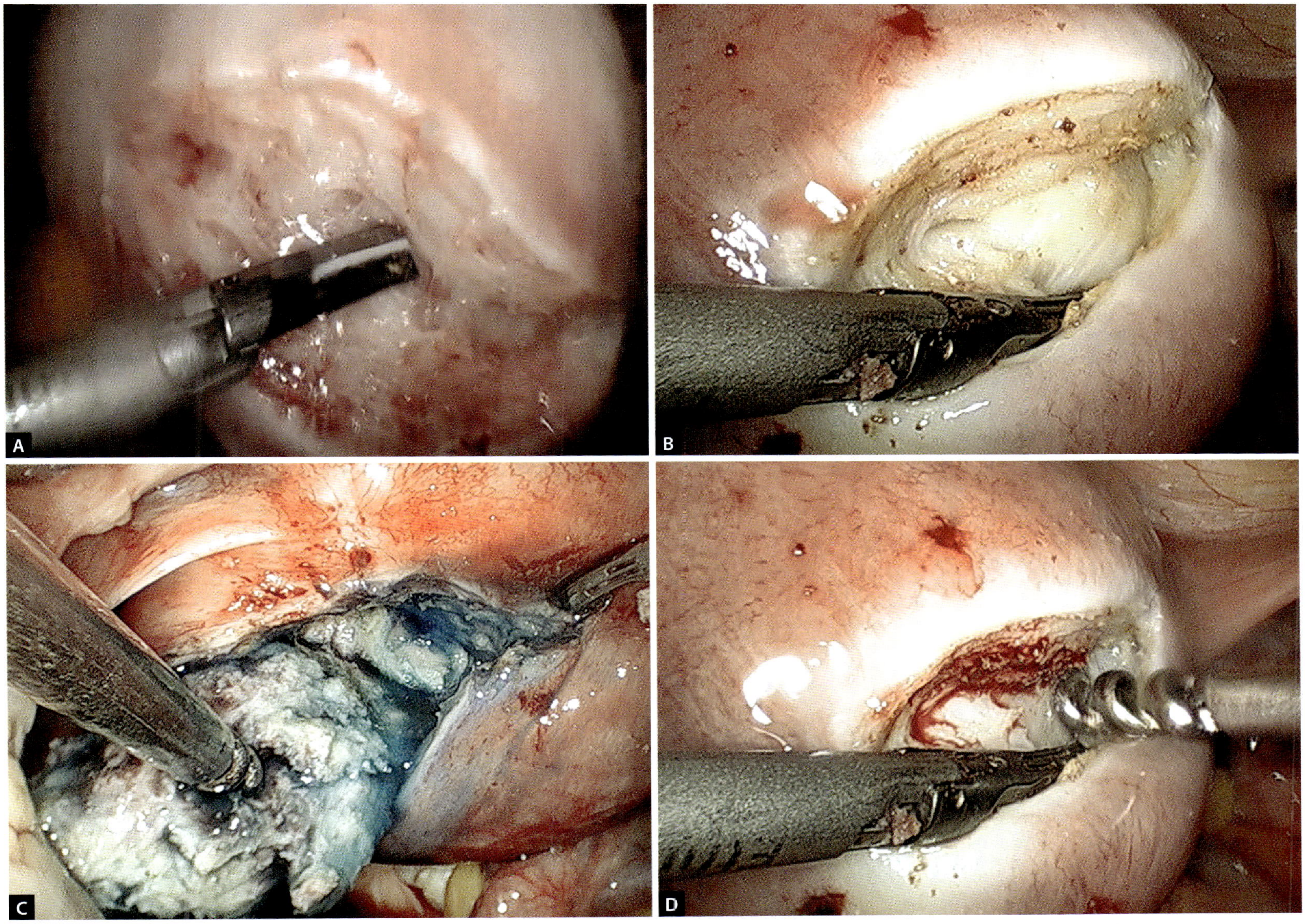

Figs. 11A to D: (A) Ragged incision of adenomyoma; (B) Clean-cut incision of myoma; (C) Difficult dissection (adenomyoma); (D) Easier dissection (myoma).

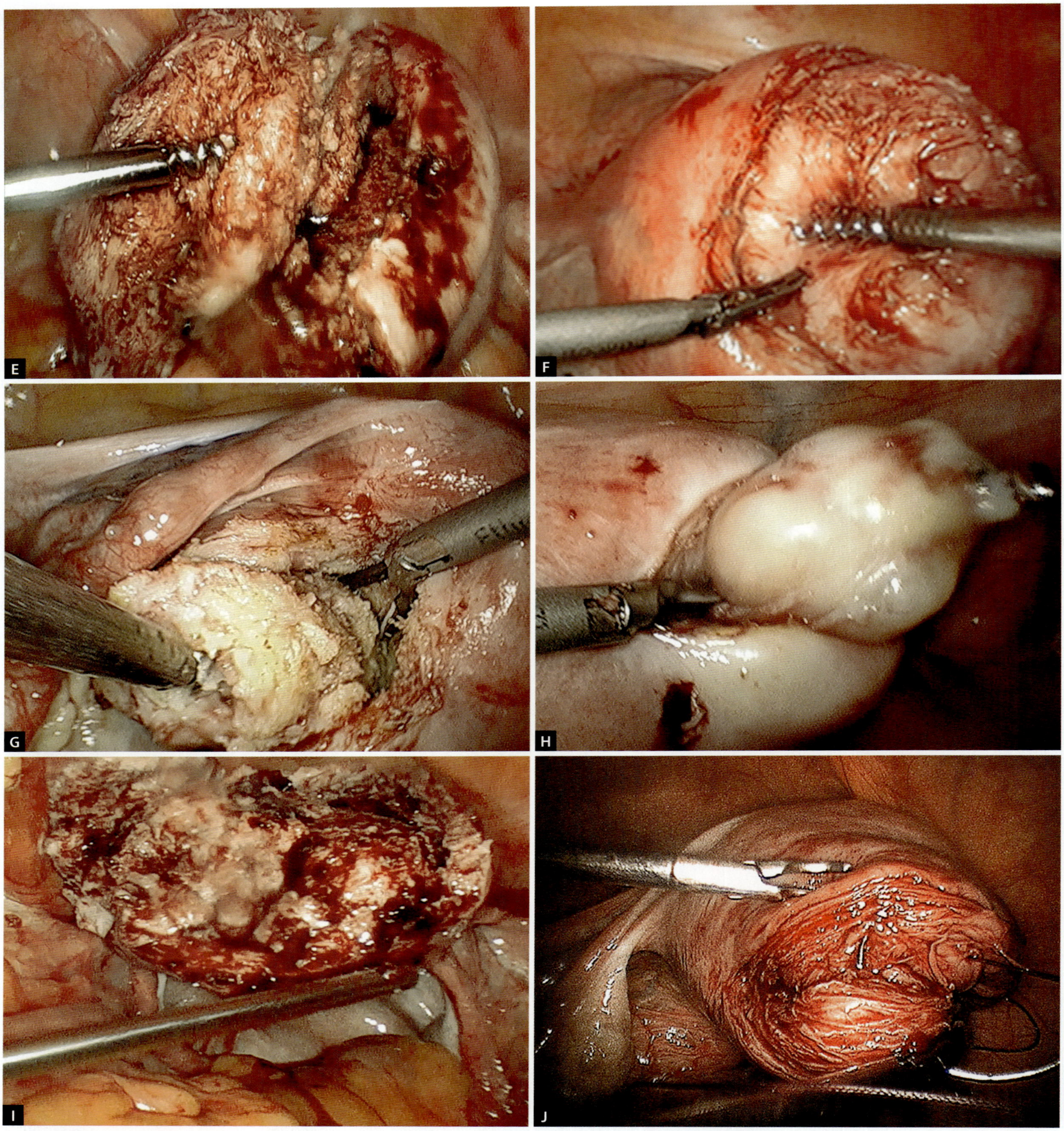

Figs. 11E to J: (E) Inconspicuous cleavage plane of adenomyoma; (F) Clear cleavage plane of myoma; (G) Pinkish white (adenomyoma); (H) Pearly white (myoma); (I) Irregular bed of adenomyoma; (J) Smooth bed of myoma.

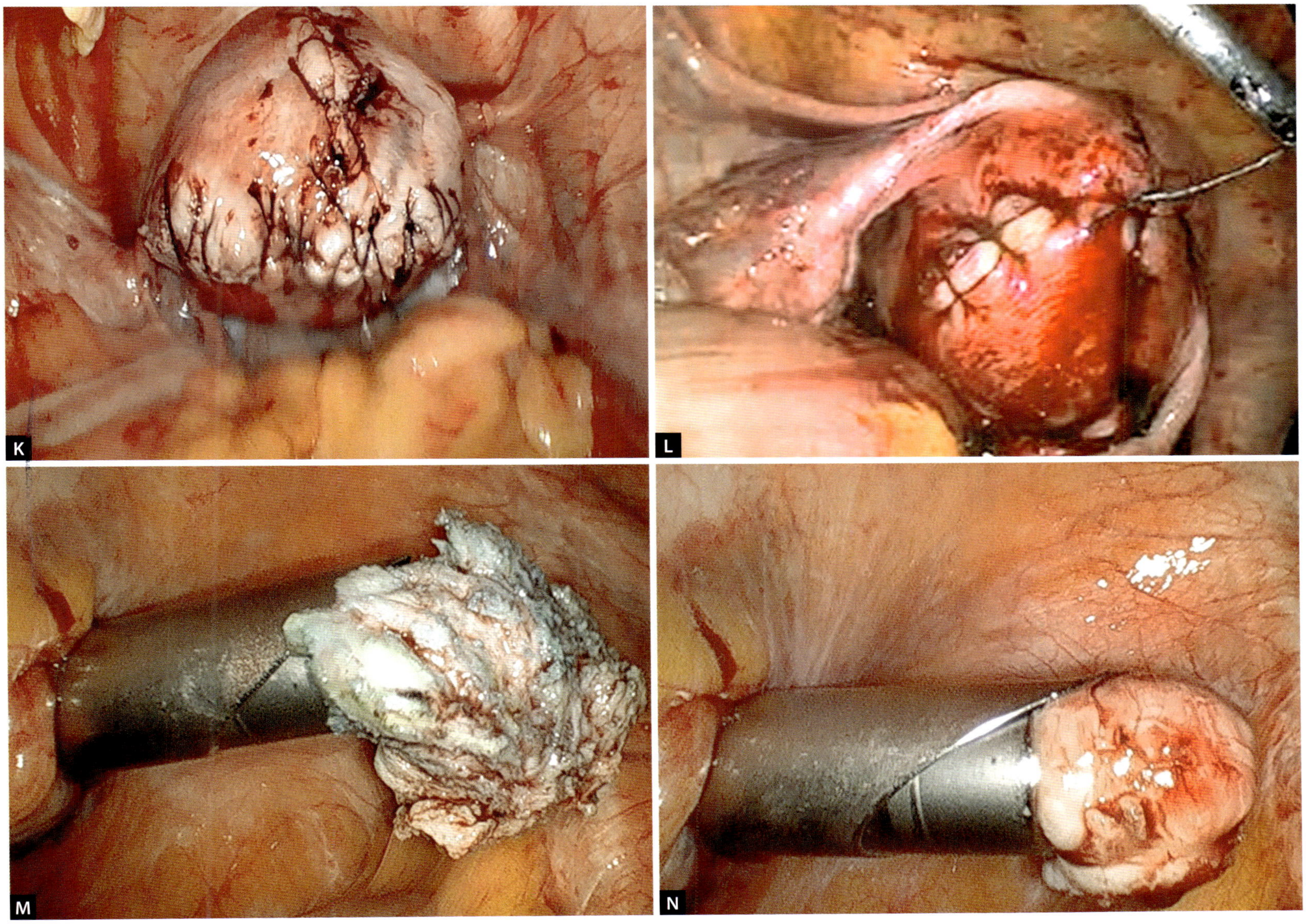

Figs. 11K to N: (K) Sutured edges in adenomyoma; (L) Even edges of myoma; (M) Difficult morcellation; (N) Easier morcellation.

Also, the possibility of tissues being cut through is more. During morcellation, process continuity is disturbed by the consistency of the adenomyoma.

However, other techniques described in literature are explained here:

Classic Technique (Figs. 12A to D)

This technique involves—(1) recognition of the lesion, (2) longitudinal incision given over adenomyoma, (3) sharp and blunt dissection of the lesion with scissors, graspers, (4) suturing of the uterine wall in a seromuscular layer or in two or more layers and suturing of the endometrial cavity with absorbable suture when necessary followed by specimen retrieval with morcellator.

Double-flap Technique (Figs. 13A to D)

An incision was made on the fundus and continued along the posterior and anterior walls of the uterus to the level of the internal os of the cervix by midline serosal incision by using scissors, monopolar or harmonic. Incision is continued until the uterine cavity was reached. Afterward, avoid damaging the endometrium and the serosal surface of the uterus, adenomyomatous tissues were excised from the surrounding myometrium and, if the myometrium appeared normal, this part was spared as much as possible. The myometrium and serosa of the bisected uterus were sutured with 2-0 Vicryl.

Modification in Wall Reconstruction (Figs. 14A to D)

- *U-shaped suturing:* The wound is approximated by U-shaped sutures at the muscle layer and seromuscular layer is closed by figure-eight sutures after removal of adenomyomatous tissue.[26]
- *Overlapping flaps*: In this laparoscopic modification, with the help of monopolar needle, transverse incision is made in the adenomyotic tissue.[27,28]

Transverse H Incision Technique[29]

Transverse incisions are given along the upper and lower edges of the uterus (H incision) and vertical incision is made over the uterine wall. The uterine serosa is opened and adenomyotic tissue is excised followed by suturing in multiple layers.

Wedge Resection of the Uterine Wall (Figs. 15A to F)

In this technique (laparoscopic), adenomyoma, which is the part of seromuscular layer, is removed by wedge resection of the uterine wall. Closure of the uterine wounds is same as described in the classic technique of partial adenomyomectomy.[30]

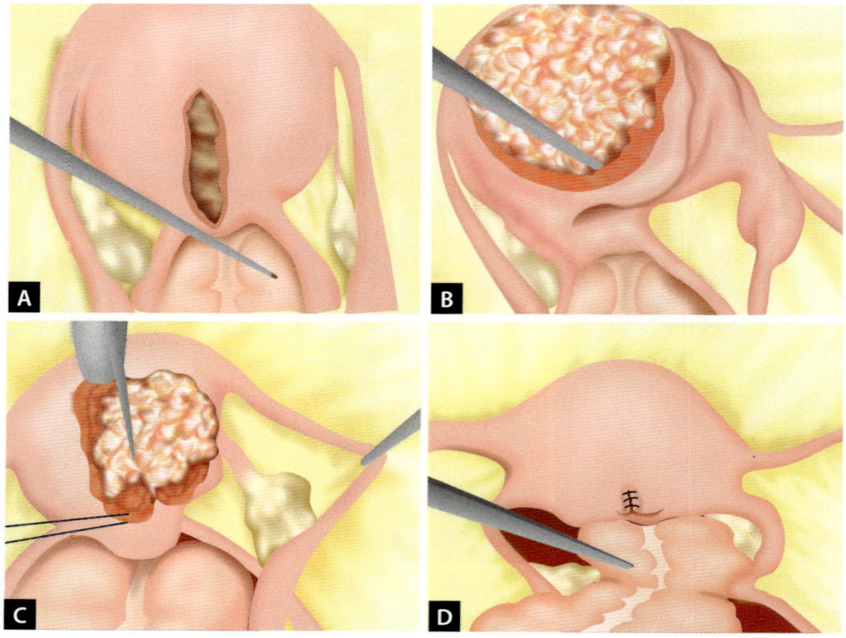

Figs. 12A to D: Classic technique of adenomyomectomy.

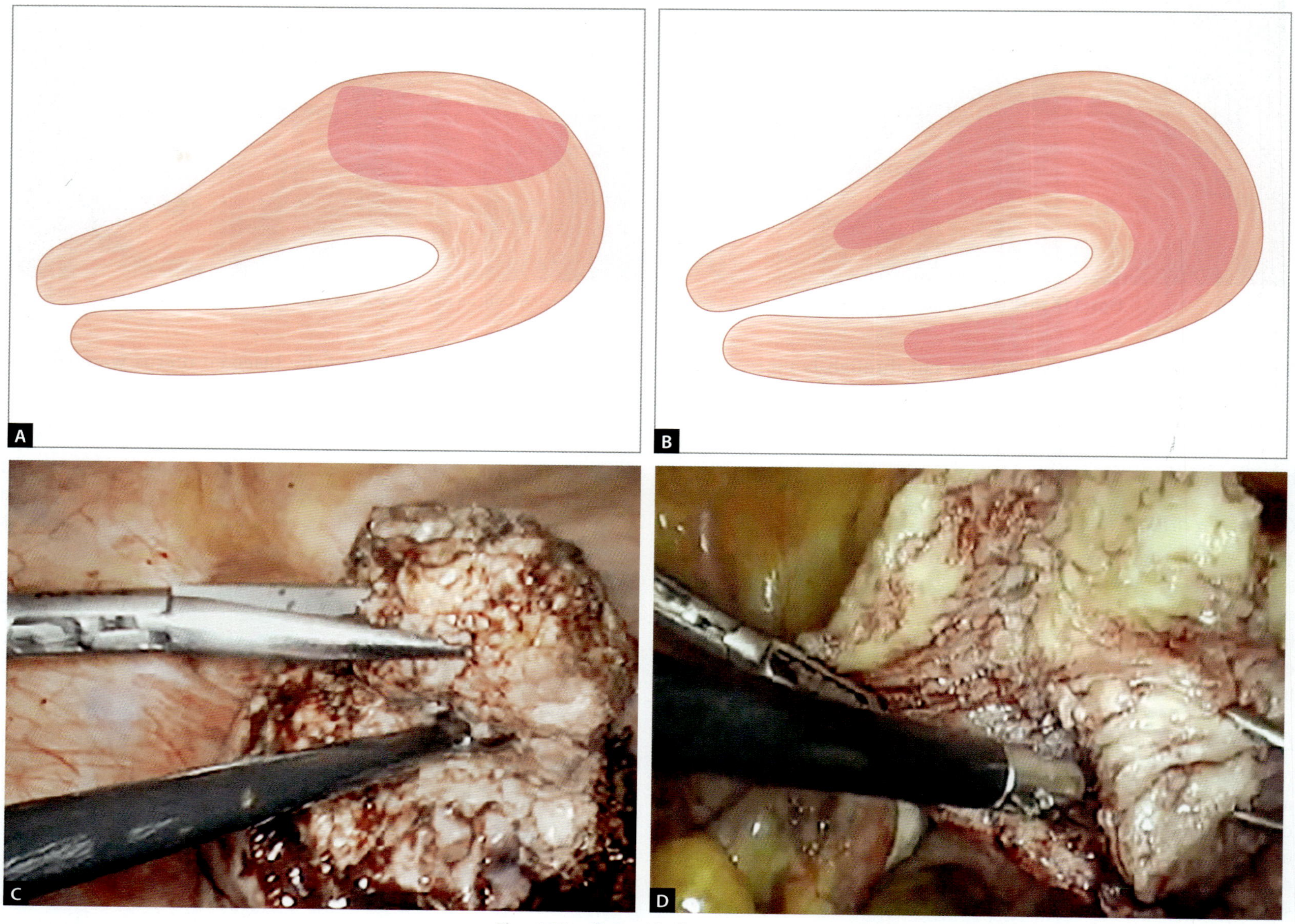

Figs. 13A to D: Double-flap technique.

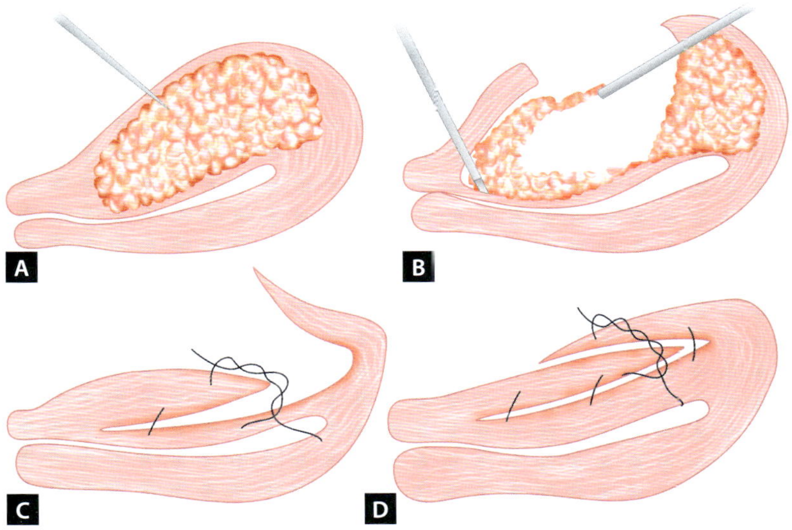

Figs. 14A to D: Overlapping flap technique.

Triple-flap Method (Figs. 16A to F)

This method as described by Osada et al. involves:

- Extraperitonealization of the uterus and rubber tourniquet placement at the level of lower segment for hemostasis.
- Bisection of the uterus in the sagittal plane (midline) until the uterine cavity is reached.
- Opening of the endometrial cavity to permit the introduction of the index finger to guide during excision of adenomyotic tissues.
- Grasp adenomyotic tissues with the help of Martin forceps, and to excise the adenomyoma from the surrounding myometrium, leaving a myometrial thickness of 1 cm from serosa above and endometrium below.
- Endometrium is closed with the help of 3-0 Vicryl suture material.
- Myometrium and serosa is approximated by flaps of the uterine wall which is in the anteroposterior plane with 2-0 Vicryl and cover the reconstructed first side by the contralateral side of the uterine wall.[31]

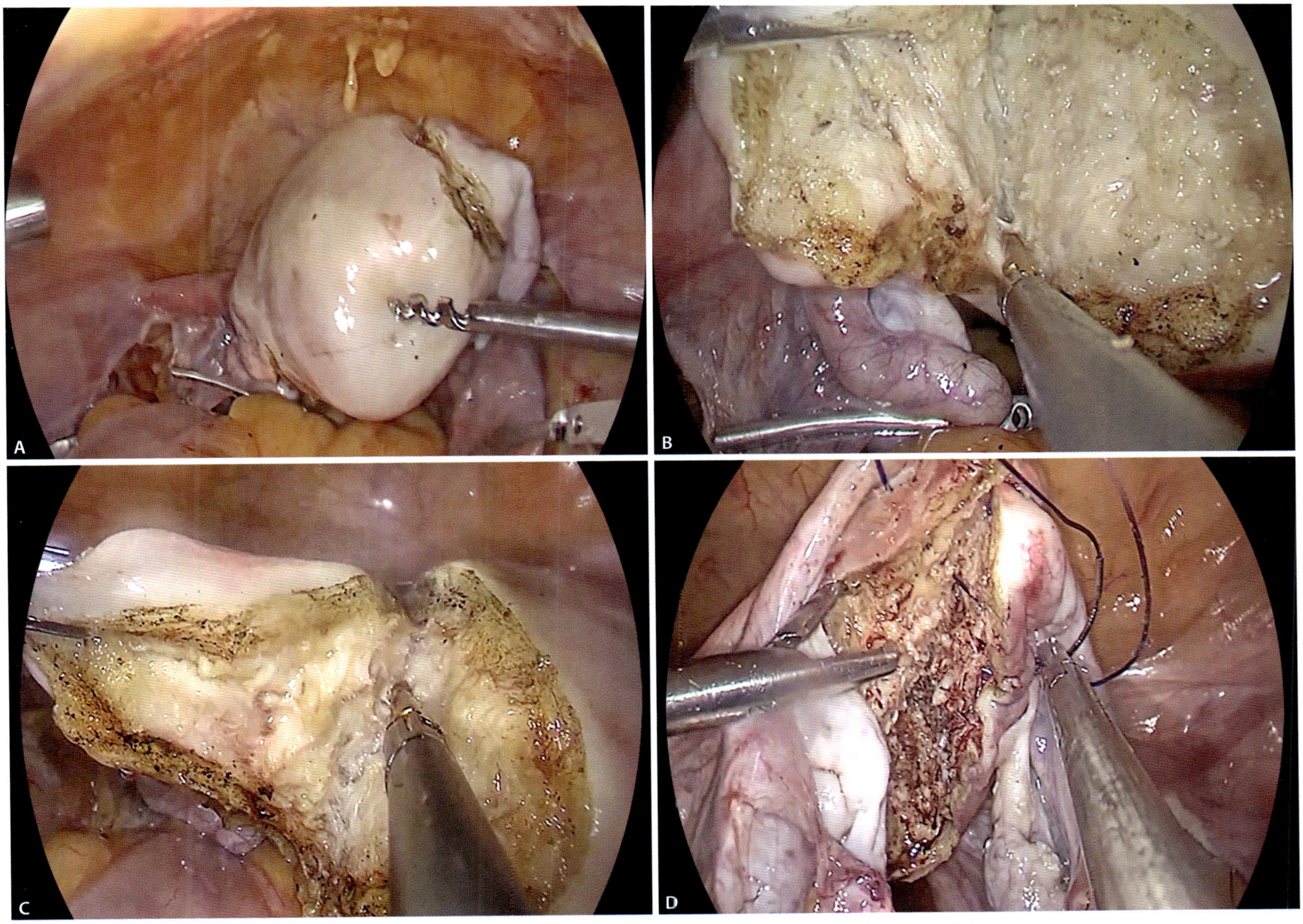

Figs. 15A to D: (A) Fixing the adenomyoma; (B) Separation of adenomyotic from normal tissues; (C) Wedge resection; (D) Suturing of adenomyoma bed.

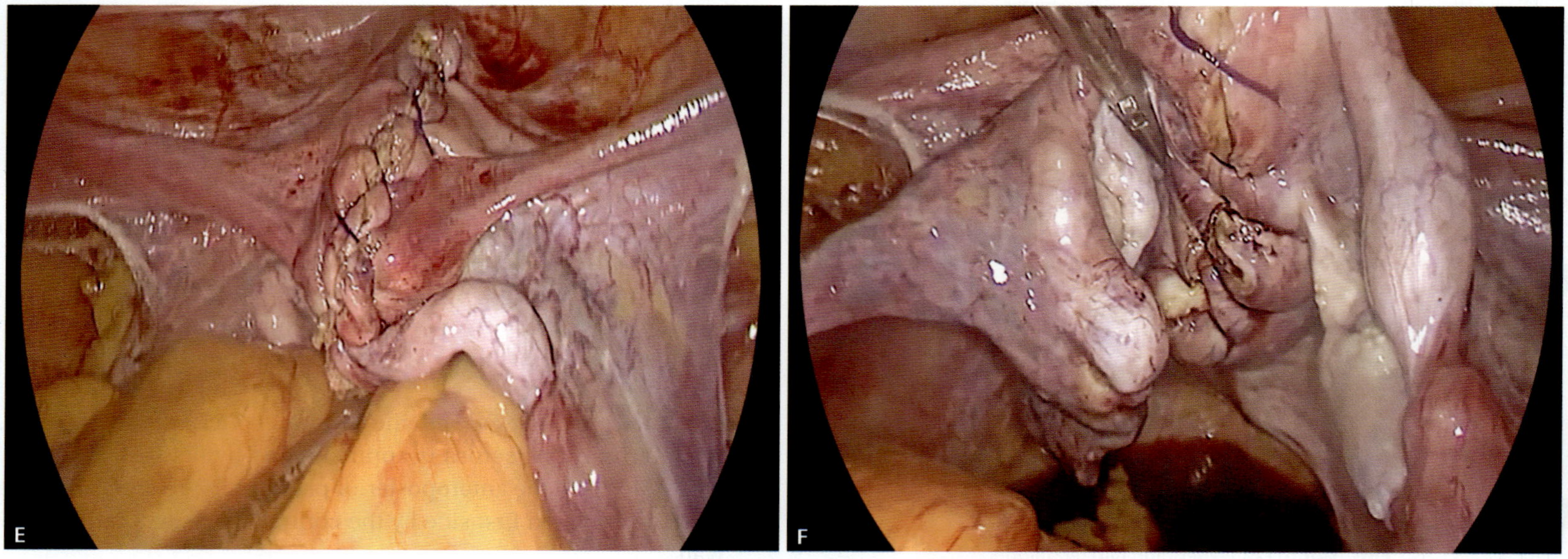

Figs. 15E and F: Suturing of adenomyoma bed (continued).

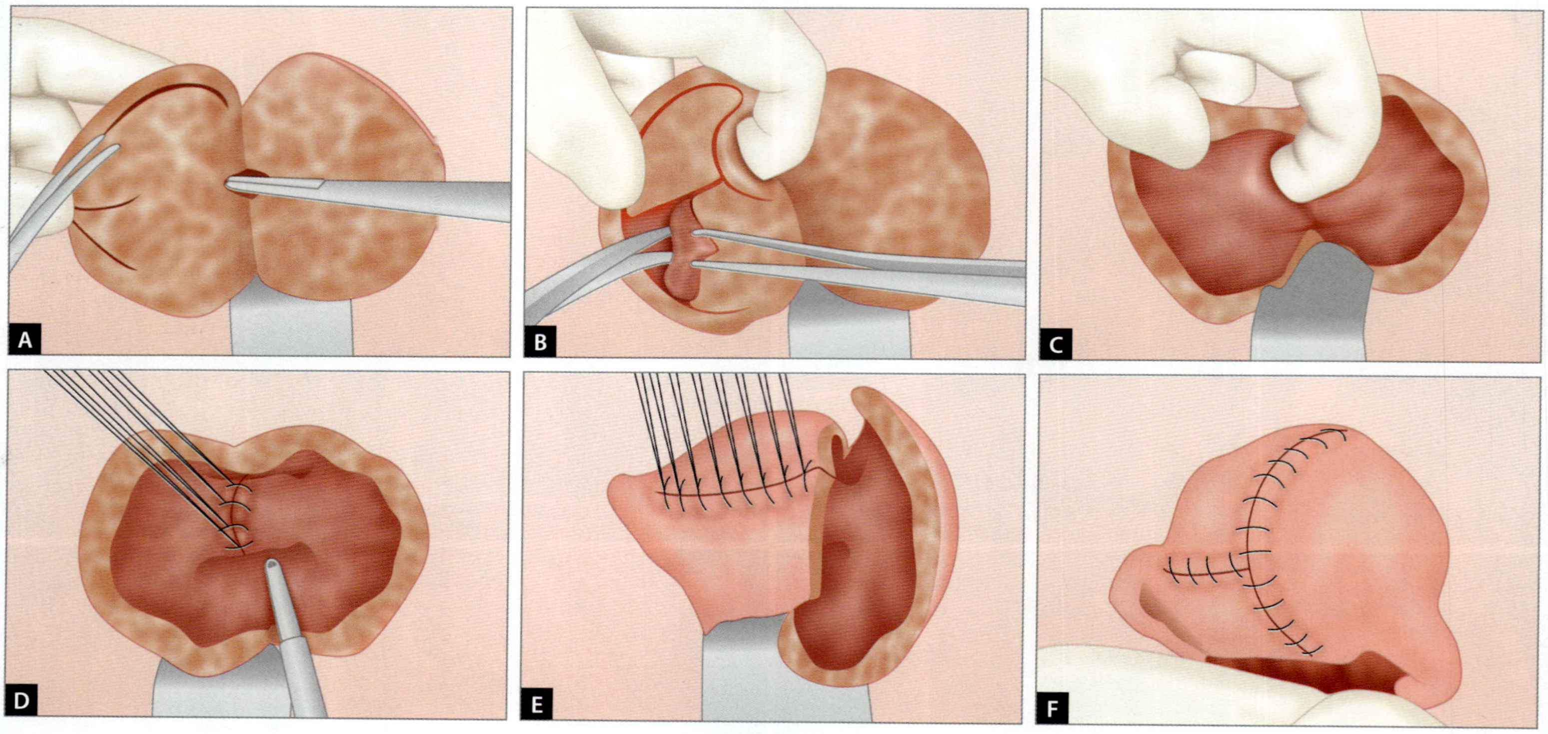

Figs. 16A to F: Osada technique.

Complications of Laparoscopic Adenomyomectomy (Box 1)

The success of laparoscopic adenomyomectomy included: (i) a 30% chances of successful pregnancy rate, (ii) reduction of heavy bleeding pattern by 65%, and (iii) a decrease in dysmenorrhea symptoms by 41%.[32]

The main complications that can occur in a laparoscopic adenomyomectomy are:

- Intraoperative and immediate postoperative
  - Hemorrhage and hematoma formation
  - Hysterectomy (very rare)
  - Morcellator injury
  - Conversion to laparotomy
  - Minor complications like pyrexia, abdominal pain, vaginitis, metrorrhagia, dysuria, etc.
  - Adhesions
- Late
  - Scar dehiscence during pregnancy
  - Recurrence
- Other complications like shoulder pain, subcutaneous emphysema, atelectasis, gas embolism, pneumothorax, rarely diaphragmatic rupture can also occur.

Pregnancy rates following adenomyomectomy were around 60%.[31] Morimatsu et al.[33] showed that the rate of uterine rupture is higher

Box 1: Complications of laparoscopic adenomyomectomy.

- Hemorrhages requiring blood transfusion
- Postoperative hematomas
- Bowel injury
- Failure to complete planned surgery/conversion to hysterectomy
- Spontaneous uterine rupture during pregnancy
- Recurrence.

after adenomyomectomy than the entire rate of uterine rupture during pregnancy, i.e., 6.0% and 0.035%, respectively.[34] Complications are more after myomectomy than cesarean section, i.e., (2.45%)[35,36] and (0.27–0.7%),[37,38] respectively.

Intervention to conception time: Most of the studies advised planning for pregnancy after 3 months of adenomyomectomy. Elective cesarean section after 37 weeks is recommended to prevent the risk of rupture uterus.

Postoperative Care

Close monitoring of vitals, along with strict vigil on input and urine output is recommended in the immediate postoperative period. Adequate analgesia should be administered. Parenteral antibiotics are administered 24–48 hours following surgery. Graded compression stockings and low molecular weight heparin are administered in patients prone to deep vein thrombosis (DVT). Patients are initially allowed clear liquids, once bowel sounds resume. If tolerated, the diet is advanced to "soft diet" for 2–3 days, followed by regular diet with ample intake of fluids. Medications taken preoperatively (stopped temporarily) are usually resumed once patient crosses the immediate postoperative period. Although minimally invasive, adenomyomectomy is considered a major surgery and patients are observed for at least 24 hours postoperatively. Once patient voids without discomfort, tolerates a regular diet and ambulates wall, she can be discharged. Postoperatively, patient is advised contraception for 3 months in the form of oral contraceptive pills or hormonal intrauterine device (IUD). Gonadotropin releasing hormone (GnRH) analogs are also advised if concomitant endometriosis is present.

REFERENCES

1. Vercellini P, Parazzini F, Oldani S, et al. Adenomyosis at hysterectomy: a study on frequency distribution and patient characteristics. Hum Reprod. 1995;10:1160-2.
2. Parazzini F, Vercellini P, Panazza S, et al. Risk factors for adenomyosis. Hum Reprod. 1997;12:1275-9.
3. Vercellini P, Cortesi I, De Giorgi O, et al. Transvaginal ultrasonography versus uterine needle biopsy in the diagnosis of diffuse adenomyosis. Hum Reprod. 1998;13:2884-7.
4. Bergholt T, Eriksen L, Berendt N, et al. Prevalence and risk factors of adenomyosis at hysterectomy. Hum Reprod. 2001;16:2418-21.
5. McCausland V, McCausland A. The response of adenomyosis to endometrial ablation/resection. Hum Reprod Update. 1998;4:350-9.
6. Farquhar C, Brosens I. Medical and surgical management of adenomyosis. Best Pract Res Clin Obstet Gynaecol. 2006;20:603-16.
7. Azziz R. Adenomyosis: current perspectives. Obstet Gynecol Clin North Am. 1989;16:221-35.
8. Benson RC, Sneeden VD. Adenomyosis: a reappraisal of symptomatology. Am J Obstet Gynecol. 1958;76:1044-57.
9. Ferenczy A, Bronsen I. Pathophysiology of adenomyosis. Hum Reprod Update. 1998;4:312-22.
10. Bergeron C, Amant F, Ferency A. Pathology and physiology of adenomyosis. Best Pract Res Clin Obstet Gynaecol. 2006;20:511-21.
11. Bird C, McElin T, Manalo-Estrella P. The elusive adenomyosis of the uterus revisited. Am J Obstet Gynecol. 1972;112:583-93.
12. Garcia L, Isaacson K. Adenomyosis: review of the literature. J Minim Invasive Gynecol. 2011;18:428-37.
13. Nishida M. Relationship between the onset of dysmenorrhea and histologic findings in adenomyosis. Am J Obstet Gynecol. 1991;165:229-31.
14. Kunz G, Leyendecker G. Uterine peristaltic activity during the menstrual cycle: characterization, regulation, function and dysfunction. Reprod Biomed Online. 2002;4 Suppl 3:5-9.
15. Tamai K, Koyama T, Umeoka S, et al. Spectrum of MR features in adenomyosis. Best Pract Res Clin Obstet Gynaecol. 2006;20(4):583-602.
16. Gordts S, Brosens JJ, Fusi L, et al. Uterine adenomyosis: a need for uniform terminology and consensus classification. Reprod Biomed Online. 2008;17(2):244-8.
17. Dueholm M. Transvaginal ultrasound for diagnosis of adenomyosis: a review. Best Pract Res Clin Obstet Gynaecol. 2006;20:569-82.
18. Bazot M, Cortez A, Darai E, et al. Ultrasonography compared with magnetic resonance imaging for the diagnosis of adenomyosis: correlation with histopathology. Hum Reprod. 2001;16:2427-33.
19. Reinhold C, Tafazoli F, Wang L. Imaging features of adenomyosis. Hum Reprod Update. 1998;4:337-49.
20. Bromley B, Shipp TD, Benacerraf B. Adenomyosis: sonographic findings and diagnostic accuracy. J Ultrasound Med. 2000;19:529-34.
21. Kepkep K, Tuncay YA, Goynumer G, et al. Transvaginal sonography in the diagnosis of adenomyosis: which findings are most accurate? Ultrasound Gynecol Obstet. 2007;30:341-5.
22. Van den Bosch T, Dueholm M, Leone FP. Terms, definitions and measurements to describe sonographic features of myometrium and uterine masses: a consensus opinion from the Morphological Uterus Sonographic Assessment (MUSA) group. Ultrasound Obstet Gynecol. 2015;6:284-98.
23. Grimbizis GF, Mikos T, Tarlatzis B. Uterus-sparing operative treatment for adenomyosis. Fertil Steril. 2014;101(2):472-87.
24. Grimbizis GF, Mikos T, Zepiridis L, et al. Laparoscopic excision of uterine adenomyomas. Fertil Steril. 2008;89:953-61.
25. Morita M, Asakawa Y, Nakakuma M, et al. Laparoscopic excision of myometrial adenomyomas in patients with adenomyosis uteri and main symptoms of severe dysmenorrhea and hypermenorrhea. J Am Assoc Gynecol Laparosc. 2004;11:86-9.
26. Sun AJ, Luo M, Wang W, et al. Characteristics and efficacy of modified adenomyomectomy in the treatment of uterine adenomyoma. Chin Med J (Engl). 2011;124:1322-6.
27. Hyams LL. Adenomyosis, its conservative surgical treatment (hysteroplasty) in young women. NY State J Med. 1952;52:2778-84.
28. Wang PH, Fuh JL, Chao HT, et al. Is the surgical approach beneficial to subfertile women with symptomatic extensive adenomyosis? J Obstet Gynaecol Res. 2009;35:495-502.
29. Takeuchi H, Kitade M, Kikuchi I, et al. Laparoscopic adenomyomectomy and hysteroplasty: a novel method. J Minim Invasive Gynecol. 2006;13:150-4.
30. Fujishita A, Masuzaki H, Khan KN, et al. Modified reduction surgery for adenomyosis: a preliminary report of the transverse H incision technique. Gynecol Obstet Invest. 2004;57:132-8.
31. Osada H, Silber S, Kakinuma T, et al. Surgical procedure to conserve the uterus for future pregnancy in patients suffering from massive adenomyosis. Reprod Biomed Online. 2011;22:94-9.
32. Saremi A, Bahrami H, Salehian P, et al. Treatment of adenomyomectomy in women with severe uterine adenomyosis using a novel technique. Reprod Biomed Online. 2014;28(6):753-60.
33. Morimatsu Y, Matsubara S, Okuchi A, et al. Shikyūsenkinshōkakushutsujutsu go no ninshin – Shikyūharetsu no literature review to sankakanrinitsuite – [Pregnancy after adenomyomectomy – literature review of uterine rupture and obstetrical management –] Sanka to fujinka [Japanese Journal of Obstetrics and Gynaecology]. 2007;74(9):1047-53. Japanese.
34. Kim MS, Uhm YK, Kim JY, et al. Obstetric outcomes after uterine myomectomy: laparoscopic versus laparotomic approach. Obstet Gynecol Sci. 2013;56(6):375-81
35. Tian YC, Long TF, Dai YM. Pregnancy outcomes following different surgical approaches of myomectomy. J Obstet Gynaecol Res. 2015;41(3):350-7.
36. Guise JM, McDonagh MS, Osterweil P, et al. Systematic review of the incidence and consequences of uterine rupture in women with previous caesarean section. BMJ. 2004;329(7456):19-25.
37. Ofir K, Sheiner E, Levy A, et al. Uterine rupture: risk factors and pregnancy outcome. Am J Obstet Gynecol. 2003;189(4):1042-6.
38. Landon MB, Hauth JC, Leveno KJ, et al. Maternal and perinatal outcomes associated with a trial of labor after prior cesarean delivery. N Engl J Med. 2004;351(25):2581-9.

Accompanying Video: Laparoscopic adenomyomectomy.

CHAPTER

26

Laparoscopic Unification of Bicornuate Uterus

Dhivya B, Aditi Rai, B Ramesh

INTRODUCTION

Incidence of Müllerian duct anomalies in about 4.3% and 13% in patient with recurrent pregnancy loss.[1] The mean incidence of bicornuate uterus in Müllerian duct anomalies is approximately 25%, and it is associated with abortion, preterm delivery and term delivery rates of 36%, 23%, and 40.6%, respectively.[2] Patient with bicornuate uterus, conventional transabdominal unification surgery has shown significant improvement in pregnancy outcomes.[3] In January 2006, laparoscopic unification of bicornuate uterus was reported for the first time in one patient with a successful outcome.[4]

SURGICAL ANATOMY (FIG. 1)

The uterus is formed by two paramesonephric ducts (Müllerian ducts). The cranial part of fusion of Müllerian duct form fundus and caudal two-thirds of the ducts form the uterus, whereas the upper lateral part of the Müllerian duct forms fallopian tubes. *At 6–9 weeks of gestation*: In Müllerian duct, caudal vertical part fused as a single solid rod of cells and further extend caudally until they make contact with the urogenital sinus. So, uterine aplasia occurs due to failure of development of the Müllerian ducts. *At 10–13 weeks of gestation*: Lateral fusion of paired Müllerian duct takes place. Any failure of lateral fusion of Müllerian ducts during this period of time leads to uterine duplications (uterus didelphys, bicornuate uterus). *At 14–18 weeks of gestation:* The uterovaginal channel is formed which is the origin of the uterine cavity and the superior two-thirds of the vagina, which is formed by resorption of the medial septum which separates the caudal parts of the Müllerian ducts. Failure of resorption of the midline septum after complete fusion of Müllerian duct leads to uterine septation (septate uterus) **(Fig. 2 and Table 1)**.

LAPAROSCOPIC UNIFICATION

Despite controversy about the role of corrective surgery, there is good evidence that live birth rates following unification of bicornuate uterus improved up to 80%.[5-8] However, complication of abdominal surgery for unification is such as adhesion (intrauterine or extra-uterine), uterine perforation, intraoperative bleeding, cervical incompetence, adherent placenta, postpartum hemorrhage, infection, and possible uterine rupture in subsequent pregnancies.[9] In January 2006, laparoscopic unification of bicornuate uterus was reported for the first time in one patient with a successful outcome.[10,11]

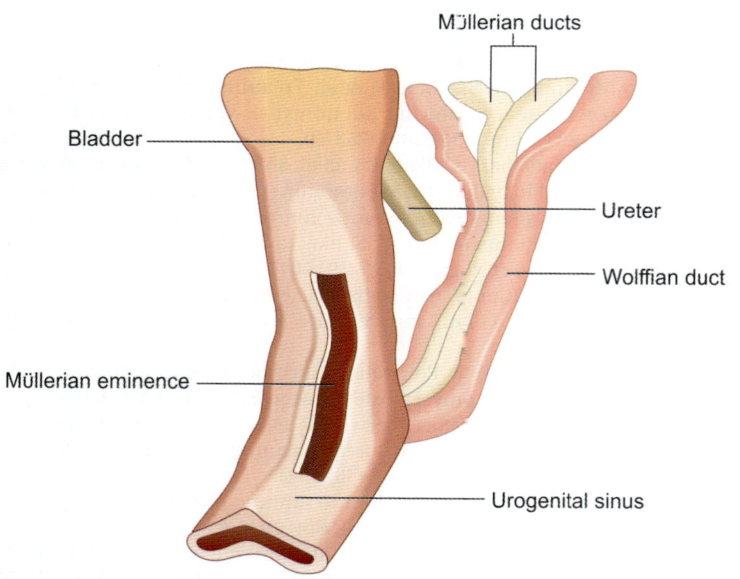

Fig. 1: Urogenital sinus of female human embryo of eight and a half to 9 weeks old (from model by Keibel).

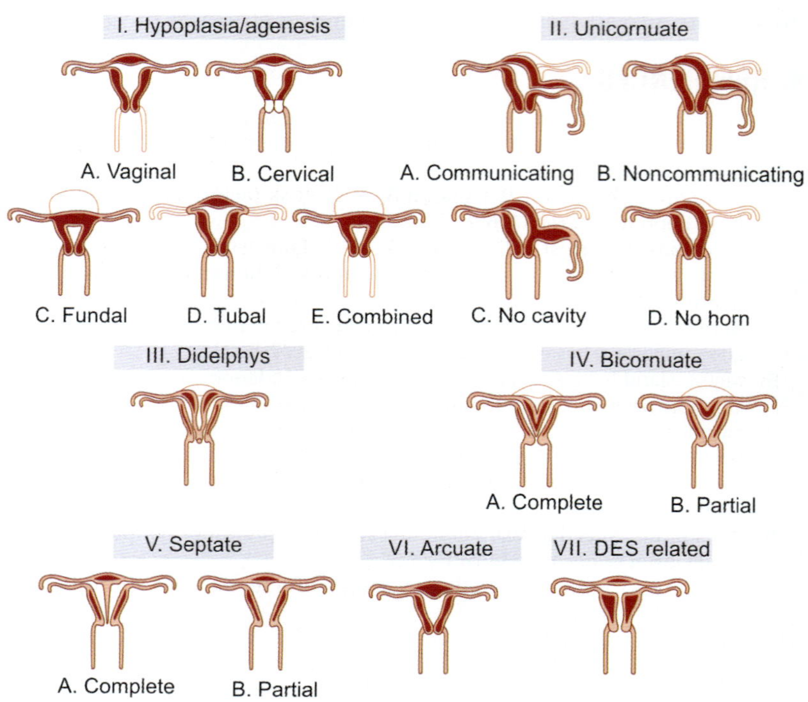

Fig. 2: ESHRE/ESGE: Classification of uterine anomalies.

Table 1: Features of bicornuate uterus.

Investigation	*Finding*	
Per speculum	Single cervix ± septa	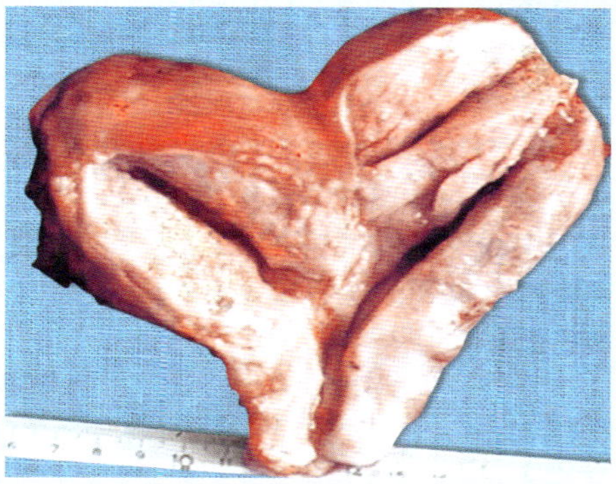
Hysterosalpingogram	Separate uterine cavities with intercornual angle >105°	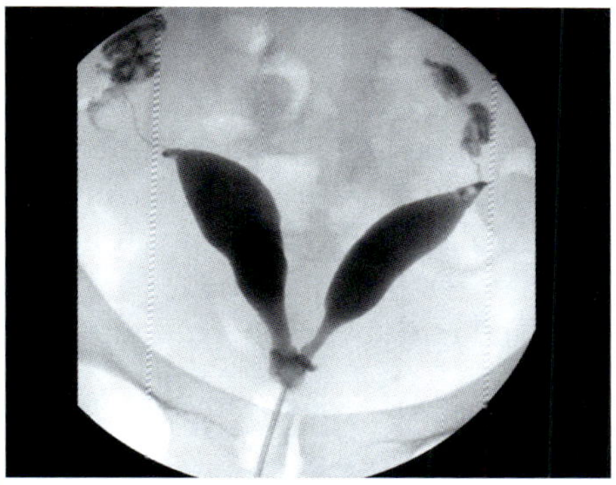
3D USG	Analysis of fundal contour and endometrial stripe in each cavity	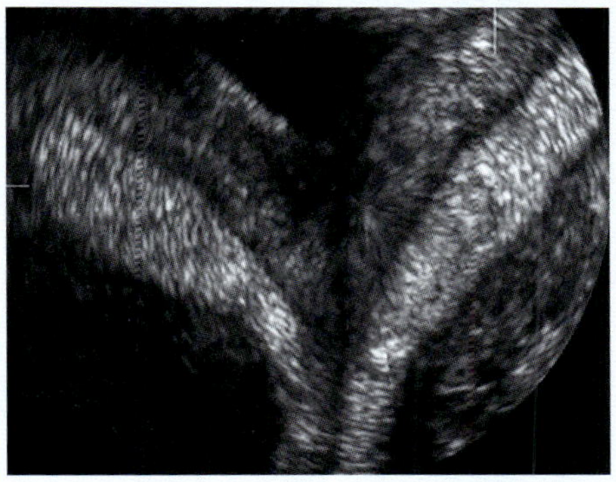
MRI	Deep (>1 cm) fundal cleft in the outer uterine contour and an intercornual distance of >4 cm	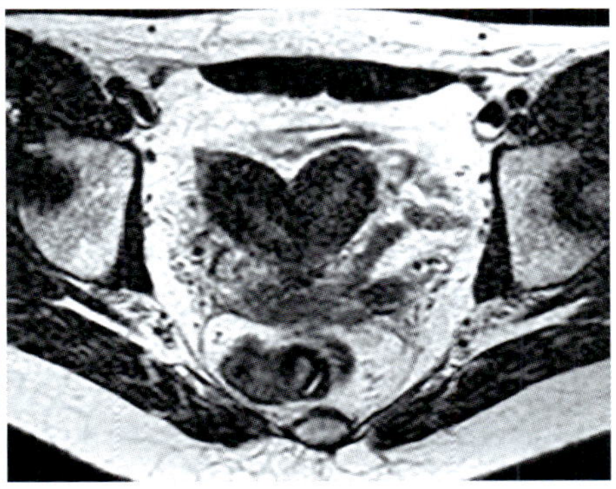
Hysteroscopy	Septate uterine cavity	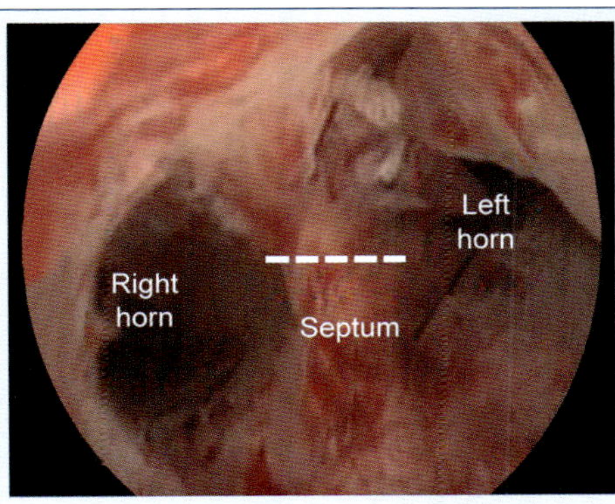
Laparoscopy	Two uterine horns fused at or above the cervix	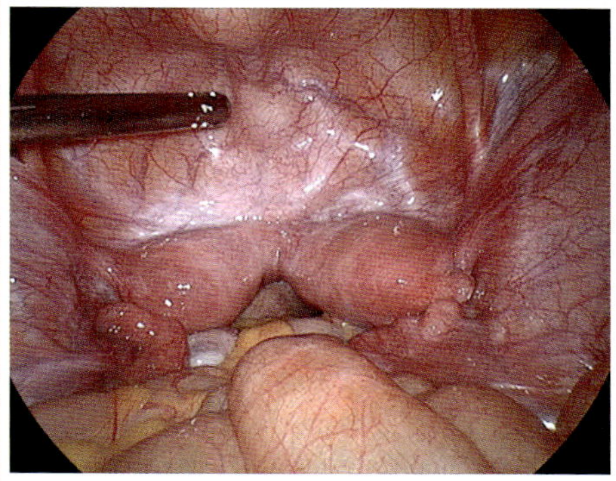

Contd...

INDICATIONS

- Recurrent abortions
- Pregnancy complications—preterm delivery, ectopic pregnancy
- Prior to in vitro fertilization (IVF)
- Endometriosis.

CONTRAINDICATION

Asymptomatic.

SURGICAL EQUIPMENT (FIGS. 3A TO C)

- A laparoscopic tower with a high-flow CO_2 insufflator, camera, and a light source
- An operating table with leg stirrups
- Vasopressin injection needle
- Hysteroscope—to rule out intrauterine structural pathology/Müllerian anomaly
- Laparoscopic toothed grasper for grasping and manipulating the uterus

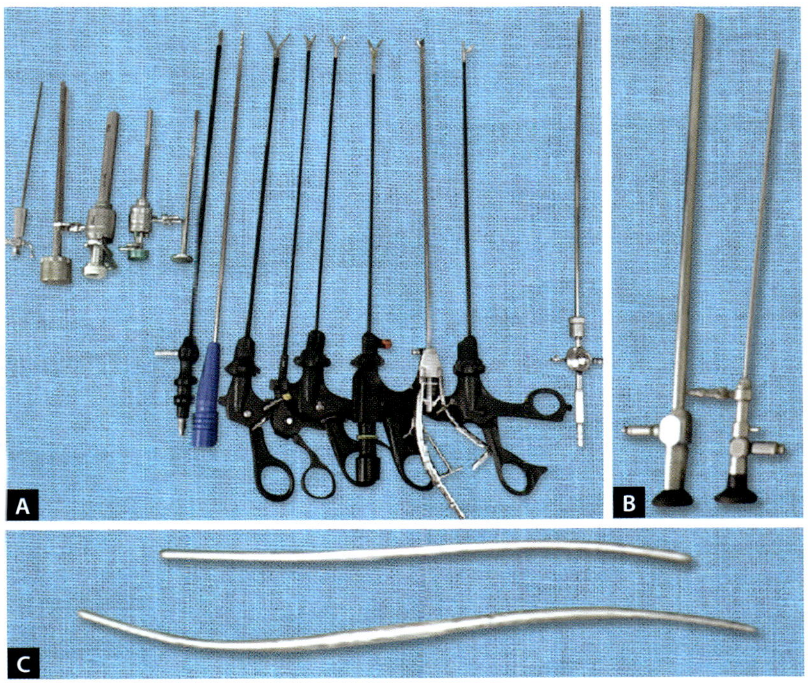

Figs. 3A to C: (A) Laparoscopic instruments; (B) Laparoscope and hysteroscope; (C) Hegar's dilators.

- Laparoscopic plain grasper to manipulate adnexal structures and bowel
- Suction irrigator is essential to clear out the smoke, blood and clots
- Uterine dilators for uterine manipulation
- Bipolar electricity generator and bipolar forceps
- Laparoscopic scissors
- A needle holder and hooked scissors is used for suturing the vault and cutting the suture respectively.

PREOPERATIVE EVALUATION

Routine preoperative tests include a complete blood count, bleeding time, clotting time, renal function tests, serum electrolytes, evaluation of thyroid status, viral markers, Pap smear, electrocardiography (ECG), and urinalysis. Preanesthetic assessment is an essential step prior to anesthesia in an attempt to decrease the morbidity and mortality related to anesthesia and surgery. Patient is advised for admission the evening prior to surgery. Informed consent is obtained from the patient after a thorough explanation of the planned operation, its risks and benefits, the possibility of laparotomy, and therapeutic alternatives. All patients are advised to eat lightly for 24 hours before surgery. Oral laxative tablets (bisacodyl) are given the night before. If adhesions or difficult surgery is contemplated, an oral mechanical bowel preparation like Coloprep or Peglec is administered. Patient is kept nil per oral 6–8 hours prior to surgery.

STEPS OF SURGERY (FIGS. 4 TO 15)

The patient is placed in dorsolithotomy position. Hysteroscopy reveals a septate uterine cavity with the septa extending from fundus to the level of internal os in a variable manner. Veress needle is inserted through the umbilicus, pneumoperitoneum created by insufflations of CO_2 gas. A 10-mm trocar is inserted in the umbilicus. A 30°, 10-mm telescope is inserted and entry injuries ruled out. Under direct vision, three 5 mm trocars are placed, two in right and left lower quadrants of the abdomen, lateral to the inferior epigastric vessels, and one in 5 mm suprapubic trocar is placed. Both Fallopian tubes and ovaries are normal.

Vasopressin solution (a dilution of 20 units in 200 mL normal saline) is infiltrated into both uterine horns. An incision is made over the superomedial aspect of each horn with cold scissors and extended inferomedially till the base of the horn guided by uterine dilators (manipulators). Both the cavities are opened along the length of the incision and the cavities merged into one. The opposing myometrial

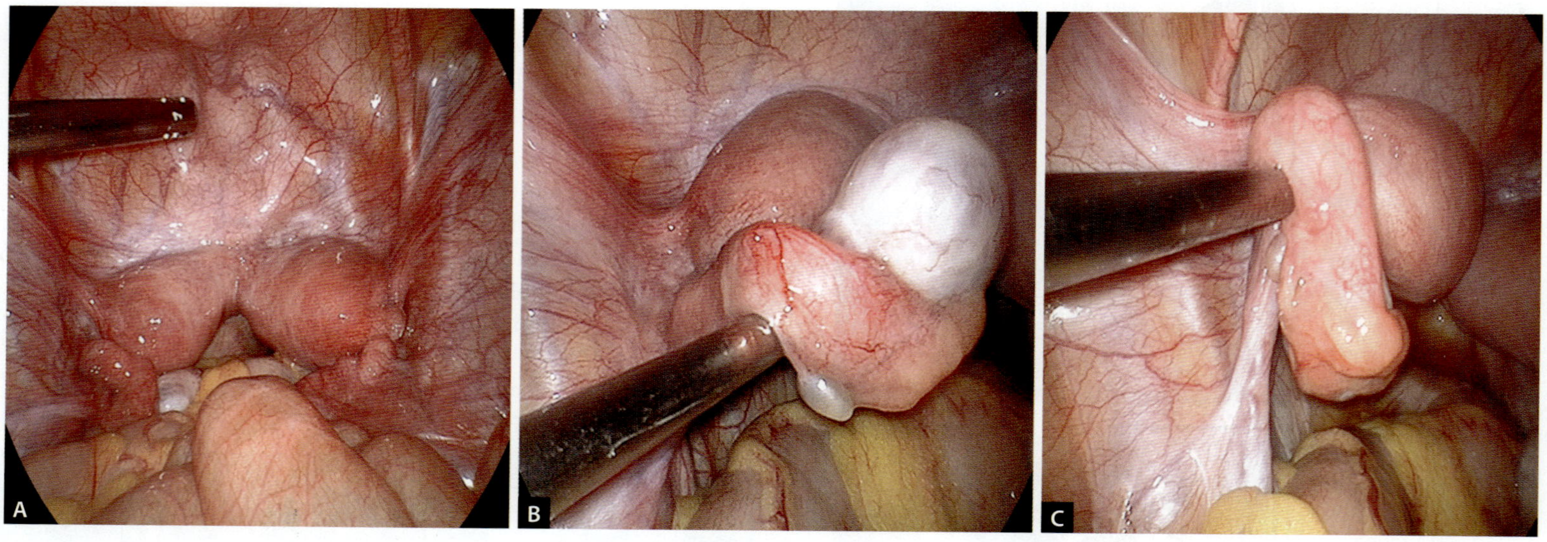

Figs. 4A to C: Appearance of bicornuate uterus.

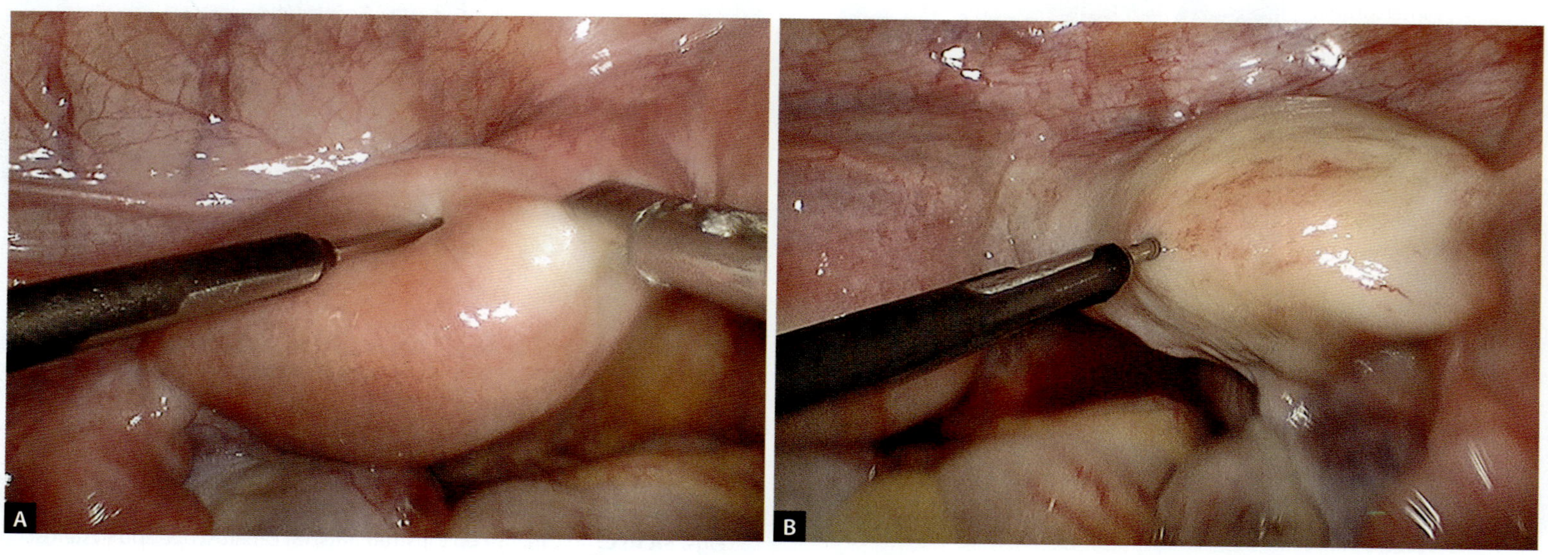

Figs. 5A and B: Vasopressin infiltration.

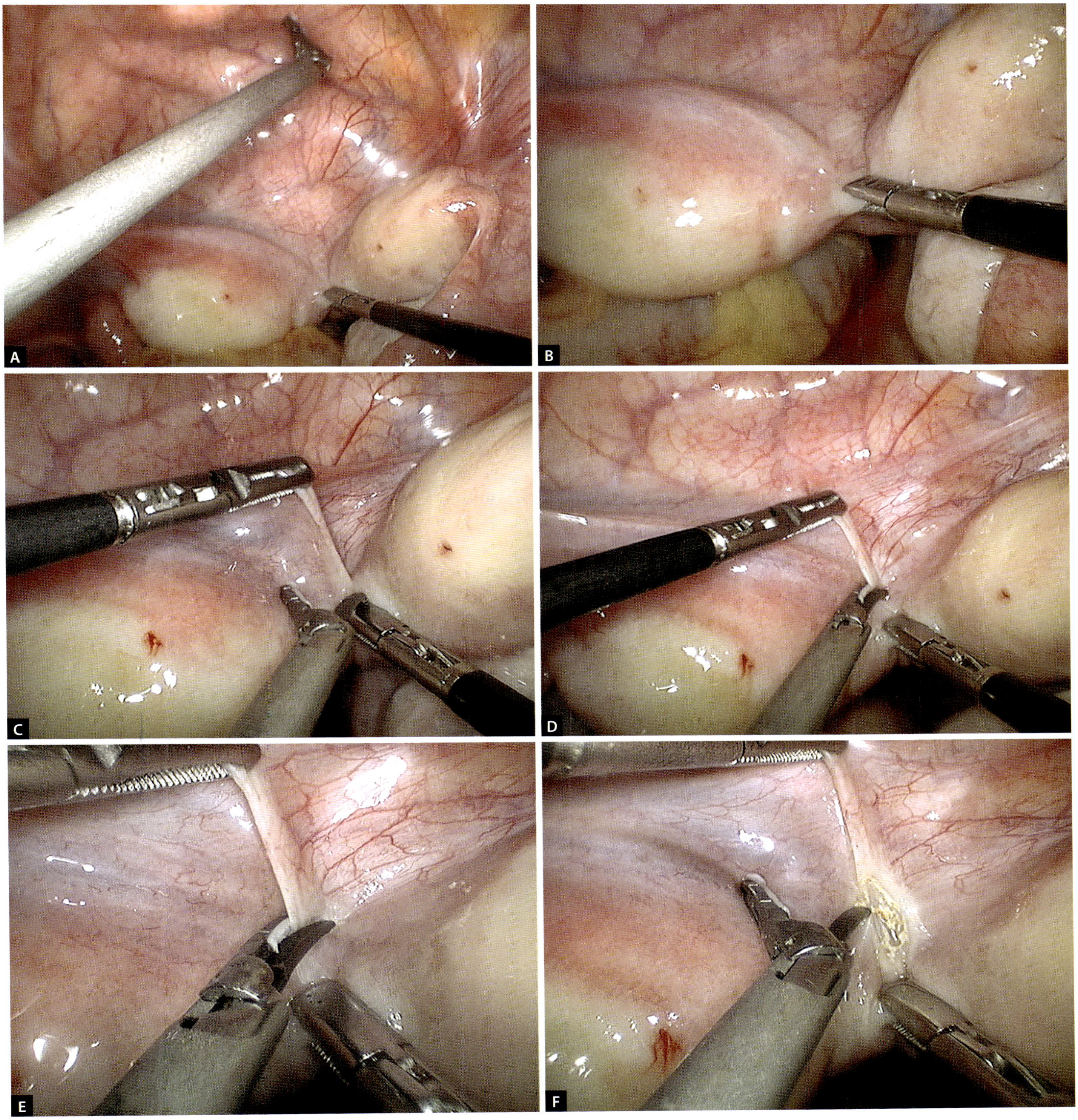

Figs. 6A to F

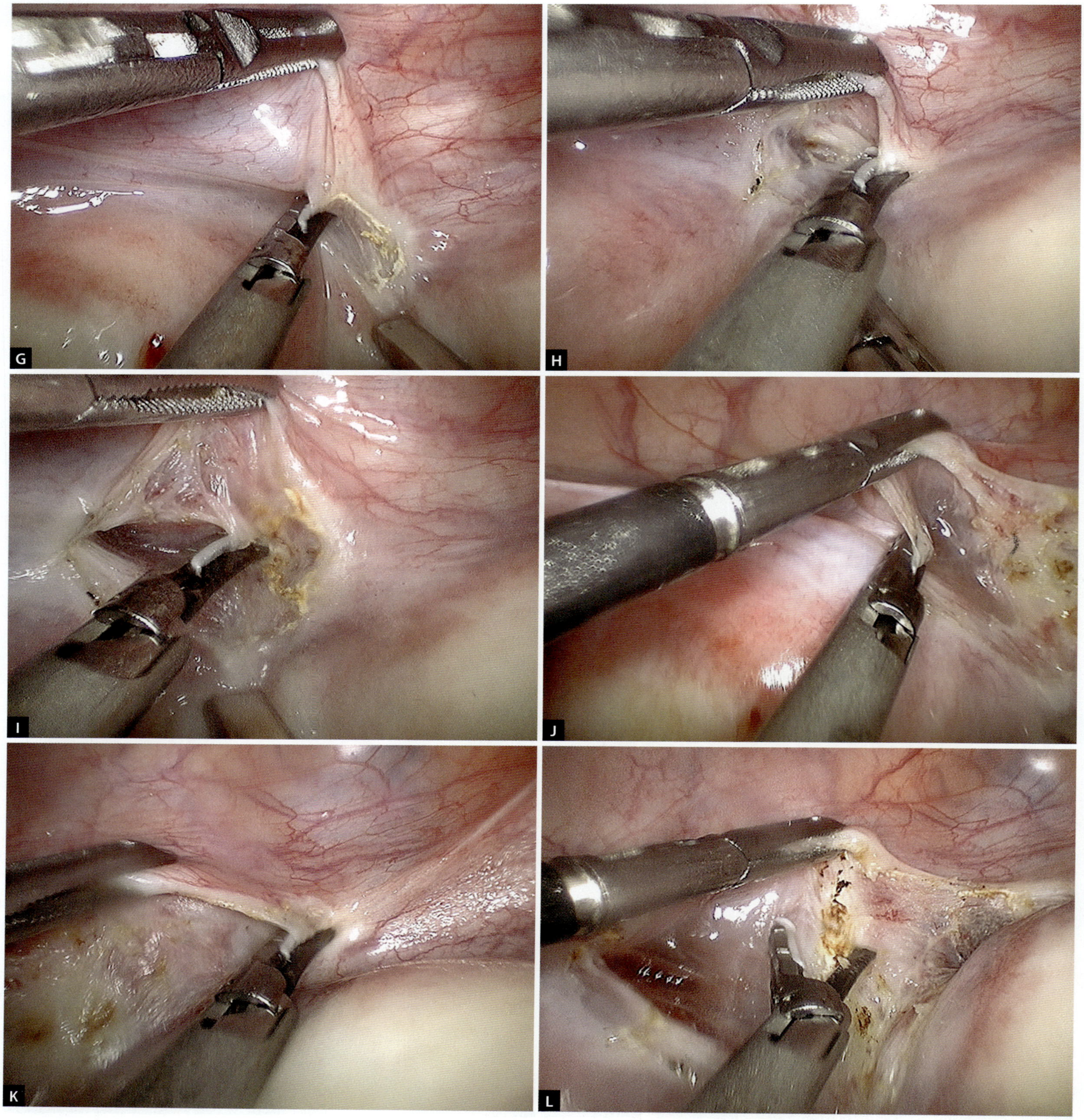

Figs. 6G to L

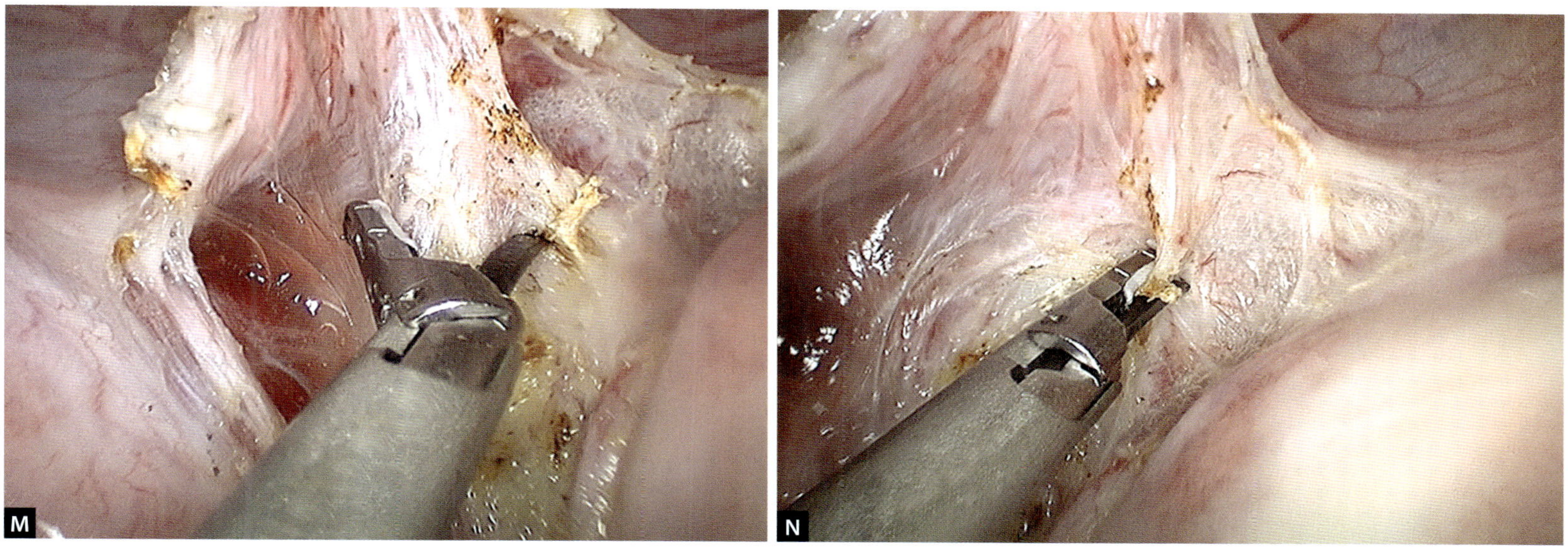

Figs. 6M and N

Figs. 6A to N: Development of bladder flap.

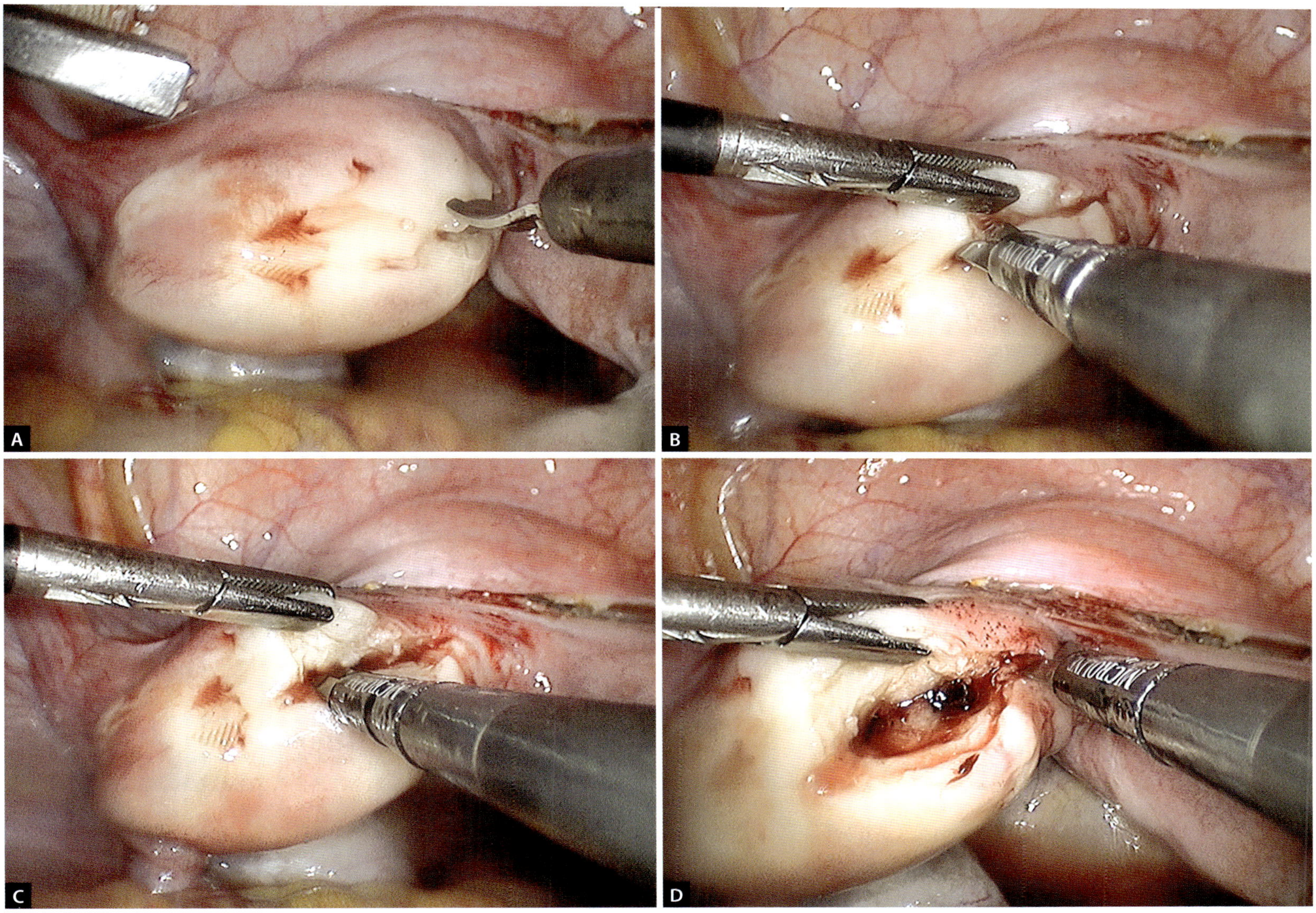

Figs. 7A to D

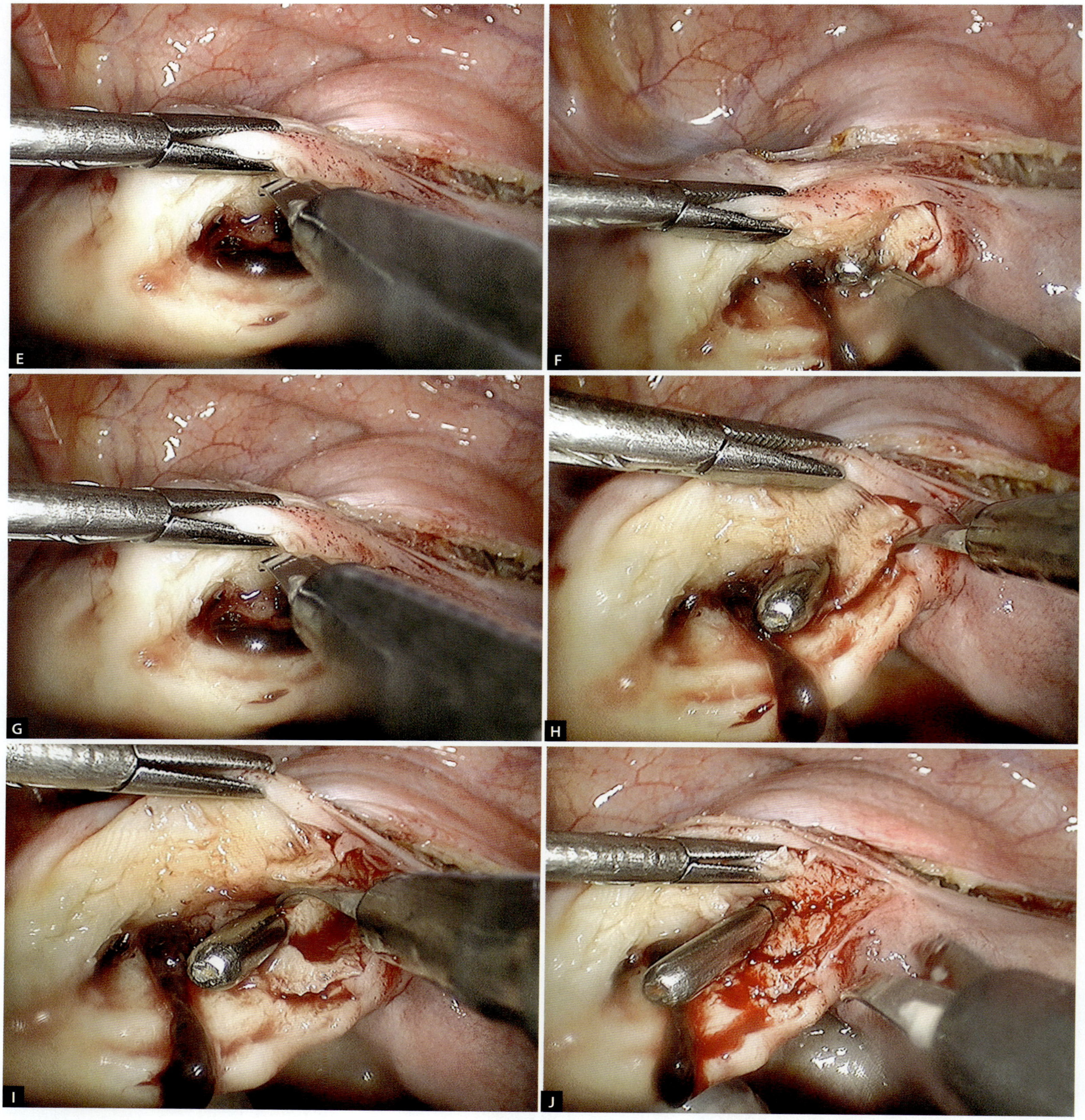

Figs. 7E to J

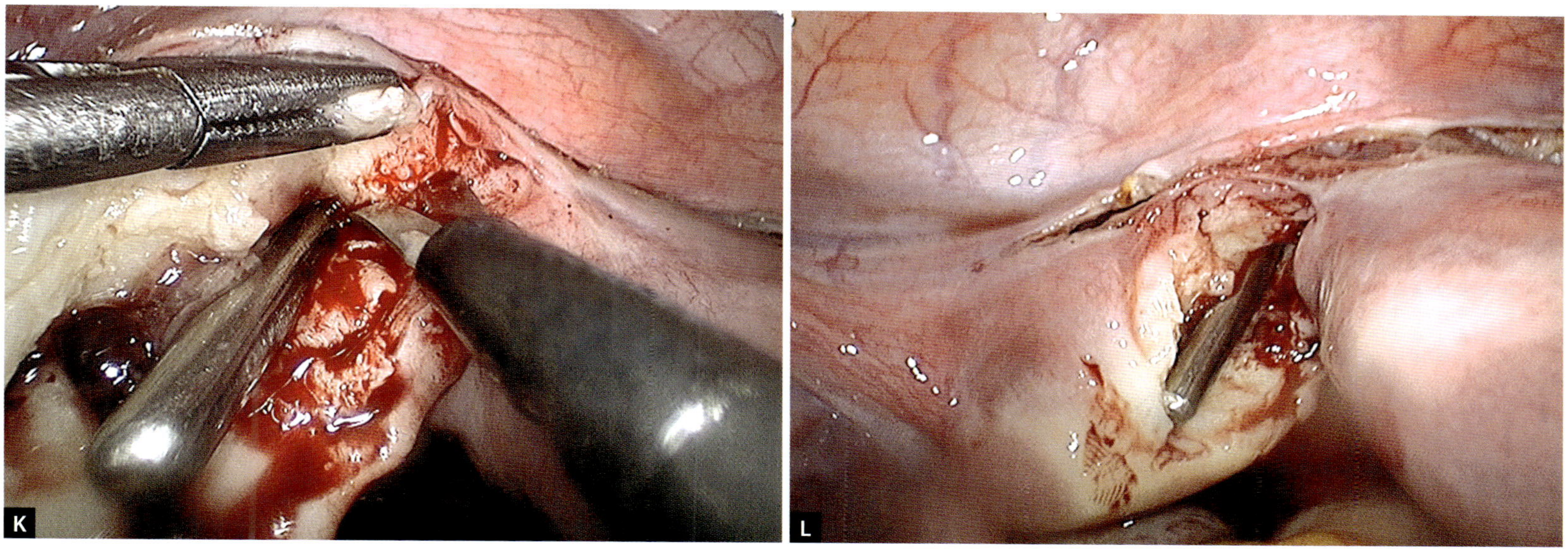

Figs. 7K and L

Figs. 7A to L: Incision on left horn.

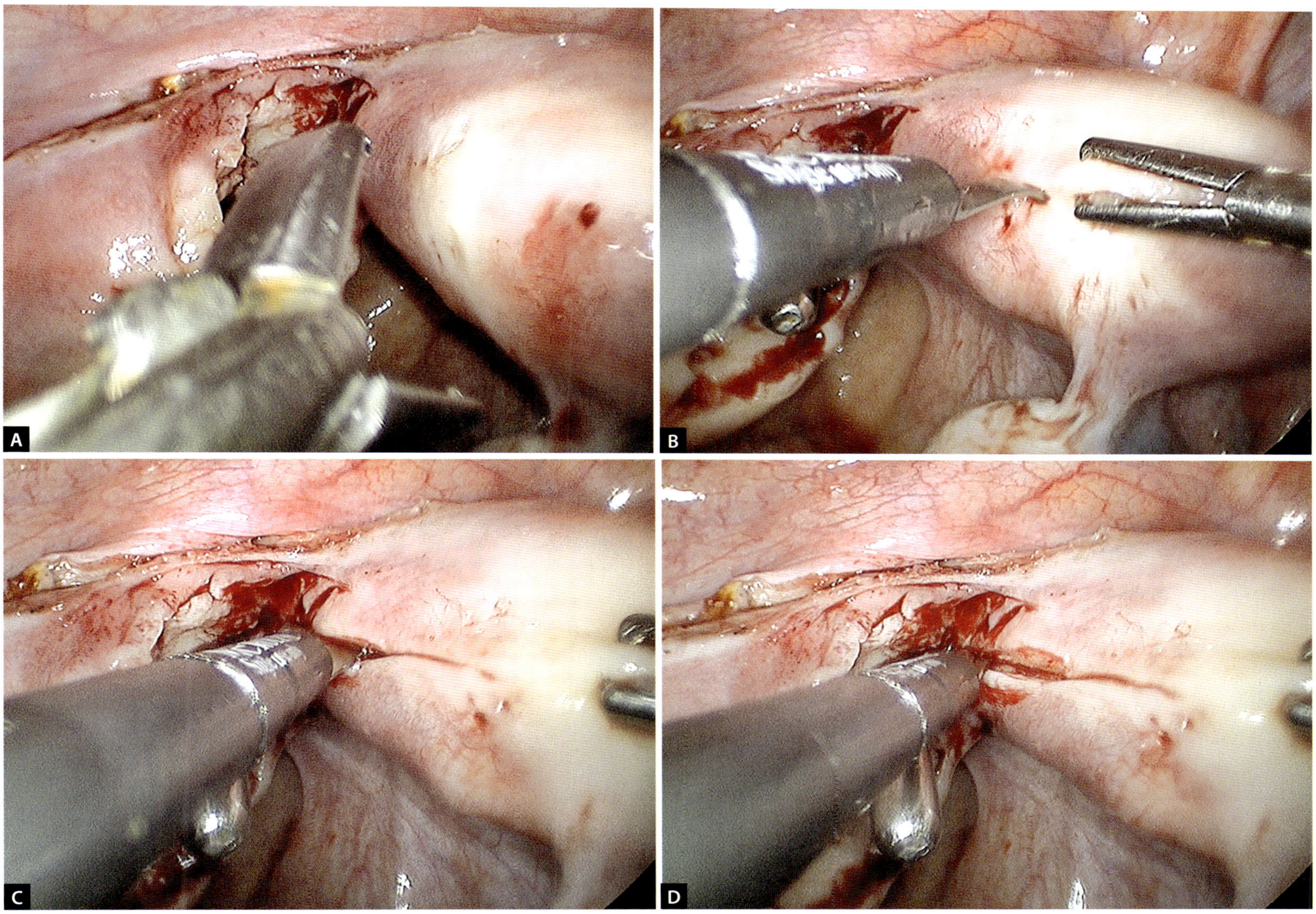

Figs. 8A to D

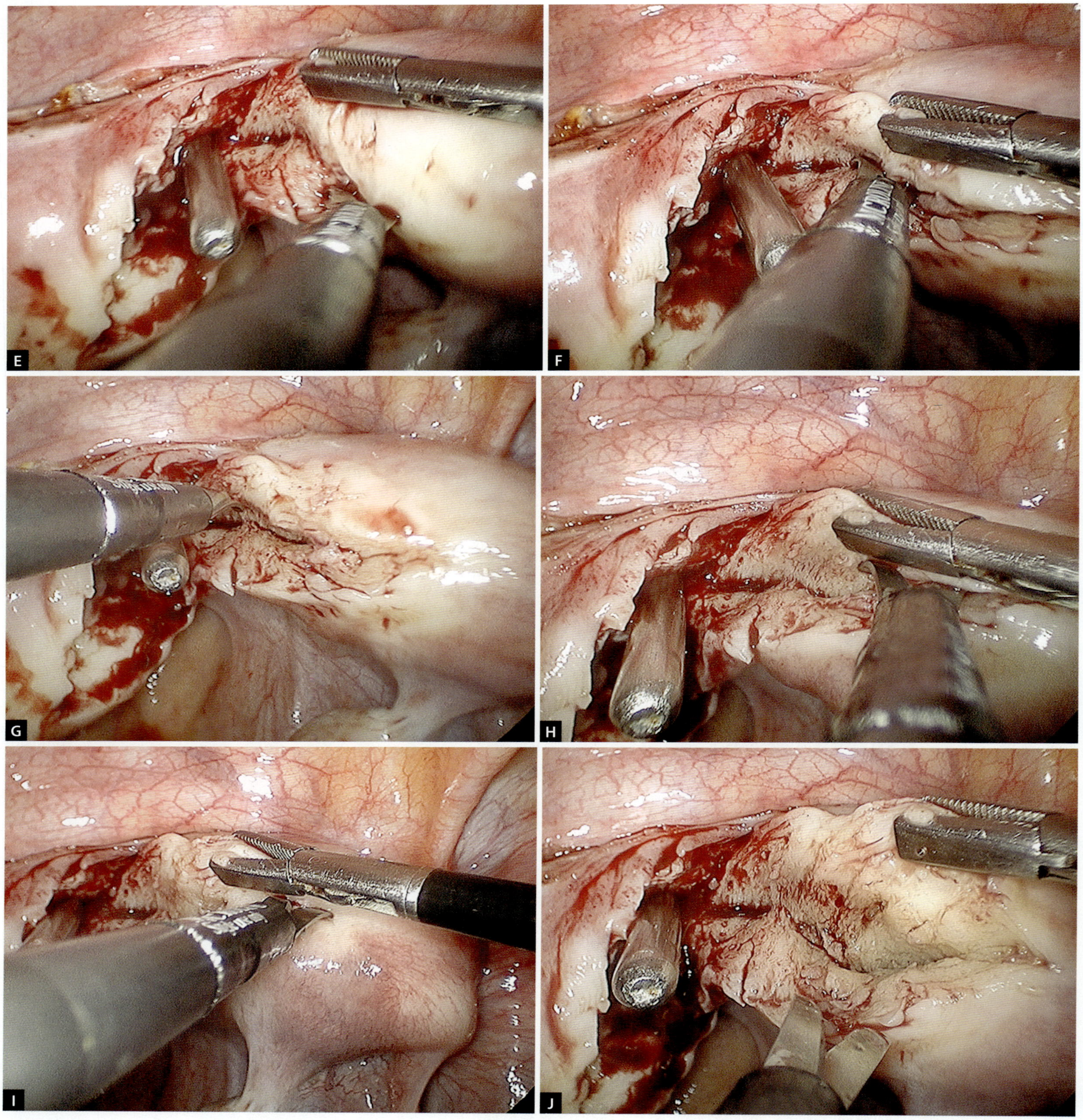

Figs. 8E to J

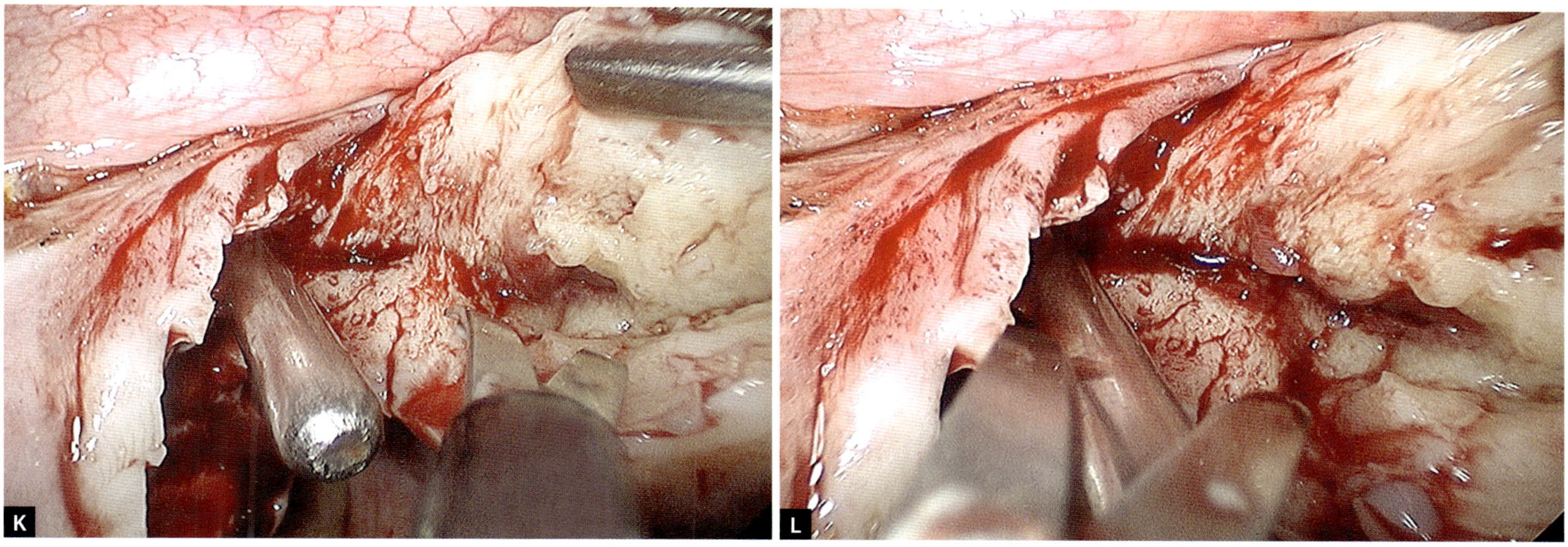

Figs. 8K and L

Figs. 8A to L: Incision on the right horn.

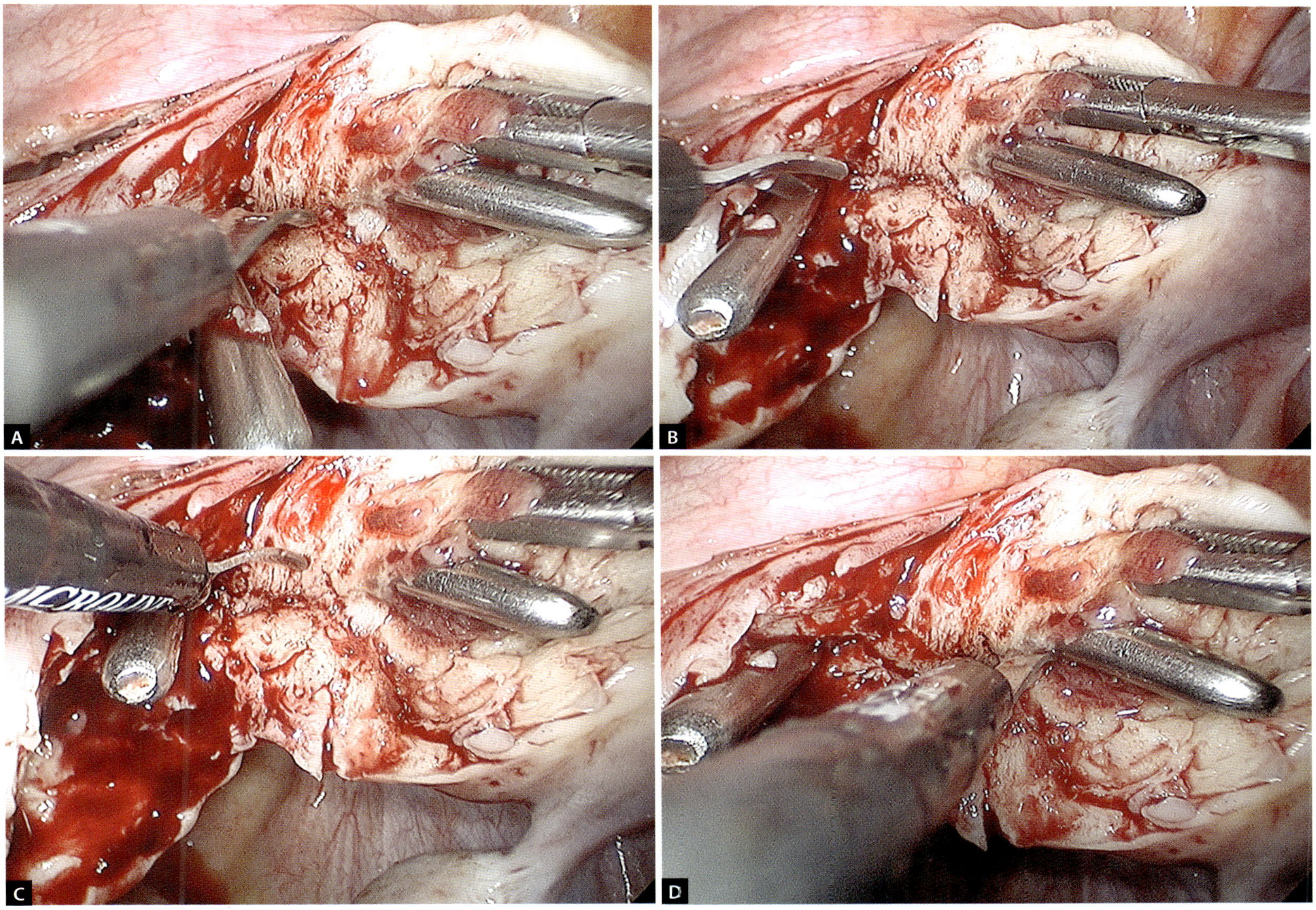

Figs. 9A to D

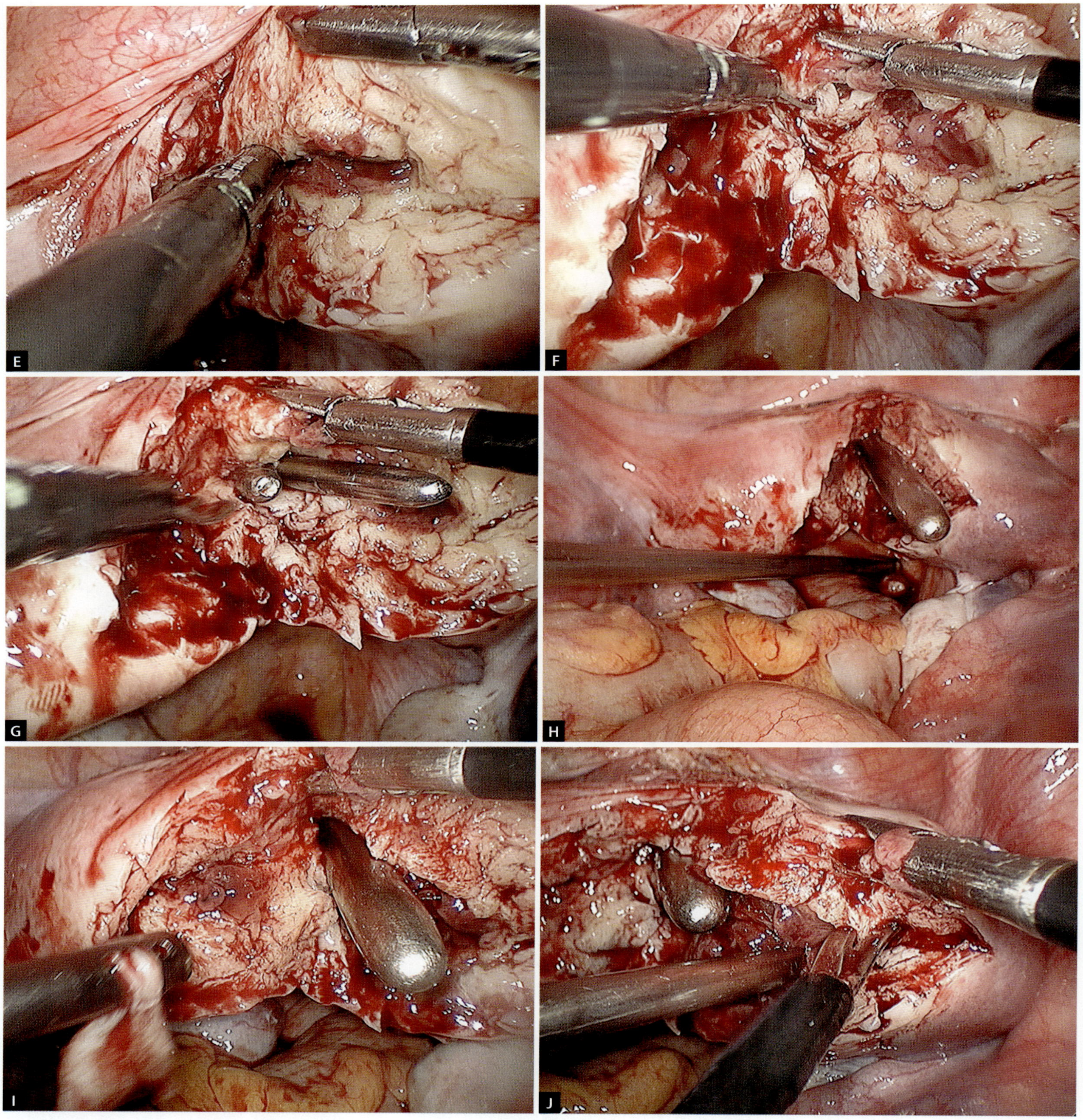

Figs. 9E to J

Figs. 9A to J: Bilateral horns being merged into a single cavity.

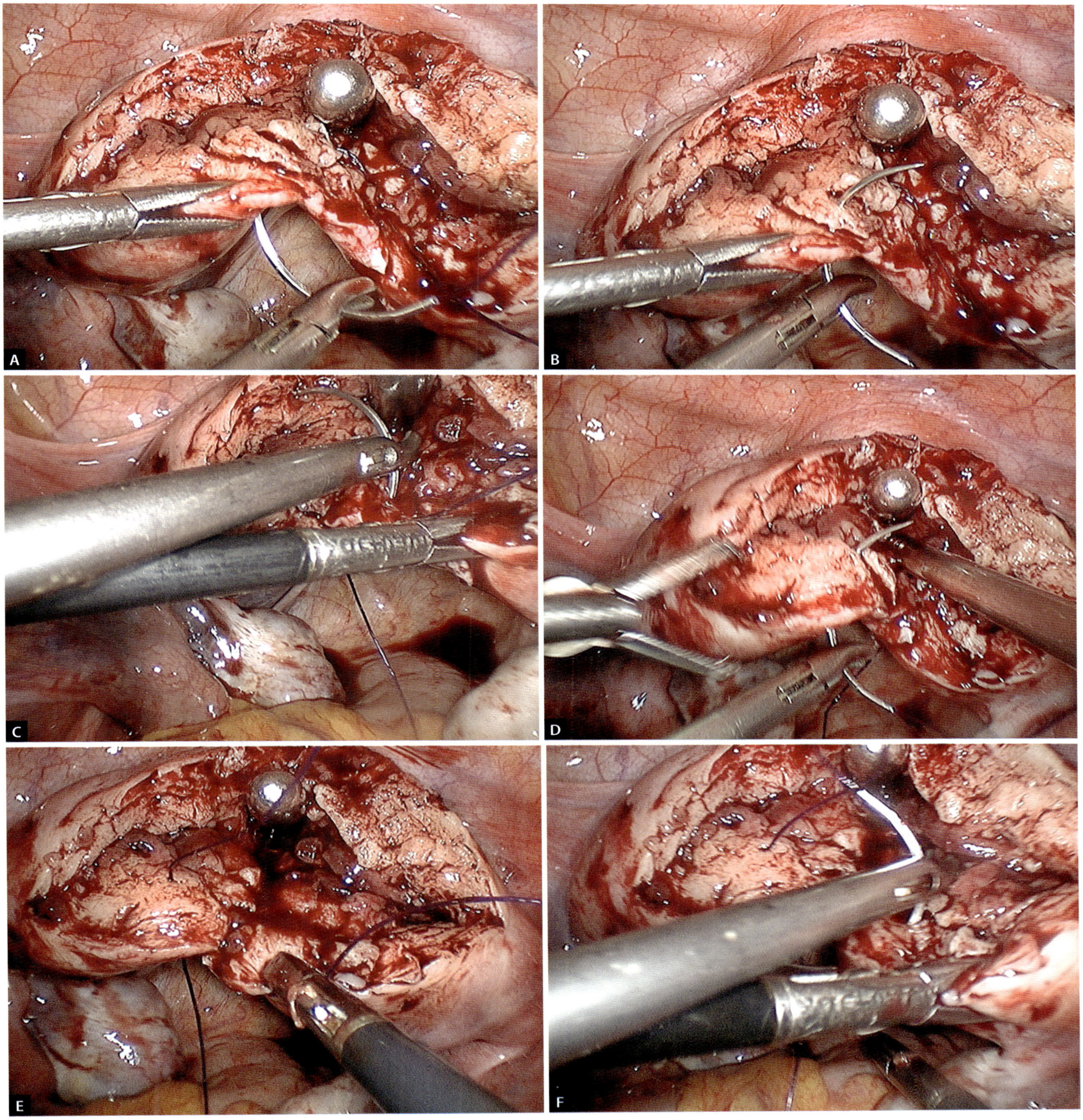

Figs. 10A to F

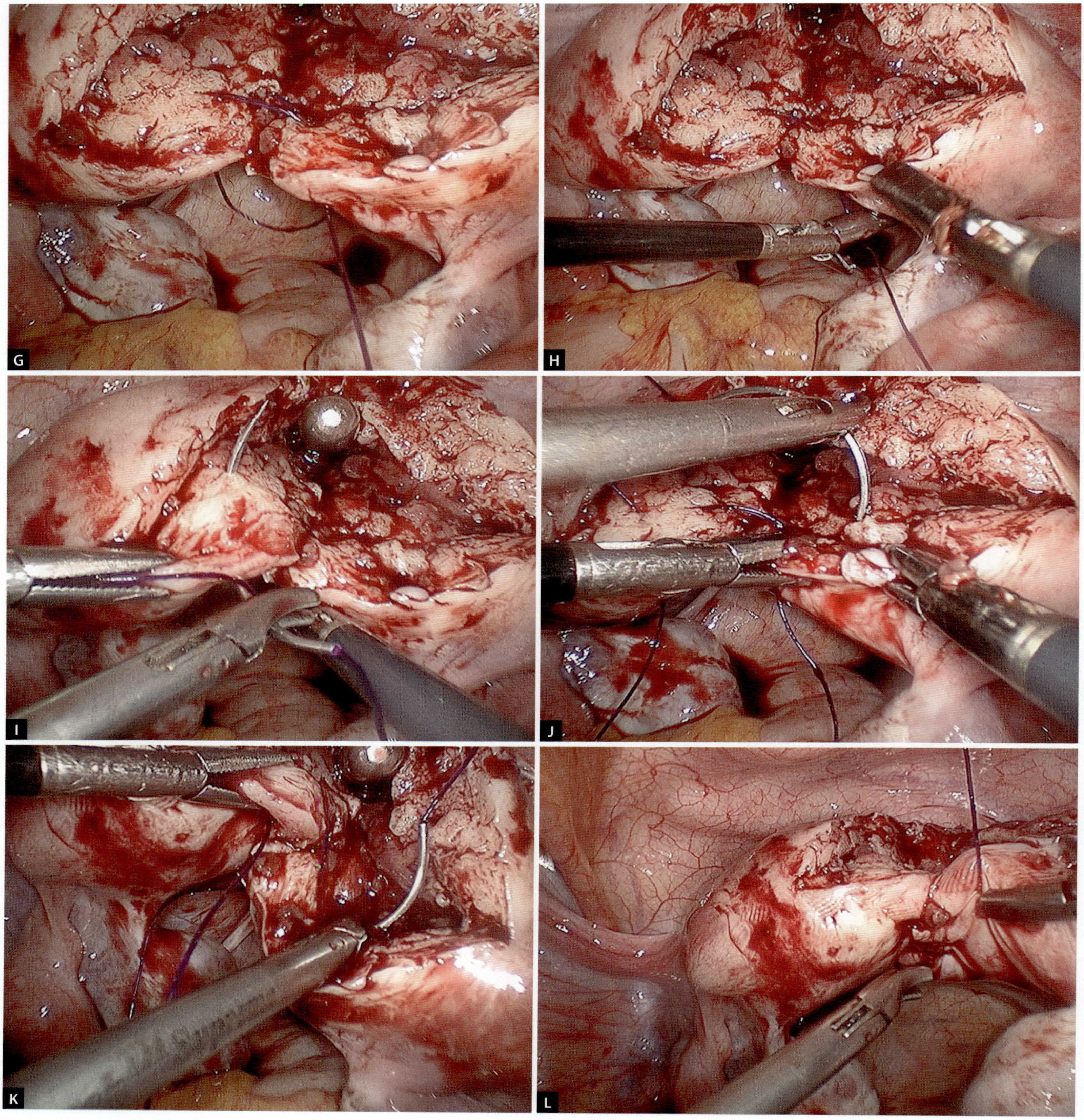

Figs. 10G to L

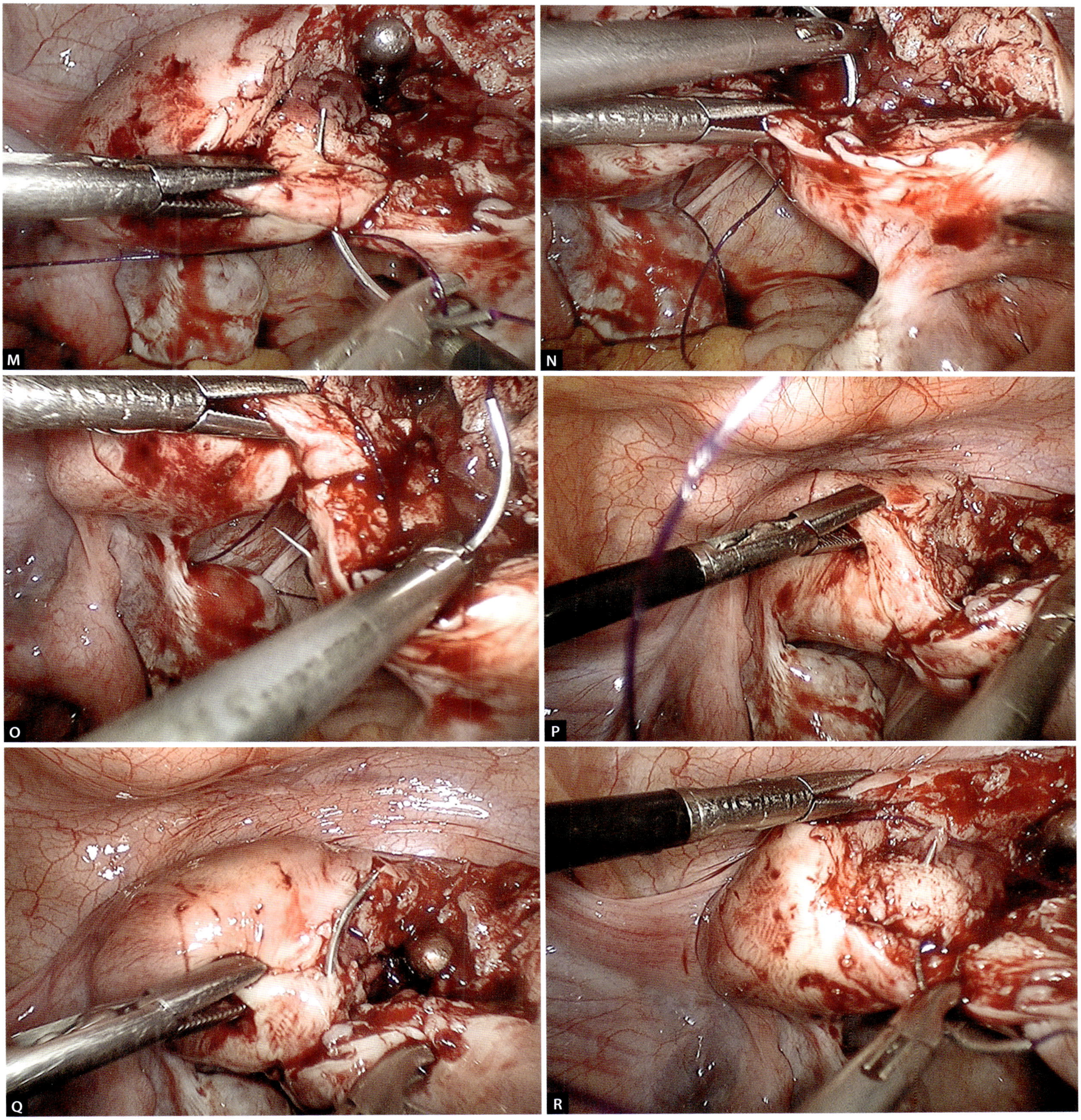

Figs. 10M to R

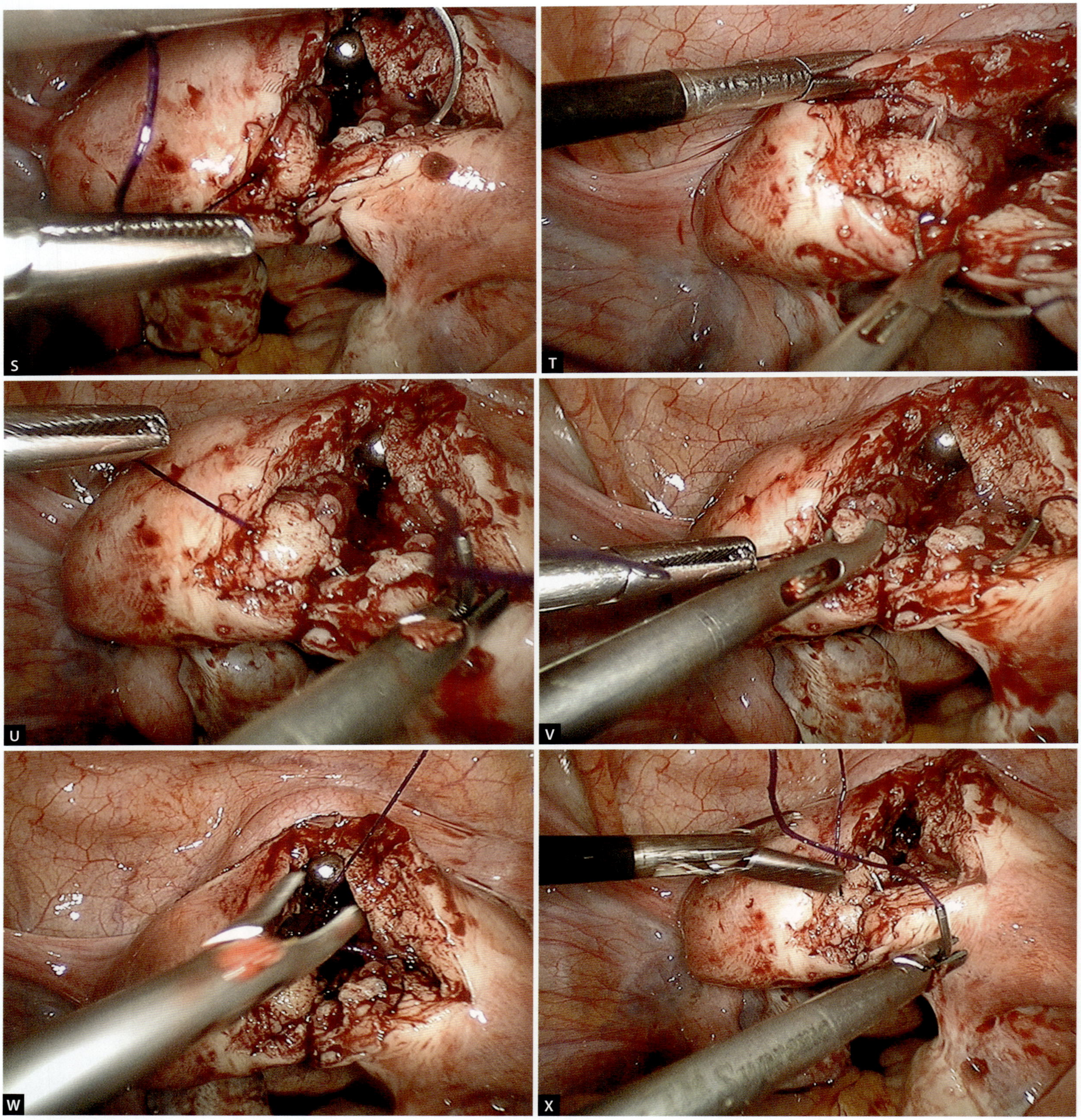

Figs. 10S to X

Figs. 10A to X: First layer of myometrial suturing posteriorly.

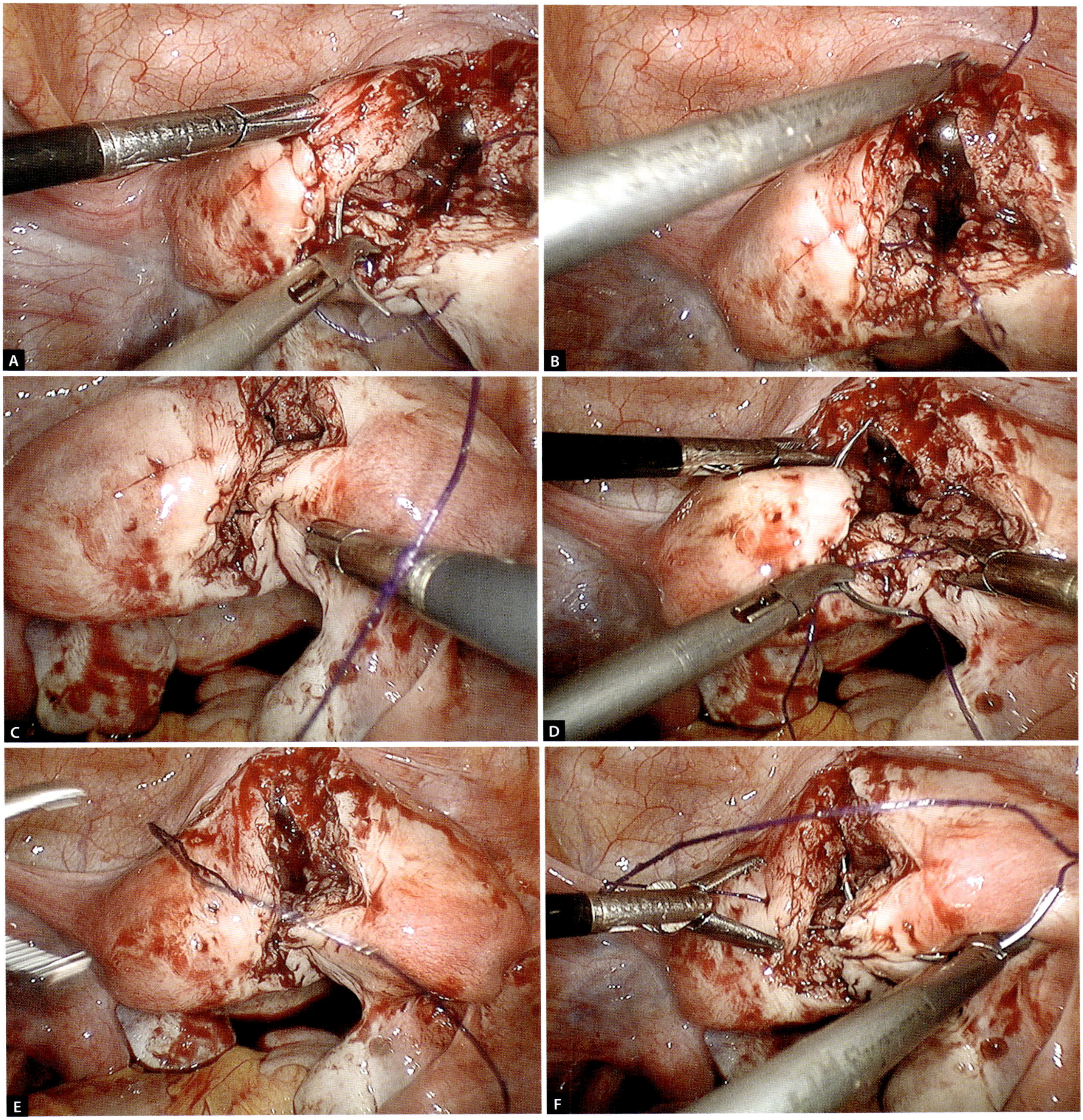

Figs. 11A to F

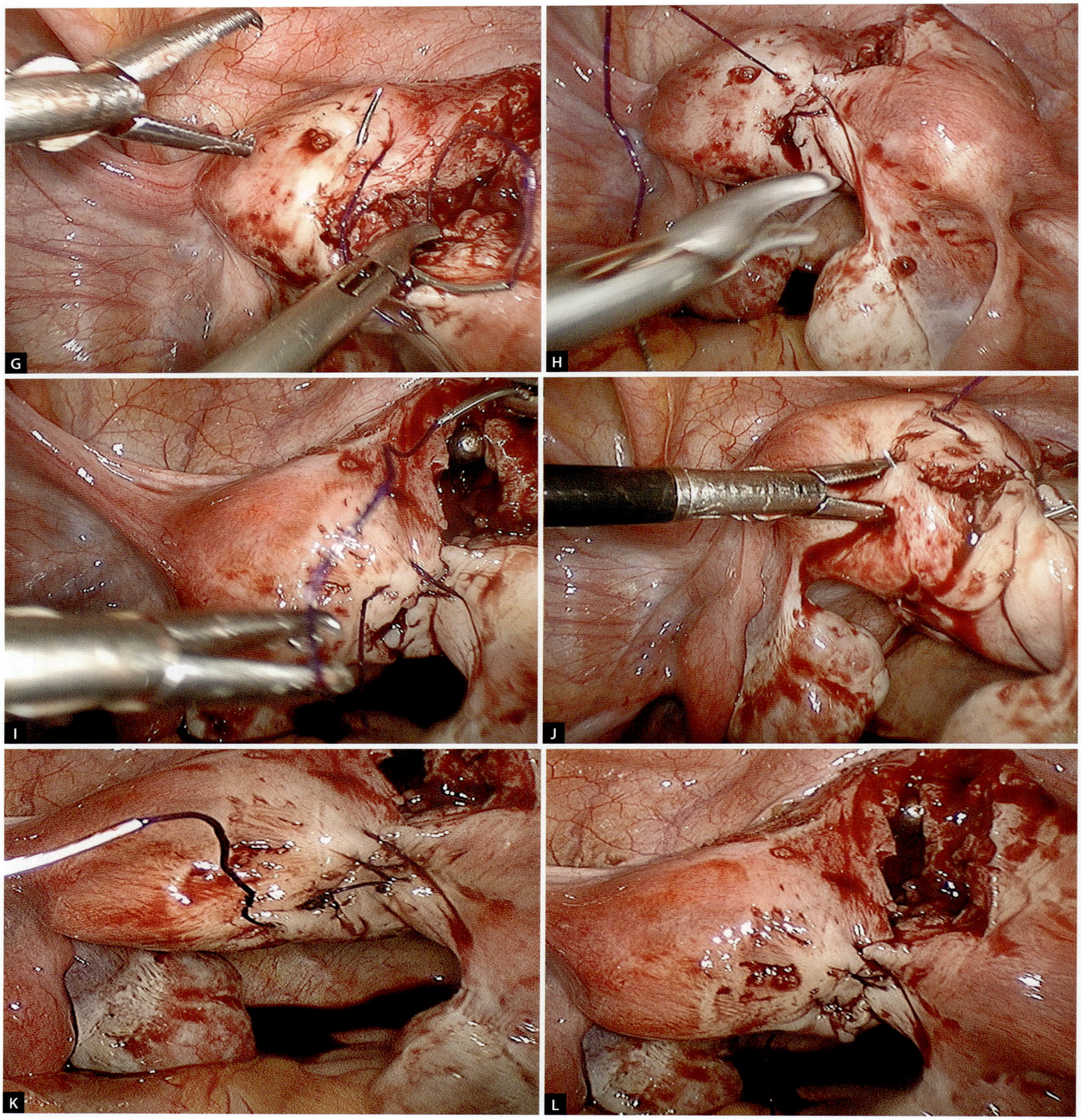

Figs. 11G to L

Figs. 11A to L: Myometrial suturing in the fundo-anterior region.

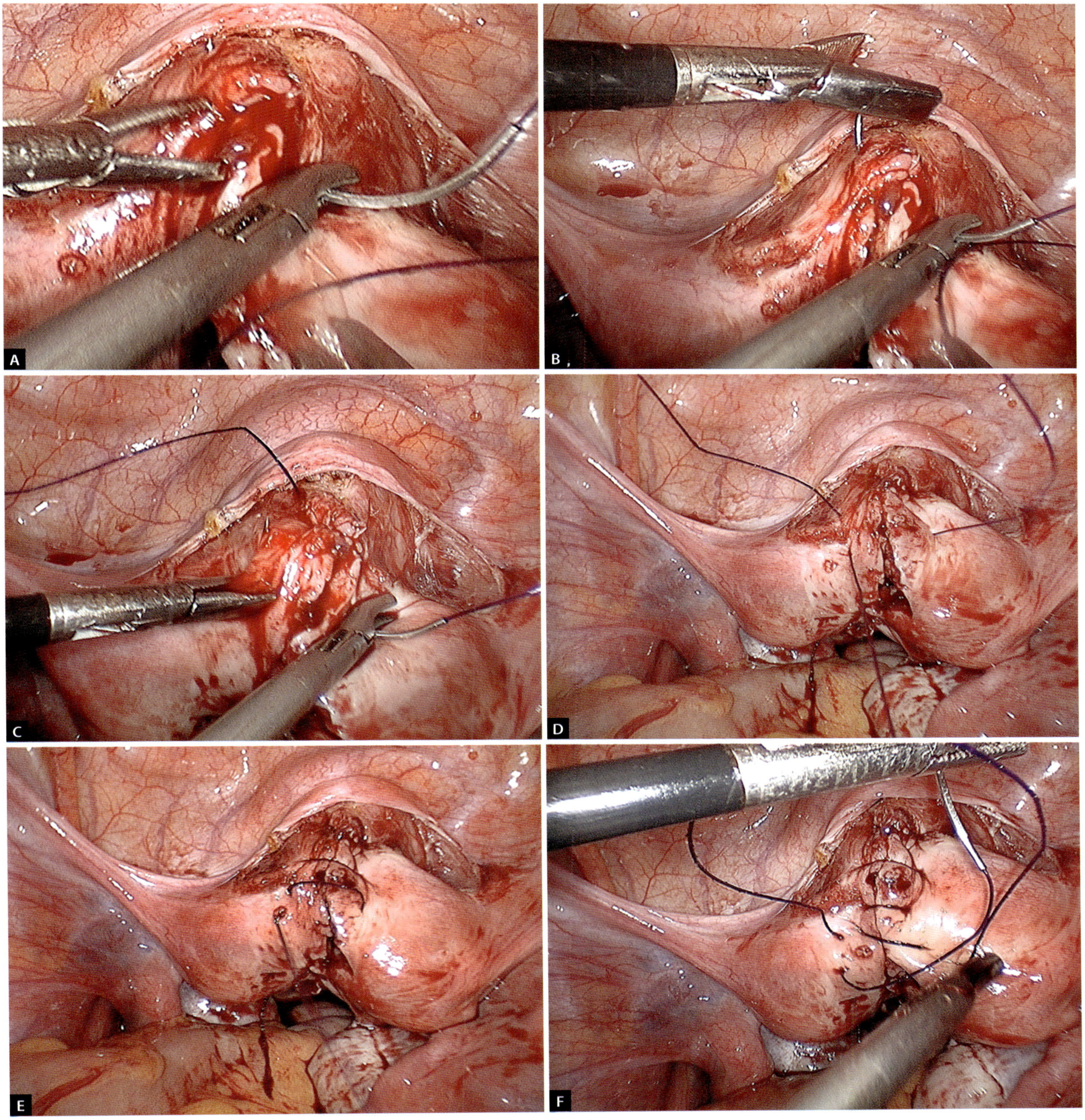

Figs. 12A to F

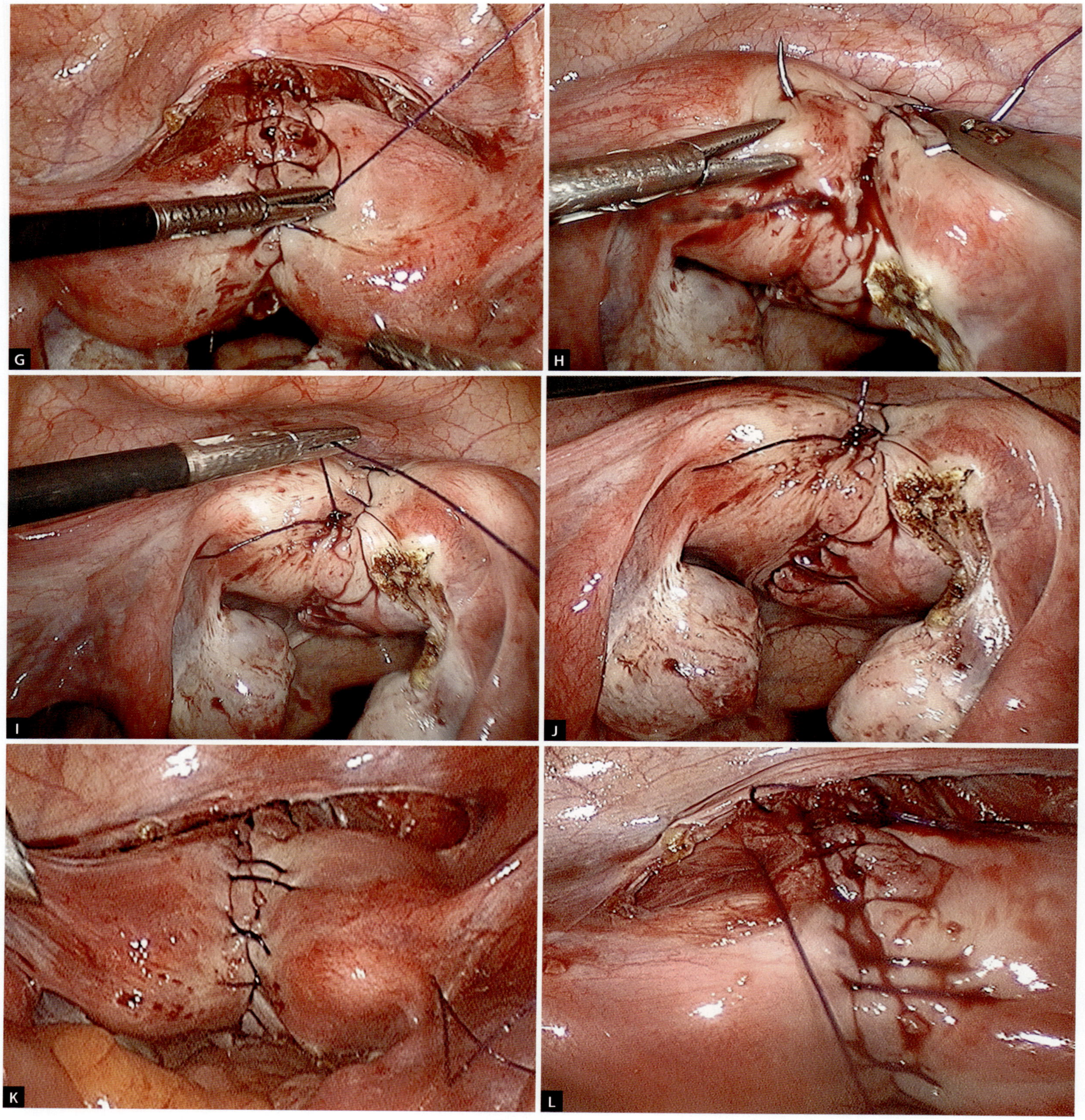

Figs. 12G to L

Figs. 12A to L: Myometrial suturing anteriorly.

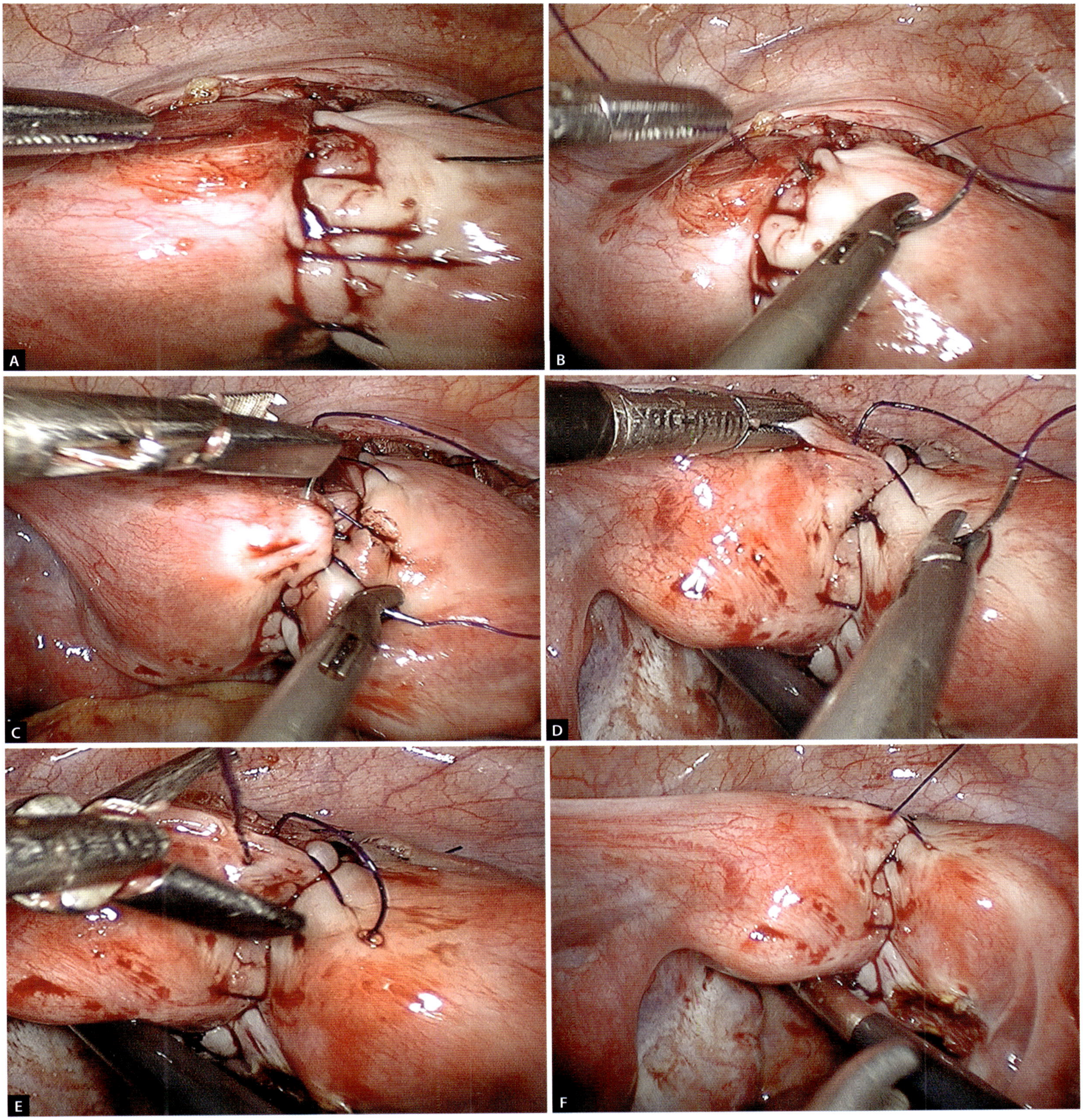

Figs. 13A to F

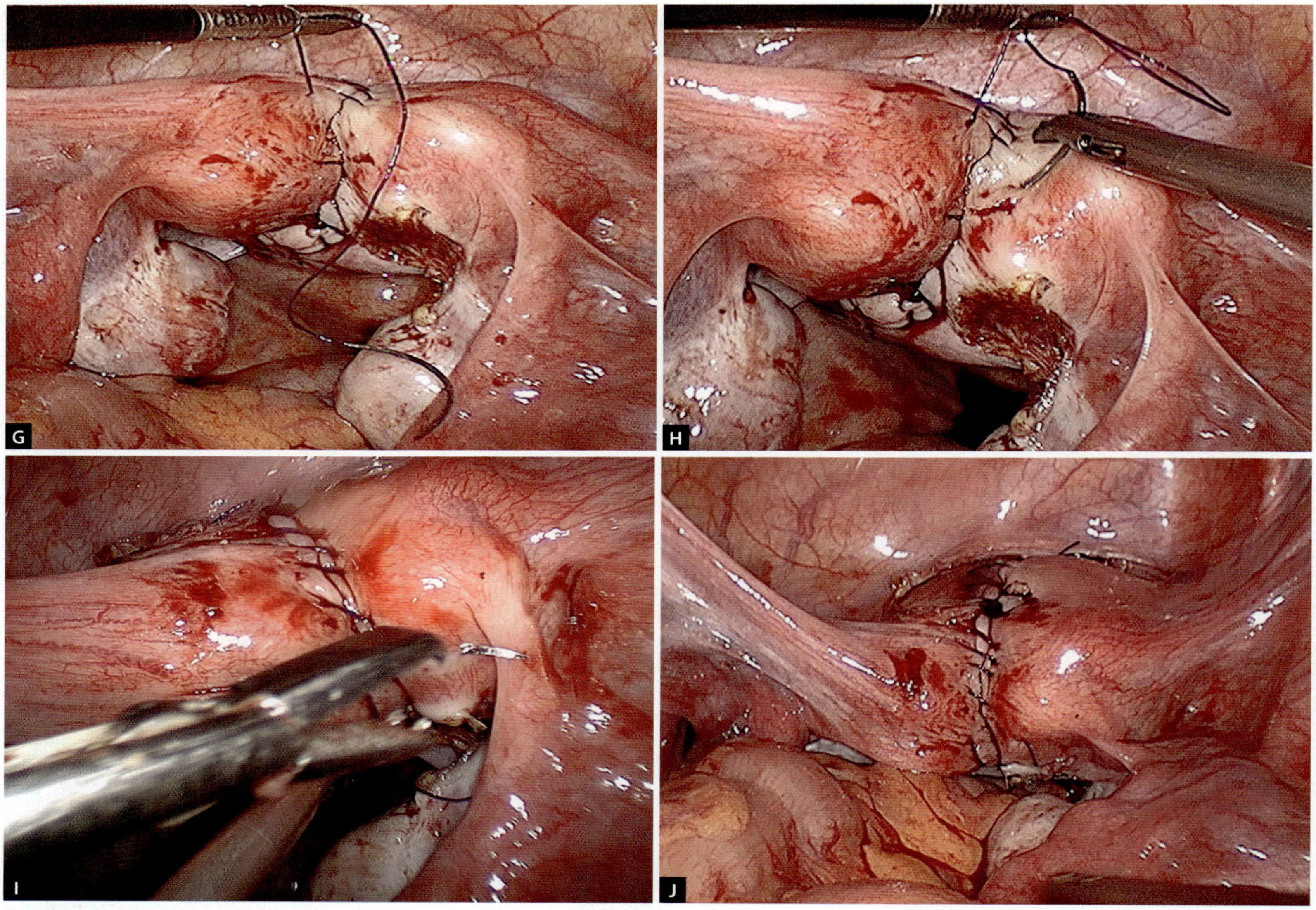

Figs. 13G to J

Figs. 13A to J: Suturing of second layer.

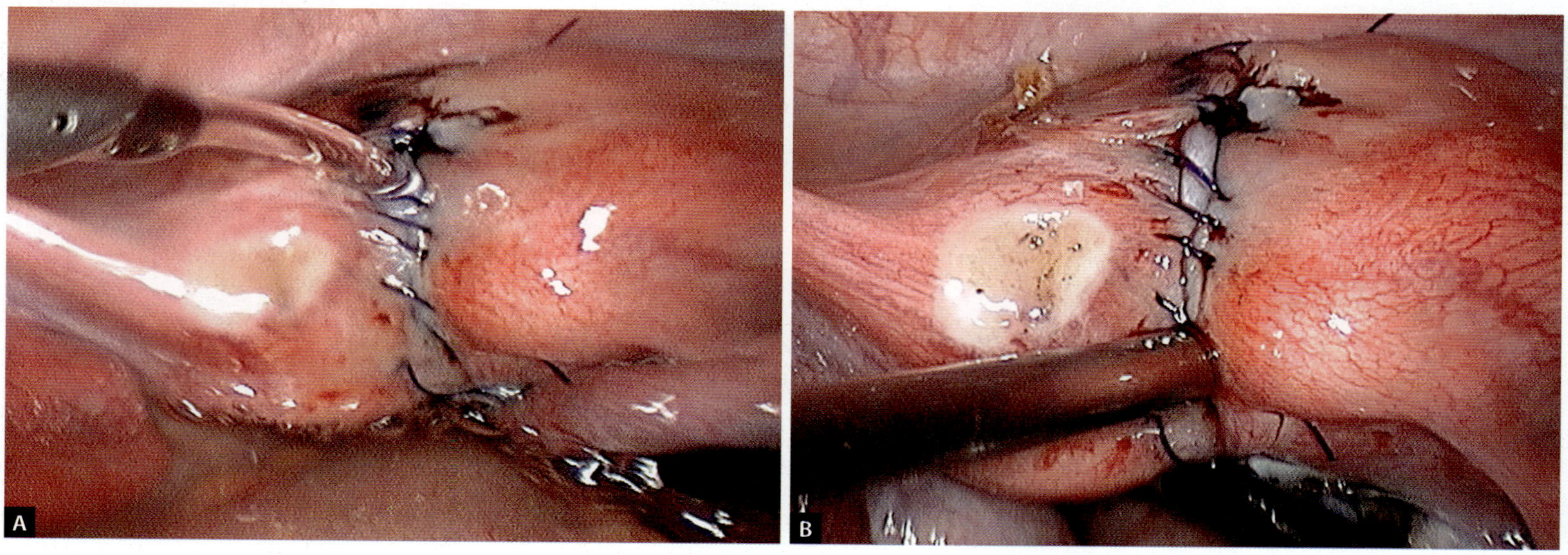

Figs. 14A and B: Final appearance of unified uterus.

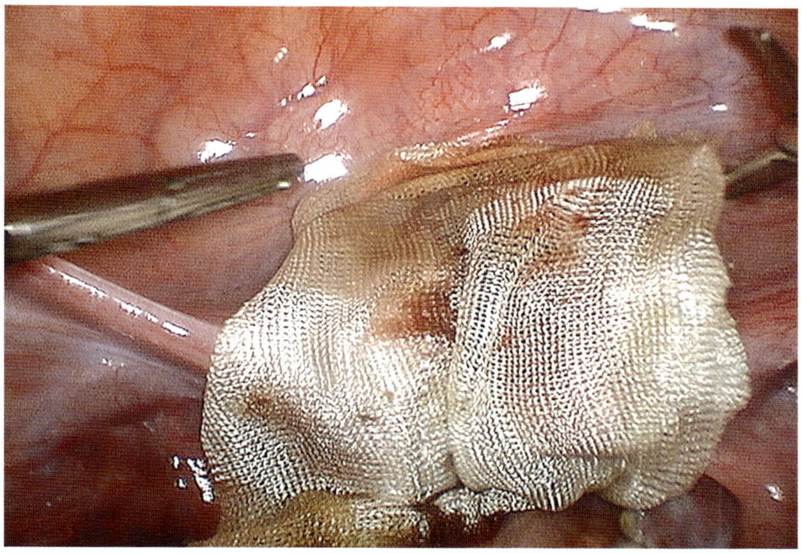

Fig. 15: Interceed placed over the unified uterus.

edges are sutured in layers continuously with Quill barbed sutures along the length of the incision. Caution is taken to exclude the endometrium.

The serosa is closed with 3-0 Prolene to prevent adhesion formation. The peritoneal surface is irrigated with saline and hemostasis is confirmed. Interceed is placed over the uterine wound. An intrauterine device is placed followed by 3 months of cyclical hormone replacement therapy (HRT).

POSTOPERATIVE CARE

Close monitoring of vitals, along with strict input and output chart is recommended in the immediate postoperative period. Adequate analgesia should be administered. Oral antibiotics are advised in most cases; however, intravenous antibiotic can be administered if necessary. Patients are initially allowed clear liquids, once bowel sounds resume. If tolerated, the diet is advanced to "soft diet" for 2–3 days, followed by regular diet with ample intake of fluids. Once patient voids without discomfort, tolerates a regular diet and ambulates wall, she can be discharged. Postoperatively, patient is advised cyclical HRT for 3 months (Tab. estradiol valerate 2 mg 2-2-2 from day 2 to day 25 of cycle, Tab. medroxyprogesterone acetate 10 mg 1-0-1 from day 16 to day 25 of cycle). Recheck hysterolaparoscopy is advised after 3 months.

SECOND-LOOK HYSTEROLAPAROSCOPY

A repeat hysteroscopy is performed 3 months later. On hysteroscopy (Bettocchi, Karl Storz), the uterus is inspected to see if a uniform spacious cavity has formed and to rule out synechiae. Tubal patency is confirmed by laparoscopy.

Cervical cerclage (interval or during pregnancy) is recommended. Elective LSCS is recommended at 37 weeks of gestation.

COMPLICATIONS (BOX 1)

With the use of good laparoscopic skills and instrumentation risk of weak scar can be significantly minimized and ensured safety in subsequent pregnancy.[12,13] Overall prevalence of adhesion formation can also be reduced to minimum by proper utilizing the laparoscopic properties such as reduced tissue handling and reduced tissue dryness.[14,15]

Box 1: Complications.

- Adhesions—intrauterine and extrauterine
- Hemorrhage
- Infection
- Cervical incompetence
- Antepartum hemorrhage
- Adherent placenta, postpartum hemorrhage
- Uterine rupture

CONCLUSION

Laparoscopic unification of bicornuate uterus surgery is comparatively safe and effective alternative to conventional abdominal unification. Advantage of laparoscopic unification surgery is less blood loss, less peritoneal adhesions, restoration of the uterine anatomy, and good scar integrity, shorter hospital stay. Despite the controversy in the literature, laparoscopic unification of bicornuate surgery should be preferred in symptomatic patients with recurrent poor reproductive outcomes over conventional abdominal surgery.

REFERENCES

1. Grimbizis GF, Camus M, Tarlatzis BC, et al. Clinical implications of uterine malformations and hysteroscopic treatment results. Hum Reprod Update. 2001;7:161-74.
2. Porcu G, Heckenroth H. Uterine abnormalities and infertility. EMC Gynecol Obstet. 2005;2:135-97
3. Papp Z, Mezei G, Gávai M, et al. Reproductive performance after transabdominal metroplasty: a review of 157 consecutive cases. J Reprod Med. 2006;51:544-52.
4. Sinha R, Mahajan C, Hedge A, et al. Laparoscopic metroplasty for bicornuate uterus. J Minim Invasive Gynecol. 2006;13:70-3.
5. Rackow BW, Arici A. Reproductive performance of women with müllerian anomalies. Curr Opin Obstet Gynecol. 2007;19:229-37.
6. Rock JA, Jones HW. The clinical management of the double uterus. Fertil Steril. 1977;28:798-806.
7. Candiani GB, Fedele L, Parazzini F, et al. Reproductive prognosis after abdominal metroplasty in bicornuate or septate uterus: life table analysis. Br J Obstet Gynaecol. 1990;97:613-7.
8. Ayhan A, Yucel I, Tuncer ZS, et al. Reproductive performance after conventional metroplasty: an evaluation of 102 cases. Fertil Steril. 1992;57:1194-6.
9. Whittaker MD, Garry R. Modern management of congenital abnormalities of the uterus. Curr Obstet Gynaecol. 1995;5:41-5.
10. Alborzi S, Asadi N, Zolghadri J, et al. Laparoscopic metroplasty in bicornuate and didelphic uteri. Fertil Steril. 2009;92:352-5.
11. Pisat S, Tas B, van Herendael B. Laparoscopic Strassman's metroplasty for bicornuate uterus. Gynecol Surg. 2009;6:153-8.
12. Jelsema RD, Wittingen JA, Vanderkolk KJ. Continuous, nonlocking, single-layer repair of the low transverse uterine incision. J Reprod Med. 1993;38:393-6.
13. Sinha R, Hedge A, Warty N, et al. Laparoscopic excision of very large myomas. J Am Assoc Gynecol Laparosc. 2003;10:461-8.
14. Sinha R, Hedge A, Warty N, et al. Laparoscopic removal of large multiple myomas with cumulative weight of 2.3 kg. J Am Assoc Gynecol Laparosc. 2003;10:403-6.
15. Stringer NH, Walker JC, Meyr PM. Comparison of 49 laparoscopic myomectomies with 49 open myomectomies. J Am Assoc Gynecol Laparosc. 1997;4:457-64.

Accompanying Video: Laparoscopic unification of bicornuate uterus.

CHAPTER 27

Ureter Relations and Injury in Gynecology

Shruti Paliwal, Isha Rani, B Ramesh

INTRODUCTION

Ureteral injury is a serious concern during abdominal and pelvic surgery and represents one of the most dreaded complications during gynecologic operations, with an overall incidence ranging from 0.5% to almost 30%.[1] Iatrogenic ureteral trauma encompasses ligature, crush, laceration, avulsion, stretch, and devascularization.[2,3] The rate of ureteral injury is increased when technically demanding laparoscopic and ureteroscopic manipulations are undertaken,[3-6] and suture ligation accounts for almost half of the cases.[7] Ureteral injury may be recognized intraoperatively and treated without any complications, or it may be overlooked and present in the immediate or late postoperative period, leading to substantial morbidity, threatening kidney viability, and justifying medicolegal litigation.[3,8,9]

COURSE OF URETER

The ureter is divided anatomically into two major components—(1) abdominal and (2) pelvic—with lengths ranging from 12 cm to 15 cm each. The ureter descends over the pelvic brim as it courses over the iliac vessels at the bifurcation of the common iliac artery into the external and internal iliac arteries **(Fig. 1)**. Deep in the pelvis, the ureter courses along the lateral aspect of the uterosacral ligament to enter the base of the broad ligament. The ureter is found 1.5 cm lateral to the cervix, passing under the uterine artery and then medially over the anterior vaginal fornix before entering the trigone of the bladder.[10] Radiologic studies have revealed that, in 10% of cases involving cervical pathology, the ureter may be only 5 mm from the cervix.[11] The most common locations of ureteral injury in pelvic surgery are at the cardinal ligament, where the ureter passes inferior to the uterine vessels, as well as the level of the infundibulopelvic (IP) ligament. The ureter can also be injured along the lateral border of the uterosacral ligament or along its course near the anterior vaginal wall. It has been suggested that during laparoscopic surgery specifically, the ureter is at greatest risk of injury at the IP ligament, in the ovarian fossa, and in the ureteric canal **(Fig. 2)**.[12]

In cases of laparoscopic adnexectomy, the ureter can be identified transperitoneally as it courses over the pelvic brim. The left ureter is often more challenging to view by this approach due to physiologic adhesions of the descending colon to the pelvic sidewall. This visualization may also be limited by the rectosigmoid colon or in cases involving inflammation, adhesions, and endometriosis. If the ureter is not clearly visualized at this level, a superficial incision in the peritoneum (taken parallel to the IP ligament) will allow for the initial development of the pararectal space; subsequent blunt dissection will identify the ureter. The rectosigmoid is then mobilized medially, which will enable a relatively easy identification of the left ureter at the pelvic brim. In severely distorted anatomy, it is best

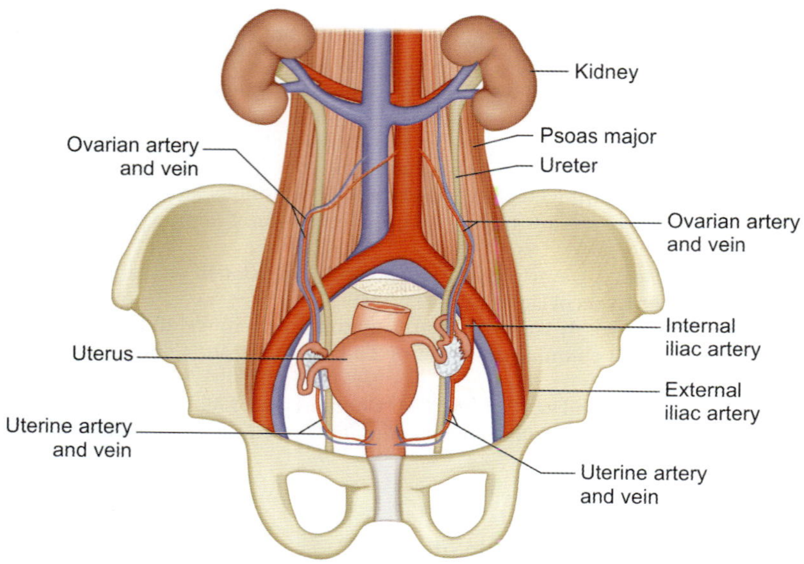

Fig. 1: Course of ureter.

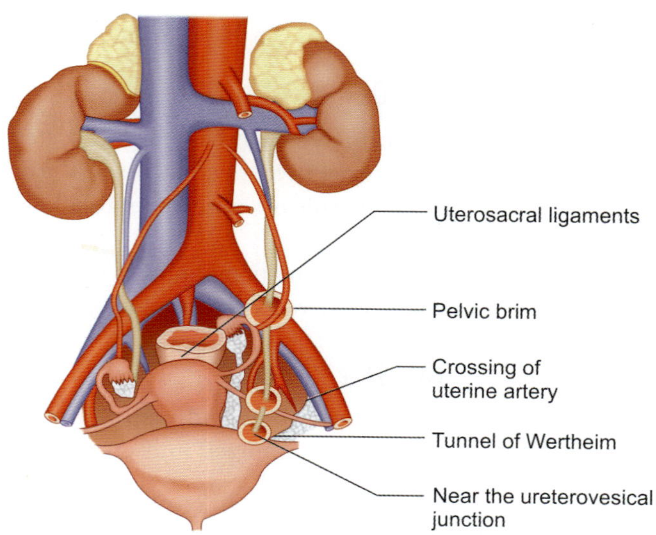

Fig. 2: Common sites of ureteral injury.

to find the ureter by making a peritoneal incision that begins just medial to the IP ligament and continues in the direction of the ischial spine. This way the ureter is found quicker than if the incision is continued parallel to the suspected course of the ureter. After ensuring that the ureter is sufficiently distant from the IP ligament, the blood supply to the ovary can be controlled. It is important to note that identification of the ureter at the pelvic brim is not adequate in cases involving significant deep pelvic adhesions, such as in severe endometriosis with rectovaginal involvement. In these cases, the ureters are often deviated more medially and the ureterolysis needs to be carried all the way down to the cardinal ligament. When approaching the cardinal ligament dissection during laparoscopic hysterectomy, a few techniques can help ensure that the ureter is sufficiently lateralized. First, sufficient skeletonization of the uterine vasculature will ensure that any peritoneal attachments involving the ureter are released. Second, it is important to maintain cranial deviation of the uterus with firm upward pressure on the uterine manipulator before cauterizing or incising the uterine vessels. Other procedures that necessitate special consideration regarding ureteral location include apical prolapse repairs (laparoscopic sacropexy or uterosacral suspension) and management of severe endometriosis or adhesive disease involving the pelvic sidewall or uterosacral ligaments. It is imperative that the ureter be identified along its entire course in these cases; ureterolysis should be performed as needed to ensure visualization or appropriate distance from the intended operative field.

DIAGNOSIS

Intraoperatively, if a ureteral injury is suspected **(Fig. 2)**, then a low threshold should be maintained for visual inspection of the ureters through meticulous dissection in an open operation or laparoscopically. The ureters may also be interrogated by cystoscopy and passage of a ureteral catheter in a retrograde fashion. When the patient is in a supine position and cystoscopy is difficult, a cystotomy may be performed, and ureteral catheters passed in a retrograde manner. The most sensitive diagnostic study for diagnosis of a ureteral injury is a retrograde pyelogram. This procedure also allows for possible treatment of a ureteral injury with retrograde indwelling stent placement.

When iatrogenic ureteral injuries present later in the postoperative course, the most common presenting signs and symptoms are abdominal pain with peritonitis, leukocytosis, and fever. Flank pain may or may not be present depending on the nature of the injury and whether the ureter is occluded, or has fistulized to the peritoneal cavity or retroperitoneal space.[13] Occasionally an urinoma may form in the confined space of the retroperitoneum and present as a flank mass. Immediate cystoscopy and retrograde pyelogram should be performed for diagnosis of a suspected ureteral injury and possible stenting. If cystoscopy and retrograde pyelogram cannot be performed then the preferred imaging technique is computed tomography with intravenous pyelogram (CT-IVP). A CT-IVP allows for visualization of the relevant anatomy and continuity of the upper urinary tract as well as the location of extravasated urine that often develops near a ureteral injury. Delayed scans using CT-IVP often reveal an enhancement of fluid collections as contrast leaks from a ureteric injury.[14]

SURGICAL MANAGEMENT

Surgical management for ureteral injury has been shown in **Figures 3A and B**.

Distal Ureteral Injuries

Ureteroneocystostomy

The majority of operative injuries occur in the distal ureter. The distal ureter is most often injured during attempts to ligate branches of the internal iliac vessels, and the injured ureter may have an even more tenuous blood supply than usual after these maneuvers. As the blood supply of the distal ureteral segment may be disrupted, ureteroneocystostomy is an ideal option for distal ureteral repair. When preparing the ureter for implantation, it should be judiciously debrided back to viable tissue and spatulated. The reimplantation site should be on the posterior or anterior dome of the bladder and not on the lateral aspects. Reimplantation of the ureter on the lateral aspects of the bladder is prone to kinking with bladder filling.[15] The reimplanted ureter should be stented and a Foley catheter maintained in the bladder perioperatively together with a Jackson-Pratt (JP) drain near the anastomosis. The Foley catheter may be removed in approximately 1 week and the JP drain removed once it is determined that the repair is not leaking. The stent is removed in 6 weeks **(Figs. 4 to 16)**.

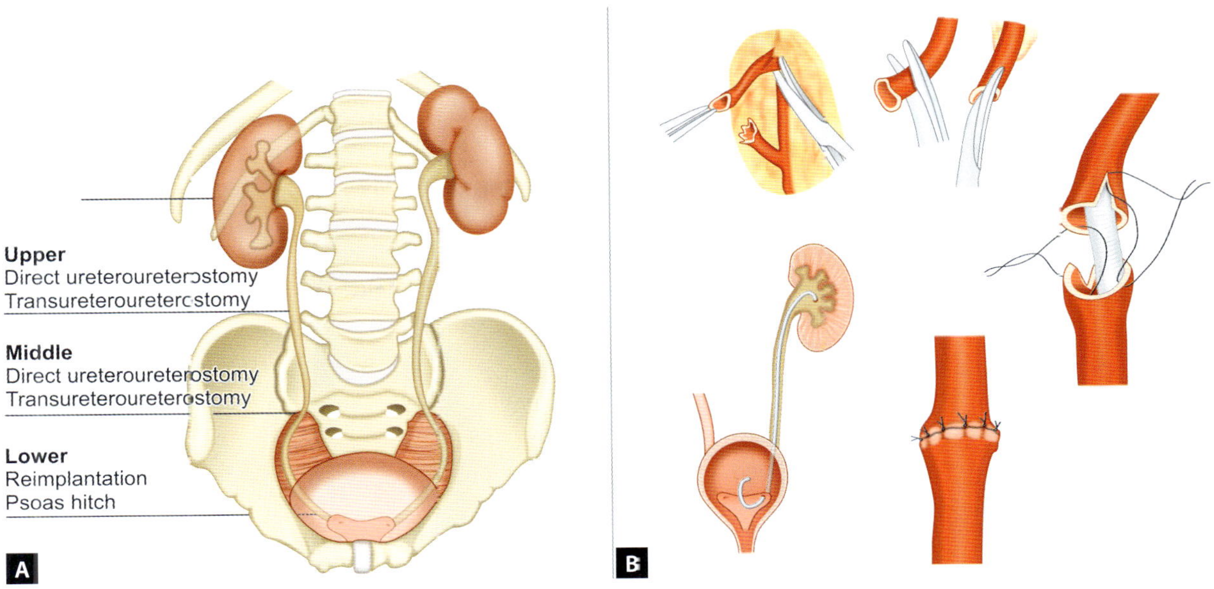

Figs. 3A and B: Surgical management for ureteral injury.

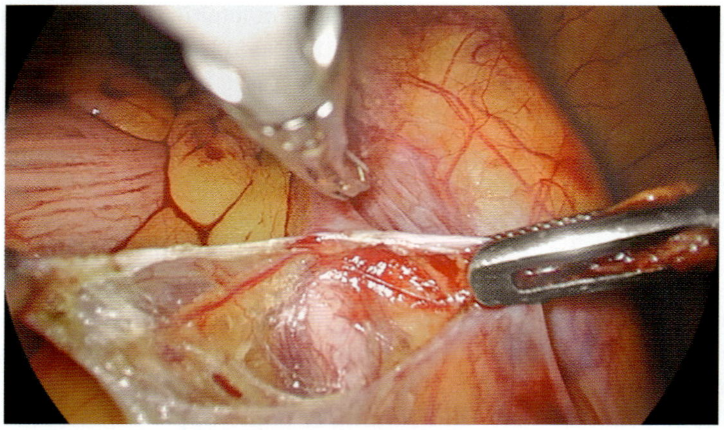

Fig. 4: Ureter exposed by dissecting overlying peritoneum.

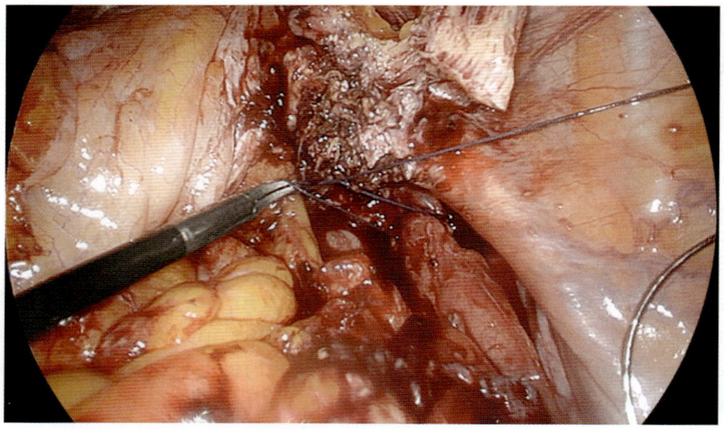

Fig. 5: Staysure placed at proximal ureteric stump.

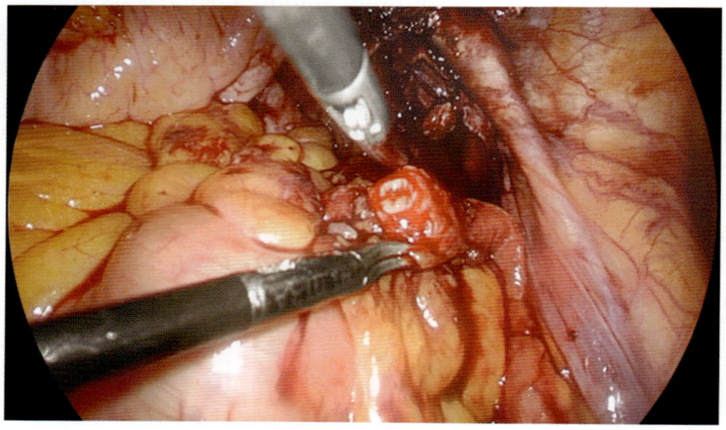

Fig. 6: Ureteric opening freshened.

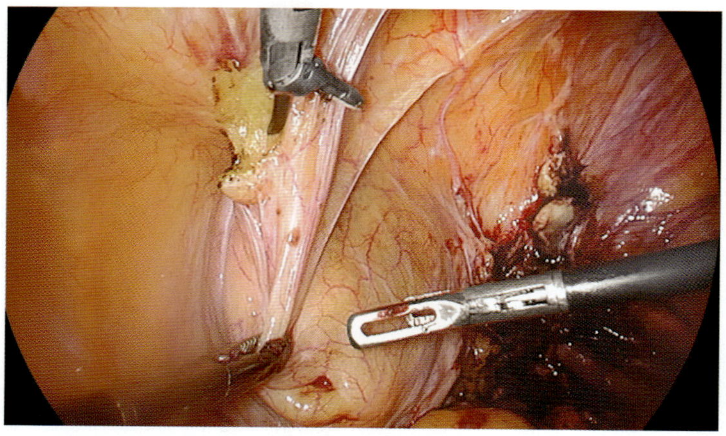

Fig. 7: Bladder mobilized.

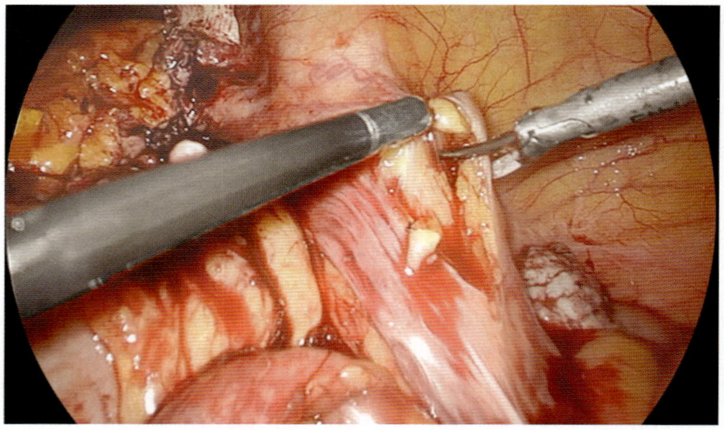

Fig. 8: Ipsilateral psoas muscle exposed.

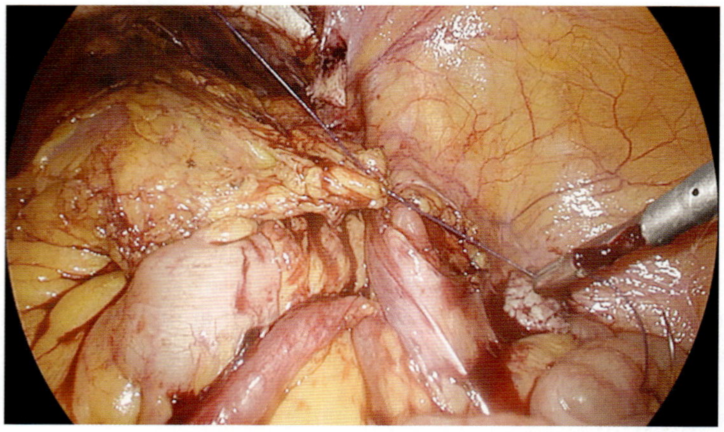

Fig. 9: Bladder fixed to ipsilateral psoas muscle.

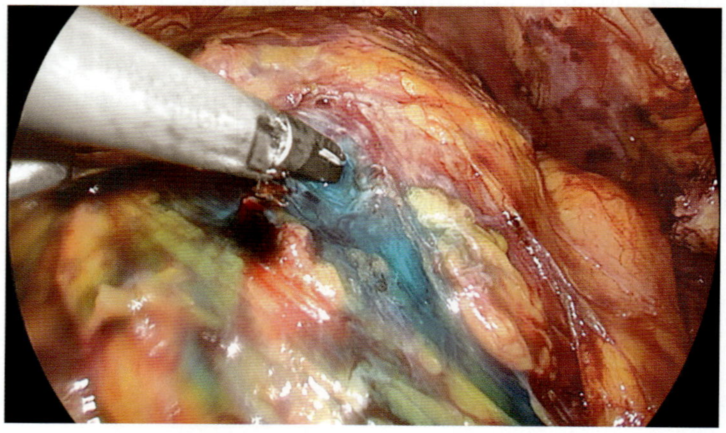

Fig. 10: New ureteric opening created in bladder.

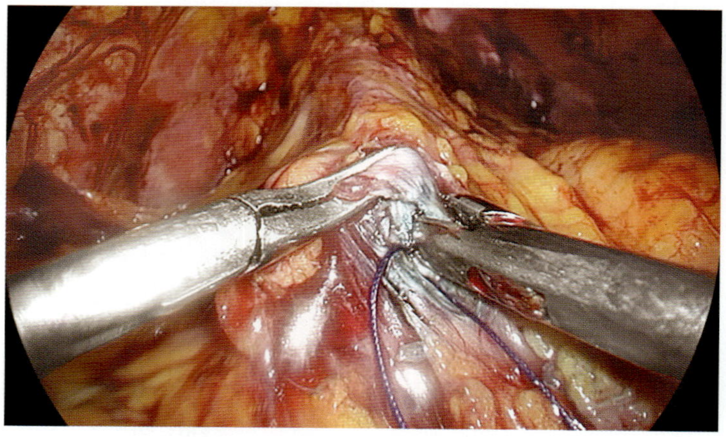

Fig. 11: Stay suture placed in bladder.

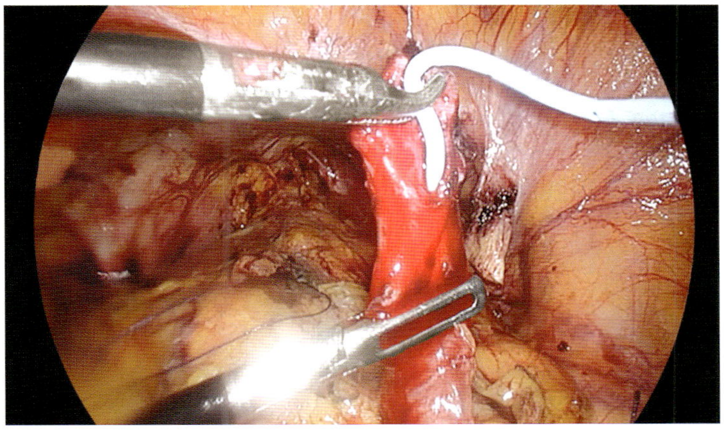
Fig. 12: Double-J (DJ) stent introduced into proximal ureteric stump.

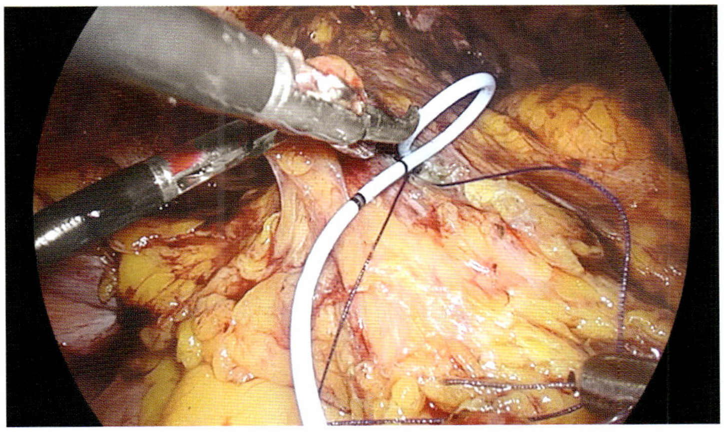
Fig. 13: Double-J stent introduced into bladder.

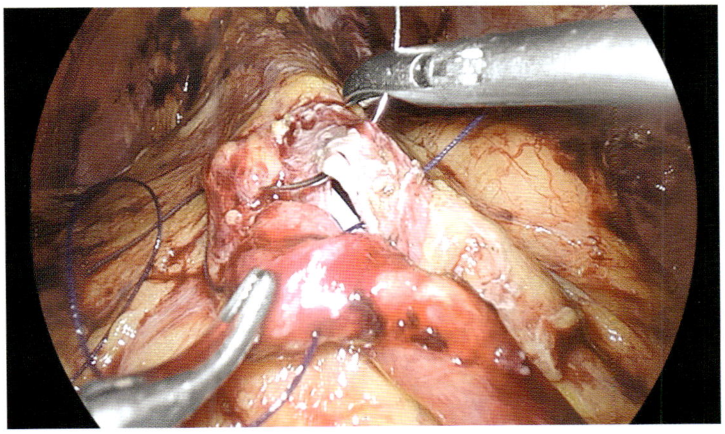
Fig. 14: New ureteric opening on bladder sutured to ureter.

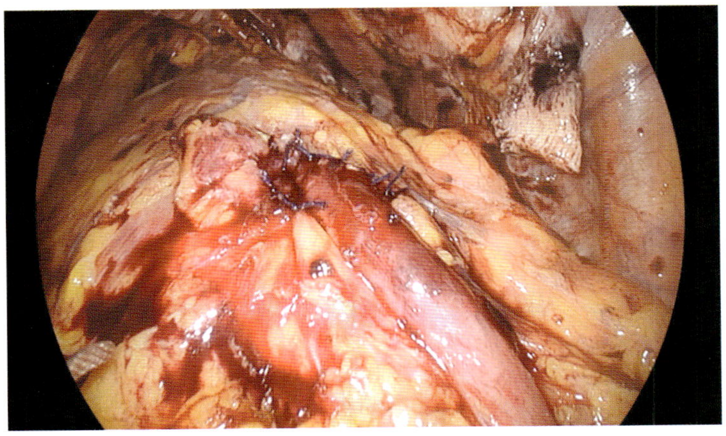
Fig. 15: Stitch placed at 12, 9, 6, and 3 o'clock position.

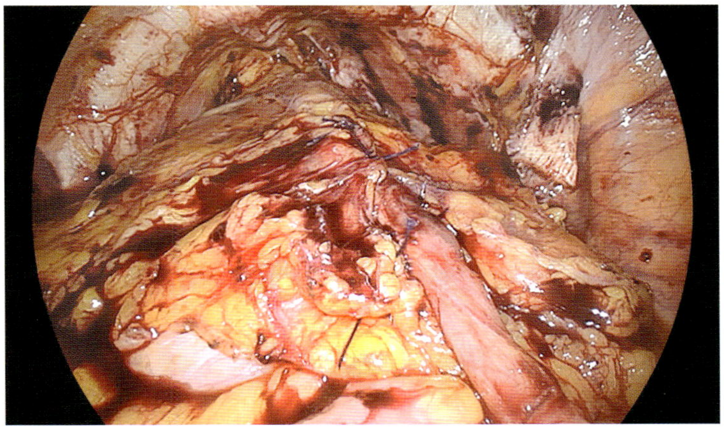
Fig. 16: Omental flap placed.

Vesicopsoas Hitch

When a lengthy defect in the distal ureter is discovered, such that performing a simple ureteroneocystostomy would result in tension on the anastomosis, often this distance can be bridged with a vesicopsoas hitch, first described by Zimmerman and colleagues.[16] Mobilization of the bladder in the space of Retzius and ligation of the contralateral bladder pedicle aids in positioning the bladder near the psoas muscle. The bladder detrusor is then "hitched" to the psoas muscle with longitudinal, nonabsorbable monofilament sutures to make up the length between the bladder and proximal ureteral stump. Care is taken to avoid the genitofemoral nerve that lies on the anterior surface of the psoas muscle. The ureter is then reimplanted into the repositioned bladder in a similar manner to the previously mentioned ureteroneocystostomy.

Upper and Midureteral Injuries

Ureteroureterostomy

Often with small (2–3 cm) defects of the midureter and upper ureter a primary ureteroureterostomy can be performed.[17] The distal and proximal ureteral ends are debrided back to viable tissue and a standard running or interrupted anastomosis is performed. The anastomosis should be stented and, if possible, covered with peritoneum or other tissue.

Boari Tubularized Bladder Flap

When a midureteral or proximal ureteral injury occurs and the distal ureteral segment is not suitable for anastomosis, a Boari tubularized bladder flap is often a viable alternative. The bladder is opened on its anterior surface, and a full thickness bladder flap is swung cranially and tubularized for anastomosis to the proximal ureteral segment **(Figs. 17A and B)**. This is a technically challenging procedure and should be referred to a center with urologic reconstruction experience if necessary.

Transureteroureterostomy

Most often the length of ureteral loss as a result of iatrogenic ureteral injury is quite short making transureteroureterostomy (TUU) unnecessary. In cases when primary reanastomosis to a distal segment is not feasible, or if an ureteroneocystostomy is precluded (i.e. rectal injury, major vascular injury, or extensive bladder injury), then TUU is an acceptable option. Contraindications to TUU include inadequate donor ureter length, which would create tension on the anastomosis, or disease of the recipient ureter such as urothelial carcinoma, urolithiasis, retroperitoneal fibrosis, or pelvic tumors with ureteral involvement.[18] The donor ureter should be extensively mobilized, but care should be taken not to disrupt the longitudinal blood supply in the adventitial layer. Very little of the recipient ureter should be mobilized so that the area of anastomosis has a sufficient blood supply. The donor ureter should be passed under the sigmoid colon through the mesentery to the location of the recipient ureter. The donor ureter is then spatulated approximately 2 cm and the recipient ureter is opened to match the donor ureter opening.[18] An end-to-side anastomosis is performed. The donor ureter should be stented with the stent passing through the distal portion of the recipient ureter down to the bladder. An attempt should be made to try to reperitonealize the ureteral anastomosis if possible **(Figs. 18 to 20)**.

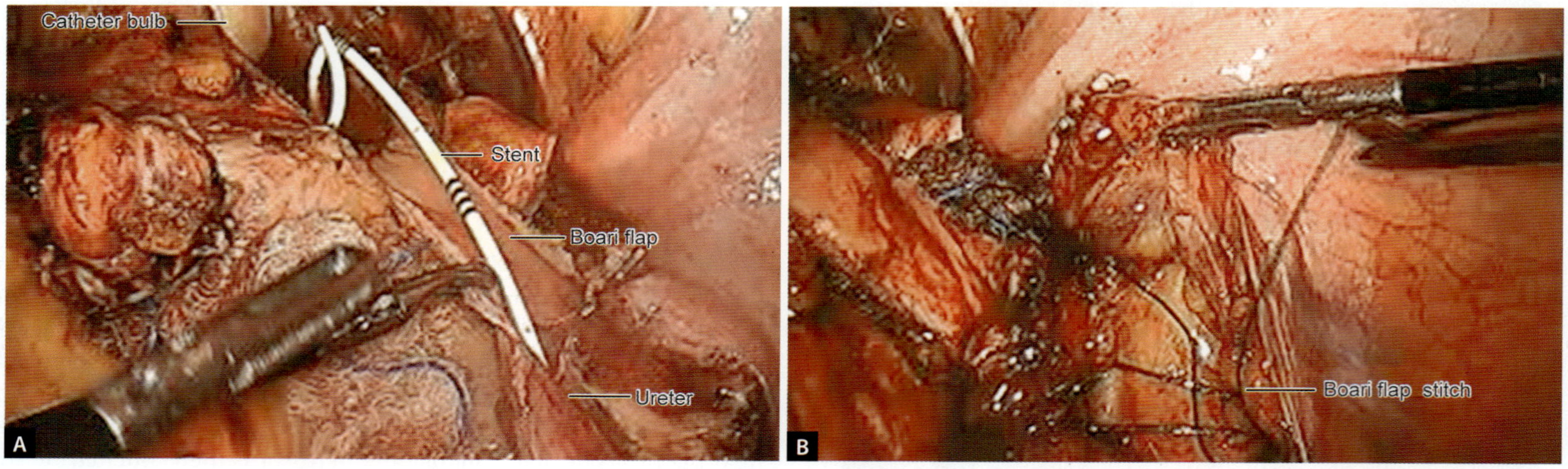

Figs. 17A and B: Proximal ureteric injury repaired by Boari flap method.

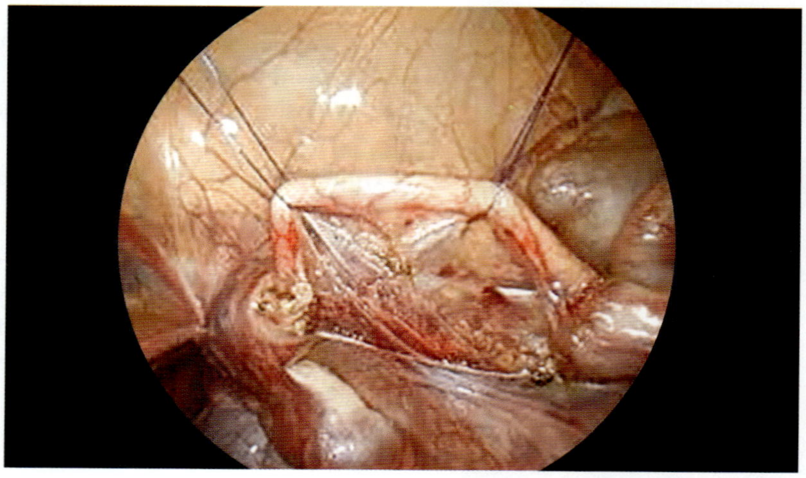

Fig. 18: Ureter held up with stay suture.

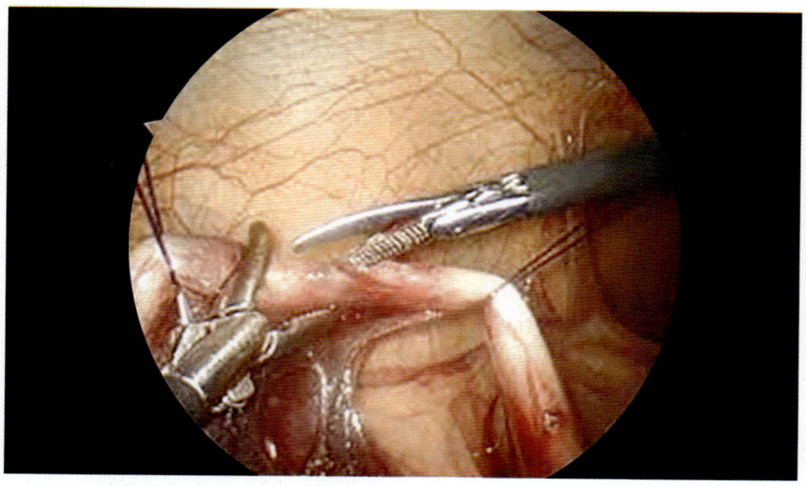

Fig. 19: Edges freshened up.

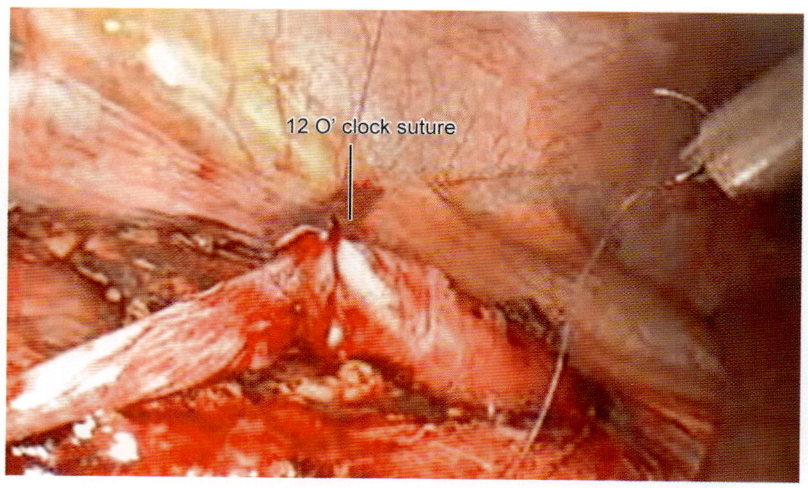

Fig. 20: Ureteric openings anastomosed to each other.

Renal Autotransplantation

Renal autotransplantation is rarely if ever indicated at the time of intraoperative consultation for ureteral injury. If an iatrogenic ureteral injury precludes ureteral reconstruction and renal autotransplantation is being considered, then the ureter should be ligated and a percutaneous nephrostomy tube placed for renal drainage.

Ureteral Substitution

The use of gastrointestinal segments, such as ileum for ureteral substitution, was first popularized in the 1950s by Goodwin and colleagues.[19] Other reported tissue sources for ureteral substitution include appendix, tubularized stomach, and colon.[20] By far the most common source of tissue for ureteral replacement is the ileum.

Laparoscopic and Minimally Invasive Treatment of Ureteral Injuries

Laparoscopy and minimally invasive surgical techniques have transformed modern surgical care. Not surprisingly the management of iatrogenic ureteral injuries also encompasses these techniques. Possibly the most minimally invasive treatment of an iatrogenic ureteral injury is cystoscopy and retrograde ureteral stent placement or antegrade placement of a ureteral stent. A recent series describes the management of iatrogenic ureteral injuries with minimally invasive techniques such as percutaneous nephrostomy tube placement, wire recanalization of the ureteral lumen, antegrade ureteral dilation, and ureteral stent placement.

Laparoscopic techniques for the management of ureteral injuries include ureteroureterostomy, ureteroneocystostomy, and Boari flap procedures. In a comparative retrospective review of patients undergoing laparoscopic and open techniques for ureteral reimplantation, patients undergoing distal ureteral reimplantation laparoscopically required less pain medication, had a shorter length of stay, and less blood loss.[21]

REFERENCES

1. Gangai MP, Agee RE, Spence CR. Surgical injury to ureter. Urology. 1976;8:22-7.
2. Drake MJ, Noble JG. Ureteric trauma in gynecologic surgery. Int Urogynecol J Pelvic Floor Dysfunct. 1998;9:108-17.
3. Utrie JW Jr. Bladder and ureteral injury: prevention and management. Clin Obstet Gynecol. 1998;41:755-63.
4. Harkki-Siren P, Sjoberg J, Tiitinen A. Urinary tract injuries after hysterectomy. Obstet Gynecol. 1998;92:113-8.
5. Assimos DG, Patterson LC, Taylor CL. Changing incidence and etiology of iatrogenic ureteral injuries. J Urol. 1994;152:2240-6.
6. Selzman AA, Spirnak JP. Iatrogenic ureteral injuries: a 20-year experience in treating 165 injuries. J Urol. 1996;155:878-81.
7. Sakellariou P, Protopapas AG, Voulgaris Z, et al. Management of ureteric injuries during gynecological operations: 10 years' experience. Eur J Obstet Gynecol Reprod Biol. 2002;101:179-84.
8. Williams TJ. Urologic injuries. Obstet Gynecol Annu. 1975;4:347-68.
9. Preston JM. Iatrogenic ureteric injury: common medicolegal pitfalls. BJU Int. 2000;86:313-7.
10. Fröber R. Surgical anatomy of the ureter. BJU Int. 2007;100:949-65.
11. Gemer O, Simonovsky A, Huerta M, et al. A radiological study on the anatomical proximity of the ureters and the cervix. Int Urogynecol J Pelvic Floor Dysfunct. 2007;18:991-5.
12. Hurt WG, Jones CM III. Intraoperative ureteral injuries and urinary diversion. In: Nichols DH (Ed). Gynecologic and Obstetric Surgery. Baltimore, MD: Mosby; 1993. pp. 900-10.
13. Grainger D, Soderstom R, Schiff S, et al. Ureteral injuries at laparoscopy: insights into diagnosis, management and prevention. Obstet Gynecol. 1990;75:839-43.
14. Gayer G, Zissin R, Apter S, et al. Urinomas caused by ureteral injuries: CT appearance. Abdom Imaging. 2002;27:88-92.
15. Hensle T, Berdon W, Baker D, et al. The ureteral "J" sign: radiographic demonstration of iatrogenic distal ureteral obstruction after ureteral reimplantation. J Urol. 1982;127:766-8.
16. Zimmerman I, Precourt W, Thompson C. Direct uretero-cysto-neostomy with the short ureter in the cure of ureterovaginal fistula. J Urol. 1960;83:113-5.
17. Coburn M. Ureteral injuries from surgical trauma. In: McAninch JW (Ed). Traumatic and Reconstructive Urology. Philadelphia, PA: Saunders; 1996.
18. Iwaszko M, Krambeck A, Chow G, et al. Transureteroureterostomy revisited: long-term surgical outcomes. J Urol. 2010;183:1055-9.
19. Goodwin W, Winter C, Turner R. Replacement of the ureter by small intestine: clinical application and results of the ileal ureter. J Urol 1959;81:406-18.
20. Moreira S, Carrion R, Seigne J, et al. Non-conventional alternatives for ureteral replacement. J Urol. 2004;171:65.
21. Rassweiler JJ, Gozen AS, Erdogru T, et al. Ureteral reimplantation for management of ureteral strictures: a retrospective comparison of laparoscopic and open techniques. Eur Urol. 2007;51:512-23.

CHAPTER

28

Laparoscopically-assisted Neovaginoplasty

Kavya Rashmi Rao, Aditi Rai, B Ramesh

INTRODUCTION

Most significant congenital anomalies of the female reproductive tract is vaginal agenesis. Neovaginal reconstruction is needed for multitude of congenital and acquired causes of partial or total absence of vaginal canal. Mayer–Rokitansky–Küster–Hauser (MRKH) syndrome (Rokitansky syndrome) is the frequent indication for neovaginoplasty. This chapter focuses on new surgical techniques in which laparoscopy has replaced traditional surgery which has been the treatment of choice in rare congenital anomalies.

Mayer–Rokitansky–Küster–Hauser syndrome is characterized by uterine and vaginal aplasia. Typically, presentation is primary amenorrhea with normal secondary sexual characters, blind vagina, absence of uterus, and cervix on ultrasonography with normal 46XX karyotype.[1] MRKH syndrome is mostly associated with renal, skeletal, and other anomalies. The exact incidence of Rokitansky syndrome is unknown, although a recent study estimated that vaginal agenesis (MRKH syndrome) affects 1 in 4,000 to 1 in 10,000 women.[2]

For creation of a neovagina, there are various techniques including using dilators (Frank method) or passive pressure applied by a bicycle seat (Ingram method).[3,4] Operative techniques include interposition of intestinal segments, such as ileum or sigmoid,[5,6] myocutaneous flaps,[7-9] grafts of skin,[10] peritoneum,[11] or amnion,[12] and even use of synthetic absorbable membranes such as oxidized regenerated cellulose (Interceed, Ethicon Endo-Surgery, Cincinnati, OH) to simulate vaginal mucosa.[13]

Vecchietti procedure is a unique surgical and nonsurgical techniques, then later modified via a laparoscopic approach and first described in 1992 (**Table 1**).[14-17] This chapter explains detail about Vecchietti laparoscopic procedure.

Table 1: Different types of neovaginoplasty method.

Author	*Methods*
Frank (1931)	Intermittent use of vaginal dilators
D'alberton (1971)	Sexual activity (functional method)
Ingram (1981)	Intermittent pressure with bicycle seat
Baldwin (1906)	Double ileal segment transplantation
Popoff (1910)	Rectal segment transplantation
Schubert (1911)	Sigmoid segment transplantation
Graves (1921)	Pedunculated skin flaps from vulva and thigh
Frank and Geist (1927)	Cylindric dermoepidermal flaps from thigh
Brindeau (1934)	Perineal dissection and transplantation of amniotic membrane and insertion of vaginal stent for continuous dilation
Wharton (1938)	Perineal dissection and insertion of balsa wood vaginal stent for continuous dilatation
McIndoe (1938)	Perineal dissection and transplantation of skin flaps and insertion of vaginal stent for continuous dilatation
William (1964)	Creation of vulvovaginal pouch
Vecchietti (1965)	Traction from above on the hymen pseudomembrane
Davydov (1969)	Perineal dissection and transplantation of peritoneum and insertion of vaginal stent for continuous dilatation

SURGICAL ANATOMY

Gonadal indifferentiation phase is 4–6 weeks and it will differentiate around 7 weeks. Reproductive ducts differentiate between 9 weeks and 11 weeks and external genitalia differentiate between 10 weeks and 12 weeks. The main events critical to the in utero development of the female gynecological tract are given in **Table 2**.

Table 2: Main events critical to the in-utero development of the female gynecological tract.

Phase of genital development	*Time of gestation (in weeks)*
Indifferent gonadal phase	4–6
Gonadal differentiation	7
Ductal differentiation	9–11
External genitalia differentiation	10–12

Relationship between the Early Fetal Genital and Urinary Systems

There are three distinct stages of renal development (**Fig. 1**): pronephros, mesonephros, and metanephros (permanent kidney). In the third fetal week, paired pronephros develop which regress by the fifth week in the cervical region. In the fourth week, mesonephros develop just below the pronephros in the thoracic region. The paired mesonephric ducts (Wolffian duct) drain the mesonephros into the cloaca (**Figs. 2A to C**). The mesonephros and mesonephric ducts regress by the third month, but vestigial structures such as the Gartner's duct, epoophoron, and the paraoophoron may persist and are described later (**Figs. 3A to D**).

Development of the Genital Tract

- Genital system is in an indifferent state till the end of the sixth week. Invagination of the coelomic epithelium to form paramesonephric ducts. The invagination takes place at the lateral most part of the coelomic epithelium. Müllerian ducts grow downward and lateral to corresponding Wolffian ducts. Caudal part, the Müllerian ducts, passes medially to the Wolffian ducts. Each side of the Müllerian ducts is fused as a single solid rod of cells. Upper lateral part of Müllerian duct → Fallopian tube.

- Cranial point of fusion of Müllerian ducts—fundus of uterus.
- Lower part fuses to each other and form uterus, cervix, and upper one-third of the vagina.

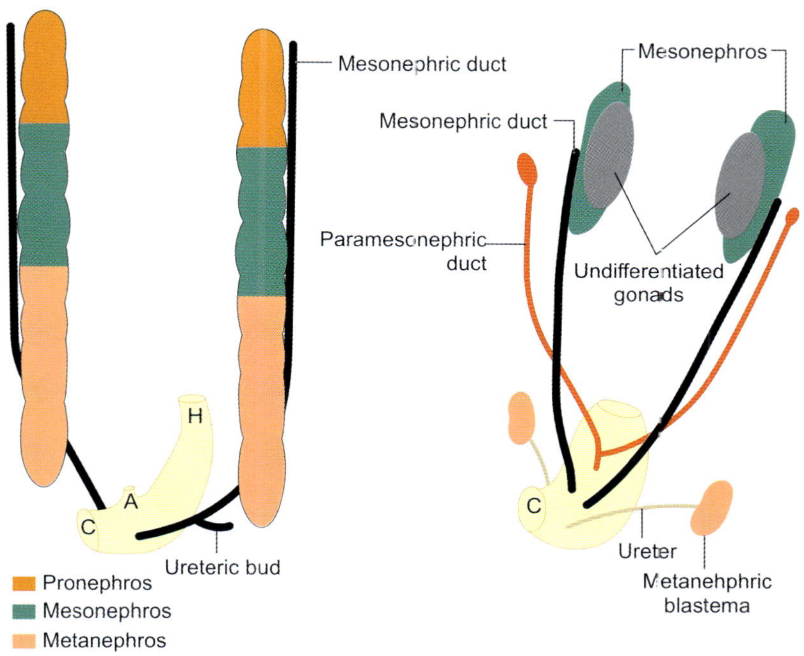

Fig. 1: Stages of renal development.

- During the third month of embryonic life, vagina develops. Vaginal plate develops from uterovaginal canal and sinovaginal bulb (develops from posterior aspect of urogenital sinus) which later canalizes to form vaginal canal.

Development of the Lower Genital Tract

The Cloaca

The hymen is formed by embryonic septum between Müllerian tubercle above and urogenital sinus proper below. Both endodermal and mesodermal origin. A membrane separating the vagina from the urogenital sinus develops and is normally perforated by birth.

In the third fetal week, cloacal membrane is formed which is under the umbilical cord **(Figs. 4A and B)**. The cloacal membrane remains imperforate at this time.

The Urogenital Sinus

During the seventh week, the urorectal septum fuses to the inner surface of the cloacal membrane, and it forms the anterior (ventral) urogenital membrane and the posterior anal membrane. Rectum proper is separated from the urogenital tract posterior anal membrane **(Fig. 4C)**.

Differentiation of the urogenital sinus: Urogenital system consists of a caudal phallic portion and a pelvic portion **(Fig. 4D)**. Vaginal introitus (vestibule) formed by the urethral groove and phallic (distal) portion of the urogenital sinus **(Fig. 4E)**. This is closed off externally by the urogenital membrane, which perforates in the seventh week. Definitive urogenital sinus forms short distal female urethra and lower third of the vagina **(Fig. 4F)**.

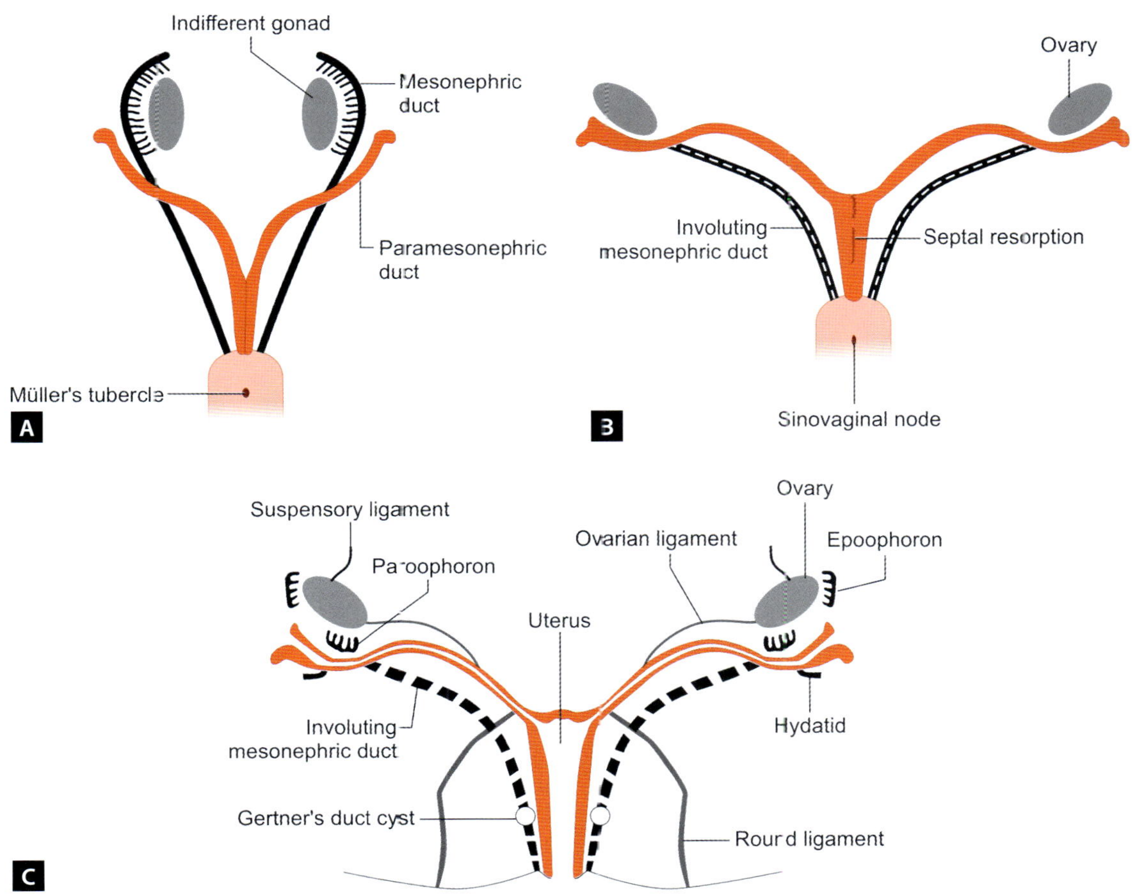

Figs. 2A to C: Mesonephric ducts drain the mesonephros into cloaca.

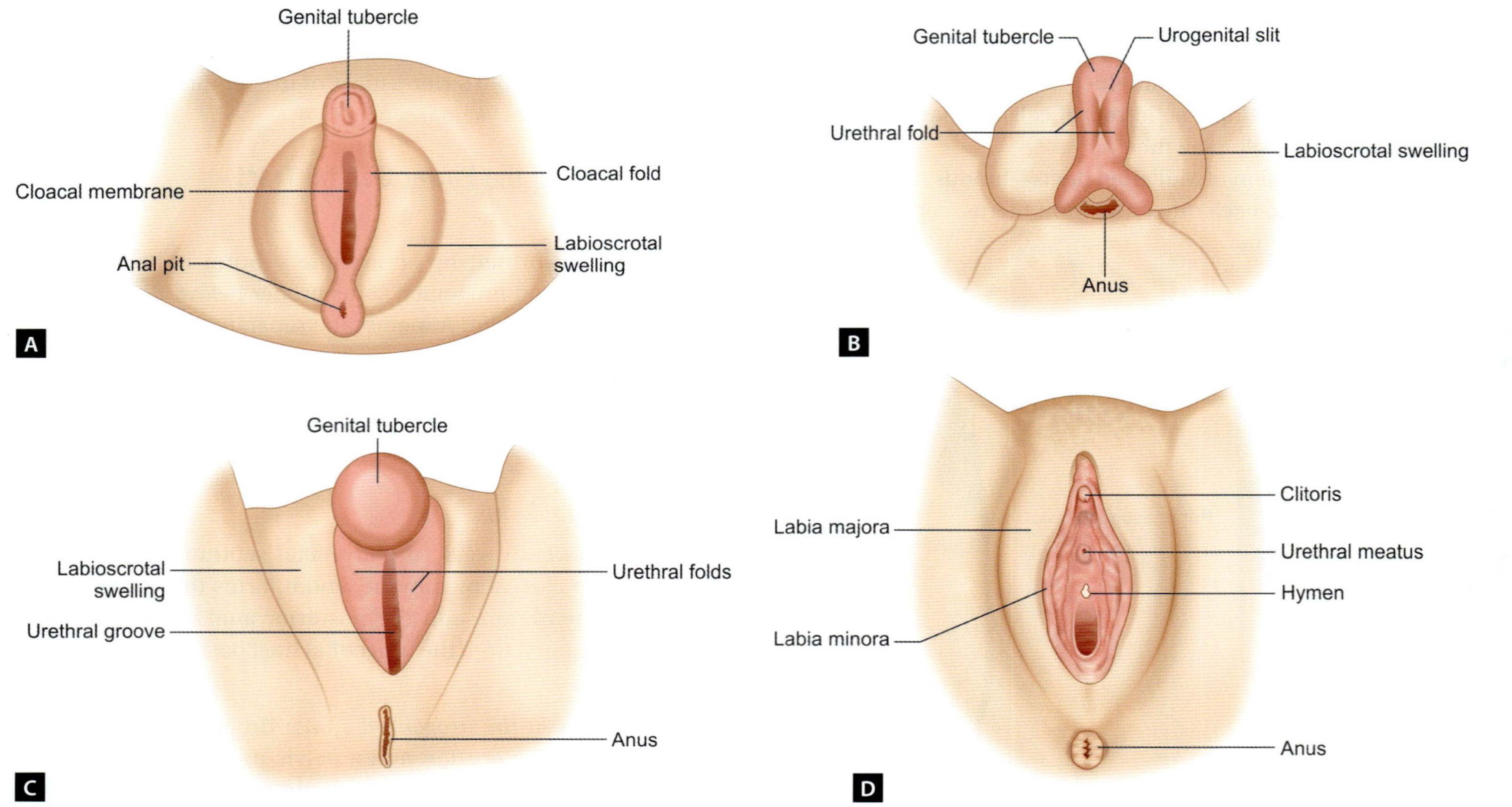

Figs. 3A to D: Differentiation of the female external genitalia. Stages of development at (A) 4 weeks (indifferent stage); (B) 6–7 weeks; (C) 9–11 weeks; (D) 12 weeks (full differentiation).

Development of the External Genitalia

Around seventh fetal week, external genitalia remain sexually undifferentiated. Sexual characteristics appear during the 10th week and around 12th week, complete differentiation occurs.

Abnormal Development of Müllerian Duct

Interruption or dysregulation in Müllerian duct development at various stages of morphogenesis **(Table 3)**.

Causes:

- Genetics
- Intrauterine elements
- Extrauterine elements
- Diethylstilbestrol (DES) and thalidomide have been associated with Müllerian duct anomalies.

Mayer–Rokitansky–Küster–Hauser Syndrome

Mayer–Rokitansky–Küster–Hauser syndrome is a rare congenital disorder characterized by uterine and vaginal aplasia. Typically, presentation is primary amenorrhea with normal secondary sexual characters, blind vagina, absence of uterus, and cervix on ultrasonography with normal 46XX karyotype. Associated abnormalities of the kidneys and other organ systems are often seen. Hippocrates described a membranous obstruction of the vagina in the book on the nature of women. A few centuries later, Celsius presented a complete description of vaginal atresia.[1] Mayer in 1829[2] and Rokitansky in 1838[3] described a syndrome that included agenesis of the uterus and vagina due to an anomalous development of the Müllerian ducts. Subsequently, Küster[4] recognized urologic

Table 3: Scheme for the classification of female genital tract anomalies according to the new ESHRE/ESGE classification system

Uterine anomaly		
	Main class	*Sub-class*
U0	Normal uterus	
U1	Dysmorphic uterus	• T-shaped • Infantilis • Others
U2	Septate uterus	• Partial • Complete
U3	Bicorporeal uterus	• Partial • Complete • Bicorporeal septate
U4	Hemi-uterus	• With rudimentary cavity (communicating or not horn) • Without rudimentary cavity (horn without cavity/no horn)
U5	Aplastic	• With rudimentary cavity (bi- or unilateral horn) • Without rudimentary cavity (bi- or unilateral uterine remnants/aplasia)
U6	Unclassified malformations	

Cervical/vaginal anomaly	
Co-existent class	
C0	Normal cervix
C1	Septate cervix
C2	Double 'normal' cervix
C3	Unilateral cervical aplasia
C4	Cervical aplasia
V0	Normal vagina
V1	Longitudinal non-obstructing vaginal septum
V2	Longitudinal obstructing vaginal septum
V3	Transverse vaginal septum and/or imperforate hymen
V4	Vaginal aplasia

U	C	V
Associated anomalies of non-Müllerian origin:		
Drawing of the anomaly		

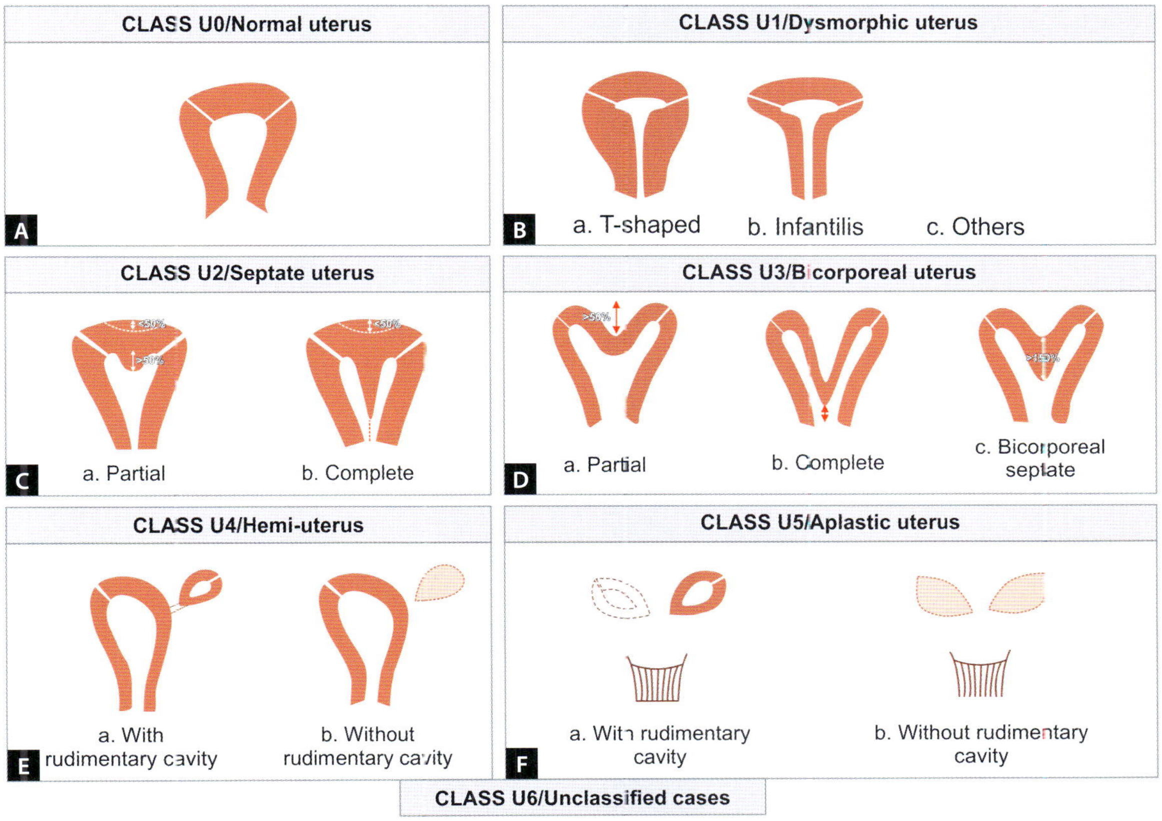

Figs. 4A to F: Vaginal agenesis, which is frequently accompanied by urinary tract anomalies, is discussed in Class I - Vaginal Agenesis.

associations whereas Hauser[5] distinguished Rokitansky syndrome from testicular feminization. Rokitansky syndrome is the major cause of primary amenorrhea.

Etiology of Rokitansky syndrome is not yet understood. It occurs sporadically but has been described in sisters with a normal karyotype and in a pair of monozygotic twins. The majority of the patients have normal female karyotype, although some shows a mosaicism of sex chromosomes (45X/46XX; 46XX/47XX). The exposure to a teratogenic agent during fourth gestational week may be responsible for Rokitansky syndrome as well as for the frequently associated anomalies of skeletal and urinary systems. Indeed, in this intrauterine stage, the pronephric duct and cervicothoracic somite blastemal are closely linked.

The genital anatomy of Rokitansky syndrome is distinguished by normal genitalia and absence of the upper two-thirds of the vagina **(Fig. 5)**.

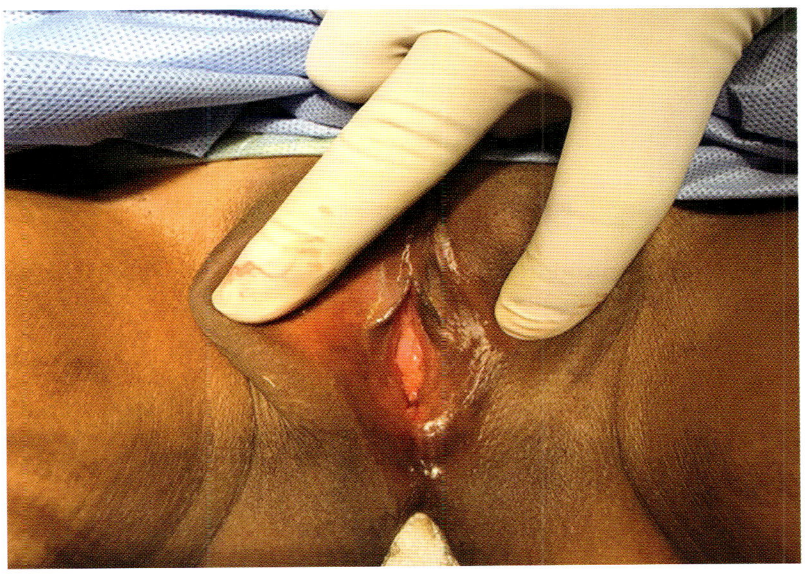

Fig. 5: Blind vaginal pouch.

Other findings:

- Blind retrohymenal pouch—up to 2 cm deep.
- Uterus absent/two fibromuscular cords are found originating from medial aspect of tubal extremities and fused along the median lines resembling a double rudimentary uterus **(Figs. 6A and B)**.
- Asymmetric and distinct rudimentary horns are seldom found and are usually of greatest size.
  Sometimes, these horns may appear hollow and lined with endometrial tissues that is generally hyporesponsive to cyclic hormonal modification. Sometimes, the horns may also rarely be site of menstruation as seen in reports of subjects with Rokitansky syndrome developing hematometra in one or both rudimentary horns.
- The salpinges and ovaries are normal with rare chance of ovarian anomalies such as unilateral agenesis.

Rokitansky syndrome is most of the times associated with malformations of the urinary and skeletal systems, with rare possibility of congenital cardiac anomalies.

Classification

Clinical Presentation

Between 70 and 80% of women present with primary amenorrhea.[9,10]

Examination reveals normal secondary sexual characteristics and a short, blind-ending vagina.[2]

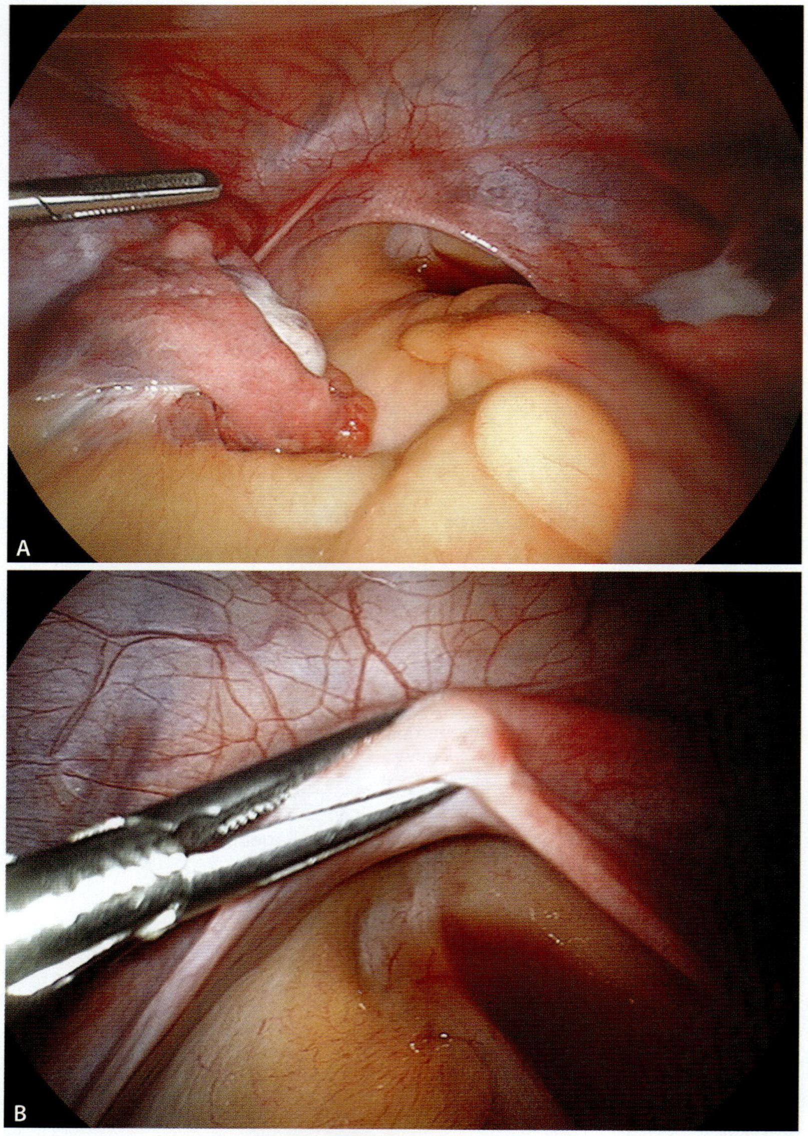

Figs. 6A and B: Rudimentary uterus.

General examination may show associated musculoskeletal abnormalities. If functioning endometrium is present, cyclical abdominal pain may be the presenting symptom, necessitating removal of the horns.[2,8]

Other rare presenting complaints are subfertility and dyspareunia.[9]

Mayer–Rokitansky–Küster–Hauser syndrome is classified into three types:

1. *Typical (type I):* Isolated symmetrical uterovaginal aplasia or hypoplasia
2. *Atypical (type II):* Asymmetrical uterovaginal aplasia or hypoplasia, hypoplasia of one or both fallopian tubes and malformation in the ovaries and/or the renal system.
3. MURCS (Müllerian duct aplasia, renal dysplasia and cervical somite anomalies) syndrome.

ANATOMICAL ABNORMALITIES

The caudal portions of the Müllerian ducts are involved, in type I MRKH syndrome. This is characterized by two rudimentary uterine buds connected by a peritoneal fold, normal Fallopian tubes with absence of the upper part of the vagina **(Fig. 7)**.

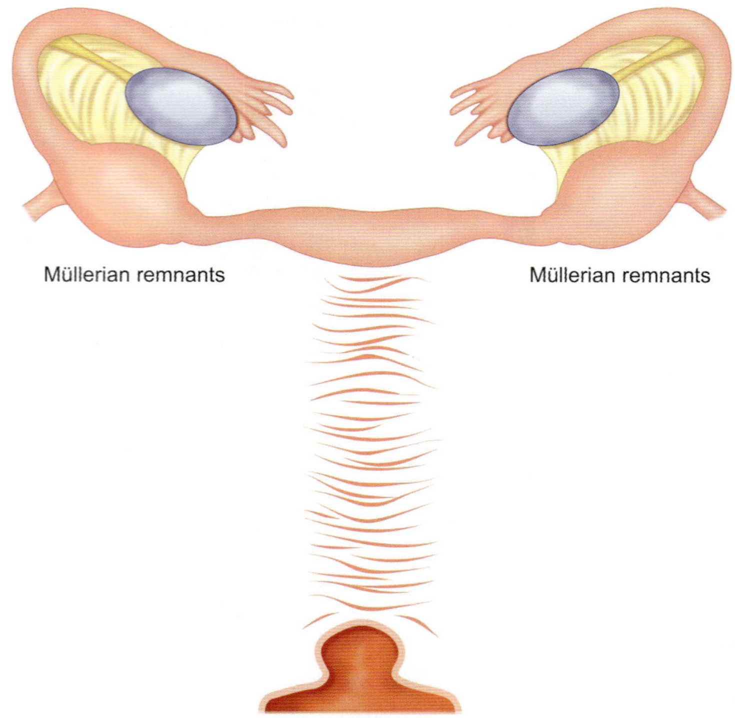

Fig. 7: Type 1 MRKH syndrome.

In type II MRKH syndrome, there is asymmetrical hypoplasia of the uterine buds with or without hypoplasia of one or both Fallopian tubes;[2,19-21] 7–10% of the women will have rudimentary uterus with functional endometrium and 25% will have cavitated Müllerian remnants.[22,23] Ovaries are absent, hypoplastic, or extrapelvic (pelvic brim) in 10–15% in cases.[2,21,22,24]

OTHER ORGAN ABNORMALITIES

Most common abnormality is renal abnormality which was reported in up to 40% of women like renal agenesis, ectopic kidney, horseshoe kidney, and ectopic ureter.[19,22,24] 12–20% of women will have skeletal abnormalities, comprising Klippel–Feil anomaly, fused vertebrae, radial aplasia, absent thumb, scoliosis, and radial hypoplasia.[19,21,22,24]

In 10–25% of cases, auditory malformations has seen. Stapedial ankylosis and sensorineural deafness are reported due to conductive deafness.[23]

Rarely, cardiac abnormality such as tetralogy of Fallot, patent ductus arteriosus and truncus arteriosus are reported.[19,22,24]

SYMPTOMS

Clinical Presentation

In 70–80% of cases, women come to OPD (outpatient department) with complaint of primary amenorrhea and sexual dysfunction but with normal endocrine workup and normal secondary sexual features.

If women have rudimentary uterine bodies with functioning endometrium, they would present with cyclical abdominal pain after development of secondary sexual characters. Sexual intercourse is almost always problematic because of blind vaginal pouch which may be problematic initially but after a certain period, sexual activity may become satisfactory due to stretching of ectodermal vaginal residue.

Differential Diagnosis

- Complete androgen insensitivity syndrome (CAIS) is characterized by no axillary or pubic hair, karyotype is 46 XY, but the phenotype is a tall female with short, blind vagina.

- Imperforate hymen and agenesis of the lower part of the vagina and transverse lower vaginal septum.

Diagnosis

Diagnosis of Rokitansky syndrome is usually apparent on a clinical examination, which demonstrates normal external genitalia and absence of the vagina. Rectal examination often confirms absence of uterus or presence of small fibrous nodule.

The presence of normal pubic and axillary hair growth permits exclusion of androgen insensitivity syndrome. A transabdominal ultrasound scan usually confirms absence of uterus and if present shows median rudimentary uterus or laterally displaced rudimentary horns.[25]

Magnetic resonance imaging (MRI) is the imaging method that best defines the anatomic features of Rokitansky syndrome, especially the subperitoneal structures and possible endometrial cavitations.

Presence of endometrium within a rudimentary horn may be confirmed during laparoscopy by endoscopic ultrasound probe **(Fig. 8)**.

Treatment

In spite of numerous surgical and nonsurgical techniques proposed in the past **(Table 1)**, standardized and internationally acknowledged treatment for correction of Rokitansky syndrome still does not exist. All surgical procedures aim at creating neovagina by means of separating the rectal-urethrovesical space as well as maintaining an open cavity, thus ensuring its reepithelization.

Nonsurgical method proposed by Frank in 1938[3] has been applied in patients with relatively deep (2–3 cm) retrohymenal pouch. Some authors observed that patients with Rokitansky syndrome were able to achieve a vagina of adequate depth and caliber solely with sexual activity. The most widely known surgical approaches are surgery proposed by McIndoe in 1938,[10] which requires surgical creation of tunnel in the rectal-urethrovesical space, which is then coated with strip of skin taken from the buttocks or from the medial aspect of the thigh. Among the surgical operations requiring dissection of rectal-urethrovesical space for creation of neovagina, the best results can be achieved by the method proposed by Davydov[11] and Rothman,[26] in which the tunnel formed by surgical dissection is coated by pelvic peritoneum that is mobilized and pulled downward toward hymen. In Europe, during the past 30 years, the most frequently used method for creation of a neovagina has been that proposed by Vecchietti in 1965.[14] This technique is essentially a surgical variant of the traditional method by Frank. Instead of applying pressure from below on the retrohymenal tissue, constant traction is maintained from above.

LAPAROSCOPIC SURGERY FOR CREATION OF NEOVAGINA

The first approach for creation of neovagina through laparoscopy was introduced by Semm in 1983;[27] the purpose was to create neovagina in the vesicorectal space stating from the perineum. In 1992, two laparoscopic versions of Vecchietti laparotomy procedure were proposed. Gauwerky et al.[15] and Popp and Ghiraradini[16] described two relatively similar approaches—a proper device producing upward traction from the retrohymen pouch on acrylic olive, which acts as a wedge through the rectovesical space, thus creating between the two viscera an adequate space that can be maintained by dilators and sexual activity. These authors' suggestions have not achieved popularity, probably because of their excessive complexity.

There are only two laparoscopic procedures that have been used sufficiently on patients and therefore be evaluated adequately: laparoscopic modification of original operation of Rothman[26] and Davydov[11] proposed by Soong et al.[18] and laparoscopic modification of original laparoscopic operation of Vecchietti[14] proposed by Fedele et al.[28]

Laparoscopic Modification of the Vecchietti Operation

Surgical Equipment (Figs. 9 to 12)

- Gas insufflators
- Light source
- Video camera unit
- Suction irrigation device
- Monitor and documentation system
- Telescopes—0° 10 mm and 30° 10 mm
- Trocars—one 5 mm and 1-5 mm
- *Operating instruments—atraumatic and traumatic graspers:*
    - Dissecting and hook scissors

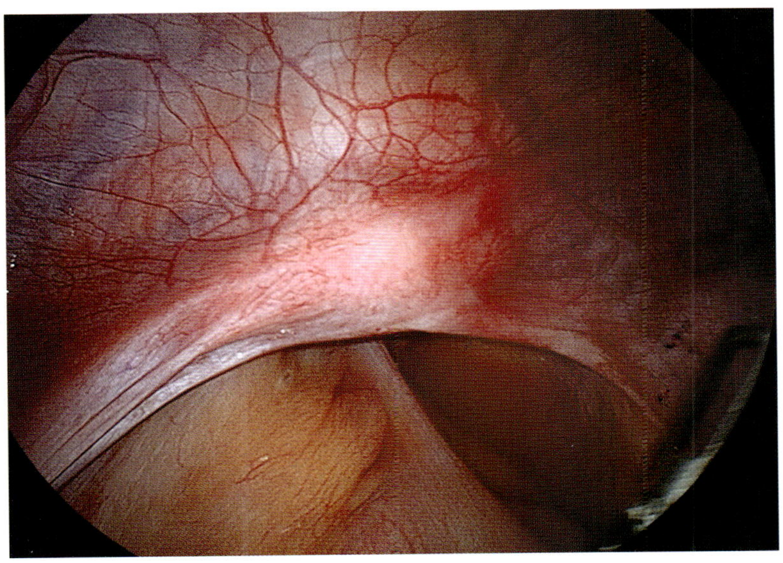

Fig. 8: Presence of endometrium within a rudimentary horn.

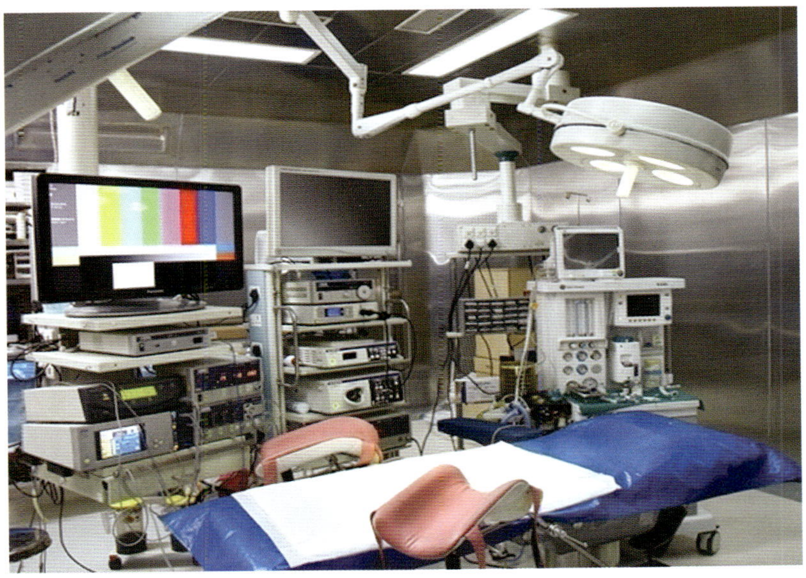

Fig. 9: Operation theater setup.

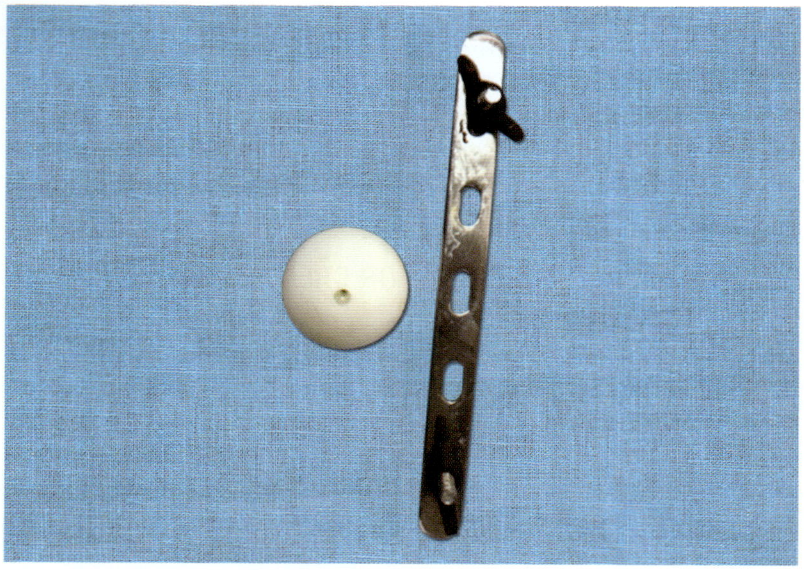

Fig. 10: Traction device and acrylic olive.

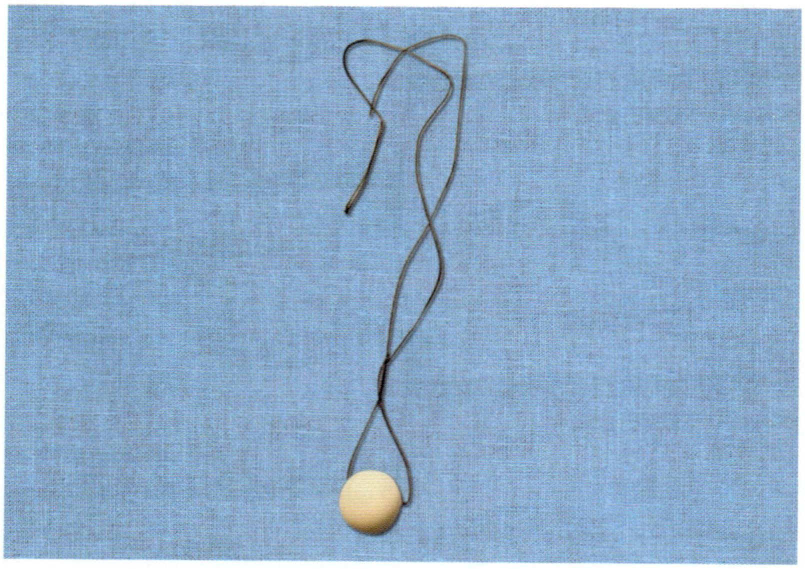

Fig. 11: Acrylic olive with silk thread within.

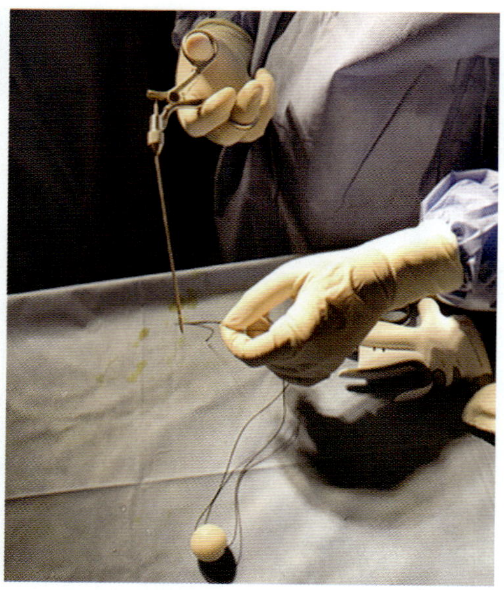

Fig. 12: Port closure needle with acrylic olive and silk thread.

    - Thread-bearing cutting needle (we used, port closure needle)
    - The traction device
    - Acrylic olive
    - Needle holder
- Energy sources—harmonic scalpel
    - Bipolar forceps
- Suture materials.

PREOPERATIVE EVALUATION

Routine preoperative tests include a complete blood count, bleeding time, clotting time, renal function tests, evaluation of thyroid status, viral markers, electrocardiography (ECG), and urinalysis. However, tests such as liver function tests, serum electrolytes, prothrombin time and international normalized ratio (PT-INR), activated partial thromboplastin time (aPTT), chest radiography, 2D-echocardiography, CT (computed tomography), MRI and contrast MRI should be done as indicated. Preanesthetic fitness is obtained.

Preanesthetic assessment is an essential step prior to anesthesia in an attempt to decrease the morbidity related to anesthesia and surgery. Patient is advised for admission the evening before the surgery. Informed consent should be taken from the patient after a thorough explanation. Aspirin and warfarin are to be stopped 5 days prior to surgery. All patients are advised to eat lightly for 24 hours before surgery. An oral mechanical bowel preparation such as Coloprep or Peglec is administered. Patient is kept nil per oral 8 hours prior to surgery and blood is kept reserved.

Procedure

In our center, the surgical technique followed predominantly for laparoscopic Vecchietti vaginoplasty is described here.

A proper device producing upward traction is placed in a retrohymenal pouch on an acrylic olive, which acts as a wedge through the rectovesical space, thus creating between the two viscera an adequate space that can be maintained by dilators and sexual activity.

Bladder should be emptied by catheterization, adequate pneumoperitoneum is created with the help of CO_2 gas, and laparoscope is introduced in supraumbilical region. The traction device along with thread is temporarily placed on the suprapubic region and marked on the skin.

Adjacent to the markings, one ancillary trocar is introduced to allow accurate exploration of the abdominal and pelvic organs. Adjacent to the trocar at the level of deep inguinal ring, we made a stab incision following which Maryland forceps is passed through the incision to reach the loose subperitoneal connective tissue downward and medially until it reaches the fold between the bladder and the uterine rudiment.

The black silk no. 4 is fed into the acrylic olive on either side and placed in retrohymenal pouch. The end of the thread is hooked on to the port closure needle with finger guiding the needle through the blind vagina, needle is retrieved through the uterine rudiment intra-abdominally under laparoscopic guidance. The edge of the silk thread is brought out onto the skin by Maryland forceps through subperitoneal tunnel and fixed to the traction device which is placed suprapubically and its tension is graduated.

When the traction device is first positioned, traction on the mobile intruder must be applied to allow the downward movement of the olive by approximately 1 cm if counter traction is applied.

The traction device and mobile intruder are removed after the neovagina has progressed to at least 6–7 cm in depth which may be obtained between 9th and 10th day after surgery.

Patients can be discharged from hospital 48–72 hours after the surgery and adjust the thread tension in every 48 hours. Adequate analgesic therapy is given on the day of traction is readjusted. In our set-up, we made the patient to stay till the traction device was out after 10 days.

We noticed an increment of 5–6 cm length in vagina after 10 days of surgery which was 1 cm preoperatively.

After this initial period, all women are instructed to use dilators and keep for approximately 8–10 hours per day during the first month. Although there are various type of dilators, we recommend those that are soft and blunt.

The dilators are made up of soft latex, measure 10 cm long, and comes in 3 diameters: 1.5, 2, and 2.5 cm. After use, they are washed and sterilized with antiseptic solution or otherwise washed with normal water and covered with condom. Intercourse is generally allowed 20 days after removal of acrylic olive **(Figs. 13 to 32)**.

In 1 weeks' hospitalization, the patient was given steady traction by adding one gauze pads beneath the traction device.

After 1 weeks' time the silk thread is cut and olive was removed.

DAVYDOV PROCEDURE

A woman's own peritoneum lining is used to created neovagina. Peritoneum graft from pouch of Douglas is dissected and mobilized. After creating vaginal space, peritoneum is reached and then mobilized peritoneum sac is opened and pulled downward to connect the vaginal epithelium with graft taken from peritoneum of pouch of Douglas. Postoperatively, a vaginal mold is inserted for 6 weeks and regular vaginal dilators are used until commencement of regular sexual activity.[11]

CONCLUSION

Mayer–Rokitansky–Küster–Hauser syndrome is characterized by uterine and vaginal aplasia. Typically, presentation is primary amenorrhea with normal secondary sexual characters, blind vagina,

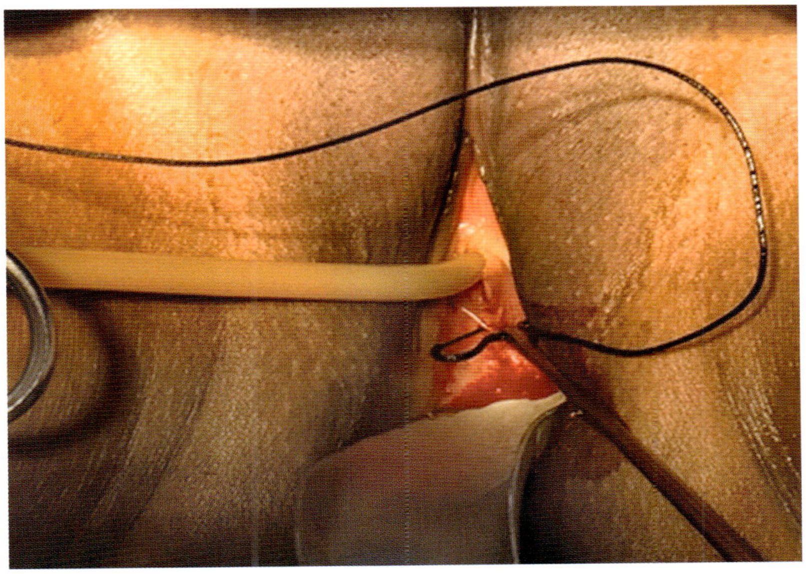

Fig. 13: Needle piercing the retrohymenal pouch.

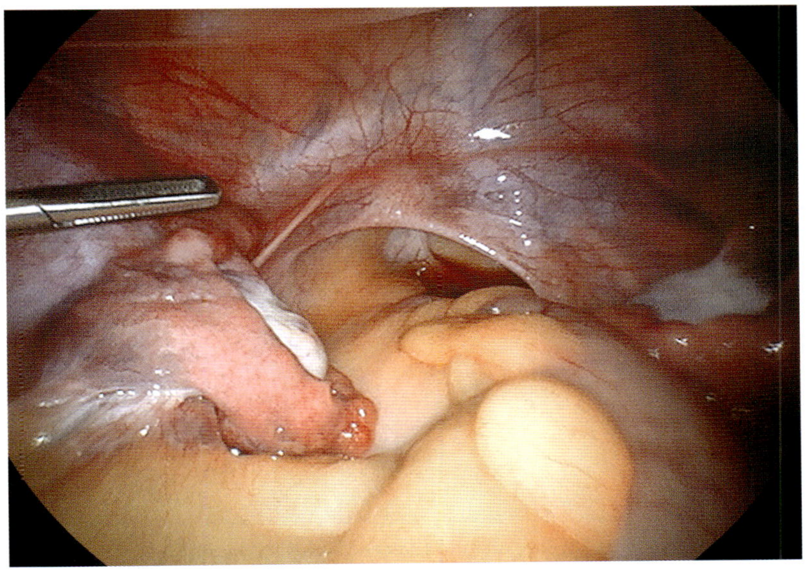

Fig. 15: Rudiment horn with bilateral tubes and ovaries.

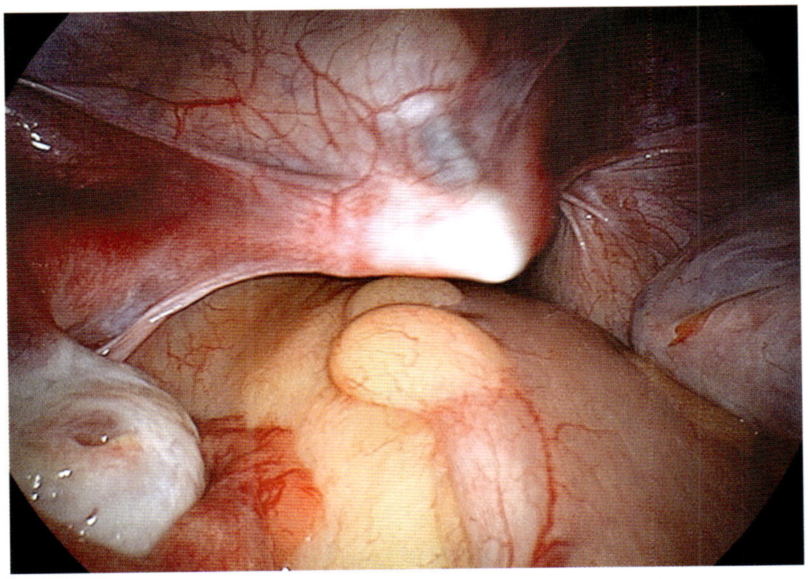

Fig. 14: Lap finding of needle piercing through rudiment horn.

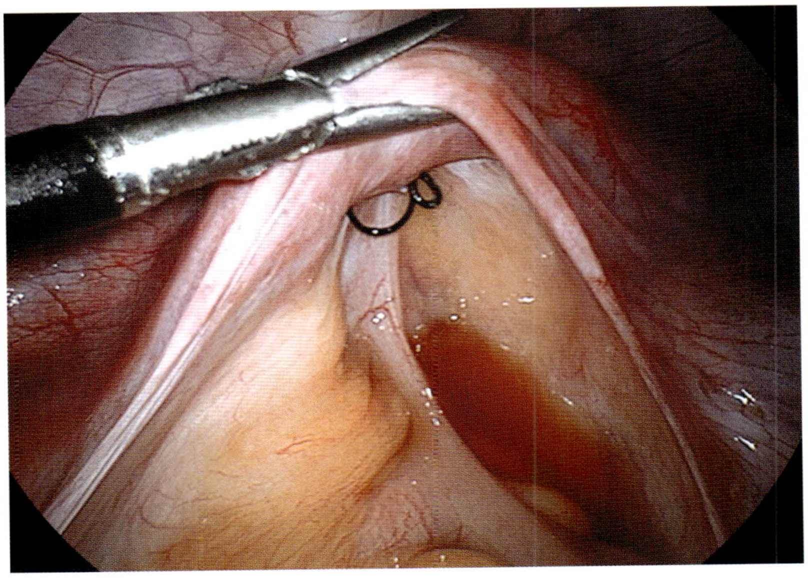

Fig. 16: Rudiment horn held with Maryland forceps.

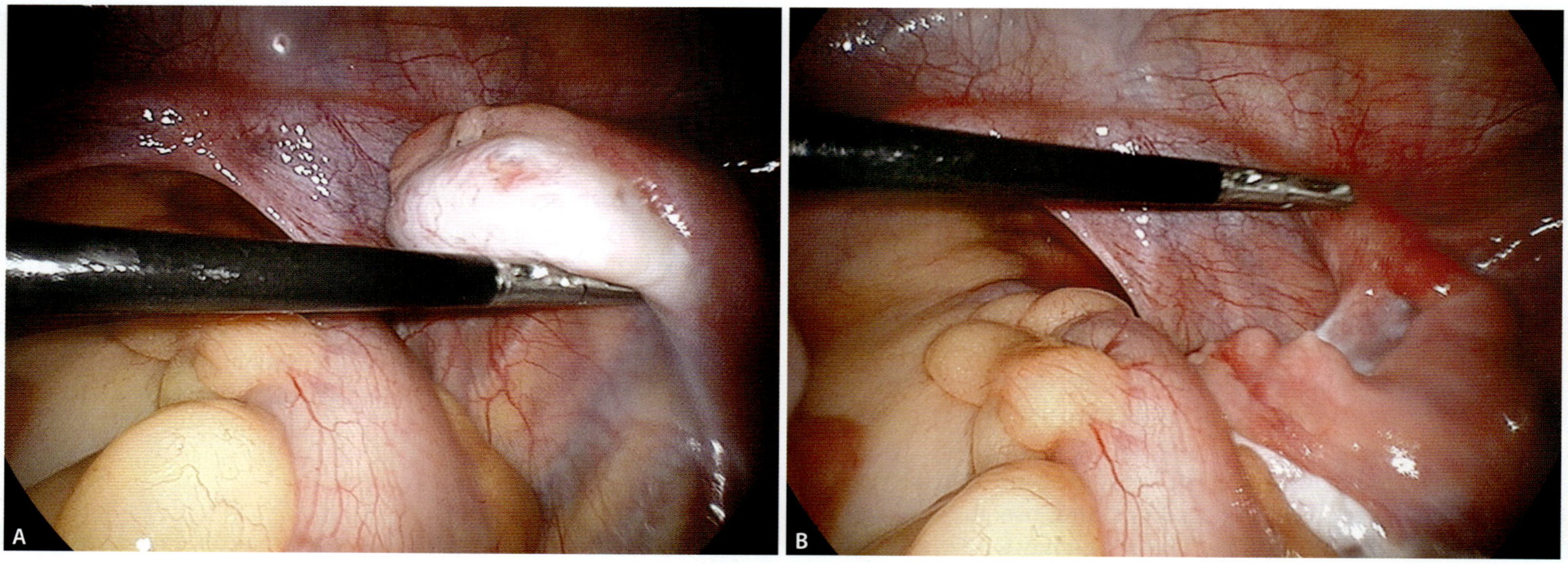

Figs. 17A and B: Bilateral normal tubes and ovaries.

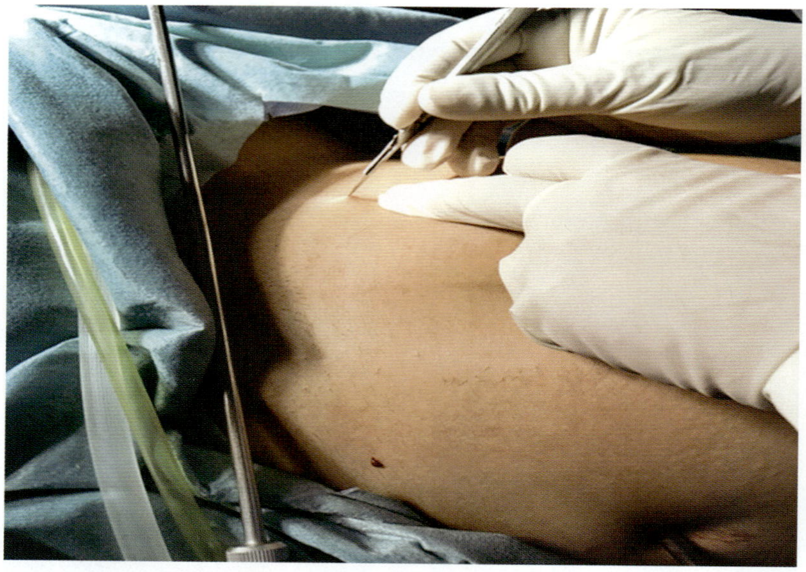

Fig. 18: Stab incision adjacent to the lateral port.

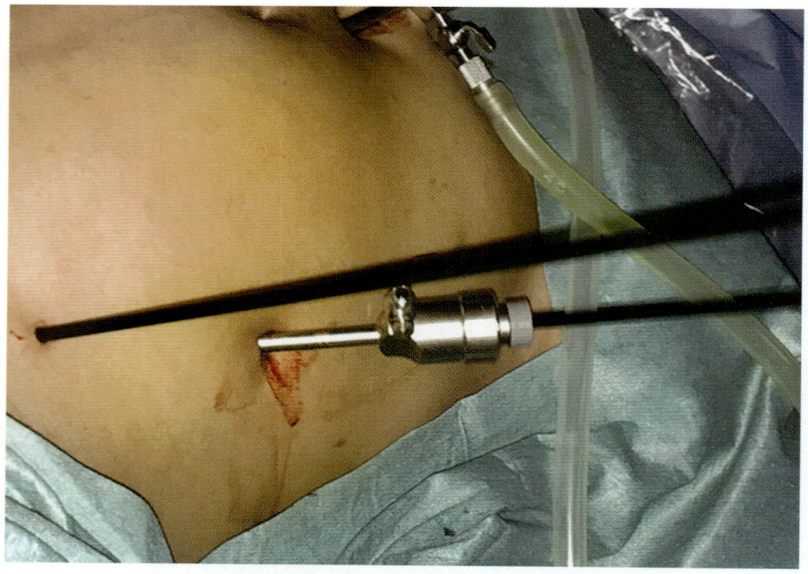

Fig. 19: Maryland forceps introduced into the incision.

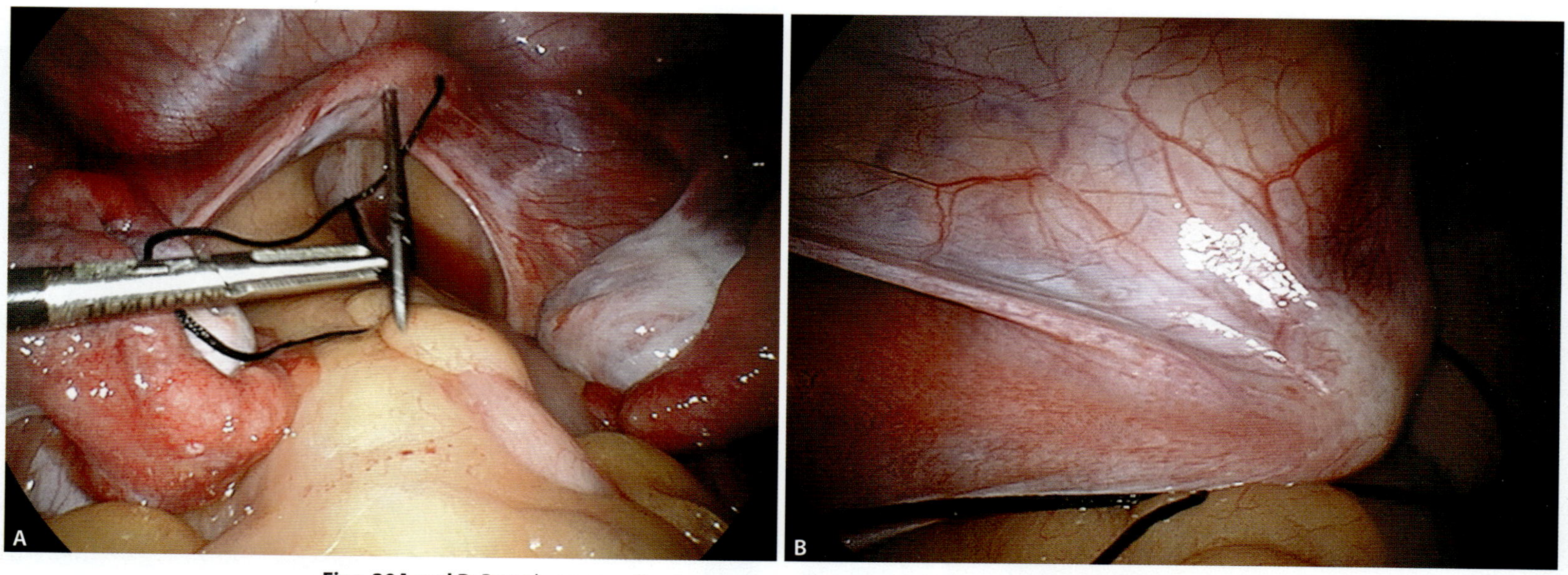

Figs. 20A and B: Port closure needle piercing the rudiment horn getting the silk into operating area.

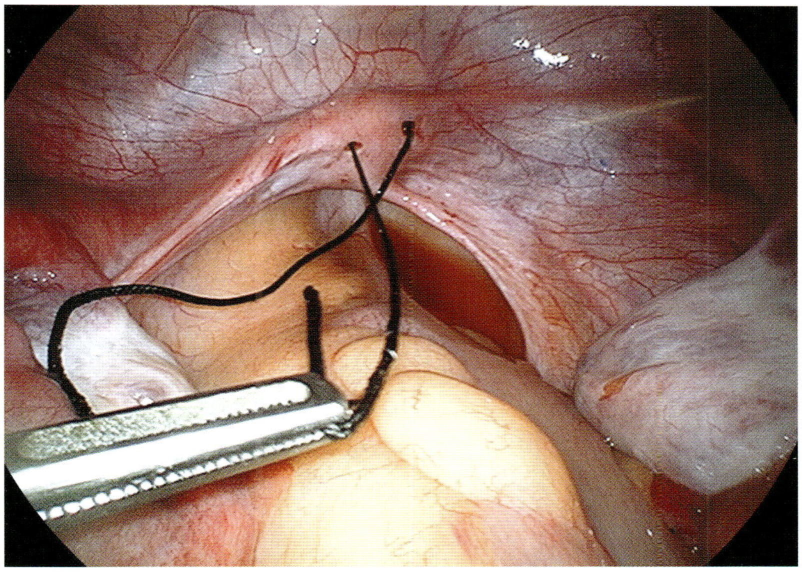

Fig. 21: Silk 4-0 held with atraumatic forceps.

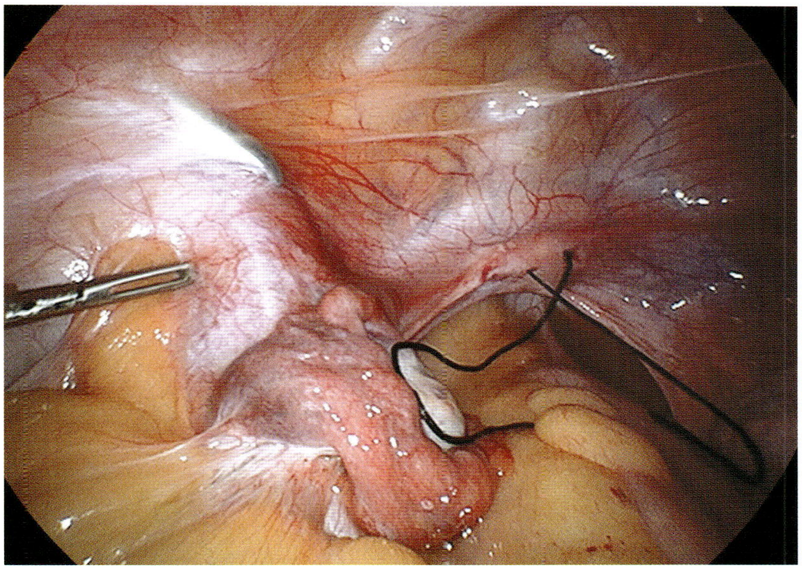

Fig. 22: Maryland tunneling through subperitoneal tissue.

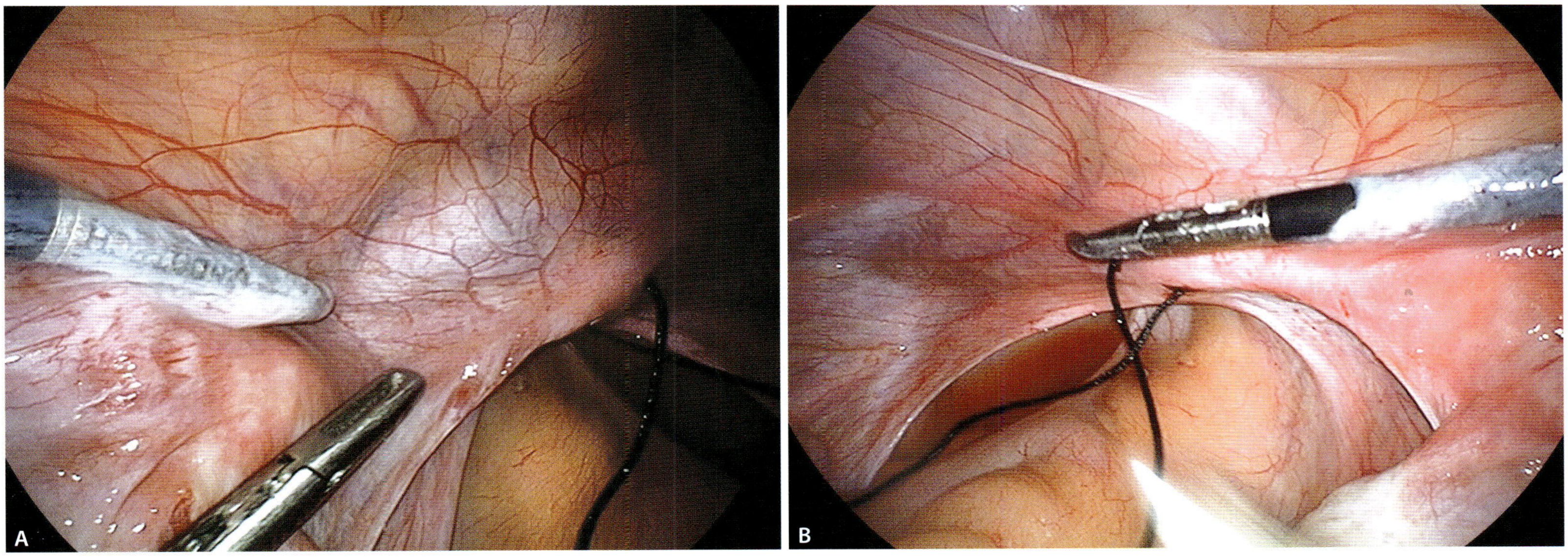

Figs. 23A and B: Maryland tunneling toward rudiment horn.

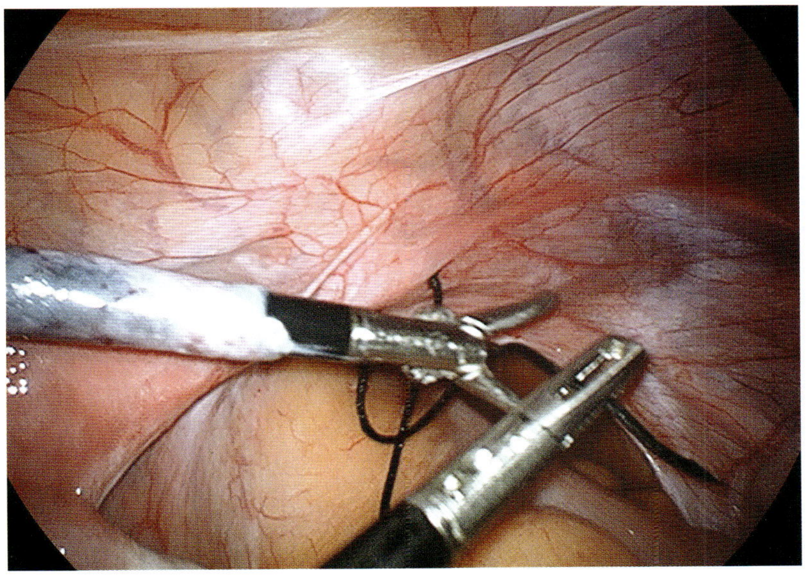

Fig. 24: Silk thread held via Maryland forceps.

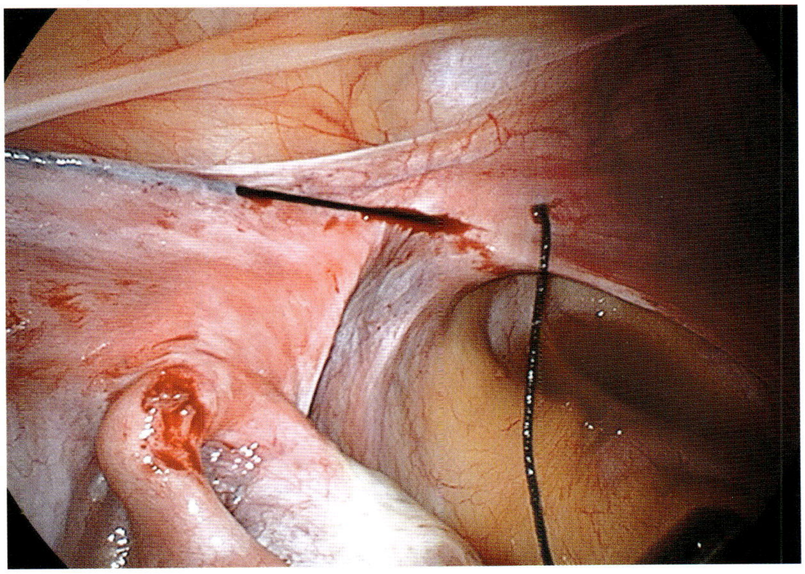

Fig. 25: End of the silk thread is brought out onto the skin by Maryland forceps through subperitoneal tunnel.

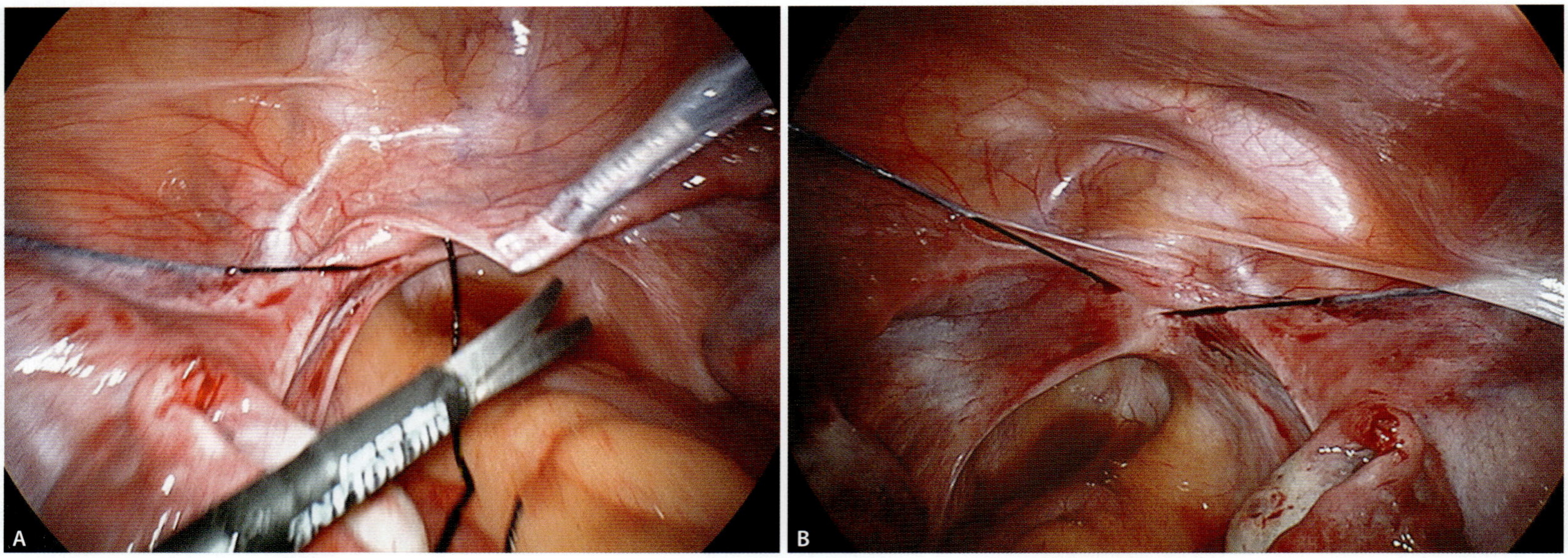

Figs. 26A and B: Bilateral end of silk thread held via Maryland and taken through the subperitoneal tissue.

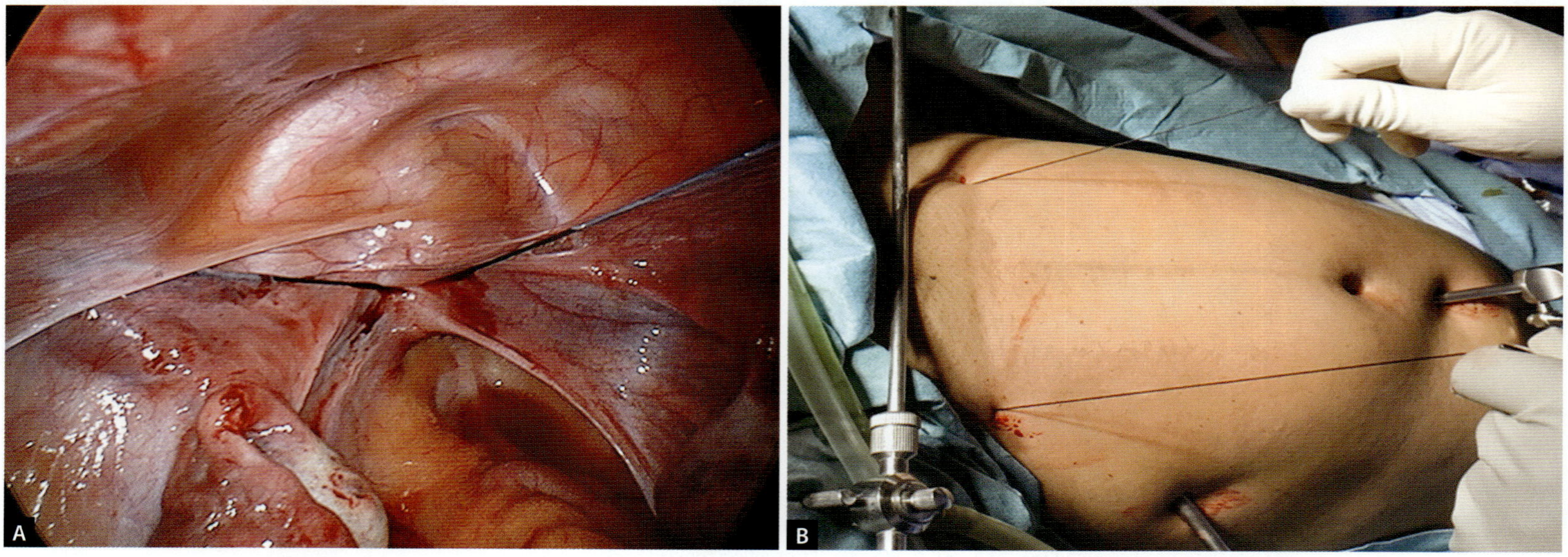

Figs. 27A and B: Silk thread taken out via subperitoneal tissue into the skin outside to get fixed into a traction device.

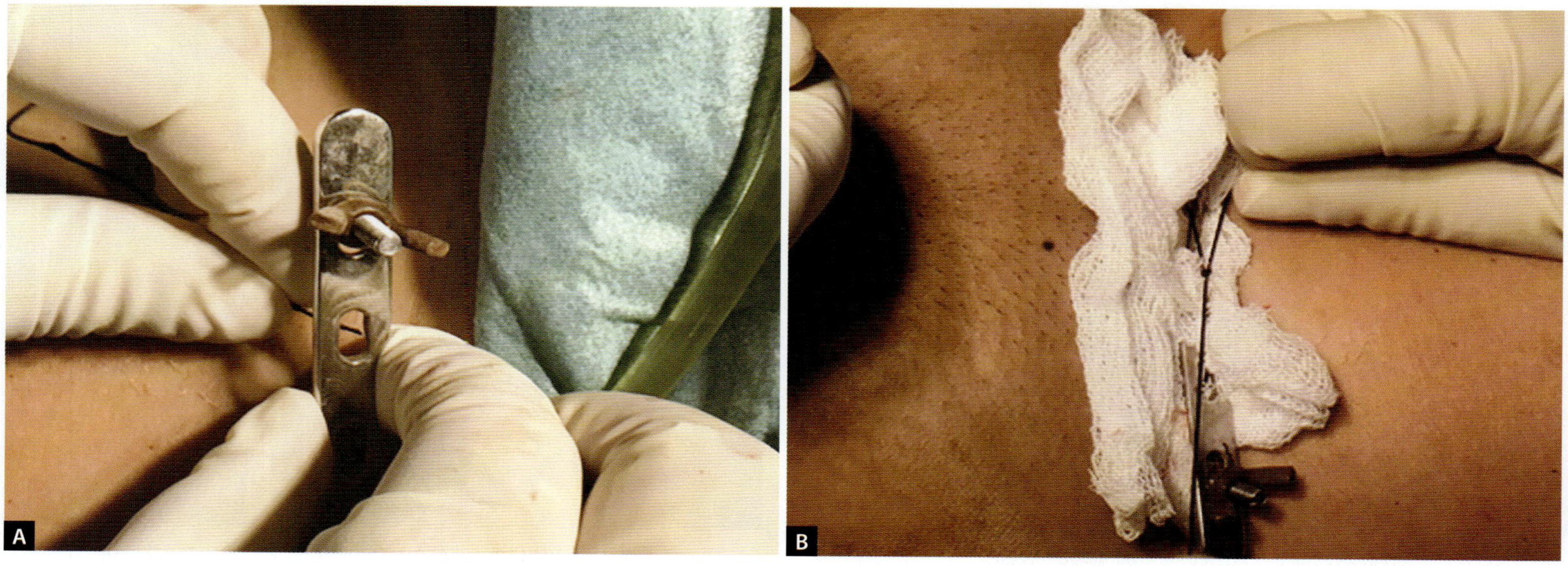

Figs. 28A and B: Silk thread fixing into the traction device.

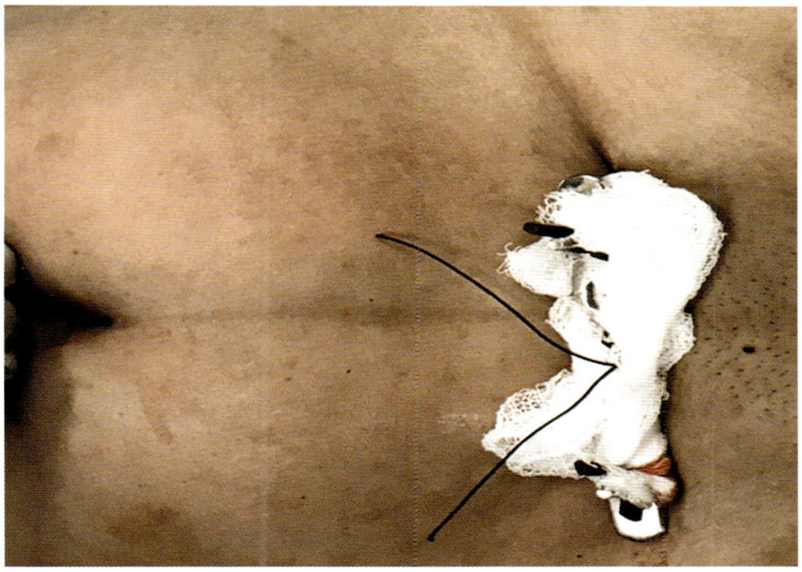

Fig. 29: Traction device fixed.

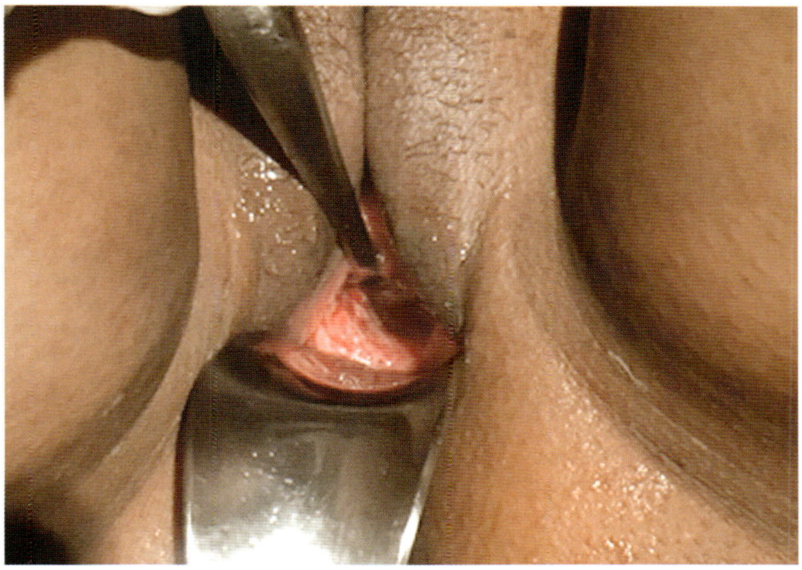

Fig. 31: Vaginal length increased by 5 cm by the end of 1 week.

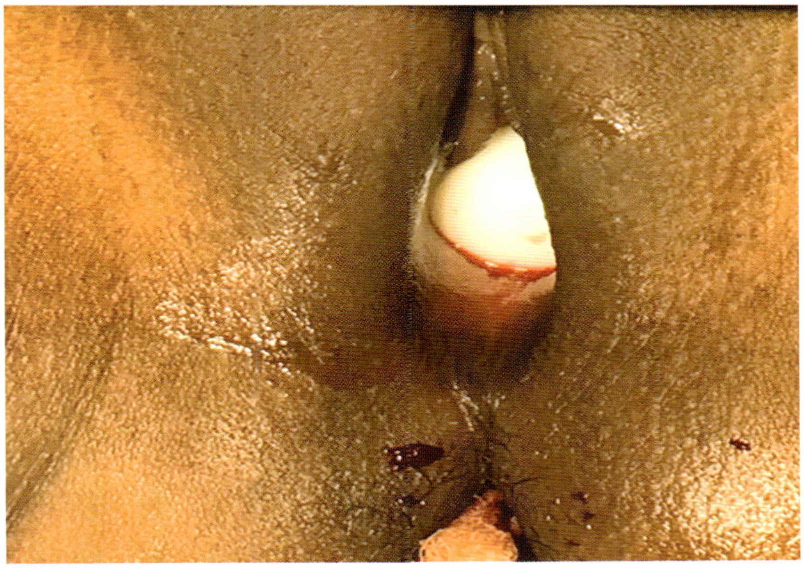

Fig. 30: Acrylic olive ball onto the blind vagina.

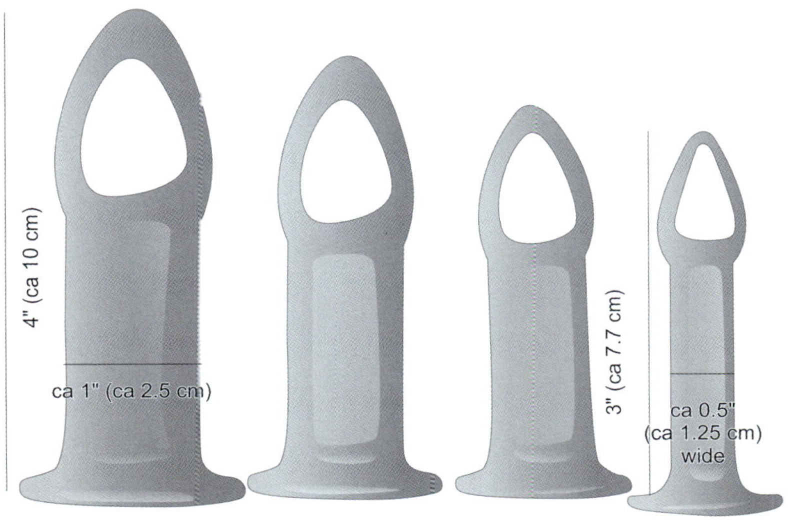

Fig. 32: The original Vecchietti dilator.

absence of uterus, and cervix on ultrasonography with normal 46XX karyotype. Patient and family need urgent psychological counseling. Neovagina is firstly created by serial vaginal dilators. In failure of nonsurgical techniques or women refusal to do so, vaginoplasty is done by either open/laparoscopic techniques. Pregnancy can be achieved by using latest in vitro fertilization techniques and surrogacy.

REFERENCES

1. Evans TN, Poland ML, Boving RL. Vaginal malformations. Am J Obstet Gynecol. 1981;141(8):910-20.
2. Fedele L, Bianchi S, Frontino G, et al. Laparoscopic findings and pelvic anatomy in Mayer-Rokitansky-Küster-Hauser syndrome. Obstet Gynecol. 2007;109(5):1111-5.
3. Frank RT. The formation of an artificial vagina without operation. Am J Obstet Gynecol. 1938;35(6):1053-5.
4. Ingram JM. The bicycle seat stool in the treatment of vaginal agenesis and stenosis: a preliminary report. Am J Obstet Gynecol. 1981;140(8): 867-73.
5. Baldwin JF. The formation of an artificial vagina by intestinal transplantation. Ann Surg. 1904;40(3):398-403.
6. Freundt I, Toolenaar TAM, Huikeshoven FJM, et al. A modified technique to create a neovagina with an isolated segment of sigmoid colon. Surg Gynecol Obstet. 1992;174(1):11-6.
7. McGraw J, Kemp G, Given F, et al. Correction of high pelvic defects with the inferiorly based rectus abdominis myocutaneous flap. Clin Plast Surg. 1988;15(3):449-54.
8. Kee JTK, Joseph VT. A new technique of vaginal reconstruction using neurovascular pudendal-thigh flaps: a preliminary report. Plast Reconstr Surg. 1989;83(4):701-9.
9. Chen ZJ, Chen MY, Chen C, et al. Vaginal reconstruction with an axial subcutaneous pedicle flap from the inferior abdominal wall: a new method. Plast Reconstr Surg. 1989;83(6):1005-12.
10. McIndoe AH, Banister JB. An operation for the cure of congenital absence of the vagina. J Obstet Gynaecol Br Emp. 1938;45(3):490-4.
11. Davydov SN. 12 years' experience with colpopoiesis using the peritoneum. Gynakologe. 1980;13:120-1.
12. Dhall K. Amnion graft for treatment of congenital absence of the vagina. Br J Obstet Gynaecol. 1984;91(3):279-82.
13. Jackson ND, Rosenblatt PL. Use of an Interceed absorbable adhesion barrier for vaginoplasty. Obstet Gynecol. 1994;84(6):1048-50.
14. Vecchietti G. Creation of an artificial vagina in Rokitansky-Küster-Hauser syndrome. Attual Obstet Gynecol. 1965;11(2):131-47.

15. Gauwerky JFH, Wallwiener D, Bastert G. An endoscopically assisted technique for construction of a neovagina. Arch Gynecol Obstet. 1992;252(2):59-63.
16. Popp LW, Ghirardini G. Creation of a neovagina by pelviscopy. J Laparoendosc Surg. 1992;2(3):165-73.
17. Fedele L, Bianchi S, Zanconato G, et al. Laparoscopic creation of a neovagina in patients with Rokitansky syndrome: analysis of 52 cases. Fertil Steril. 2000;74(2):384-9.
18. Soong YK, Chang FH, Lee CL, et al. Vaginal agenesis treated by laparoscopically assisted neovaginoplsty. Gynecol Endosc. 1994;3:217-20.
19. Morcel K, Camborieux L, Guerrier D. Programme de Recherches surles Aplasies Müllériennes, Mayer-Rokitansky-Küster-Hauser (MRKH) syndrome. Orphanet J Rare Dis. 2007;2:13.
20. Pittock ST, Babovic-Vuksanovic D, Lteif A. Mayer-Rokitansky-Küster-Hauser anomaly and its associated malformations. Am J Med Genet A. 2005;135(3):314-6.
21. Varner RE, Younger JB, Blackwell RE. Müllerian dysgenesis. J Reprod Med 1985;30(6):443-50.
22. Strübbe EH, Willemsen WN, Lemmens JA, et al. Mayer-Rokitansky-Küster-Hauser syndrome: distinction between two forms based on excretory urographic, sonographic, and laparoscopic findings. Am J Roentgenol 1993;160(2):331-4.
23. Sultan C, Biason-Lauber A, Philibert P. Mayer-Rokitansky-Kuster-Hauser syndrome: recent clinical and genetic findings. Gynecol Endocrinol. 2009;25(1):8-11.
24. Oppelt P, Renner SP, Kellermann A, et al. Clinical aspects of Mayer-Rokitansky-Kuester-Hauser syndrome: recommendations for clinical diagnosis and staging. Hum Reprod. 2006;21(3):792-7.
25. Griffin JE, Edwards C, Madden JD, et al. Congenital absence of the vagina. The Mayer-Rokitansky-Küster-Hauser syndrome. Ann Intern Med. 1976; 85(2):224-36.
26. Rothman D. The use of peritoneum in the construction of a vagina. Obstet Gynecol. 1972;40(6):835-8.
27. Semm K. Pelviskopische Kontrolle der neovaginalen operatiostechnik uber eine Gliederopik. Alete wissenschaftlicher Dienst. 1983;93:24-7.
28. Fedele L, Busacca M, Candiani M, et al. Laparoscopic creation of neovagina in Mayer-Rokitansky-Küster-Hauser syndrome by modification of Vecchietti's operation. Am J Obstet Gynecol. 1994;171(1):268-97.

CHAPTER

29

Urological Injury in Laparoscopic Surgery

Shruti Paliwal, Aditi Rai, B Ramesh

INTRODUCTION

The female genital and urinary tracts are anatomically closely related; therefore, the potential for injury to one must always be considered when operating on the other. Owing to improvements in gynecological and obstetric techniques that help to prevent urinary tract injury and an emphasis on immediate recognition and repair should any injury occur, long-term complications are less frequent nowadays. The risk of damage increases when the normal anatomy is altered by primary pathologic factors or when it is insufficiently identified during intraoperative complications, such as severe bleeding or pelvic adhesions. Urinary tract injury complicates an estimated 0.2–1% of all gynecologic procedures during pelvic operations.[1] Eighty-two percent of ureter injuries occur during pelvic surgery,[2] and 75% of urinary tract injuries are due to gynecologic surgery.[3] Not only it is associated with the morbidity of vesicovaginal fistula and ureteric stenosis, but also long-term complications like hydronephrosis with variable degrees of renal impairment and failure may ensue. Urological injury is also the basis of medico-legal suits. Urinary tract injuries due to obstetric and gynecologic surgery are normally divided into two categories: (1) acute complications such as bladder laceration or ureter laceration that can be identified immediately during the operation, and (2) chronic complications such as vesicovaginal fistula, ureterovaginal fistula, and ureter stricture, which can occur later on.

INJURY TO THE URINARY TRACT

Bladder

If a bladder lesion is not obvious or not immediately recognized, the finding of gas and/or blood in the urethral catheter bag should cause the laparoscopic surgeon to look for any laceration in the bladder **Figure 1**. Irrigation of the bladder via the urethral catheter can help to locate the lesion.[4] Once detected, any defect in the bladder wall can be closed with an absorbable single-layer running suture **(Fig. 2)**, which most endourological surgeons will be able to complete laparoscopically. Depending on the size of the lesion, the Foley catheter should be left to continuously drain the repaired bladder for up to 10 days postoperatively. An easy and effective measure to prevent intraoperative bladder injuries is the routine preoperative placement of a Foley catheter in all patients undergoing laparoscopic procedure **(Fig. 3)**. Injury to the bladder may result from a secondary suprapubic trocar or from dissection of the bladder during the course of laparoscopic surgery, e.g. laparoscopic hysterectomy or colposuspension. If bladder injury is suspected, methylene blue dye may be instilled into the bladder to establish if there is any leakage of dye **(Fig. 4)**. Perforation of the bladder may also result in the escape of gas into the Foley catheter (drainage bag). Bladder injury recognized during laparoscopy may be sutured in a single layer, followed by bladder drainage for 7–10 days. Bladder injury not recognized during laparoscopy may present a few days later, the patients having lower abdominal discomfort and blood biochemistry results not dissimilar to those of someone in acute renal failure. The diagnosis may be confirmed with a retrograde cystogram. A small defect may be managed conservatively by continuous drainage with a Foley catheter,[5] whereas a larger defect would require repair. A case of vesicovaginal fistula was reported to present 2 months after total laparoscopic hysterectomy.[6]

Bladder Repair (Figs. 1 to 7)

Case 1

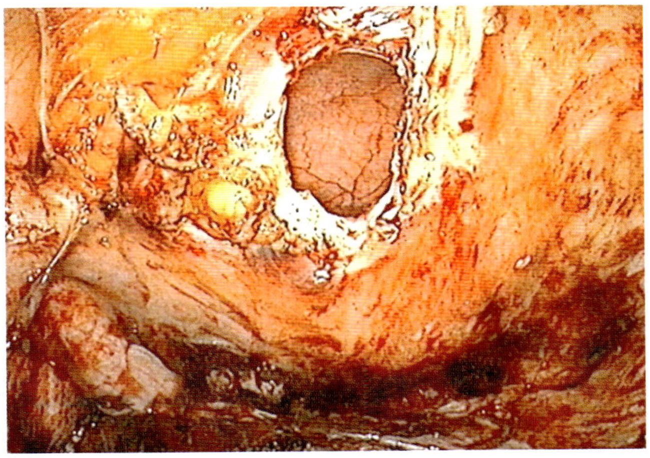

Fig. 1: Bladder rent identified

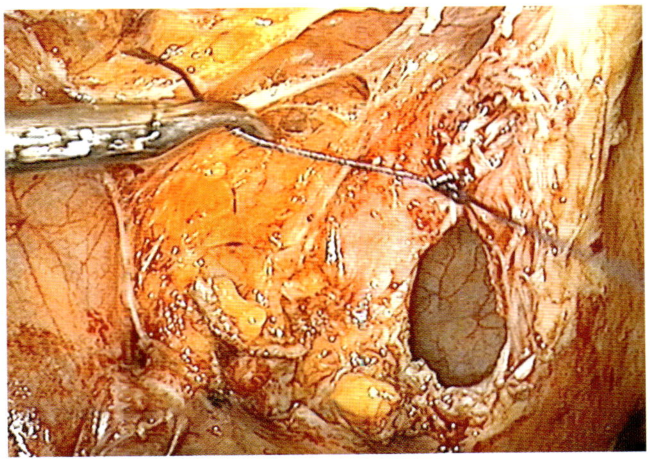

Fig. 2: Bladder repair with Vicryl suture.

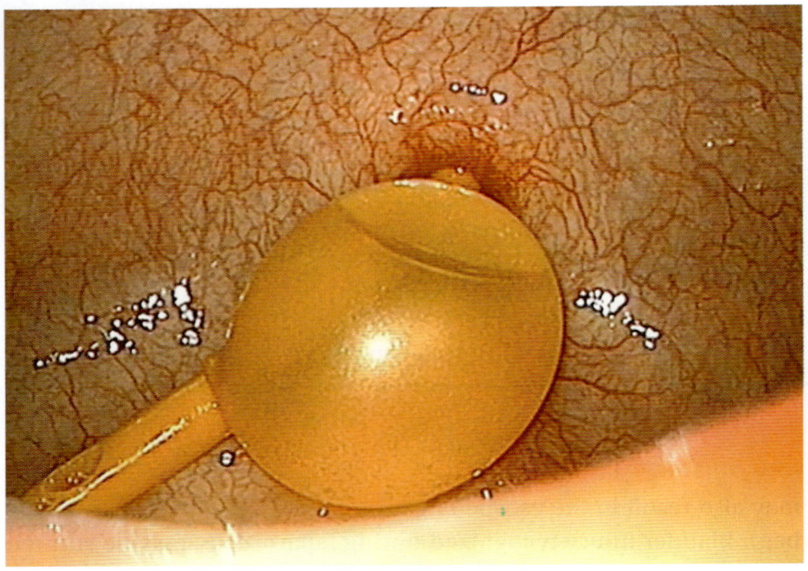

Fig. 3: Foley's bulb seen.

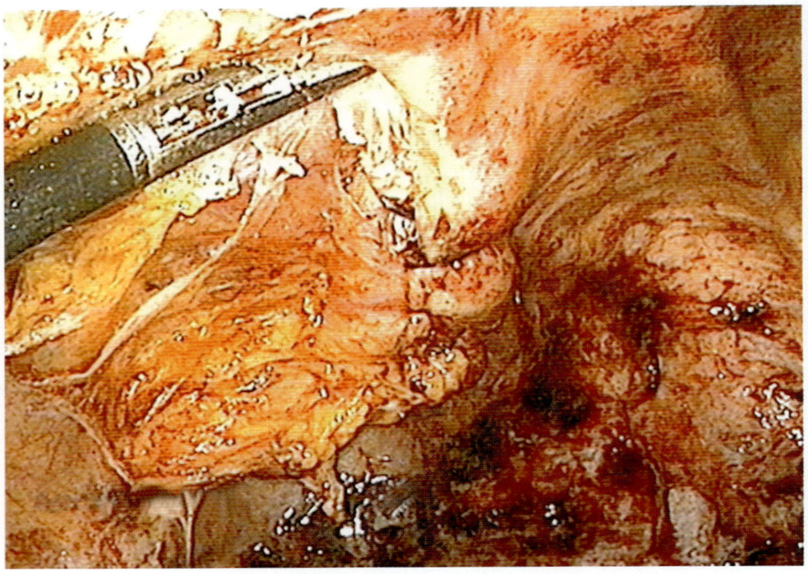

Fig. 4: No leak noted postbladder repair.

Case 2

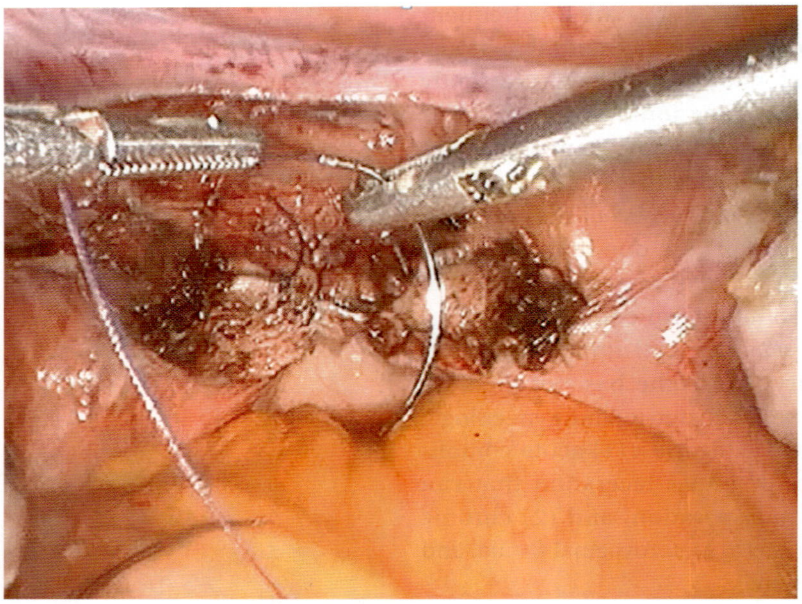

Fig. 5: Bladder suture with Vicryl continuous suture.

Case 3

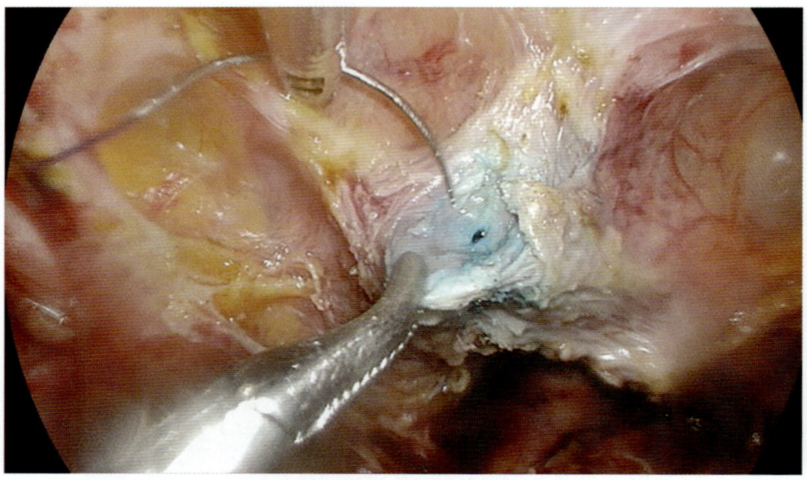

Fig. 6: Bladder defect identified.

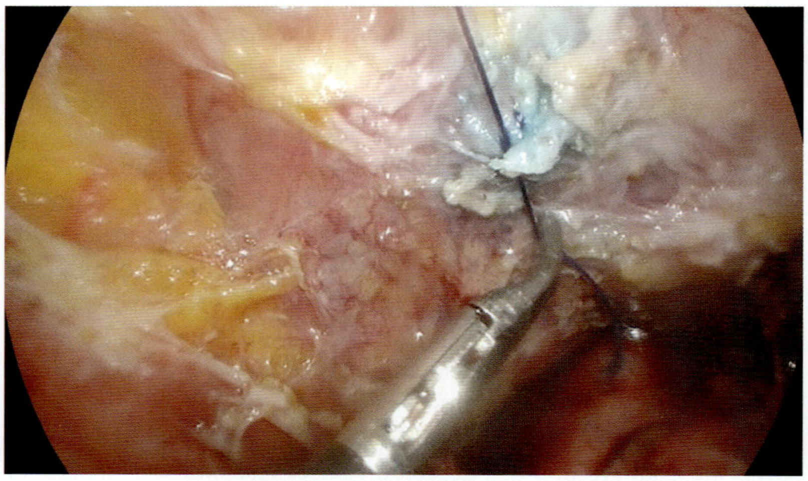

Fig. 7: Bladder defect sutured with figure of 8 Vicryl suture.

Prevention

To prevent injury of the bladder at laparoscopy, it is important that the bladder is catheterized before the patient is tilted head downward. During a long operation, urine may reaccumulate in the bladder, hence an indwelling Foley catheter is advisable in all cases of laparoscopic surgery other than simple ones such as laparoscopic sterilization. There is a natural tendency for gynecologists to direct the suprapubic trocar toward the retropubic space of Retzius and this should be avoided. This is particularly important if a large trocar is inserted in those who have had a previous cesarean section, or in those who have undergone multiple pelvic surgery, distorting the peritoneal anatomy.

Ureter

Recognition of Ureteric Injury

Delay in presentation:

- Extravasation of urine may follow laceration of the ureter or, less commonly, thermal injury complicated by tissue necrosis. The presentation of the latter injury may be delayed by several days or weeks. The urine leaking into the peritoneal cavity may be absorbed. The presentation is variable and consists of nonspecific symptoms such as nausea, vomiting, malaise, leakage of fluid via the trocar sites, abdominal distension and ileus. Blood tests show a characteristic increase in creatinine levels. X-ray of the abdomen may reveal a ground-glass appearance indicative of fluid collection. The diagnosis should be confirmed by intravenous urogram.
- Obstructive uropathy may follow accidental stapling of the ureter, or thermal injury resulting in a stricture leading to hydroureter and hydronephrosis. Superimposed infection may result in pyonephrosis.

MANAGEMENT

Surgical Management

Distal Ureteral Injuries

Ureteroneocystostomy: The majority of operative injuries occur in the distal ureter. The distal ureter is most often injured during attempts to ligate branches of the internal iliac vessels. As the blood supply of the distal ureteral segment may be disrupted, ureteroneocystostomy is an ideal option for distal ureteral repair. When preparing the ureter for implantation, it should be judiciously debrided back to viable tissue and spatulated. The reimplantation site should be on the posterior or anterior dome of the bladder and not on the lateral aspects. Reimplantation of the ureter on the lateral aspects of the bladder is prone to kinking with bladder filling **(Fig. 12)**.[7] The reimplanted ureter should be stented and a Foley catheter maintained in the bladder perioperatively together with a Jackson–Pratt (JP) drain near the anastomosis. The Foley catheter may be removed in approximately 1 week and the JP drain removed once it is determined that the repair is not leaking. The stent is removed in 6 weeks.

Vesicopsoas hitch: When a lengthy defect in the distal ureter is discovered, such that performing a simple ureteroneocystostomy would result in tension on the anastomosis, often this distance can be bridged with a vesicopsoas hitch, first described by Zimmerman and colleagues.[8] Mobilization of the bladder in the space of Retzius and ligation of the contralateral bladder pedicle aids in positioning the bladder near the psoas muscle **(Fig. 18)**. The bladder detrusor is then "hitched" to the psoas muscle with longitudinal, nonabsorbable monofilament sutures to make up the length between the bladder and

Ureteric Injury Repair (Figs. 8 to 24)

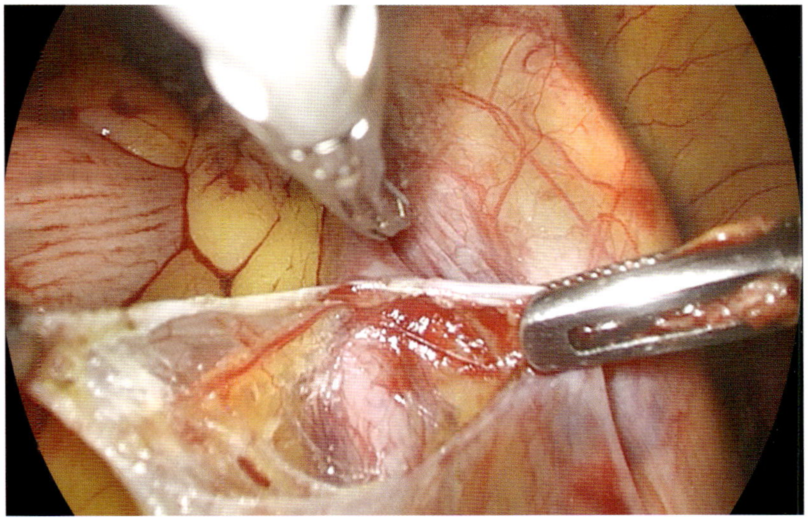

Fig. 8: Ureter exposed by dissecting overlying peritoneum.

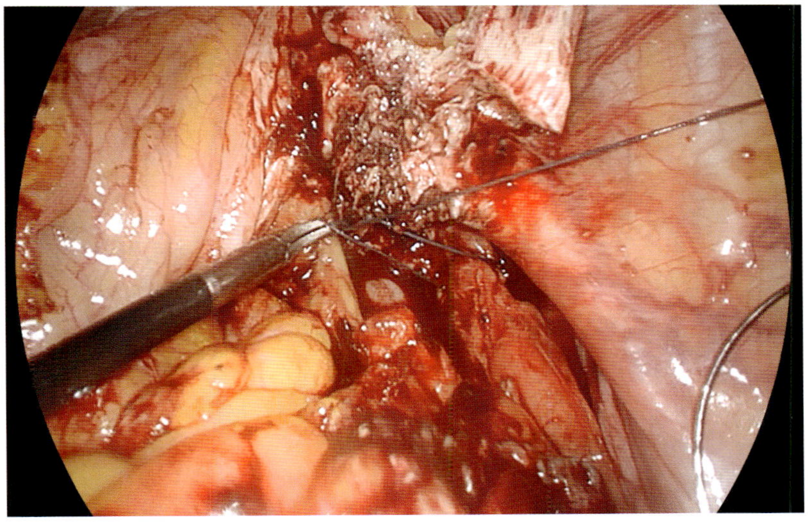

Fig. 9: Stay sure placed at proximal ureteric stump.

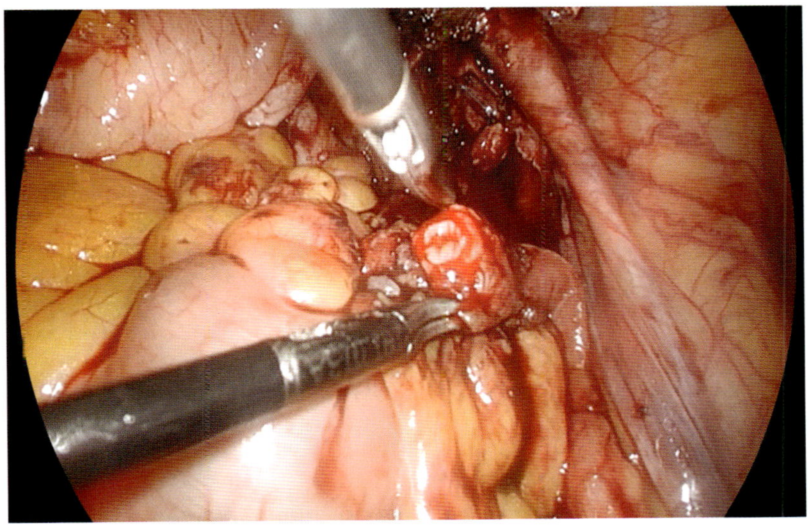

Fig. 10: Ureteric opening freshened.

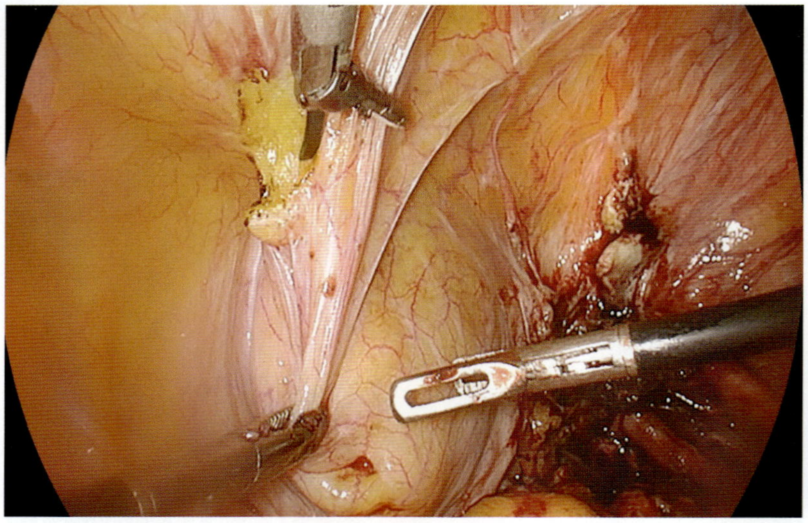

Fig. 11: Bladder mobilized.

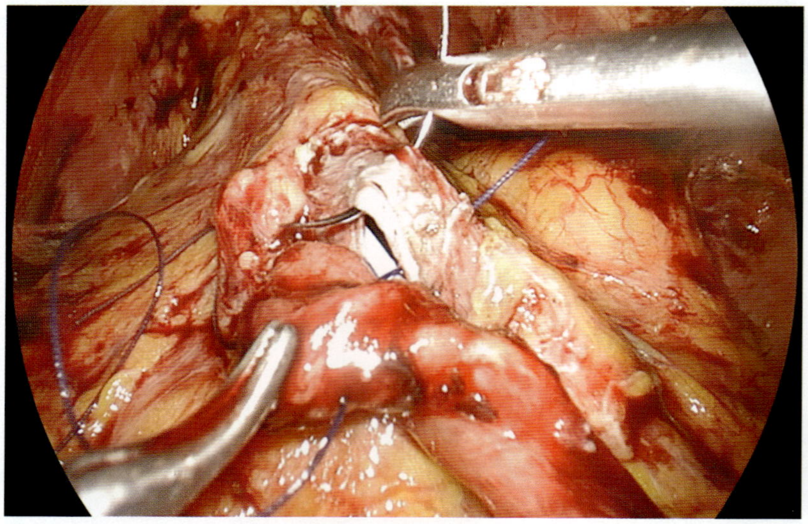

Fig. 12: New ureteric opening on bladder sutured to ureter.

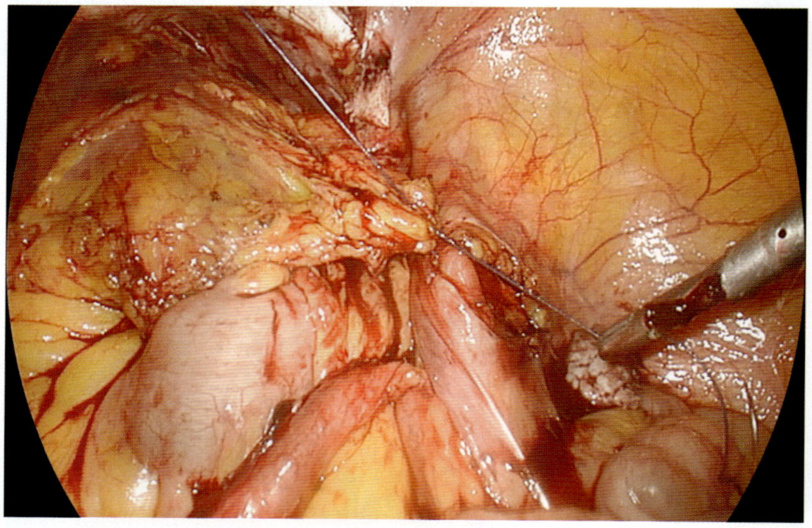

Fig. 13: Bladder fixed to ipsilateral psoas muscle.

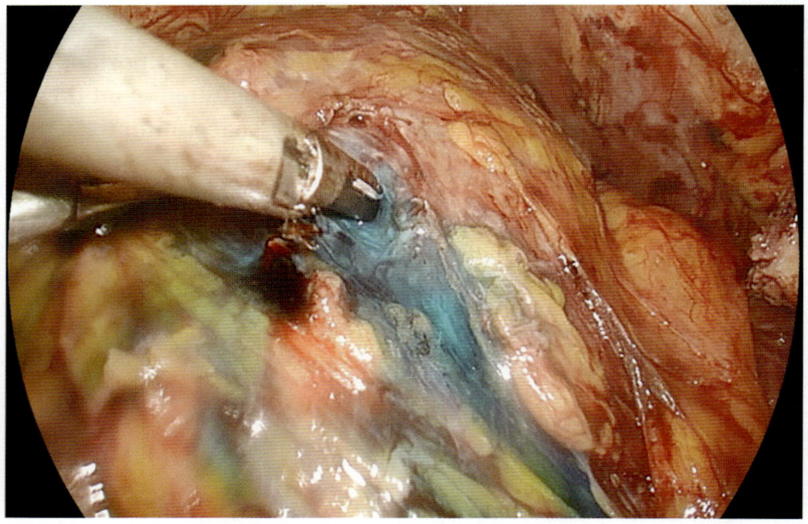

Fig. 14: New ureteric opening created in bladder.

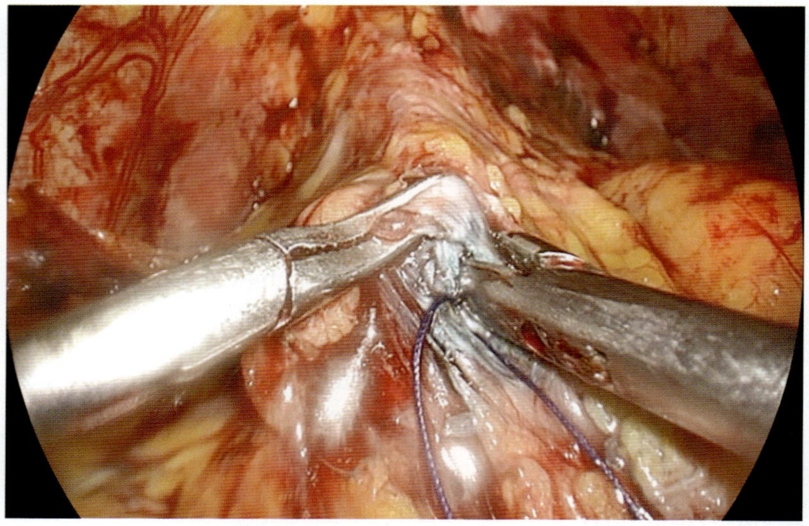

Fig. 15: Stay suture placed in bladder.

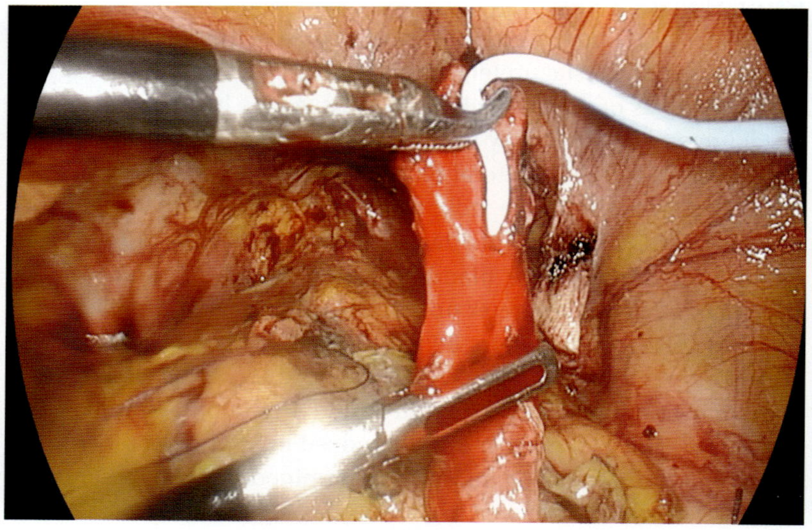

Fig. 16: DJ stent introduced into proximal ureteric stump.

proximal ureteral stump. Care is taken to avoid the genitofemoral nerve that lies on the anterior surface of the psoas muscle. The ureter is then reimplanted into the repositioned bladder in a similar manner to the previously mentioned ureteroneocystostomy. Some authors have advocated the routine use of a vesicopsoas hitch for ureteral reimplantation because it provides a long, fixed, and straight submucosal tunnel that is unlikely to be affected by the degree of bladder filling.[9]

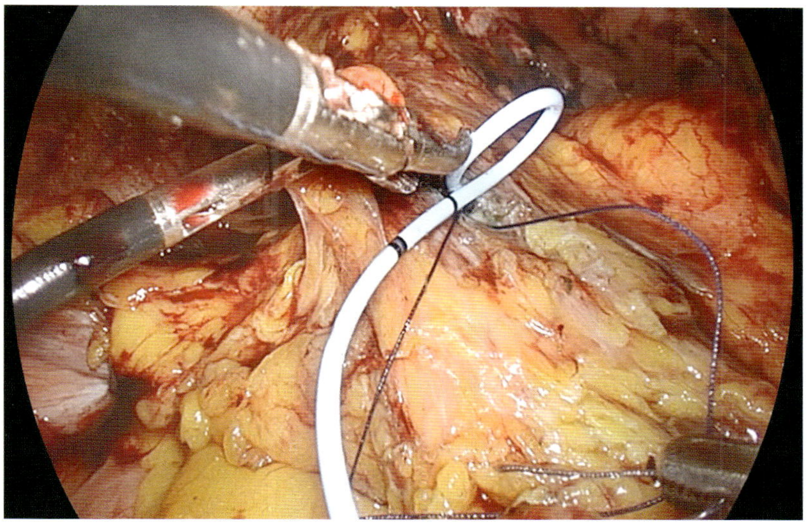

Fig. 17: DJ stent introduced into bladder.

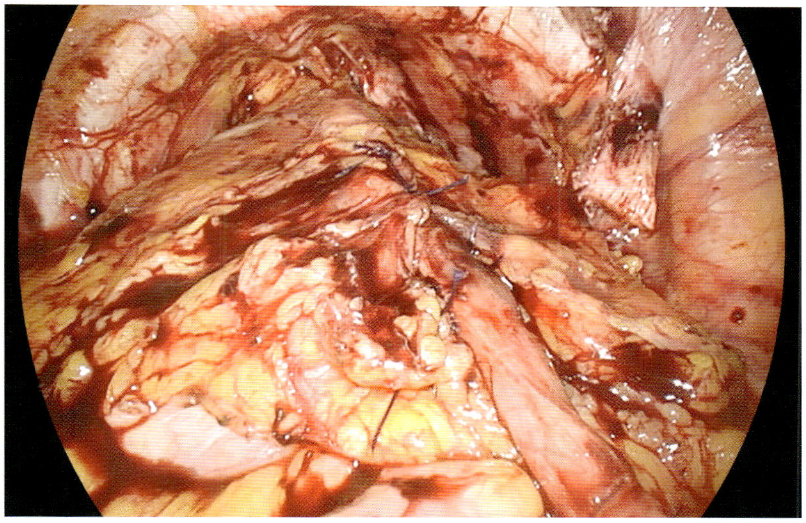

Fig. 20: Omental flap placed.

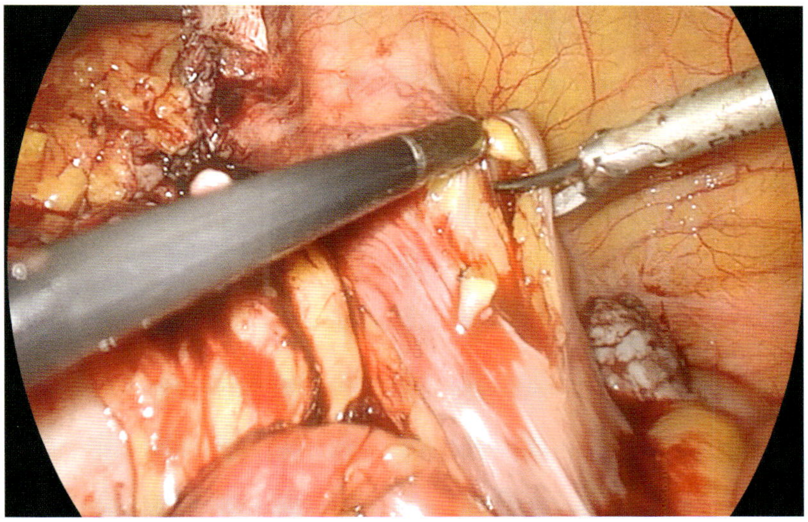

Fig. 18: Ipsilateral psoas muscle exposed.

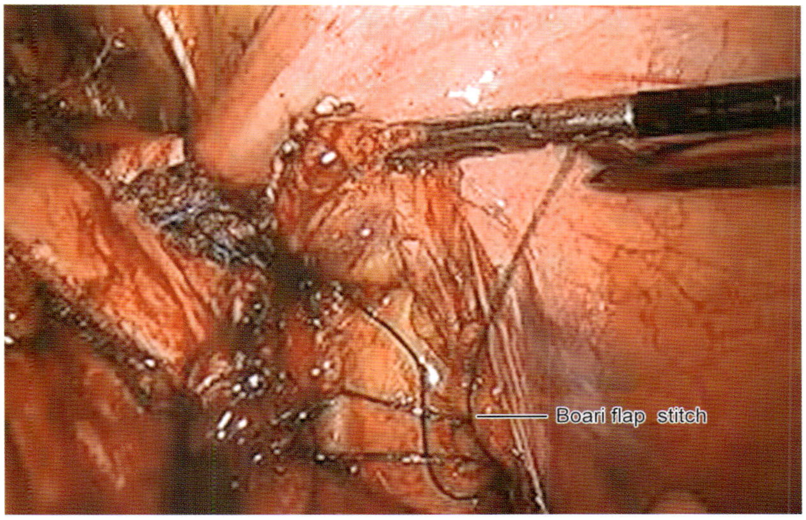

Fig. 21: Proximal ureteric injury repaired by Boari flap method.

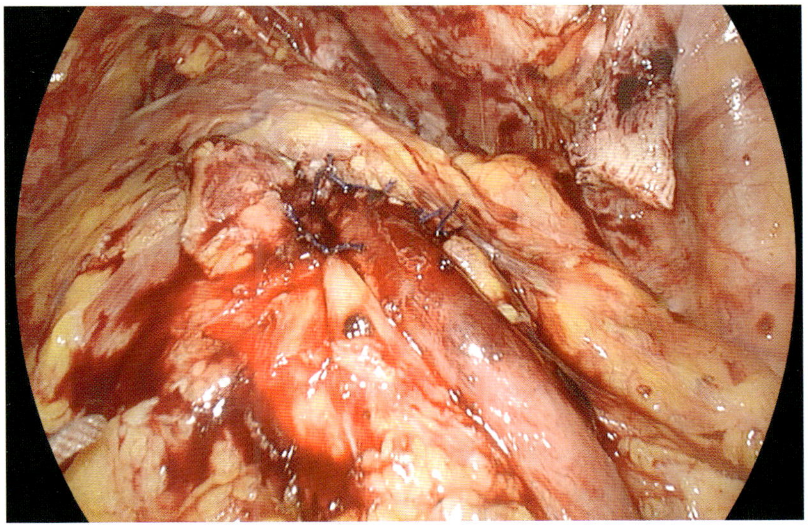

Fig. 19: Stitch placed at 12, 9, 6, and 3 o, clock position.

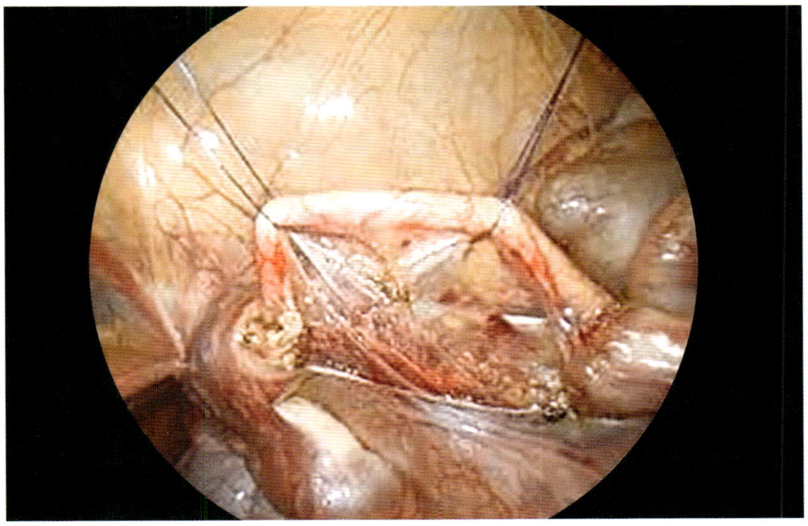

Fig. 22: Ureter held up with stay suture.

Boari tubularized bladder flap: When a midureteral or proximal ureteral injury occurs and the distal ureteral segment is not suitable for anastomosis, a Boari tubularized bladder flap is often a viable alternative **(Fig. 21)**. The bladder is opened on its anterior surface, and a full thickness bladder flap is swung cranially and tubularized for anastomosis to the proximal ureteral segment as shown. This is a technically challenging procedure and should be referred to a center with urologic reconstruction experience if necessary.

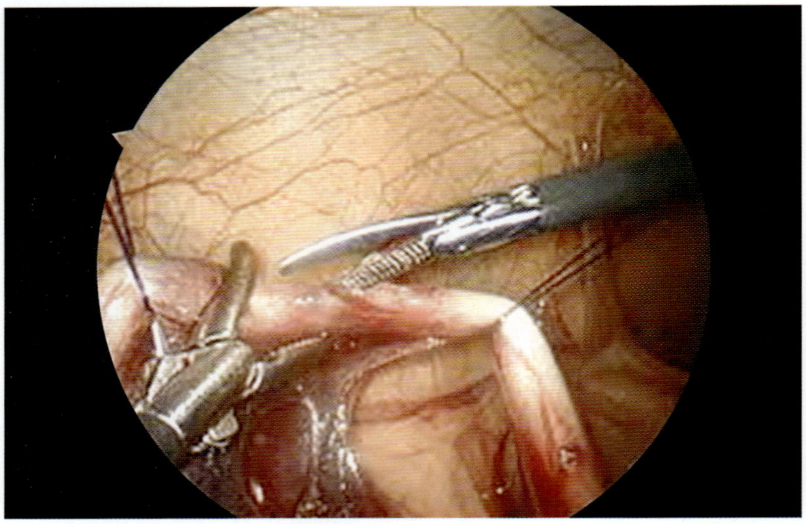

Fig. 23: Edges freshened up.

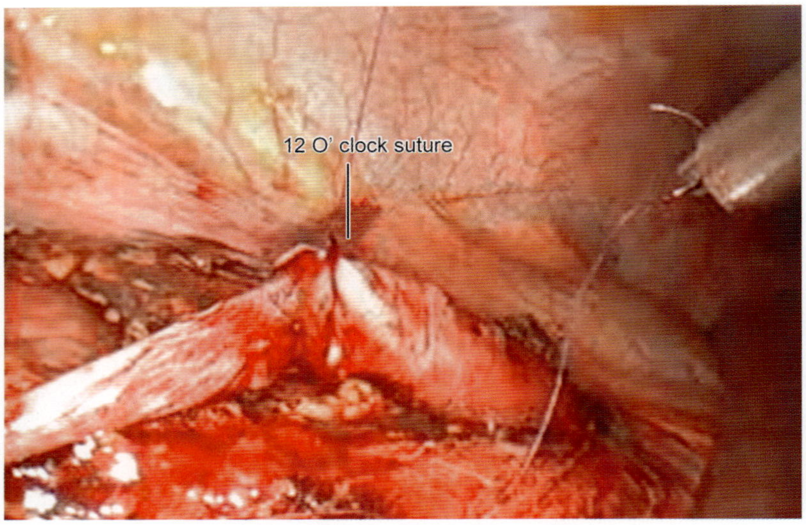

Fig. 25: Ureteric openings anastomosed to each other.

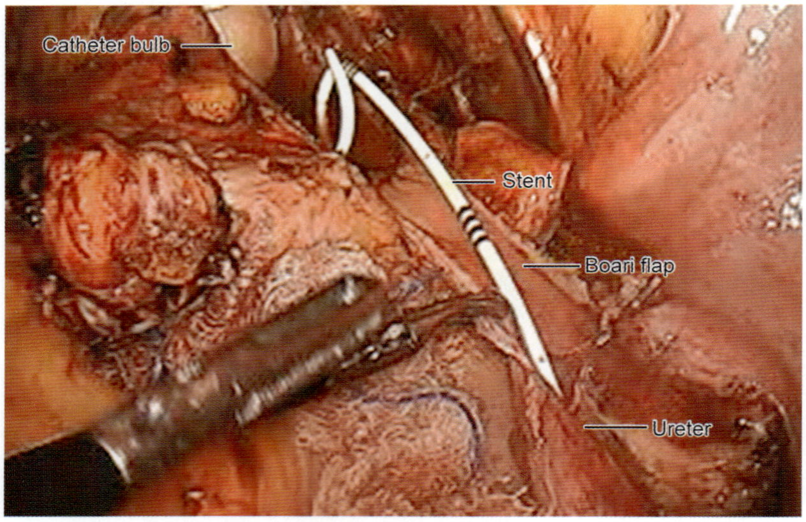

Fig. 24: DJ stent introduced.

Upper and Midureteral Injuries

Ureteroureterostomy: Often with small (2–3 cm) defects of the mid-ureter and upper ureter, a primary ureteroureterostomy can be performed.[10] The distal and proximal ureteral ends are debrided back to viable tissue and a standard running or interrupted anastomosis is performed. The anastomosis should be stented and, if possible, covered with peritoneum or other tissue.

Transureteroureterostomy: Most often, the length of ureteral loss as a result of iatrogenic ureteral injury is quite short making transureteroureterostomy (TUU) unnecessary. In cases when primary reanastomosis to a distal segment is not feasible, or if an ureteroneocystostomy is precluded (i.e. rectal injury, major vascular injury, or extensive bladder injury), then TUU is an acceptable option. Contraindications to TUU include inadequate donor ureter length, which would create tension on the anastomosis, or disease of the recipient ureter such as urothelial carcinoma, urolithiasis, retroperitoneal fibrosis, or pelvic tumors with ureteral involvement.[11] The donor ureter should be extensively mobilized, but care should be taken not to disrupt the longitudinal blood supply in the adventitial layer. Very little of the recipient ureter should be mobilized so that the area of anastomosis has a sufficient blood supply. The donor ureter should be passed under the sigmoid colon through the mesentery to the location of the recipient ureter. The donor ureter is then spatulated approximately 2 cm and the recipient ureter is opened to match the donor ureter opening.[12] An end-to-side anastomosis is performed **(Fig. 24)**.

Many reconstructive techniques have been performed laparoscopically and reconstruction of the ureter after iatrogenic injury is no exception. Laparoscopic techniques for the management of ureteral injuries include ureteroureterostomy, ureteroneocystostomy, and Boari-flap procedures. In a comparative retrospective review of patients undergoing laparoscopic and open techniques for ureteral reimplantation, patients undergoing distal ureteral reimplantation laparoscopically required less pain medication, had a shorter length of stay, and less blood loss.[13]

PREVENTION

- *Generous irrigation of pelvic side wall:* Diathermy of the pelvic side walls, e.g. following ovariolysis to achieve hemostasis, should be accompanied by generous fluid irrigation to cool down the tissue to minimize thermal injury.
- *Hydroprotection:* To diathermize endometriotic deposits adjacent to the ureter, 10–20 mL of normal saline solution or Hartmann's solution may be injected via a long needle (e.g. long spinal needle) just beneath the parietal peritoneum, at a point above the ureter, creating a pseudospace and lifting the peritoneum off the pelvic side wall. The water-filled space so created serves to protect the ureter from thermal injury.
- When oophorectomy is to be carried out, avoid the use of staples. Some reports suggest a high incidence of ureteric injury with staples, especially when used by those not familiar with the instrument.
- The use of a transilluminating ureteric stent, e.g. in laparoscopic hysterectomy.
- Most commonly, the ureter is injured near the uterosacral ligaments, as it cannot be identified reliably in this area. Therefore, special attention is required when performing laparoscopic procedures in this anatomical region, particularly in the presence of endometriosis or adhesions.

REFERENCES

1. Gilmour DT, Dwyer PL, Carey MP. Lower urinary tract injury during gynecologic surgery and its detection by intraoperative cystoscopy. Obstet Gynecol. 1999;94(5 Pt 2):883-9.
2. Aronson MP, Bose TM. Urinary tract injury in pelvic surgery. Clin Obstet Gynecol. 2002;45:428-38.
3. Thompson JD. Operative injuries to the ureter: prevention, recognition, and management. In: Rock JA, Thompson JD (Eds). TeLinde's Operative Gynecology, 8th edition. Philadelphia, PA: Lippincott Williams & Wilkins; 1997. pp. 1135-74.
4. Gilll S, Kerbl K, Meraney AM, et al. Basic principles techniques, and equipment of laparoscopic surgery. In: Walsh PC, Retik AB, Vaughan ED, Wein AJ (Eds). Campbell's Urology. Philadelphia: Saunders; 2002. p. 3455.
5. Saravelos H, Lee C, Li TC. Delayed presentation of inadvertent perforation of the bladder during laparoscopic surgery. Gynaecol Endosc. 1996;5:45-7.
6. Chapron CM, Dubuisson J, Ansquer Y. Is total laparoscopic hysterectomy a safe surgical procedure? Hum Reprod. 1996;11:2422-4.
7. Hensle TW, Berdon WE, Baker DH, et al. The ureteral "J" sign: radiographic demonstration of iatrogenic distal ureteral obstruction after ureteral reimplantation. J Urol. 1982;127:766-8.
8. Zimmerman IJ, Precourt WE, Thompson CC. Direct uretero-cysto-neostomy with the short ureter in the cure of ureterovaginal fistula. J Urol. 1960;83:113-5.
9. Middleton RG. Routine use of the psoas hitch in ureteral reimplantation. J Urol. 1980;123:352-4.
10. Coburn M. Ureteral injuries from surgical trauma. In: McAninch J (Ed). Traumatic and Reconstructive Urology. Philadelphia, PA: Saunders; 1996.
11. Iwaszko MR, Krambeck AE, Chow GK, et al. Transureteroureterostomy revisited: long-term surgical outcomes. J Urol. 2010;183:1055-9.
12. Barry JM. Surgical atlas transureteroureterostomy. BJU Int. 2005;96:195-201.
13. Rassweiler J, Gozen A, Erdogru T, et al. Ureteral reimplantation for management of ureteral strictures: a retrospective comparison of laparoscopic and open techniques. Eur Urol. 2007;51:512-23.

Accompanying Video: Laparoscopic bladder injury repair.

CHAPTER

30

Ureteric Injuries

Supriya Raina, Minal Kumbhalwar, B Ramesh

INTRODUCTION

Ureteric injury while performing various obstetric as well as gynecological procedures are the most common mode of iatrogenic ureteric injury comprising approximately 1.75% of ureteric injury cases.

INCIDENCE

During any abdominopelvic surgery, incidence of ureteric injuries is found to be 0.2–1.0%, among which gynecological and obstetric operations contribute for 50% of these injuries approximately.[1,2]

However, the incidence tends to rise up to 11% as in sacrocolpopexy, bladder neck suspension, urethropexy, and vaginal vault suspension surgeries.

The prevalence is higher mainly after surgery for gynecological malignancy. In spite of decline in the trend of major complications associated with minimally invasive surgery, the percentage of ureteric injury has been constant almost at 1%.[3] 38% of injuries to ureters occur during operative laparoscopy for endometriosis.[4]

Injury to left ureter is more common than right side, particularly at the pelvic part of the ureter.

Chianakwana et al. reported ligation as the common mode of injury comprising 87% cases; while Oboro et al. and Ozumba and Attah stated transection as common mode in 58% and 60% of cases, respectively.

ETIOLOGY

The ureter is closely attached to the peritoneum, which makes it vulnerable for injury during surgery.

Factors listed below enhances the risk more:

- Uterine enlargement[5,6]
- Prior single/multiple pelvic surgery[5,6]
- Ovarian malignancies[5,6]
- Endometriosis[5]
- Pelvic adhesions[5,7]
- Distorted pelvic anatomy[5,7]
- Concomitant bladder injuries
- Massive intraoperative bleeding.[8]

SITES OF INJURY

Most frequently affected part is lower third of ureter (51%), followed by upper (30%) and middle third (19%).[9] Typical site of injuries are:

- Lateral aspect of uterine artery
- The ureterovesical junction area nearer to Mackenrodt's ligament
- At the ovarian fossa where ureters crosses the pelvic brim at base of the infundibulopelvic ligament
- Adjacent to uterosacral ligament.

Different studies reported the most common site of injury as the lateral part of the uterine vessels,[10] but Daly et al. stated ovarian fossa as common area for injury. In case of laparoscopic surgeries, most frequent location is at the level of uterosacral ligaments.[9]

TYPES OF INJURY

Different mechanisms through which injury can happen are ligation, kinking, clamp crush injury, transection either partial or complete, division, diathermy-related, or devascularization.

The incidence in decreasing order reported are: complete transection 61%, excision 29%, ligation 7%, and partial transection 3%.[11]

After the surgery, avascular necrosis can also occur if extensive dissection is done around periureteric region hampering the anastomotic blood supply of ureter. Another mechanism is via kinking or obstruction due to lymphocele or large hematoma.

CLASSIFICATION

The Committee of American Association for Surgery of Trauma devised the Organ Injury Scaling System for classifying ureteric injuries.[12]

- Grade I—contusion/hematoma with or without devascularization
- Grade II—laceration but <50% transection
- Grade III—laceration with 50% transection
- Grade IV—laceration with complete transection but <2 cm of devascularization
- Grade V—laceration/avulsion with >2 cm of devascularization.

However, above anatomical classification does not have prognostic implications.

DIAGNOSIS

Ureteric injuries can be diagnosed intraoperatively or postoperatively. Most of the ureteric injuries nearly 70% which occurs in gynecological surgeries are diagnosed postoperatively.[9]

INTRAOPERATIVE DIAGNOSIS

Intraoperative identification helps in immediate repair and also decreases morbidity.[13] Attempts should be made to verify ureteric integrity constantly during any pelvic surgery. There exists no definitive mechanism for diagnosing intraoperative devascularization.

Whenever it is not possible to visualize the ureters, intravenous injection of indigo carmine dye (5 mL) or methylthioninium chloride is given for confirming patency of ureter.[14] Intraoperative telescopy through cystotomy via abdominal route or transurethral cystoscopy can be performed to check release of dye-stained urine from bilateral ureteric orifices.

Appearance of bubbles or blood-stained urine through the ureteric orifices indicates ureteric injury. Using cystoscopy and telescopy intraoperatively during urogynecology surgeries has shown increased incidence of ureteric injury to 2.6–8%.[15,16] However, its use in benign gynecological operations found undetected damage in 0.4% cases.[17]

The cystoscopy performed routinely will be cost-effective only if ureteric injury incidence exceeds 1.5% for abdominal and 2% for vaginal or lap-assisted vaginal hysterectomy.[10]

PREVENTIVE MEASURES TO DECREASE URETERIC DAMAGE

- Adequate operative technique
- Proper exposure
- No blind clamps to be applied in case of bleeding
- Direct visualization and dissection of ureter **(Figs. 1 and 2)**
- Mobilizing the bladder from operative field **(Fig. 4)**
- Minimal use of diathermy.

POSTOPERATIVE PRESENTATION

Signs and symptoms of ureteric injury postoperatively are:

- Fever associated with flank pain is the most common symptom.
- Hematuria, definitive indicator of renal injury, may not be there in almost 30% cases.[18,19]

Rarely, patient may come with retroperitoneal urinoma[20] (local urine collection), detected by ultrasonography. Postoperative anuria is the key indicator for immediate evaluation. Leakage of urine from site other than urethra clinches diagnosis for fistula. In few cases, hypertension can be late presentation owing to obstructive uropathy. However, typical symptoms may be found only in 50% of ureteric injuries.

INVESTIGATIONS TO DIAGNOSE URETERIC INJURIES

Intravenous Urogram

Ureteric continuity, drainage, or any leak as well as hydronephrosis (series of sagittal images) is usually seen on intravenous urogram (IVU). Dye extravasation is a hallmark of ureteric injury, but subtle features may be present as delayed functioning to normal findings sometimes in spite of injury.

Computed Tomography

A computed tomography (CT) scan with contrast can be used for determining ureteric patency. Extravasation of contrast mainly in medial perirenal space is a characteristic feature.[21] The disappearance of contrast in the distal part of ureter on delayed CT visuals confirms complete transection of ureter.

As CT scan is a series of cross-sectional images, checking ureteric continuity with CT is more complicated than with an IVU. Rapid-sequence spiral CT cannot demonstrate it, hence delayed images are required explicitly.[22]

Retrograde Ureterogram

Whenever IVU and CT gives inconclusive diagnosis, a retrograde ureterogram can be performed to evaluate the ureteric course. It helps to identify exact anatomical position of injury/obstruction, in spite being missed by IVU/CT scan, by delivering greater density of contrast at the site of injury. But retrograde ureterogram is definitely invasive modality than IVU/CT scan as it requires prior cystoscopy also.

Renal Ultrasound

Renal ultrasonography is the best noninvasive imaging to visualize kidney but it fails to assess renal function or continuity of ureter. However, hydronephrosis and retroperitoneal urinomas are shown with great sensitivity.

Cystoscopy

Postoperative anuria **(Fig. 6)**, suggestive of bilateral ureter blockage, needs cystoscopic analysis. Spurting of urine from bilateral ureteric openings confirms ureteric patency. Retrograde ureterogram helps whenever doubt arises.

Contrast-dye Tests

Contrast-dye tests are done with cystoscopy specifically if urinary fistula is suspected. The fistulous tract is detected with concomitant injection of indigo carmine dye and Congo red dye in bladder via transurethral catheter.

The complete blood count (guide to infection) with serum electrolytes must be done in ureteric injuries. Postoperative serum urea, creatinine, and sodium levels help in diagnosis. Analyzing creatinine on postoperative day 2 aids in evaluating ureteric integrity. Unilateral ureteric obstruction is suspected if there is an increase in creatinine by >0.2 mg/dL. Normally, if bilateral ureters are patent, creatinine elevations will be <0.3 mg/dL.[23] Apart from ureteric obstruction, creatinine levels are also affected due to causes such as intraoperative bleeding/hemorrhage, replacement of fluids, and using nephrotoxic drugs such as aminoglycosides, furosemide, and nonsteroidal inflammatory drugs.

Postoperative uremia happens when there is total urinary obstruction as in bilateral ureter injury or injury to single functioning kidney. Anuria is the hallmark sign of impending uremia and such patient requires urgent intervention for preventing further damage and preserving residual renal function.

Hyponatremia is common after ureteric injury[24] due to spillage of urine in the retroperitoneum. Reabsorption of free water from such dilute urinoma decreases osmolality and serum sodium levels, leading to sodium-sparing and free water-excreting reaction by kidney.

MANAGEMENT

Most of the time injuries occur due to failure of anticipating primary hemorrhage, distorted anatomy/altered ureteric course as seen in pelvic adhesions, and malignancy.

The better prognosis depends on the interval between the injury and repair, longer interval has worst outcome. Prompt intraoperative diagnosis and immediate correction decreases morbidity as well as mortality.

Unfortunately, lots of cases are diagnosed postoperatively presenting with urinary leakage from vagina, surgical site, or wound drain site. Other presenting signs and symptoms include loin pain, anuria, azotemia, uremia, pyelonephritis, or accidently during radiological imaging for an unrelated medical case.

Prior stenting of ureter does not decreases ureteric injury but has increased chances of diagnosing eventual injury intraoperatively. Before proceeding, repair definitive nature of the injury should be determined. The complete renal assessment and delineation of ureteric course are obtained by laboratory and radiological investigations, respectively. Medical management is not useful for ureteric injury, except treating coexisting infection and renal failure.

All ureteric transections require stent to increase urinary diversion, e.g. double-J stent. Urinoma formation can be prevented by using passive drain retroperitoneally such as Penrose drain because active drain prolongs leakage by providing negative pressure and hence avoided. The bladder is emptied by using Foley or Malecot catheter. Even if ureteric injury is diagnosed delayed, one should not delay the repair except in sepsis, hemodynamic instability, large hematoma, or pus collection at the site. In above scenarios, retrograde ureteric stenting or percutaneous nephrostomy followed by drainage is done and surgery is delayed till complications are dealt with.

Management Options for Ureteric Injury

- *Needle injury:* No action needed till bleeding or leakage
- *Partial transection:* Stenting
- *Complete transection but without loss of length:*
  - Less than 5 cm from vesicoureteric junction—ureteroneocystostomy **(Fig. 7)**
  - Greater than 5 cm from vesicoureteric junction—uretero-ureterostomy **(Fig. 5)**
- *Complete transection with loss of length: Psoas hitch:*
  - Boari flap with a psoas hitch
  - Transureteroureterostomy
  - Ureteroileocystostomy
  - Ureterocalycostomy
  - Renal autotransplantation.

PRINCIPLES OF URETERIC REPAIR

- Adequate ureteric mobilization and tension-free anastomosis
- Careful ureteric **(Figs. 1, 2 and 9A to F)** dissection preserving adventitia and vascular supply
- Watertight closure by reducing use of fine absorbable suture
- Using peritoneal or omental covering around the anastomosis **(Figs. 8A to R)**
- Keeping passive drain at the repair site to prevent urinoma formation
- Stenting with a ureteric catheter **(Fig. 3)**
- Considering proximal diversion.

CONCLUSION

Berard (1841) and Simon (1869) documented earliest ureteric injury surgical repairs in gynecological and obstetric surgery.[25,26] The ureteric anatomy and its course were difficult to understood that time but various contributions have been made to enhance understanding etiology, prevention, diagnosis, and treatment of iatrogenic ureteric injuries.

If postoperative recovery is poor, the diagnosis of ureteric injury should be kept in mind. Radiological imaging forms the base of diagnosis since laboratory investigations and symptoms are nonspecific. It must be performed as early as possible if there is suspicion of ureteric injury.

Postoperative Complications of Ureteric Injury Repair

- Stricture formation
- Excess drainage
- Stent and stoma-related issues
- Recurrent urinary tract infection **(Figs. 11A to H)**
- Ureteric reflux/obstruction
- Complications of Boari flap
- Wound infection
- Hematoma formation.

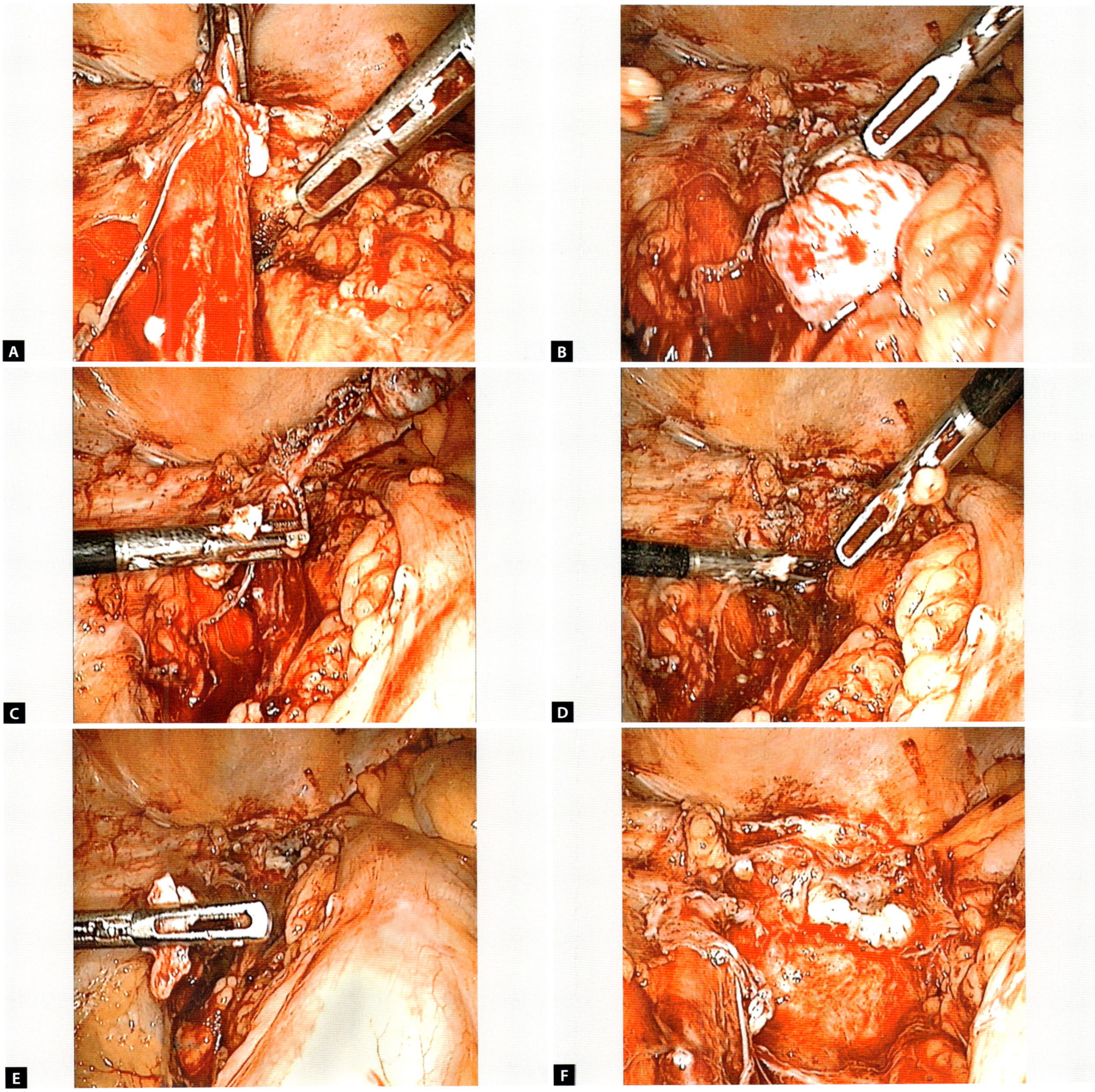

Figs. 1A to F: Stepwise ureteric dissection.

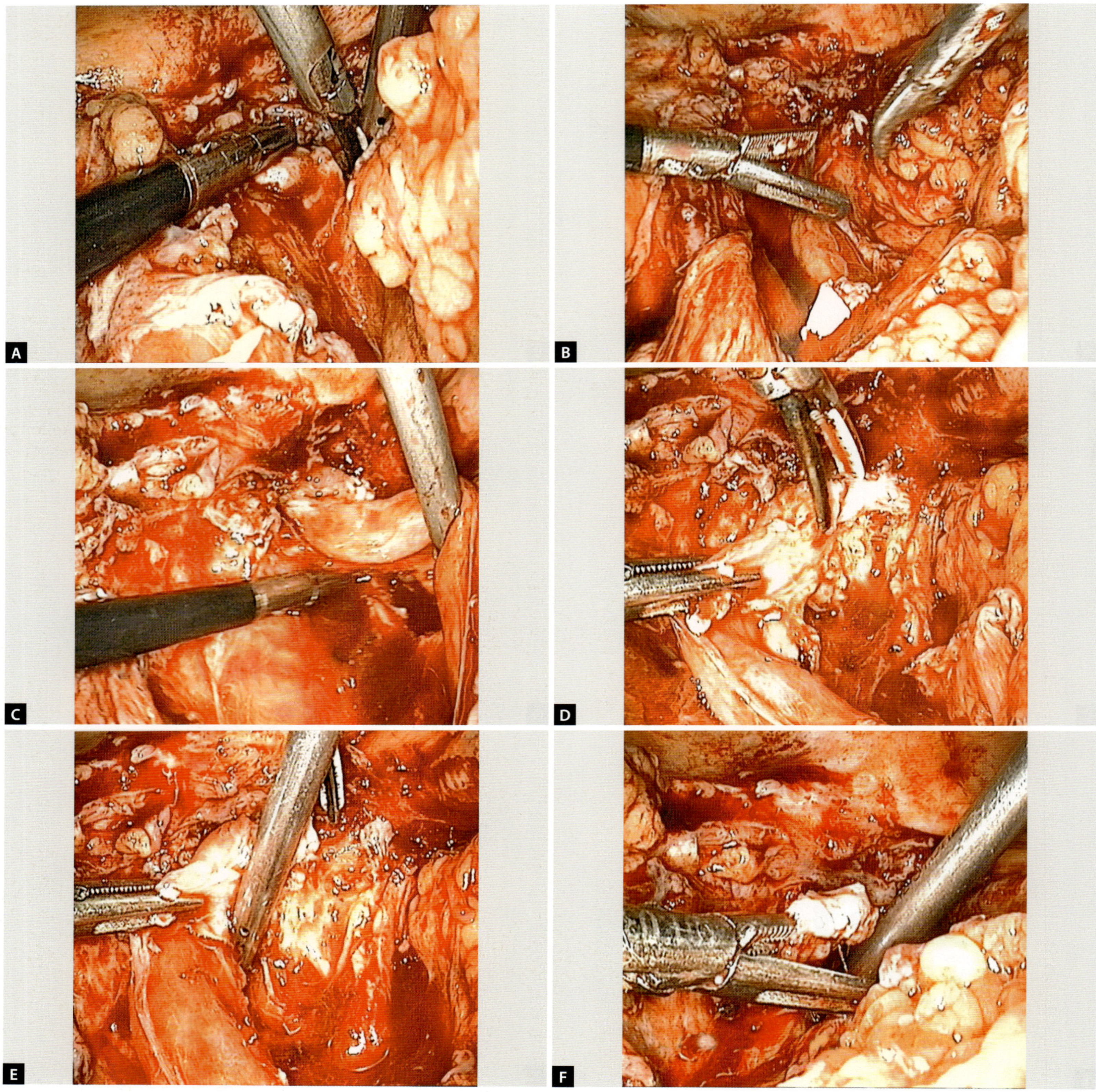

Figs. 2A to F: Steps of ureteric dissection.

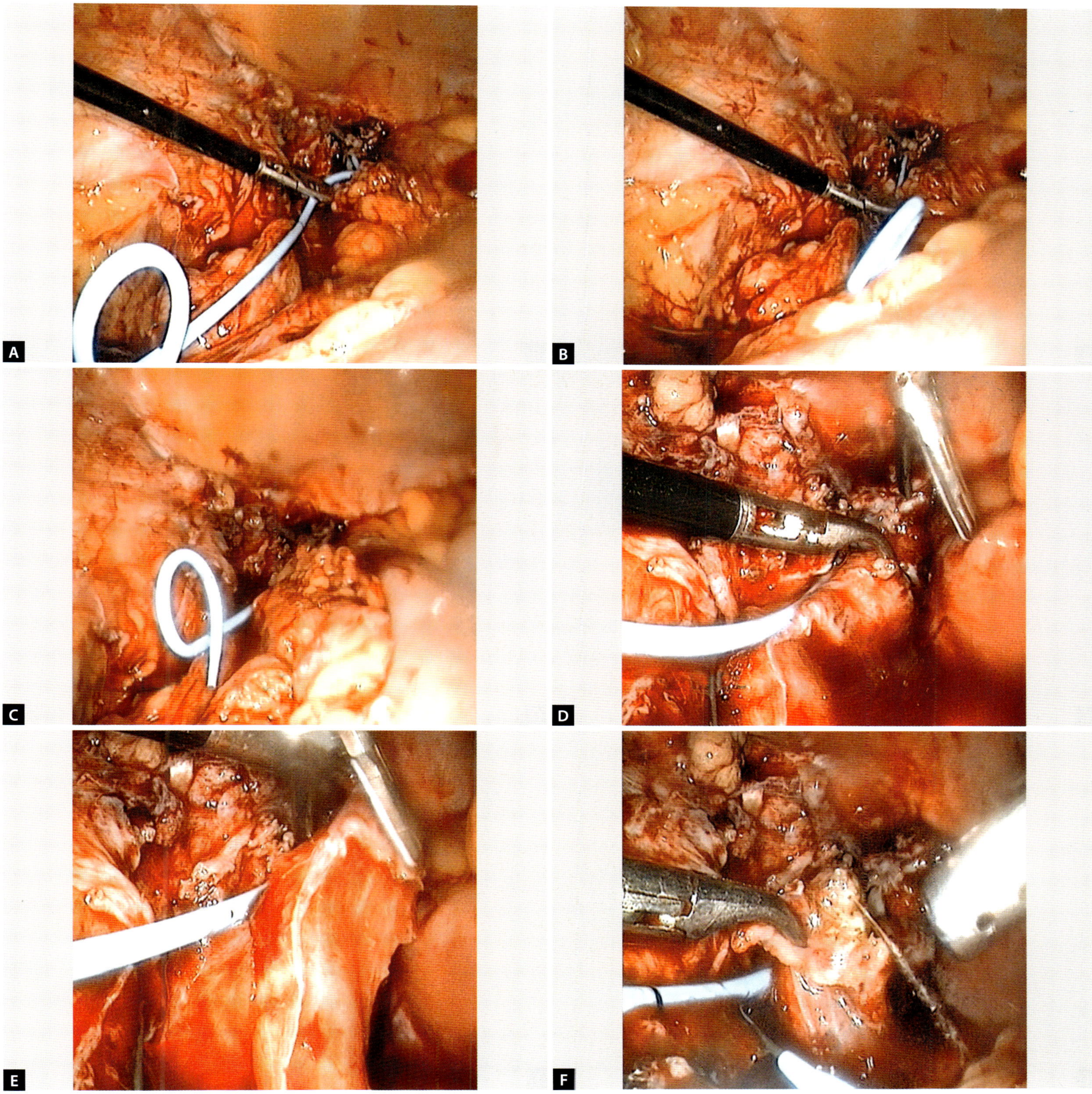

Figs. 3A to F: Steps of ureteric stenting.

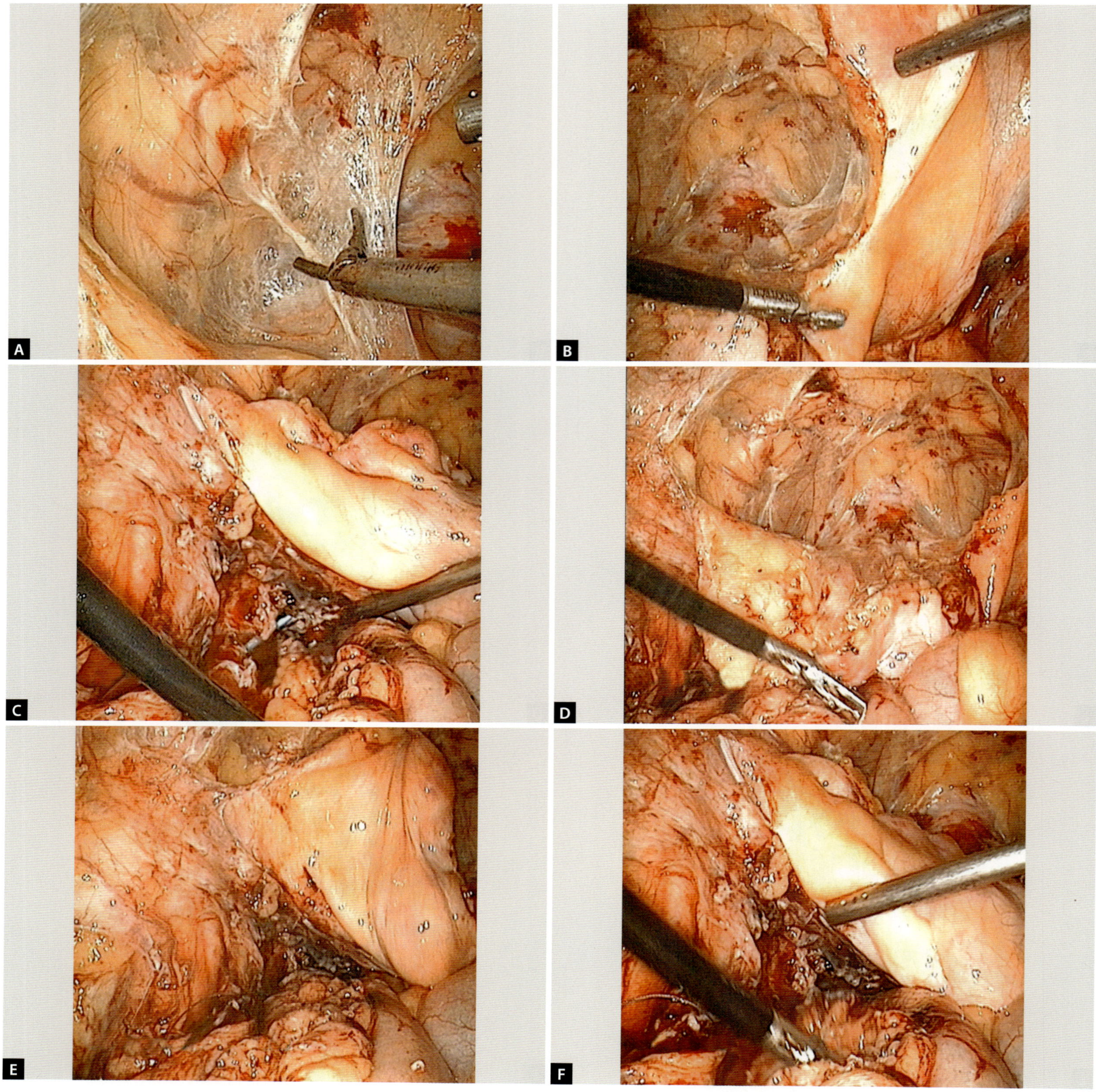

Figs. 4A to F: Bladder dissection done after dissecting the ureter and placing the stent in it.

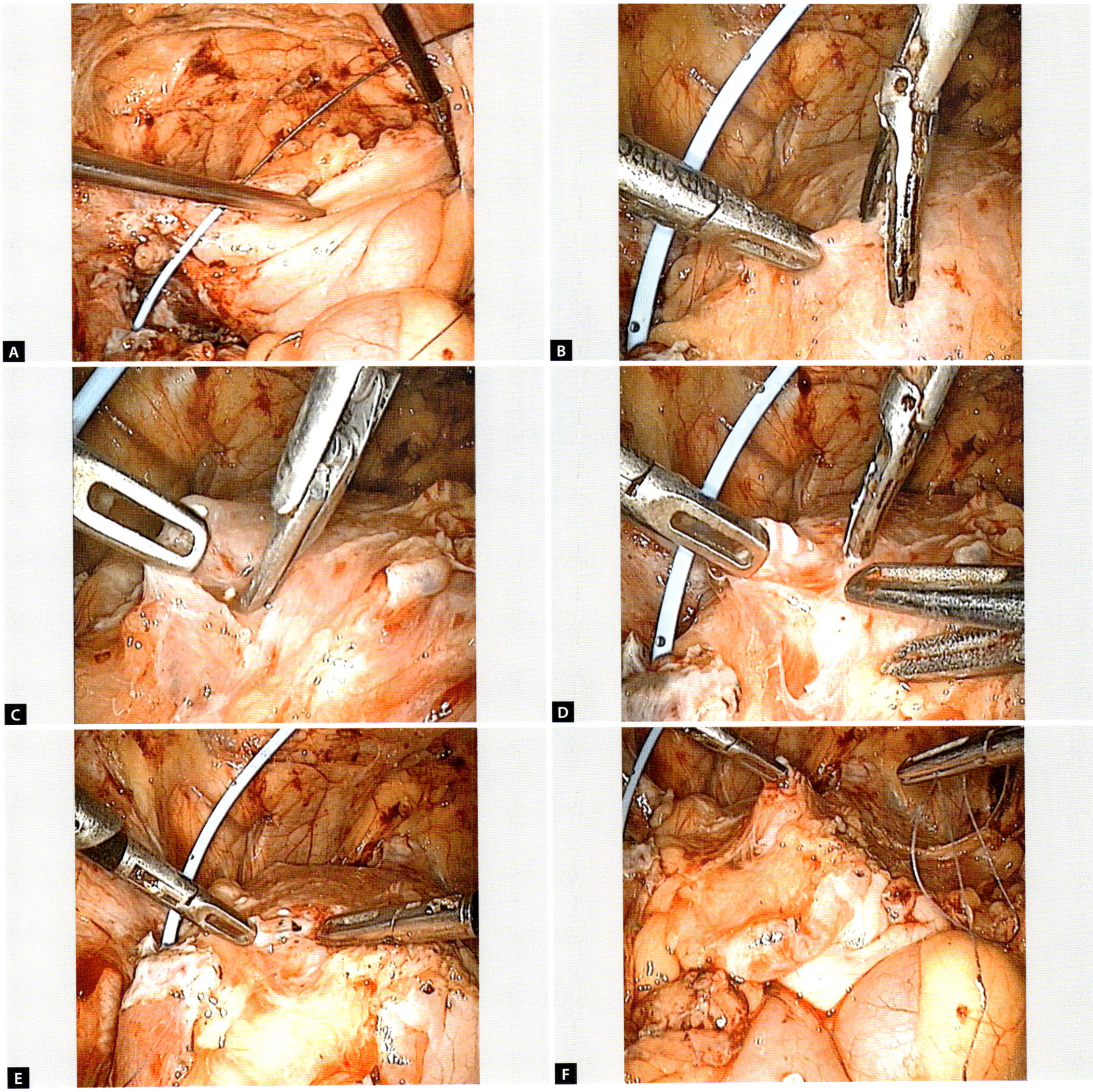

Figs. 5A to F: Neostoma made in the bladder wall for ureteric reimplantation.

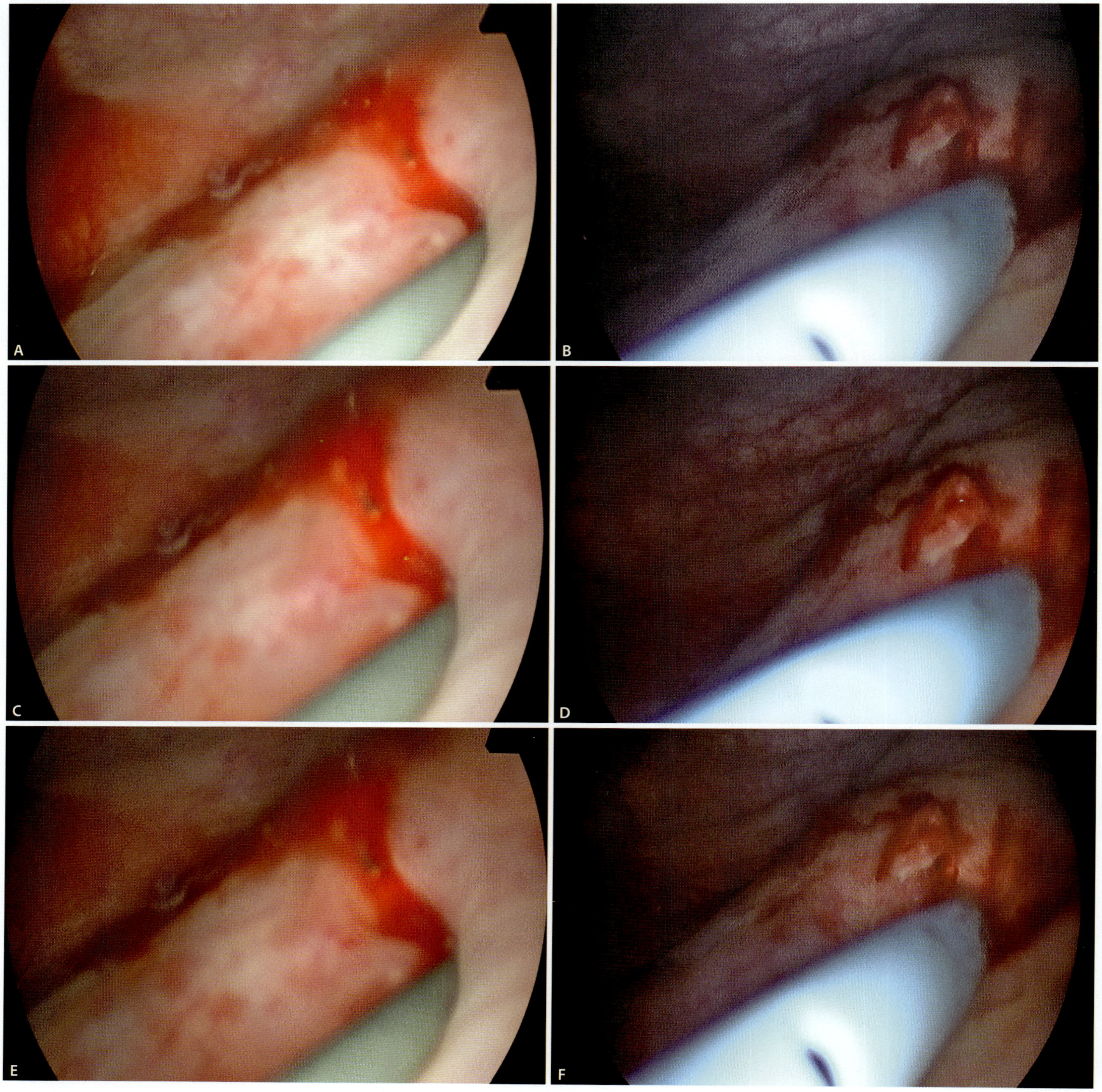

Figs. 6A to F: Ureteric stenting as seen on cystoscopy.

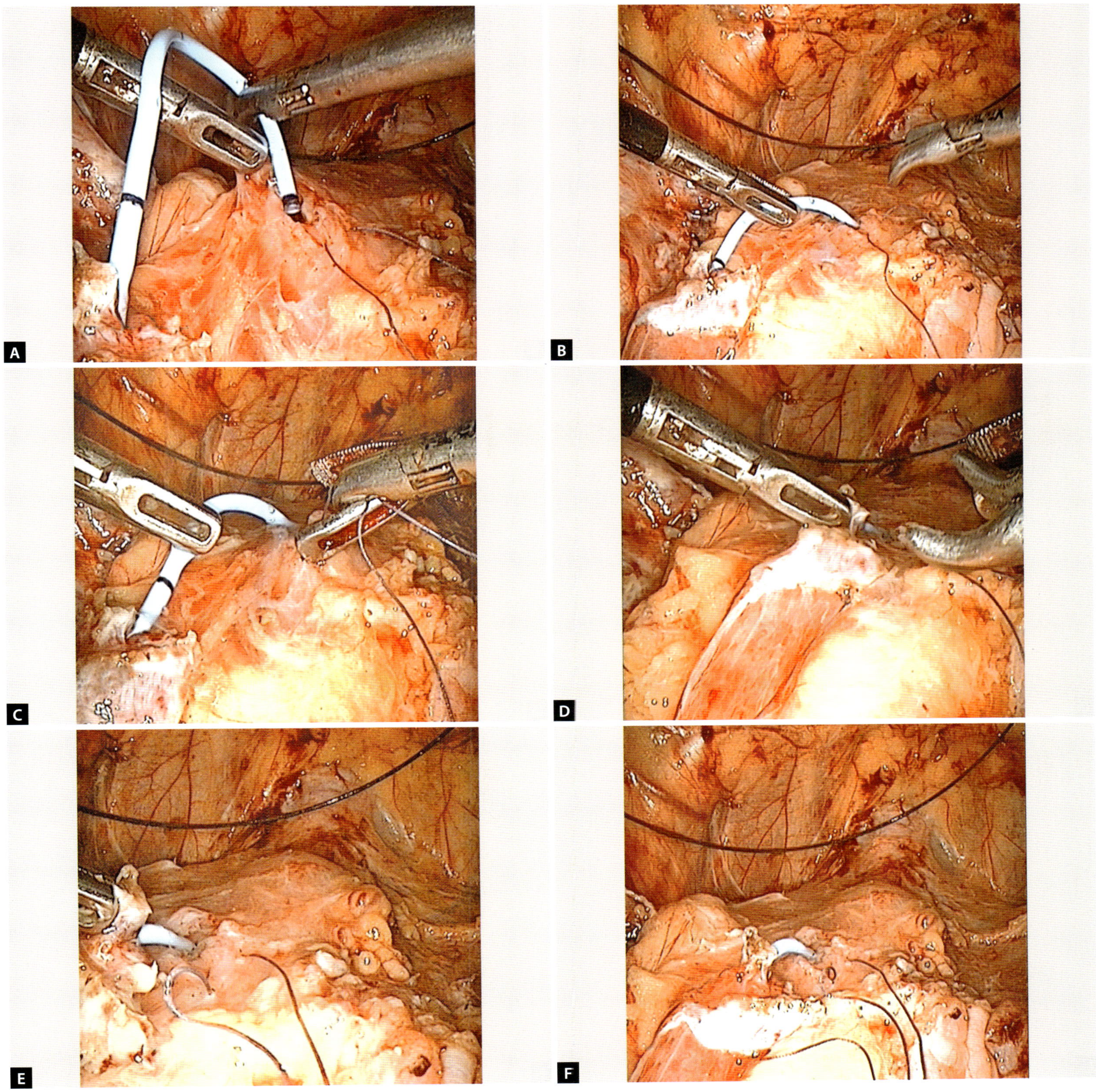

Figs. 7A to F: Ureteric reimplantation into the bladder over the ureteric stent.

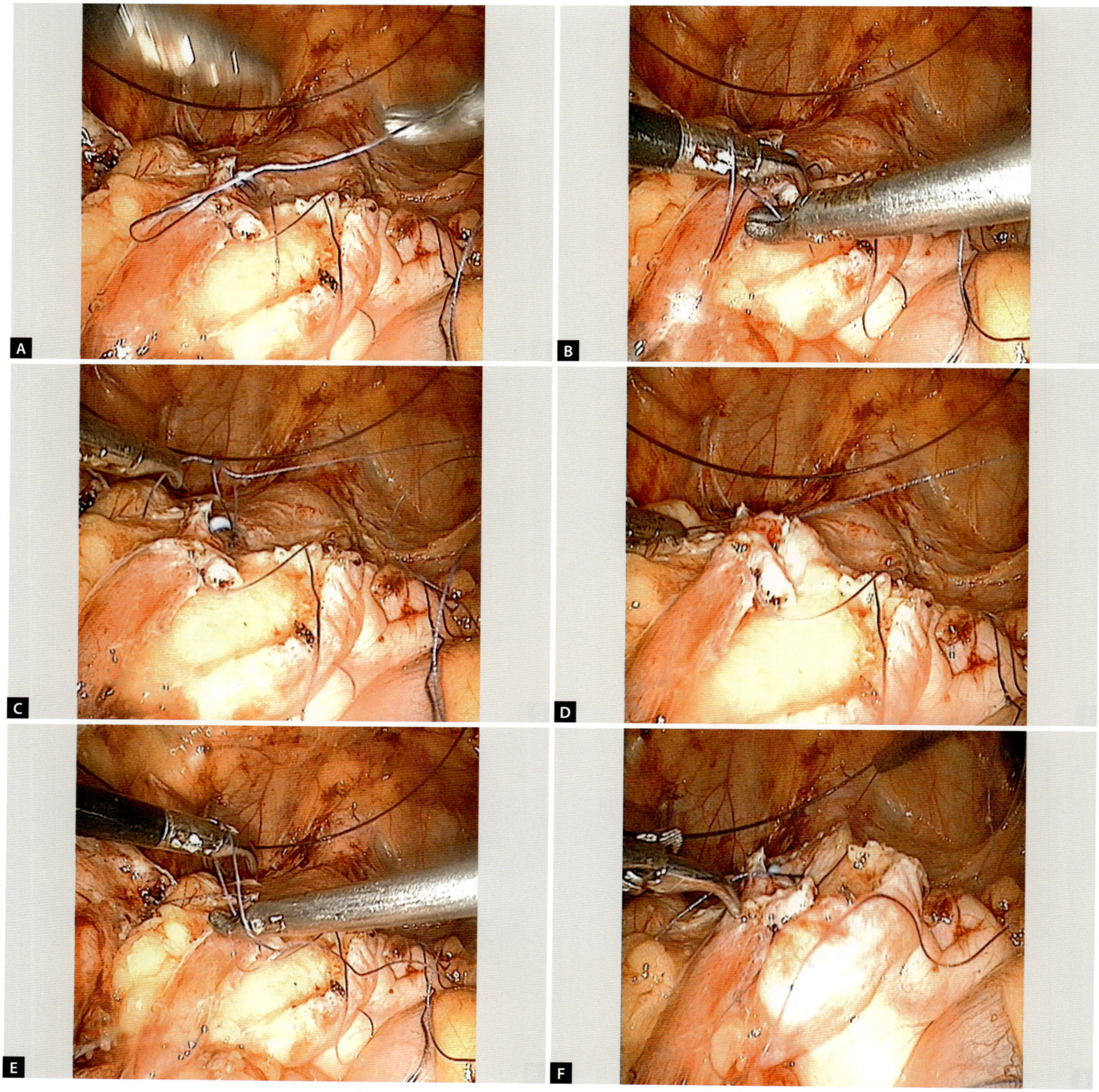

Figs. 8A to F: Layer-by-layer closure of uretric reimplantation.

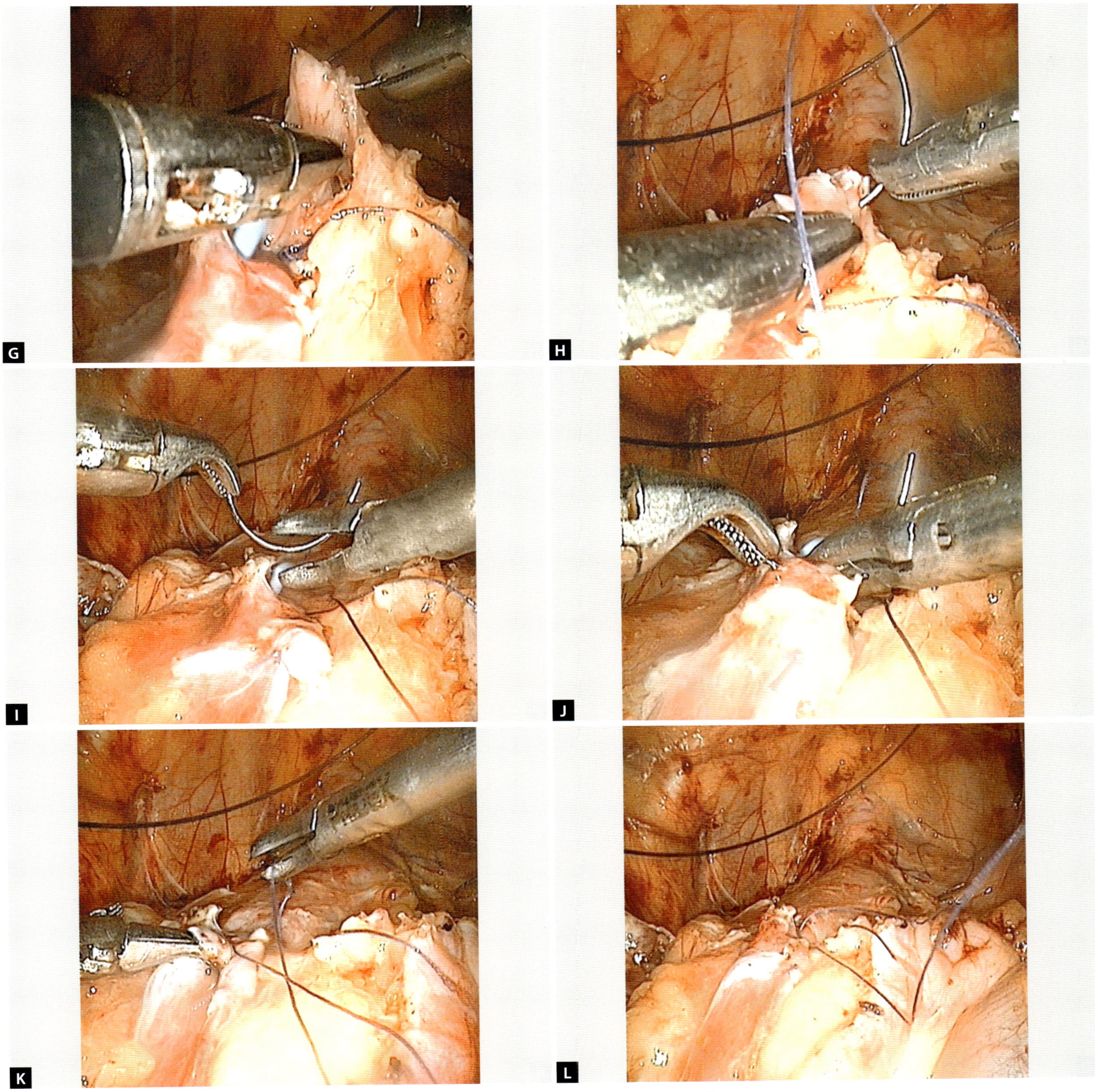

Figs. 8G to L: Approximating layers of bladder wall.

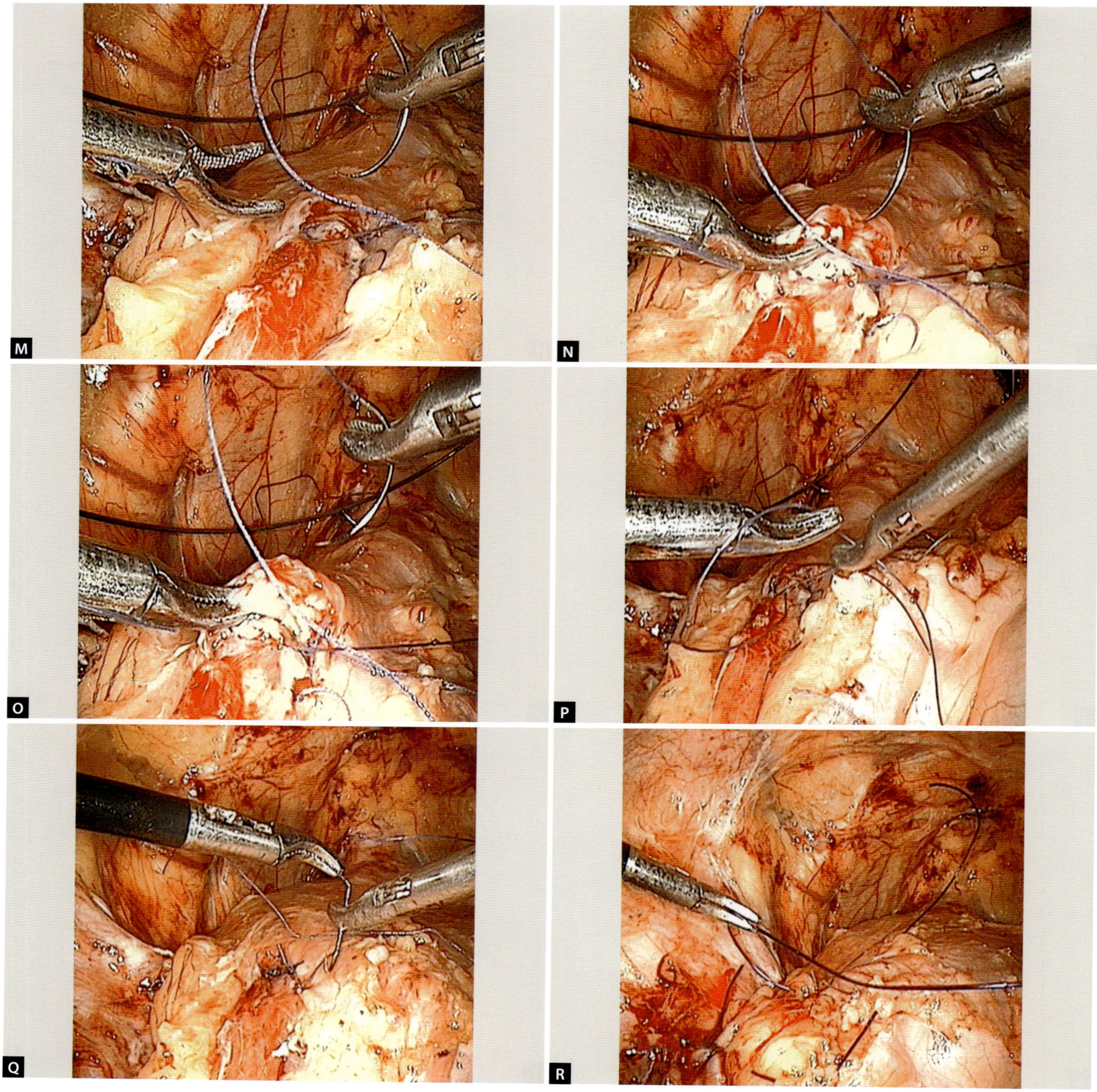

Figs. 8M to R

Figs. 8A to R: Bladder wall closed in layers after ureteric reimplantation.

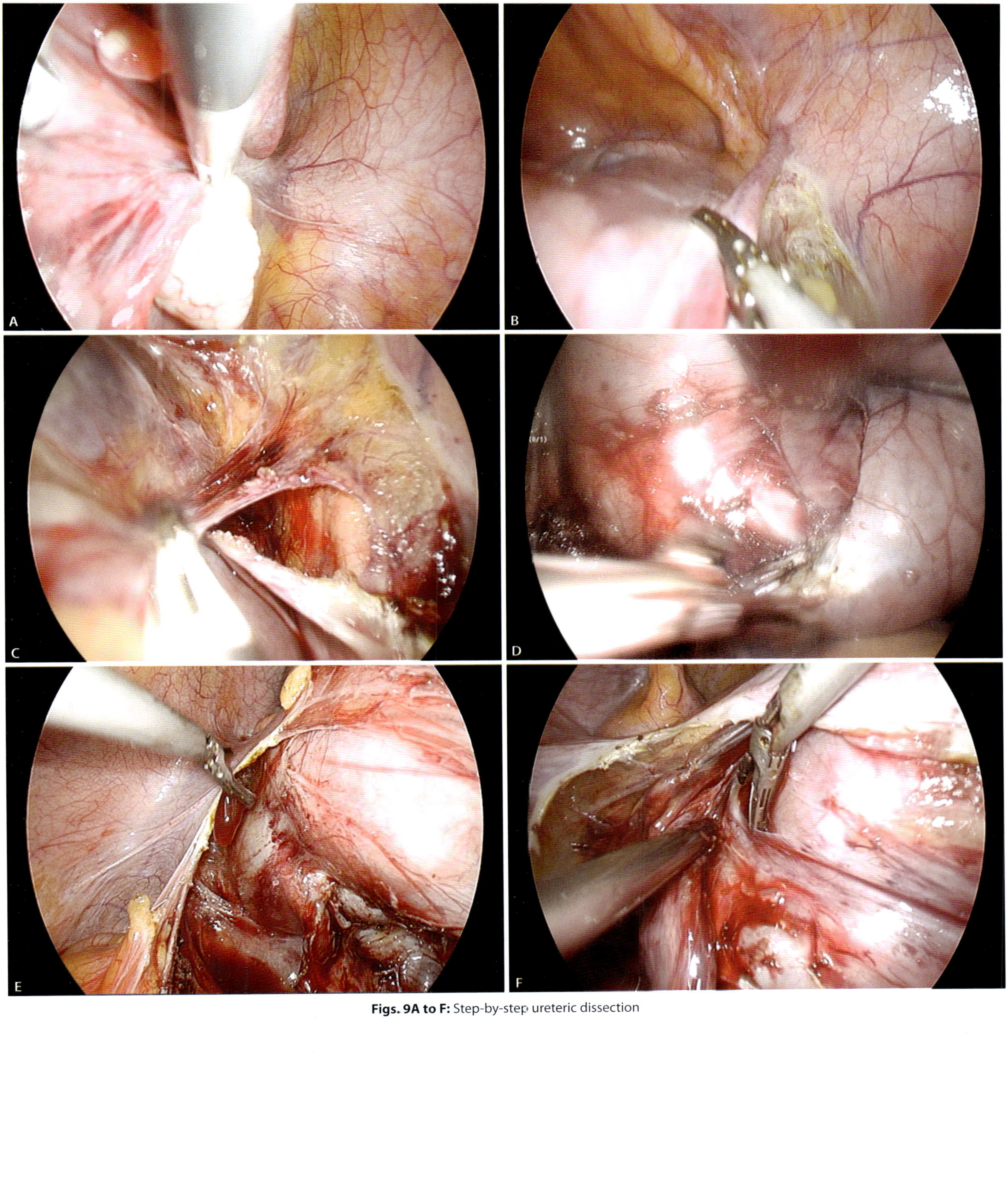

Figs. 9A to F: Step-by-step ureteric dissection

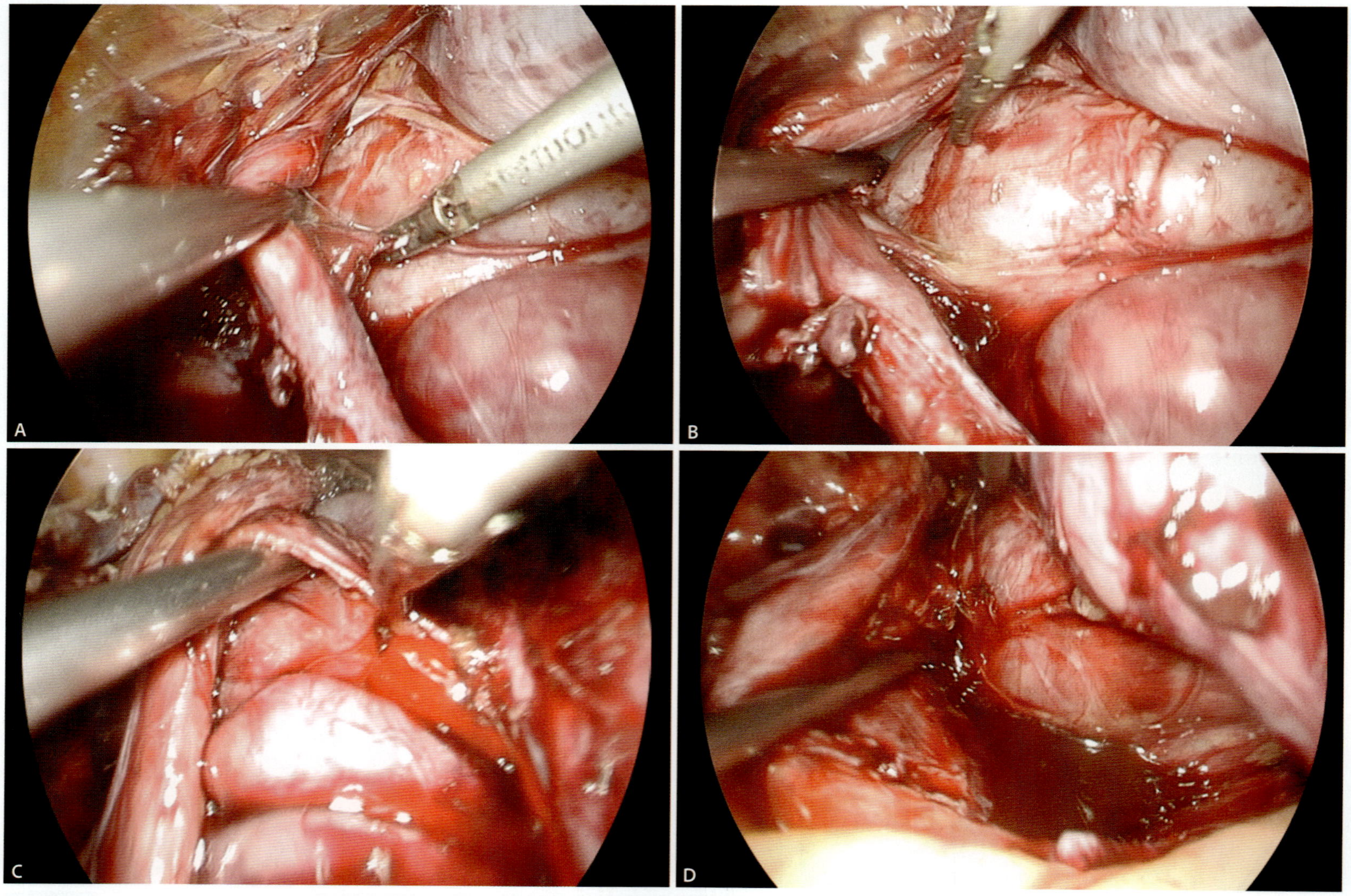

Figs. 10A to D: Ureterolysis done in a patient of total laparoscopic hysterectomy.

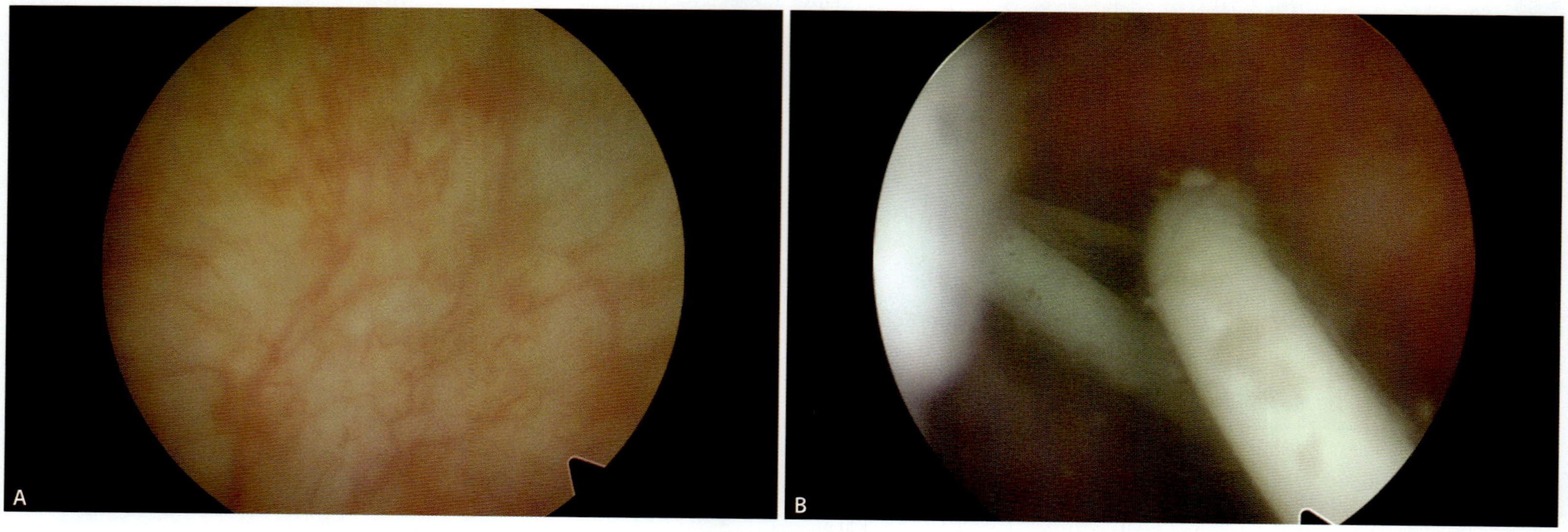

Figs. 11A and B

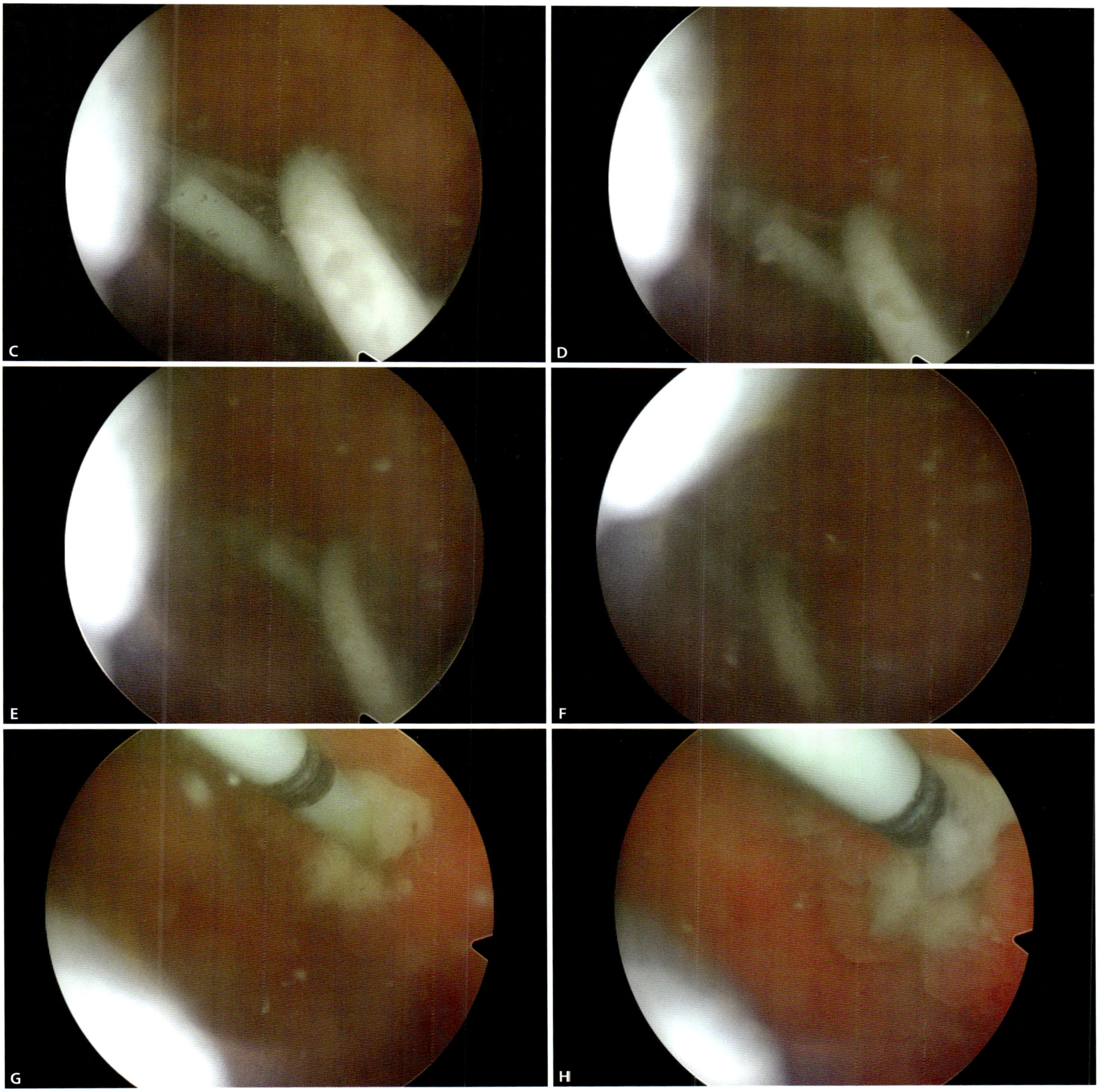

Figs. 11C to H

Figs. 11A to H: Hysteroscopic appearance of the stent.

REFERENCES

1. Chan JK, Morrow J, Manetta A. Prevention of ureteral injuries in gynecologic surgery. Am J Obstet Gynecol. 2003;188(5):1273-7.10.
2. Barber MD, Visco AG, Weidner AC, et al. Bilateral uterosacral ligament vaginal vault suspension with site-specific endopelvic fascia defect repair for treatment of pelvic organ prolapse. Am J Obstet Gynecol. 2000;183(6): 1402-10.
3. Eke N. Iatrogenic urological trauma: a 10 year experience from Port Harcourt. West Afr J Med. 2000;19(4):246-9.
4. Aghaji AE, Odoemene C. Ureteric injuries in Enugu, Nigeria. East Afr Med J. 1999;76(4):184-8.
5. Ozumba BC, Attah CA. Ureteral injury in obstetric and gynecologic operations in Nigeria. Int J Gynaecol Obstet. 1991;36(2):131-5.
6. Liapis A, Bakas P, Giannopoulos V, et al. Ureteral injuries during gynecological surgery. Int Urogynecol J Pelvic Floor Dysfunct. 2001;12(6):391-3.
7. Mensah J, Klufio G, Ahiaku F, et al. Delayed recognition of bilateral ureteral injury after gynaecological surgery. Ghana Med J. 2008;42(4):133-6.
8. Kim JH, Moore C, Jones JS, et al. Management of ureteral injuries associated with vaginal surgery for pelvic organ prolapse. Int Urogynecol J. 2006;17(5):531-5.
9. Mann WJ, Arato M, Patsner B, et al. Ureteral injuries in an obstetrics and gynecology training program: etiology and management. Obstet Gynecol. 1988;72(1):82–5.
10. Visco AG, Taber KH, Weidner AC, et al. Cost effectiveness of universal cystoscopy to identify ureteral injury at hysterectomy. Obstet Gynecol. 2001;97(5 pt 1):685-92.
11. Ghali AM, El Malik EM, Ibrahim AL, Ismail G, Rashid M. Ureteric injuries: diagnosis, management and outcome. J Trauma 1999 Jan;46(1): 150-8.
12. Chou MT, Wang CJ, Lien RC. Prophylactic ureteral catheterization in gynecologic surgery: a 12-year randomized trial in a community hospital. Int Urogynecol J Pelvic Floor Dysfunct. 2009;20(6):689-93.
13. Gill EJ, Elser DM, Bonidie MJ, et al. The routine use of cystoscopy with the Burch procedure. Am J Obstet Gynecol. 2001;185(2):345-8.
14. Stanhope CR, Wilson TO, Utz WJ, et al. Suture entrapment and secondary ureteral obstruction. Am J Obstet Gynecol. 1991;164(6 Pt 1):1513-7.
15. Pettit PD, Petrou SP. The value of cystoscopy in major vaginal surgery. Obstet Gynecol. 1994;84(2):318-20.
16. Tulikangas PK, Weber AM, Larive AB, et al. Intraoperative cystoscopy in conjunction with anti-incontinence surgery. Obstet Gynecol. 2000; 95(6 Pt 1):794-6.
17. Onwudiegwu U, Makinde OO, Badejo OA, et al. Ureteric injuries associated with gynaecologic surgery. Int J Gynaecol Obstet. 1991;34(3):235-8.
18. Wiskind AK, Thompson JD. Should cystoscopy be performed at every gynecologic operation to diagnose unsuspected ureteral injury? J Pelvic Surg. 1995;1:134-7.
19. Armenakas NA. Current methods of diagnosis and management of ureteral injuries. World J Urol. 1999;17(2):78-83.
20. Sharfi AR, Ibrahim F. Ureteric injuries during gynaecological surgery. Int Urol Nephrol. 1994;26(3):277-81.
21. Kenney PJ, Panicek DM, Witanowski LS. Computed tomography of ureteral disruption. J Comput Assist Tomogr. 1987;11(3):480-4.
22. Mulligan JM, Cagiannos I, Collins JP, et al. Ureteropelvic junction disruption secondary to blunt trauma: excretory phase imaging (delayed films) should help prevent a missed diagnosis. J Urol. 1998;159(1):67-70.
23. Walter AJ, Magtibay PM, Morse AN, et al. Perioperative changes in serum creatinine after gynecologic surgery. Am J Obstet Gynecol. 2002;186(6):1315-9.
24. Lukacz ES, Nager CW. Ureteral injury presenting with hyponatremia. Obstet Gynecol. 2001;98(5 Pt 2):974-6.
25. Grace PA, Murphy DM, Butler MR. Surgical injury to the ureter: a report on 21 injuries in 19 patients. Ir Med J. 1983;76:418-20.
26. Medscape. (2018). Vasavada SP. Ureteral injury during gynecologic surgery. [online] Available from: http://www.emedicine.com/med/topic3320.htm. [Last accessed January, 2020].

Accompanying Video: Laparoscopic ureteric stenting and re-implantation.

CHAPTER

31

Tubal Recanalization

Sowmya MS, Aditi Rai, B Ramesh

INTRODUCTION

Tubal sterilization is a most widely used method for contraception throughout the world. The most common reasons for reanastomosis are regret on sterilization at a young age, loss of a child, remarriage, and low level of education. Rather than reanastomosis, some couples prefer in vitro fertilization (IVF). The demand for reanastomosis has been reported as 14.3% with operations carried out at the rate of 1.1%.[1]

Gomel V in 1974 reported first time tubal reanastomosis procedures with laparotomy and with laparoscopy by Sedbon E et al. in 1989.[2,3]

Microsurgical tubal recanalization is the gold standard technique for recanalization through the laparotomy route. The advantage of microsurgical tubal recanalization is shorter hospital stay, minimal tissue handling, and less postoperative adhesions.[4]

INDICATIONS FOR LAPAROSCOPIC TUBAL REANASTOMOSIS

- Reversal of sterilization
- Midtubal block secondary to various pathologies
- Tubal occlusion secondary to postectopic pregnancy management
- Salpingitis isthmica nodosa
- Failed tubal cannulation for proximal block.

Tubal sterilization is a most reliable method, but regret may be encountered afterward. The strongest factors are the woman's age.[5] In the Carotid Revascularization Endarterectomy versus Stenting Trial (CREST) study, the possibility of feeling cumulative regret after the procedure was reported as 4%, 8%, and 13% in 3rd year, 7th year, and 14th year,[6] respectively.

PREOPERATIVE CONSIDERATIONS

Factors affecting pregnancy success following MTR include:

- More than 4 cm remaining tubal length
- Different methods of sterilization (Pomeroy, clip, and ring sterilization best)
- Site of reanastomosis (isthmic-isthmic best)
- Time lag from sterilization (the less time the better)
- Techniques employed (microsurgical technique best)
- Younger age
- Associated with other infertility factors.

There are 60–80% chances of intrauterine pregnancy rates in well-selected patients after microsurgical tubal recanalization. Before MTR, following things should be noticed, include an operative note of tubal ligation (tubal interruption) and the associated pathology, along with couple's fertility potential followed by other tests like ultrasonographic assessment of the uterine anatomy, semen analysis, and ovulation monitoring. In women who are >35 years old, or who started experiencing premature ovulation insufficiency symptoms, a more comprehensive evaluation is required.

TYPES OF ANASTOMOSIS

- *Isthmic-isthmic segments:* The distal stump should be prepared and opened in the same manner as the proximal isthmic stump, if both the proximal and distal tubal segments are isthmic.
- *Ampullary-ampullary segments:* Adhesions are released from the occluded ampullary stump. Surrounding ostia is applied by digital pressure; through the IV catheter, sleeve surgeon can inject indigo carmine into the occluded distal ampullary segment.
- *Ampullary-isthmic segments:* If the distal segment is ampullary and the proximal segment is isthmus, adhesions are released from occluded ampullary stump and the tension between the two stumps is tested.

SURGICAL PROCEDURE

Setup

Pneumoperitoneum was created with the help of carbon dioxide (CO_2) gas, systematically explored the abdominopelvic cavity and the adnexa was inspected (Gomel, 1980; Dubuisson et al., 1995).[8] Three 3-mm trocars (Surgiport; USSC, Elancourt, France) were inserted suprapubically; these were placed high, so easy access to see the Fallopian tube.

Stump Preparation and End Marking

When using Hulka clips, Li et al. (1996) showed that the microvilli and cilia of the epithelium which was 1.0 cm from the ligated scar were normal on the mucosa and numerous microvilli and cilia were even lost at a distance of 0.5 cm away from the ligated scar (Li et al., 1996).[9]

SURGICAL TECHNIQUE

Bladder should be emptied by Foley catheter, uterus mobilized by the uterine manipulator.

The intrauterine balloon is inflated with 3 mL normal saline. Pneumoperitoneum was created with the help of CO_2 gas; under direct visualization, the 3- or 5-mm secondary ports are then placed **(Fig. 4)**. Following this, the uterus is mobilized to inspect the pelvis.

If all criteria are fulfilled for anastomosis, the operation proceeds **(Fig. 5)**. The instruments described are all part of the complete Storz "KOH Ultramicro Series™" set **(Figs. 1 to 3)**. The dilute Pitressin (1:100) is injected into the terminal serosa of the proximal tube **(Figs. 6A and B)**. Next the operator introduces the microneedle electrode/scissors **(Figs. 7A and B)** used to circumscribe the serosa of the proximal tube. We can avoid cautery close to the tube, to avoid mesosalpingeal vessels from damage **(Figs. 8A and B)**, which may compromise the blood supply to the Fallopian tube. Chromopertubation is performed later **(Figs. 9A and B)**.

With the help of intracorporeal knot, mesosalpinx is sutured together and tying around 5 mm away from the Fallopian tube with

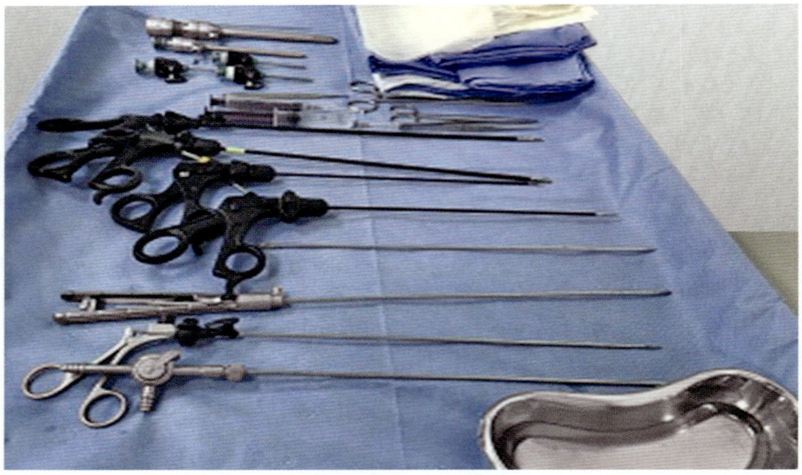

Fig. 1: Trolley with instruments.

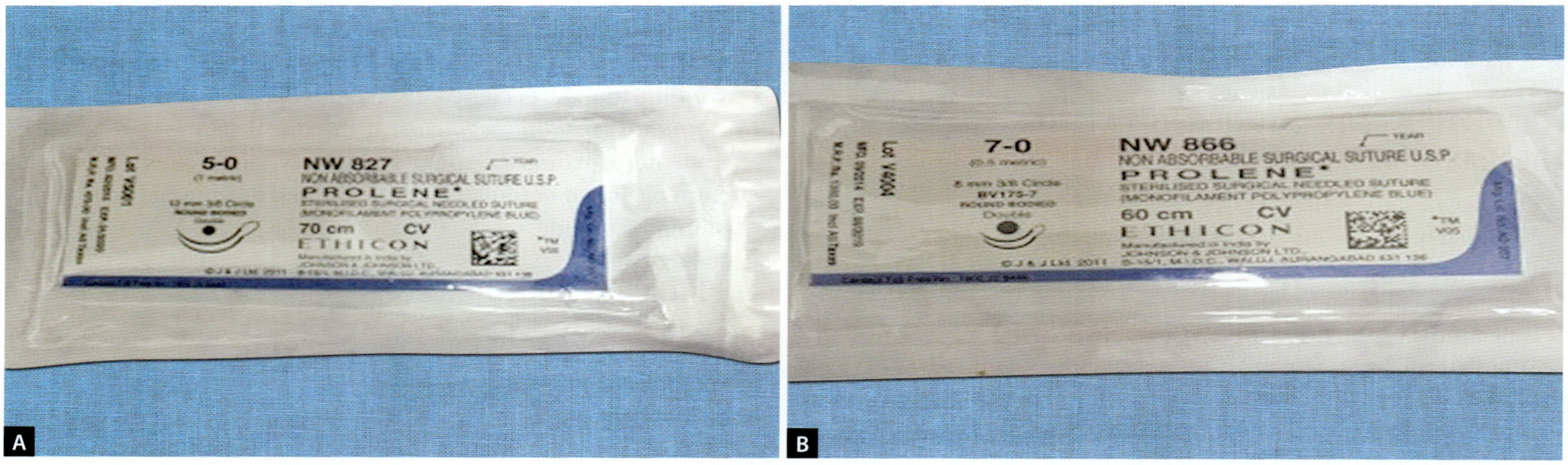

Figs. 2A and B: Suture materials used.

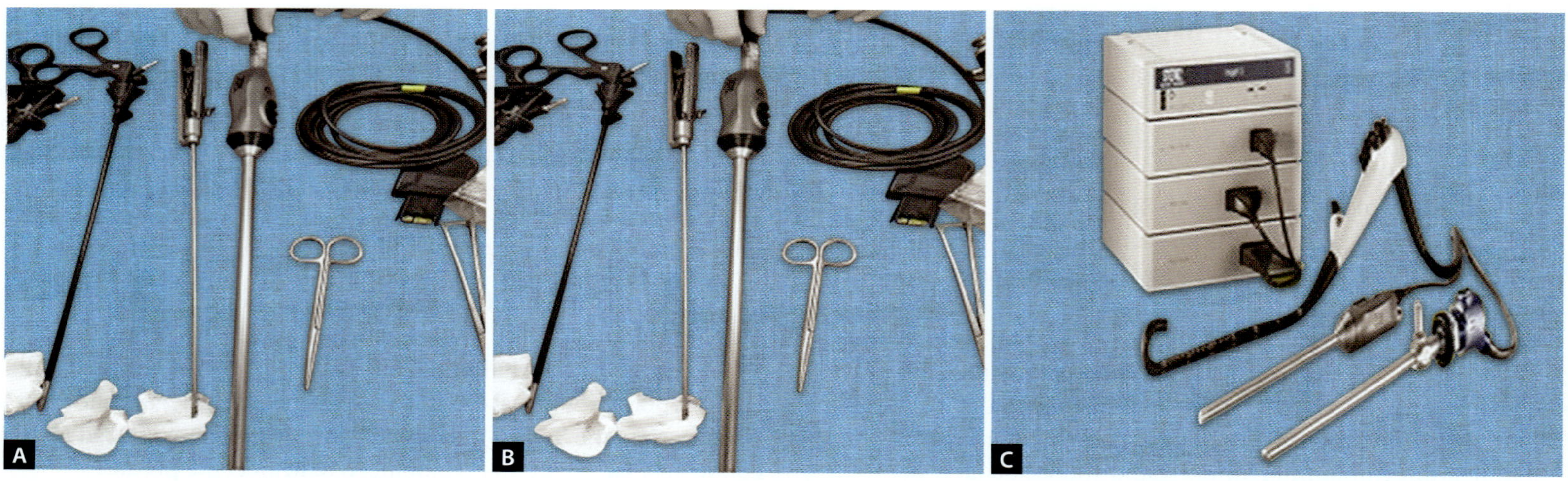

Figs. 3A to C: Three-dimensional (3D) camera.

the help of 5-0 Polydioxanone (PDS) or Prolene suture material. We should avoid not to approximate the mesosalpinx too near the tube, as it will hinder subsequent anastomosis.

6-0 suture of 6 cm length is introduced and at 6 o'clock position of distal tube, mucosa and muscularis layers are included **(Figs. 10 and 11)**. The needle is then inserted at 6 o'clock position of the proximal tube from mucosa through muscularis **(Fig. 12)**. Intracorporeal knot is placed by throwing three knots **(Figs. 13A to C)**. Intracorporeal knotting can be facilitated by using curved grasper. Sutures are cut using ultramicrosuture cutting scissors. Second suture is placed at 12 o'clock position of the proximal tube with needle piercing muscularis to submucosa or mucosa then to 12 o'clock position of distal tube from muscularis to mucosa/submucosa **(Figs. 14A and B)**.

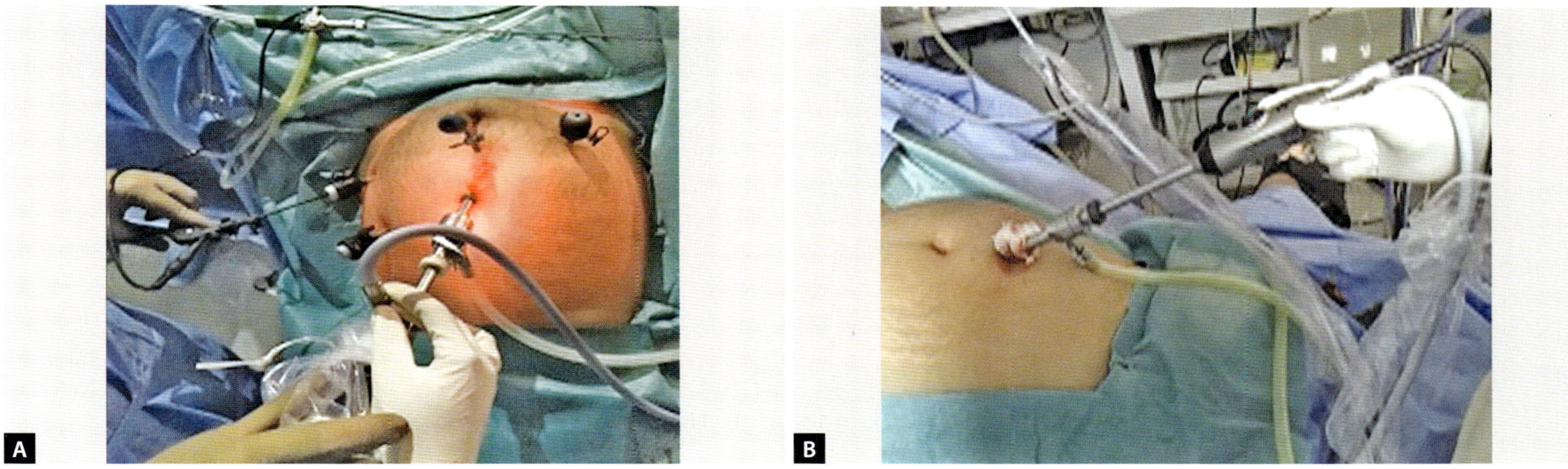

Figs. 4A and B: Ports placement.

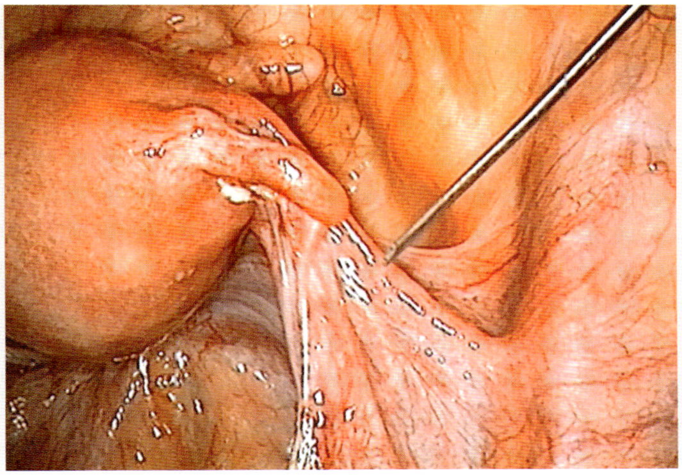

Fig. 5: Panoramic view of right-sided Fallopian tube in post-tubectomy status by Pomeroy method during cesarean section.

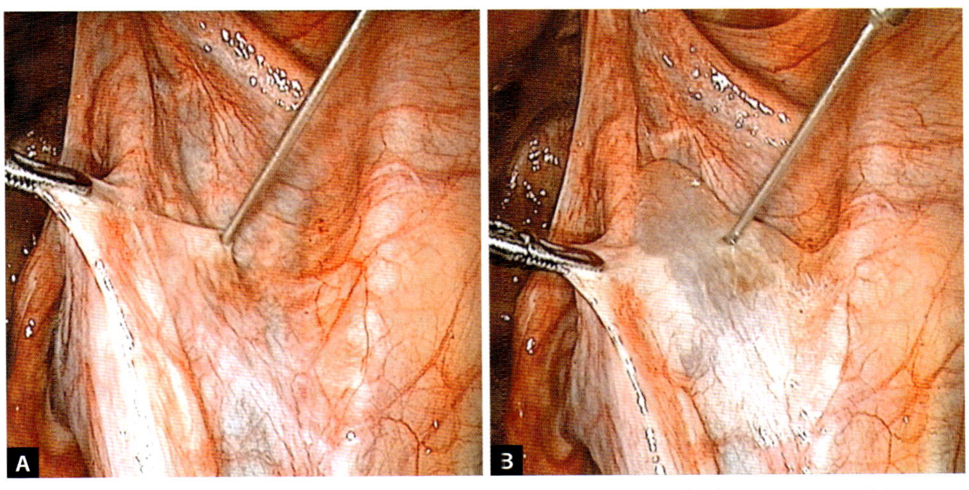

Figs. 6A and B: Injection vasopressin 20 U diluted in 200 mL normal saline into mesosalpinx.

These are placed next and tied and at last 12 o'clock suture is tied **(Figs. 15 to 17)**. At the end in order to demonstrate patency of the tube, chromopertubation is performed **(Fig. 19)**. One or two interrupted serosal sutures are placed by 6-0 or 7-0 Prolene or PDS suture material. Mesosalpinx is then searched for any gaps, if found is closed using 6-0 Nylon **(Fig. 20)**. The opposite tube is then treated in the same manner.

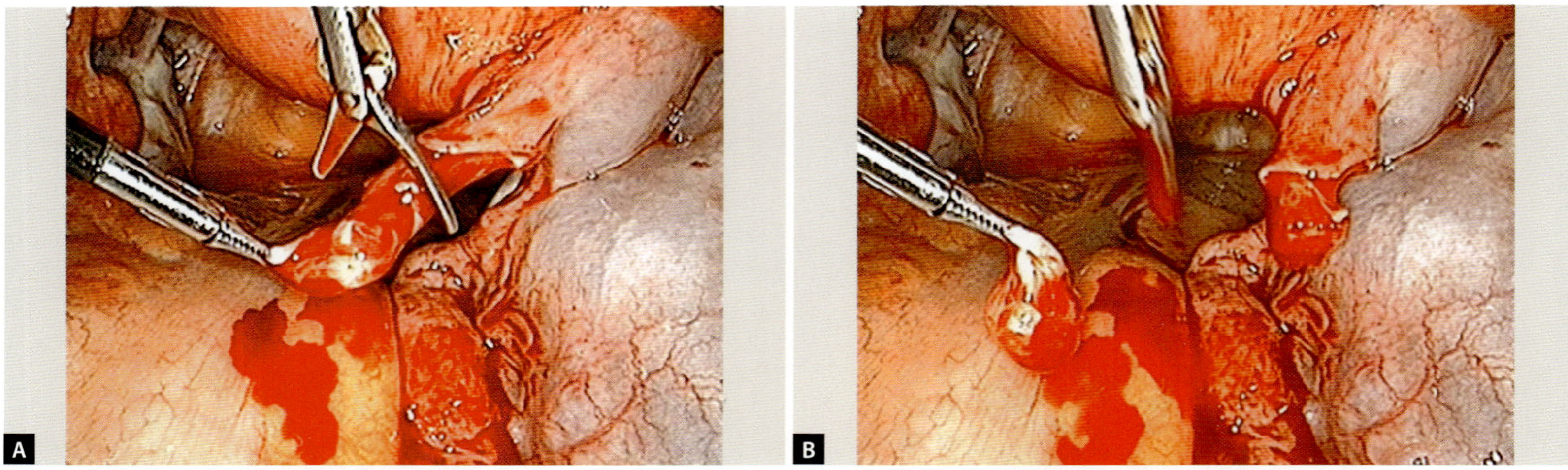

Figs. 7A and B: By using scissors, right angled cut is made on the proximal tube.

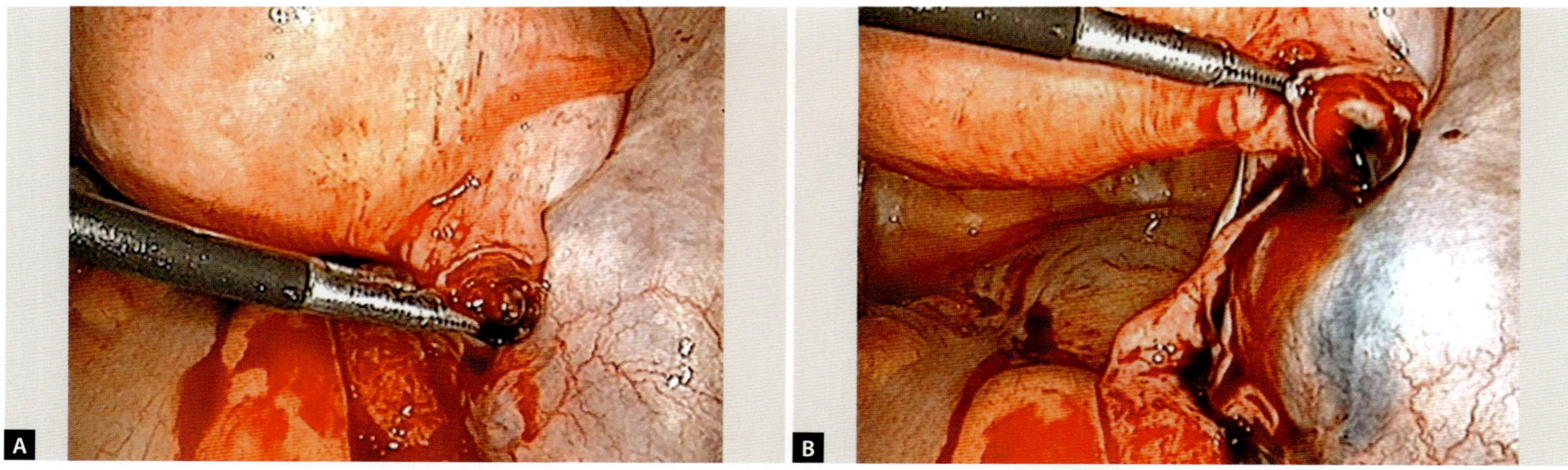

Figs. 8A and B: Patency of proximal end of tube checked and confirmed by free spill of dye.

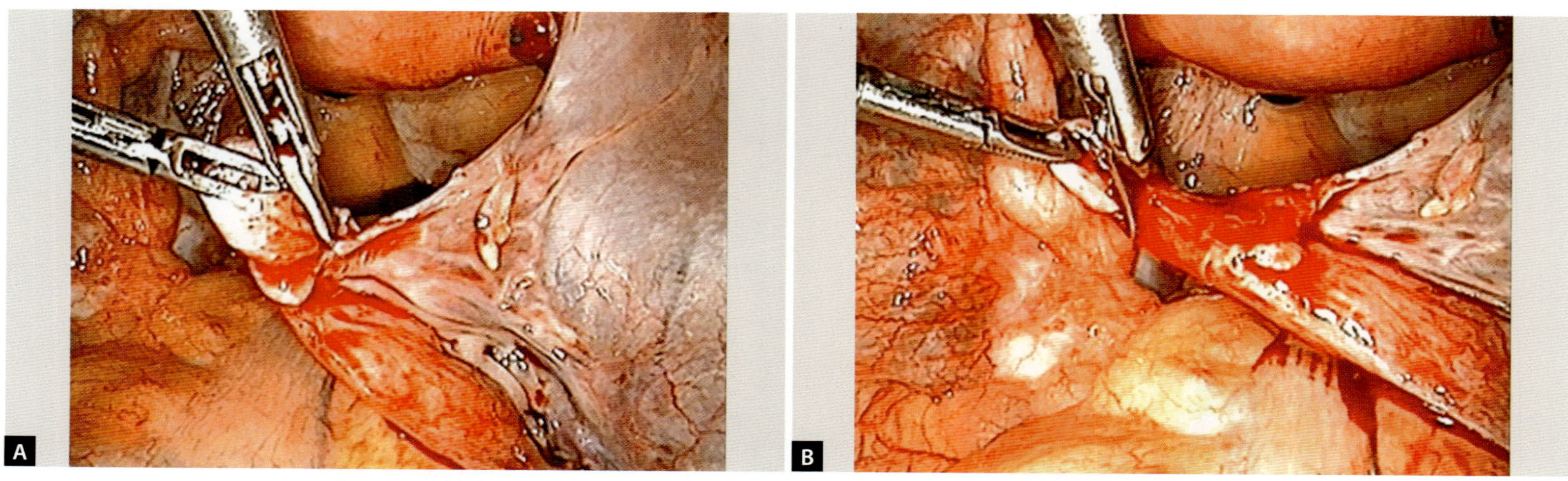

Figs. 9A and B: Dissection of proximal end of distal tube, scissors are used to make right angled cut.

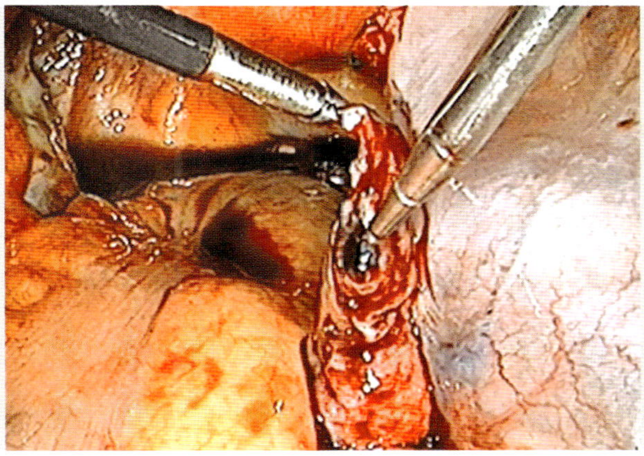

Fig. 10: Patency of distal tube confirmed.

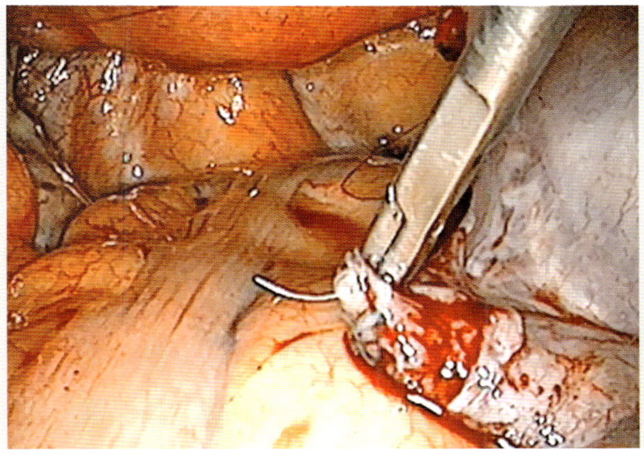

Fig. 11: Using 6-0 polydioxanone (PDS), muscularis and mucosa pierced at 6 o'clock position of distal tube.

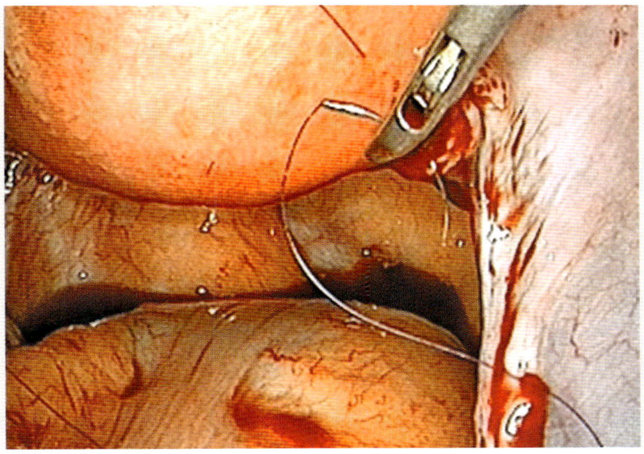

Fig. 12: Proximal tube pierced at 6 o'clock position.

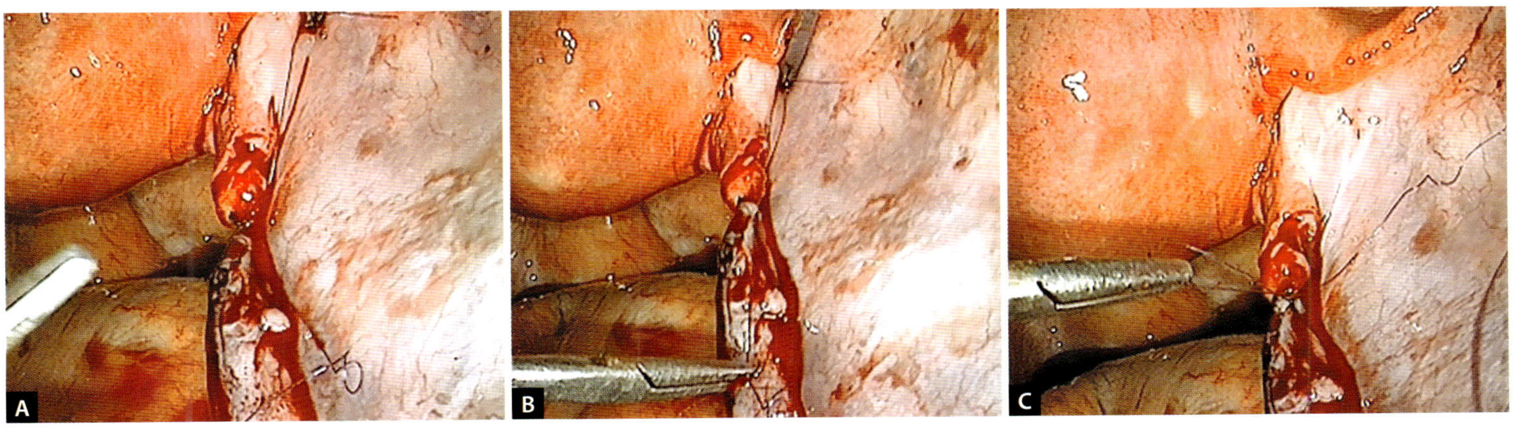

Figs. 13A to C: Intracorporeal knot tying.

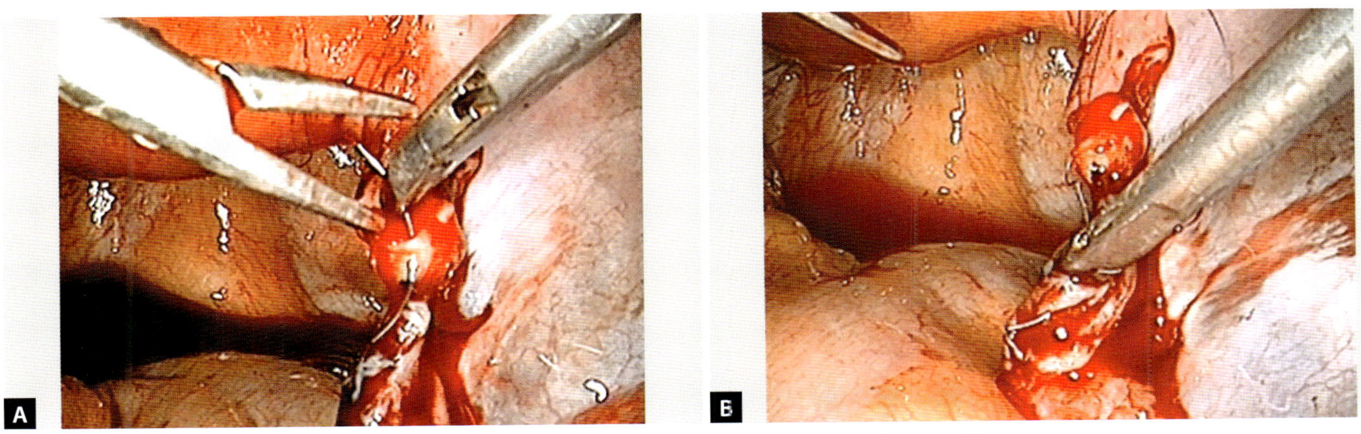

Figs. 14A and B: Another 6-0 suture placed at 2 o'clock position.

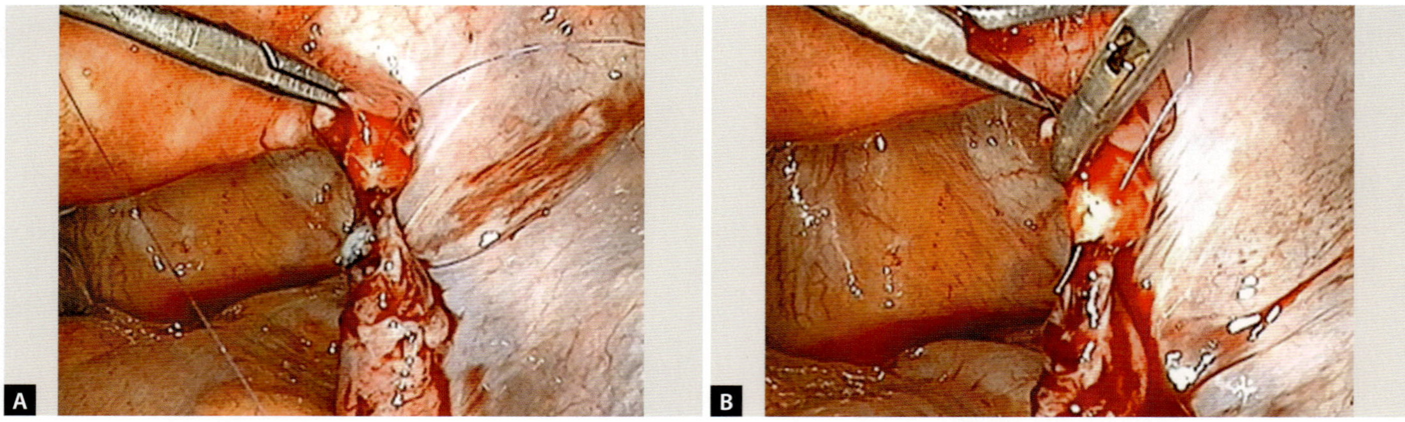

Figs. 15A and B: Sutures taken at 2 o'clock position.

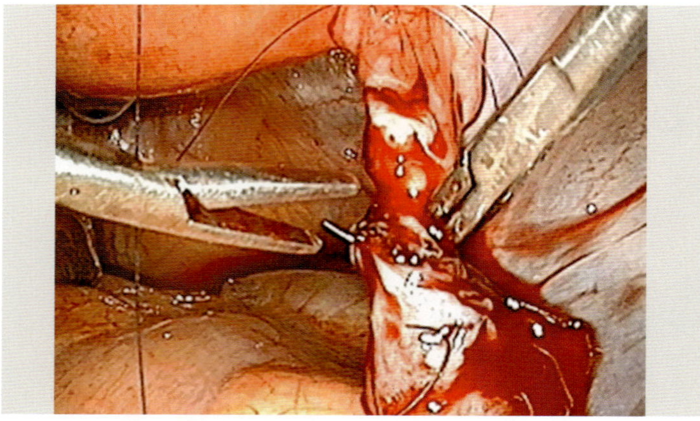

Fig. 16: Sutures at 10 o'clock position.

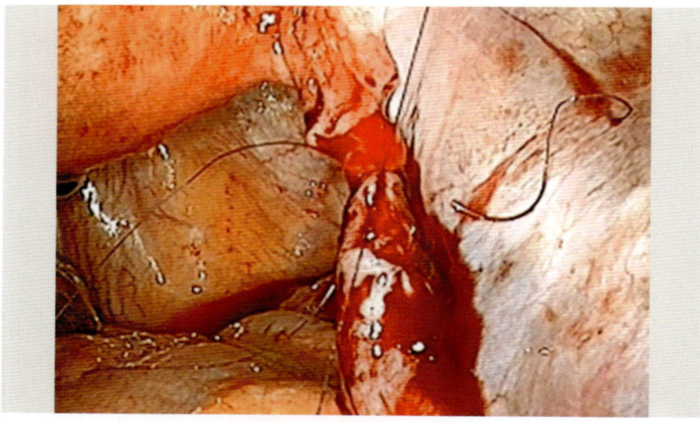

Fig. 17: 2 o'clock suture tied.

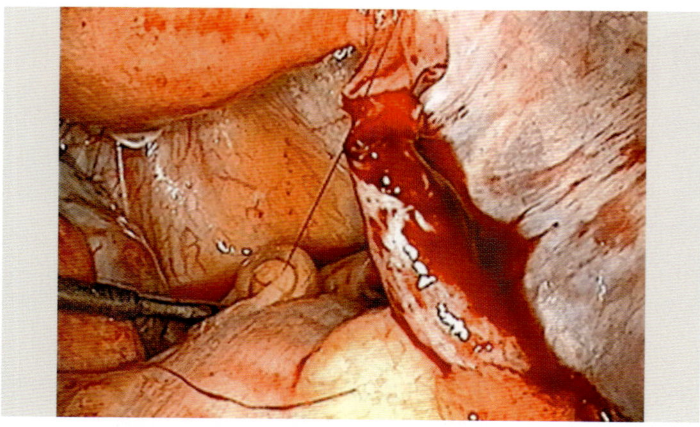

Fig. 18: 10 o'clock suture tied.

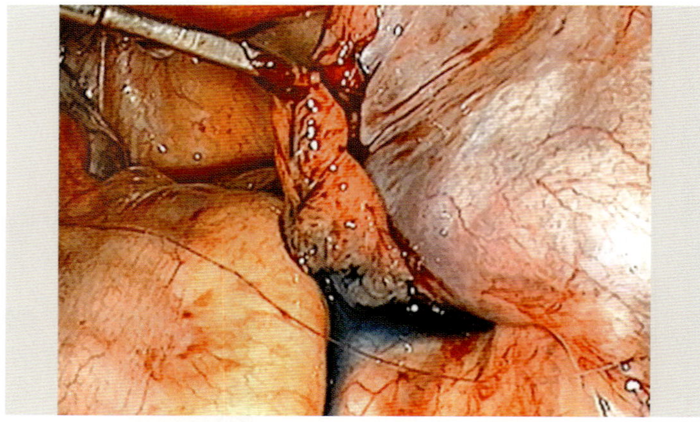

Fig. 19: Ampulloisthmic anastomosis with free spill of dye suggesting good anastomosis.

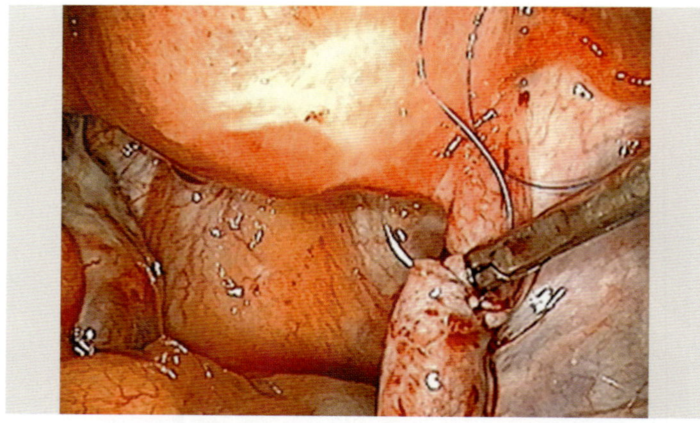

Fig. 20: Mesosalpinx sutures of right tube [5-0 polydioxanone (PDS)].

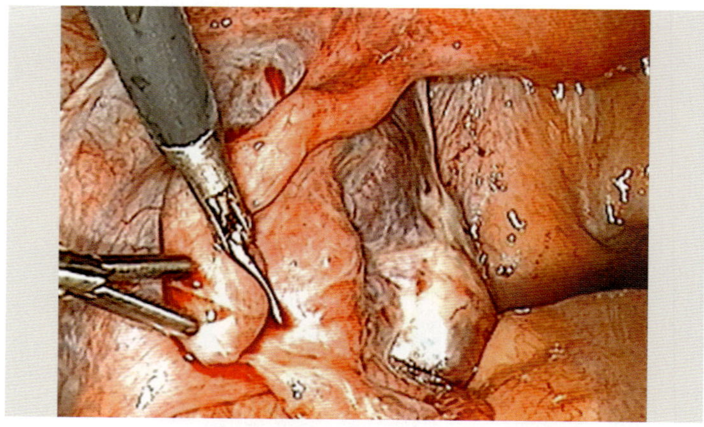

Fig. 21: Left-sided Fallopian tube.

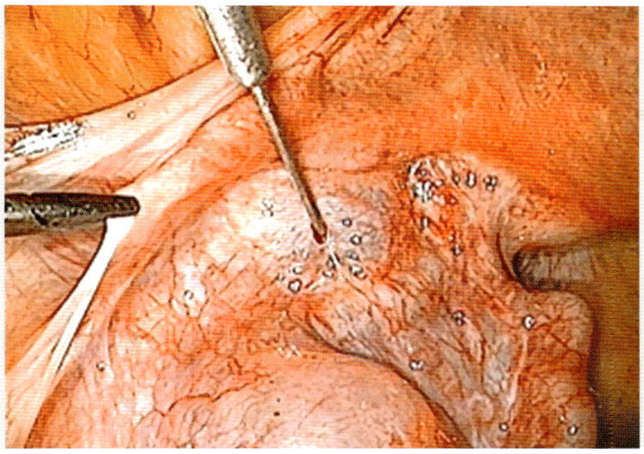

Fig. 22: Diluted vasopressin injected to mesosalpinx.

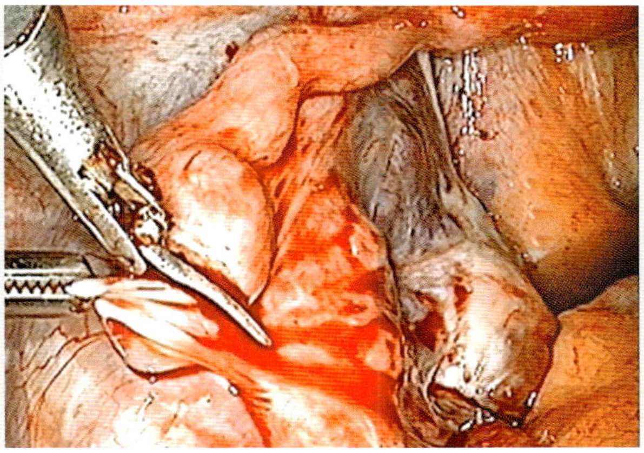

Fig. 25: Right-angled cut is made into proximal tube.

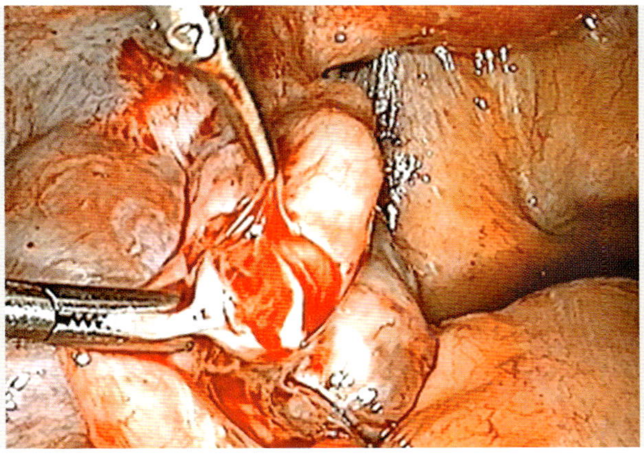

Fig. 23: Preparation of proximal stump in two layers.

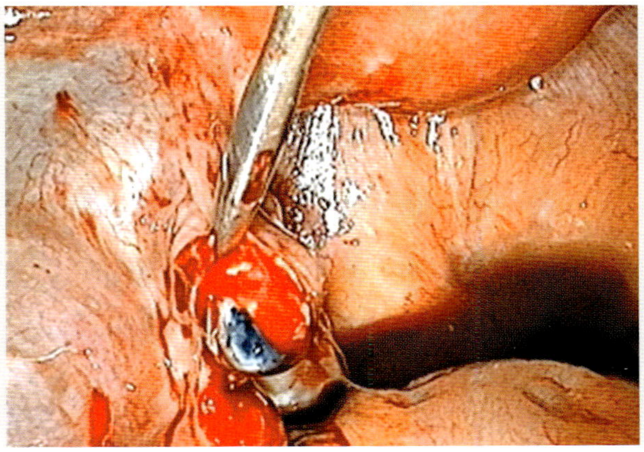

Fig. 26: Patent proximal tube with spill.

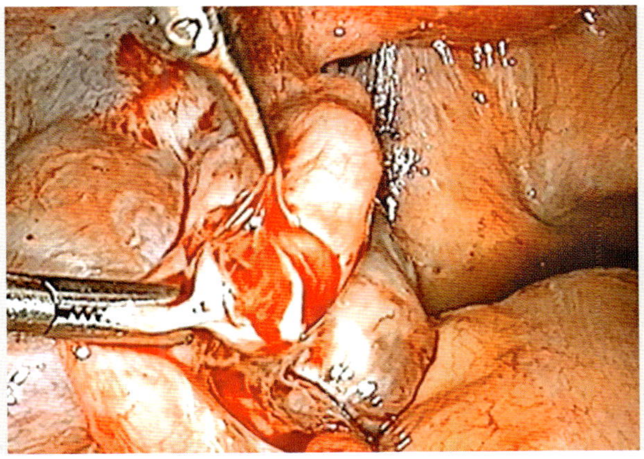

Fig. 24: Adhesiolysis.

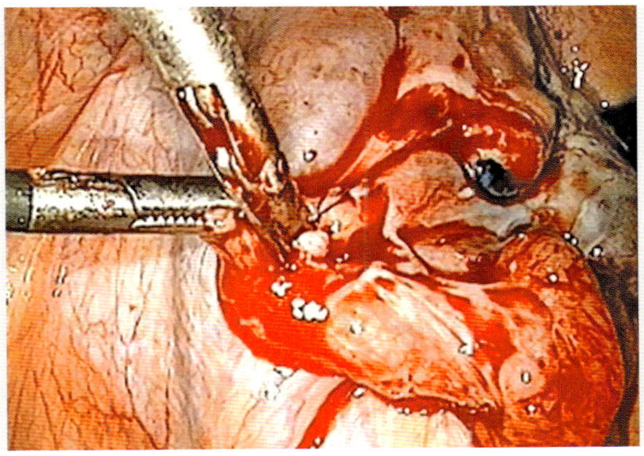

Fig. 27: Adhesiolysis of distal tube serosa pushed from muscularis.

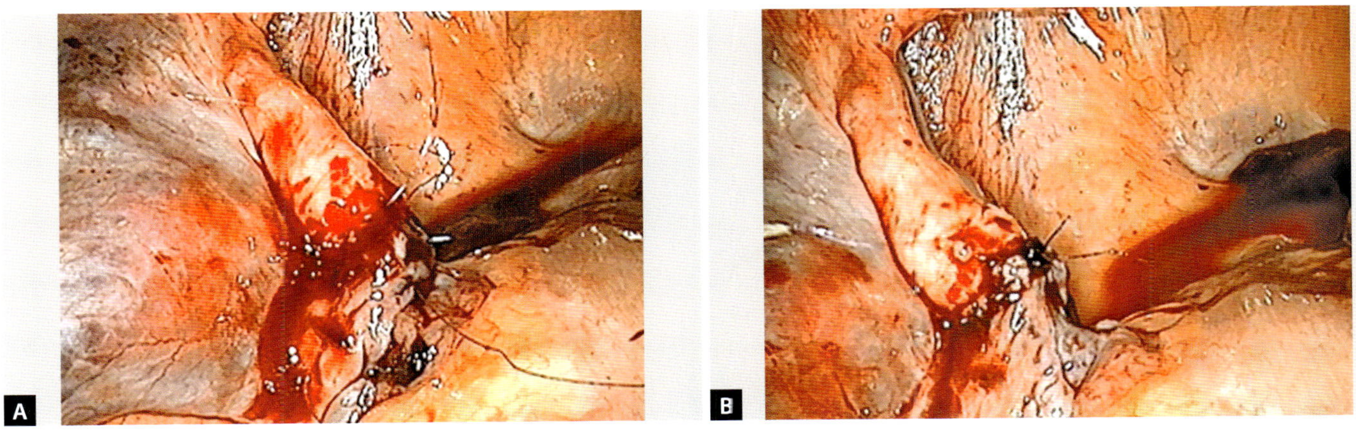

Figs. 28A and B: Ampullo-ampullary anastomosis.

Suture

First stitch is placed in the mesosalpinx by Vicryl no. 1.5 by intra-abdominal knot. Initial knot is placed to approximate both stump and also to permit tension-free anastomosis. Through serosa, extra-mucosal stitches are taken in a triangular fashion with Vicryl 6-0 at the anterior and posterior sides and at the antimesenteric edge of the Fallopian tube. Catheter was then removed under visual control once the sutures had been tied up.

The patient was discharged 48 hours after the procedure. Hysterography should be advised within 2 months after the operation.[7]

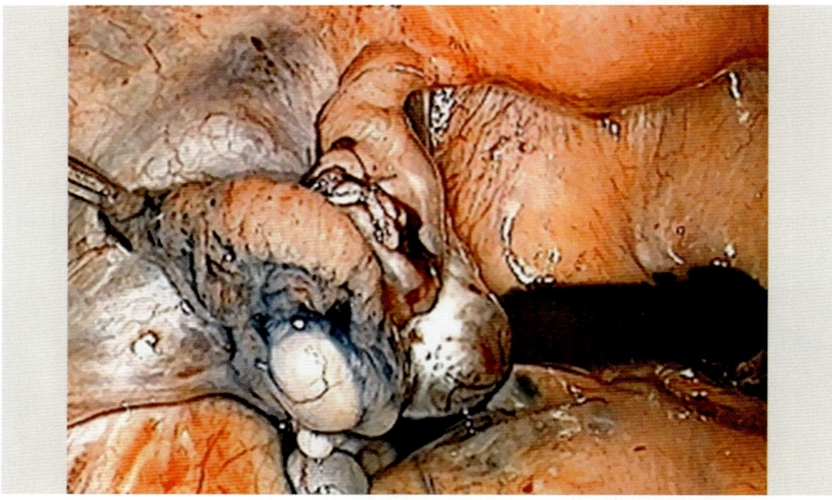

Fig. 29: Free spill with patent tube.

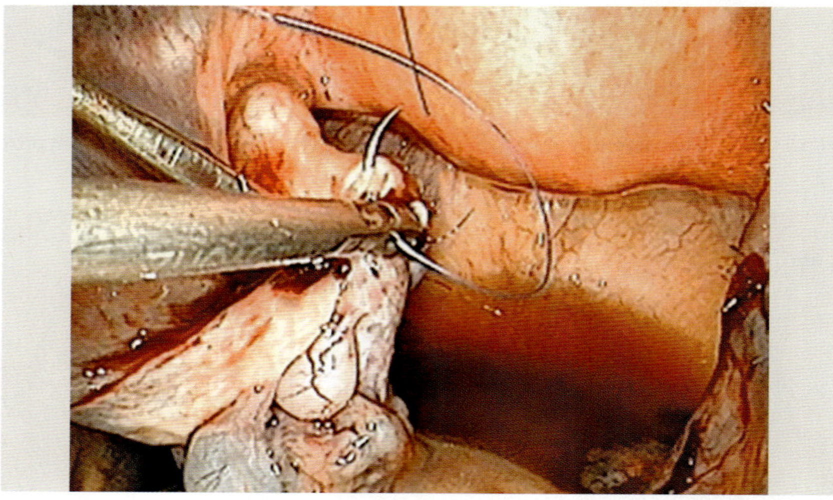

Fig. 30: Approximation of mesosalpinx.

UNFEASIBLE FALLOPIAN TUBES

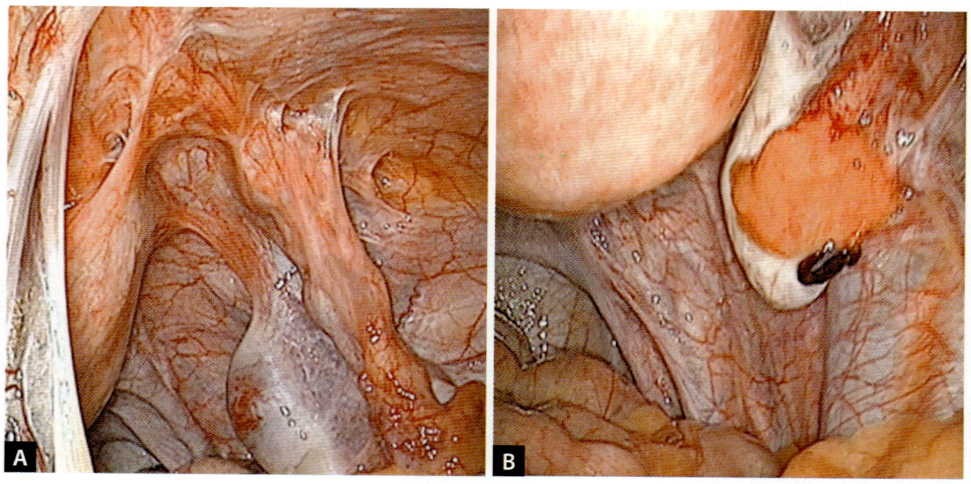

Figs. 31A and B: Unfeasible Fallopian tubes.

RESUTURING OF FAILED PRIMARY ANASTOMOSIS

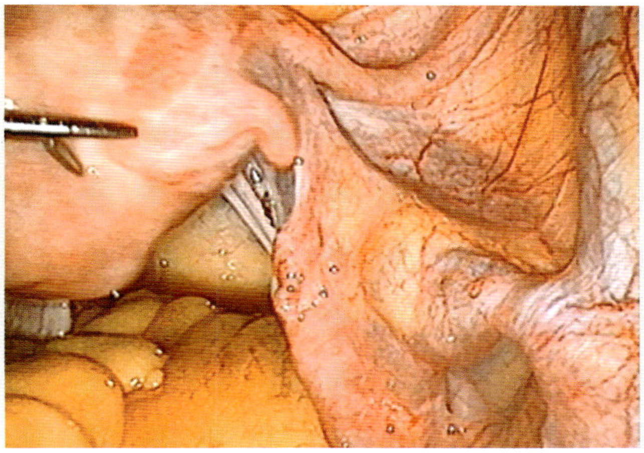

Fig. 32: Panoramic view post-tubectomy status.

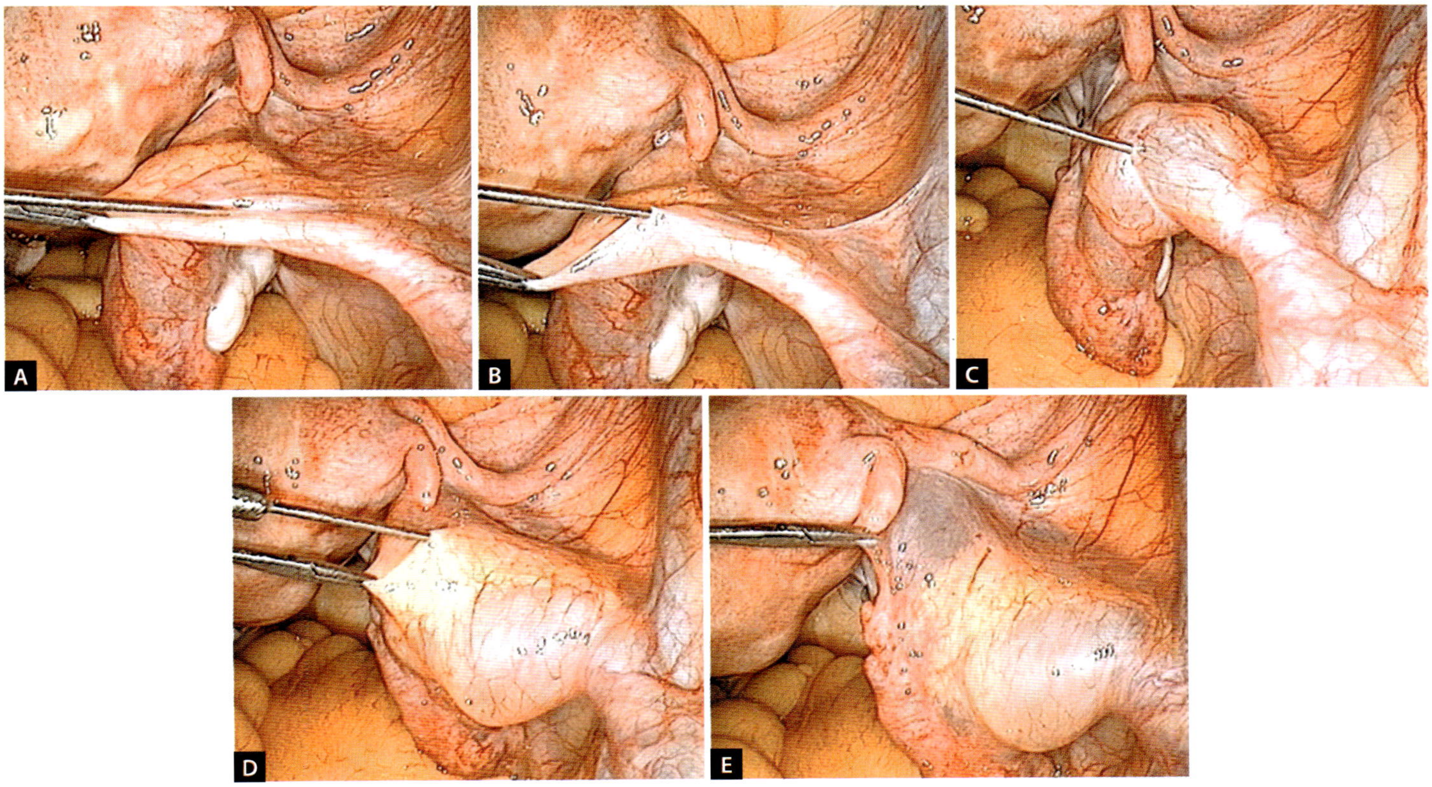

Figs. 33A to E: Injection of diluted vasopressin into mesosalpinx.

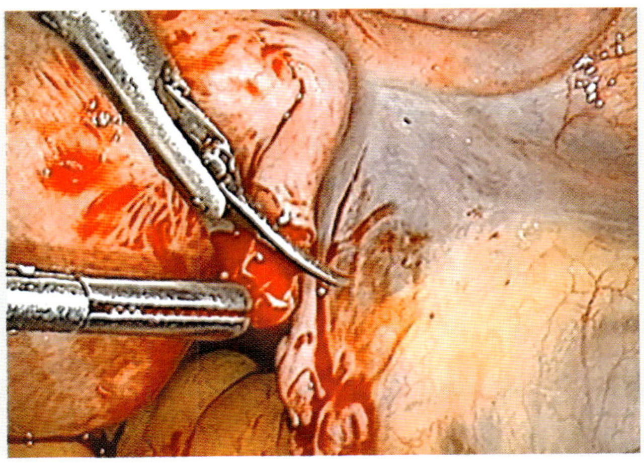

Fig. 34: Right angle cut of proximal tube.

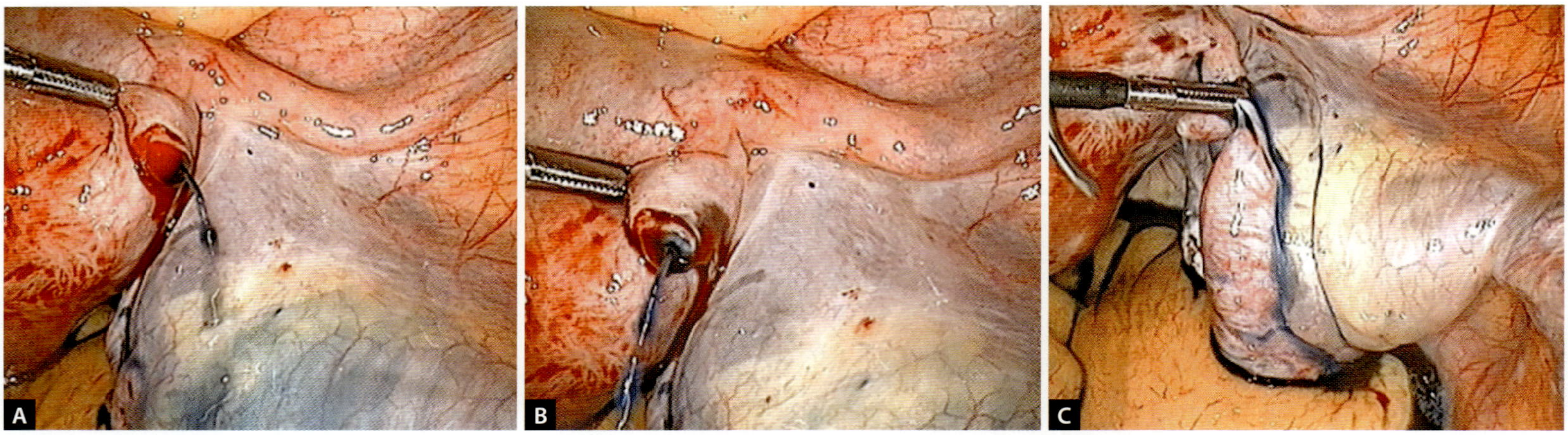

Figs. 35A to C: Free spill of dye from proximal end.

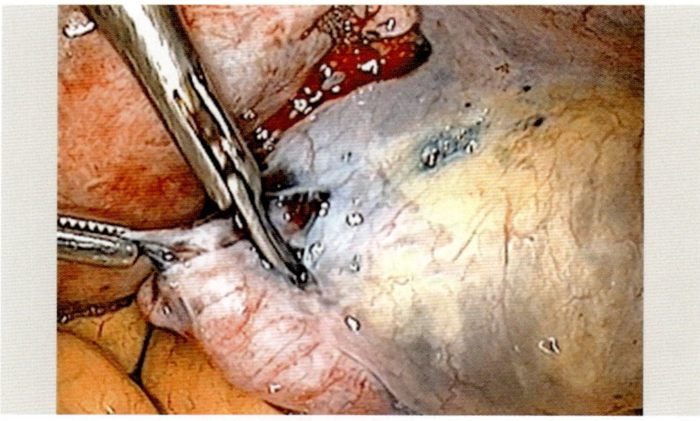

Fig. 36: Adhesiolysis with scissors.

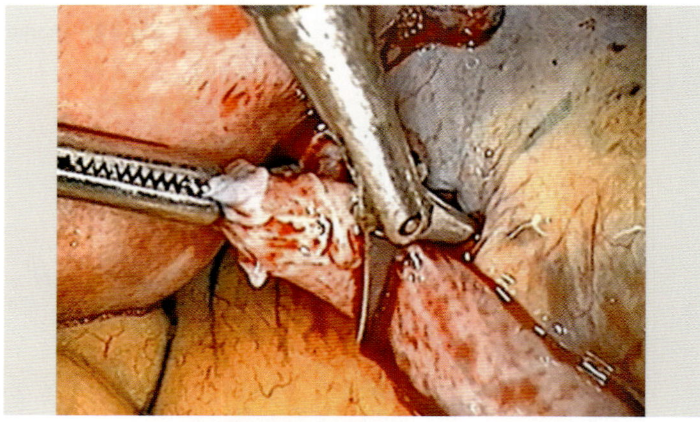

Fig. 37: Right angle cut to distal tube.

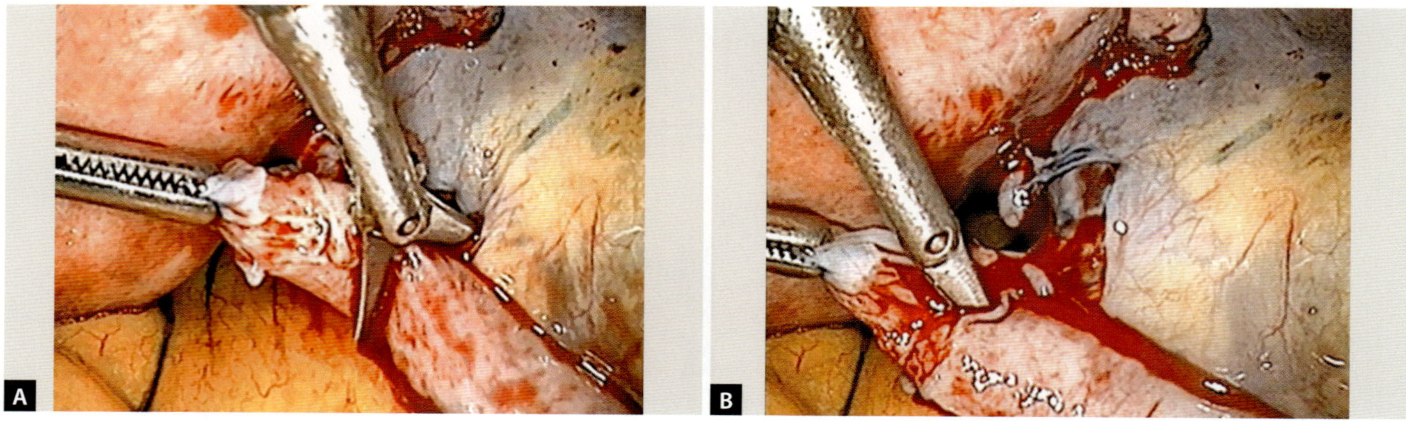

Figs. 38A and B: Dissection of proximal end of distal tube, scissors are used to make right angled cut.

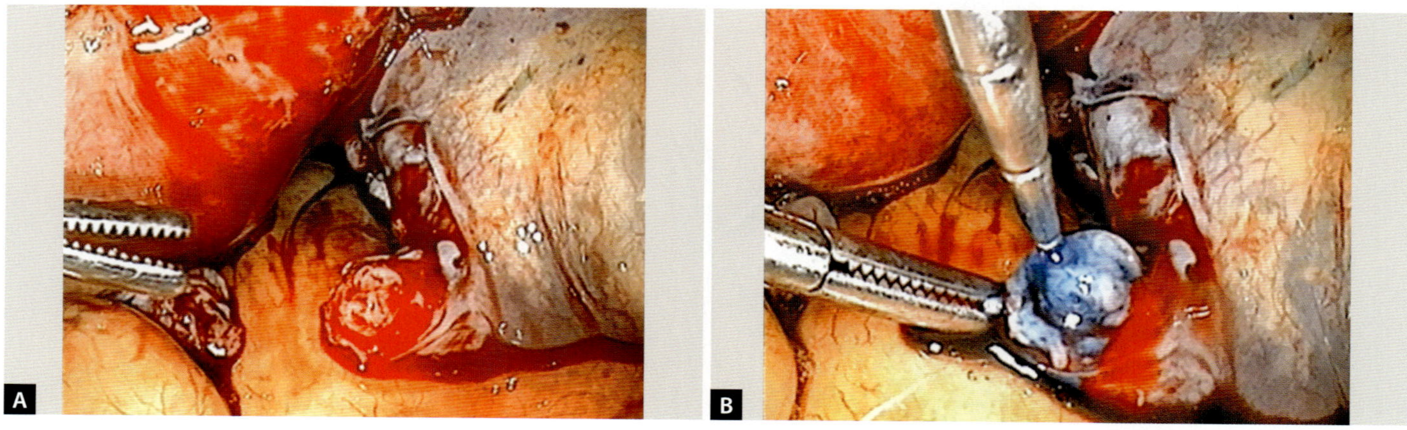

Figs. 39A and B: Adhesiolysis of distal tube, serosa pushed from muscularis.

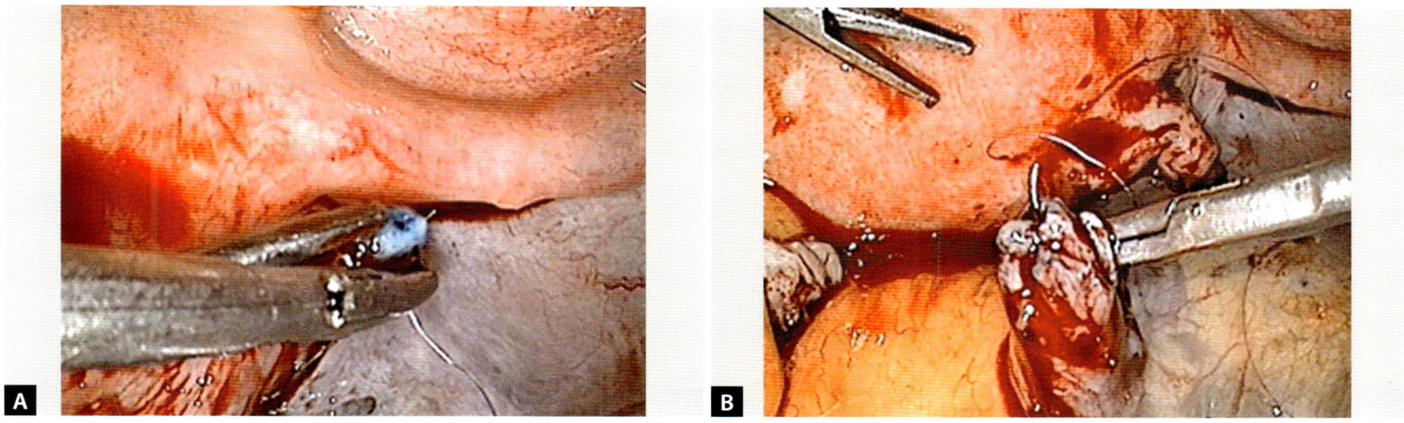

Figs. 40A and B: 5-0 Polydioxar one (PDS) sutures taken at 6 o'clock position from proximal tube.

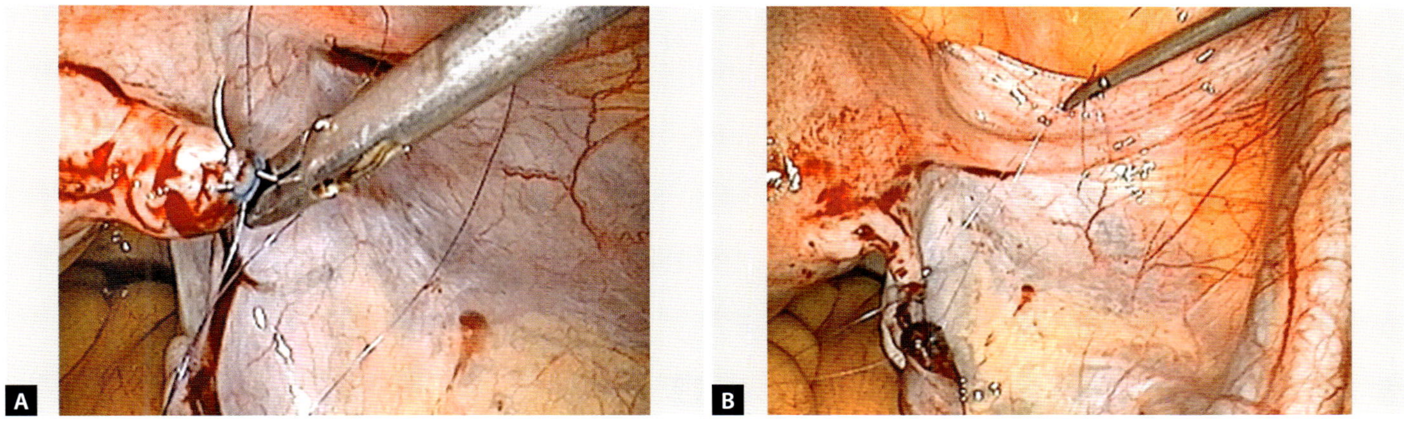

Figs. 41A and B: 5-0 Polydioxanone (PDS) sutures taken at 12 o'clock position on both sides of tube.

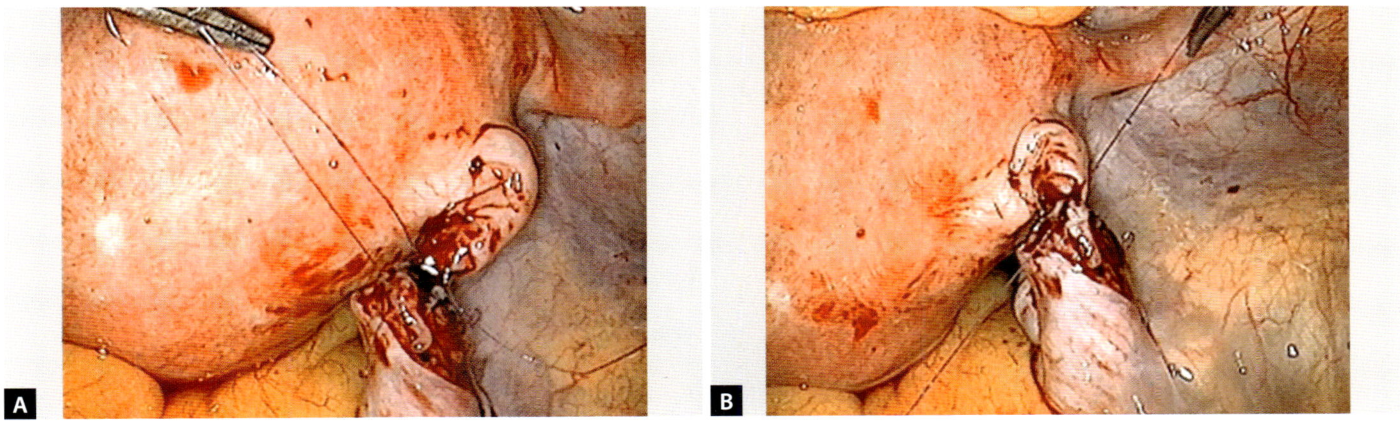

Figs. 42A and B: Approximation and tying of sutures at 6 o'clock position.

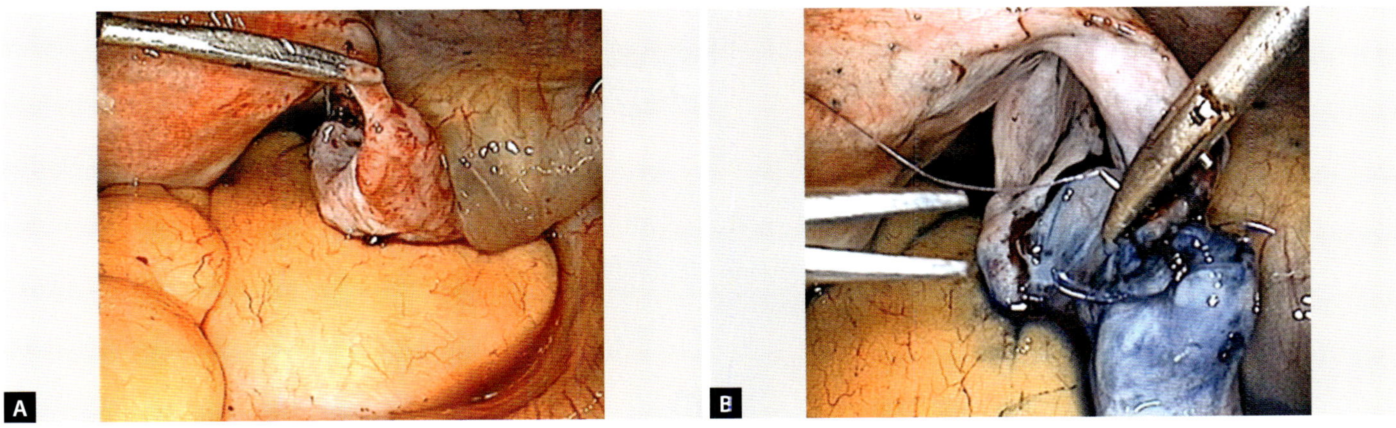

Figs. 43A and B: Sutures taken over 2 and 10 o'clock positions.

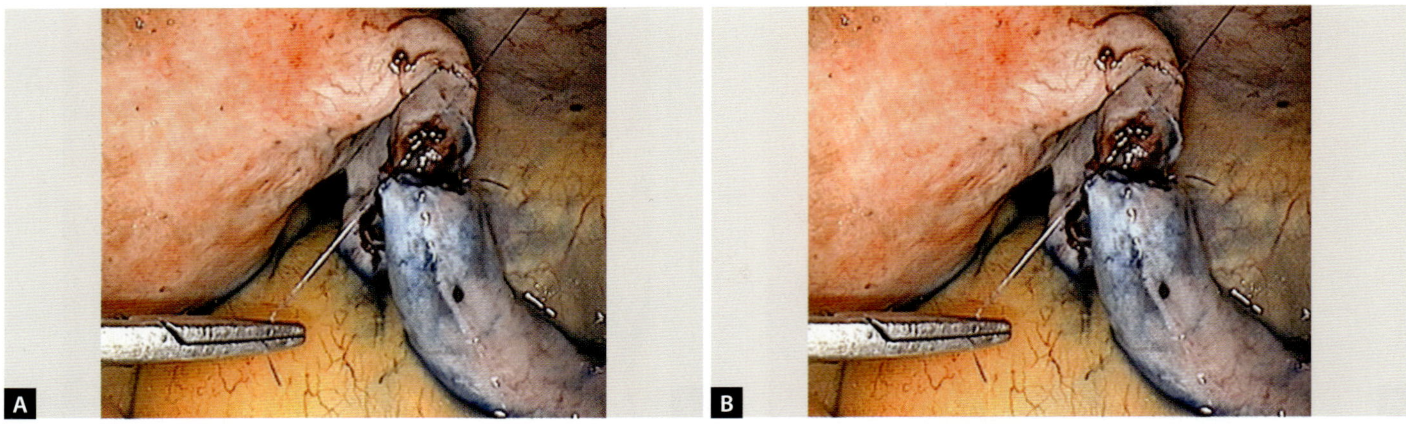

Figs. 44A and B: Approximation of sutures at 2 and 10 o'clock positions.

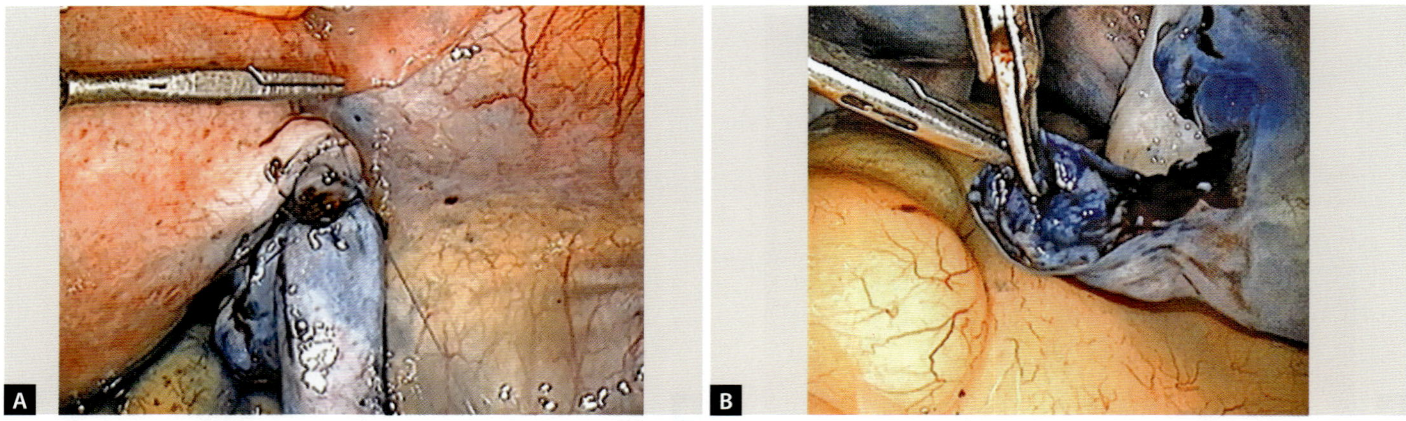

Figs. 45A and B: No free spill of dye after final reanastomosis.

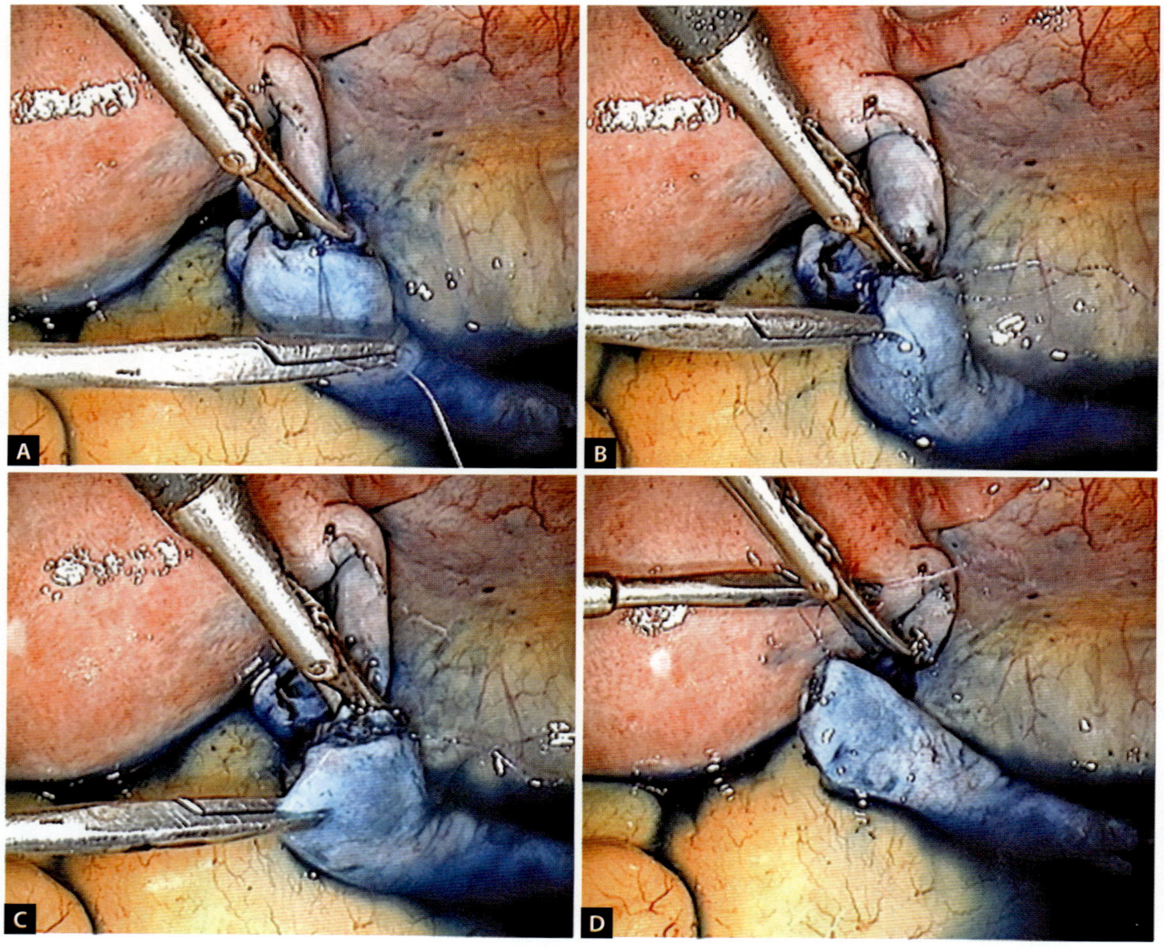

Figs. 46A to D: Approximated sutures are cut due to absence of free spill of dye.

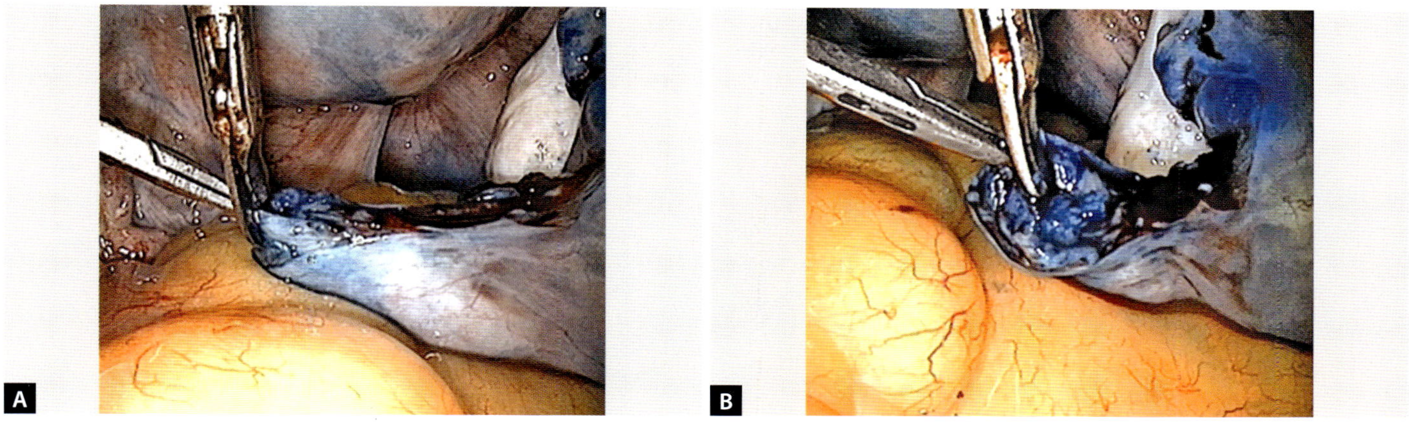

Figs. 47A and B: Freshening of mucosal edges of proximal part of distal tube.

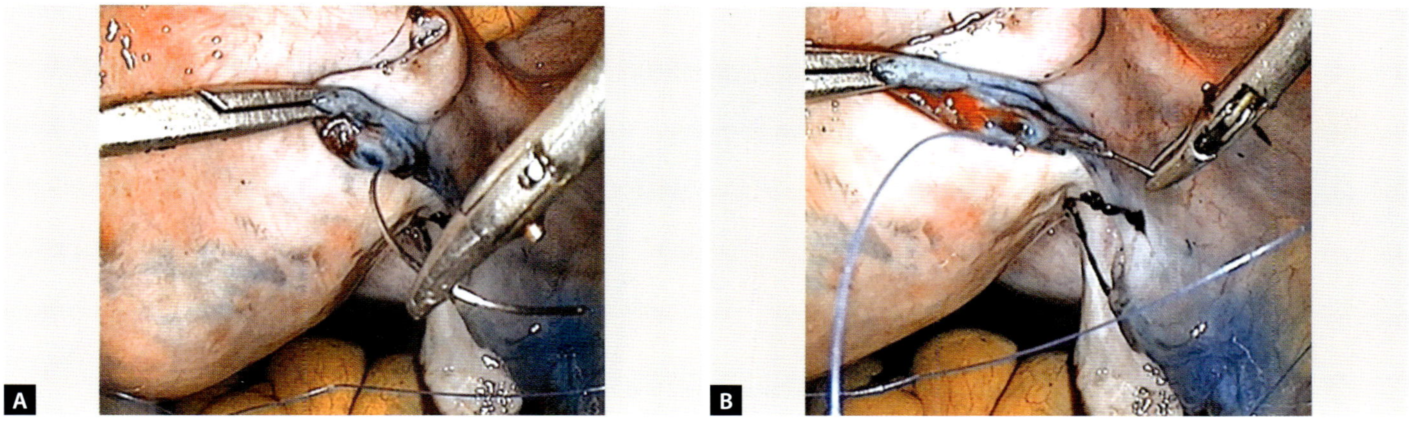

Figs. 48A and B: 6-0 Prolene used sutures taken at 6 o'clock position of proximal tube.

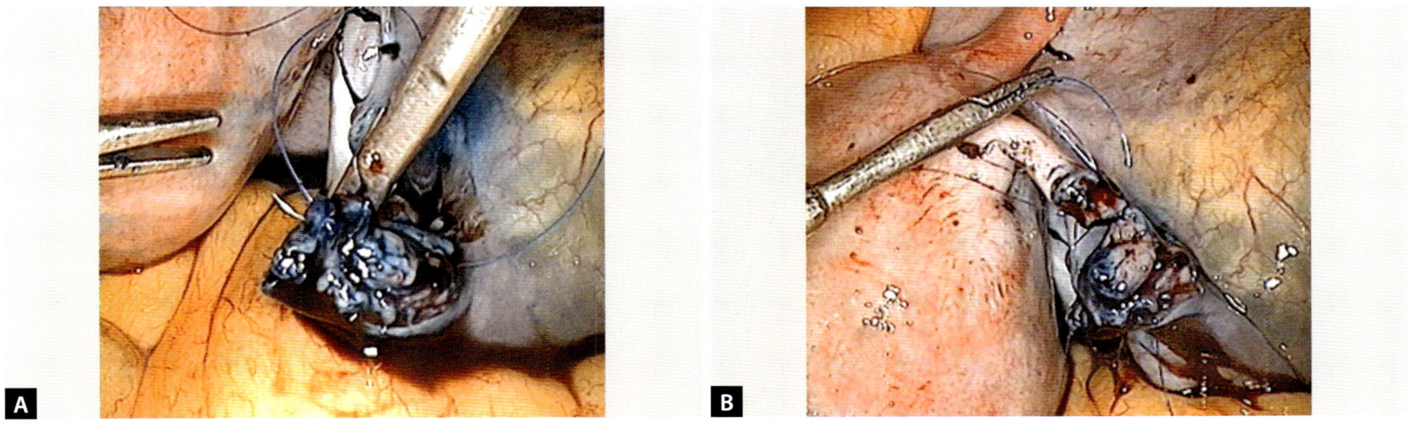

Figs. 49A and B: 6-0 Prolene used sutures taken at 6 o'clock position of distal tube.

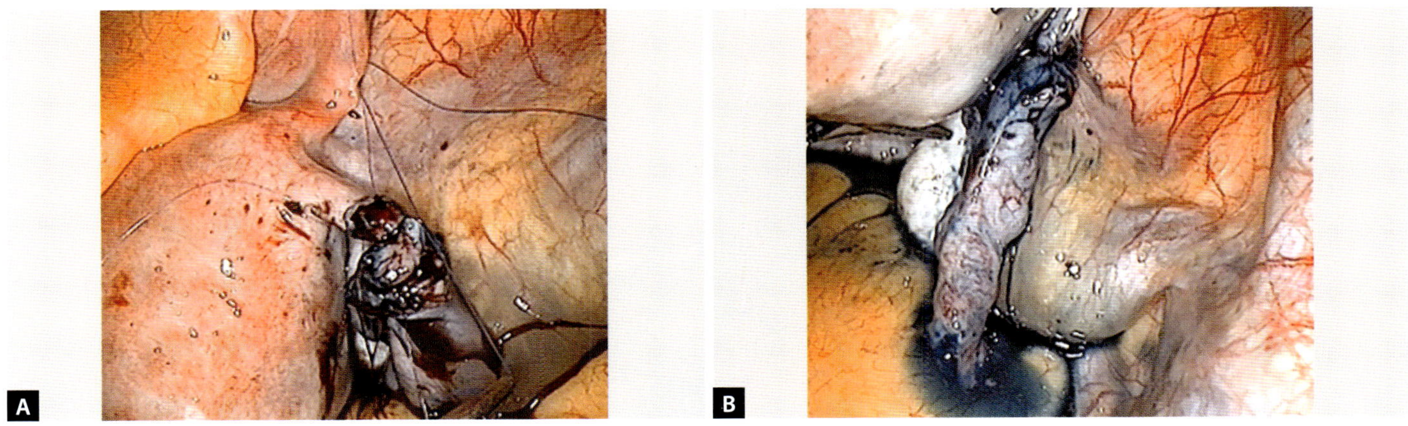

Figs. 50A and B: 6-0 Polydioxanone (PDS) used to take sutures at 12 o'clock position, free spill of dye seen after reapproximation.

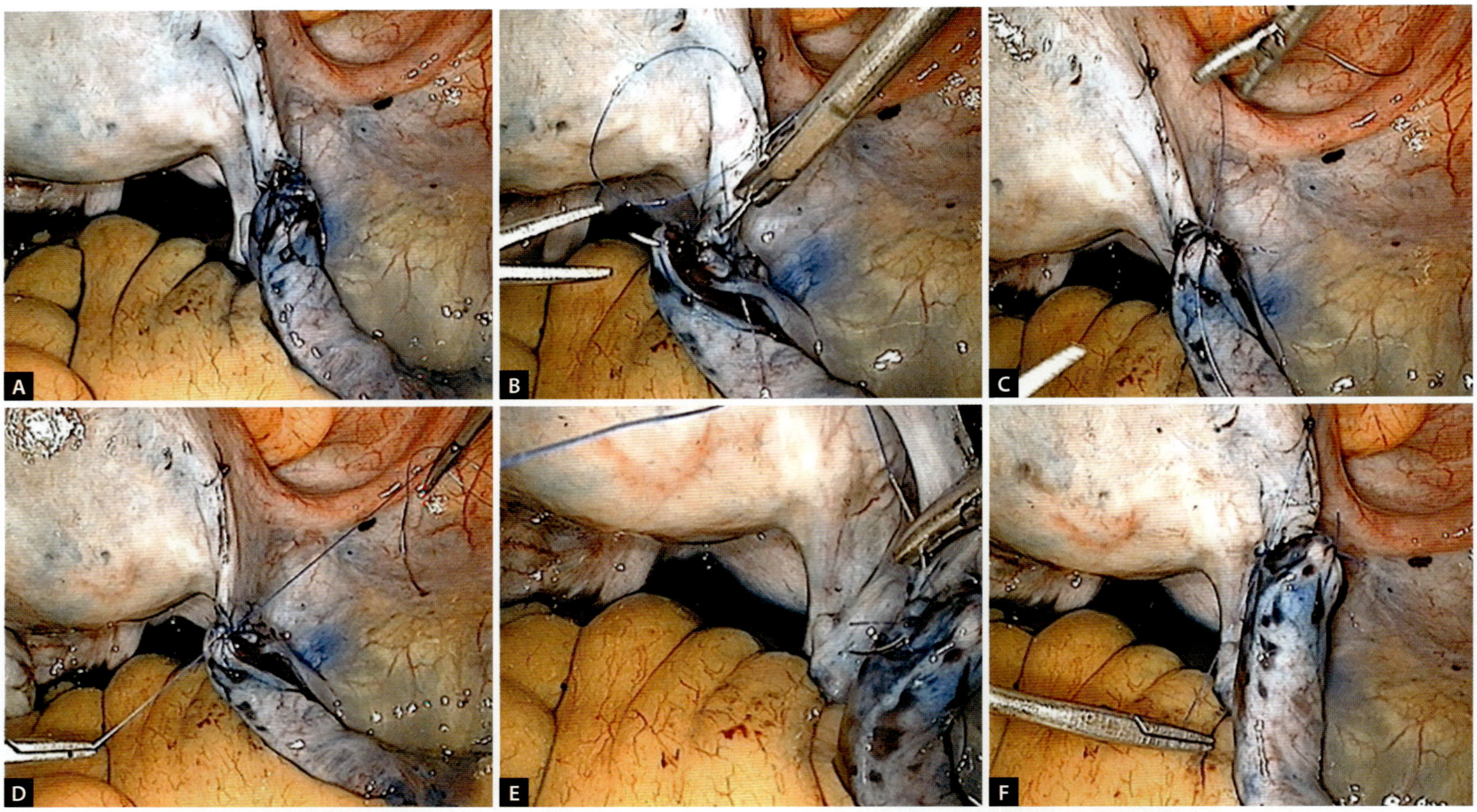

Figs. 51A to F: Using 6-0 Prolene sutures taken over 2 and 10 o'clock position and reapproximated.

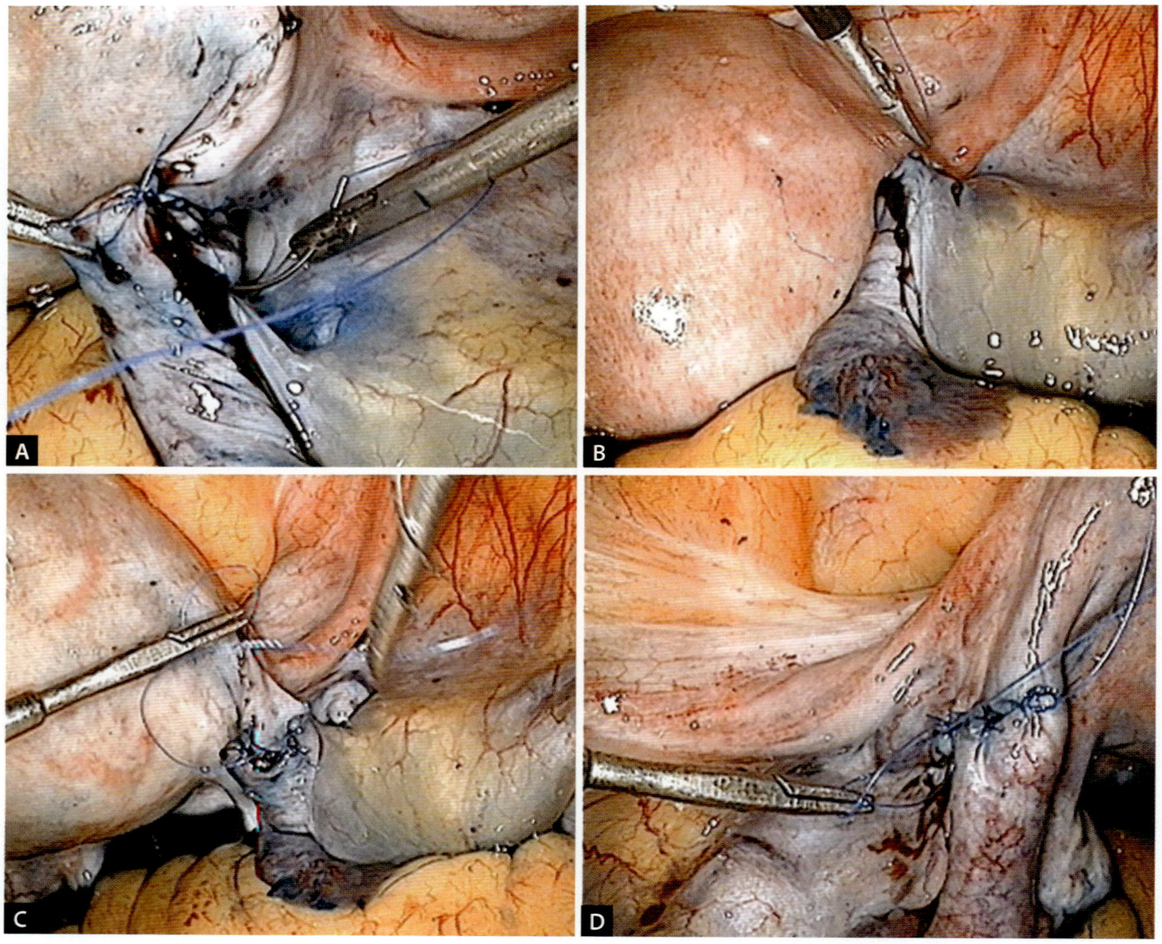

Figs. 52A to D: Continuous sutures taken over serosa using 6-0 Prolene.

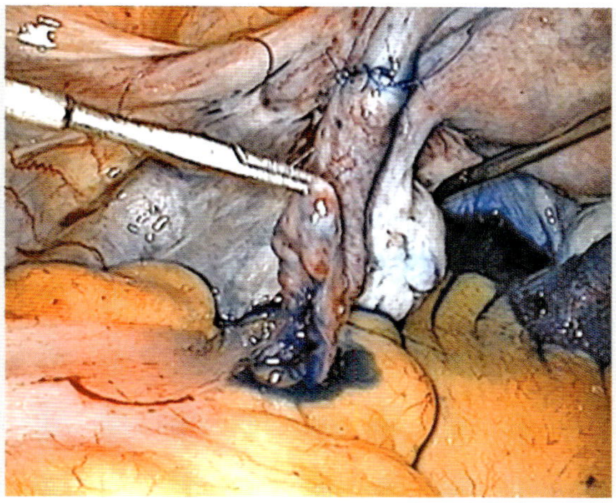

Fig. 53: Free spill of dye following reanastomosis.

UNFEASIBLE TUBAL RECANALIZATION

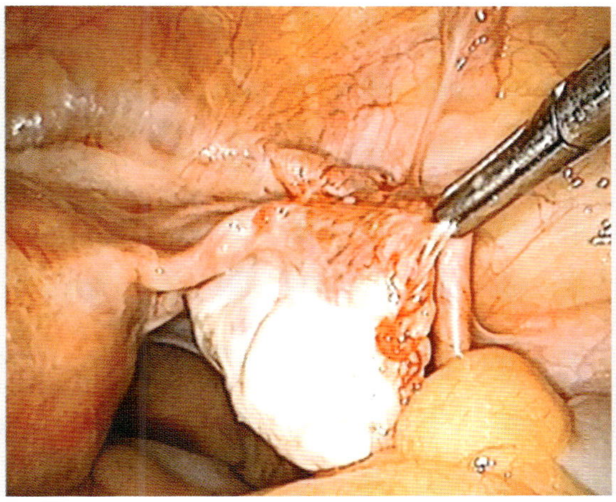

Fig. 54: Absence of distal end of tube.

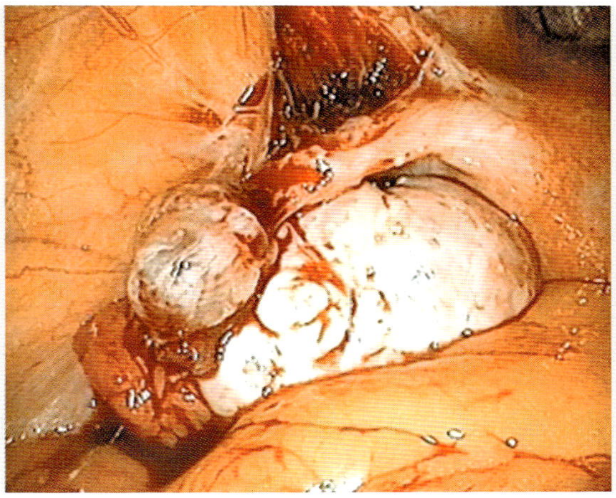

Fig. 56: Unfeasible Fallopian tube due to hydrosalpinx.

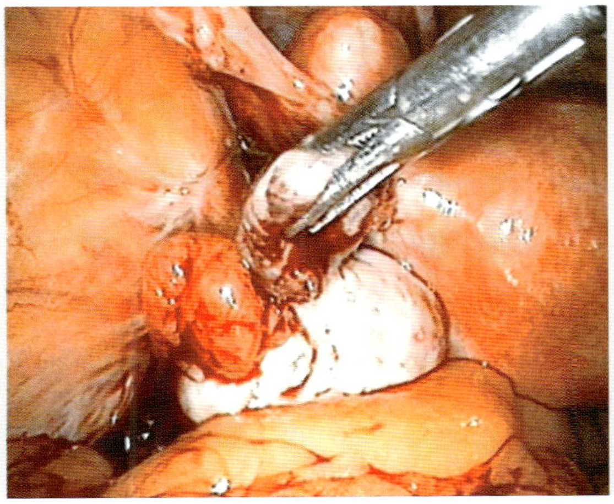

Fig. 55: Proximal and distal tube parallel to each other.

REFERENCES

1. Seyfettinoğlu S, Arıer S, Adıgüzel FI, et al. Fertility outcomes after reversal of tubal sterilisation. J Clin Anal Med. 2016;7(1):85-8.
2. Gomel V. Microsurgical reversal of female sterilization: a reappraisal. Fertil Steril. 1980;33 587-97.
3. Sedbon E, Delajolinieres JB, Boudouris O, et al. Tubal desterilization through exclusive laparoscopy. Hum Reprod. 1989;4(2):158-9.
4. Jayakrishnan K, Baheti SN. Laparoscopic tubal sterilization reversal and fertility outcomes. J Hum Reprod Sci. 2011;4(3):125-9.
5. Wilcox LS, Chu SY, Eaker ED, et al. Risk factors for regret after tubal sterilization: 5 years of follow-up in a prospective study. Fertil Steril. 1991;55(5): 927-33.
6. Peterson HB, Xia Z, Hughes JM, et al. The risk of pregnancy after tubal sterilization: findings from the U.S. Collaborative Review of Sterilization. Am J Obstet Gynecol. 1996;174(4):1161-8.
7. Barjot PJ, Marie G, Von Theobald P. Laparoscopic tubal anastomosis and reversal of sterilization. Hum Reprod. 1999;14(5):1222-5.
8. Dubuisson JB, Chapron C, Nos C. et al. Sterilization reversal: fertility results. Hum Reprod. 1995;(10):1145-51.
9. Li J, Chen X, Zhou J. Ultrastructural study on the epithelium of ligated Fallopian tubes in women of reproductive age. Ann Anat. 1996;178:317-20.

Accompanying Video: Laparoscopic tubal recanalization.

CHAPTER

32

Laparoscopic Umbilical Hernia Repair

Sowmya MS, Aditi Rai, B Ramesh

INTRODUCTION

Umbilicus represents a midline opening in the linea alba. Umbilical hernia occurs when the umbilical scar closes incompletely in the child or fails and stretches in later years in the adult patient. A hernia becomes readily apparent once the abdominal contents move through the umbilical opening given the relative lack of soft tissue in the anterior body wall at the site of the umbilicus.

Prevalence of umbilical hernia is 2% in adult population and is much more common in cirrhotic patients and obese middle-aged multiparous women. Adult umbilical hernias have an acquired origin and aggravating factor is increased in pressure (pregnancy, ascites, etc.), the pull of the abdominal muscles, and the deterioration of connective tissue. During laparoscopic trocar insertion, if trocar sites larger than 10 mm there is increase chances of umbilical hernia development, it should be properly closed after operation. The possibility of the application of biomaterials to the surgical correction of umbilical hernias that have been successfully used in the inguinal canal opens a new field for further clinical investigation.[1]

HISTORY

Umbilical hernias have been documented throughout history with the first references dating back to the ancient Egyptians with the first known record of a surgical repair by Celsus in the first century AD. Mayo in 1901 reported the first series of patients to undergo the classic overlapping fascia operation through a transverse umbilical incision using nonabsorbable suture.[2]

INCIDENCE

The incidence of umbilical hernia in the adult is largely unknown but most cases are thought to be acquired rather than congenital. It is known to occur more commonly in adult females with a female:male ratio of 3:1. Umbilical hernia is also more commonly found in association with processes that increase intra-abdominal pressure, such as pregnancy, obesity, ascites, persistent or repetitive abdominal distention in bowel obstruction, or peritoneal dialysis. The etiology of umbilical hernia in the adult may be multifactorial, with increased intra-abdominal pressure working against a weak or incomplete umbilical scar.

CLINICAL EXAMINATION

A diagnosis of umbilical hernia is not difficult to make. A condition presents with a soft bulge located anterior or adjacent to the umbilicus. In most cases, the bulge will be readily reducible so that the actual fascial defect can be easily defined by palpation. A patient may provide a history of vague abdominal pain associated with herniation and reduction. A list of differential diagnoses is short and includes abdominal wall varices associated with advanced cirrhosis, umbilical granulomas, and metastatic tumor implants in the umbilical soft tissue (Sister Joseph's node). In clinical practice, there is usually little doubt as to the diagnosis of umbilical hernia on physical examination.

The hernia in the adult is often symptomatic and does not show a tendency to close without intervention. As the hernia contents increase in size, the overlying umbilical skin may become thin and ultimately ulcerated by pressure necrosis. The umbilical hernia with incarcerated omentum may present with significant tenderness on examination, despite the fact that bowel integrity is not at risk. Alternatively, an umbilical hernia may be found incidentally in the adult on physical examination. This hernia is usually small and any hernia contents are usually readily reducible. The small, asymptomatic, reducible hernia in the adult can be observed without the need for immediate intervention. Patients with umbilical hernia secondary to chronic, massive ascites require special consideration. The repair of such hernias is associated with significantly increased morbidity and mortality. Fluid shifts leading to hemodynamic instability, infection, electrolyte imbalance, and blood loss are all considerable risks for the patient in this clinical scenario. Umbilical hernia recurrence is also common in this setting because of increase intra-abdominal pressure. Thus, hernia repair in this population should be reserved for those with progressively symptomatic or incarcerated umbilical hernias.

TREATMENT

In the adult patient, most small umbilical hernia repairs are performed using local anesthesia with the possible addition of intravenous sedation. The approach is also through a curvilinear incision, placed transversely on the inferior border of the umbilicus or vertically on one curved edge of the umbilicus. A skin flap is raised to elevate the umbilicus of the hernia sac. The sac is again dissected free of its fascial attachments to isolate the sac for complete reduction and to allow for an adequate width of fascia for suture closure. The sac contents are then reduced into the abdominal cavity and any excess sac can be excised. The defect is then closed with a strong, non-absorbable suture (such as 0 polypropylene or nylon), usually in an interrupted fashion. The fascial edges are approximated through this technique. A traditional "vest-over-pants" technique originated by Mayo is less commonly utilized since overlapping fascial closures have been shown to weaken the overall wound strength in hernia repair. In large defects that may close only with a significant degree of tension, a cone of polypropylene mesh can be fitted to fill the umbilical defect in place of a tissue repair. The mesh is then sutured circumferentially to the surrounding umbilical fascia to prevent migration. Newer mesh products contain polypropylene mesh or polyester mesh in combination with a bioabsorbable layer so that they can be placed in contact with the bowel without the formation of significant adhesions. These products can be very useful in the treatment of umbilical and other ventral hernias where mesh adherence to bowel is a concern.[3]

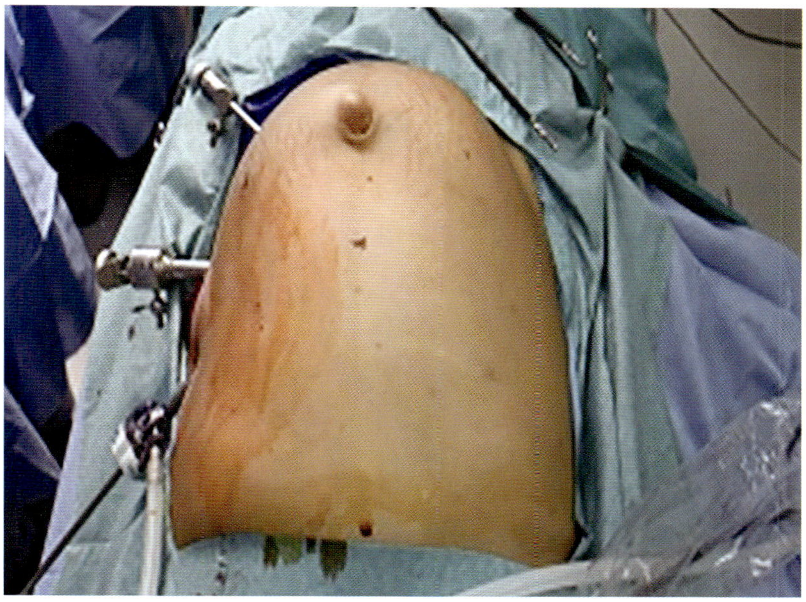

Fig. 2: Port placement.

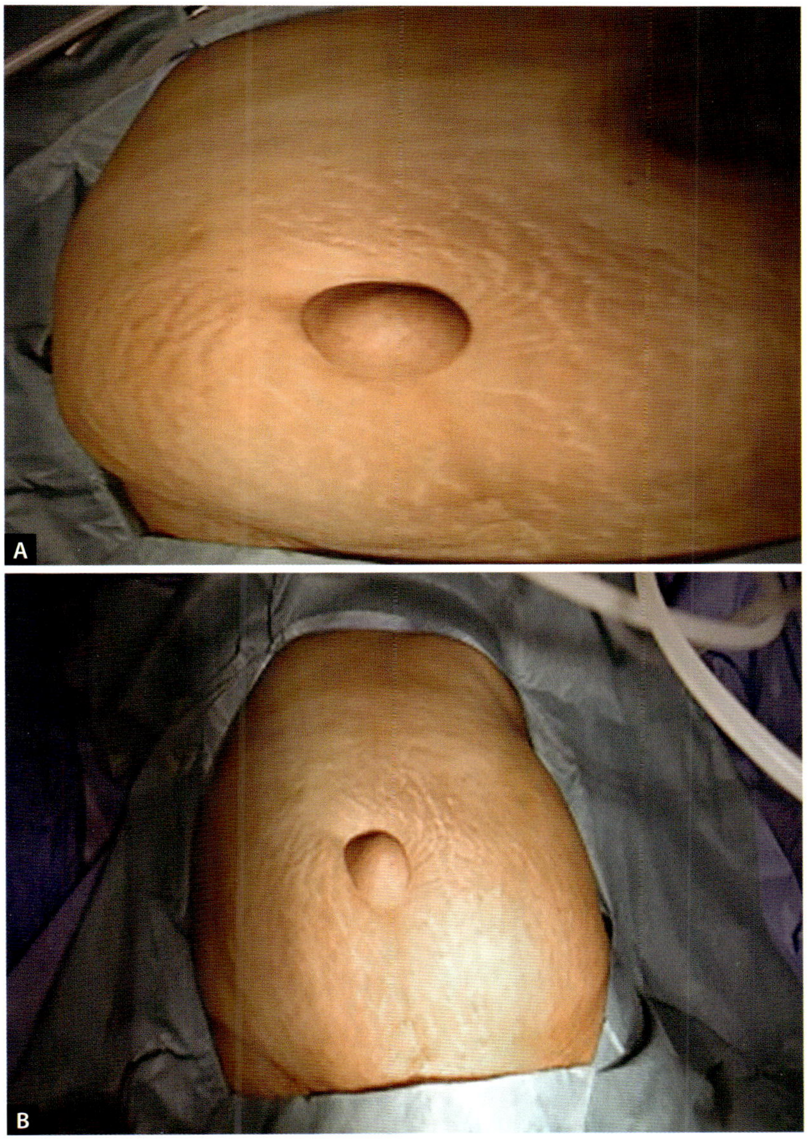

Figs. 1A and B: 3 × 3 cm umbilical hernia in 42-year-old in 88 kg women.

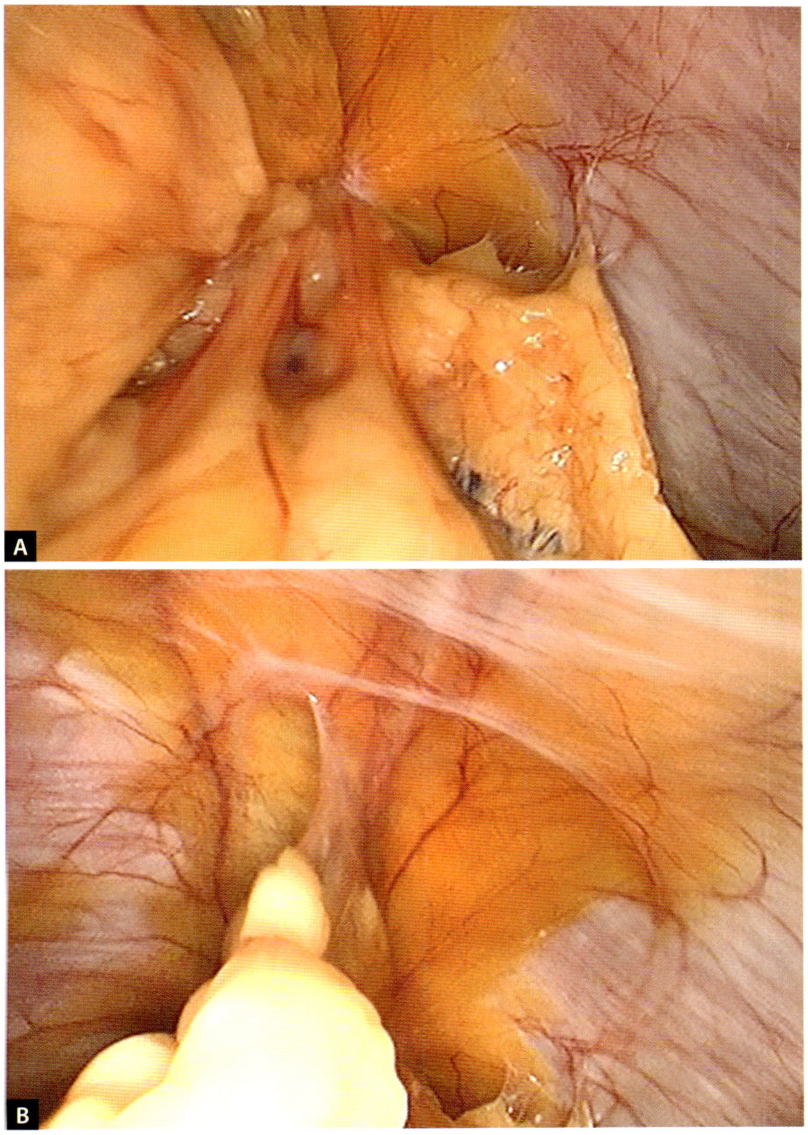

Figs. 3A and B: Omentum as hernial content.

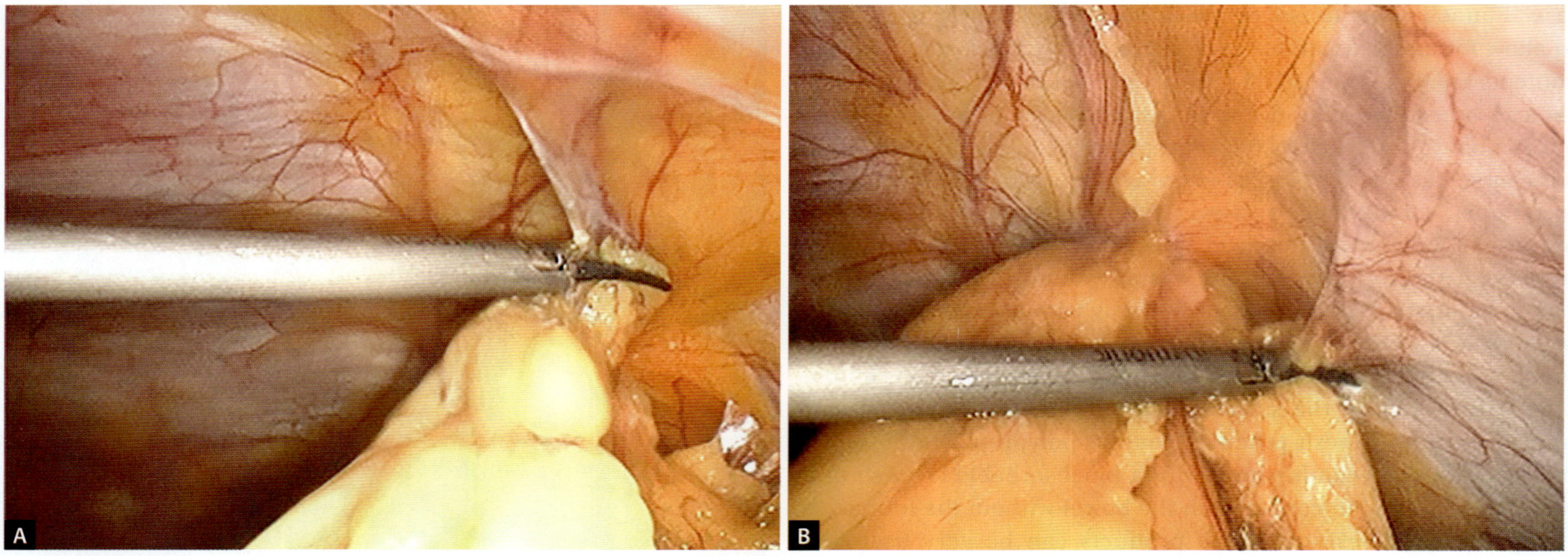

Figs. 4A and B: Adhesiolysis of omentum using harmonic.

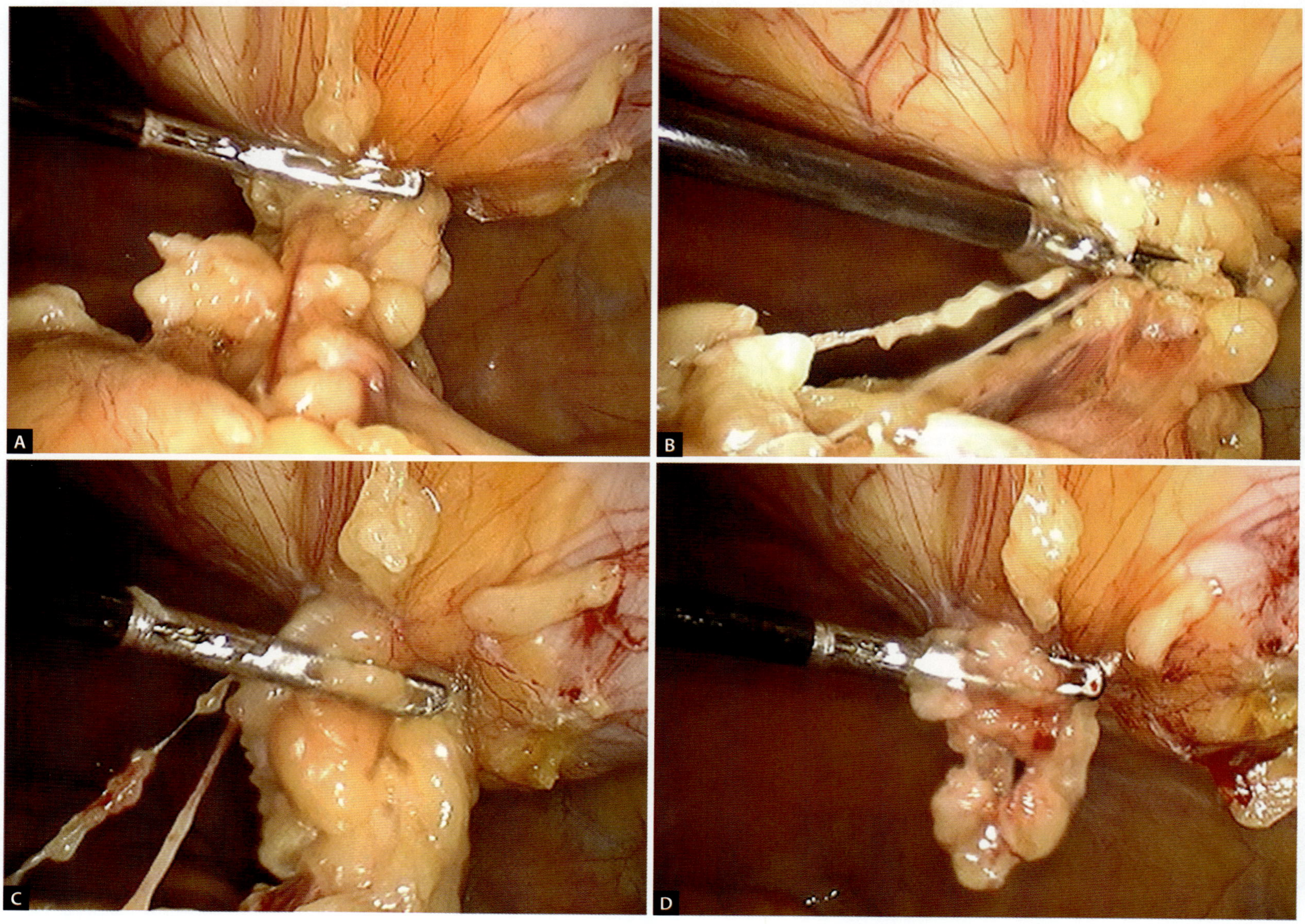

Figs. 5A to D: Blunt dissection of omentum by non-tooth grasper.

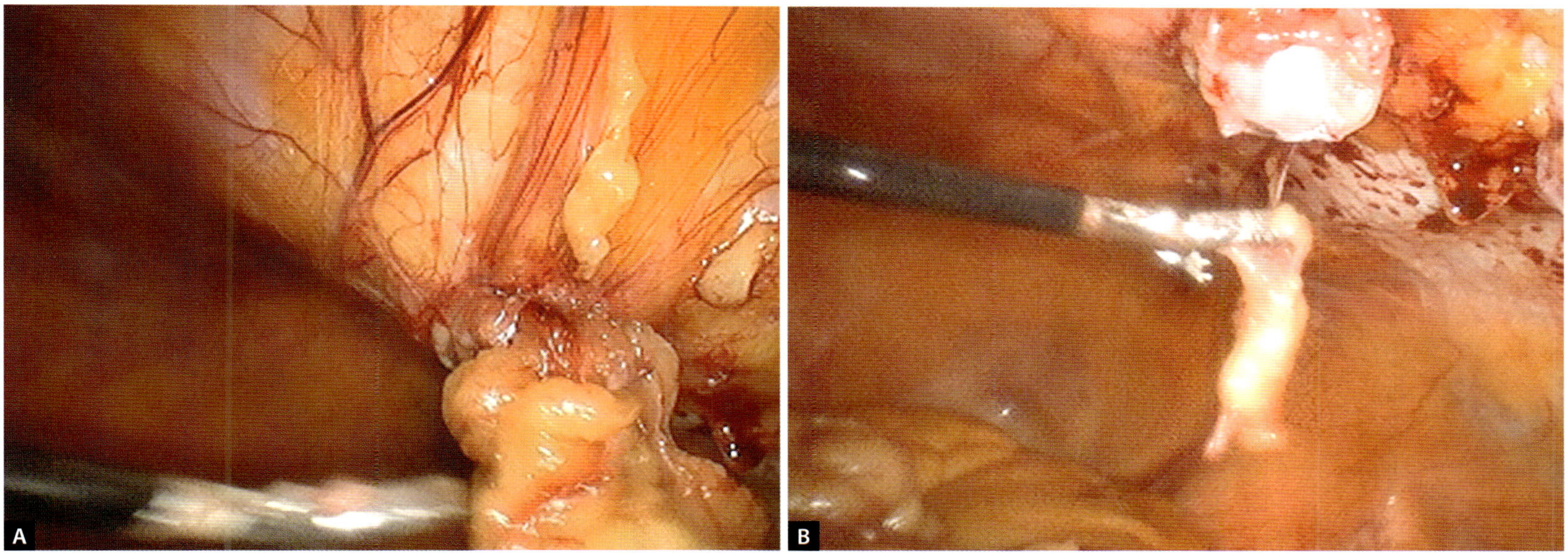

Figs. 6A and B: Visualization of hernia sac after releasing omentum from sac.

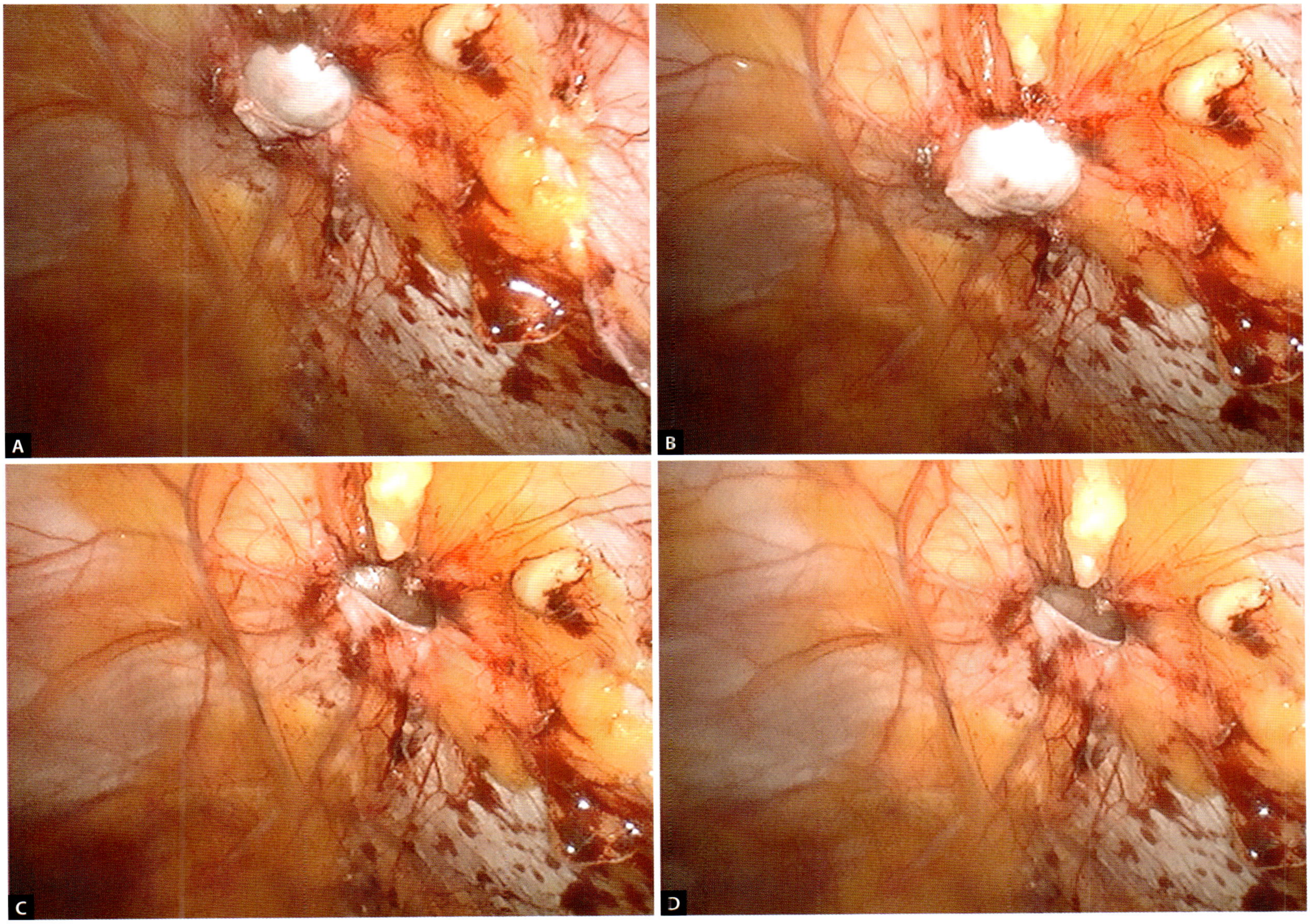

Figs. 7A to D: 3 × 3 cm laparoscopic view of hernial defect.

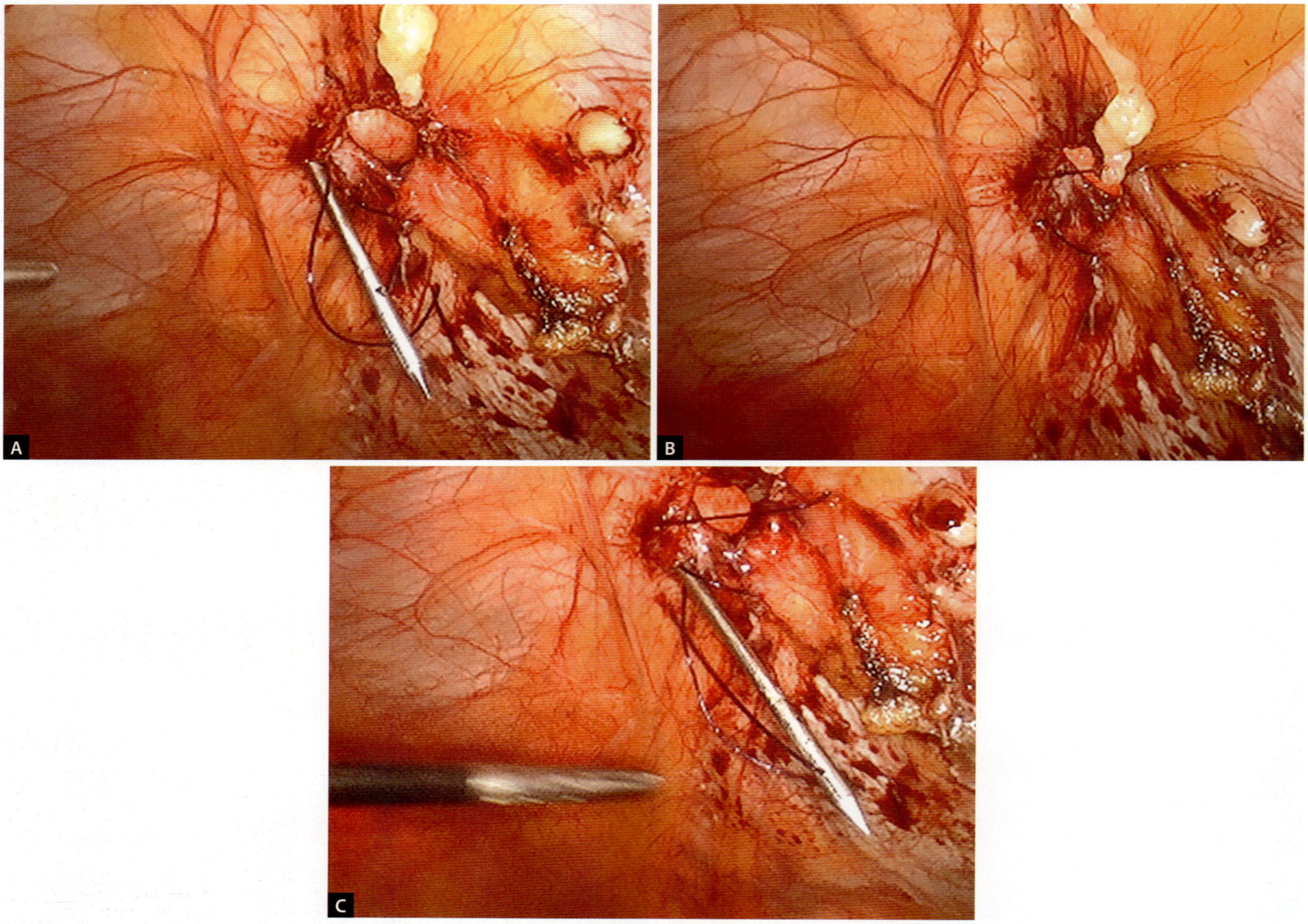

Figs. 8A to C: Using with the help of cobblers needle and no. 1 prolene ,hernia defect sutured on either side.

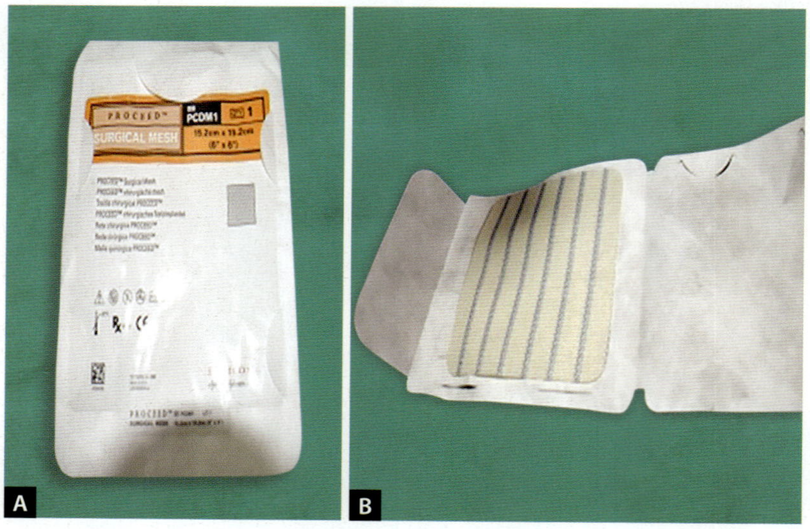

Figs. 9A and B: 10 × 15 cm polypropylene mesh. They have two sides, one is polypropylene and the other side is a non-adherent material to face viscera.

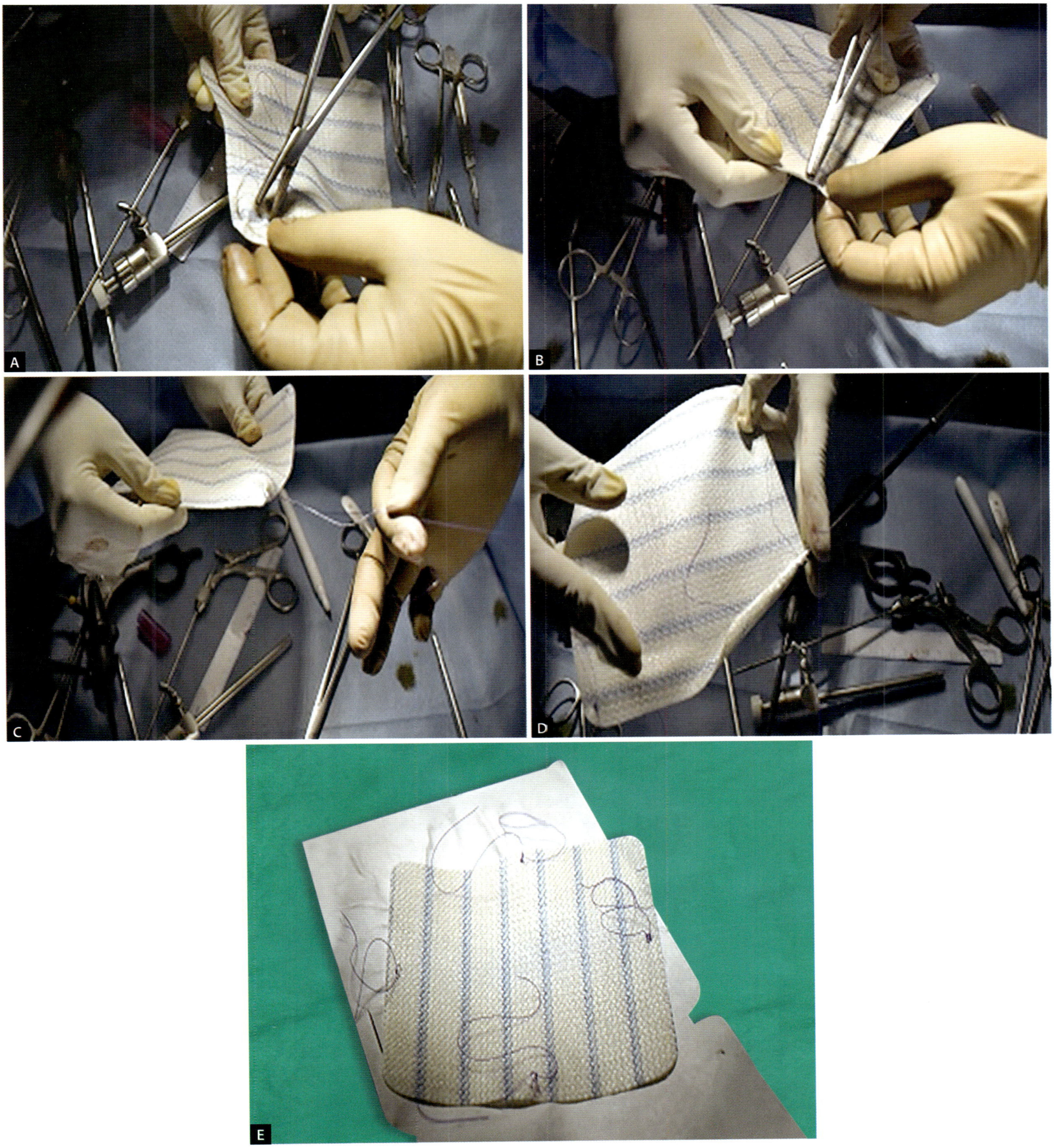

Figs. 10A to E: Using PDS 3-0 ends of mesh sutured on four sides which is used later to be fixed to skin.

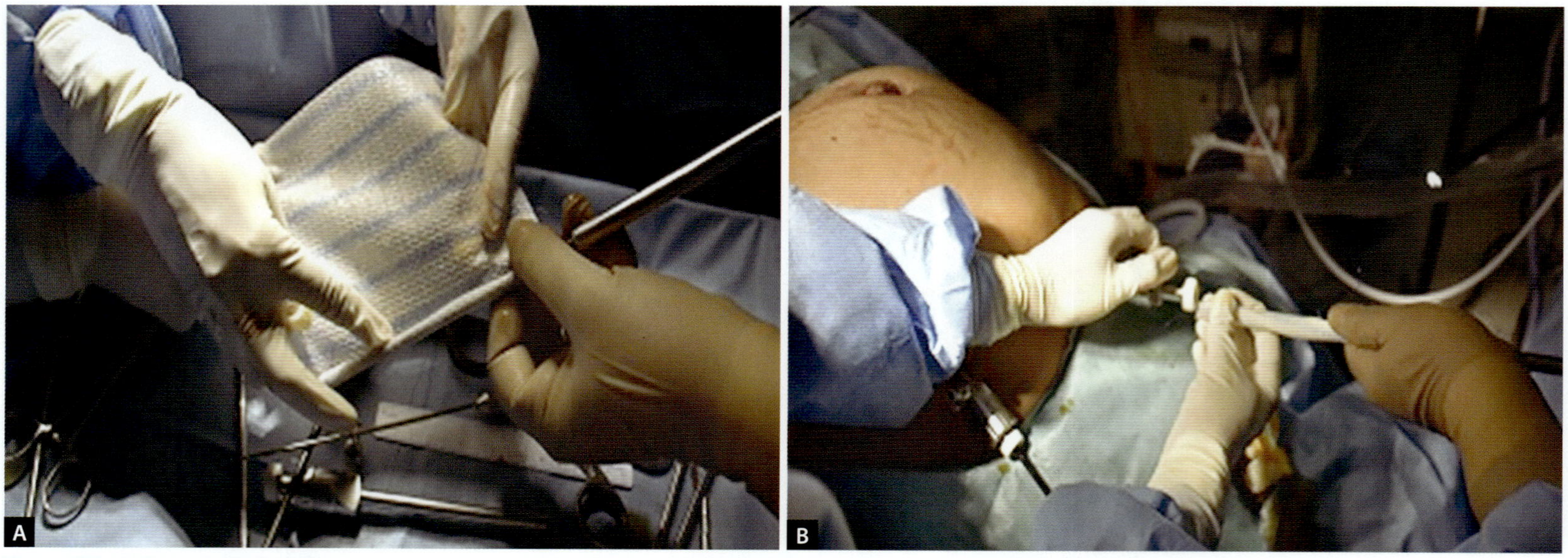

Figs. 11A and B: Introduction of mesh through primary trocar.

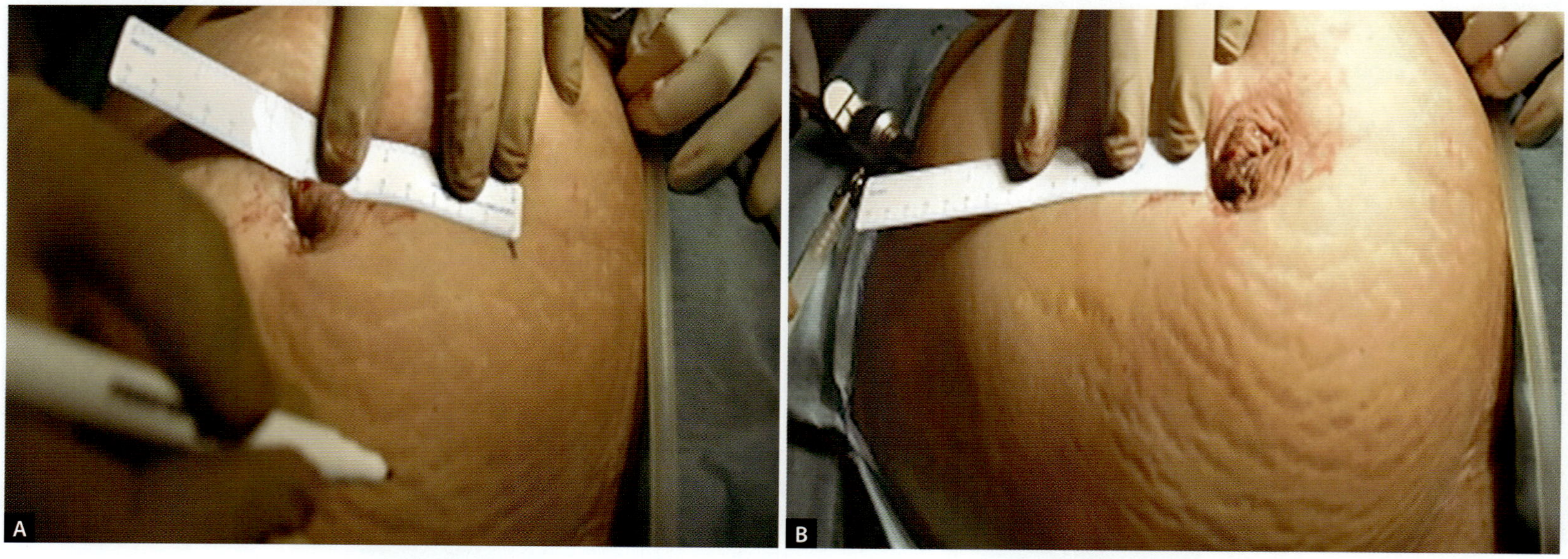

Figs. 12A and B: Surface marking on abdomen 2.5 cm on four sides of defect for fixation of mesh.

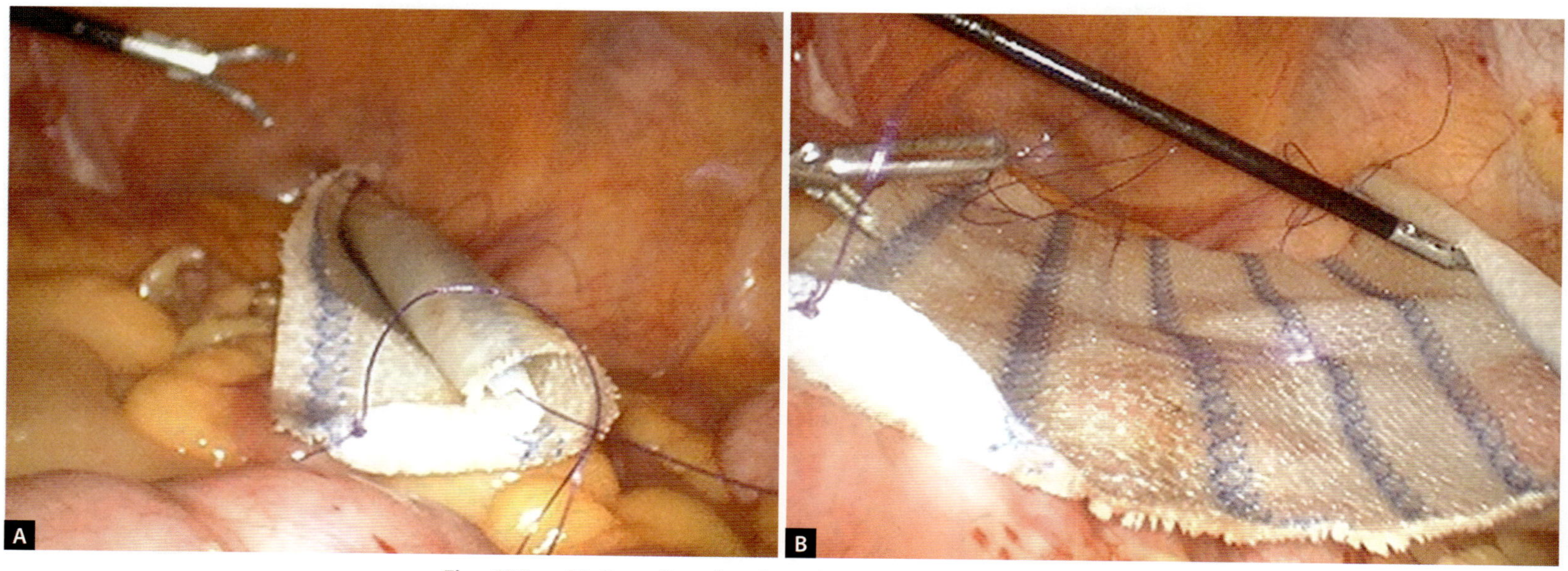

Figs. 13A and B: Spreading of mesh inside abdomen using plain graspers.

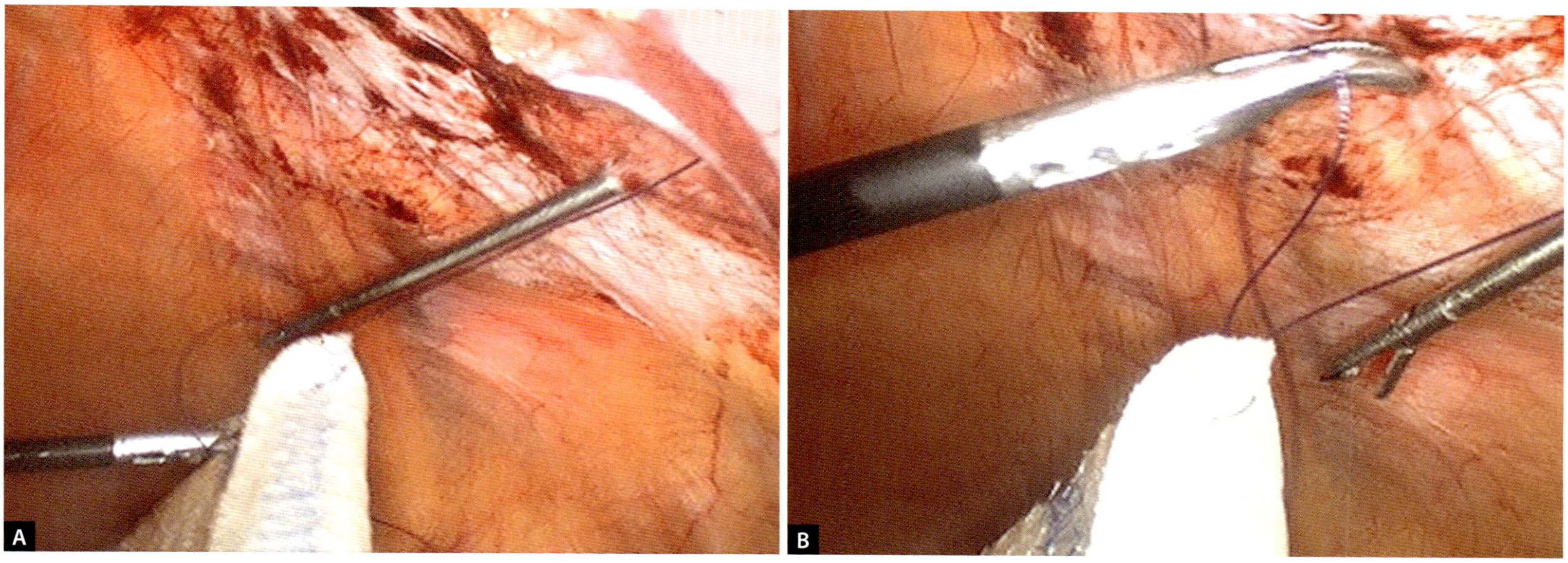

Figs. 14A and B: Bringing together each suture end of mesh using plain graspers and Cobbler's needle introduced through surface marking.

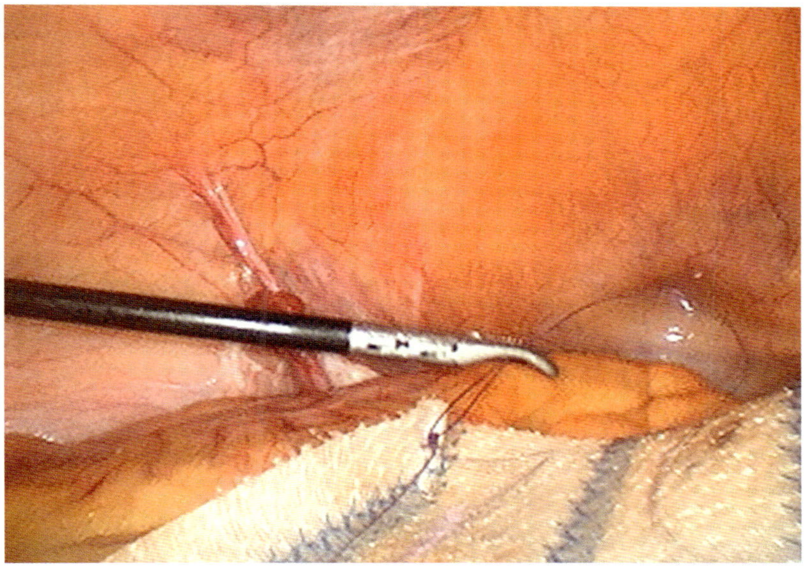

Fig. 15: Holding mesh end sutures through Maryland grasper.

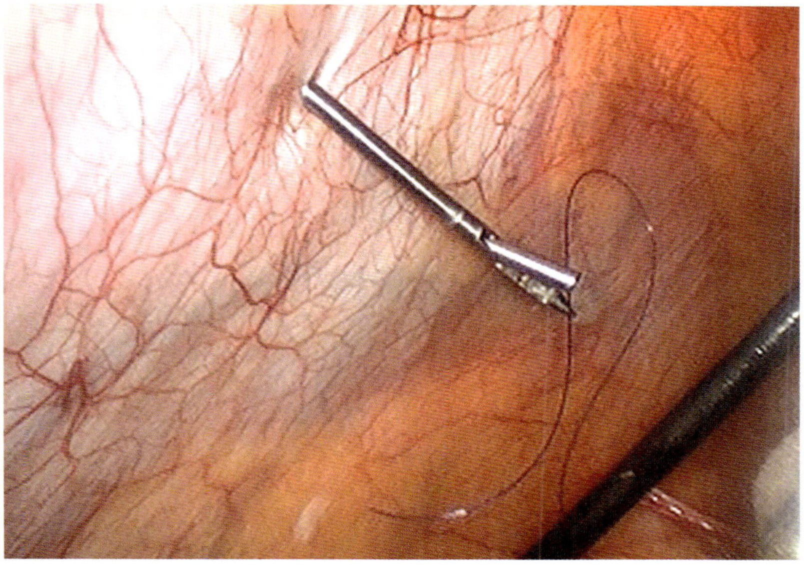

Fig. 16: Cobbler's needle introduced from surface marking which holds suture and is brought to abdominal wall.

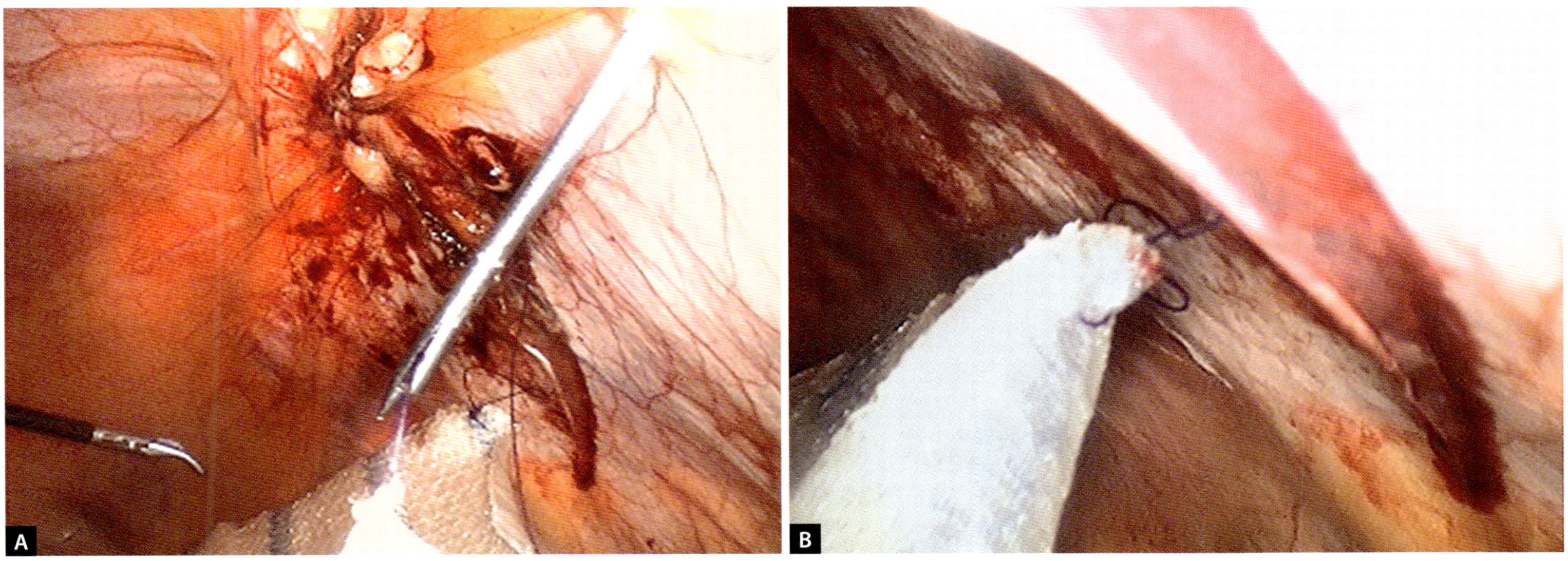

Figs. 17A and B: Gradual pulling of Cobbler's needle holding mesh end with suture to abdominal wall.

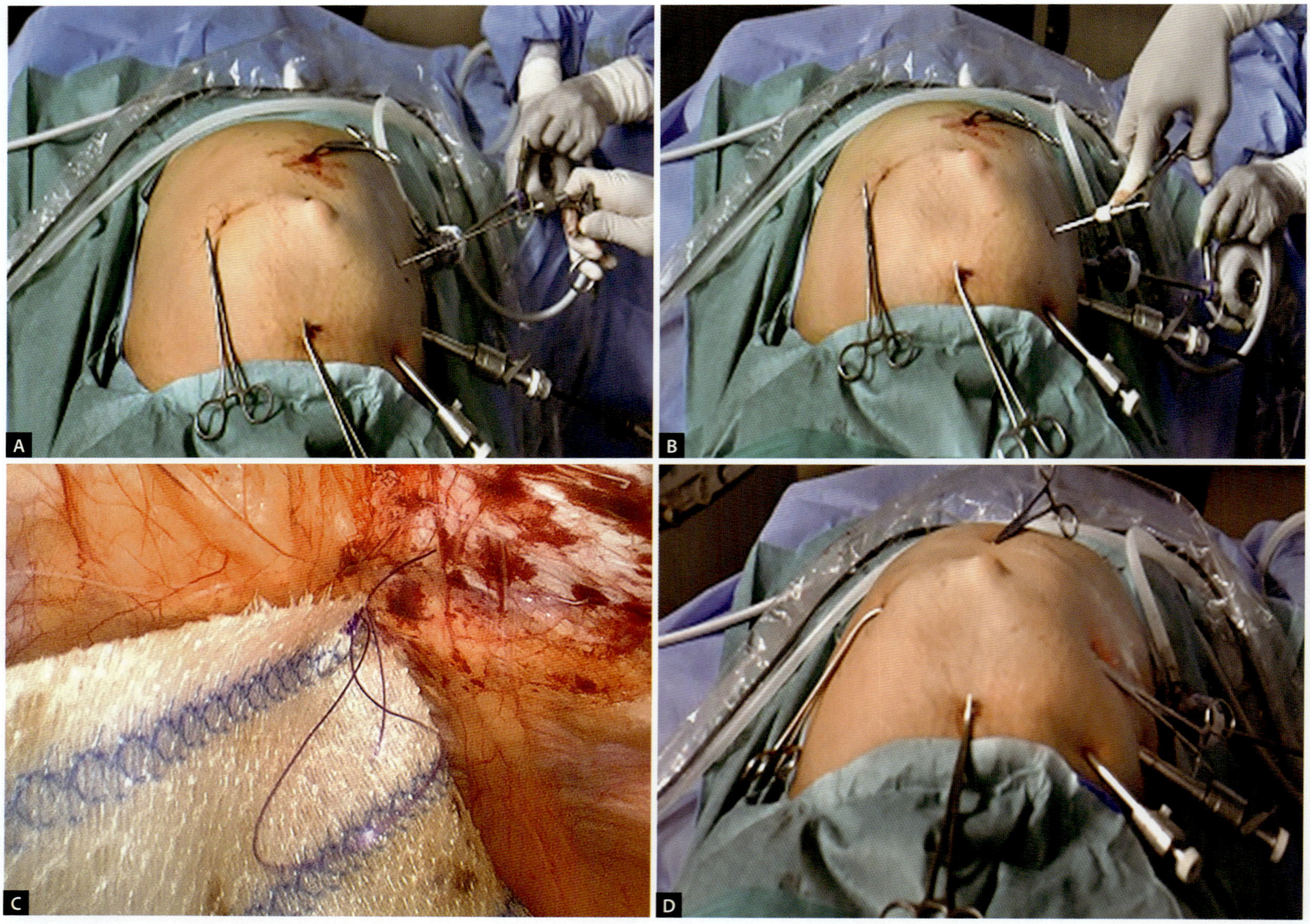

Figs. 18A to D: Externally sutures are held with artery forceps over skin, which are tied at the end of procedure.

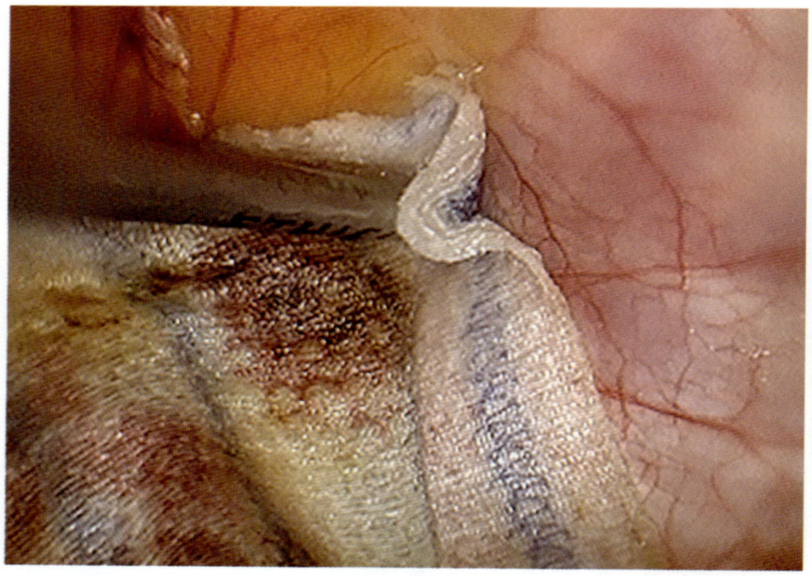

Fig. 19: Fixation of mesh with tackers.

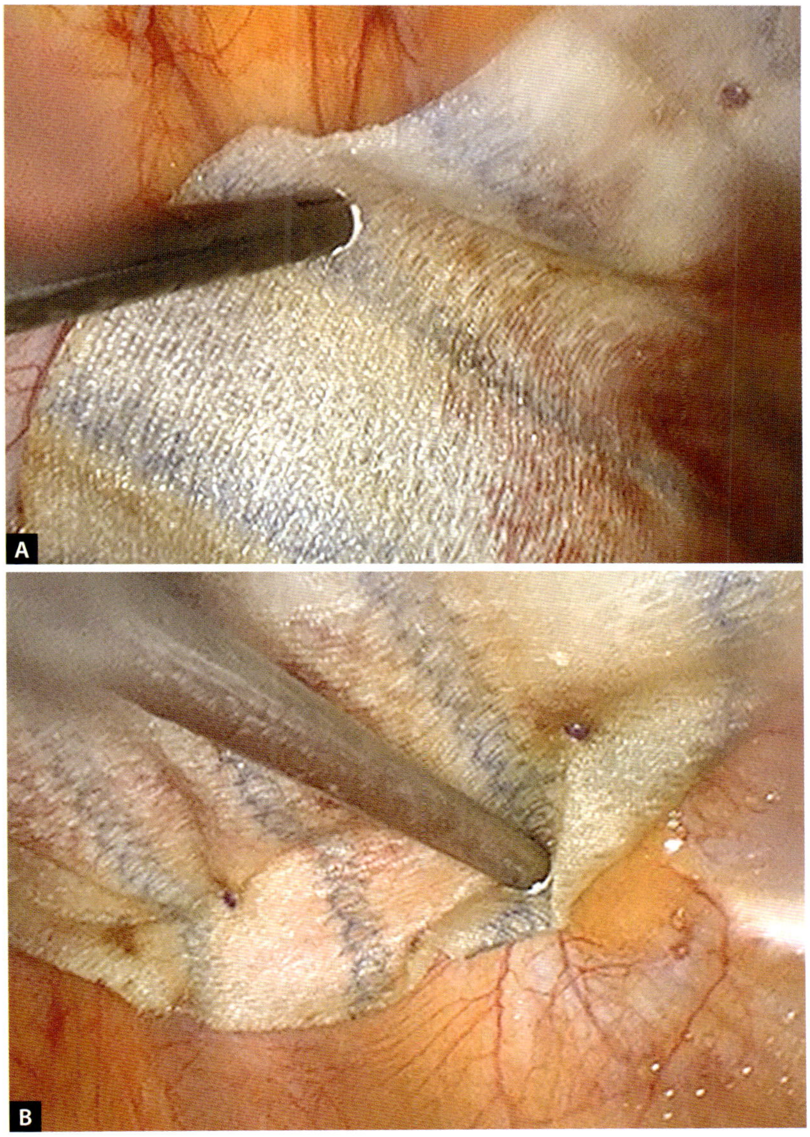

Figs. 20A and B: Circumferential fixation of mesh to abdominal wall using Secure Strap.

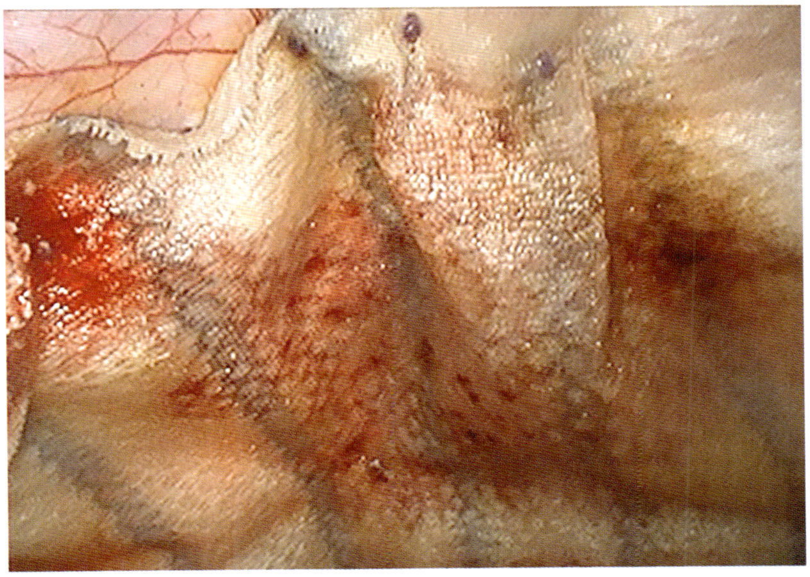

Fig. 21: Fixation of mesh to support fascial defect.

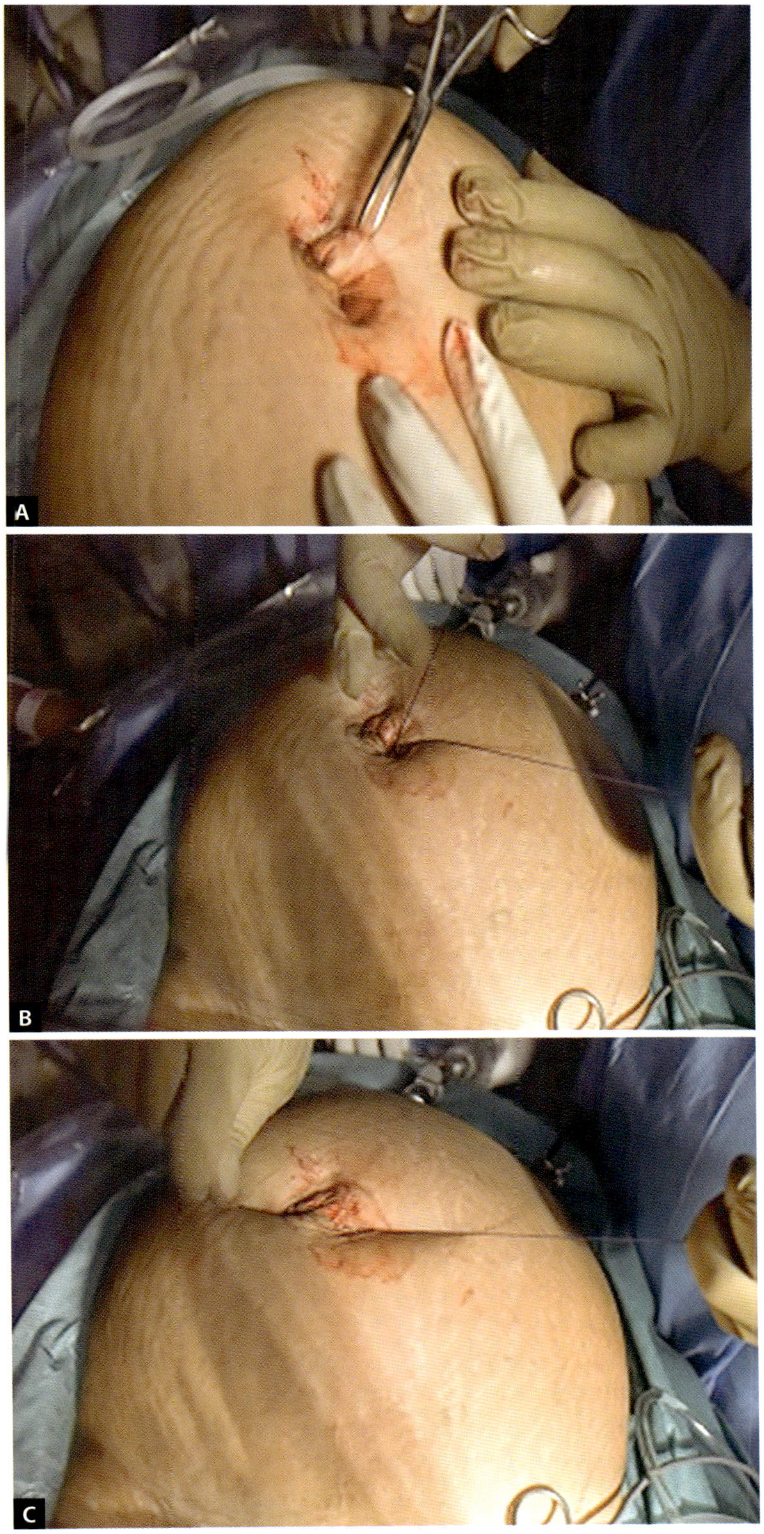

Figs. 22A to C: Final transfixation of sutures which was taken in Figures 7D and 8A which can also be done while anatomical closure of defect.

REFERENCES

1. Velasco M, Garcia-Ureña MA, Hidalgo M, et al. Current concepts on adult umbilical hernia. Hernia. 1999;3(4):253-9.
2. Mayo WJ. VI. An operation for the radical cure of umbilical hernia. Ann Surg. 1901;31:276-30.
3. Javid PJ, Greenberg JA, Brooks DC. Chapter7: Hernias. In: Zinner MJ, Ashley SW (Eds). Maingot's Abdominal Operations, 12th edition. New York: McGraw-Hill Companies, Inc.; 2013.

CHAPTER

33

Laparoscopic Pectopexy

Sushila Saini, Minal Kumbhalwar

Pelvic organ prolapse (POP) affects women all over the world posing health issue for more than 50% of women aged beyond 50 years.[1] Prolapse surgeries are the most commonly performed procedures of benign gynecological surgery. Various surgical procedures have been mentioned in the literature over time for rectifying the prolapse.[2] Although difficult to decide finest surgical method, different surgical techniques have been performed, with or without using mesh. Randomized trials depicting the use of mesh versus native tissue repair in prolapse surgery showed better anatomical but similar functional outcomes with mesh. Laparoscopic sacrocolpopexy/sacrohysteropexy is most widely accepted procedure for apical compartment prolapse and hence considered the gold standard.[3] As per the Cochrane review, abdominal sacrocolpopexy has higher long-term success rates as compared with sacrospinous ligament fixation vaginally.[3]

Being most effective surgery over the time, sacrocolpopexy poses few complications mainly including defecation problems and urinary incontinence [stress urinary incontinence (SUI)].[4] Prior studies reported gastrointestinal complications like paralytic ileus, small bowel obstruction, and defecation disorders in 0.1–5% of sacrocolpopexy surgeries approximately. The mesh interposed between sacrum and vagina (cervix) narrows the pelvis leading to defecation disorders also reduced space in the pelvis, outlet obstruction, adhesions, and hypogastric nerve injury contributes more.[4-6,7] However, presacral hemorrhage is the life-threatening intraoperative complication of sacrocolpopexy.[8]

Banerjee and Noé presented newer laparoscopic surgery for prolapse named pectopexy designed specifically for obese women.[9] In this procedure, iliopectineal ligament lateral sides are used for fixation of mesh with prolapsed organs on both sides, and then the mesh follows broad ligaments and round ligaments without crossing the ureter and bowel.[9]

The iliopectineal ligament named after Astley Cooper known as Cooper's inguinal ligament, is an extension of lacunar ligament which is attached to pectineal line on pubic bone[10] **(Fig. 1)**, Cooper's ligament is more stronger than sacrospinous ligament as well as arcus tendineus of the pelvic fascia[11] and holds suture well. There is enough space for suture in the lateral aspect of iliopectineal ligament, thus facilitating pelvic floor reconstruction.[12] This part of ligament is located at the second sacral vertebra (S2) level which is the anchor point for physiological axis of vagina.[12]

Recent literature suggests laparoscopic pectopexy as an alternative technique for patients with difficult promontory dissection in surgery.[9-11]

CHOOSING PECTOPEXY

- The main factor for deciding surgery technique is increasing laparoscopic surgical experience over the years.[9]
- The laparoscopic pectopexy can be selected for patients with body mass index (BMI) >30 and other comorbidities.[9]
- In patients with difficult dissection of promontory due to a
  - Presacral fat deposition
  - Bony deformities at promontory
  - Dense bowel adhesions at promontory
  - Unexpected vascular anomalies or variations
  - Restricted mobility or thickened sigmoid colon or
- Previous failed sacropexy
- Vault prolapses
- Associated anterior compartment defect with apical descent
- Pectopexy can be chosen by beginners also as laparoscopic suturing in anterior compartment is much easier than in posterior compartment.

Laparoscopic Pectopexy Method

- Patient laid in supine with lithotomy position.
- The standard laparoscopic preparation done.
- We operate from left of patient side.
- Primary 10 mm trocar inserted supraumbilically 3 cm above the umbilicus in midline for laparoscope, three accessory 5 mm ports were inserted under laparoscopic vision on lower abdominal area, two on left, and one port on right, approximately 2 cm and 8 cm medial and superior aspect of anterior superior iliac crest. Right port is mirror image of 2nd secondary port on left side.
- After insertion of endoscope, checking proper placement of trocar, pneumoperitoneum created.
- Complete inspection of peritoneal cavity done along with pelvic area done.
- Straight uterine manipulator placed into uterus or sponge on holder into vagina in cases of vault prolapse for placing prolapsed part into pelvis.
- After pushing uterus or vault inside and exposing uterovesical fold or apex of vault, uterovesical fold incised and bladder pushed down by blunt and sharp dissection till urethral attachment so that associated cystocele part also can be taken care of.
- In case of vault prolapse, posterior dissection also performed for making space for mesh placement between rectum and vagina. We can extend dissection till levator ani according to need for correction of rectocele.

- Peritoneal incision extended laterally toward lateral pelvic wall along with round ligament on both sides.
- On lateral pelvic wall, peritoneum over the triangle **(Figs. 1A and B)** formed by round ligament, obliterated umbilical artery and lateral pelvic wall, opened and at base of triangle **(Fig. 2)**, external iliac vein **(Figs. 4 to 6)** (EIV) found after blunt dissection of overlying fatty tissue and just adjacent and medial to EIV, iliopectineal ligament **(Figs. 3A to C)** (Cooper's ligament) identified near insertion of iliopsoas muscles.
- After proper dissection, monofilament polypropylene type 1 mesh (15 × 15 cm) inserted into the abdomen. Mesh should always be prepared according to need and defect present **(Figs. 7A and B)**.
- We design the mesh with a tongue shape process approximately 4 cm long at midpoint of mesh so that it can be placed below bladder to take care of cystocele and same 3–4 cm posteriorly also to place between rectum and vagina to correct rectocele in cases of vault prolapse **(Figs. 8 to 10)**.
- Mesh first fixed to uterus or vaginal apex and then end parts of mesh will be sutured to bilateral iliopectineal **(Fig. 12)** ligaments using nonabsorbable sutures with intracorporeal suture technique using polyester suture Ethibond 2-0, 26 mm needle or with help of tackers and apex of vagina or uterus **(Fig. 11)** will provide hammock-like fixation.
- While placement of mesh, we should always take care that mesh should not be crumpled, folded or wrinkled and mesh should not be too loose or too tight. Mesh placement should always be tension free and flat, not folded or crumpled.

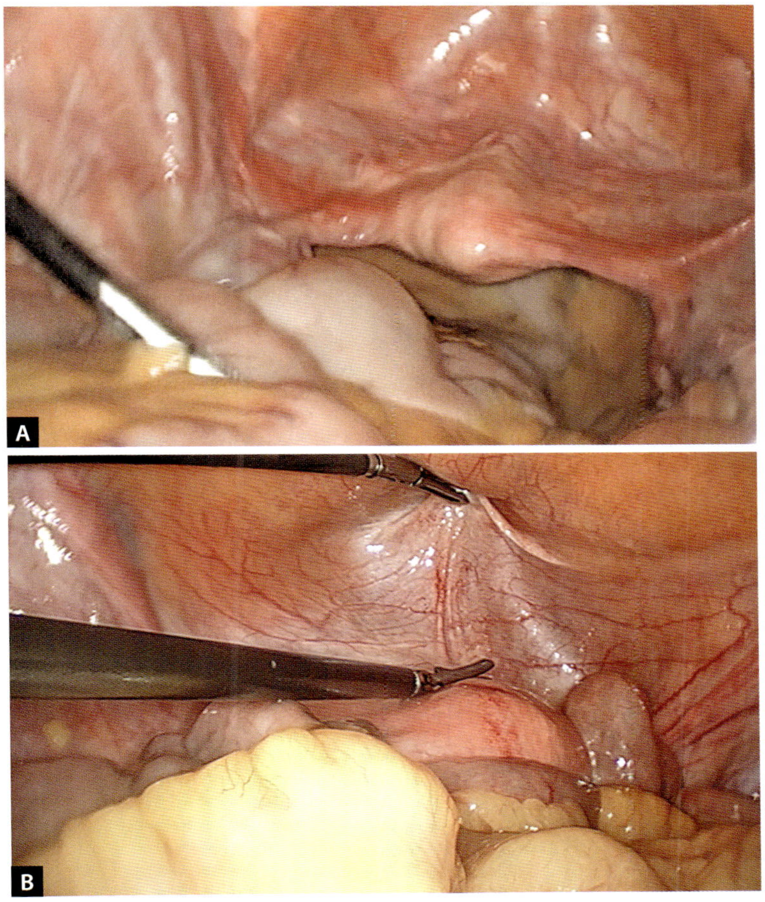

Figs. 1A and B: Opening of peritoneum over the triangle formed by round ligament, obliterated umbilical artery and lateral pelvic wall.

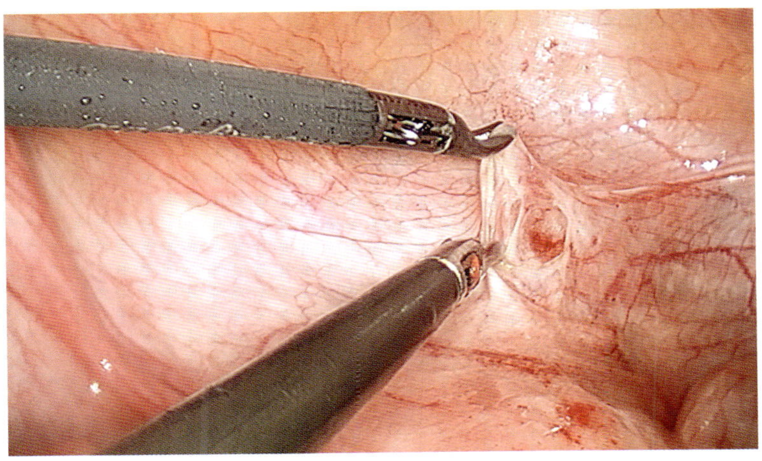

Fig. 2: Further dissection continued till base of triangle is reached.

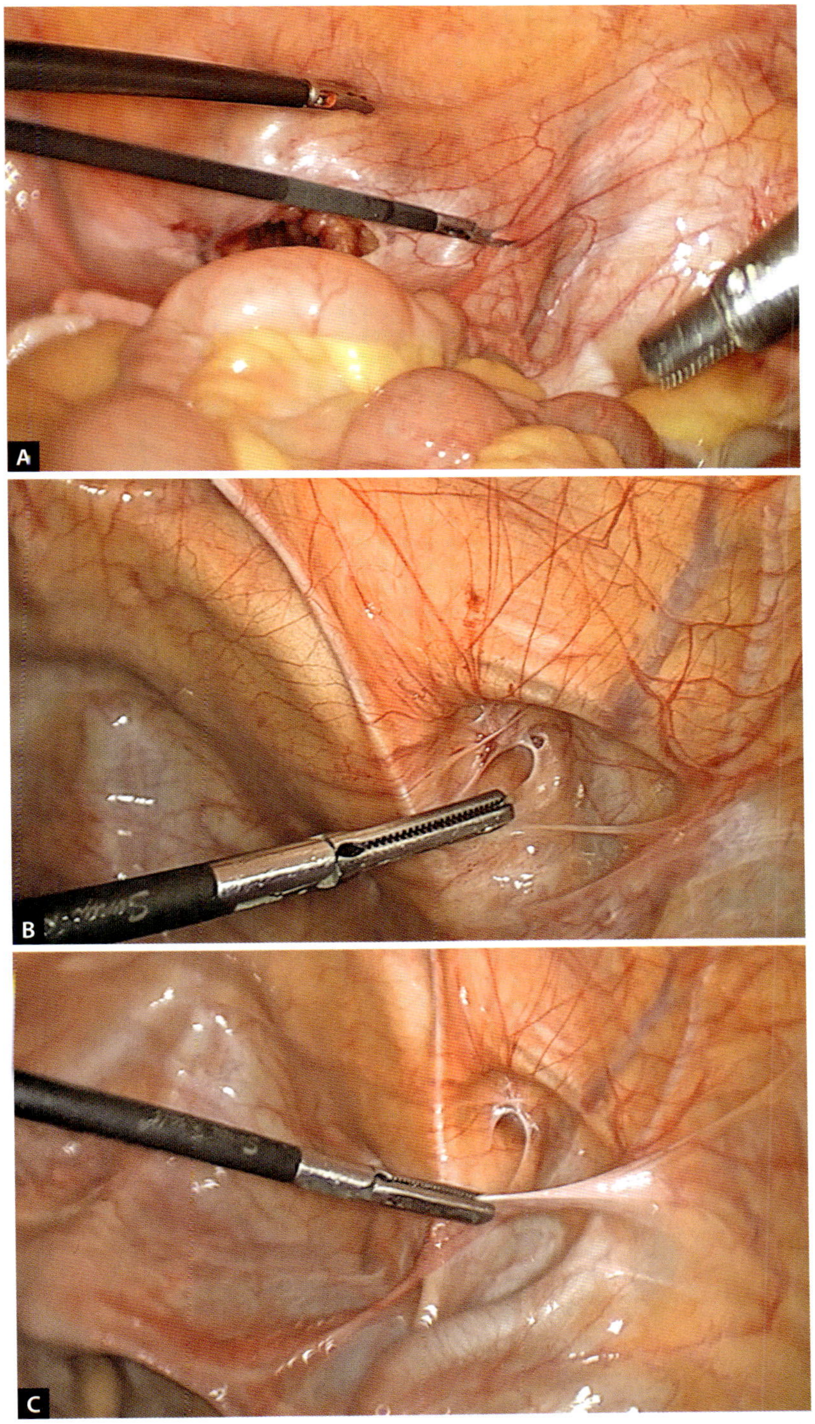

Figs. 3A to C: Overlying fatty tissue dissected out.

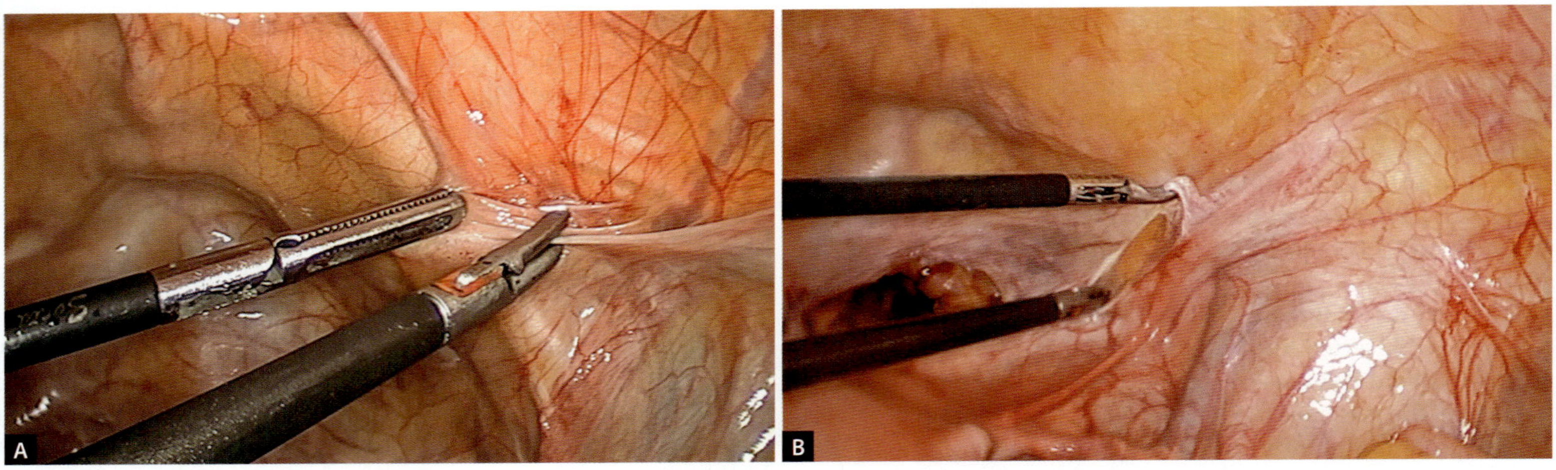

Figs. 4A and B: Further dissection continued.

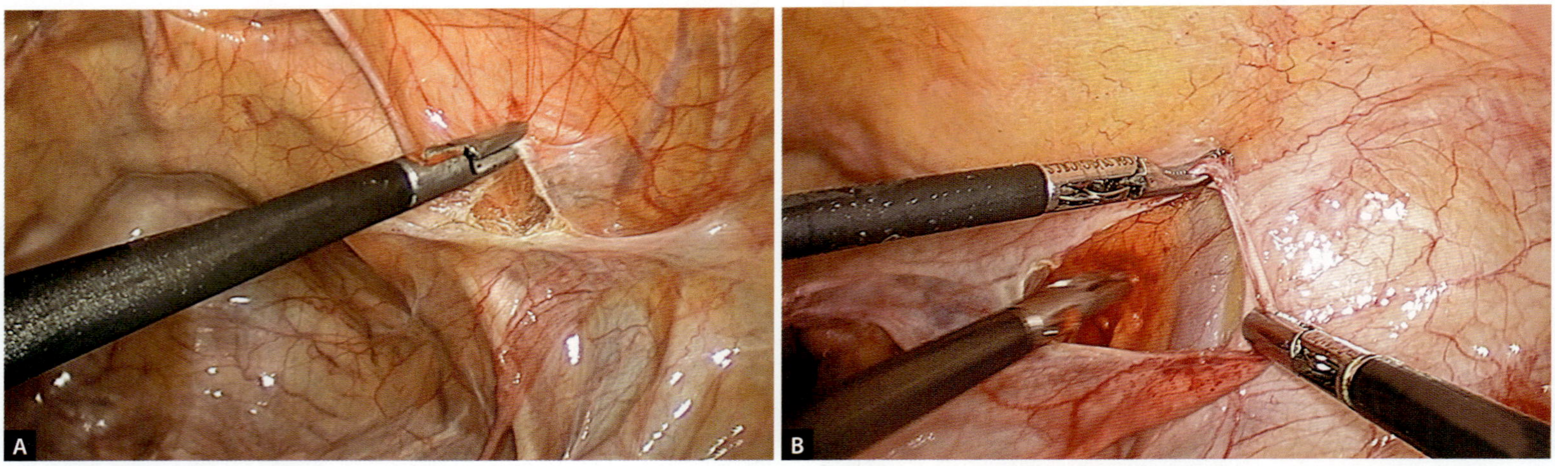

Figs. 5A and B: Blunt dissecton continued till external iliac vein (EIV) found.

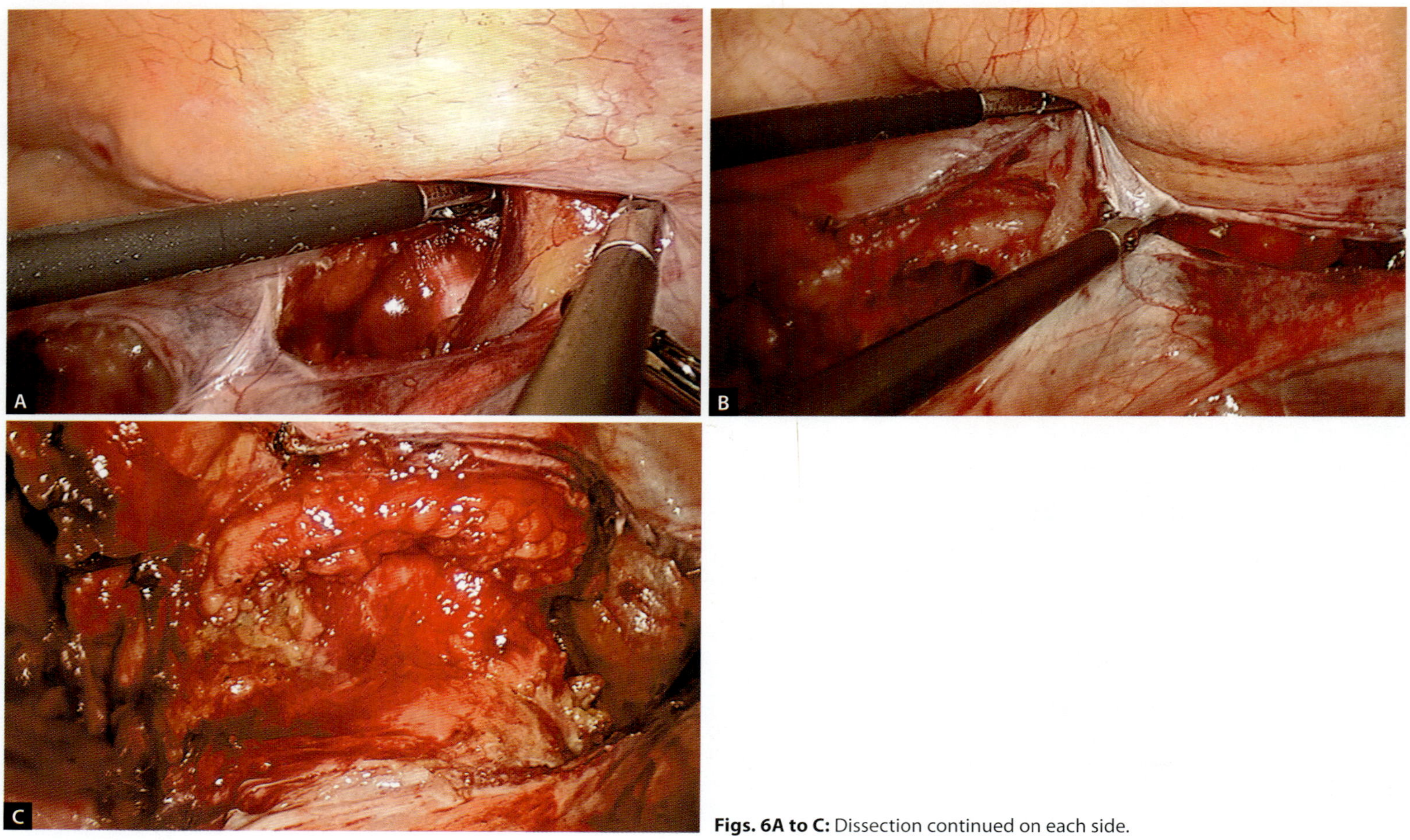

Figs. 6A to C: Dissection continued on each side.

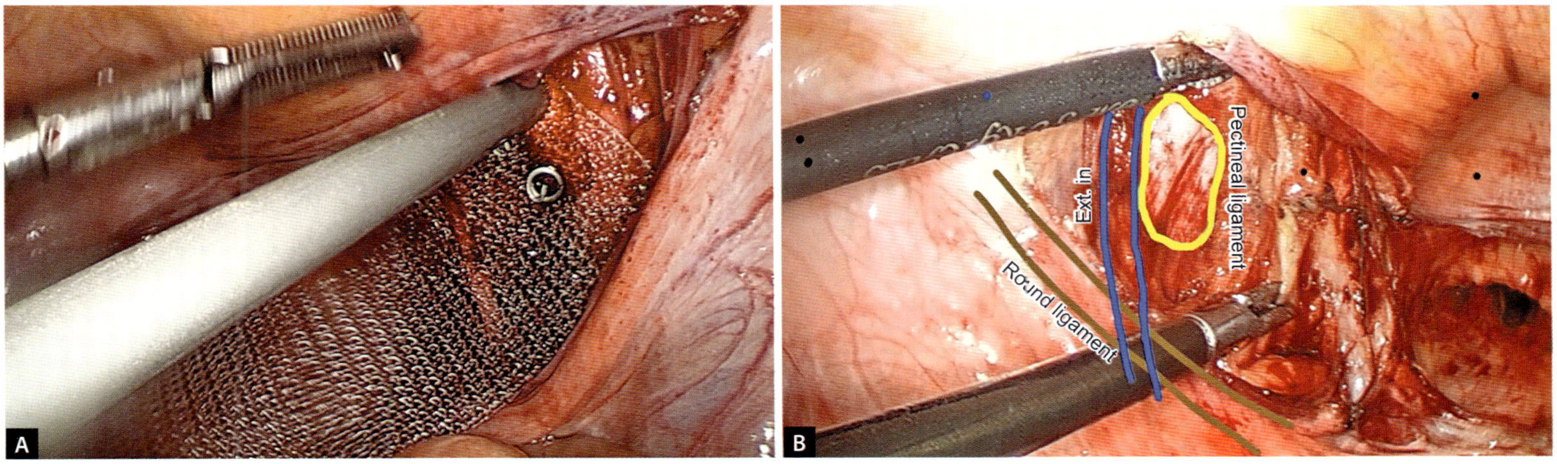

Figs. 7A and B: Monofilament polypropylene type 1 mesh (15 × 15 cm) inserted into the abdomen.

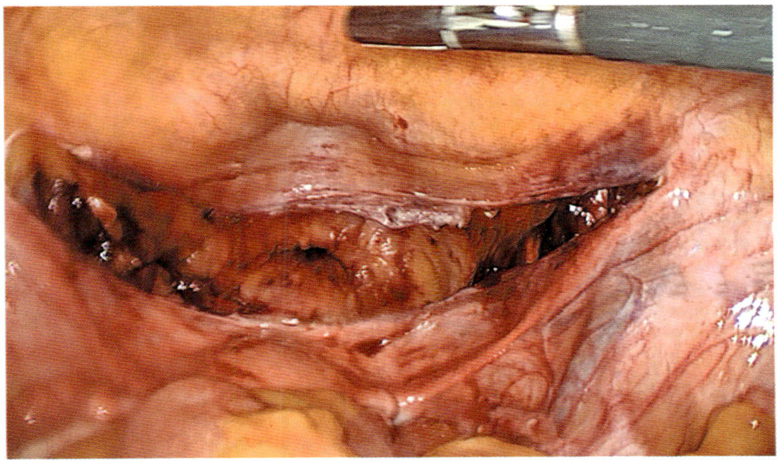

Fig. 8: Bilateral dissection done prior to mesh placement.

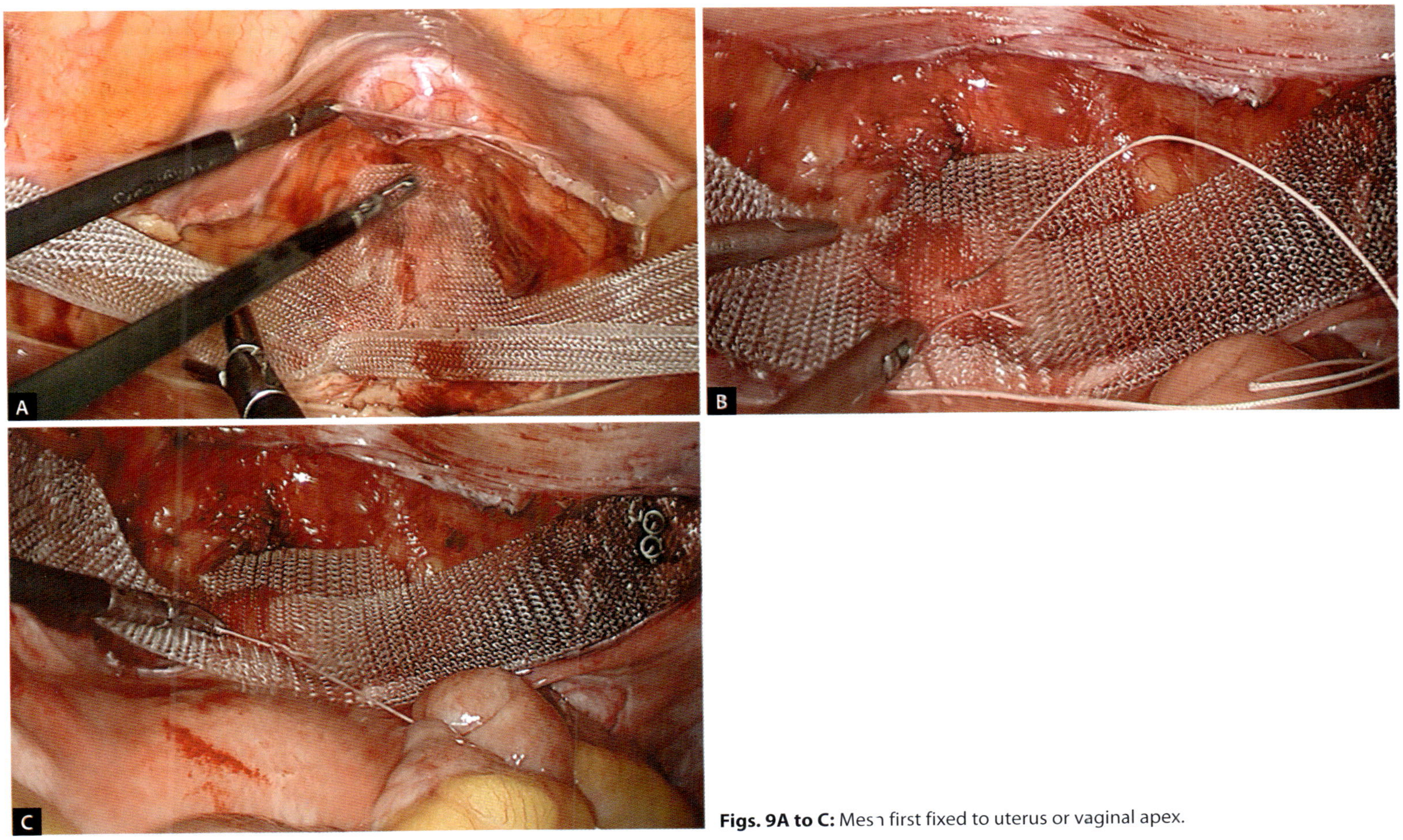

Figs. 9A to C: Mesh first fixed to uterus or vaginal apex.

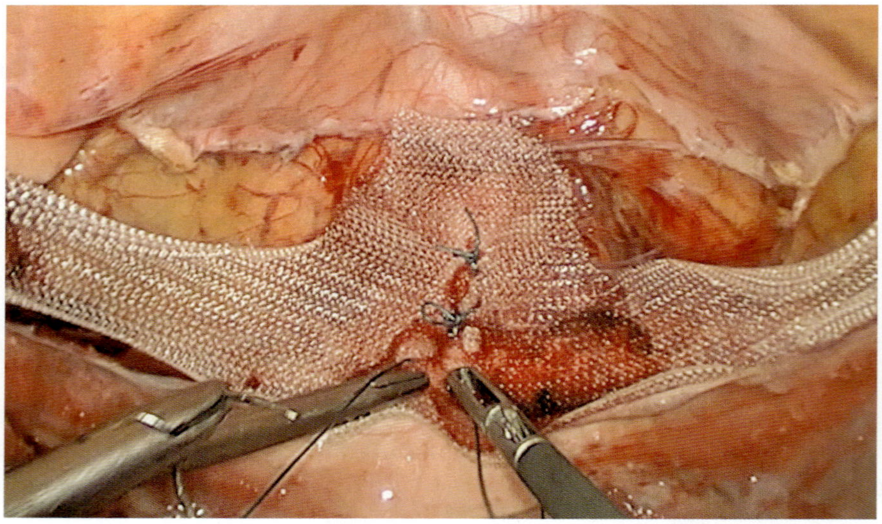

Fig. 10: Fixing of mesh to posterior aspect of uterus.

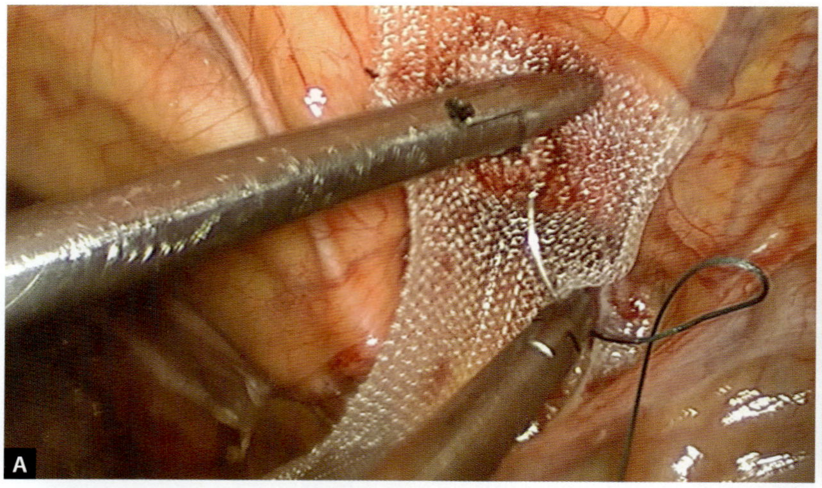

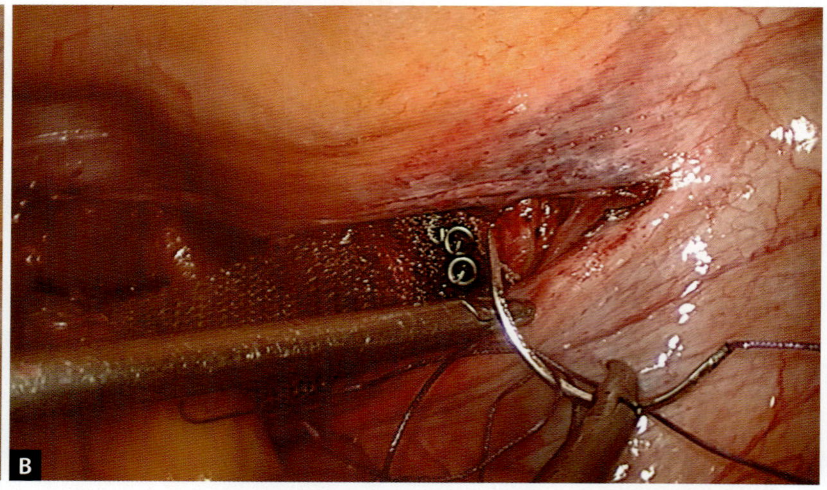

Figs. 11A and B: Suturing done using nonabsorbable sutures with intracorporeal suture technique using polyester suture ethibond 2-0, 26 mm needle.

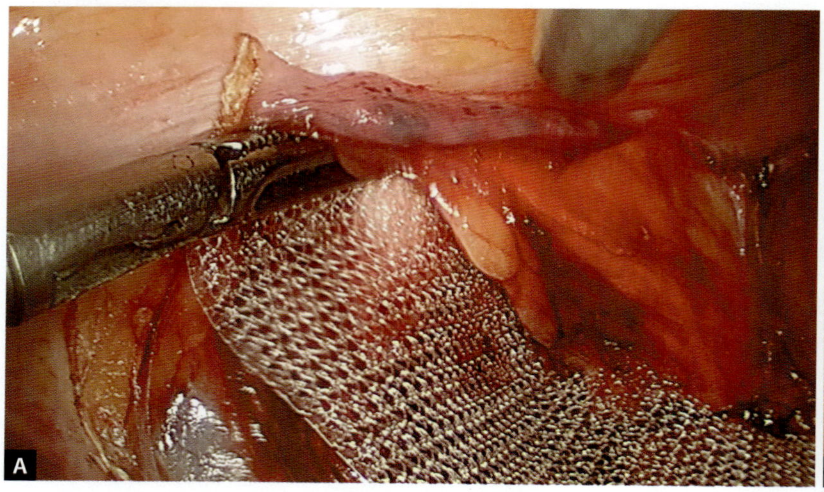

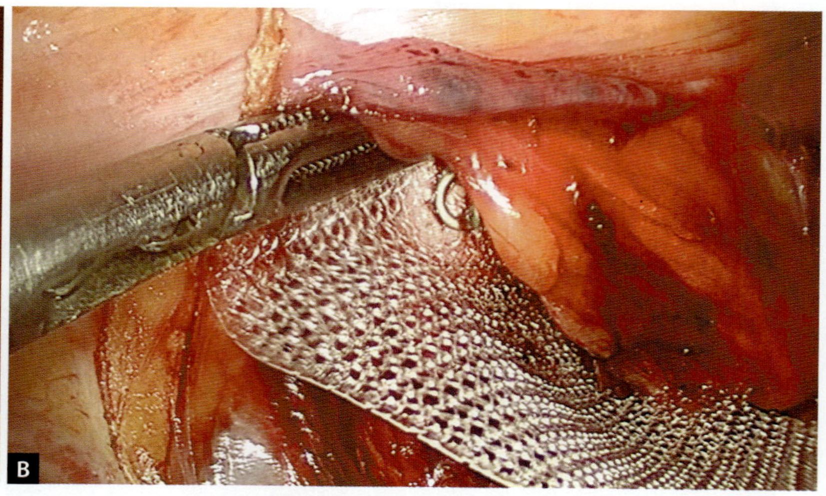

Figs. 12A and B: End parts of mesh sutured to bilateral iliopectineal ligaments.

- At last, the peritoneum above mesh is sutured with absorbable suture material **(Figs. 13 and 14)**.

Major risk involved in procedure is to injury to EIV as we have to place suture near to it. For prevention to unintended injury to vein, needle size should be 26 mm only, larger size of needle carries higher risk of laceration of vein.

Perioperative Complications

- That may happen intraoperatively or postoperatively in 6–10 weeks includes bowel, bladder, ureteric, or external iliac vessels injury
- Hematoma, abscess
- Wound infection
- Urinary tract infection

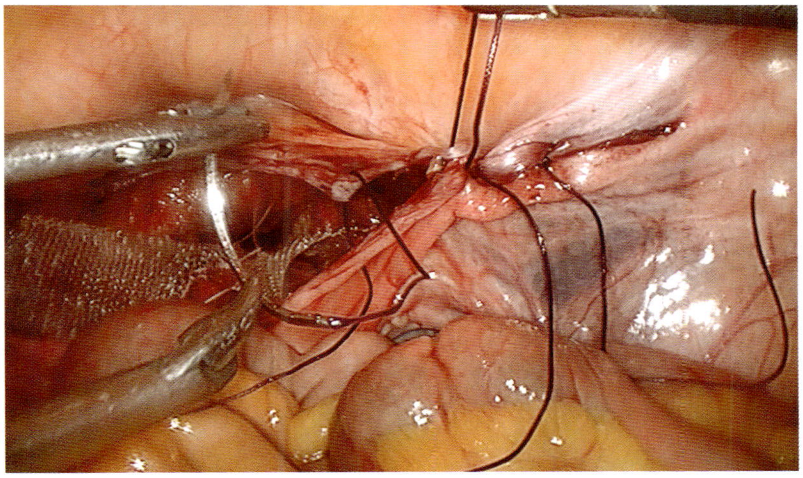

Fig. 13: Peritoneum above mesh sutured with absorbable suture material.

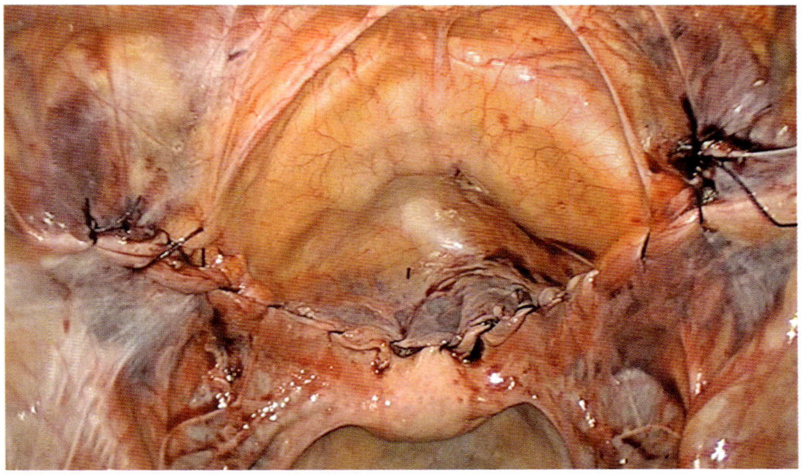

Fig. 14: Retroperitonization of mesh done.

- Paralytic ileus, bowel obstruction; and
- Infection of mesh.

Short-term complications within 6-month duration after surgery include:

- Recurrence of problem or
- Mesh erosion.

Laparoscopic Pectopexy Offers Various Advantages[13]

1. It allows the surgeon to operate in wide area of pelvis, more satisfactorily in complex surgeries.
2. The mesh placement does not interfere with pelvic structures and so minimizes the risk of bowel infection and disorders.
3. As iliopectineal ligament is too strong, there will be lesser chance of postoperative recurrence of apical prolapse.
4. The iliopectineal ligament fixation of apical prolapse maintains the physiologic axis of the vagina as S2 level is the anchor point for the physiological axis of the vagina.
5. The iliopectineal ligament is at far location from ureter, intestines, and presacral veins. Hence, lesser chances of injury to these structures during surgery, proving it safe area for apical prolapse reconstructive surgery.
6. In pectopexy, there may be added protective influence over anterior compartment also.

The pectopexy technique enhances surgeon's technical portfolio. In case of challenges due to anatomic variations, laparoscopic pectopexy acts as best alternative to sacral colpopexy. Multicenter investigations need to be considered to prove the worth of laparoscopic pectopexy in clinical practice.

OUR EXPERIENCE

We have done 35 pectopexy from April 2018 to march 2019 at our center, Jaipur Doorbeen Hospital which is a tertiary level academic institute in Jaipur.

Thirty-one cases are done mainly for 3rd-degree uterovaginal prolapse associated with cystocele mainly and four cases are of vault prolapse.

The subjective satisfaction rates were tremendously high in patients at 1 week and at 6 months postoperatively. After 6-month follow-up, no occurrences of de novo apical prolapse, lateral defect or anterior defect cystoceles or mesh infection/erosion/exposure has been observed.

Out of 31 cases, one that shows rectocele after 3 months of surgery for which posterior repair done vaginally.

Out of four cases of vault prolapse, one patient shows 2nd-degree cystocele and rectocele with vault at 0 level after 2 months of surgery.

Results are promising with 94% all over success rate and 98% after excluding one case of rectocele which is actually not addressed in primary repair.

CONCLUSION

The laparoscopic pectopexy is better alternative for laparoscopic sacropexy. It is equally effective and shows no defecation problems, backache or neuralgia in the long-term follow-up.

REFERENCES

1. Subak LL, Waetjen LE, van den Eeden S, et al. Cost of pelvic organ prolapse surgery in the United States. Obstet Gynecol. 2001;98:646-51.
2. Barbalat Y, Tunuguntla HS. Surgery for pelvic organ prolapse: a historical perspective. Curr Urol Rep. 2012;13:256-61.
3. Maher C, Feiner B, Baessler K, et al. Surgical management of pelvic organ prolapse in women. Cochrane Database Syst Rev. 2013;4:CD004014.
4. Nygaard IE, McCreery R, Brubaker L, et al. Abdominal sacrocolpopexy: a comprehensive review. Obstet Gynecol. 2004;104:805-23.
5. Sarlos D, Brandner S, Kots L, et al. Laparoscopic sacrocolpopexy for uterine and post-hysterectomy prolapse: anatomical results, quality of life and perioperative outcome: a prospective study with 101 cases. Int Urogynecol J Pelvic Floor Dysfunct. 2008;19:1415-22.
6. Akladios CY, Dautun D, Saussine C, et al. Laparoscopic sacrocolpopexy for female genital organ prolapse: establishment of a learning curve. Eur J Obstet Gynecol Reprod Biol. 2010;149:218-21.
7. Whitehead WE, Bradley CS, Brown MB, et al. Gastrointestinal complications following abdominal sacrocolpopexy for advanced pelvic organ prolapse. Am J Obstet Gynecol. 2007;197:78.e1-7
8. Kumar S, Malhotra N, Chumber S, et al. Control of presacral venous bleeding, using thumbtacks. Arch Gynecol Obstet. 2007;276:385-6.
9. Banerjee C, Noé KG. Laparoscopic pectopexy: a new technique of prolapse surgery for obese patients. Arch Gynecol Obstet. 2011;284:631-5.
10. Faure JP, Hauet T, Scepi M, et al. The pectineal ligament: anatomical study and surgical applications. Surg Radiol Anat. 2001;23:237-42.
11. Cosson M, Boukerrou M, Lacaze S, et al. A study of pelvic ligament strength. Eur J Obstet Gynecol Reprod Biol. 2003;109:80-7.
12. Noé KG, Schiermeier S, Alkatout I, et al. Laparoscopic pectopexy: a prospective, randomized, comparative clinical trial of standard laparoscopic sacral colpocervicopexy with the new laparoscopic pectopexy—postoperative results and intermediate-term follow-up in a pilot study. J Endourol. 2015;29:210-5.
13. Kale A, Biler A, Terzi H, et al. Laparoscopic pectopexy: initial experience of single center with a new technique for apical prolapse surgery. Int Braz J Urol. 2017;43:903-9.

CHAPTER

34

Conservative Surgeries for Pelvic Organ Prolapse (Shirodkar and Sling)

Tanvi Desai, Aditi Rai, B Ramesh

ETIOLOGY

In India, there is high incidence of pelvic organ prolapse in view of poor socioeconomic status, anemia, malnutrition, and one or more vaginal deliveries at home.

In view of high incidence of nulliparous prolapse in India, Indian gynecologists have devised various conservative sling operations for women who want to preserve the uterus.

Selection criteria for sling surgeries:
- Young nulliparous/multiparous women with second/third-degree uterocervical prolapse
- UCL < 5 inches
- Absent/minimal cystocele/rectocele
- Not recommended for patients with hypertrophied, infected, lacerated cervix
- If moderate/large cysto/rectocele is present, it should be repaired from below at the same sitting before proceeding with sling procedure.

SHIRODKAR'S SLING SURGERY (FIG. 1)

One end of tape is attached to anterior longitudinal ligament, then passed subperitoneally along the right pelvic wall, between the leaves of the broad ligament and transfixed to isthmus posteriorly. It passes posteriorly through left broad ligament, then through the psoas loop, through sigmoid mesentery, and finally fixed back to sacral promontory.

Laparoscopic Shirodkar's Sling Surgery

1. Peritoneal incision taken between uterosacral ligaments and ureter.

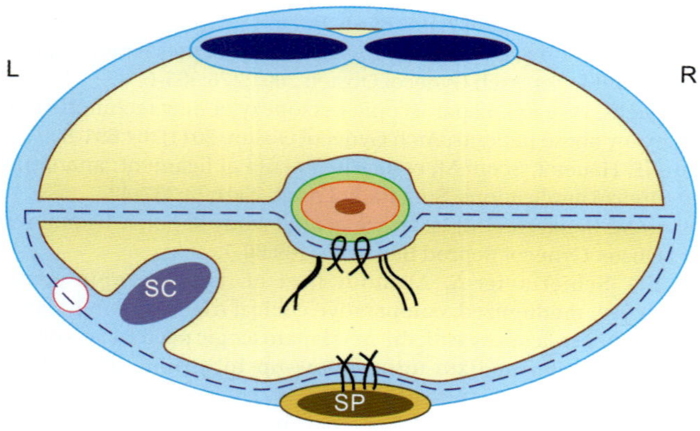

Fig. 1: Shirodkar's sling surgery.
(SC: sigmoid colon; SP: sacral promontory)

2. Ureter lateralized.
3. Peritoneum over sacral promontory opened **(Fig. 2)**.
4. Anterior longitudinal ligament exposed **(Fig. 3)**.
5. Left side psoas muscle exposed, lateral to external iliac vessels **(Fig. 4)**.
6. Artificial psoas loop created with Mersilene tape **(Fig. 5)**.
7. 30 cm Mersilene tape with two needles introduced into the peritoneum.
8. Uterus anteverted with manipulator, and posterior surface exposed.

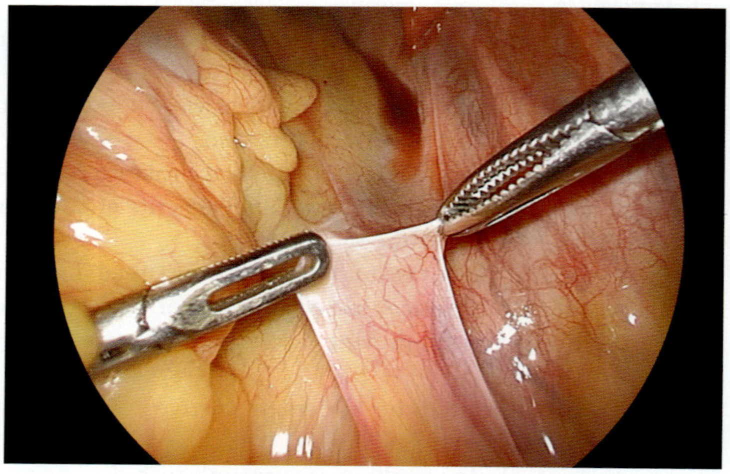

Fig. 2: Peritoneum over sacral promontory opened.

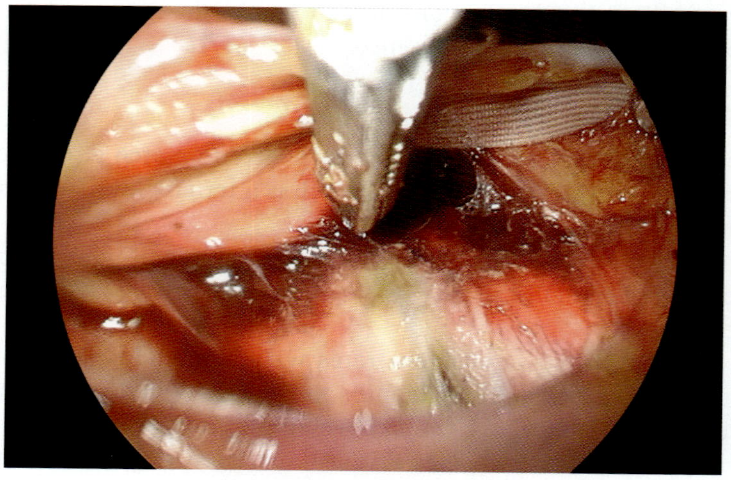

Fig. 3: Anterior longitudinal ligament exposed.

9. Thick bite taken on posterior surface of cervix. Center of the tape anchored to cervix firmly **(Fig. 6)**.
10. Right side needle tunneled through the peritoneum between ureter and uterosacral ligament, and needle brought out in front of sacral promontory **(Fig. 7)**.
11. Left side needle tunneled and tape brought out needle passed through psoas loop and tunnel created through sigmoid mesocolon close to sacrum **(Fig. 8)**.
12. Tape brought in front of sacral promontory.
13. Needle passed through anterior longitudinal ligament **(Fig. 9)**.
14. Both needles cut. Mersilene tape tied on to the promontory after adjusting the tension on the tape optimally and verifying correction of prolapse by per speculum examination **(Fig. 10)**.
15. After satisfactory correction, both sides of tape tied on sacral promontory.
16. All peritoneal openings closed **(Fig. 11)**.

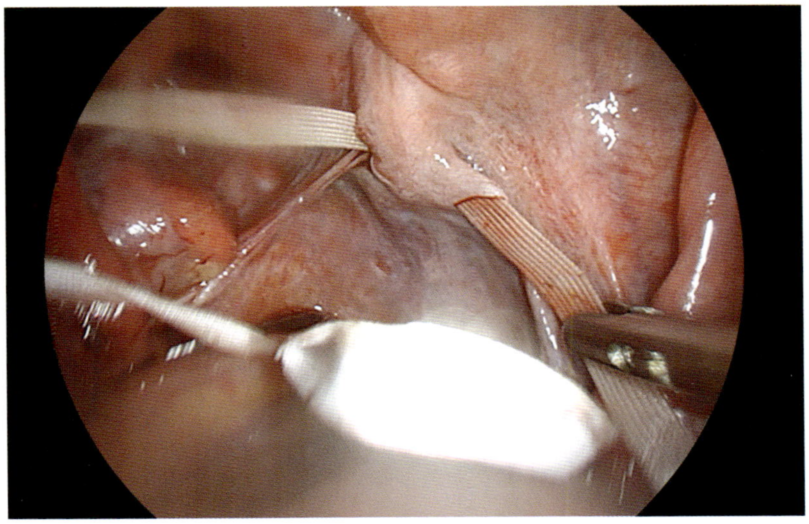

Fig. 6: Thick bite taken on posterior surface of cervix. Center of the tape anchored to cervix firmly.

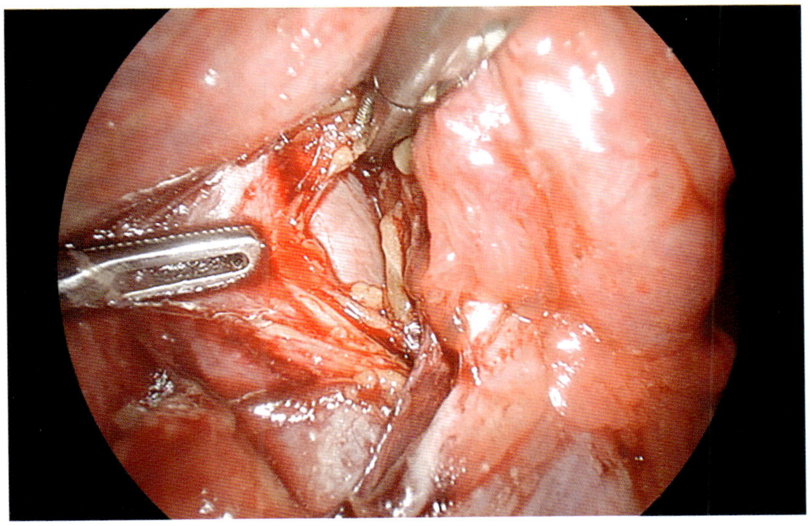

Fig. 4: Left side psoas muscle exposed, lateral to external iliac vessels.

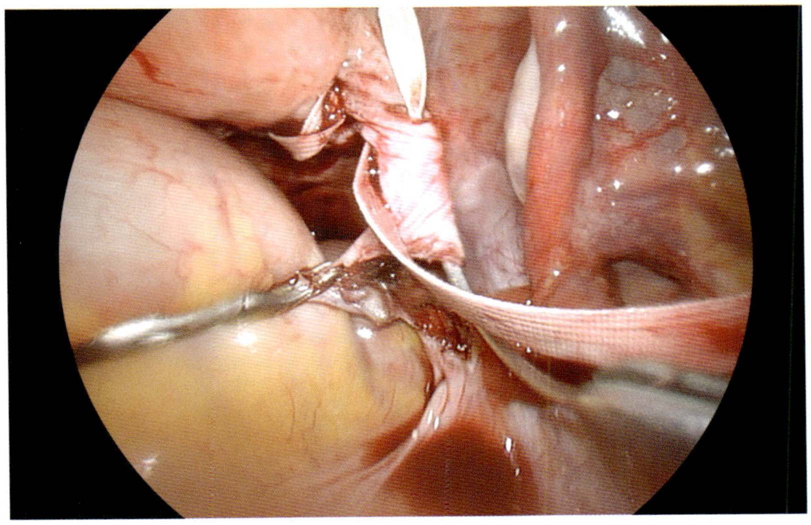

Fig. 7: Right side needle tunneled through the peritoneum between ureter and uterosacral ligament, and needle brought out in front of sacral promontory.

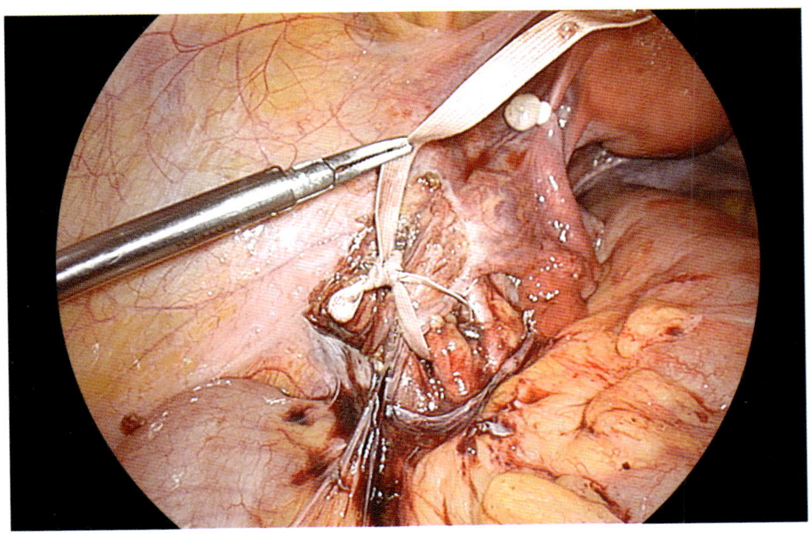

Fig. 5: Artificial psoas loop created with Mersilene tape.

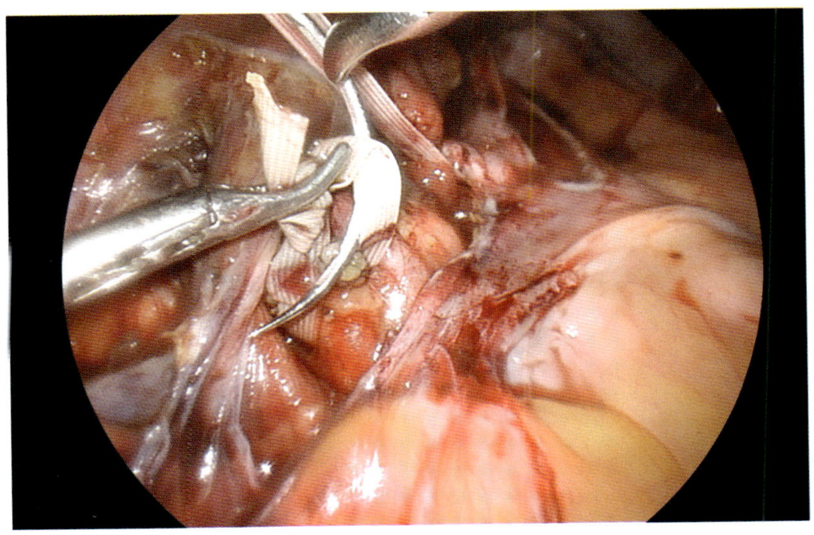

Fig. 8: Left side needle tunneled and tape brought out needle passed through psoas loop and tunnel created through sigmoid mesocolon close to sacrum.

Advantages

- Fixed to sacral promontory which is a firm structure
- Tape is on both sides, so no deviation of uterus to one side

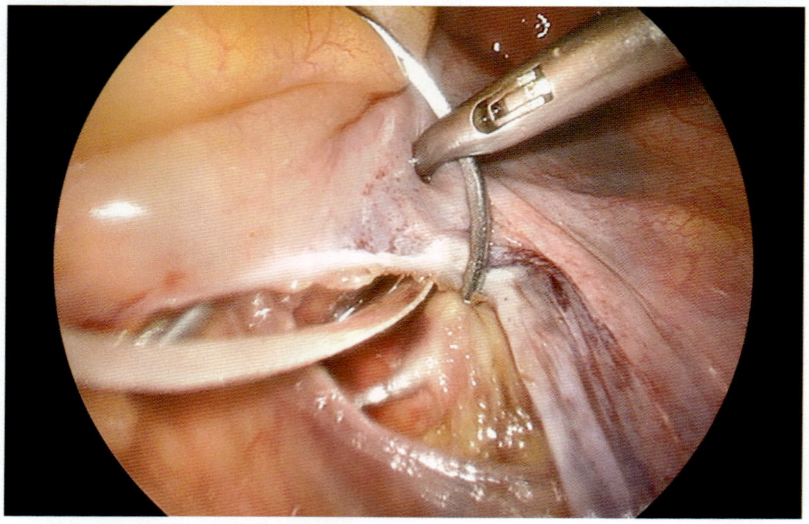

Fig. 9: Needle passed through one side of anterior longitudinal ligament

- Strong support to uterus
- Less failure rates.

Disadvantages

- Higher skill required
- Psoas loop needs to be created
- Compression of sigmoid colon can result in constipation, obstruction
- Too tight suspension may cause pain and backache
- Risk of injuries to bowel, ureter, and major vessels.

LAPAROSCOPIC SACROHYSTEROPEXY

Sacrohysteropexy is a simple and effective procedure in the conservative surgery for prolapse.

1. Peritoneum over the sacral promontory is incised and anterior longitudinal ligament exposed **(Fig. 12)**.
2. Posterior peritoneum in the pouch of Douglas incised and posterior cervicoisthmic junction exposed.
3. Bilateral levator ani muscles exposed **(Fig. 13)**.
4. Y-shaped mesh introduced **(Fig. 14)**.

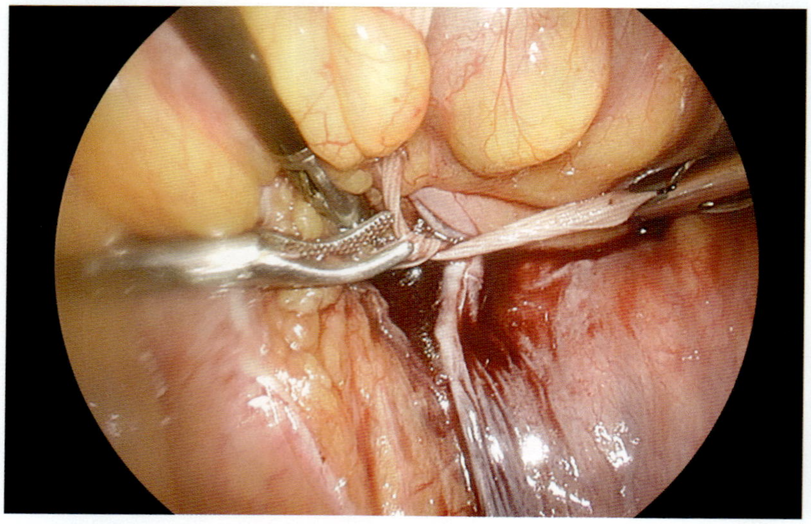

Fig. 10: Both needles cut. Mersilene tape tied on to the promontory after adjusting the tension on the tape optimally and verifying correction of prolapse by per speculum examination.

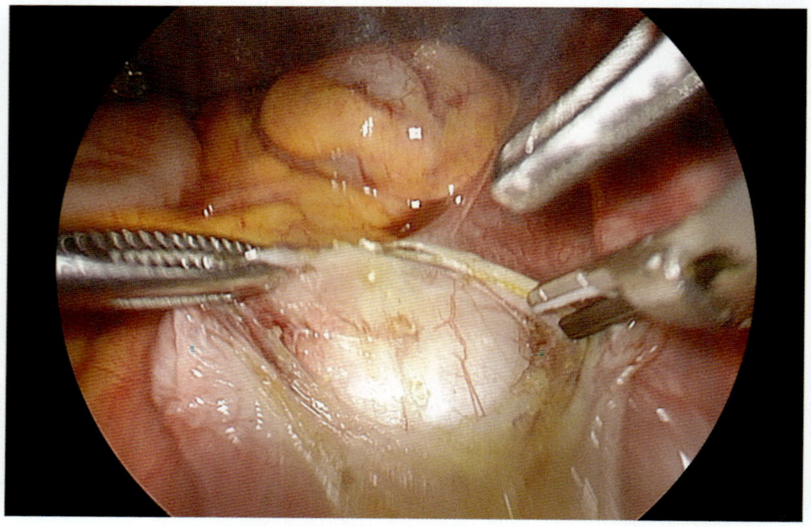

Fig. 12: Peritoneum over the sacral promontory is incised and anterior longitudinal ligament exposed.

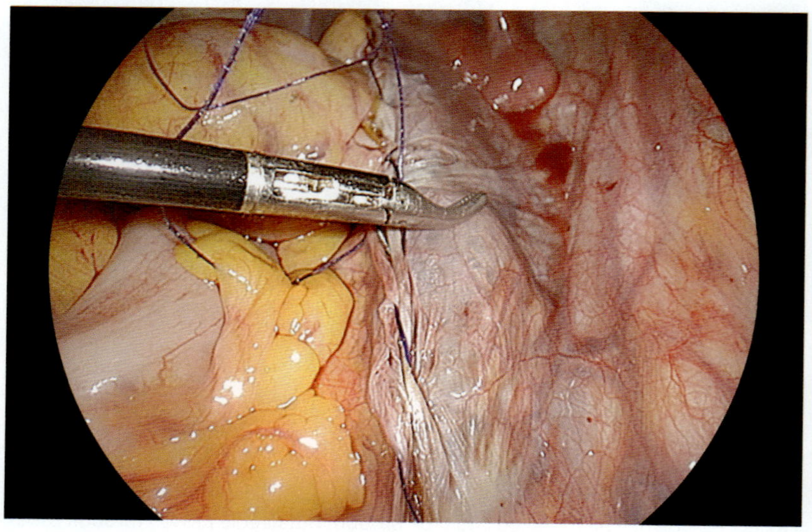

Fig. 11: Peritoneum opening closed.

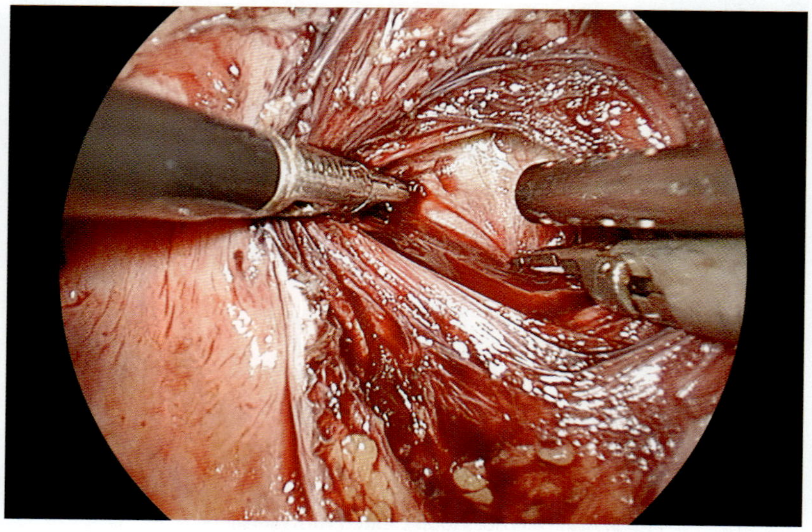

Fig. 13: Bilateral levator ani muscles exposed.

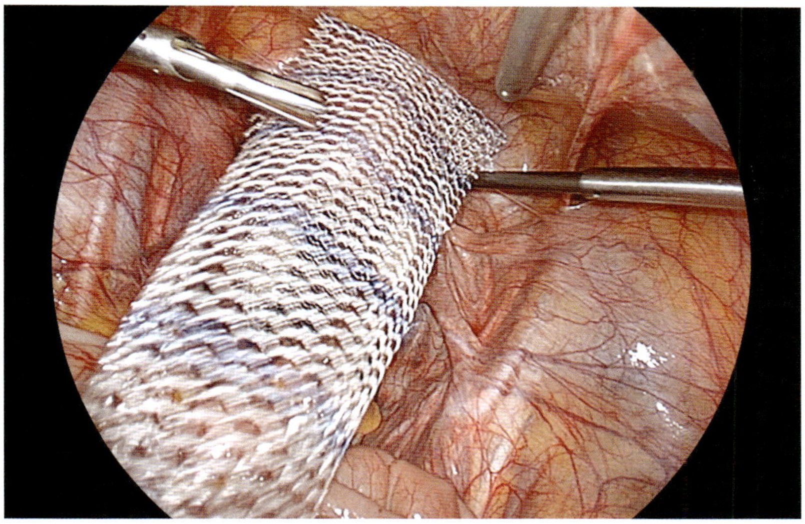

Fig. 14: Y-shaped mesh introduced.

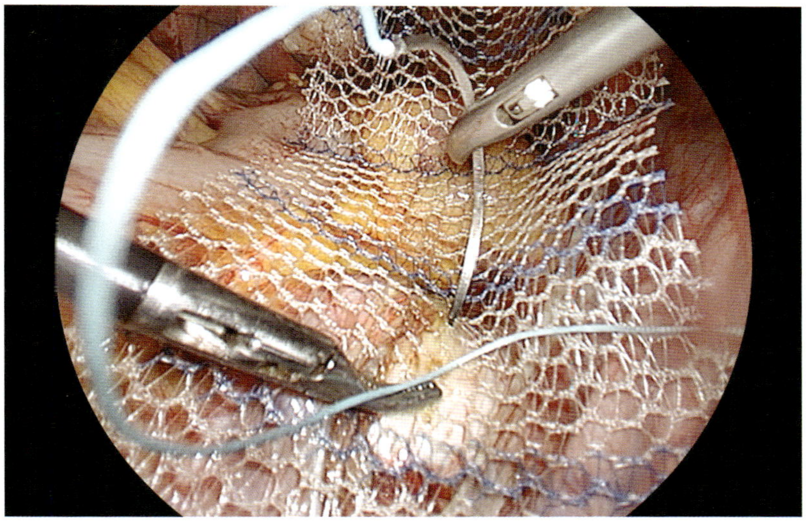

Fig. 17: After correction of the prolapse, stem of the Y-mesh fixed to anterior longitudinal ligament.

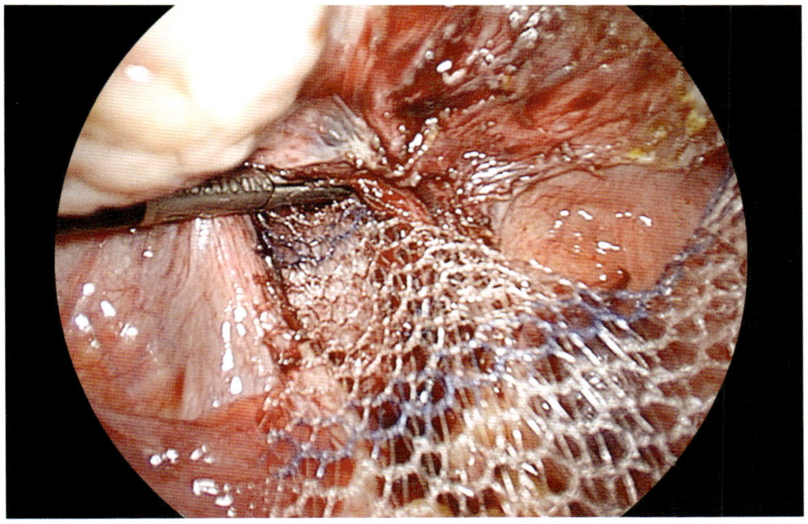

Fig. 15: Both horizontal arm of the Y-mesh fixed to levator ani muscle.

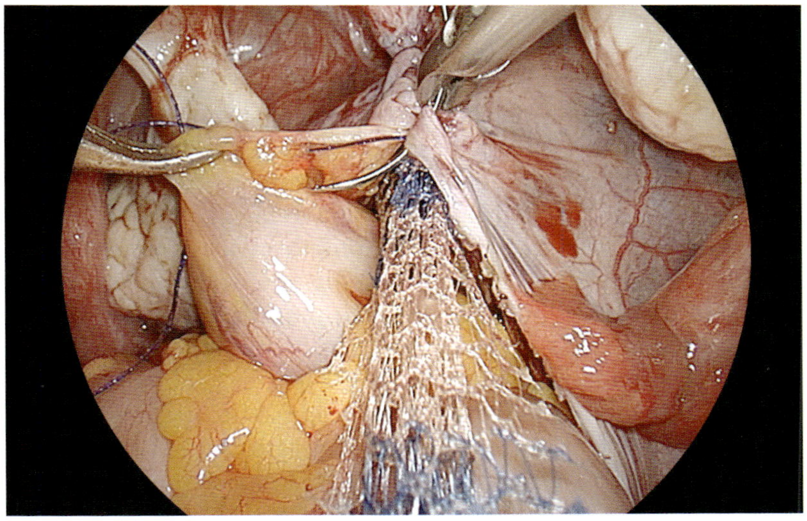

Fig. 18: Peritoneum opening closed.

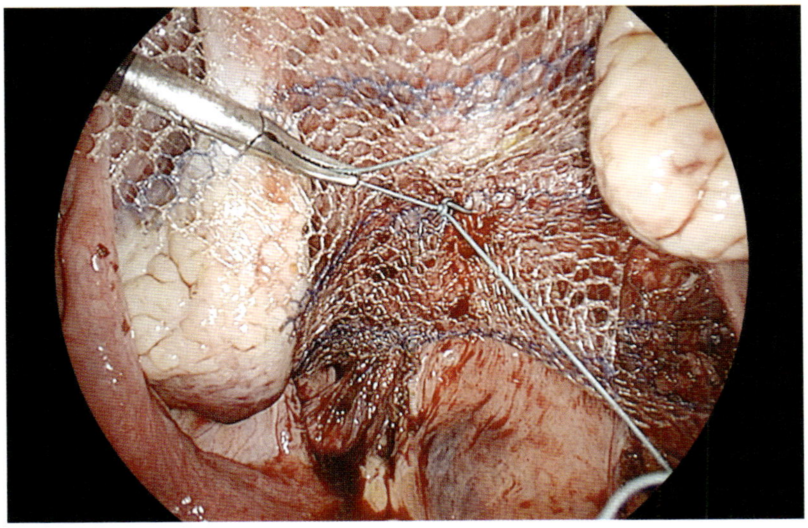

Fig. 16: Upper part of the Y-mesh fixed to posterior surface of cervicoisthmic junction.

5. Both arms of the "Y" fixed to the levator ani muscle using Ethibond **(Fig. 15)**.
6. Upper part of the Y-mesh fixed to posterior surface of cervicoi-sthmic junction **(Fig. 16)**.
7. The stem of the Y-mesh fixed to anterior longitudinal ligament after adjusting the tension on the tape optimally and verifying correction of prolapse by per speculum examination **(Fig. 17)**.
8. All peritoneal openings closed **(Fig. 18)**.

Advantages

- Fixed to sacral promontory, which is a firm structure.
- Tape is on both sides, so no deviation of uterus to one side.
- Strong support to uterus.

Accompanying Video: Laparoscopic sling and Shirodkar's repair.

CHAPTER

35

High Uterosacral Ligament Fixation

Priyanka HK, Aditi Rai, Isha Rani, B Ramesh

INTRODUCTION

Laparoscopic uterosacral ligament suspension is one effective minimally invasive surgical option for repair of DeLancey level 1 support defects of the *posthysterectomized* cervix or vaginal vault as well as for in situ uterus. The uterosacral ligament complex can be utilized in the treatment of existing defects as well as for prophylaxis of iatrogenic defects created during hysterectomy.

The 2013 Cochrane database review suggests that sacrocolpopexy has superior outcomes to uterosacral colpopexy as well as other vault suspension procedures; however, many women and surgeons are migrating back to native tissue repair and trying to avoid biologic or synthetic mesh and their potential complications. The uterosacral ligament suspension is the native tissue equivalent to the mesh-augmented sacrocolpopexy. The cardinal-uterosacral ligament complex supports the upper vertical axis of the vagina, it holds the pelvic viscera in horizontal plane on the levator plate. The skeletal matrix of the endopelvic fascia that comprise the uterosacral ligament starts at the sacrum on the lateral aspect of S2, S3, and S4, extending down to fuse on the levator ani muscles and posterior cervicovaginal ring. Avulsions of these attachments lead to herniation or prolapse of the uterus or vaginal vault through the urogenital levator hiatus. The goal of uterosacral ligament suspension is to reattach these natural ligamentous avulsions in order to pulley the uterus or vaginal vault back up to its original level at the ischial spine.

PREOPERATIVE PROCEDURE

Maximum vaginal estrogenization with at least 6 weeks of therapy is recommended prior to any repair.

Steps

The patient is placed in a low semilithotomy position which allowing the laparoscopic instruments to be rotated 360° around the abdomen after anesthetic induction. Sequential compression device are placed to reduce blood clotting. Before starting the surgery examination is done under anesthesia to reassess all site-specific defects that need to be addressed. A Foley catheter is placed in urinary bladder for continuous drainage.

At first primary port is created for camera, a vertical incision is taken just above the umbilicus and introducing a 5 mm or 10–12 mm trocar. Three ancillary ports are recommended: one just in between the suprapubic hairline area and umbilicus (5 mm), and the other two just lateral to transversalis fascia and around the level of McBurney point (1–12 and 1–5 mm). Patient is then placed in a steep Trendelenburg position. Once abdomen has been insufflated, trocars should be placed, an abdominal survey completed, and the bowel moved out of the pelvis by atraumatic instrumentation. Then the ureters should be clearly identified as they cross the bifurcation of the common iliac vessels.

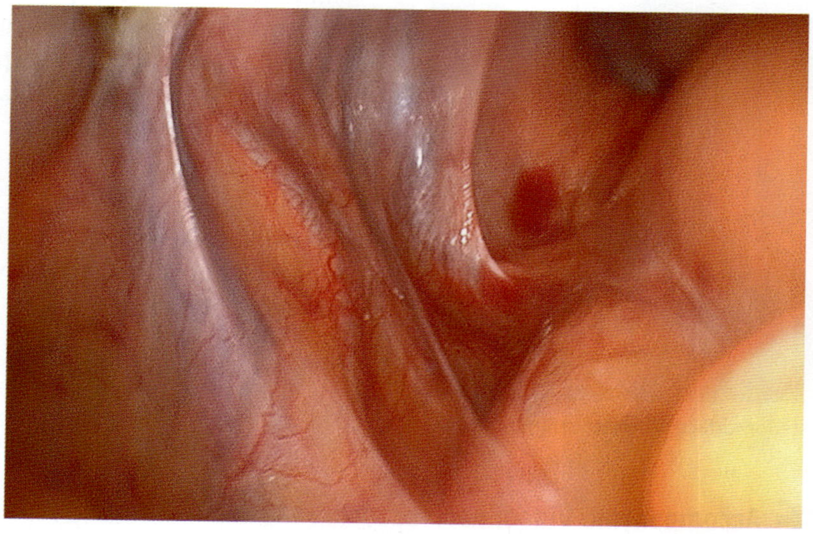

Fig. 1: Identification of ureters.

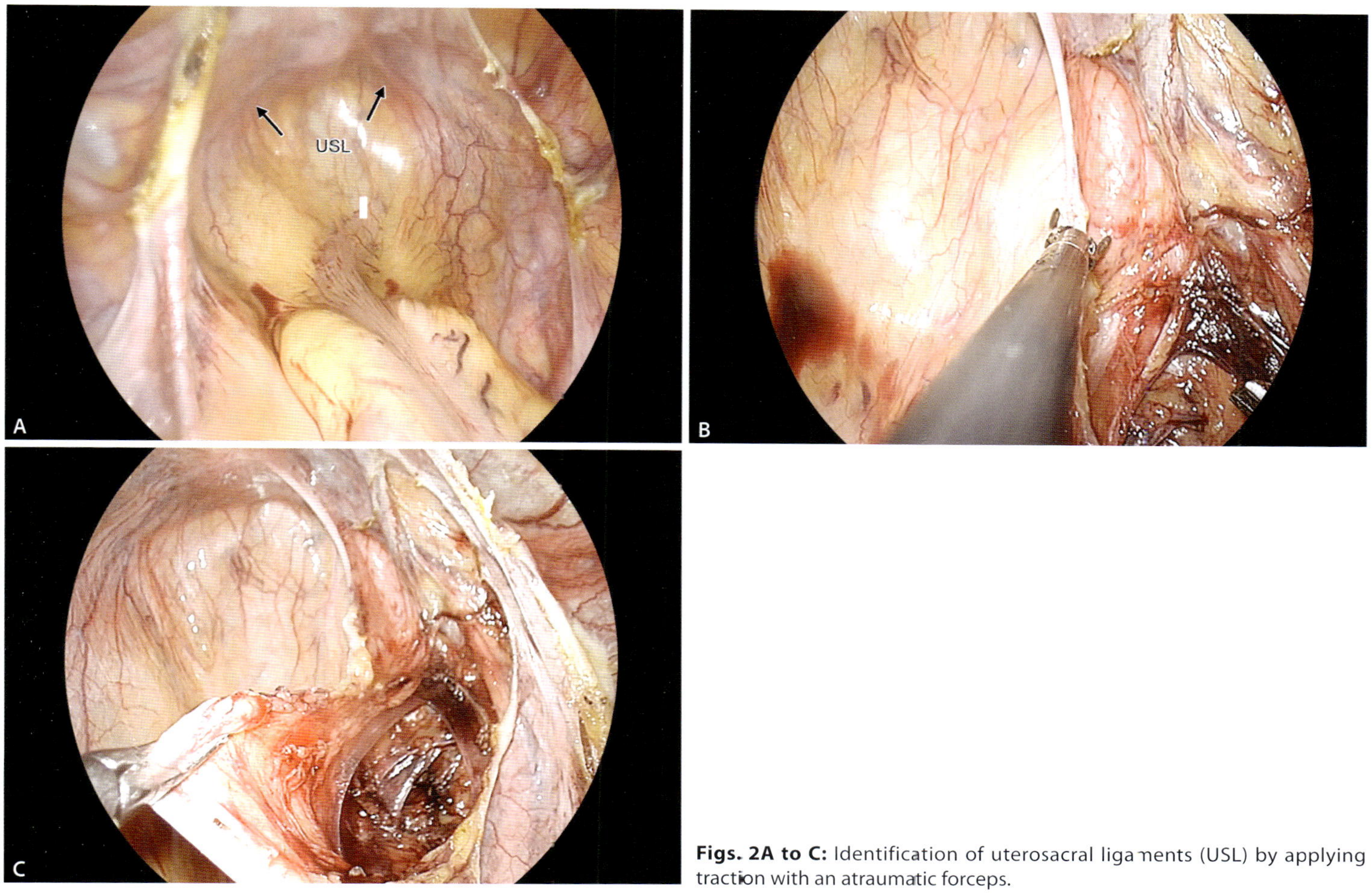

Figs. 2A to C: Identification of uterosacral ligaments (USL) by applying traction with an atraumatic forceps.

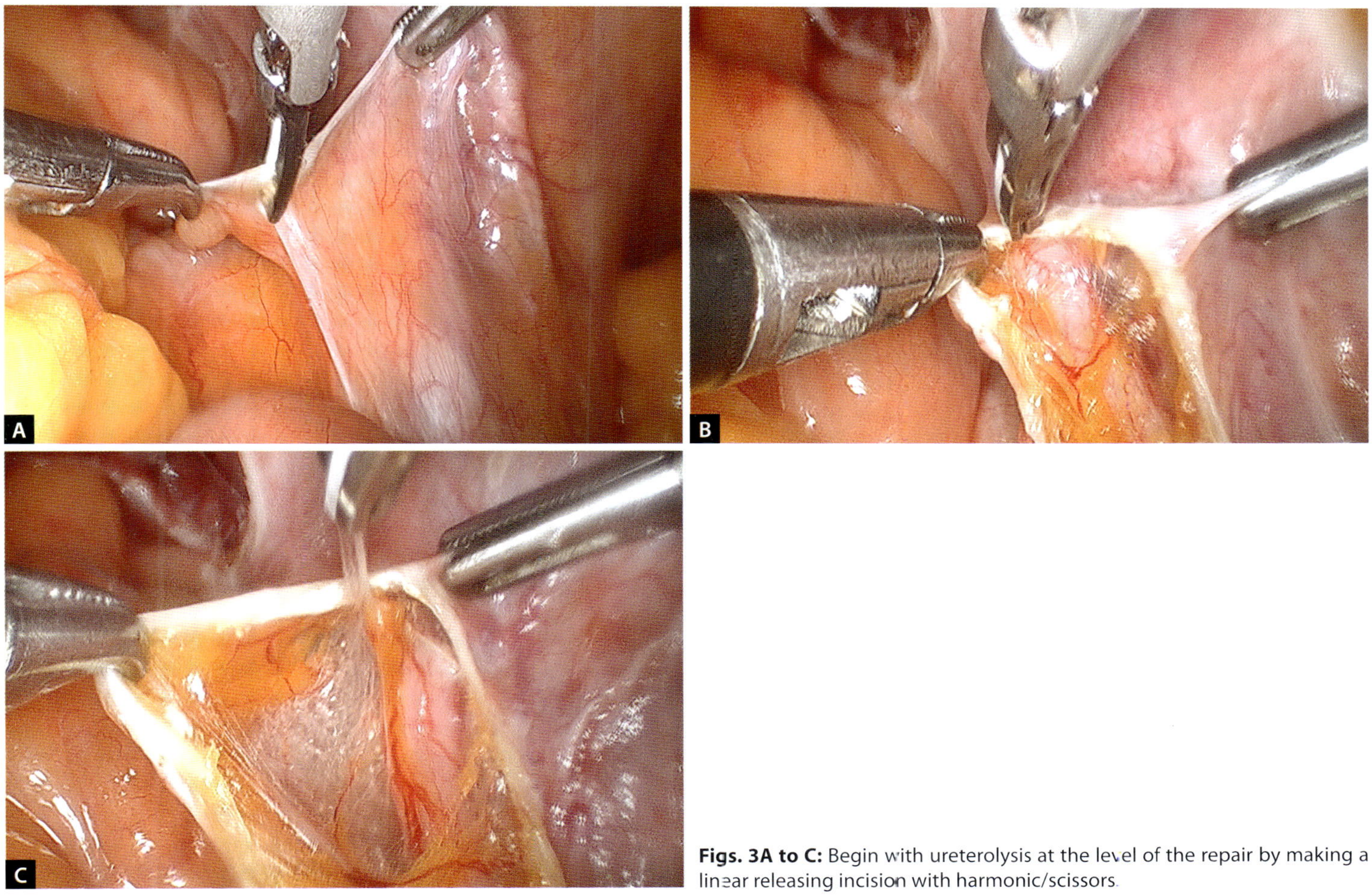

Figs. 3A to C: Begin with ureterolysis at the level of the repair by making a linear releasing incision with harmonic/scissors.

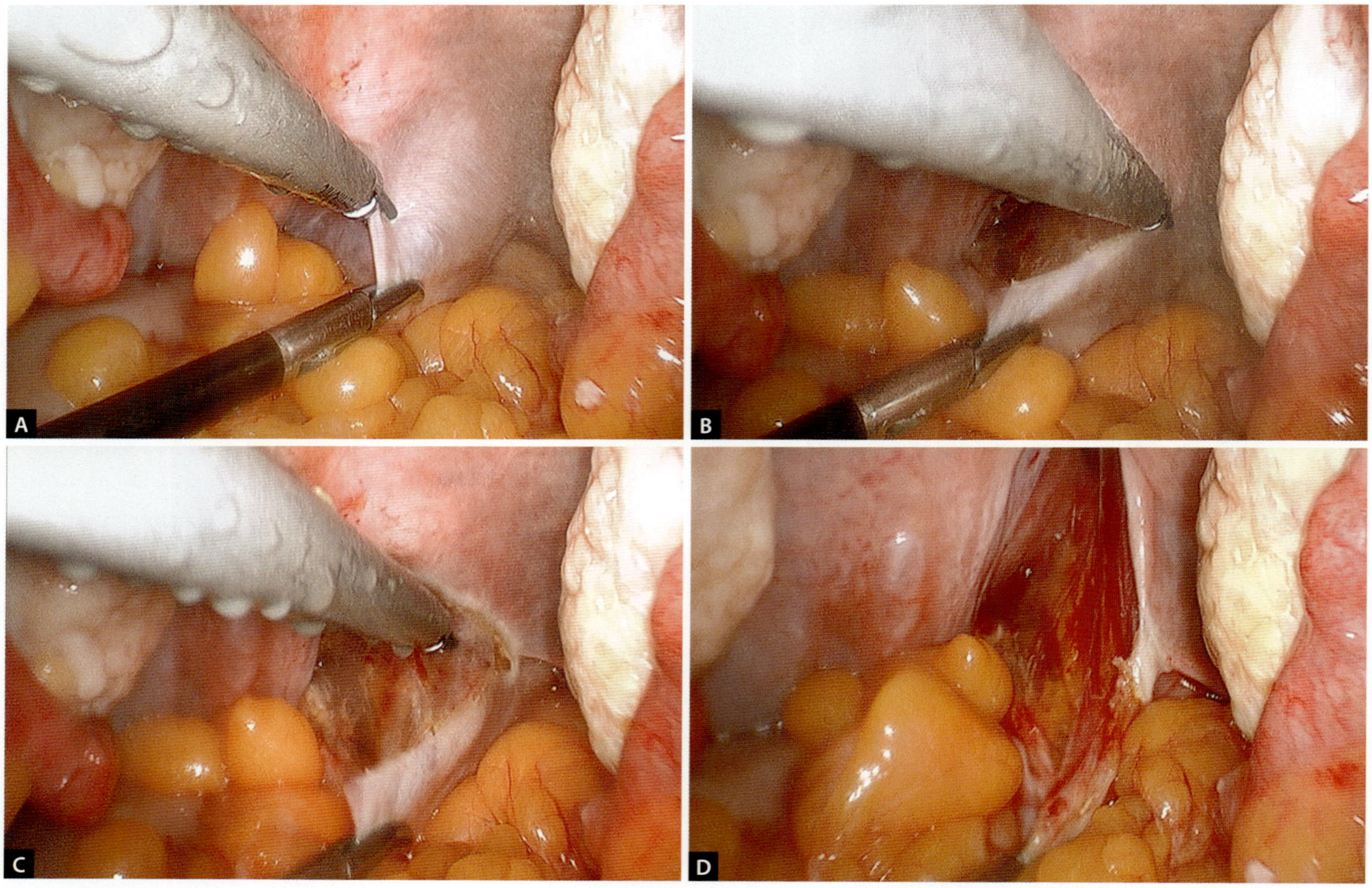

Figs. 4A to D: Posteriorly incision is made with harmonic and peritoneum is entered and dissection is conducted to identify the rectovaginal (RV) septum. Before proceeding uterosacral ligament fixation, rectovaginal septal defect should be ruled out.

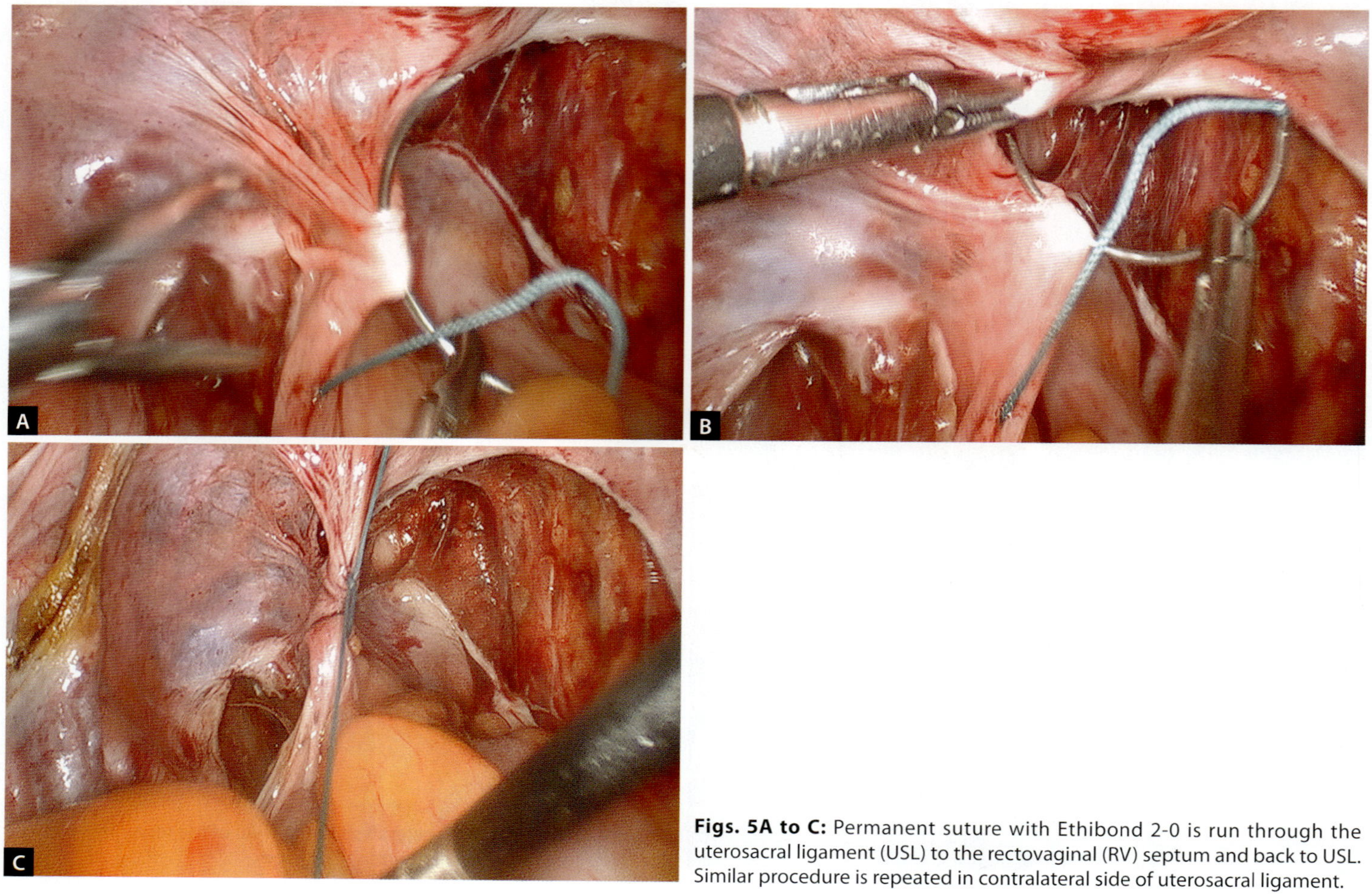

Figs. 5A to C: Permanent suture with Ethibond 2-0 is run through the uterosacral ligament (USL) to the rectovaginal (RV) septum and back to USL. Similar procedure is repeated in contralateral side of uterosacral ligament.

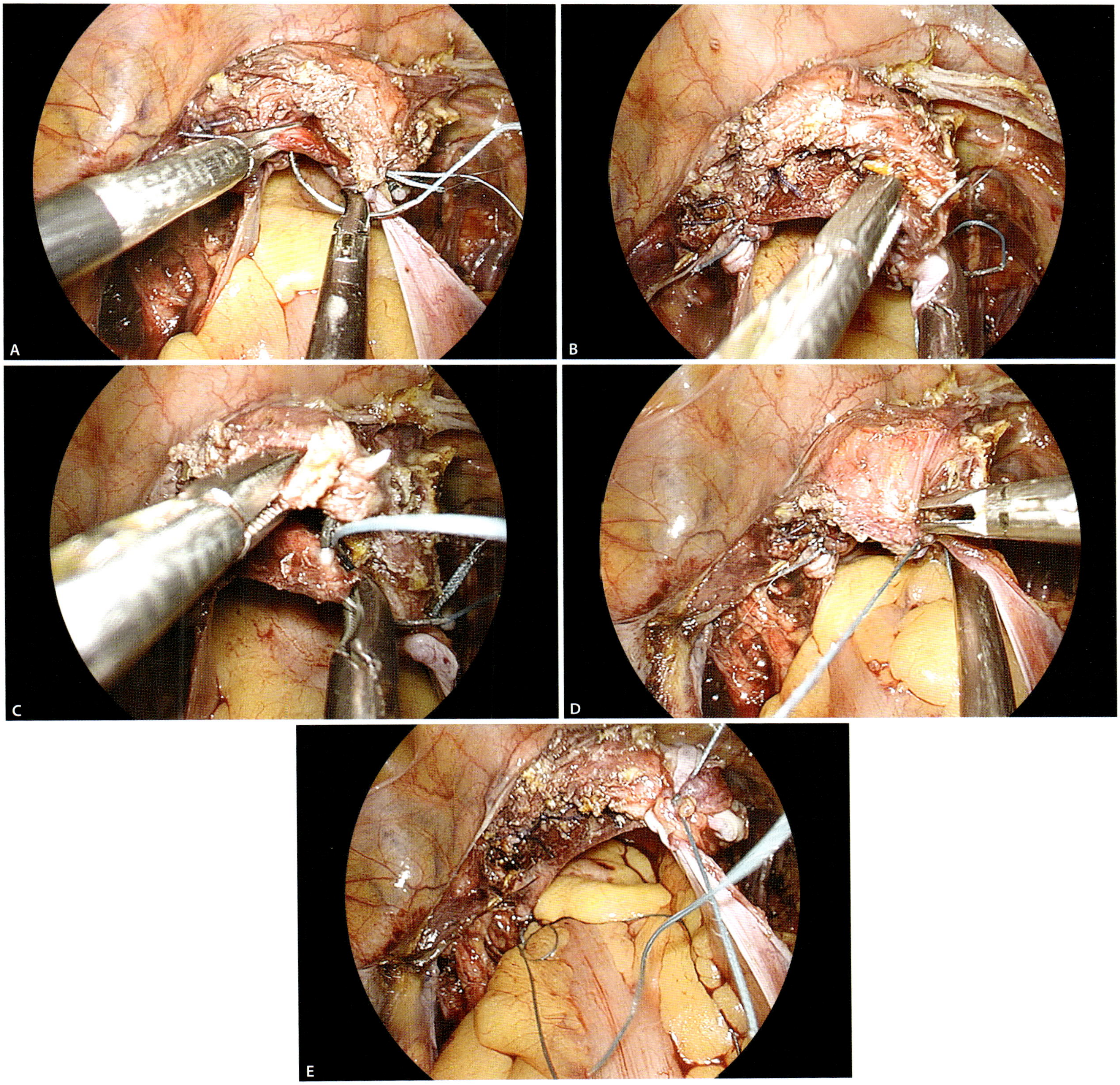

Figs. 6A to E: A second stitch is then placed through the uterosacral ligament 1 cm proximal to the previous suture continuing onto the pubocervical fascia anteriorly, rectovaginal septum posteriorly, and then back to the uterosacral ligament.

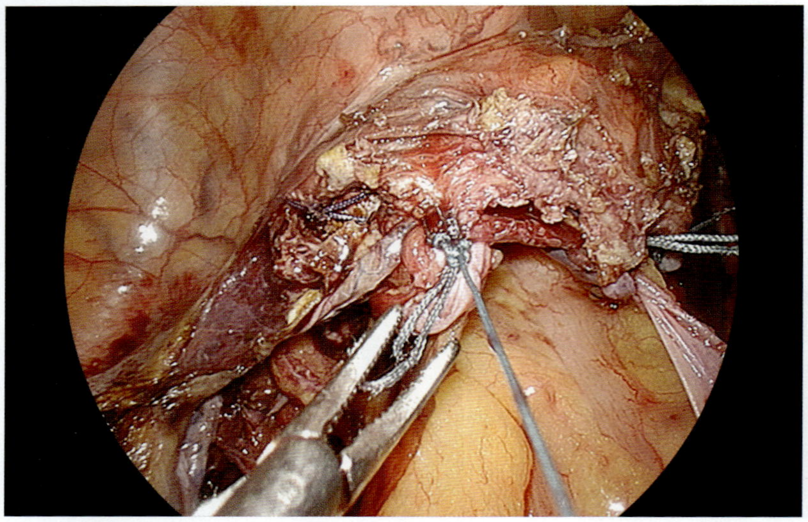

Fig. 7: Perform the sutures bilaterally before tying them down.

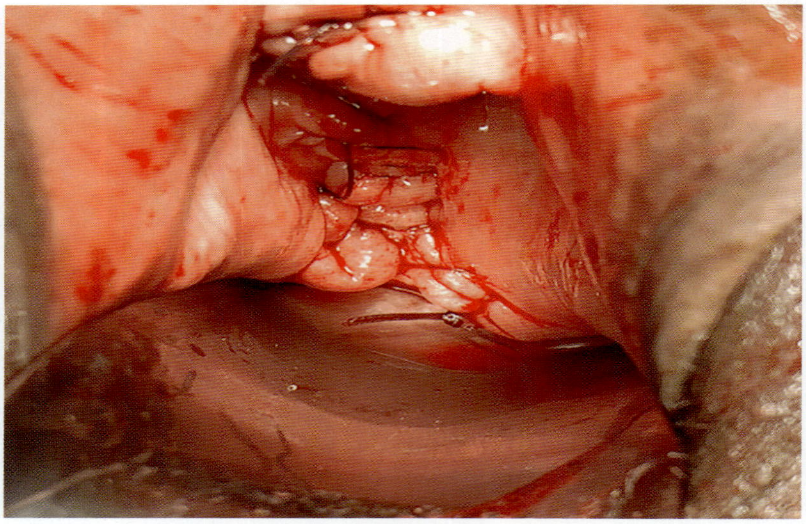

Figs. 8: Vaginal inspection of vault postlaparoscopic high uterosacral fixation.

POSTOPERATIVE CARE

The patient is transferred to postoperative ward with Foley catheter in place and is removed once patient starts ambulating, advanced to oral analgesia as quickly as tolerated.

Accompanying Video: Laparoscopic high uterosacral suspension.

CHAPTER

36

Cesarean Scar Defect and Diverticulum

Minal Kumbhalwar, Supriya Raina, B Ramesh

ISTHMOCELE

Isthmocele **(Figs. 1A and B)**, the deficient uterine scars or dehiscence of scar after cesarean section is a pouch defect on the anterior surface of the uterus at isthmic junction situated at prior cesarean scar,[1] reported by Morris for the first time[2] while analyzing hysterectomies of women with prior cesarean deliveries. Cesarean scar defect (CSD), i.e. isthmocele usually detected incidentally as a wedge-shape anechoic area at previous scar site in transvaginal ultrasound.[1] Cesarean scar syndrome (CSS) presents with postmenstrual bleeding or spotting, dysmenorrhea, and sometimes infertility also.

PATHOGENESIS OF THE CESAREAN-INDUCED ISTHMOCELE

Isthmocele involves breach in myometrial integrity at previous cesarean scar, frequently found in women with previous cesarean section exhibiting anatomical abnormalities in the lower uterine segment.[2] Cesarean section is commonly performed uterine surgery in the fertile women,[3] with low transverse incision as preferred incision.[4,5] Lower uterine segment incisions are made because it is rich in fibrous tissue allowing the scar to heal properly, reducing dehiscence risk in future. Repair can be done in a single or multiple layers.[4] There are differences in myometrial contraction on each side of the incision, the superior edge being thicker than the inferior edge. This discrepancy enhances with successive cesarean sections. Reapproximation of incision edges with differing thickness probably contributes to the development of the lower segment defects. The reason, certain patients have anatomic defects after cesarean section whereas other women do not, is unclear. Probably, the surgical technique based on the single-layer uterine closure may not be able to guarantee an accurate alignment of the uterine edges.[6] Alternatively, the most ischemic technique and slowest reabsorbable suture would be the worst combination, and thus likely to produce a CSD. In a randomized prospective study of 78 patients, Yazicioglu et al.[7] analyzed two different techniques (full-thickness, including the endometrial layer, and split-thickness, excluding the endometrial layer) and found that by selecting a full-thickness suturing technique, one may significantly lower the incidence of incomplete healing of the uterine incision after cesarean section. The occurrence of a defective uterine scar after cesarean section depended on multiple factors, including the degree of cervical dilatation and possibly the contractile effort of the uterine musculature, resulting in thinning at the uterine incision site. It was also presumed that the occurrence of chronic inflammation or, the particular arrangement of myometrial fibers in the site of uterine closure, could contribute to create a discrepancy at level of the incision.[2,8] Nevertheless, the presence of an anatomic uterine defect

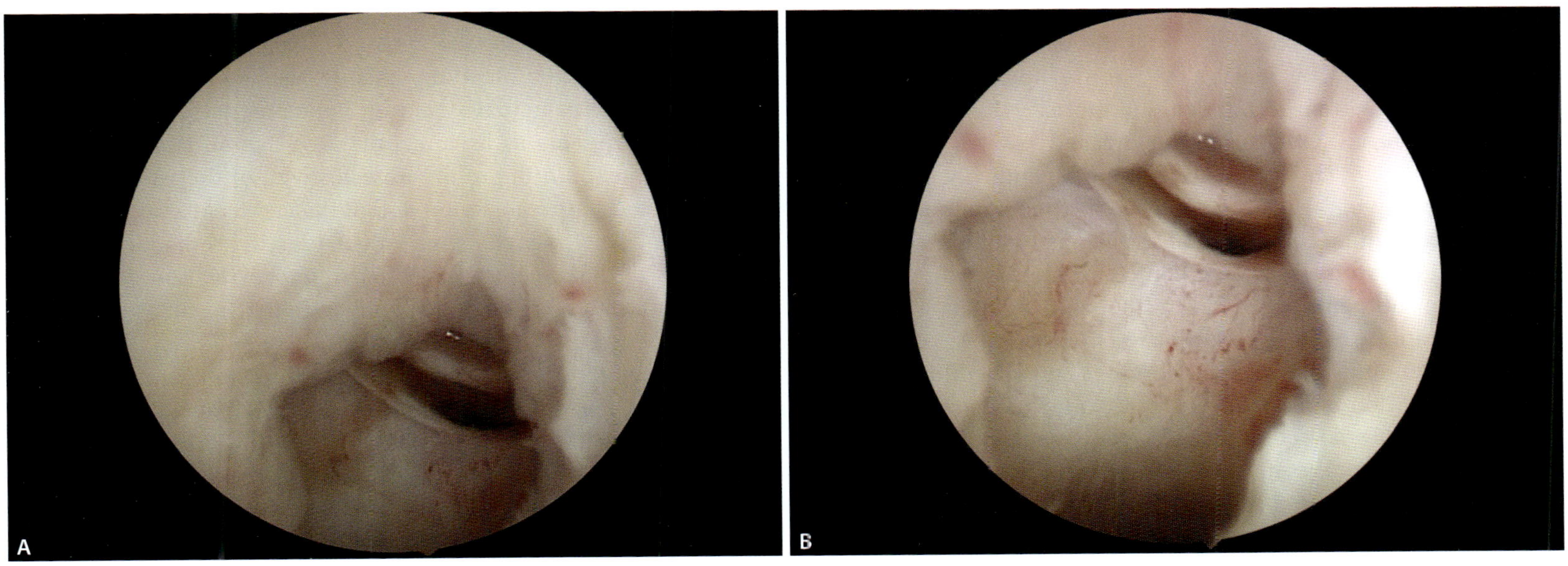

Figs. 1A and B: Isthmocele.

in patients with a history of cesarean section is a common, expected finding: the thickness of the myometrium at the level of the isthmus uteri decreases and the prevalence of scar defects and large scar defects increases with the number of cesarean sections.[7-11] Moreover, it was noted that large and total scar defects are more common in uteri in retroflexion than in anteflexion (the chance of a woman with a retroflexed uterus having a deficient scar is more than twice that of a woman with an anteflexed uterus), and that scars with defects are located lower in the uterus than intact scars.[7]

The reason by which this occurs may rely in the evidence that the flexion point of the uterus is at the level of the internal os, and therefore the lower segment of the uterus in a retroflexed uterus is under a degree of tension, which may compromise healing of a cesarean section scar. This anatomical traction to the scar and the associated reduced vascular perfusion caused by stretching of the lower uterine segment may cause impaired tissue perfusion and reduced wound oxygen tension, which has been reported to delay wound healing by slowing the production of collagen.[7]

In a prospective study of 137 women undergoing cesarean section, a double-layer closure of the uterus combining the surgical approximation of decidua with decidua followed by the approximation of myometrium with myometrium was associated with a 13-fold reduction in uterine scar defects compared with a single-layer closure including the decidua into the suture.[5] With cesarean section being one of the most frequently performed surgical procedures, there is an urgent need for appropriate clinical research and evidence-based consensus in the field of uterus closure techniques.

SYMPTOMS: FROM ABNORMAL UTERINE BLEEDING TO INFERTILITY

Isthmocele was reported to be associated with several anatomical and functional alterations, such as distortion and widening of the lower uterine segment, congested endometrium over the scar recess, lymphocytic infiltrations, capillary dilatation, and free red blood cells in the endometrial stroma of the scar were found.[1] These anatomical defects resulting from previous cesarean surgery may cause abnormal uterine bleeding, postmenstrual abnormal uterine bleeding (PAUB), chronic pelvic pain, and infertility.

In fact, the flow of menstrual blood through the cervix may be slowed by the presence of isthmocele, as the blood may accumulate in the niche due to the presence of fibrotic tissue that reduces the uterus contractility around the scar.[1,2,7,8,11,12] Or the blood may be produced in situ, as suggested by Morris[2] who found histological signs of recent hemorrhage in the stroma around the scar. Dense and viscous mucus-like material, which was not drained entirely, is found in the reservoir-like pouch.[1,2,11] This condition depends not so much on the size or location of the isthmocele as on the poor contractility of the uterine muscle around the scar, which may obstruct menstrual blood drainage and determine how much blood accumulates on the defect. Whatever the source of the blood in the isthmocele, its persistence after menstruation, together with the increased local mucus secretion because of the abnormal vascularization, may contribute to PAUB. PAUB is a condition because of discharge after menstruation of the dark thematic material accumulated in the scar defect for a variable numbers of days after the menstruation because isthmocele slows the escape of blood from the uterus. The presence of a cesarean section scar has been implicated as an under-recognized cause of PAUB in premenopausal women; therefore, awareness of the presence of a cesarean section scar may help referring clinicians with diagnostic information that can elucidate the cause of abnormal uterine bleeding. PAUB might be the most typical and distracted symptom, as in these women, the presence of a pouch-like defect will be present on the lower anterior uterine wall at the site of a previous cesarean delivery scar through transvaginal ultrasound and/or hysteroscopy.[5] Anyway, the surgical treatment of the pouch under hysteroscopic vision resects the fibrotic tissue that overhangs underneath the triangular pouch, facilitating blood drainage through the cervix and fulguration of endometrial glands and/or dilated blood vessels. The final net effect is the improvement of menstrual drainage, avoiding blood accumulation.[1,7,8,11,12]

Moreover, recent reports have indicated an association between CSS and infertility, which might be due to the isthmocele substances negatively affecting the mucus and sperm quality and interfering with embryo implantation.[12] However, reports have suggested that resection of the isthmocele **(Figs. 2 to 6)** and reconstruction of the uterine wall through laparotomy or laparoscopic surgery might restore fertility **(Fig. 6)**.[13] Recently, hysteroscopic ablation of the uterine lining at the site of isthmocele has been reported to be at least equal to or more effective, and less invasive than other surgical procedures for restoration of fertility.[12,14]

DIAGNOSIS OF ISTHMOCELE

Isthmocele is often detected incidentally in patients presenting with clinical symptoms such as postmenstrual spotting, dysmenorrhea, dyspareunia, chronic pelvic pain or dull sensation following menstruation, and infertility. The prevalence of isthmocele has been reported to be as high as 52% after a cesarean delivery,[10,15] thus patients who have undergone multiple cesarean sections have been observed to have larger scar defects, and often experience one or more of the symptoms mentioned above.[10]

Different imaging modalities, from hysterography to ultrasonographic evaluation, have been used to evaluate the integrity of the anterior uterine wall. They allow good visualization of the depth and width of the dehiscence at the level of the cesarean scar.[16,17]

The diagnosis of isthmocele is based on ultrasound.

Transvaginal sonography (TVS) with high-resolution transducers and the recent introduction of sonohysterography have proved to be useful tools in the study of intrauterine lesions **(Figs. 7 and 8)**.[18-20]

The best time during the cycle to identify the pouch with sonography is during the bleeding episode, usually a few days after the menses, as the principal symptom is postmenstrual spotting.[6] The isthmocele appears as an anechoic area like an isosceles triangle, with the apex pointing to the anterior wall of the isthmus and the base directed to the posterior wall of the cervical canal. Larger scars corresponded to heavier and longer bleeding episodes.[1,7,20,21] The diagnosis of this defect by TVS had 100% correlation with hysteroscopy, and both positive and negative predictive values were similar for both methods.[18,19]

Transvaginal sonography is a very simple, noninvasive, low-cost examination that should be considered as the first choice for screening because it highly correlates (100%) with hysteroscopy in the diagnosis of isthmocele and may help rule out other causes.[6]

Although isthmocele was valued in the same way using sonographic and hysteroscopic techniques, the importance of hysteroscopic evaluation as a diagnostic phase only recently emerged.

Hysteroscopic Resection of Isthmocele

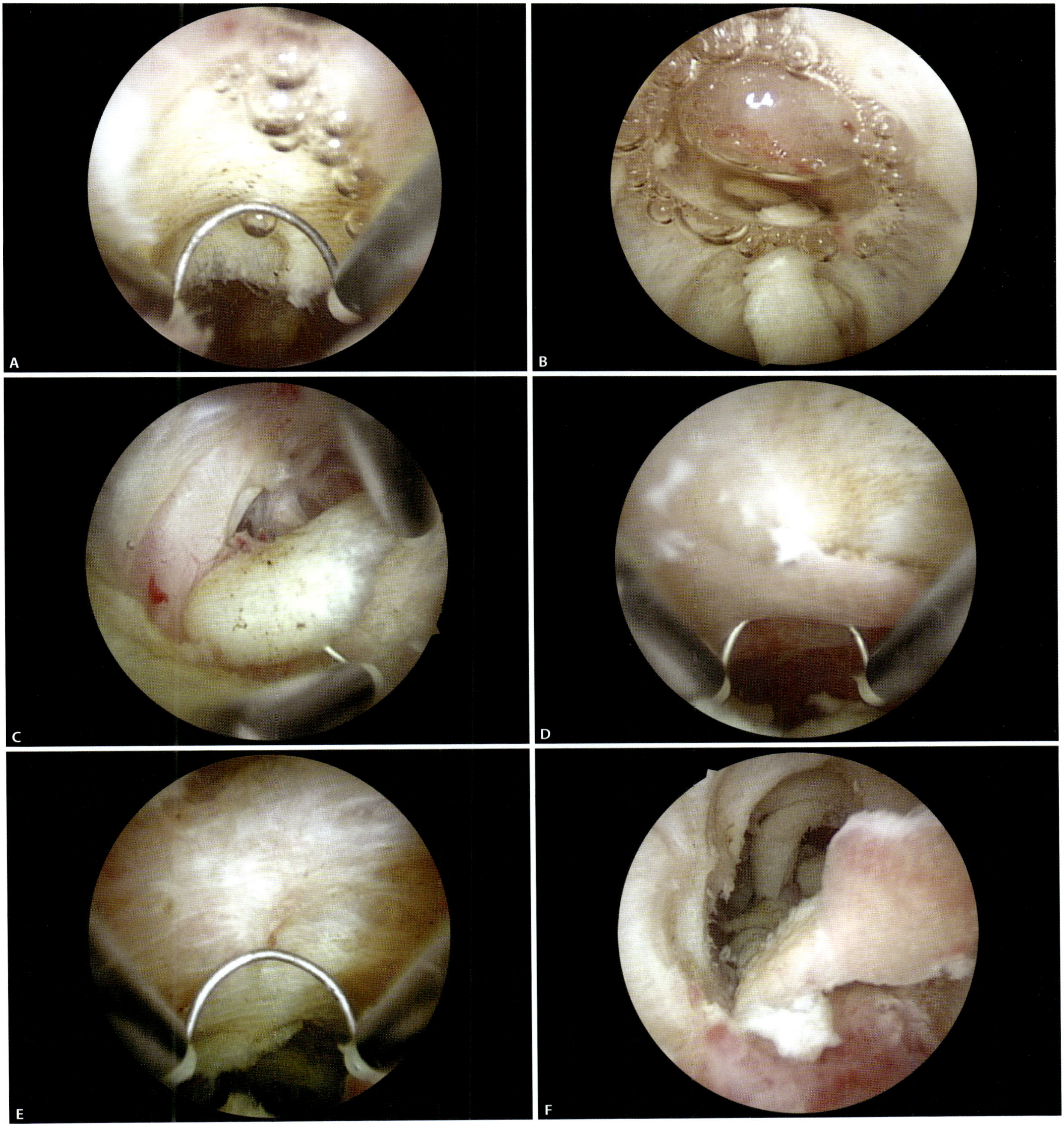

Figs. 2A to F: Resection of superior margin of isthmocele.

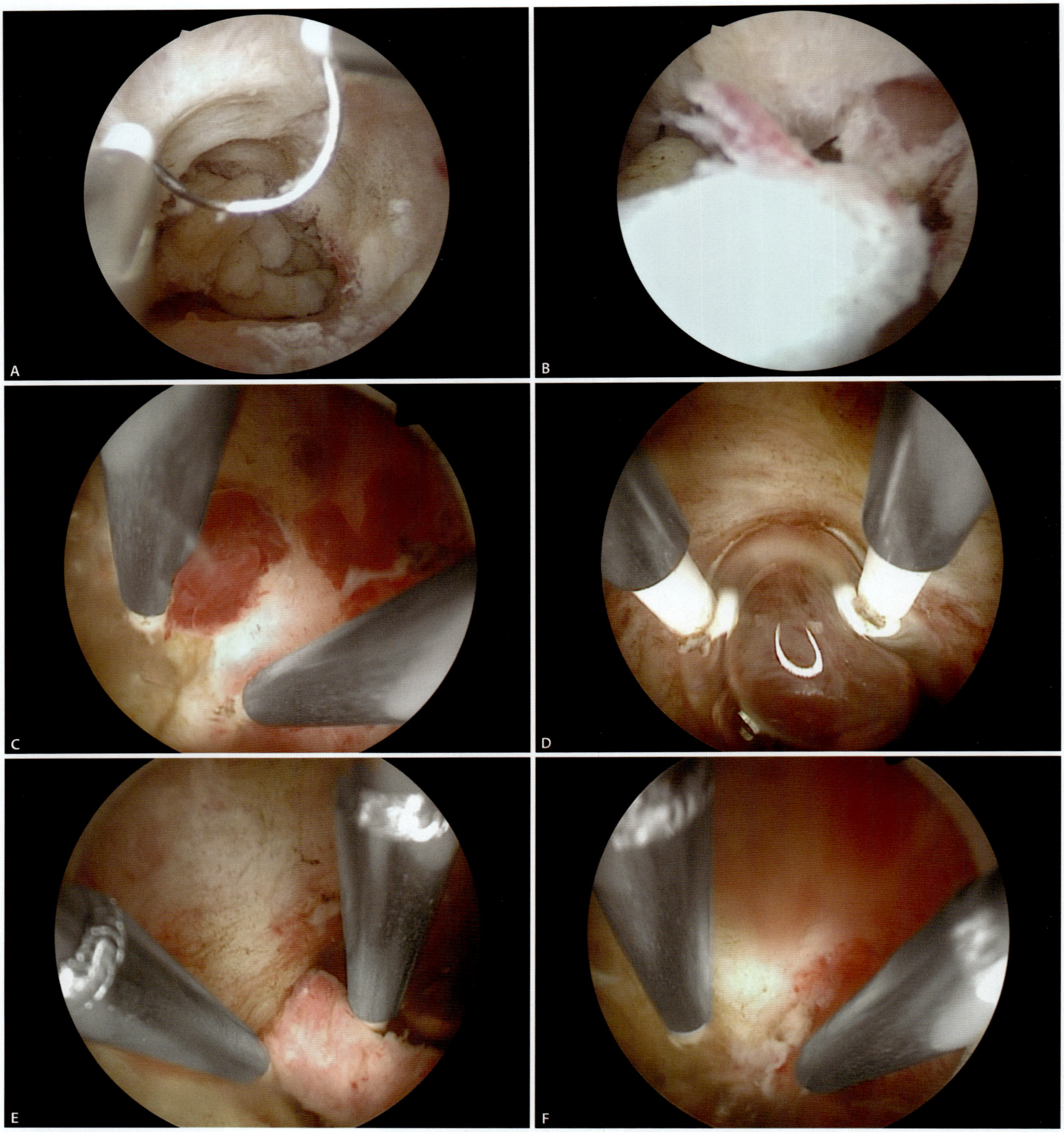

Figs. 3A to F: Resection of lower margin of isthmocele.

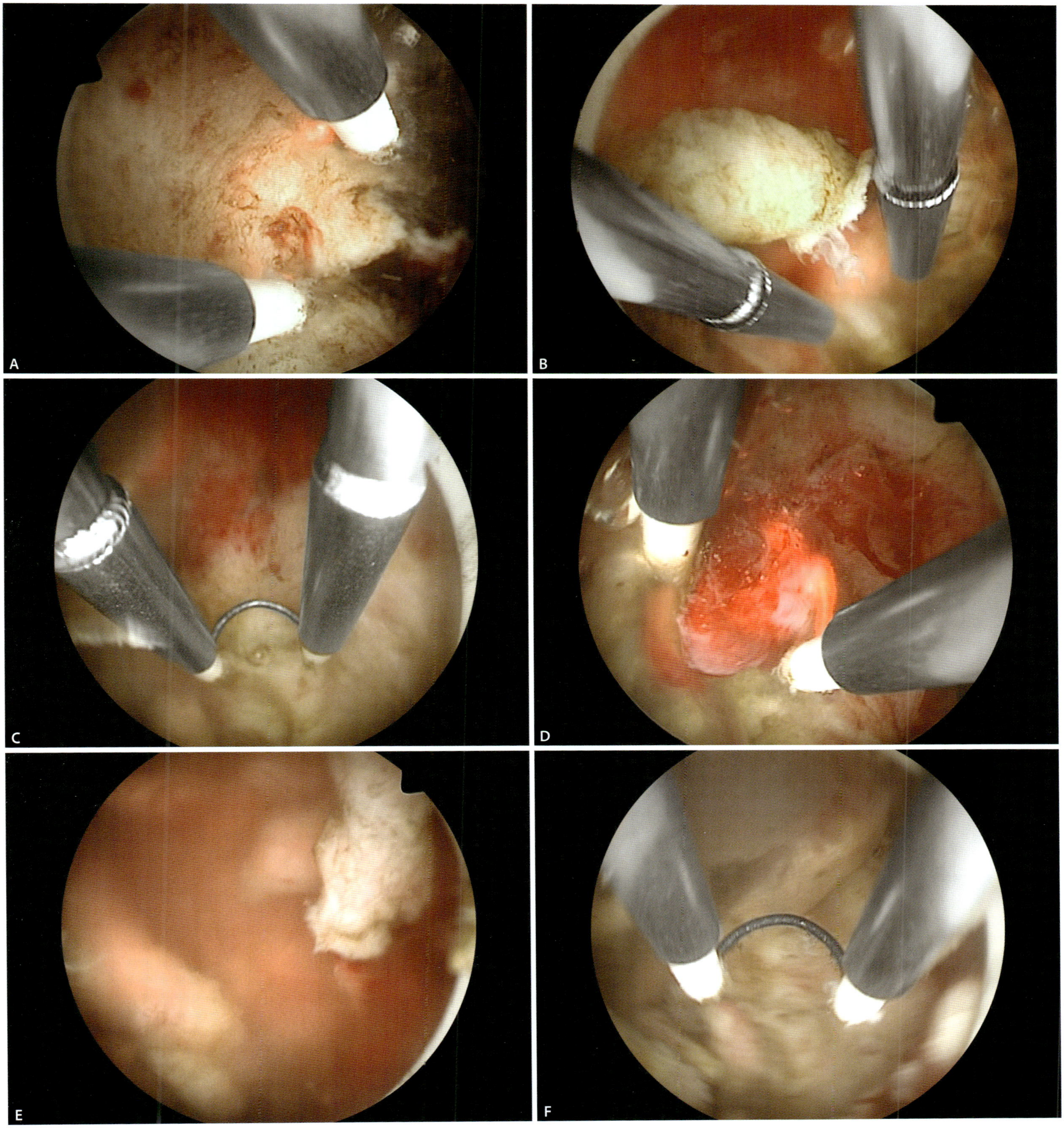

Figs. 4A to F

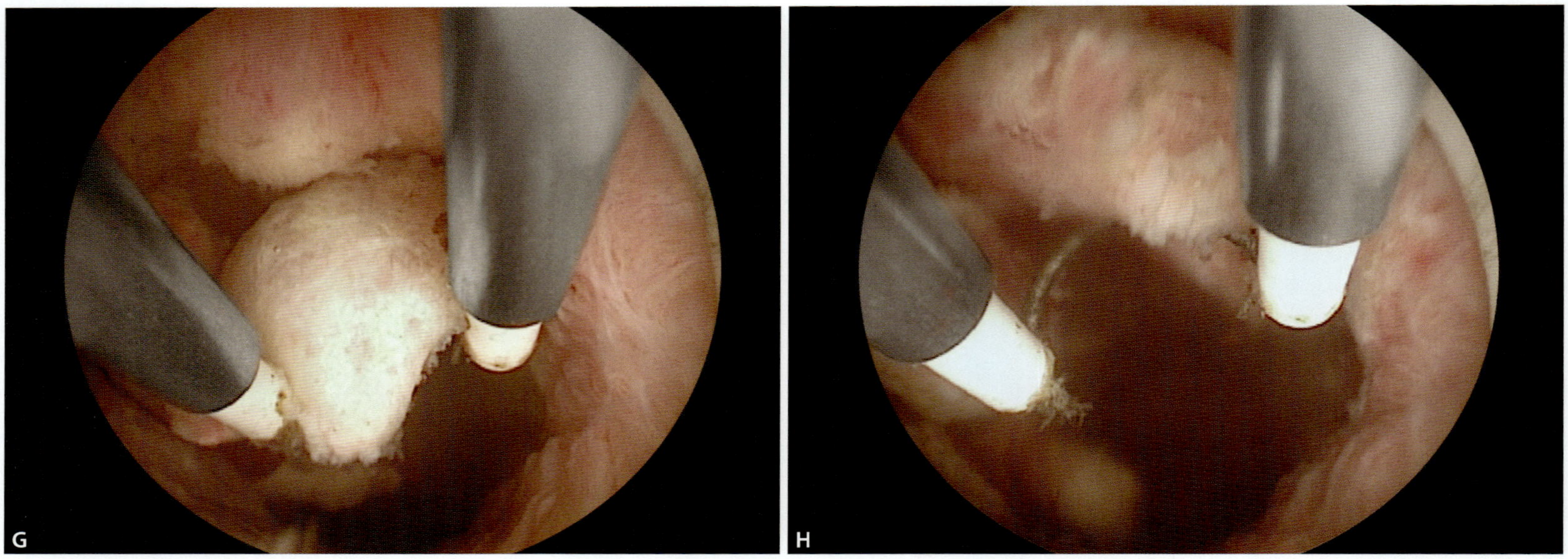

Figs. 4G and H

Figs. 4A to H: Resection of lateral fibrotic margins of isthmocele.

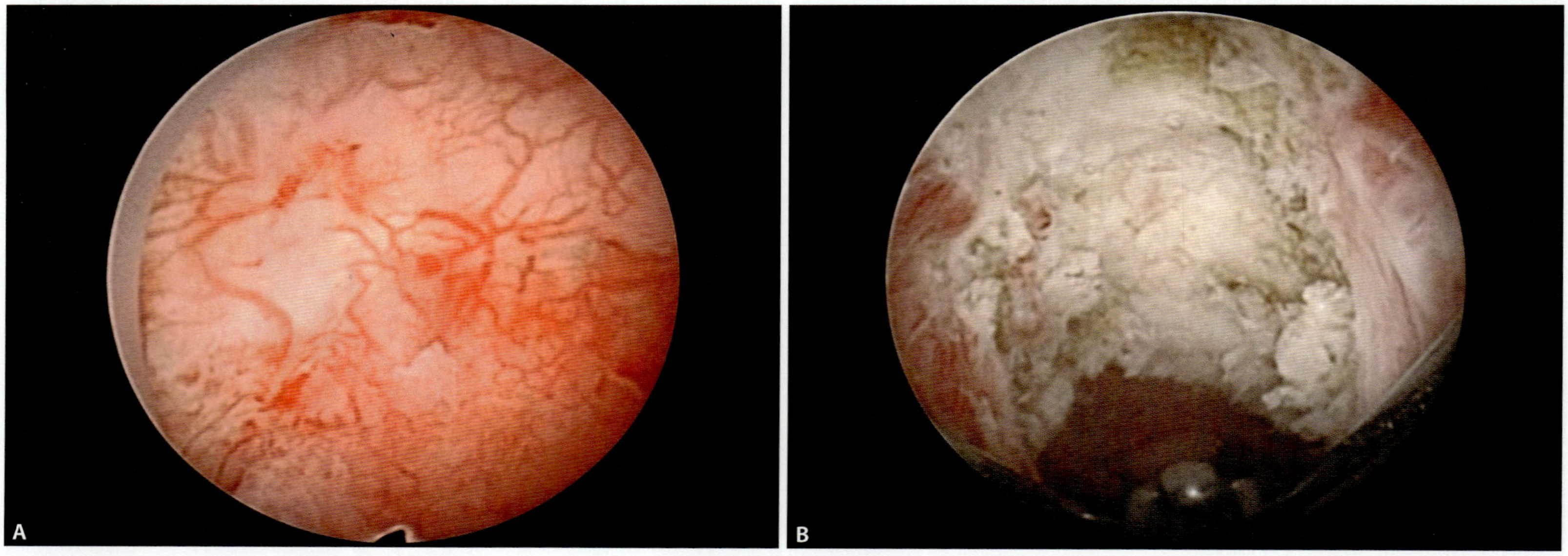

Figs. 5A and B: Dendritic vessels seen at surface of isthmocele, coagulated with roller ball electrocautery.

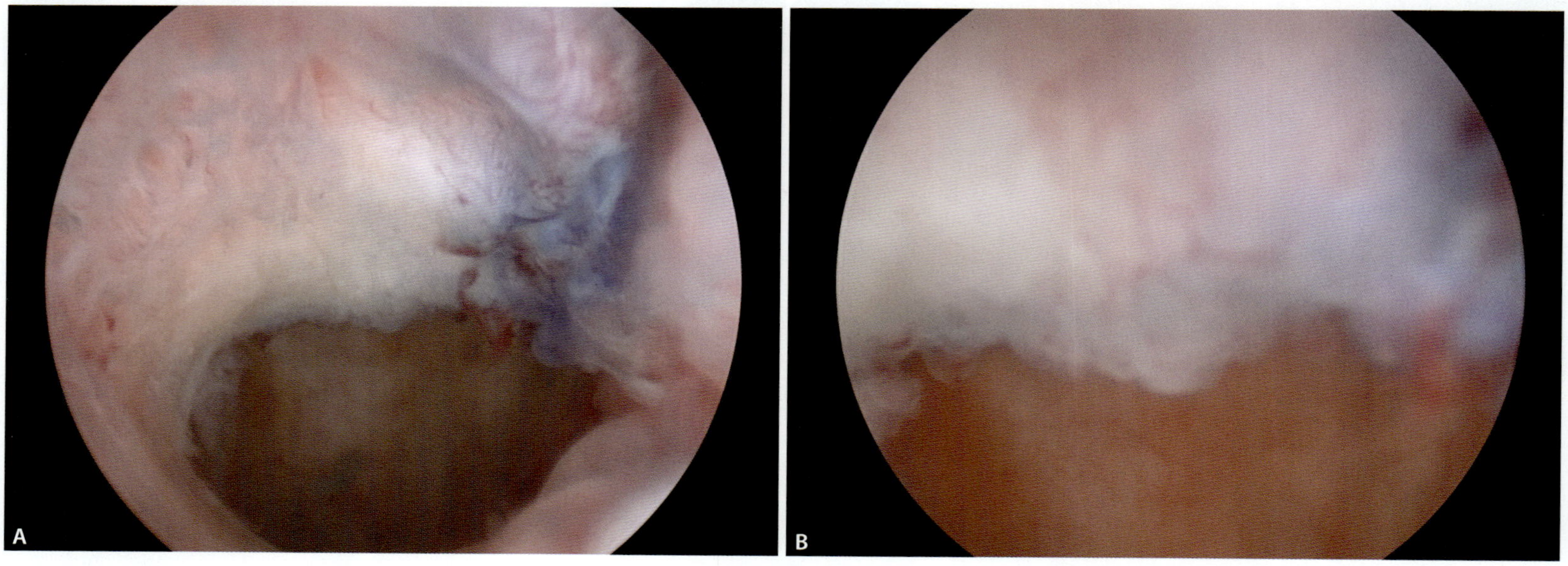

Figs. 6A and B

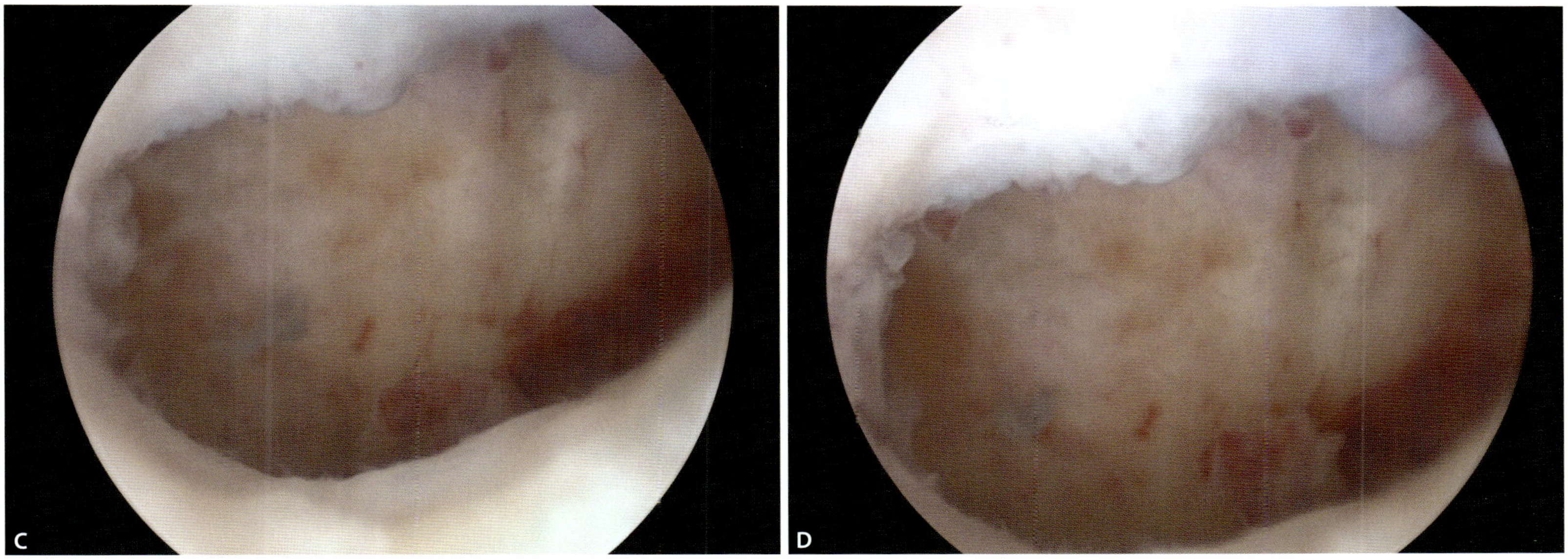

Figs. 6C and D

Figs. 6A to D: Panoramic view after hysteroscopic repair.

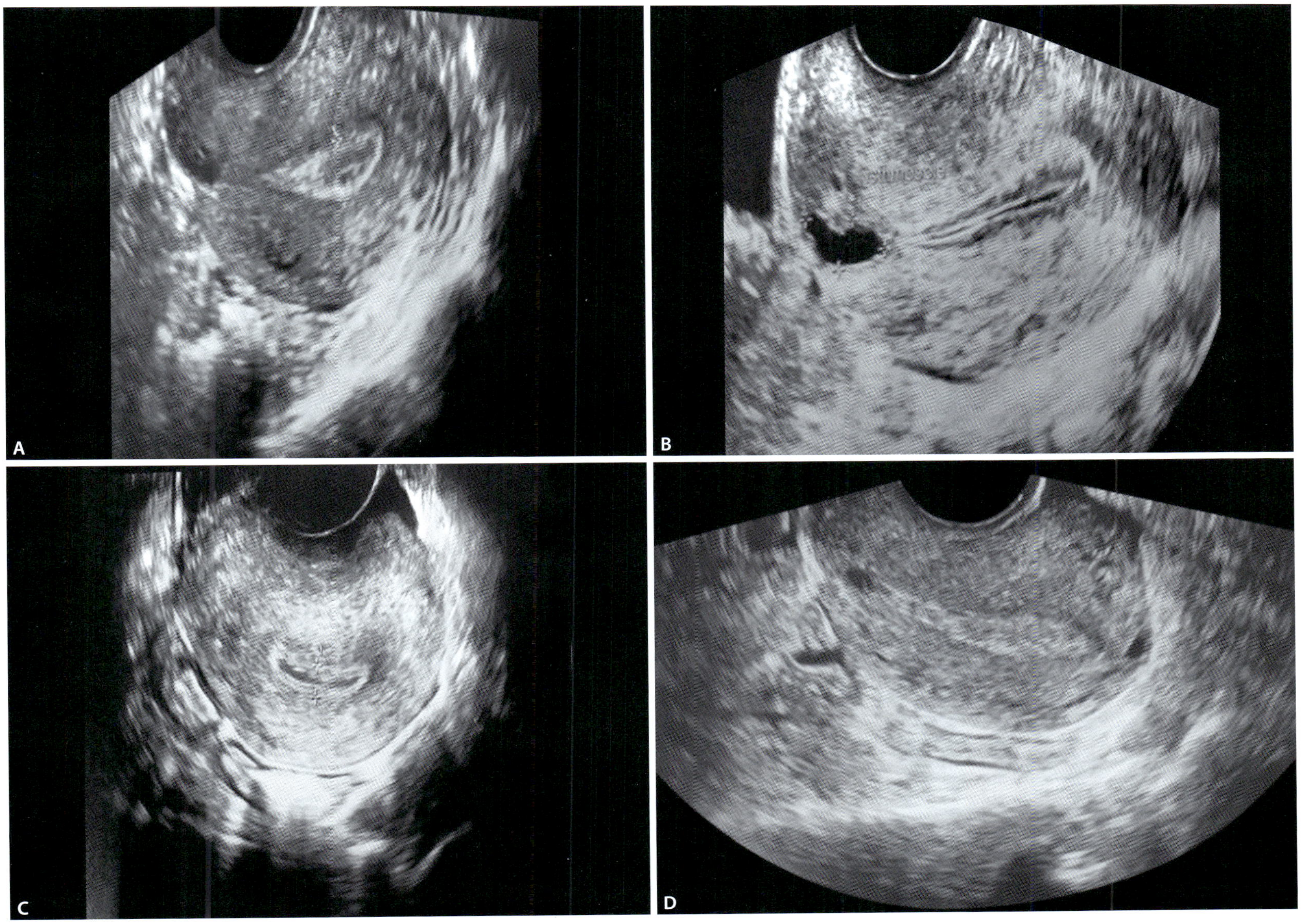

Figs. 7A to D: Ultrasonological images of isthmocele.

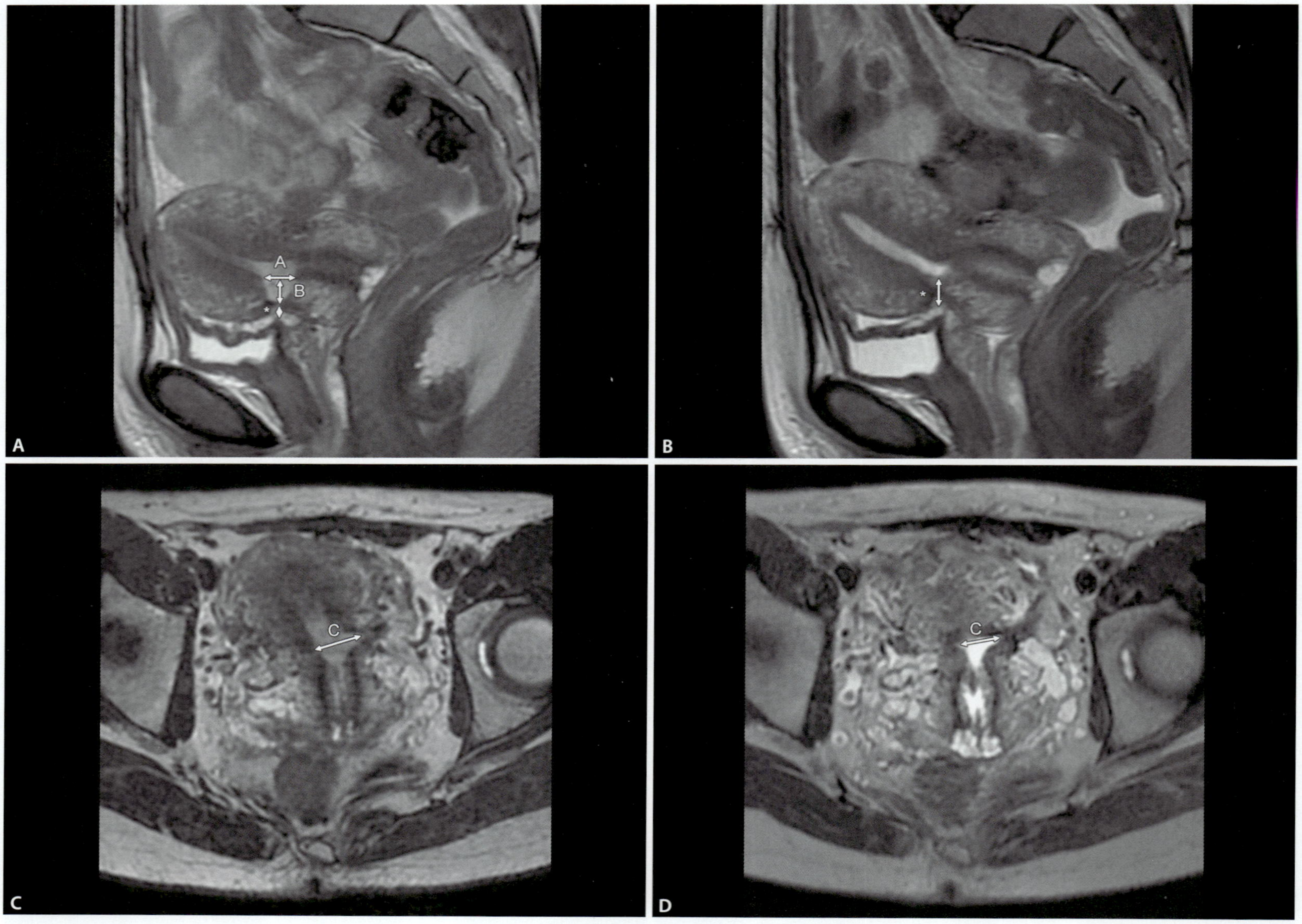

Figs. 8A to D: Radiographic images of an isthmocele.

Laparoscopic Repair of Isthmocele

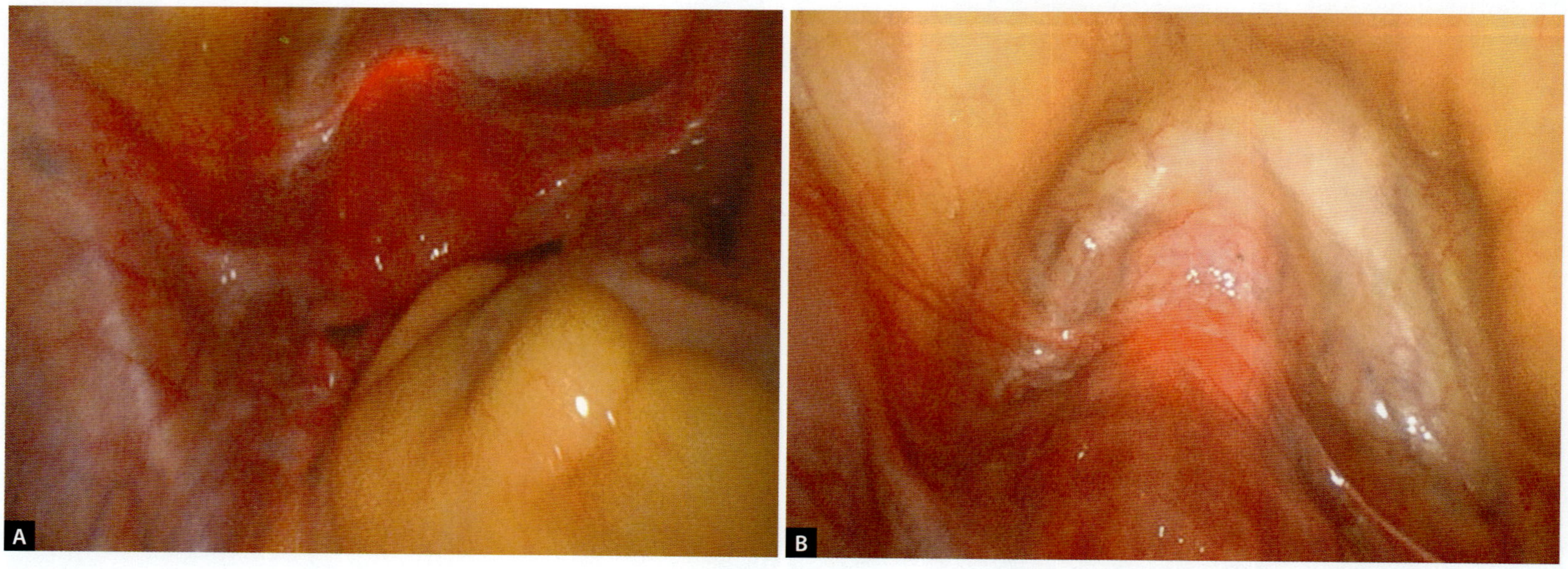

Figs. 9A and B

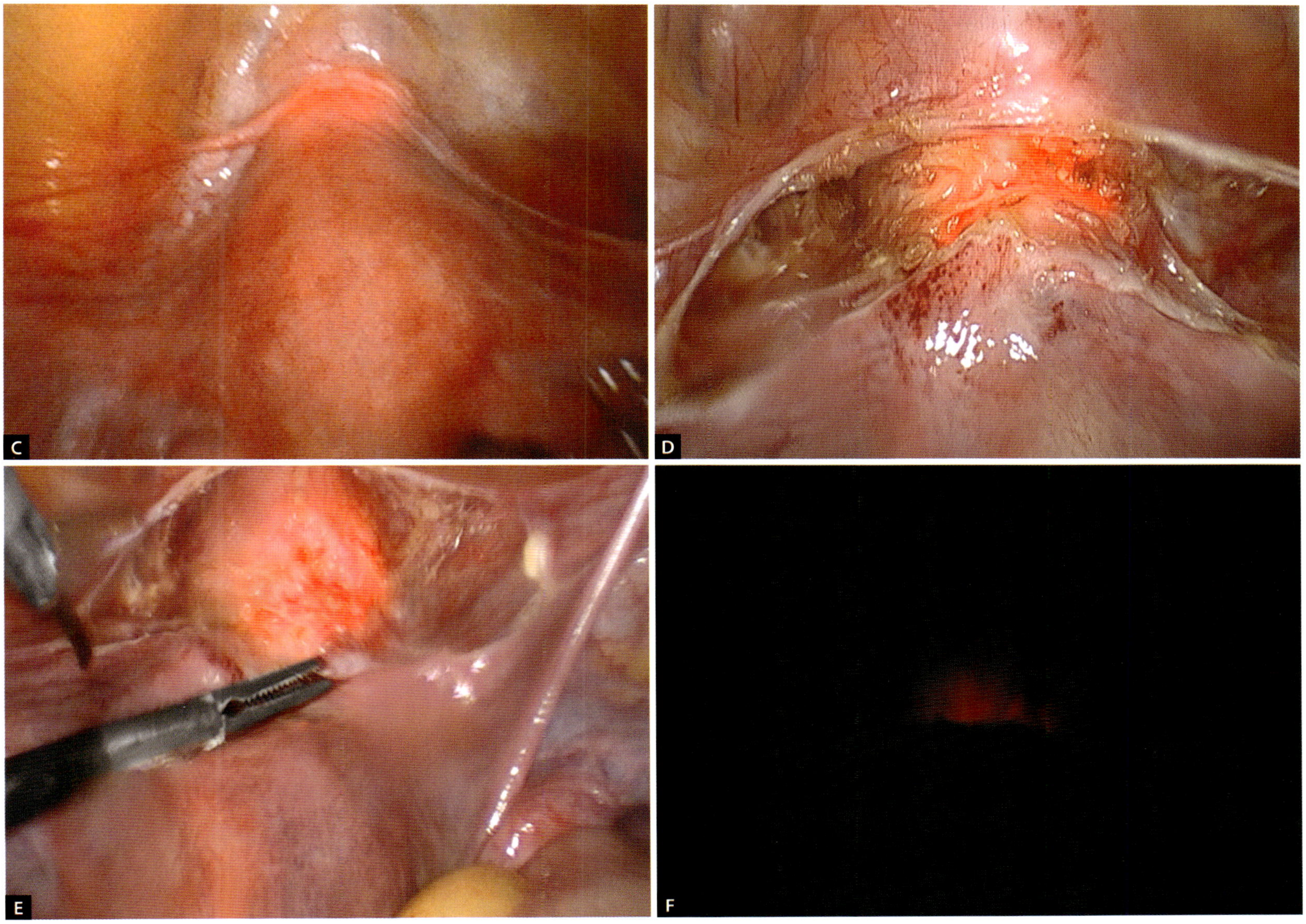

Figs. 9C to F

Figs. 9A to F: Isthmocele seen on transillumination with hysteroscopy as seen on laparoscopy.

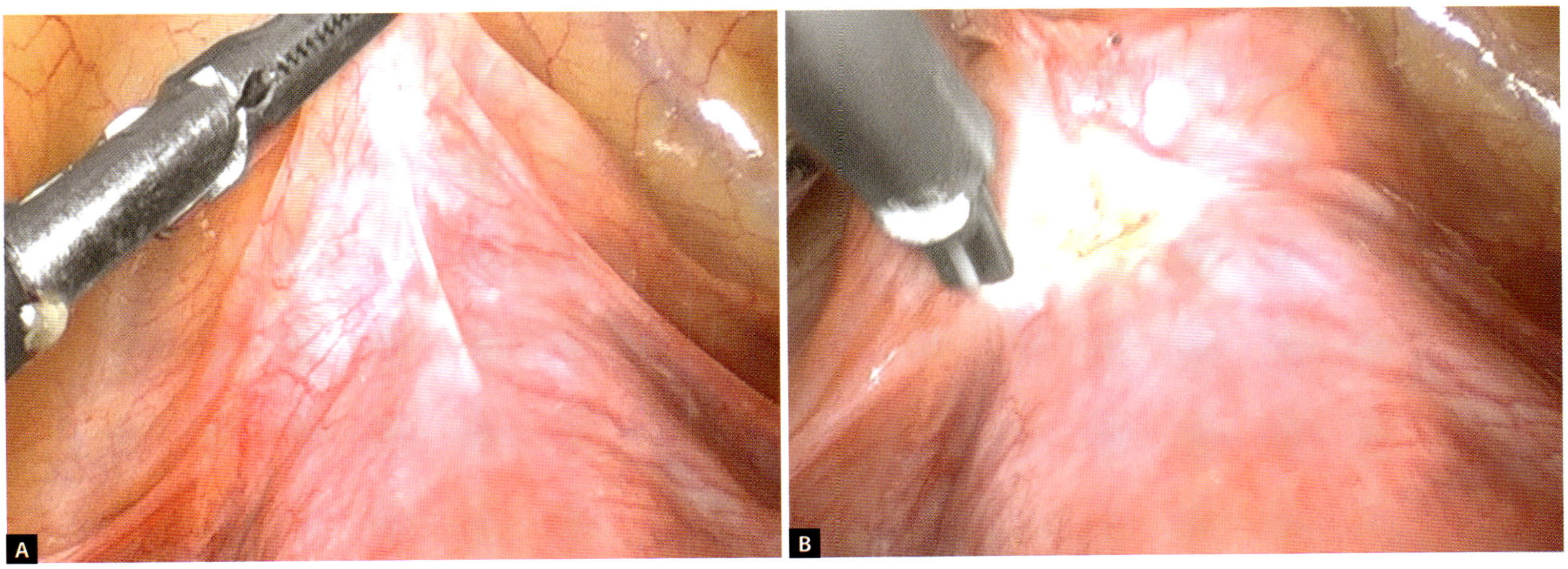

Figs. 10A and B

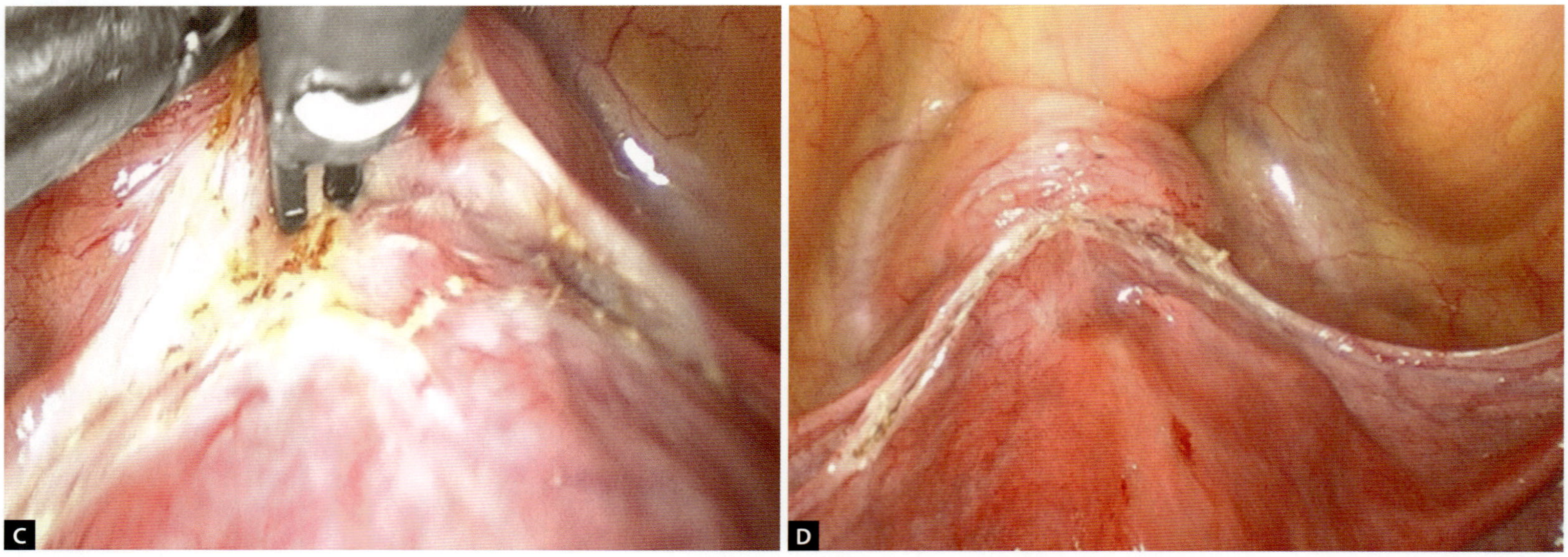

Figs. 10C and D

Figs. 10A to D: Incision made at the level of isthmocele with harmonic.

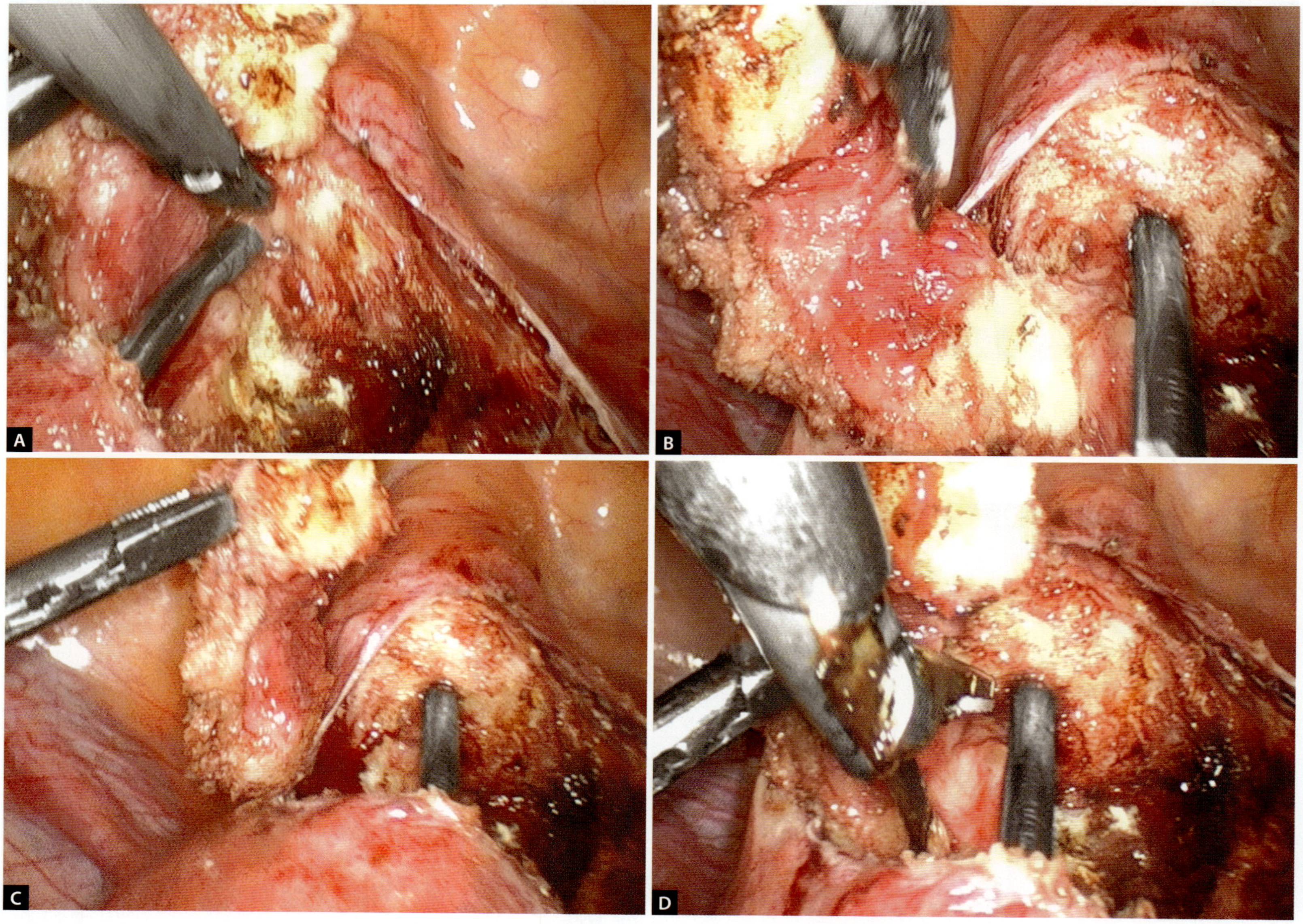

Figs. 11A to D: Fibrous tissue excised at the level of isthmocele.

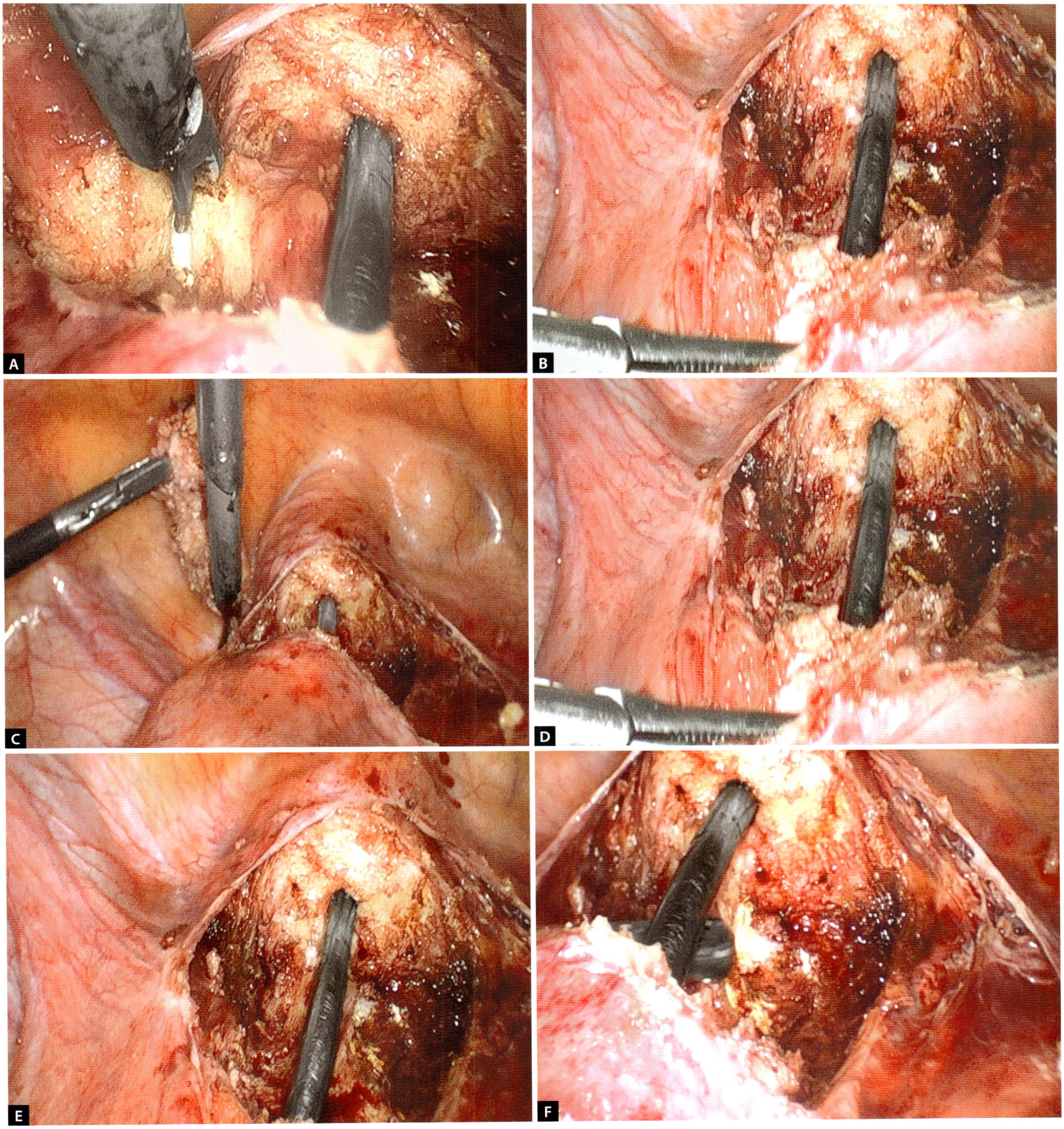

Figs. 12A to F: Lower uterine segment after excision of fibrous tissue at the site of isthmocele.

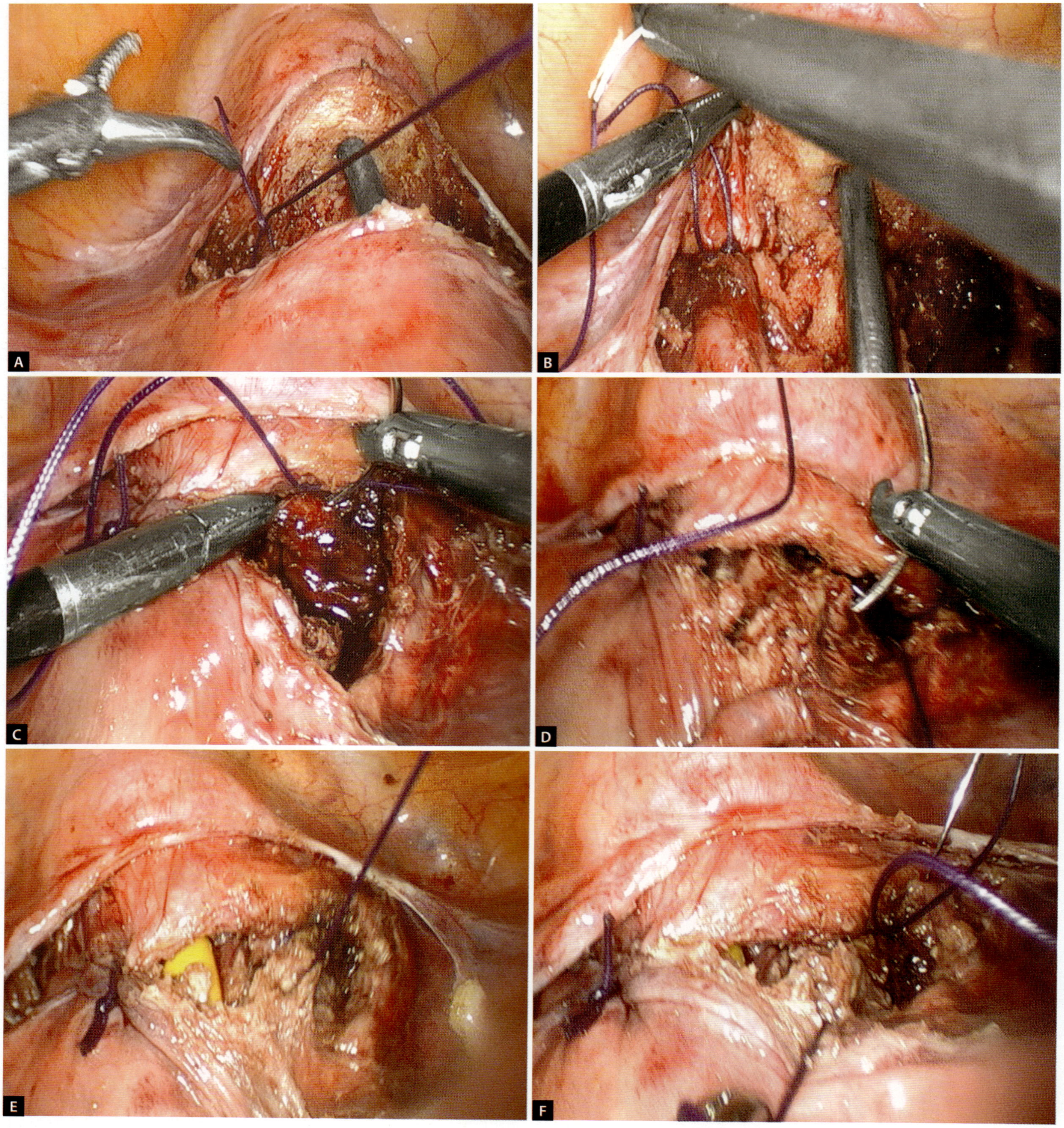

Figs. 13A to F

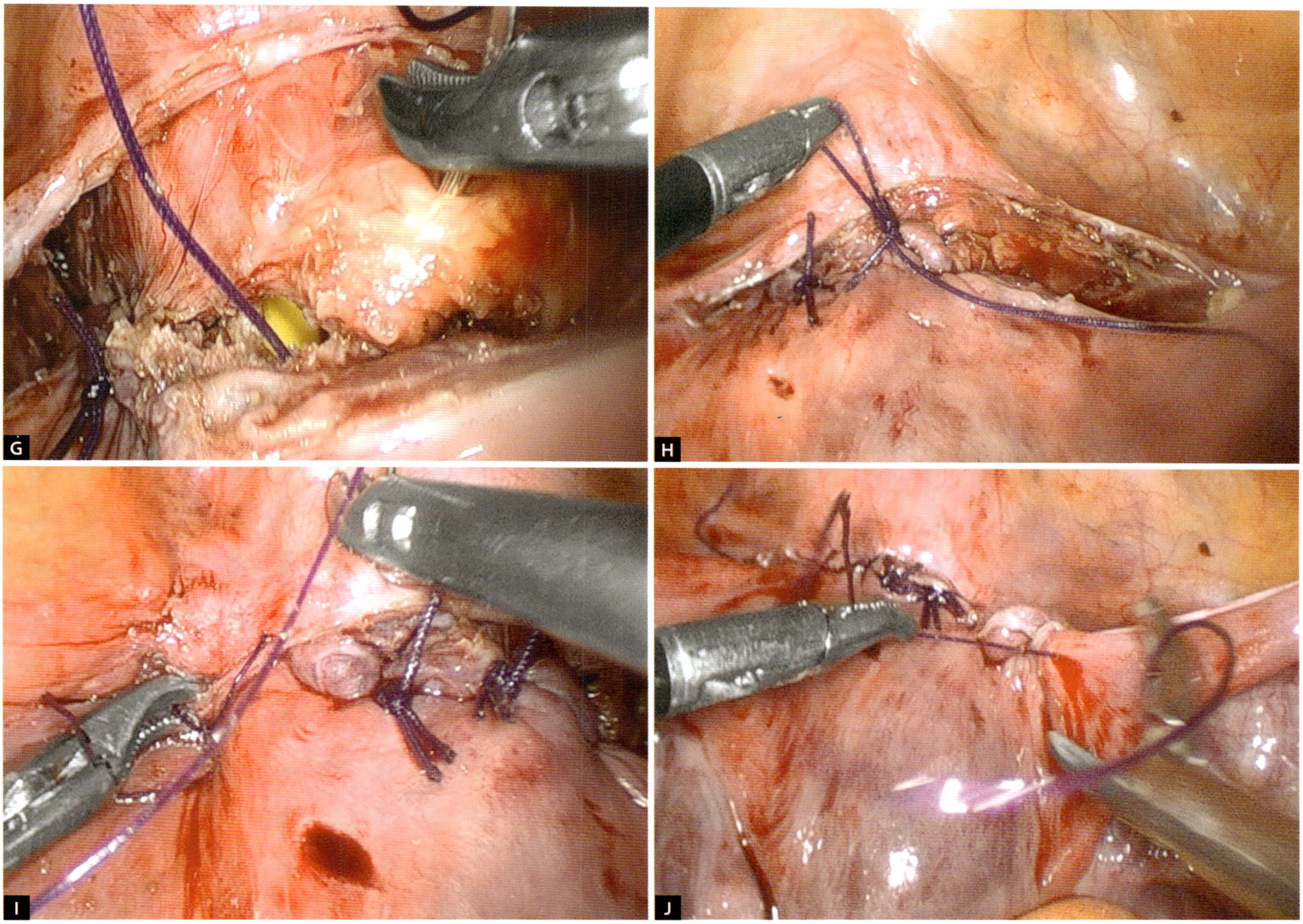

Figs. 13G to J

Figs. 13A to J: Closure of isthmus in layers after excision of fibrous tissue of cesarean scar defect 3 × 1 cm over Foley's catheter.

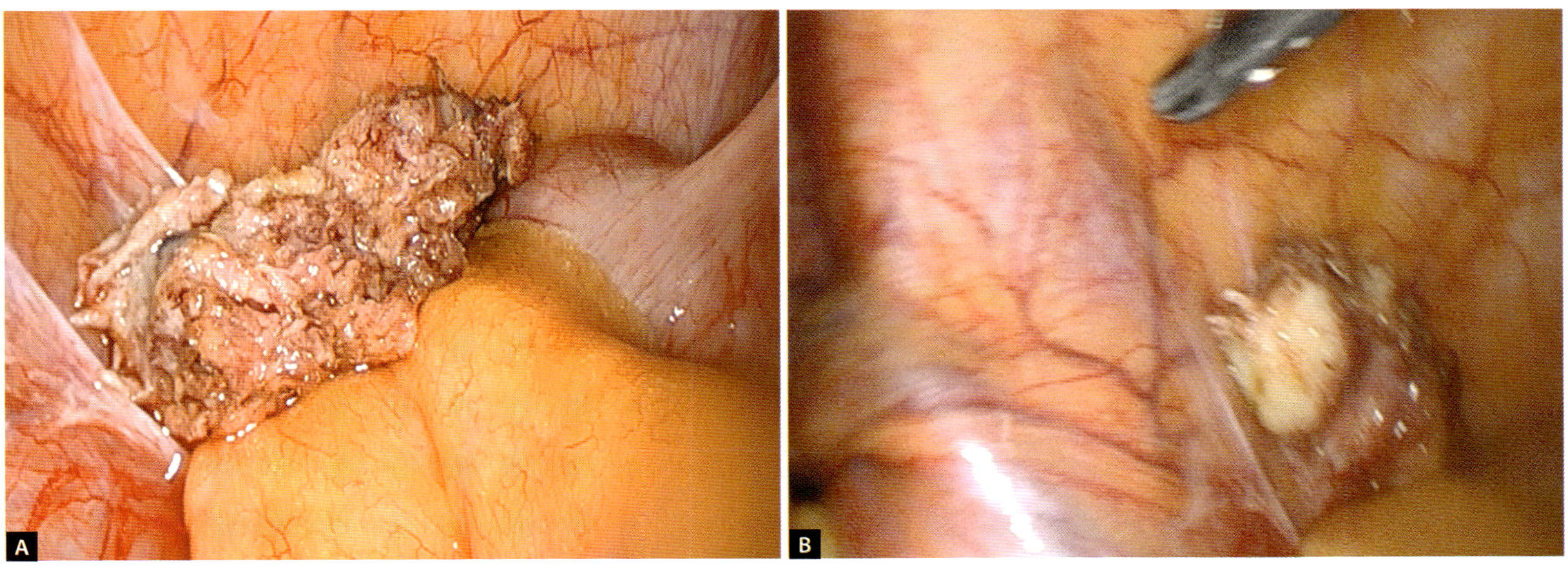

Figs. 14A and B

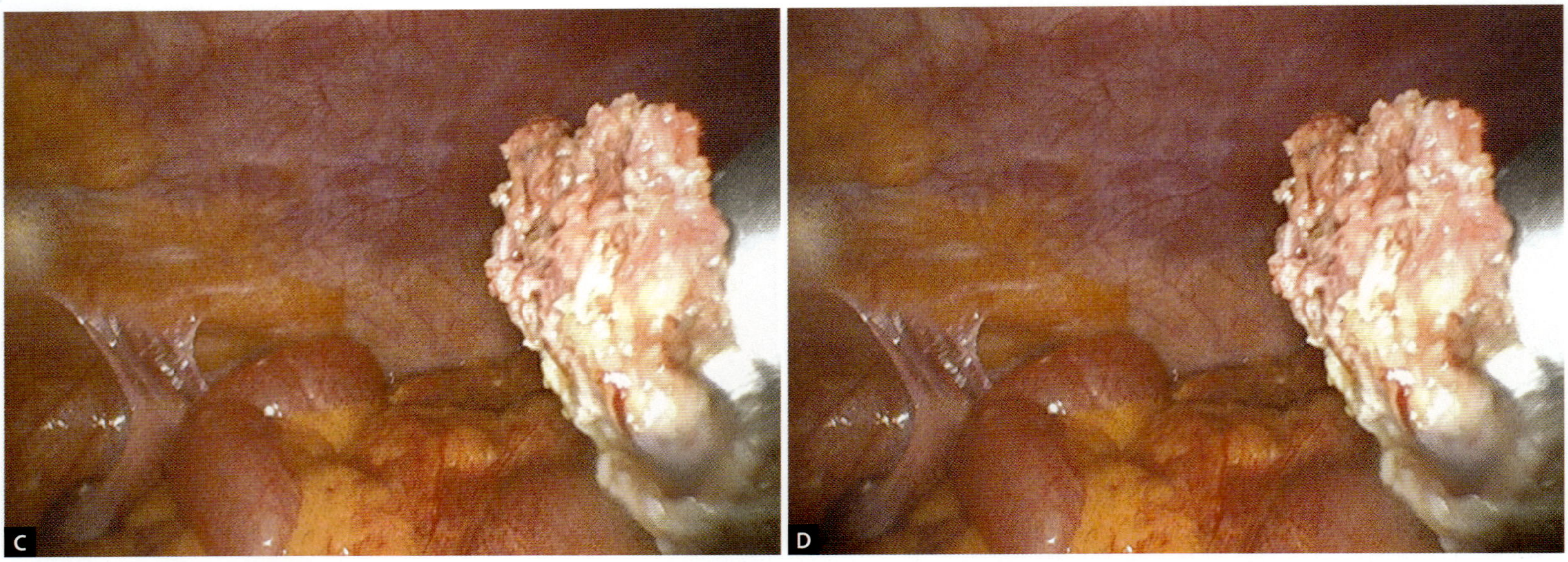

Figs. 14C and D

Figs. 14A to D: Retrieval of scar tissue through left lateral port with electromechanical morcellation.

Diverticulum Repair

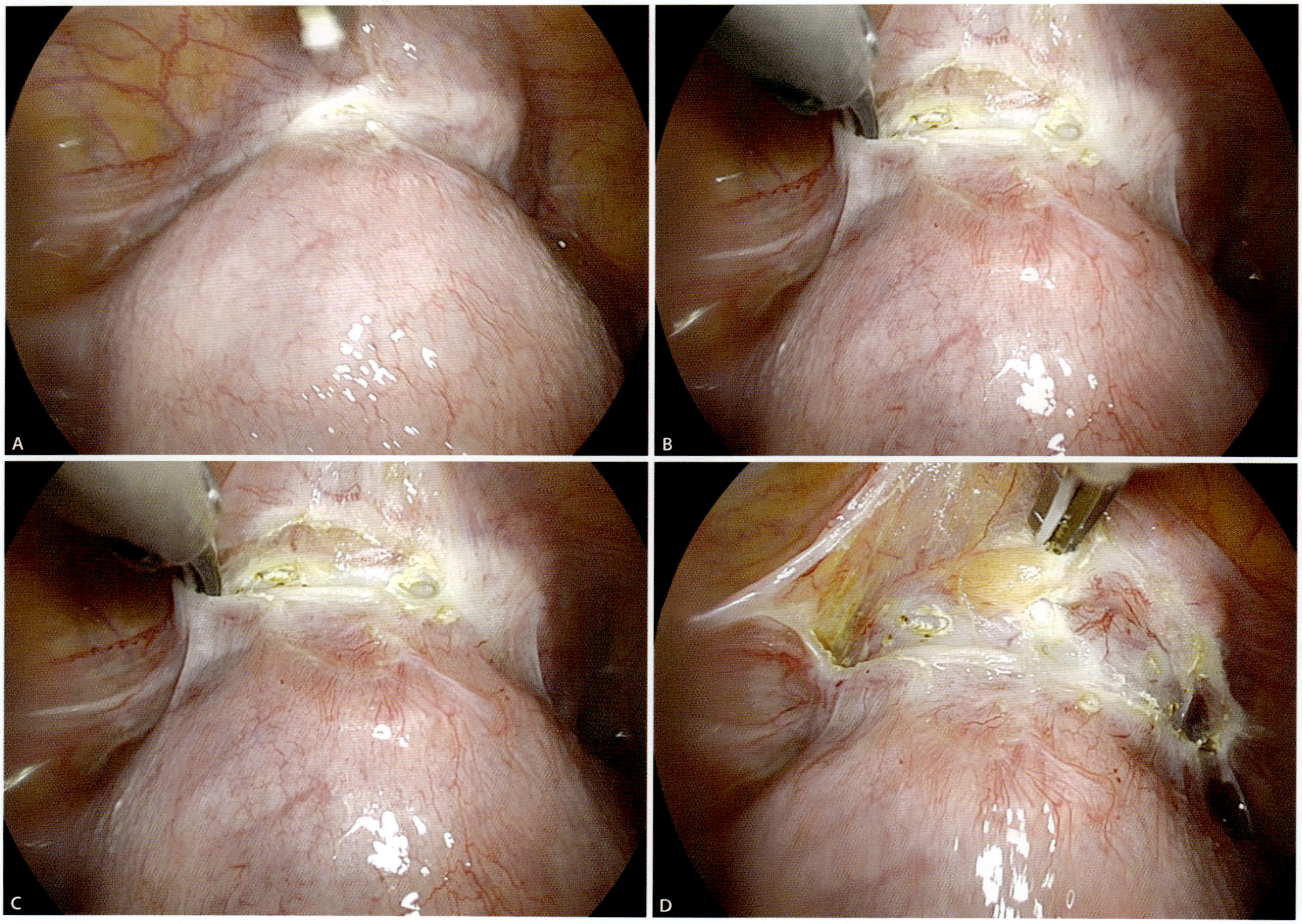

Figs. 15A to D

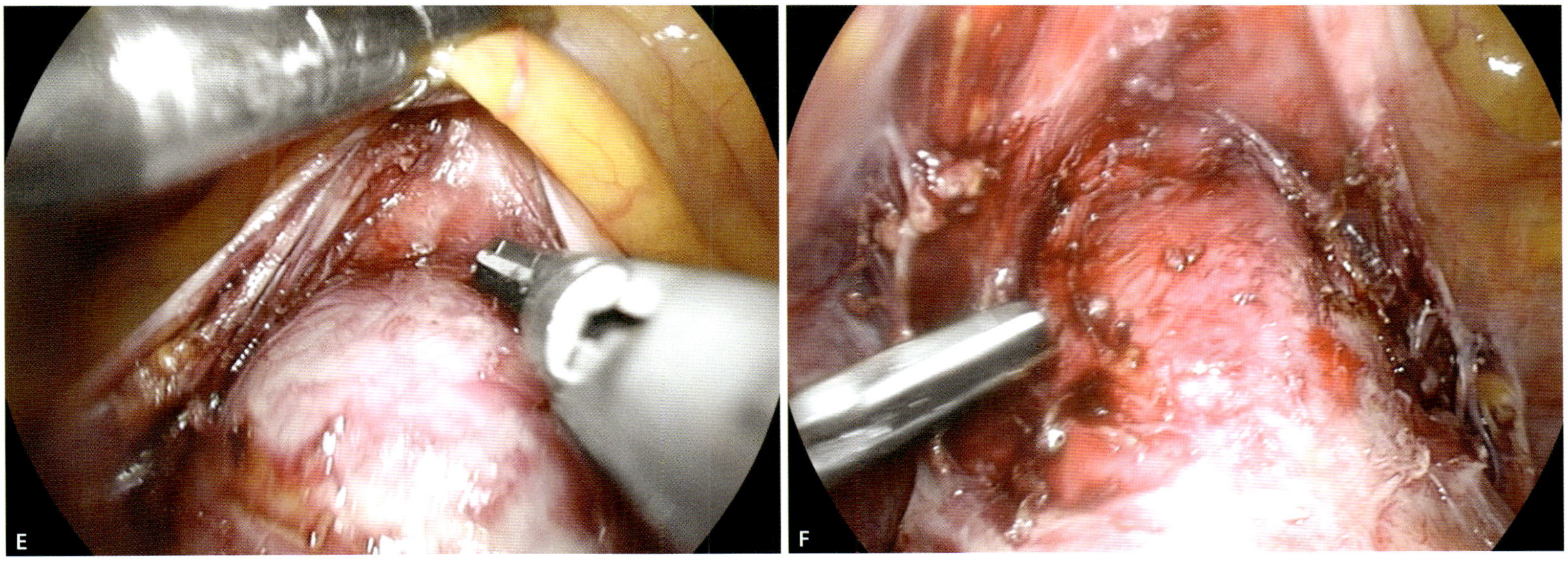

Figs. 15E and F

Figs. 15A to F: Incision made in the lower uterine segment at the level of diverticulum and bladder dissected down.

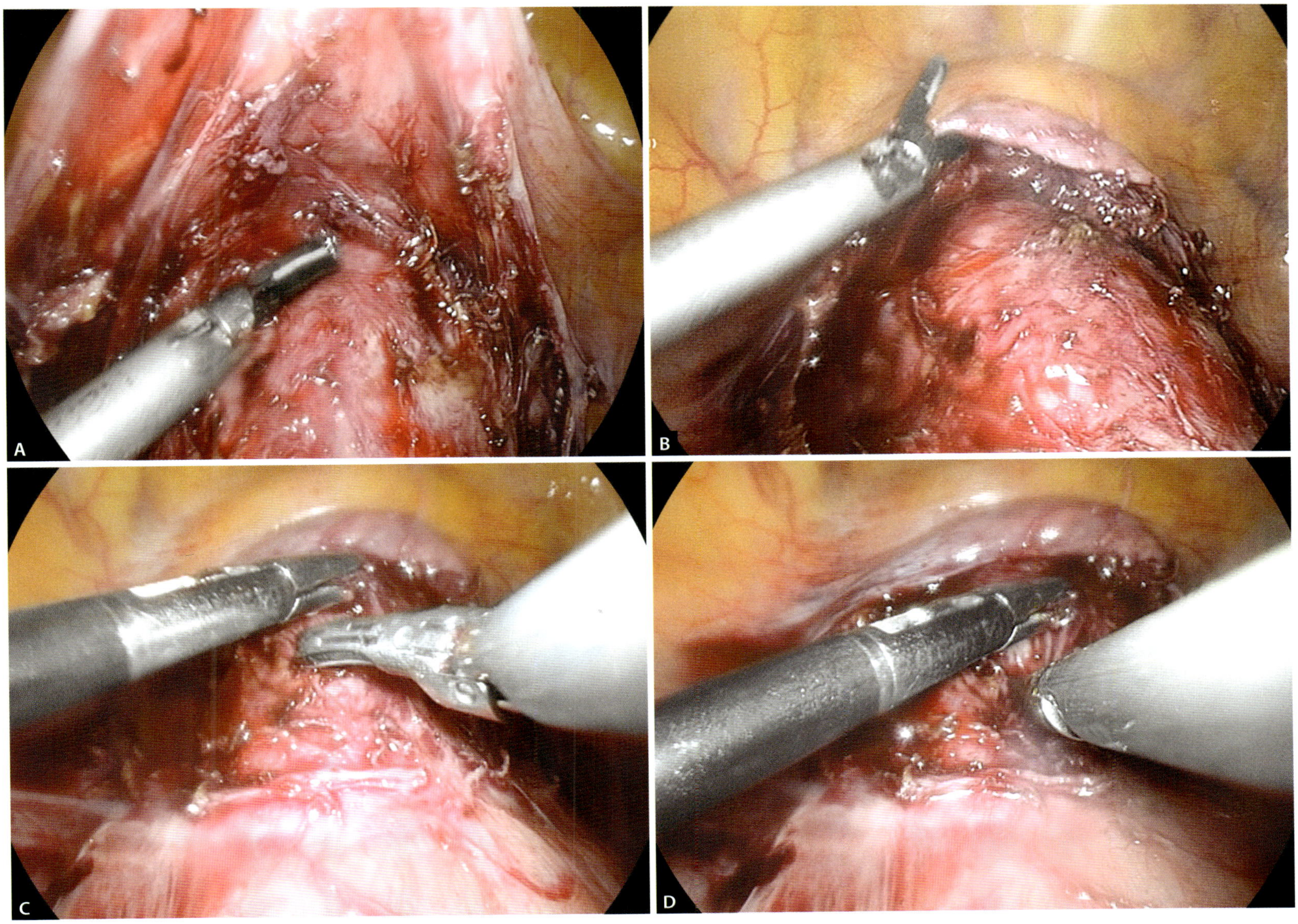

Figs. 16A to D

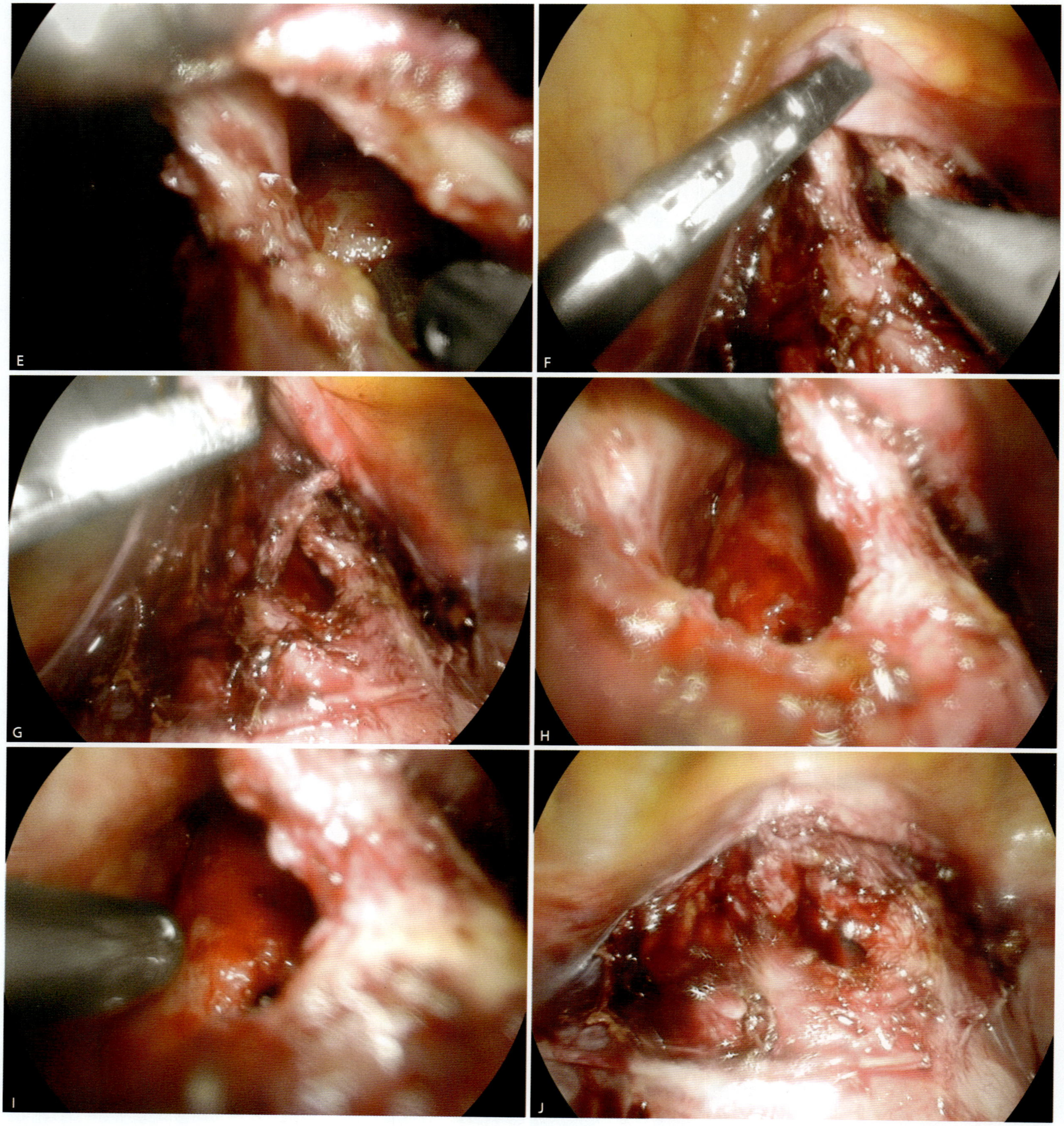

Figs. 16E to J

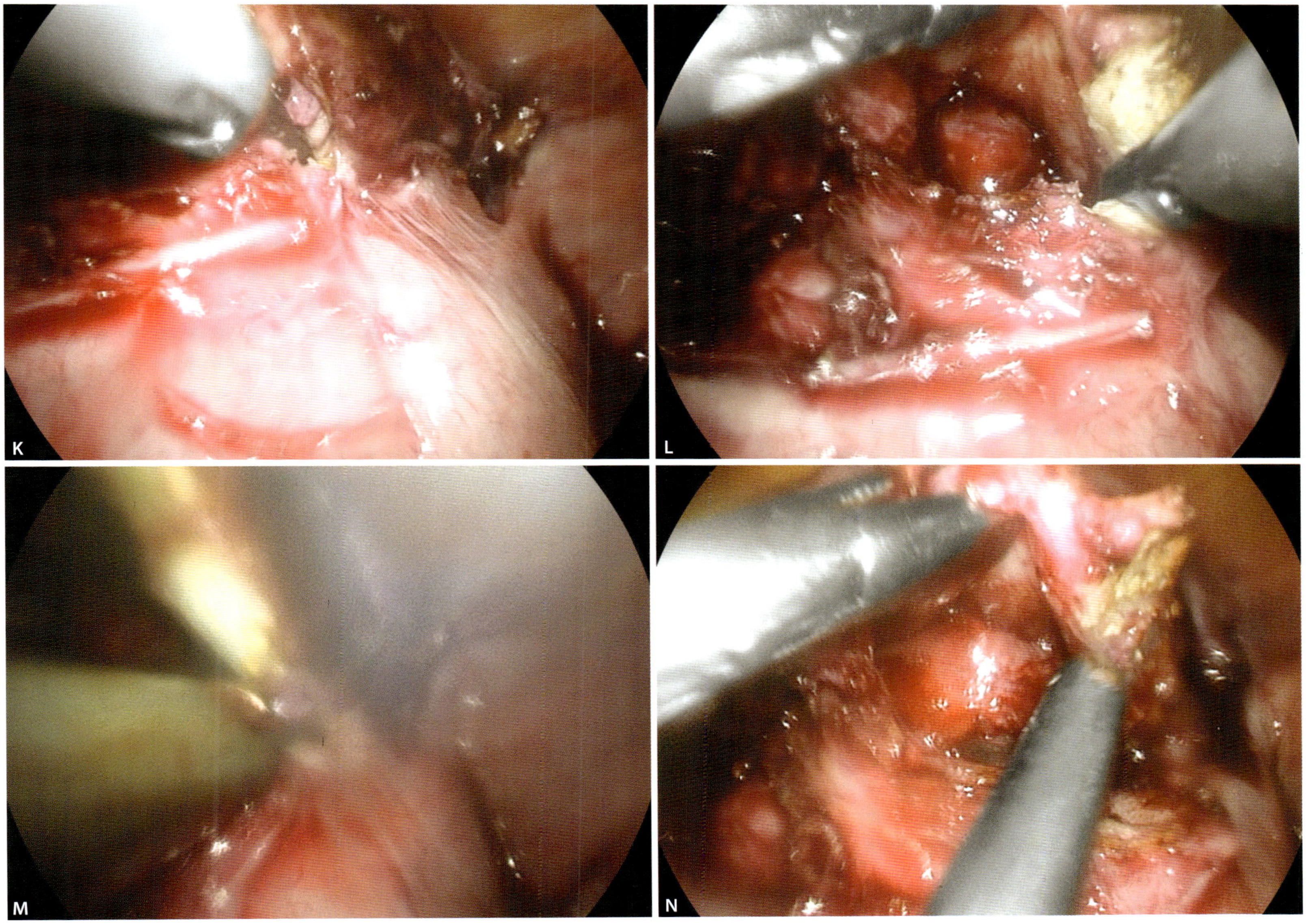

Figs. 16K to N

Figs. 16A to N: Resection of fibrous tissue at the level of diverticulum.

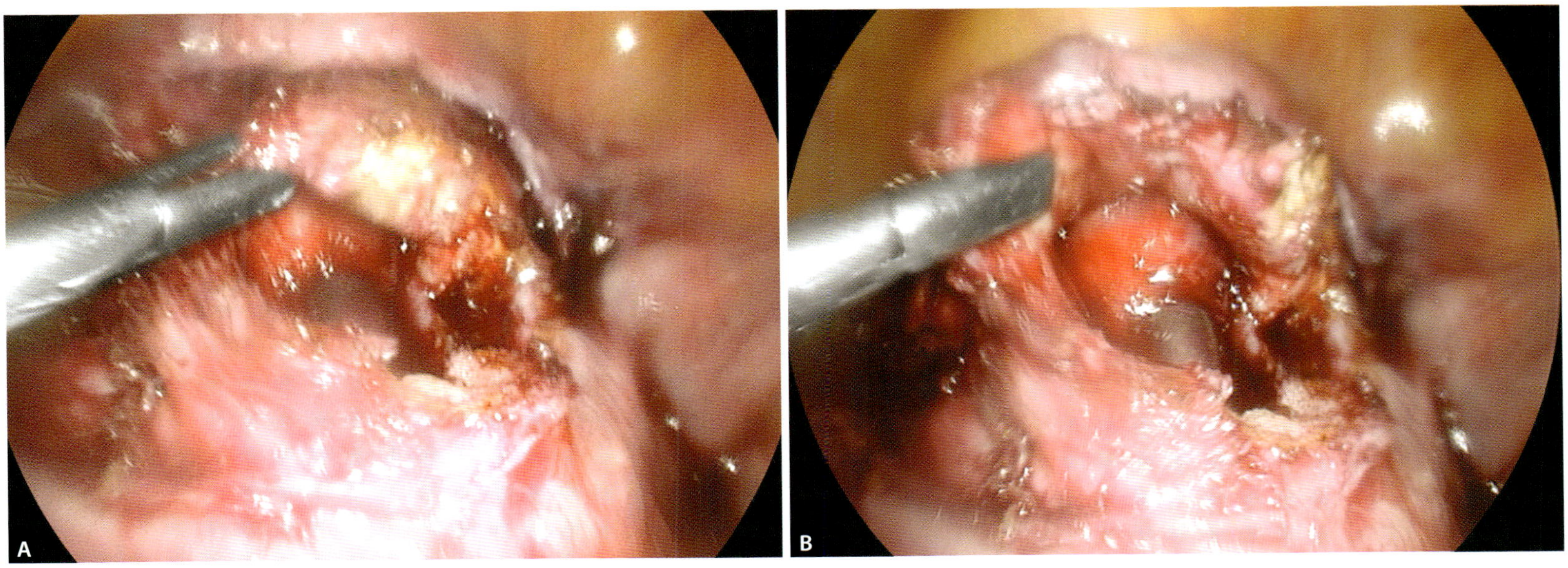

Figs. 17A and B

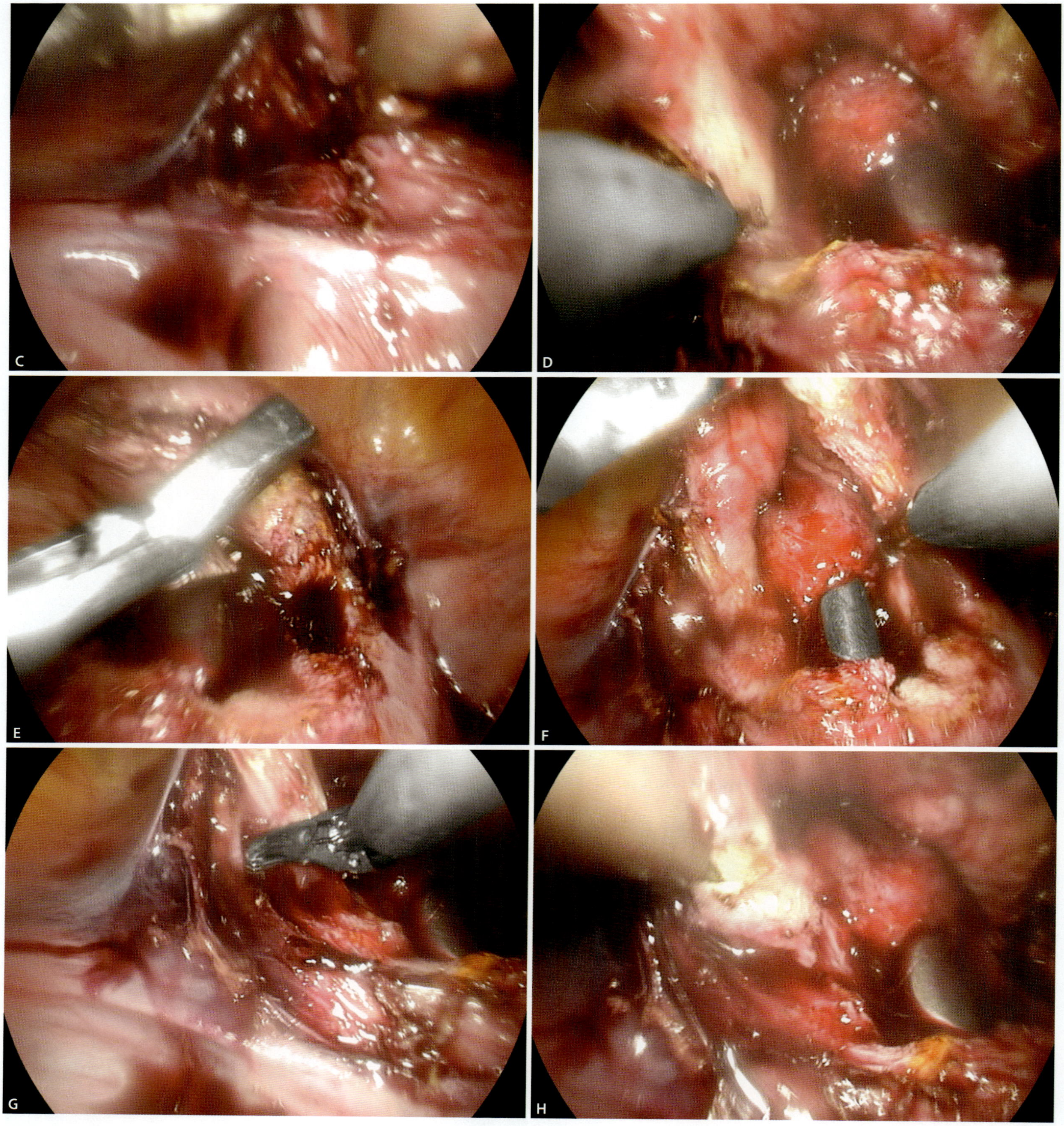

Figs. 17C to H

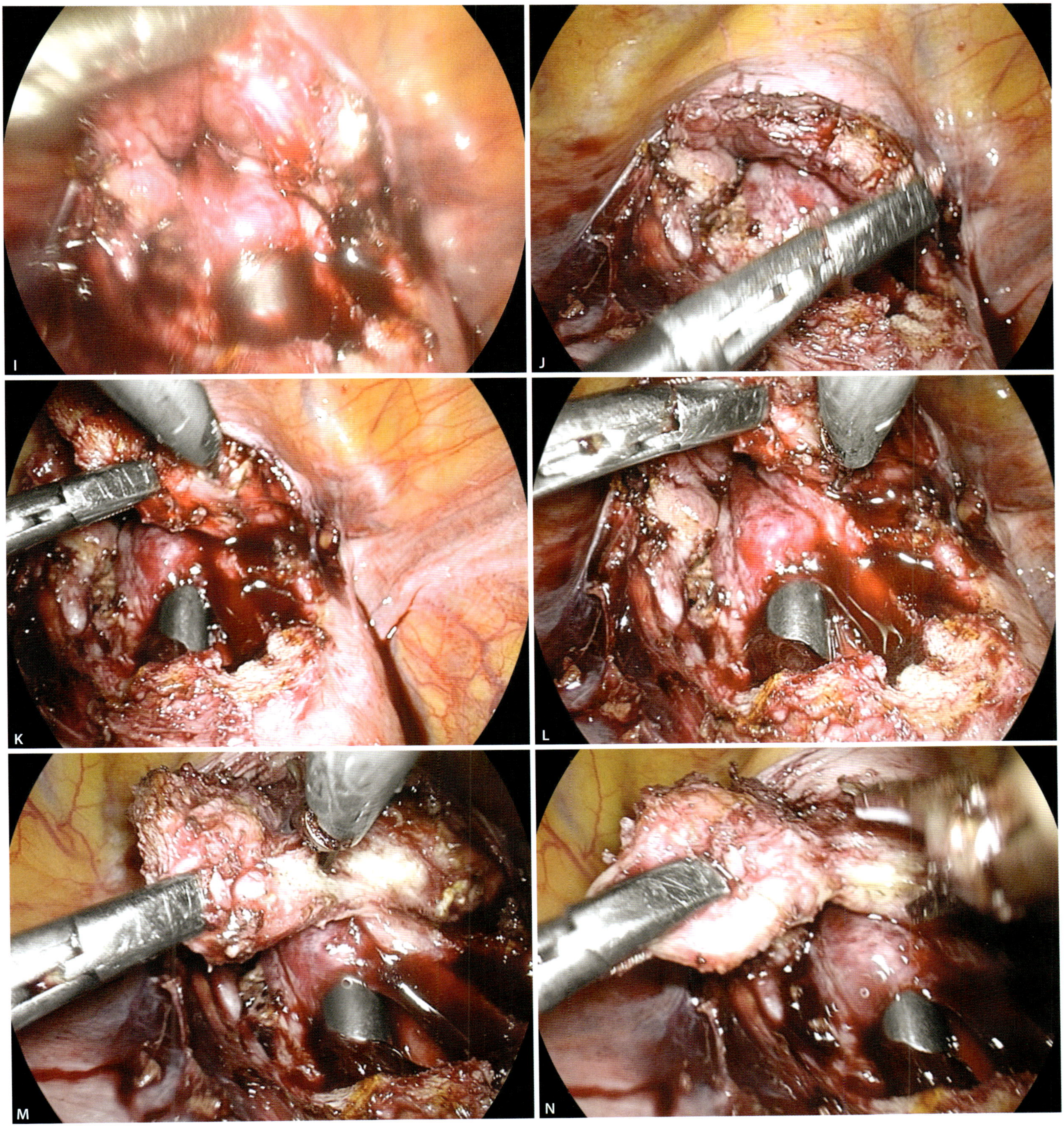

Figs. 17I to N

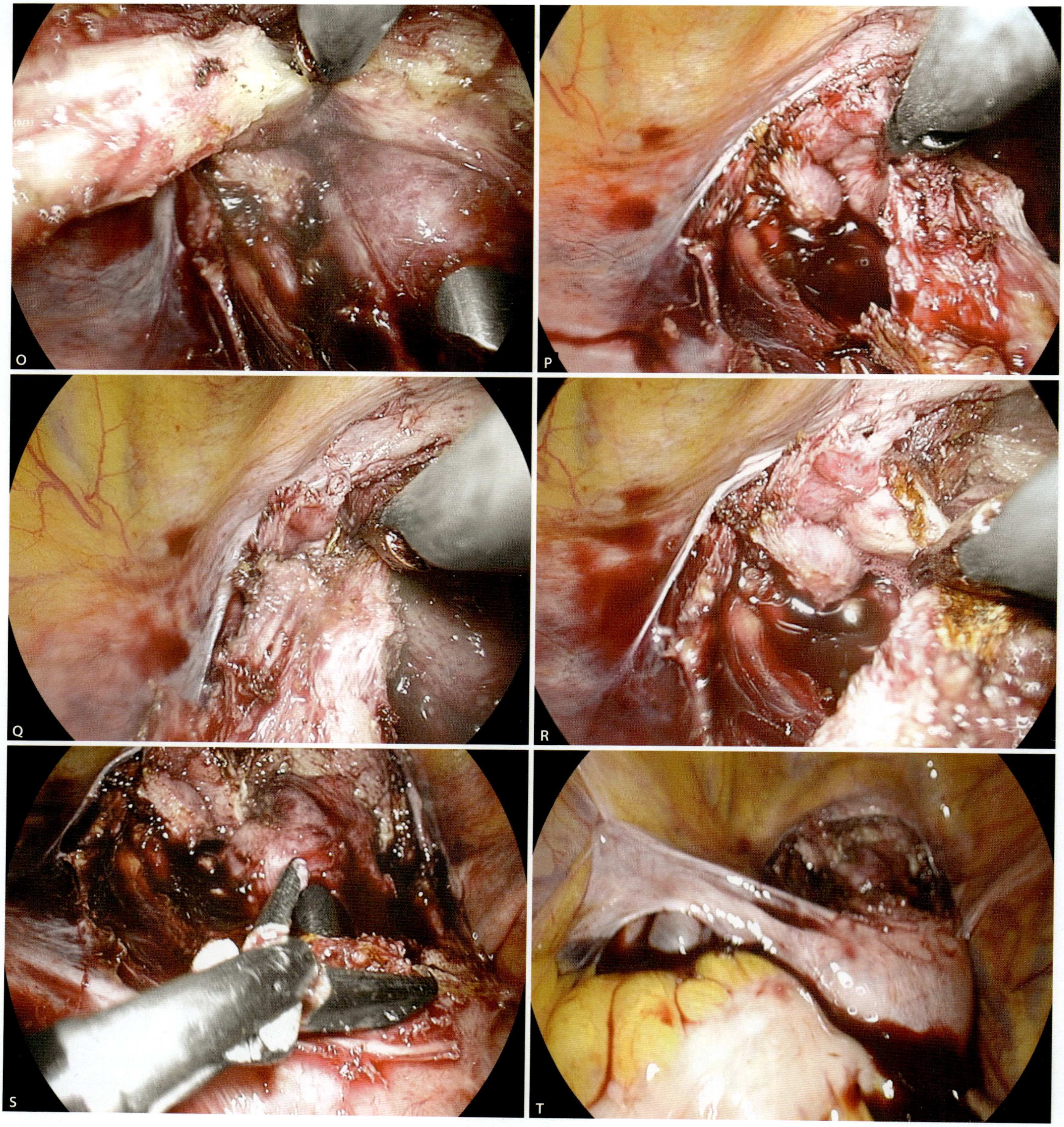

Figs. 17O to T

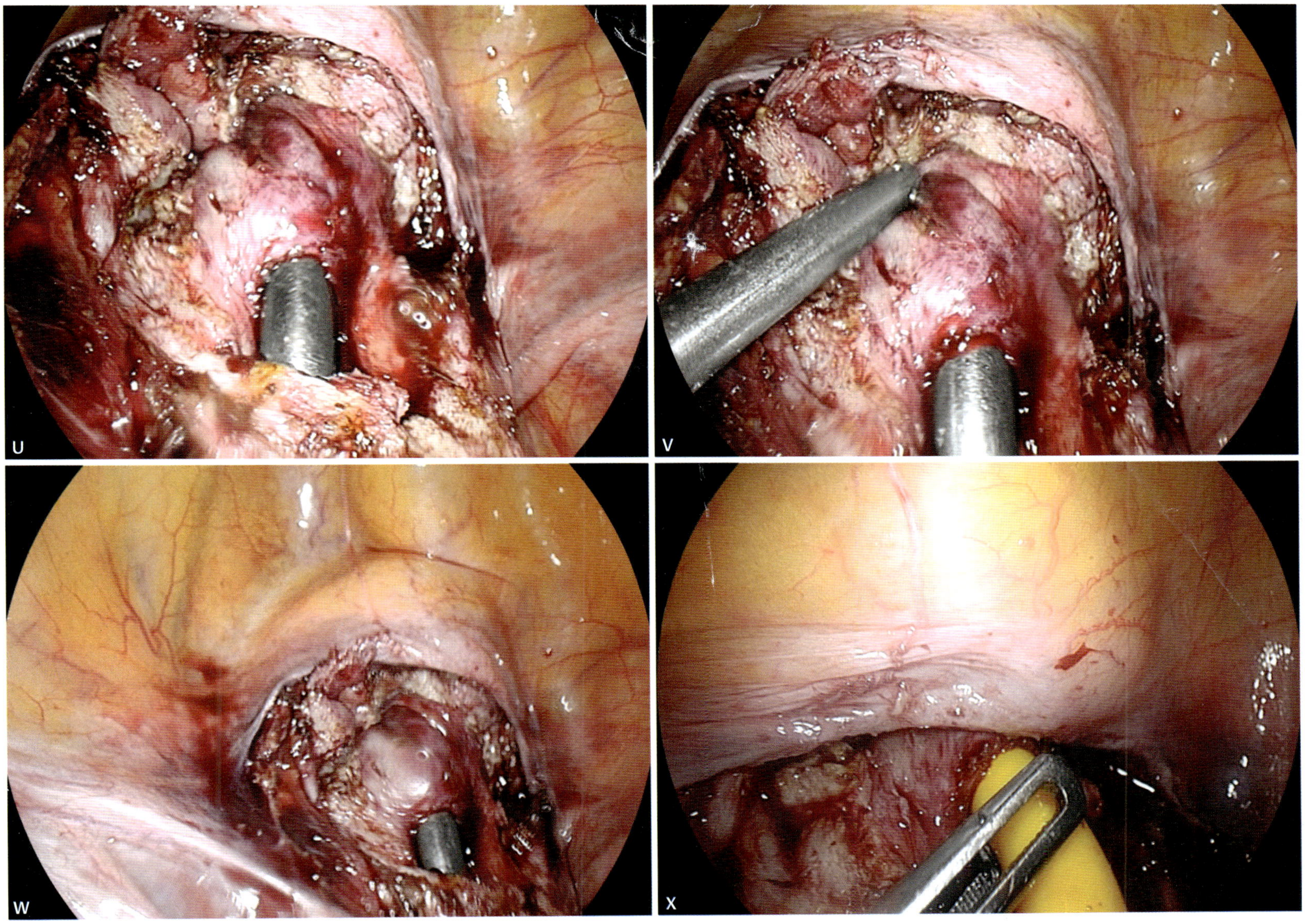

Figs. 17U to X

Figs. 17A to X: Lower uterine segment seen postresection of diverticulum.

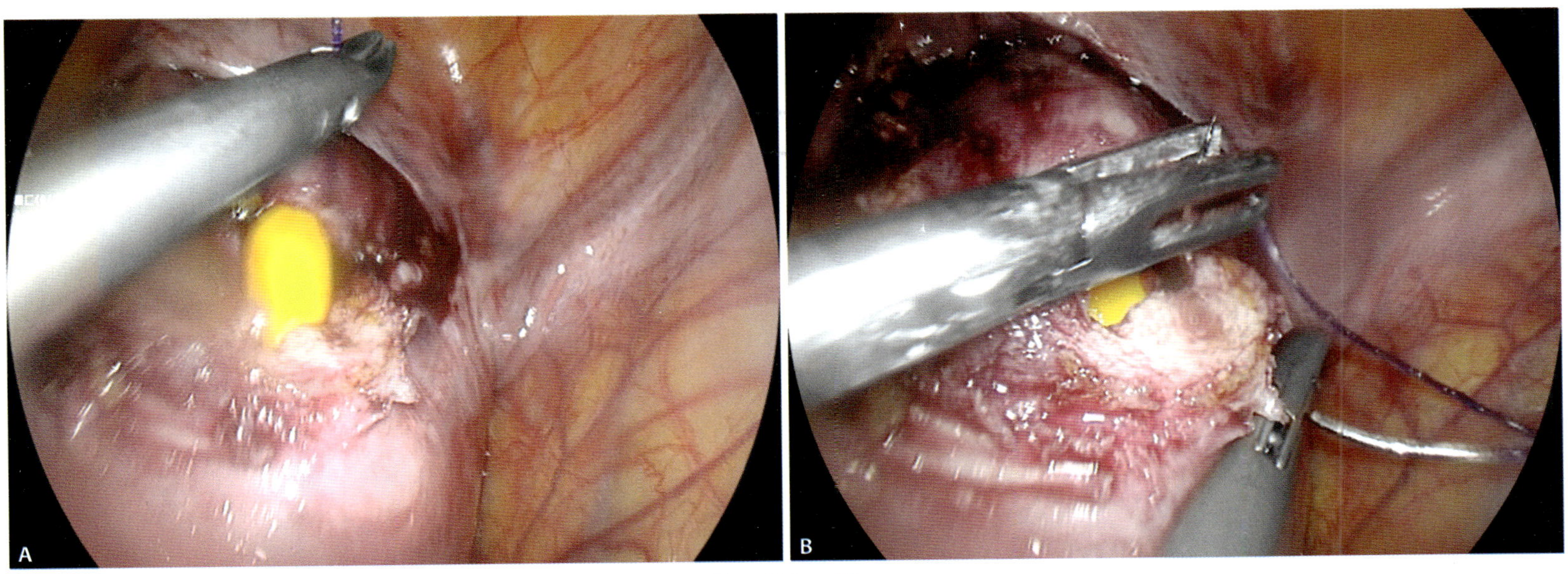

Figs. 18A and B

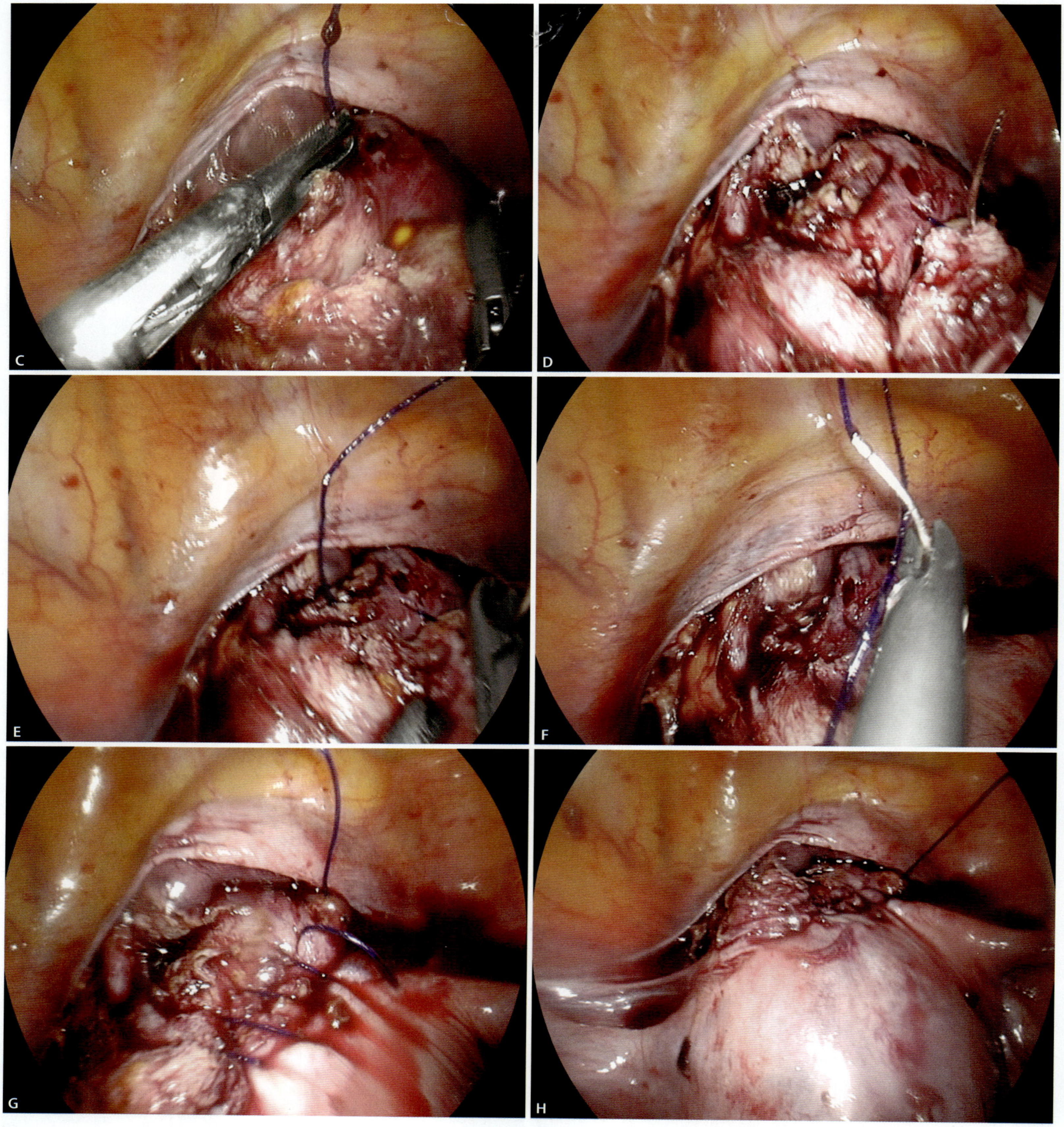

Figs. 18C to H

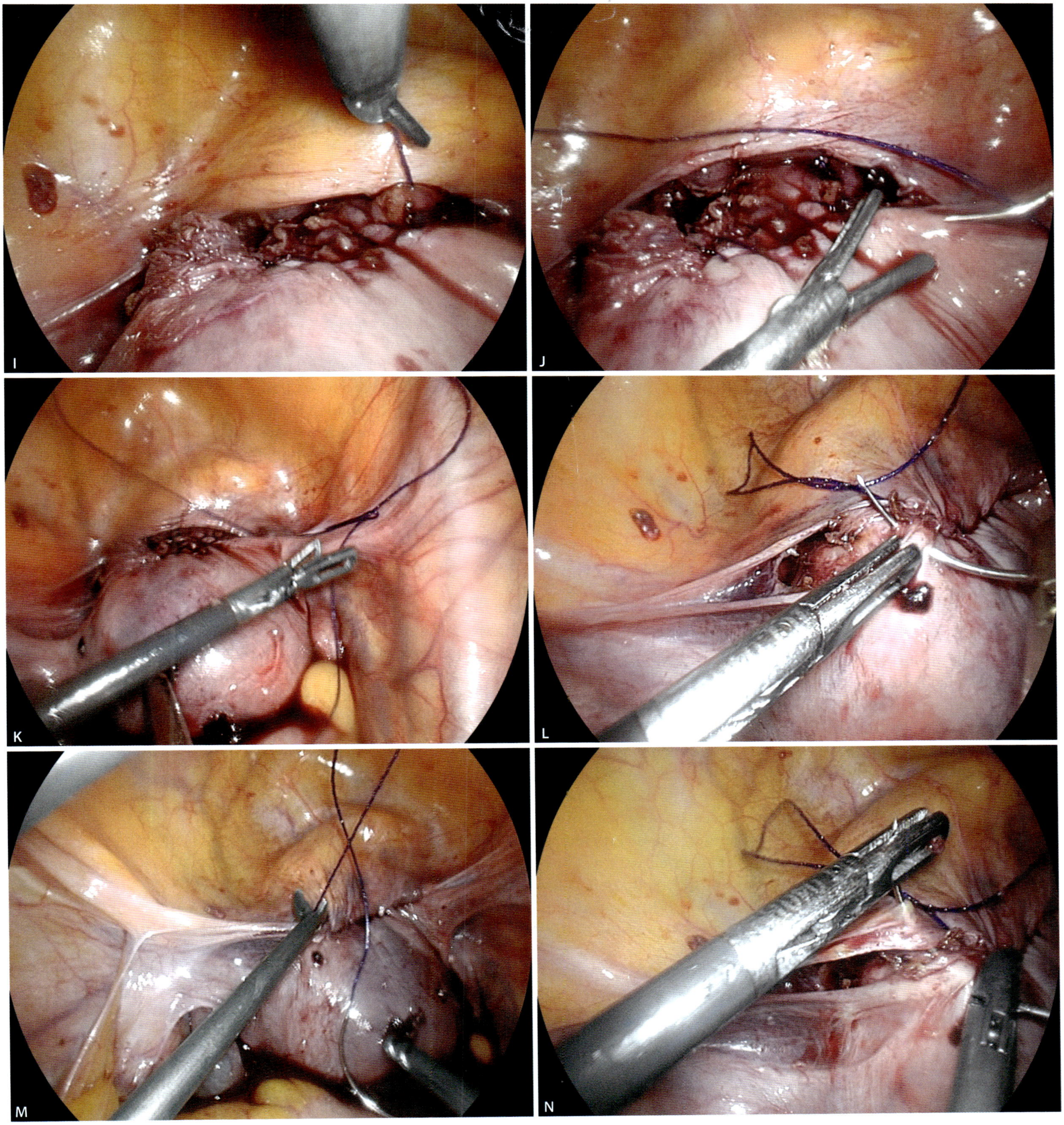

Figs. 18I to N

Figs. 18A to N: Postresection—uterus sutured back in layers at the level of diverticulum.

Through diagnostic hysteroscopy isthmocele appears as a pouch-like anatomic defect on the anterior wall of the isthmus or of the cervical canal at its superior third or less frequently at its inferior third **(Fig. 3)**. More precisely, the defect appeared anteriorly near the right as an outcome of the physiological uterine involution after delivery, and its location essentially depends on the site of the cesarean section, as patients with the defect in the higher part of the cervix previously underwent elective cesarean section, whereas in those in whom cesarean section was done in presence of cervical modifications, isthmocele is localized in the lower part of the cervical canal.[1,20,21]

In comparison with hysterosalpingographic diagnosis of CSDs, Regnard et al.[15] detected a similar rate of cesarean section scars (57.5%) via saline contrast sonohysterography. One clear limitation of hysterosalpingography is the inability to precisely measure myometrial thickness and the size of the scar, both of which can be readily characterized via sonohysterography.

Multiple techniques have been used for CSD treatment: reconstructive therapies including laparoscopic or robot-assisted laparoscopic excision, vaginal repair and channel-like resectoscopic treatment[3-6,12] All these procedures excise or ablate the fibrotic tissue of niche, suggesting that the removal of the local inflamed tissue may contribute to the improvement of symptoms. Since the aim of CSD repair in women with symptoms is to facilitate the drainage of menstrual blood through the cervix, the hysteroscopic approach, flattening the CSD and restoring the continuity of the cervical canal area, results to be effective and less invasive comparing to laparoscopic excision and vaginal repair.[22]

HYSTEROSCOPIC ISTHMOPLASTY

A channel-like hysteroscopic treatment with 16-Fr resectoscope (Gubbini system, Tontarra, Medizintechnik, GmbH, Germany) was planned immediately at the end of menstrual period. Before beginning the procedure, the bladder was filled with methylene blue solution to enable early identification of bladder injuries. With vaginoscopic approach **(Figs. 15 to 18)**, the isthmocele was localized and a bipolar loop was used to resect the fibrotic tissue of the proximal and distal part of the niche with 360° resection (endocervical ablation) of the all residual cervical canal inflamed tissue surrounding the diverticulum. The entire niche surface was superficially coagulated with a roller ball electrode in order to replace it with mono-stratified cubic cell-type epithelium. The procedure was ended controlling eventual endocervical vessel bleeding by reducing inflow and pressure of the distending medium.

Hysteroscopic isthmoplasty flattening the CSD area, restores the continuity of the cervical canal and improves menstrual drainage reducing blood accumulation in the niche and reflux into the uterine cavity. The hysteroscopic repair is performed, with small variations among authors, by resecting only the inferior/distal rim of the niche or with superior/proximal edge of the defect using a 26-Fr or 27-Fr resectoscope. The procedure is ended with or without superficial coagulation of vessels in the niche surface with the aim at reducing blood loss from these fragile vessels.[20-22]

Isthmoplasty, using a 16-Fr resectoscope with vaginoscopic approach to resect the fibrotic tissue of the distal and proximal part of the niche as well as all residual cervical canal inflamed tissue surrounding the diverticulum (360° "endocervical ablation") in order to replace it with mono-stratified cubic cell-type epithelium is an excellent method. The mini-resectoscope allows us to perform standard maneuvers of resectoscopic CSD repair according to the anatomy with the advantages of miniaturized instrumentation and without the complications related to cervical dilation.[20]

It is important to emphasize that not all CSD cause symptoms or infertility, and as the treatment is predominantly performed to relieve symptoms isthmocele without symptoms should not be treated. Since CSD treatment is to improve menstrual drainage rather than to increase the myometrial thickness, in symptomatic women a cutoff of 2–3 mm of the overlying myometrium has not been suggested for vaginal or laparoscopic repair with a multiple-layer closure.[23]

Laparoscopic repair **(Figs. 9 to 14)** was first described by Dr Olivier Donnez, who rightly pointed out that the laparoscopic approach offers an optimal view from above during dissection of the vesicovaginal space. Dr Donnez used a CO_2 laser to excise fibrotic tissue.

We have had success with a laparoscopic approach that uses concomitant hysteroscopy. The vesicouterine peritoneum is incised over the anterior uterine wall, and the bladder is backfilled so that its boundaries may be identified prior to further dissection. With the area exposed, we perform a hysteroscopy to determine the exact location of the isthmocele. As the hysteroscope enters the thinned out isthmocele, the light will be more visible via laparoscopic visualization.

When performing conventional laparoscopy, the isthmocele is excised with harmonic scalpel. We use this instrument because it enables precise tissue dissection in multiple planes. With harmonic energy, we can limit tissue desiccation and destruction, lowering the risk of future pregnancy-related complications. Monopolar scissors are best when a robotic approach is used.

Once the isthmocele is resected reddish healthy *myometrium* is visualized, the clean edges are sutured together in two layers. The first layer is sutured in an interrupted mattress-style fashion, to prevent tissue strangulation and necrosis. We use a monofilament nonbarbed delayed-absorbable 3-0 PDS suture on a CT-1 needle—a choice that limits tissue trauma and postoperative inflammation. Finally, the visceral *peritoneum* defect was closed, with the aim of restoring the physiologic uterine anatomy. In this case, multiple peritoneal endometriotic implants were also identified and excised.

CONCLUSION

Good reproductive outcomes have been reported after hysteroscopic treatment of uterine isthmocele. Laparoscopy allows thorough repair of the uterine defect, thus restoring a normal myometrial thickness. Therefore, as demonstrated in this case, a laparoscopic approach might be considered to be the procedure of choice for the repair of a large uterine isthmocele with extreme thinning of the residual myometrium.

REFERENCES

1. Gubbini G, Casadio P, Marra E. Resectoscopic correction of the isthmocele in women with postmenstrual abnormal uterine bleeding and secondary infertility. J Minim Invasive Gynecol. 2008;15:172-5.
2. Morris H. Surgical pathology of the lower uterine segment caesarean section scar: is the scar a source of clinical symptoms? Int J Gynecol Pathol. 1995;14:16-20.
3. Joseph KS, Young DC, Dodds L, et al. Changes in maternal characteristics and obstetric practice and recent increases in primary cesarean delivery. Obstet Gynecol. 2003;102:791-800.
4. Rayburn WF, Schwartz WJ 3rd. Refinements in performing a cesarean delivery. Obstet Gynecol Surv. 1996;51:445-51.
5. Hofmeyr GJ, Mathai M, Shah A, et al. Techniques for caesarean section. Cochrane Database Syst Rev. 2008;(1):CD004662.

6. Fabres C, Aviles G, De La Jara C, et al. The cesarean delivery scar pouch: clinical implications and diagnostic correlation between transvaginal sonography and hysteroscopy. J Ultrasound Med. 2003;22:695-700.
7. Yazicioglu F, Gokdogan A, Kelekci S, et al. Incomplete healing of the uterine incision after caesarean section: is it preventable? Eur J Obstet Gynecol Reprod Biol. 2006;124:32-6.
8. Hayakawa H, Itakura A, Mitsui T, et al. Methods for myometrium closure and other factors impacting effects on cesarean section scars of the uterine segment detected by the ultrasonography. Acta Obstet Gynecol Scand. 2006;85:429-34.
9. Ofili-Yebovi D, Ben-Nagi J, Sawyer E, et al. Deficient lower-segment cesarean section scars: prevalence and risk factors. Ultrasound Obstet Gynecol. 2008;31:72-7.
10. Wang CB, Chiu WW, Lee CY, et al. Cesarean scar defect: correlation between cesarean section number, defect size, clinical symptoms and uterine position. Ultrasound Obstet Gynecol. 2009;34:85-9.
11. Osser OV, Jokubkiene L, Valentin L. Cesarean section scar defects: agreement between transvaginal sonographic findings with and without saline contrast enhancement. Ultrasound Obstet Gynecol. 2010;35:75-83.
12. Florio P, Filippeschi M, Moncini I, et al. Hysteroscopic treatment of the cesarean-induced isthmocele in restoring infertility. Curr Opin Obstet Gynecol. 2012;24(3):180-6.
13. Tsuji S, Murakami T, Kimura F, et al. Management of secondary infertility following cesarean section: report from the Subcommittee of the Reproductive Endocrinology Committee of the Japan Society of Obstetrics and Gynecology. J Obstet Gynaecol Res. 2015;41:1305-12.
14. Tanimura S, Funamoto H, Hosono T, et al. New diagnostic criteria and operative strategy for cesarean scar syndrome: endoscopic repair for secondary infertility caused by cesarean scar defect. J Obstet Gynaecol Res. 2015;41:1363-9.
15. Regnard C, Nosbusch M, Fellemans C, et al. Cesarean section scar evaluation by saline contrast sonohysterography. Ultrasound Obstet Gynecol. 2004; 23:289-92.
16. Poidevin LO, Bockner VY. A hysterographic study of uteri after cesarean section. J Obstet Gynaecol Br Emp. 1958;65:278-83.
17. Bockner V. Hysterography and ruptured uterus. J Obstet Gynaecol Br Emp. 1960;67:838-9.
18. Fabres C, Alam V, Balmaceda J, et al. Comparison of ultrasonography and hysteroscopy in the diagnosis of intrauterine lesions in infertile women. J Am Assoc Gynecol Laparosc. 1998;5:375-8.
19. Chang Y, Tsai EM, Long CY, et al. Resectoscopic treatment combined with sonohysterographic evaluation of women with postmenstrual bleeding as a result of previous cesarean delivery scar defects. Am J Obstet Gynecol. 2009;200:370.e1-4.
20. Gubbini G, Centini G, Nascetti D, et al. Surgical hysteroscopic treatment of cesarean-induced isthmocele in restoring fertility: a prospective study. J Minim Invasive Gynecol. 2011;18:234-7.
21. Florio P, Gubbini G, Marra E, et al. A retrospective case-control study comparing hysteroscopic resection versus hormonal modulation in treating menstrual disorders due to isthmocele. Gynecol Endocrinol. 2011;27:434-8.
22. Fabres C, Arriagada P, Fernandez C, et al. Surgical treatment and follow-up of women with intermenstrual bleeding due to cesarean section scar defect. J Minim Invasive Gynecol. 2005;12:25-8.
23. Api M, Boza A, Gorgen H, et al. Should cesarean scar defect be treated laparoscopically? A case report and review of the literature. J Minim Invasive Gynecol. 2015;22(7):1145-52.

Accompanying Video: Laparoscopic repair of cesarean scar defect.

CHAPTER

37

Laparoscopic Management of Adhesions and Prevention

Divyesh V Shukla, Shilpi D Shukla, G Hemasree

INTRODUCTION

It is expected more than 50% of patients who undergo gynecological surgery and surgical trauma will develop adhesions. The risk after laparotomy is high up to 95% and following laparoscopic surgery where the risk varies from 50% to 100%.[1-3] Others express a very low incidence of 5% adhesion risk following laparoscopic surgery. In similar way women undergoing laparotomy *via* a midline incision had a 50% incidence of umbilical adhesions, whereas women undergoing laparoscopy had only a 1.6% incidence of umbilical adhesions.[4] Certain gynecological diseases, infection and inflammation will result in adhesions and in patients who receive radiation can be the cause of adhesion formation in them. Some of such examples are pelvic inflammatory disease (PID), endometriosis, pelvic bleeding, genital tuberculosis, genital malignancies, and following pelvic irradiation. Surgeons' learning curve is also associated with more risk of adhesion in the beginning.[5]

Adhesions represent nonfunctional scar tissue and are highly cellular, vascularized, and innervated.

The adhesion formation leads to many morbidities as pelvic pain related to menstruation, infertility, abdominal pain, symptoms of bowel obstruction, chronic pelvic pain, and/or decreased quality of life.[6,7] It should be clear after adhesiolysis the readhesion formation rate are as high as 80–90%. In this circumstance, every effort should be made to minimize this risk. Despite of seriousness of this problem less success have been achieved for its prevention and limited research has been made so far.[8,9]

PATHOGENESIS

Adhesions are defined as abnormal fibrous connections between anatomic surfaces. They develop as a result of inflammatory processes but most frequently secondary to surgical trauma (incision, cauterization, suturing, foreign material, drying of peritoneal surface, blood clots in peritoneal cavity, etc.). Adhesions are more likely when contacting surface of peritoneum is injured.

Injury to peritoneal surfaces initiates repair response and inflammatory process and bleeding results in local hypoxia and increased endothelial permeability results in serosanguineous exudation and lymphatic leakage.

The disruption of stromal mast cells will cause release of vasoactive substances including histamines, kinins, growth factors, and inflammation and finally this results in the foundation of a fibrin clot overlying the injured tissue.

Fibrin is deposited that contains exudates of cells, leukocytes, and macrophages. This process occurs within 3 hours after injury this is degraded by fibrinolysis within 72 hours.

Normal tissue repair is facilitated by this exudate, which attracts invading fibroblasts and angiogenesis. With complete fibrinolysis and reabsorption of degradation products, reepithelialization will result without evidence of adhesions.

Adhesions are the result of tissue trauma after which fibrinolytic activity that is compromised, fibrinous mass persisting, and fibroblast ingrowth occurring with deposition of extracellular matrix (ECM) material.

Tissue injury leads to a hypoxic state, which is an important advocate to modifying the cascade of responses that ultimately progresses to the development of postoperative adhesions.[10-13]

A reduction in plasmin promotes increased adhesion establishment by altering fibrinolysis.

Plasminogen activator activity (PAA), which is represented by the ratio of tissue plasminogen activator to its plasminogen activator inhibitor-1, resides in both the peritoneal mesothelial cells and the underlying fibroblasts. PAA endures typically with dissolution of the fibrinous mass by fibrinolysis for 72 hours.

The activated fibroblasts are removed by apoptosis allowing tissue to heal without inappropriate attachments to other tissues.

When fibrinolytic activity is compromised, the fibrinous structure remains, and fibroblast ingrowth occurs with deposition of ECM material including collagen, which forms atypical connections between tissue to form adhesions. Imbalance between fibrin deposition and fibrinolysis is the key driver in the development of postoperative adhesions.[14-17]

Role of hypoxia induced release of reactive oxygen species (ROS) such as superoxide seems to be a major factor in the development of postoperative adhesions. Reactive nitrogen species (RNS) as well as antioxidant enzymes such as superoxide dismutase, catalase, and glutathione peroxidase, which when optimal have the potential to abrogate the abnormal milieu, preventing the cascade of events leading to the development of adhesions in injured peritoneum have been extensively studied.[18]

Under normal physiological conditions, eukaryotic cells are under aerobic conditions and have an innate defense system against ROS which contributes to the maintenance of the balance between prooxidants (free radical species) and the body's scavenging ability (antioxidants).

Reactive oxygen species and RNS are also known to contribute to vascular dysfunction and remodeling through oxidative damage by reducing the bioavailability of NO, impairing endothelium-dependent vasodilatation and endothelial cell growth, causing apoptosis, stimulating endothelial cell migration, and activating adhesion molecules. These functions are strictly linked with the mediators of the inflammatory pathways.[19,20]

Adhesion Score

To have uniformity in description of adhesions this scoring appears relevant.[21,22] Almost every preoperative and intraoperative points are covered in this scoring system. This scoring or similar such scoring may help in uniform pattern in reporting. The authors say, "we encourage gynecological surgeons to use the adhesion risk score to evaluate the risk of adhesions in their patients in a consistent fashion and thus assist in making both better informed decisions and justification for use of appropriate preventive measures in high-risk patients, especially in younger women identified as at high risk of adhesions who wish to conceive" We agree to their statement.

DIAGNOSIS

A history of previous surgery, having diagnosis of pelvic or bowel pathology of have undergone irradiation is important. Note presenting symptoms of the patient include points to find out primary disease. On abdominal examination, scar over the abdomen, distension, tympanic percussion notes, tenderness indicated obstructive disease or peritonitis. Per speculum and prevaginal examination help in finding out uterine mobility, pelvic pathology, and adhesions with anterior abdominal wall. Rectal examination to find out fibrosis or induration of adnexal region, rectovaginal disease, and adhesion with uterus.

Laboratory investigations are targeted to find out primary or secondary etiology.

Imaging is valuable to rule out etiologies for a patient's symptoms and give an indication of extent of adhesions between organs. This includes abdominal and pelvic sonography, MRI, and required CT scan. Sliding organ test on transvaginal sonography (TVS) is for identifying pelvic adhesions.

NONSURGICAL TREATMENT

Various drugs are used for symptomatic treatment for pain in patients with adhesions.

Dyspepsia may be treated by simethicone, proton pump inhibitors, and nortriptyline with variable efficacy, depending on the extent to which symptoms are attributable to adhesions as well as their severity.

High fiber supplementation to treat constipation is not recommended. Instead non-bulking, non-stimulant agents such as polyethylene glycol along with low residue diet may be used. For cramp-like symptoms, smooth muscle relaxants such as dicyclomine may be indicated. In gynecology disease specific drugs, if available, may be given which could be the cause of adhesion. Dienogest is used in cases of pelvic endometriosis if the criteria are fulfilled for its indication of its use. This is for pain relief and its efficacy of treating the disease. For pelvic pain because of adhesions, anti-inflammatory drugs are used with varying success.

SURGICAL TREATMENT

Laparoscopic or Robotic Adhesiolysis

Laparoscopy is commonly used for adhesiolysis because of the shorter recovery time, lower incidence of pain, infection, and readhesion formation in comparison with laparotomy.

One may use mechanical bowel preparation or may not. In case extensive bowel adhesions are expected it may help to simultaneous deal with bowel injury. Primary pneumoperitoneum may be carried out through umbilicus or alternative sites as Palmer's point. In our unpublished data of more than 10 years have shown adhesions at exact umbilical site are very rare except in some cases of umbilical hernia, operated for umbilical hernia and previous laparotomy for gastrointestinal complications. The rates are in <1%.[23] Although literature reports contradictory findings and mentions very high rates of infraumbilical adhesions and not umbilical site.[24] Visual method of entry should be used in all cases where adhesions are expected. In patients with past history of surgery/surgeries either laparotomy or laparoscopy, same approach is selected. Primary trocar is usually inserted above 3–4 cm of upper margin of umbilicus after creating pneumoperitoneum.

Surgeons may prefer open method of primary trocar insertion in these cases or otherwise. All other ancillary trocars are inserted under vision. If possible, removal of omental adhesions is done by adhesiolysis through upper abdominal additional port to facilitate ancillary trocar entry at regular pelvic site of insertion. At times these pelvic site trocars might be inserted through adherent omentum with parietal peritoneum. Make sure there is no bowel loop between omentum and abdominal wall.

Laparoscopic adhesiolysis provides short and long-term therapeutic benefits. Laparoscopic surgery in experienced hand is highly successful, however, complex, and/or dense adhesions are present. Traction on both organ and peritoneal surface is essential to divide adhesion in correct tissue plane. Patient counseling regarding co existing pathology treatment and chance of readhesion formation should be done. All intraperitoneal adhesions or bowel adhesions cannot be removed or may not be removed. Some asymptomatic adhesions detected may not be lysed.

Surgery is simultaneously aimed to treat the pathology causing adhesion.

When attempt to separate firm bowel adhesions is made, it may risk bowel injury. If diagnosis is not sure with respect of suspected adhesions laparoscopy can confirm or modify the diagnosis and change management and outcome. The risk of laparoscopic surgery may be higher in the acutely obstructed bowel compared to the elective setting.

All energy sources are suitable for adhesiolysis, monopolar, bipolar electrosurgery, scissors, and ultrasound energy during laparoscopy or laparotomy. Peritoneal adhesions with omentum and bowel are cut identifying the line of adhesion. Flimsy avascular adhesions get separated by blunt dissection. Injury to serosa or peritoneal surface is avoided. Adhesion bands are excised from both surfaces instead of dividing them. Most complicated adhesions can be lysed by using scissors. In majority of cases my preference is scissors. Start dividing superficial adhesions and later the deeper ones. Scissors remain as the first choice for adhesiolysis. When adhesiolysis is performed in proper anatomical planes generally there is no bleeding. Some thin

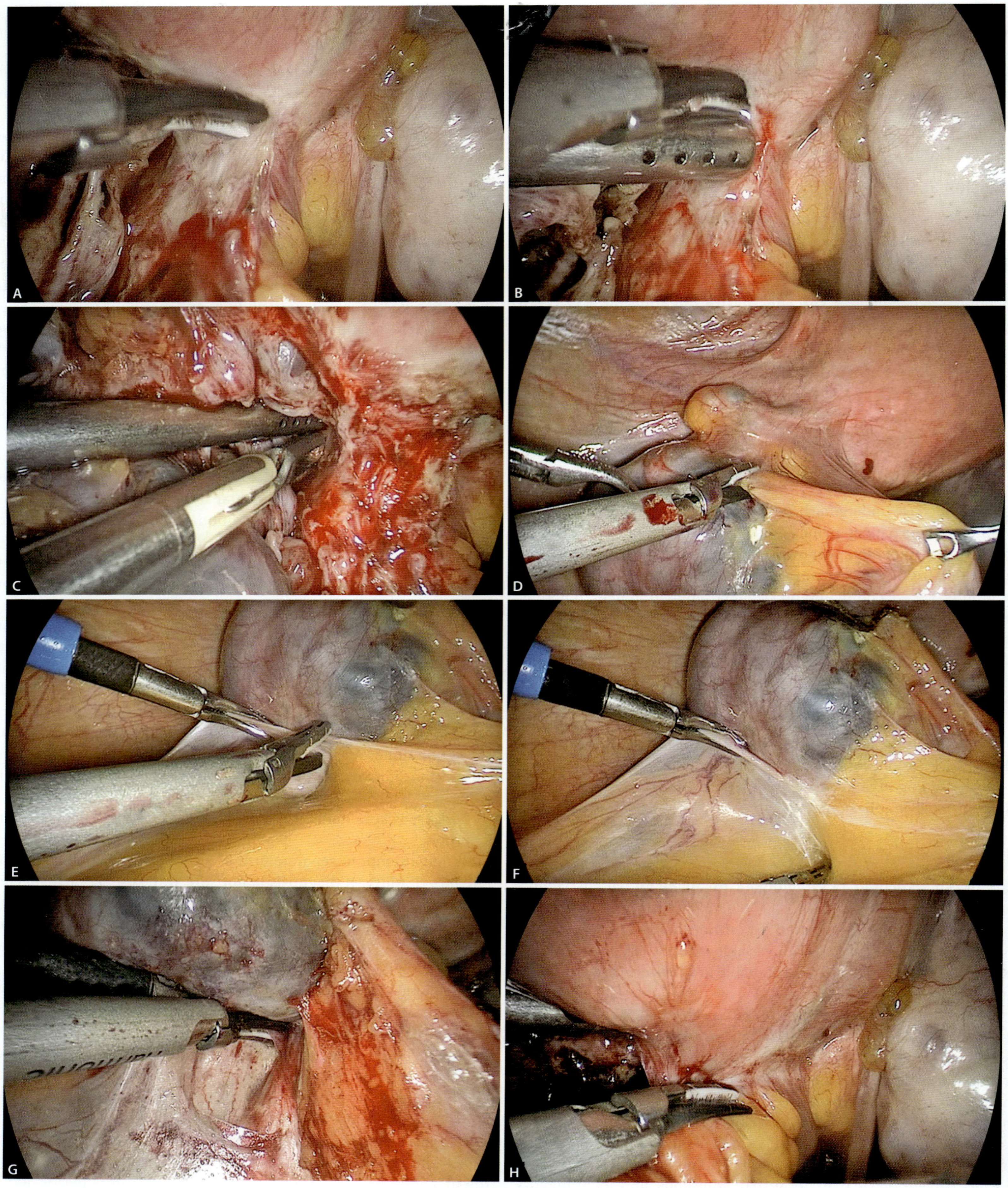

Figs. 1A to H: Sigmoid adhesion with left adnexa and uterus.

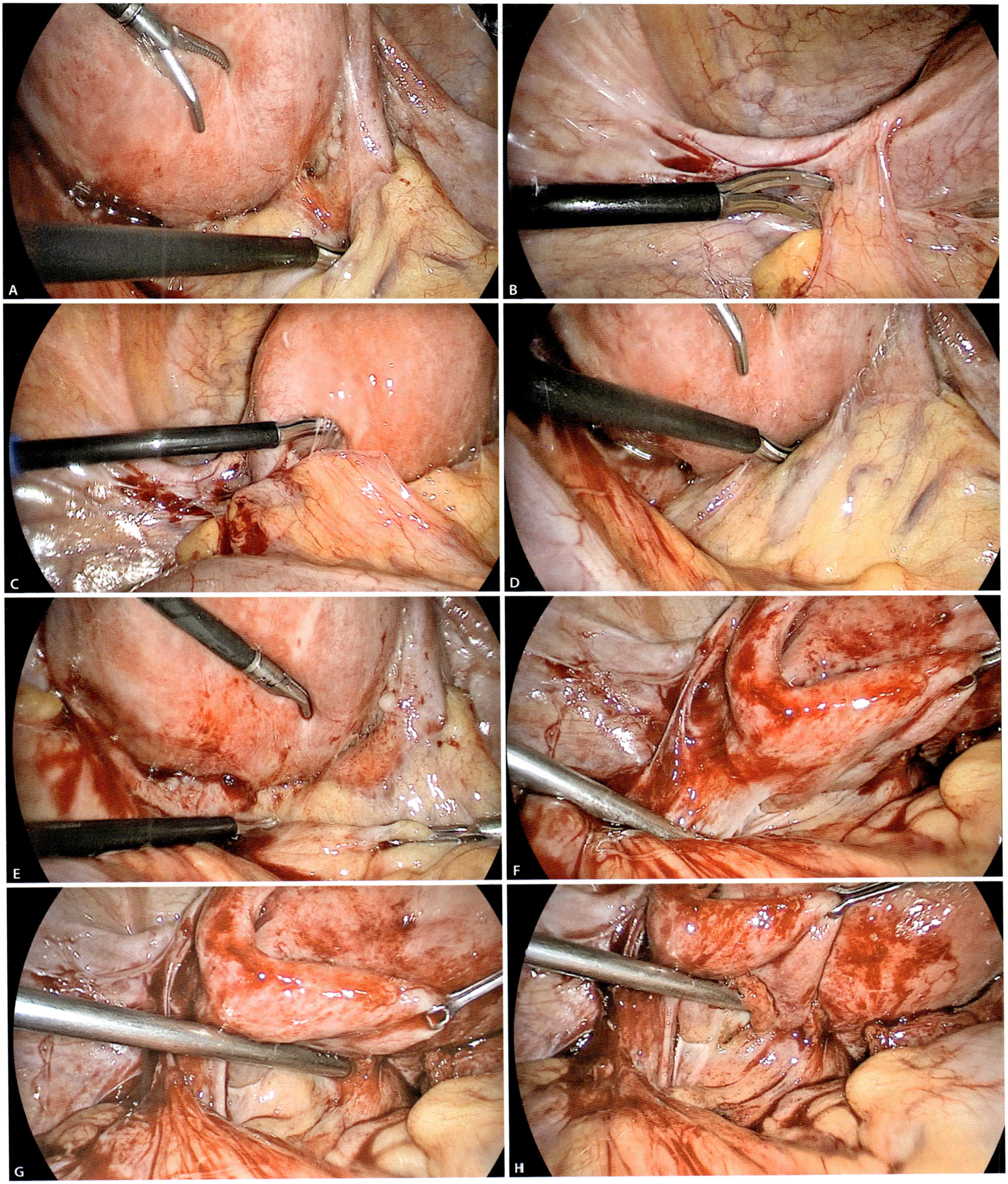

Figs. 2A to H: Sigmoid adhesiolysis with scissors.

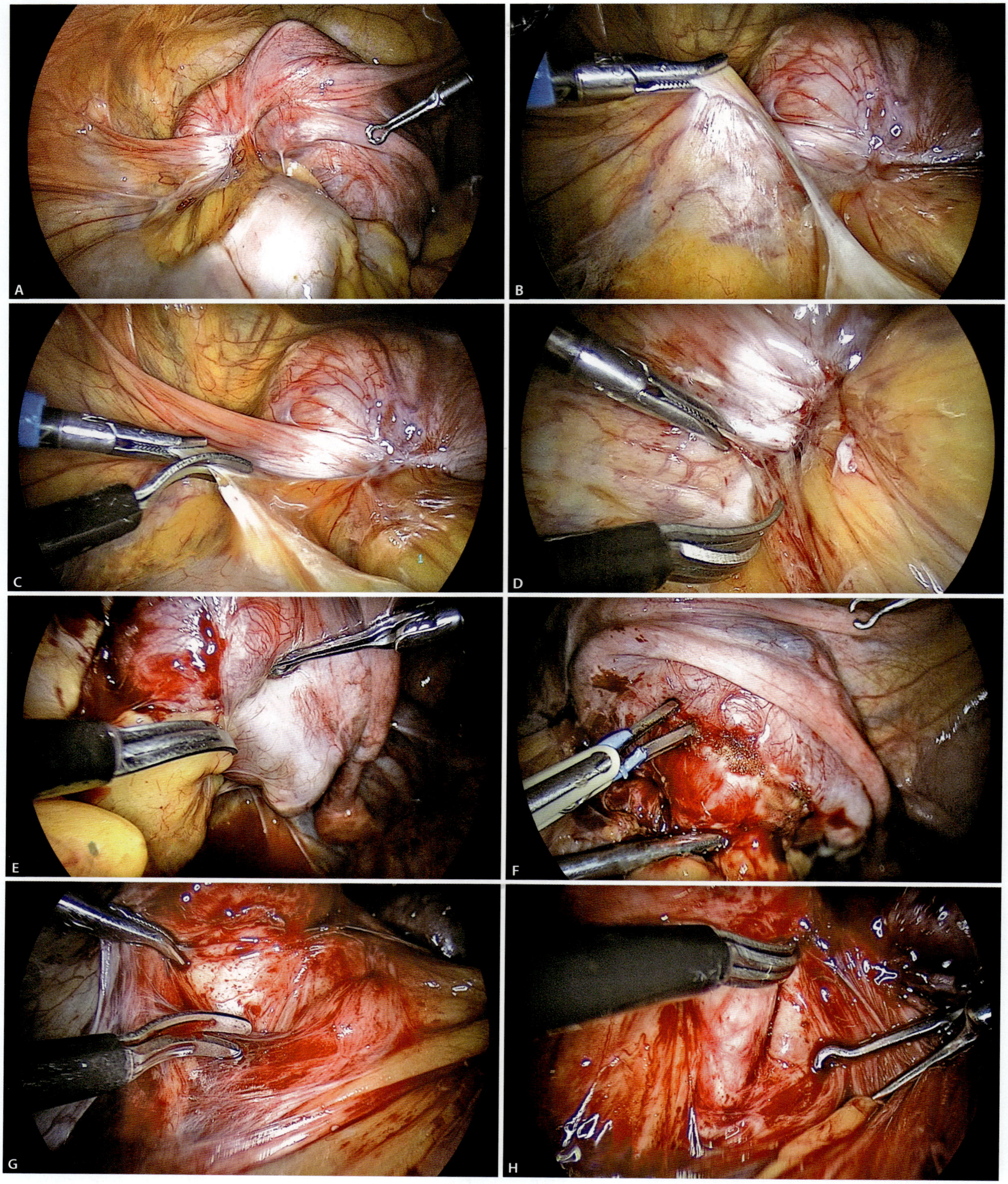

Figs. 3A to H

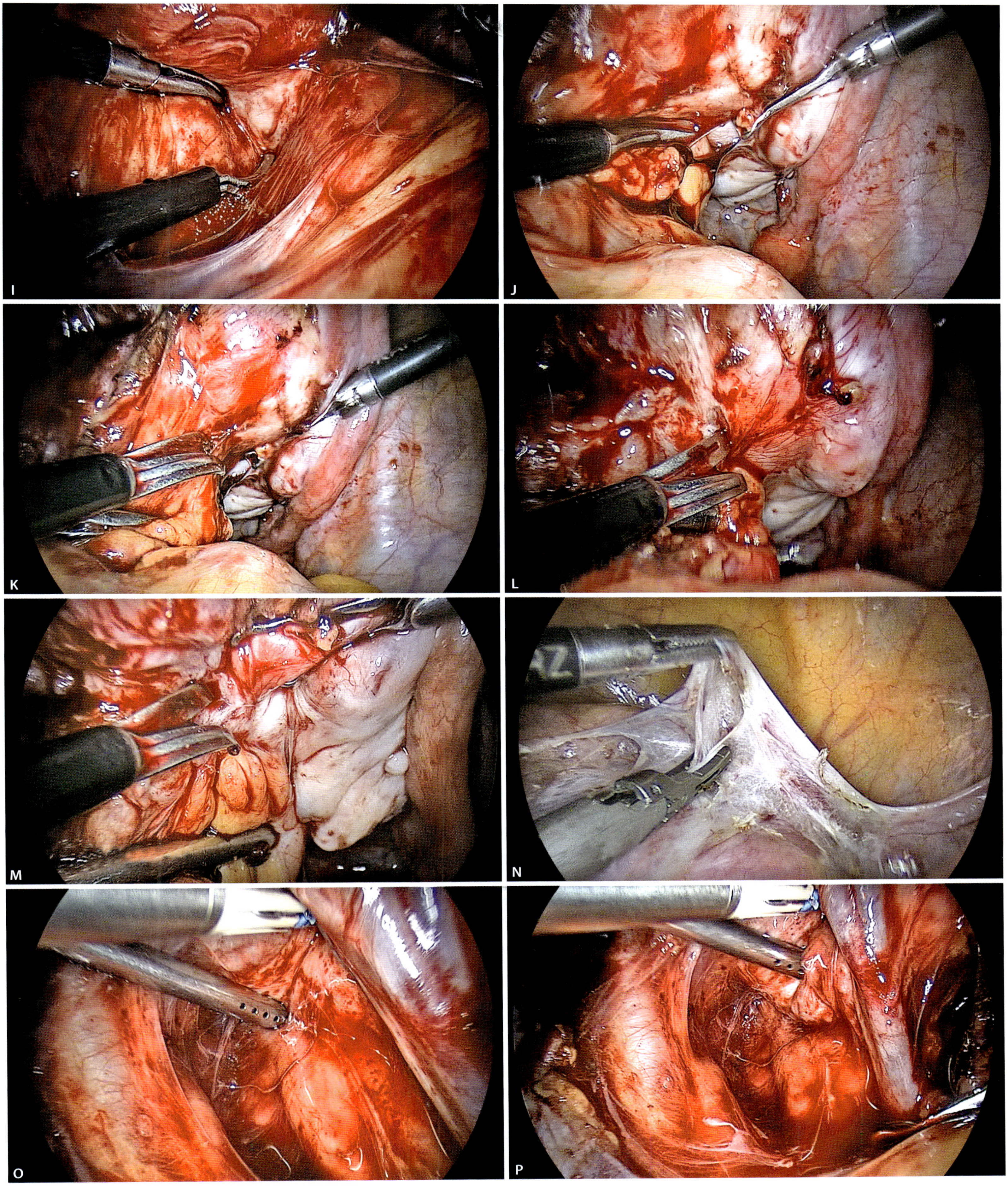

Figs. 3I to P

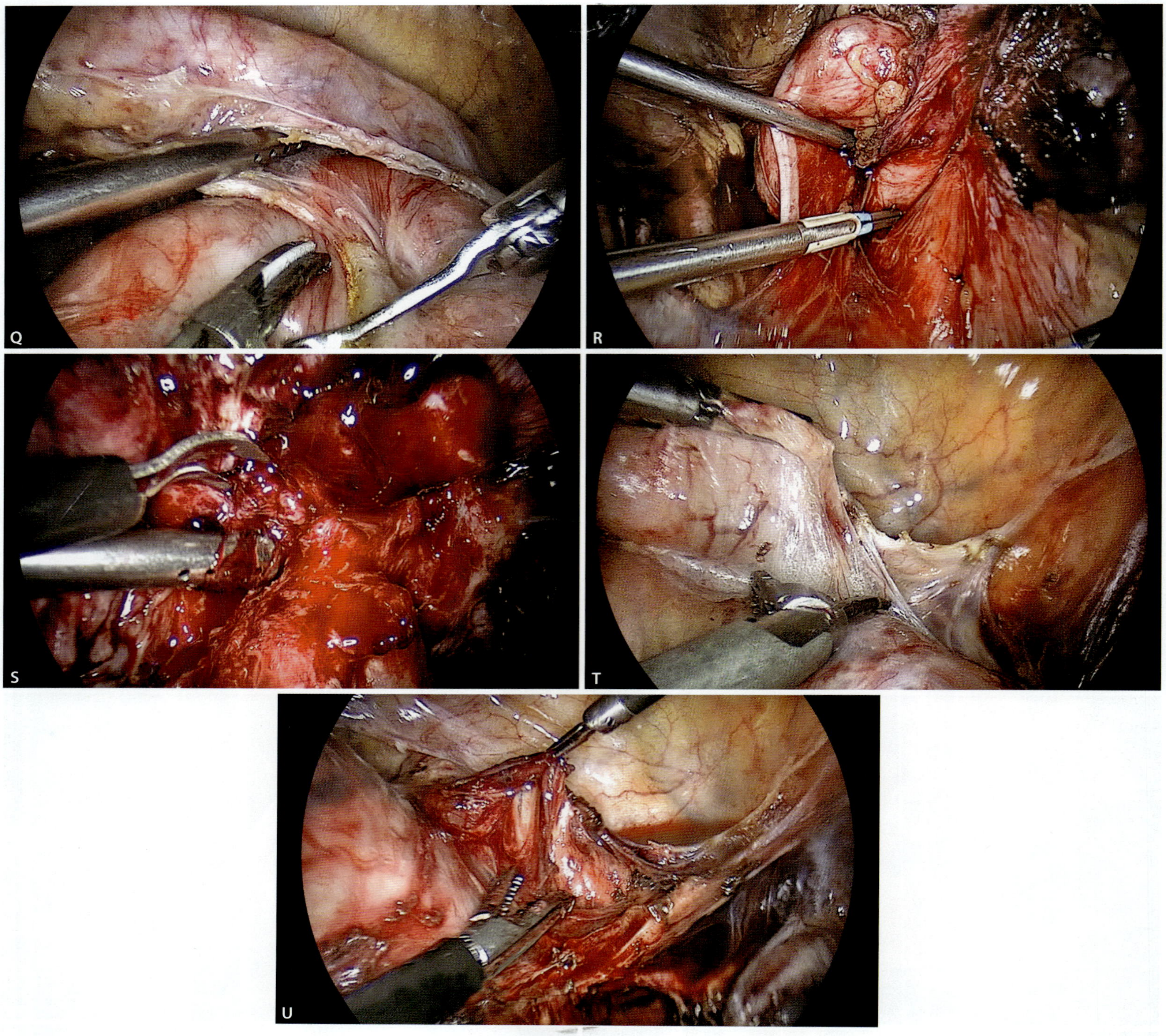

Figs. 3Q to U

Figs. 3A to U: Sigmoid adhesions with uterus, adnexa, and obliterated pouch of Douglas (POD).

transparent wide film of adhesions uniting two surfaces also requires dividing from both surfaces and removing them instead of just dividing them. Copious irrigation may be used as required. This also helps in preventing dryness of the surfaces. Complete hemostasis is achieved following dissection. Other microsurgical principles are followed.

Elective laparoscopic adhesiolysis in those with chronic GI symptoms, 70% achieved complete adhesiolysis, and 80% experienced complete resolution of symptoms suggesting that even partial adhesiolysis was effective; also, none of the cases required conversion to open surgery.[25]

Laparotomy Adhesiolysis

Alternatively, laparotomy is performed for adhesiolysis in case the surgeon is not a laparoscopic surgeon. The rate of conversion from laparoscopic to open adhesiolysis for a small-bowel obstruction has been reported to be as high as 32%. Some authors recommend early conversion to laparotomy adhesiolysis in cases of difficult laparoscopic adhesionlysis as there can be increased rates of unrecognized sharp, blunt, or energy-related bowel injury during laparoscopic adhesiolysis. All other principles of surgery would remain same as mentioned earlier.

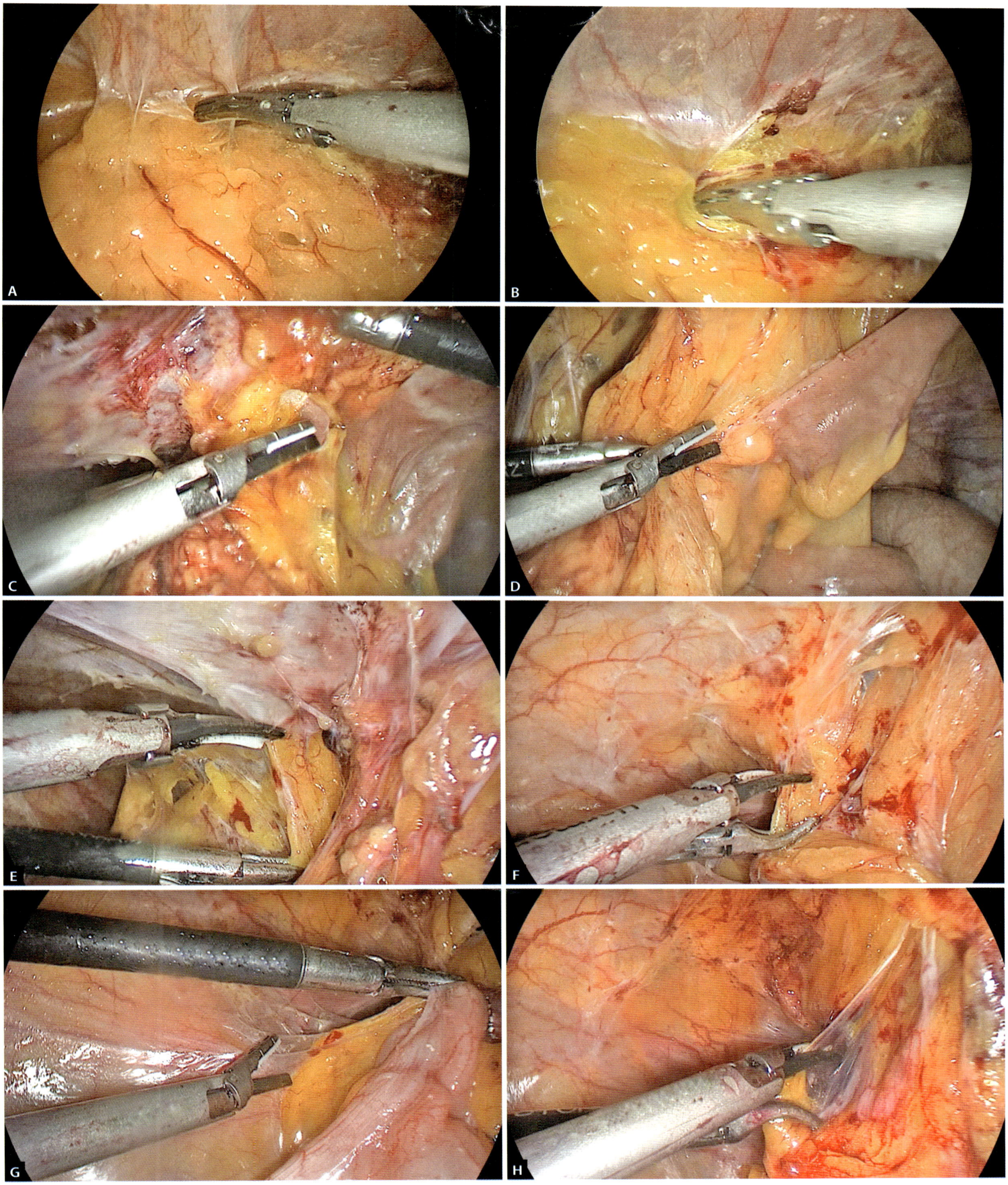

Figs. 4A to H

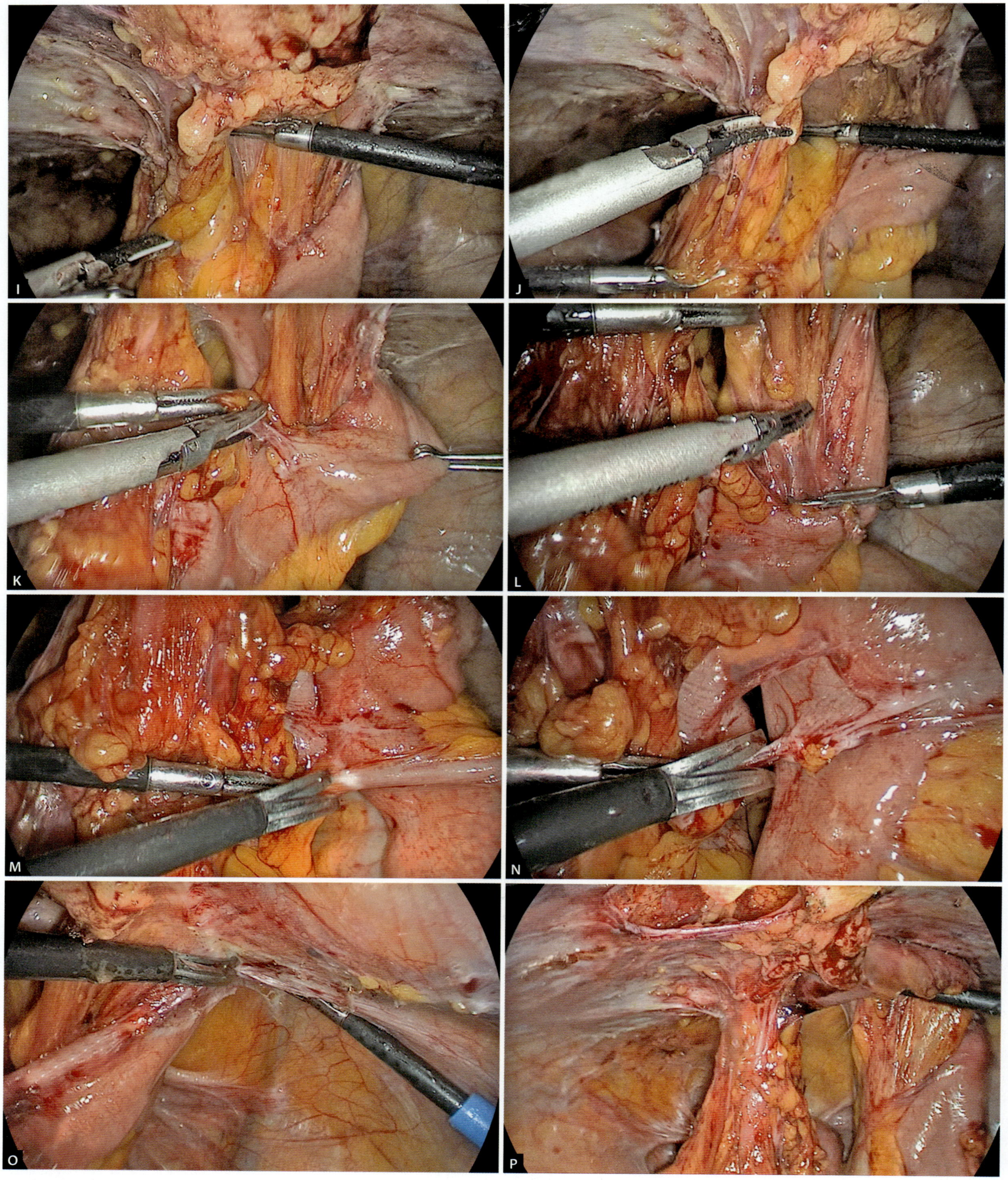

Figs. 4I to P

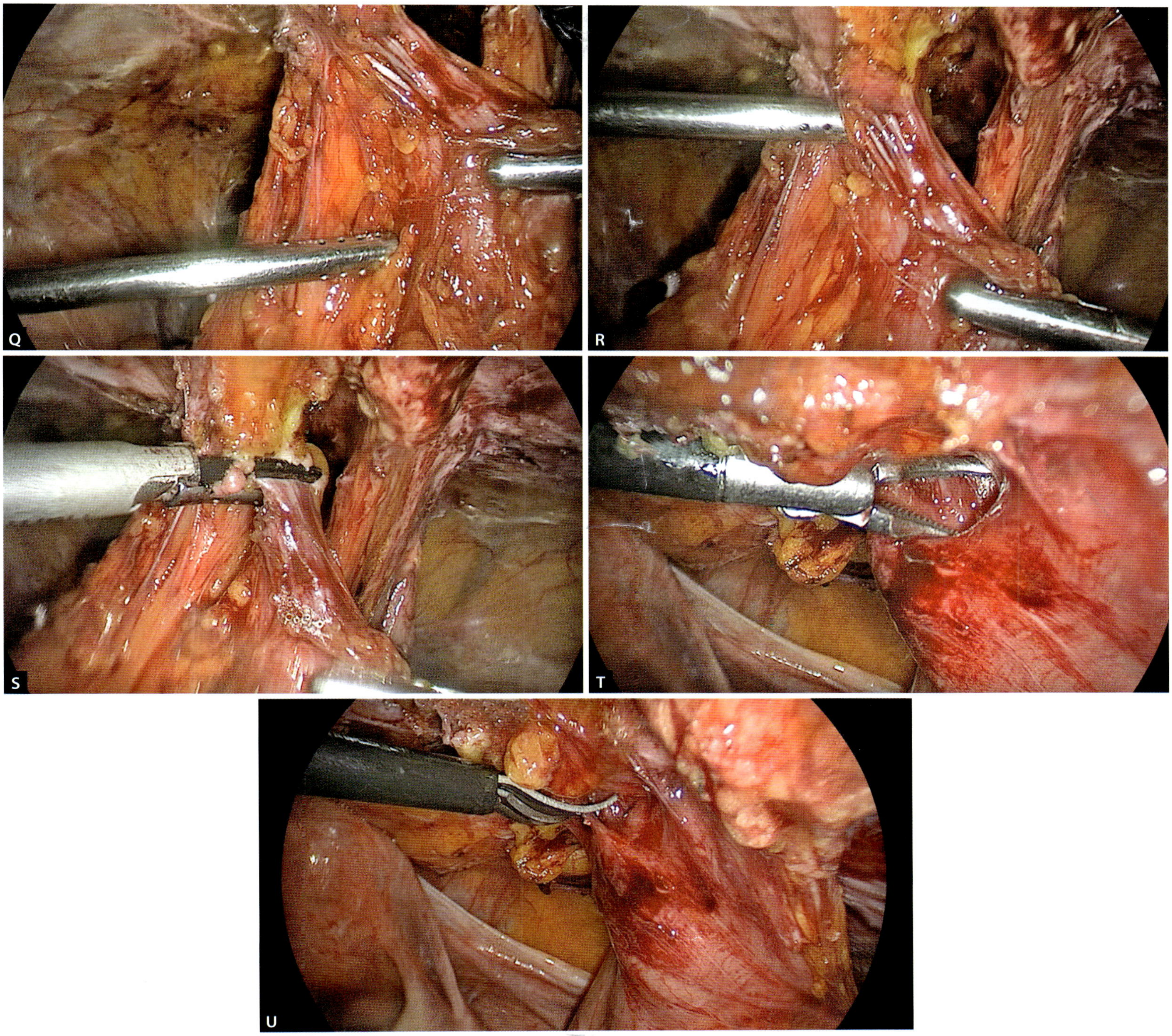

Figs. 4Q to U

Figs. 4A to U: Omental and bowel adhesions with anterior abdominal wall.

Adhesion Prevention

Strategies including the reduction of peritoneal damage, prevention of coagulation of serous exudate, resolution of fibrin deposits, inhibition of fibroblast activities, prevention of collagen deposits, and separation of peritoneal surfaces during formation of mesothelium again have been proposed to reduce adhesion risk. Meticulous surgical techniques and observing microsurgical principles of surgery are best for adhesion prevention. They include gentle and less handling of tissues, keeping peritoneal and surface of abdominal organs moist, preserving blood supply, proper use of electrocautery, complete hemostasis, placing less braided sutures in peritoneal cavity, etc. In case barbed sutures are used to close vaginal vault or otherwise, some authors recommend peritoneal closure over it or use of adhesion prevention barrier to cover them. This is to prevent incidental entanglement of soft tissue with them.

We additionally practice early intake of liquid and solid food in the postoperative period (4–6 hours) in low-risk patients along with early ambulation.

Various drugs and injectable (anti-inflammatory, fibrinolytic, anti-coagulants, corticosteroids, low dose intraperitoneal heparin, etc.) studied does not reduce the adhesion risk.[26]

Constant irrigation to moisten tissues, accuracy of hemostasis at the end of surgery, the suturing technique, correct and minimal placement of sutures, and attention to maintaining vascularity mainly depend on the surgeon's experience. Surgeons very often underestimate the clinical problems of adhesions and their complications

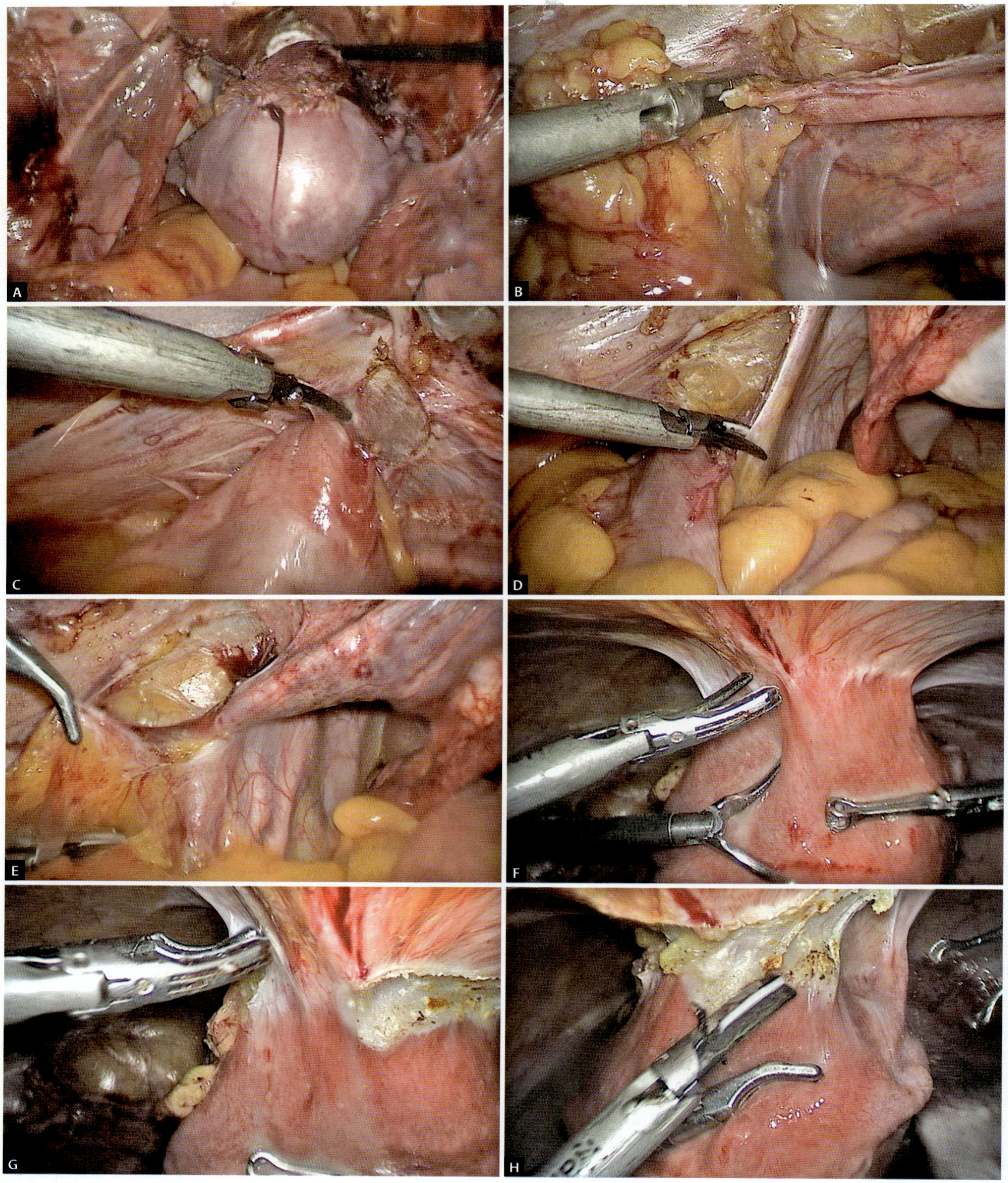

Figs. 5A to H

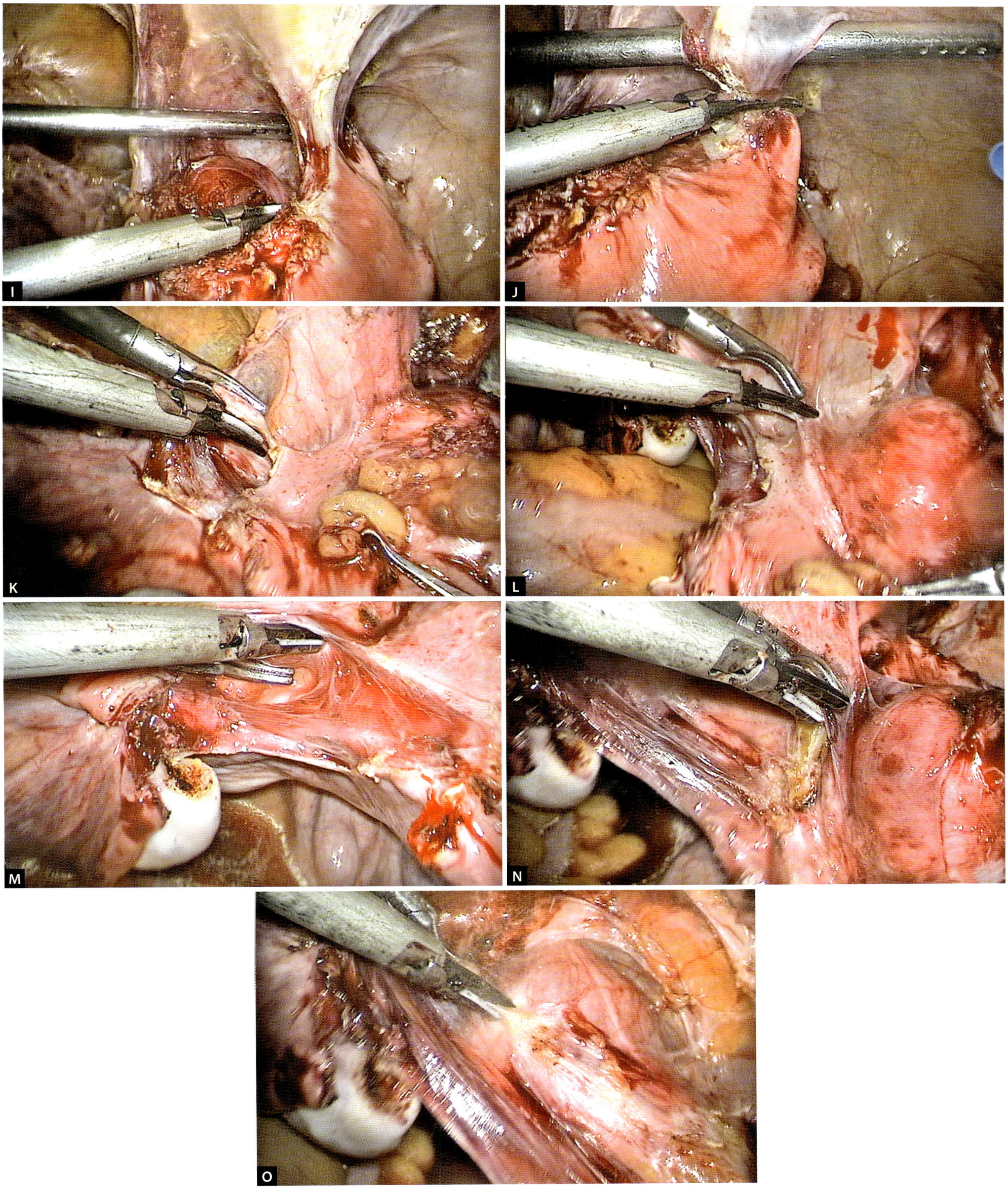

Figs. 5I to O

Figs. 5A to O: Adhesion of uterus with anterior abdominal wall.

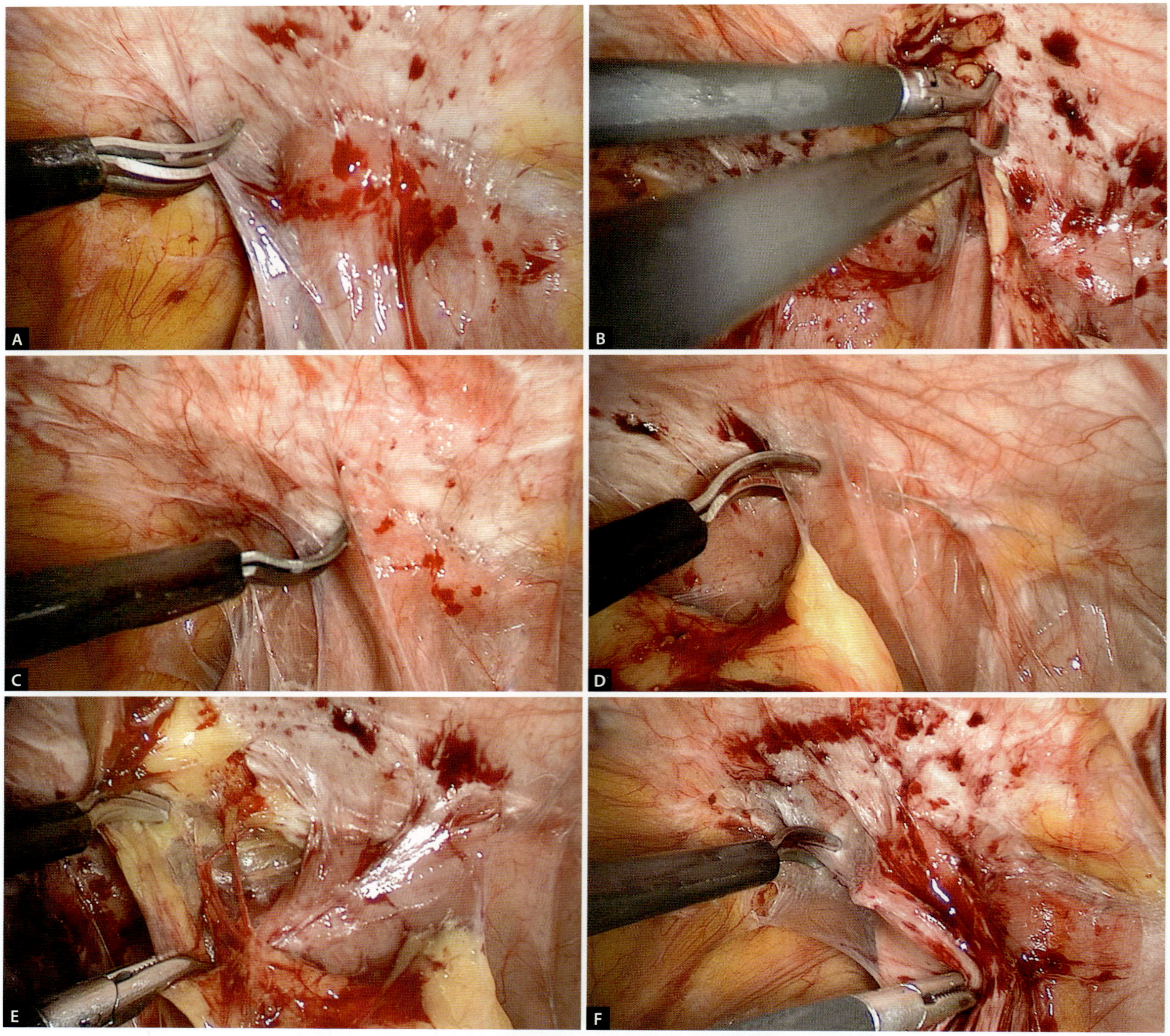

Figs. 6A to F: Bowel adhesions with anterior abdominal wall.

and only surgeons with the proper perception and knowledge of the problem of adhesions are likely to undertake adhesion prevention during surgery. And so, with an expert surgeon likelihood of adhesion are low.[27]

A systematic review and meta-analysis of randomized, controlled trials evaluated the efficacy of and side effects experienced with the intraperitoneal application of four antiadhesion barriers (an oxidized regenerated cellulose absorbable barrier, a sodium hyaluronate/carboxymethylcellulose absorbable barrier, a polyethylene glycol sprayable barrier, and icodextrin 4% solution) after abdominal surgery.

None of the barriers showed serious side effects compared to controls. Both the oxidized regenerated cellulose absorbable barrier and the sodium hyaluronate/carboxymethylcellulose absorbable barrier significantly reduced peritoneal adhesion formation.

The sodium hyaluronate/carboxymethylcellulose absorbable barrier reduced the incidence of small-bowel obstruction.[28] Currently here are some gels being tried in experimental study for adhesion prevention.

Polyethylene glycol has been evaluated in three clinical trials investigating laparoscopic myomectomy. This sprayable barrier seems to be efficacious in reducing de novo peritoneal adhesion development.[27] Luckily, I was witness to this study as during the same time we were enrolled for fellowship program with the University of Kiel hospital, Kiel Germany, in the year 2000.

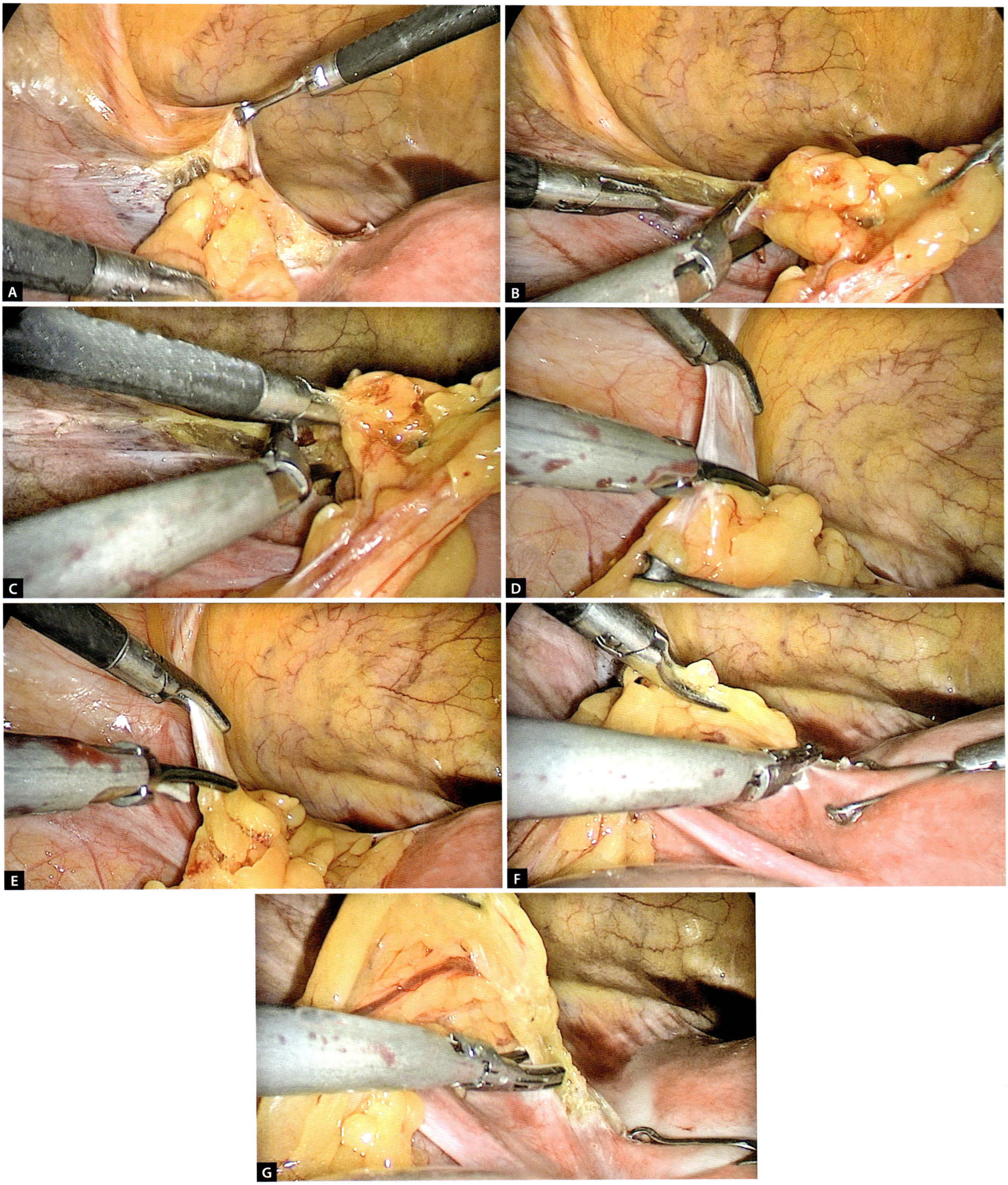

Figs. 7A to G: Omental adhesion with vesical per toneum.

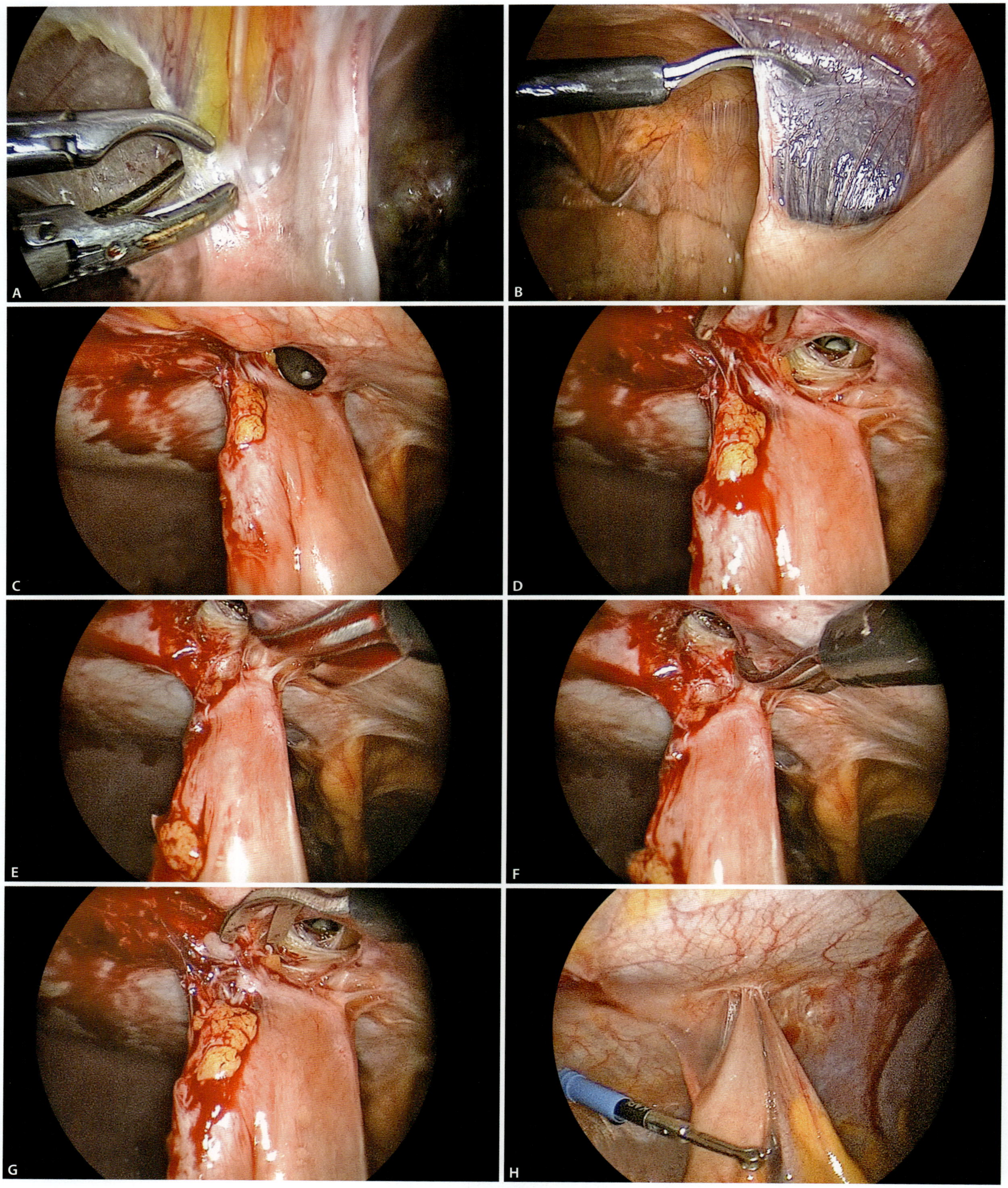

Figs. 8A to H

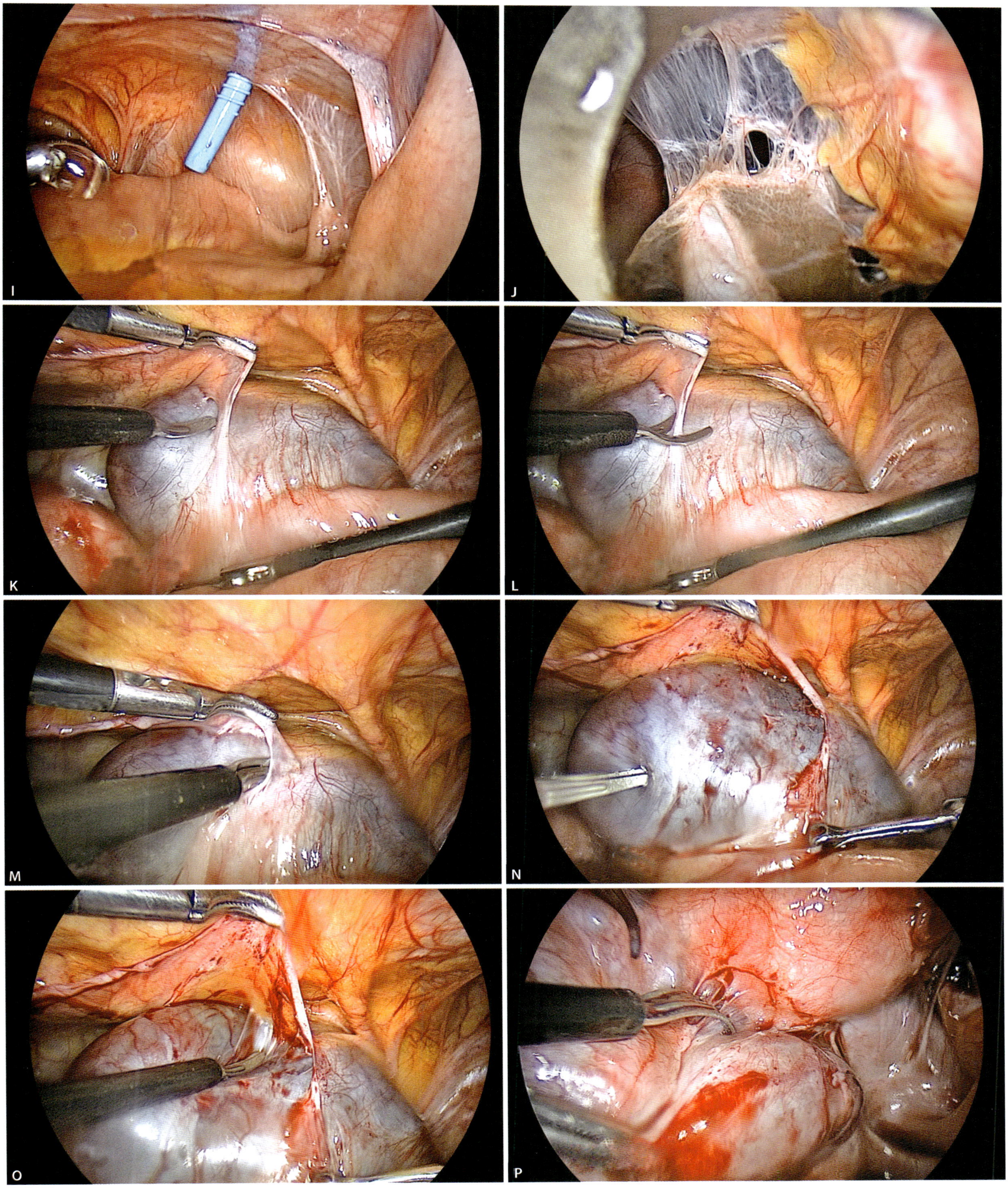

Figs. 8I to P

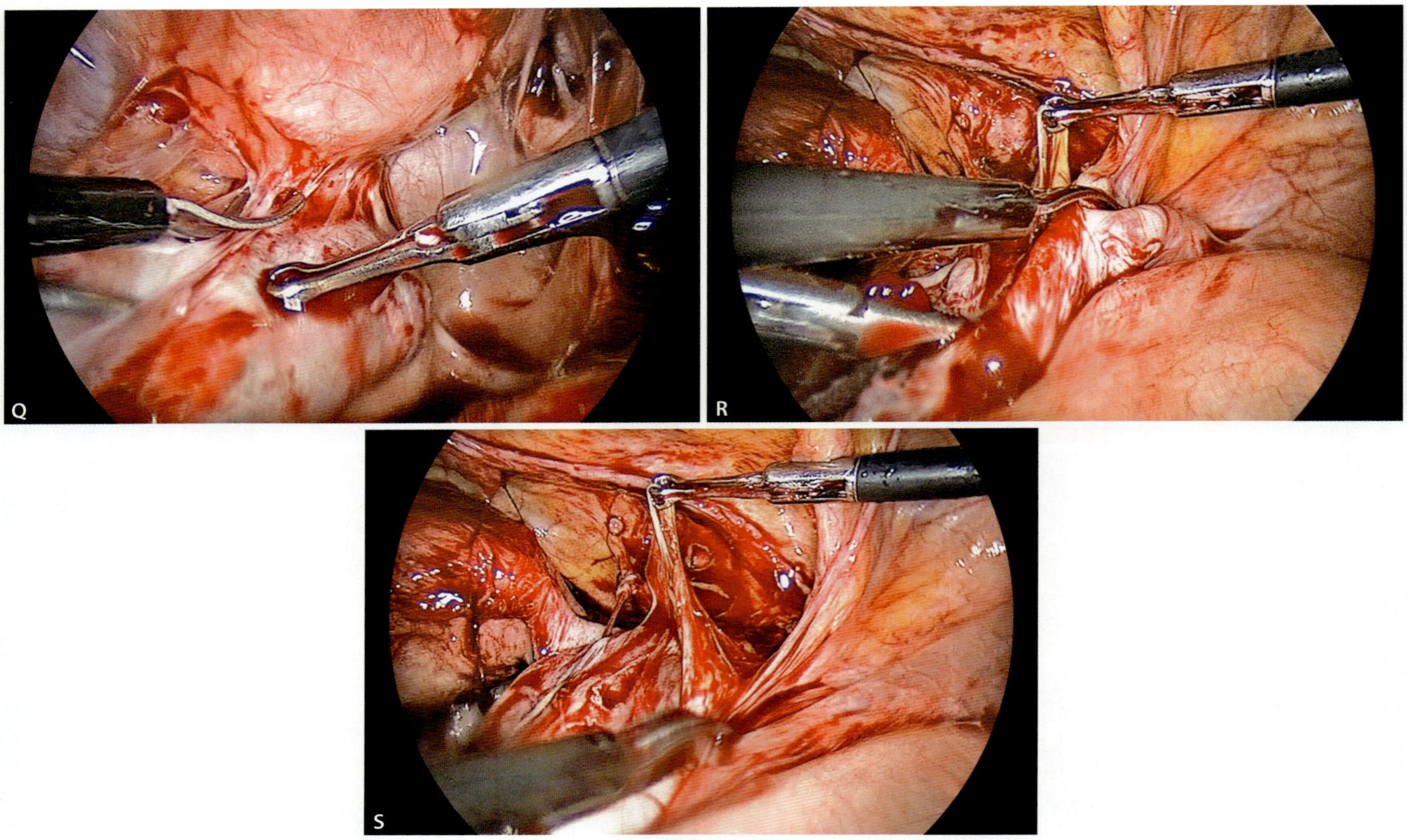

Figs. 8Q to S

Figs. 8A to S: Pelvic adhesions and anterior abdominal wall adhesions.

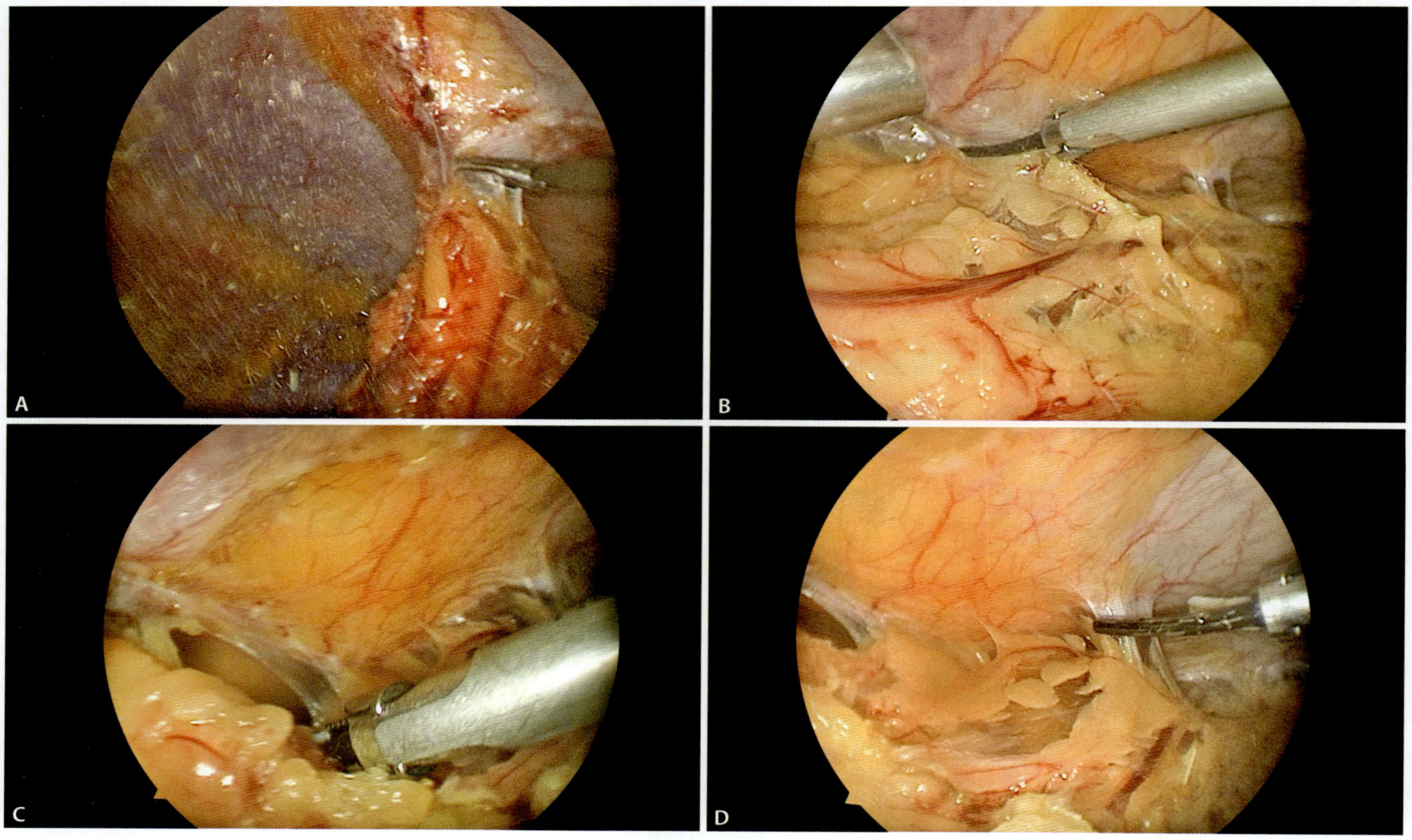

Figs. 9A to D

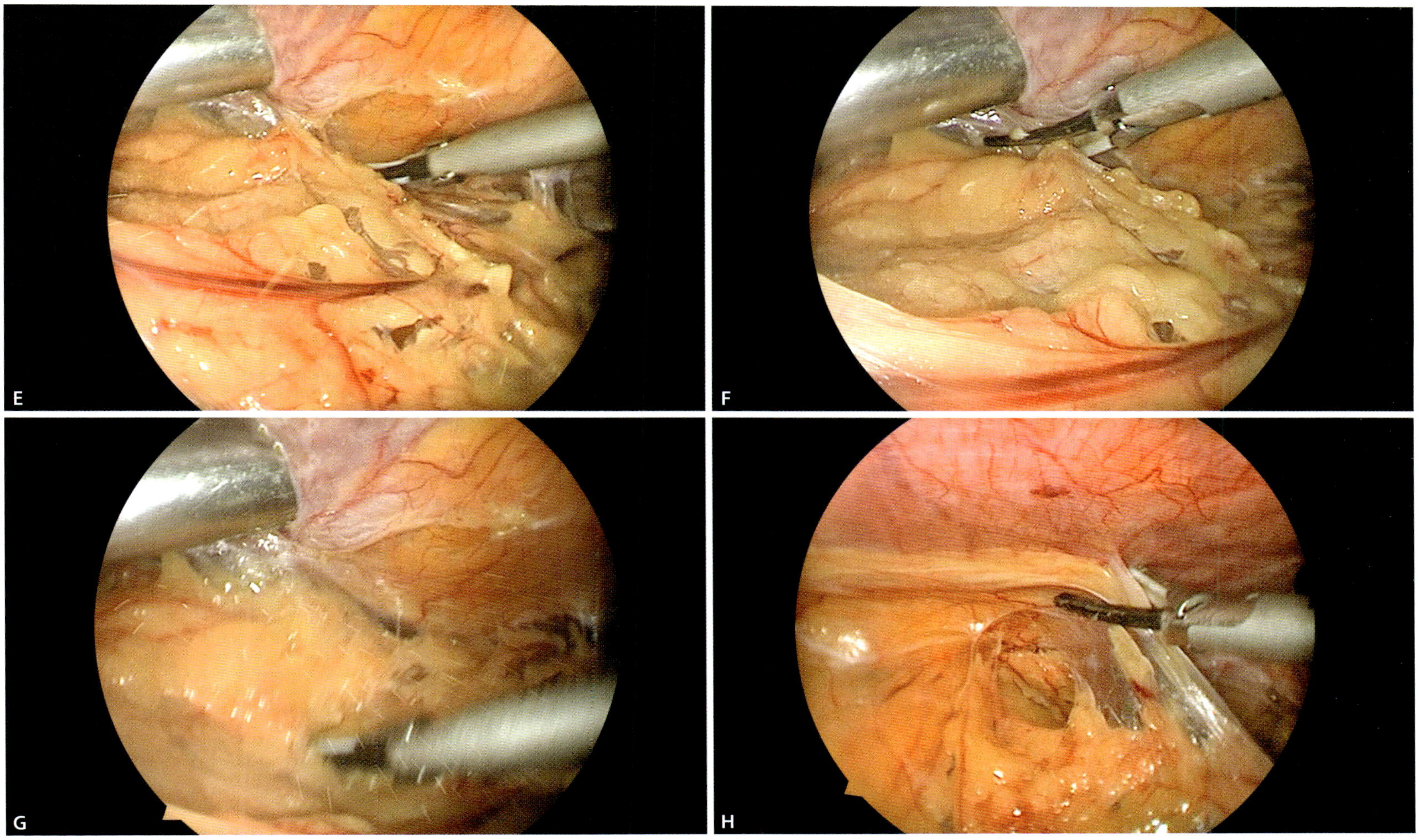

Figs. 9E to H

Figs. 9A to H: Omental adhesion around primary trocar site.

SUMMARY

Adhesion and readhesion formation are cause of morbidity and infertility. Adhesions should be taken seriously as they can cause significant discomfort, complicate future operative procedures by altering anatomy, increase risk for bowel obstruction, and affect fertility in women. The satisfactory reduction of postsurgical adhesions and its adverse sequelae is challenge despite a large number of scientific researches in the topic available.

REFERENCES

1. Ellis H. The magnitude of adhesion related problems. Ann Chir Gynaecol. 1998;87:9-11.
2. diZerega GS. Biochemical events in peritoneal tissue repair. Eur J Surg Suppl. 1997;577:10-6.
3. Ellis H, Moran BJ, Thompson JN. Adhesion related hospital admissions after abdominal and pelvis surgery: a retrospective cohort study. Lancet. 1999;353:1476-80.
4. Audebert AJ, Gomel V. Role of microlaparoscopy in the diagnosis of peritoneal and visceral adhesions and in the prevention of bowel injury associated with blind trocar insertion. Fertil Steril. 2000;73:631-5.
5. Mais V, Ajossa S, Piras B, et al. Prevention of de-novo adhesion formation after laparoscopic myomectomy: a randomized trial to evaluate the effectiveness of an oxidized regenerated cellulose absorbable barrier. Hum Reprod. 1995;10:3133-5.
6. Porpora MG, Koninckx PR, Piazze J, et al. Correlation between endometriosis and pelvic pain. J Am Assoc Gynecol Laparosc. 1999;6:429-34.
7. The American Fertility Society classifications of adnexal adhesions, distal tubal occlusion, tubal occlusion secondary to tubal ligation, tubal pregnancies, müllerian anomalies and intrauterine adhesions. Fertil Steril. 1988;49:944-55.
8. Ray NF, Denton WG, Thamer M, et al. Abdominal adhesiolysis: inpatient care and expenditures in the United States in 1994. J Am Coll Surg. 1998; 186:1-9.
9. De Wilde RL, Brölmann H, Koninckx PR, et al. Prevention of adhesions in gynaecological surgery: the 2012 European field guideline. Gynecol Surg. 2012;9:365-8.
10. Saed GM, Diamond MP. Molecular characterization of postoperative adhesions: the adhesion phenotype. J Am Assoc Gynecol Laparosc. 2004; 11:307-14.
11. Vipond MN, Whawell SA, Thompson JN, et al. Peritoneal fibrinolytic activity and intra-abdominal adhesions. Lancet. 1990;335:1120-2.
12. Dunn RC, Buttram VC Jr. Tissue-type plasminogen activator as an adjuvant for post-surgical adhesions. Prog Clin Biol Res. 1990;358:113-8.
13. Desmouliere A, Redard M, Darby I, et al. Apoptosis mediates the decrease in cellularity during the transition between granulation tissue and scar. Am J Pathol. 1995;146:56-66.
14. Saed GM, Diamond MP. Hypoxia-induced irreversible up-regulation of type I collagen and transforming growth factor-beta1 in human peritoneal fibroblasts. Fertil Steril. 2002;78:144-7.
15. Hellebrekers BW, Emeis JJ, Kooistra T, et al. A role for the fibrinolytic system in postsurgical adhesion formation. Fertil Steril. 2005;83:122-9.
16. Shavell VI, Fletcher NM, Jiang ZL, et al. Uncoupling oxidative phosphorylation with 2,4-dinitrophenol promotes development of the adhesion phenotype. Fertil Steril. 2012;97:729-33.

17. Berra E, Pages G, Pouyssegur J. MAP kinases and hypoxia in the control of VEGF expression. Cancer Metastasis Rev. 2000;19:139-45.
18. Awonuga AO, Belotte J, Abuanzeh S, et al. Advances in the pathogenesis of adhesion development: the role of oxidative stress. Reprod Sci. 2014;21:823-36.
19. Yung LM, Leung FP, Yao X, et al. Reactive oxygen species in vascular wall. Cardiovasc Hematol Disord Drug Targets. 2006;6:1-19.
20. Crimi E, Ignarro LJ, Napoli C. Microcirculation and oxidative stress. Free Radic Res. 2007;41:1364-75.
21. Meuleman T, Schreinemacher MH, van Goor H, et al. Adhesion awareness: a nationwide survey of gynaecologists. Eur J Obstet Gynecol Reprod Biol. 2013;169:353-9.
22. Lundorff P, Brölmann H, Koninckx PR, et al. Predicting formation of adhesions after gynaecological surgery: development of a risk score. Arch Gynecol Obstet. 2015;292:931-8.
23. Kumakiri J, Kikuchi I, Kitade M, et al. Potential risk of port-site adhesions in patients after laparoscopic myomectomy using radially expanding trocars. Int J Gynaecol Obstet. 2015;128:5-9.
24. Sepilian V, Ku L, Wong H, et al. Prevalence of infraumbilical adhesions in women with previous laparoscopy. JSLS. 2007;11:41-4.
25. Onders R. Laparoscopy Effective for Management of Chronic Abdominal Pain. Gastroenterology and Endoscopy News; 2001. pp. 14-5.
26. Arung W, Meurisse M, Detry O. Pathophysiology and prevention of postoperative peritoneal adhesions. World J Gastroenterol. 2011;17:4545-53.
27. Mettler L, Audebert A, Lehmann-Willenbrock E, et al. Prospective clinical trial of SprayGel as a barrier to adhesion formation: an interim analysis. J Am Assoc Gynecol Laparosc. 2003;10:339-44.
28. Ten Broek RPG, Stommel MWJ, Strik C, et al. Benefits and harms of adhesion barriers for abdominal surgery: a systematic review and meta-analysis. Lancet. 2014;383:48-59.

CHAPTER

38

General Complications in Laparoscopy

Shruti Paliwal, Aditi Rai, B Ramesh

INTRODUCTION

Laparoscopy has become a standard and accepted surgical option for many surgical and gynecologic conditions, replacing open surgery. The advances in technology and equipment coupled with the improvement in skill acquisition have enabled more and more complex procedures to be performed laparoscopically. There is a steep learning curve associated with laparoscopy with a need for high degree of expertise and precision. Therefore, risk of complications exists over and above that associated with open surgery. Complications can occur in any case and by any operating surgeon. But it is necessary to recognize high-risk cases. Anticipation and appropriate preparedness is of utmost importance. The knowledge of how to prevent complications is as important as how to manage them.[1] It is important for every surgeon to understand the mechanism of complications associated with laparoscopic surgery as it is essential for their prevention, early detection and management **(Box 1)**.

Box 1: Classification of complications (mechanism).

- *Anesthetic complications:*
  - *Patient position (Trendelenburg position):*
    - Raised intraocular and intracranial pressure
  - *Reverse Trendelenburg position:*
    - Deep venous thrombosis
  - *Pneumoperitoneum:*
    - Respiratory acidosis (hypercarbia)
    - Deep venous thrombosis (calf and axial)
    - Subcutaneous emphysema
    - Pneumomediastinum
    - Pneumothorax
    - Pneumopericardium
    - Preperitoneal insufflation
- Patient positioning—nerve injuries
- *Entry complications—access related:*
  - Injury to vessels
  - Abdominal wall hematoma
  - Wound infection
  - Injury to small bowel/large bowel
  - Injury to retroperitoneal organ
  - Injury to liver/spleen
- *Intraoperative complications:*
  - Mechanical injuries
  - Electrosurgical injuries
  - Postoperative morbidity—shoulder pain/infection
- *Late complications:*
  - Fascial dehiscence
  - Herniation (umbilical)
  - Port site metastasis

CLASSIFICATION OF COMPLICATIONS (MECHANISM)

Anesthesia-related Complications

In case of prolonged ventilation followed by difficult intubation, there is high chance of stomach being distended with gas making it prone to Veress or trocar injury. Simple deflation of stomach by Ryle's tube before insertion of Veress needle or trocar is recommended. For gynecological procedures, the patient is placed in the Trendelenburg position (head down) which causes upward displacement of the diaphragm[2] and aggravates the pulmonary effects of tension pneumoperitoneum, producing high intrathoracic pressure, alveolar atelectasis and hypoxemia. Alveolar dead space however is reduced because of the decrease in hydrostatic gradient in the lung and the increase in cardiac output from augmented venous return from the lower half of the body. The latter also minimizes the deleterious cardiovascular effects of tension pneumoperitoneum.[3] However, venous congestion of the head and neck region may compromise cerebral perfusion and produce intracerebral and intraocular hypertension.[4] For upper abdominal surgery such as cholecystectomy, the patient is placed in the reverse Trendelenburg (foot down) position. A reverse of the physiological changes described above can be expected and improved pulmonary function occurs at the expense of less favorable cardiovascular changes. Obese patients with greater omental and intestinal fat require more extreme positioning to expose the surgical site making them even more prone to respiratory complications such as hypoxemia during surgical positioning.[5] Similar to what happens during other operations; cardiac arrhythmias including bradycardia, sinus tachycardia, ventricular tachycardia, and arrest related to anesthesia are also reported in laparoscopy.

EXTRAPERITONEAL GAS INSUFFLATIONS

Subcutaneous Emphysema (Fig. 1)

Subcutaneous emphysema occurs when carbon dioxide is insufflated into the subcutaneous spaces. Subcutaneous emphysema has been noted in 0.3–3.0% of laparoscopic procedures.[6,7] Commonly, the gas passes through any disruption of the peritoneum into the subcutaneous tissue and into the retroperitoneal tissue. It is rarely the consequence of inadvertent placement of trocars and direct insufflation into the subcutaneous tissue. It can extend further on larger areas and even to the mediastinum and pleura, thus being the cause of pneumomediastinum and pneumothorax. The reverse situation is also possible, i.e. the extension of a pneumomediastinum into the subcutaneous tissue. It may result from placement of the Veress needle into the extraperitoneal space of the abdominal wall and/or the omentum; a condition that is usually not discovered until the surgeon places the laparoscope for visualization. When this occurs, the gas should be disconnected allowing the extraperitoneal gas to escape. Fortunately, carbon dioxide is absorbed rapidly and the subcutaneous emphysema begins to resolve by the time the patient transferred in the recovery room. Subcutaneous emphysema may secondarily occur during prolonged laparoscopic procedures as gas gains access through enlargement of the trocar incision in the parietal peritoneum and extraperitoneal surgery. It is important for the surgeon to warn the patient's companions when facial swelling is significant. Subcutaneous emphysema usually dissolves in 12–24 hours.

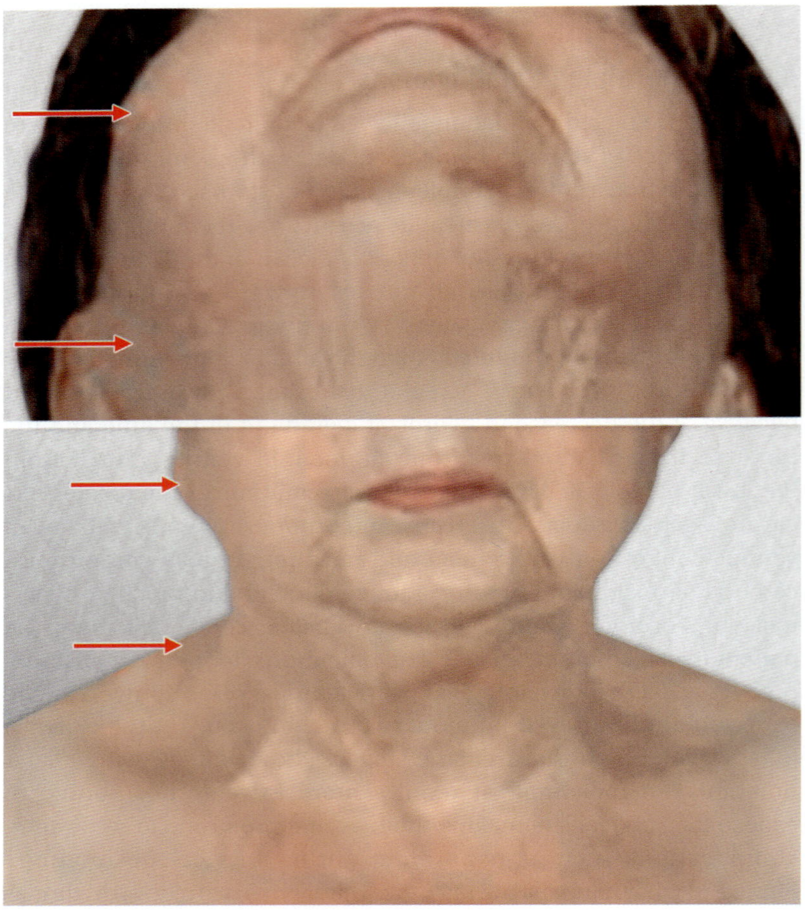

Fig. 1: Subcutaneous emphysema.

PATIENT POSITIONING

For gynecological laparoscopic procedures, patients are placed in Trendelenburg and dorsal low lithotomy position, often for several hours. Nerve injuries are uncommon but avoidable complications. Slender patients (body mass index less than 20 kg/m^2) are more vulnerable as their peripheral nerves are less protected by subcutaneous fat. Diabetics have a higher risk of nerve injury.

To decrease the risk of brachial plexus injuries during laparoscopy, the arms should be tucked at the side of the patient. If the arms are extended on arm boards, they should be abducted less than 90°.[8]

The lithotomy position is associated with lower limb nerve injuries. Four important elements of correct position are: (1) hip flexion of 60–170°; (2) knee flexion of 90–120°; (3) hip abduction of 90° or less; and (4) minimal external hip rotation.

Use of Boot Stirrups[8]

Long nerves and those that course superficially are especially vulnerable to injury under general anesthesia. These include the brachial plexus, ulnar, femoral, and common peroneal nerves. Prognosis depends on the amount of stretching and the duration of compression.[1] Postoperative numbness or tingling usually resolves by the fifth day; but symptoms that persist beyond 5 days require neurological consultation. Motor deficits, too, should be assessed by a neurologist.

Procedures lasting more than 2 hours appear to put patients at increased risk of position-related nerve injury, although injuries have been reported after procedures as short as 35 minutes.[9] Altering lithotomy position during long duration surgeries is recommended however not followed due to decrease incidence of nerve injuries.[10] The risk of lower extremity nerve injury appears to be reduced by avoiding patient positioning that puts strain on various nerves and by the use of boot stirrups, especially during lengthy procedures. Boot stirrups are used which are adjustable so that the pressure can be avoided on the lateral and posterior aspect of the calf. Laparoscopic surgeons should have a working knowledge of the nerves at risk of injury during laparoscopy and preventing neurological complications **(Fig. 2)**.[8]

AIR EMBOLISM

Although rare, air embolism the most feared and dangerous complication of laparoscopy. Intravascular injection of gas insufflation may follow direct needle or trocar placement into a blood vessel

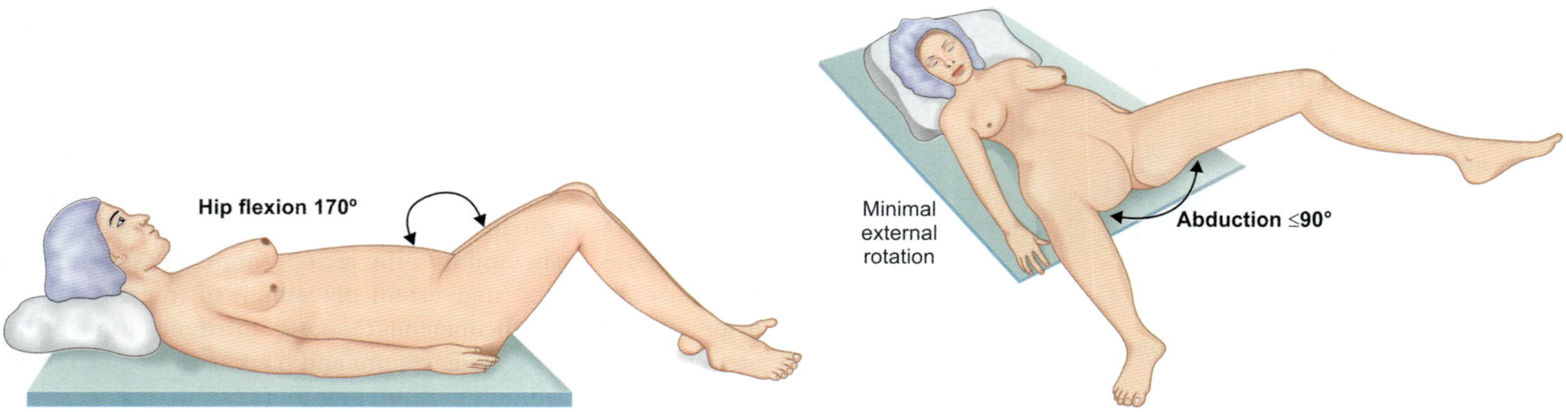

Fig. 2: Ideal patient positioning at laparoscopy.

or it may occur as a consequence of gas insufflation into an abdominal organ. This complication develops principally during the induction of pneumoperitoneum, particularly with previous abdominal surgery. Air embolism may also occur later during surgery. CO_2 is used most frequently for laparoscopy because it is more soluble in blood than either air, oxygen or N_2O. Rapid elimination also increases the margin of safety in case of intravenous injection of CO_2. All these characteristics explain the rapid reversal of the clinical signs of CO_2 embolism with treatment. The lethal dose of CO_2 emboli is approximately five times greater than that of air.[11] The pathophysiology of gas embolism is also determined by the size of the bubbles and the rate of intravenous entry of the gas. During laparoscopy, the rapid insufflation of gas under high pressure probably causes a "gas lock" in the vena cava and the right atrium; obstruction to venous return with a fall in cardiac output or even a circulatory collapse can result. Acute right ventricular hypertension may open the foramen ovale, allowing paradoxical gas embolism. Paradoxical embolism can occur even without patent foramen ovale. Volume preload reduces the risk of gas embolism and of paradoxical embolism. During gas embolism, ventilation-perfusion mismatch develops with increase in physiologic dead space and hypoxemia.[11] The diagnosis of gas embolism depends on the detection of gas emboli in the right side of heart or on recognition of the physiological changes from embolism. Early events occurring with 0.5 mL/kg of air or less include changes in Doppler sounds and increased mean pulmonary artery pressure. The low incidence of gas embolism during laparoscopy precludes the use of invasive or expensive monitors to detect embolism of small quantities of air. When the size of embolus increases (2 mL/kg of air) tachycardia, cardiac arrhythmias, hypotension, increased CVP, alteration in heart tones (mill-wheel murmur) cyanosis and ECG changes of right heart strain can develop. All these changes are rarely consistently positive. Pulmonary edema can also develop and may be an early sign of gas embolism.[11] Although pulse oximetry is helpful in recognizing hypoxemia, capnometry and capnography are more valuable in providing early diagnosis of gas embolism and determining the extent of embolism. $PETCO_2$ decreases in the case of embolism due to fall in cardiac output and the enlargement of physiological dead space.[11] Aspiration of gas or foamy blood for central venous line establishes the diagnosis. However, routine use of central venous line for a healthy patient in laparoscopic surgery is not warranted. Treatment for CO_2 embolism consists of immediate cessation of insufflation and release of the pneumoperitoneum. The patient is placed in steep head-down and left lateral decubitus (Durant) position. The amount of gas that advances through the right side of heart to the pulmonary circulation is less in this position, because the buoyant foam is displaced laterally and away from the right ventricular outflow tract. Ventilation with 100% oxygen to correct hypoxemia. Hyperventilation increases CO_2 excretion. If these simple measures do not succeed then a central venous or pulmonary artery catheter may be introduced for aspiration of the gas. Cardiopulmonary resuscitation must be initiated, if necessary. External cardiac massage may be helpful in fragmenting CO_2 emboli into small bubbles. The high solubility of CO_2 in blood results in rapid absorption from the blood stream and a rapid reversal of clinical signs of CO_2 embolism occur with the treatment. However, CO_2 embolism can be fatal. Cardiopulmonary bypass has been used successfully to treat massive CO_2 embolism **(Figs. 3 to 5)**.

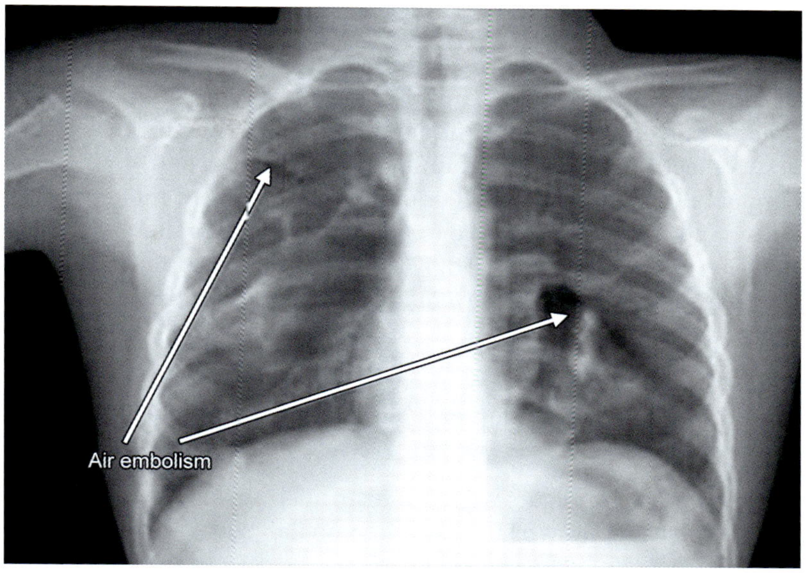

Fig. 3: Chest X-ray showing air embolism hyperechoic area.

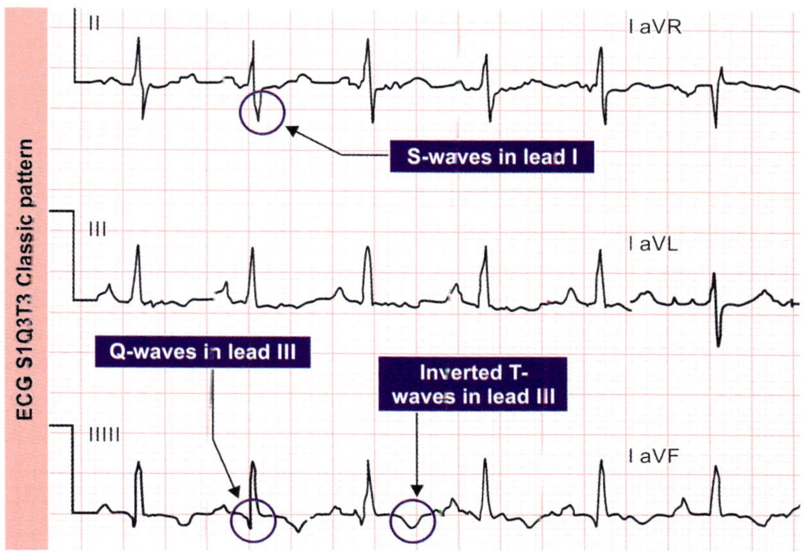

Fig. 4: ECG changes in gas embolism.

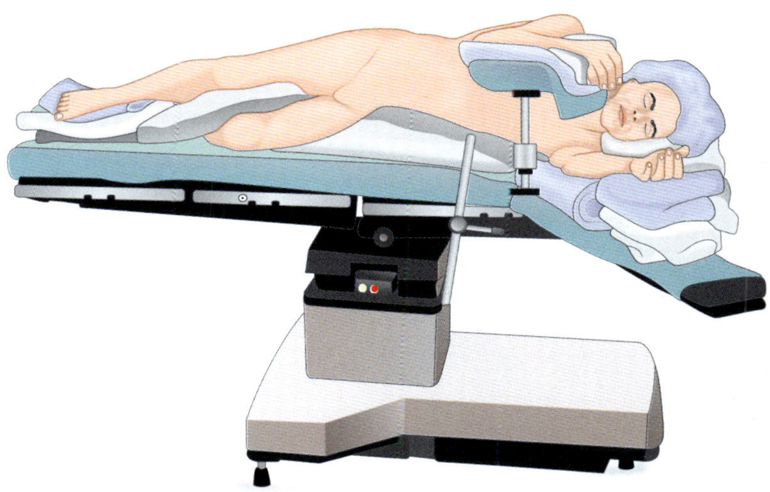

Fig. 5: Positioning after air embolism.

ELECTROSURGICAL INJURIES

Electrical and thermal burns to patient are usually predictable and usually preventable. Two pathways of current, i.e. monopolar and bipolar current are used. In monopolar mode, the current is from active electrode to tip to grounding plate (return pad) to electrosurgical unit (generator) to complete the cycle. In bipolar circuit, current flows from one paddle to another and acts on the tissue held between the two paddles. High voltage monopolar current seeks pathway to the ground, however if there is an interruption it results in unwanted effects.

Insulation failure: Any break in insulation results in thermal injury. Always check the insulation of the instrument before beginning the surgery **(Fig. 6)**.

Direct coupling: It occurs when an instrument makes a contact with another instrument. When using a monopolar cautery all instrument tips and trocar tips, which are close, should be visualized **(Fig. 7)**.

Capacitive coupling: In monopolar mode, an alternate current may induce a counter current through the insulation to an instrument in close proximity. Capacitively coupled currents are eliminated in bipolar cords since they travel in opposite directions and cancel each other **(Fig. 8)**.

Dispersive electrode pad: Although the dispersive electrode pad provides a pathway of low impedance for returning current to the generator, its misapplication can result in catastrophic thermal insult that is usually undetected at the time of injury.

The rules for proper usage seek to minimize impedance while providing the greatest surface area for current return. Impedance is primarily minimized by choosing a site with adequate water content for conduction. Areas of skin with hyperkeratosis or hair and those that overlie dense fat deposits (e.g. buttocks) should be avoided, while hair-free or shaved skin over larger muscles is preferred (e.g. upper thigh). Impedance is further reduced by choosing a site as close as possible to the active electrode **(Fig. 9)**. The surface area of the return electrode must be large enough to permit the returning current to be widely dispersed. Tissue heating is intimately related to current density; current density is inversely related to the square of the surface area, and the rise in tissue temperature is directly proportional to the square of the current. Therefore, small decrements in the surface area between the dispersive pad and the skin can dramatically result in injurious thermal effects to the underlying tissues. A large surface area is guaranteed by a uniform and unalterable application. Areas with bony prominences are prone to movement on patient repositioning

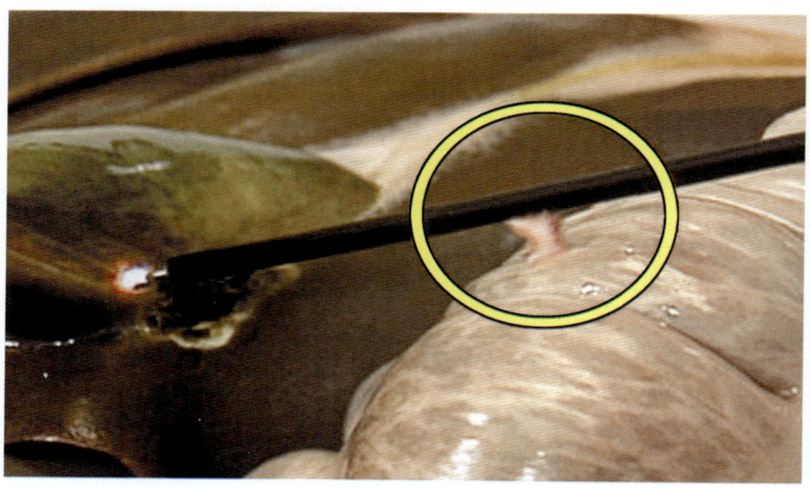

Fig. 6: Bowel injury due to insulation failure.

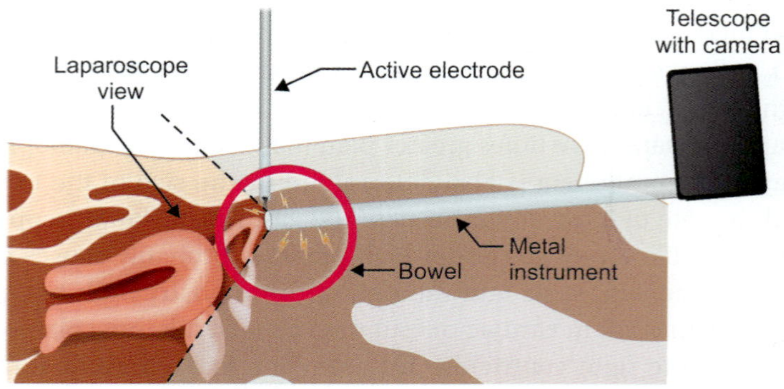

Fig. 7: Injury due to direct coupling.

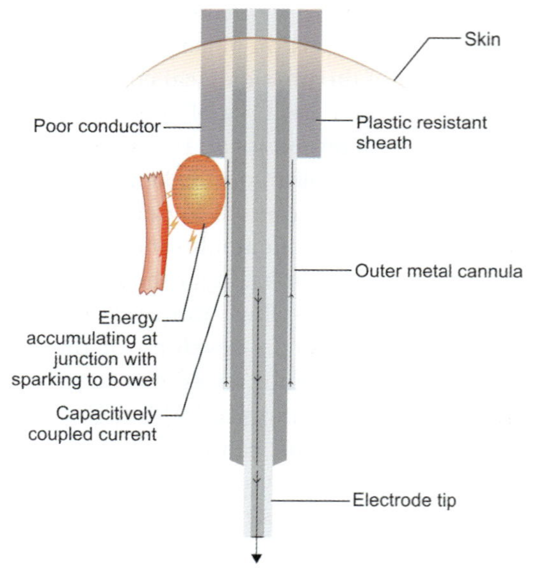

Fig. 8: Injury due to capacitive coupling.

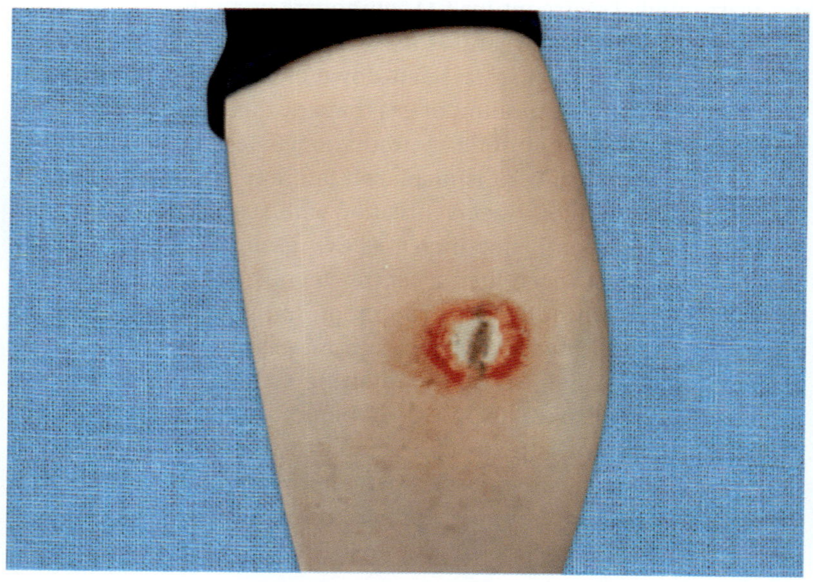

Fig. 9: Burn at site of grounding pad.

(such as the back and buttocks) and should be avoided. Since the edge of the dispersive electrode pad closest to the active electrode tends to concentrate the current, the longer edge of the pad should be placed toward the operative site.

POSTOPERATIVE SHOULDER PAIN

It is commonly felt due to irritation of the diaphragm through phrenic nerves or rarely stretched falciform ligament or CO_2 gas caught between liver and diaphragm due to the Trendelenburg position and inappropriate CO_2 removal. The CO_2 gas should be completely removed before the end of the procedure. Also importantly, heating and humidifying the insufflation gas prevents cellular death and results in less shoulder pain.[12] Intraperitoneal normal saline infusion has been reported to reduce the incidence of postoperative shoulder pain.[13] Local analgesics and pain killers help in alleviating the pain.

PORT SITE HERNIA

Incisional Hernia

Incisional hernia rarely occurs at the umbilical trocar site. It may occur at an extraumbilical site if the trocar size is >5 mm.

Recognition

The patient presents with pain and a tender swelling over the hernia site, often within 2 weeks of the operation. Other presentations include vomiting, diarrhea, and colicky pain, and may mimic gastro-enteritis.[14] There may be features of partial bowel obstruction, e.g. hyperactive bowel sounds,[15] because the herniation involves only a portion of the small bowel. The diagnosis may be established with the help of an X-ray of the abdomen (which may show bowel dilatation and fluid levels), ultrasonographic studies or computerized tomography. A loop of bowel may be seen herniating through the fascia **(Fig. 10)**. A common mistake is to consider an abdominal hernia as a wound hematoma.

Management

The hernia may be confirmed by laparoscopy, following which it may be reduced and the rectus sheath defect repaired.

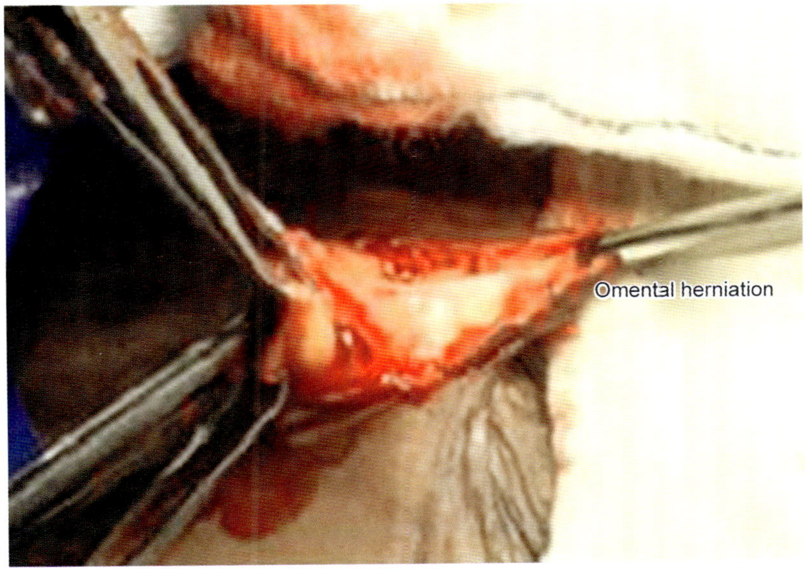

Fig. 10: 5-mm port site omental herniation.

Prevention

- Careful closure of the fascia whenever a ≥10-mm trocar is used at an extraumbilical site. When inserting the suture it is important that the edge of the rectus sheath is carefully identified with a clamp (e.g. Littlewood clamp) to ensure that the sheath is included in the suture. After the placement of the suture, the rectus sheath should be checked digitally to ensure adequate closure. Several other methods of closing the port defect have been described: a "J" needle, which is disposable;[13] a Veress needle;[17] and a reusable Reverdin needle.[18] In all cases, the closure site should be inspected carefully using the laparoscope to ensure that the bowel or omentum has not been trapped in the suture.
- Keeping the trocar valve closed while it is being withdrawn. A possible mechanism whereby the small bowel is trapped in the abdominal wall is as follows: if the trocar (especially >5 mm) is removed hastily while the valve is open, it would create a suction effect at the intra-abdominal end of the trocar, bringing along with it part of the bowel or omentum to the abdominal wall as it is being withdrawn. It is therefore advisable that all trocars should be removed with the valve closed.
- The trocars in the secondary ports should be removed first, whereas the primary trocar should be removed last. This permits visual inspection of the peritoneal surface of each secondary port for any unusual findings such as bleeding or entrapment of the bowel or omentum.
- The use of small (5 mm) trocars whenever possible.[19]
- Insertion of a trocar in a "Z" fashion.[20]
- Muscle relaxation is frequently integral to the anesthetic techniques employed. It is essential that the recovery of muscle tone by antagonizing the effect of the muscle relaxants should not occur until after all trocars have been removed.

PORT SITE HEMATOMA

Large life-threatening intra-abdominal and intramuscular abdominal wall hematoma is a rare presentation of trocar insertion-related injury. Massive bleeding from trocar insertion sites can occur with any laparoscopic procedure. Deep and superficial epigastric vessels arise from the external iliac and femoral artery, respectively. Topography of the deep circumflex iliac artery is also important to avoid abdominal wall hematoma induced by trocar insertion.[21] Abdominal wall transillumination increases superficial abdominal wall vessels' visibility even in colored skin normal weight women[22] but can be problematic in patients with a high body mass index.[23] Although it cannot be effectively located by transillumination, port insertion under direct vision, by laparoscope, decreases the chance of damage to deep abdominal wall vessels. The inferior epigastric artery could be identified in some patients by direct vision, after laparoscope insertion through a midline trocar, and finding of a raised fold of peritoneum overlying it, named the lateral umbilical fold.[22] Control of bleeding by direct pressure by port or Foley catheter balloon or full-thickness abdominal wall suture ligation may be beneficial when bleeding is detected during laparoscopy. Delayed bleeding in a stable patient may respond to conservative management.[24] Treatment with selective arterial transcatheter embolization is also reported.[25] An unstable patient needs emergent wound exploration or formal laparotomy.[26]

Venous Thrombosis

Although venous thrombosis is relatively uncommon following laparoscopic surgery because of earlier mobilization, venous thrombosis and pulmonary embolism do occur following laparoscopic pelvic surgery. Apart from the use of stockings and subcutaneous heparin for prophylaxis in those having major laparoscopic surgery, the filling pressure of carbon dioxide should be set at ≤13 mm. If the filling pressure rose significantly >15 mm mercury, it would impede venous return from the vena cava and consequently would cause venostasis predisposing to deep vein thrombosis.

PORT SITE METASTASIS

With the increase in number of laparoscopic oncological procedures the incidence of port site metastasis is present though not higher than open surgery. Studies show that recurrence of tumor at the port site probably can be avoided by the use of plastic bags or wound protectors to avoid direct contact between the tumor and the wound. It is also essential that extraction of the specimen is done through an abdominal incision wide enough to allow easy passage of the specimen.

REFERENCES

1. Philosophe R. Avoiding complications of laparoscopy surgery. Sexuality, Reproduction and Menopause. 2003;1:30-9.
2. Prentice JA. The Trendelenburg position: anesthesiologic considerations. In: Martin JT (Ed). Positioning in Anesthesia and Surgery. Philadelphia: WB Saunders; 1978. pp. 99-115.
3. Lenz RJ, Thornas TA, Wilkins DG. Cardiovascular changes during laparoscopy: studies of stroke volume and cardiac output using impedance cardiography. Anaesthesia. 1976;31:4-12.
4. Wilcox S, Vandam LD. Alas, poor Trendelenburg and his position! A critique of its uses and effectiveness. Anesth Analg. 1988;67:574-8.
5. Vaughan RW, Wise L. Postoperative arterial blood gas measurement in obese patients: effect of position on gas exchange. Arm Surg. 1975;182:705-9.
6. Bonjer HJ, Hazebroek EJ, Kazemier G, et al. Open versus closed establishment of pneumoperitoneum in laparoscopic surgery. Br J Surg. 1997;84: 599-602.
7. Hashizume M, Sugimachi K. Needle and trocar injury during laparoscopic surgery in Japan. Surg Endosc. 1997;11:1198-201.
8. Barnett JC, Hurd WW, Rogers RM, et al. Laparoscopic positioning and nerve injuries. J Minimal Invasive Gynecol. 2007;14:664-72.
9. Warner MA, Warner DO, Harper CM, et al. Lower extremity neuropathies associated with lithotomy positions. Anesthesiology. 2000;93:938-42.
10. Hopper CL, Baker JB. Bilateral femoral neuropathy complicating vaginal hysterectomy. Obstet Gynecol. 1968;32:543-7.
11. Yacoub OF, Cardona I Jr, Coveler LA, et al. Carbon dioxide embolism during laparoscopy. Anesthesiology. 1982;57: 533-5
12. Demco L. Painless Laparoscopy? J Int Soc Gynecol Endosc. 2001;7(1).
13. Tsai H, Chen Y, Ho C, et al. Maneuvers to decrease laparoscopy-induced shoulder and upper abdominal pain: a randomized controlled study. Arch Surg. 2011;146:1360-6.
14. Trehan AK. Richter's hernia following operative laparoscopy. Gynaecol Endosc. 1996;5:353-4.
15. Beck DH, McQuillan PJ. Fatal carbon dioxide embolism and severe haemorrhage during laparoscopic salpingectomy. Br J Anaesth. 1994;72: 243-5.
16. Phipps JH, Taranissi M. Laparoscopic peritoneal closure needle for prevention of port hernias and management of abdominal wall vessel injury. Gynaecol Endosc. 1994;3:189-91.
17. Tsaltas J, Lolatgis N, Lawrence AS, et al. A novel approach for the repair of an incisional hernia following laparoscopic hysterectomy. Gynaecol Endosc. 1996;5:39-41.
18. Dosoky M EI. A simple method for fascial and peritoneal repairs in operative laparoscopy. Gynaecol Endosc. 1996;5:37-8.
19. Chapron CM, Dubuisson J, Ansquer Y. Is total laparoscopic hysterectomy a safe surgical procedure? Hum Reprod. 1996;11:2422-4.
20. Whitelaw MJ, Nale VF. 'Z' procedure for laparoscopy. Am J Obstet Gynecol. 1973;116:864.
21. Balzer KM, Witte H, Recknagel S, et al. Anatomic guidelines for the prevention of abdominal wall hematoma induced by trocar placement. Surg Radiol Anat. 1999;21:87-9.
22. Epstein J, Arora A, Ellis H. Surface anatomy of the inferior epigastric artery in relation to laparoscopic injury. Clin Anat. 2004;17:400-8.
23. Bhatti AF, Iqbal S, Lee TC. Variation in surface marking of superior epigastric vessels. A guide to safe laparoscopic port insertion. Surgeon. 2008;6:50-2.
24. Fernández EM, Malagón AM, Arteaga I, et al. Conservative treatment of a huge abdominal wall hematoma after laparoscopic appendectomy. J Laparoendosc Adv Surg Tech A. 2005;15:634-7.
25. Martín-Malagón A, Arteaga I, Rodríguez L, et al. Abdominal wall hematoma after laparoscopic surgery: early treatment with selective arterial transcatheter embolization. J Laparoendosc Adv Surg Tech A. 2007;17:781-3.
26. Bakshi GK, Agrawal S, Shetty SV. A giant parietal wall hematoma: unusual complication of laparoscopic appendectomy. JSLS. 2000;4:255-7.

CHAPTER

39

Bowel Injury in Laparoscopic Surgery

Shruti Paliwal, Isha Rani, Chandramouli MS

INTRODUCTION

Small bowel obstruction (SBO) is a leading cause of acute hospital admission. Bowel injury is thought to be a rare complication of laparoscopy but carries a high rate of morbidity and mortality, particularly when diagnosed postoperatively.[1] Bowel injury is one of the most important complications of laparoscopic surgery because it is potentially life-threatening, especially if the injury is not recognized at the time of operation. Some studies suggest that the mortality rate associated with delayed diagnosis bowel injury may be as high as 21%.[2,3] Obtaining abdominal access is a high-risk segment of laparoscopic procedures. Approximately 55% of bowel injuries occurred during abdominal access and insufflation, either as a result of the Veress needle or a trocar. Until recently, previous abdominal operations were viewed as a relative contraindication to laparoscopy. However, with advances in laparoscopic skills and experience, various studies have reported laparoscopic management of SBO.[4-9]

CAUSATION

- *Laceration:* This is most commonly sustained during the insertion of the Veress needle or the primary trocar.
- *Thermal injury:* The bowel may be injured as a consequence of direct burn, direct coupling or capacitive coupling.

RECOGNITION

- *Perforation by Veress needle or trocar:* If the tip of the Veress needle or the trocar has entered the bowel lumen, foul smelling gas or greenish fluid may be detected from the open end of the needle/trocar. If in doubt, use a syringe to aspirate. If the injury is not detected at this stage, the laparoscope may be inserted and the characteristic features of the bowel mucosa will establish the diagnosis.
- *Through and through trocar perforation:* This may result if a segment of the bowel is adherent to the anterior abdominal wall at the trocar insertion site. The injury may then escape detection. To verify that this type of injury has not occurred, the laparoscope is withdrawn into the trocar and the trocar sleeve is then retracted slowly until the edges of the peritoneum can be visualized. If a through and through injury has occurred, the bowel lumen, instead of the edges of the peritoneum, will be evident. Such a maneuver is more likely to detect bowel injury than moving the laparoscope to another site.
- During the course of laparoscopic surgery, if bowel injury is suspected, laparotomy should be strongly considered because it is much more difficult to exclude bowel injury via the laparoscope. It is possible to carry out the "sterile milk test", by injecting sterile milk into the lumen to confirm the integrity of the bowel wall.

MANAGEMENT

- *Veress needle perforation:* Injury caused by the Veress needle may be managed expectantly.[10]
- *Trocar injury:* Bowel injury sustained by a trocar should be managed by laparotomy. If the injury is diagnosed while the tip of the trocar is still in the bowel lumen, it should be left in situ to facilitate localization of the site of injury at laparotomy. The bowel wall should then be carefully inspected for an additional "exit" injury. If the small bowel is involved, primary closure in two layers is adequate. If the large bowel is involved, the treatment options include primary repair, colostomy or segmental resection. The decision is influenced by the extent of the injury and whether the bowel has been prepared. It is wise to seek the assistance of a general surgeon in case of doubt.
- *Thermal injury:* Thermal injury of the bowel necessitates segmental resection with a wide margin around the site of injury because thermal damage may extend for a considerable distance from the site of thermal contact (several centimeters).
- *Laceration sustained during laparoscopic surgery:* Small bowel injury is usually sustained during laparoscopic adhesiolysis. The laceration may be oversewn either laparoscopically or via laparotomy, depending on the experience of the surgeon. A large bowel laceration may be repaired laparoscopically if the laceration is small and there is minimal soiling (e.g. involving the rectum, and the bowel has been prepared), otherwise it is advisable to proceed to laparotomy and repair. The management of laparoscopic bowel injury has been reviewed by Reich et al.[11]

Delayed Presentation

Bowel injury sustained during laparoscopy is often missed at the time of surgery. Zaki et al.[12] reported two cases of intestinal perforation (one laparoscopic sterilization, one diagnostic laparoscopy for infertility), both of which were missed at the time of surgery, which presented a few days later. Unrecognized perforation usually presents within 24–48 hours. On the other hand, unrecognized thermal injury often presents later, around 4–10 days.

The clinical picture may be varied. Initially, the symptoms may be nonspecific, e.g. vomiting, abdominal pain, distension, and malaise. Later on, there may be additional features, such as a localized peritoneal abscess or generalized peritonitis. Fever and leukocytosis are usually present. In some cases, the patient may present with features of septic shock. It must be emphasized that the prognosis for undiagnosed bowel injury depends very much on prompt diagnosis. Soderstrom[13] reviewed 66 cases of missed intestinal perforation and concluded that if the diagnosis is made after 72 hours there is a significant increase in mortality rate.

A high index of suspicion in any patient who presents with persistent abdominal pain, nausea, or feeling generally unwell within 2 weeks of laparoscopic surgery is advisable. It requires thorough investigation and careful observation as an inpatient to exclude bowel injury. Of paramount importance is the education of patients and general practitioners to report symptoms early (including persistence or increase in abdominal pain, nausea, vomiting, temperature, deterioration in general well-being) and to return to hospital promptly to avoid delay in diagnosis and management of the condition.

Small bowel injuries can be sutured repaired. Alternately, if the hole is confined to the antimesenteric portion, the bowel can be closed with interrupted 3-0 Vicryl tied either externally or with intracorporeal instrument ties. All enterotomies are suture repaired transversely to reduce the risk of stricture. If the hole involves greater than 50% of the bowel circumference, resection is done. An extracorporeal segmental enterectomy with side-to-side stapled anastomosis is preferred.

BOWEL INJURY DIAGNOSED AT THE TIME OF SURGERY

Case 1 (Figs. 1 to 5)

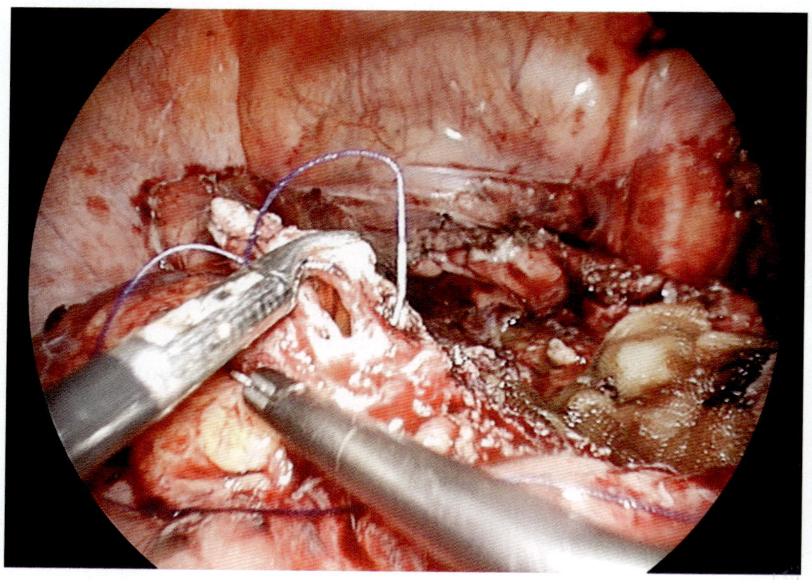

Fig. 1: Bowel rent recognized intraoperative.

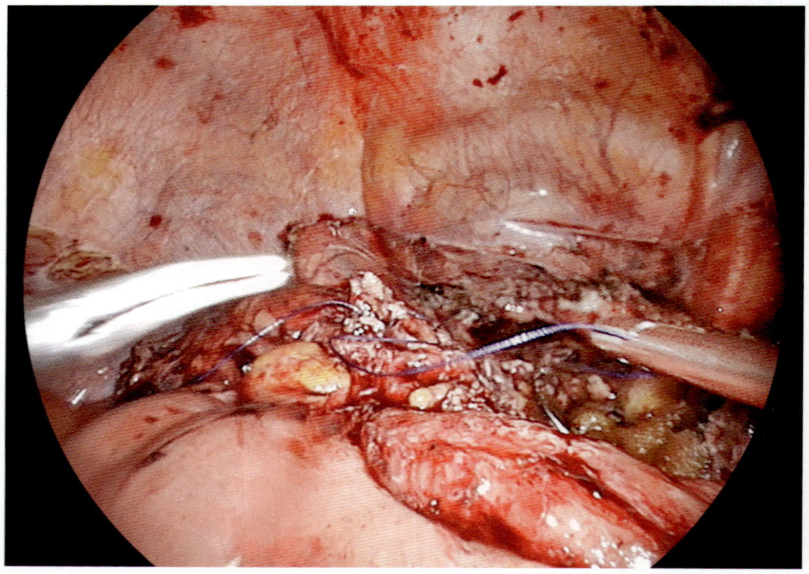

Fig. 2: Bowel rent repaired with Vicryl 3-0 suture.

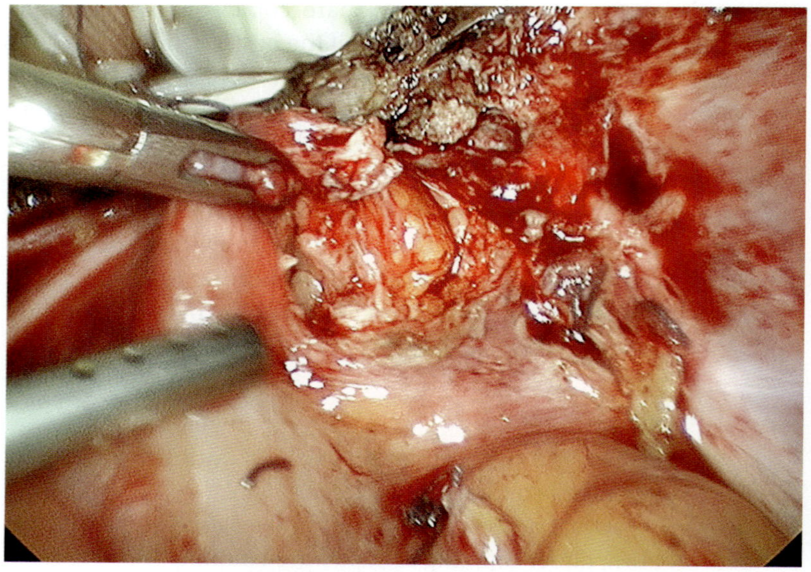

Fig. 3: Bowel injury recognized.

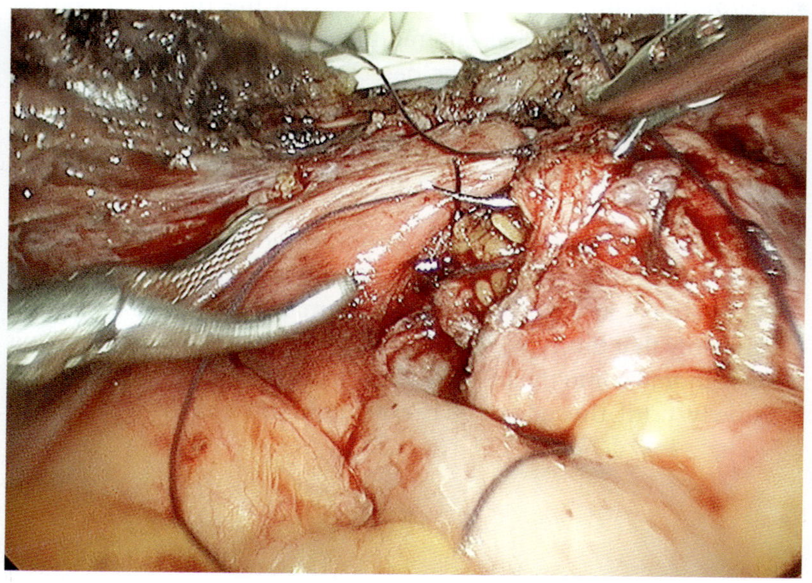

Fig. 4: Bowel repaired in continuous suture with Vicryl 3-0.

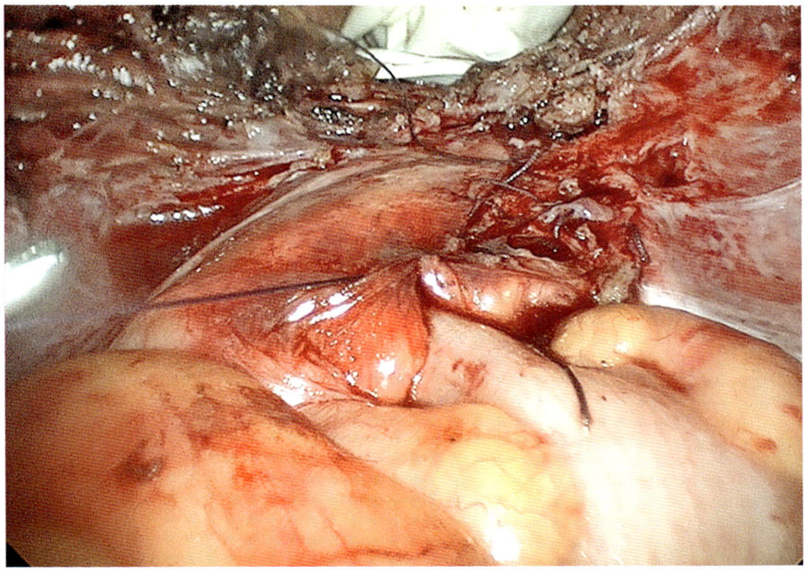

Fig. 5: Double layer bowel repair done.

Case 2 (Figs. 6 to 19)

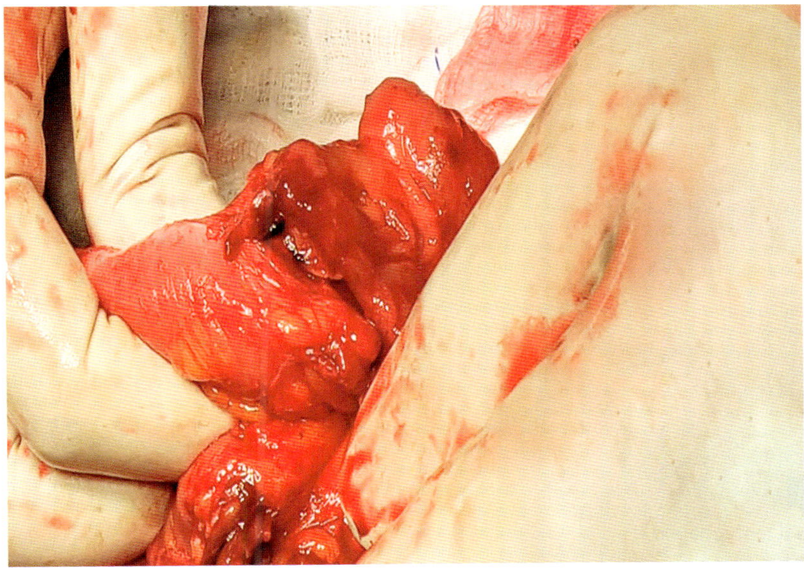

Fig. 6: Bowel laceration identified.

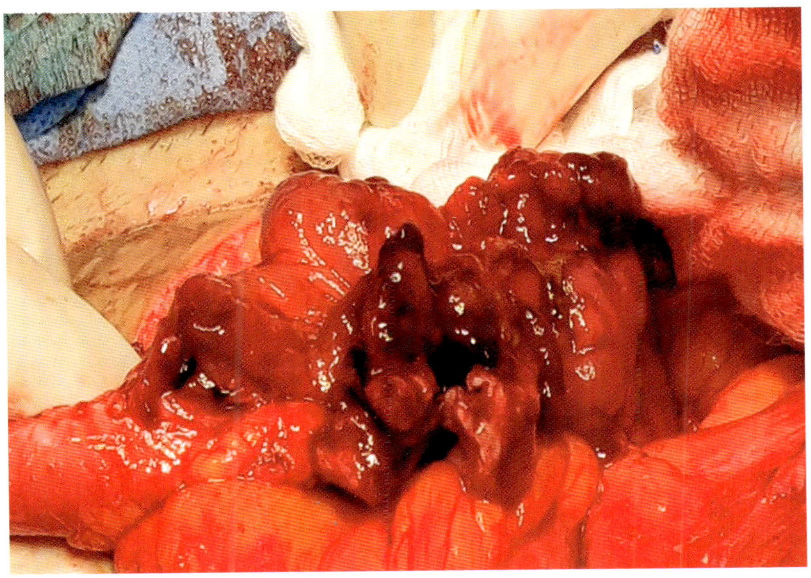

Fig. 7: Bowel injury diagnosed.

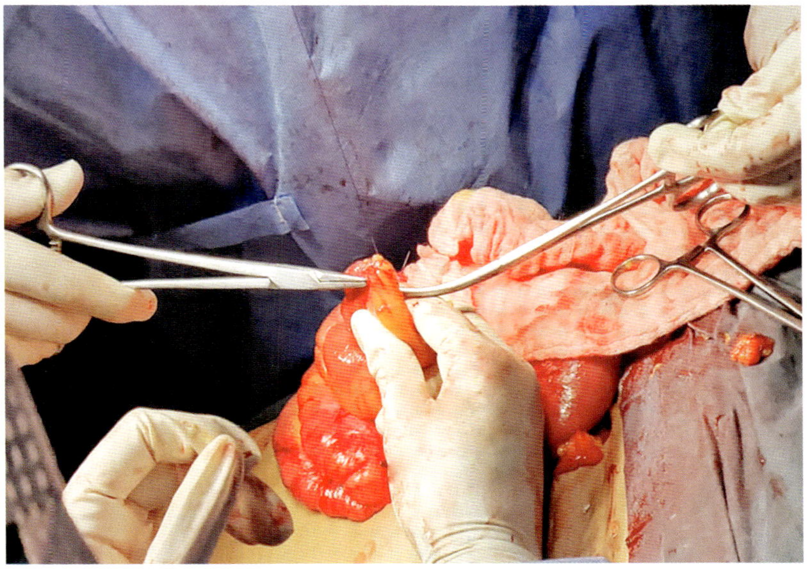

Fig. 8: Bowel repaired with interrupted suture.

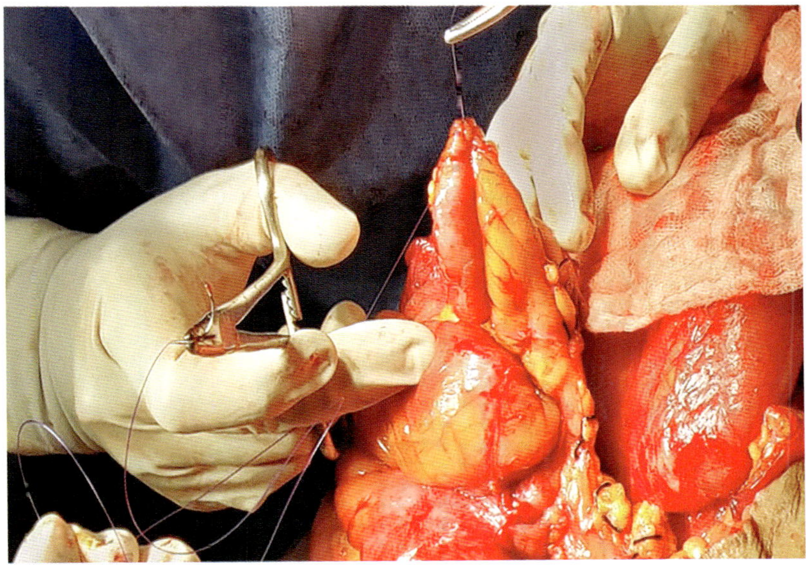

Fig. 9: Bowel injury repaired with Vicryl suture.

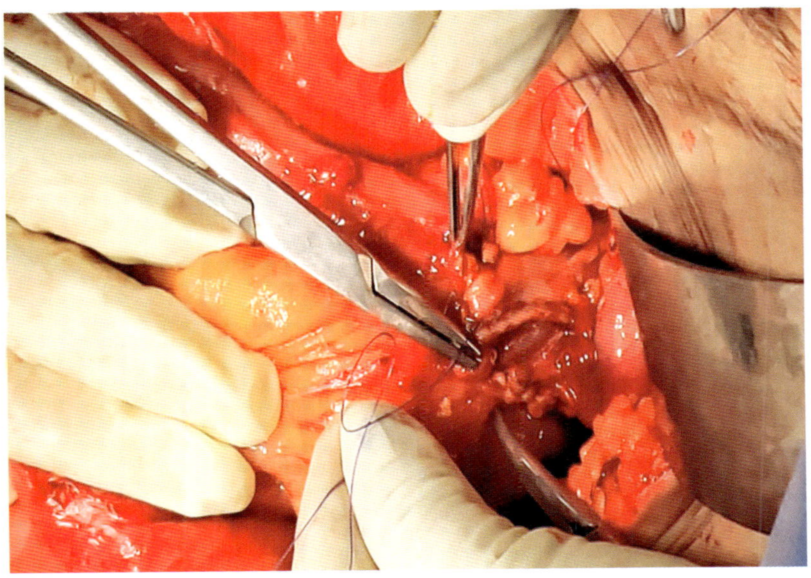

Fig. 10: Bowel injury repaired.

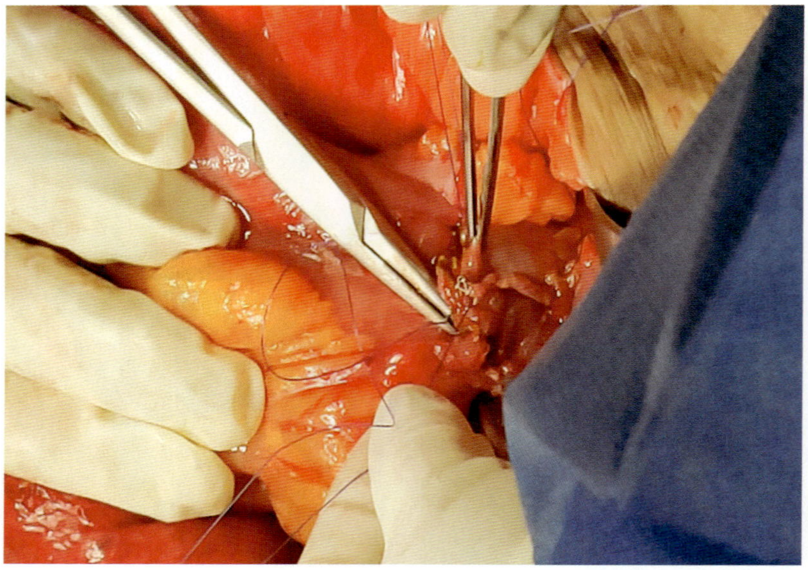

Fig. 11: Bowel repaired with Vicryl suture.

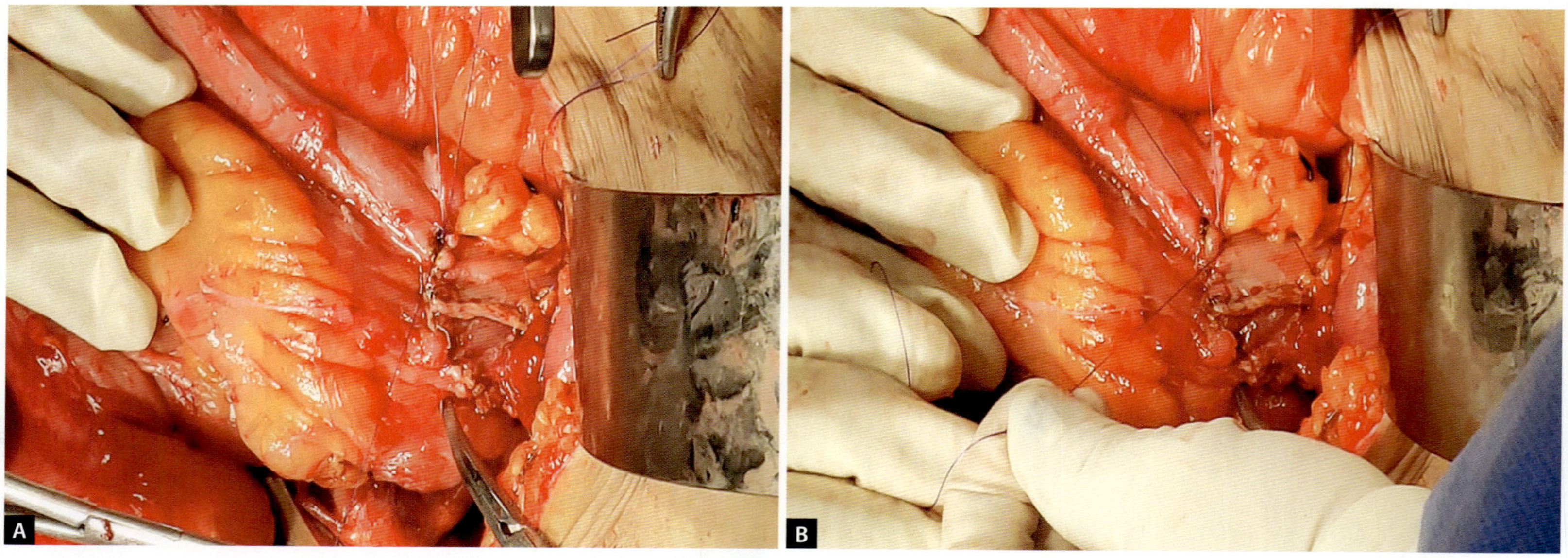

Figs. 12A and B: Bowel rent repaired.

Delayed Presentation

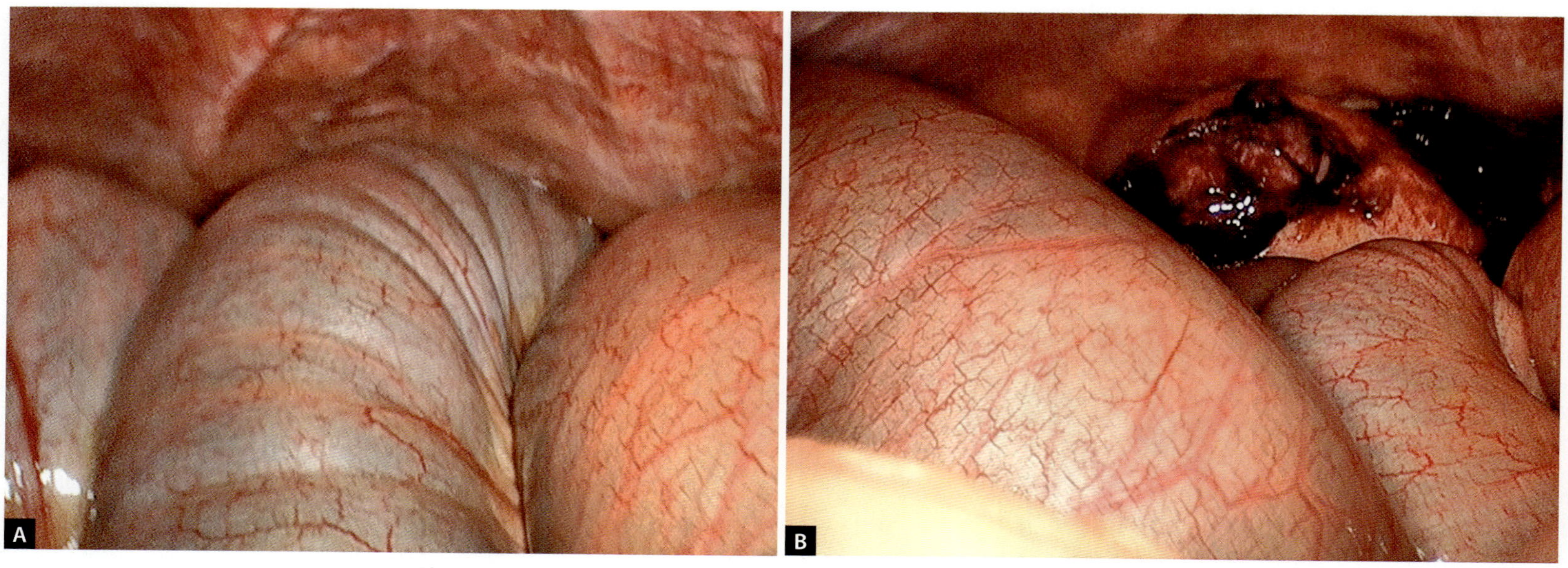

Figs. 13A and B: Intraoperative laparoscopic view after acute small obstruction.

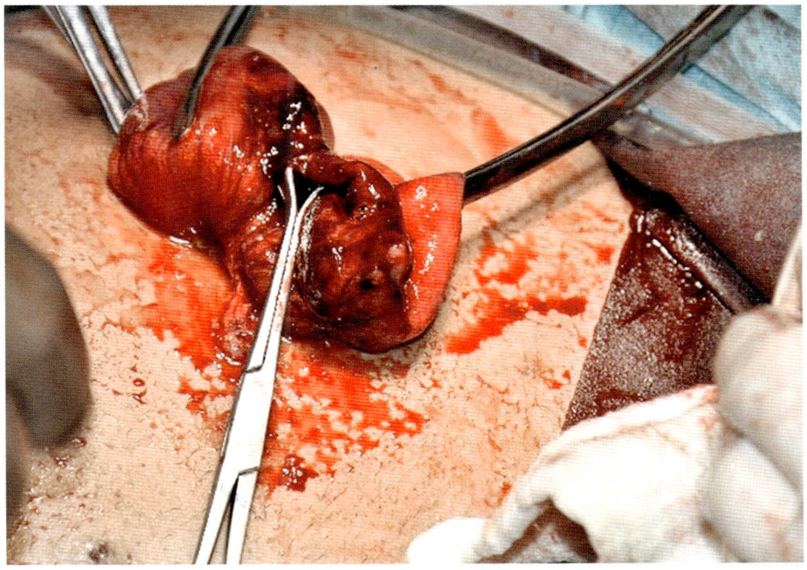

Fig. 14: Bowel necrosed a: site of obstruction.

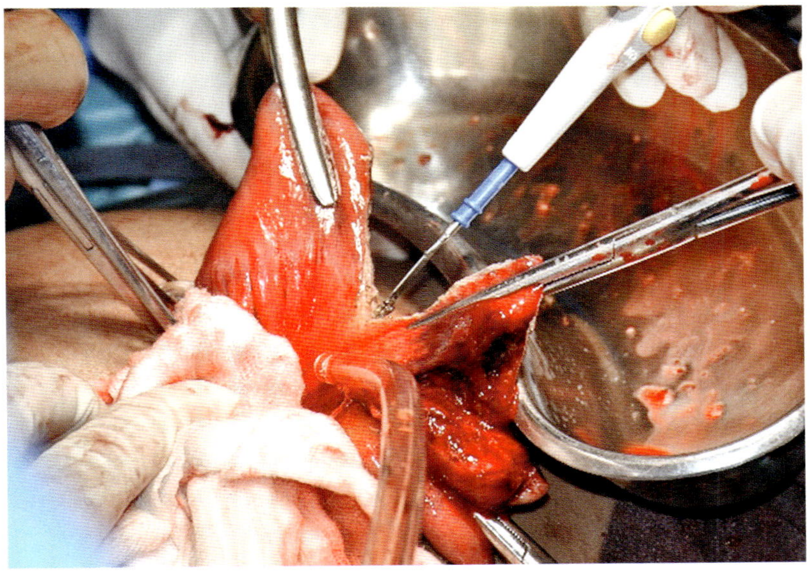

Fig. 15: Bowel ends freshened up.

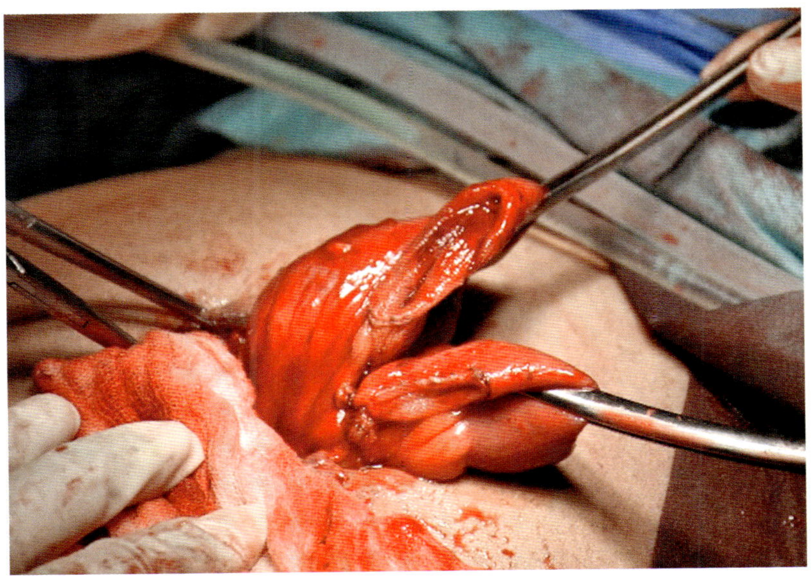

Fig. 16: Freshed bowel edges held with intestinal clamp.

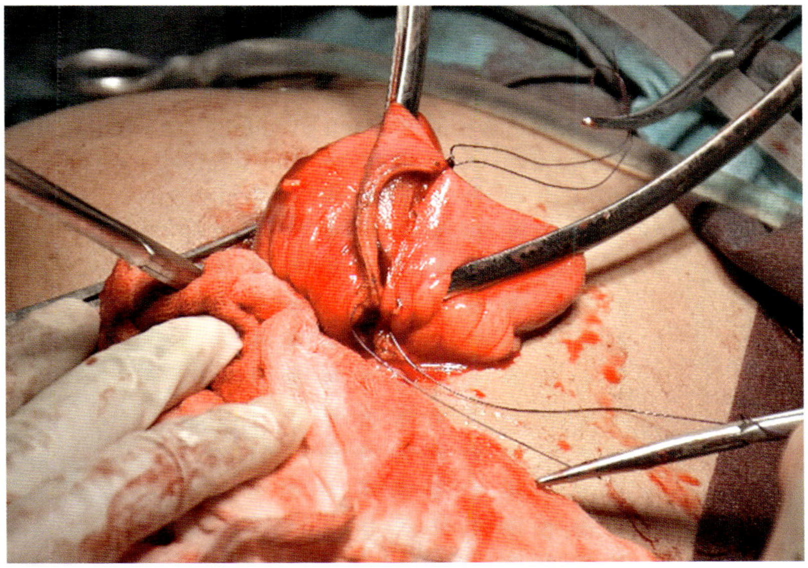

Fig. 17: Bowel ends anastomosed to each other.

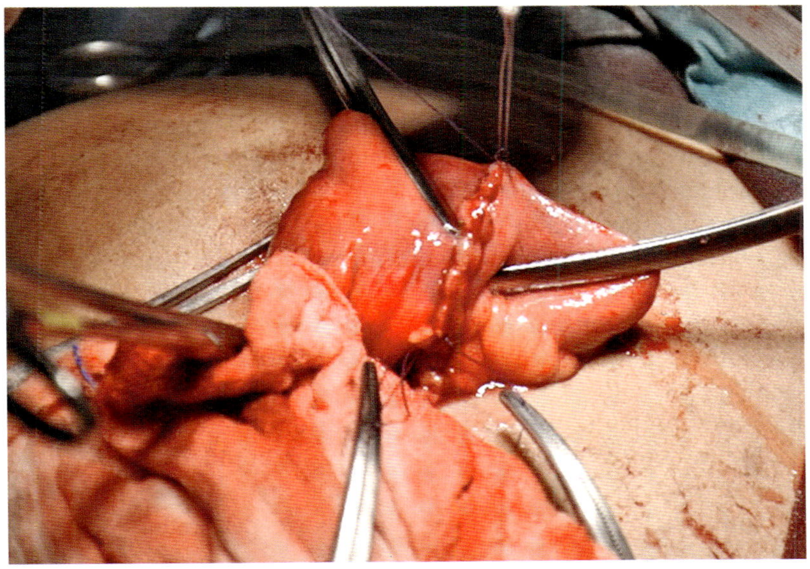

Fig. 18: 3owel anastomosis done with continuous suture.

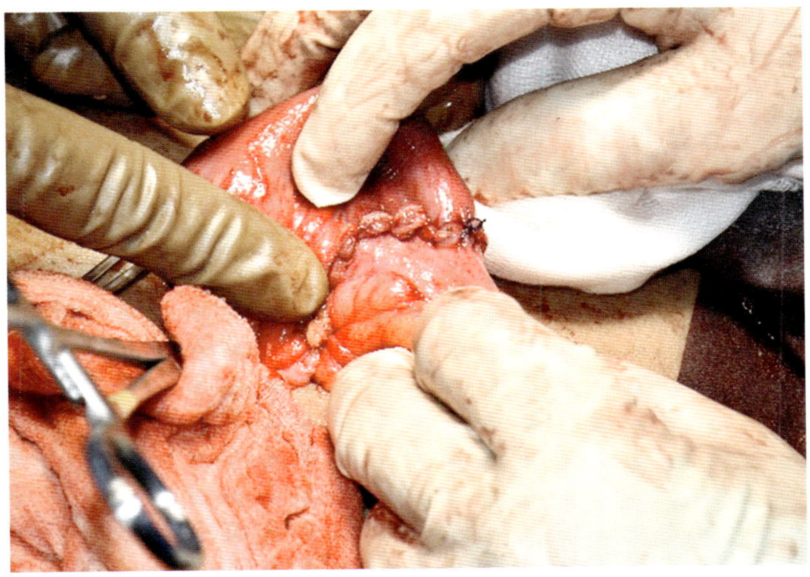

Fig. 19: Bowel integrity restored.

PREVENTION

- Use safety techniques when performing laparoscopy in patients who are presumed to have anterior abdominal wall adhesions: a number of techniques may be used to reduce the likelihood of significant bowel injury, including (i) the establishment of the pneumoperitoneum through the left ninth intercostal space;[14] (ii) the use of a minilaparoscope to help to identify an alternative, safe site for introduction of the primary trocar; (iii) use of the open laparoscopy method introduced by Hassan[15] may reduce the likelihood of bowel injury in patients who are likely to have anterior wall adhesions; and (iv) performance of transumbilical puncture of the abdominal wall under direct vision with a 5 mm optically equipped trocar, as described by Semm.[16]
- The routine use of a nasogastric tube to empty the stomach reduces the risk of injury to the stomach. Gaseous distension of the stomach may be due to assisted positive pressure ventilation before intubation or aerophagia. However, nasogastric tube insertion may be complicated by esophageal injuries, which could have severe consequences. For the latter reason, very few centers in Britain employ the routine use of a nasal gastric tube to empty the stomach. It is, however, desirable to identify a patient at risk of undue gaseous distension. Gaseous distension is a particular feature of assisted positive pressure ventilation prior to intubation in a paralyzed patient. This problem is exacerbated in those patients where airway management in the anesthetized state is a problem and consequently higher inflation pressures are required. For these patients, it must be decided preoperatively to use an alternative technique not requiring positive pressure ventilation with high inflation pressure prior to intubation. Alternatively, if high inflation pressure were indeed used prior to intubation in these patients, then a nasogastric tube must be passed to decompress the stomach.
- Bowel preparation facilitates operative maneuvers by increasing intraperitoneal free space and reducing inadvertent bowel trauma. Additionally, bowel preparation reduces the severity of complications, which may occur after bowel perforation.
- Extensive adhesiolysis should be classified as advanced laparoscopic surgery and should be performed only by experienced laparoscopic surgeons.[17]

REFERENCES

1. Härkki-Sirén P, Sjoberg J, Mäkinen J, et al. Finnish national register of laparoscopic hysterectomies: a review and complications of 1165 operations. Am J Obstet Gynecol. 1997;176:118-22.
2. Jansen FW, Kapiteyn K, Trimbos-Kemper T, et al. Complications of laparoscopy: a prospective multicentre observational study. Br J Obstet Gynaecol. 1997;104:595-600.
3. Brosens I, Gordon A. Bowel injuries during gynaecological laparoscopy: a multinational survey. Gynaecol Endosc. 2001;10:141-5.
4. Adams S, Wilson T, Brown AR. Laparoscopic management of acute small bowel obstruction. Aust NZ J Surg. 1993;63:39-41.
5. Bailey IS, Rhodes M, O'Rourke N, et al. Laparoscopic management of acute small bowel obstruction. Br J Surg. 1998;85:84-7.
6. Navez B, Arimont JM, Guiot P. Laparoscopic approach in acute small bowel obstruction. A review of 68 patients. Hepatogastroenterology. 1998;45:2146-50.
7. Strickland P, Lourie DJ, Suddleson EA, et al. Is laparoscopy safe and effective for treatment of acute small-bowel obstruction? Surg Endosc. 1999;13:695-8.
8. Agresta F, Piazza A, Michelet I, et al. Small bowel obstruction—laparoscopic approach. Surg Endosc. 2000;14:154-6.
9. Wullstein C, Gross E. Laparoscopic compared with conventional treatment of acute adhesive small bowel obstruction. Br J Surg. 2003;90:1147-51.
10. Bateman BG, Kolp LA, Hoeger K. Complications of laparoscopy—operative and diagnostic. Fertil Steril. 1996;66:30-5.
11. Reich H, McGlynn F, Budin R. Laparoscopic repair of full-thickness bowel injury. J Laparoendoscopic Surg. 1991;1:119-22.
12. Zaki H, Penketh R, Newton J. Gynaecological laparoscopy audit: Birmingham experience. Gynaecol Endosc. 1995;4:251-7.
13. Soderstrom RM. Bowel injury ligation after laparoscopy. J Am Assoc Gynecol Laparosc. 1993;1:74-7.
14. Reich H, Levie M, McGlynn F, et al. Establishment of pneumoperitoneum through the left ninth intercostal space. Gynaecol Endosc. 1995;4:141-3.
15. Hassan HM. Window for open laparoscopy. Am J Obstet Gynecol. 1990;137:869-70.
16. Semm K. History. In: Sanfilippo JS, Levine RL (Eds). Operative Gynecologic Endoscopy. New York: Springer Verlag; 1989. pp. 1-18.
17. Querleu D, Chevallier L, Chapron C, et al. (1993) Complications of gynaecological laparoscopic surgery. A French multicentre collaborative study. Gynaecol Endosc. 1993;2:3-6.

CHAPTER

40

Vascular Injury

Shruti Paliwal, G Hemasree, B Ramesh

INTRODUCTION

Vascular injury may involve abdominal wall vessels or large retroperitoneal vessels.

ABDOMINAL WALL VESSELS

Injuries involving the inferior epigastric vessel are the most common type of vascular complication. The true incidence is unknown, but it is likely to exceed 3/1,000 operative laparoscopies **(Fig. 1)**.[1]

Recognition

Bleeding from the inferior epigastric vessels is often obvious during the course of laparoscopic surgery. Occasionally, it may not be apparent until after the trocar has been removed at the end of the operation, because the increased intra-abdominal pressure and retroperitoneal hematoma formation may tamponade even a large vessel injury. This may remain unnoticed until the pressure is gradually reduced at the conclusion of the procedure. It is good practice to inspect all secondary trocar sites for active bleeding before the laparoscope is finally withdrawn. The inspection should be carried out when the intra-abdominal pressure has been lowered following the release of carbon dioxide from the intra-abdominal cavity.

Management

Bleeding from the inferior epigastric vessels may be managed by (i) bipolar coagulation, (ii) tamponade, or (iii) suturing **(Fig. 2)**.

1. *Bipolar coagulation:* This may produce quick and adequate hemostasis, provided the vessel has not retracted into the abdominal wall.
2. *Tamponade:* This may be achieved by (i) rotating the trocar sleeve through 360° and, if bleeding is successfully arrested, the tamponade should be applied for at least 5 min; (ii) upsizing the port; (iii) using a Foley catheter: a size 14 Foley catheter may be inserted through the cannula, the balloon is then inflated with 15–30 mL of normal saline. The cannula is then removed and the balloon is pulled up to produce pressure on the bleeding vessel. If the bleeding is successfully stopped, the tamponade may be sustained by clamping the Foley catheter close to the abdominal wall. If bleeding continues, or recurs after the tamponade is released (at the end of 5 min, or at the end of the operation), suturing is necessary to stop the bleeding. Some laparoscopic surgeons advocate continuing the tamponade for up to 24 hours, and removing the Foley catheter after the patient has returned to the ward.[2] The concern in this situation is that, following the removal of the catheter, one may not be certain whether the bleeding has recurred and if it does, the diagnosis may be delayed and the patient would need to return to the operating theater for suturing **(Fig. 3)**.
3. *Suturing:* (i) A through and through suture may be applied by using a large curved needle; however, this may be difficult if the patient is obese. (ii) If a straight needle is used, the entry and exit of the needle through the abdominal wall is achieved with the help of a laparoscopic needle holder/grasper, under direct laparoscopic control. (iii) A specially designed "J"-shaped peritoneal

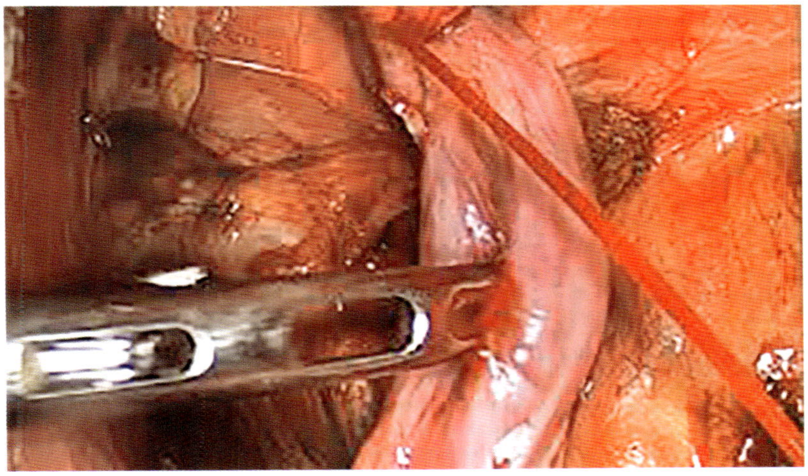

Fig. 1: Inferior epigastric artery injury.

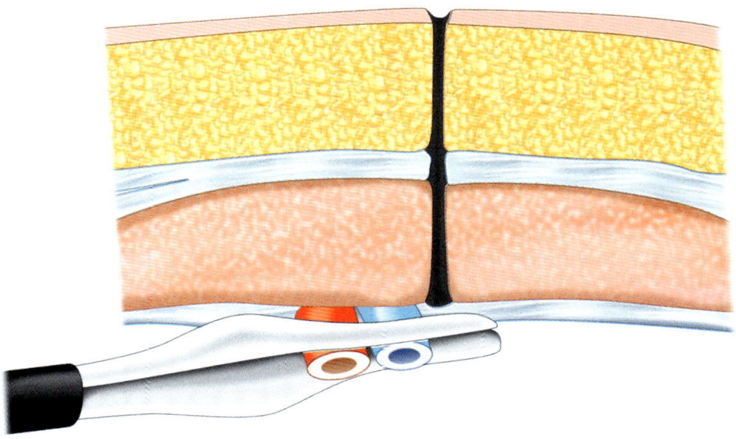

Fig. 2: Bipolar cauterization of inferior epigastric vessels.

closure needle has been described by Phipps and Taranissi (1994). The needle (Rocket of London, Watford, UK), has a leading-end fenestration for carrying the closure suture, and the round-bodied, pointed tip can be shielded by an integral guard sheath. (iv) If the bleeding is significant, or if there is doubt that the above measures have achieved satisfactory hemostasis, a small abdominal incision (~3 cm) should be made over the bleeding site, which would then permit the identification of the bleeder, following which the bleeder is clamped and ligated **(Figs. 4A to C)**. Similarly, an enlarging hematoma is best managed by minilaparotomy.[3]

Prevention

- Insert the trocar in the lower quadrant, lateral to the rectus sheath, above a line joining the anterior superior iliac spine.
- Transillumination of the anterior abdominal wall will help to identify the superior epigastric vessel.
- Careful visual inspection of the peritoneum below an arcuate line (where the vessels enter the rectus sheath) will locate the position of the lower part of the inferior epigastric vessel.

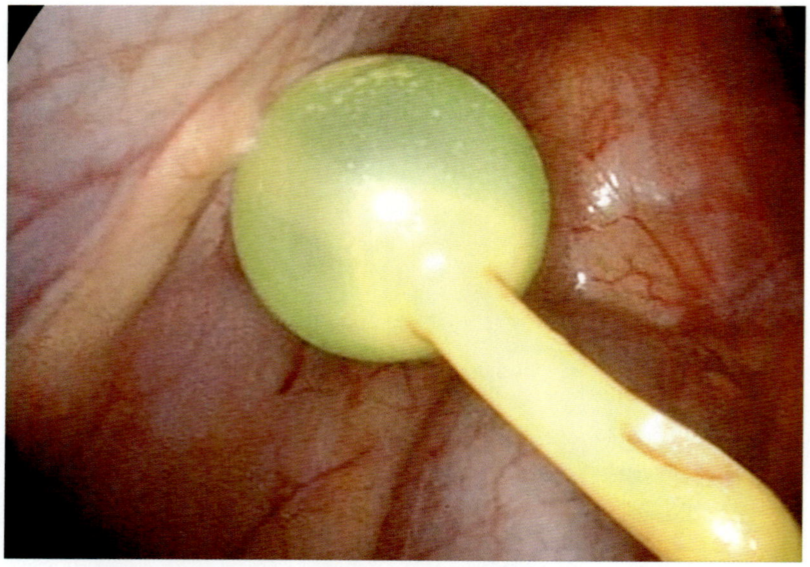

Fig. 3: Foley catheter tamponade for injury to inferior epigastric artery.

- For lateral ports, identify obliterated hypogastric vessels intraperitoneally in the anterior abdominal wall and ensure puncture remains lateral to it.
- Use a small (5 mm) trocar in lateral ports.[4]

LARGE RETROPERITONEAL VESSELS

These include the aorta, vena cava, and iliac vessels. In most cases, the injury is sustained during the insertion of the Veress needle or the primary trocar **(Fig. 5)**.

Presentation

- *Hemorrhage detected immediately following insertion of the Veress needle or primary trocar:* After the Veress needle has been inserted, prior to connecting the tubing and introducing carbon dioxide into the abdominal cavity, with the tap open, blood may ooze out from the open end of the Veress needle. In this situation either the aorta, vena cava, or, more commonly, the common iliac vessel has been traumatized. In the case of the primary trocar, the removal of the primary trocar from the cannula may similarly be associated with a gush of blood through the cannula; in either case, one must never remove the perforating/traumatizing instrument (Veress needle or cannula).
- *Hemorrhage detected following the insertion of the laparoscope:* There may be signs of peritoneal or retroperitoneal bleeding, the latter almost always in the form of a hematoma. It is good practice as soon as the laparoscope has been introduced into the abdominal cavity to survey the abdominal cavity, especially the area just beneath the umbilicus, before attention is focused on the pelvis **(Figs. 6 to 8)**.
- Sudden drop in blood pressure.

Management

Firstly, the Veress needle or the trocar/cannula must not be removed, because the tip of the instrument may act as a plug to prevent catastrophic bleeding. Instead the tip of the instrument should be pushed slightly in. In the case of blood oozing out through the cannula, the assistant should be asked to place his/her finger over the open end of the cannula. If the cannula is removed, it may

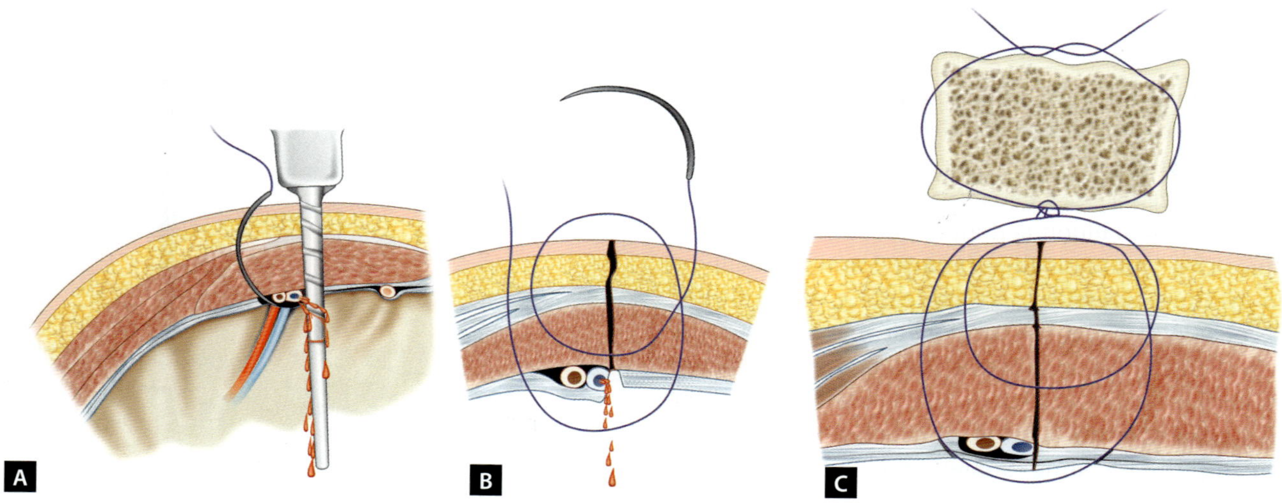

Figs. 4A to C: Suture ligation of inferior epigastric vessels.

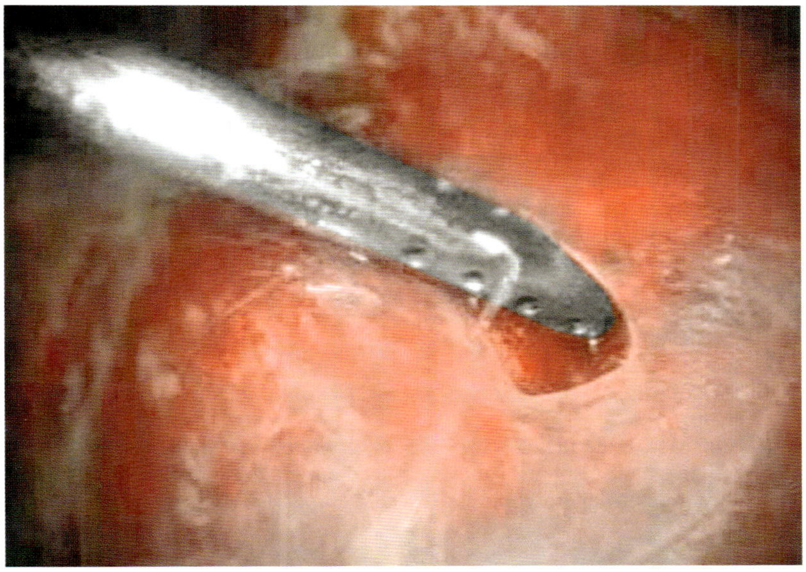

Fig. 5: Retroperitoneal hematoma post-venous injury.

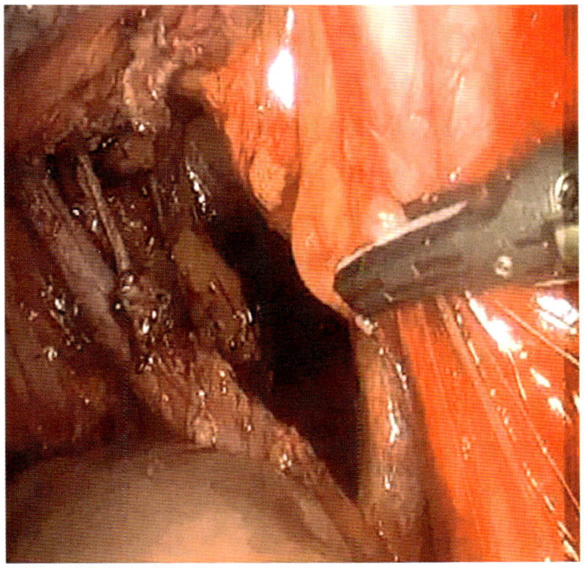

Figs. 7: External iliac vein injury.

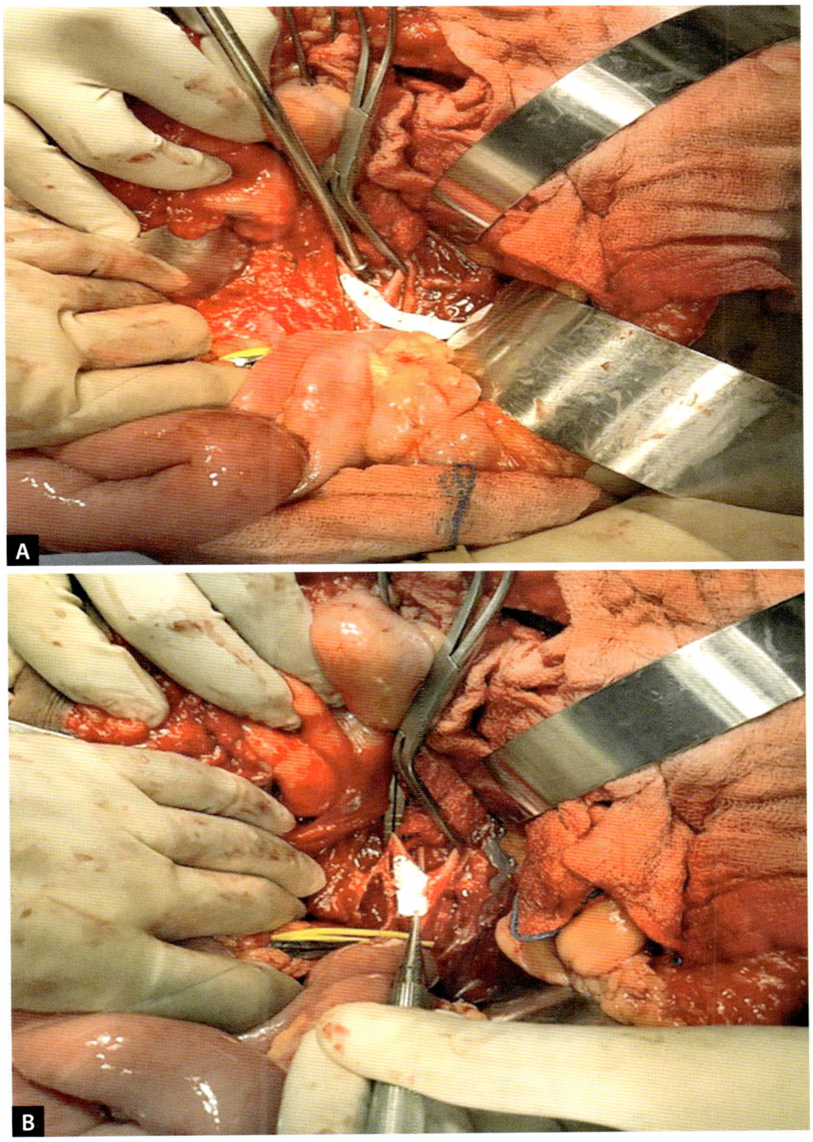

Figs. 6A and B: Aortic repair by placement of vascular graft.

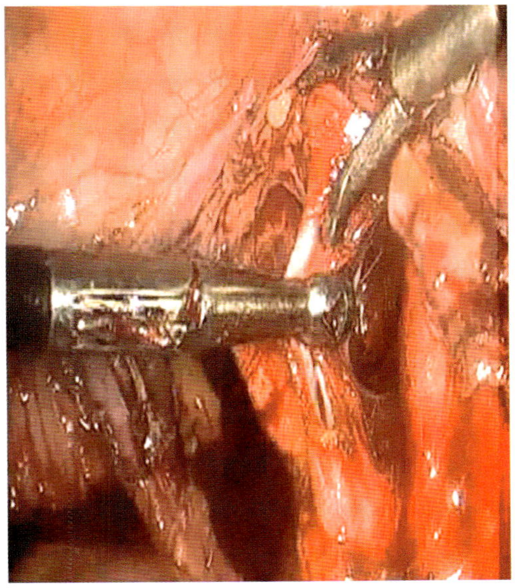

Fig. 8: Laparoscopic repair of external iliac vein.

produce massive blood loss either intraperitoneally or retroperitoneally. In the latter situation, it may be difficult to identify the exact site of injury. An immediate midline laparotomy should be carried out and pressure applied either digitally or with the help of a large pack over the site of the vascular defect. Sometimes a large hematoma makes the identification of the exact site of injury difficult. In such a case, compression may be applied over the aorta. The assistance of a vascular surgeon should have been sought at this stage. Resuscitative measures should already have been initiated by the anesthetic staff. One should never attempt to put a hemostatic clamp over a large vessel because it may produce further crushing injury to the vessel wall and complicate the subsequent repair procedure.

Prevention

- Adhere to safe laparoscopic entry techniques.
- Prior to insertion of the Veress needle/primary trocar, palpate the abdominal wall carefully for any pelvic mass.
- The trocar must be sharp, preferably with a safety shield.
- Ensure that the skin incision is adequate. There should be gentle and controlled entry of the trocar. Remember that the

greater the force required to insert the trocar, the higher the risk of injury.

- The Veress needle and primary trocar should be inserted in the direction of the hollow of the sacrum. The tip should be kept to the midline and should not be allowed to wander off sideways (risk of injury to the iliac vessels).
- There is no evidence to suggest that disposable trocars are safer than reusable ones provided the latter are not blunt.
- All secondary trocars must be placed under direct vision.
- Very occasionally, accidental vascular injury may result during the course of laparoscopic surgery from sharp instruments, e.g. diathermy needle or scissors, so it is important that the tip of any sharp instrument is kept under vision at all times and not be allowed to "wander" within the abdominal cavity. If the instrument is not in active use, it ought to be removed.
- One should be aware that thin patients may be at greater risk of major vessel injury, as the aorta may lie only 3 cm below the umbilicus.[5]

REFERENCES

1. Zaki H, Penketh R, Newton J. Gynaecological laparoscopy audit: Birmingham experience. Gynaecol Endosc. 1995;4:251-7.
2. Aharoni A, Condea A, Leibovitz Z, et al. A comparative study of Foley catheter and suturing to control trocar-induced abdominal wall haemorrhage. Gynaecol Endosc. 1997;6:31-2.
3. Bateman BG, Kolp LA, Hoeger K. Complications of laparoscopy—operative and diagnostic. Fertil Steril. 1996;66:30-5.
4. Saidi MH, Vancaillie TG, White AJ, et al. Complications and cost of multi-puncture laparoscopy: a review of 264 cases. Gynaecol Endosc. 1994;3:85-90.
5. Hurd WH, Bude RO, DeLancey JO, et al. Abdominal wall characterization with magnetic resonance imaging and computed tomography. The effects of obesity on the laparoscopic approach. J Reprod Med. 1991;36:473-76.

CHAPTER

41

Abdominal Hysterectomy

B Ramesh, Shwetha Kamath, G Hemasree

INTRODUCTION

Hysterectomy can be done by various techniques and approaches including abdominal, vaginal, laparoscopic, and robotic hysterectomy. In most cases, a total hysterectomy with removal of the uterine corpus and cervix is done. The ovaries and tubes may be or may not be removed along with the uterus depending on the patient's age and other factors.

INDICATIONS FOR ABDOMINAL HYSTERECTOMY

Common indications are fibroids, abnormal uterine bleeding (AUB), adenomyosis, endometriosis, pelvic inflammatory disease (PID), and pelvic malignancies. Although today most of the hysterectomies can be done vaginaly for prolapsed, AUB and benign conditions. Beyond 14 weeks, vaginal hysterectomy (VH) becomes difficult then abdominal hysterectomy (AH) is indicated.

TECHNIQUE OF ABDOMINAL HYSTERECTOMY

Patient under anesthesia, incision is taken depending on the pathology **(Fig. 1)**. In most instances Pfannenstiel incision is sufficient, whenever exposure of abdomen is required vertical midline incision may be taken. Once the abdomen is opened, the pelvic pathology is carefully evaluated and abdomen explored **(Fig. 2)**.[1]

The bowels are packed away, elevating the uterus out of pelvis **(Fig. 3)**. The round ligaments and utero-ovarian ligaments and Fallopian tube are grasped with a Kocher clamp on each side of the uterus for uterus manipulation **(Fig. 4)**. Any adhesions to the adjacent bowel or omentum are freed.

The round ligament on one side is ligated, divided and transfixed with absorbable suture material (Vicryl 1-0) **(Fig. 5)**. If the ovaries are to be preserved the utero-ovarian pedicle is clamped, divided, and ligated. If the ovaries are to be removed the infundibular ligament is clamped, divided, and ligated. The same steps are repeated on the opposite side.

The bladder is then dissected free from the anterior wall of the lower uterine segment and cervix. So that the anterior vaginal wall is exposed. The uterine vessels are clamped, divided, and suture ligated on each side.

The bladder and rectum are disserted further down to expose the vagina. The remaining portion of the broad ligament on each side of the cervix is then clamped, divided and ligated with strong traction on the uterus **(Fig. 6)**. Right angle clamps are placed across the vaginal just below the cervix on each side with the tips meeting in the middle. The vagina is divided with scissors above the clamps and the specimen is removed. The vagina is closed incorporating the uterosacral and cardinal ligaments into the cuff for support and prevention of future vault prolapse.

Hemostasis is active and abdomen is closed in layers.

Common complications of AH include, hemorrhage, injuries to adjacent organs, and infection.

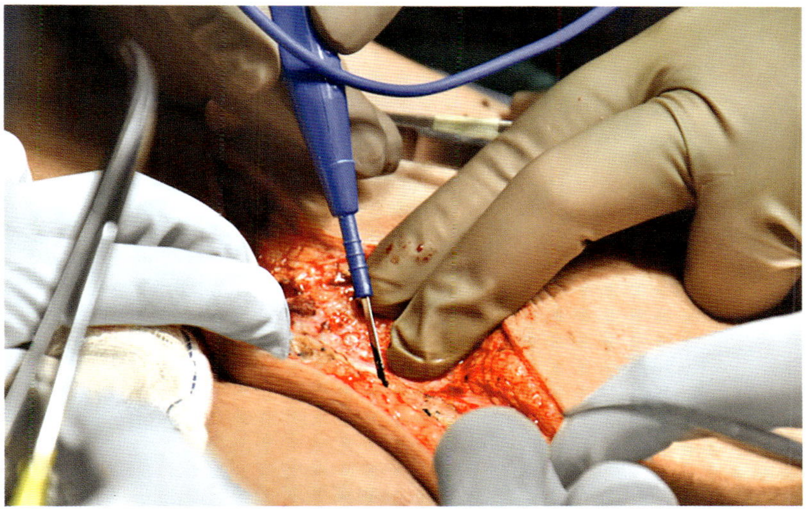

Fig. 1: Pfannenstiel incision.

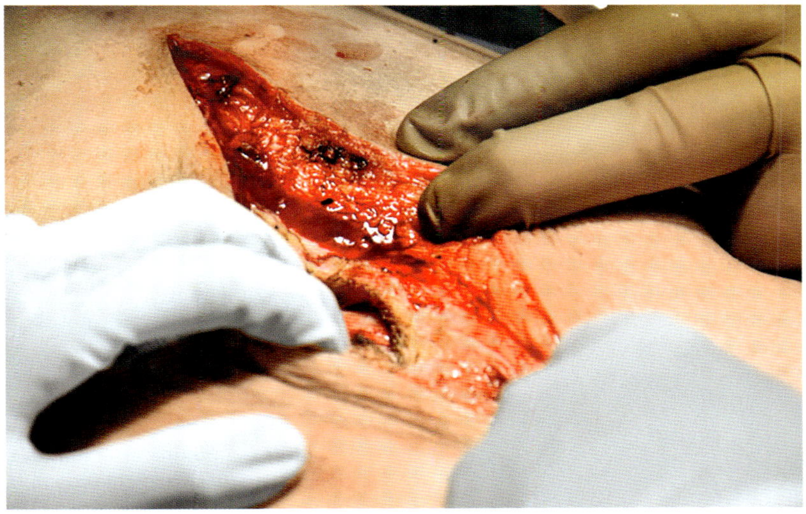

Fig. 2: Abdomen opened in layers.

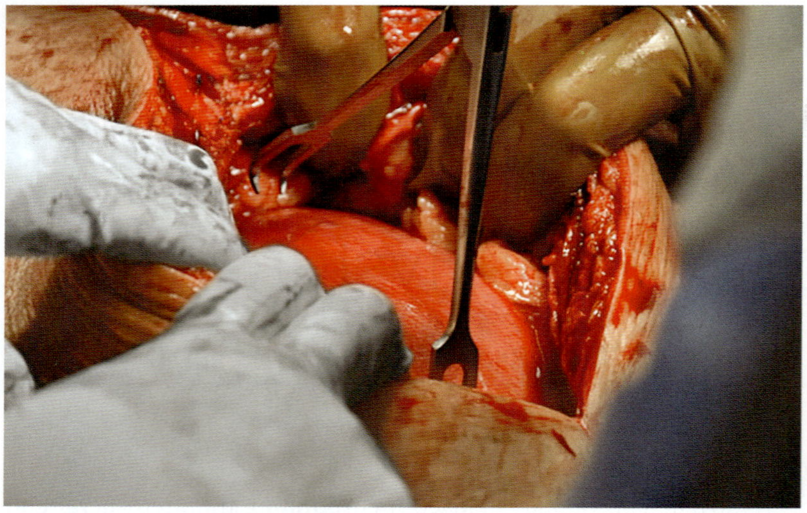

Fig. 3: Elevating the uterus out of pelvis.

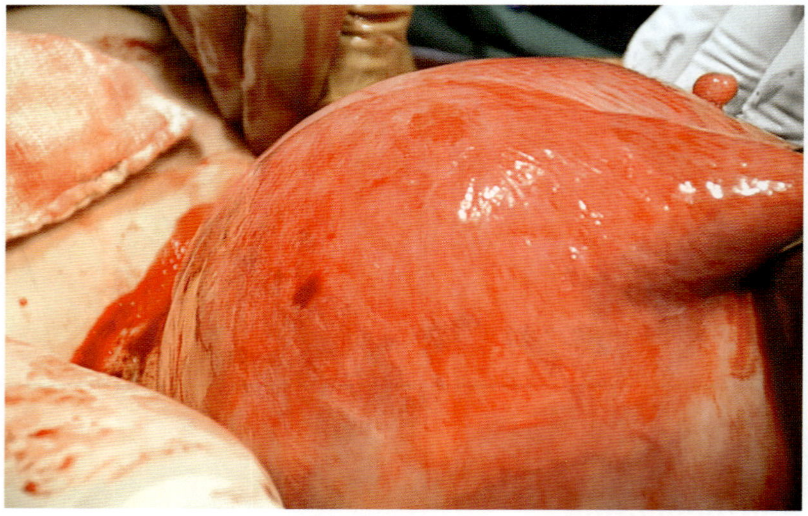

Fig. 5: Bilateral upper pedicle's clamp, cut and ligated.

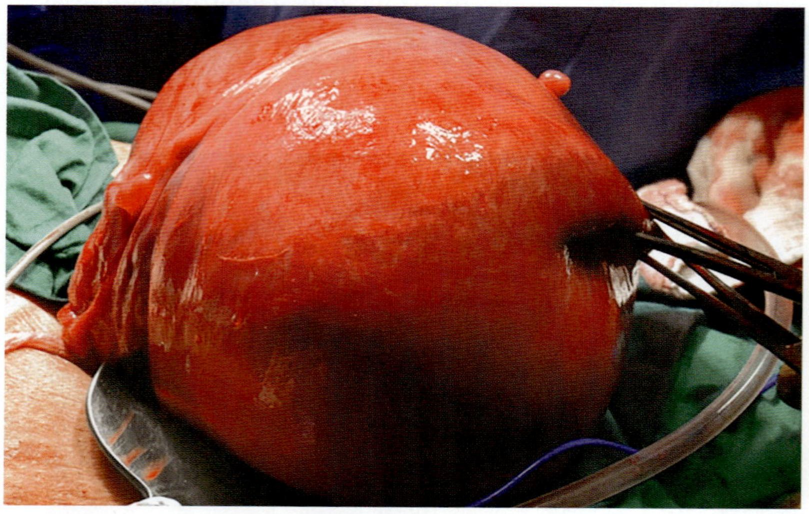

Fig. 4: Kocher clamp on each side of the uterus.

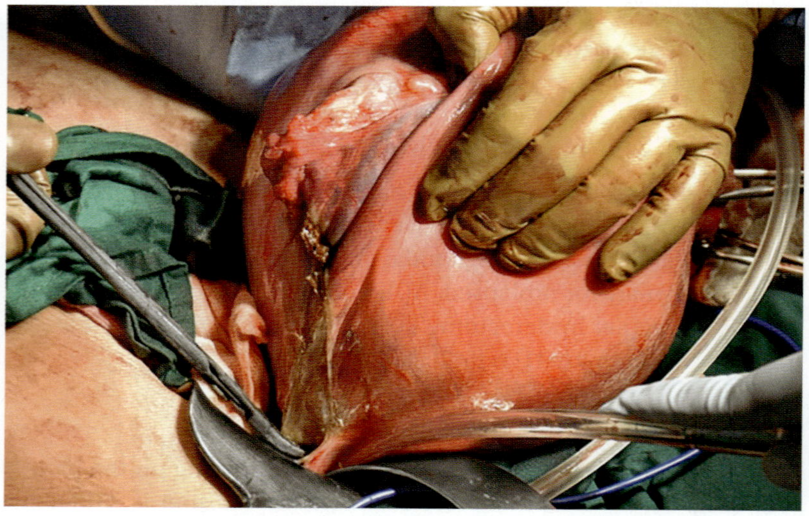

Fig. 6: Broad ligament is clamped with a series of straight clamps.

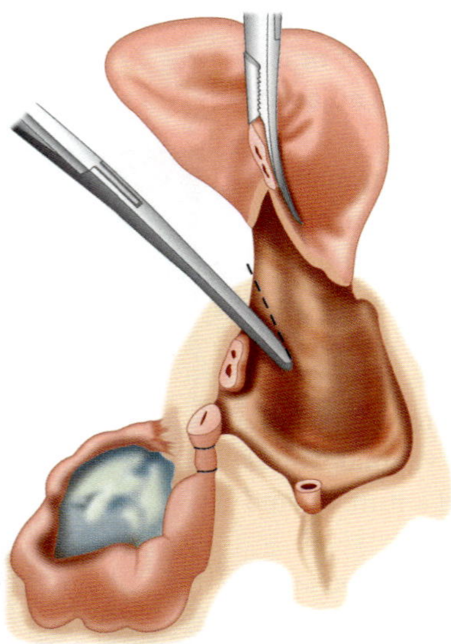

Fig. 7: After the uterine artery and vein have been ligated, the remaining lower portion of the broad ligament is clamped with a series of straight clamps. The tips are placed on the edge of the cervix and the back of the jaw immediately adjacent in the previous pedicle.

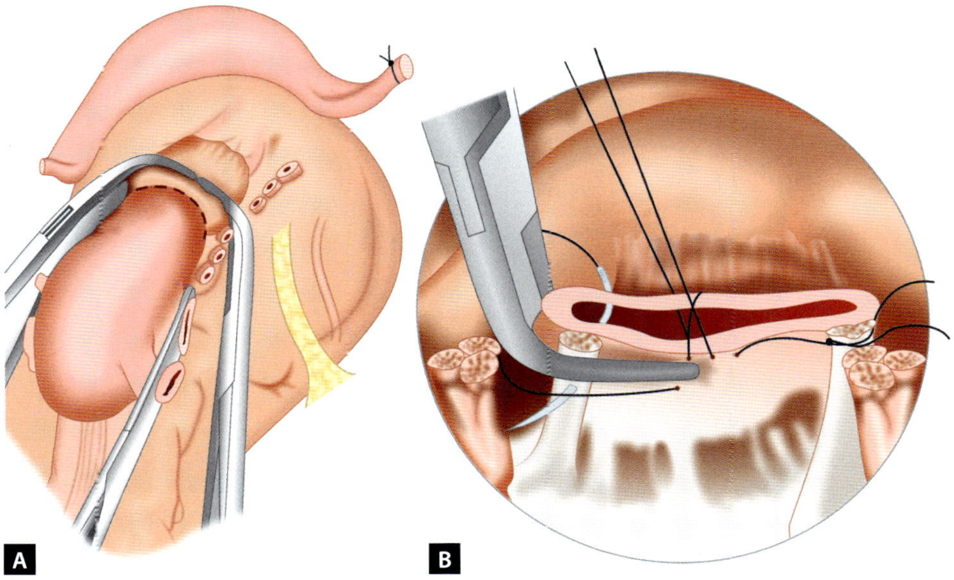

Figs. 8A and B: (A) After checking to be sure the bladder and rectum are clear, the vagina is cross clamped with long, sharply curved Zeppelin clamps just below the cervix (dotted line). The vagina is divided just above the clamps with a knife or angled scissors; (B) The vaginal cuff then is closed with a figure-of-eight suture in the middle and Heaney suture ligatures on the angles, including the uterosacral and cardinal ligaments for support.

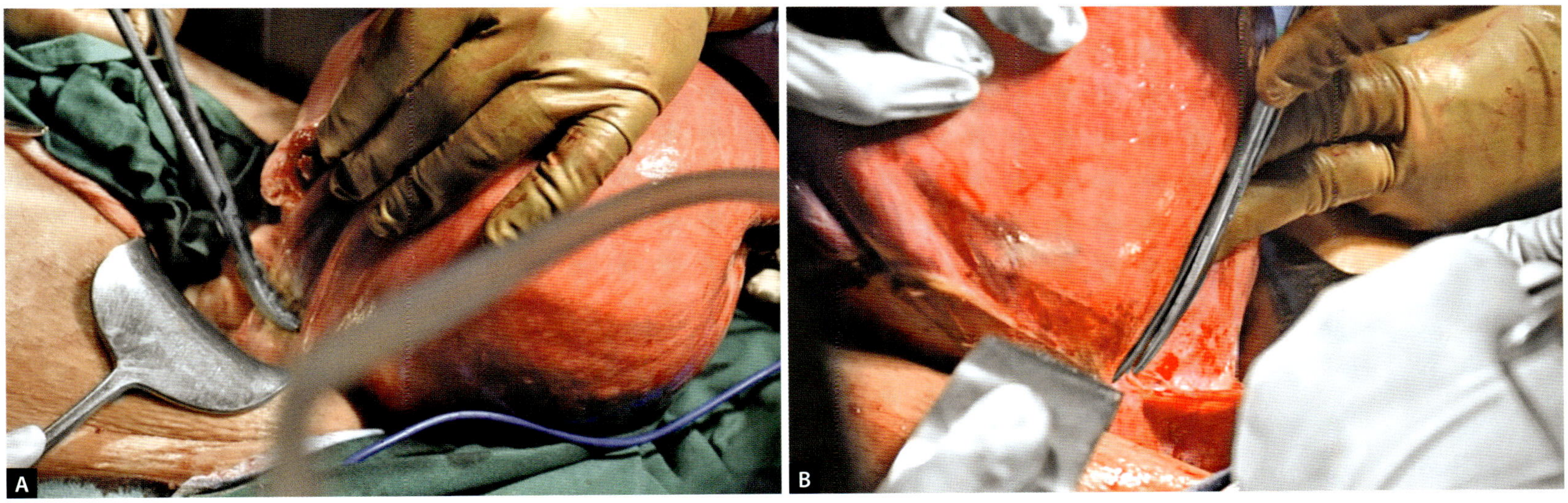

Figs. 9A and B: Bladder dissection with sharp scissors.

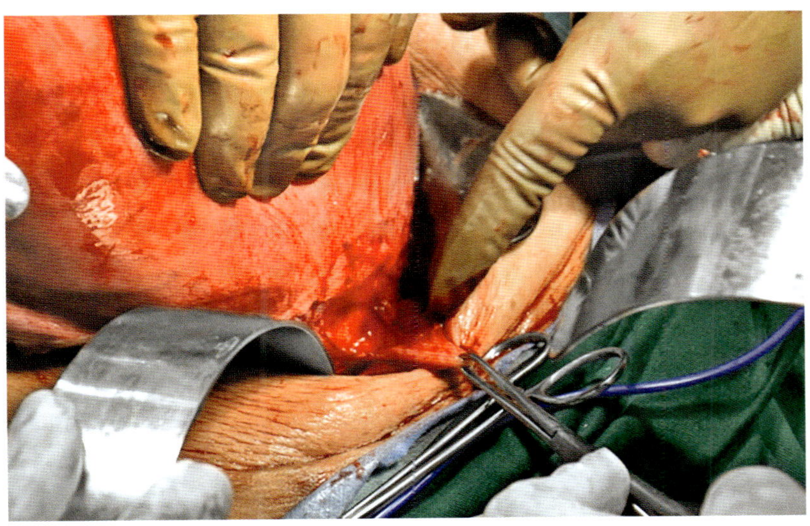

Fig. 10: Bladder dissection is continued.

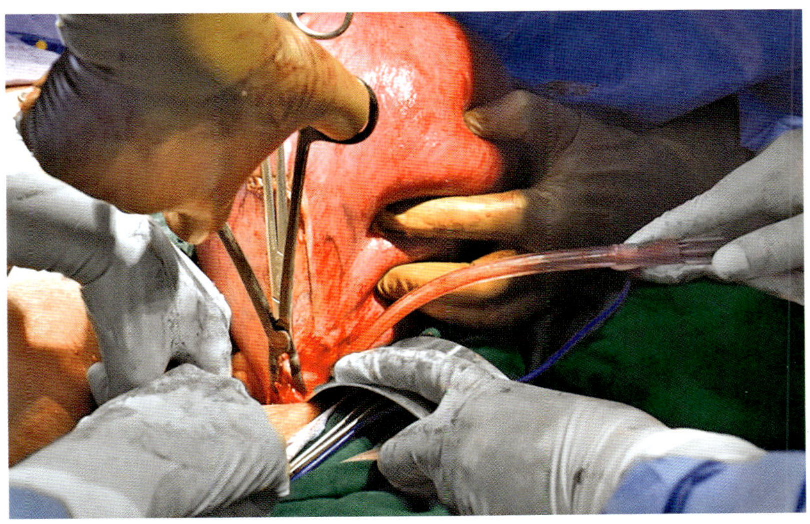

Fig. 11: Ligation litigation of the uterine artery.

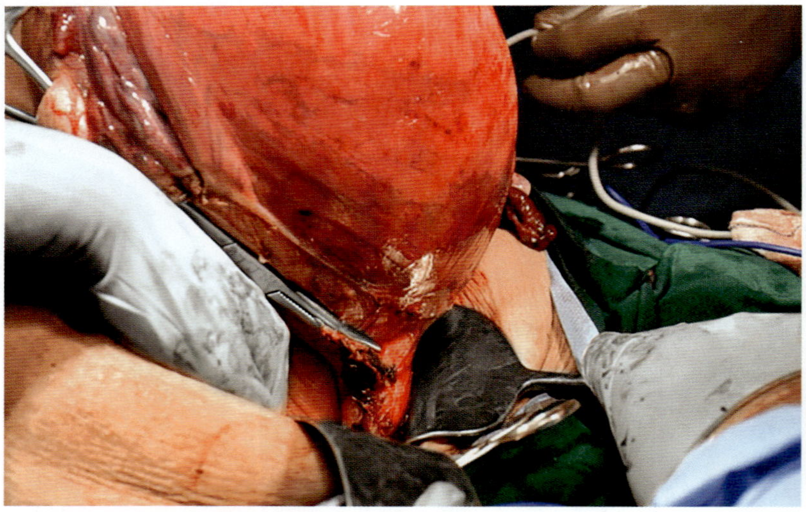

Fig. 12: Exposure of cervix and vagina.

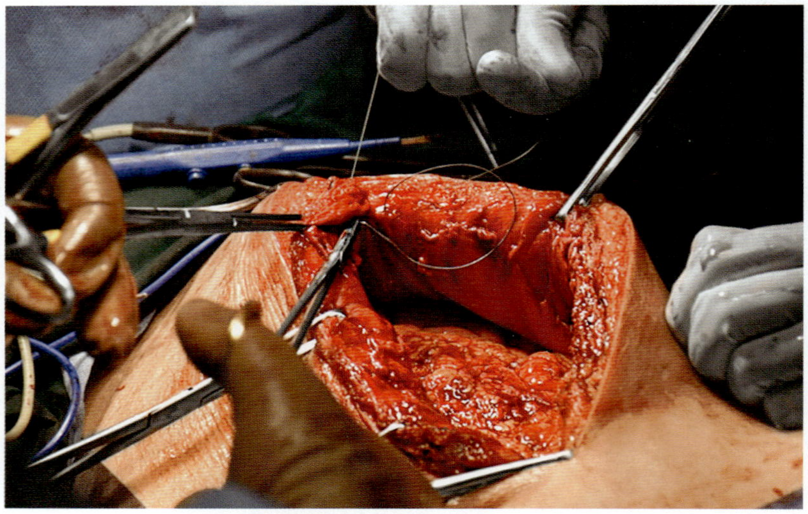

Fig. 14: Closure of layers.

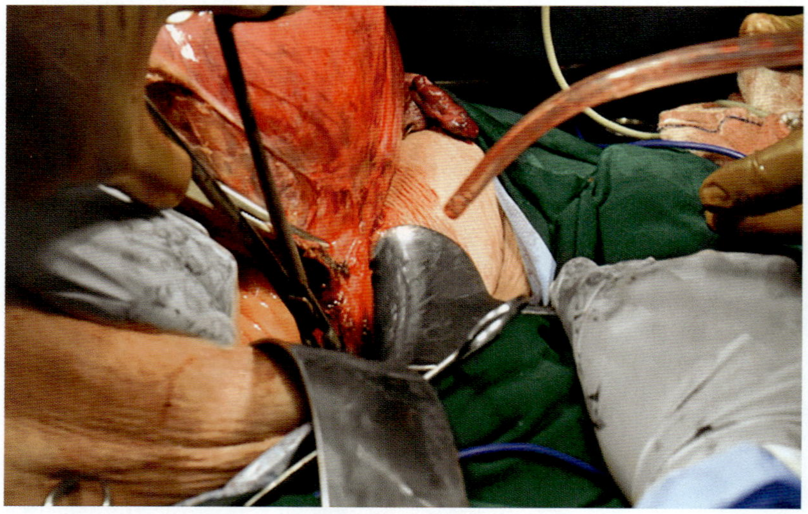

Fig. 13: Ligation of the cervical ligament.

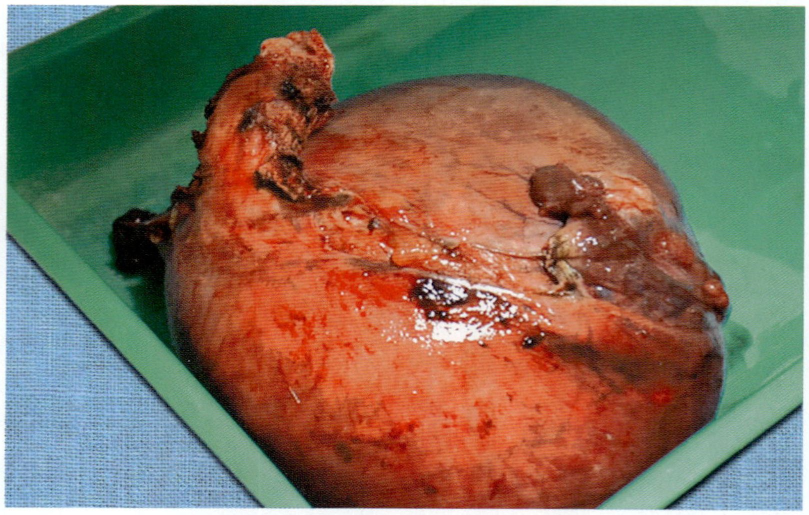

Fig. 15: Specimen delivered out.

REFERENCE

1. Jones HW. Abdominal hysterectomy. In: Jones HW, Rock JA (Eds). Te Linde's Operative Gynecology, 11th edition. Philadelphia, PA: Wolters Kluwer Health; 2016. p. 703, 709-10.

CHAPTER

42

Transobturator Tape

Supriya Raina, Minal Kumbhalwar, B Ramesh

MIDURETHRAL SLINGS

Tension-free slings are procedures for supporting midurethra using a polypropylene mesh without tension. This surgery was first invented by Ulmsten and colleagues. 85% cure rates have been found with long-term follow-up. Initially retropubic approach was used, but the transobturator approach is now widely used tension-free sling technique for primary stress urinary incontinence (SUI). The advantage of a tension-free sling is that it is minimally invasive effective technique using local anesthetic and intravenous sedation in a daycare setting.

Procedure

The anesthetic for the procedure is injected as a solution of lidocaine hydrochloride diluted to 0.25% (1/4%) strength. Because the approximate maximum safe dose is 30 mL of a 1% solution, the 0.25% (1/4%) solution will provide 120 mL. Epinephrine may be used in the mixture and with an original concentration of 1/100,000, the dilution ends up as 1/400,000. Alternatively, bupivacaine hydrochloric acid (HCl) may be used for local infiltration.

The transobturator approach [transobturator tape (TOT)] theoretically has safety factors that may make it preferable to the original transvaginal tape (TVT) approach **(Table 1)**.

It is placed more horizontally and does not interfere with voiding. Local infiltration of dilute lidocaine is carried out along the tracks of needle. There are two basic types of transobturator surgeries for stress incontinence. One is an outside-in technique, which emphasizes speed, safety, and ease of placement. The vaginal incision needs to be large enough to insert a finger to reach to the ischiopubic ramus and same hand thumb grasps the ramus in the genitofemoral fold between labia majora and thigh. A point in the groin fold level with the clitoris is selected and a 5-mm incision made on each side. The needle passer is introduced perpendicularly and guided with finger till it perforates the obturator membrane. The needle is then rotated under the ramus and the vaginal index finger guides it inside the vaginal incision. The tightening of the sling is the same as the TVT.

The inside-out TOT starts with local infiltration of dilute anesthetic. The incision may be slightly smaller than the outside-in TOT. Scissor dissection proceeds on one side until the obturator membrane is penetrated with the scissor tips. A metal winged guide is placed into the defect in the obturator membrane. The needle passer is placed along the direction of the winged guide and then rotated while the handle is moved inferiorly to a vertical position. The needle passer exits 1 cm lateral to the groin fold about 2 cm superior to the urethral meatus and parallel to the clitoris. The tape is retrieved and tightening follows the same pattern as with the technique described above. The same day patient attempts to void in recovery; if unsuccessful, she uses self-catheterization or has a Foley placed overnight.

Advantages

- As there is no retropubic passage, TOT avoids the major complications like retroperitoneal vessel injury, bladder and bowel injury.
- Postoperative voiding dysfunction is also less with TOT tape.

Disadvantages

- During insertion of needle, obturator vessels and nerve may get injured
- There are few case reports of bladder perforation with TOT, hence it is preferred to perform cystoscopy at the end of procedure with urethral inspection mainly for women with significant prolapse
- Complications of bleeding, hematoma, dysuria, urgency, and bladder infections. Uncommonly abscess formation in the ischiorectal fossa
- Occasionally, there is persisting groin pain or irritation with movement.

The tension-free sling is thought to work by forming a solid buttress under the midurethra, allowing the mobile bladder neck to descend and rotate with increased intra-abdominal pressure and compress the urethra against the sling. Most efficacy reports are in the 85% range for both TVT and TOT procedures and this can safely be quoted to patients in preoperative discussion.

When the tension-free tape procedures are done in conjunction with other pelvic floor surgery, order in which things are done does not matter. The tape can be laid in position initially and then the rest of the procedures completed and the tape tightened at the end of the case. If there is a lot of bleeding from dissection for the tape, this can cause some delay and interference with the rest of the case. The other way is to do all the other procedures and then place the tape at the end. Any anterior vaginal wall dissection should not extend closer than 2 cm to the urethral meatus, thus leaving room for the tape dissection. If a colpocleisis is performed, the tape has to be placed before obliterating the anterior wall.

Table 1: Differentiating features between transobturator tape and transvaginal tape.

Transobturator tape	*Transvaginal tape*
It does not have a retropubic passage	It has a retropubic passage
Chances of injury to the vessels, bladder, and viscera are less	Chances of injury to vessels, bladder, and viscera are more
Possibility of damage to obturator nerve and vessels is more	No risk of damage to obturator nerve and vessels
The incidence of voiding dysfunction with TOT is less.	The incidence of voiding dysfunction with TVT is more.

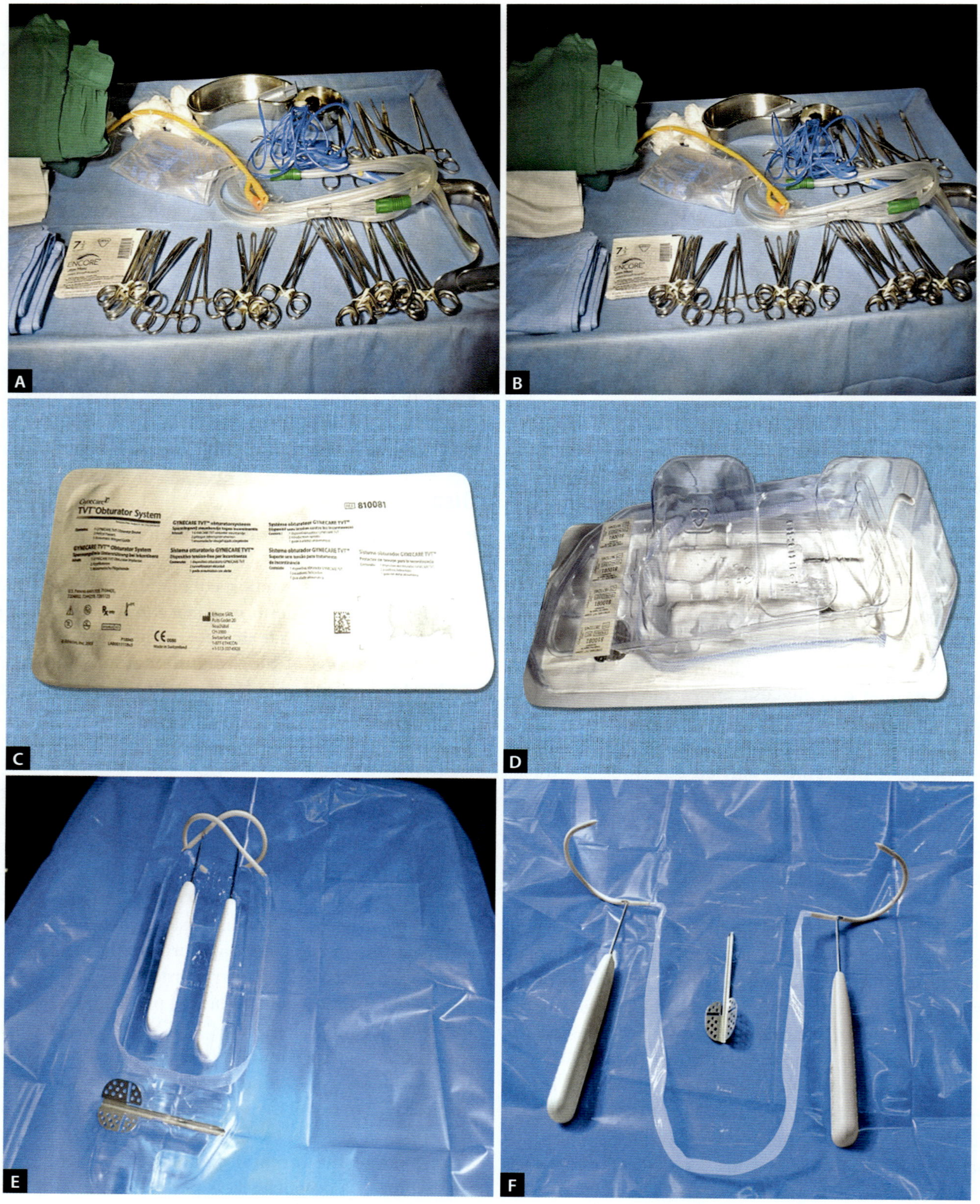

Figs. 1A to F: Instruments for transobturator tape placement.

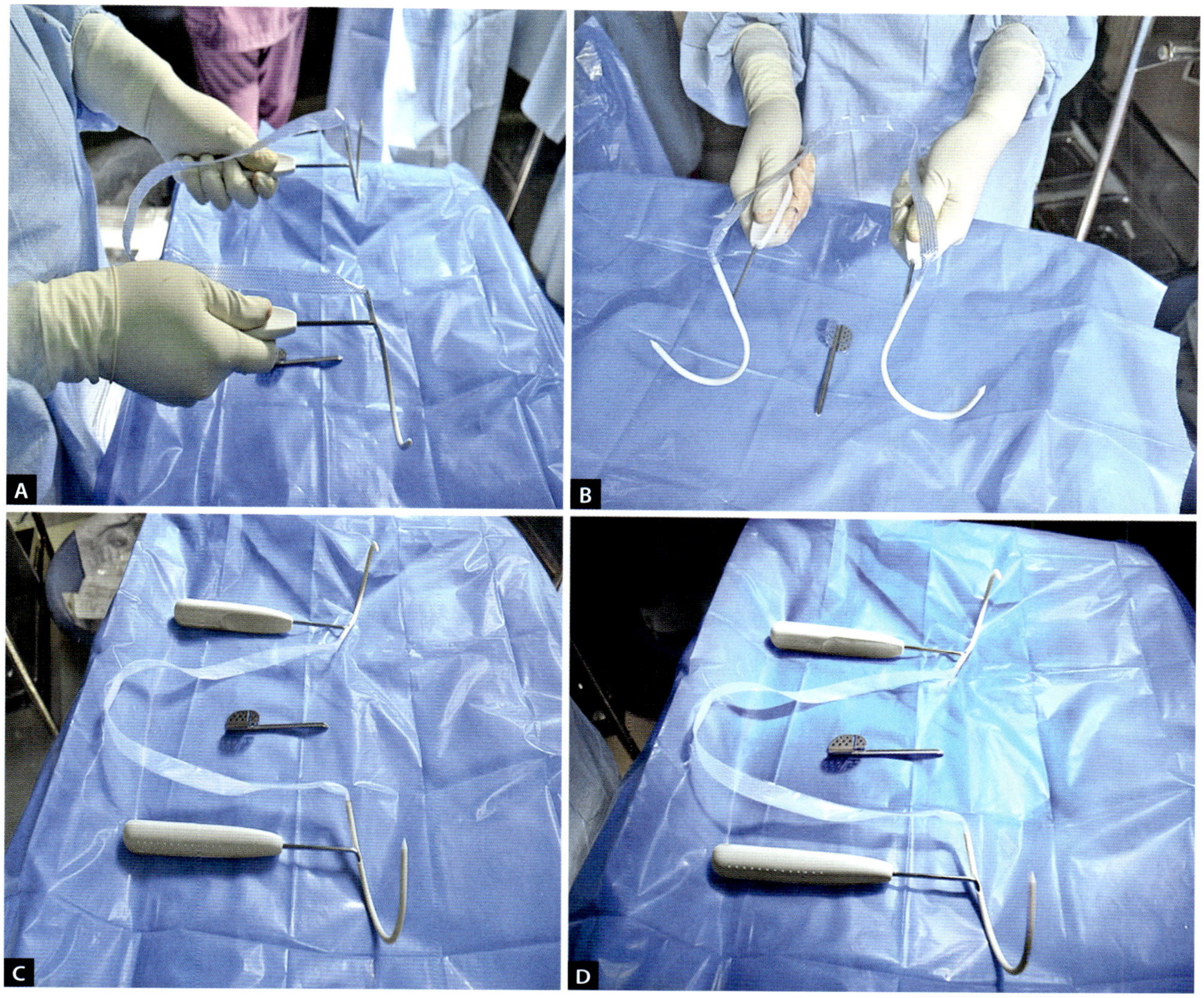

Figs. 2A to D: Transobturator tape.

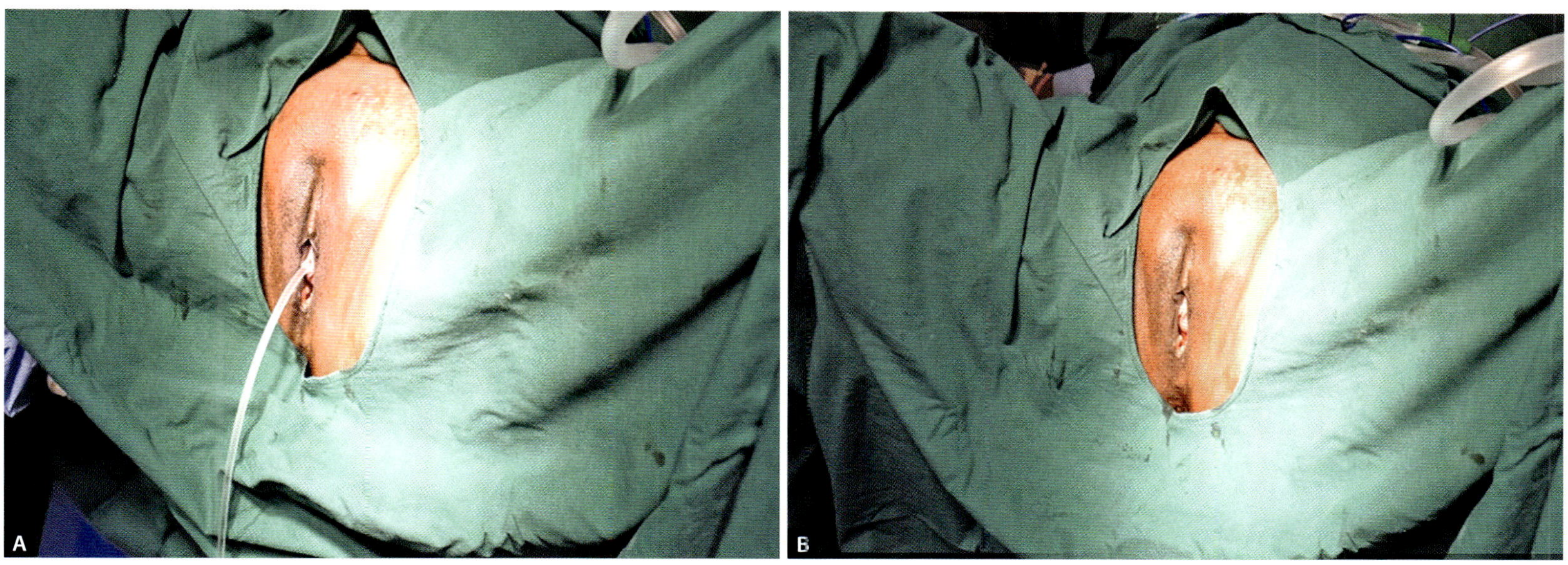

Figs. 3A and B: Painting and draping the parts.

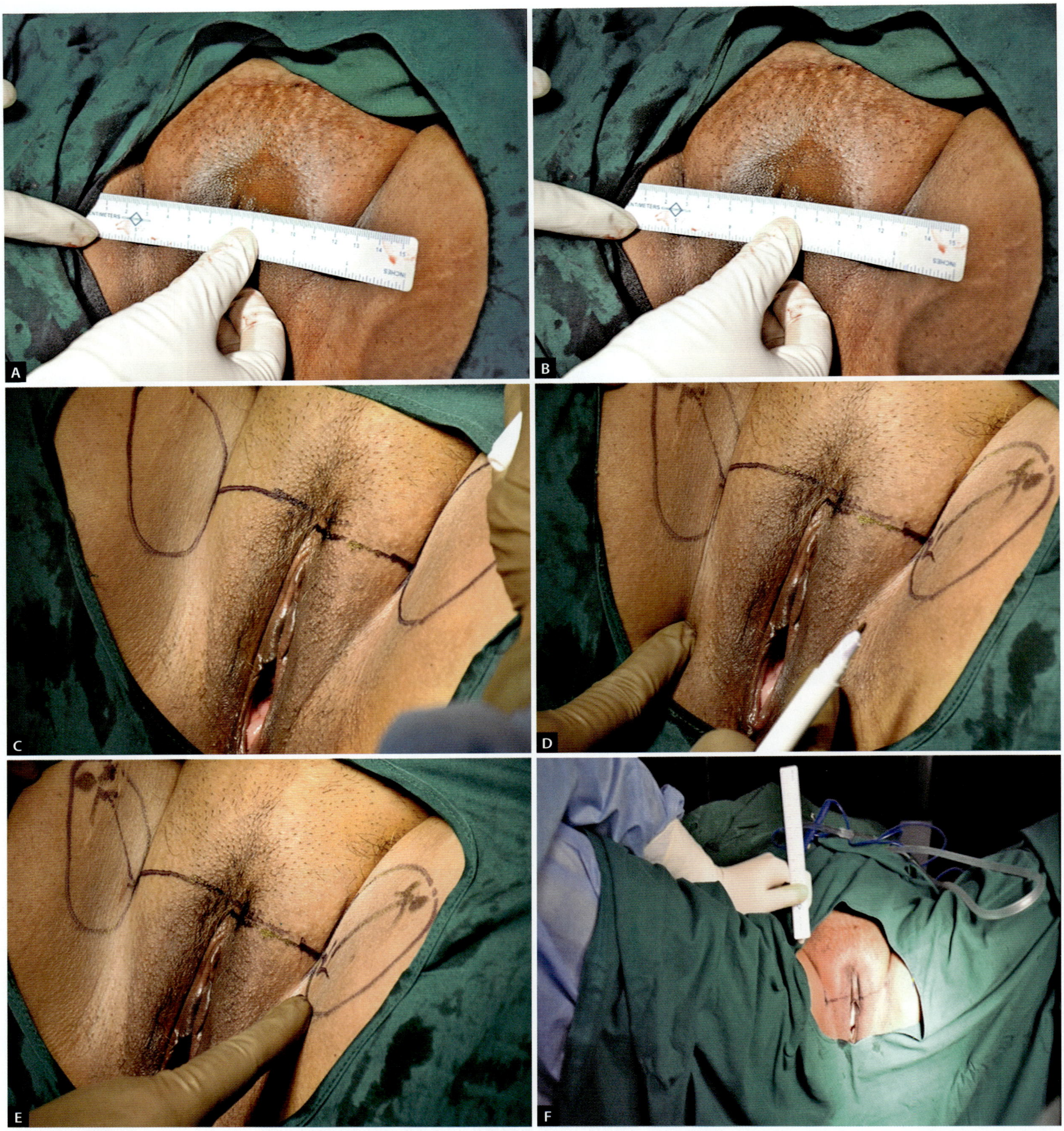

Figs. 4A to F: Marking the line at the level of clitoris to make incisions.

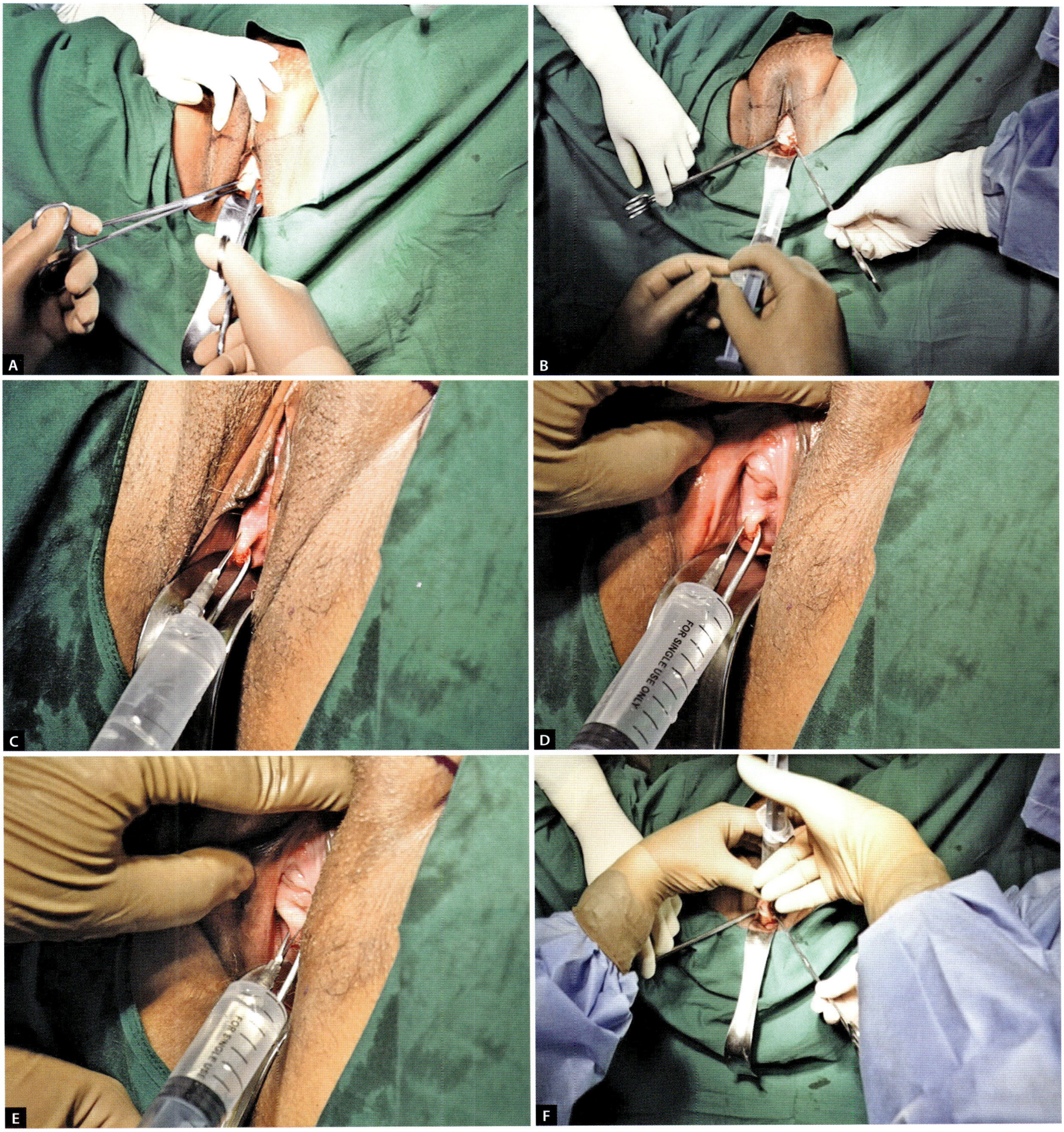

Figs. 5A to F: Infraurethrally held with Ellis forceps and vasopressin injected.

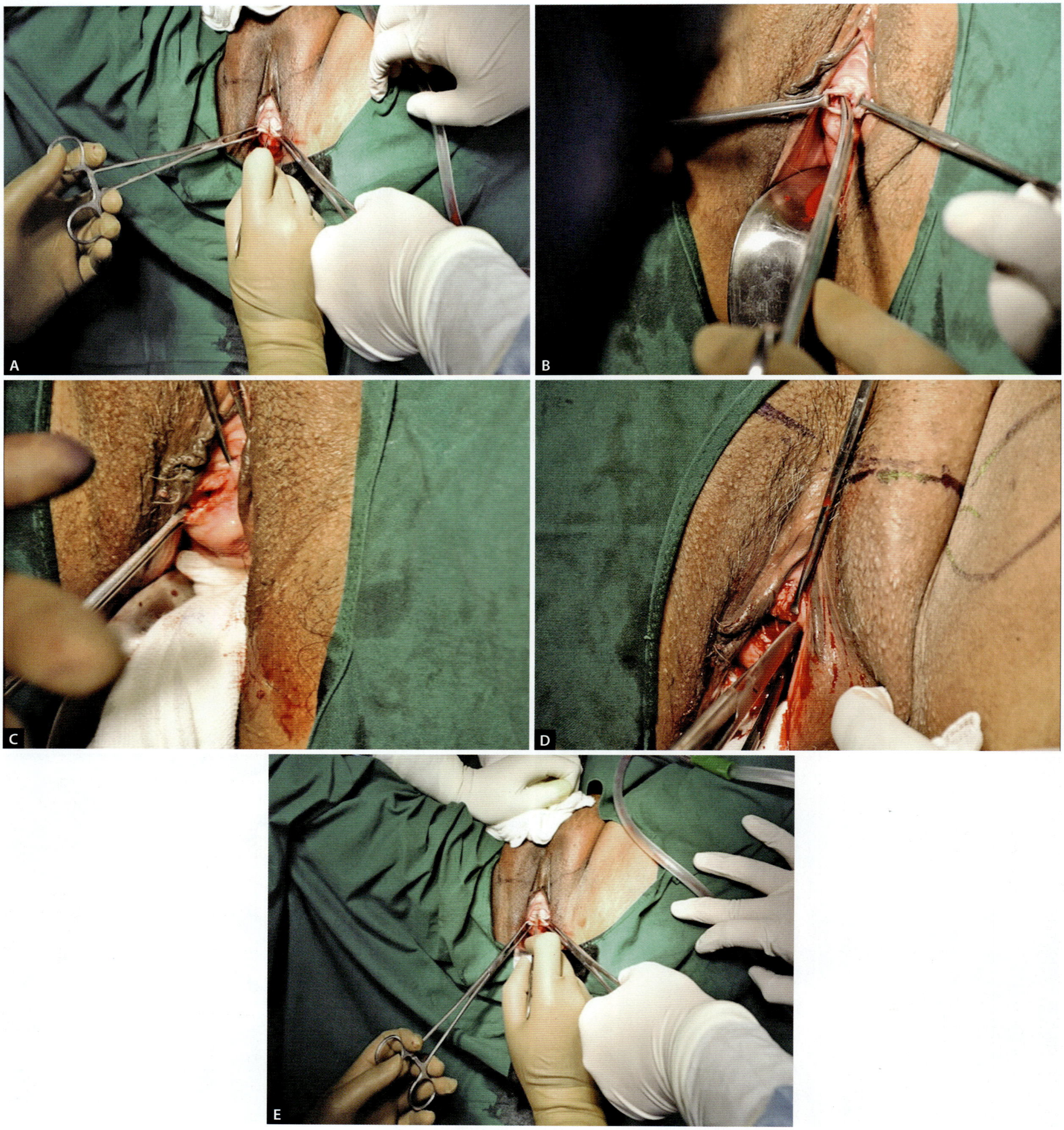

Figs. 6A to E: Vertical incision made in infraurethral area.

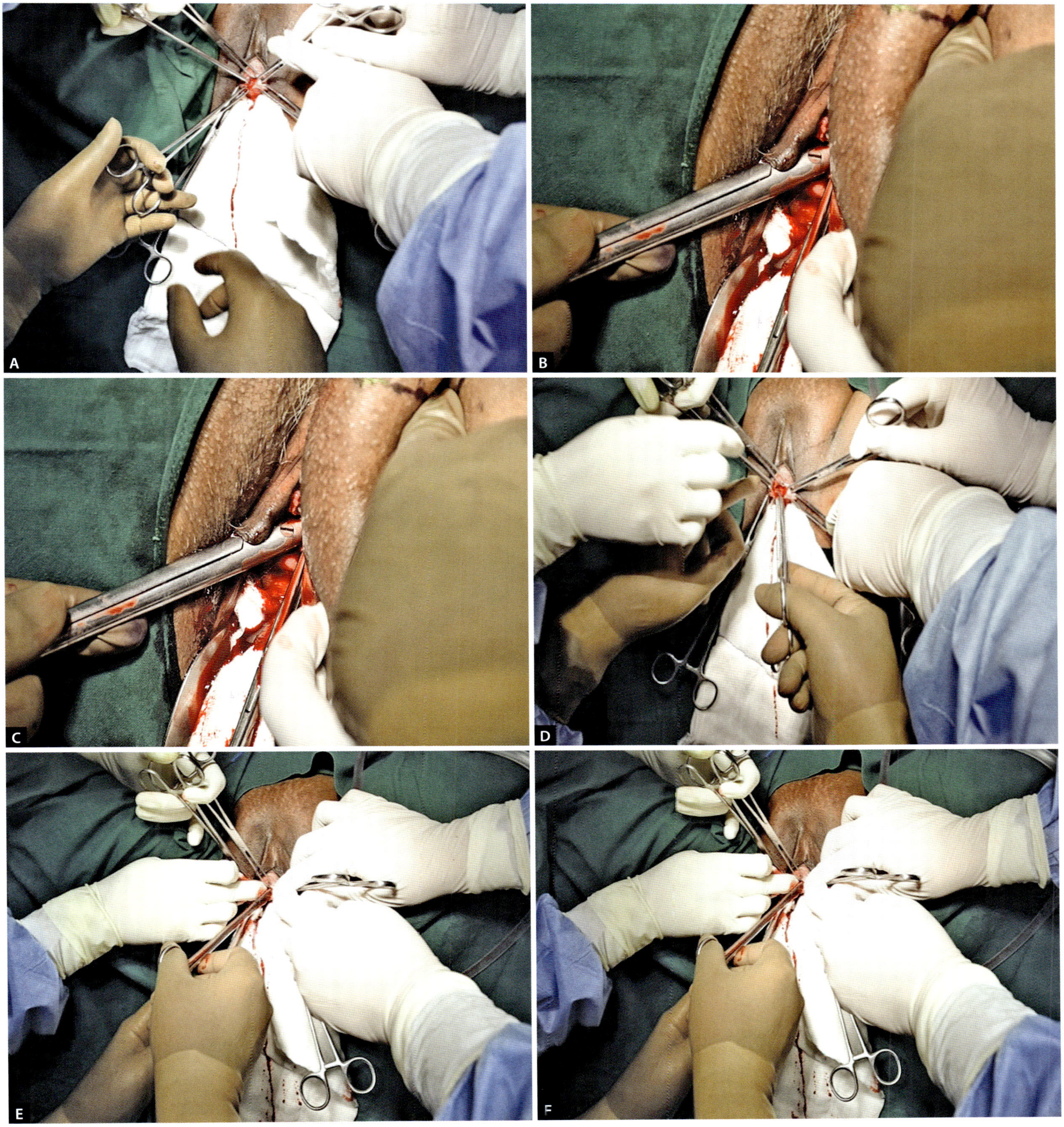

Figs. 7A to F: Passage created on both sides with artery forceps for introducing tape.

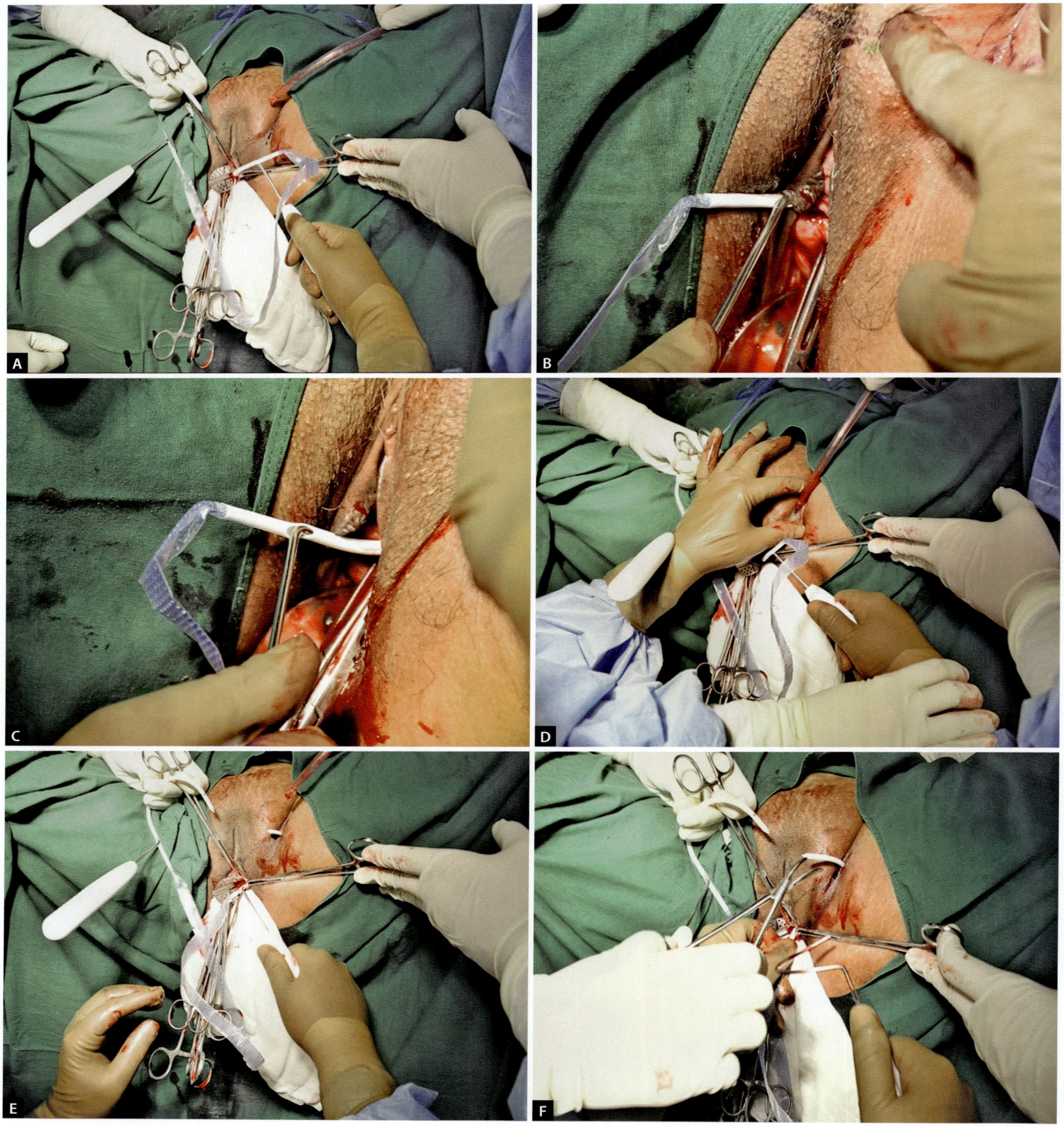

Figs. 8A to F

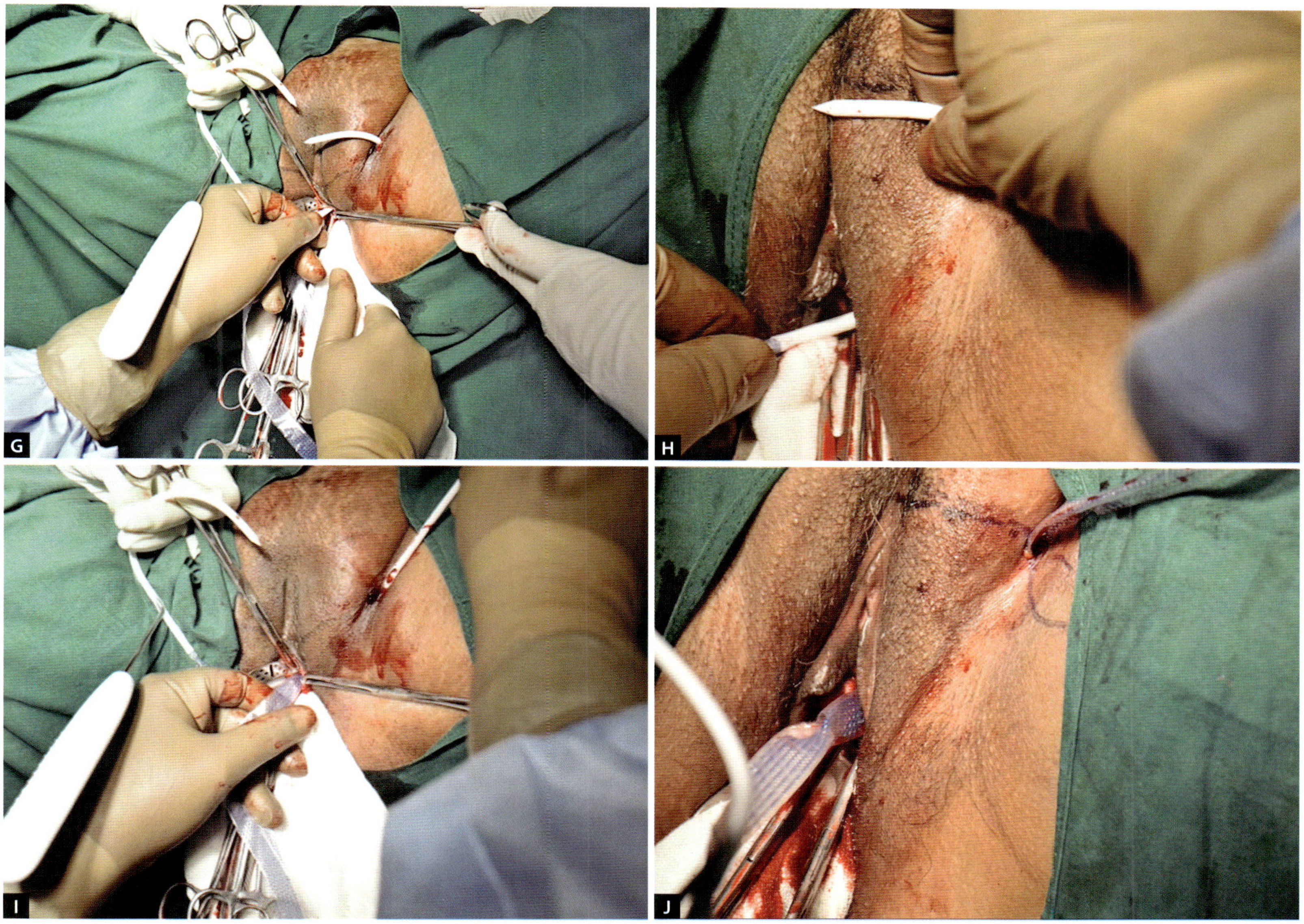

Figs. 8G to J

Figs. 8A to J: Tape introduced from medial to lateral side infraurethrally to incision in the groin.

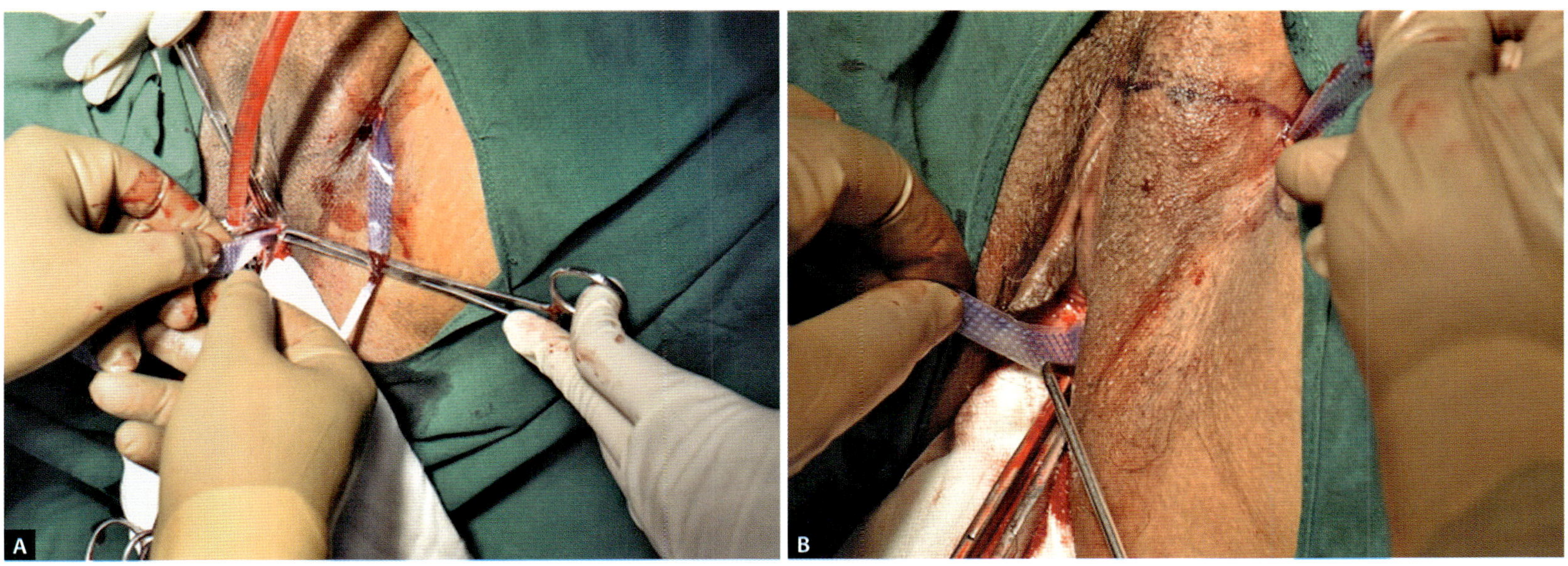

Figs. 9A and B

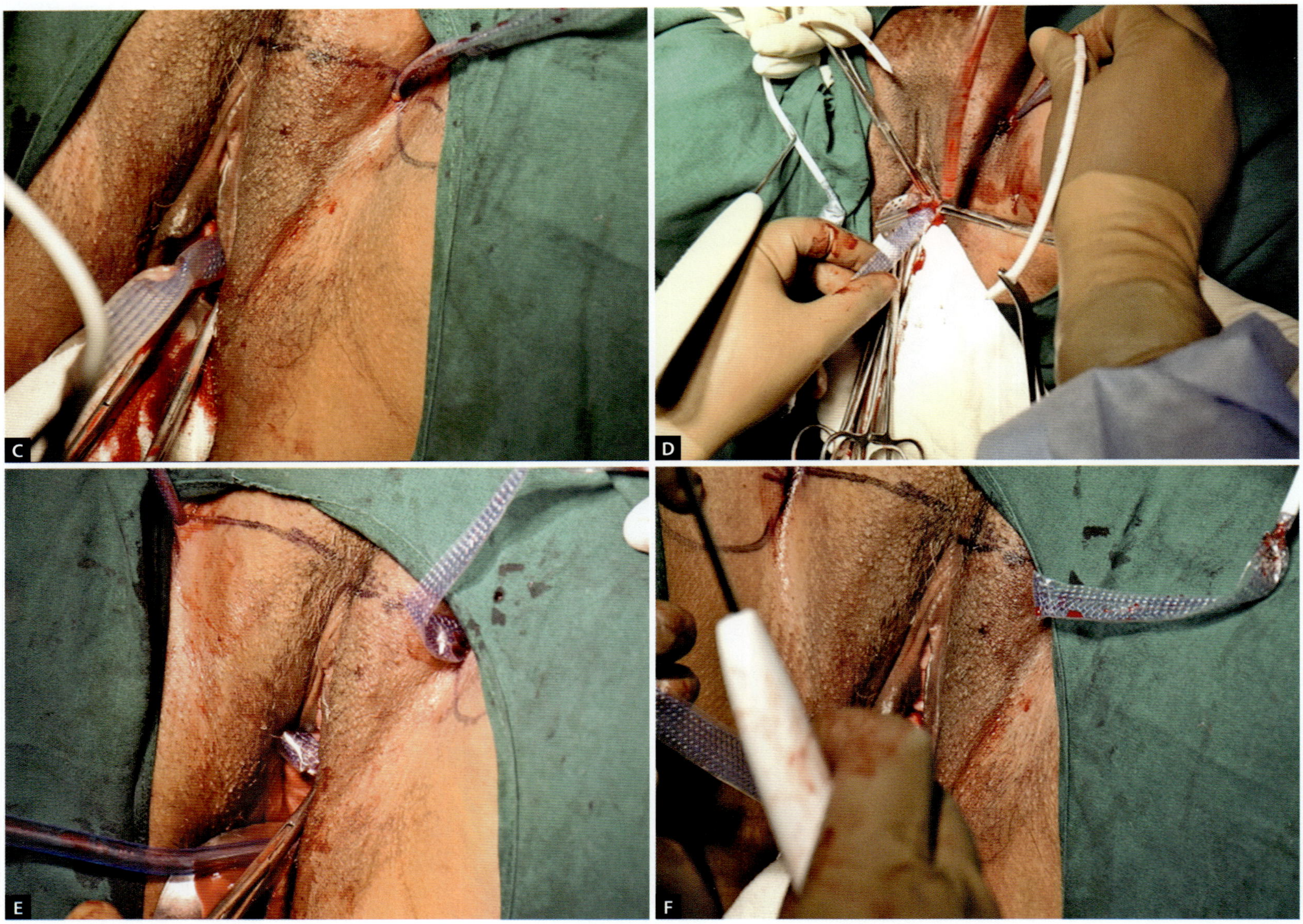

Figs. 9C to F

Figs. 9A to F: Tape introduced from medial to lateral side infraurethrally to incision in the groin on left side.

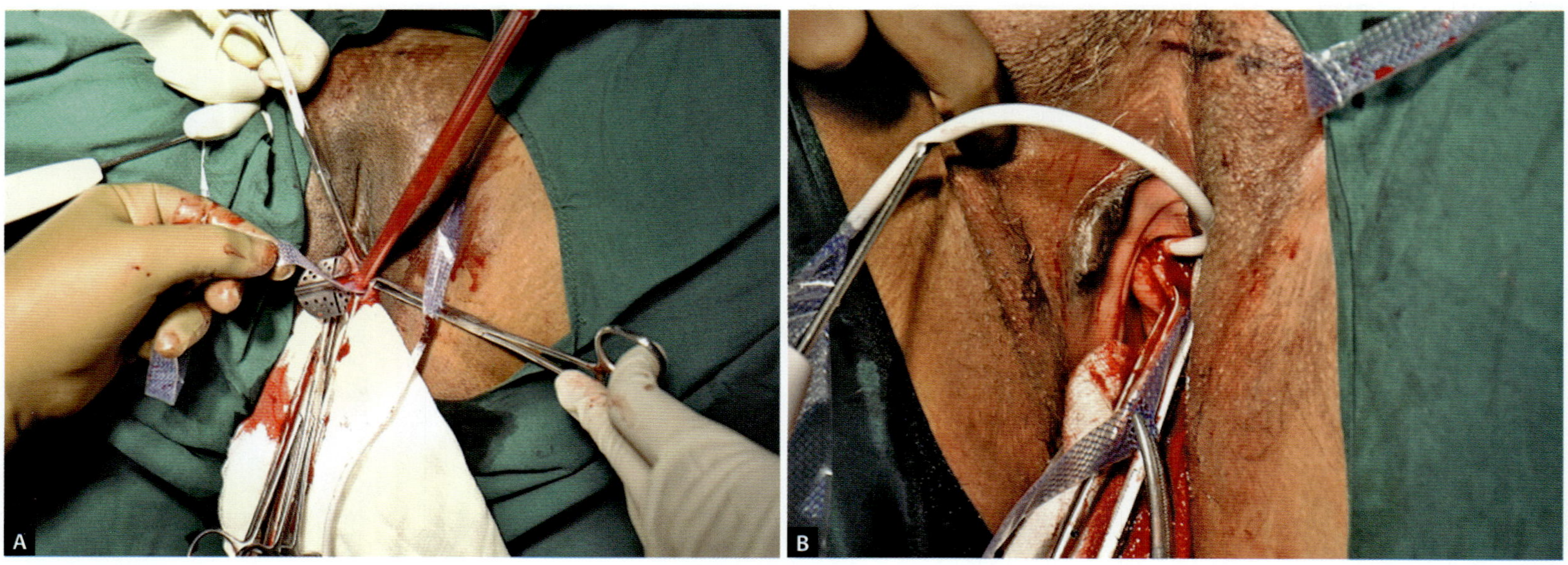

Figs. 10A and B

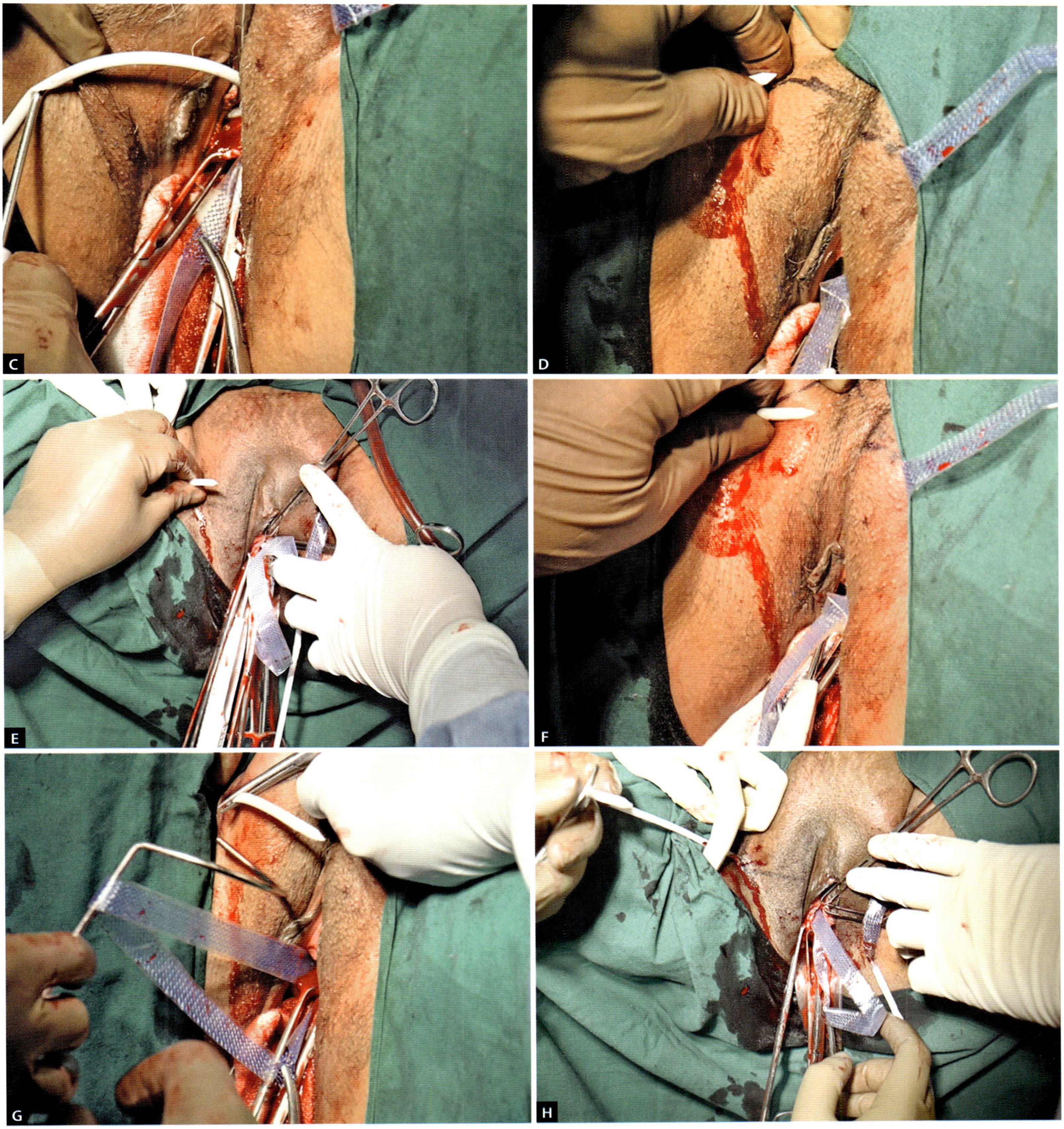

Figs. 10C to H

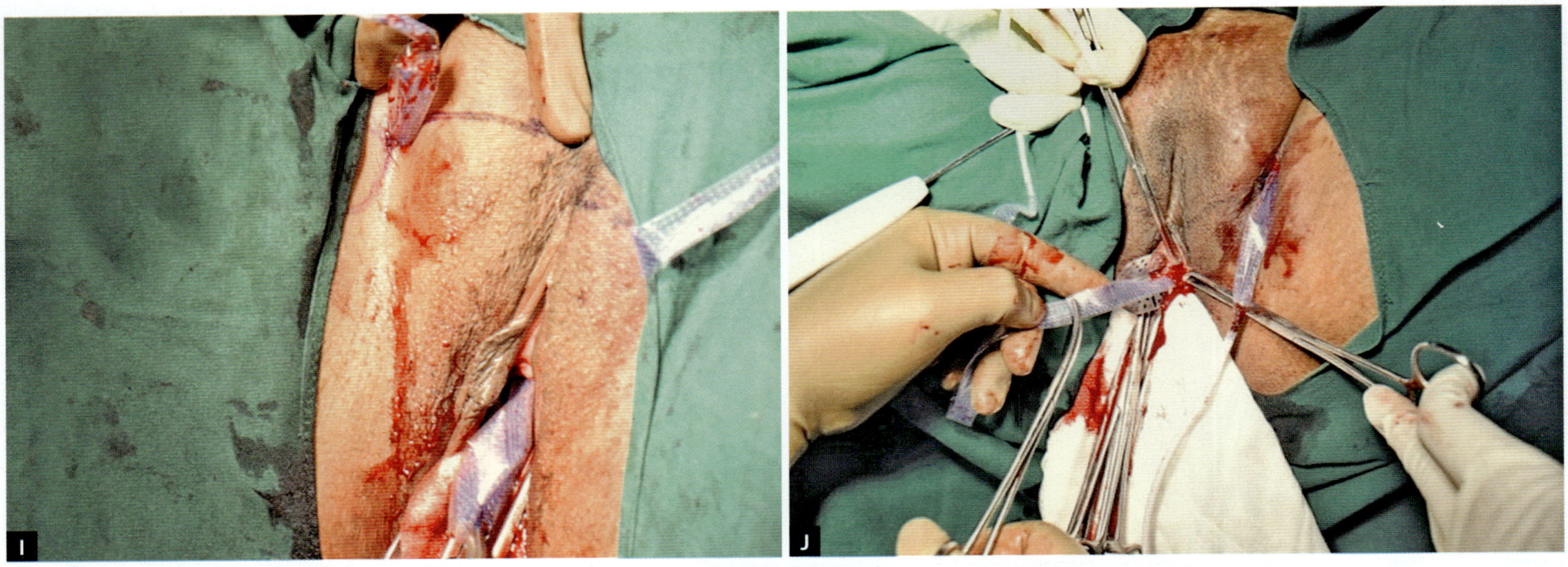

Figs. 10I and J

Figs. 10A to J: Tape introduced from medial to lateral side infraurethrally to incision in the groin on right side.

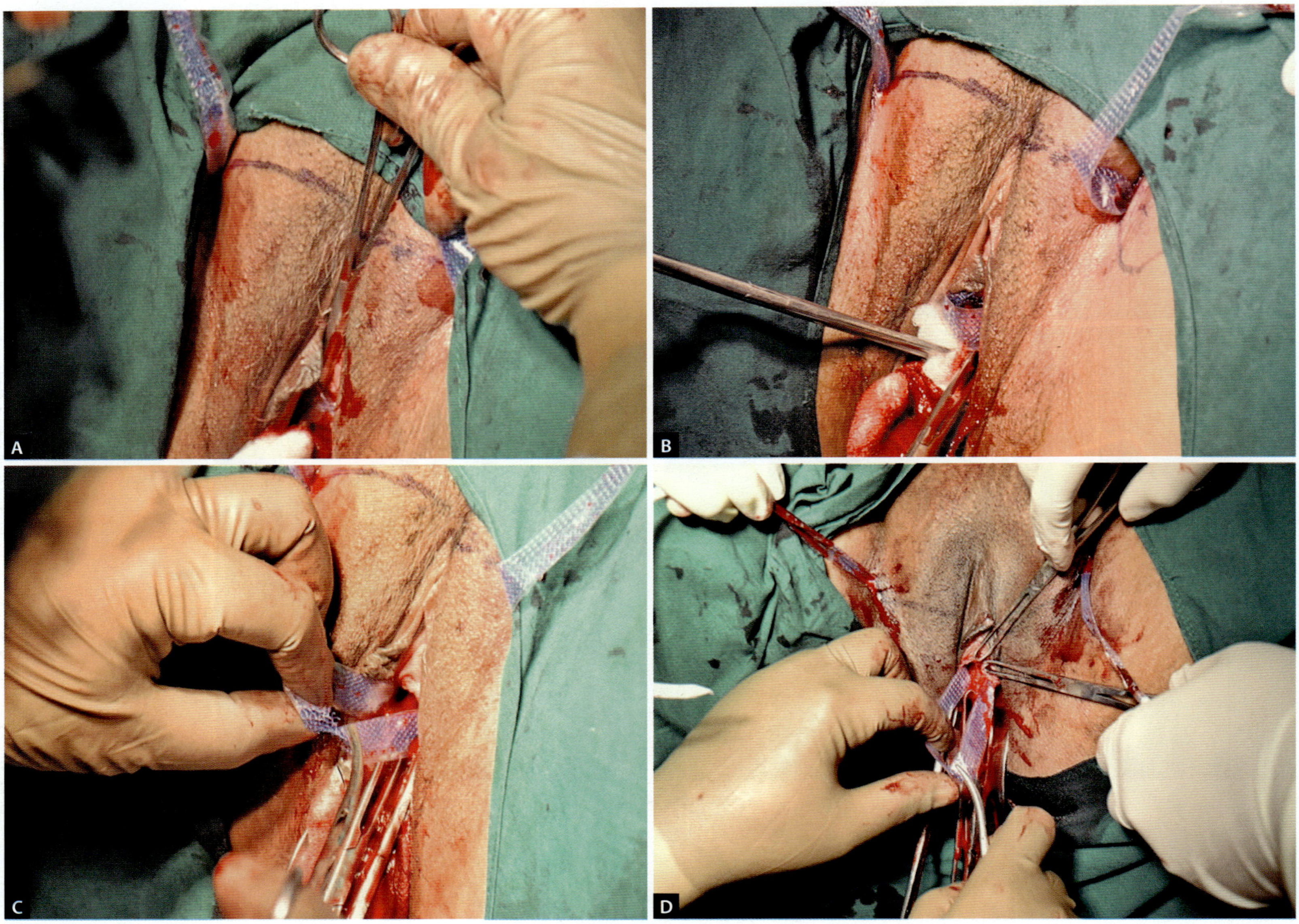

Figs. 11A to D

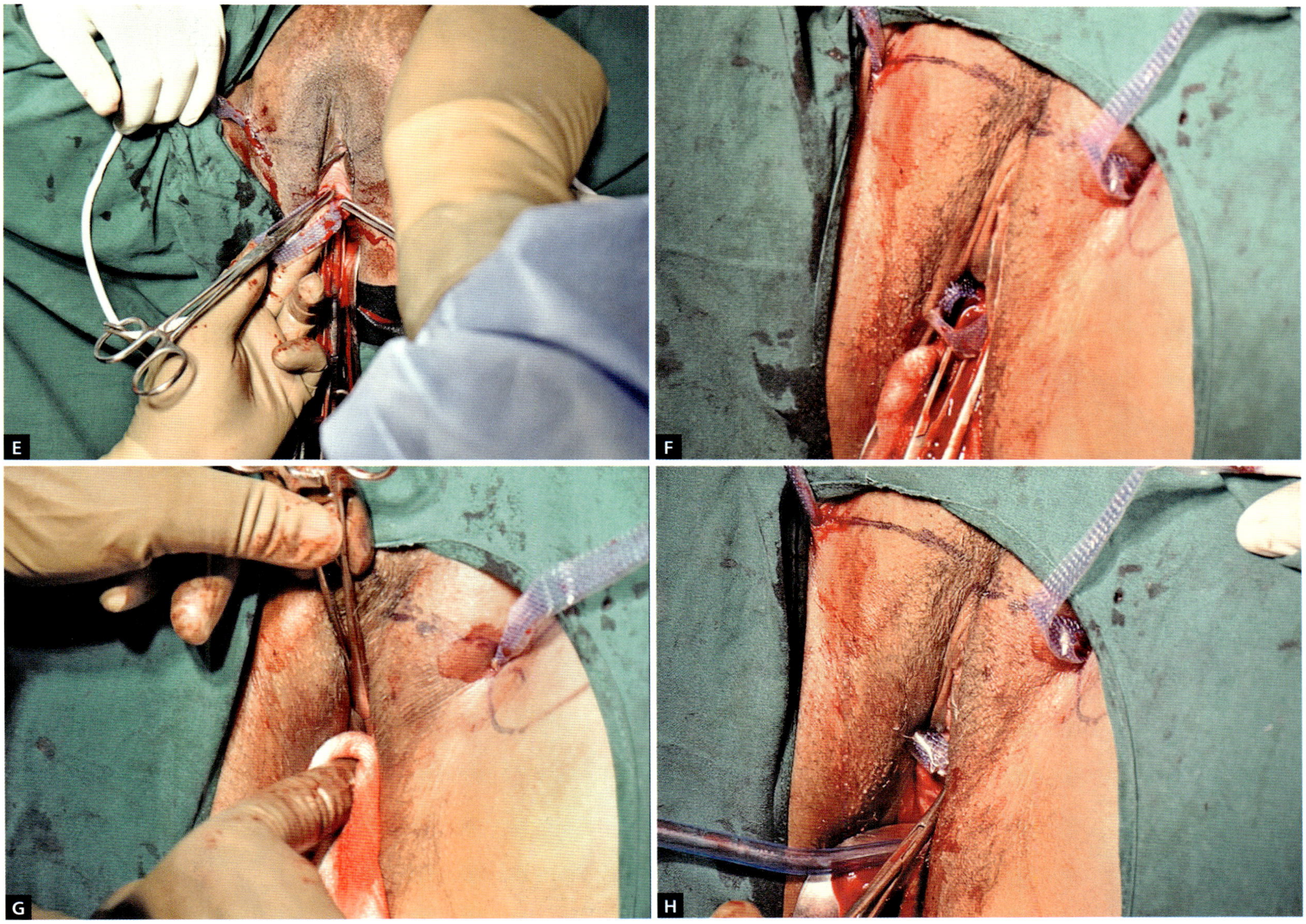

Figs. 11E to H

Figs. 11A to H: Adjusting the tape infraurethrally.

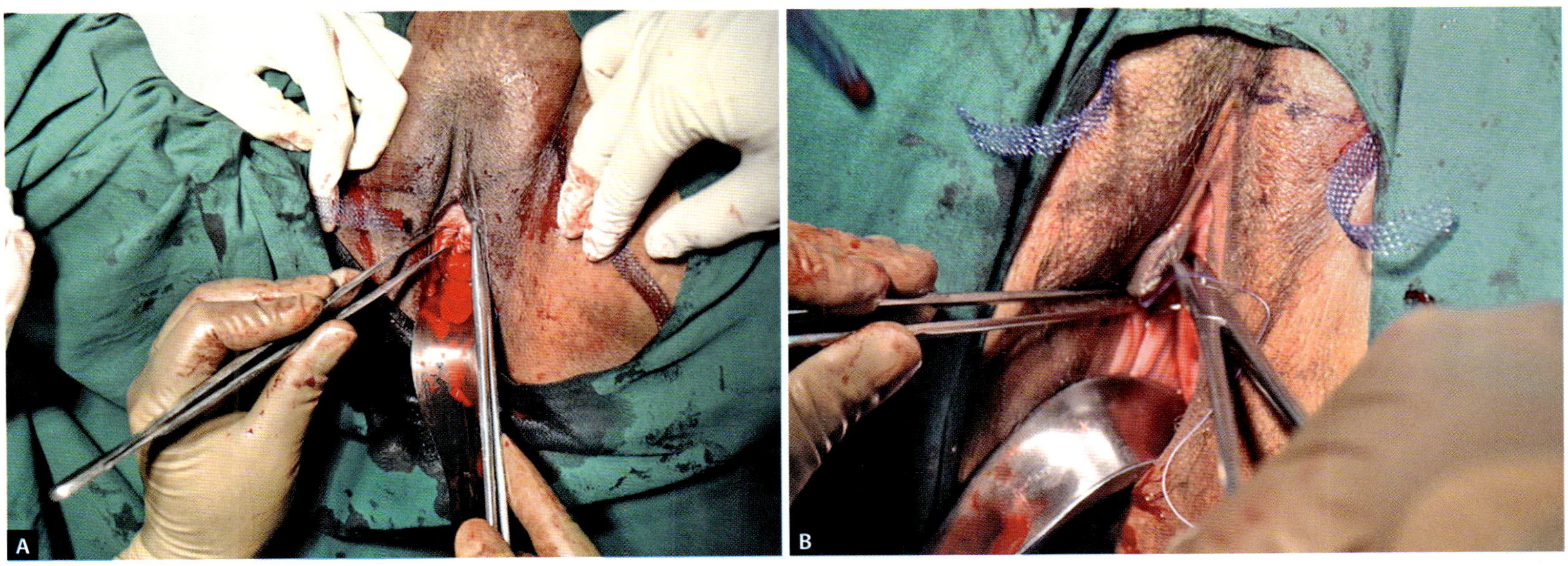

Figs. 12A and B

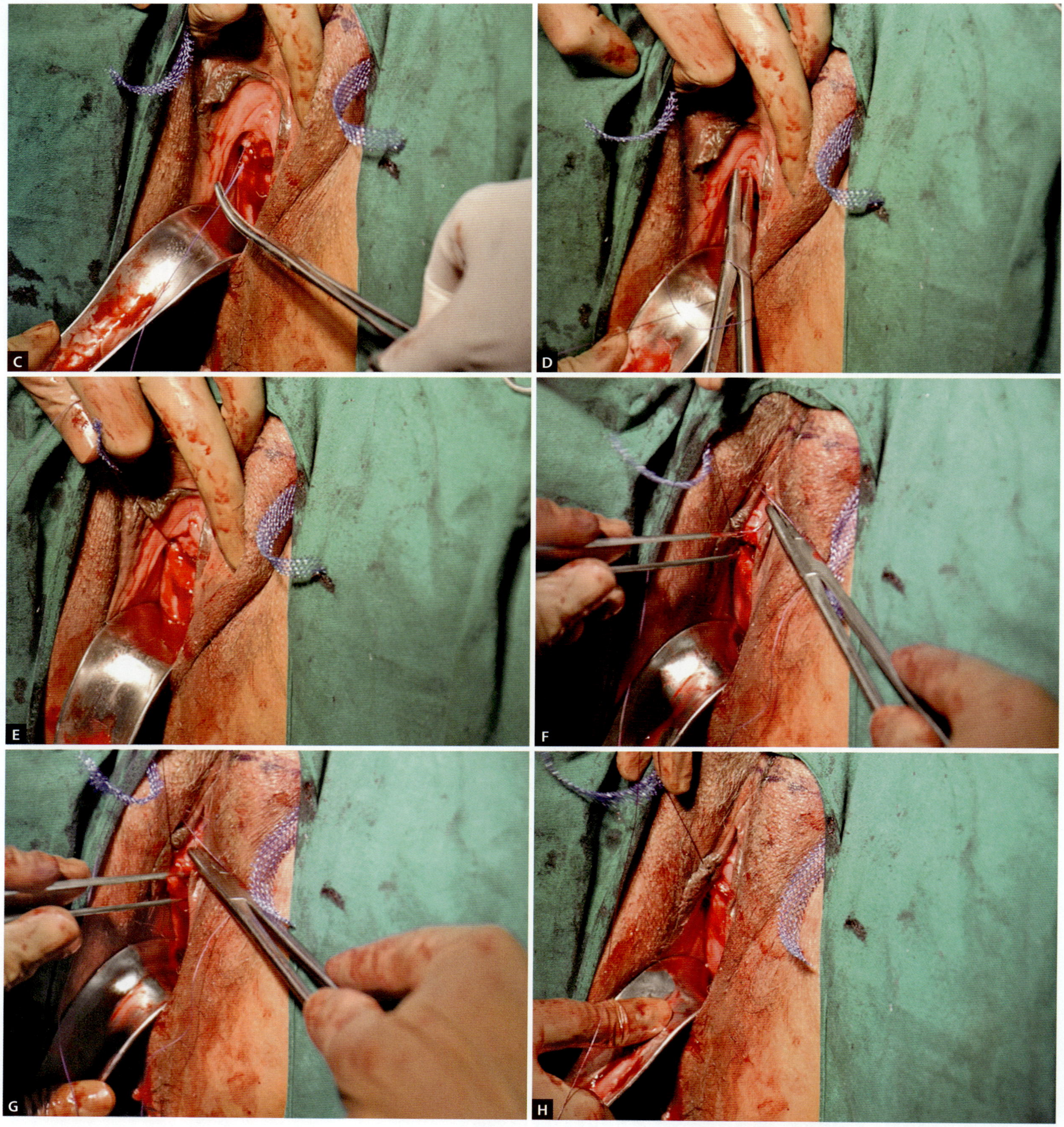

Figs. 12C to H

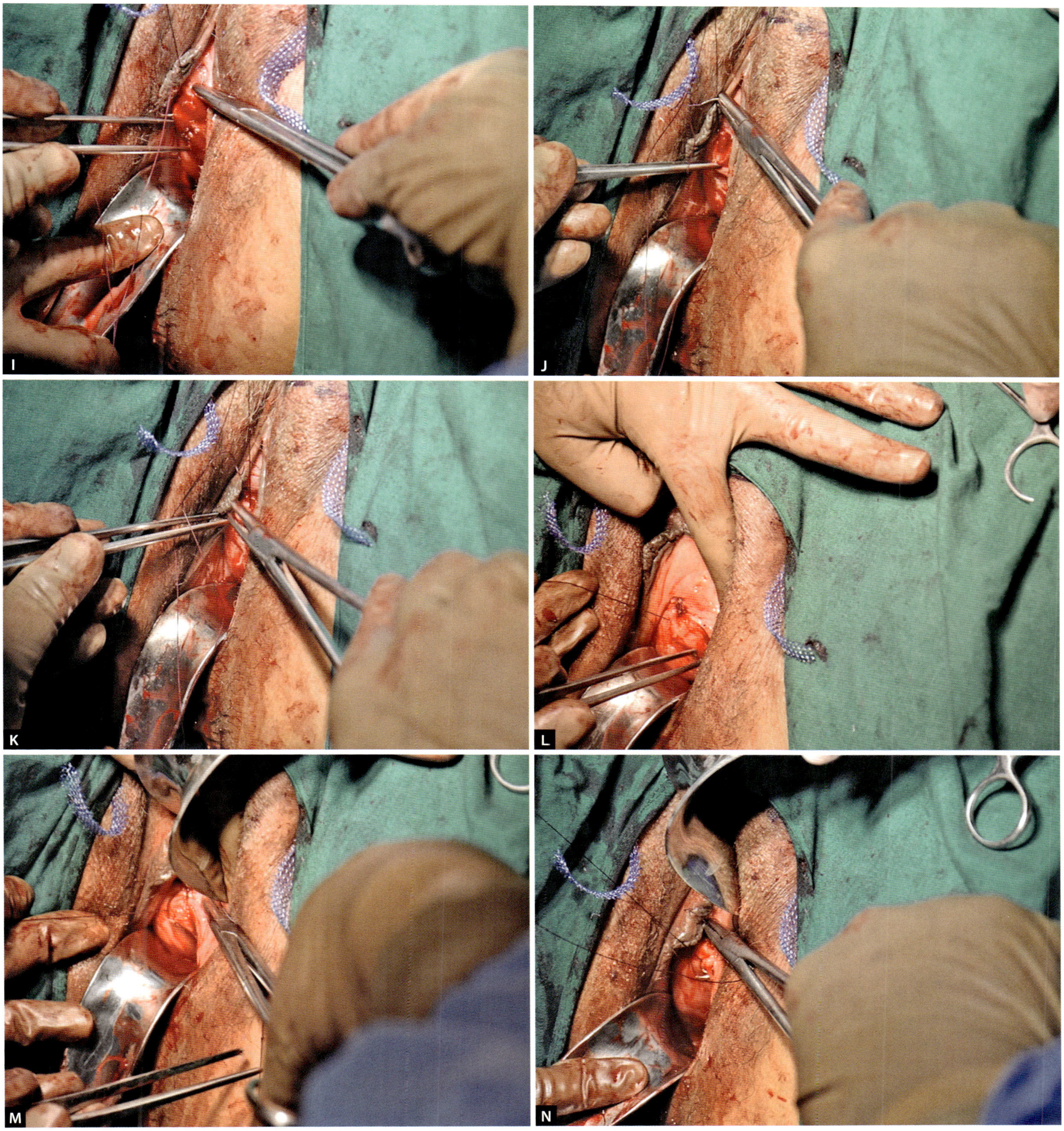

Figs. 12I to N

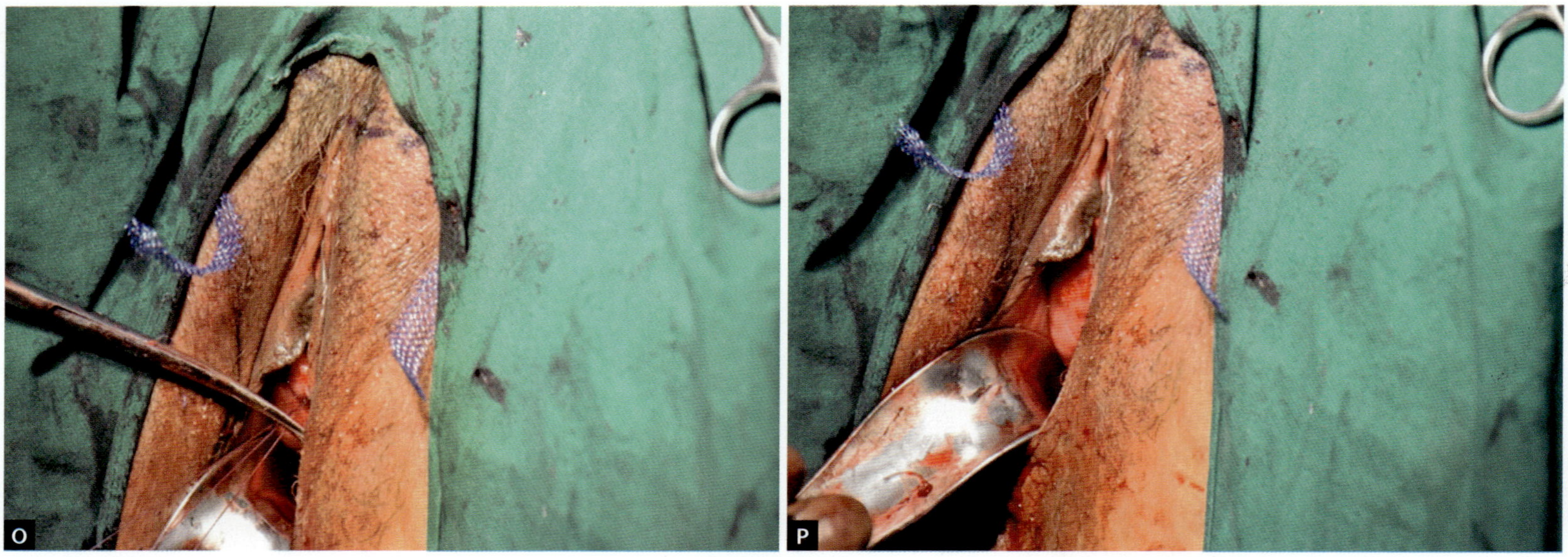

Figs. 12O and P

Figs. 12A to P: Suturing infraurethral incision after fixing the transobturator tape.

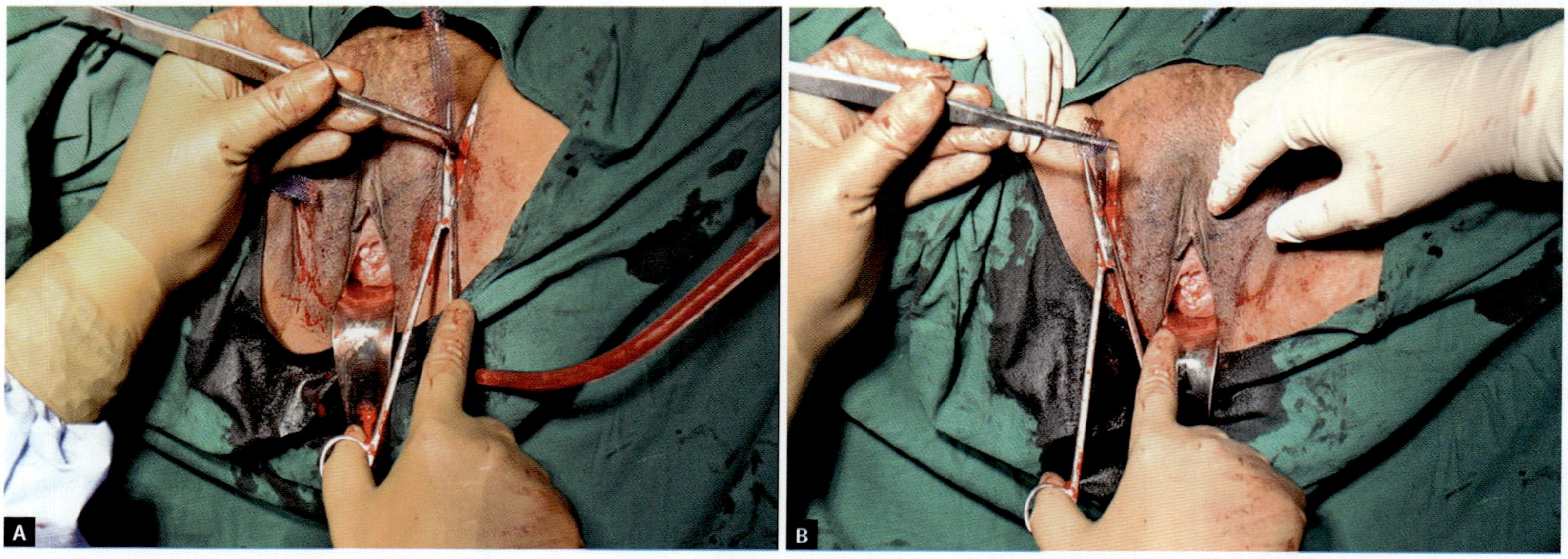

Figs. 13A and B: Cutting the ends of tape in both groin folds.

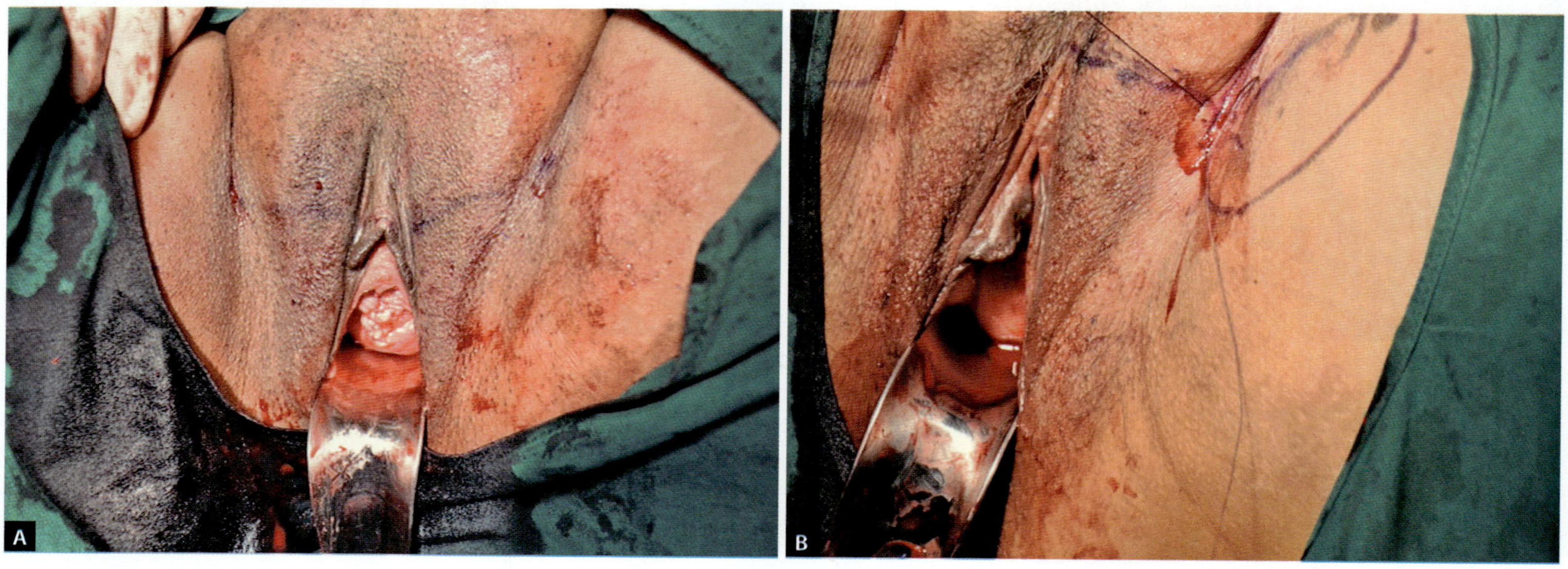

Figs. 14A and B

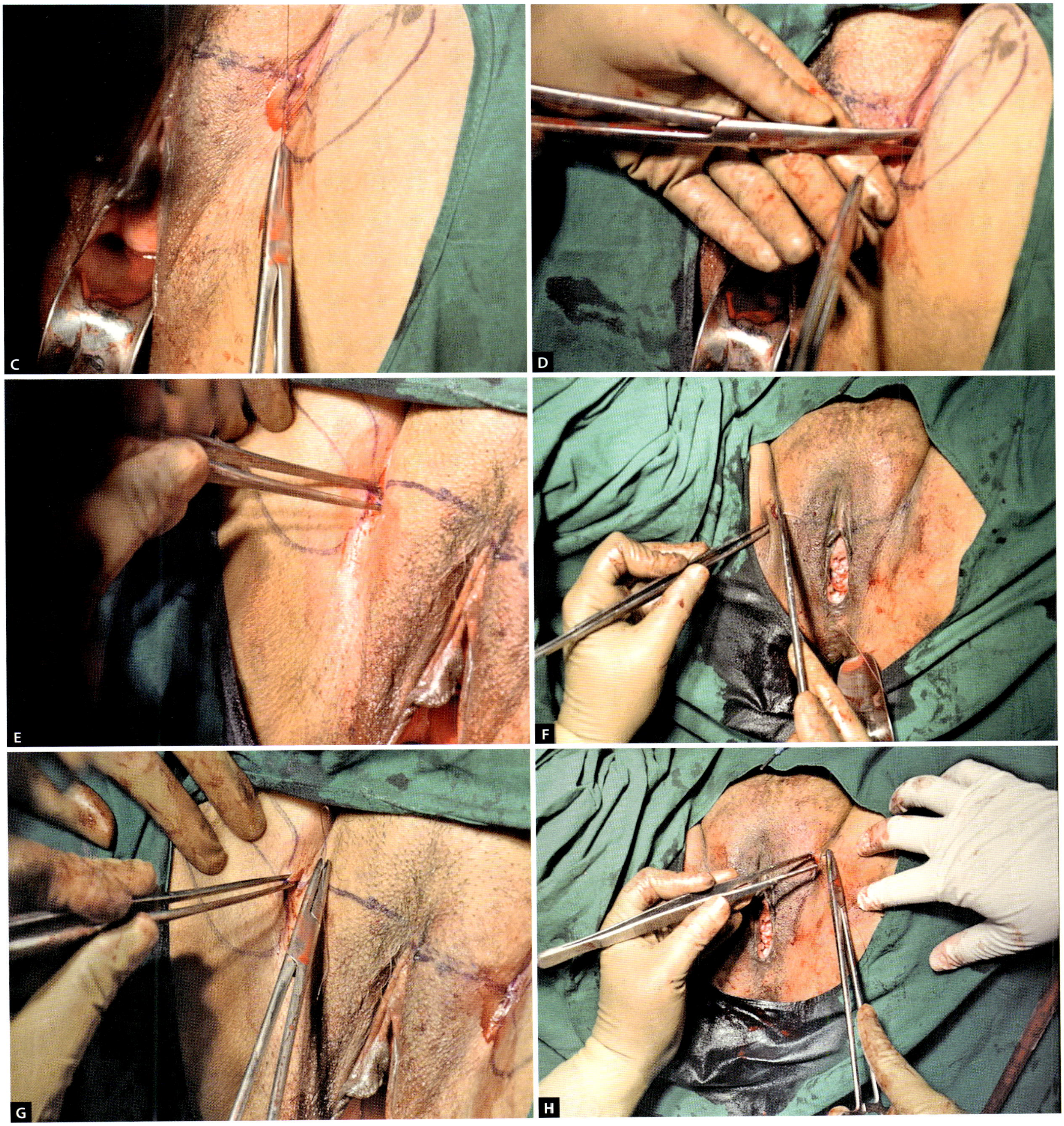

Figs. 14C to H

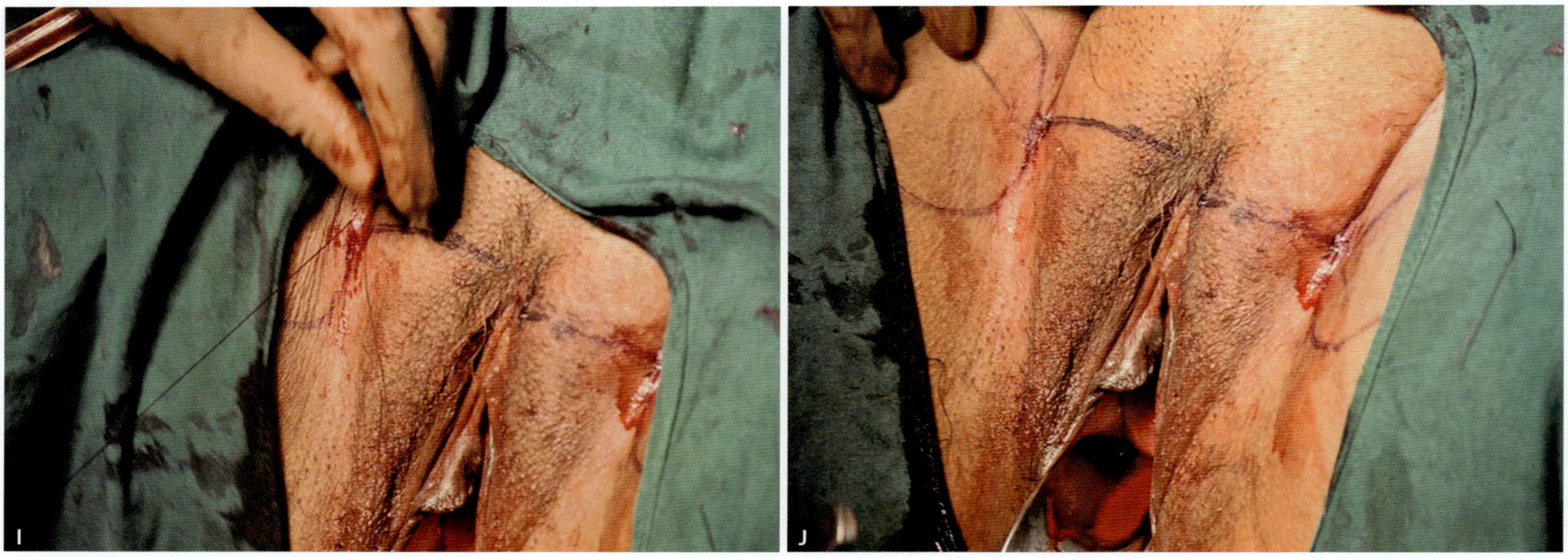

Figs. 14I and J

Figs. 14A to J: Suturing the incisions in the groin folds after cutting the tape ends tension free.

CHAPTER

43

Management of Male Varicocele

R Niranjana Radhakrishnan, Aditi Rai, B Ramesh

INTRODUCTION

A varicocele is considered one of the most common causes of male infertility, a condition in which there is abnormal dilation of the pampiniform plexus in the scrotum, often described as a "bag of worms". The valvular incompetence of the internal spermatic vein (IVS) results in dilation of the pampiniform plexus causing varicocele. The prevalence of varicocele among men is as high as 15%. Among these, approximately 10–15% are subfertile.[1,2] Varicocele is the most common surgically correctable cause of subfertility in men. Varicoceles are more severe on the left side (90%) and a recent study suggests that 80% of patients can have bilateral presentation. It is to be noted than when varicocele present unilaterally, a high suspicion for retroperitoneal pathologies has to be kept.

ANATOMY

Venous blood drains from each testes into venous sinuses called *pampiniform plexus* or *spermatic venous plexus*. This plexus coalesces at the level of the femoral head to form the ISV, the primary draining vein. Classically, the left ISV drains into the left renal vein, and the right ISV drains directly into the inferior vena cava (IVC). Three other veins arise within the pampiniform plexus: (1) the external pudendal, (2) vasal, and (3) cremasteric veins. The external pudendal vein forms at the level of the superior pubic ramus and drains into the great saphenous vein. The vasal or ductus deferens vein forms just above the testicle and joins the inferior or superior vesicle vein, and ultimately drains into the internal iliac vein. The cremasteric (external spermatic) vein forms at the level of the superior pubic ramus and drains via the inferior epigastric vein into the external iliac vein. The number of valves in spermatic veins varies between zero and three.

In addition to drainage to the systemic circulation through the external pudendal, vasal, and cremasteric veins, additional collateral communication between testicular venous drainage and the systemic circulation exists in men. These collaterals communicate with the retroperitoneal, peritoneal, ureteral, and adrenal veins and with the portal circulation through the splenic, superior mesenteric, and sigmoid colonic veins.

TYPES OF VARICOCELE

There are two types of varicoceles

Primary (Idiopathic)

The primary or idiopathic varicocele is caused by incompetent valves in the ISV, which results in impaired drainage of blood from the spermatic vein. This type of varicocele is common on the left side in the adult age group. This "sidedness" is probably because the left testicular vein has venous drainage into the left renal vein at a right angle, as opposed to the right spermatic vein, which drains directly into the IVC. There is no obstruction to the venous drainage and hence easily decompresses on lying down position and increases in size during Valsalva maneuver due to uninhibited transmission of abdominal pressure.

Secondary

Secondary varicoceles result from increased pressure on the spermatic vein or its tributaries due to obstructed venous drainage. Few of the common causes are listed in **Box 1**.

The appearance of secondary varicoceles is not affected by patient position.

PATHOPHYSIOLOGY

Several theories have been proposed for the etiology of a left varicocele on the ipsilateral testicular function such as scrotal hyperthermia, reflux of toxic agents, increased oxidative stress, autoimmunity, DNA fragmentation and apoptosis. Of these theories, increased testicular temperature is thought to induce this effect by elevating scrotal temperature through incompetent valves. The elevated intrascrotal temperature results in reduction in testosterone synthesis and reduced Sertoli cell secretory function. The observation that resulted in the hypothesis that the hypothalamo-pituitary-gonadal axis is not affected by a varicocele.

The reflux of renal venous blood to the spermatic vein results in increased concentrations of prostaglandin E and prostaglandin F in spermatic venous blood in varicocele patients, which may impair spermatogenesis. Other theories investigated high concentrations of adrenal products such as catecholamines, prostaglandins, serotonin, and adrenomedullin in spermatic veins. Anti-sperm antibodies have multiple effects on fertilization, acrosome reaction capacitation, and fertilization.

Box 1: Causes for secondary varicocele.

- Hydronephrosis
- Hepatomegaly
- Abdominal neoplasms
- Retroperitoneal mass
- Nutcracker syndrome (compression of left renal vein by superior mesenteric artery)

Another main theory is that the increased levels of reactive oxygen species and decreased antioxidant capacity levels in the semen are associated with varicocele. These changes may be related to functional sperm abnormalities and the infertility. Oxidative stress is considered to be pathogenic mechanism for testicular damage in infertile patients with varicocele.

DIAGNOSIS

Varicocele is diagnosed initially by clinical presentation and physical examination. Mostly men with varicocele are asymptomatic. Scrotal pain is associated with 2–10% of patients. Some patients presents with dull, nagging ache in the scrotum. It is imperative that the examination to detect a varicocele be done with the patient in an upright standing position, because the dilated veins will collapse when the patient lies down and even a large varicocele will remain undetected. A Valsalva maneuver should be requested (cough or abdominal straining or both); this will produce a "tapping" sensation, representing transmission of increased abdominal pressure in the scrotally palpated dilated veins.

The simple grading system of Dubin and Amelar is most commonly used ***(Table 1)***.

Even small varicoceles may be associated with a subfertility effect. High-resolution real-time ultrasound and color-flow Doppler ultrasound may be used to either confirm the diagnosis or detect subclinical (nonpalpable) varicoceles. In USG, a varicocele consists of multiple, serpentine, anechoic structures more than 2 mm in diameter, creating a tortuous, multicystic collection located adjacent or proximal to the upper pole of the testis and head of the epididymis. Ultrasonography may also be useful in diagnosing a subclinical varicocele. Other techniques for diagnosing varicocele, such as preoperative ISV venography and scrotal thermography. These not routinely utilized. Similarly, semen analysis is an integral component of varicocele evaluation in adults for fertility related issues. Endocrine evaluation using measurements of serum follicle-stimulating hormone (FSH) and luteinizing hormone (LH) levels is done.

The diagnostic ability to detect testicular dysfunction in these circumstances would be especially helpful clinically, because we could then differentiate those with normal-size testes.

TREATMENT

Even though varicocele is the common cause for male infertility, aim of treatment is to restore and improve testicular function.

The primary indications for treatment of a varicocele are:

1. Subfertility in adult men
2. Varicocele and testicular atrophy
3. Scrotal pain
4. Nonobstructive azoospermia.

Table 1: Grading system of Dubin and Amelar classification.

Grade	Description
0 (subclinical)	Not visible or palpable; identified only by ultrasound
I	Not visible; palpable in upright position with Valsalva only
II	Not visible; palpable in upright position without Valsalva
III	Visualized and palpable without Valsalva

Criteria for treatment in this group should include:

1. Abnormal semen parameters
2. Absence of any other identifiable or correctable causes of male infertility
3. A female partner with normal fertility or treated infertility
4. Adult men with a palpable varicocele and abnormal semen analysis.

Treatment Modalities

Medical Management

Combination of L-carnitine and cinnoxicam has been used to treat varicocele and infertility. Oral supplementation of N-acetylcysteine and micronutrients and vitamins and minerals for 3 months improves the sperm count. Daily intake of folic acid, pentoxifylline zinc compounds showed improvement in semen morphology after 1 month.

Surgical Management (Historical)

Surgical management was first described by Celsus, who applied crude ligatures and thin cauterizing irons to manage dilated scrotal veins. The first series in the modern era was published by Barwell in 1885. Numerous other surgical approaches have been described, each with benefits and drawbacks.

Open Surgical Approaches

Scrotal approach: A variety of open surgical techniques have been described. Due to a high rate of testicular artery damage leading to testicular ischemia and hydrocele formation, the scrotal approach is a historical operation that is rarely employed in the modern era and has been replaced by safer and more.

The retroperitoneal high ligation technique, known as the Palomo approach described in 1949. It is muscle splitting technique performed at the level of internal inguinal ring. A horizontal incision medial to the anterior superior iliac spine is made and extended medially. Both external and internal oblique muscles are split. This approach enables identification of the ISV lateral to ureter. The spermatic veins are double ligated with sutures or hemoclips. The transversalis and internal oblique muscles are closed with absorbable sutures. The external oblique muscle is closed in interrupted manner.

Difficulty in identification of the lymphatics in this approach may lead to their ligation and increase risk of postoperative hydrocele formation and pain reliable approaches. Disadvantages include: increased pain due to the additional necessary tissue dissection, higher hydrocele rates, and an inability to identify the external spermatic veins resulting in increased recurrences.

Inguinal approach: The inguinal (also known as Ivanissevich) approach is a traditional surgical dissection in familiar anatomy, but the inguinal canal dissection requires fascial incision and increases the risk of pain and hernia formation, as well as inadvertent damage to the ilioinguinal nerve. A 3 cm incision is made at the level of external ring and extended laterally. Scarpa's fascia opened and external oblique is incised in fiber directions. Spermatic cord is delivered out. Ilioinguinal and genital branch of genitofemoral nerve are excluded and then cremasteric fascia opened and vessels are exposed. Testicular artery and lymphatics should be preserved. All veins are double ligated. After hemostasis cremasteric muscle is closed and spermatic cord is put in position. Scarpa's fascia is reapproximated, skin is closed and dressing is applied.

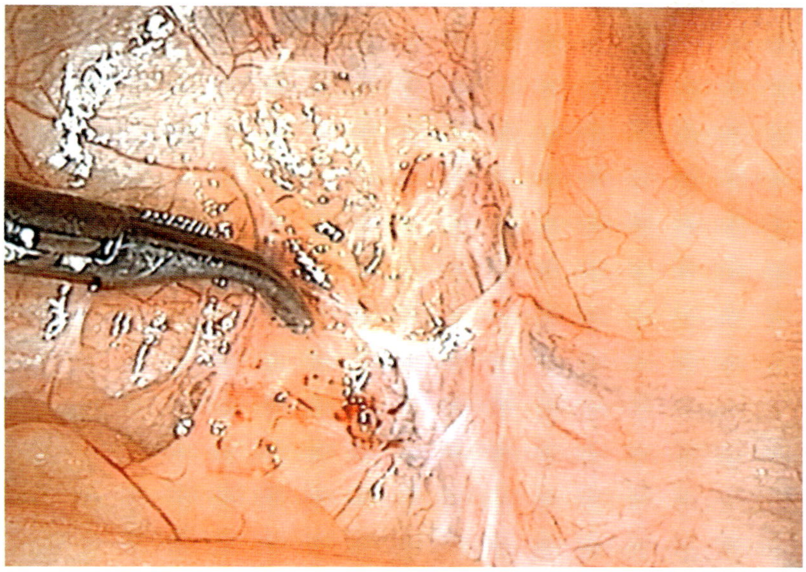

Fig. 1: Identification of the peritoneum.

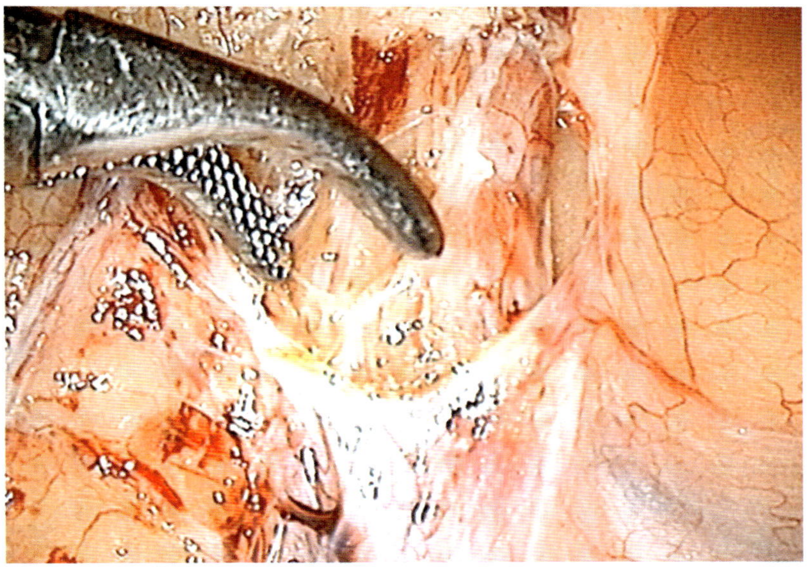

Fig. 2: Peritoneum is sharply excised to identify the structures.

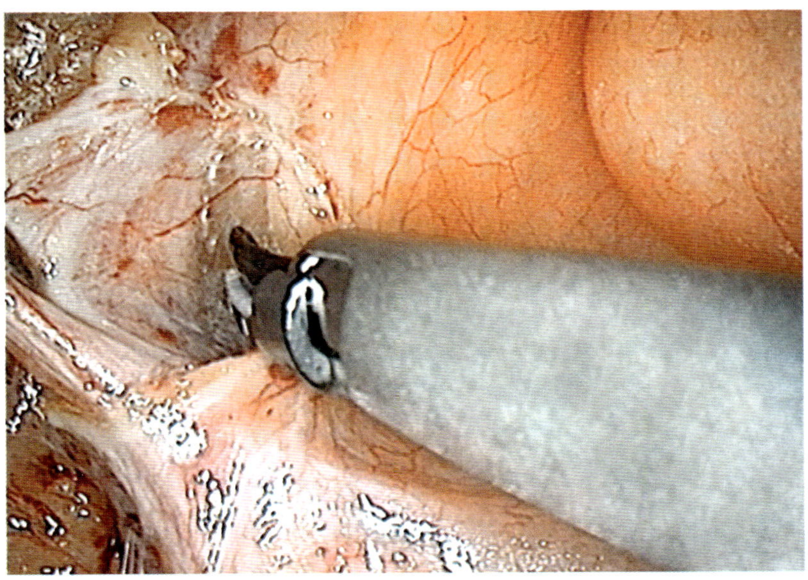

Fig. 3: Connective tissue between vessels separated.

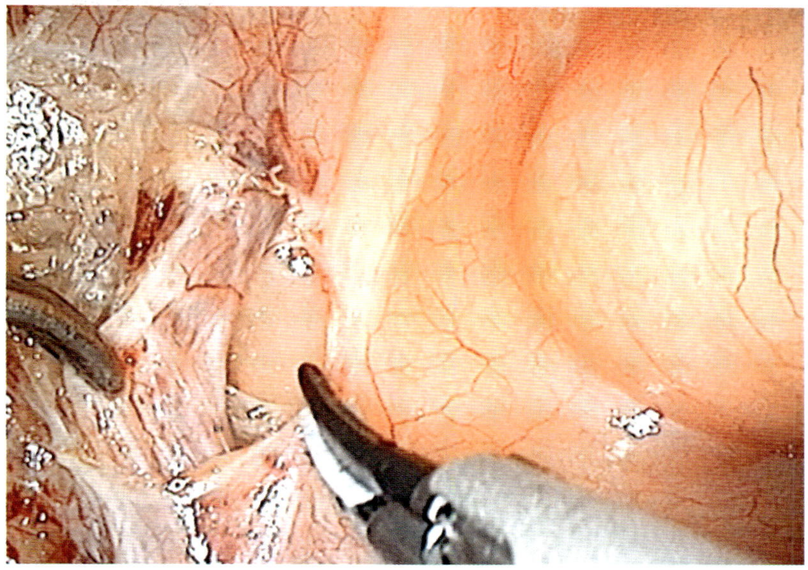

Fig. 4: Testicular vascular bundle identified on each side.

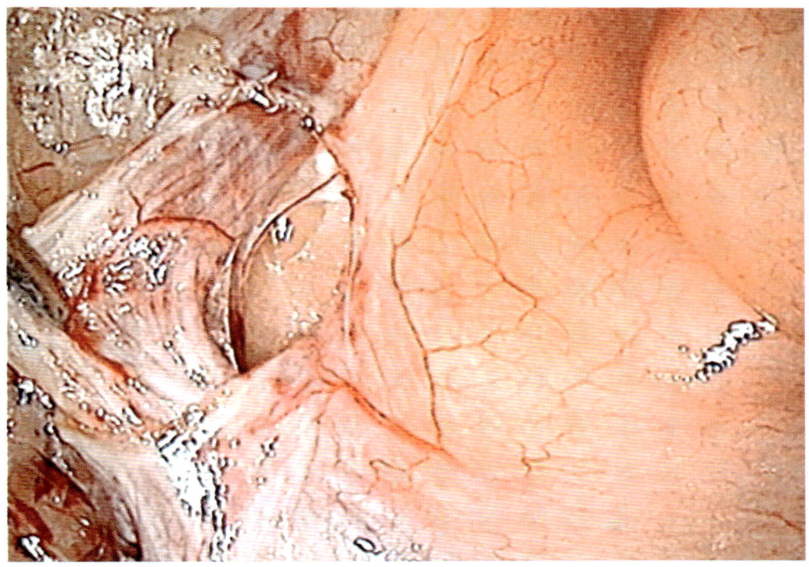

Fig. 5: Testicular artery identified and isolated.

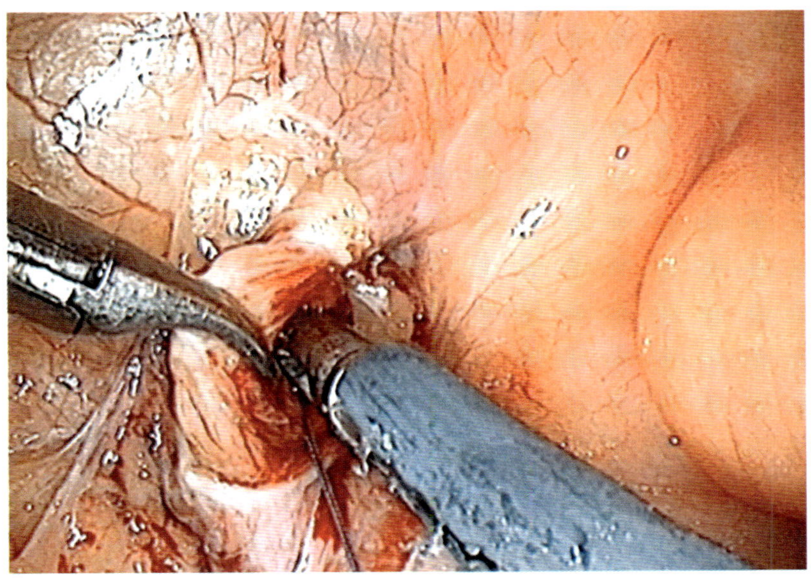

Fig. 6: Testicular veins exposed.

Subinguinal Goldstein approach: This approach has gained popularity as a safe and effective operation. Benefits include a shorter recovery and less pain than the inguinal approach (probably due to the lack of fascial violation). Disadvantages include a longer operative time.

A 2.5 cm incision is made at external inguinal ring. Scarpa's fascia is opened and exposed. The spermatic cord is mobilized and delivered through wound. Cremasteric fascia is opened and testicular artery is identified by vision or USG probe. All spermatic veins expect basal vein are ligated with silk or hemoclips. Testicular artery is identified. After hemostasis spermatic cord is put back in position. Scarpa's fascia is reapproximated, skin is closed.

Microsurgical technique: The microscopic approach, first published by Marmar et al. in 1985 and further refined by Goldstein et al., involves a subinguinal approach or inguinal approach with use of surgical microscope which gives 25 times magnification. This magnification will help the surgeon to ligate and better outcome. It is also efficacious and cost-effective procedure. It also takes a long operative time compared to other approaches.

Endovascular approach: In stark contrast to surgical management, the Tauber approach utilizes antegrade injection of a sclerosing agent directly into the pampiniform plexus via a small incision. This technique is straightforward, relatively painless, and carries relatively minimal risk. The retrograde sclerotherapy or coil embolization approach avoids surgical incisions entirely and instead relies on retrograde cannulation of the testicular vein and injection of the appropriate agent to cause venous obstruction. Disadvantages to these techniques include a relatively high rate of recurrence of up to 15% and the necessity for experienced interventional radiology or urology providers.

Laparoscopic approach: This approach is similar to retroperitoneal approach and allows identification and ligation of IVSs and preservation of testicular artery before it branches. It is usually performed transperitoneally but extraperitoneal approach has been performed as well. Retroperitoneal laparoscopic varicocelectomy is performed to avoid serious complications of transperitoneal approach. The approach involves placement of laparoscopic ports in the abdomen, identifying the inguinal ring and the spermatic cord contents, and selectively ligating the gonadal veins, while leaving the arterial blood supply intact. However, this approach is an intra-abdominal procedure and carries a small added risk for complications, e.g. visceral injury from trocar placement.

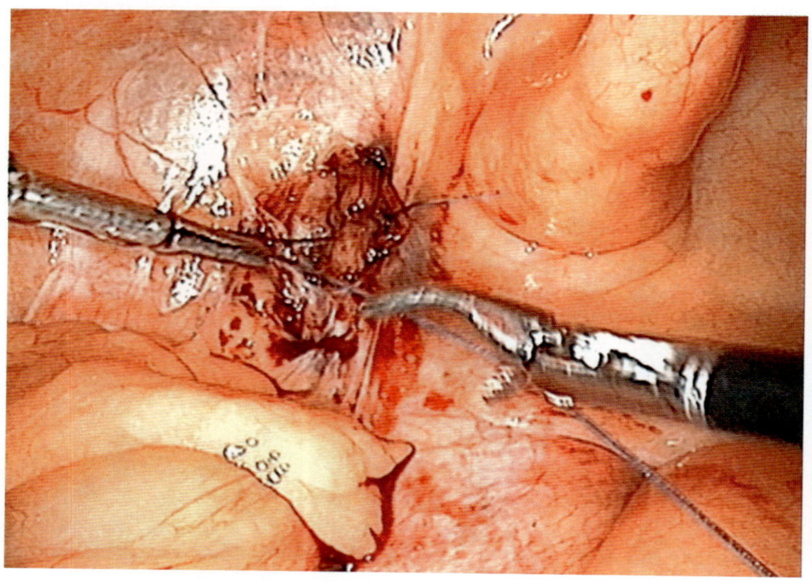

Fig. 7: Testicular vein marked and suture thread passed underneath.

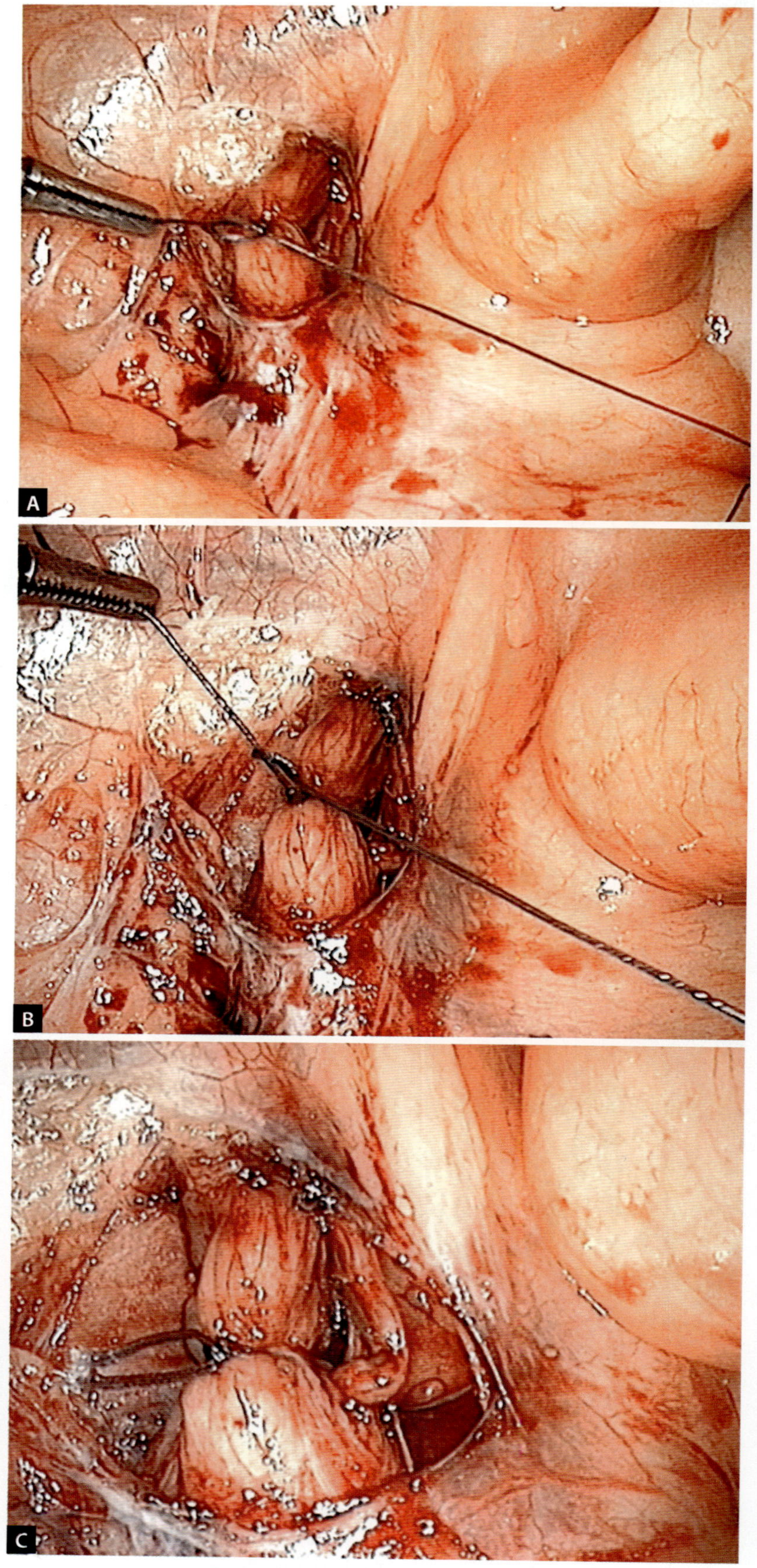

Figs. 8A to C: Dilated veins are ligated.

Procedures performed under general anesthesia with the patient in a supine, slightly head-down position. After the 10-mm camera port was inserted below the umbilicus under direct vision, the pneumoperitoneum was inflated by carbon dioxide to a maximum of 12 mm Hg. The laparoscope was subsequently introduced and used to monitor the insertion of two 5-mm ports. Finally, the three ports were placed in a triangle formation with one of the 5-mm trocars placed at the flank of the affected side and the other beside the contralateral rectus. If needed, the adhesion between the intestine and the peritoneum was dissected to expose the area of varicoceles, and the peritoneum overlying the enlarged vessels was incised approximately 3 cm superior to the internal inguinal. Slight blunt dissection was used to mobilize and preserve the artery. If the artery was not obvious, the recognizable lymphatic vessels were spared, and any other tortuous veins around the internal ring were dissected and clipped. The ipsilateral testicle was squeezed to identify if all of the varicose veins were clipped before the laparoscope was removed. The incision was closed layer-by-layer, and the skin closure was performed with subcuticular absorbable sutures. Patients were discharged on the second postoperative day, and a telephone follow-up regarding the incision occurred after 7 days.

Surgical Complications

Regardless of the approach, the complications after surgical or percutaneous intervention are relatively similar.

- Postoperative pain and hematoma can occur to varying degrees but typically improve or resolve over time.
- Hydrocele formation, typically attributed to the ligation of lymphatics.
- Testicular artery injury.
- Recurrence of the varicocele can occur.

REFERENCES

1. Kim HH, Goldstein M. Adult varicocele. Curr Opin Urol. 2008;18:608-12.
2. Masson P, Brannigan RE. The varicocele. Urol Clin North Am. 2014;41:129-44.

CHAPTER

44

Robotics in Gynecology

Meenakshi Sundaram, Abdul Basith, G Hemasree

INTRODUCTION

Laparoscopy has revolutionized modern gynecological practice. Now, it is no longer needed to have large, cosmetically displeasing wounds on the abdomen and the attendant morbidity due to them. Naturally, the next innovation that came about after laparoscopy was robotic surgery. Initially Da Vinci robotic surgical system was developed at the Stanford Research Institute along with the defense department to operate on wounded soldiers by surgeons sitting away remotely from the battlefield. It was then rapidly adopted into general surgical and gynecological practice and has assumed an important position now. The US FDA approved the system for gynecological surgeries in 2005.

PARTS OF THE SURGICAL ROBOT (FIGS. 1 AND 2)

The Da Vinci surgical system comprises three components: (a) a surgeon console where the surgeon sits in an ergonomically built device, unscrubbed, away from the actual patient and operates it, (b) robotic cart with three or four arms that articulate instruments through trocars in the patient's abdomen. The articulating arms are attached to the trocars externally with a binder device, (c) camera and vision system: through this a high definition three-dimensional (3-D) picture is relayed to the surgeon in the console. Four to five trocars are used. One additional port is placed for the assistant surgeon to allow him to help.

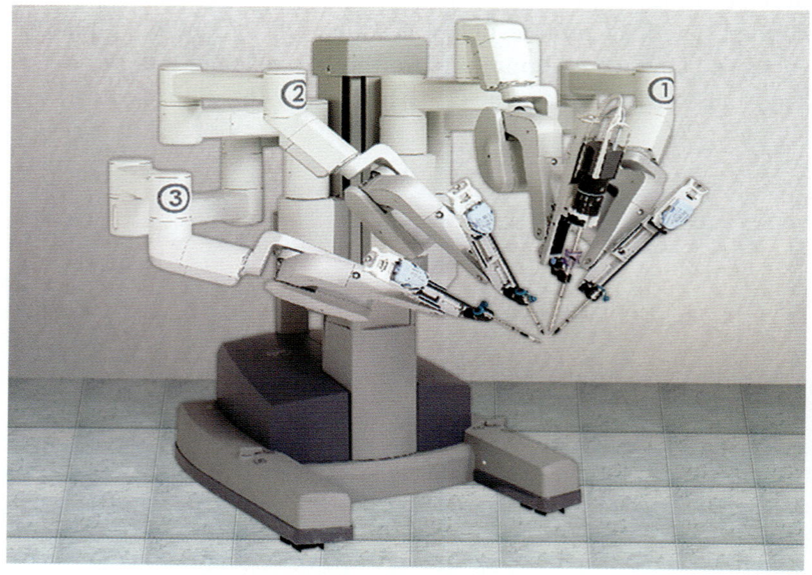

Fig. 1: Parts of the surgical robot—patient robotic cart.

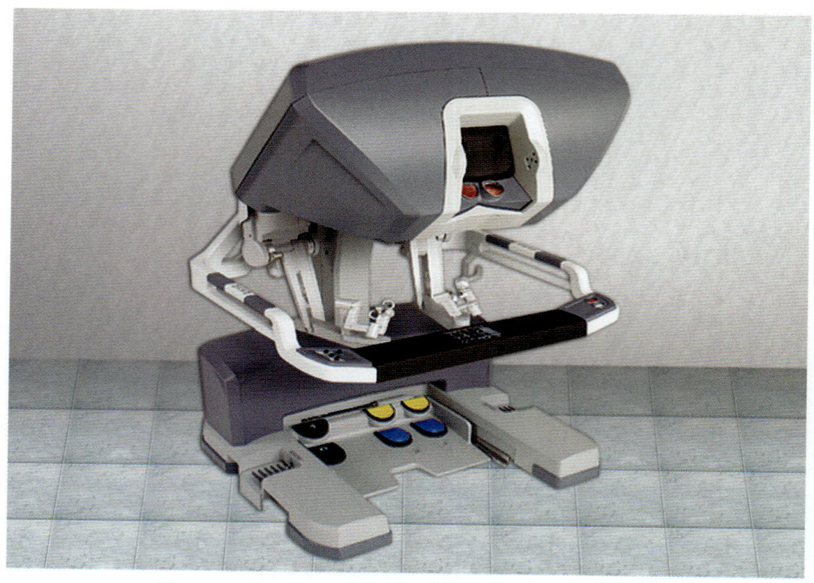

Fig. 2: Parts of the surgical robot—surgeon console.

ADVANTAGES OF ROBOTIC SURGERY OVER OTHER MODE OF SURGERIES

1. Console provides magnified, 3-D imaging and good depth perception, far superior to open surgeries and 2-D laparoscopic surgeries.
2. Surgeon has autonomous control of the camera and the instruments unlike in laparoscopy where the surgeon is dependent on the assistant for the camera.
3. Robotic arm has a wristed joint (Endowrist), i.e. 6° of movement is possible which allows for greater dexterity.
4. With the robotic arms, there is a massive reduction in the hand tremors.
5. Endowrist movement allows precise suturing and allows surgical maneuvers that are similar to open surgeries in places, which require extensive dissection, e.g. iliac node dissection.
6. Easier for surgeons with less advanced laparoscopic skills to learn, as the learning curve is small compared to laparoscopy.
7. Lower morbidity, less postoperative pain and shorter hospital stays compared to open surgeries.

PORT PLACEMENT FOR A ROBOTIC GYNECOLOGICAL SURGERY AND DOCKING

Patient is placed in a low lithotomy position with legs padded in the stirrups. Arms are tucked and padded. Proper port placement is necessary to successfully complete the surgery without any complications. We have the option of using either the two-arm system or the three-arm system. We usually prefer using the two-arm system. The camera port is always 12-mm supraumbilical port in the midline depending on the size of the pathology in the pelvis. The two robotic ports are placed about 8–10 cm away from the camera port on either side in the middle quadrants. The two assistant ports are placed about 6–8 cm away from the robotic arms in the upper quadrants on either side and slightly below the camera port. The entire configuration of the ports looks like an inverted "U" around the pathology in the pelvis **(Fig. 3)**.

Initially after Veress insufflation of carbon dioxide in the Palmer's point, a 5-mm assistant port is taken on the left upper quadrant. Using a conventional laparoscope, the abdomen is surveyed and pathology is identified. Port configurations are then marked with a surgical marker on the abdomen and under vision all the other ports are placed in succession. Once the port placement is done, the robot is docked. Docking is the process of attachment of the robotic arms to the robotic ports. Usually in the gynecological procedures, we prefer a side docking at the patient's hip. The robot can also be "straight docked" with the platform placed between the patient's legs.

We prefer to use the bipolar grasper on the left side, i.e. non-dominant side of the surgeon and a monopolar spatula/scissior or harmonic scalpel on the right side, for dissection. The assistant utilizes the assistant port on either side. The vaginal assistant is seated at the vaginal end and uses the uterine manipulator to maneuver the uterus and the adnexa.

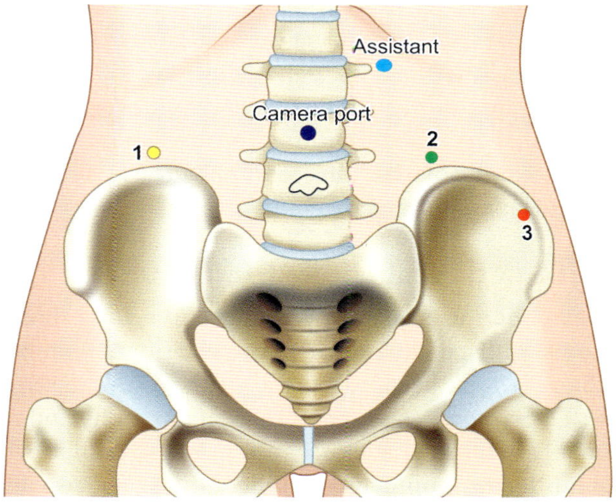

Fig. 3: Robotic port placement.

DISADVANTAGES OF ROBOTIC SURGERY

- Absence of tactile feedback as the operating surgeon is far away from the patient. This can lead to increased trauma due to excessive pull and tear or increased bleeding or give way of tissues due to faulty knot tying.
- Surgeon depends on an assistant to change instruments and accessory tasks like suctioning, etc.
- Increased cost to the patient. With more advanced robotic surgical systems and more companies developing their own devices, this may come down in the future.

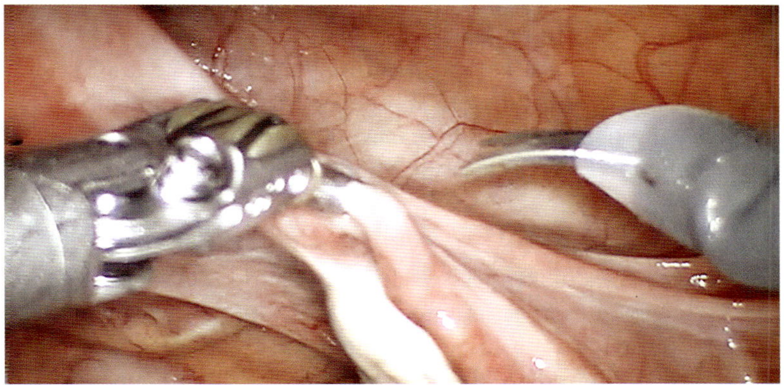

Fig. 4: Robotic hysterectomy performed on right cornual structures. Bipolar grasper is shown on the left and monopolar scissors on the right.

SPECIFIC SURGERIES

Robotic Hysterectomy for Benign Disease (Figs. 4 to 6)

The most common operation in gynecology is hysterectomy. There is a hesitancy to adopt minimally invasive approaches toward performing a hysterectomy due to various reasons such as lack of training, lack of resources, and lack of patient education. Of importance is the complex technical expertise needed to perform a laparoscopic hysterectomy, which needs endosuturing skills and limited motion inside the abdomen. This can be overcome by adopting robotics to perform a hysterectomy.

Is robotic hysterectomy better than laparoscopy?

There are two randomized controlled trials (RCTs) comparing laparoscopic and robotic hysterectomy for benign conditions. There were no differences between groups in complication rates, estimated blood loss and hospital stay. Similar conversion to laparotomy rates was observed. The longer operative times observed with robotic surgery were probably due to preoperative robot docking and lack of volumes by the operating surgeons and these surgeons were more

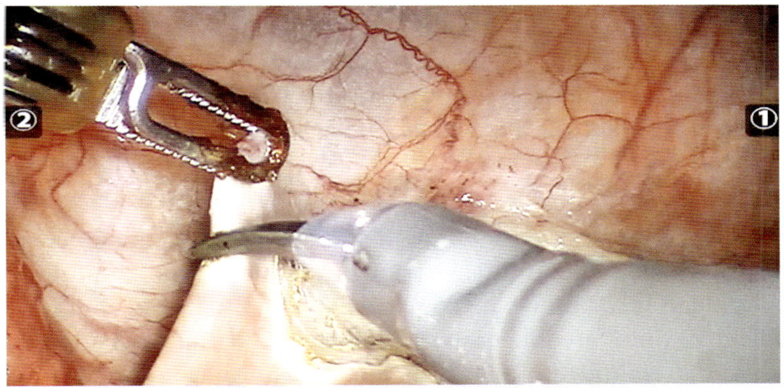

Fig. 5: Dissection of uterovesical fold of peritoneum.

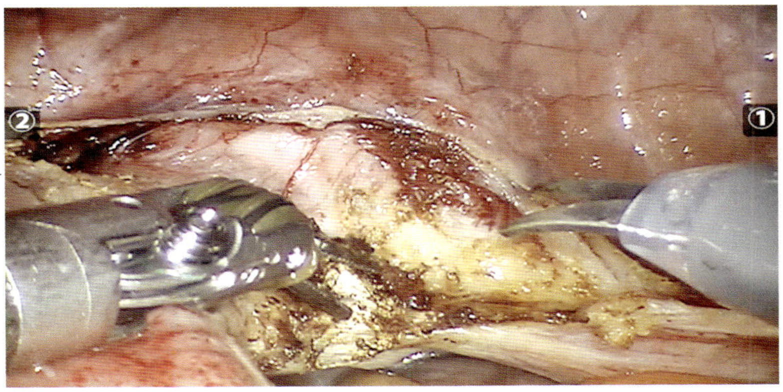

Fig. 6: Dissection of uterine vessels.

used to either the laparoscopic or the vaginal route. Number of hysterectomies performed robotically was 263,000 in the US in 2015.

For women with extensive pelvic adhesions, advanced endometriosis and large uteruses, the hysterectomies would be a more challenging surgery. Observational studies report that rate of intraoperative and postoperative complications were low and no conversions to laparotomy were required.

ROBOTICS IN GYNECOLOGICAL ONCOLOGY

There is evidence to say that learning curve for robotic radical hysterectomy with pelvic and or para-aortic lymphadenectomy is shorter than for laparoscopy. Especially in women with high BMI (>35 kg/m^2) laparotomy has highest rates of morbidity and restriction of movements in straight stick surgeries. A systematic review comparing open, laparoscopic and robotic surgery for cervical cancer showed that mean blood loss, postoperative infectious morbidity and hospital stay was lower with robotic and laparoscopic approaches. Other studies have shown robotic radical hysterectomy and pelvic lymphadenectomy to be feasible, safe and comparable in both early and advanced cancer cervix. Another additional advantage with robotics is that procedures which are technically difficult with laparoscopy may be performed quite easily, like radical trachelectomy and removal of bulky pelvic tumors and nodes **(Fig. 7)**.

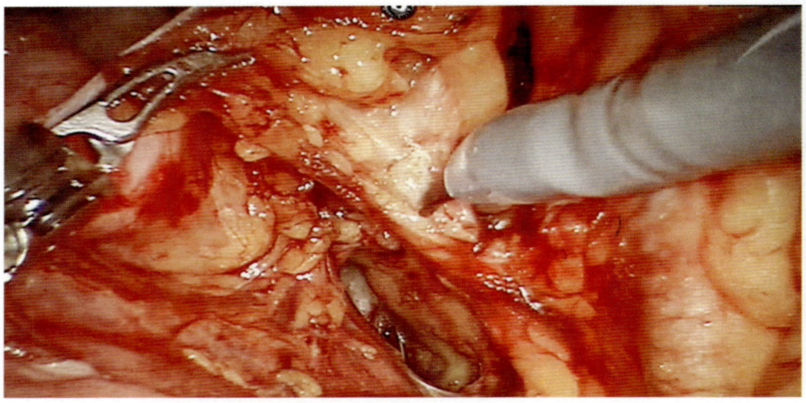

Fig. 7: Retroperitoneal pelvic lymph node dissection.

ROBOTICS IN UROGYNECOLOGY

Cochrane reviews in 2013 concluded that abdominal sacrocolpopexy was the gold standard for the treatment of vault prolapse. Numerous studies found comparable outcomes with laparoscopic sacrocolpopexy compared to abdominal approach. However, technical aspects hamper the laparoscopic approach from adopting it by the gynecologists. So, there is much interest in robotic sacrocolpopexy. A systematic review by Hallock et al. showed similar outcomes, operative time, blood loss, and complications. Robotic surgery for repairing vesicovaginal fistula was reported by Melamud et al. Other observational studies have shown that robotic repair of genitourinary fistula to be a very safe alternative to open repair.

ROBOTIC MYOMECTOMY

Compared to abdominal myomectomy, robotic myomectomy has shown less blood loss, shorter stay in the hospital and fewer complications. But when compared to laparoscopic route, the operative times are longer. With large myomas there is inadequate counter traction due to insufficient torque during enucleation. Another alternative to this could be a hybrid surgery. Robotic surgery could also impede manipulation outside the pelvis into the upper abdomen. One of the advantages of robotic myomectomy is the ability to remove oddly located myomas and suturing of the defects thereafter due to the complex Endowrist movements **(Fig. 8)**.

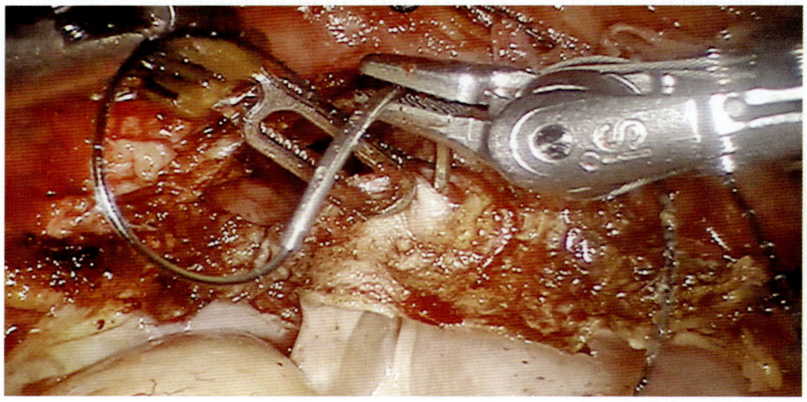

Fig. 8: Robotic endowrist suturing.

CONVERSION RATES

Most of the studies show a very small incidence of conversion (8–10%) to laparotomy and complications in robotic surgery. The reasons for conversion to laparotomy were due to poor visualization due to adhesions, patients who could not tolerate the steep Trendelenburg, very large uteruses and bowel injury.

PAIN RELIEF

Pain relief requirement after robotic surgery is said to be less. This could be due to the fulcrum of movement being at the abdominal wall level for laparoscopies whereas for robotic surgeries the fulcrum of movement is at the Endowrist.

SUGGESTED READING

1. American College of Obstetricians and Gynecologists. (2017). Committee opinion. Robotic surgery in Gynaecology. [online] Available from: https://www.acog.org/Clinical-Guidance-and-Publications/Committee-Opinions/Committee-on-Gynecologic-Practice/Robotic-Surgery-in-Gynecology?IsMobileSet=false [Last accessed December, 2019].
2. Nair R, Kilicoat K, Thomas EJ. Robotic surgery in gynaecology. Obstet Gynaecol. 2016;18:221-9.
3. Puntambekar SP, Kathya N, Mallireddy C, et al. Indian experience of robotics in gynaecology. J Minim Access Surg. 2014;10(2):80-3.
4. Sinha R, Sanjay M, Rupa B, et al. Robotic surgery in gynaecology. J Minim Access Surg. 2015;11(1):50-9.
5. Weinberg L, Rao S, Escobar PF. Robotic surgery in gynaecology: an updated systematic review. Obstet Gynaecol Int. 2011;2011:852061 .

CHAPTER 45

Staging Laparotomy for Ovarian Cancer including Pelvic and Para-aortic

Praveen Rathod, Minal Kumbhalwar

Box 1: World health organization histological classification of ovarian carcinoma.[1]

- Serous adenocarcinoma
- Mucinous adenocarcinoma
- Endometrioid adenocarcinoma
- Clear cell adenocarcinoma
- Malignant Brenner tumor
- Mixed epithelial and mesenchymal
- Adenosarcoma
- Carcinosarcoma
- Squamous cell carcinoma
- Mixed carcinoma
- Undifferentiated carcinoma
- Small cell carcinoma

Source: Adapted from Tavassoli, 2003.

Table 1: FIGO staging classification for cancer of the ovary, fallopian tube, and peritoneum.

Stage	*Characteristics*
I	**Tumor confined to ovaries or fallopian tube(s)**
	T1-N0-M0
IA	Tumor limited to 1 ovary (capsule intact) or fallopian tube; no tumor on ovarian or fallopian tube surface; no malignant cells in the ascites or peritoneal washings
	T1a-N0-M0
IB	Tumor limited to both ovaries (capsules intact) or fallopian tubes; no tumor on ovarian or fallopian tube surface; no malignant cells in the ascites or peritoneal washings
	T1b-N0-M0
IC	Tumor limited to 1 or both ovaries or fallopian tubes, with any of the following:
IC1	Surgical spill
	T1c1-N0-M0
IC2	Capsule ruptured before surgery or tumor on ovarian or fallopian tube surface
	T1c2-N0-M0
IC3	Malignant cells in the ascites or peritoneal washings
	T1c3-N0-M0
II	**Tumor involves 1 or both ovaries or fallopian tubes with pelvic extension (below pelvic brim) or peritoneal cancer**
	T2-N0-M0
IIA	Extension and/or implants on uterus and/or fallopian tubes and/or ovaries
	T2a-N0-M0
IIB	Extension to other pelvic intraperitoneal tissues
	T2b-N0-M0
III	**Tumor involves 1 or both ovaries or fallopian tubes, or peritoneal cancer, with cytologically or histologically confirmed spread to the peritoneum outside the pelvis and/or metastasis to the retroperitoneal lymph nodes**
	T1/T2-N1-M0
IIIA1	Positive retroperitoneal lymph nodes only (cytologically or histologically proven):
	IIIA1(i) Metastasis up to 10 mm in greatest dimension
	IIIA1(ii) Metastasis more than 10 mm in greatest dimension
IIIA2	Microscopic extrapelvic (above the pelvic brim) peritoneal involvement with or without positive retroperitoneal lymph nodes
	T3a2-N0/N1-M0
IIIB	Macroscopic peritoneal metastasis beyond the pelvis up to 2 cm in greatest dimension, with or without metastasis to the retroperitoneal lymph nodes

Contd...

Contd...

Stage	*Characteristics*
	T3b-N0/N1-M0
IIIC	Macroscopic peritoneal metastasis beyond the pelvis more than 2 cm in greatest dimension, with or without metastasis to the retroperitoneal lymph nodes (includes extension of tumor to capsule of liver and spleen without parenchymal involvement of either organ)
	T3c-N0/N1-M0
IV	**Distant metastasis excluding peritoneal metastases**
IVA	Pleural effusion with positive cytology
IVB	Parenchymal metastases and metastases to extra-abdominal organs (including inguinal lymph nodes and lymph nodes outside of the abdominal cavity)
	Any T, any N, M1

STEPS FOR THE STAGING LAPAROTOMY FOR THE OVARIAN CANCERS

Early Stage Tumors: Clinically and Radiologically Stage I Tumor (Figs. 1 to 28)

1. Midline vertical incision.
2. Inspection of pelvic and abdominal organs.
3. Palpation of the pelvic, abdominal and retroperitoneal structures.
4. Washings with 200 mL normal saline with eight drops of heparin, collecting fluid samples from pelvis, paracolic gutters, diaphragmatic area for cytology study.
5. Ovarian tumor debulking; total abdominal hysterectomy with bilateral salpingo-oophorectomy, pelvic and para-aortic lymphadenectomy, omentectomy and suspicious peritoneal biopsies.
6. Frozen section study needs to be done after the primary tumor debulking and further staging depending on the frozen histopathology.
7. Fertility preservation surgeries need to be done in the young patients desiring child bearing.
8. The fertility preservation generally involves sparing uterus, other normal ovary without applying any clamps to prevent the Fallopian tubal injury.

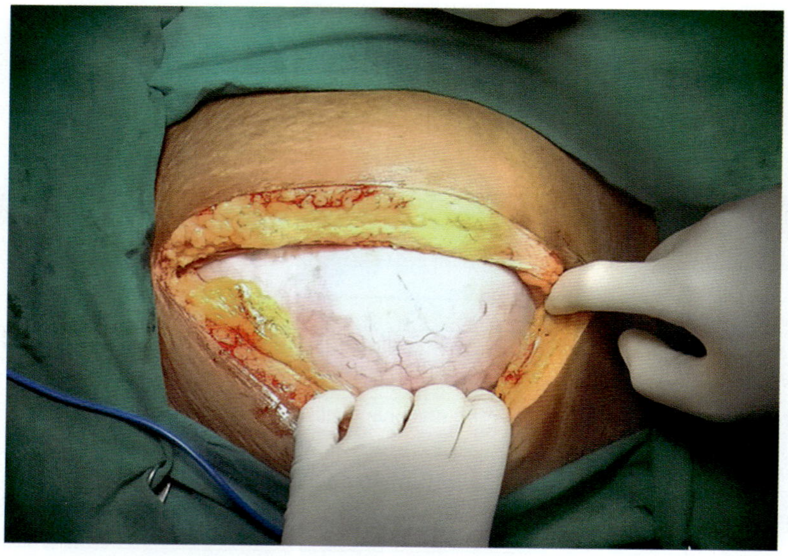

Fig. 1: Ovarian epithelial tumor with intact capsule.

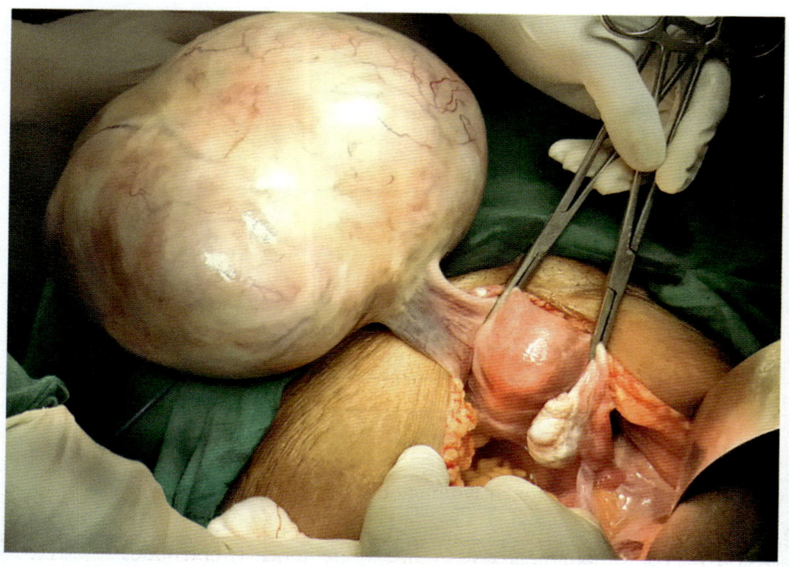

Fig. 2: Ovarian tumor with intact capsule and other normal ovary.

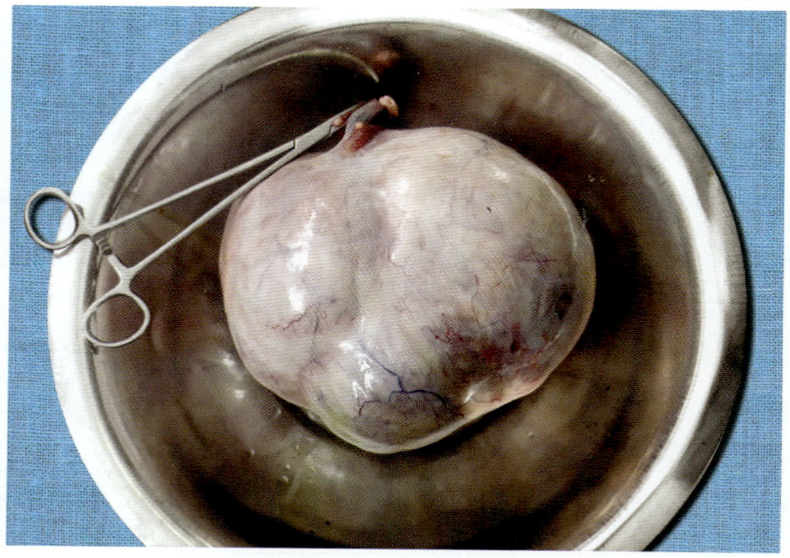

Fig. 3: Ovarian epithelial tumor with intact capsule after removal.

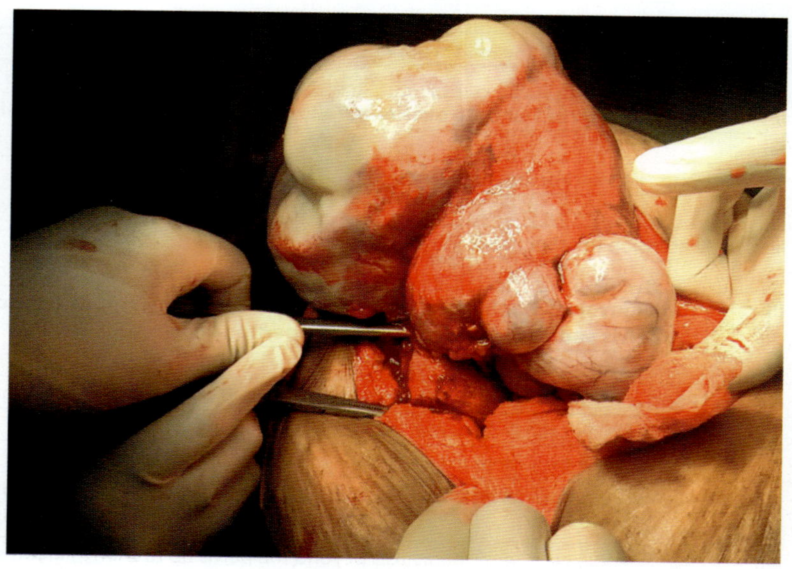

Fig. 4: Early stage epithelial ovarian cancer.

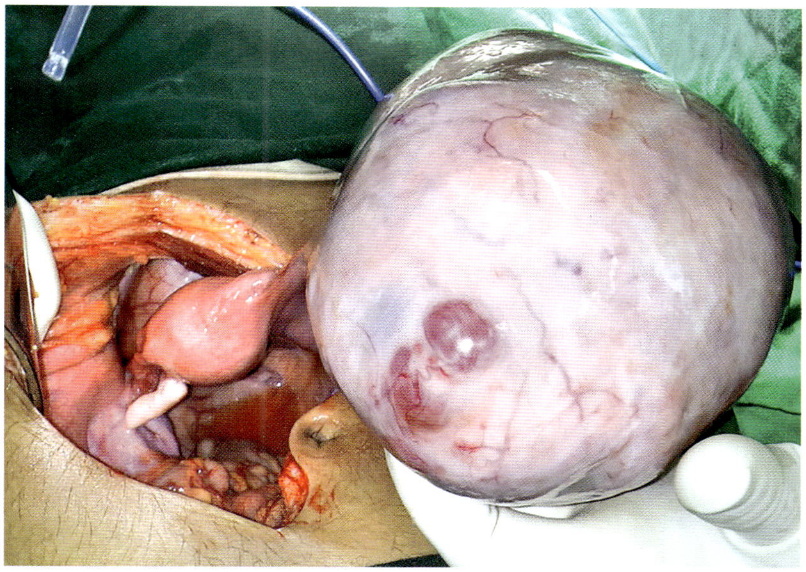

Fig. 5: Early stage granulosa cell tumor ovary.

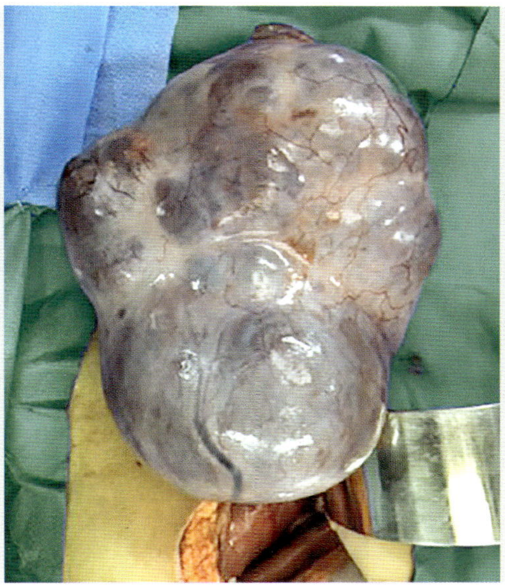

Fig. 6: Early stage immature teratoma.

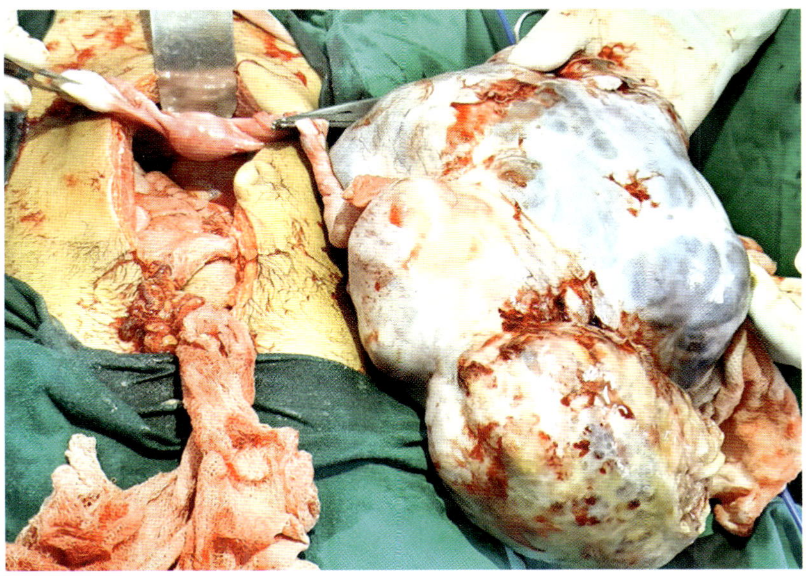

Fig. 7: Stage IC immature teratoma.

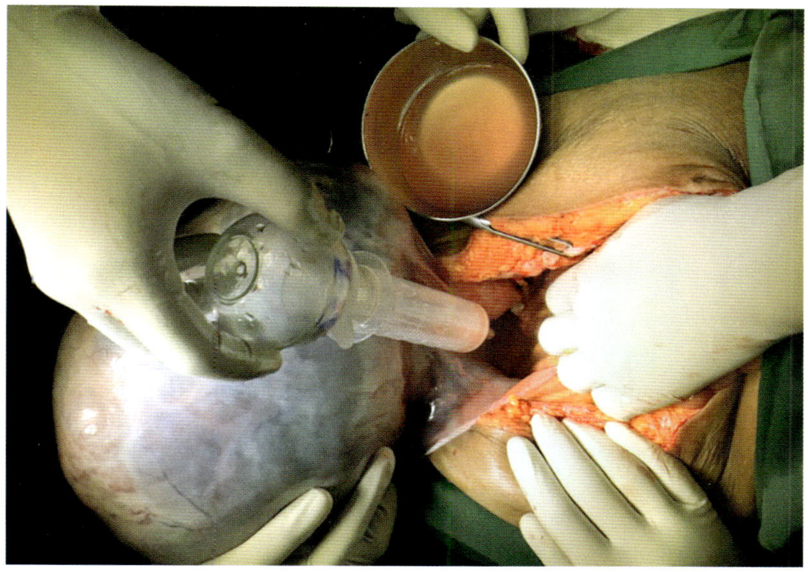

Fig. 8: Cytology collection in early stage ovarian cancer.

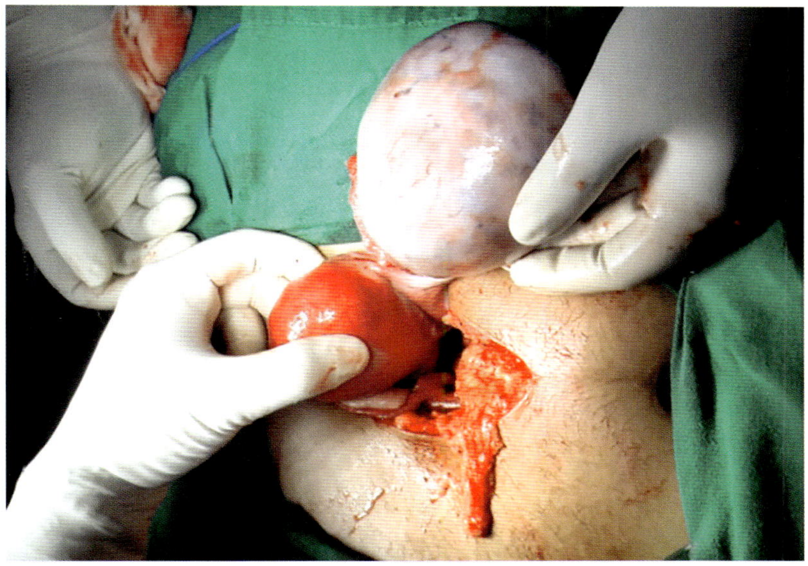

Fig. 9: Early stage dysgerminoma.

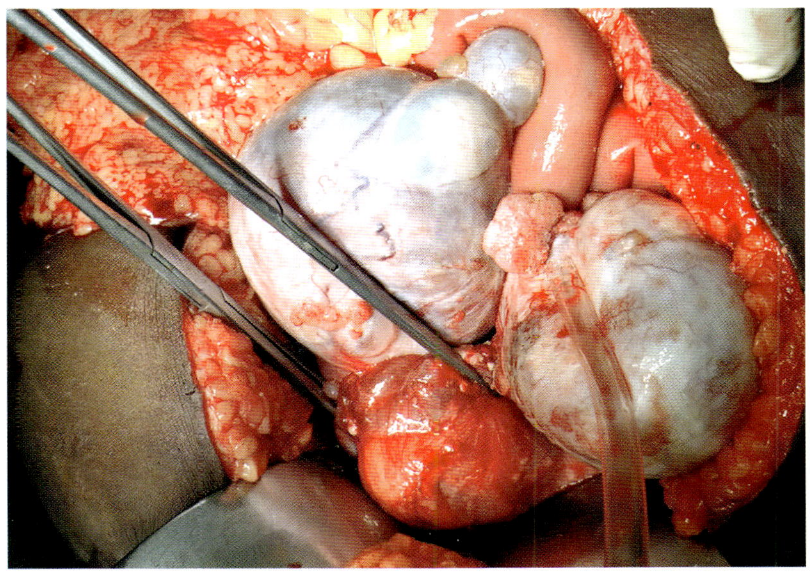

Fig. 10: Bilateral borderline ovarian tumor.

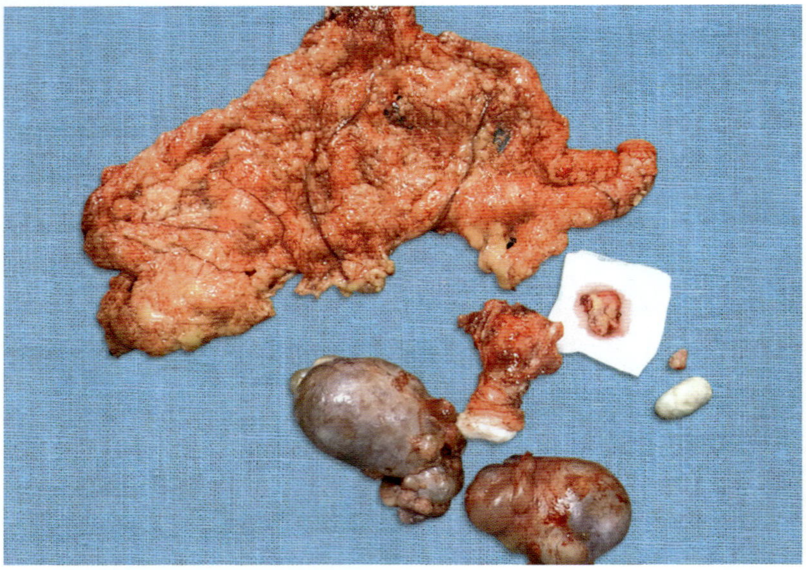

Fig. 11: Bilateral borderline ovarian tumor, staged with omentectomy.

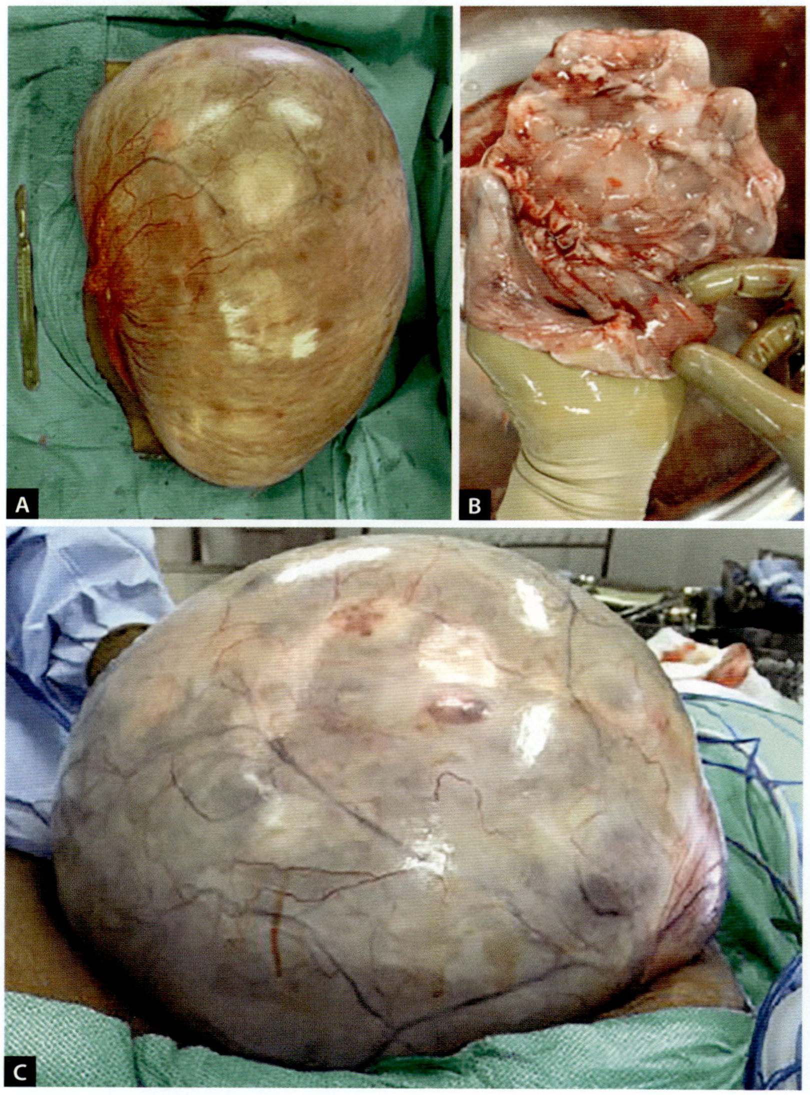

Figs. 12A to C: Borderline mucinous ovarian tumor.

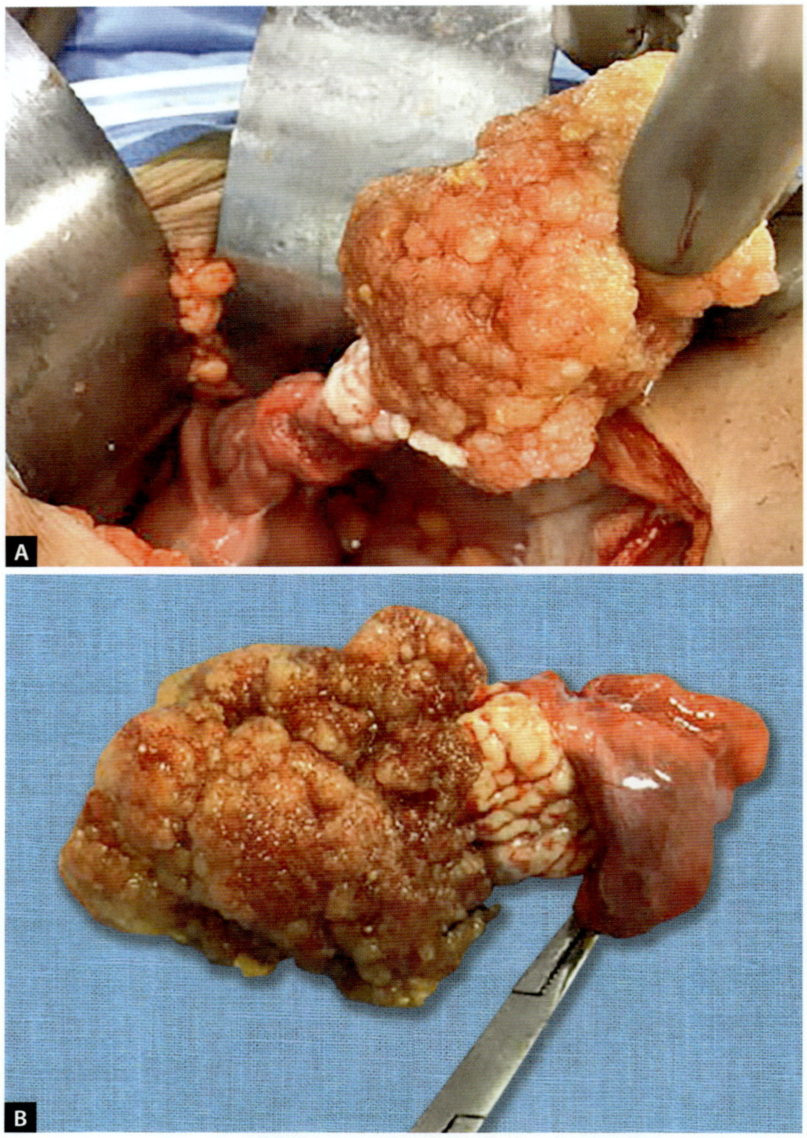

Figs. 13A and B: The borderline serous ovarian tumor, characteristically part of normal ovary is seen with it.

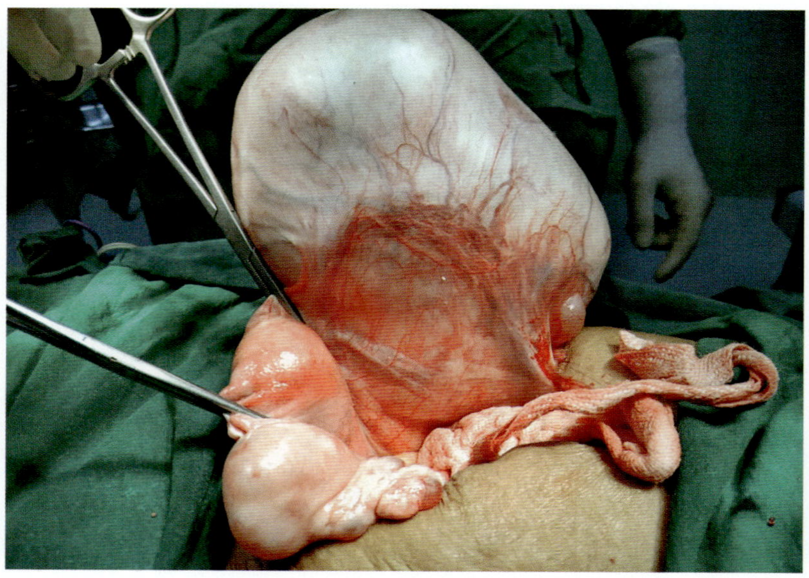

Fig. 14: Benign ovarian tumor cystadenoma with other normal ovary.

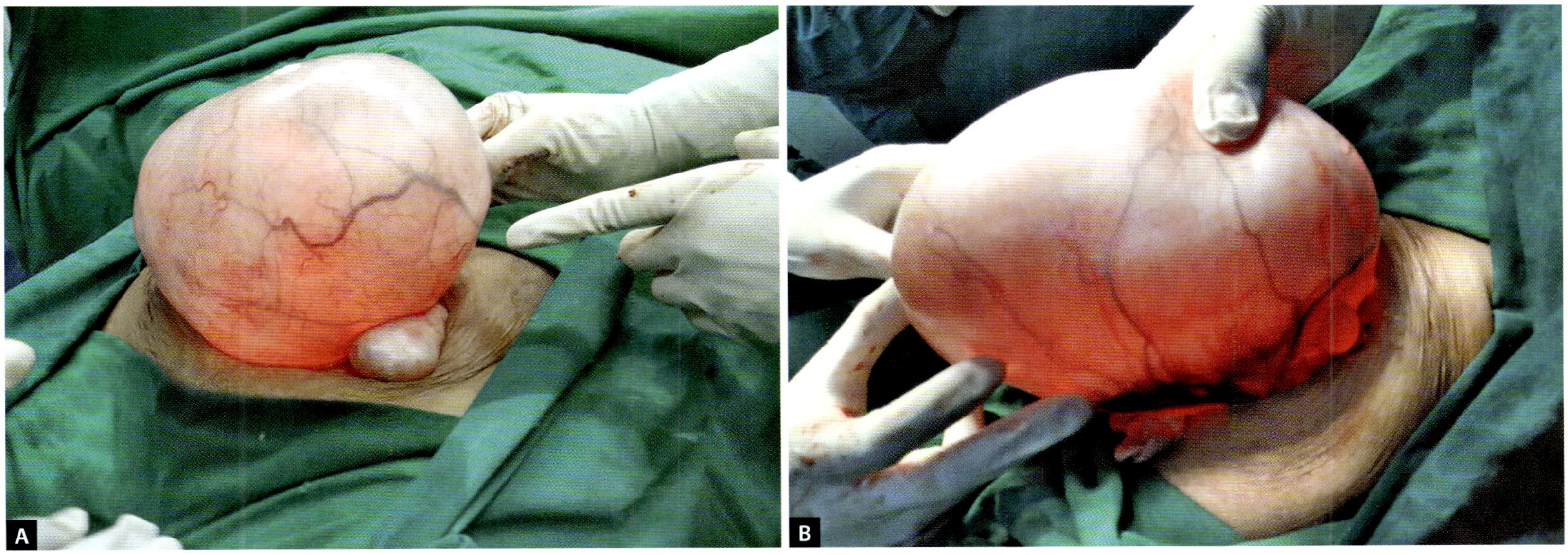

Figs. 15A and B: Benign ovarian tumor cystadenoma, having transillumination.

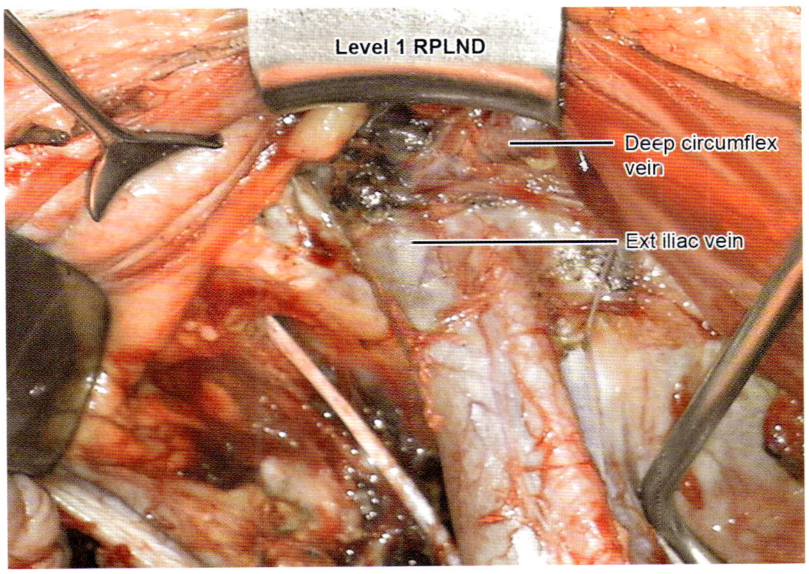

Fig. 16: Distal limit of pelvic lymphadenectomy.
(Ext: external; RPLND: retroperitoneal lymph node dissection)

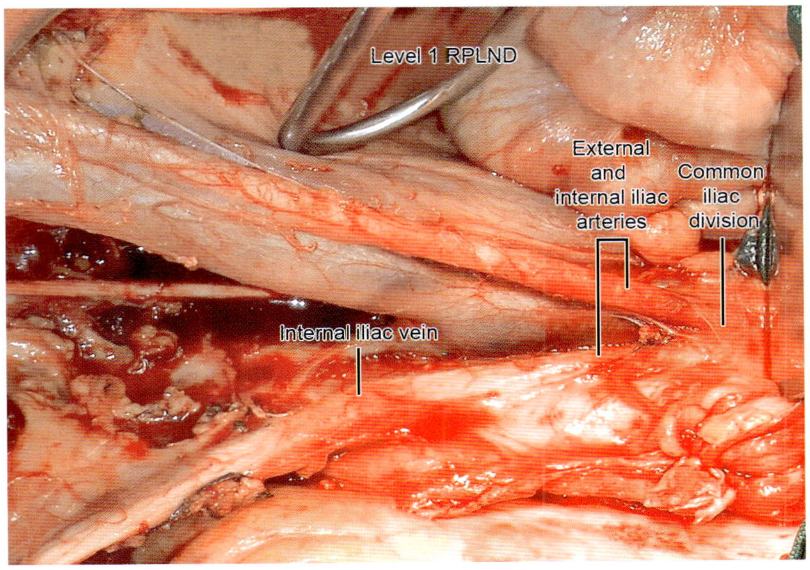

Fig. 17: Upper limit of level 1 pelvic lymphadenectomy.
(RPLND: retroperitoneal lymph node dissection)

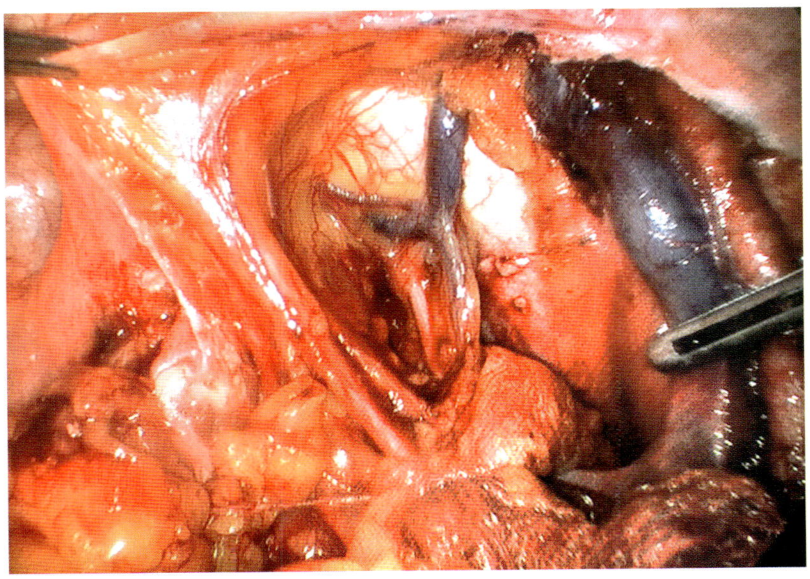

Fig. 18: Descending circumflex vein a tributary of external iliac vein usually found in anterior aspect of obturator fossa.

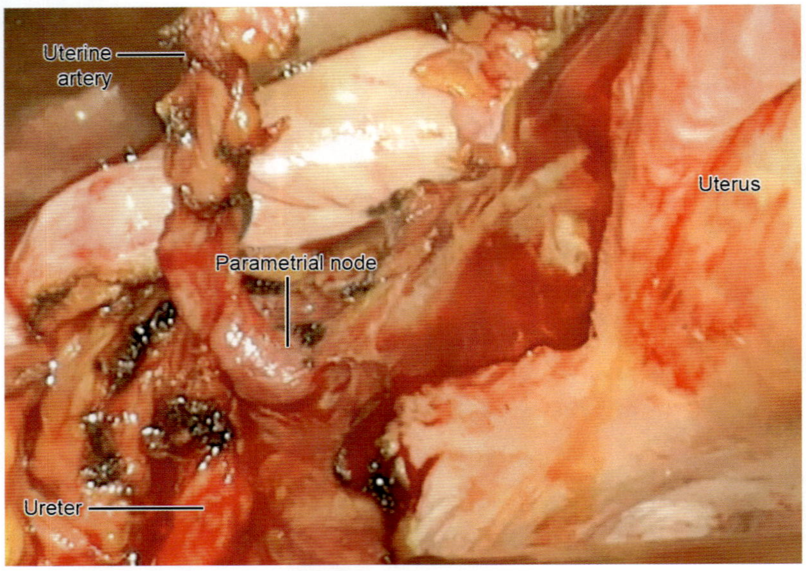

Fig. 19: Parametrial node.

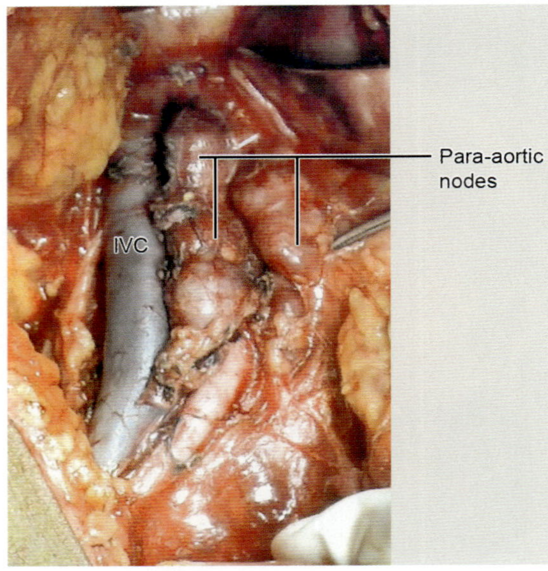

Fig. 22: Significantly enlarged para-aortic nodes. (IVC: inferior vena cava)

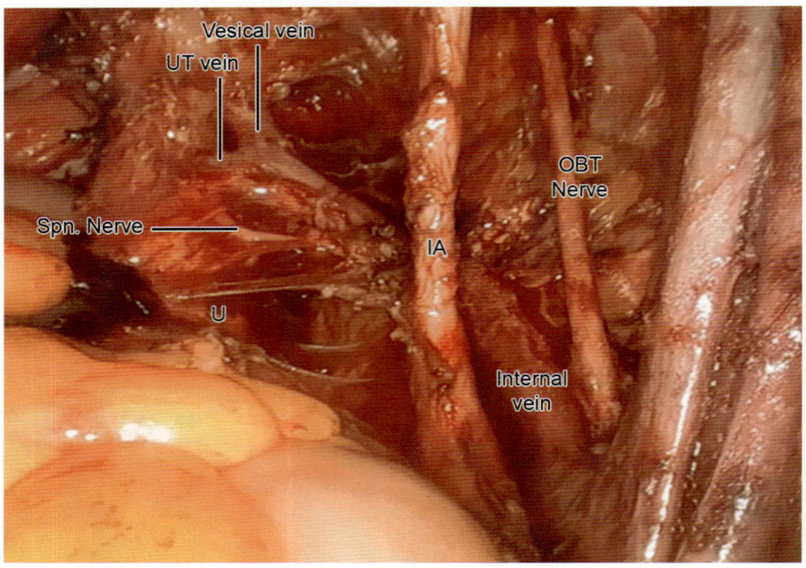

Fig. 20: Lateral parametrial neuroanatomy. (Spn: superficial peroneal; OBT: obturator)

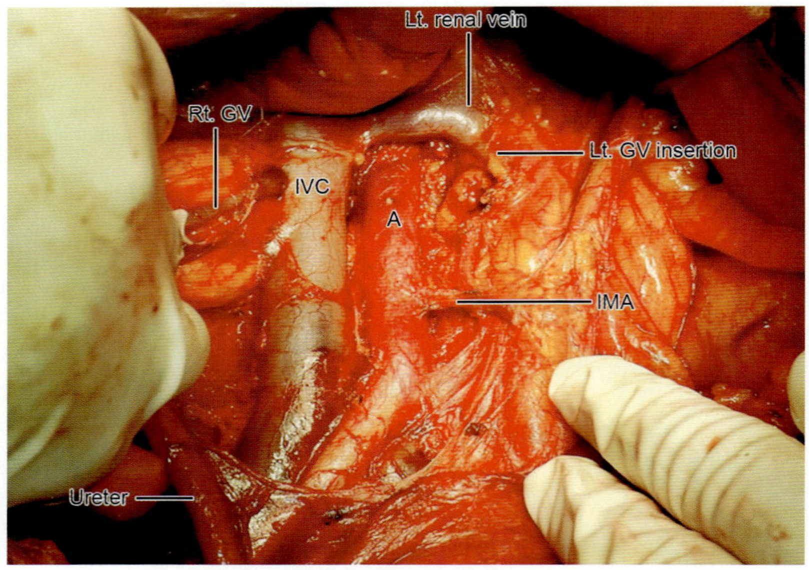

Fig. 23: Para-aortic anatomy after the nodal removal.

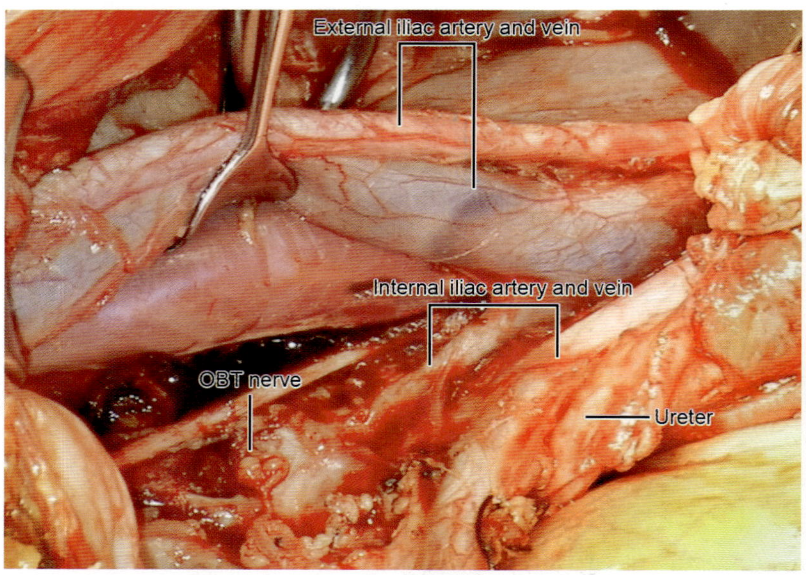

Fig. 21: Pelvic nodes dissection and pelvic iliac veins. (OBT: obturator)

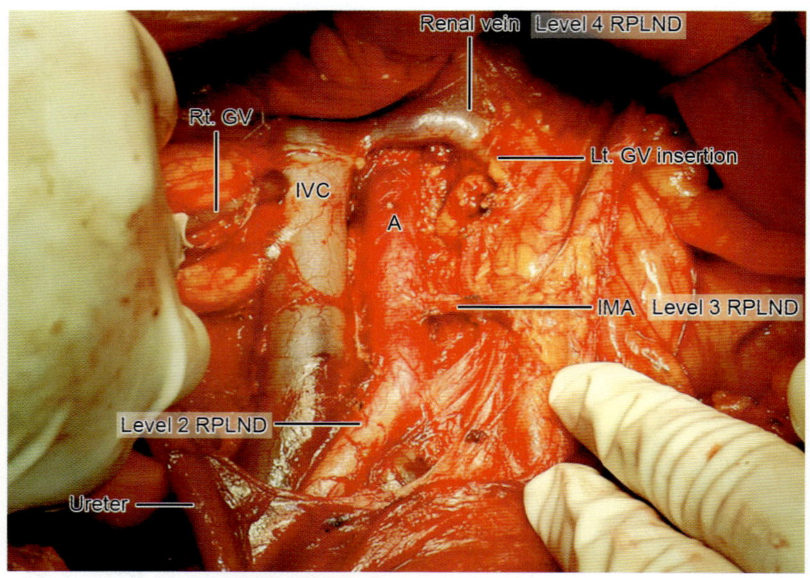

Fig. 24: Renal vein exposure level 4 retroperitoneal para-aortic nodal dissection. (IVC: inferior vena cava; RPLND: retroperitoneal lymph node dissection)

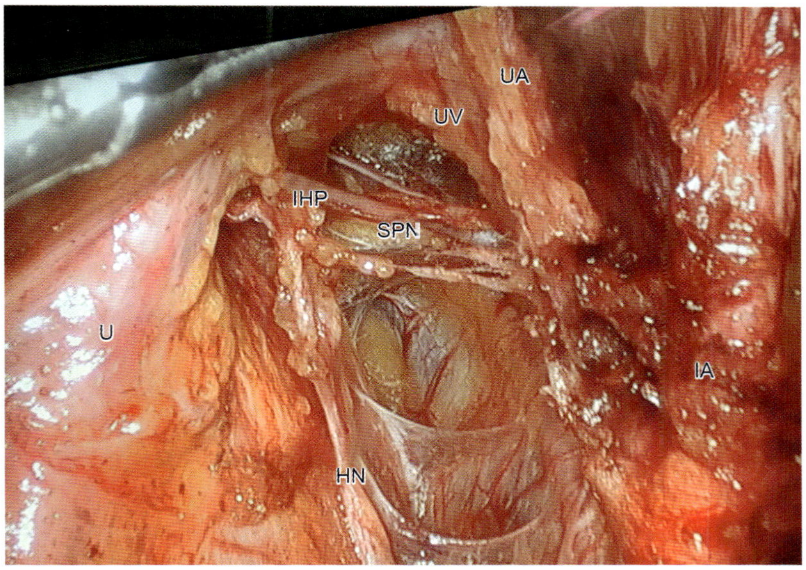

Fig. 25: Pelvic autonomic nerve plexus forming inferior hypogastric plexus. (UA: uterine artery; UV: uterine vein; IHP: inferior hypogastric plexus; SPN: superficial peroneal nerve; U: ureter; HN: hypogastric nerve)

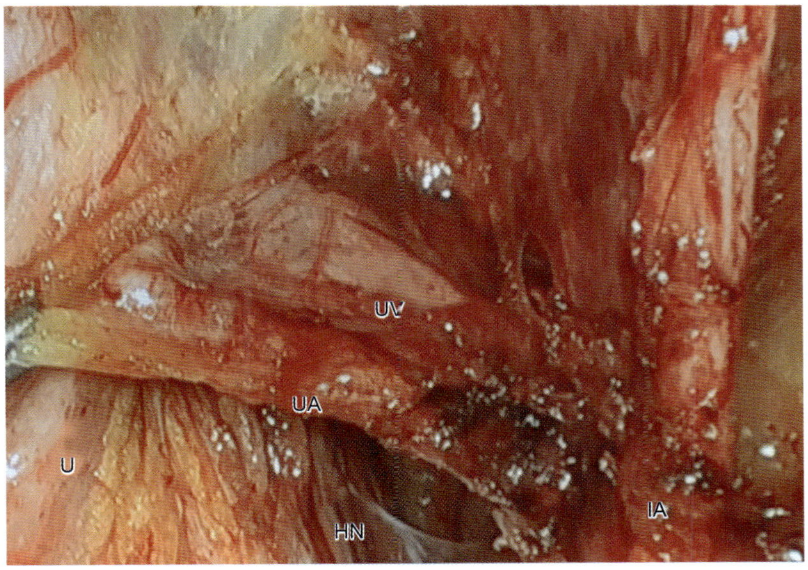

Fig. 26: Uterine artery and vein. (UA: uterine artery; UV: uterine vein; IA: iliac artery; U: ureter; HN: hypogastric nerve)

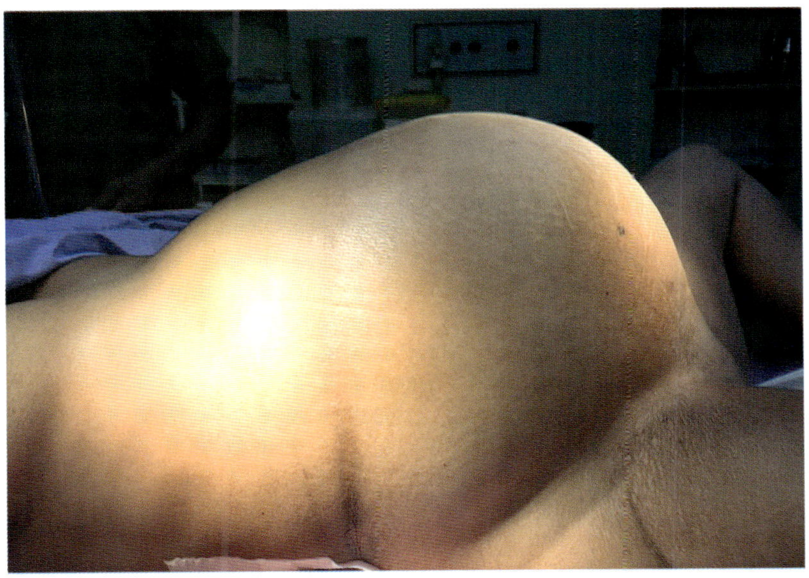

Fig. 27: Huge ovarian mucinous tumor.

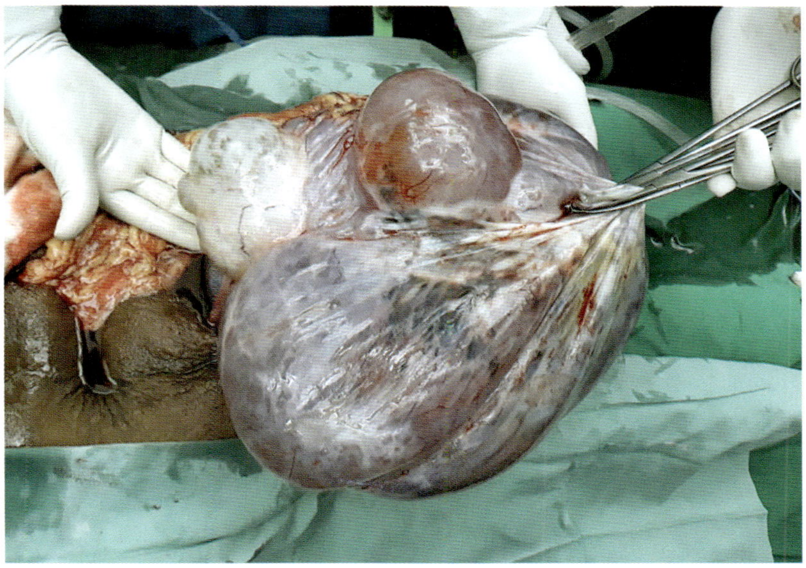

Fig. 28: Mucinous bigger tumor.

Advanced Stage Tumors; Clinically and Radiologically Advanced Tumor (Figs. 29 To 68)

1. Midline vertical incision may extend from pubic symphysis to xiphisternum.
2. Inspection of pelvic, abdominal organs and assessment of optimal tumor resectability.
3. Clinical or peritoneal carcinomatosis index (PCI) calculation.
4. Tumor cytoreduction includes, ovarian tumor removal, total abdominal hysterectomy with bilateral salpingo-oophorectomy, excision of the involved peritonectomy, pelvic and abdominal deposits excision, total omentectomy, removal of the enlarged (>1 cm) retroperitoneal lymph nodes, and additional organ resection like bowel resection/diaphragm stripping/splenectomy depending on the individual case requirements to achieve optimal cytoreduction (residual tumor nil or at least <1 cm in size).
5. Intraperitoneal chemotherapy and/or hyperthermic intraperitoneal chemotherapy depending on the discretion of case attending gynecological oncologist.
6. Abdominal drain insertion is needed in bowel resection and in extensive peritonectomy cases.

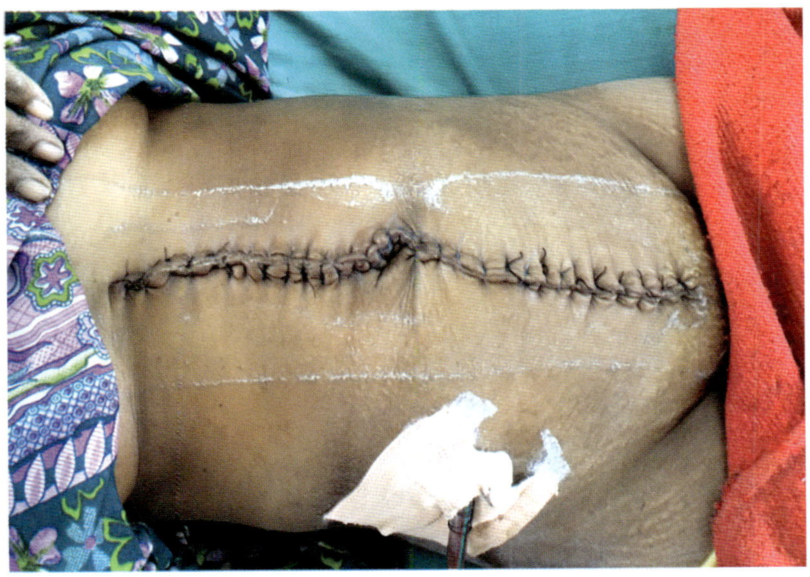

Fig. 29: Incision for the advanced ovarian cancer.

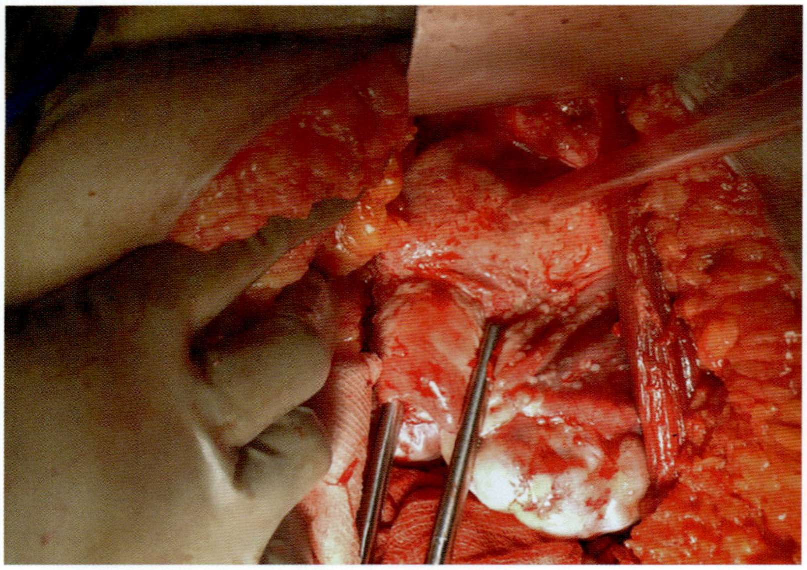

Fig. 30: Bladder peritoneal tumor deposits in advanced stage ovarian cancer.

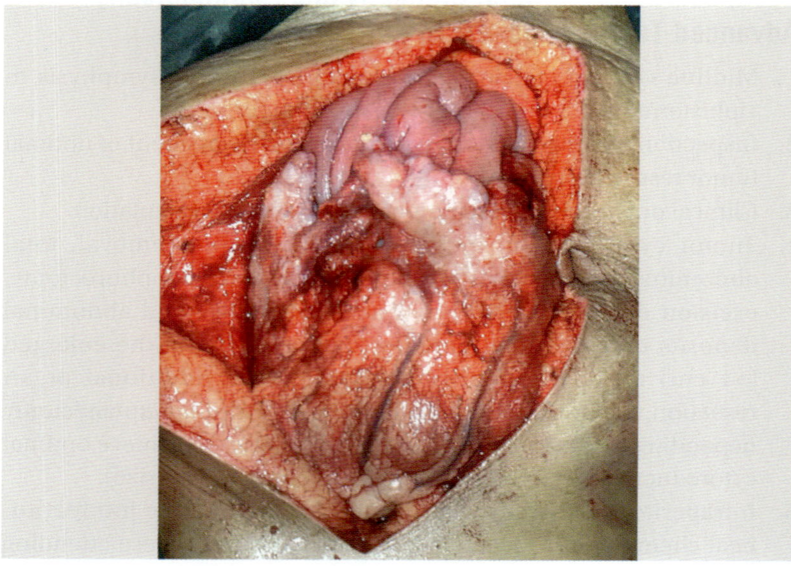

Fig. 31: Omental cake, stage 3 ovarian cancer.

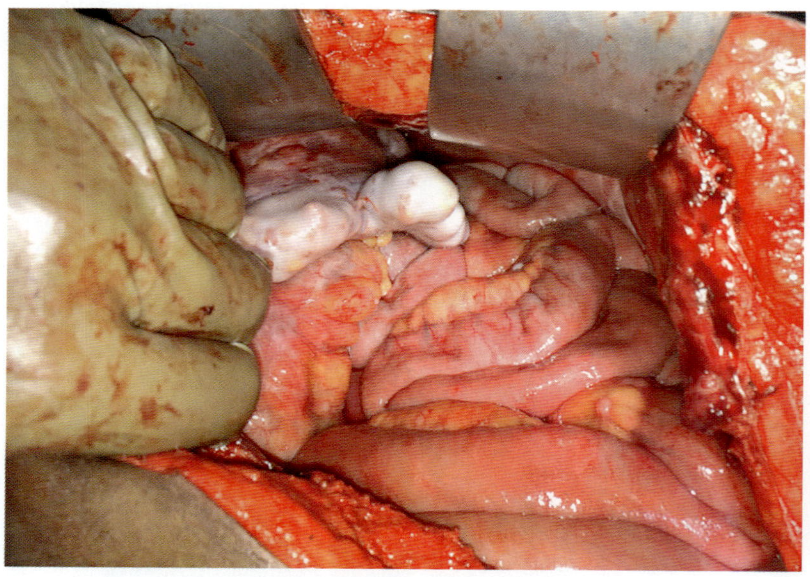

Fig. 32: Caked up omentum with tumor deposits.

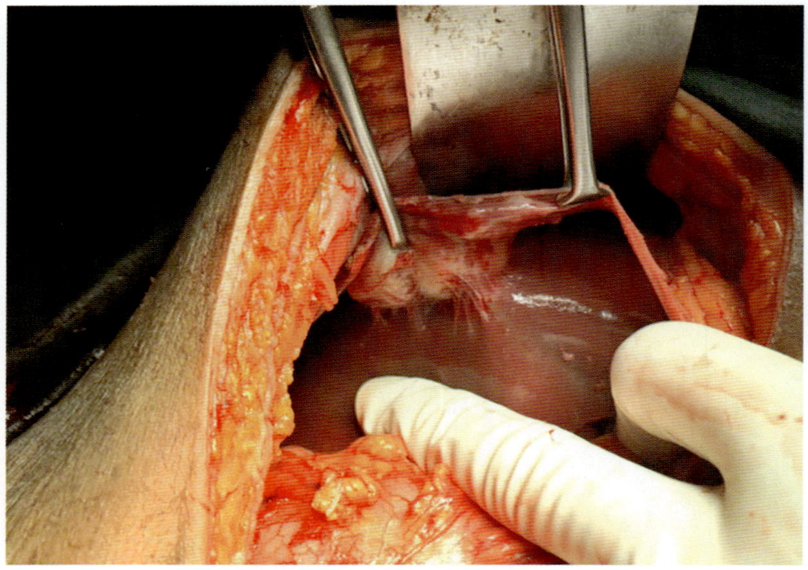

Fig. 33: Perihepatic deposit.

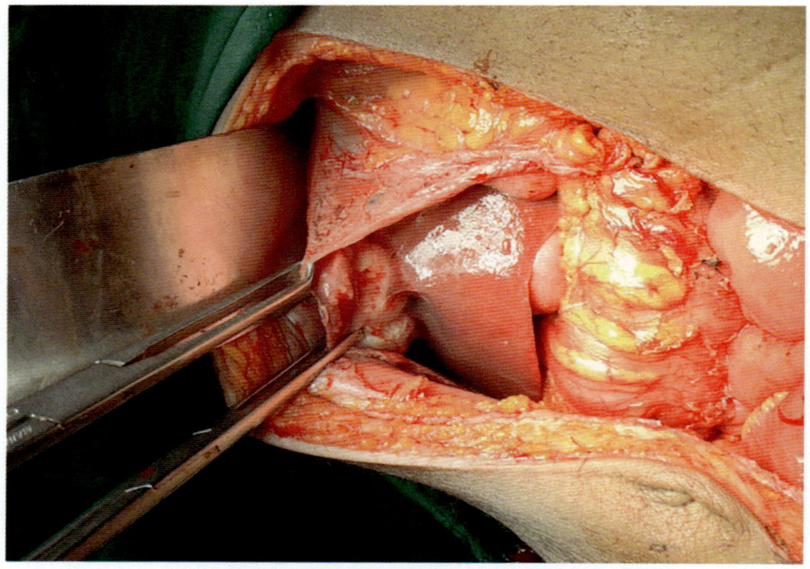

Fig. 34: Perihepatic deposit excisable.

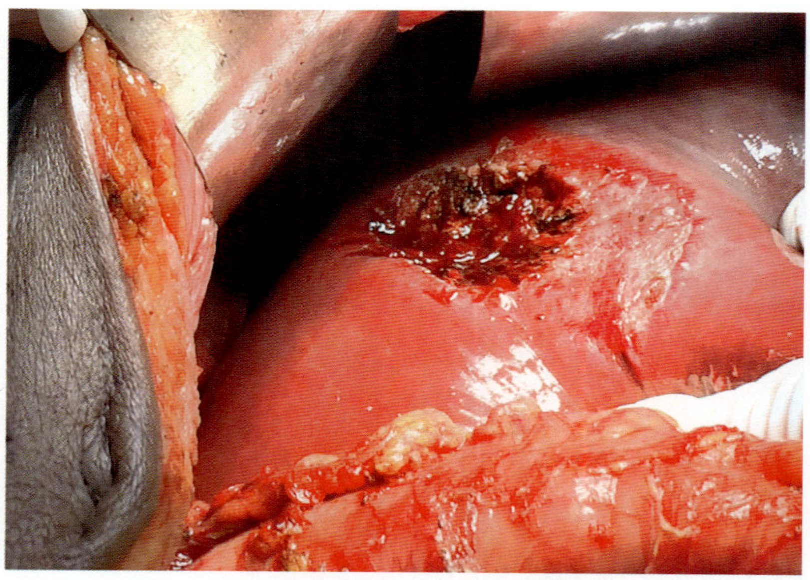

Fig. 35: Perihepatic deposit excision.

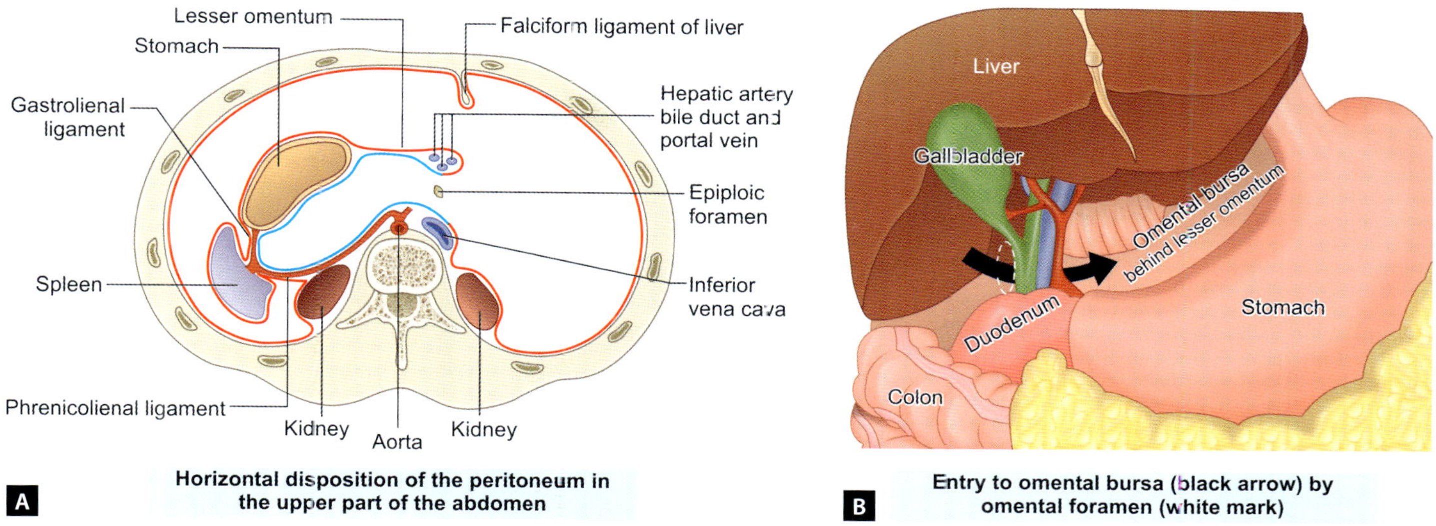

Figs. 36A and B: Foramen of Winslow and porta hepatis—diagram.

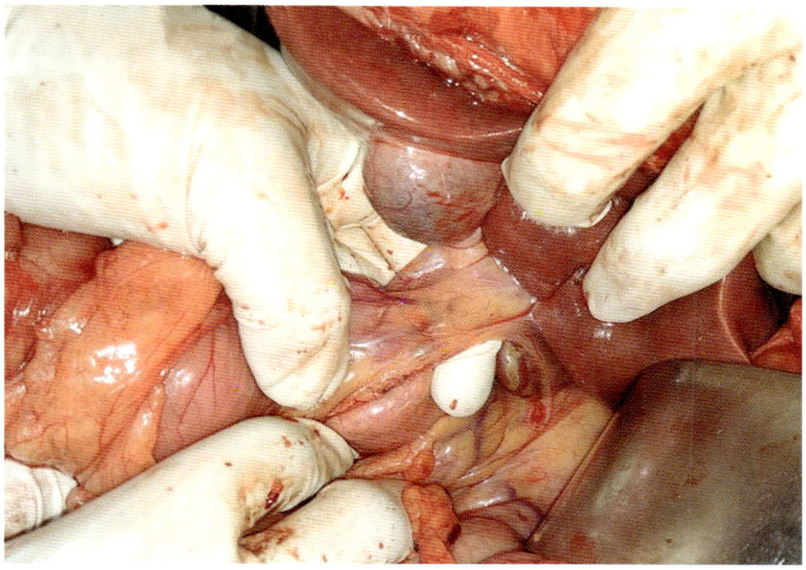

Fig. 37: Foramen of Winslow and porta hepatis.

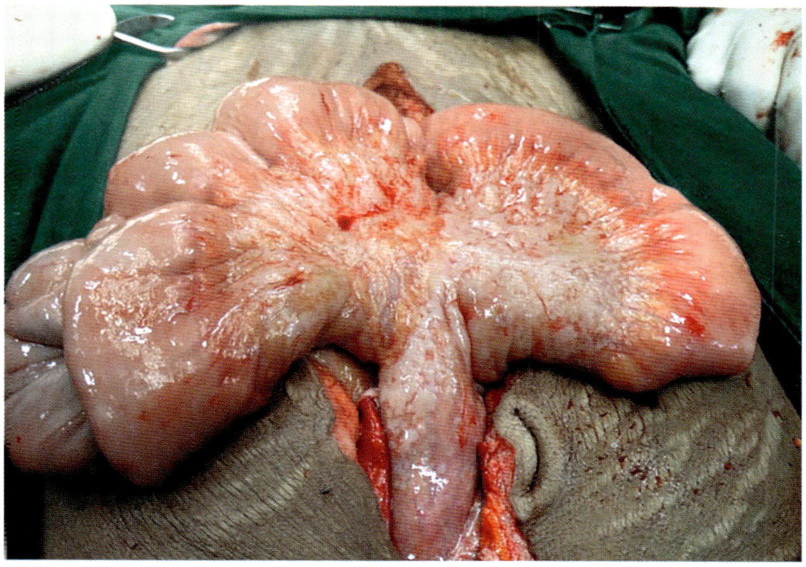

Fig. 39: Miliary deposits on the mesentery.

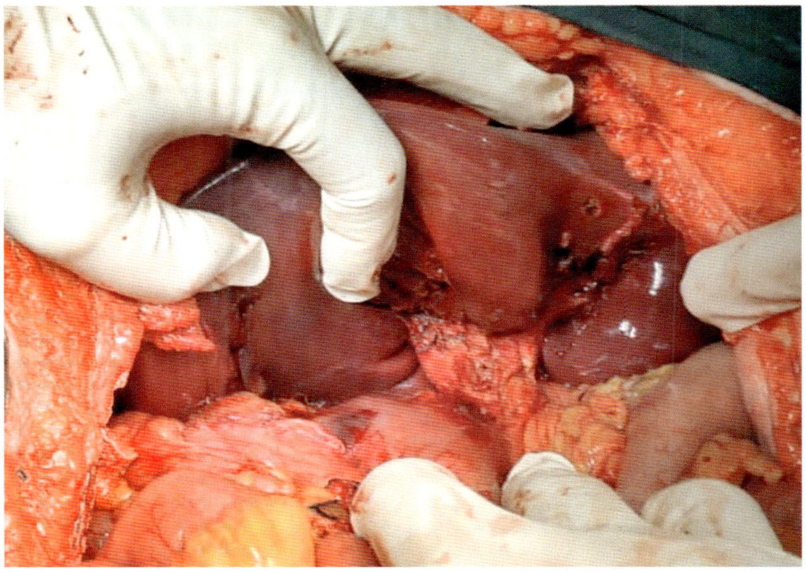

Fig. 38: Porta hepatic deposit excision following cholecystectomy.

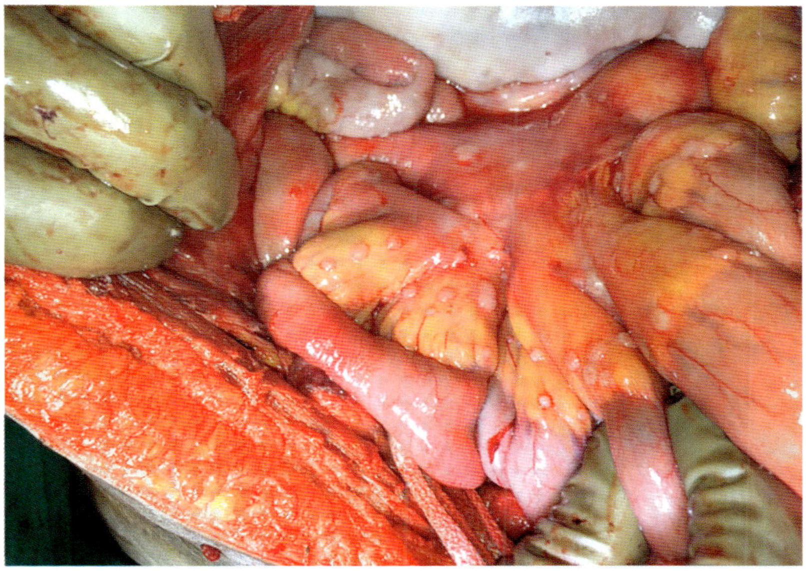

Fig. 40: Multiple bowel mesenteric tumor deposits in advanced ovarian cancers.

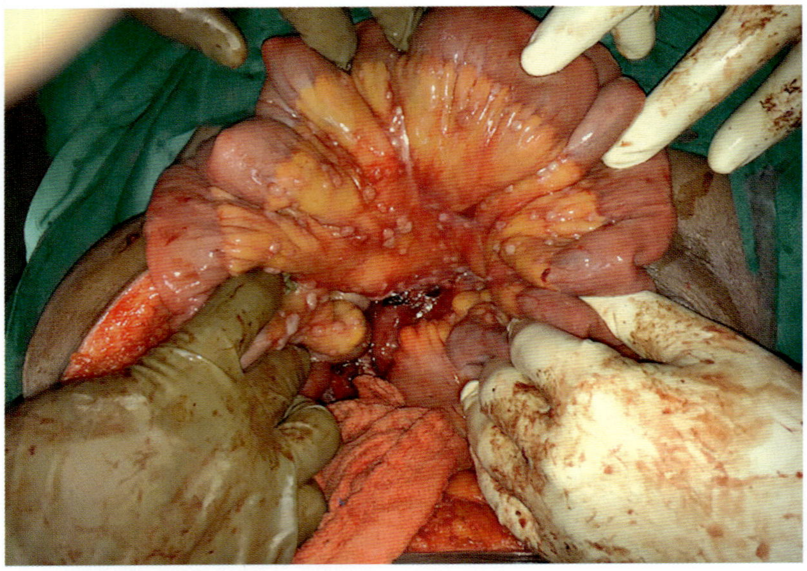

Fig. 41: Multiple small bowel mesenteric tumor deposits in advanced ovarian cancers up to the root.

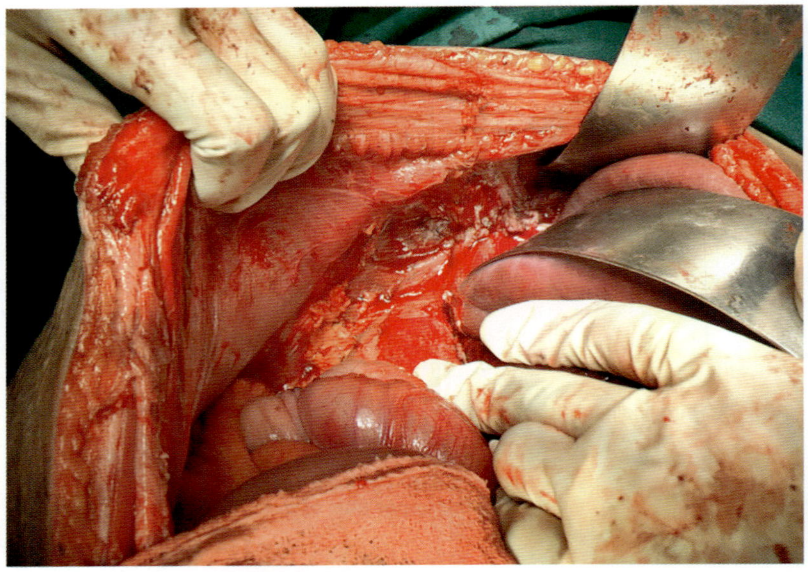

Fig. 44: Diaphragm peritoneal stripping with tumor deposit.

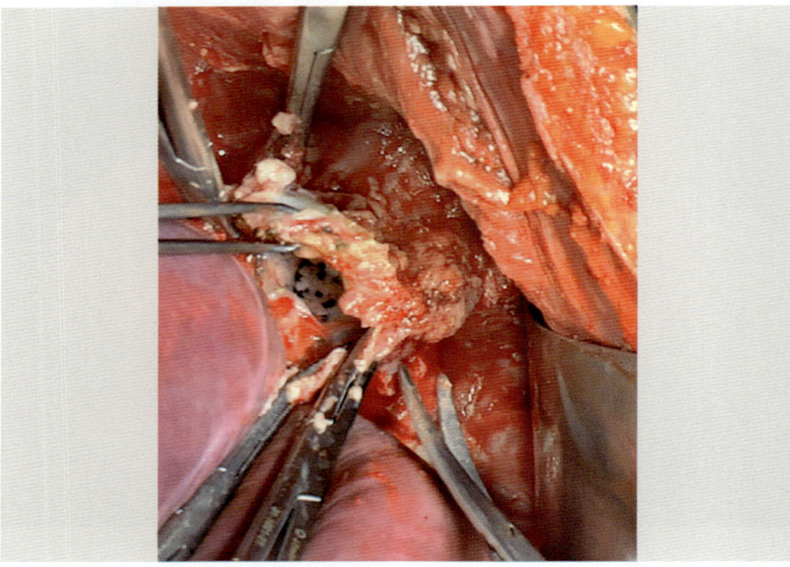

Fig. 42: Diaphragm central tendon excision with a deposit.

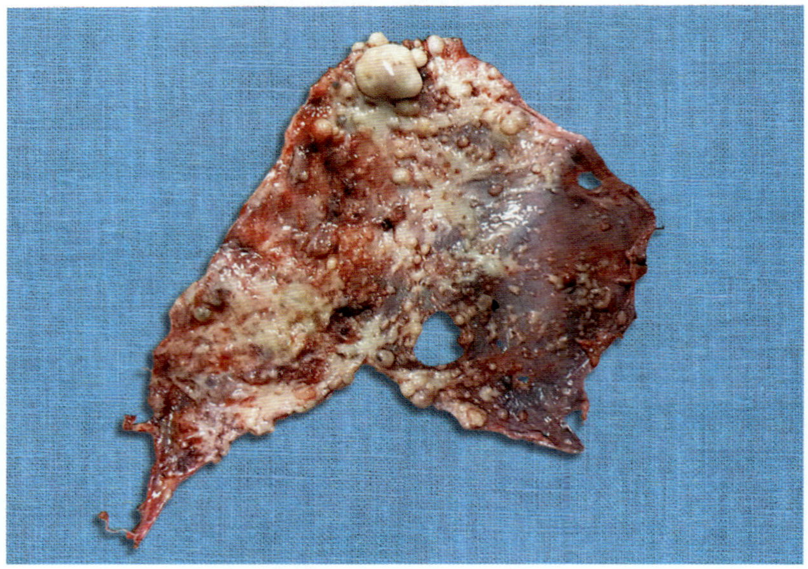

Fig. 45: Diaphragm peritoneal stripped peritoneum with tumor deposits.

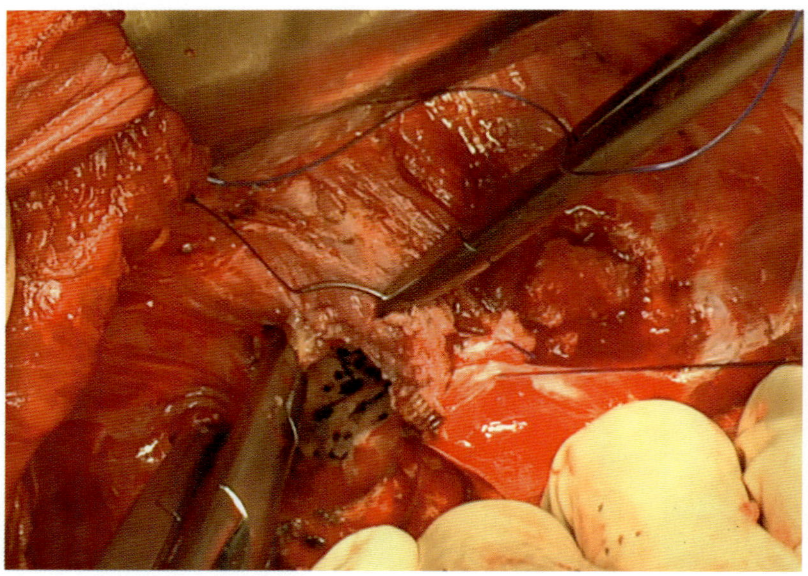

Fig. 43: Diaphragm repair after the excision.

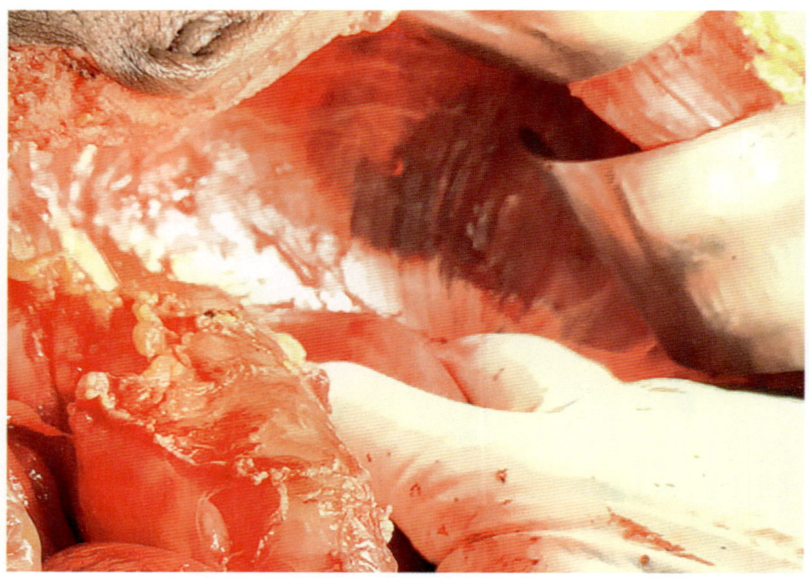

Fig. 46: Diaphragm after peritoneal stripping.

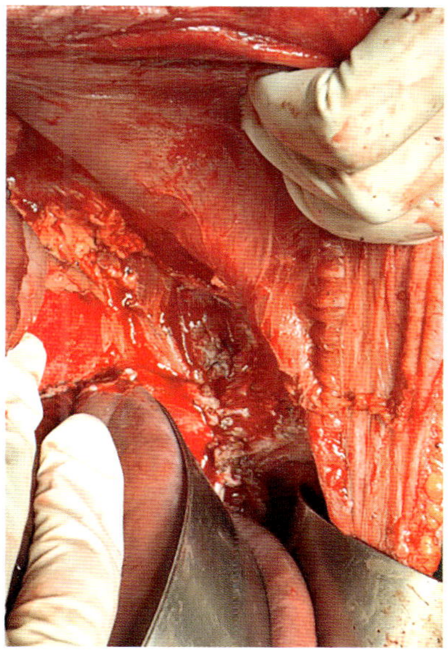

Fig. 47: Diaphragm after central tendon deposit excision and repaired with Prolene no 1.

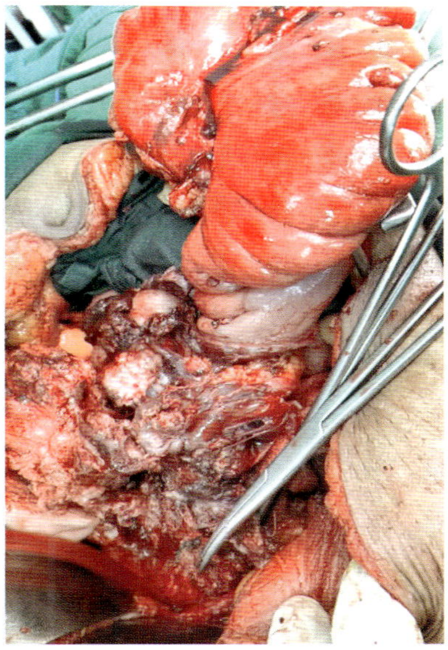

Fig. 48: En bloc resection of uterus with ovarian tumor and rectosigmoid in an ovarian cancer infiltrating rectosigmoid mesentery.

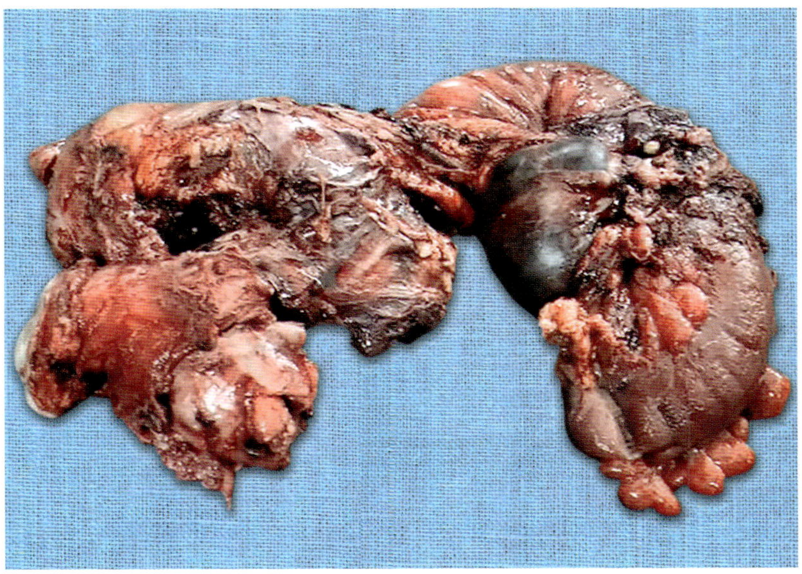

Fig. 49: En bloc resection of uterus with ovarian tumor and rectosigmoid in a ovarian cancer infiltrating rectosigmoid mesentery—specimen.

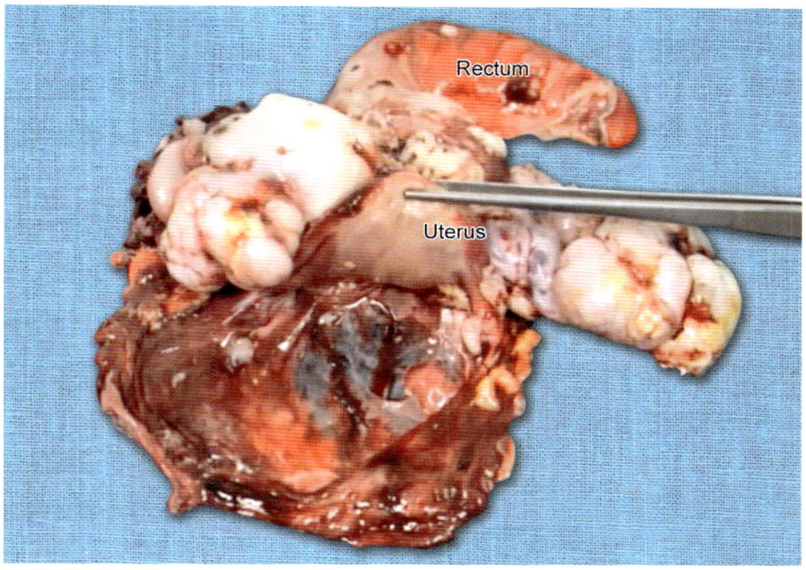

Fig. 50: En bloc resection of uterus with ovarian tumor and rectosigmoid in an infiltrating ovarian cancer.

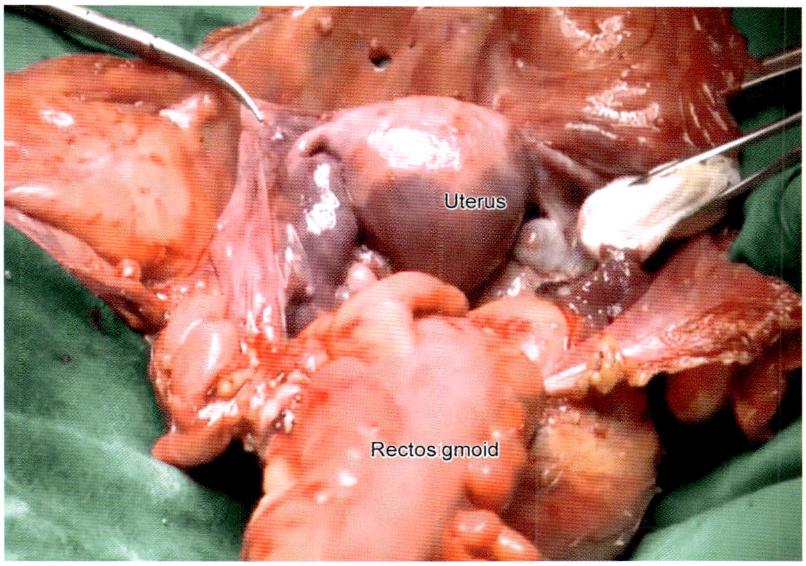

Fig. 51: En bloc resection of uterus with ovarian tumor and rectosigmoid in an infiltrating ovarian cancer—retroperitoneal approach.

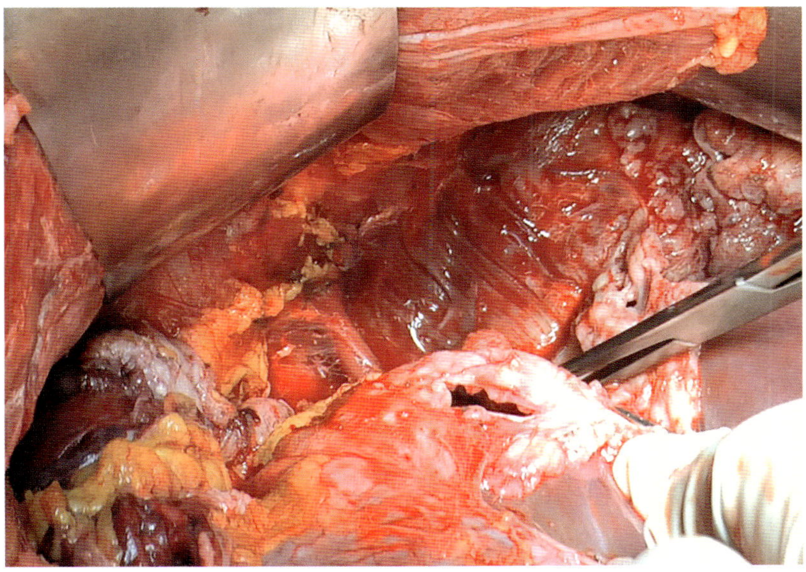

Fig. 52: Diaphragm deposit excision.

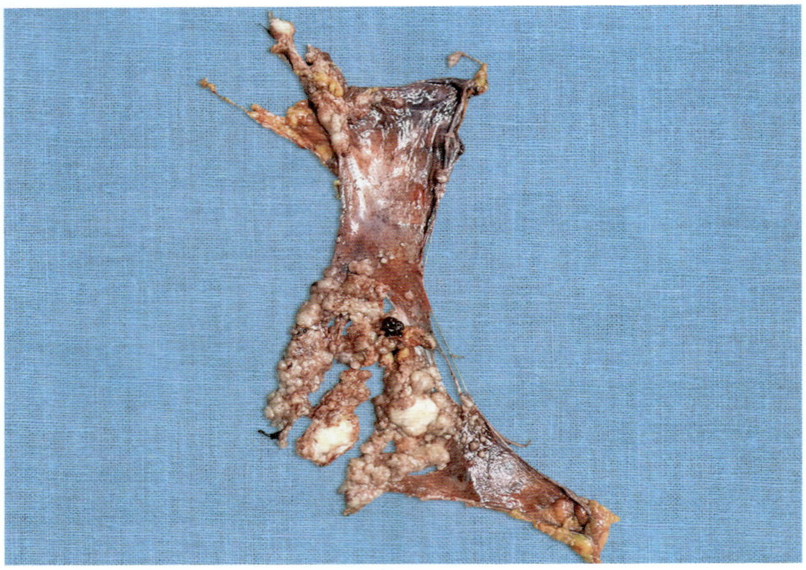

Fig. 53: Diaphragm peritoneal deposit excision.

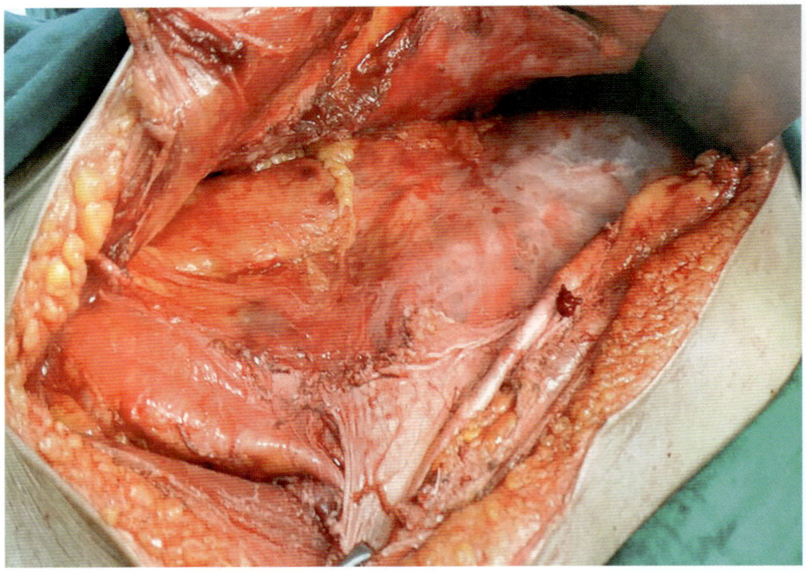

Fig. 54: En bloc abdominal peritonectomy for a primary peritoneal cancer.

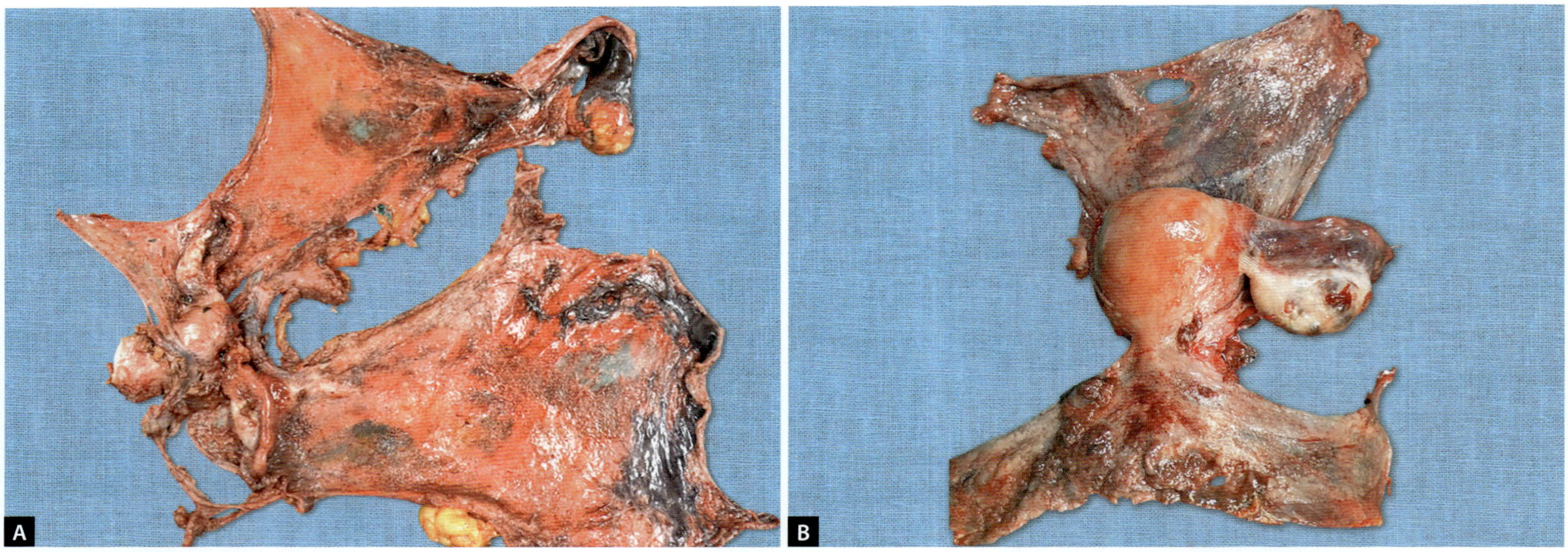

Figs. 55A and B: En bloc pelvic and abdominal peritonectomy for a primary peritoneal cancer specimen with uterus and ovaries.

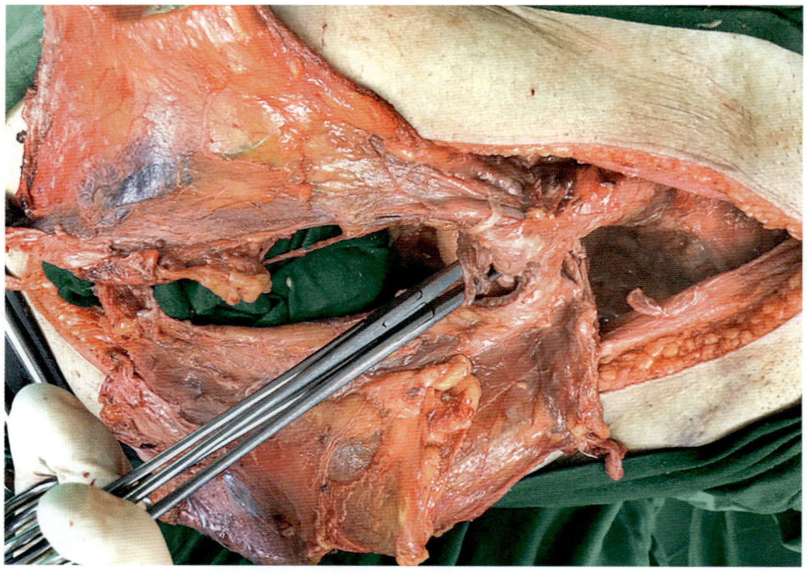

Fig. 56: En bloc pelvic and abdominal peritonectomy for a primary peritoneal cancer.

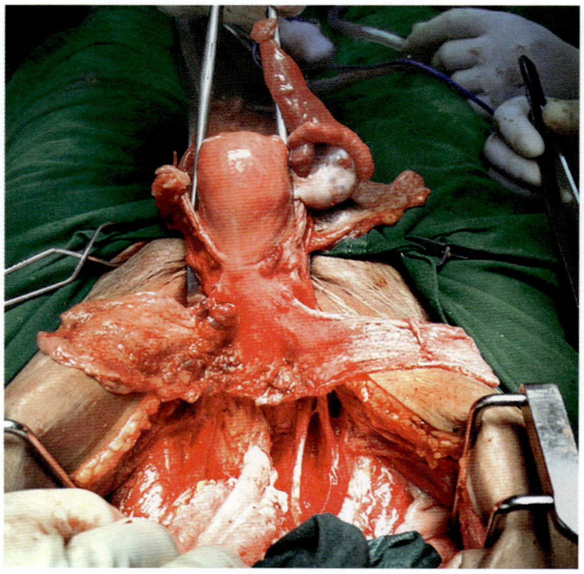

Fig. 57: En bloc pelvic and abdominal peritonectomy for a primary peritoneal cancer pouch of Douglas (POD) clearance.

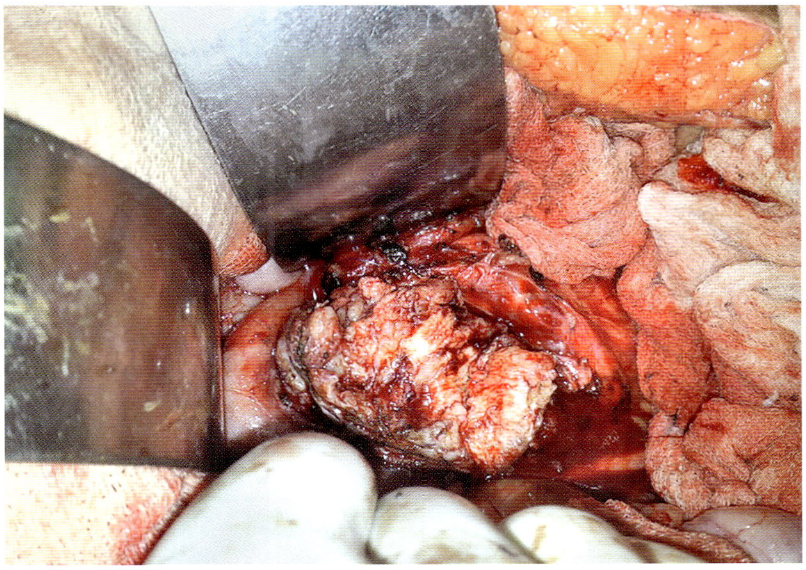

Fig. 58: A big para-aortic node.

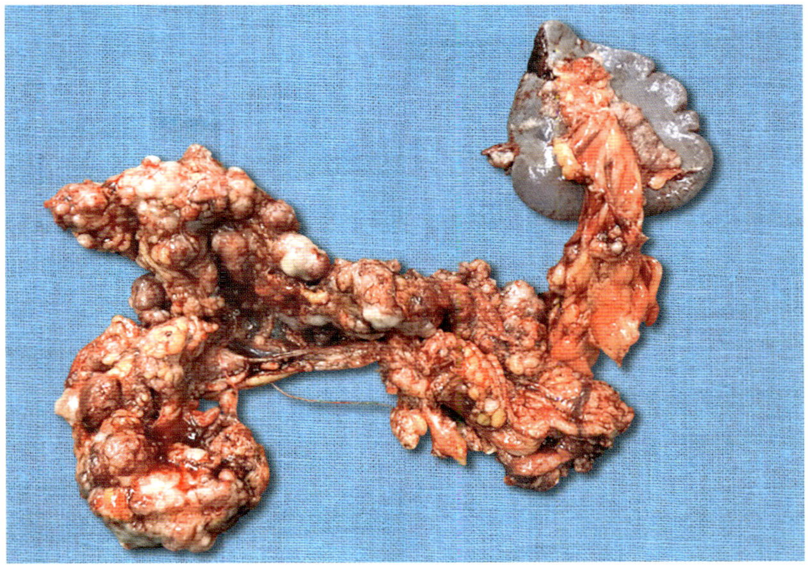

Fig. 61: Omental cake and splenectomy en bloc excision.

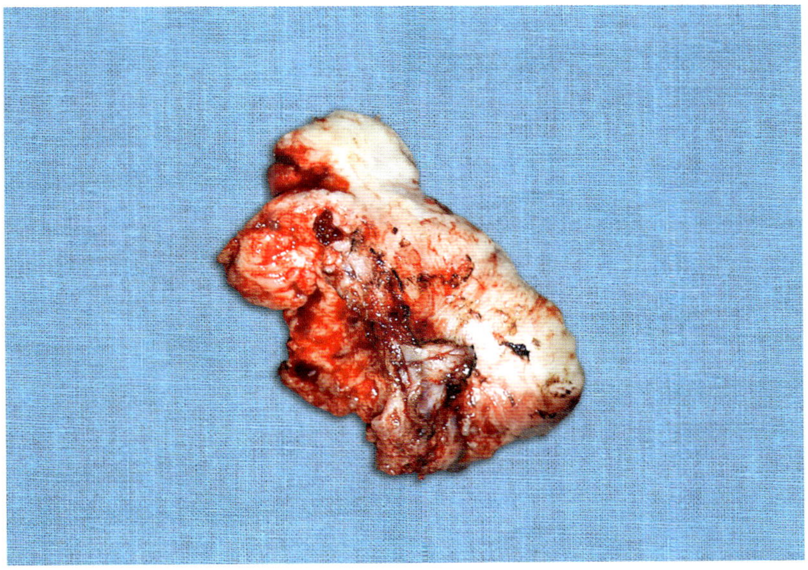

Fig. 59: A big para-aortic node debulked.

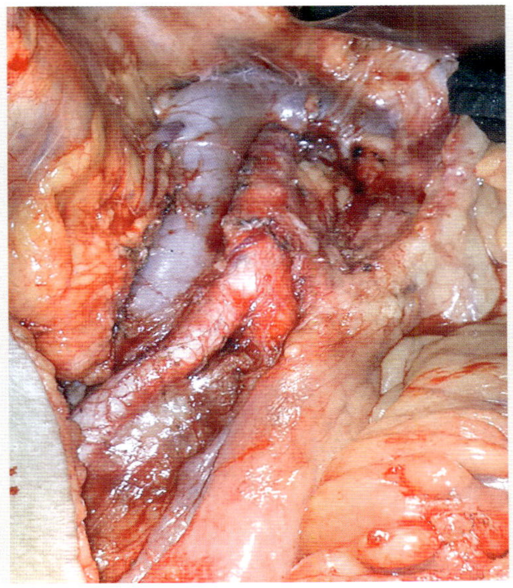

Fig. 62: Para-aortic nodal clearance.

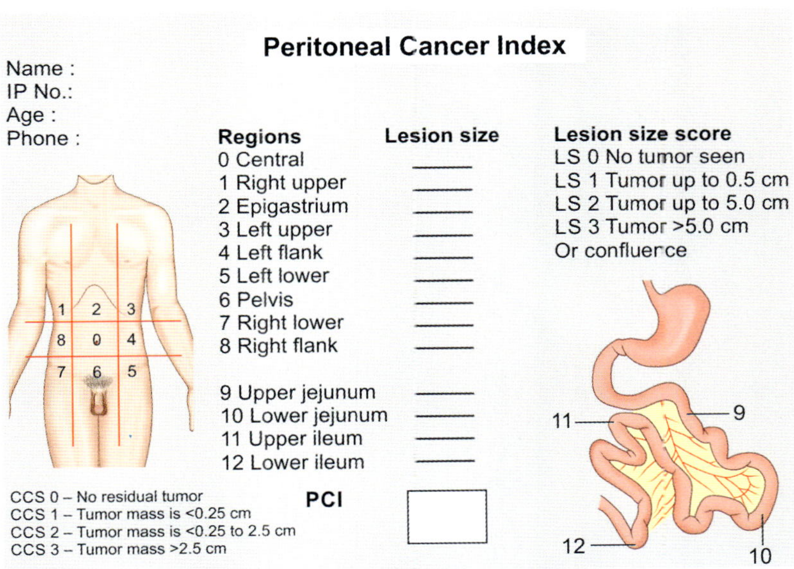

Fig. 60: Peritoneal carcinomatosis index chart.

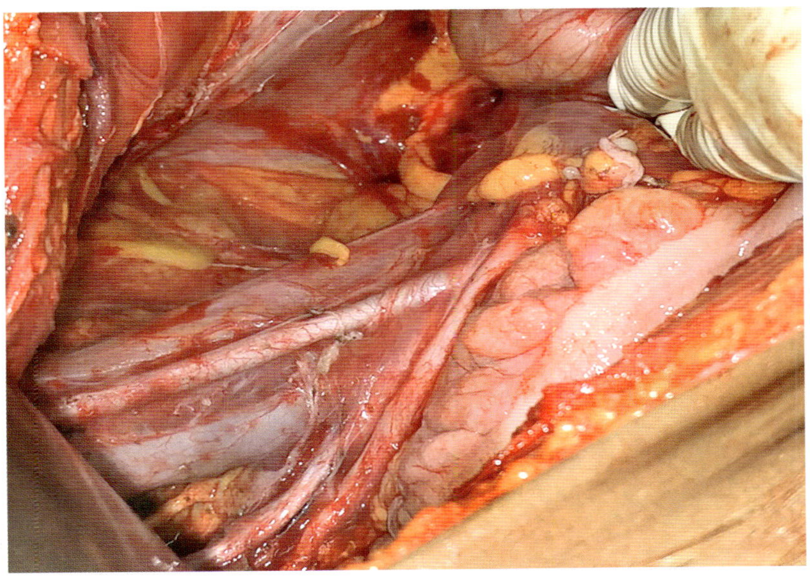

Fig. 63: Paracolic gutter after peritonectomy.

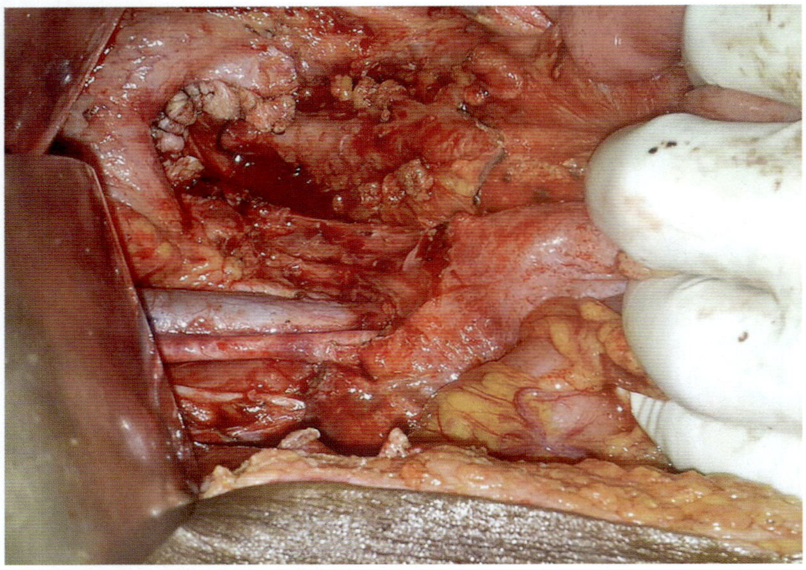

Fig. 64: Pelvic anatomy after the pelvic tumor excision and pelvic peritoneal excision.

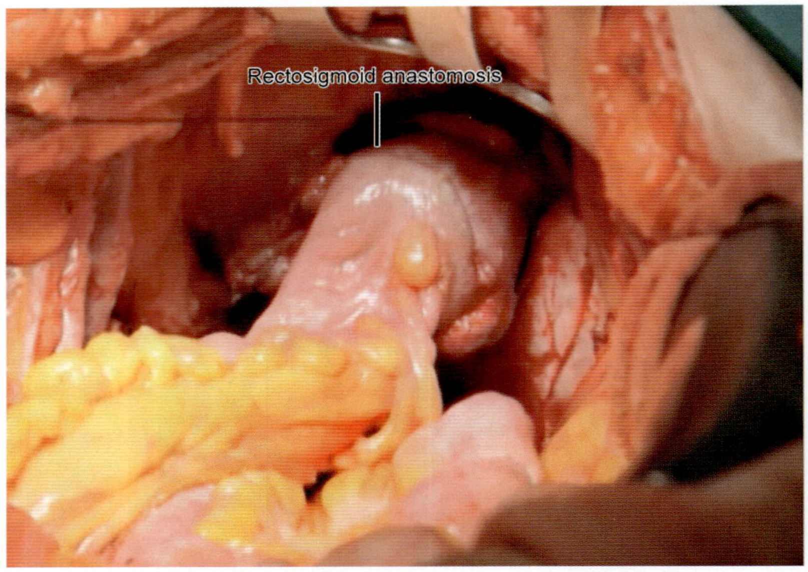

Fig. 66: Rectosigmoid resection anastomosis as part of primary cytoreductive surgery.

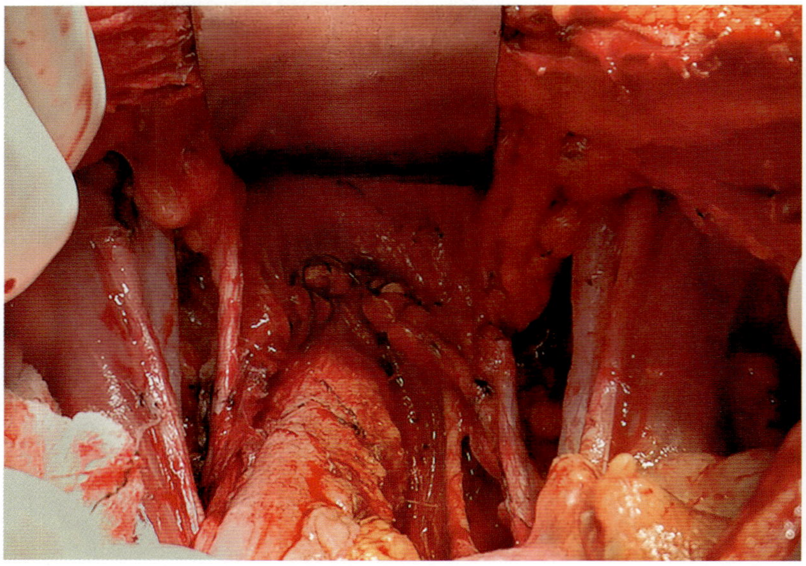

Fig. 65: Pelvis after peritonectomy.

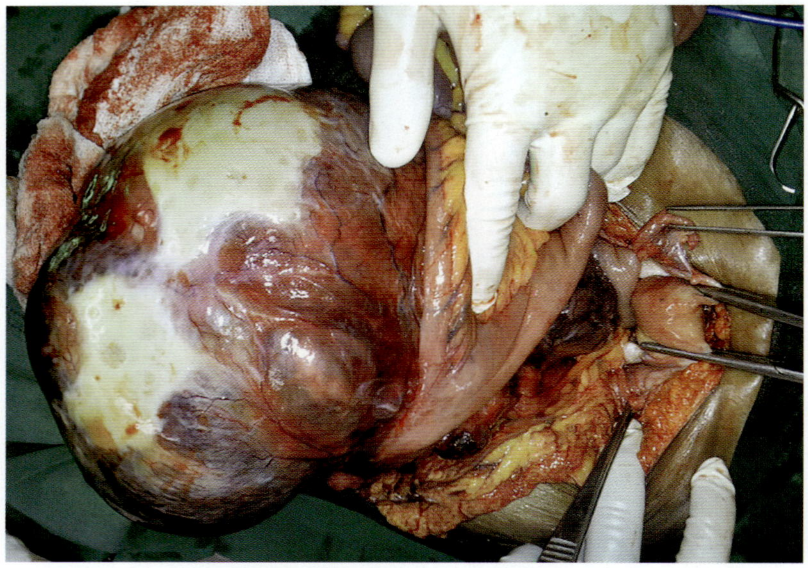

Fig. 67: Gastrointestinal stromal tumor intraoperative surprise, ovaries normal.

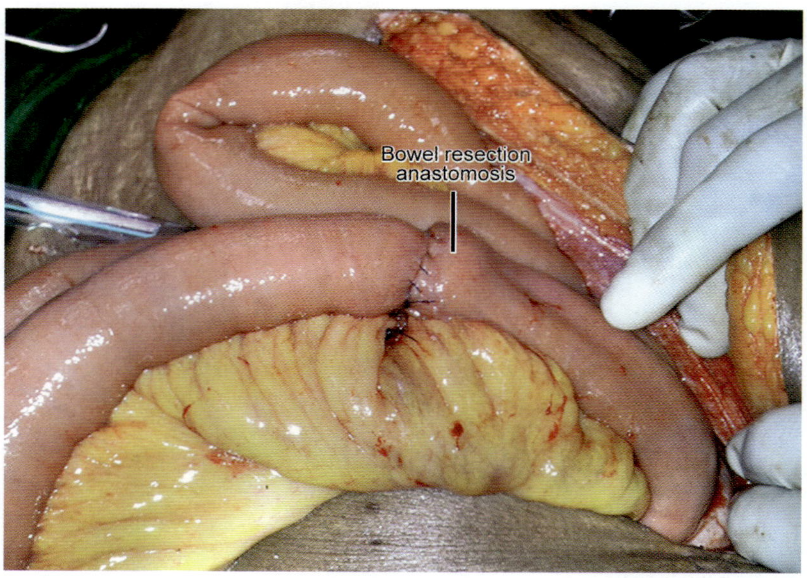

Fig. 68: Small bowel resection anastomosis.

RARE TUMORS OF OVARIES

Metastatic Ovarian Cancers Krukenberg's Tumors (Figs. 69 to 73)

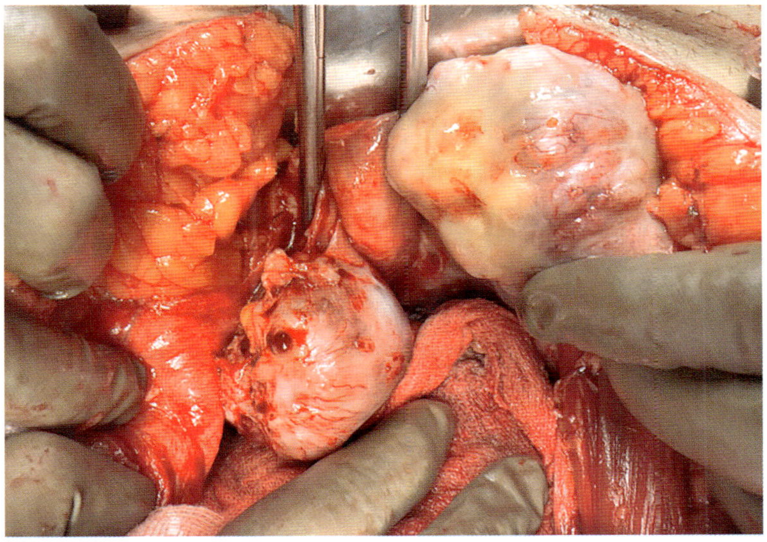

Fig. 69: Krukenberg's tumor ovary.

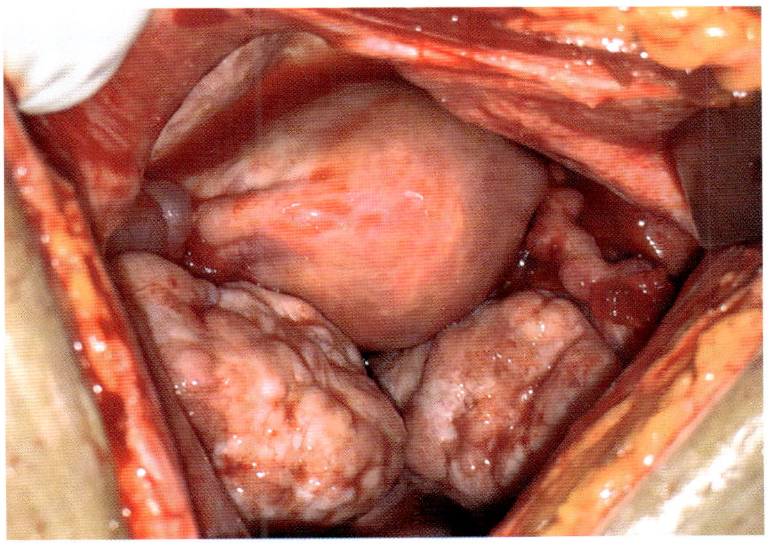

Fig. 70: Krukenberg's tumor ovary, the surface ovarian contour is maintained.

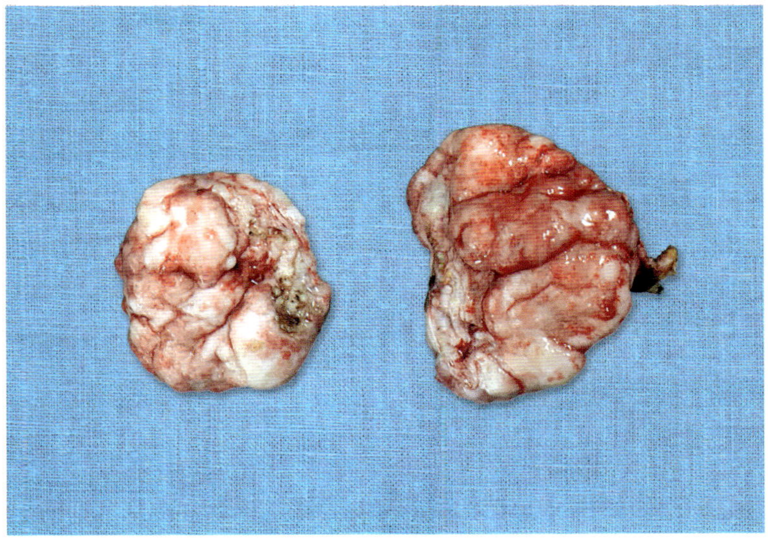

Fig. 71: Specimen Krukenberg's tumor ovaries, the surface ovarian contour is maintained.

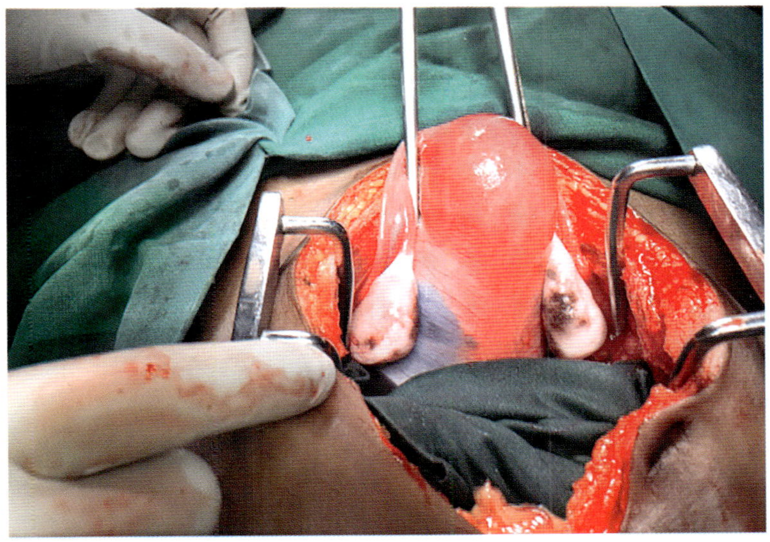

Fig. 72: A rare melanoma deposit in the ovary.

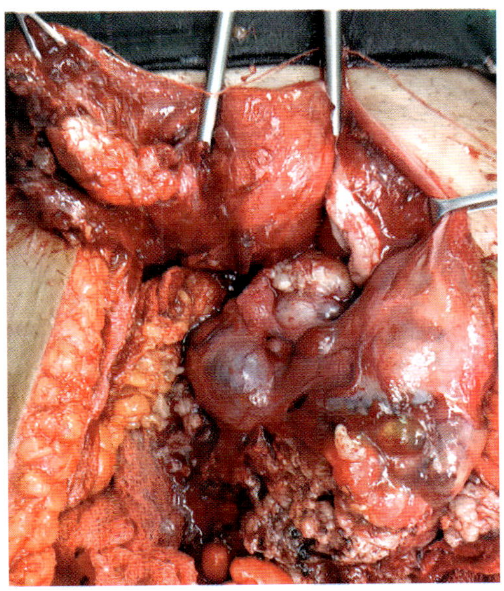

Fig. 73: Fallopian tube cancer involving sigmoid.

Case 1: Recurrent Immature Teratoma Presenting as Growing Teratoma Syndrome (Figs. 74 to 78)

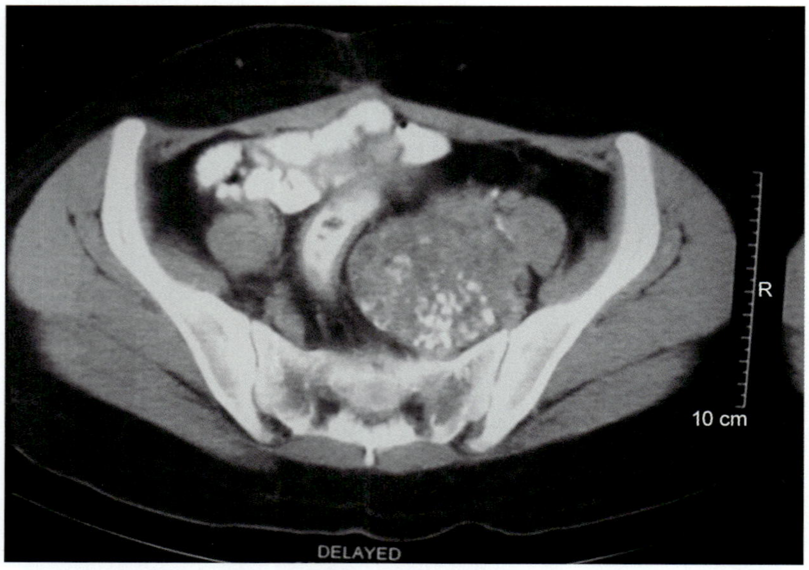

Fig. 74: Immature teratoma recurrence in pararectal space.

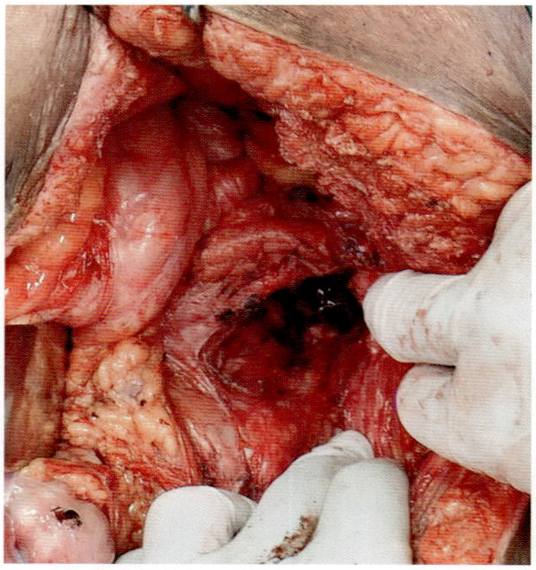

Fig. 76: Pararectal space after the excision recurrent immature teratoma.

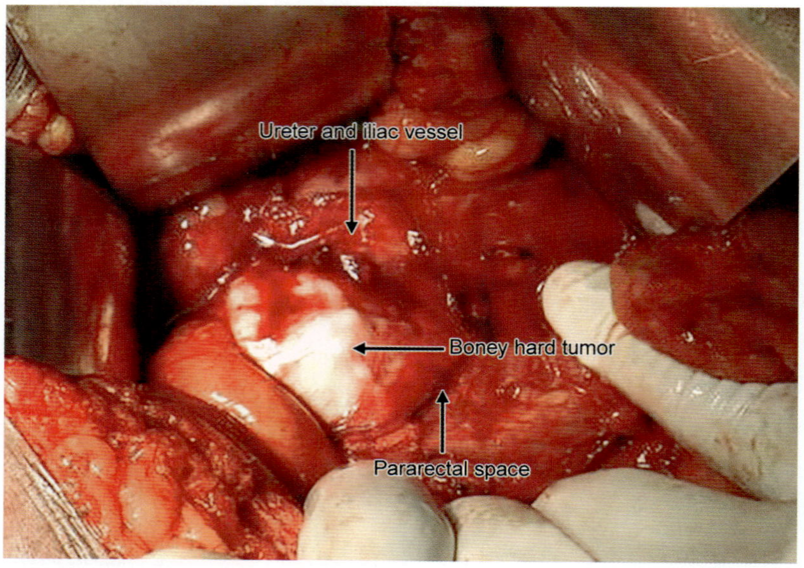

Fig. 75: Boney hard immature teratoma recurrence in pararectal space.

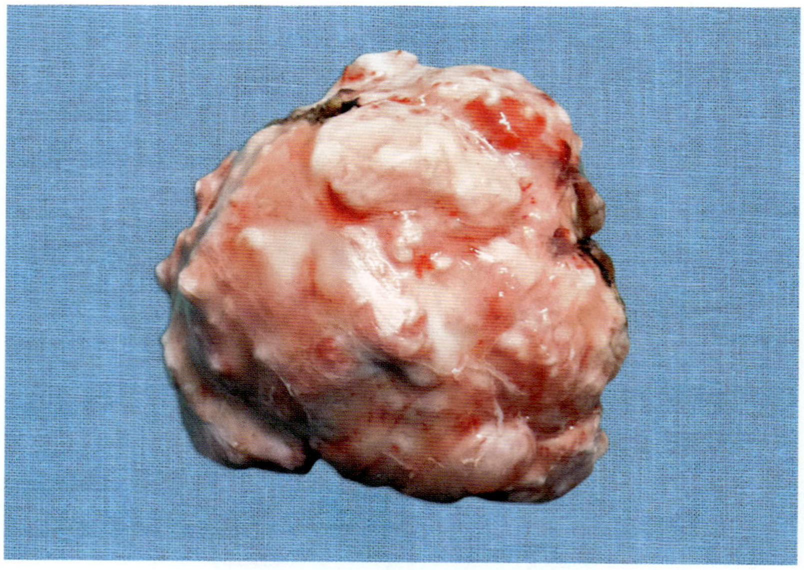

Fig. 77: Recurrent immature teratoma.

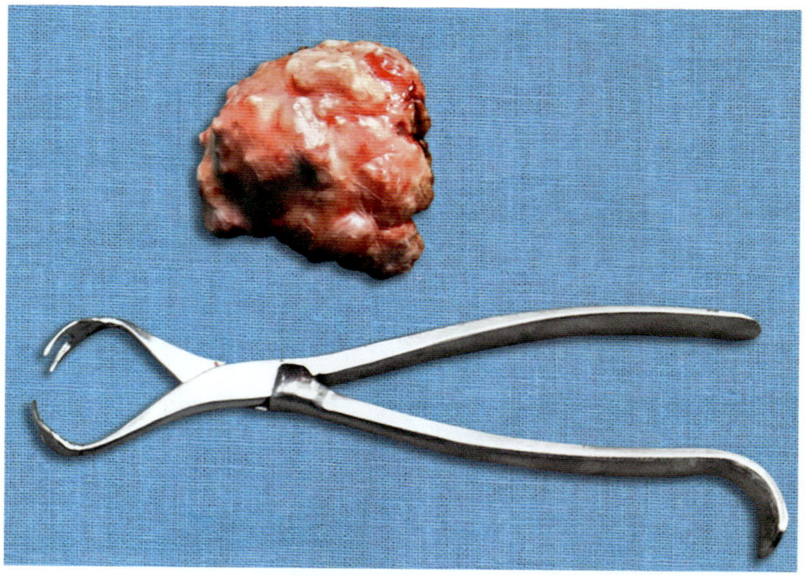

Fig. 78: Boney hard recurrent immature teratoma needed a bone cutter instrument for the excision.

Case 2: Recurrent Immature Teratoma Presenting as Growing Teratoma Syndrome (Figs. 79 To 85)

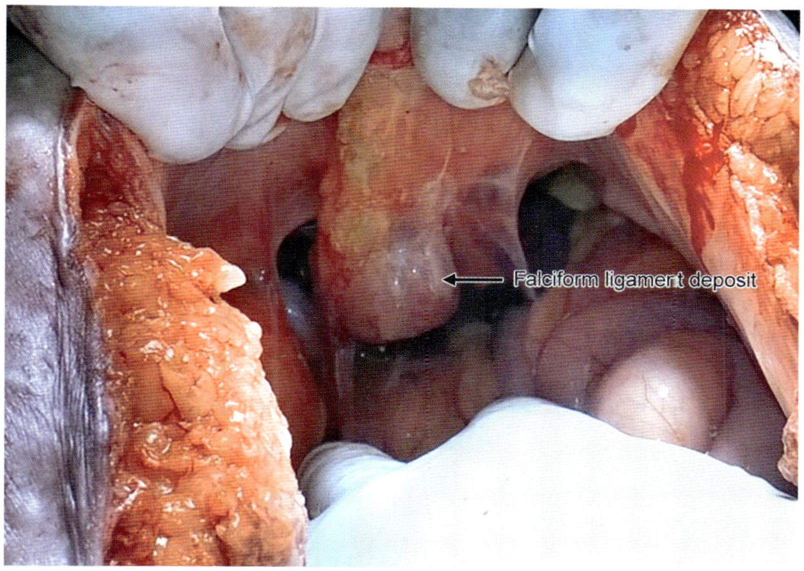

Fig. 79: Growing teratoma syndrome falciform ligament deposit.

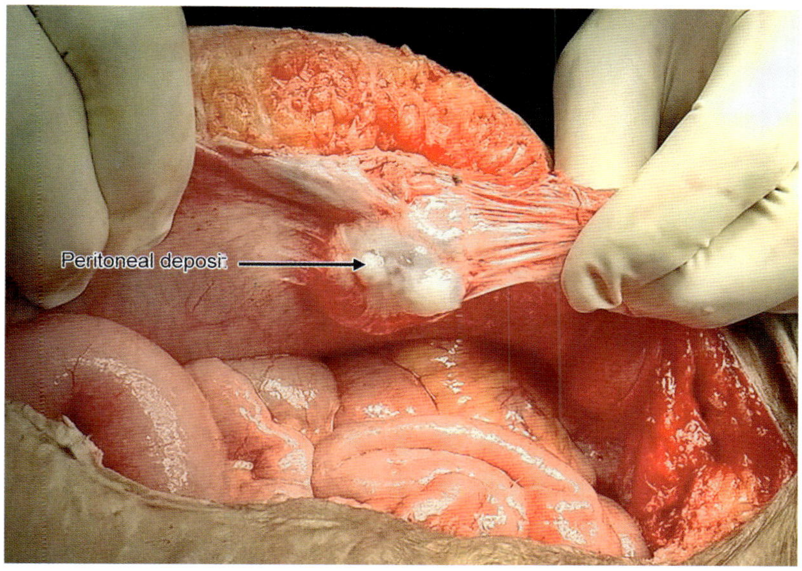

Fig. 82: Growing teratoma syndrome peritoneal deposit.

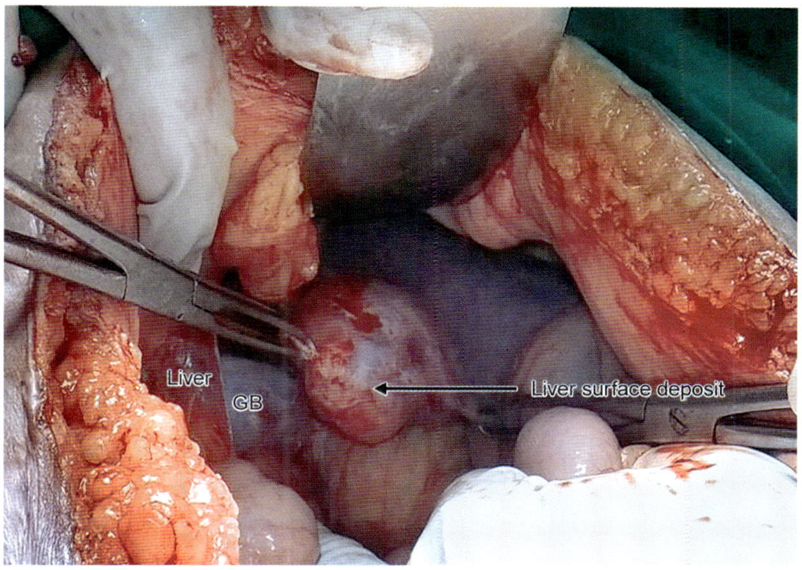

Fig. 80: Growing teratoma syndrome liver deposit.

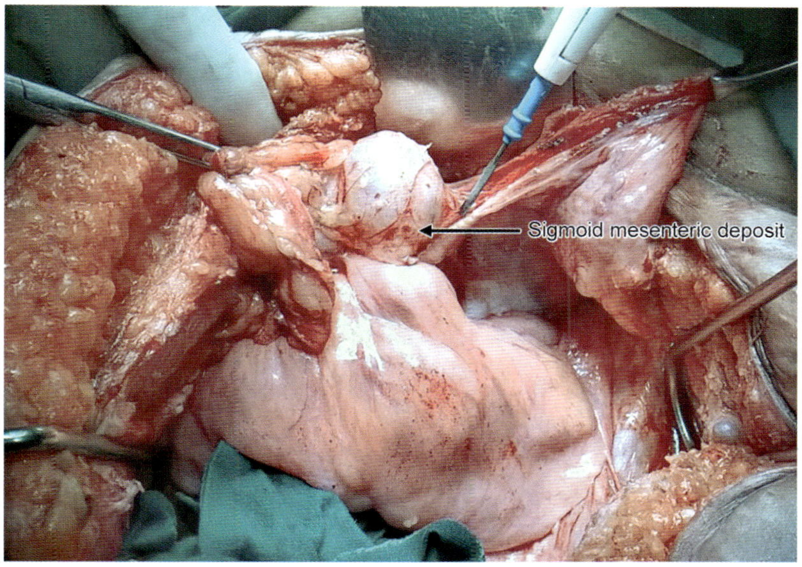

Fig. 83: Growing teratoma syndrome pelvic peritoneal deposit.

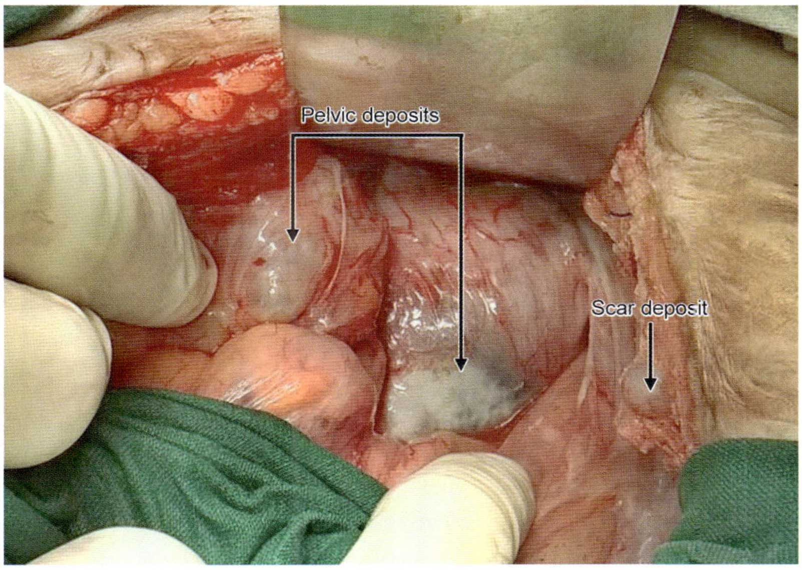

Fig. 81: Growing teratoma syndrome pelvic deposits.

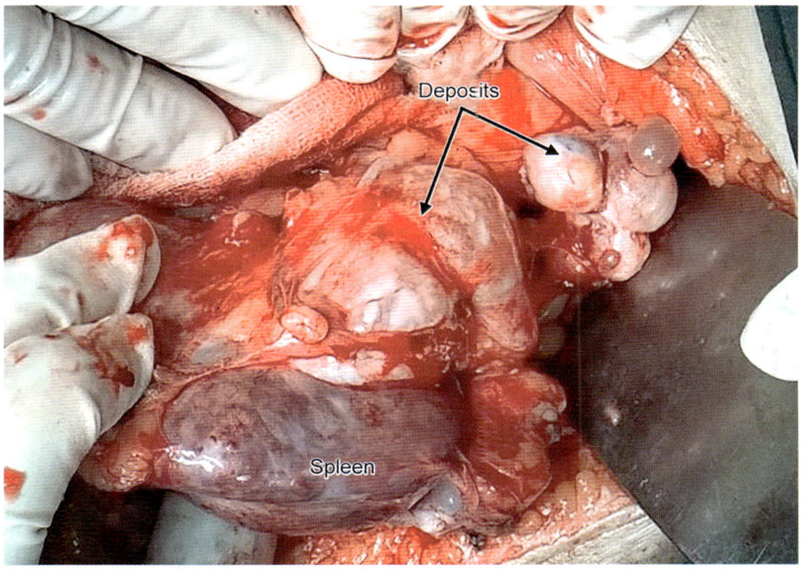

Fig. 84: Growing teratoma syndrome spleen deposit.

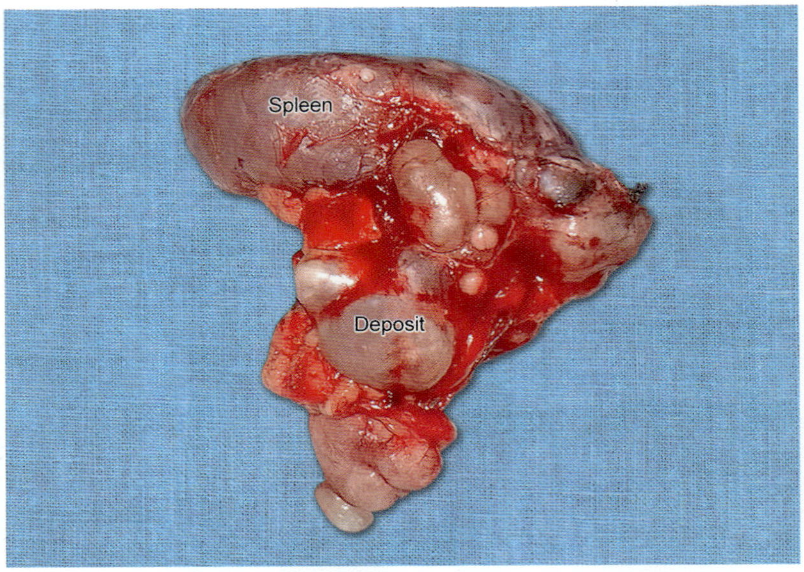

Fig. 85: Growing teratoma syndrome—spleen deposit specimen.

Recurrent Dysgerminoma (Figs. 86 to 88)

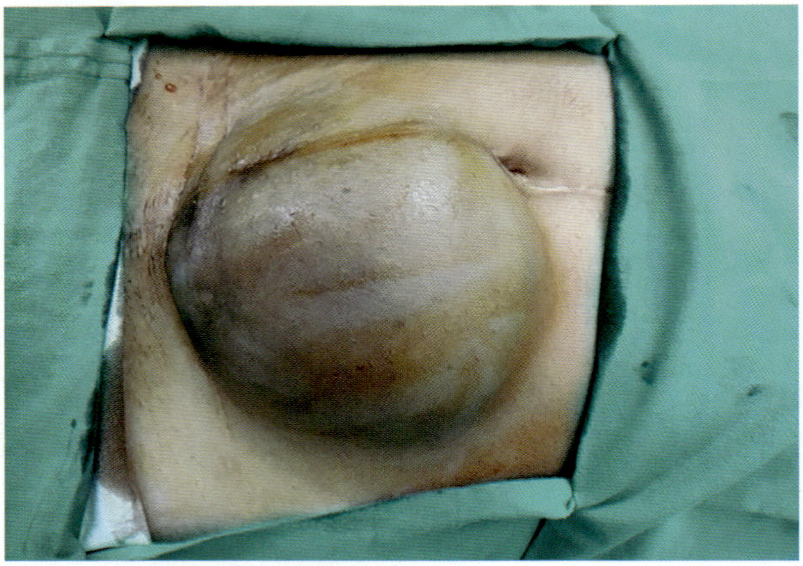

Fig. 86: Recurrent dysgerminoma in the abdominal wall.

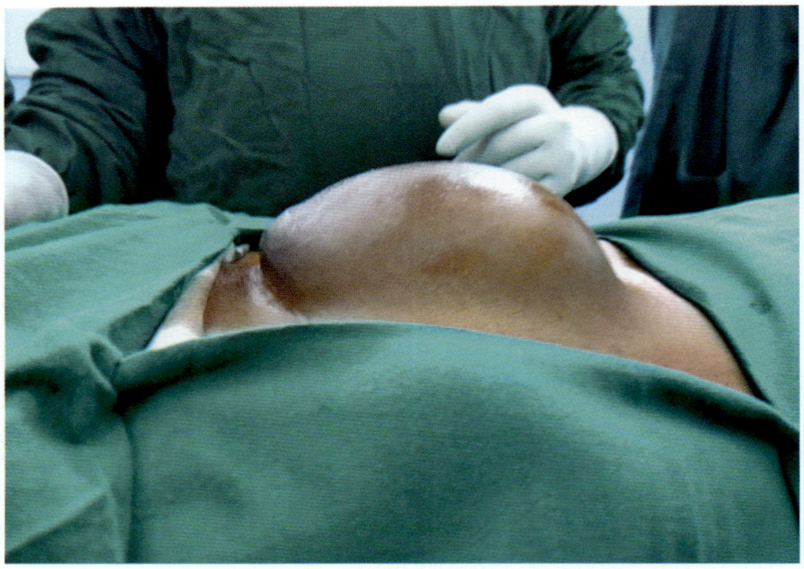

Fig. 87: Recurrent dysgerminoma in the abdominal wall for secondary cytoreduction.

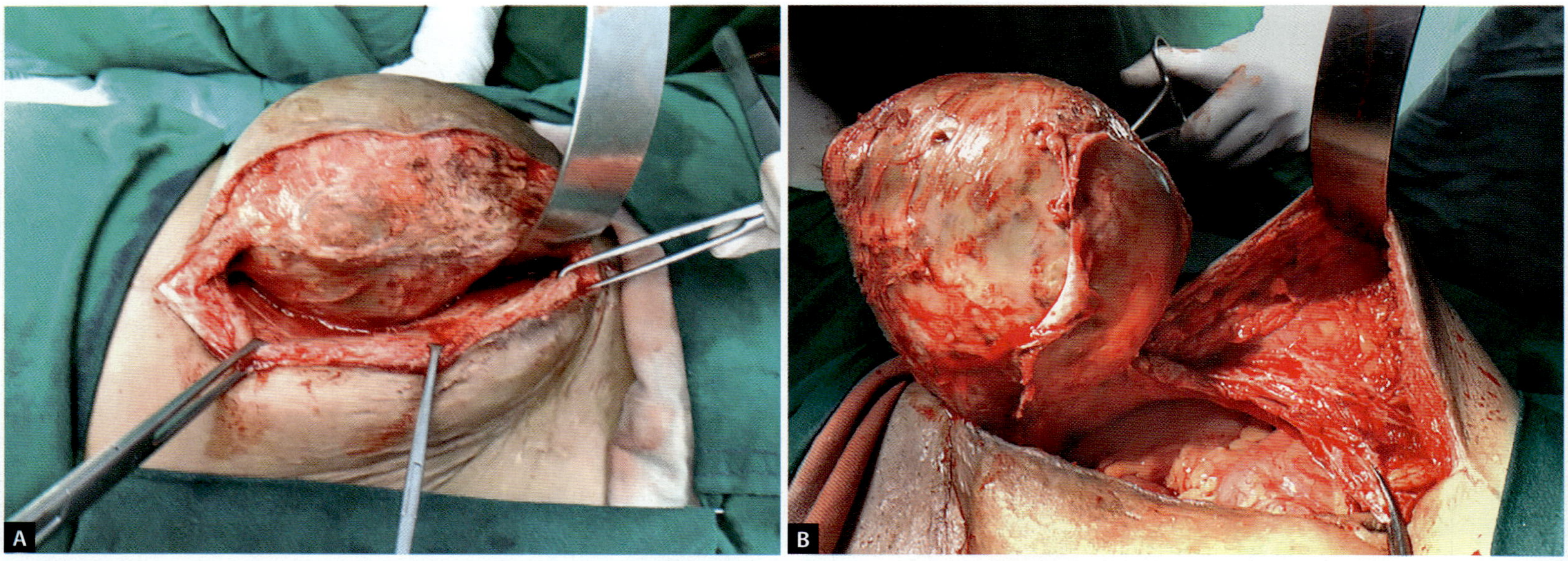

Figs. 88A and B: Resection of recurrent dysgerminoma in the abdominal wall.

Extragenital Sacrococcygeal Teratoma (Figs. 89 to 100)

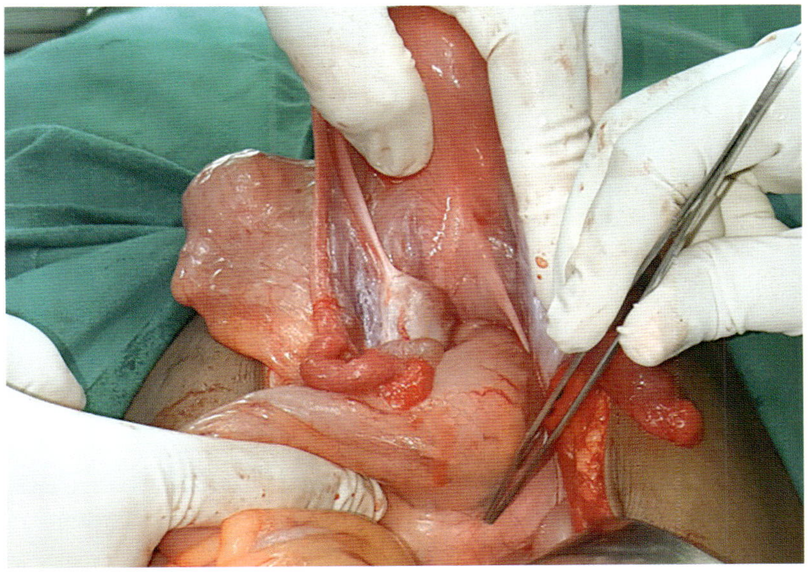

Fig. 89: Presacral teratoma.

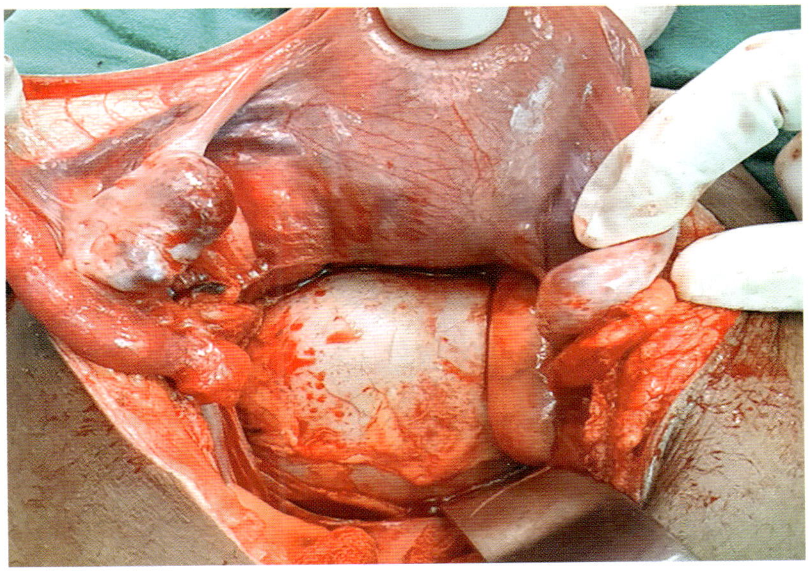

Fig. 90: Extragenital presacral teratoma.

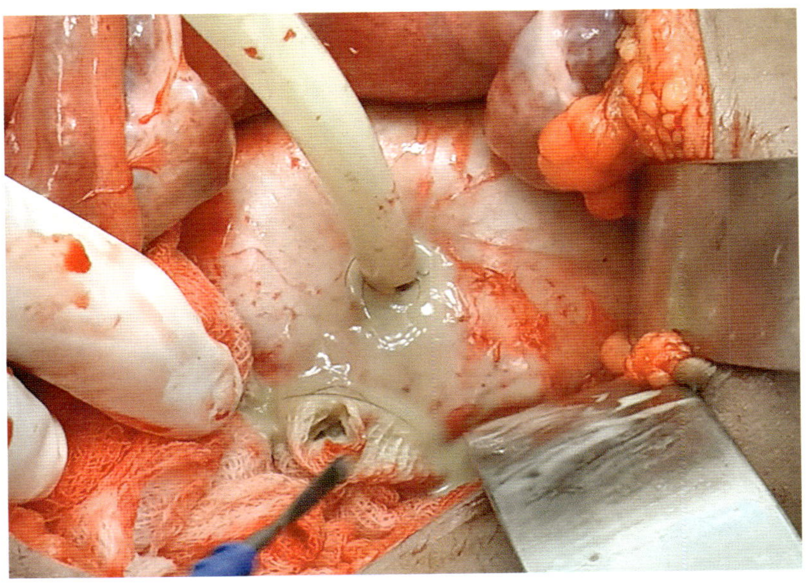

Fig. 91: Extragenital presacral teratoma decompression.

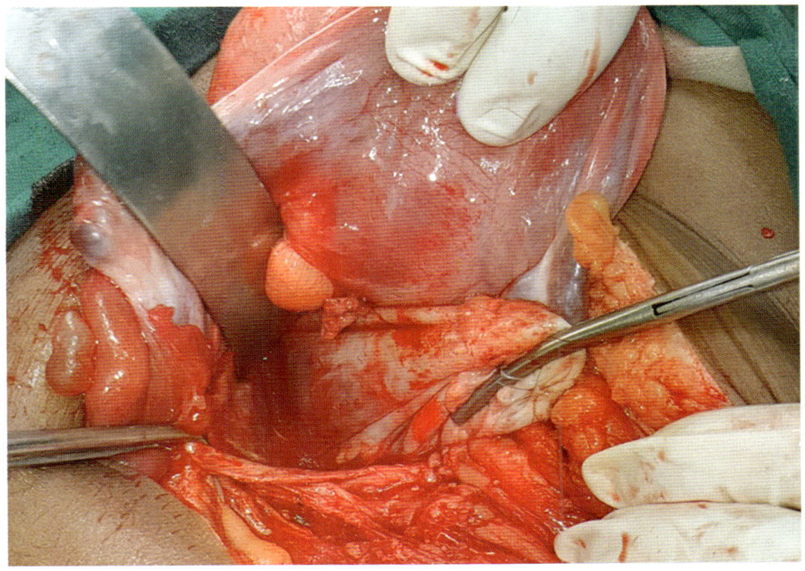

Fig. 92: Extragenital presacral teratoma excision after the decompression.

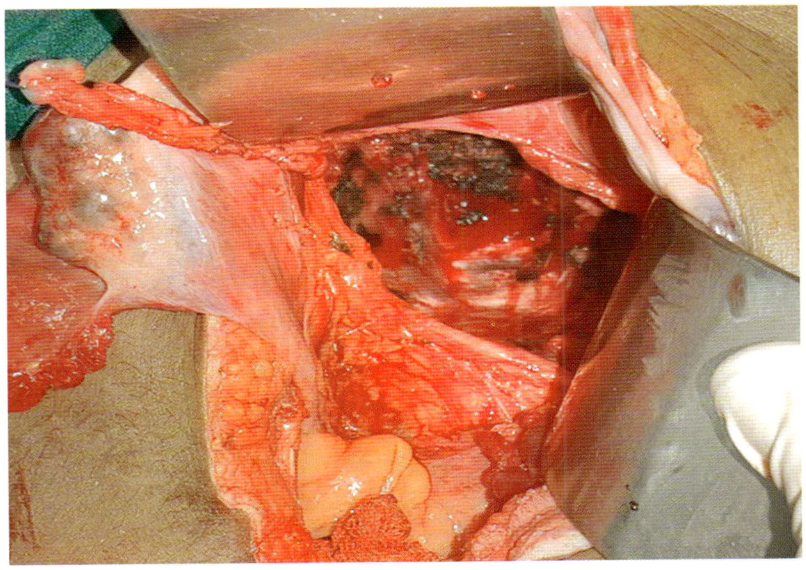

Fig. 93: Extragenital presacral teratoma excision and the remnant presacral dead space.

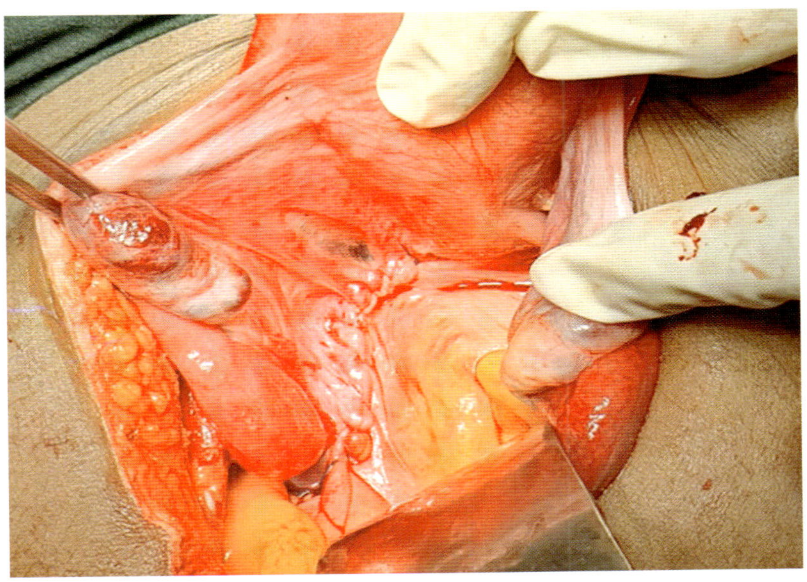

Fig. 94: Peritoneal closure after the excision of extragenital sacrococcygeal teratoma.

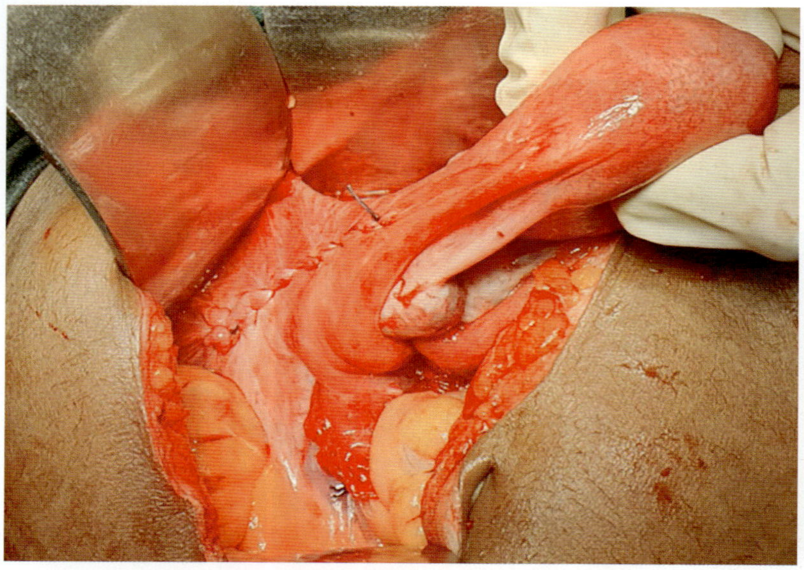

Fig. 95: Broad ligament peritoneal closure after the excision of extragenital sacrococcygeal teratoma.

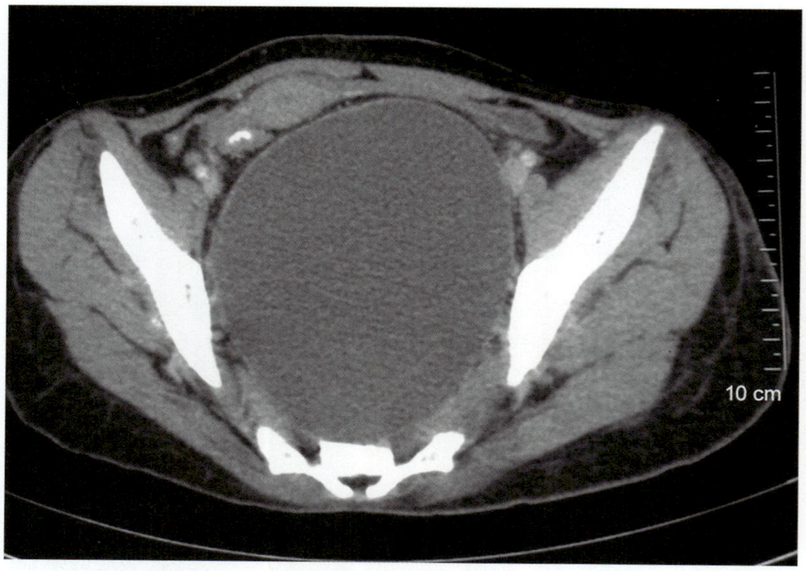

Fig. 96: Computed tomography scan showing presacral tumor.

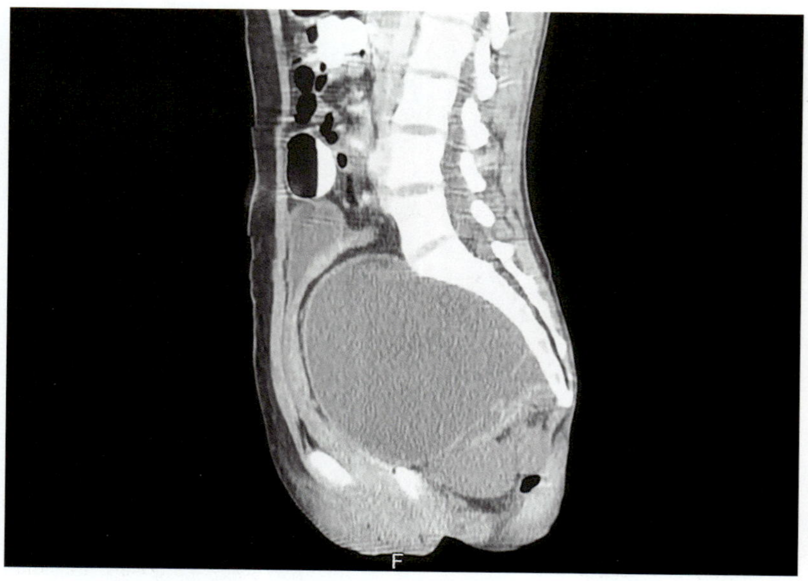

Fig. 97: Magnetic resonance imaging showing presacral tumor.

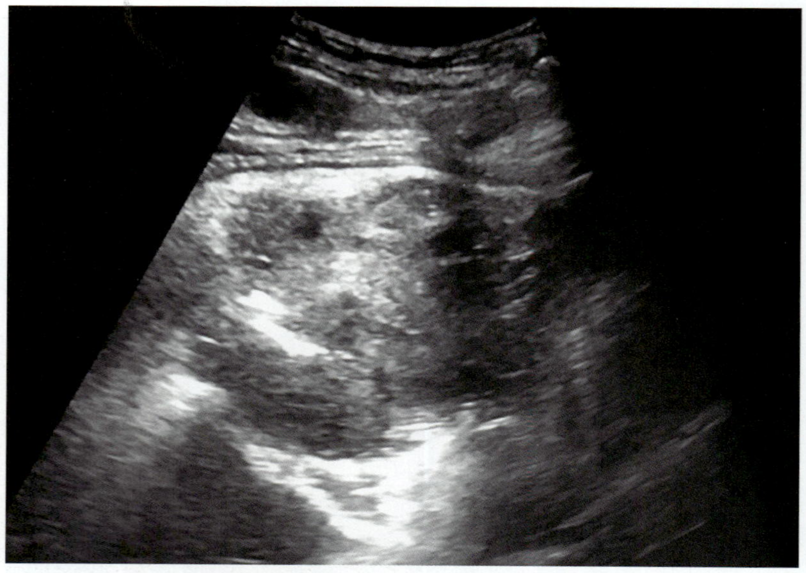

Fig. 98: Ultrasonography revealing a big hematoma in the presacral area on the postoperative site on 3rd postoperative day.

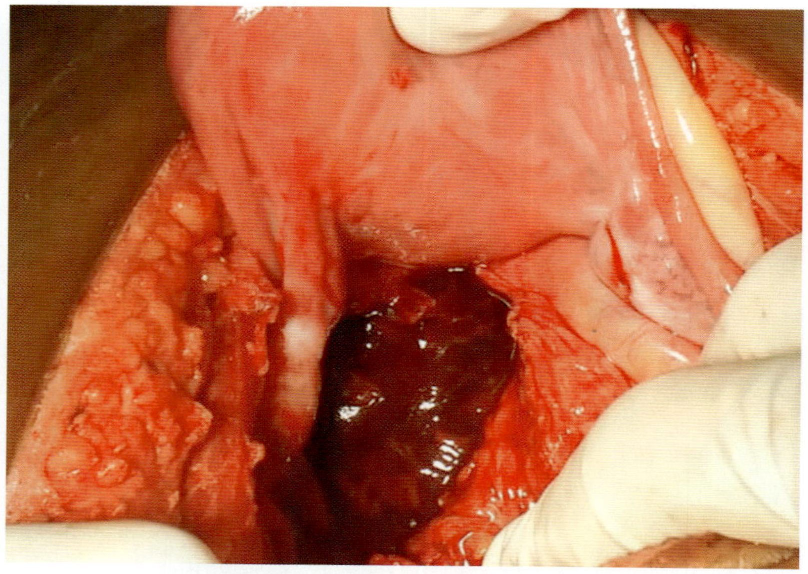

Fig. 99: Hematoma formation on 3rd postoperative day after excision of extragenital sacrococcygeal teratoma.

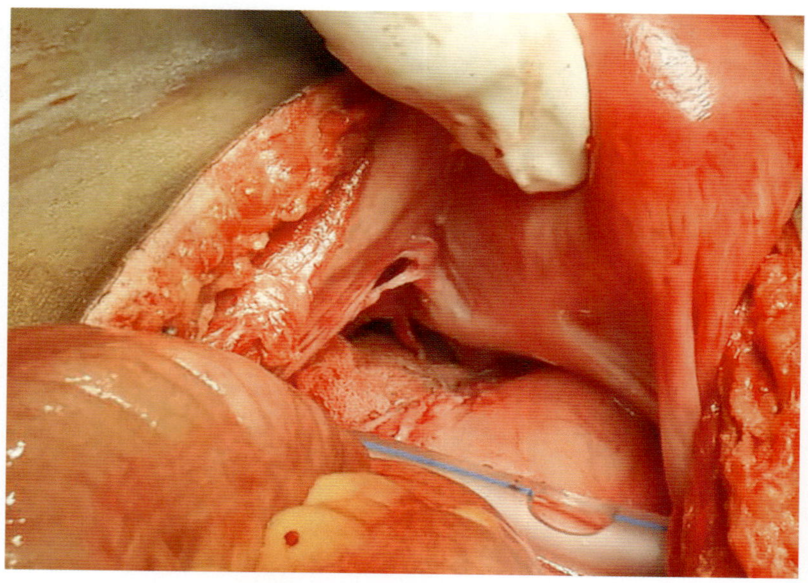

Fig. 100: The prophylactic packing the dead space after excision of sacrococcygeal hematoma and keeping the drain.

Mayer-Rokitansky-Küster-Hauser (MRKH) Syndrome with Ovarian Tumor (Figs. 101 and 102)

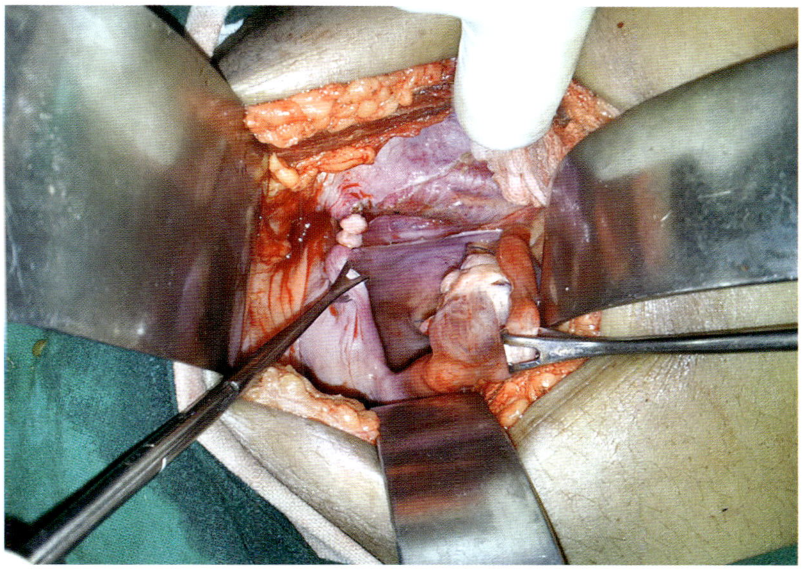

Fig. 101: Mayer-Rokitansky-Küster-Hauser syndrome with ovarian tumor and absent uterus.

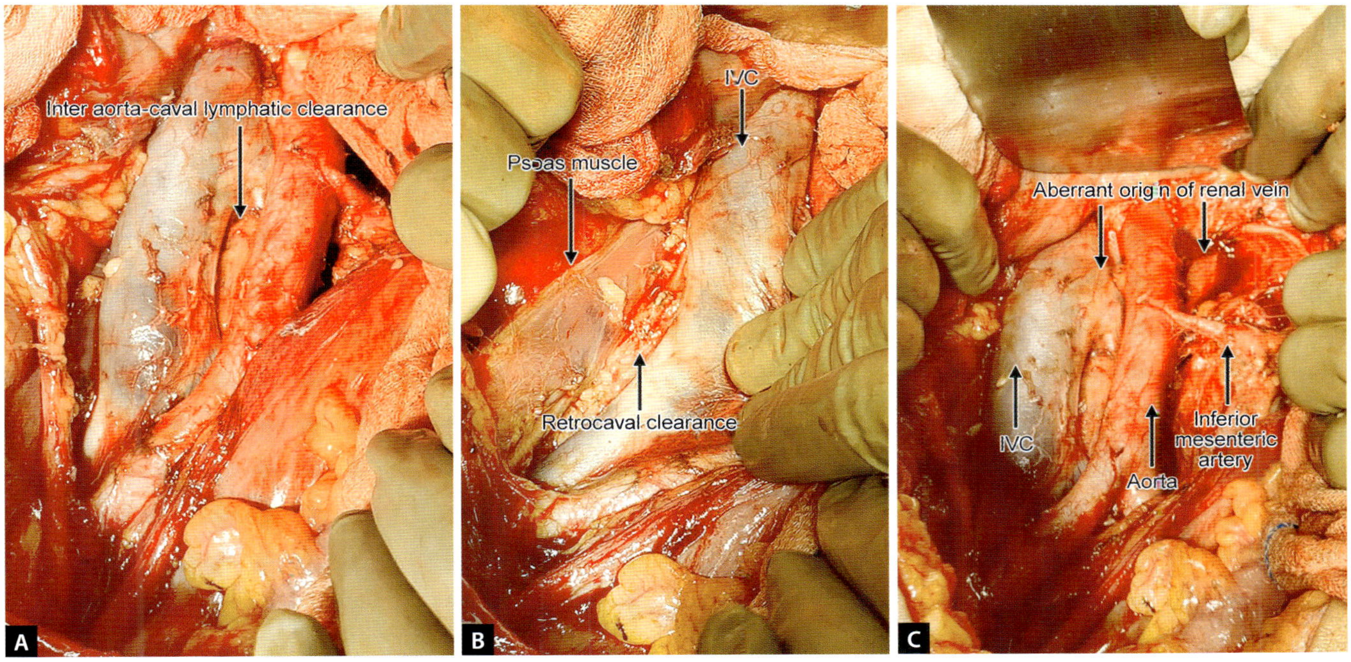

Figs. 102A to C: Para-aortic lymphadenectomy.
(IVC: inferior vena cava)

REFERENCE

1. Hoffman BL, Schorge JO, Schaffer JI, Halvorson LM, Bradshaw KD, Cunningham FG, Calver LE (Eds). Williams Gynecology, 2nd edition. Epithelial Ovarian Cancer (Chapter 35). New York, NY: McGraw-Hill Education; 2012. pp. 863, 869.

CHAPTER

46

Fibroadenoma of Breast

Tanvi Desai, Aditi Rai, B Ramesh

WHAT IS FIBROADENOMA?

Fibroadenomas are benign tumors of the breast. Fibroadenomas are usually seen fully developed breasts between the age group of 15–25 years.[1] They arise from hyperplasia of single lobule of breast and are 2–3 cm in size. Occasionally they may be larger in size. They are well demarcated and surrounded by a capsule. Hence, they can be easily enucleated.

Fibroadenomas require excision only when there is any suspicious pathology, size is rapidly growing, or patients have any symptoms and requests for excision.

SYMPTOMS

Usually fibroadenomas do not cause any symptoms. They may be incidentally detected as a lump in the breast while having bath. Sometimes they may be detected on routine mammogram or ultrasound. Occasionally they may cause some mild pain.

ETIOLOGY

Development of fibroadenomas may be related to hormonal changes occurring during puberty or pregnancy.

DIAGNOSIS

- *Clinical examination:* Palpation of both breasts needs to be done to look for lumps/masses. Fibroadenomas are usually firm to palpate, well-demarcated, and freely mobile.[2]
- Mammography or sonomammography may be done to evaluate the breast lump.
- Fine needle aspiration biopsy or core needle biopsy may be done and tissue from the lump may be sent for histopathological examination in order to confirm the diagnosis.

TREATMENT

In small asymptomatic fibroadenomas, no treatment will be required. However if fibroadenoma is big in size or for cosmetic reasons, woman might want removal of fibroadenoma:

- *Nonsurgical management:* If fibroadenoma is left alone, without doing anything, patient will require periodic evaluation/mammogram to rule out any increase in size or changes in nature of the breast lump.
- *Cryoablation:* A thin needle like probe is inserted through the skin to the fibroadenoma under ultrasound guidance and gas is used to freeze the tissue and destroy the fibroadenoma. But prerequisites for this procedure are that diagnosis of fibroadenoma should be confirmed, no malignant component should be there, it should not be more than 4 cm in size and not more than 3 in number, patient should not have any local skin infections or bleeding disorders.[3]
- *Excision of fibroadenoma:* The fibroadenoma can be excised through a cosmetic incision under general anesthesia and sent for histopathological examination **(Figs. 1 to 8)**.

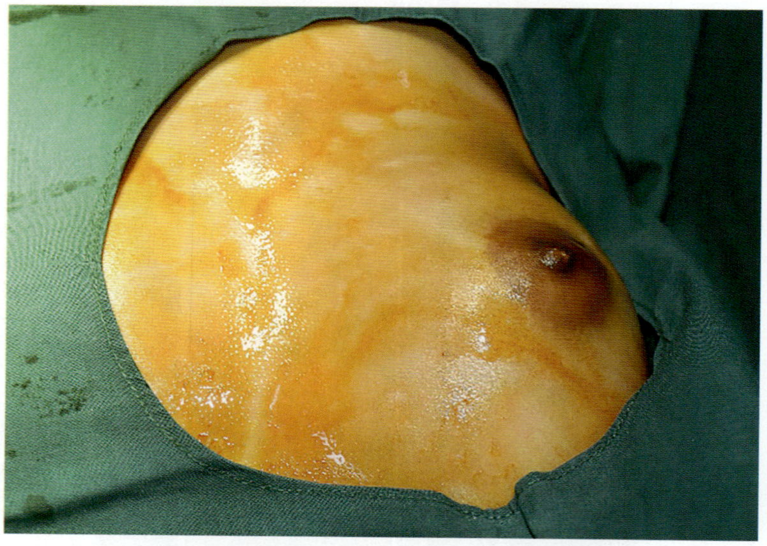

Fig. 1: Painting and draping for excision of fibroadenoma of breast.

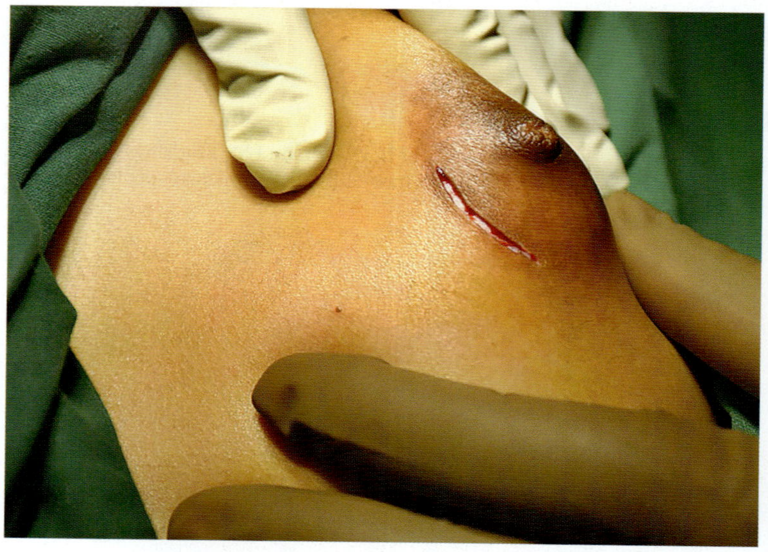

Fig. 2: Curvilinear incision taken above the areola, over the site of fibroadenoma.

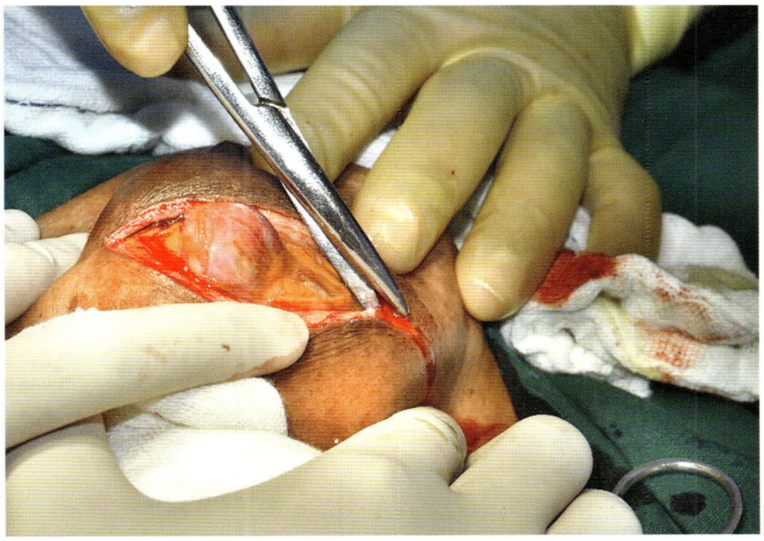

Fig. 3: Layers over the fibroadenoma dissected away.

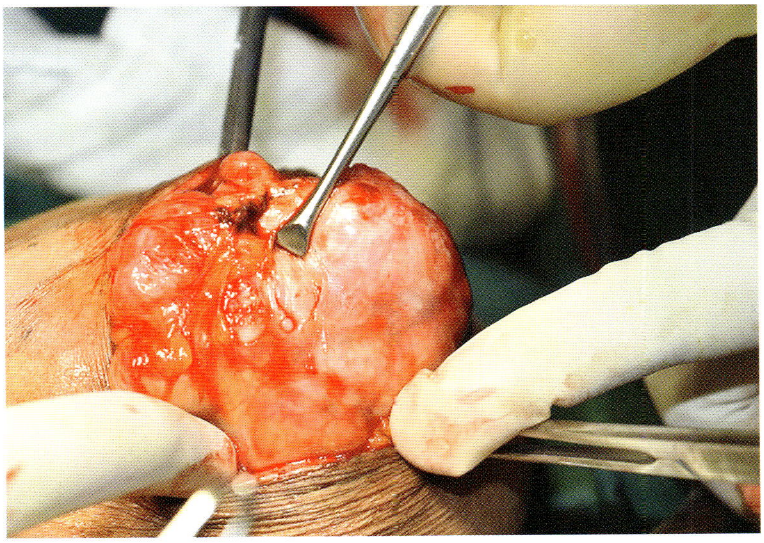

Fig. 4: Fibroadenoma enucleated using Allis' forceps and scissors.

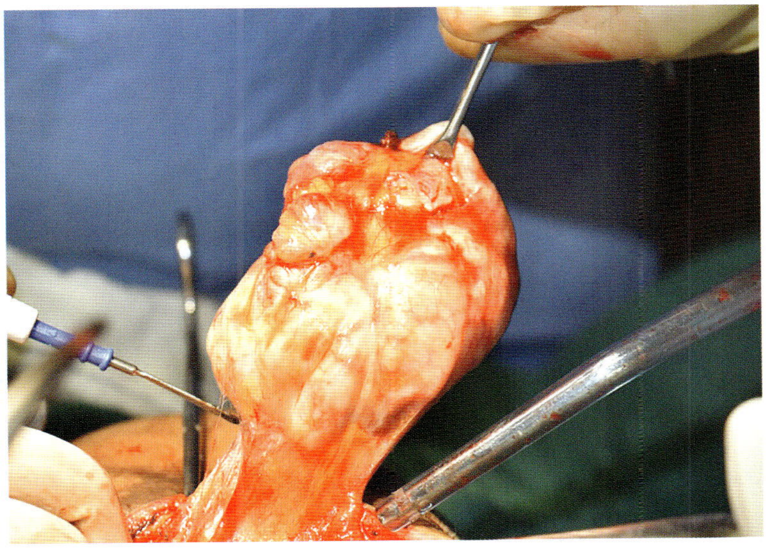

Fig. 5: Fibroadenoma being released from it base using hand cautery.

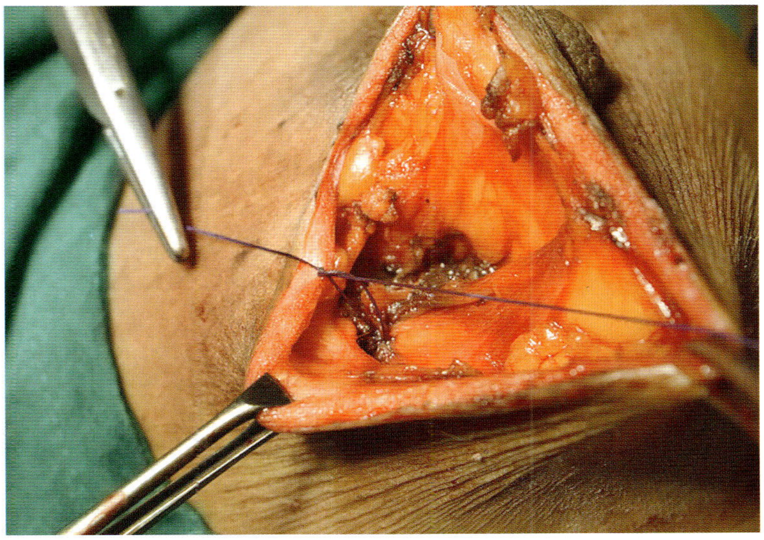

Fig. 6: Fibroadenoma bed obliterated using 2-0 Vicryl.

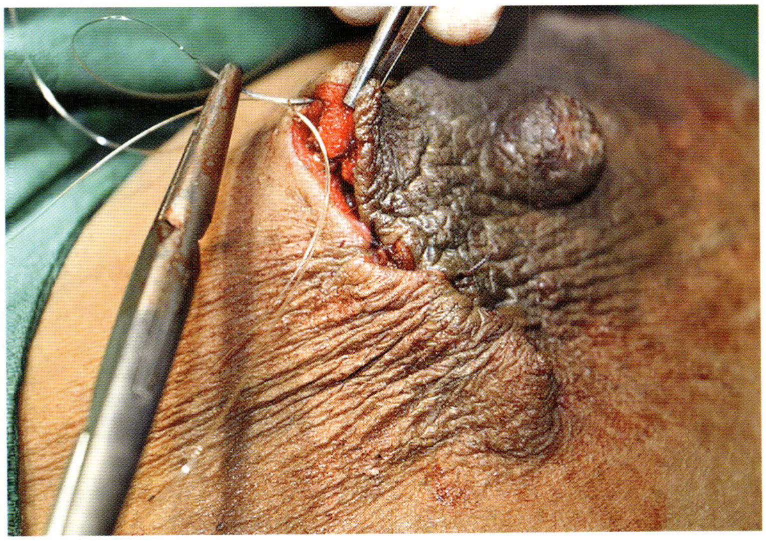

Fig. 7: Skin incision being closed with subcuticular sutures using 3-0 Monocrly.

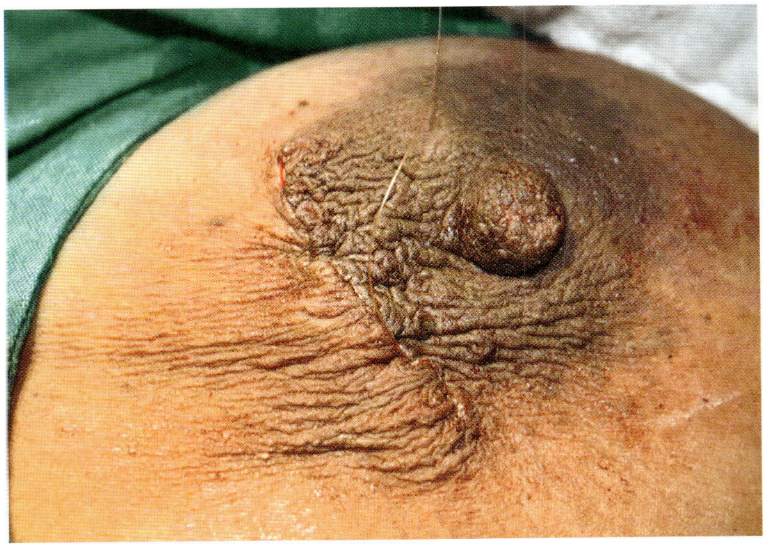

Fig. 8: Appearance at the end of skin closure.

REFERENCES

1. Williams N, O'Connell PR, McCaskie A (Eds). Bailey and Love, Short Practice of Surgery, Diseases of Breast, 27th edition. New York: CRC Press; 2018.
2. Mayoclinic. (2018). Fibroadenoma. [online] Available from: https://www.mayoclinic.org/diseases-conditions/fibroadenoma/diagnosis-treatment/drc-20352756 [Last accessed January, 2020].
3. Niu L, Wu B, Xu K. Cryosurgery for breast fibroadenomas. Gland Surg. 2012;1:128-31.

CHAPTER

47

Laparoscopic Radical Hysterectomy

Deepak Limbachiya, R Niranjana Radhakrishnan, G Hemasree, B Ramesh

INTRODUCTION (FIG. 1)

A laparoscope is introduced via supraumbilical port with intra-abdominal pressure of 18 mm Hg after creating pneumoperitoneum with carbon dioxide (CO_2). The accessory ports three 5 mm trocars are introduced in the abdomen under direct visualization medial to iliac crest in the suprapubic area. After deep Trendelenburg position, bowels are cleared away from the pelvis.

UTERINE FIXATION (FIGS. 2A AND B)

Myoma screw is placed through 5 mm port and the uterus is fixed. It is not placed deep into endometrium placed till the myometrium.

BILATERAL ADNEXAL DISSECTION

After visualizing the whole abdomen and pelvis, if any adhesions present are released. Adnexa is excised with bipolars and harmonic for clear vision.

Figures 3A to H show that proximal tube, round ligament, and utero-ovarian ligament of the right side are coagulated and cut.

The proximal tube, round ligament, and utero-ovarian ligament of the left side are coagulated and cut **(Figs. 4A to D)**.

DEVELOPMENT OF RECTOVAGINAL SPACE

U-shaped incision is made in the posterior wall, i.e posteromedial aspect to infundibulopelvic ligament (IPL) on the right side and incision continued up to pouch of Douglas (POD), same incision is done on the left side and U shape is created.

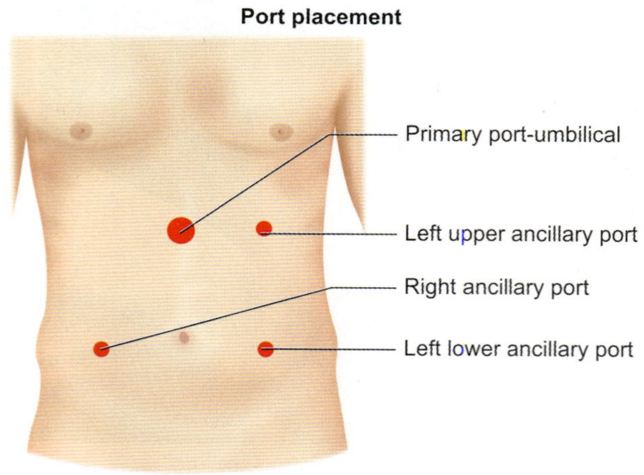

Fig. 1: Port placement.

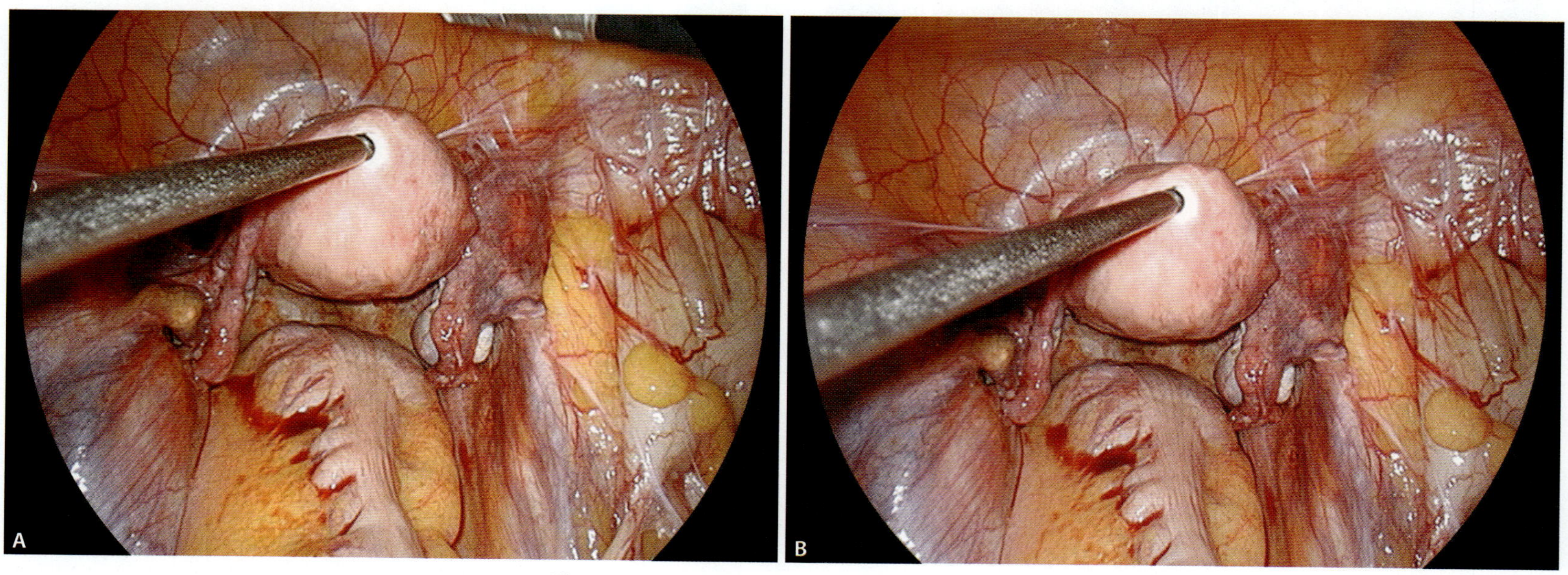

Figs. 2A and B: Uterine fixation with myoma screw.

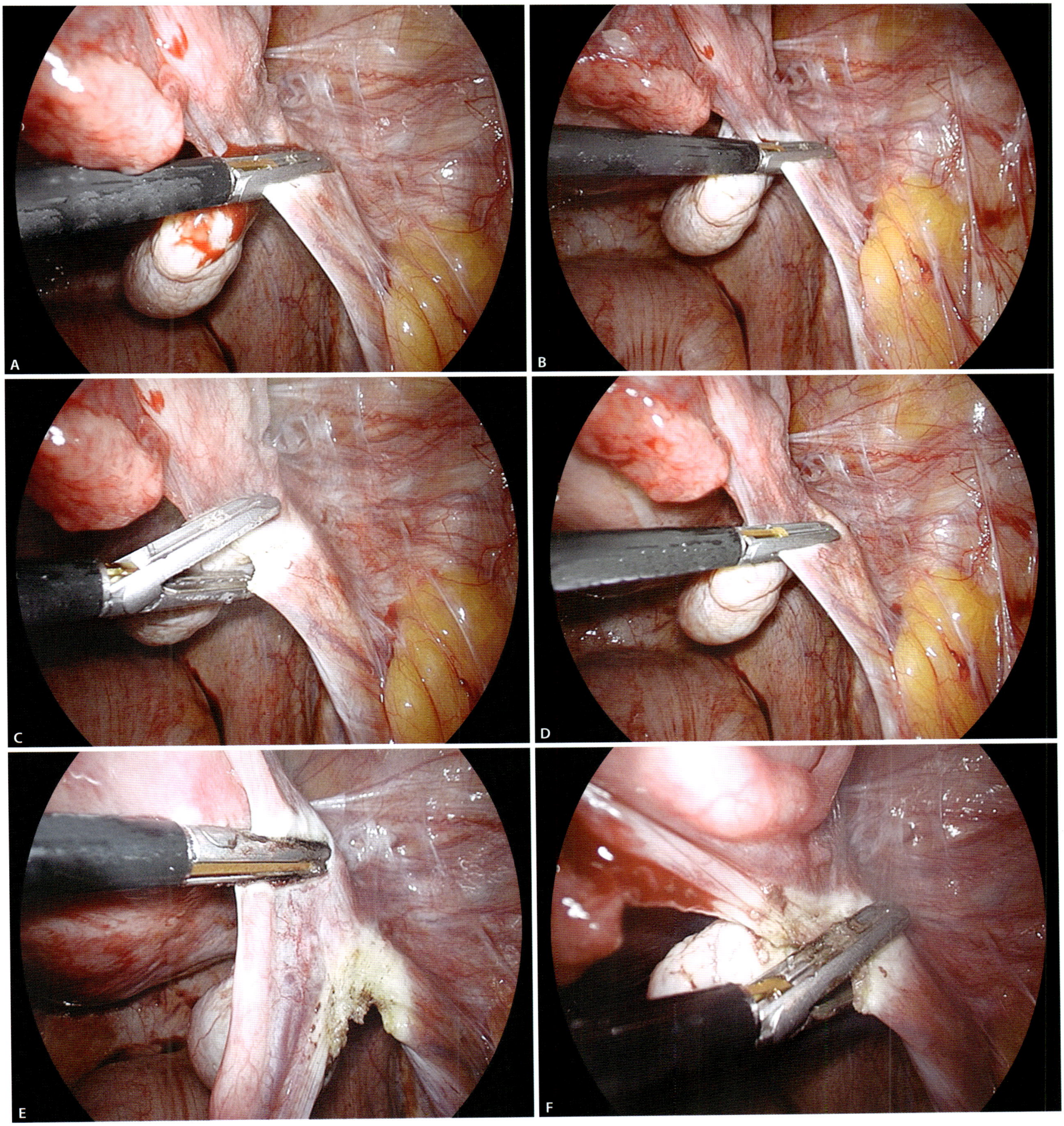

Figs. 3A to F

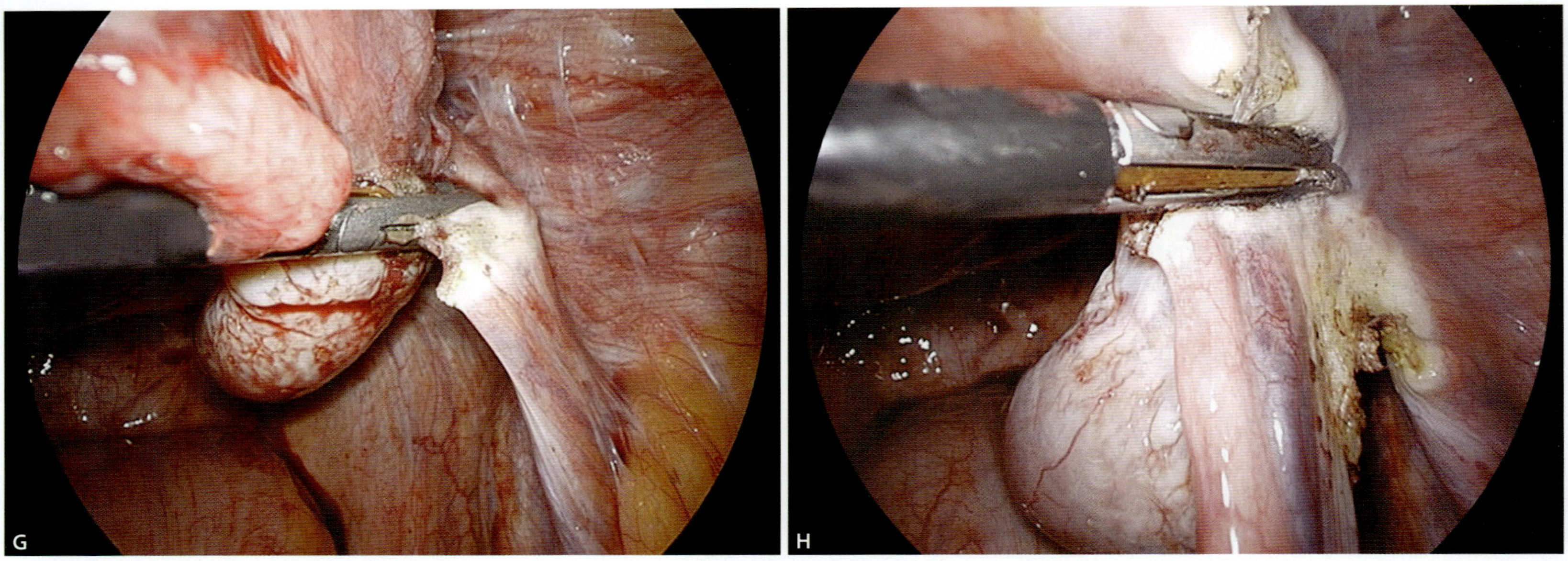

Figs. 3G and H

Figs. 3A to H: Proximal tube, round ligament, and utero-ovarian ligament of the right side are coagulated and cut.

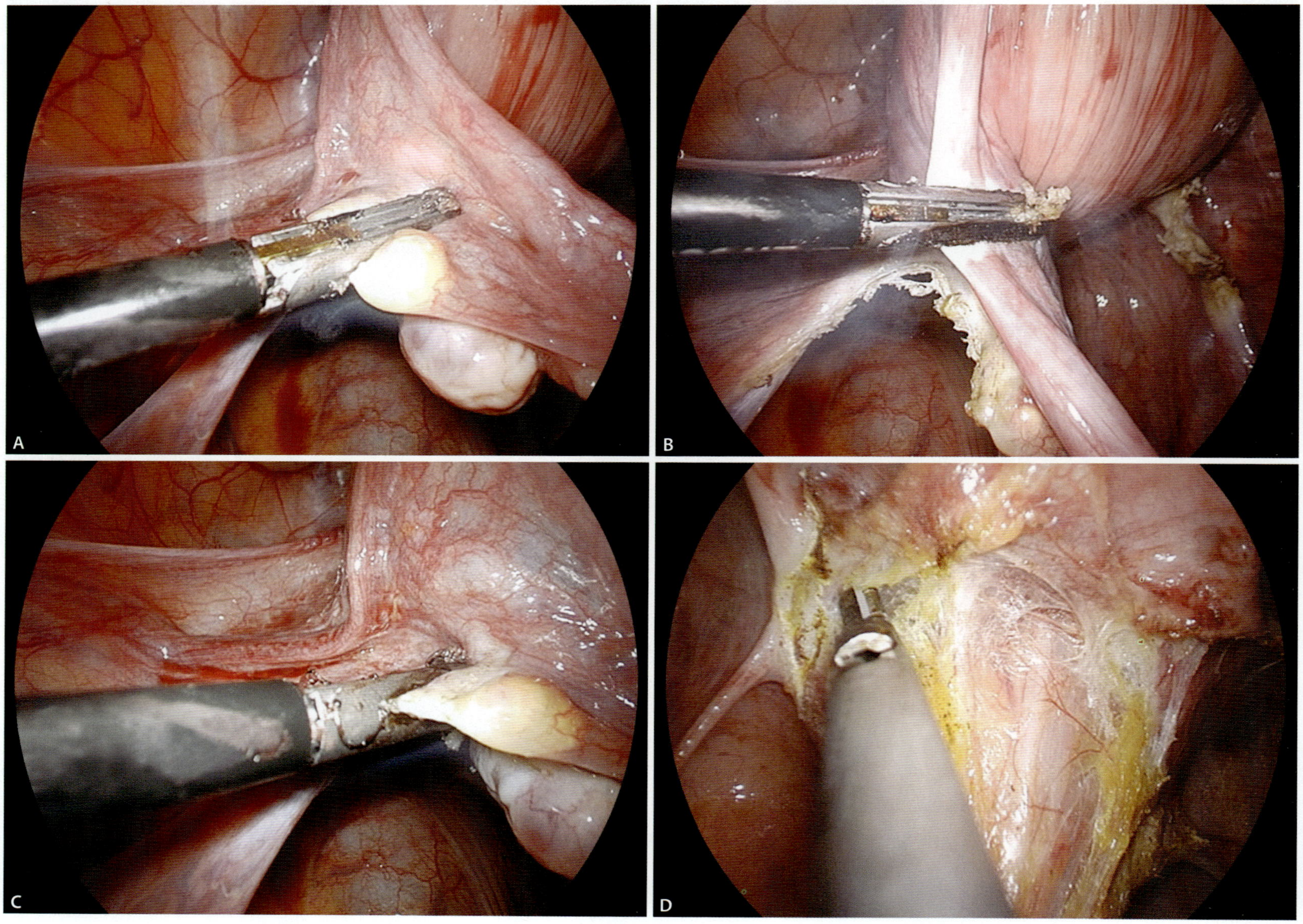

Figs. 4A to D: Proximal tube, round ligament, and utero-ovarian ligament of the left side are coagulated and cut.

Figures 5A to F show incision in the posteromedial aspect of IPL ligament in the right side and dissection is continued.

The dissection is continued in the left side and U shape is created in the posterior aspect and rectovaginal space is entered **(Figs. 6A to E)**.

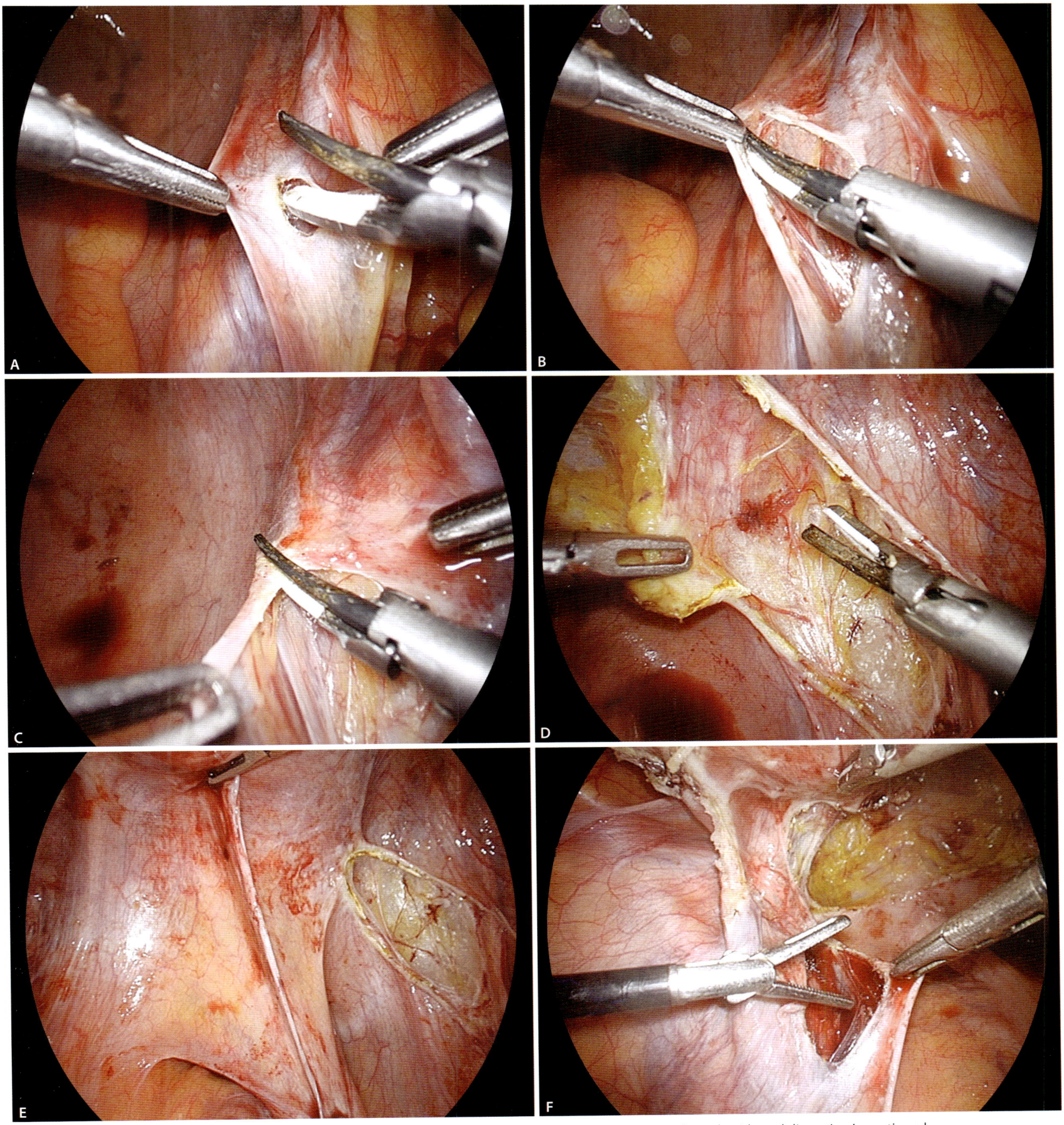

Figs. 5A to F: Incision in the posteromedial aspect of infundibulopelvic ligament (IPL) in the right side and dissection is continued.

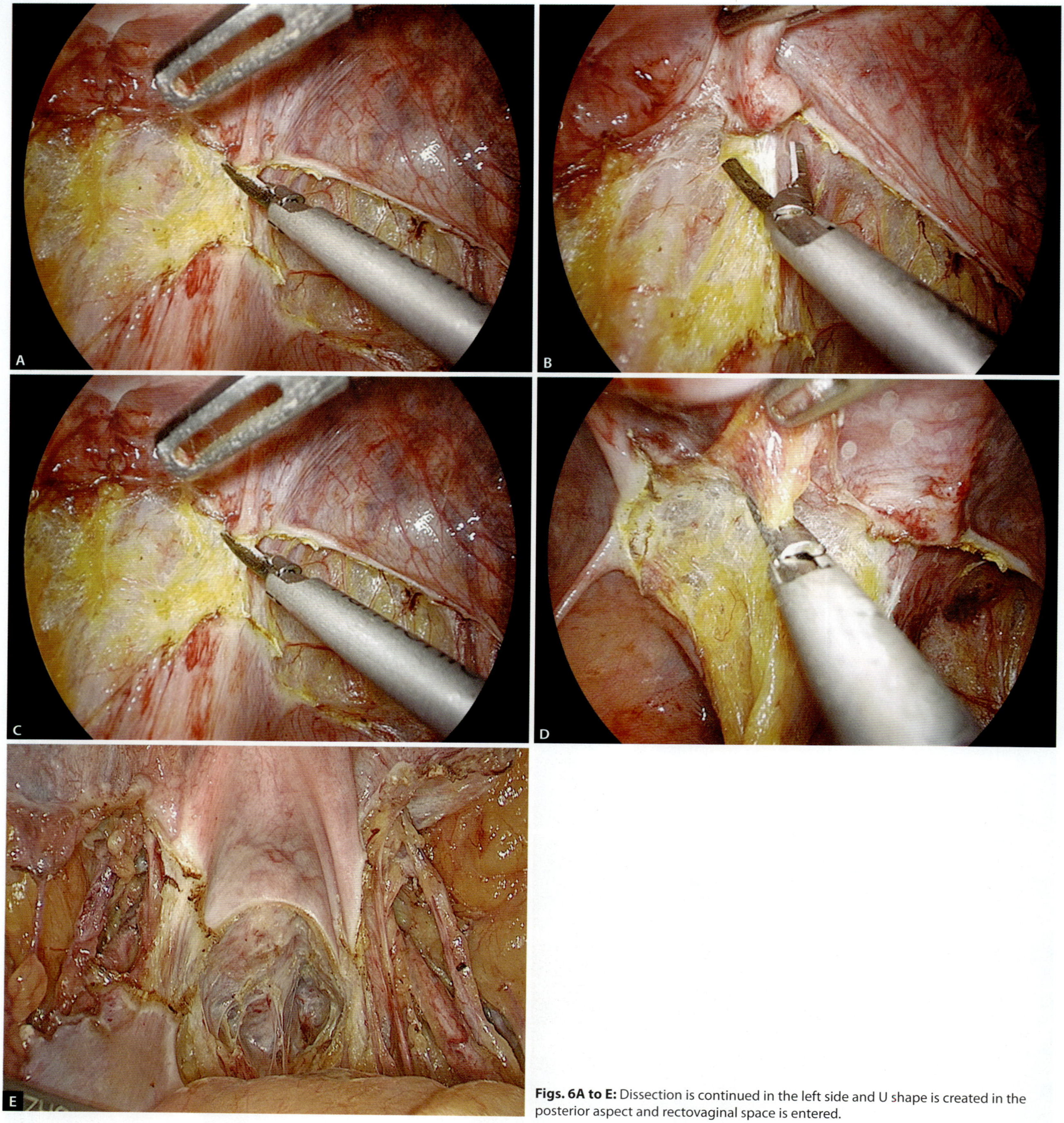

Figs. 6A to E: Dissection is continued in the left side and U shape is created in the posterior aspect and rectovaginal space is entered.

DISSECTION AND IDENTIFICATION OF URETER (FIGS. 7 AND 8)

Ureter is identified as it crosses the iliac vessels at the pelvic brim and ureter is dissected laterally with harmonic.

Pararectal space is dissected and entered with harmonic where the uterine vessels crossing pararectal space from lateral to medial. These vessels are skeletonized and cauterized and cut at the origin. Dissection is continued in pararectal space fossa till levator ani is reached. Inferior hypogastric plexus is identified and lateralized. Uterosacral ligament is transected 2.5 cm away from insertion.

The space between ureter and uterosacral ligament is called Okabayashi space **(Fig. 9)**.

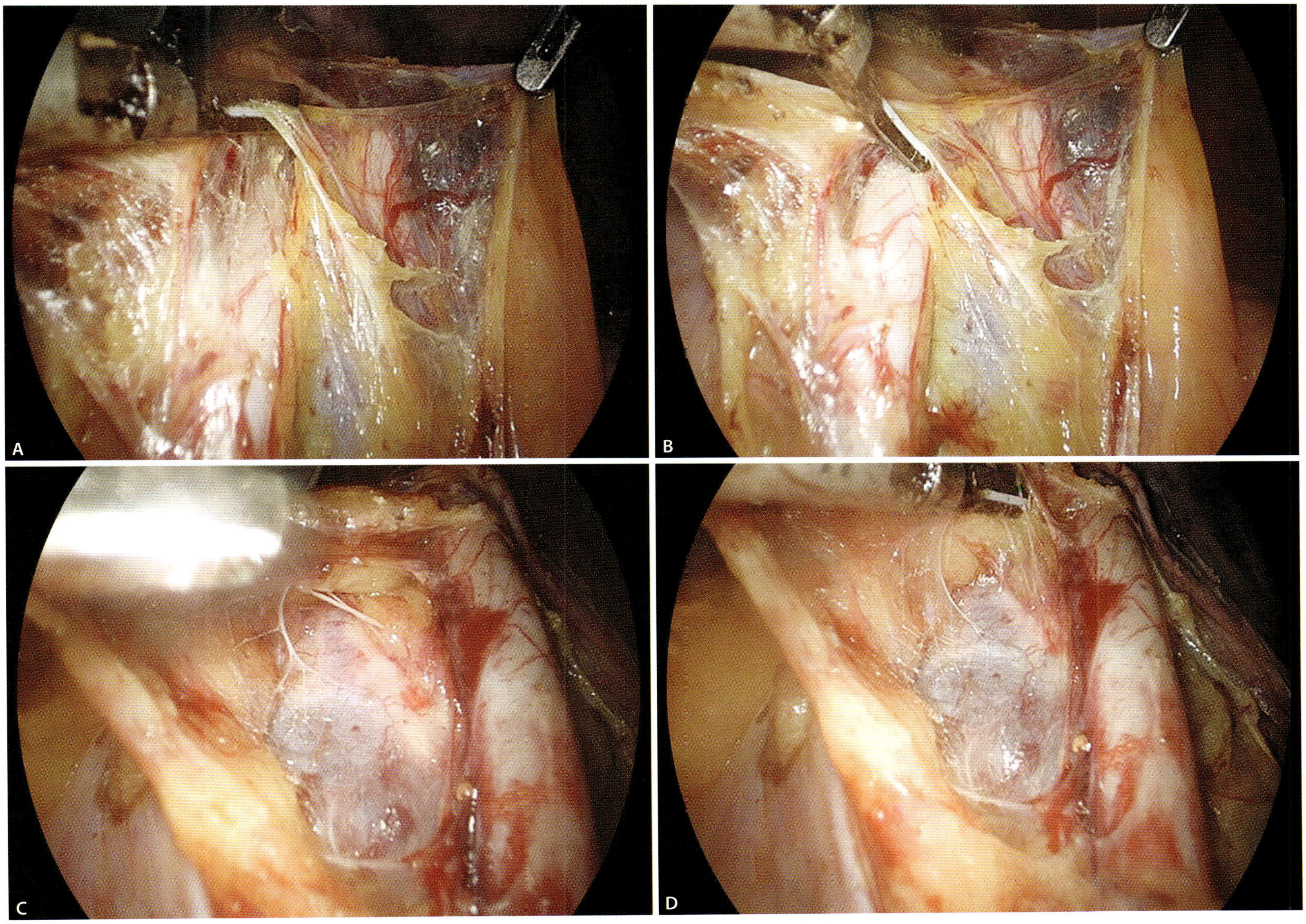

Figs. 7A to D: Identification and lateral dissection of right ureter.

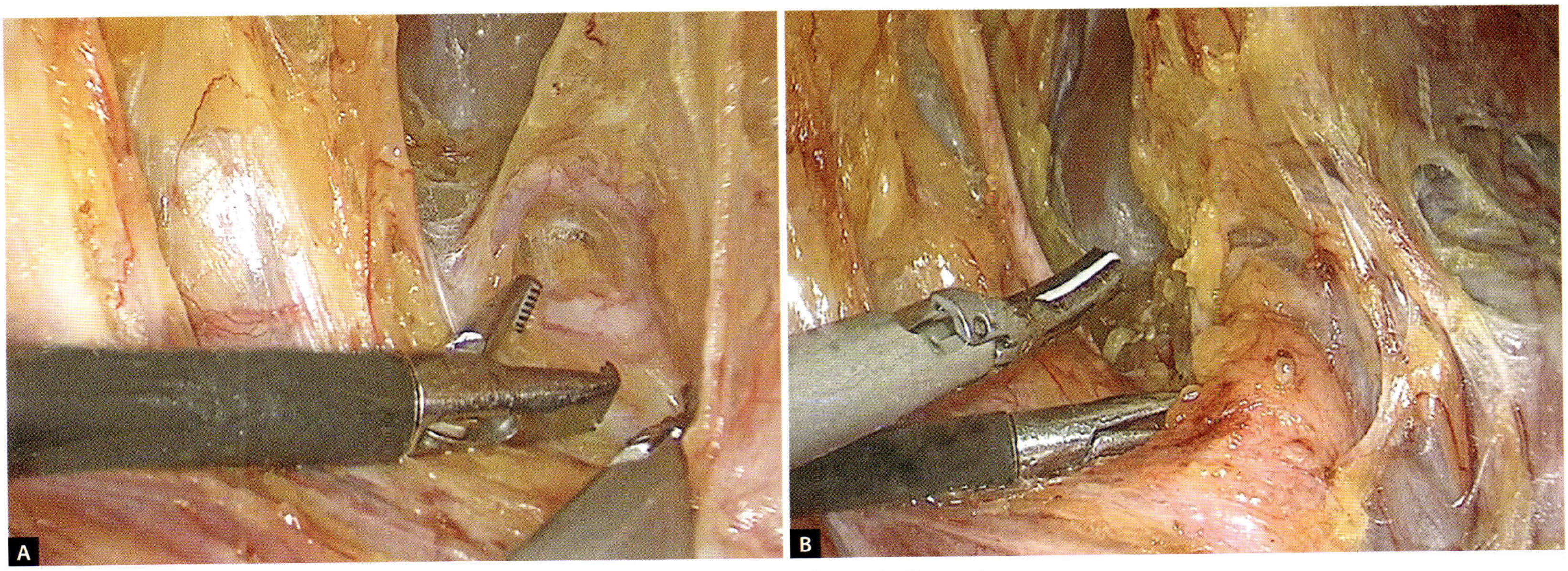

Figs. 8A and B: Pararectal space is dissected.

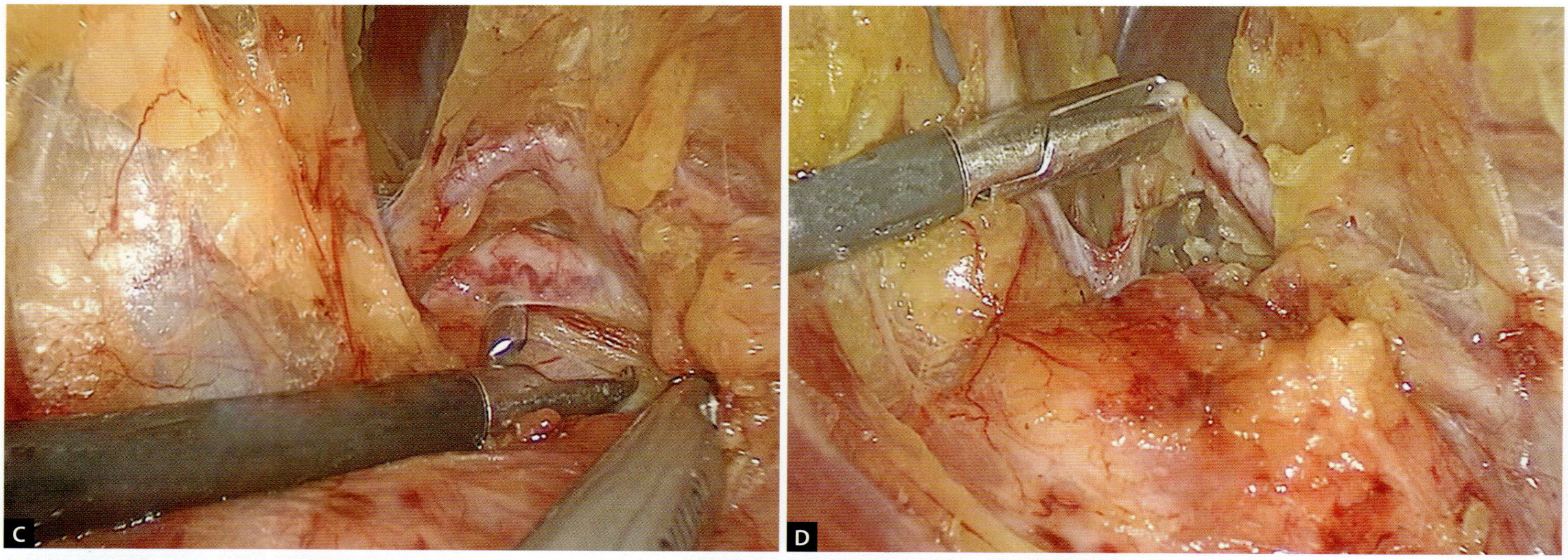

Figs. 8C and D: These vessels are skeletonized and cauterized and cut.

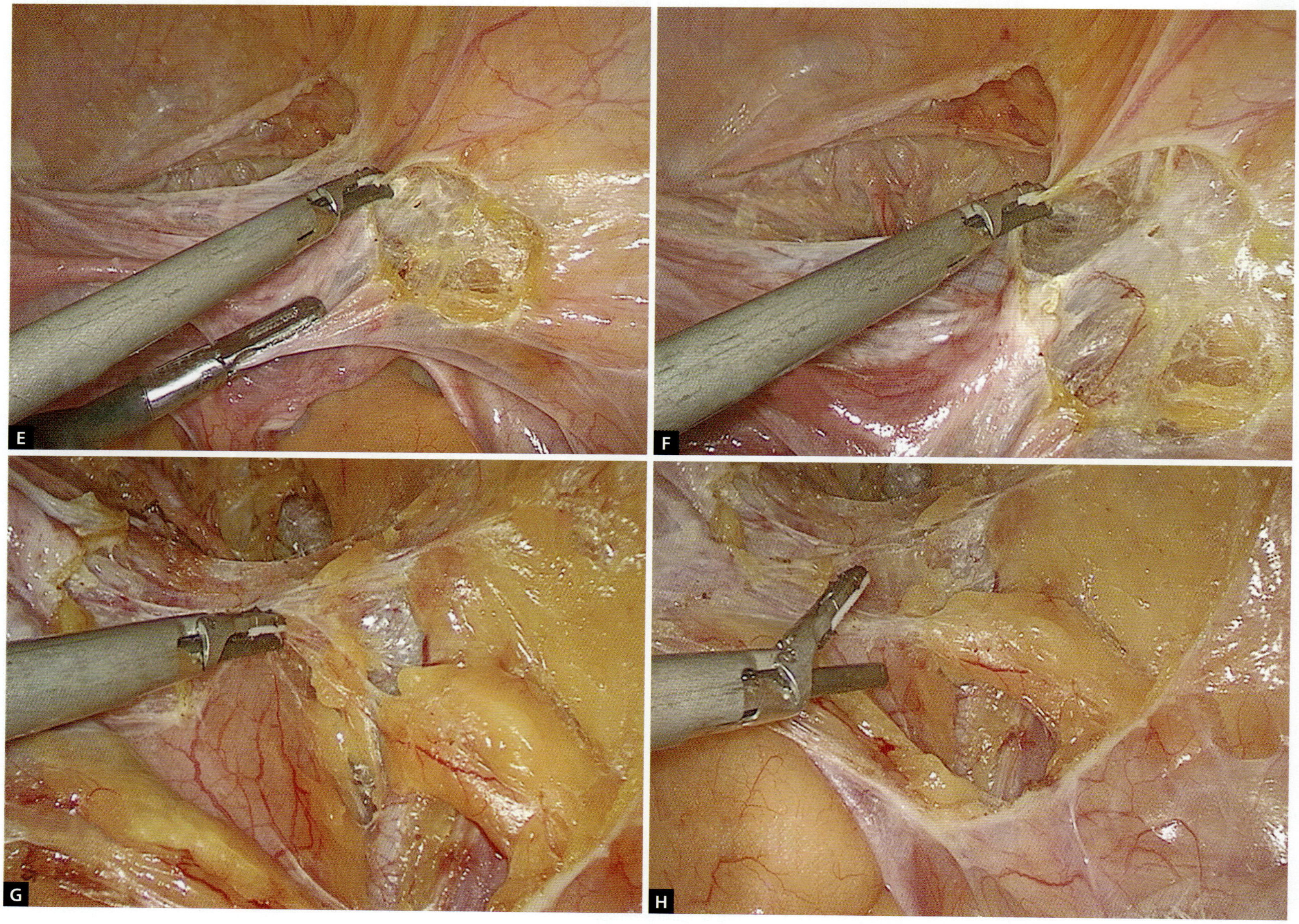

Figs. 8E to H

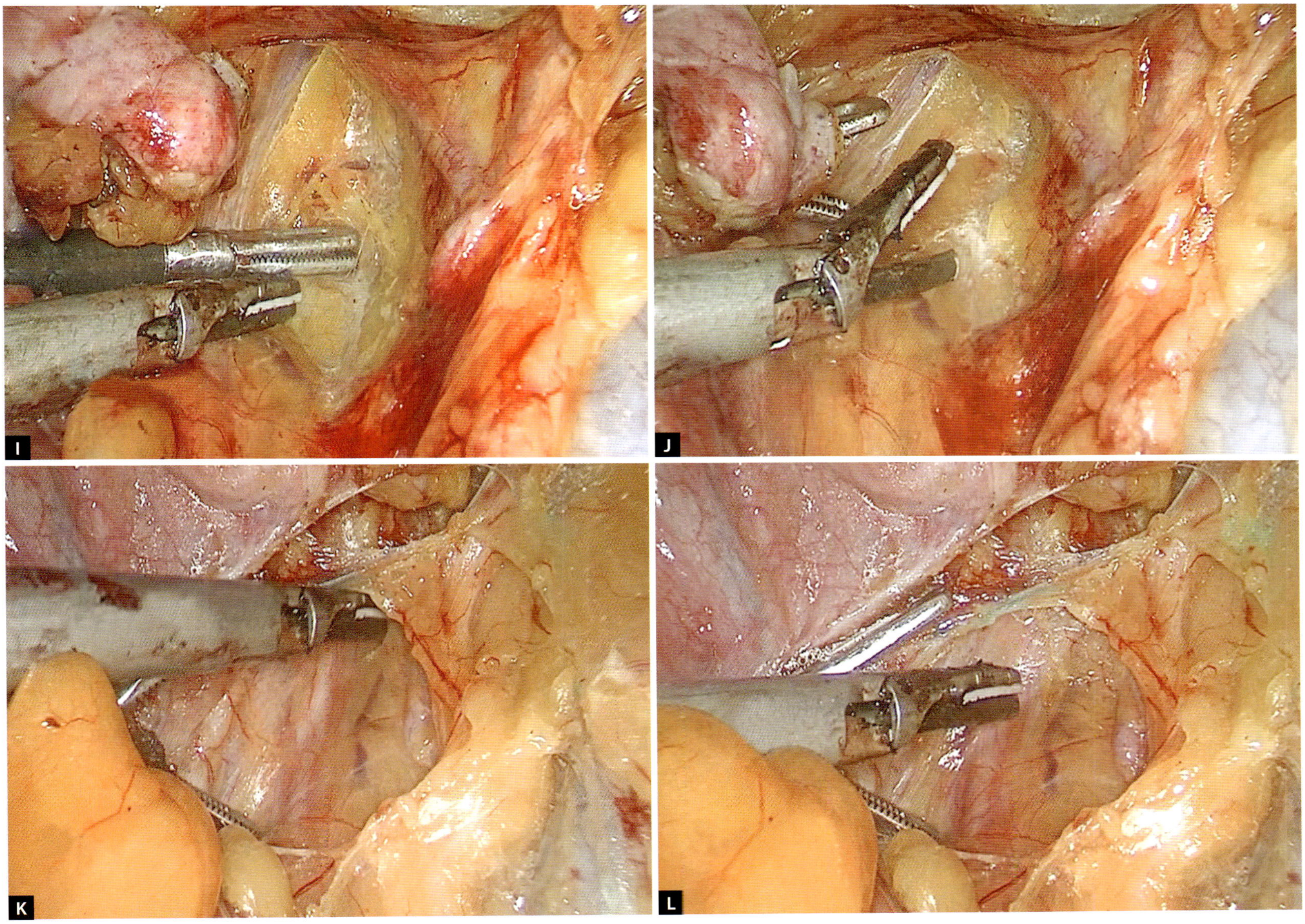

Figs. 8I to L

Figs. 8E to L: Right pararectal space entry and ligation of uterine vessels.

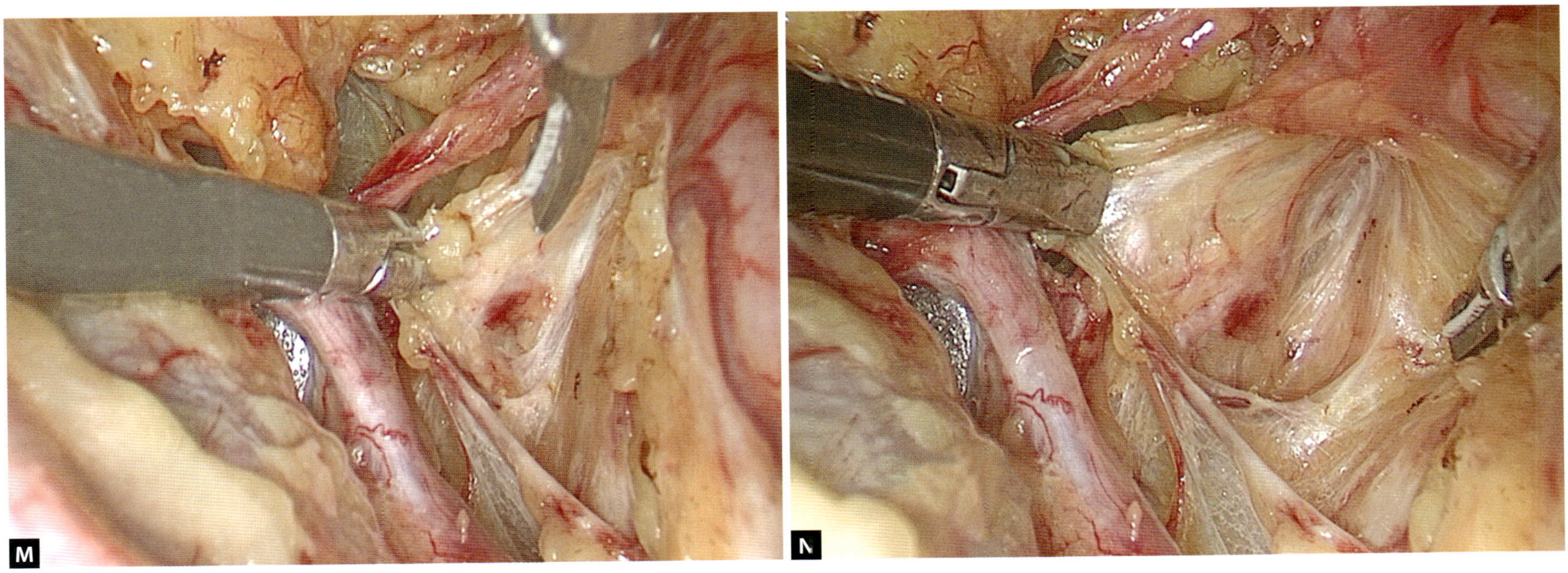

Figs. 8M and N

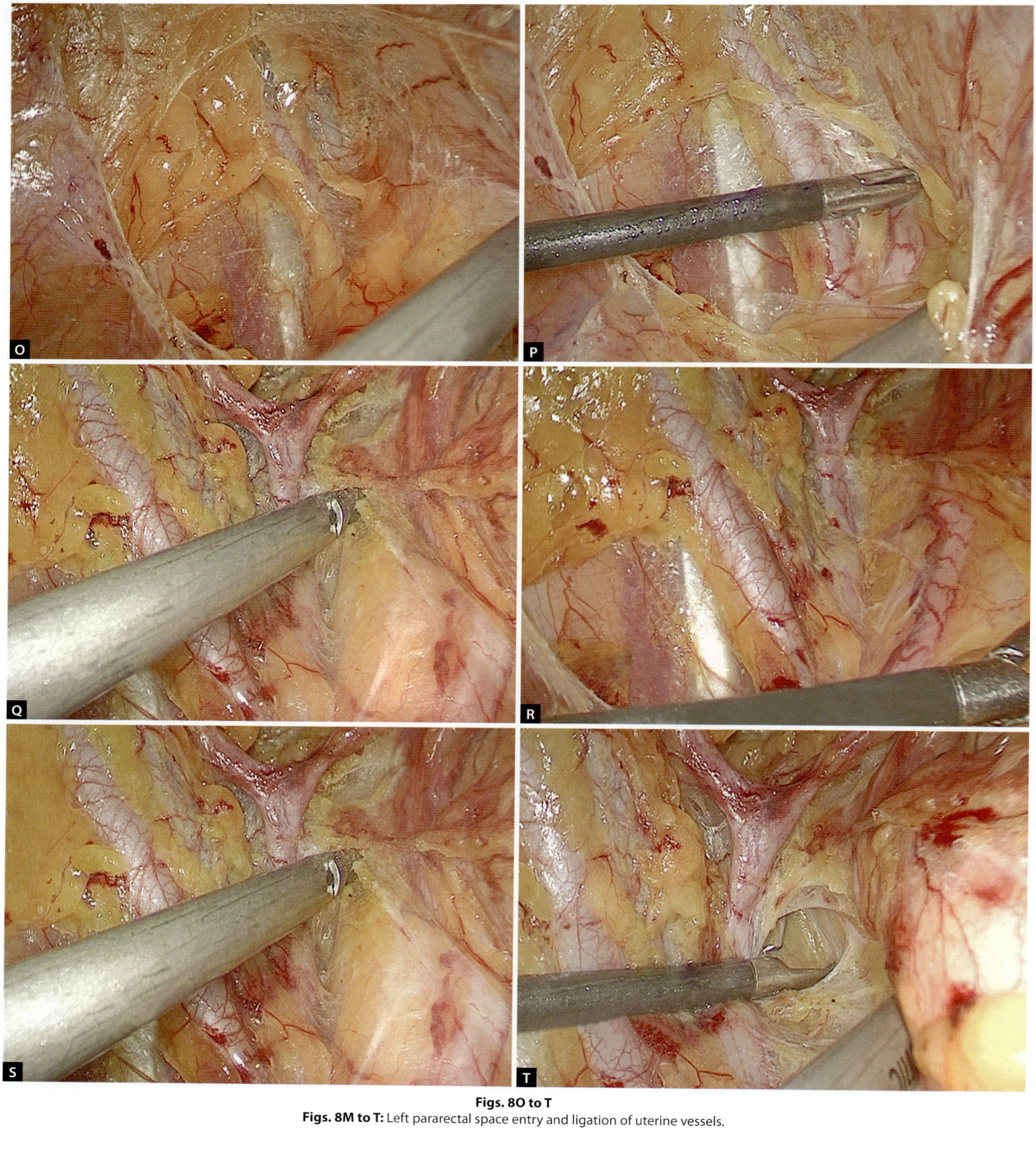

Figs. 8O to T

Figs. 8M to T: Left pararectal space entry and ligation of uterine vessels.

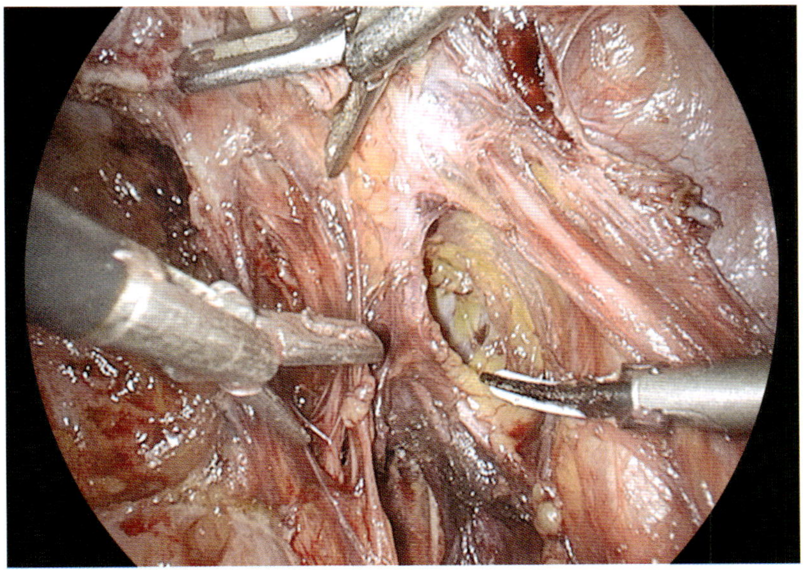

Fig. 9: Okabayashi space.

BLADDER DISSECTION (FIGS. 10A TO G)

Anteriorly UV is incised and bladder is completely dissected from cervix and vagina in the vesicovaginal space.

Window is created in the broad ligament and ureter is traced to ureteric tunnel **(Figs. 11 and 12)**.

URETERIC TUNNEL DISSECTION (FIGS. 13A TO F)

Roof of ureteric tunnel is opened with right-angled grasper and it is clipped and cut. Ureter is separated from lateral and posterior attachment dissected away from the tunnel. Parametrium is visible after ureter moves laterally and paracolpos is taken with harmonic/vessel sealer. Bladder is pushed further down to free upper one-third of vagina.

COLPOTOMY (FIGS. 14A TO I)

Bladder is pushed further down to free upper third of vagina. Colpotomy is done using harmonic, taking upper one-third of vagina

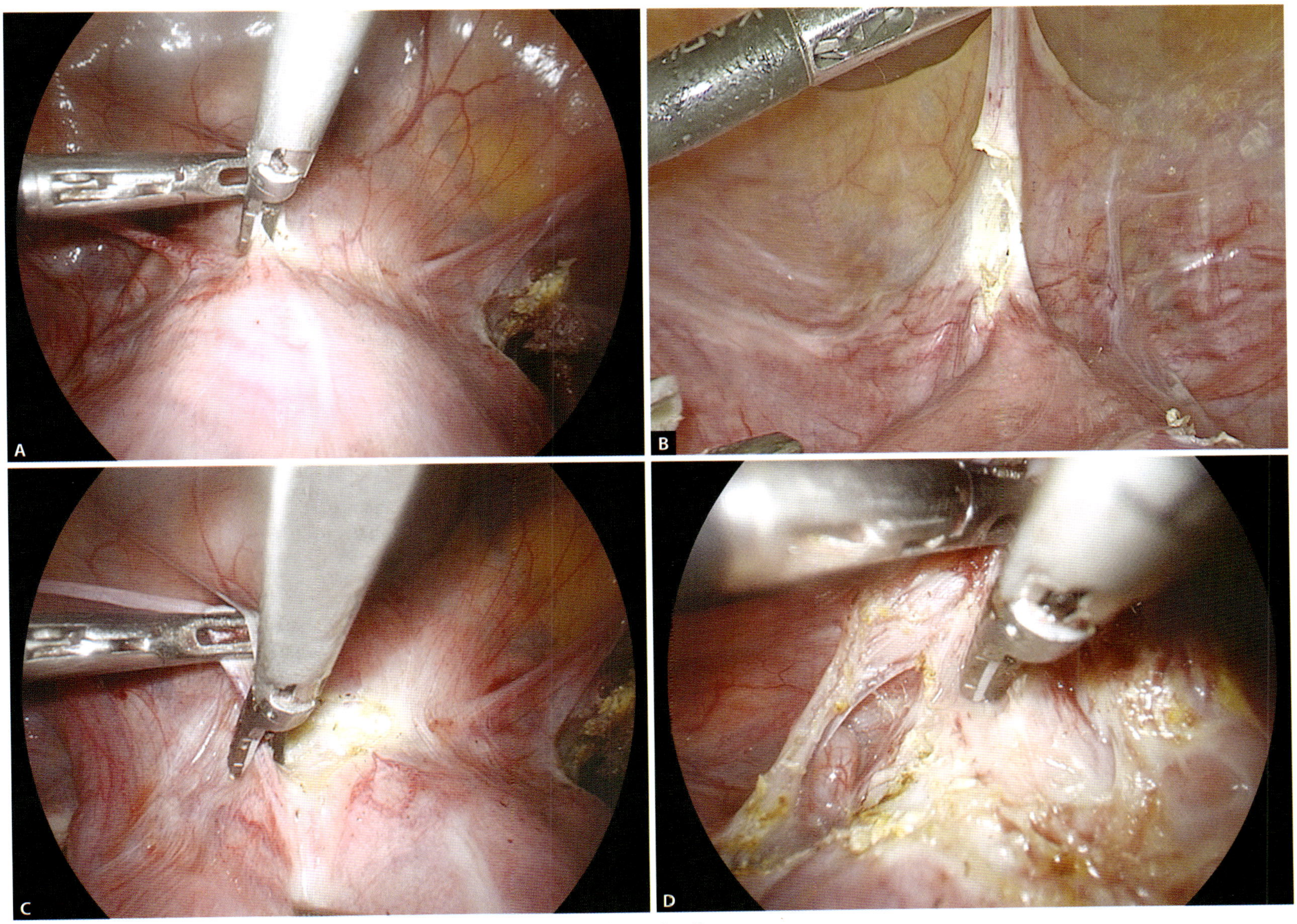

Figs. 10A to D

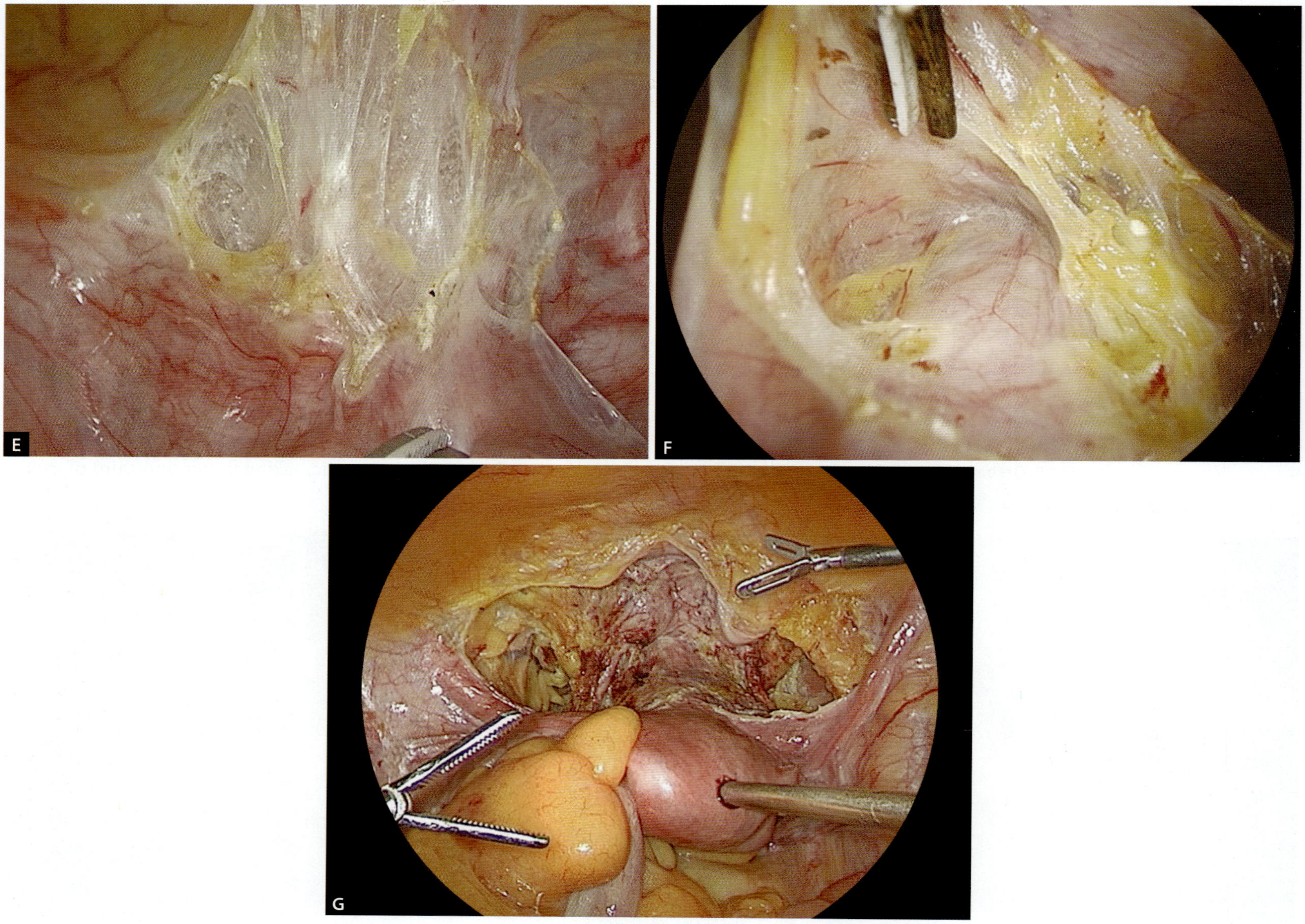

Figs. 10E to G

Figs. 10A to G: Bladder dissection.

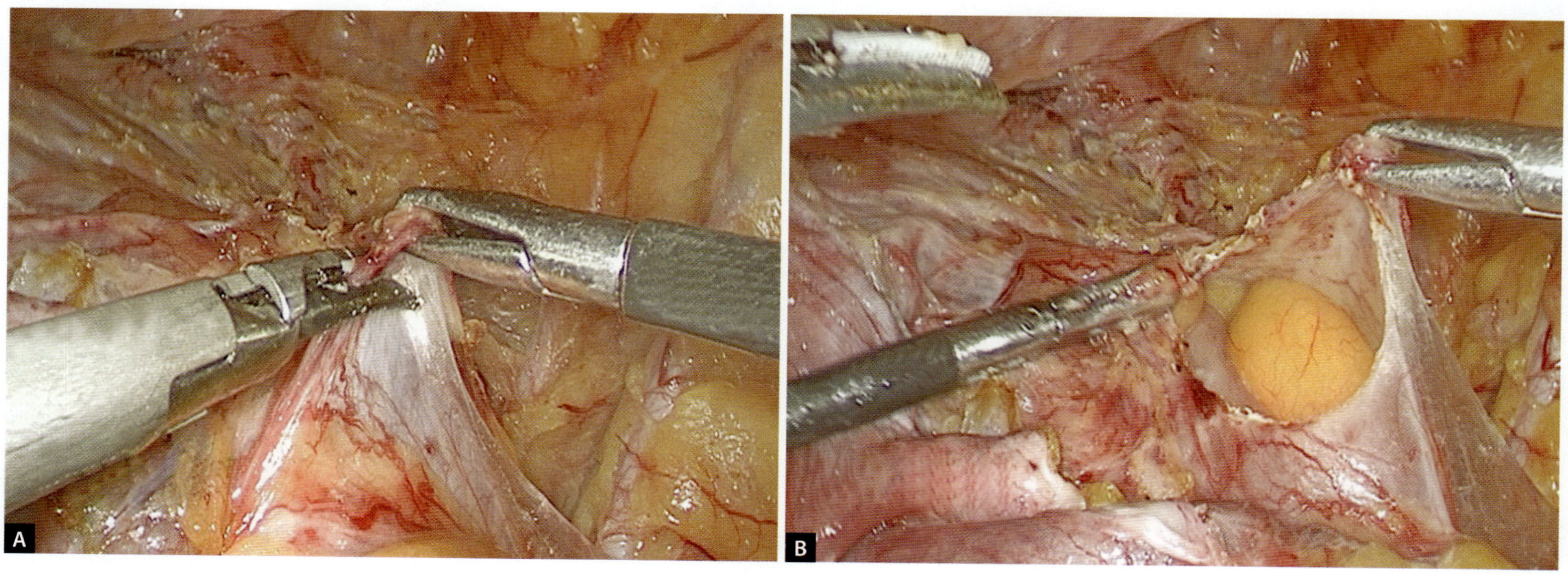

Figs. 11A and B

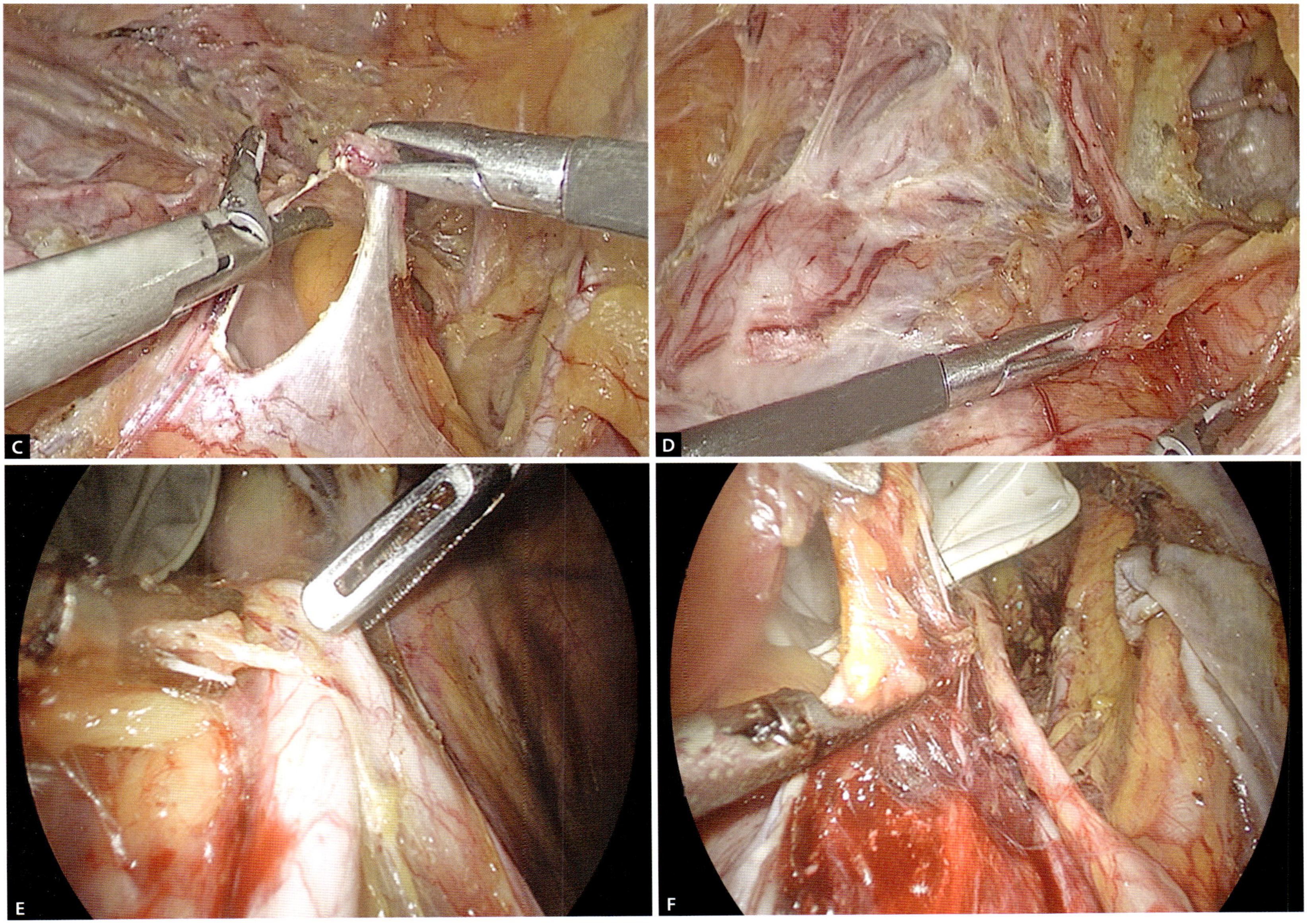

Figs. 11C to F

Figs. 11A to F: Right side ureteric tunnel.

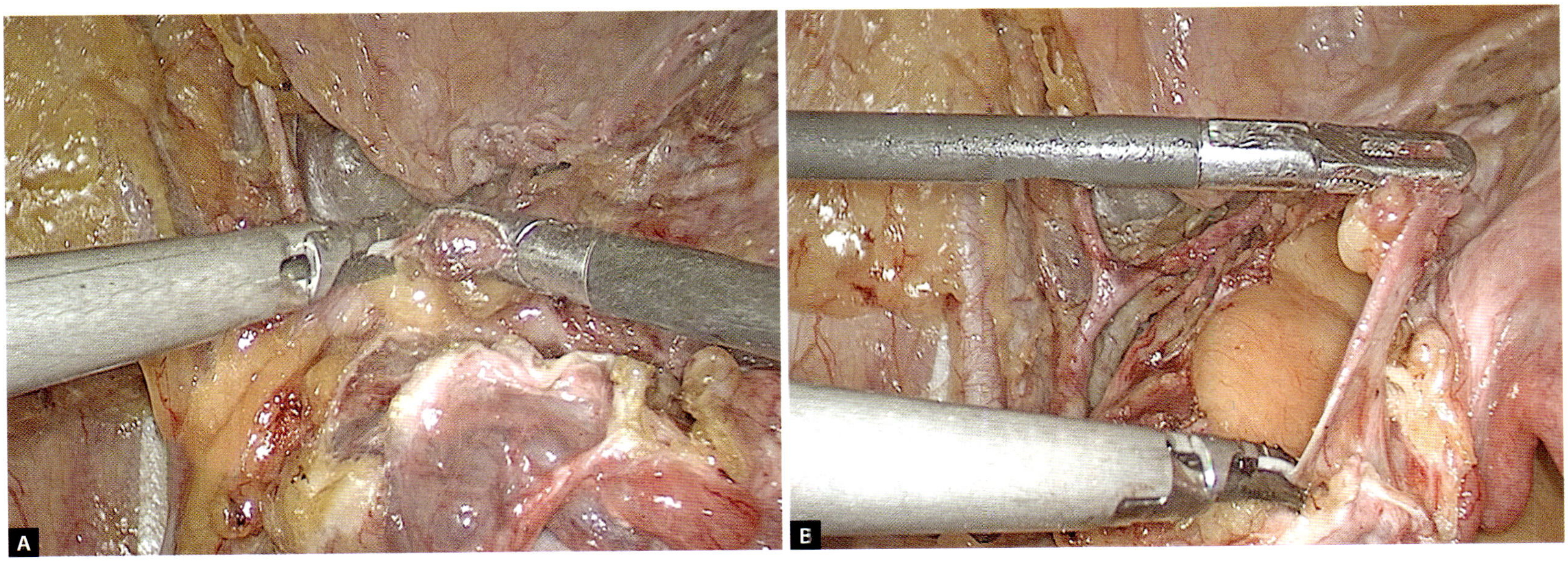

Figs. 12A and B

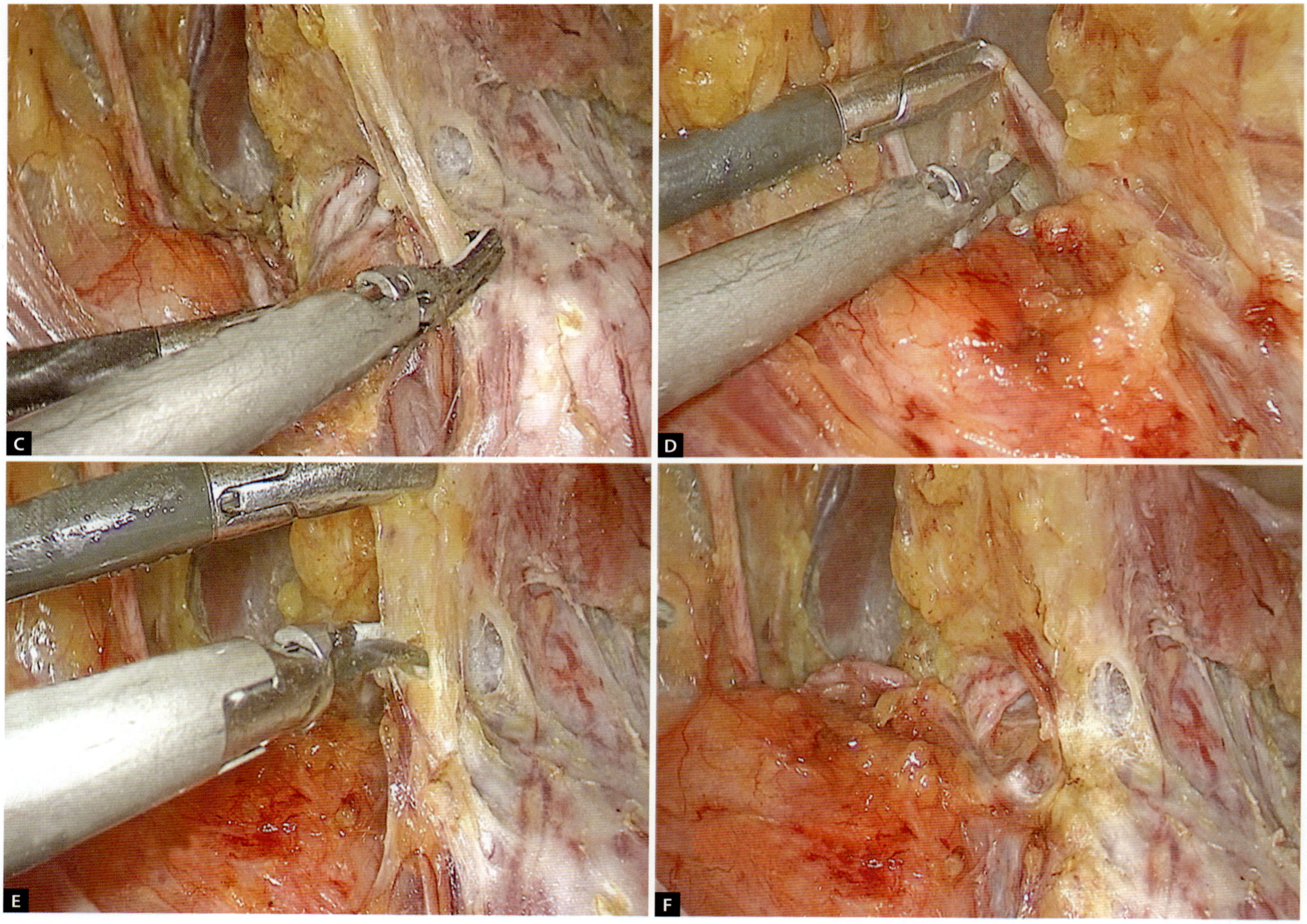

Figs. 12C to F

Figs. 12A to F: Left side ureteric tunnel.

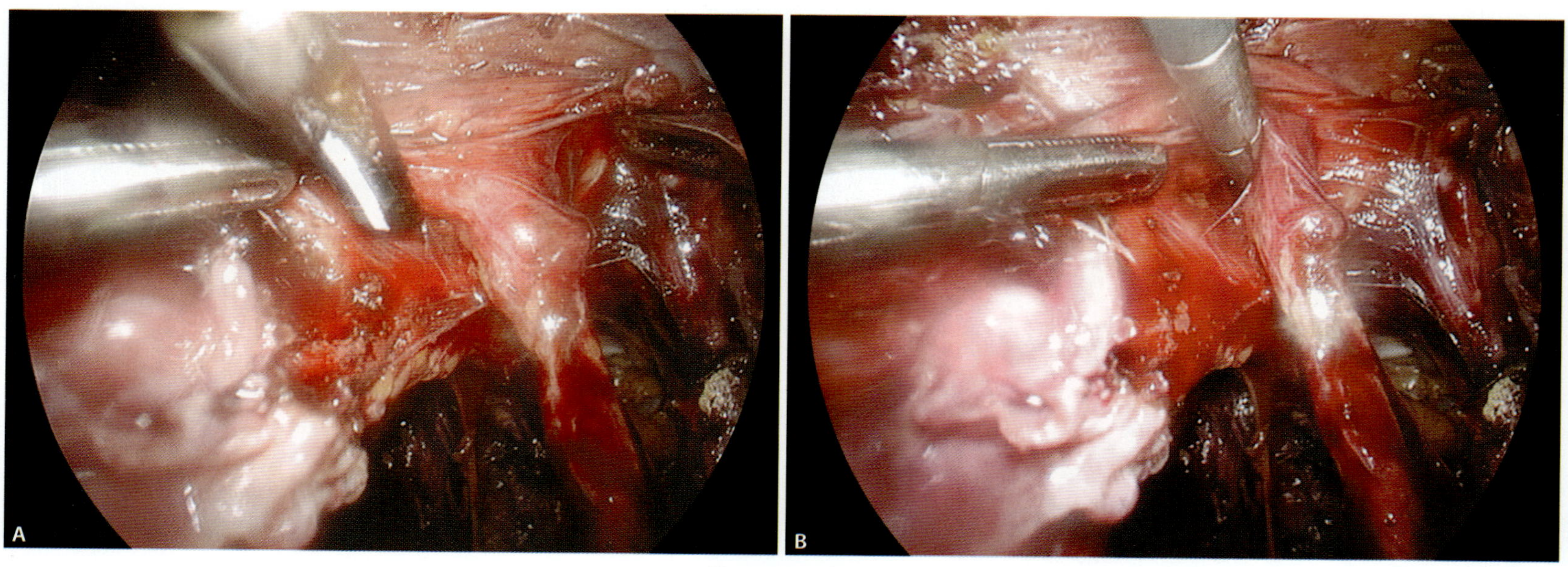

Figs. 13A and B

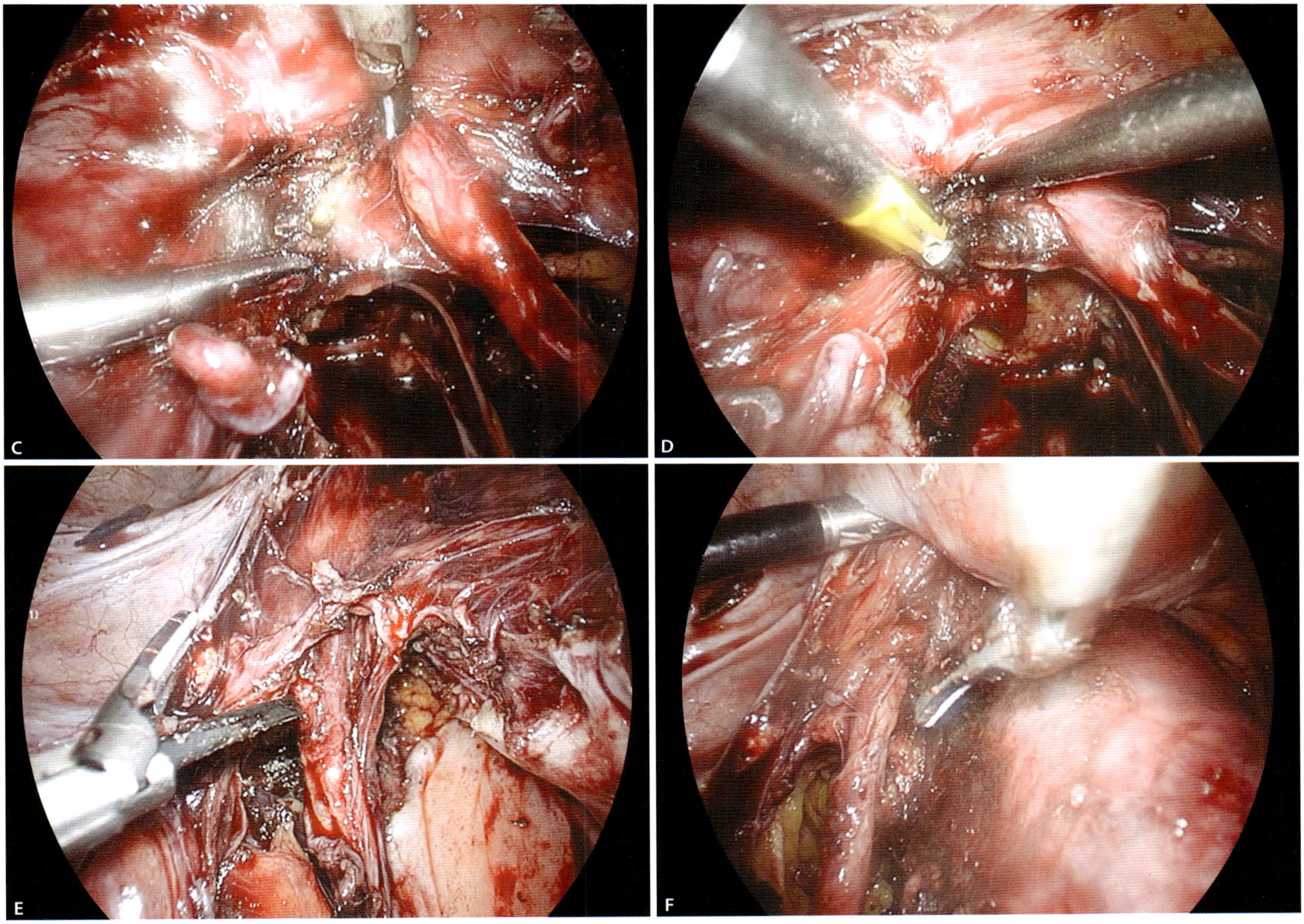

Figs. 13C to F

Figs. 13A to F: Ureteric tunnel dissection.

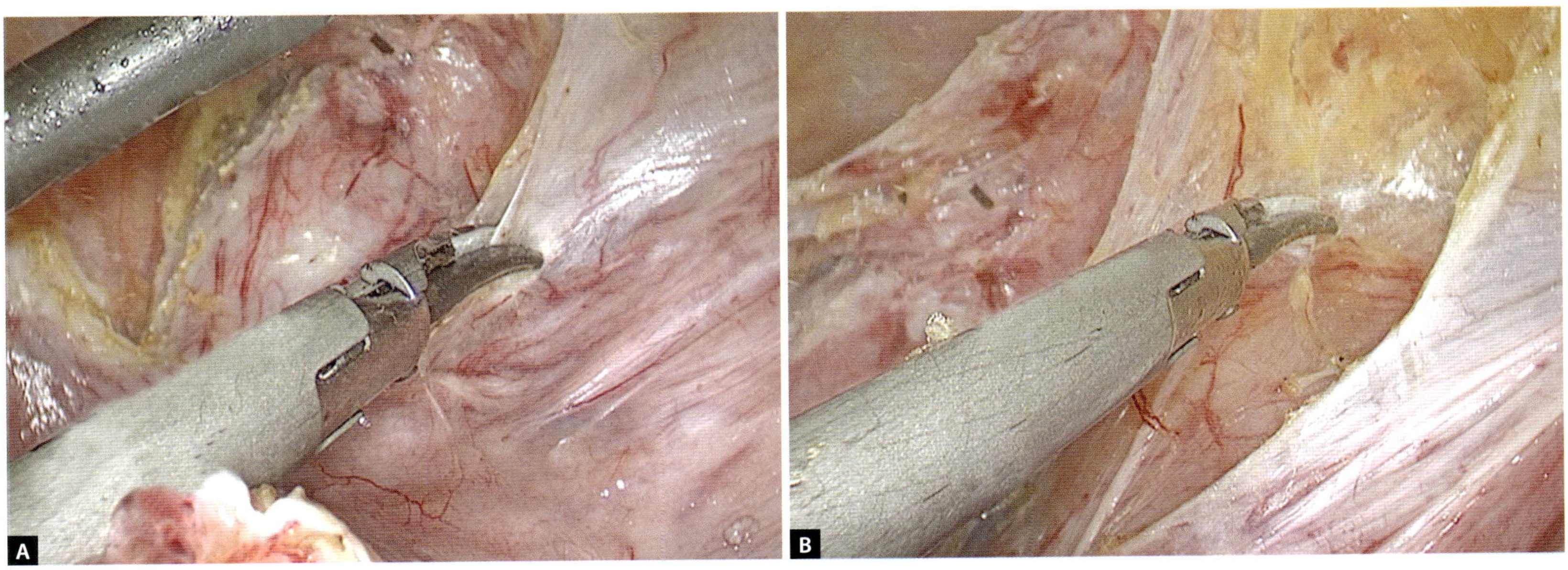

Figs. 14A and B

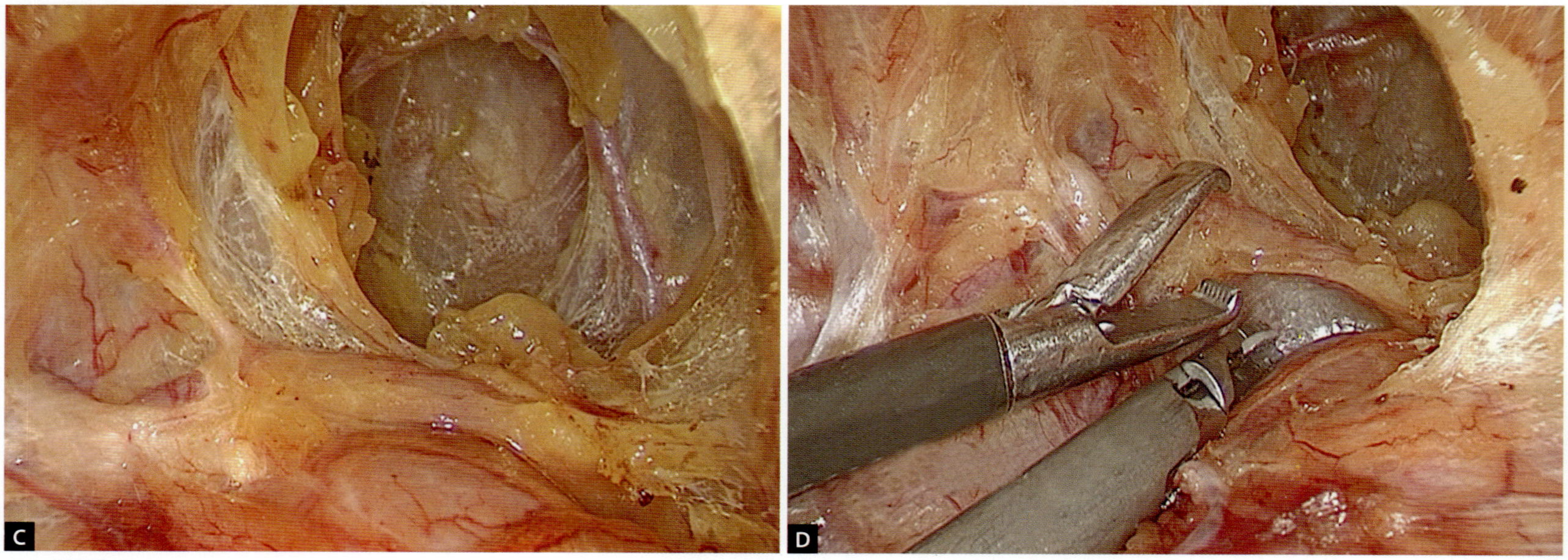

Figs. 14C and D

Figs. 14A to D: Bladder is pushed further down to free upper third of vagina.

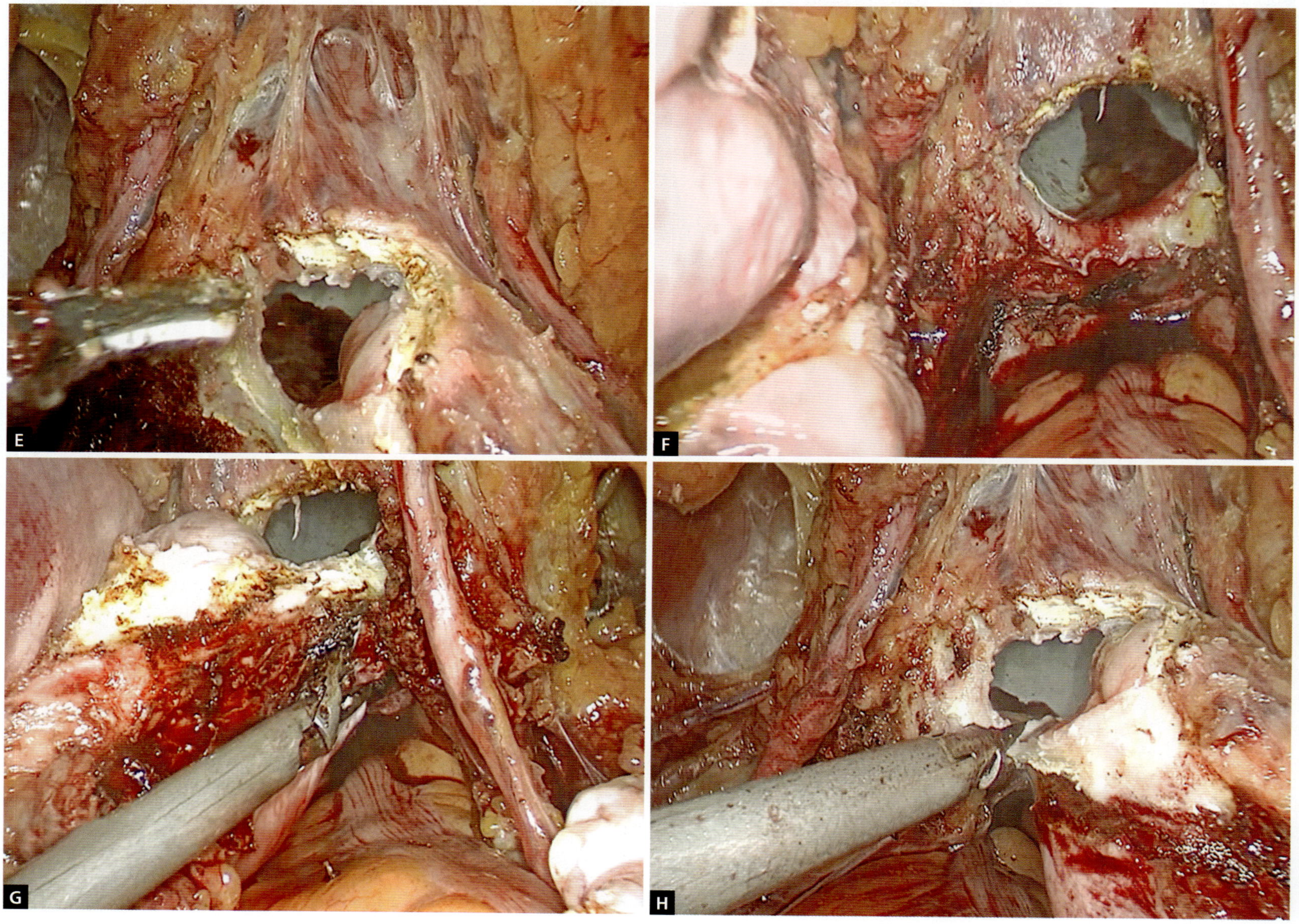

Figs. 14E to H

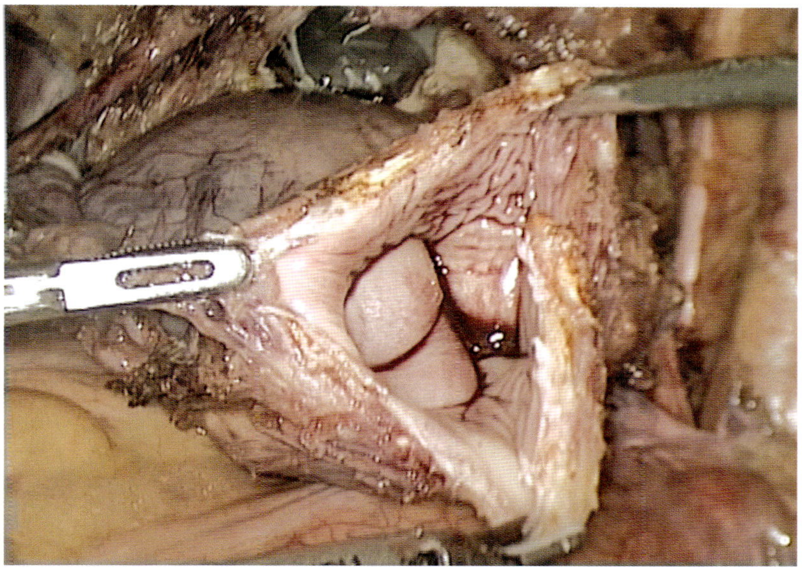

Fig. 14I

Figs. 14E to I: Colpotomy.

with specimen in cancer of cervix and not removed in case of cancer of endometrium. Specimen is removed vaginally. Vault is closed laparoscopically with barbed sutures.

VAULT SUTURING

The vault suturing is described in **Figures 15A to F**.

PELVIC LYMPHADENECTOMY

The commonly performed pelvic lymphadenectomy involves removal of external iliac, internal iliac, and common iliac group of nodes. The lymph node dissection starts at the bifurcation of common iliac artery. Incision is made parallel to external iliac vessels in the posterior peritoneum which is extended up to inguinal ligament. Peritoneum is lifted and the underlying structures are exposed laterally as far as psoas muscle. The fibrofatty tissue over psoas muscle is excised till the inguinal ligament. Now, external iliac artery and vein are traced. Lymphatics, fibrofatty tissue around external iliac vessels are separated from the vessels wall. Dissection is done till external iliac artery gives circumflex iliac branch. The fibrofatty tissue along the external iliac vein is dissected. The obturator fossa is exposed by retracting external iliac vessels laterally. The nodes in the obturator fossa are visualized by stretching of the peritoneum. The obturator nerve is exposed and all the nodes anterior to the nerve are cleared. The dissection should not go below obturator nerve as there can be dangerous bleeding. The dissection is done up to the main trunk of the internal iliac vessels. The entire fibrofatty tissues are cleared from the internal iliac vessels. The external iliac artery, vein, and obturator fossa should be devoid of fibrofatty tissue at the end of dissection. The psoas muscle and the genitofemoral nerve are the lateral end of the dissection. The entire nodal tissue is placed in an Endobag and removed through vagina. This avoids port metastasis. Hemostasis is achieved and irrigated with normal saline.

- Peritoneum over external iliac vessels is incised **(Figs. 16A to F)**.
- The fibrofatty tissues over the external iliac vessels are excised **(Figs. 17A1 to V2)**.
- Nodes in the obturator fossa are excised along with the fibrofatty tissue. The dissection is done only up to the obturator nerve **(Figs. 18A and B)**.
- Internal iliac vessels are exposed **(Figs. 19A to D)**.

AORTIC NODE DISSECTION

The transperitoneal approach is preferred since it provides adequate space for dissection. Initially, the left colon is mobilized. The splenic flexure is cut to achieve better visualization. The colon is reflected till the lateral border of the inferior vena cava (IVC) is seen clearly. The ureter and psoas muscle are identified and the dissection first involves removing the nodes along the common iliac artery and then proceeding along the anterior and lateral border of the aorta. The fibrofatty tissues between the lateral border of the aorta and the ureter are removed. The lumbar arteries are to be protected during this nodal dissection. The dissection proceeds cranially upward till the left renal vein is identified. Now, a clear plane along the Gerota's fascia is identified. The nodes between the Gerota's fascia need not to be opened. These nodes are collected separately (para-aortic group). The next step is removal of preaortic group of lymph nodes for which dissection starts from the bifurcation of aorta. The hypogastric plexus, which starts at the bifurcation of aorta, should be identified and carefully avoided. The nodes are then swept cranially along the anterior border of the aorta. In the midportion, the inferior mesenteric artery is visualized and preserved. The entire fibrofatty tissue is removed up to the renal vein. This entire group of nodes is separately preserved as preaortic group of lymph nodes.

The interaortocaval lymph nodes are then slowly removed by dissecting the fibrofatty tissue between the aorta and IVC. The lumbar veins are encountered during the dissection and care should be taken to avoid any damage to this. These are collected separately as interaortocaval lymph nodes. After the final wash, the aorta should be devoid of all the fibrofatty tissue.

- Peritoneum is dissected and nodes are removed in caudocranial direction **(Figs. 20A to O)**
- Para-aortic lymph nodes are removed **(Figs. 21A to P)**.

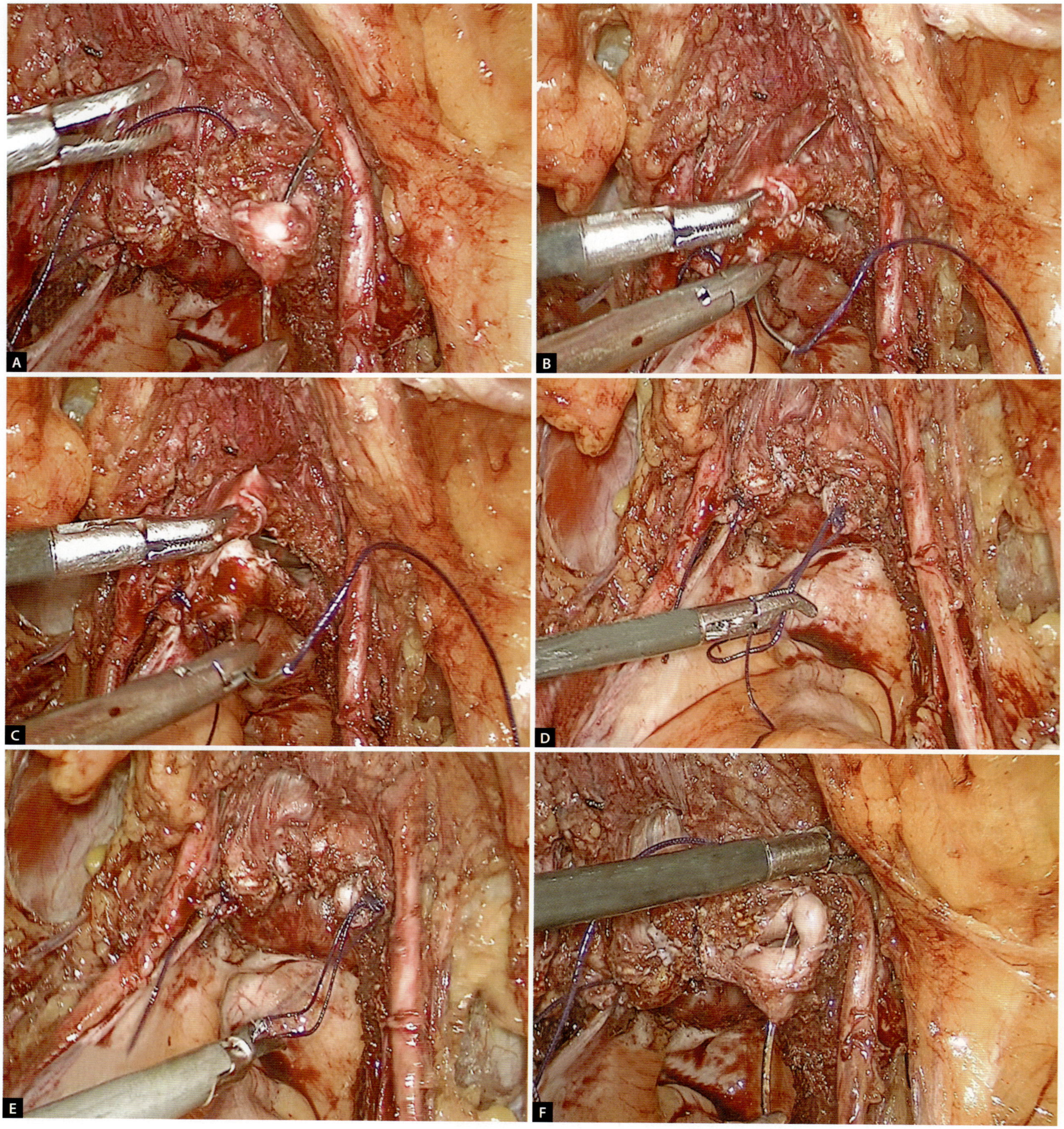

Figs. 15A to F: Vault suturing.

Pelvic and Para-aortic Lymphadenectomy

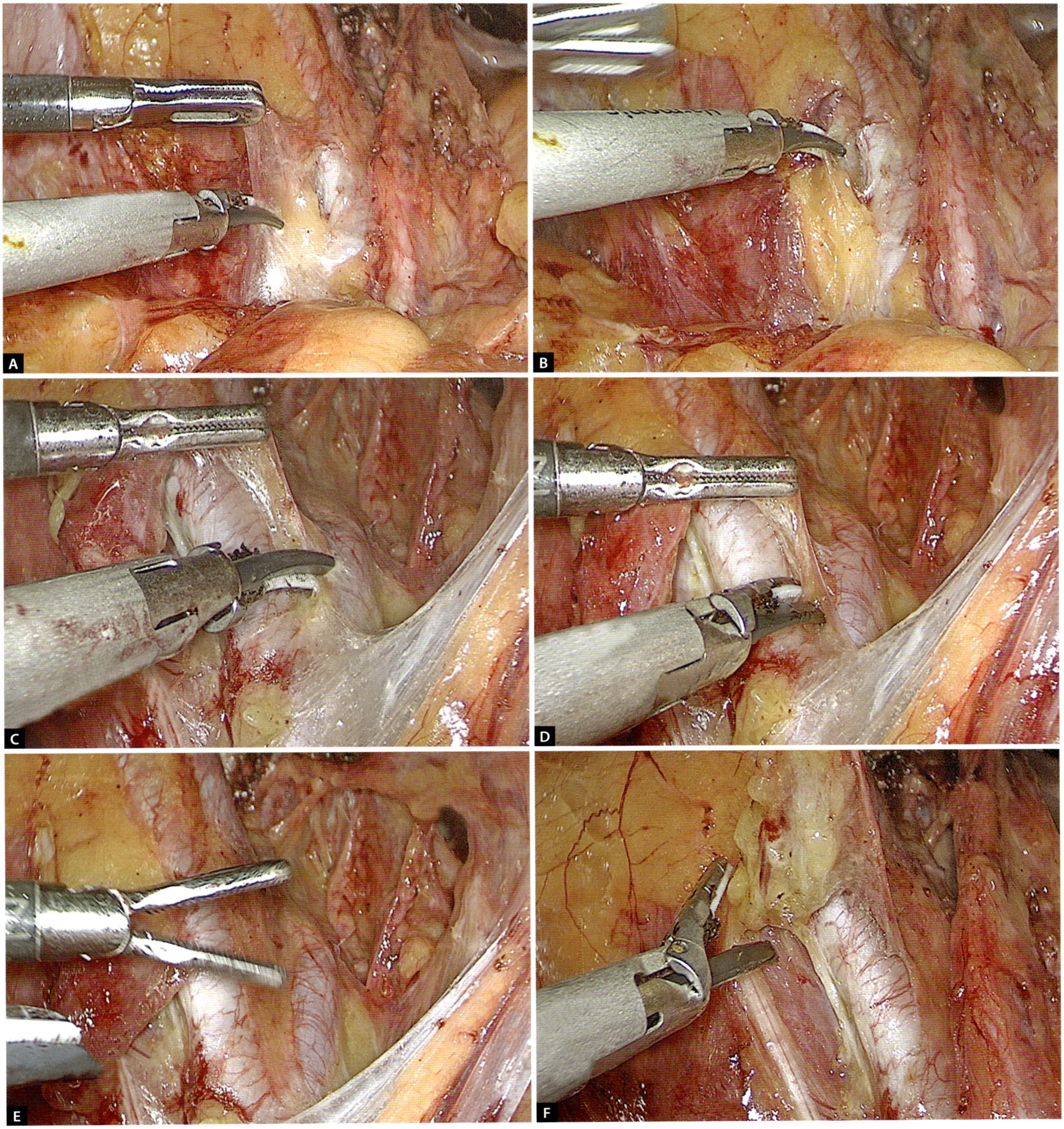

Figs. 16A to F: Peritoneum over external iliac vessels is incised.

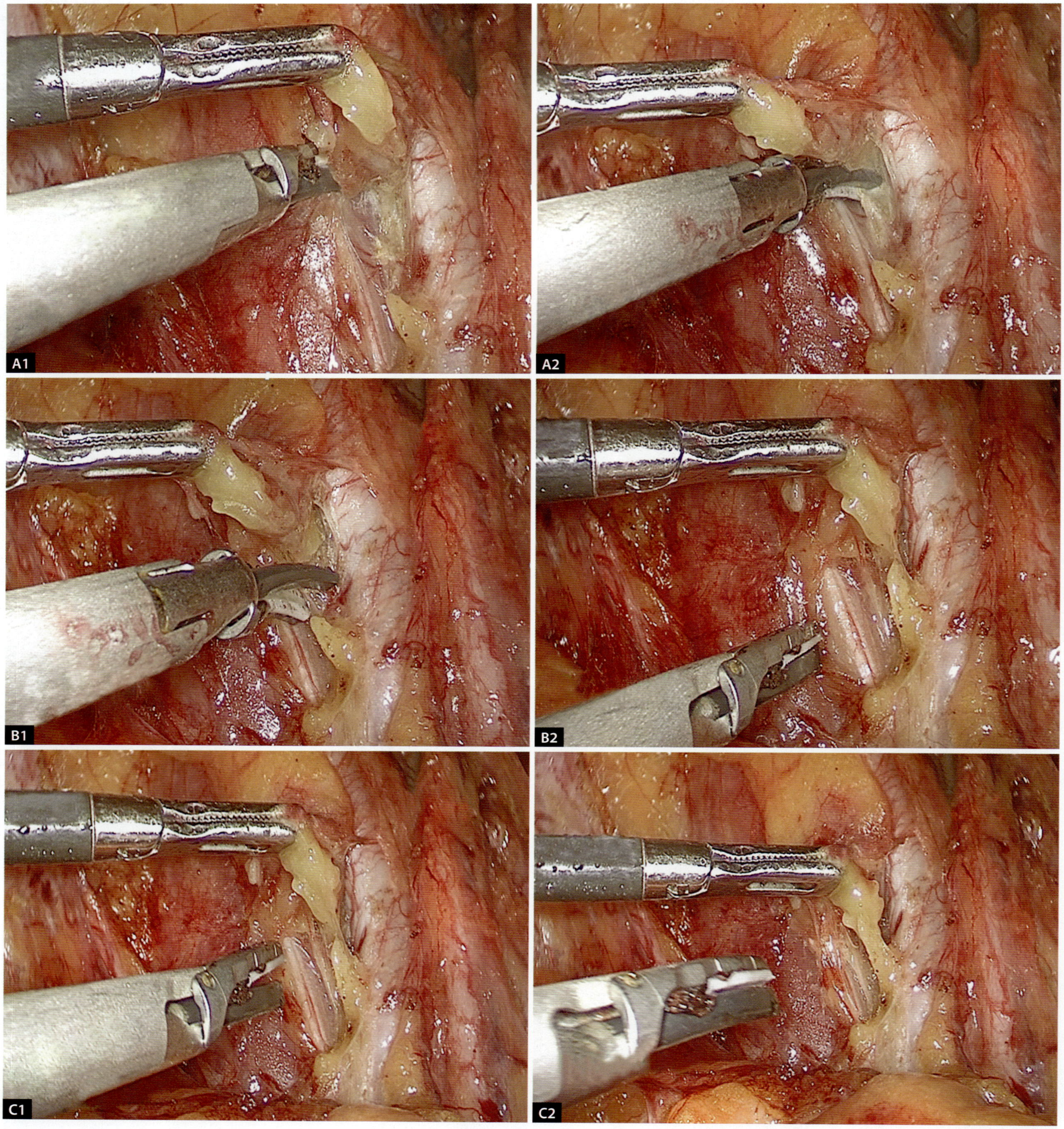

Figs. 17A1 to C2

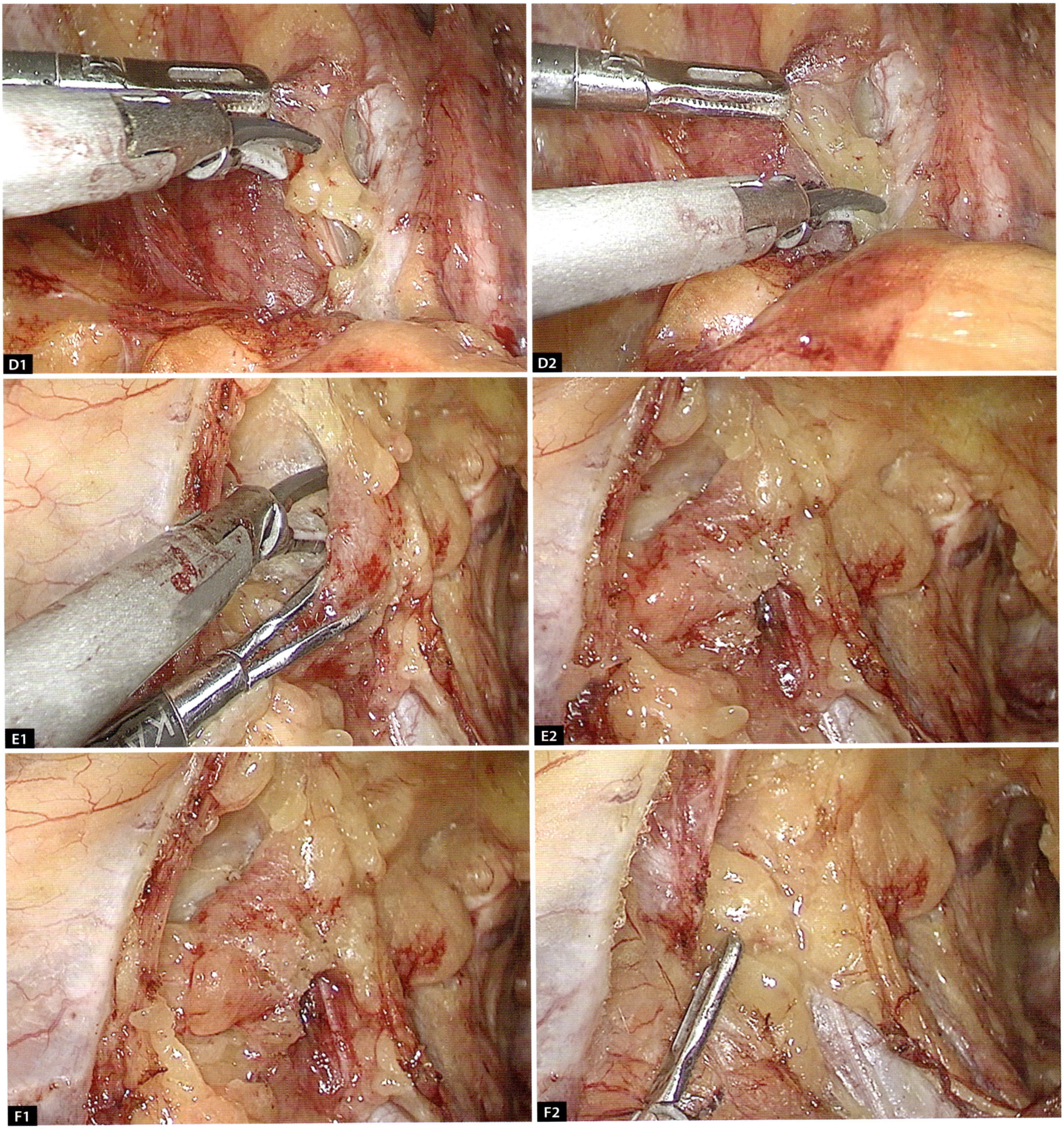

Figs. 17D1 to F2

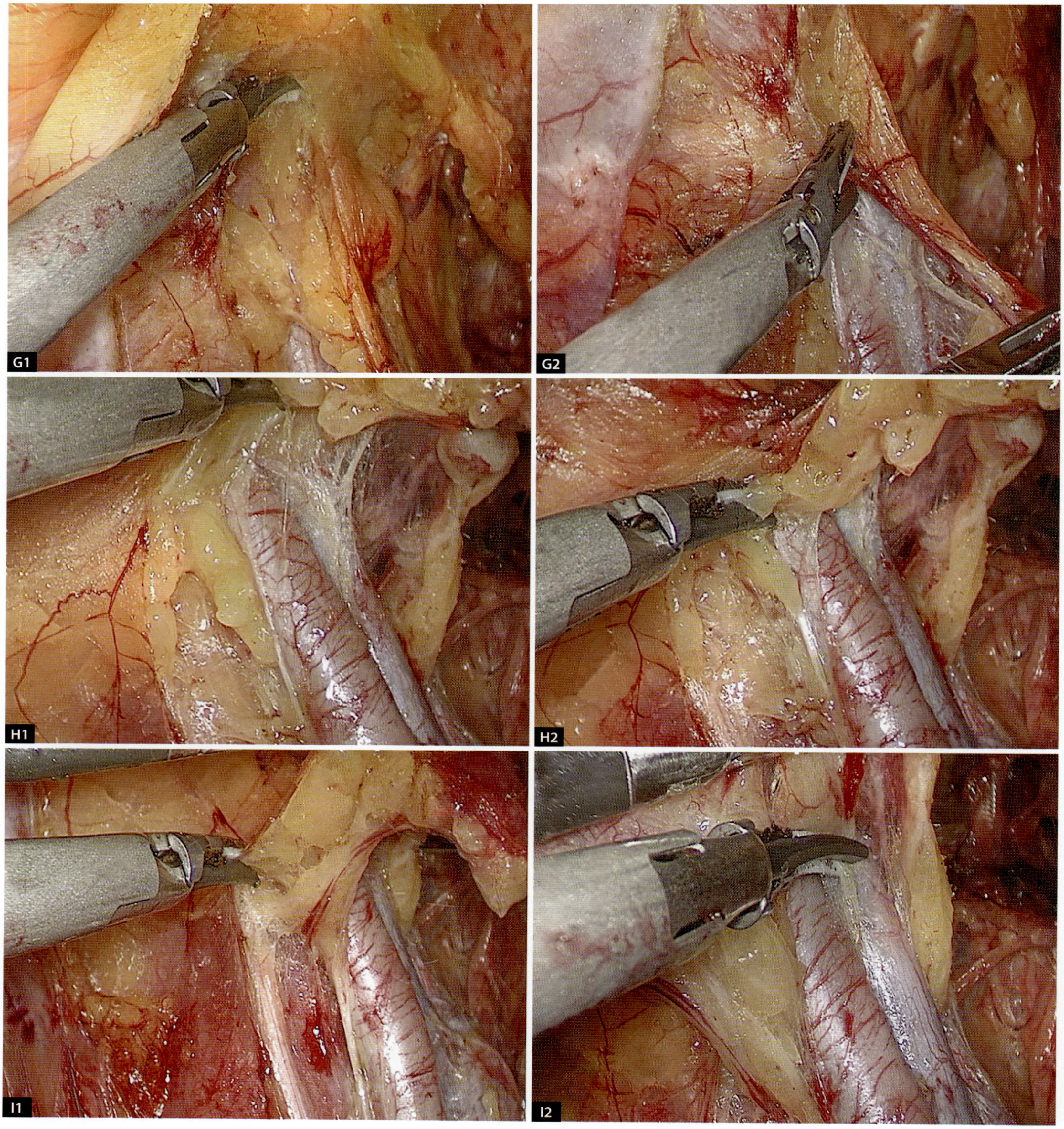

Figs. 17G1 to I2

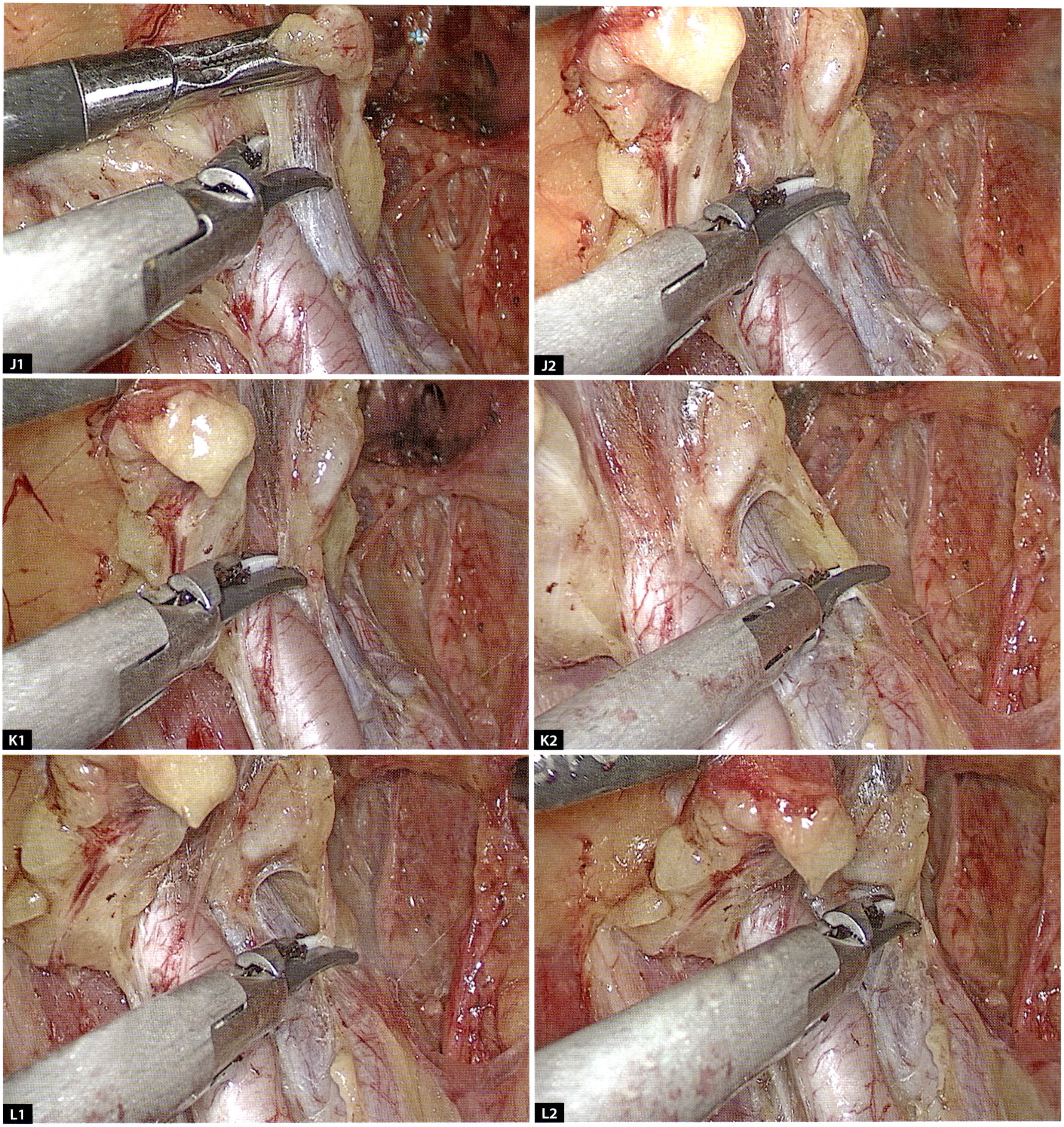

Figs. 17J1 to L2

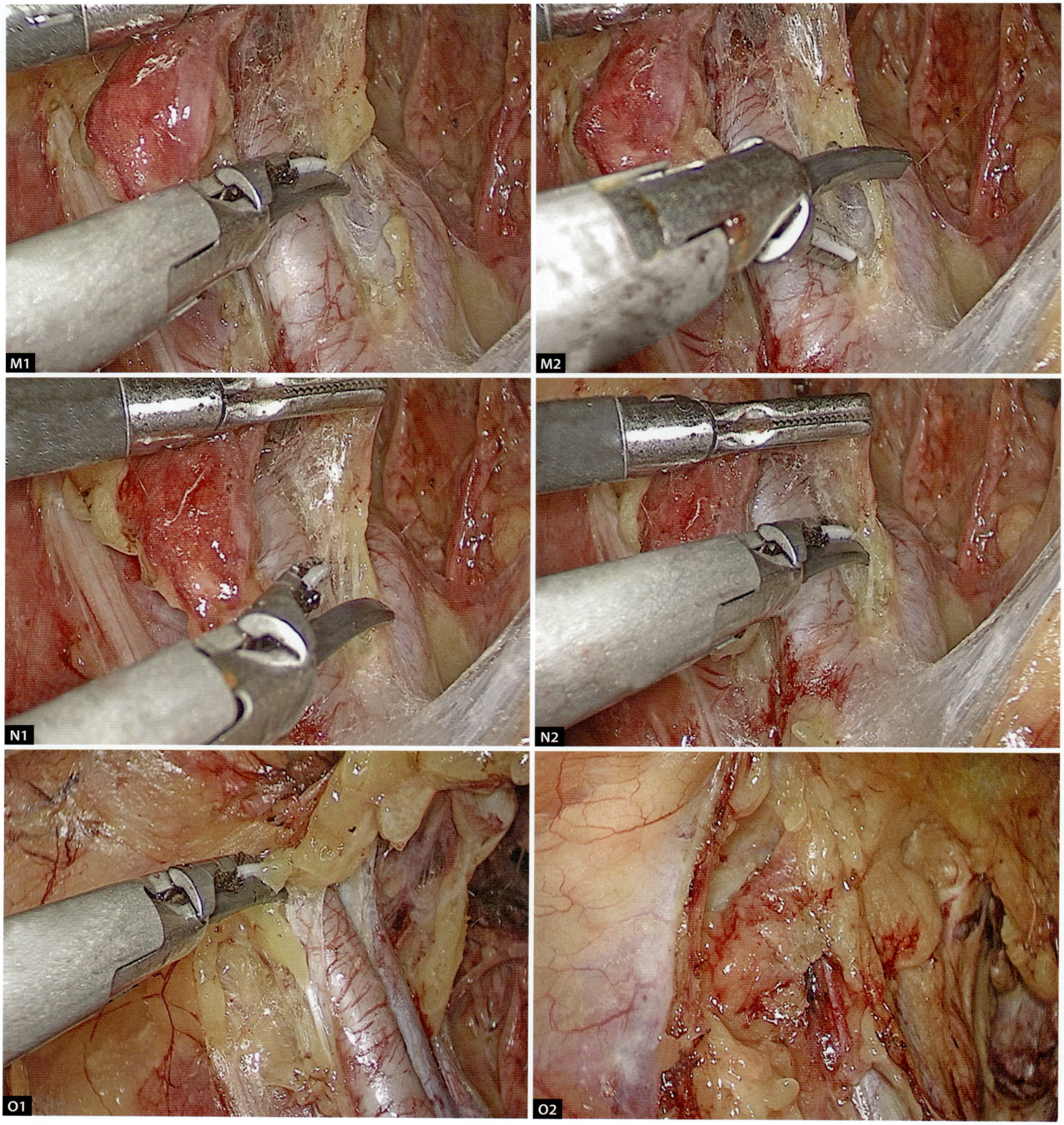

Figs. 17M1 to O2

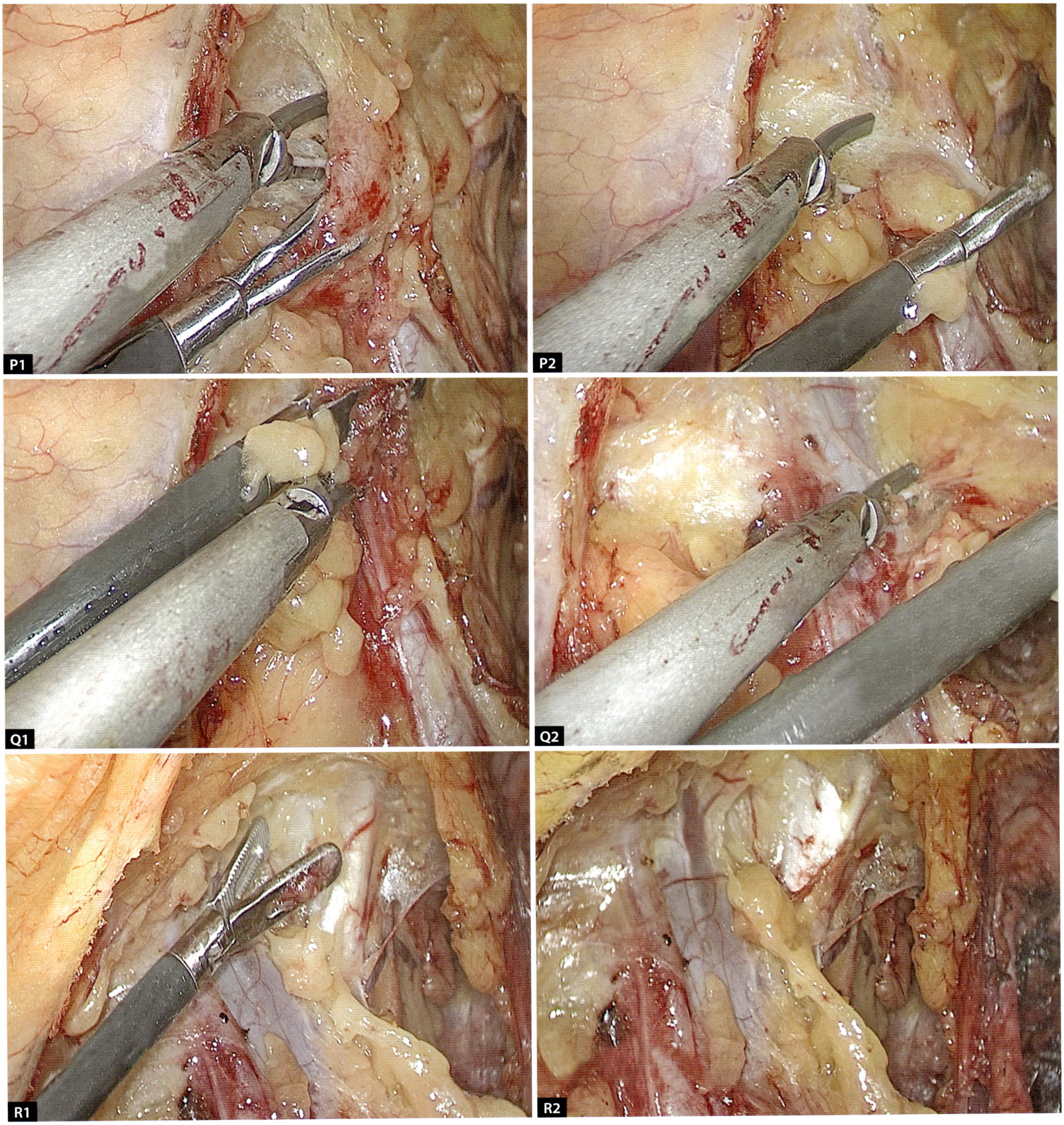

Figs. 17P1 to R2

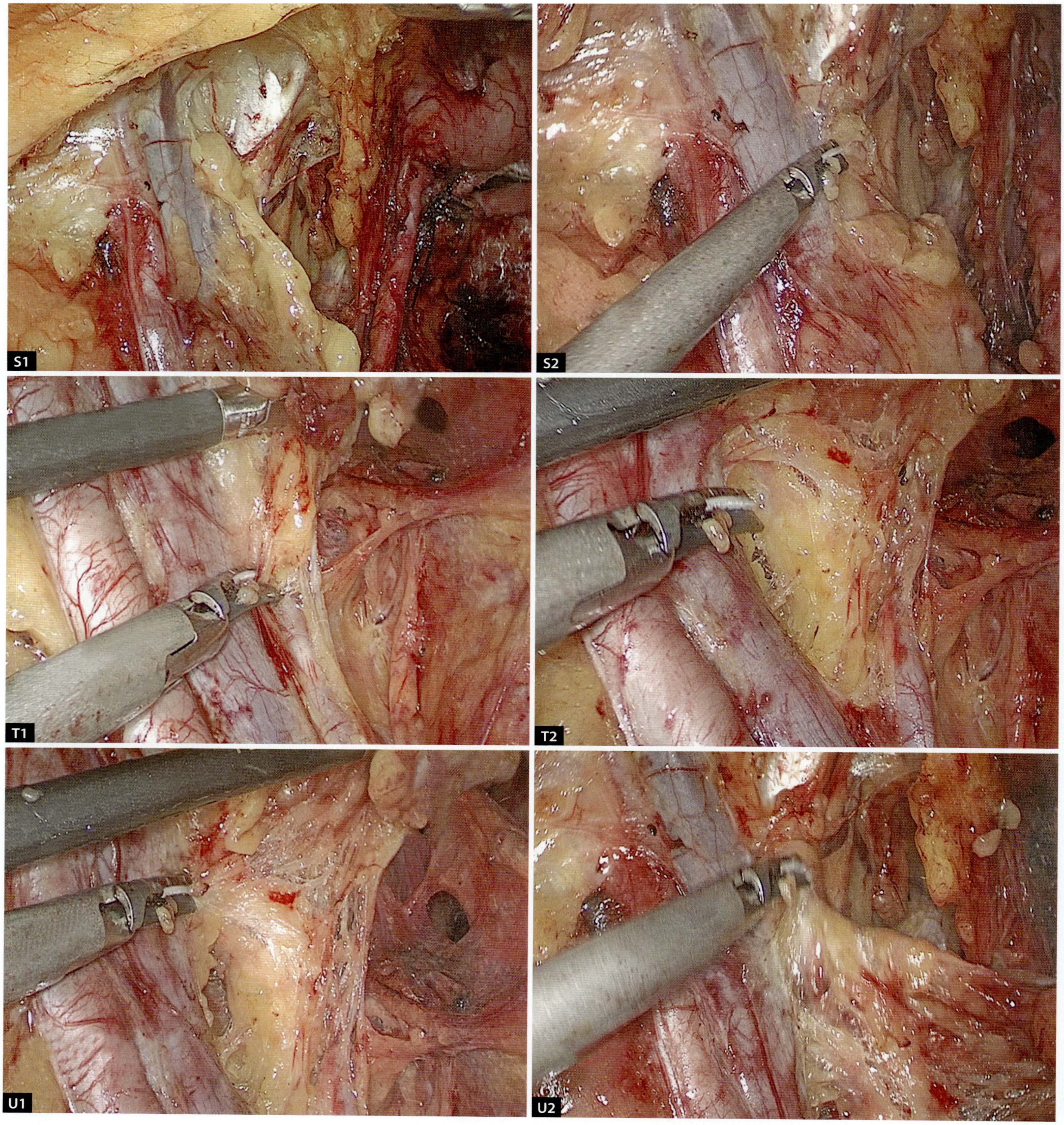

Figs. 17S1 to U2

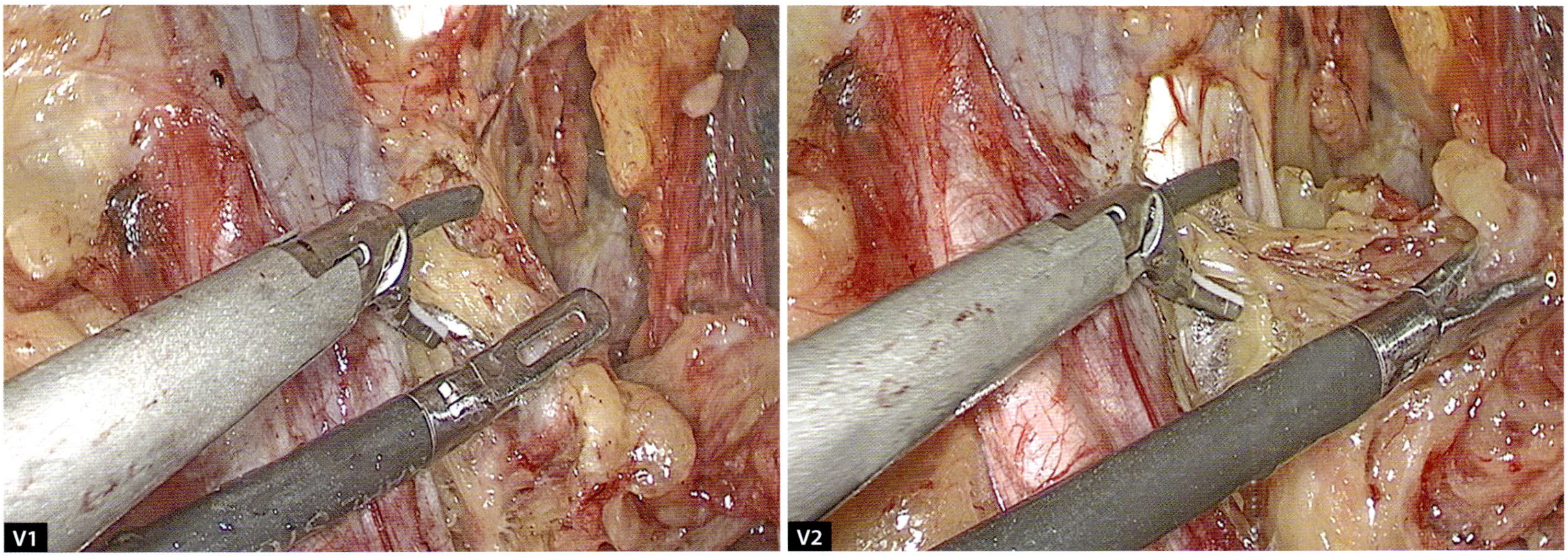

Figs. 17V1 and V2

Figs. 17A1 to V2: The fibrofatty tissues over the external iliac vessels are excised.

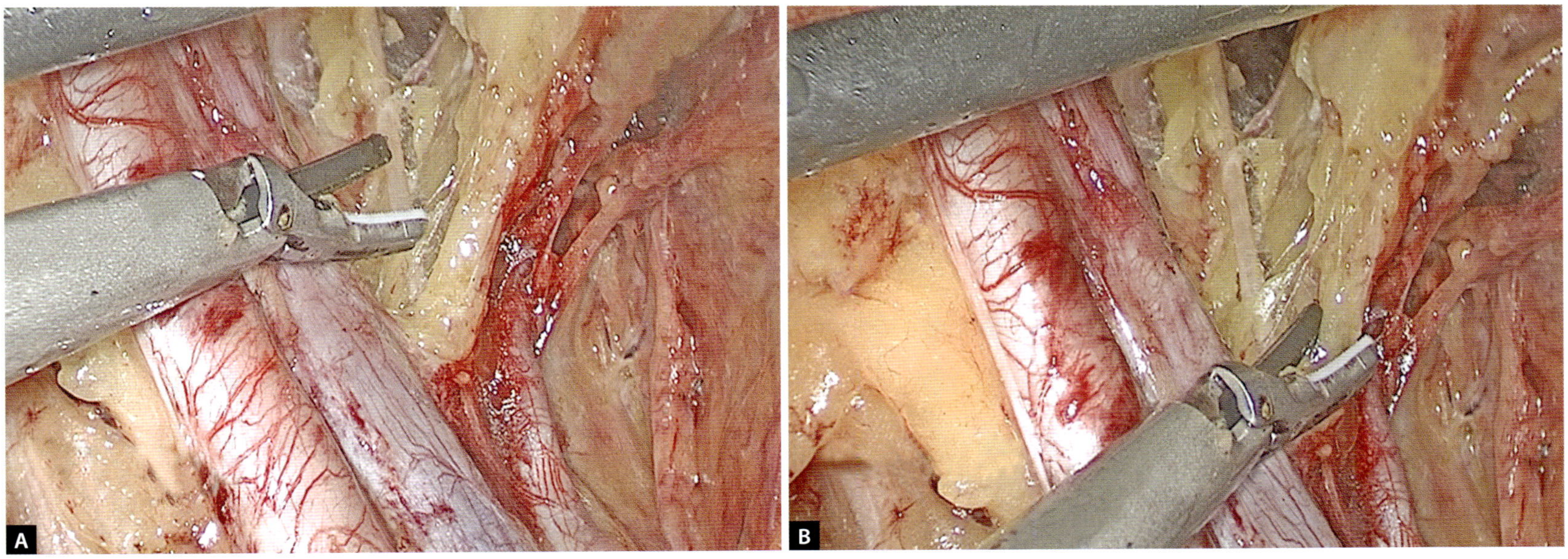

Figs. 18A and B: Nodes in the obturator fossa are excised along with the fibrofatty tissue only up to the obturator nerve.

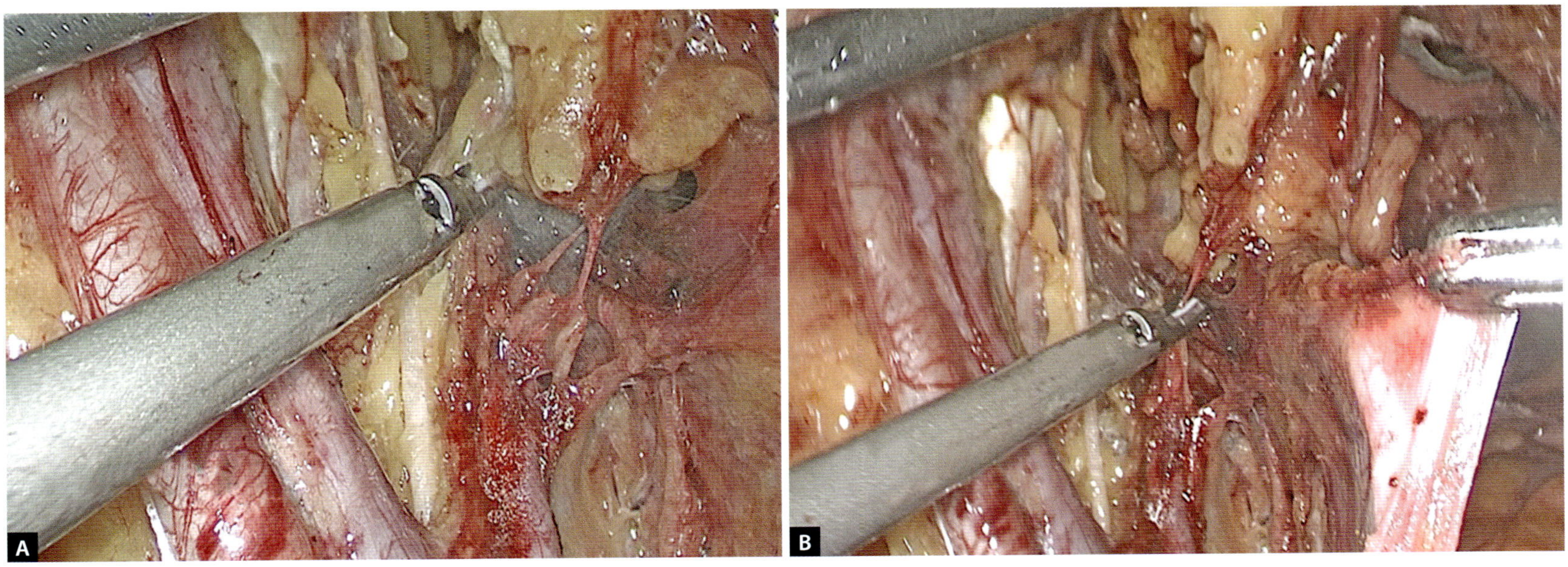

Figs. 19A and B

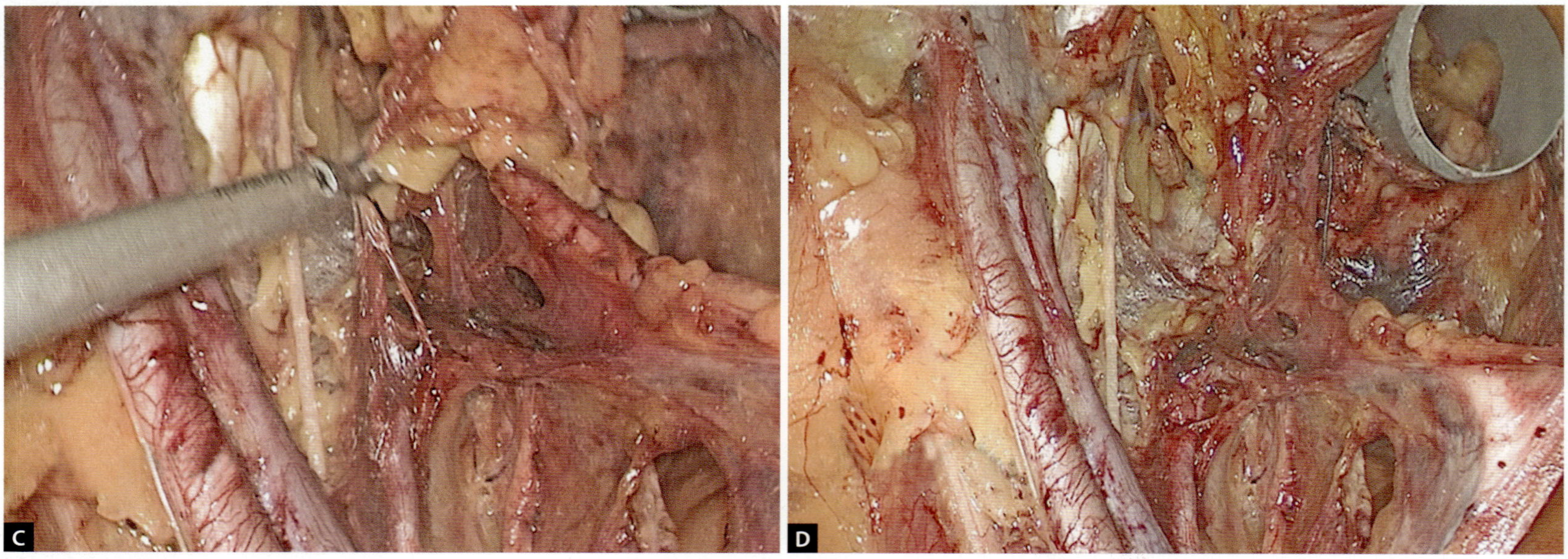

Figs. 19C and D

Figs. 19A to D: Internal iliac vessels are exposed.

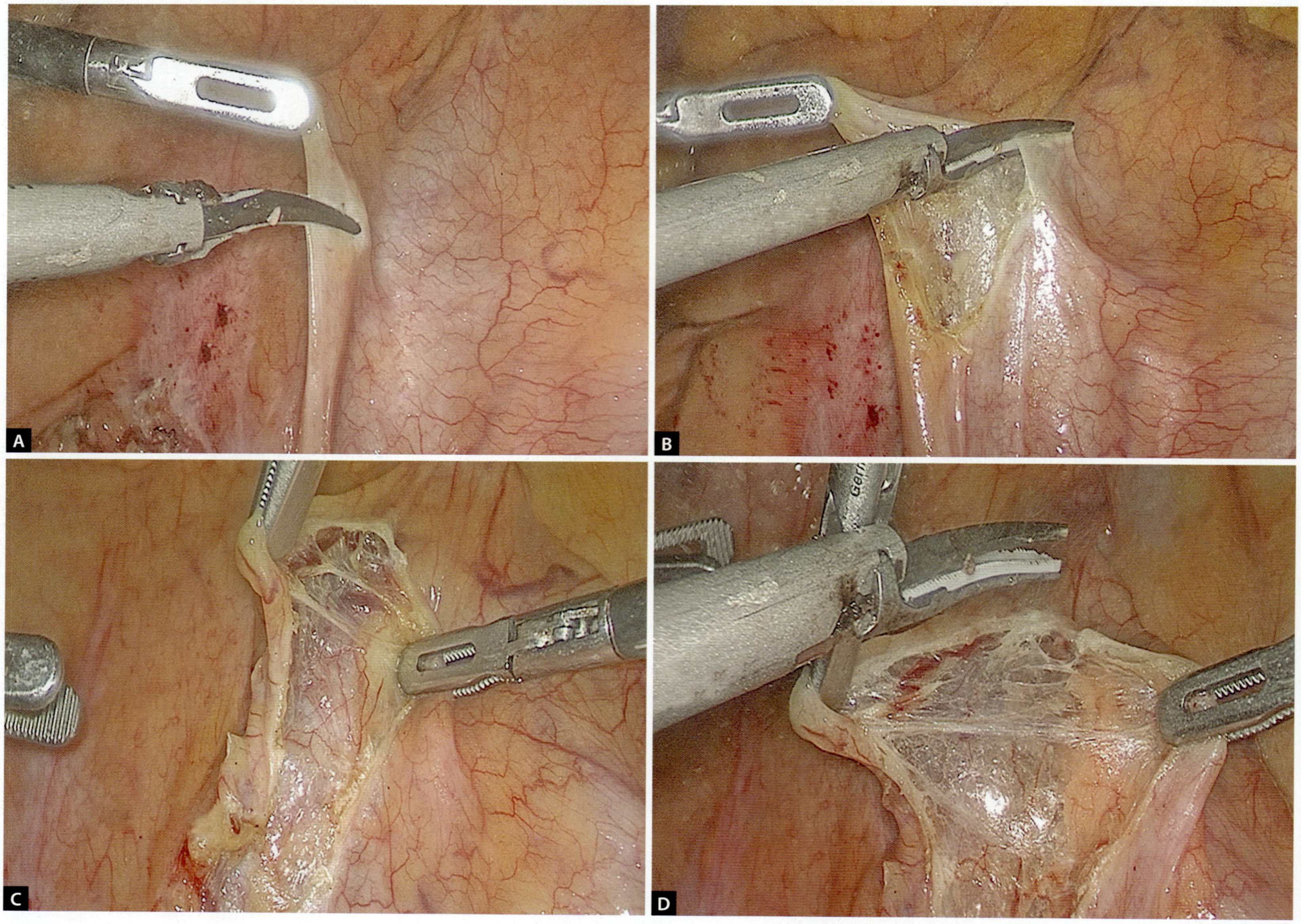

Figs. 20A to D

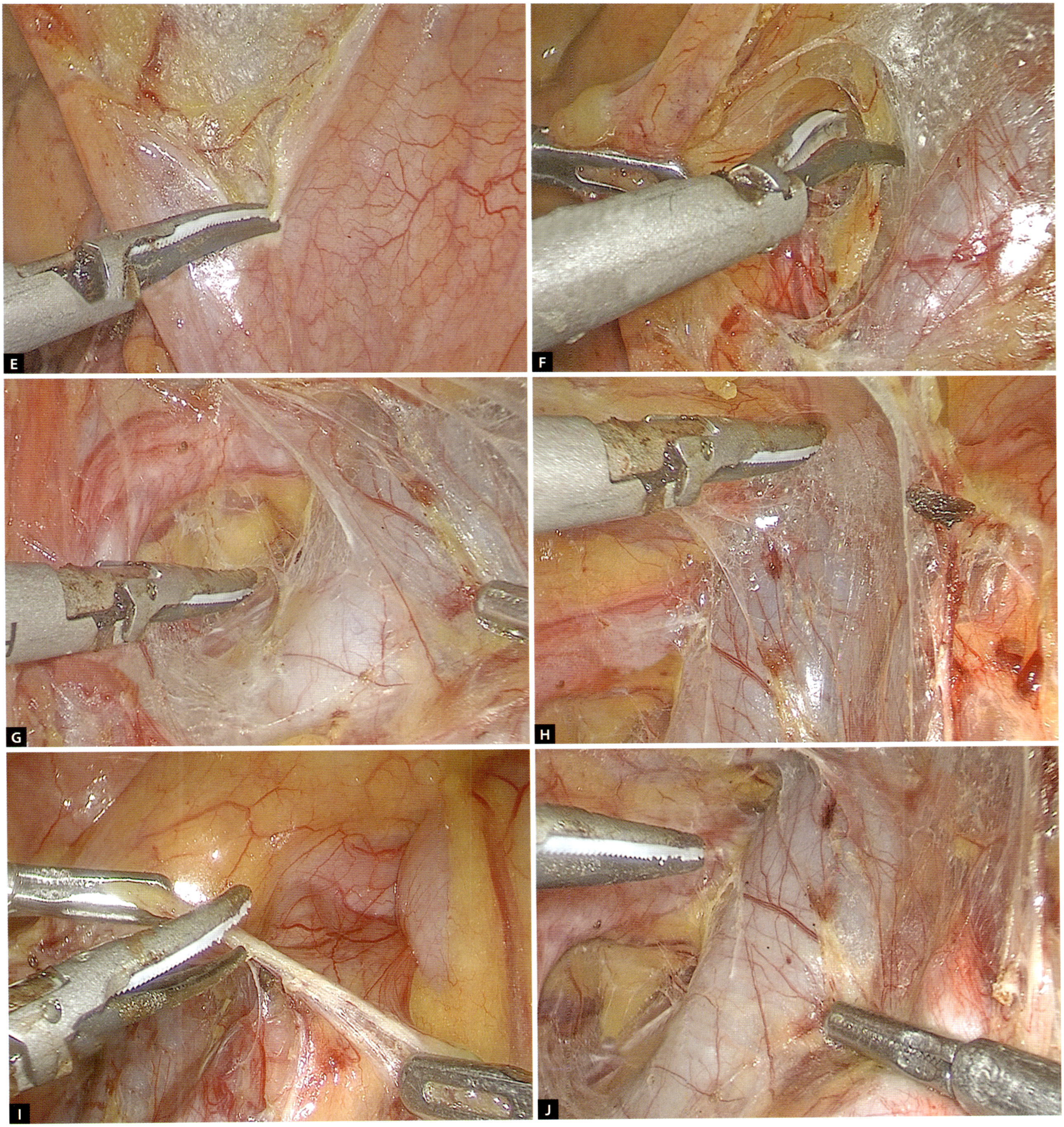

Figs. 20E to J

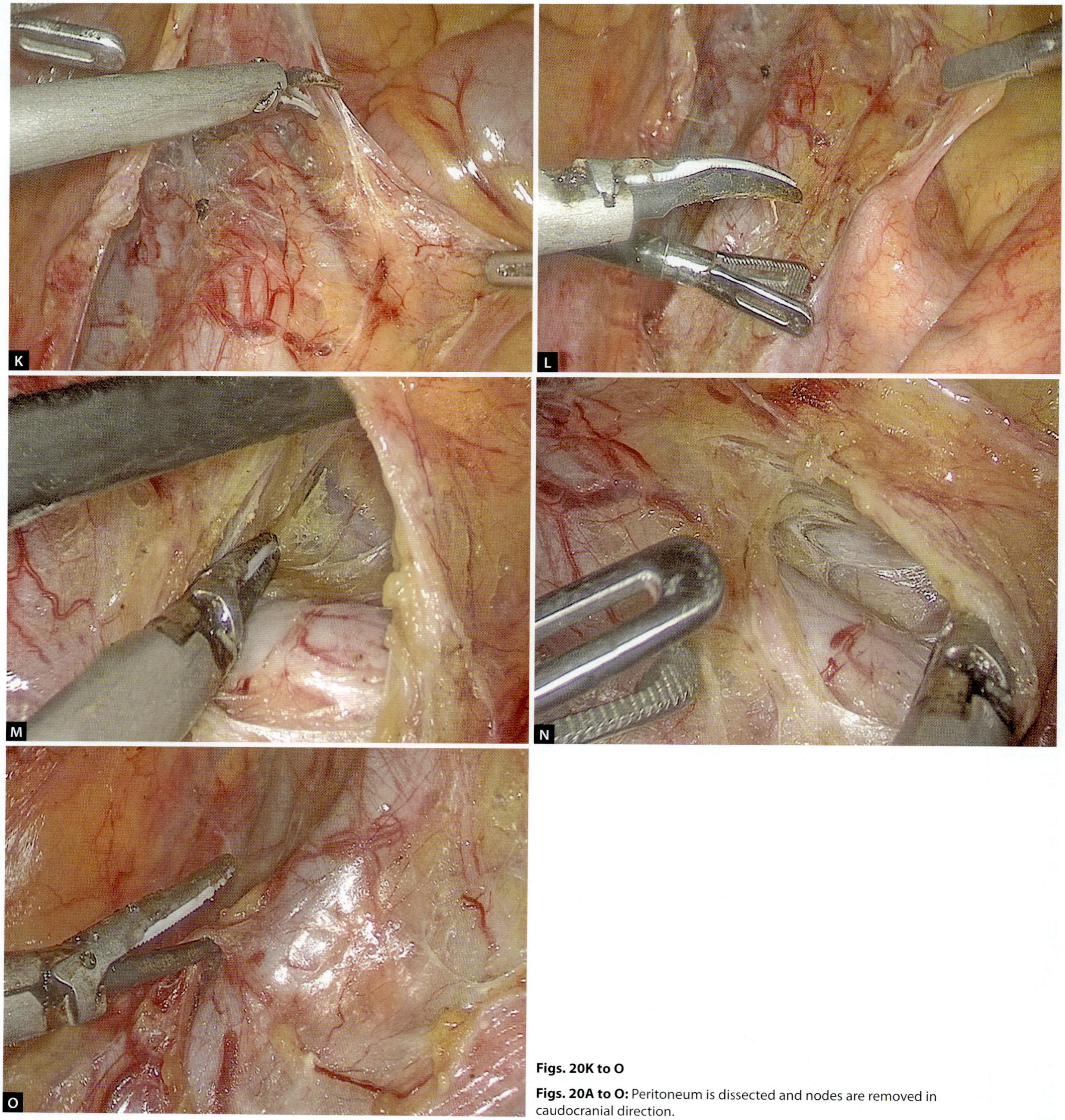

Figs. 20K to O

Figs. 20A to O: Peritoneum is dissected and nodes are removed in caudocranial direction.

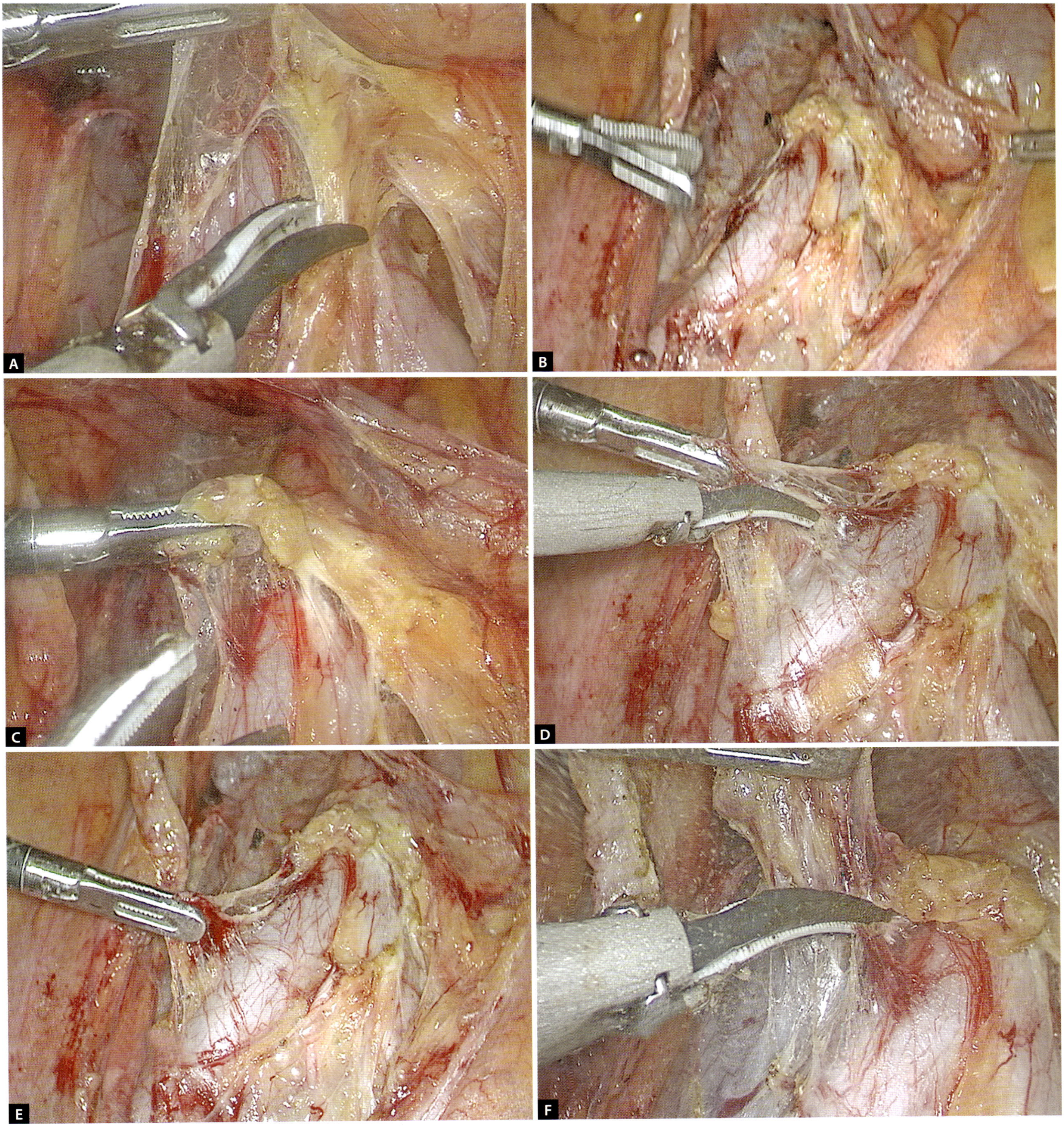

Figs. 21A to F

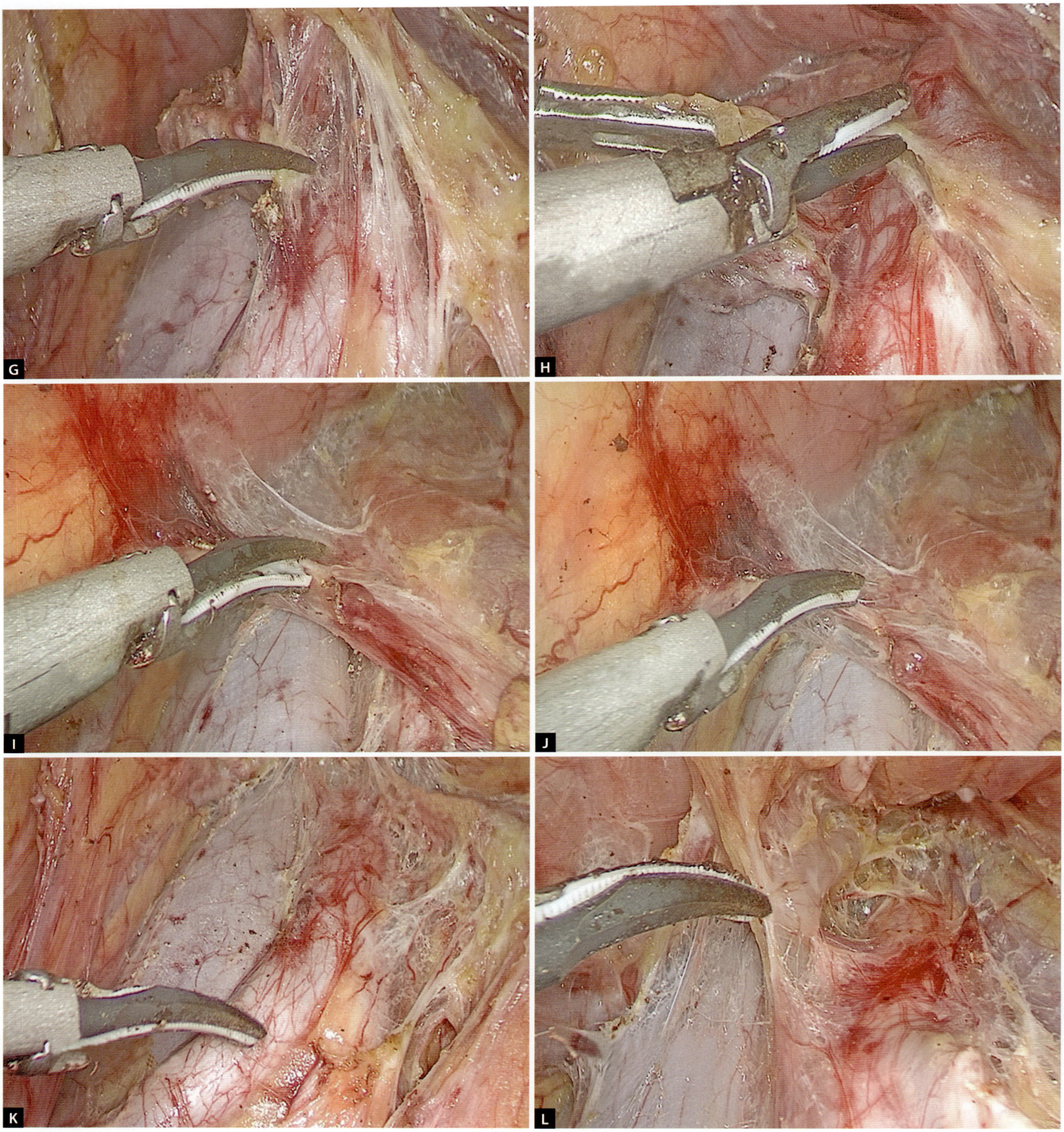

Figs. 21G to L

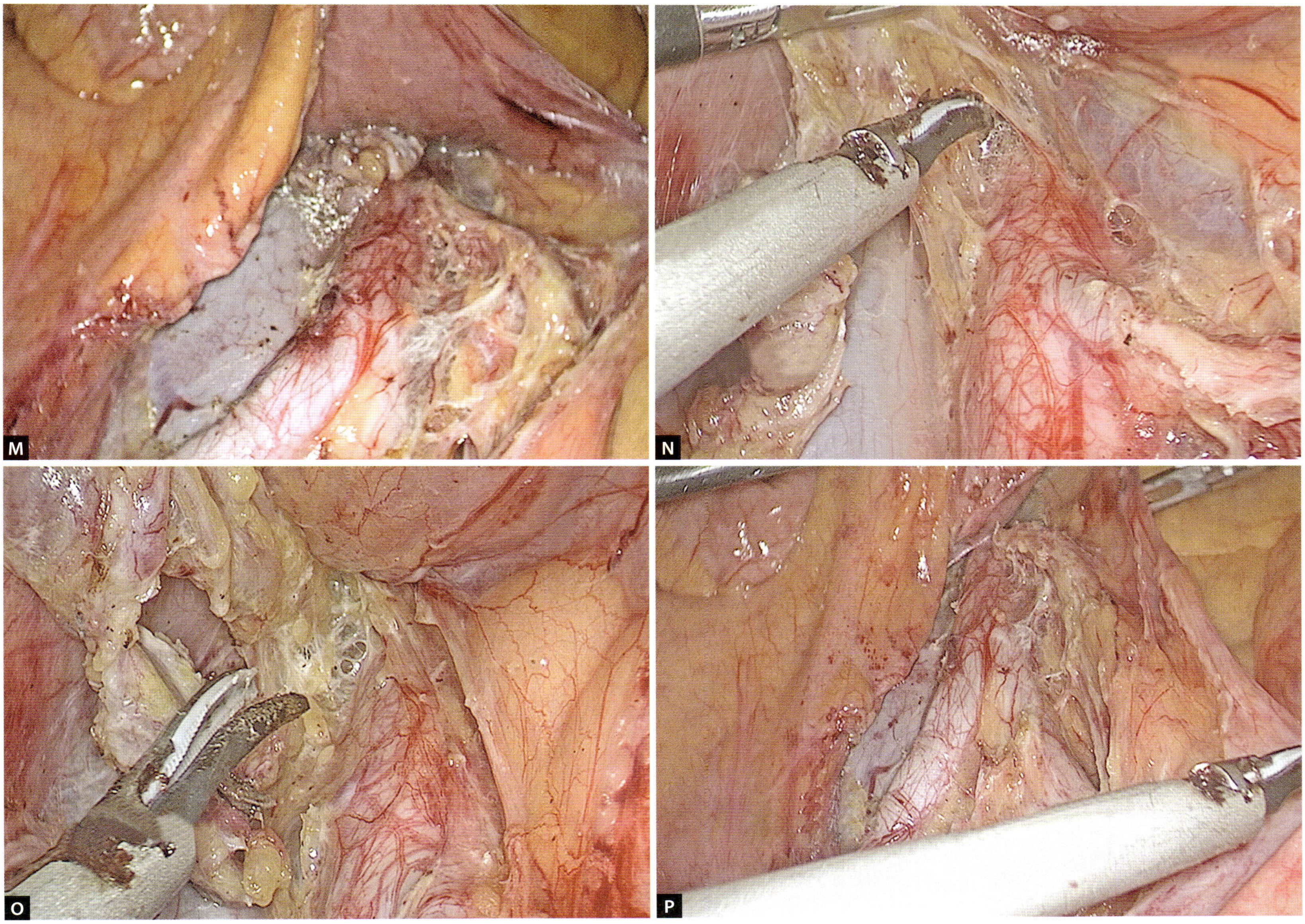

Figs. 21M to P

Figs. 21A to P: Para-aortic lymph nodes are removed

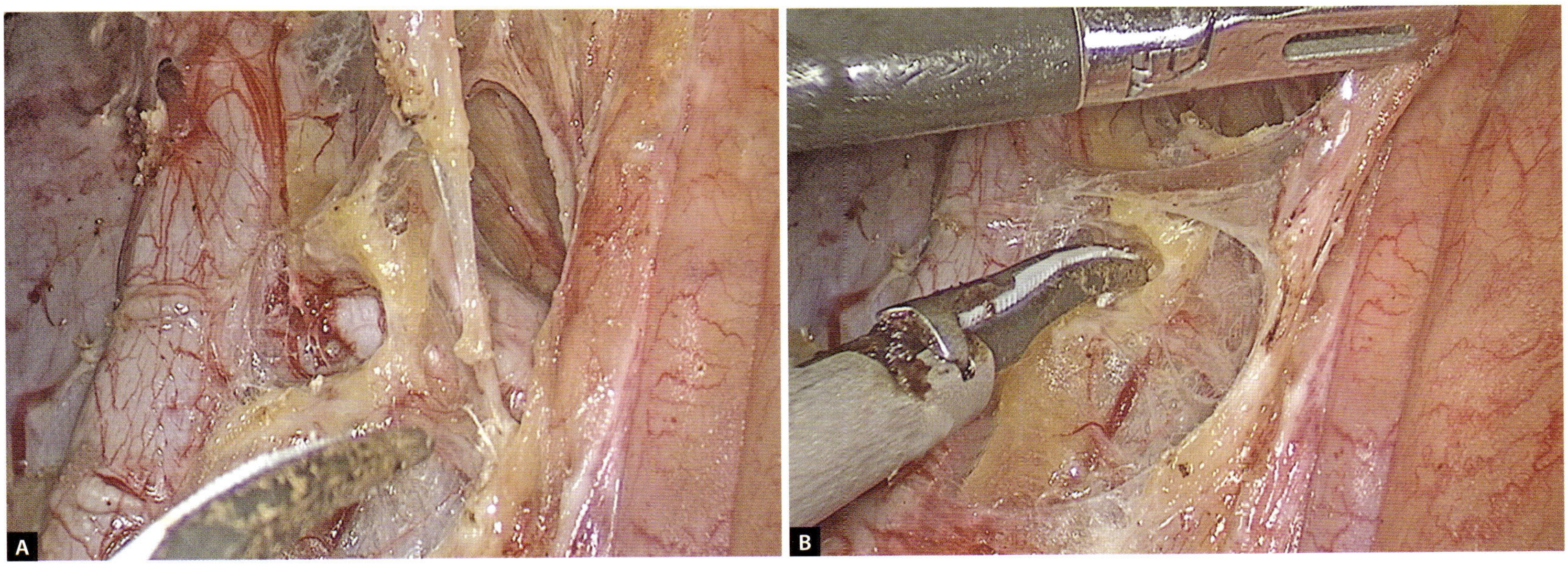

Figs. 22A and B

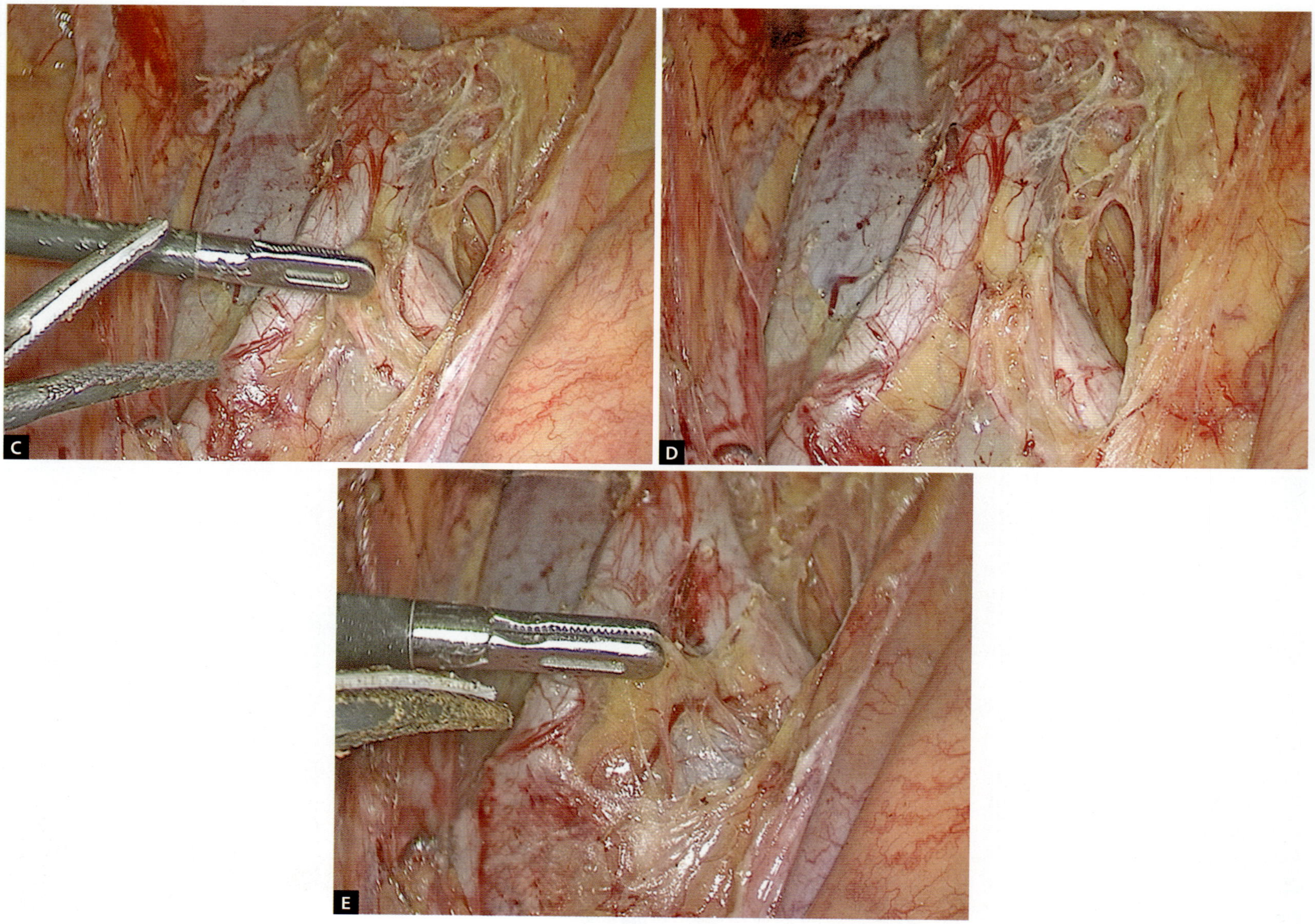

Figs. 22C to E

Figs. 22A to E: Preaortic group of lymph nodes are dissected in craniocaudal direction.

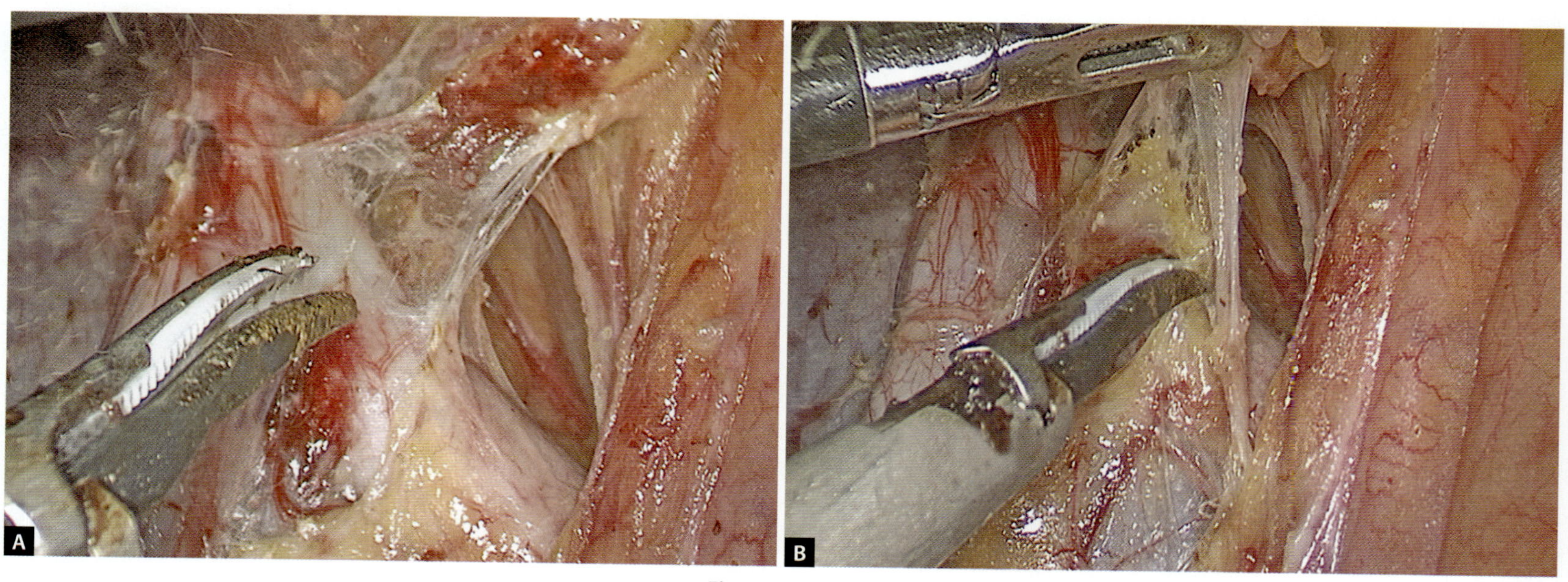

Figs. 23A and B

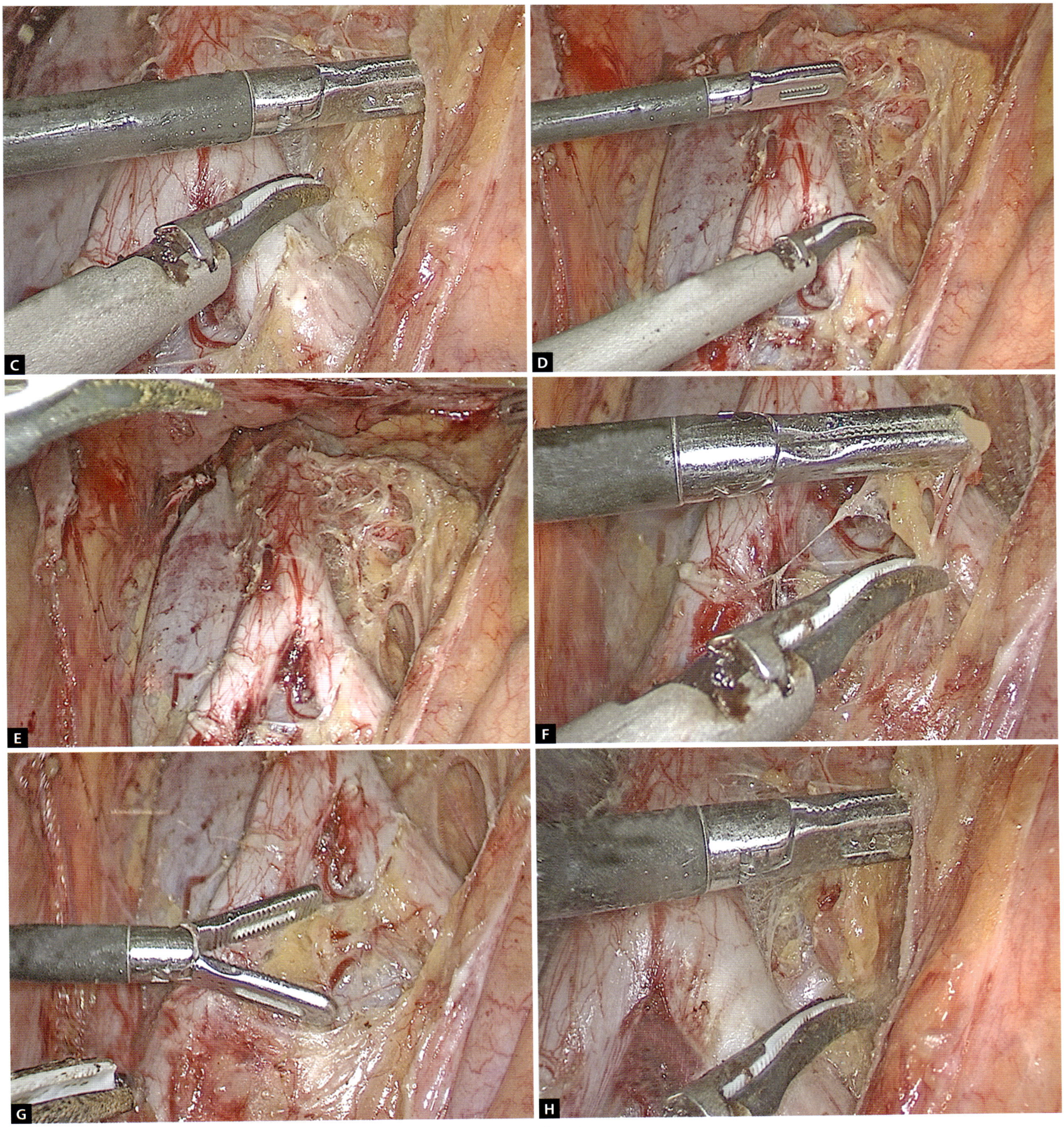

Figs. 23C to H

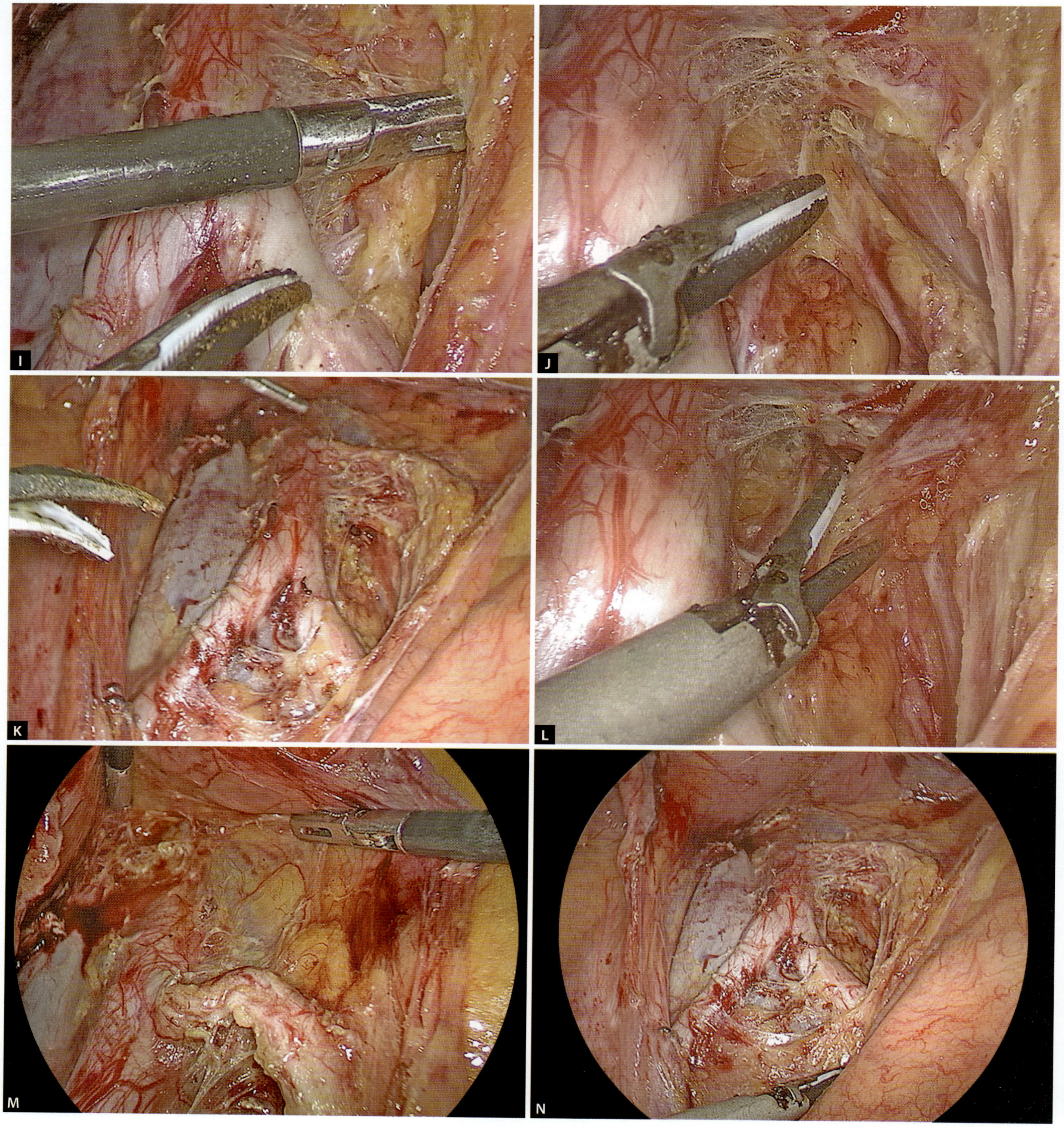

Figs. 23I to N

Figs. 23A to N: Aortocaval lymph nodes are dissected separate.

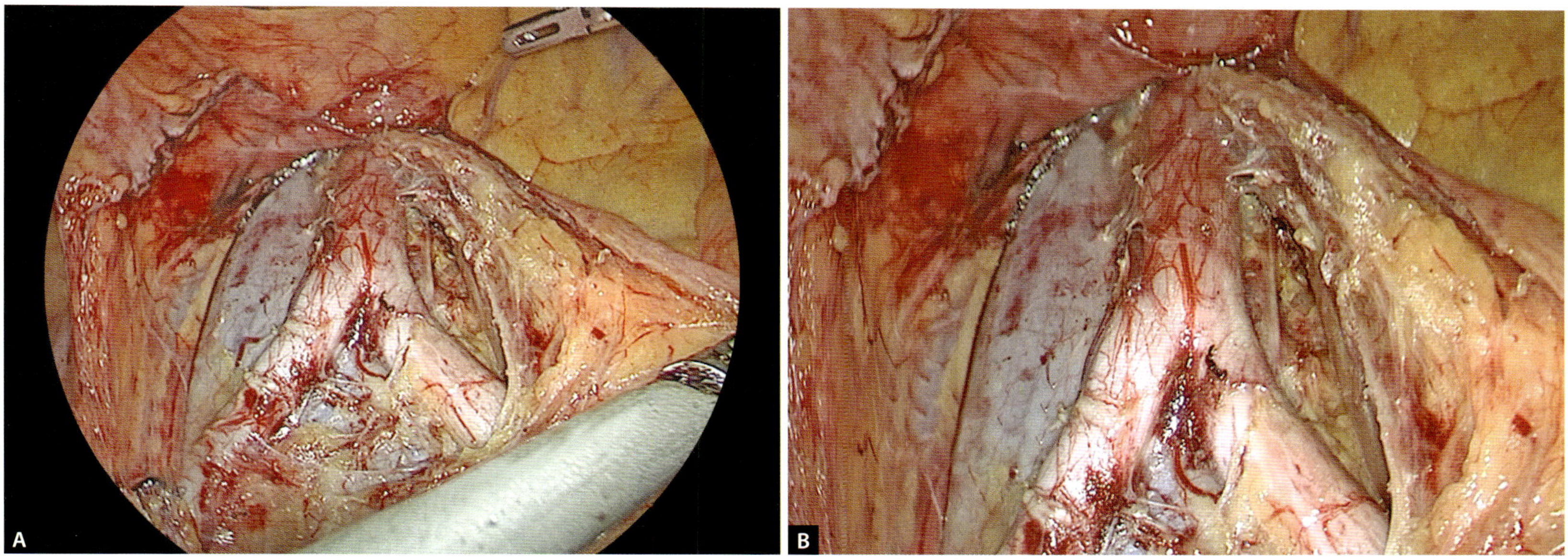

Figs. 24A and B: Bare aorta after complete dissection.

- Preaortic group of lymph nodes are dissected in craniocaudal direction **(Figs. 22A to E)**.
- Aortocaval lymph nodes are dissected separate **(Figs. 23A to N)**.
- The bare aorta after complete dissection **(Figs. 24A and B)**.

Accompanying Video: Laparoscopic radical hysterectomy.

CHAPTER

48

Pelvic Abscess

Tanvi Desai, Isha Rani, B Ramesh, Usha Rani G

DEFINITION

Pelvic abscess is a condition in which there is collection of purulent fluid walled off by inflammatory tissues in any part of the pelvis. In females it lies between the uterus and posterior fornix of vagina anteriorly and rectum posteriorly. In women of reproductive age group, as a complication of pelvic inflammatory disease, tubo-ovarian abscess may form. Tubo-ovarian abscess is an inflammatory mass involving the Fallopian tube and ovary.

EPIDEMIOLOGY

Following may be the predisposing factors for development of pelvic abscess:

- Childbirth or septic abortions
- Following operative interventions such as hysterectomy, dilation, and curettage, cervical cautery or surgery for ruptured tubal ectopic pregnancy
- Acute cervicitis or vaginitis
- Long-standing pelvic inflammatory disease
- Investigations for infertility like salpingogram
- Conditions involving the alimentary tract such as appendicitis, perforated peptic ulcer, Crohn's disease
- Diabetes mellitus, immunodeficiency.

SIGNS AND SYMPTOMS

- Bilateral pelvic and abdominal pain
- Foul smelling vaginal discharge
- Vaginal bleeding
- Pain increased on intercourse
- Malaise and high-grade fever (≥ 103°F)
- Nausea, vomiting, and anorexia
- Guarding and tenderness
- Cervical motion tenderness
- Diarrhea, tenesmus, discharge of mucus per rectum
- Rectal examination may reveal bulging of anterior rectal wall
- Increased frequency of micturition, dysuria
- Tachycardia
- Prostration
- Increased WBC count.

DIFFERENTIAL DIAGNOSIS

- Acute appendicitis
- Ectopic pregnancy
- Diverticulitis
- Perforated peptic ulcer
- Septic abortion.

INVESTIGATIONS

- CBC: Leukocytosis
- USG
- CT/MRI: These may be extremely useful in finding the origin of the abscess.

MANAGEMENT

- Requires urgent admission to hospital.
- Broad-spectrum anaerobic antibiotic coverage to be given, along with rest, fluid and electrolyte replacement.
- In case of failure of medical management as indicated by persistent fever, increasing size of abscess, persistent ileus surgical management will be required **(Figs. 1 to 10)**.
- Posterior colpotomy is preferred to laparotomy **(Figs. 2 and 4 to 8)**.
- Aspiration and drainage of abscess under ultrasound guidance can be done in females vaginally **(Fig. 3)**.
- Percutaneous transgluteal aspiration and drainage of abscess can be done under CT guidance.
- Evidence supporting drainage of abscess by endoscopic approach under ultrasound guidance is increasing.

PROGNOSIS

It is almost impossible to preserve function of Fallopian tubes in developing tubal abscess.

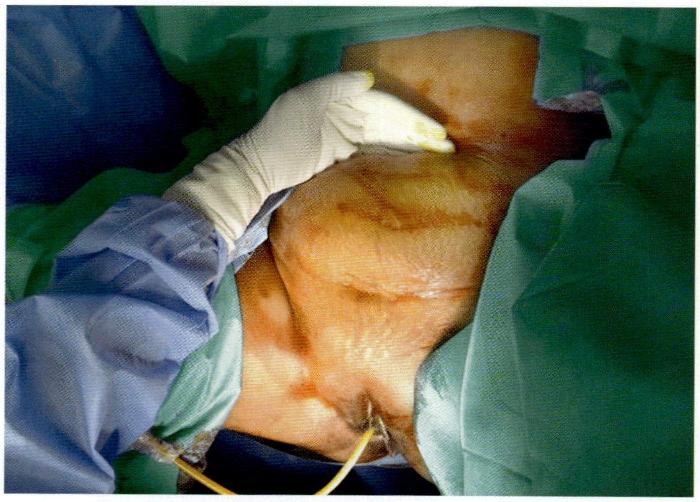

Fig. 1: Per abdomen examination in a patient with POD abscess.

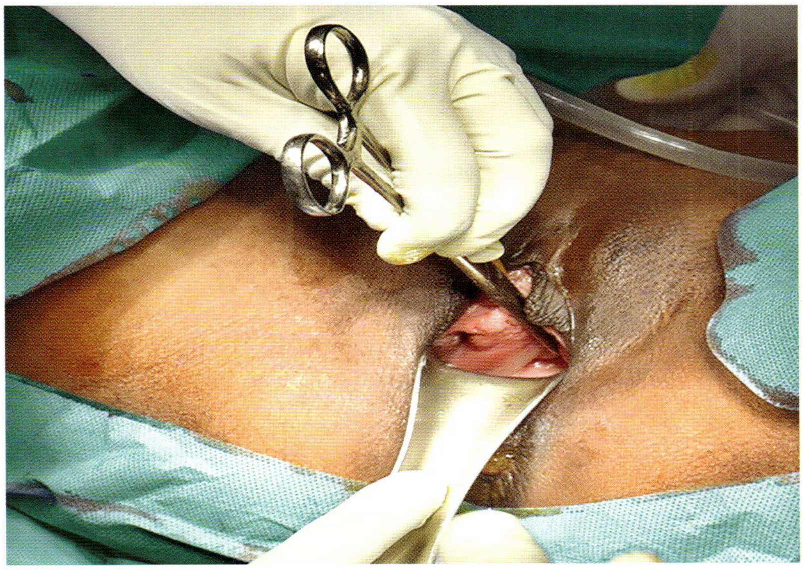

Fig. 2: Per speculum examination to plan for colpotomy.

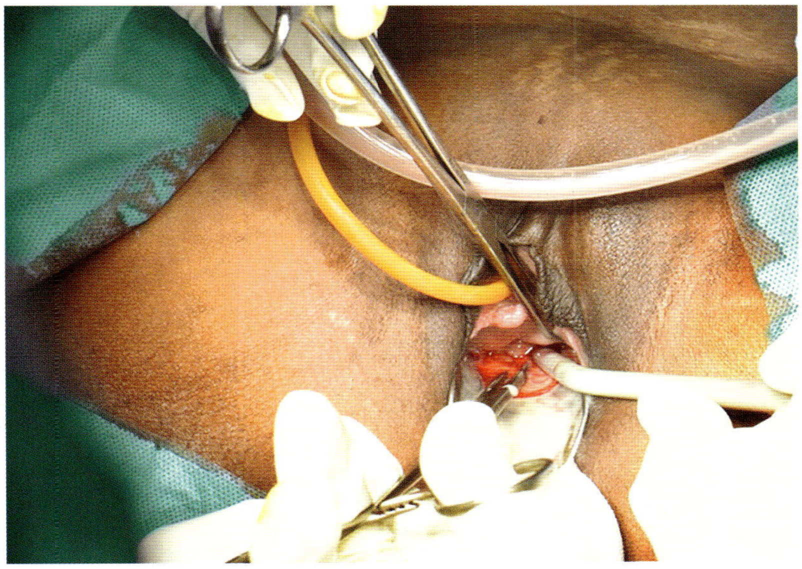

Fig. 5: The POD abscess being drained through posterior colpotomy using suction cannula.

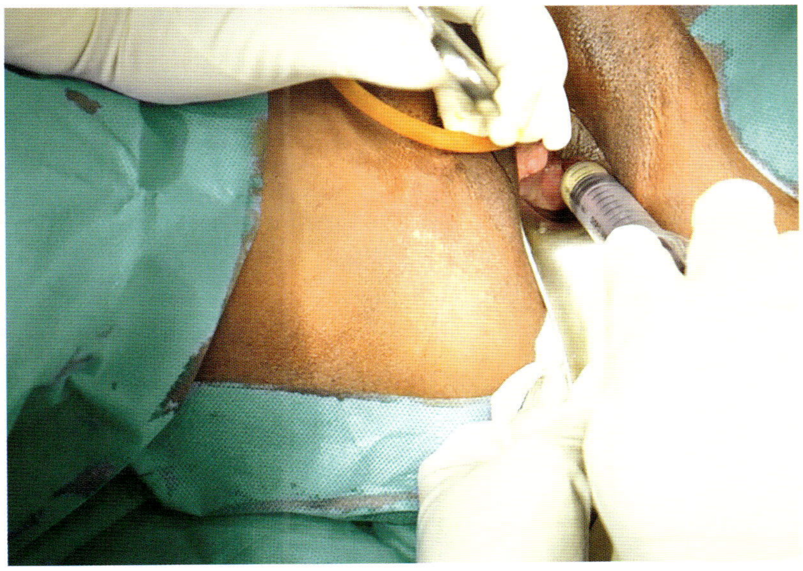

Fig. 3: Aspiration of polycystic ovarian disease (POD) abscess through posterior vaginal fornix.

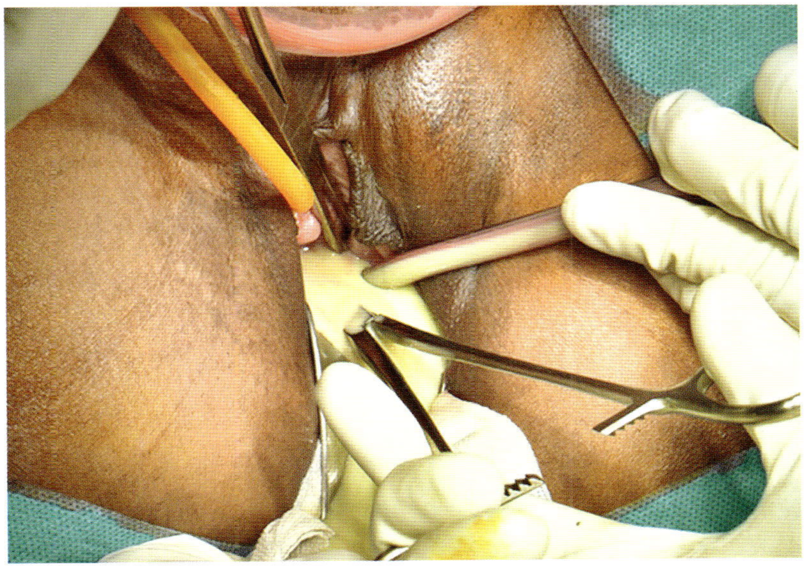

Fig. 6: Colpotomy incision being extended with artery forceps to drain the abscess.

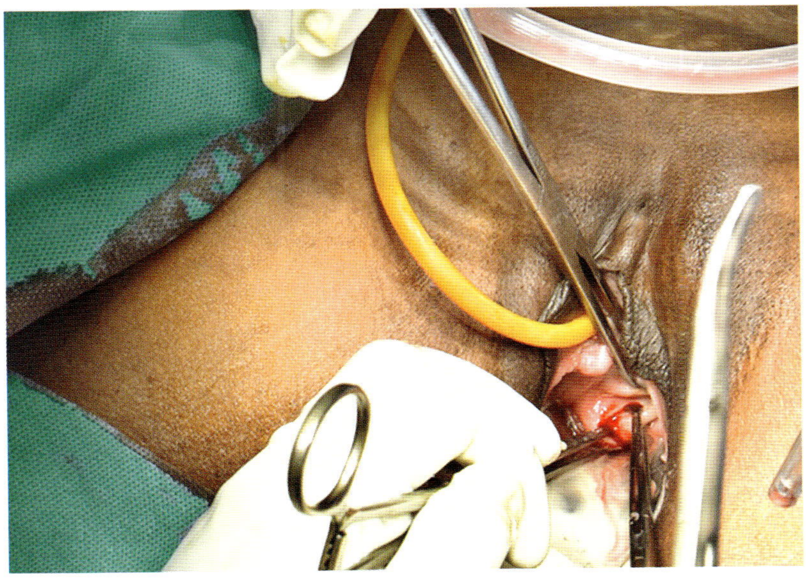

Fig. 4: Posterior colpotomy being done.

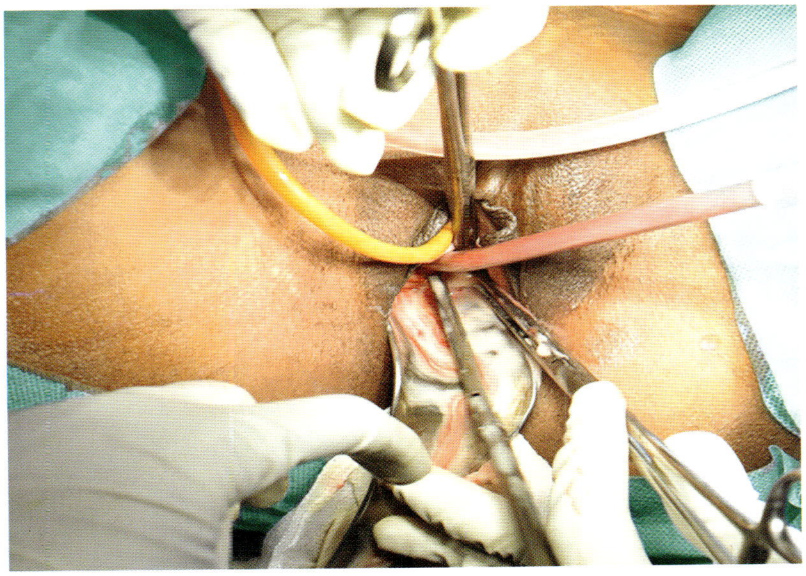

Fig. 7: The POD abscess being drained.

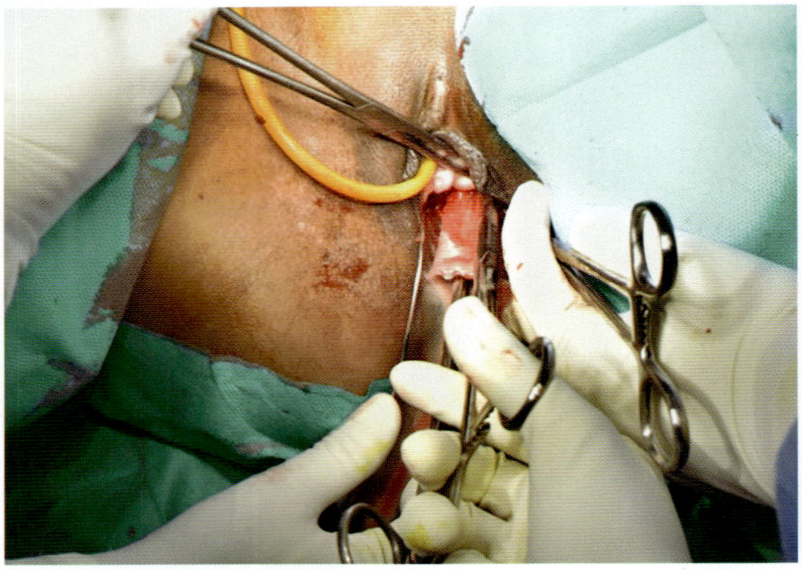

Fig. 8: Drain kept in POD through posterior colpotomy incision.

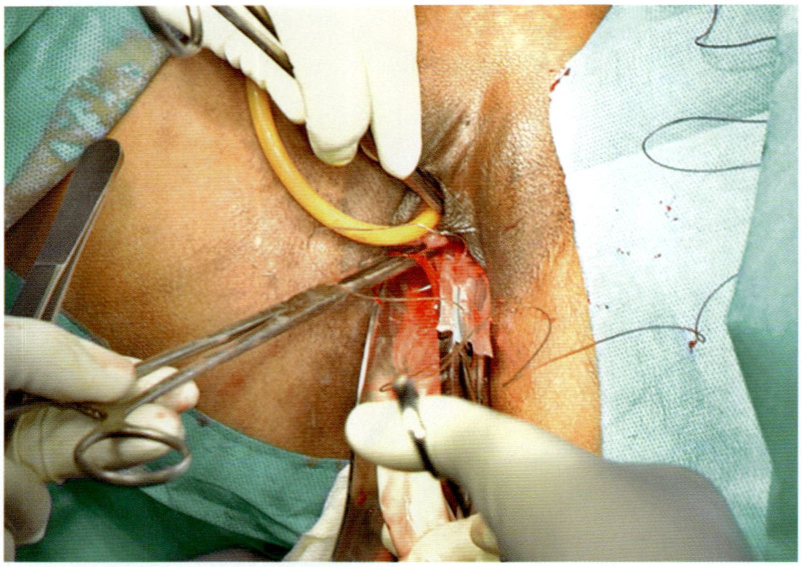

Fig. 9: Drain being sutured in place.

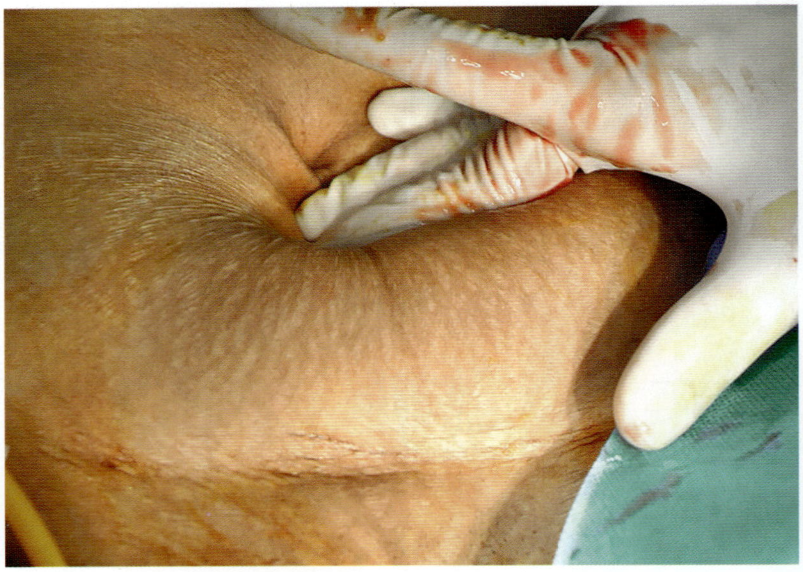

Fig. 10: On per abdomen examination—decrease in size of abdominal mass noted.

SUGGESTED READING

1. Benigno BB. Medical and surgical management of the pelvic abscess. Clin Obstet Gynecol. 1981;24(4):1187-97.
2. Gervais DA, Brown SD, Connolly SA, et al. Percutaneous imaging-guided abdominal and pelvic abscess drainage in children. Radiographics. 2004;24(3):737-54.
3. Hadithi M, Bruno MJ. Endoscopic ultrasound-guided drainage of pelvic abscess: a case series of 8 patients. World J Gastrointest Endosc. 2014; 166(8):373-8.
4. Prasad GA, Varadarajulu S. Endoscopic ultrasound-guided abscess drainage. Gastrointest Endosc Clin N Am. 2012;22(2):281-90.
5. Robert B, Chivot C, Fuks D, et al. Percutaneous, computed tomography-guided drainage of deep pelvic abscesses via a transgluteal approach: a report on 30 cases and a review of the literature. Abdom Imaging. 2013;38(2): 285-9.
6. Saokar A, Arellano RS, Gervais DA, et al. Transvaginal drainage of pelvic fluid collections: results, expectations, and experience. AJR Am J Roentgenol. 2008;191(5):1352-8.
7. Sudakoff GS, Lundeen SJ, Otterson MF. Transrectal and transvaginal sonographic intervention of infected pelvic fluid collections: a complete approach. Ultrasound Q. 2005;21(3):175-85.

CHAPTER

49

Uterus Transplant

B Ramesh, Shailesh Puntambekar, Aditi Rai

INTRODUCTION

Patients with absolute uterine factor infertility have only option of adoption or surrogacy, with the advent of uterine transplant these patients can have legal and gestational motherhood.

Uterine transplant surgery is a complex procedure involving harvesting and retrieval of uterus from donor, graft preparation and fixation, and vascular anastomosis in the recipient. An end-to-end anastomosis between donor and recipient internal iliac arteries increases the chances of success.[1]

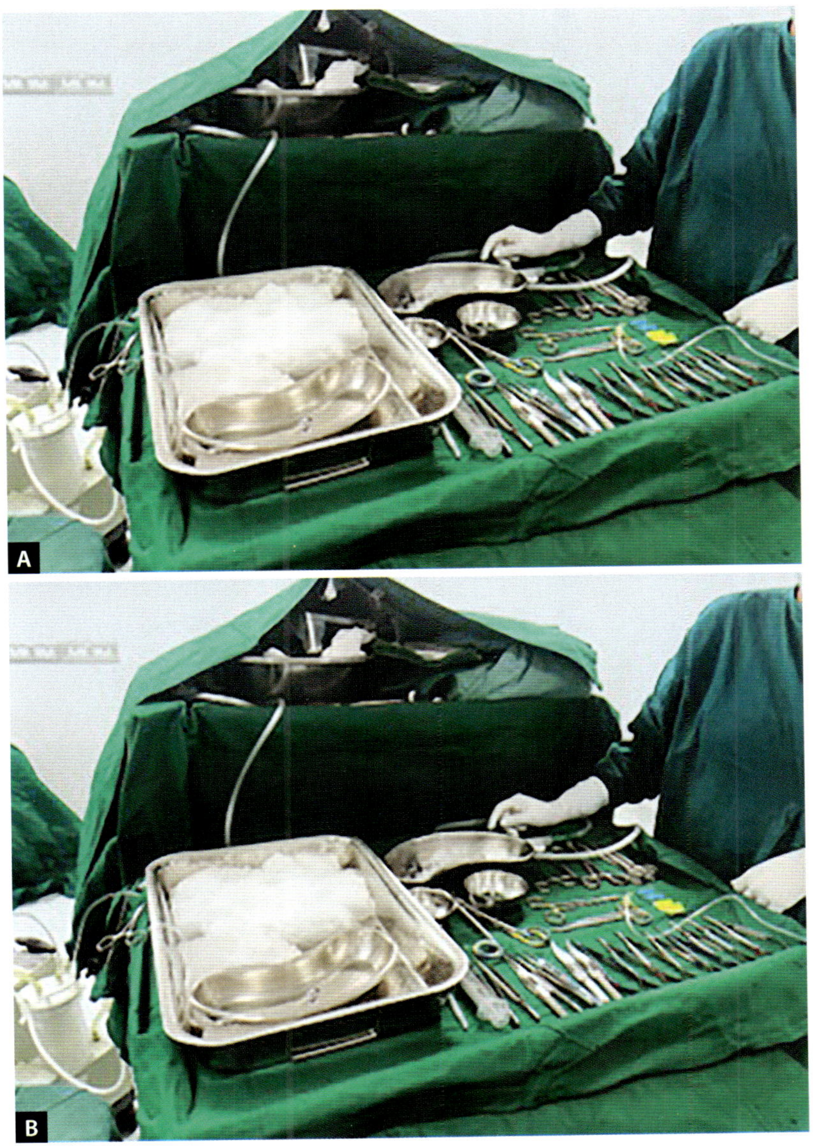

Figs. 1A and B: Instruments for transplant.

RECIPIENT SELECTION

- Less than 35 years
- Absolute uterine factor infertility
- Healthy hormone profile
- Psychological well-being.

DONOR SELECTION

- Less than 50 years and menstruating
- Absence of vascular disorders
- Good uterine blood flow.

TECHNIQUE

Organ Harvest Surgery

Dissection is done laparoscopically and at the end, the uterus is retrieved by open method. Three-dimensional (3D) laparoscope gives best vision and depth for dissection and four to five 5-mm ports are placed in the lower abdomen.

A stitch with Vicryl 1-0 is placed on the fundus for manipulation. First infundibular pelvic ligaments are isolated retroperitoneally and ovarian artery and veins are separated from the surrounding tissue. Next pararectal and paravesical spaces are dissected uterine to the

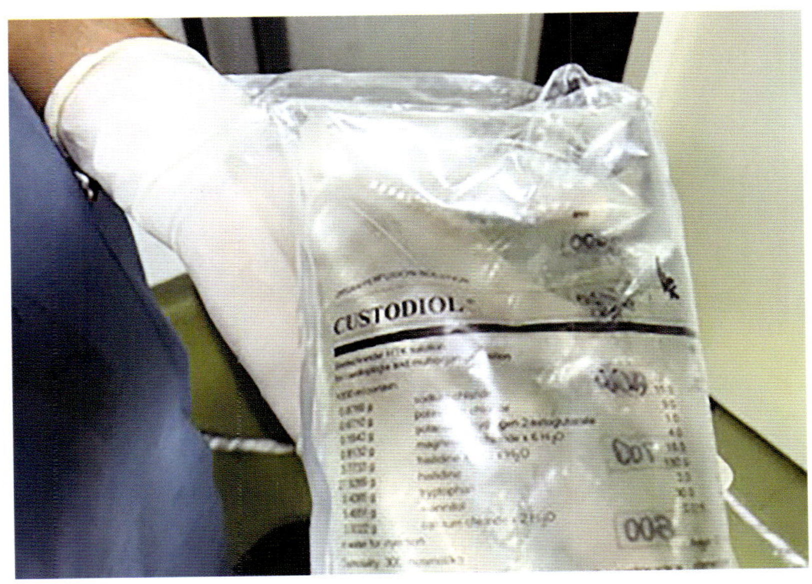

Fig. 2: HTK solution.

levator ani muscle by opening the broad ligament. The uterine artery was traced from its origin up to its insertion in the uterus. All the small branches of the uterine artery were dissected and clipped. The rectovaginal space was opened up to the pelvic floor. The bladder is completely dissected from the uterus and the cervix. Uterine veins were identified and clipped. The ureter is completely dissected from the pelvic brim to its entry into the bladder. The anterior branch of internal iliac artery is dissected from its origin. The internal iliac artery distal to the origin of the uterine artery was clipped and cut, the endopelvic fascia or the ligaments were then cut, and the uterosacral ligaments

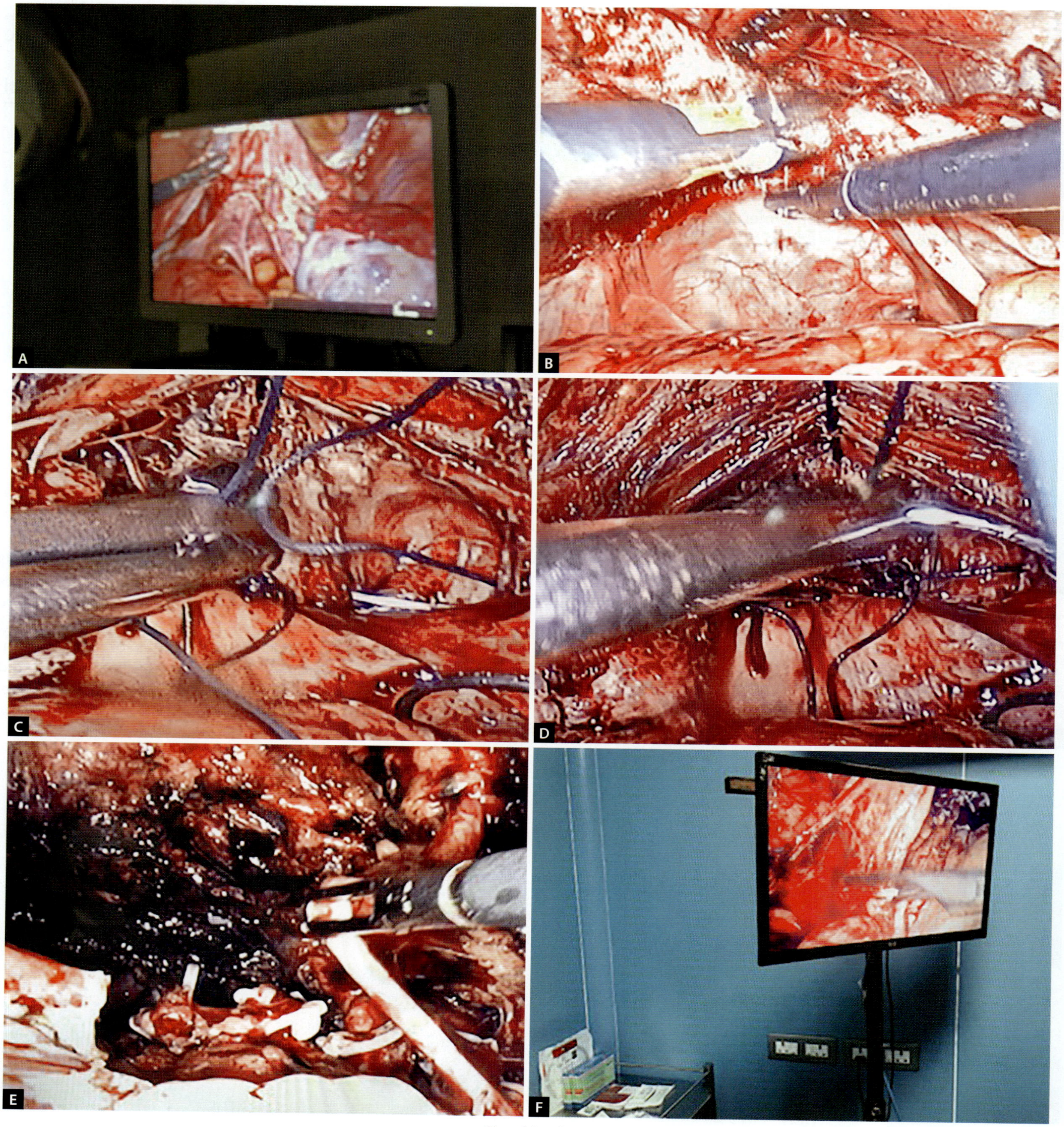

Figs. 3A to F

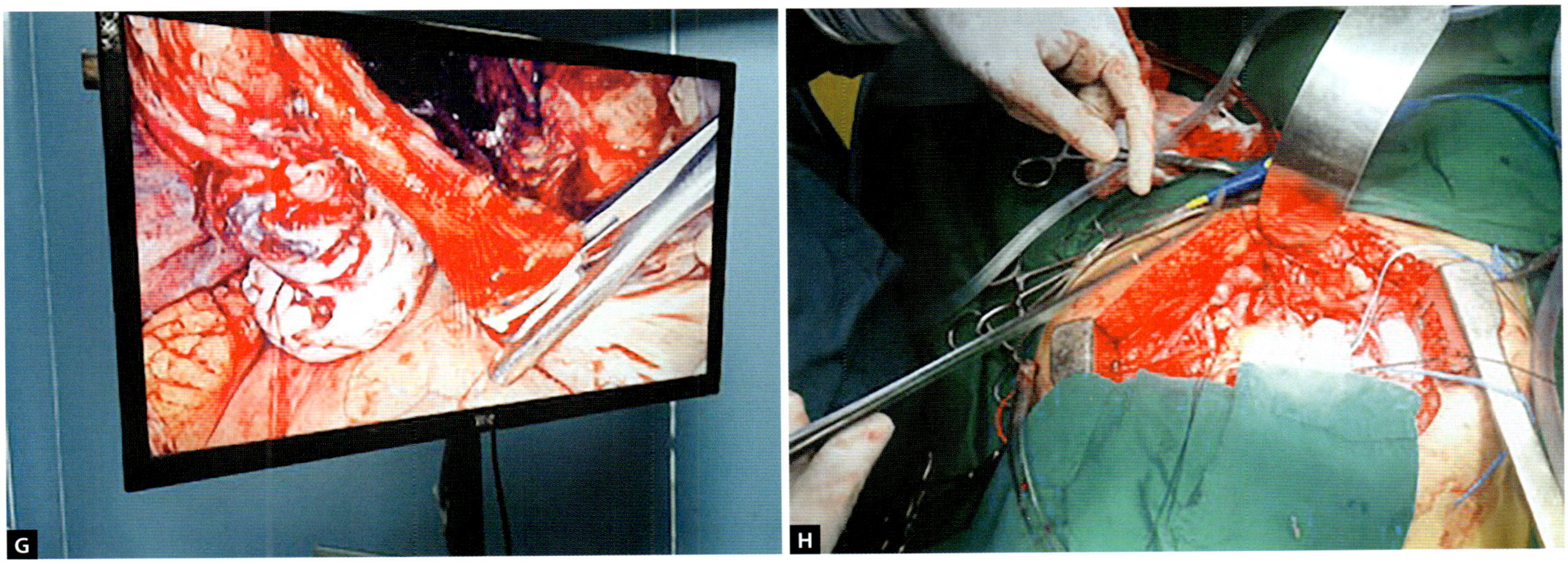

Figs. 3G and H

Figs. 3A to H: Donor surgery.

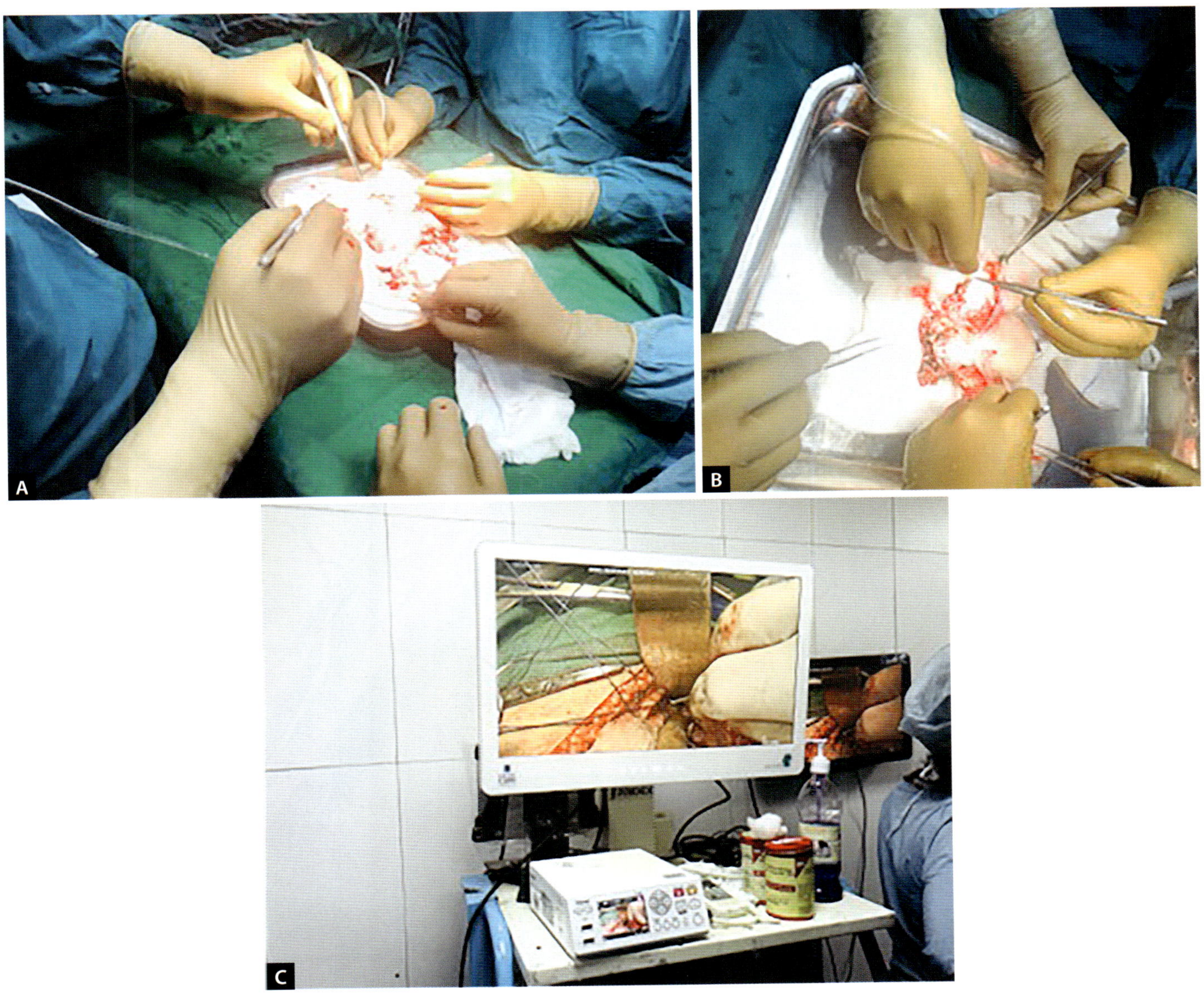

Figs. 4A to C: Bench surgery.

were cut approximately 2 cm away from the attachment of the uterus. Adequate length of the vagina is obtained by dissection. Colpotomy is done circumferentially. Small Pfannenstiel incision done and infundibulopelvic (IP) ligament clipped and cut and uterus retrieved. The retrieved uterus along with vascular pedicles was transported on a tray of ice for bench surgery. The abdomen was closed.

Recipient Surgery

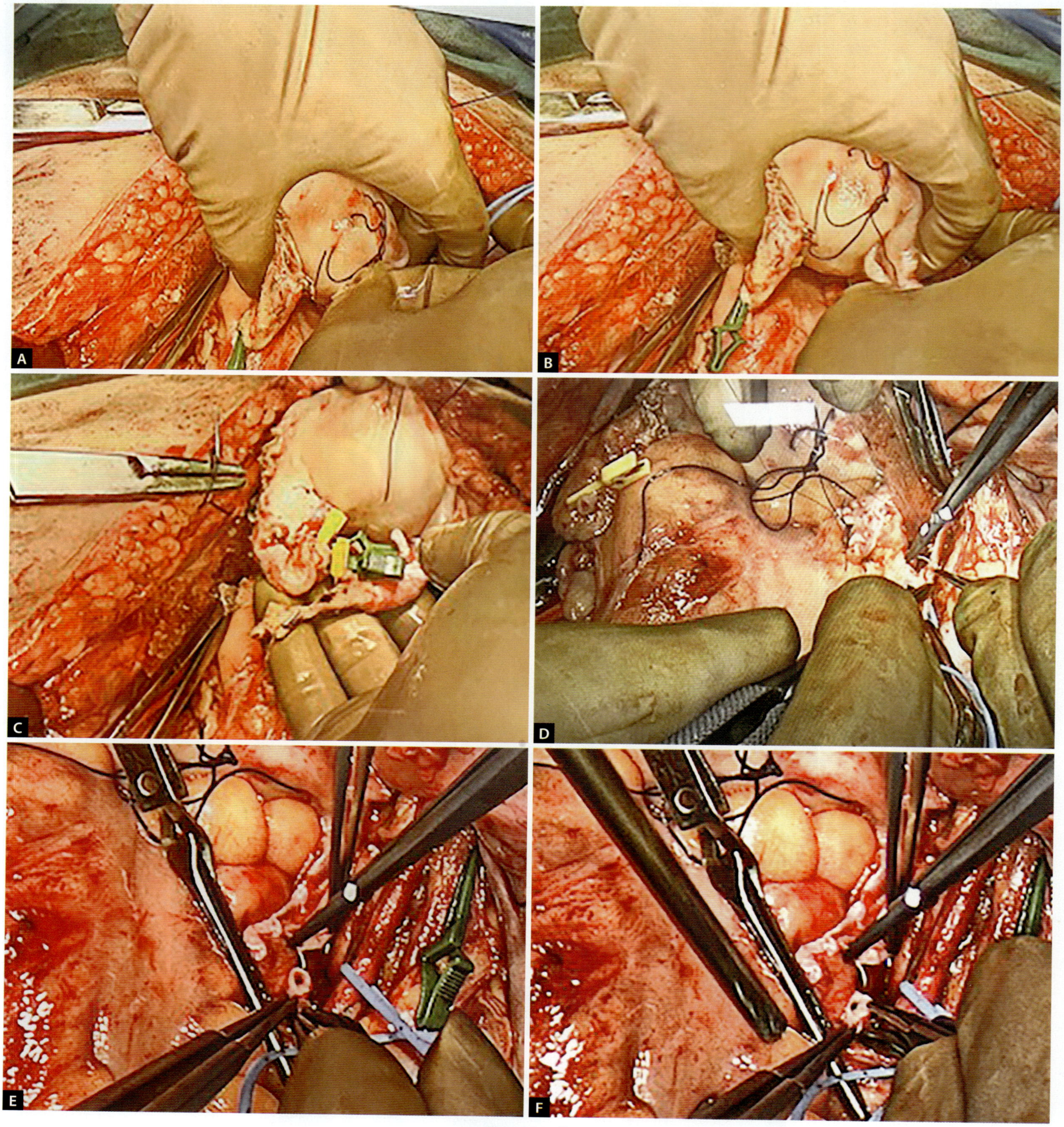

Figs. 5A to F

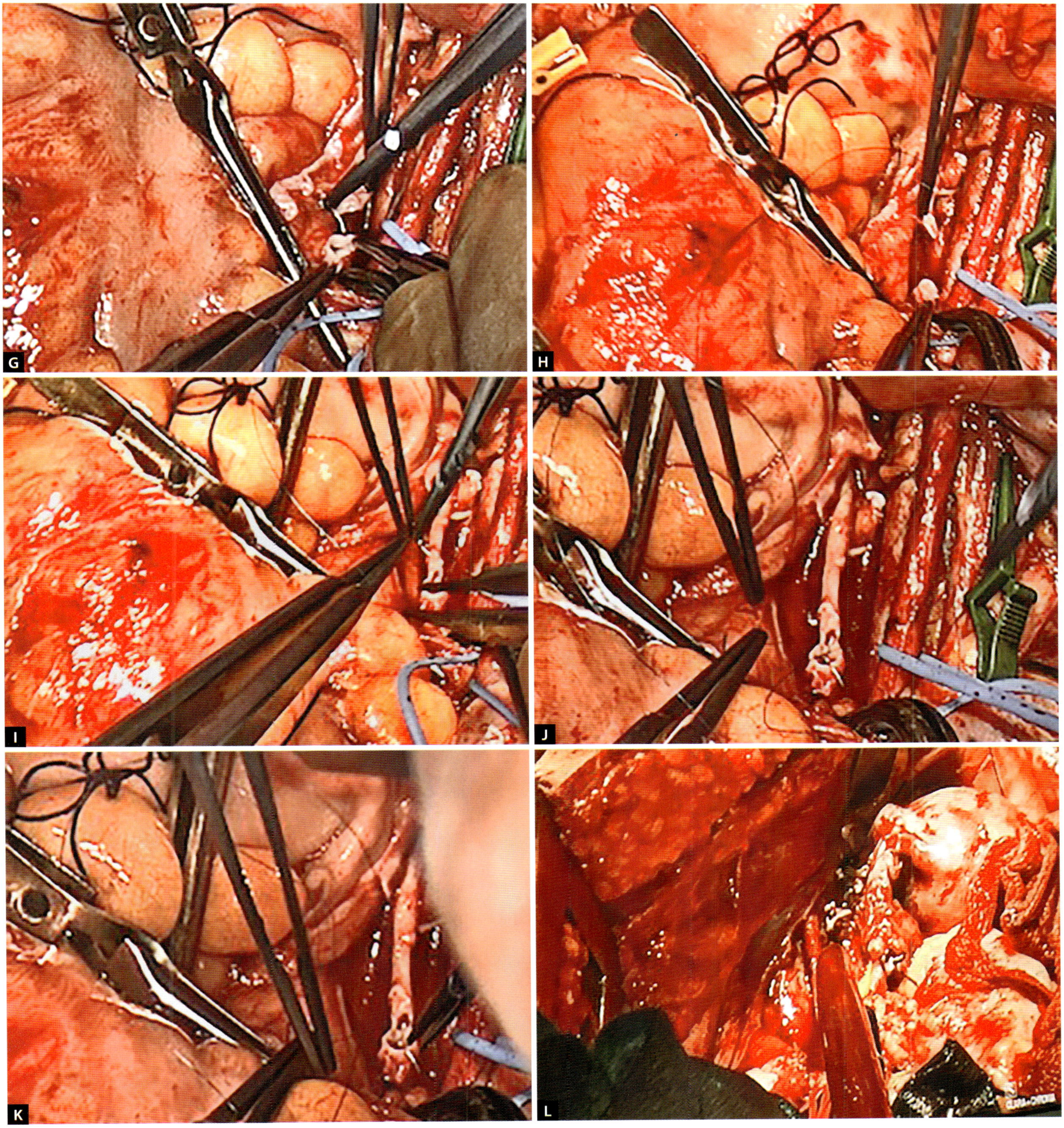

Figs. 5G to L

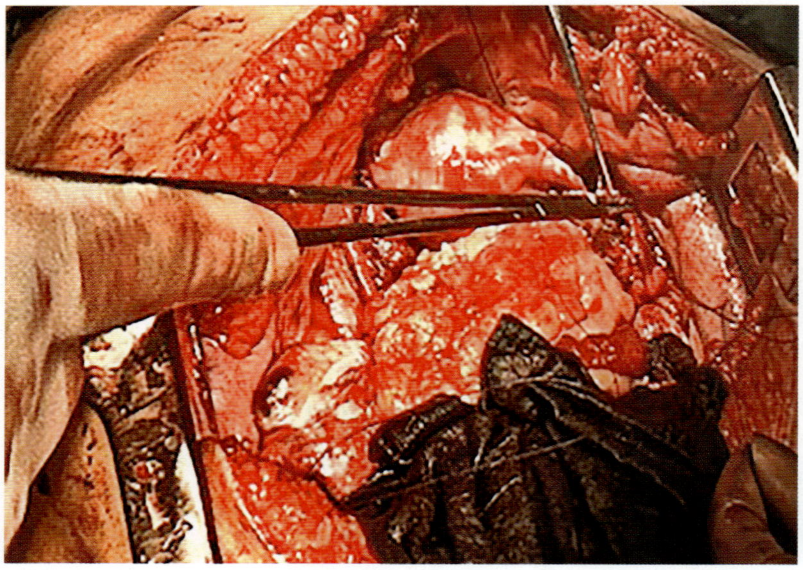

Fig. 5M

Figs. 5A to M: Recipient surgery.

Bench Surgery

The uterus was cleaned and washed with cold histidine-tryptophan-ketoglutarate (HTK) solution. The vessels were cannulated and blood flushed and all vessel leaks sealed.

Transplant Surgery

Recipient pelvis is prepared laparoscopically, with harmonic peritoneal incision made for one round ligament to other, the bladder and rectum separated from the midline creating space, uterine buds were excised. Ureters are dissected and external iliac vessels and internal iliac are dissected. Now laparotomy is done and donor uterus was placed in the pelvic cavity in an orthotropic position. The ovarian veins were anastomosed to external iliac veins in an end to side manner using prolene 7.0 continuous suture under operating loupe. End-to-end anastomosis between donor and recipient internal iliac arteries was performed with prolene 7.0 bilaterally. All soft tissues and ligaments are correspondingly sutured and approximated.

POSTOPERATIVE CARE OF RECIPIENT

Monitoring in ICU, blood texts, uterine Doppler, inspection of cervix, and cervical biopsy are done to rule out rejection. Appropriate immunosuppressants administered.

REFERENCE

1. Puntambekar S, Puntambekar S, Telang M, et al. Novel anastomotic technique for uterine transplant using utero-ovarian veins for venous drainage and internal iliac arteries for perfusion in two laparoscopically harvested uteri. J Minim Invasive Gynecol. 2019;26(4):628-35.

2

SECTION

Hysteroscopy

CHAPTER

50

Hysteroscopy Instruments

Shubhanjali Sen, G Hemasree, B Ramesh

These **Figures 1A and B** are depicting the evolution of the hysteroscopic approach and the ease of video hysteroscopy which helps in seeing the pathology and treating the pathology at one sitting with a proper documentation, i.e. "see and treat".

EQUIPMENT

Hysteroscope (Figs. 2 and 3)

Hysteroscopes come in two main configurations: (1) rigid and (2) flexible.

Stainless steel barrel houses a series of rod lens system. It consists of distal objective lens that captures and focuses the image and proximal set of lens prepares the image for final viewing.

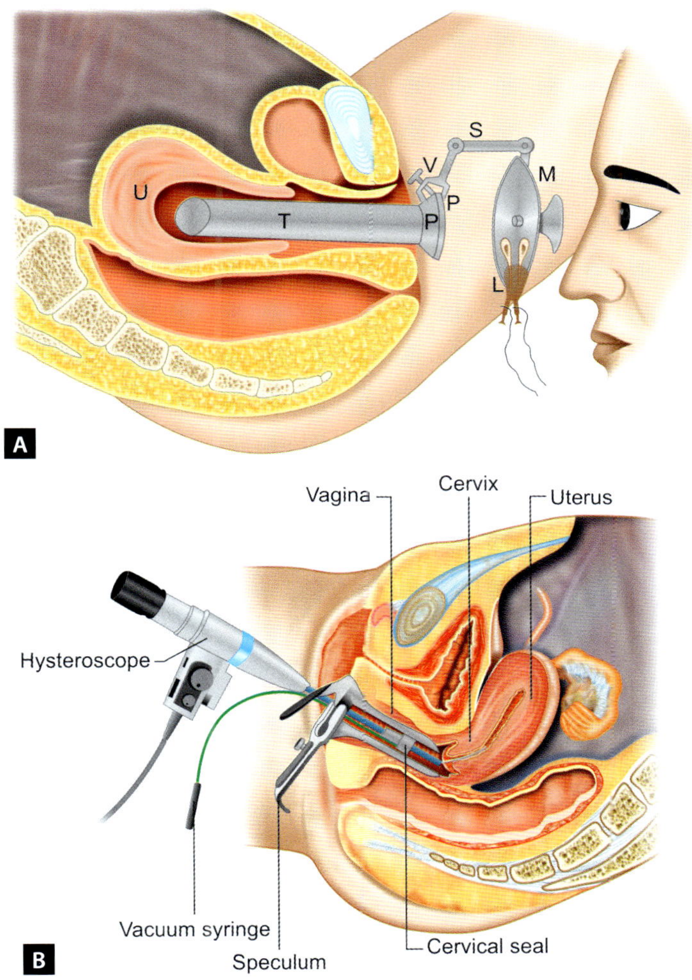

Figs. 1A and B: Evolution of the hysteroscopic approach and the ease of video hysteroscopy.

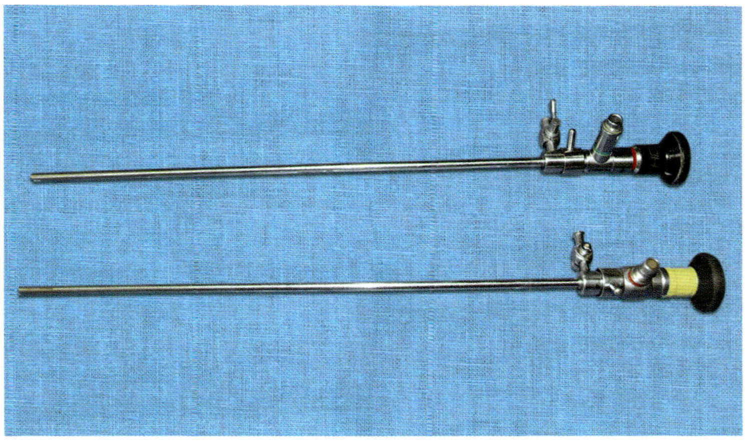

Fig. 2: Rigid hysteroscope with 30° viewing angle.

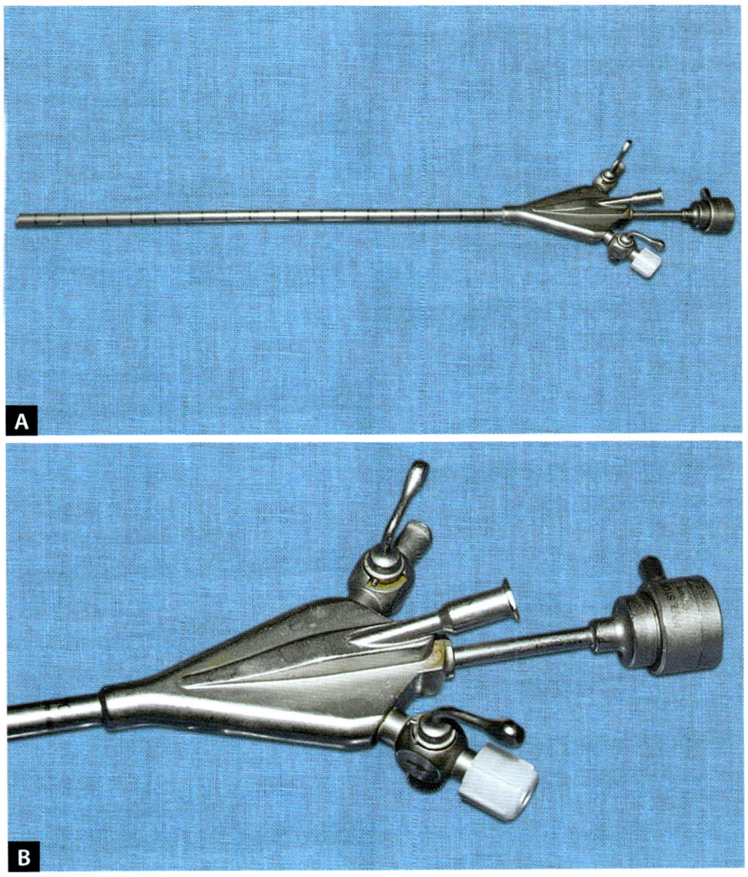

Figs. 3A and B: Hysteroscope with integrated inner and outer sheath.

It includes outer sheath which surrounds channels for telescope, distending media inflow and outflow and operative instruments. Operative sheaths have single ports or dual ports which have a continuous laminar flow of distending media to clear blood and thus it improves the visualization, and irrigation channel.

Advanced operative sheaths have three channels, two for operative instruments and one for instilling distention media.

Office Hysteroscope

- 2.9 mm Bettocchi hysteroscope
- 2 mm trophyscope (Campo contact hysteroscope)
- Campo Trophyscope 2.9 mm with office continuous flow operative sheath 4.4 mm (Karl Storz)
- Bettocchi Integrated Office Hysteroscope (BIOH)
- Modified Bettochi 1.9 mm.

Optics

Hysteroscopes are monocular optical system, hence lack depth perception. Telescope has three parts:

1. Eyepiece
2. Barrel
3. Objective lens.

Light Source

Illumination is a very important requirement for hysteroscopy. A cold light source like xenon is commonly used and very effective. They have high content of blue spectral light. This light is classified as cold referring not to its temperature, but its location on the blue (cold) end of the light spectrum. Though light is extremely hot at it source and can cause thermal injury. Light is transmitted through fiberoptics or fluid light cables with a diameter of 3.5–5 mm and a length of 180–350 cm.

Hysteroscopic Sheaths (Figs. 4 to 7)

There are two basic types of hysteroscopic sheaths: (1) single channel and (2) dual channel sheaths. Simple diagnostic sheaths have one port for entry of distention media. Single channel sheath does not allow for active flushing of the uterine cavity.

Modern hysteroscopic sheaths are multichannel minimum of three ports with stopcocks for the passage of hysteroscopic instruments and the instillation and drainage of distention media.

Diagnostic Hysteroscopes: Varying Outer Diameters

- 2.9 mm hysteroscope
- 2 mm microhysteroscope.

Distending Media

Hysteroscopy performed using a distention medium. The distention media used are high molecular weight liquids or low molecular weight liquids.

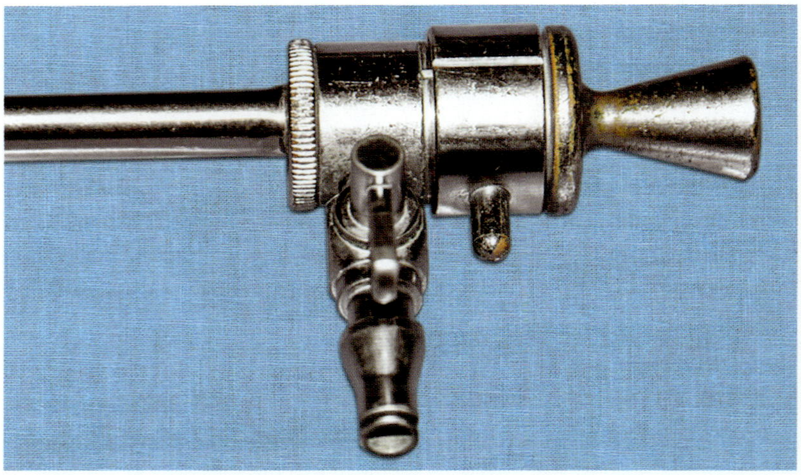

Fig. 5: Outlet port in operative sheath.

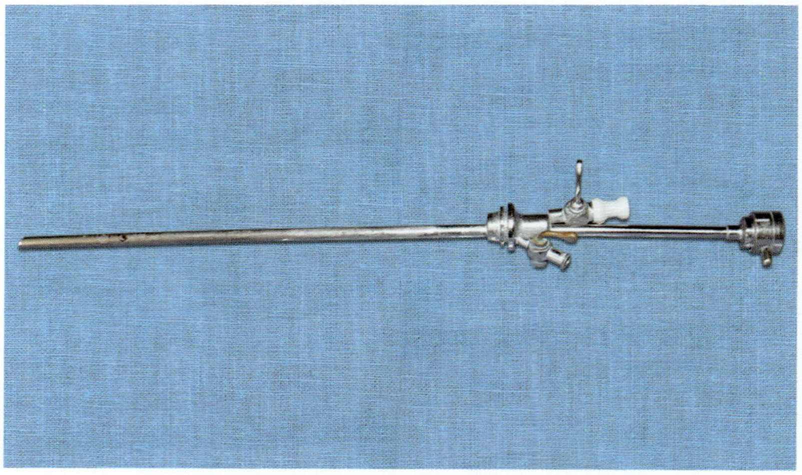

Fig. 6: Sheath with working channel for cold (mechanical) instruments of 5 Fr.

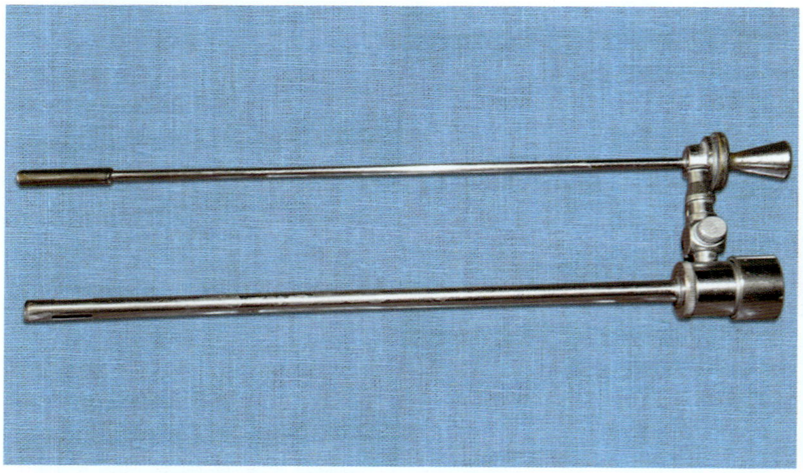

Fig. 4: Operative sheath with obturator.

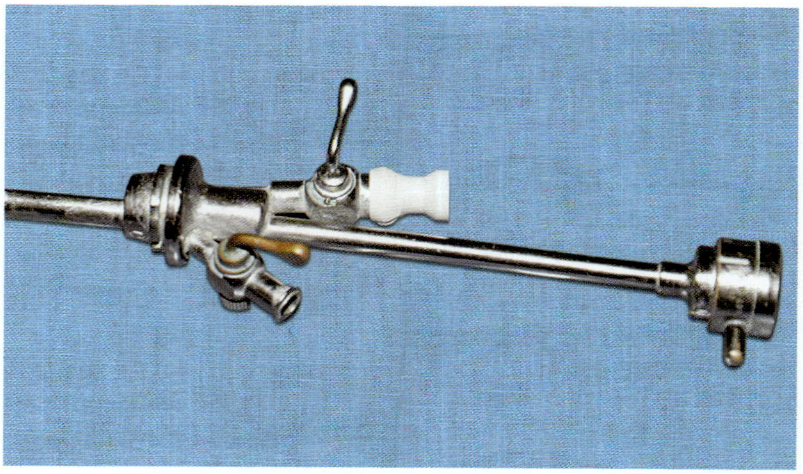

Fig. 7: Sheath with working channel for cold (mechanical) instruments of 5 Fr with irrigation inflow port.

High molecular weight medium is Hyskon 32% with advantage of low miscibility with blood. Low molecular weight medium is Ringer's lactate.

Delivery System

- *Gravity fall of liquid:* The bag is suspended at a height of 90–100 cm from the patient's perineum to achieve a pressure of 70 mm Hg
- *Pressure cuff:* Devices similar to sphygmomanometer are applied around the bag and the pressure in the cuff is raised and maintained at 80 mm Hg
- *Electronic suction and irrigation pump* ***(Fig. 8)****:* These allow to control flow rate as well as suction and irrigation pressure and are operated at a flow rate of approximately 200 mL/min with irrigating pressure at 75 mm Hg and a suction pressure of 0.25 lb.

MECHANICAL INSTRUMENTS (FIGS. 9 TO 12)

- Scissors
- Alligator grasping forceps
- Spoon biopsy forceps
- Punch biopsy forceps
- Punctate electrode.

RESECTOSCOPES (FIGS. 13 TO 18)

Resectoscopes have a continuous flow design, which allow constant inflow and outflow of the distending media helping in visualization of by rinsing the debris and blood. Traditional resectoscopes have monopolar electrode and require a nonconductive distention medium to allow completion of the electrical circuit. Bipolar resectoscope requires use of the conductive media like normal saline.

The diameter is 7–8 mm. Radiofrequency electrical energy is used for monopolar or bipolar.

In a monopolar resectoscope, the patient must be grounded and a nonconducting medium is used (glycine).

Components of the Resectoscope

- Hysteroscope with a diameter 2–4 mm with 30° angular view
- Cutting loop operated by passive spring mechanism
- Two sheath of continuous irrigation and suction of the distending media
- Instruments of 22 Fr and 26 Fr with respective resectoscope.

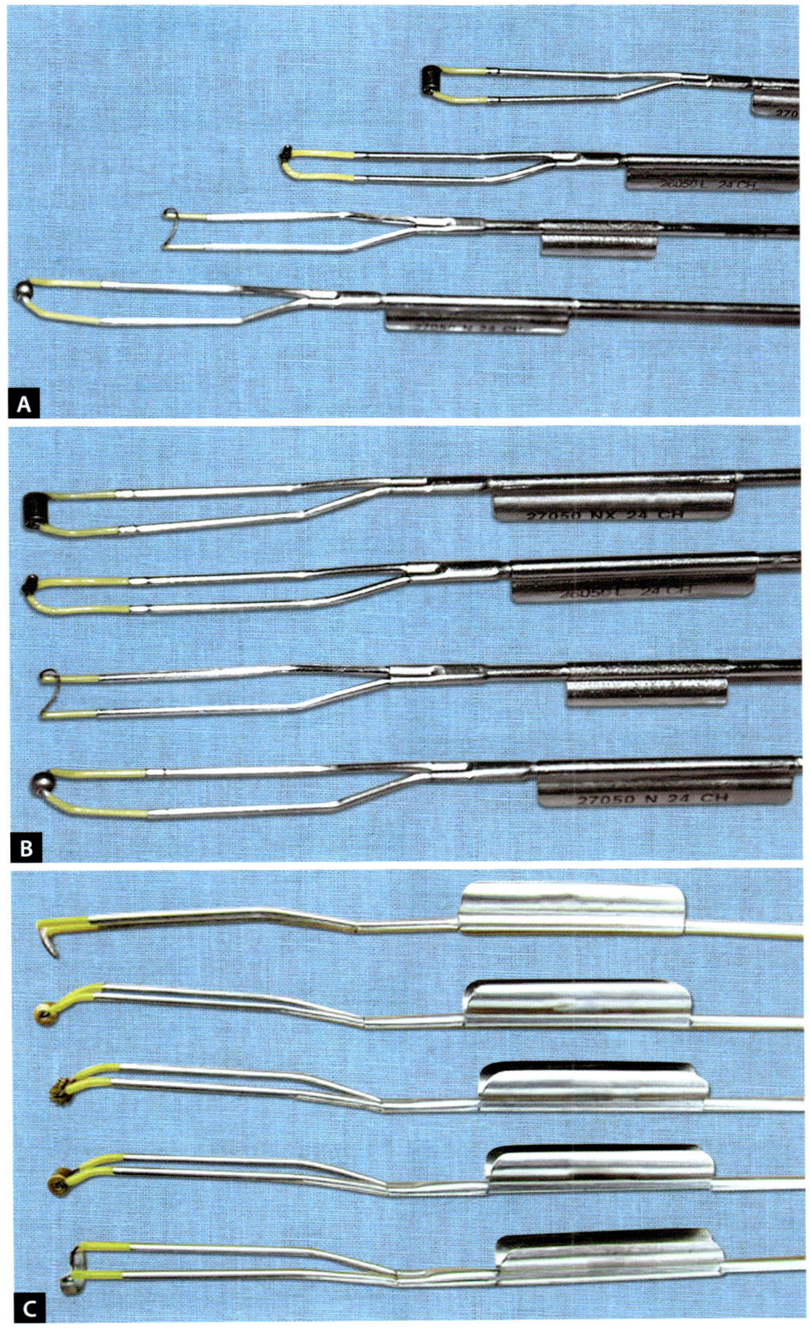

Figs. 9A to C: Electrode: 26 Fr roller ball, loop electrode, Collin's knife, vaportrode.

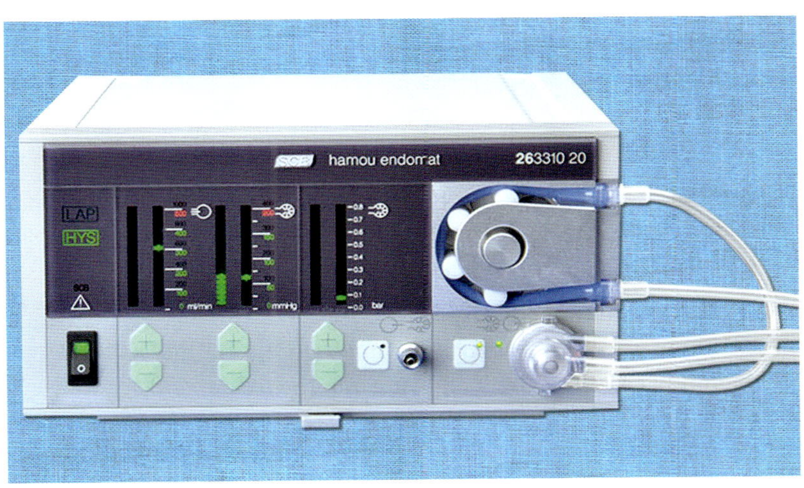

Fig. 8: Encomat.

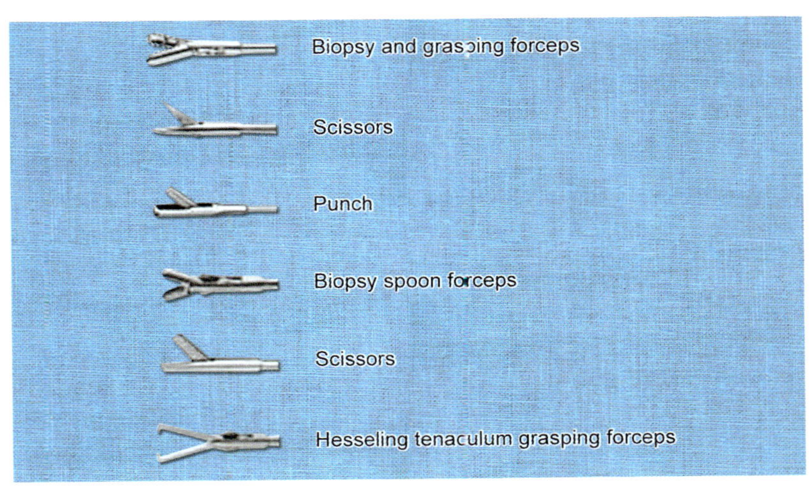

Fig. 10: Some mechanical instruments.

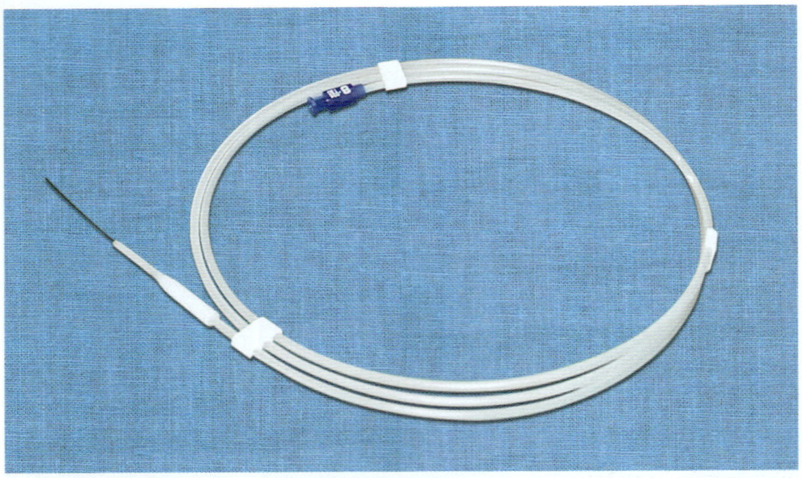

Fig. 11: Guidewire for hysteroscopic cannulation.

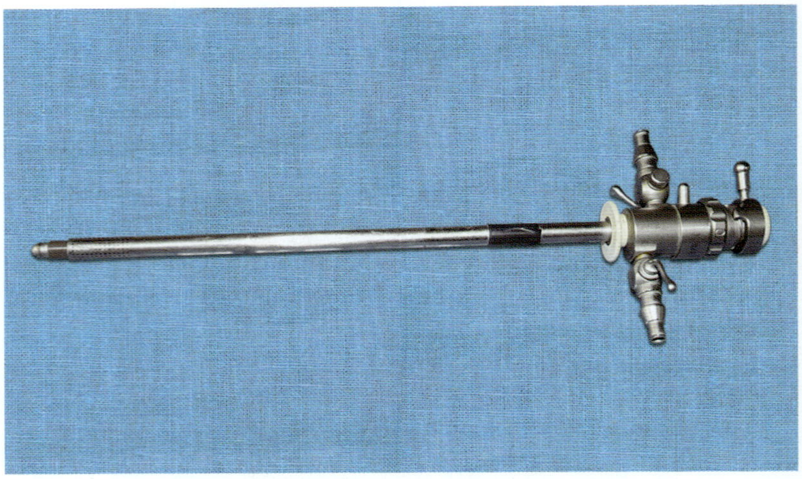

Fig. 14: Assembled resectoscope sheath with obturator.

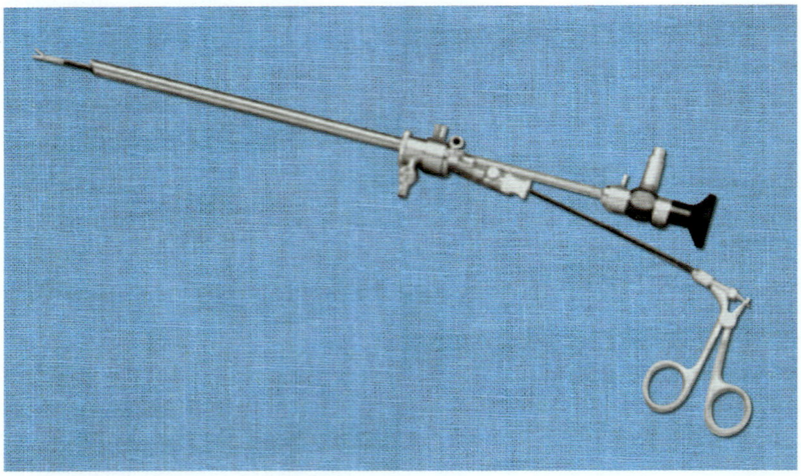

Fig. 12: Assembled mechanical instrument with hysteroscopy and operative sheath.

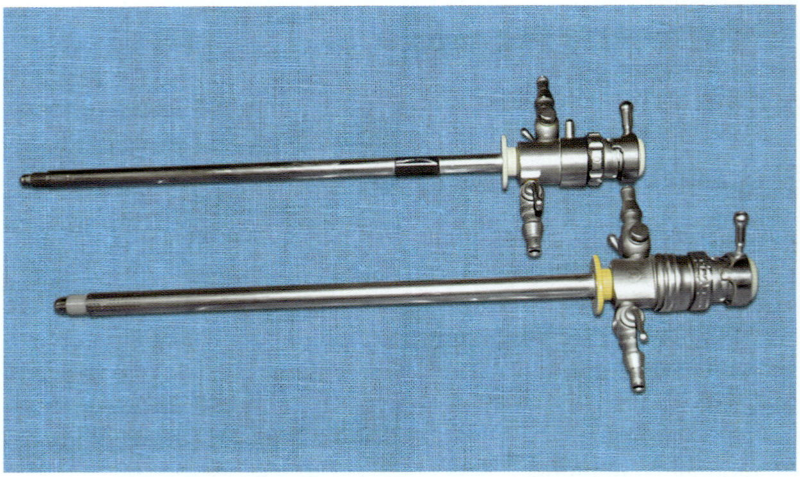

Fig. 15: Different sizes of the resectoscope sheath.

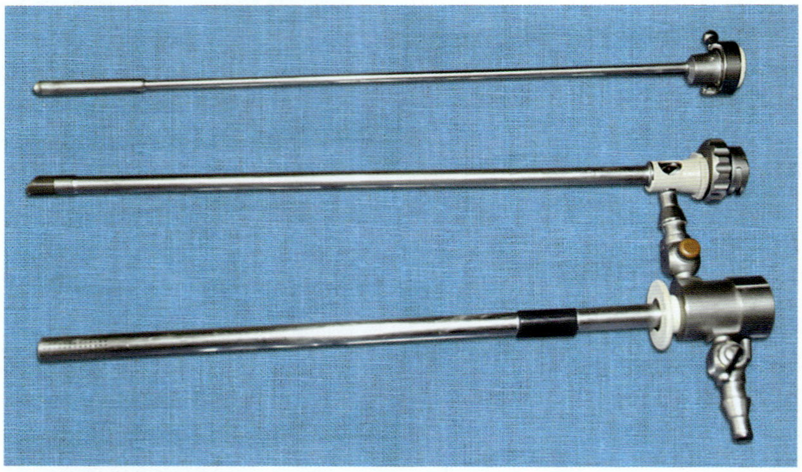

Fig. 13: Resectoscope outer sheath with obturator with outflow and inflow irrigation.

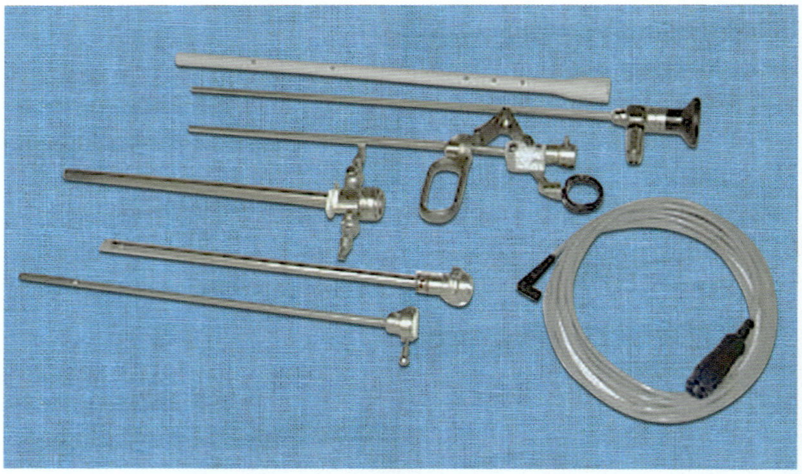

Fig. 16: Unassembled resectoscope.

Bipolar Surgery (Figs. 19 to 21)

Versapoint bipolar electrosurgical system contains two types of electrode.

1. Twizzle electrode which has a precise controlled vaporization
2. Spring electrode which has a diffuse tissue vaporization effect.

Every electrode has active electrode at tip and tissue will vaporize, return electrode is at the shaft.

There are different waveforms:

- Vapor cut waveform which is cut mode (VC1, VC2, and VC3). VC3 is the mildest flowing energy flowing into the tissue.
- Blend waveform (BL1 and BL2)
- Desiccation waveform which is a coagulation mode (DES).

The Versapoint bipolar electrosurgical generator automatically sets to VC1 and 100 W.

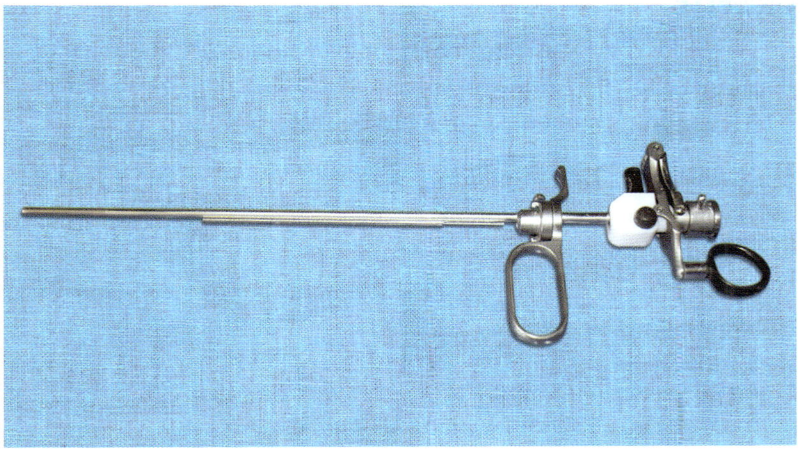

Fig. 17: Monopolar resectoscope.

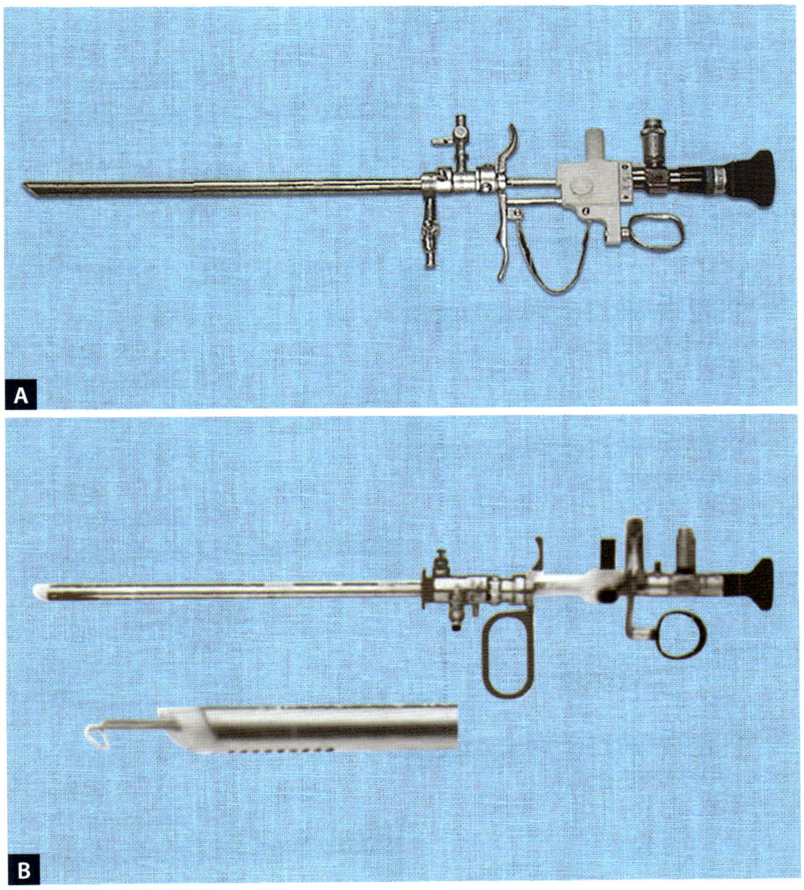

Figs. 18A and B: Assembled monopolar resectoscope.

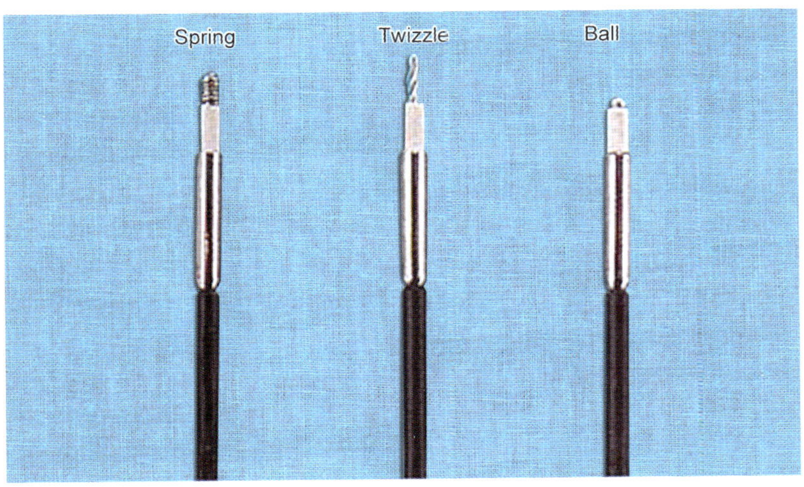

Fig. 19: Bipolar electrodes.

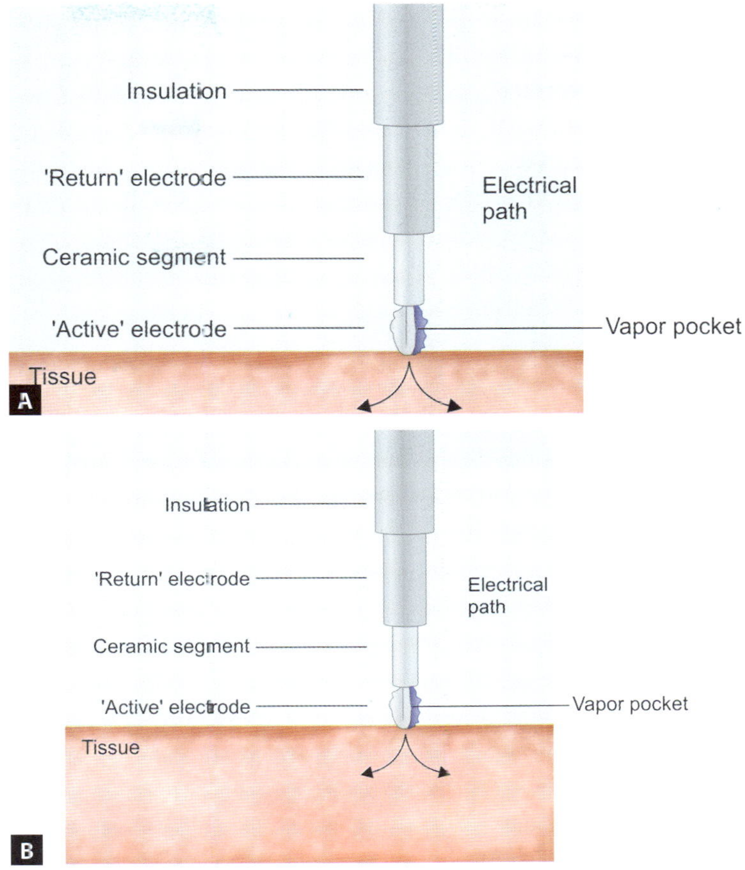

Figs. 20A and B: Active electrode at tip and tissue will vaporize; return electrode is at the shaft.

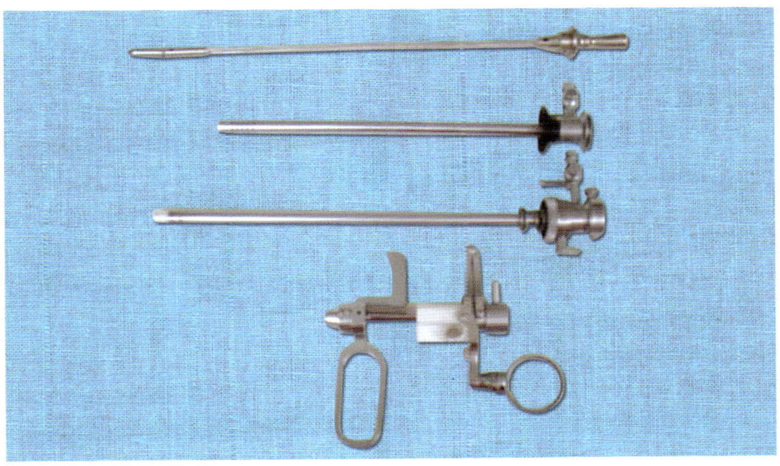

Fig. 21: Bipolar resectoscope.

CHOICE OF INSTRUMENTS

- Choose instruments which are sturdy and have long life.
- Buy instruments from a standard company which has a proven track record.
- Use flattened sheaths than the round once as they are according to the shape of the cervical canal.

MAINTENANCE AND STERILIZATION OF THE INSTRUMENTS

Hysteroscope can carry vaginal infection to the uterine cavity. Hysteroscopy should be preceded with proper disinfection of the vagina. After completion of the procedure, the hysteroscopic set should be disassembled and each part should be washed with water and detergent.

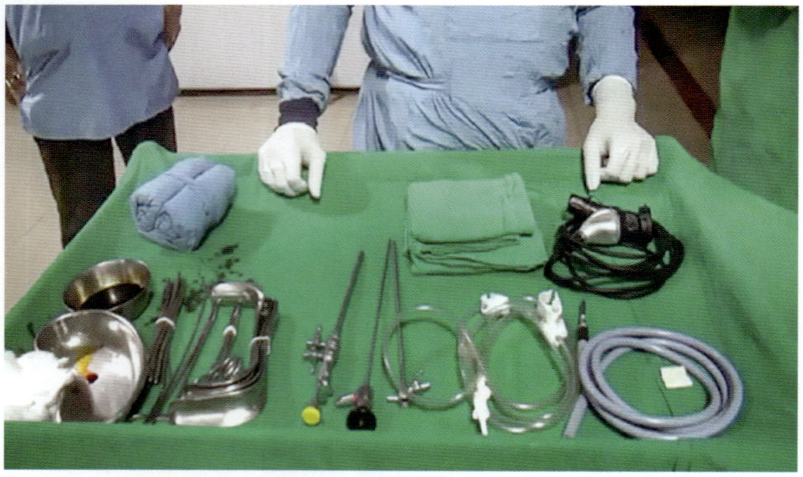

Fig. 22: An assembled table for hysteroscopic procedure.

Glutaraldehyde (2%) is proved as an effective agent against all vegetative bacteria, fungi and microorganism. Before use the clean and dried instruments should be soaked for 20 minutes in solution. It is removed and washed with distilled water before use.

Ethylene oxide sterilization takes 8–12 hours for completely sterilized.

Autoclave sterilization: It is cheapest system, with diffusion of steam. It cleans even the smallest gap and openings. Instruments may be sterilized with 20 minutes at 121°C or 7 minutes for 134°C. Autoclave sterilization of the telescope can be hazardous so should be done by self or with trained staff. Telescope should be placed in perforated metal container, wrapped in suitable gauze. Lenses can be cleaned with 90% alcohol and then dried with cotton balls.

An assembled table for hysteroscopic procedure has been shown in **Figure 22.**

CHAPTER

51

Fibroid Polyp

Shubhanjali Sen, Minal Kumbhalwar, B Ramesh

INTRODUCTION

According to PALM-COEIN classification, the FIGO classification is abnormal uterine bleeding-polyp (AUB-P).

CHARACTERISTICS

Polyps can be an isolated finding or with endometrial hyperplasia or may be in association with malignancy. Polyps can occur at various sites in uterine cavity. Commonly arise from the fundal aspect of endometrium. Polyps may be single or multiple in number with or without stalk, sessile or pedunculated.

Normally, polyps have a broad base or they may have a stalk. Usually, a feeding vessel can be demonstrated, especially if it is of significant size. If it grows with the stalk in its size, it may protrude through the cervical canal. The location can be variable. Often it is located in the lateral walls, but sometimes it may be near ostium. When polyps are near the ostia, sometimes they may obstruct the ostia leading to false interpretation for primary infertility. They may measure from a few millimeters to a few centimeters in size. They normally consist of endometrial stroma, glands, and blood vessels.

Polyps can be recurrent due to underlying hormonal cause. They are mostly noted in the reproductive age group, but if they are observed in the perimenopausal and postmenopausal age group, then they should be treated with caution.

Polyps can be leiomyomatous in nature; over transvaginal scan, its echotexture, definite margins, and whorl-like appearance are suggestive of polyp.

Endometrial polyps which are benign have smooth margin and vascular markings are neat and regular. Biopsy of such a polyp identifies it being benign or malignant in nature. Very occasionally, they are complicated by malignant hyperplasia of endometrium.

Polyp can be picked up frequently over a routine transvaginal scan. Polyps, which are very small and asymptomatic, can be left untreated. When menstrual irregularities such as menorrhagia, intermenstrual spotting, premenstrual spotting, or postmenopausal bleeding are chief complaints, then any size polyp should be removed. Polyps are also seen with polycystic ovaries who have a prolonged period of amenorrhea and endometrial hyperplasia due to hormonal imbalance. In cases of recurrent abortions also if polyps are accidently found, then resection is considered without second thought.

Medications such as use of tamoxifen may induce endometrial hyperplasia leading to formation of the polyp causing irregular bleeding.

A progestogen with high antiestrogenic activity as well as the use of oral contraceptive pills may have a protective effect on the development of endometrial polyps.

ETIOLOGY

During the pre- and postmenstrual phase, the endometrial polyp loses the apoptotic regulation and thus leads to overexpression of estrogen and progesterone receptors, thus avoiding the usual control mechanism.

DIAGNOSTIC MODALITY

- Hysterosalpingography (HSG) has high sensitivity and low specificity as compared to hysteroscopy.
- Ultrasonography (USG), saline infusion sonohysterography (SIS), or hysteroscopy are widely used for diagnosing the endometrial polyp.

GUIDELINES FOR THE DIAGNOSIS OF ENDOMETRIAL POLYP

- Transvaginal ultrasound (TVUS) provides reliable information for the detection of endometrial polyp and should be the investigation of choice.
- Color Doppler increases the capacity of TVUS to diagnose endometrial polyp.
- Adding intrauterine contrast to sonography improves the diagnostic capacity for endometrial polyp.
- Blind dilation and curettage or biopsy should not be used for diagnosis of the endometrial polyp.

MANAGEMENT

- Conservative management
- Medical management
- Conservative surgical management
- Hysteroscopic resection
- Radical surgical outcome.

Most endometrial polyps are blindly avulsed and followed by blind curettage. The drawbacks of blind avulsion and curettage is that malignant cells at the base of the polyp can be missed. Polypectomy may be incomplete and recurrence rate is high.

Hysteroscopic resection of the polyp is the gold standard treatment followed by histopathological evaluation of the polyp. Though, for hysteroscopy, cervical dilatation is required, but many studies have proved that there are no recurrences of the polyp after hysteroscopic resection.

As hysteroscopy is all about see and treat.

Hysteroscopic Resection

Hysteroscopy with guided biopsy is the most common technique to diagnose polyp as it offers the highest sensitivity and specificity for the conservative measures.

Diagnostic hysteroscopy alone only allows subjective assessment of the size and characteristics of the lesion with reported sensitivity of 58–99%, a specificity of 87–100%, positive predictive value (PPV) of 21–100%, and net present value (NPV) of 66–99% when compared with hysteroscopy with guided biopsy.

The resection is usually carried out postmenstrually under general anesthesia. Broad-antibiotic coverage should be administered before and after the procedure. All required blood test should be done. Preanesthetic check is very important and utmost required.

Lithotomy position is given. The cervix is then loaded on the hysteroscope and during gentle withdrawal of the hysteroscope, the cervical canal moves in the field of vision. After allowing the time for cervical hydrodilatation, the scope is gently navigated through the cervical canal with minimal lateral movement and no tissue contact should happen, else the tissues might bleed and obstruct the view field. Once the endometrial polyp is visualized, then operating channel is introduced through the cervix.

When there is a thin stalk of the polyp, then cold scissors are used, polyp is grasped, and pulled out and sent for histopathological evaluation.

Electrosurgical units required can be monopolar current or bipolar current. The disadvantage of the monopolar current is the use of glycine as the distention media.

In bipolar current, the distending media is normal saline and intrauterine flow pressure should be 70–100 mm Hg and it can be controlled by electronic irrigation suction device. A 5-mm 30° sheathed hysteroscope supplied with a 5F working channel using 50 W power.

Failures of the Procedure

Success depends on polyp size and patient parity. Failure can happen due to pain, polyp size, vasovagal syndrome, and incomplete removal due to technical cervical stenosis, obscured vision causing bleeding.

What is Required?

Adequate patient selection, psychological support, a competent operator, and setting that creates a private, caring, and calm environment are prerequisites.

PREVENTION OF RECURRENCE OF POLYP

Three to six cycles of progesterones to be given to prevent recurrence.

SUBMUCOSAL FIBROID POLYP (FIGS. 1 TO 22)

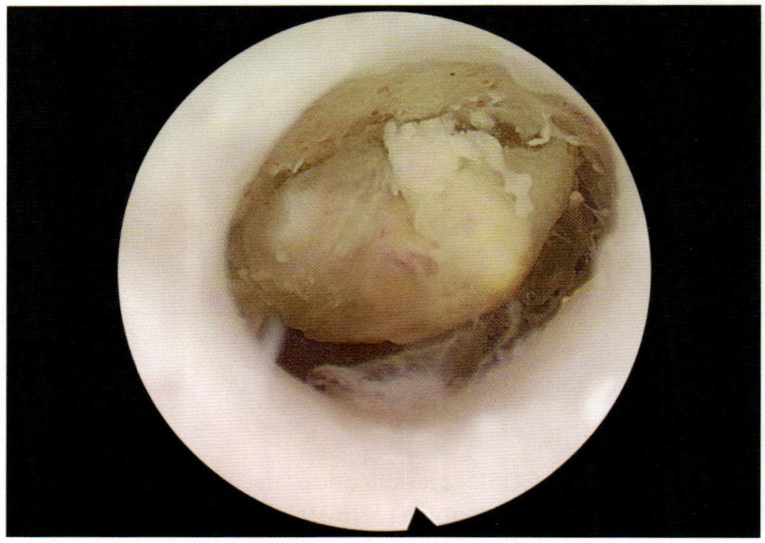

Fig. 1: Polyp.

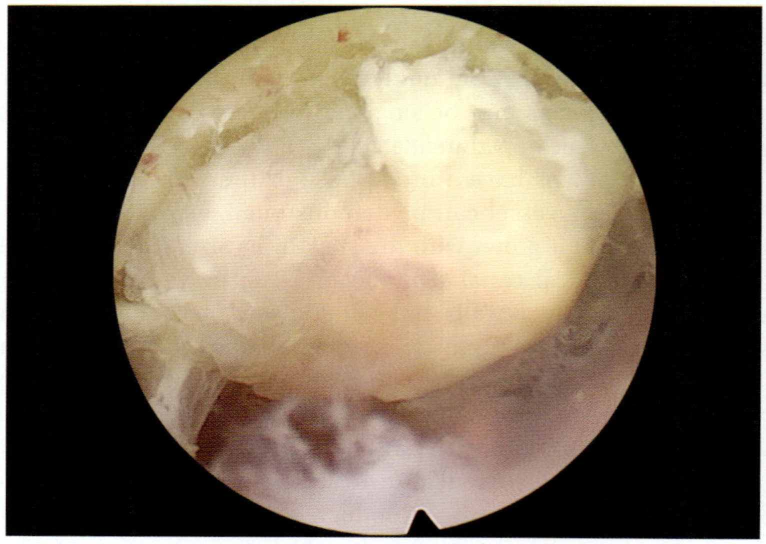

Fig. 2: Sessile polyp in endocervical canal.

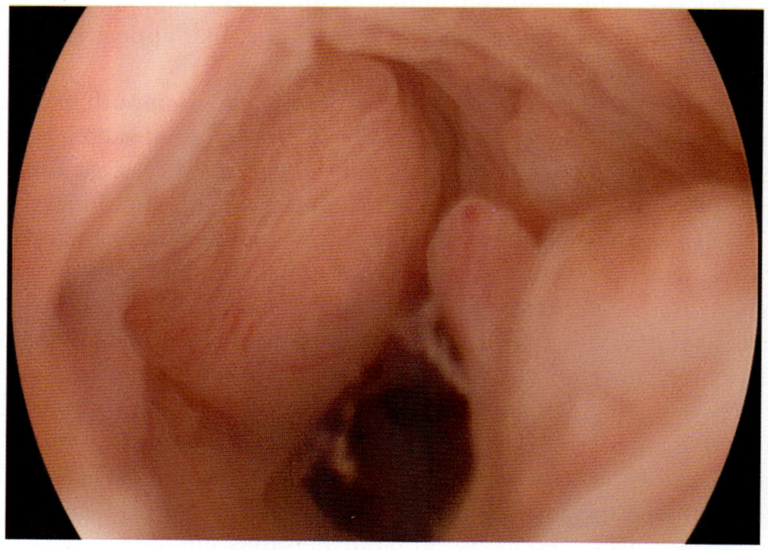

Fig. 3: Sessile polyp in cervical canal.

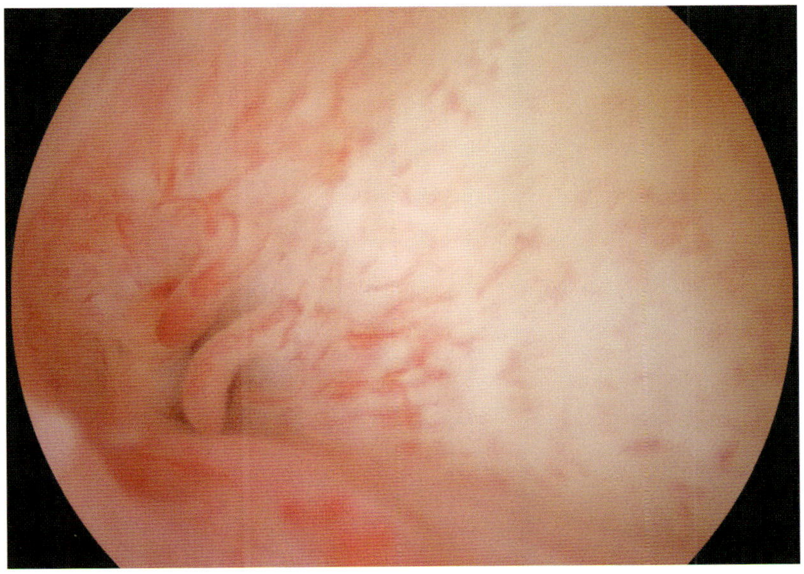

Fig. 4: Polyp at the ostia.

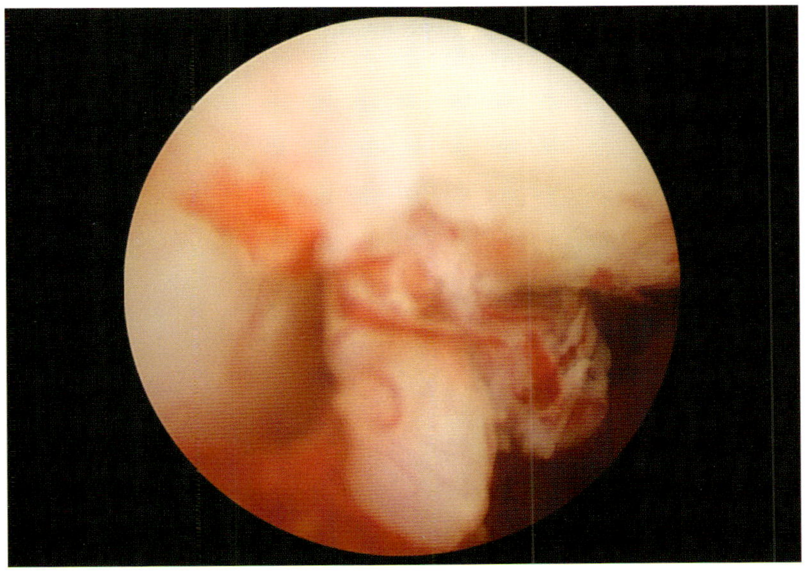

Fig. 7: Cervical polyp.

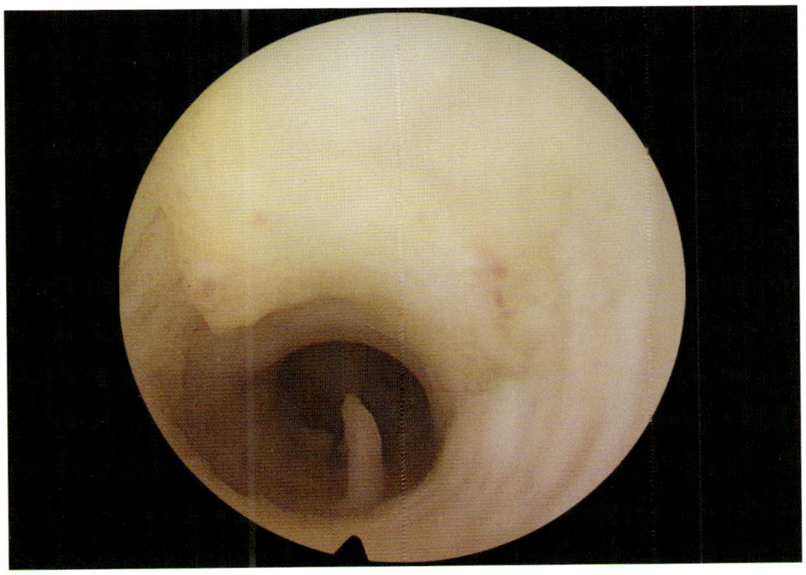

Fig. 5: Endocervical polyp.

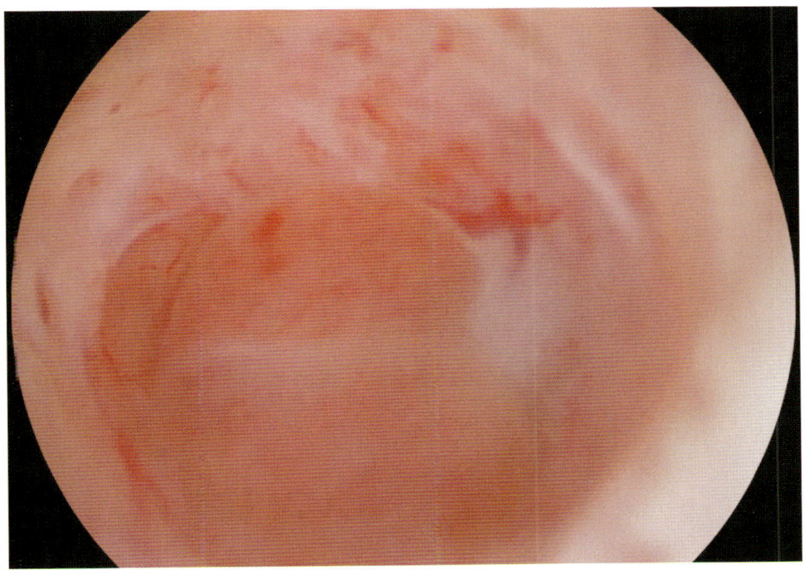

Fig. 8: Polyp at the cornua.

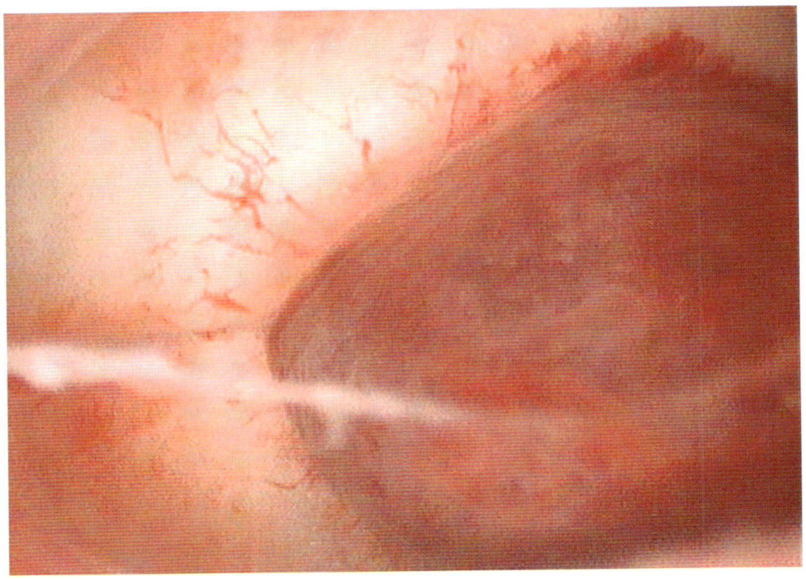

Fig. 6: Sessile fundal polyp.

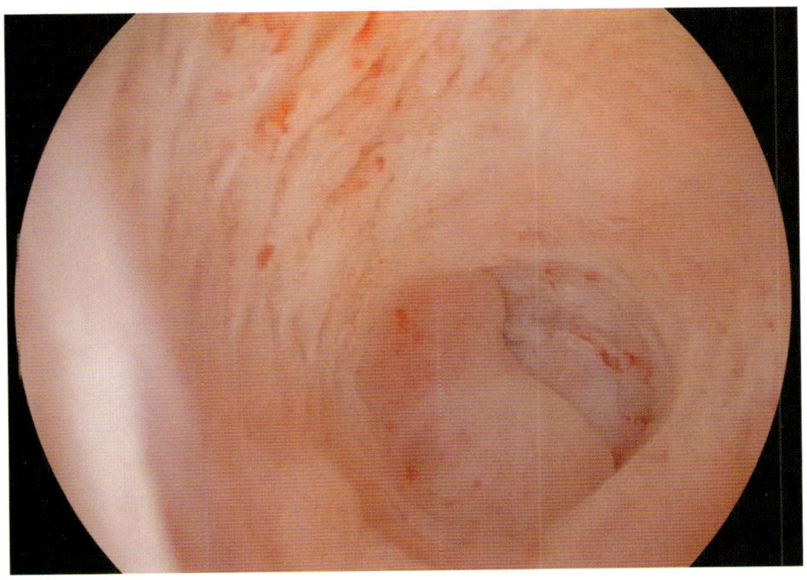

Fig. 9: Endocervical polyp.

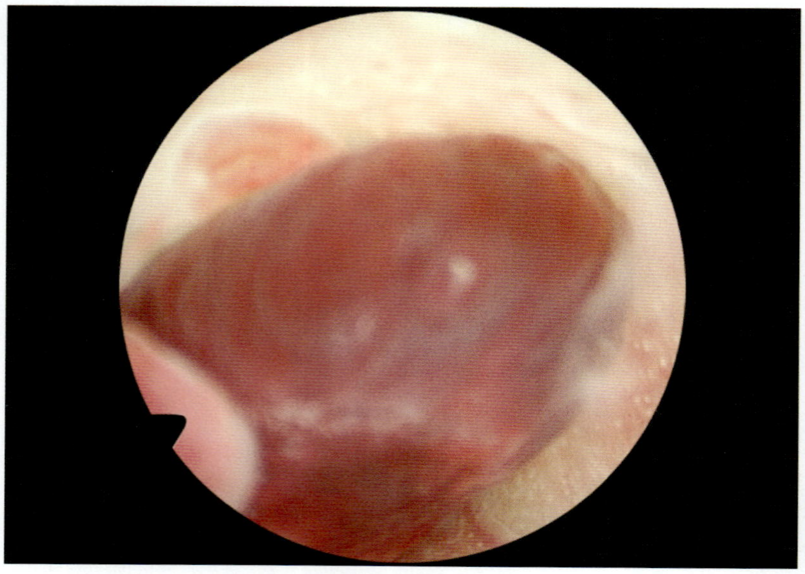

Fig. 10: Fundal polyp.

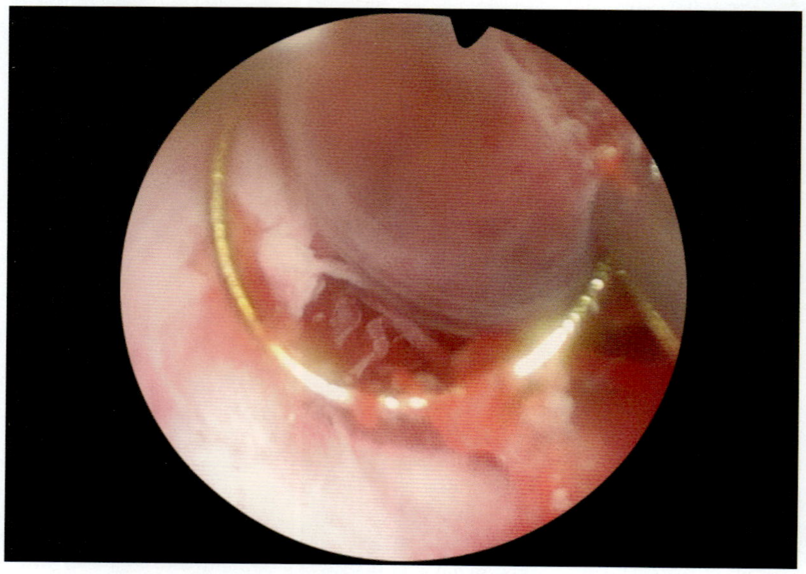

Fig. 11: Polyp being resected with loop using glycine as distending media.

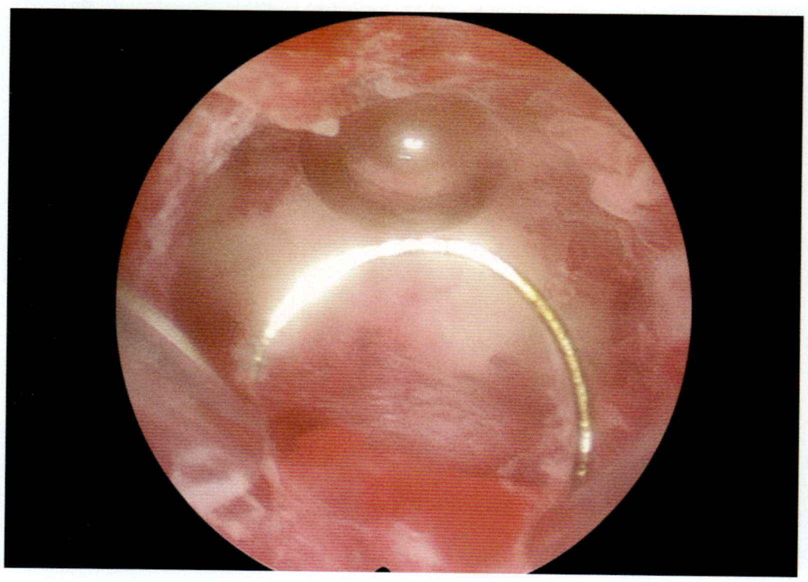

Fig. 12: Postpolypectomy view of the uterine cavity.

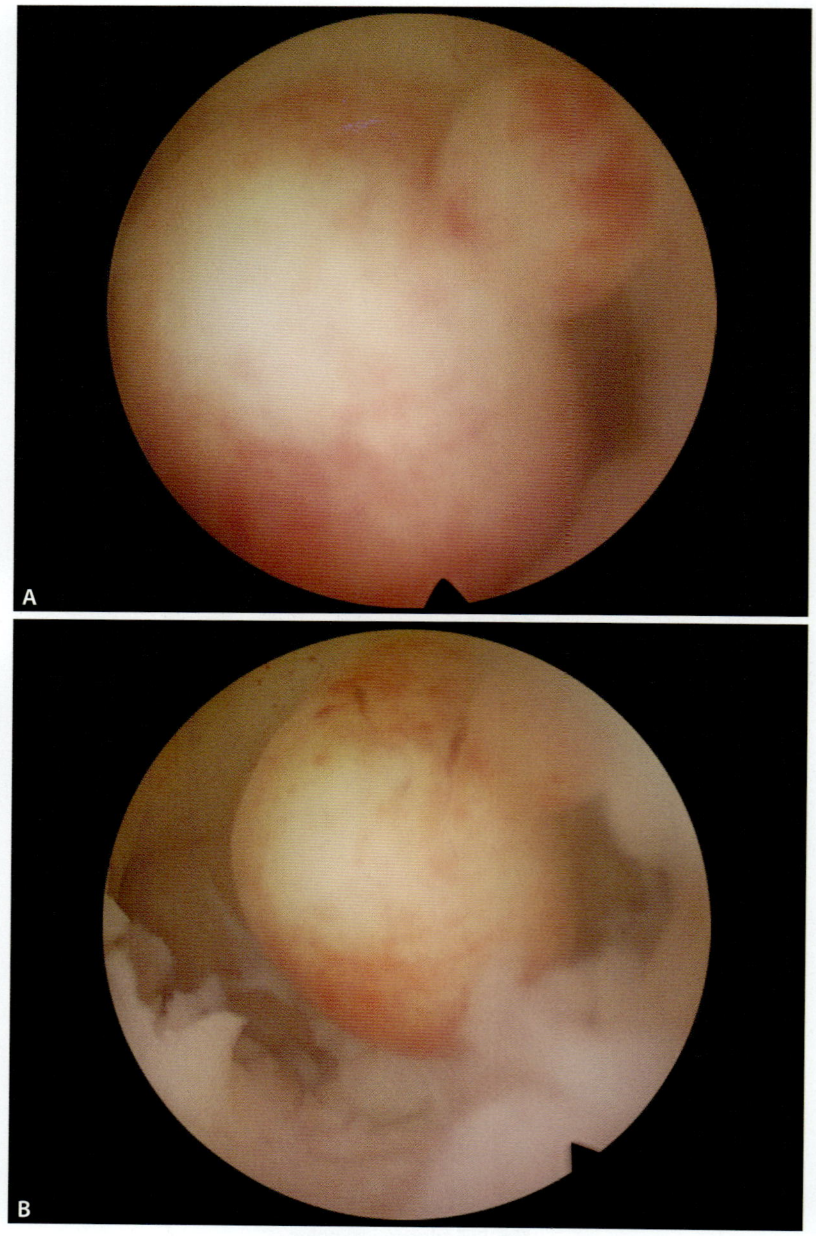

Figs. 13A and B: Fundal polyp.

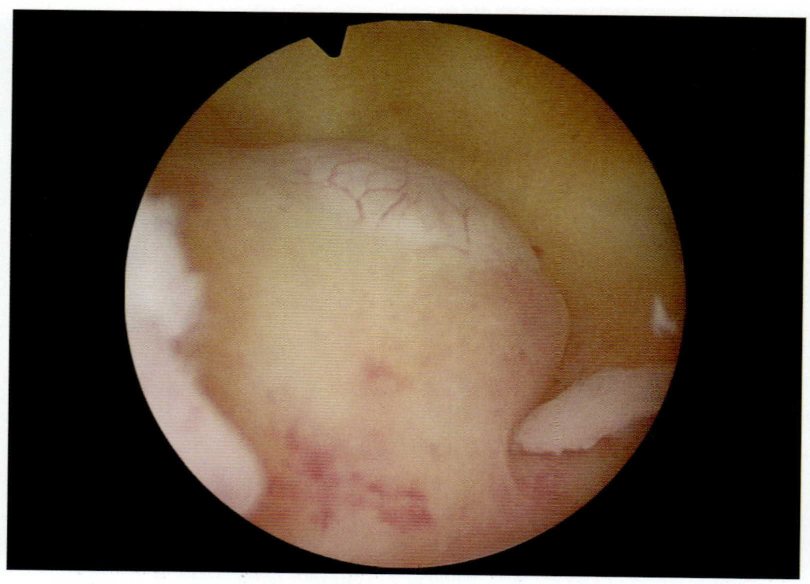

Fig. 14: Polyp being resected with the loop using glycine as distending media.

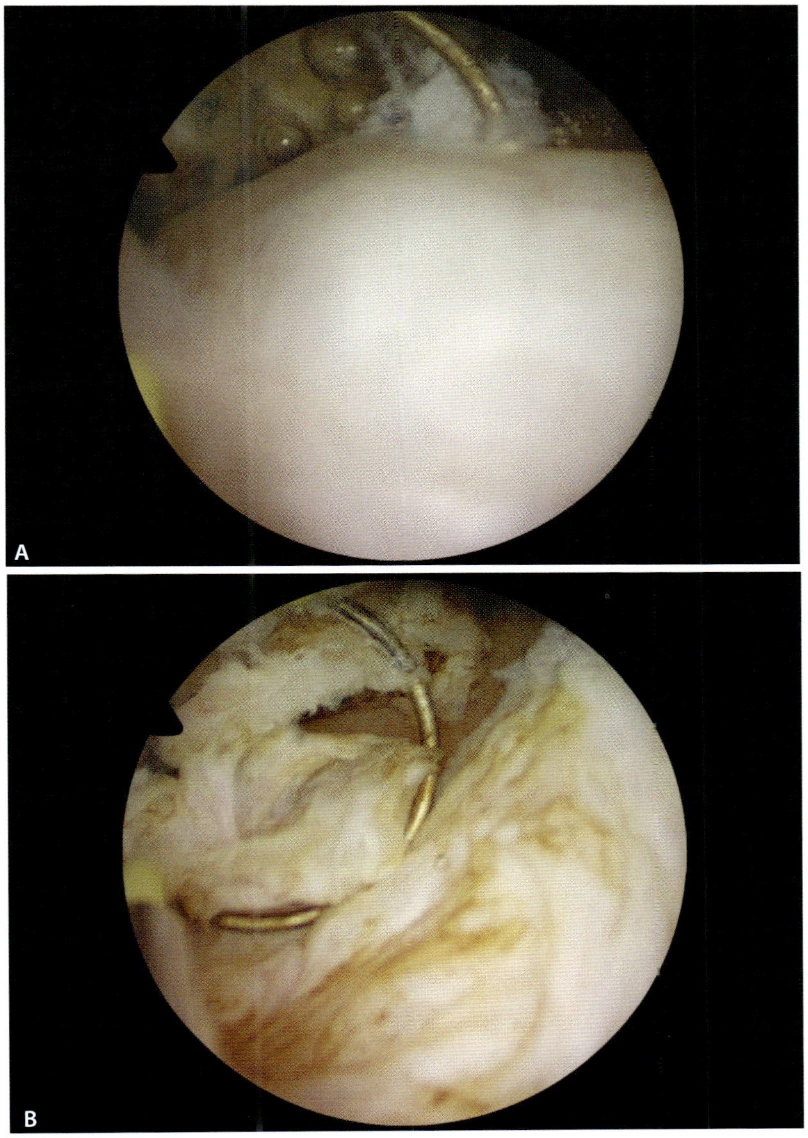

Figs. 15A and B: Resected base of polyp.

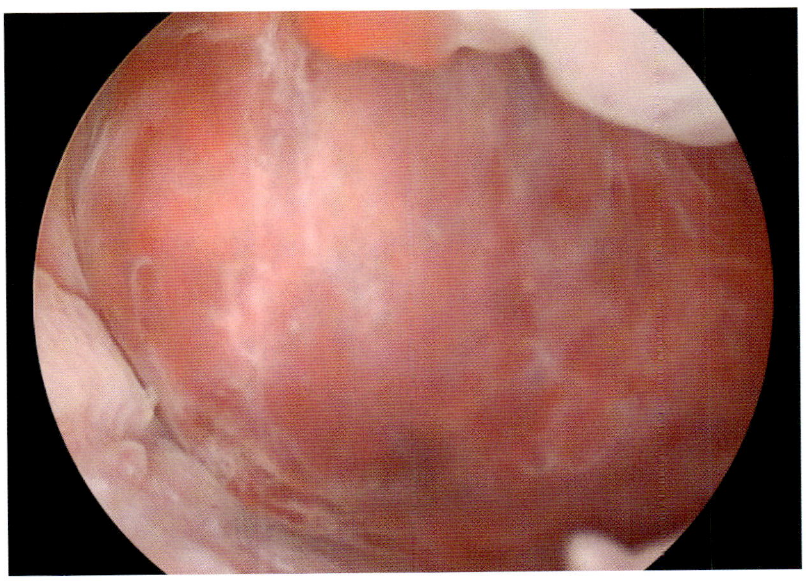

Fig. 16: Fundal polyp.

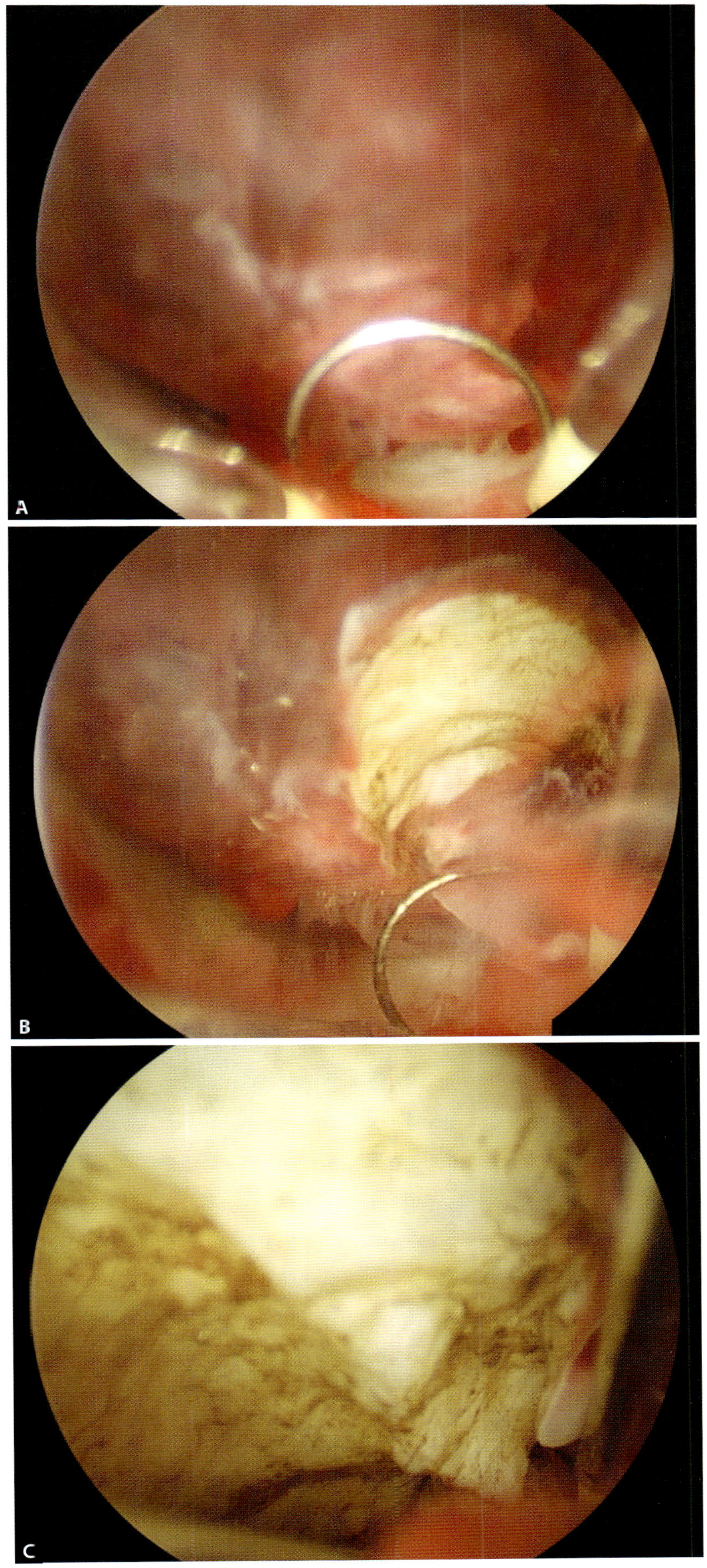

Figs. 17A to C

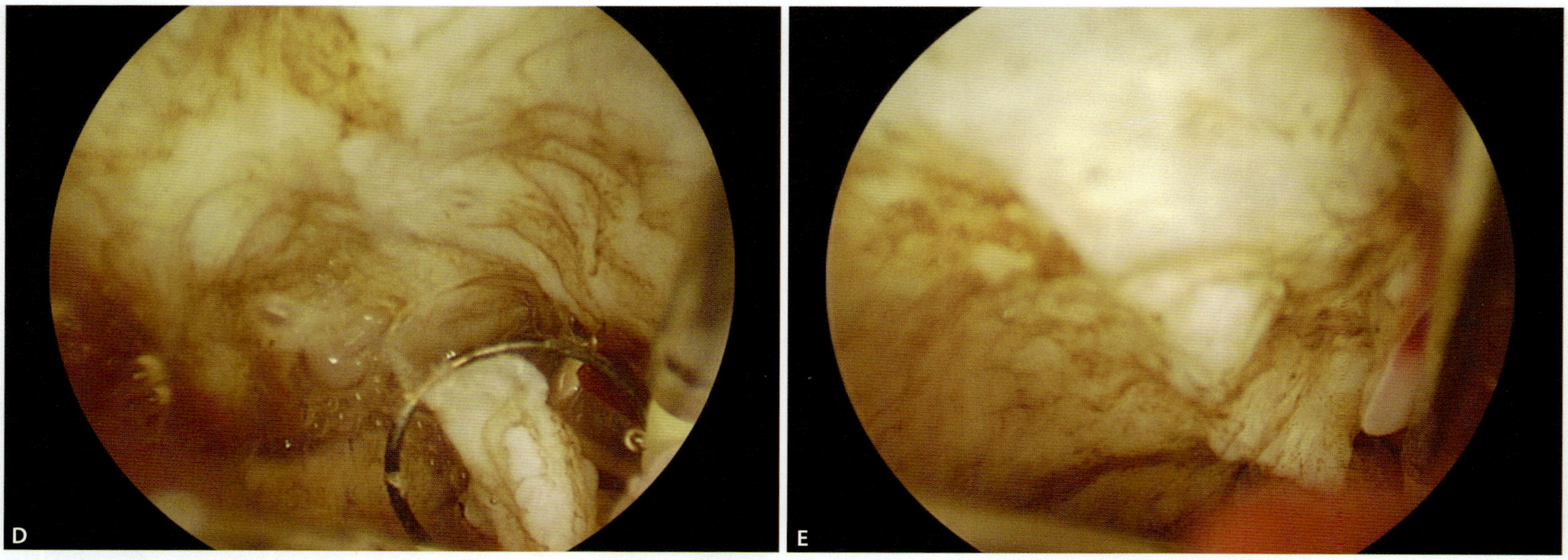

Figs. 17D to E

Figs. 17A to E: Fundal polyp resection with loop using glycine as distension media.

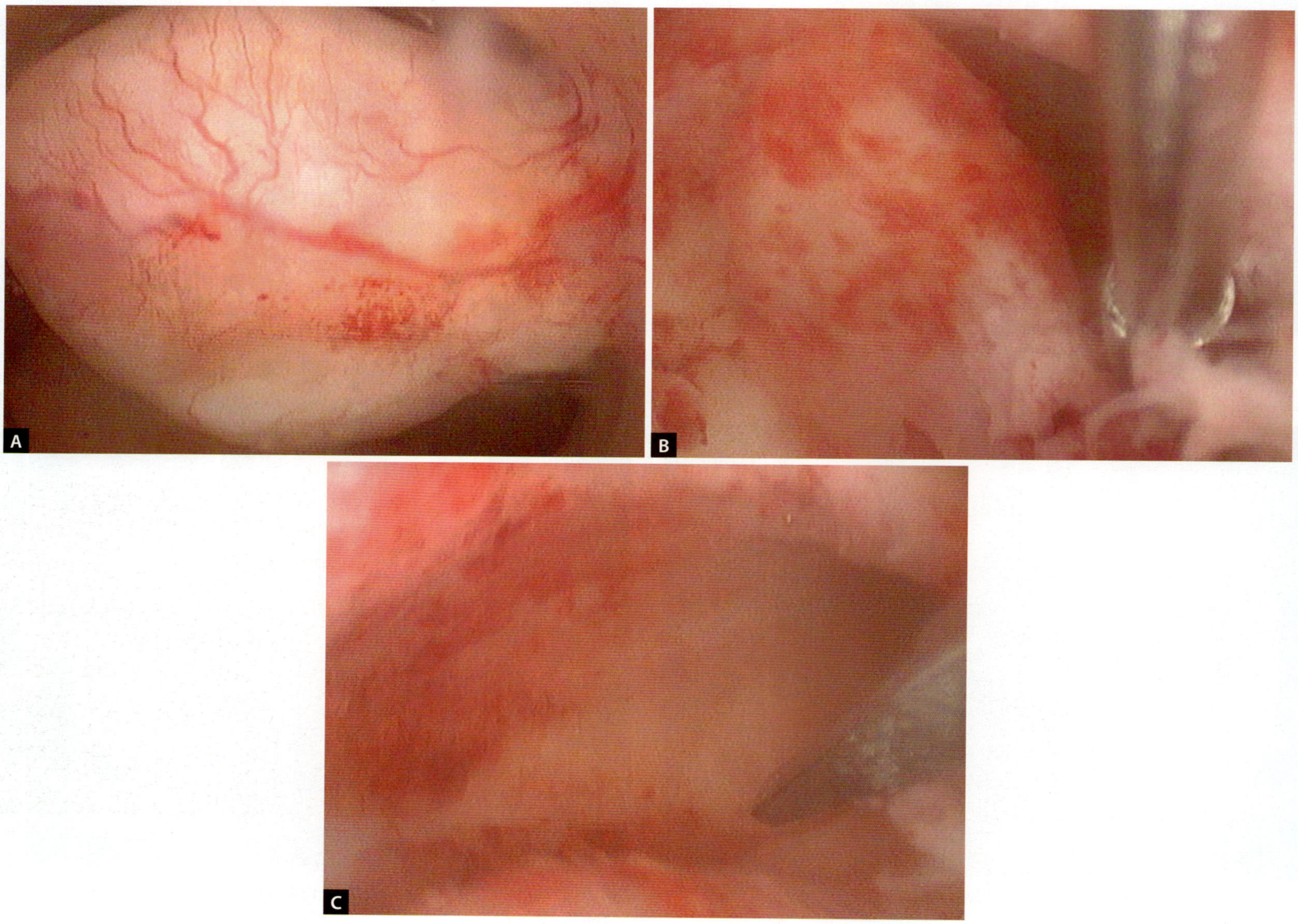

Figs. 18A to C: Pedunculated polyp resection with cold scissors.

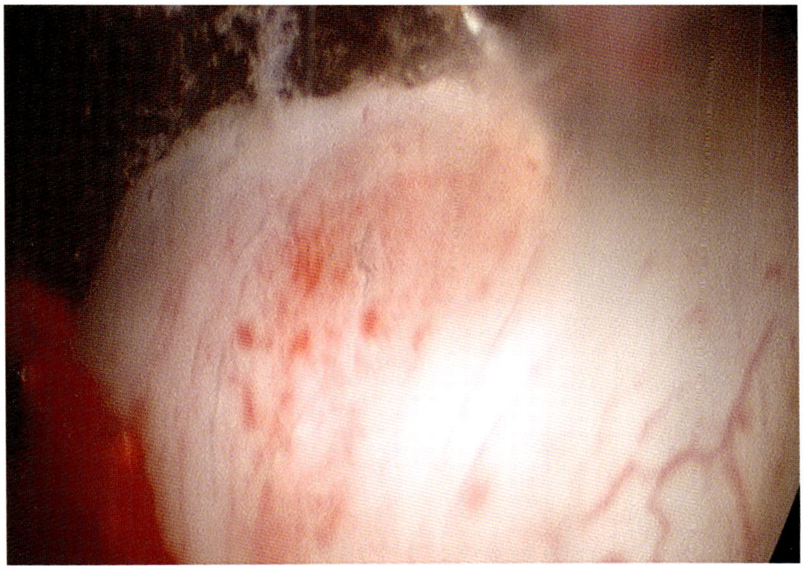

Fig. 19: Activated loop wh le polyp resection.

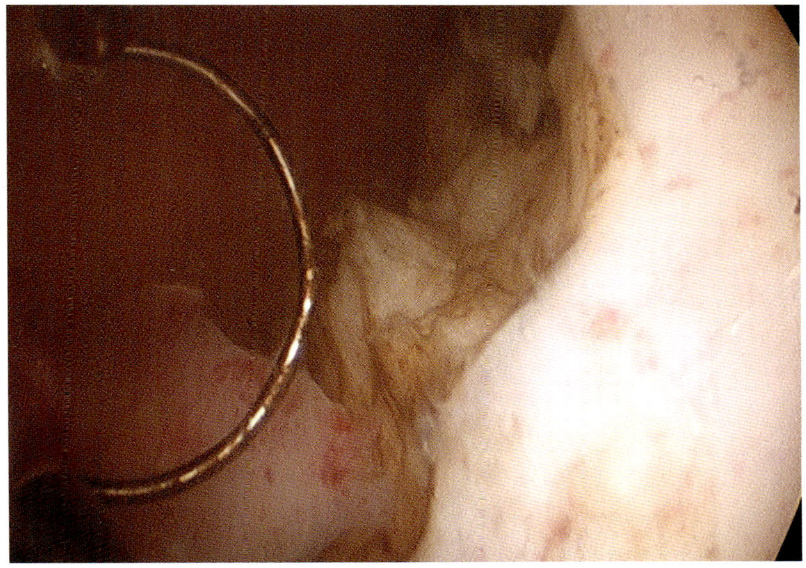

Fig. 20: Resection at base of polyp.

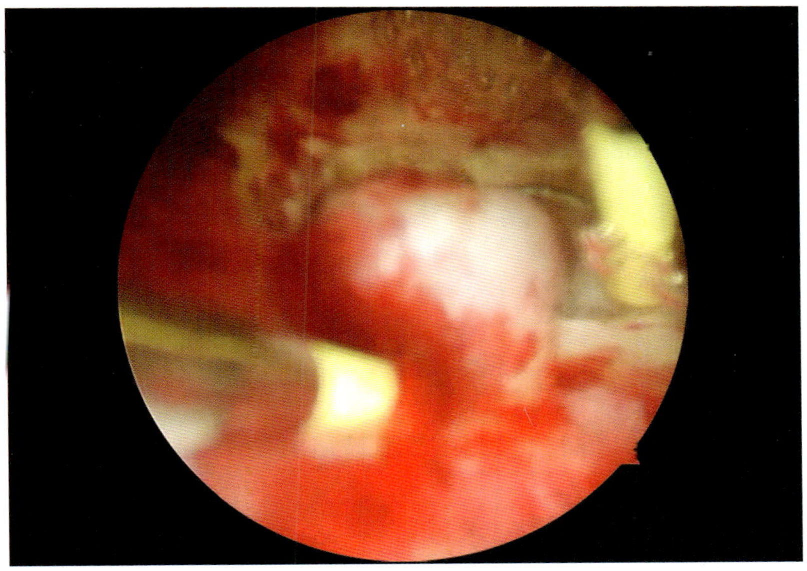

Fig. 21: Fibroid base resected with loop.

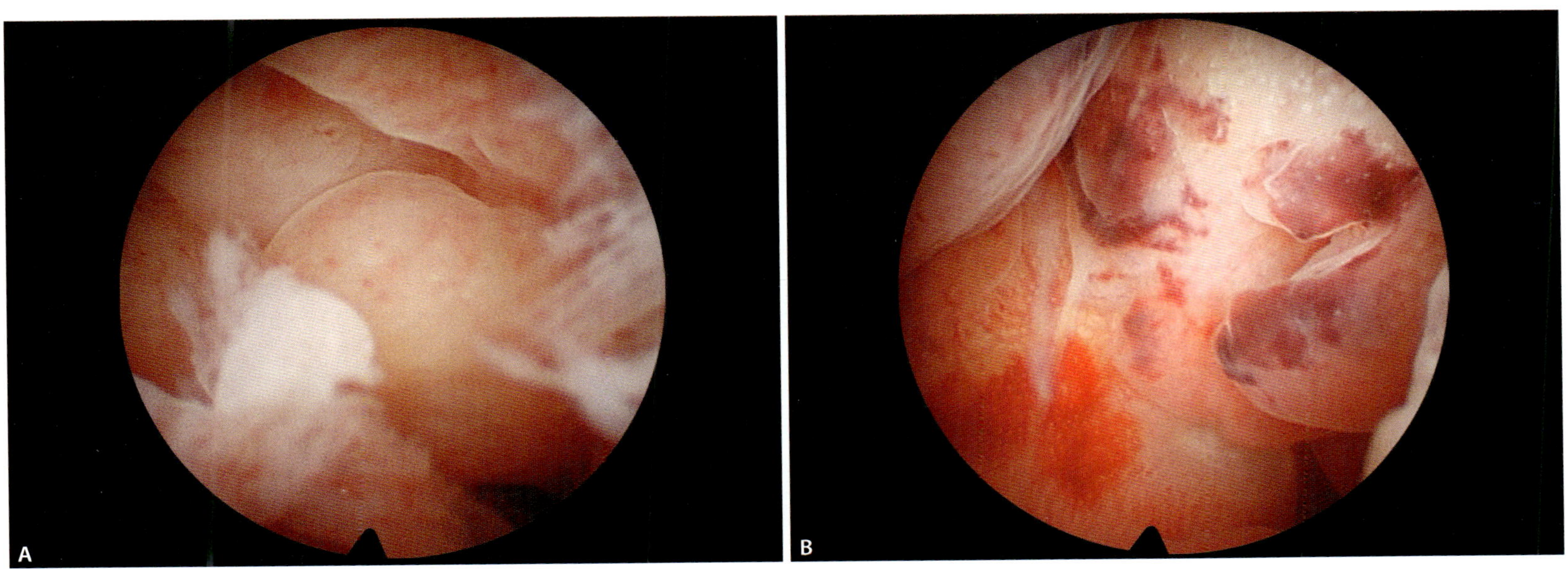

Figs. 22A and B

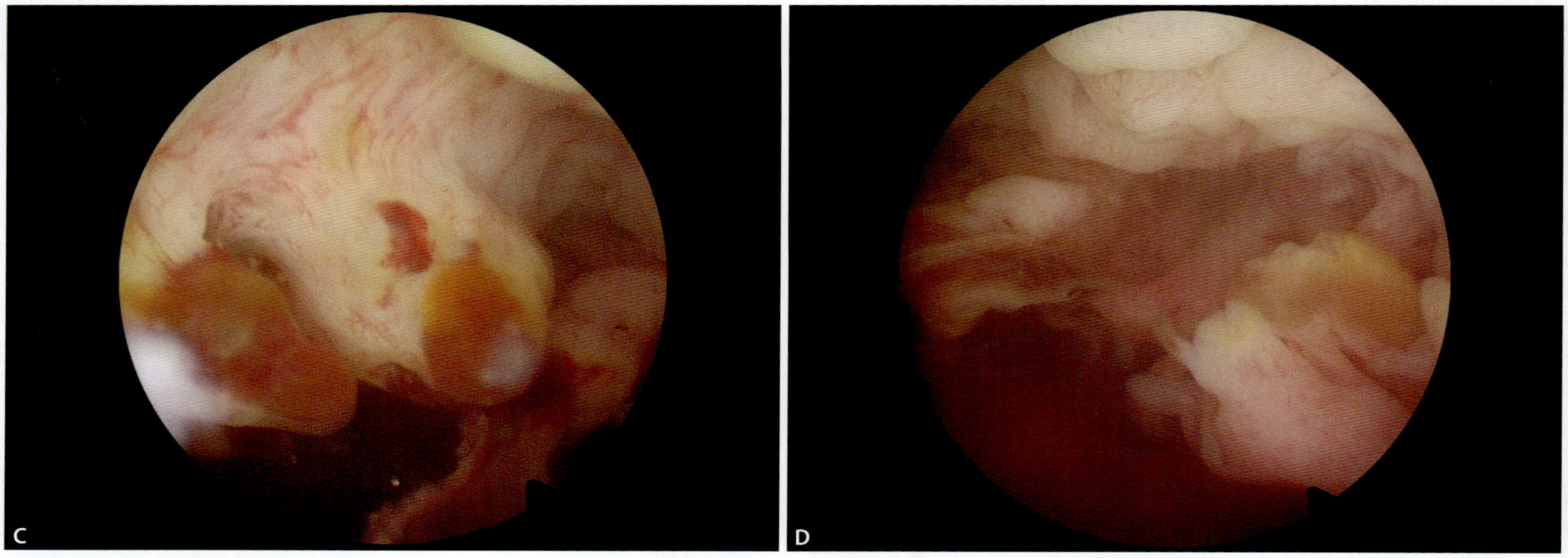

Figs. 22C to D

Figs. 22A to D: Polypoidal endometrium.

SUGGESTED READING

1. AAGL Practise Report: Practise Guidelines for the diagnosis and management of endometrial polyp. J Minim Invasive Gynecol. 2012;19(1):3-10.
2. Annan JJ, Aquilina J, Ball E. The management of endometrial polyps in 21st century. RCOG. 2012;33-8.
3. Lieng M, Istre O, Sandvik L, et al. Prevalence, 1-year regression rate, and clinical significance of asymptomatic endometrial polyps: cross sectional study. J Minim Invasive Gynecol. 2009;16(4):465-71.
4. Vilodre LC, Bertat R, Petters R, et al. Cervical polyp as risk factor for hysteroscopically diagnosed endometrial polyps. Gynecol Obstet Invest. 1997;44(3):191-5.

CHAPTER

52

Hysteroscopic Cannulation

Shubhanjali Sen, Minal Kumbhalwar, B Ramesh

INTRODUCTION

Fallopian tubes are an important site for the sperm-egg binding, and their normal functioning serve as a prerequisite for natural conception. Obstruction of Fallopian tubes a kind of common disease which is a main cause of infertility. Obstruction is of two types physiological and pathological.

Physiological obstruction is caused by debris, mucous, endometrial tags, etc. Pathological obstructions are mainly caused by inflammation, caused due to infection with *Chlamydia trachomatis, Ureaplasma urealyticum, Mycoplasma hominis*, and protozoan. About 30–40% of infertile patient are having obstruction in Fallopian tube.

EXAMINATION AND DIAGNOSIS

- *Hysterosalpingography (HSG):* This is primary radiological examination recommended for the diagnosis of Fallopian tubal obstruction. Though it is very low cost and useful in preliminary diagnosis but with this test we cannot identify pelvic inflammatory disease and endometriosis.
  Diagnostic criteria are:
  - *Tubal patency:* No resistance while injecting the contrast, X-ray result will show normal morphology with engorged contrast agent which is evenly distributed.
  - *Tubal partial obstruction:* Some resistance while injecting contrast oviduct seems tortuous, narrow, sticky, and acute sometimes. And contrast is sometimes unevenly distributed.
  - *Fallopian tube obstruction:* Oviduct no contrast outflow from tubes and appears crumby structure.
- *Hysterosalpingocontrast sonography (HyCoSy):* It is a diagnostic modality but it cannot reveal the interior of the Fallopian tubes, especially the diseased tubal mucosa and pelvic adhesions.
- *Gynecological endoscopy:*
  - *Laparoscopy:* Golden criterion for the diagnosis of tubal infertility with high sensitivity and specificity in evaluation of abdominal cavity and other pelvic structure. It is improper to use as a primary tool for diagnosis due to its high cost and invasive nature.
  - *Hysteroscopy:* One of the primary strength of the hysteroscopy is to directly look inside the uterine cavity and make an accurate diagnosis.

  Some studies point out that the combined examination of hysteroscopy and laparoscopy could improve significantly the accurate diagnosis.
- *Serological chlamydia examination: Chlamydia trachomatis* is one of the major cause of the Fallopian tube mucositis and perisalpingitis after pelvic inflammatory disease.

MANAGEMENT

The most effective therapy for proximal tubal obstruction is hysteroscopic cannulation using Terumo guidewire or various types of catheter.

Wire Guided Proximal Tubal Cannulation Under Hystero-laparoscopic Guidance (Figs. 1 to 13)

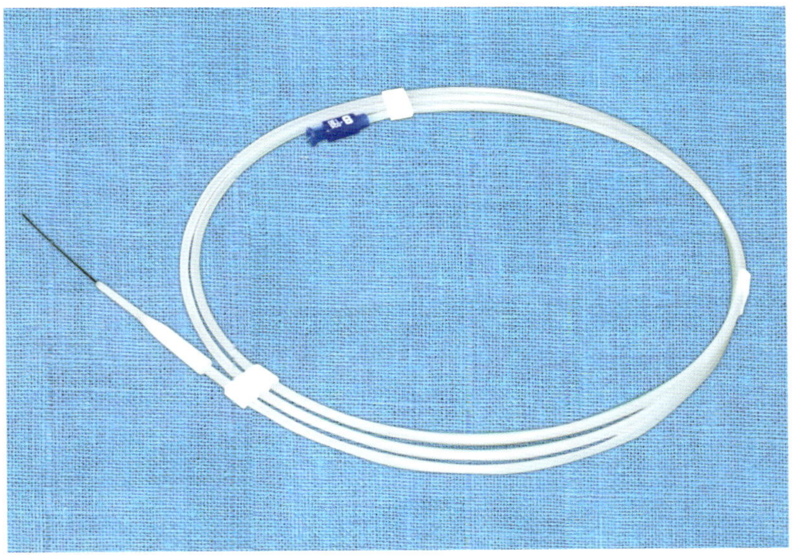

Fig. 1: Terumo guidewire.

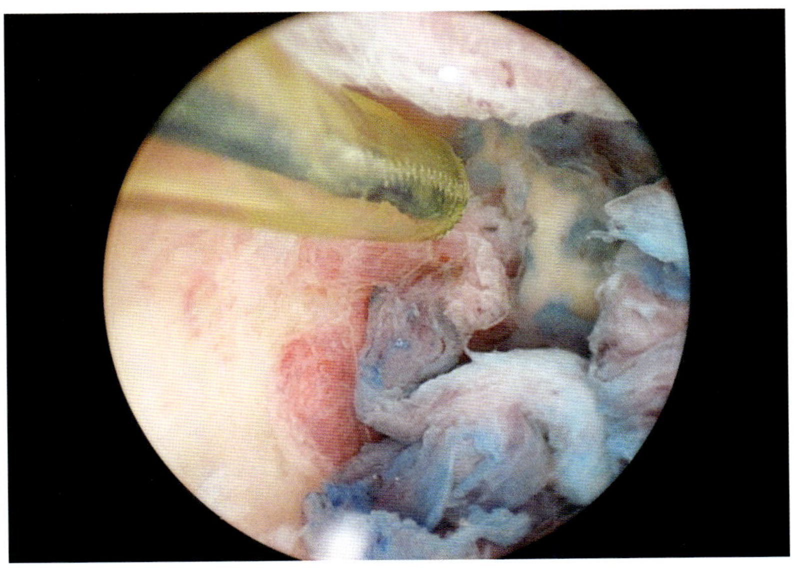

Fig. 2: Terumo guidewire. Endometrium is obstructing the vision, negotiation between endometrial tags.

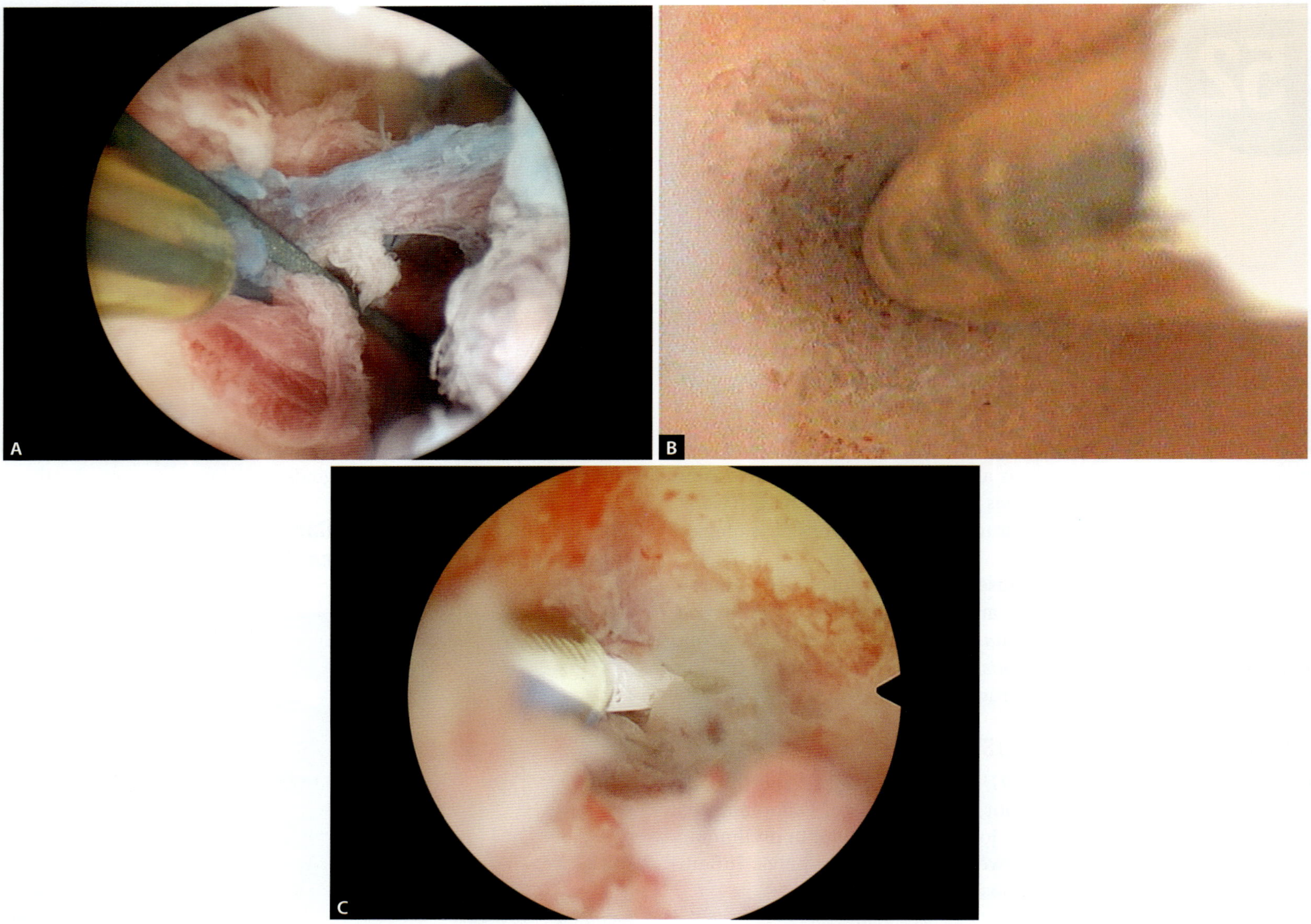

Figs. 3A to C: Ostia being cannulated with Terumo guidewire.

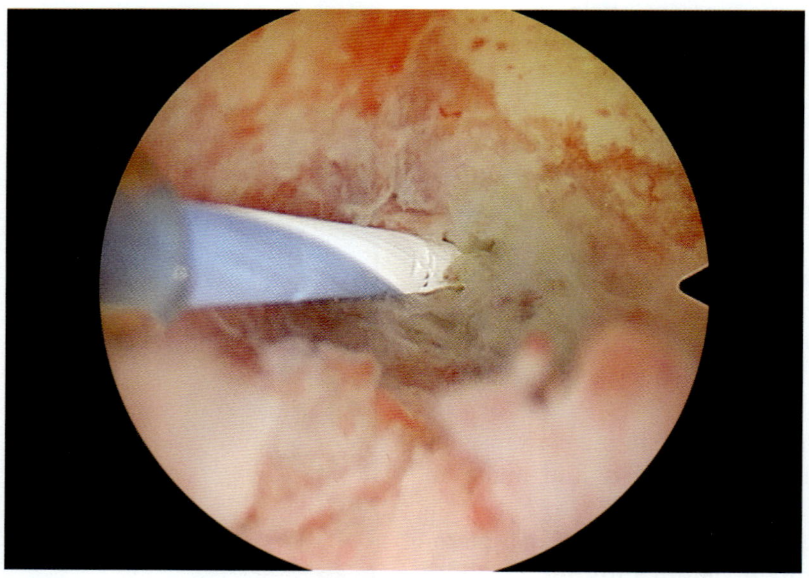

Fig. 4

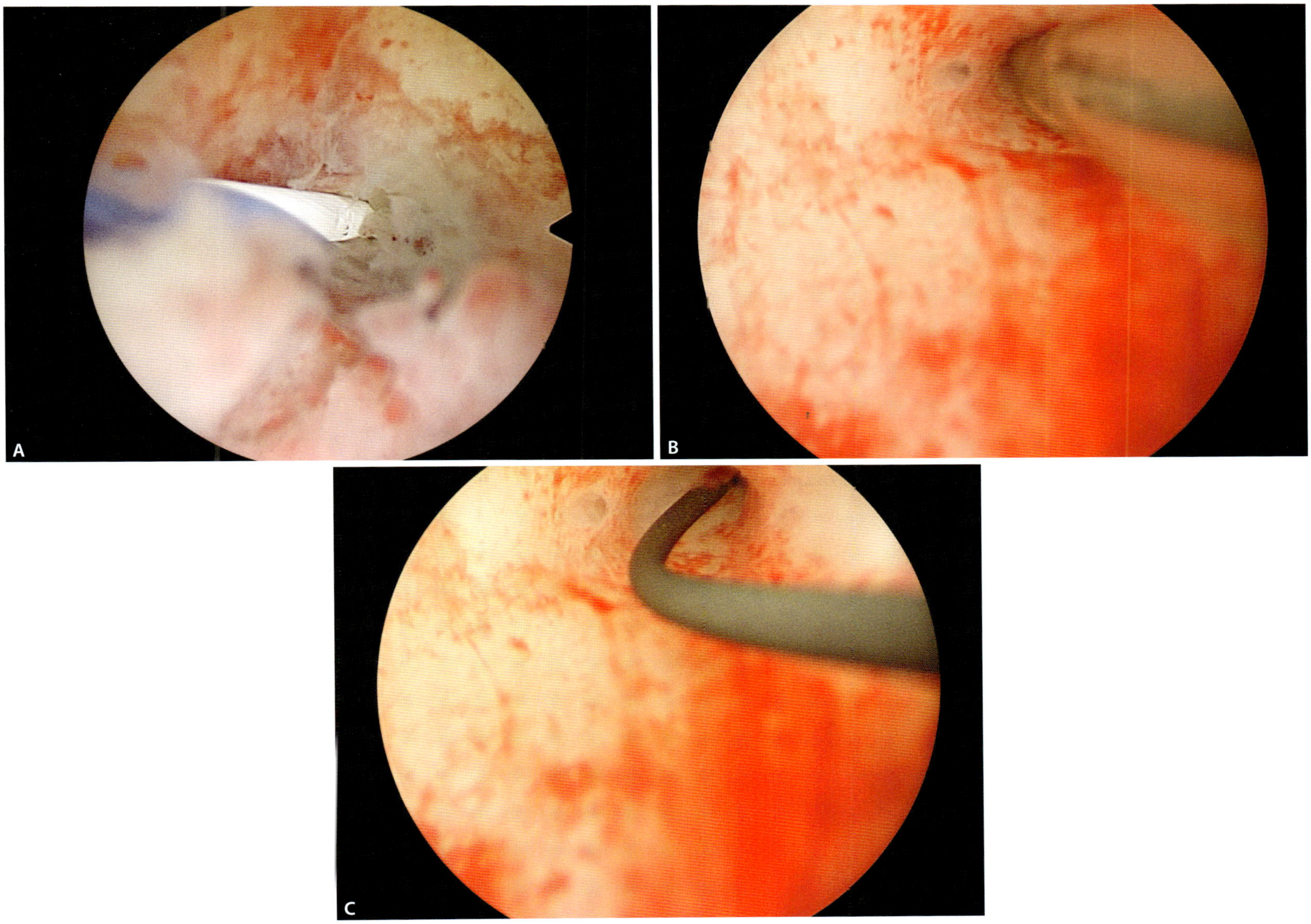

Figs. 5A to C: Guidewire is directed toward the ostium.

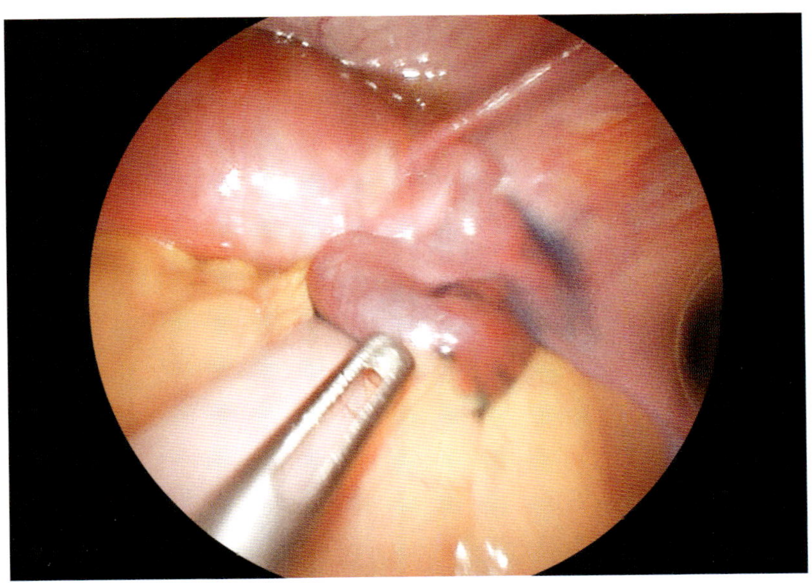

Fig. 6: Postguidewire cannulation chromopertubation observed.

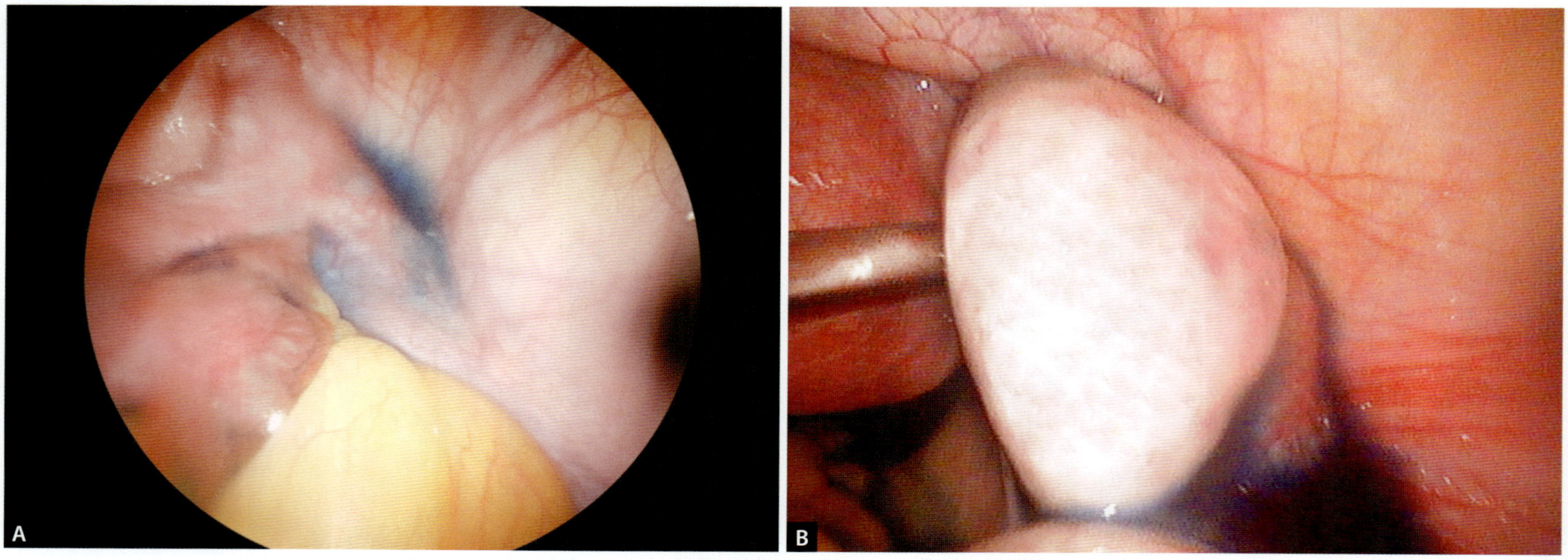

Figs. 7A and B: Postcannulation chromopertubation seen.

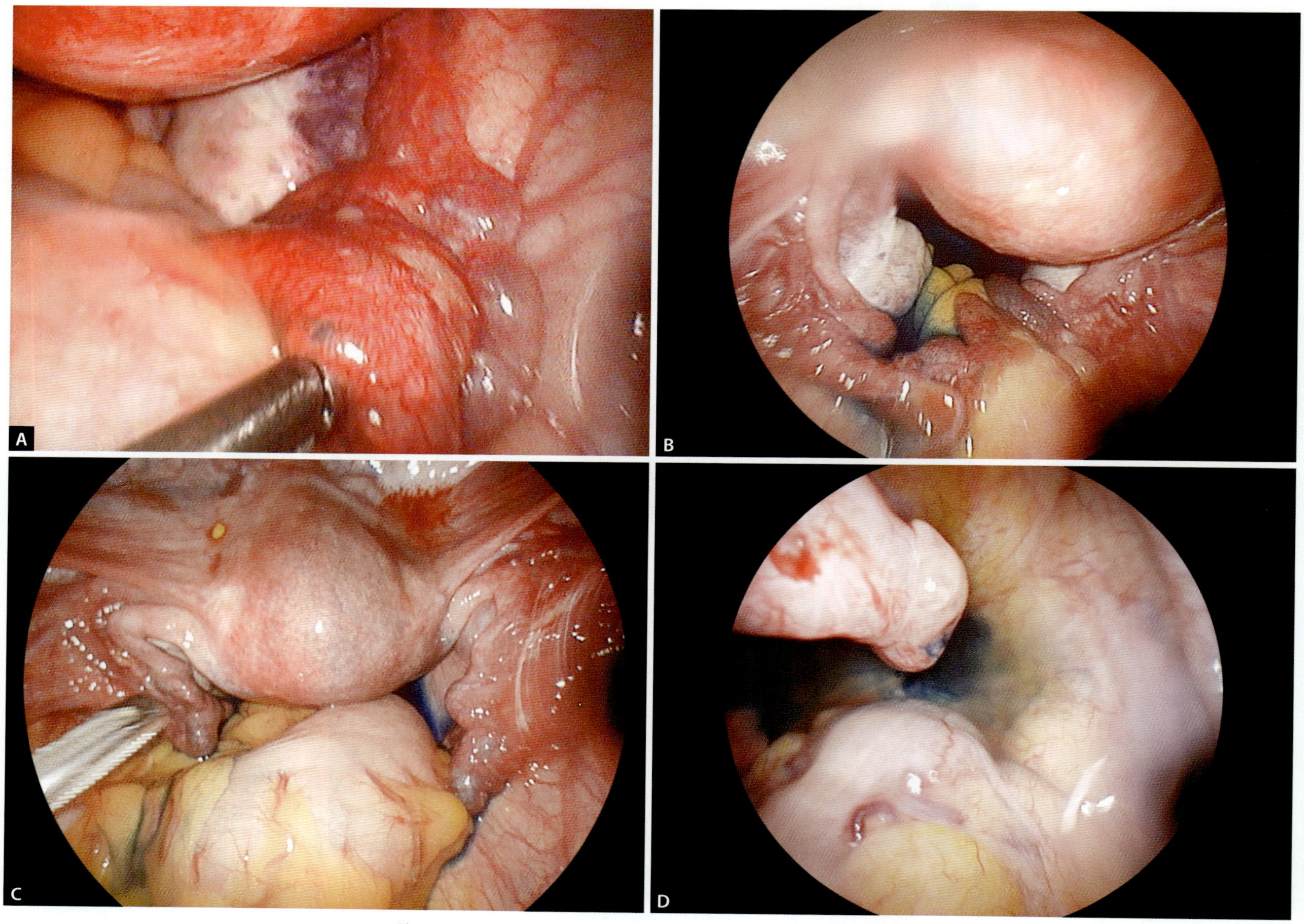

Figs. 8A to D: Postcannulation free spillage of dye from both sides.

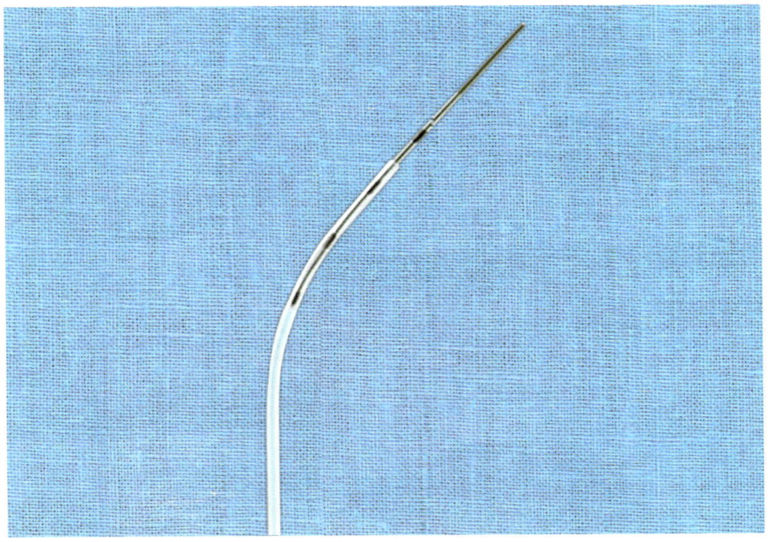

Fig. 9: Novy Cook catheter.
The Novy cornual cannulation set is intended for use through the operating channel of a hysteroscope or other uterine access device, for hysteroscopic cannulation of the proximal Fallopian tube. The introduction of chromotubation solution for the evaluation of tubal patency is checked. The guidewire in the Novy cornual cannulation set is intended only to facilitate placement of the inner catheter. It is not intended for tubal recanalization and should not be advanced beyond the tubal isthmus.

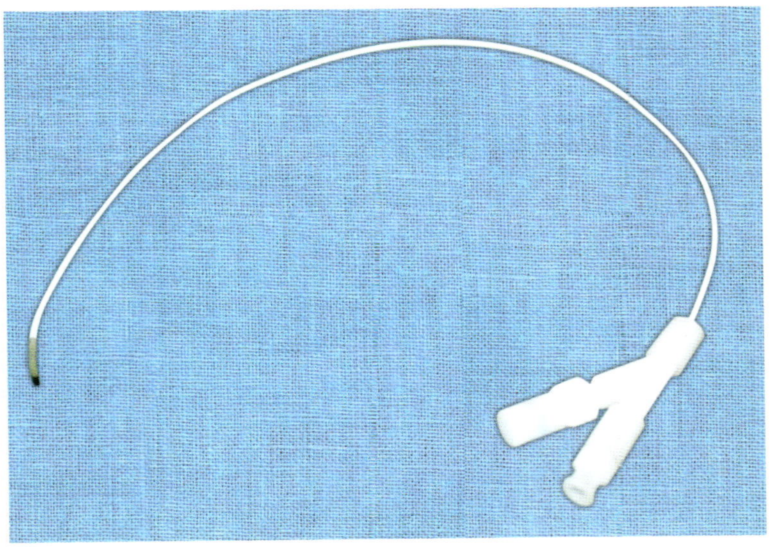

Fig. 10: 5 Fr catheter used for cannulation.

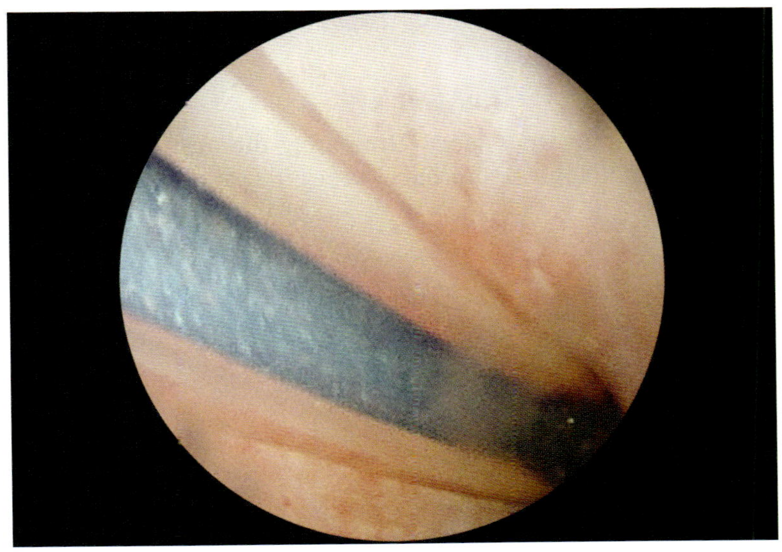

Fig. 12: Instrumentation for cannulation and completely inserted inside the ostia followed by which selective salpingography done.

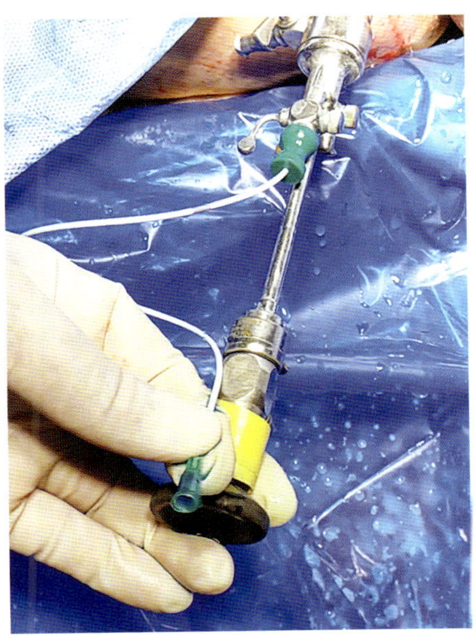

Fig. 11: Selective cannulation and salpingography.

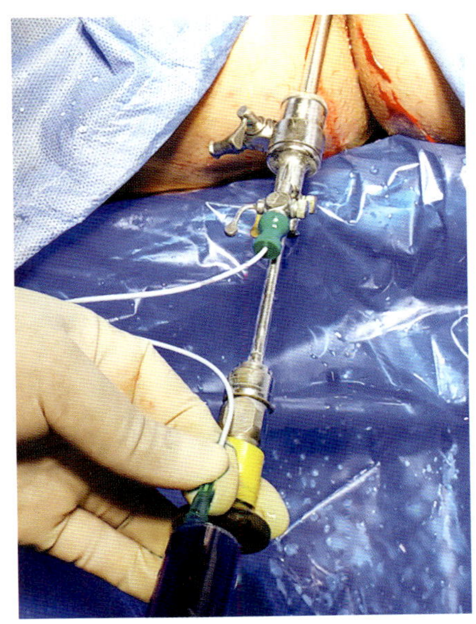

Fig. 13: Selective salpingography and chromotubation. Cannula is flushed into selective ostia and direct chromopertubation done.

PROCEDURE

The procedure takes up the lithotomy position and tracheal intubation is performed under general anesthesia.

Laparoscope is inserted into the abdominal cavity to detect the shape, size, and location of the pelvic cavity, uterus and ovary, and find out whether the Fallopian tube is functioning, presence of adhesions or distortion. If needed operative procedures are performed like pelvic adhesiolysis and restoration of pelvic anatomy is performed. Fimbrial adhesions should be treated with adhesiolysis and neostomy. Mesosalpinx cyst if present should be enucleated. In cases of endometriosis electrocoagulation should be done.

On hysteroscopy endometrial thickness and shape is evaluated. Later the methylene blue dye is injected through Leech-Wilkinson cannula and spill through the tubes noted. This procedure helps in the detailed identification of the obstructed site in Fallopian tube.

Tube cannulation is done by inserting the Terumo guidewire under hysteroscopic vision into the cornual end and the obstruction is relieved, and after the cannulation the patency of tube is checked by injecting the methylene blue dye seen with the help of laparoscope.

A successful cannulation no doubt increases the chances of pregnancy to happen. Post-cannulation the pregnancy rate varies from 30% to 60%.

INTERVENTIONAL TREATMENT

It is a minimal invasive approach treating the obstructed tube by combining radiological approach with imaging equipment to do intervention.

CONCLUSION

The tubal diseases serve as a common factor including female infertility and pose a task for the infertility treatment. The pathogenesis for tubal block can be pathological or physiological. The physiological block in proximal tubal occlusion is very common cause of infertility which can be released through hysteroscopic cannulation. There is remarkable increase in the percentage of the pregnancy happening after tubal cannulation. If in any circumstances the catheter is difficult to pass, force should not be applied else false passage can be formed or any perforation may occur.

SUGGESTED READING

1. Chung JP, Haines CJ, Kong GW. Long term reproductive outcome after hysteroscopic proximal tubal cannulation—an outcome analysis. Aust N Z J Obstet Gynaecol. 2012;52:470-5.
2. Das S, Nardo LG, Seif MW. Proximal tubal disease: the place for tubal cannulation. Reprod Biomed Online. 2007;15(4):383-8.
3. Hou HY, Chen YQ, Li TC, et al. Outcome of laparoscopy-guided hysteroscopic tubal catheterization for infertility due to proximal tubal obstruction. J Minimal Invasive Gynecol. 2014;21:272-8.
4. Ikechebelu JI, Eleje GU, Bhamare P, et al. Fertility outcomes following laparoscopy-assisted hysteroscopic fallopian tube cannulation: a preliminary study. Obstet Gynecol Int. 2018;2018:7060459.
5. Liu X, Cui H, Chen W, et al. Diagnosis and treatment of fallopian tube obstruction: a literature review. Int J Clin Exp Med. 2017;10(12): 15950-9.
6. National Collaborating Centre for women's and children health (UK). fertility: assessment and treatment for people with fertility problem. RCOG Press 2013;1:21-28.

CHAPTER

53

Hysteroscopic Septal Resection

Shubhanjali Sen, Minal Kumbhalwar, B Ramesh

INTRODUCTION

Septate uterus has found to be associated with many risks like miscarriage, premature delivery, malpresentations, and even infertility. Several studies reported that operating a uterine septum is associated with an improved outcome in live birth rates in women with a history of preterm deliveries, recurrent pregnancy loss (RPL), or dealing with infertility. When the uterine septum is implicated in RPL, second trimester loss, malpresentation, or preterm delivery, then hysteroscopic approach is preferred option owing to its safety, simplicity, and excellent posttreatment results.

Hysteroscopic septal resection significantly improves the live birth rates and decreases miscarriage rates to approximately 80–15%, respectively.

DEVELOPMENT OF THE UTERINE SEPTUM

A uterine septum is developed as a result of the failure of resorption of the tissue in between the two paramesonephric ducts before 20th embryonic week. Arcuate uterus is the mildest form of the resorption failure. The incidence is 1–2 in every 1,000 to as high as 15 in 1,000 cases.

TYPES OF THE SEPTATE UTERUS

Partial/incomplete septate uterus: Single fundus and cervix with uterine septum extending from the top of the cavity toward the cervix.

DIAGNOSTIC DEFINITIONS ACCORDING TO DIFFERENT SOCIETIES

- *European Society of Human Reproduction and Embryology (ESHRE)-European Society for Gynecological Endoscopy (ESGE):* Internal indentation extending; 50% of the myometrial wall thickness
- *American Society for Reproductive Medicine (ASRM):* No strict parameter to identify the septate uterus
- *American Fertility Society (AFS):* Morphologic criteria to differentiate a septate uterus from arcuate uterus.

The center point of the septum is at the acute angle and the length of the septum is more than 1.5 cm in partial septum.

If there is fundal invagination between 1 cm and 1.5 cm, then it is considered to be arcuate uterus.

Buttram classification criteria says if the septum originates at the fundus but is not reaching till the internal os and dividing the endometrial cavity partially, then it will be a partial septum.

COMPLETE SEPTATE UTERUS

It has a single fundus with a septum arising from the top of the endometrial cavity and continuing up till the cervix. Sometimes, it may be associated with the longitudinal vaginal septum.

Buttram classification criteria states that if the septum extends from the fundal zone to the internal os, or even to external cervical os, dividing the endometrial cavity into two units completely, it will be labeled as a complete septum.

Diagnosis of the Septate Uterus

Gold standard diagnostic modality is by direct visualization of the uterine cavity externally by laparoscope and internally by hysteroscope.

Radiological modalities like hysterosalpingogram (HSG) can be the initial test for identification, but it does not give an accurate diagnosis between the septate uterus and bicornuate uterus. Disadvantage is that there is lack of the knowledge of the external contour of the uterus and exposure to the ionizing radiation.

Saline infusion sonography (SIS), three-dimensional (3D) ultrasonography (USG), and two-dimensional (2D) USG are a sensitive modality for the septum diagnosis.

Information like morphology, external contour, and vascularization of the septum is very well-elicited. Only fallacy is to obtain a coronal section of the uterus.

Magnetic resonance imaging (MRI) is an excellent noninvasive diagnostic modality to differentiate septate uterus with bicornuate uterus before surgical correction.

So, the ASRM proposes that 3D USG, sonohysterography, and MRI are better diagnostic tools for differentiating a septate from bicornuate uterus when compared with laparoscopy and hysteroscopy.

The diagnostic accuracy for USG, MRI, HSG, hysteroscopy, and laparoscopy is 93%, 48%, 53%, 98%, and 100%, respectively.

SURGERY FOR THE SEPTAL RESECTION

Principle of the Surgery

Hysteroscopy is the gold standard for resecting septum. Various modalities are used through hysteroscope to remove septum.

Transverse incision of the uterine septum. Incision is given in the midline of the septum equidistant from anterior and posterior uterine walls. Tubal ostia help to align in the right plane.

Methodologies are resection that can be performed with scissors, resectoscope, laser metroplasty, and bipolar electrode. None of them is superior to another. Transcervical septal resection has quicker operating time, decreased surgical trauma, and minimal complications hence, it is increasingly becoming popular.

Preoperative Preparation

Ideal time for doing septal surgeries is early follicular phase of the menstrual cycle to have good operational visibility. Systemic evaluation is done including cardiac evaluation and physician fitness. Blood tests like complete blood count (CBC), coagulation profile, renal function test (RFT), liver function test (LFT), thyroid function test (TFT), serology [human immunodeficiency virus-I (HIV-I) and antibody-mediated prevention-II (AMP-II), hepatitis B and C, and venereal disease research laboratory (VDRL)], and urine routine microscopy are done to exclude any pathology. Chest X-ray, electrocardiogram (ECG) and ECHO are routinely performed. Previous night light diet and two tablets Dulcolax are orally given for bowel preparation. Tablet Cytotec 200 µg PV kept 1 hour prior to the procedure.

Procedure

Diagnostic evaluation of the thickness and length of septum, ostia location, and approximate size of the two subcavities is done. Along with that, associated pathologies such as fibroids, polyps, or intrauterine adhesions are to be ruled out. Initially if any myoma, adhesion, or polyp is present, then it should be corrected followed by septoplasty.

First of all, the uterus should be brought to midaxial position with the use of tenaculum to correctly and adequately visualize the uterine septum along with cavities. Septum is gradually resected while the tissues will retract anteriorly and posteriorly automatically. While incising the septum, it is important to stay in midline.

Microscissors do not require prior cervical dilatation; also there is no thermal injury to adjoining tissue.

It also reduces the risk of water intoxication. However, the drawback is relatively long time for the surgery, excessive equipment wear, and regular scissors replacement.

Laser surgery has a shorter operating time, minimal bleeding, adequate hemostasis, and no injury to nearby tissues. Lasers can use any type of the uterine distention fluids. Disadvantages are high cost, longer surgery time, and higher incidence of gas embolism.

Hysteroscopic electrosurgical excision is widely accepted. A 26 Fr resectoscope is used with glycine as the distention media along with either cutting knife monopolar electrode or cutting wire (Collins) loop electrode. Cutting current is set at 80–100 W and coagulation current is set at 50–70 W. A continuous instillation of glycine medium is used for uterine distention and also for draining purpose at 70–100 mm Hg inflow pressure. The inflow and outflow fluid volume difference should not exceed 1,500 mL.

Nowadays, 21 Fr resectoscopes are also available. The advantage over 26 Fr is that there is no trauma over the cervix and we need not dilate the cervix.

Nowadays, bipolar resectoscope is also very popular in use, the biggest advantage is that the normal saline is used instead of glycine and all hazards of glycine can be avoided.

When to stop the resection?

While performing the septal resection when the two ostia are seen in panoramic view and the presence of vascularization with increased blood flow at the fundus is seen, then the junction of the septum and myometrium has reached. When visualization of the myometrial fibers and typical triangular cavity is seen, then the resection should be stopped. After metroplasty, even if <1 cm residual septum is left, it will not hamper the reproductive outcome. The required distance among the upper limit of resection and fundal serosal surface should be around 10 mm.

POSTOPERATIVE TREATMENT

Antibiotics are administered for 5 days to prevent the infection. Hormone replacement therapy (HRT) should be substituted to the patients for minimum of three cycles for the endometrial regeneration (i.e. estradiol valerate 2 mg thrice a day from day 2 to day 25 and tablet Meprate 10 mg twice a day from day 16 to day 25).

POSTOPERATIVE OUTCOME

Hysteroscopic metroplasty done either for small or large septate uterus improves reproductive outcome, shortens the conception time, and reduces the spontaneous miscarriage rates. Implantation rates become better and birth rates are similar to normal uterus.

In postseptal resection, there are no harmful effects for the spontaneous conception followed by labor to happen without complications.

Cesarean section is not necessary to be done.

Steps of Hysteroscopic Septal Resection (Figs. 1 to 13)

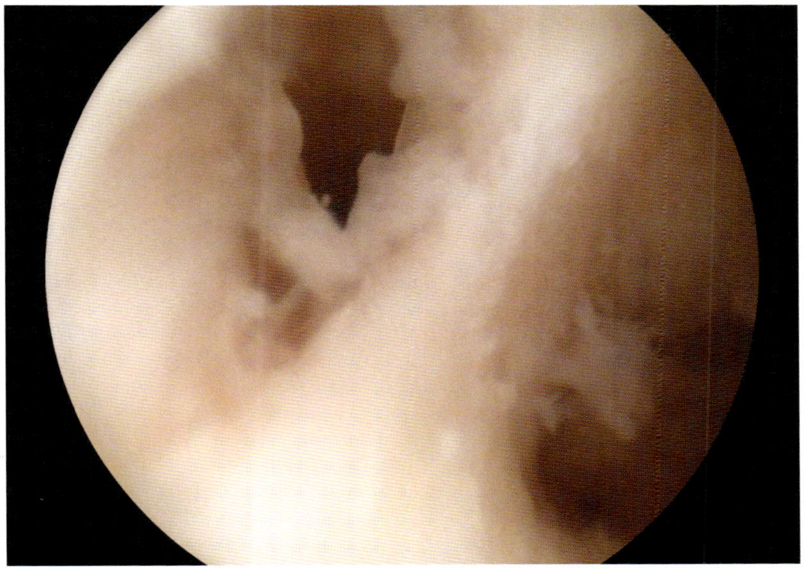

Fig. 1: Hysteroscopic appearance of the typical septum.

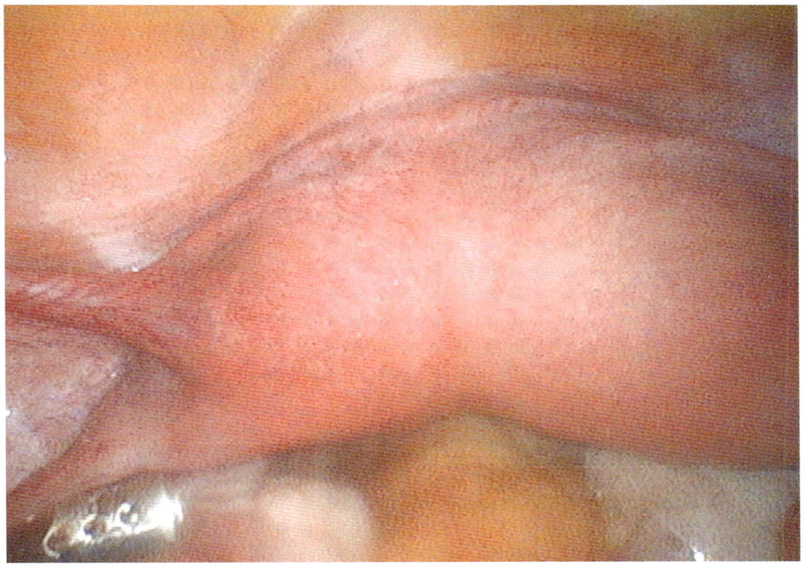

Fig. 2: Laparoscopic view of septate uterus with broad fundus and fundal depression.

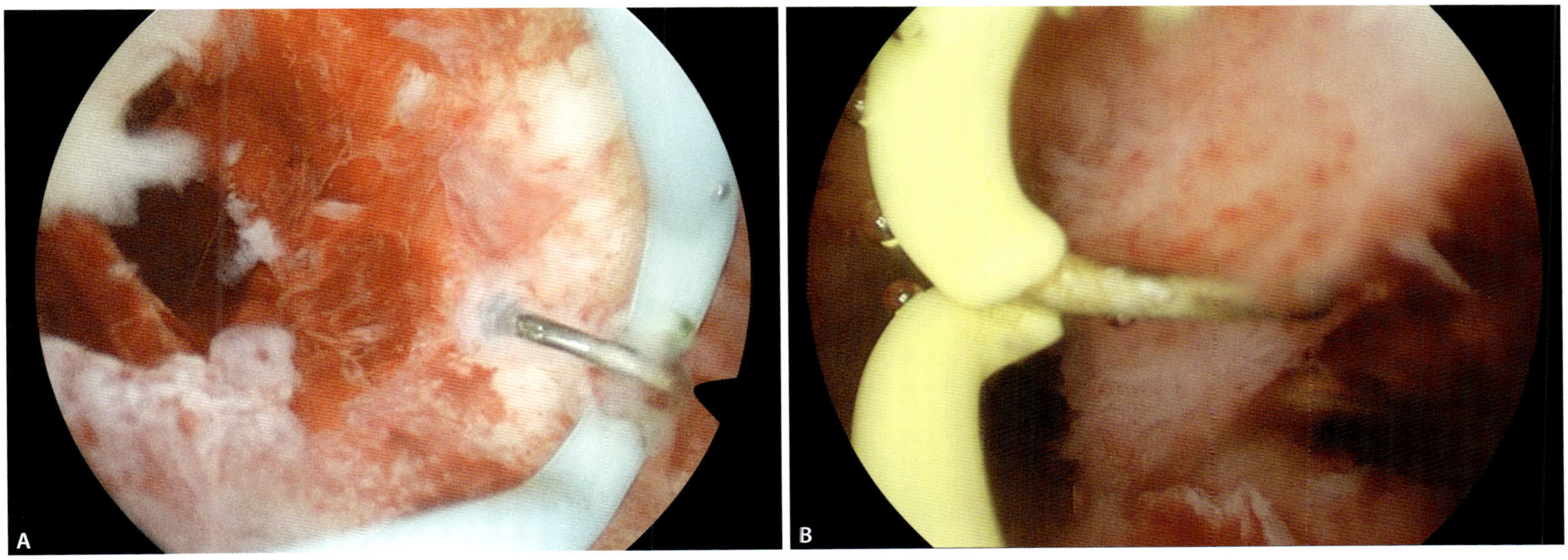

Figs. 3A and B: Beginning of the septum from the center of the resection. Collins knife is perpendicular to the septum.

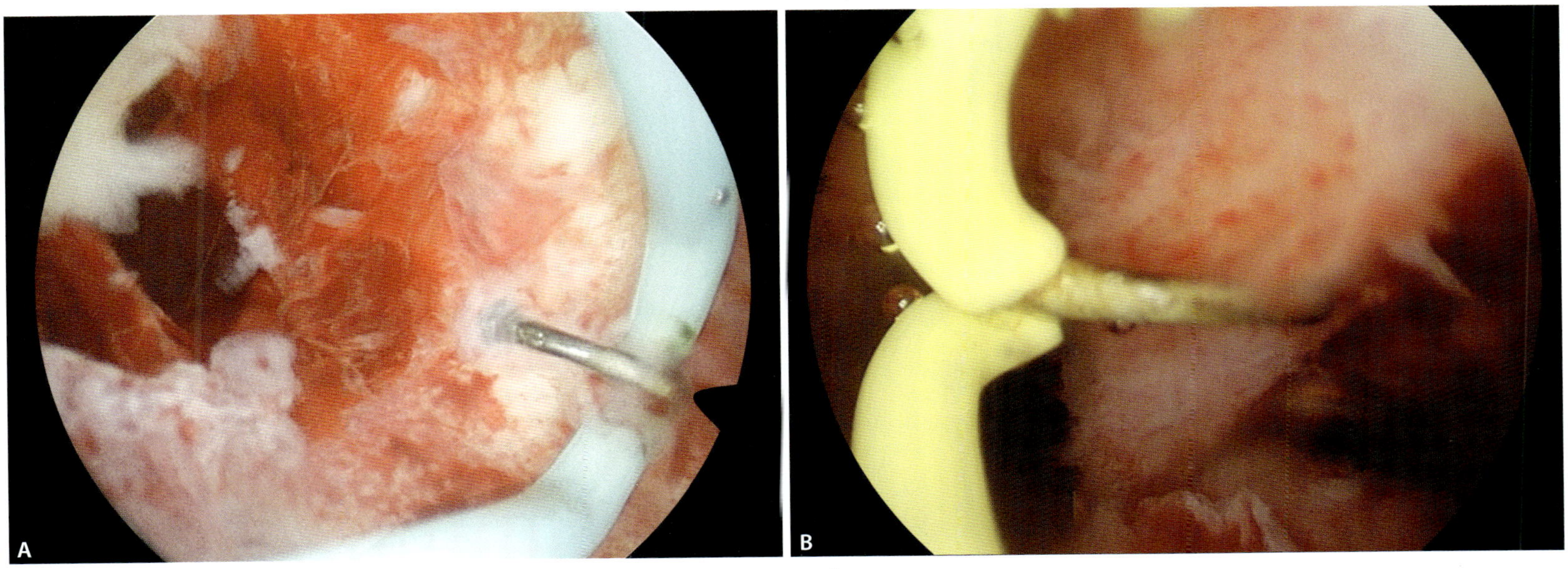

Figs. 4A and B

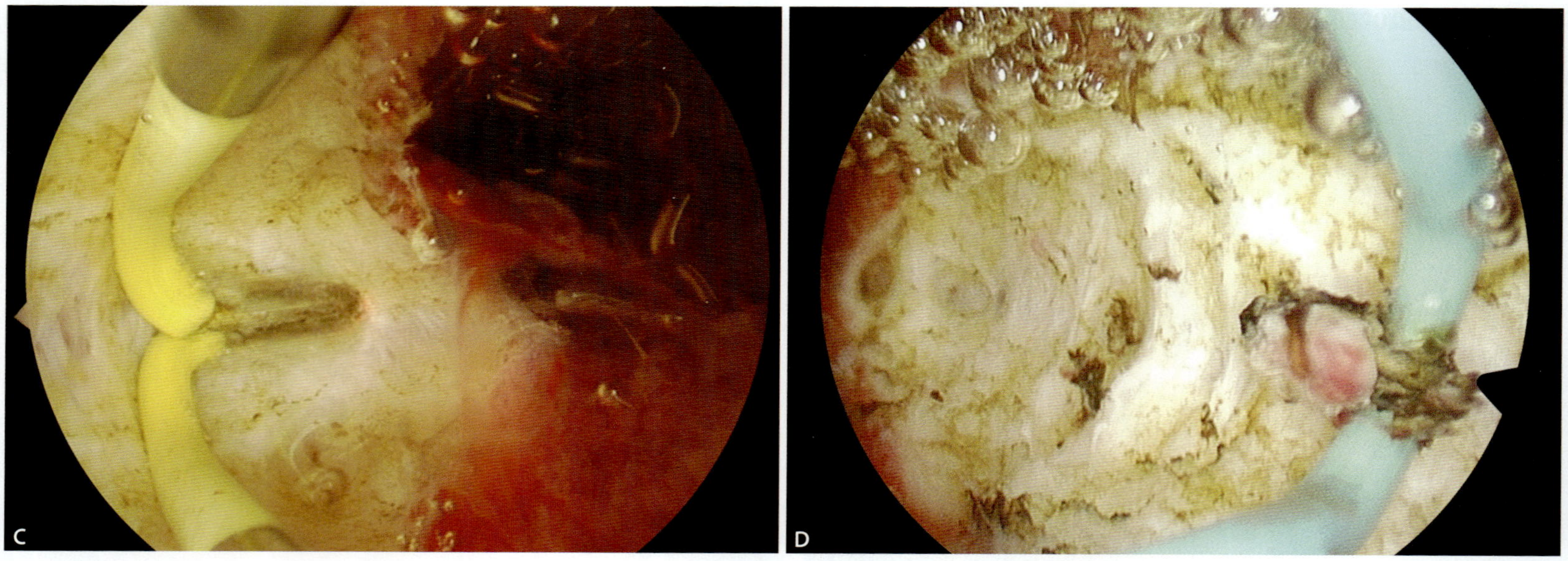

Figs. 4C and D

Figs. 4A and D: Collins knife is used for resection.

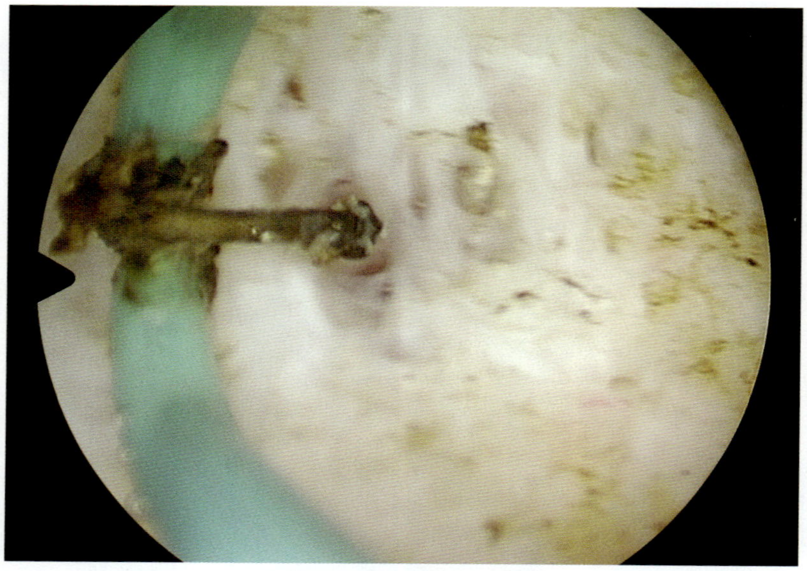

Fig. 5: Resection continued

Note: Septum is avascular with no bleeding during resection.

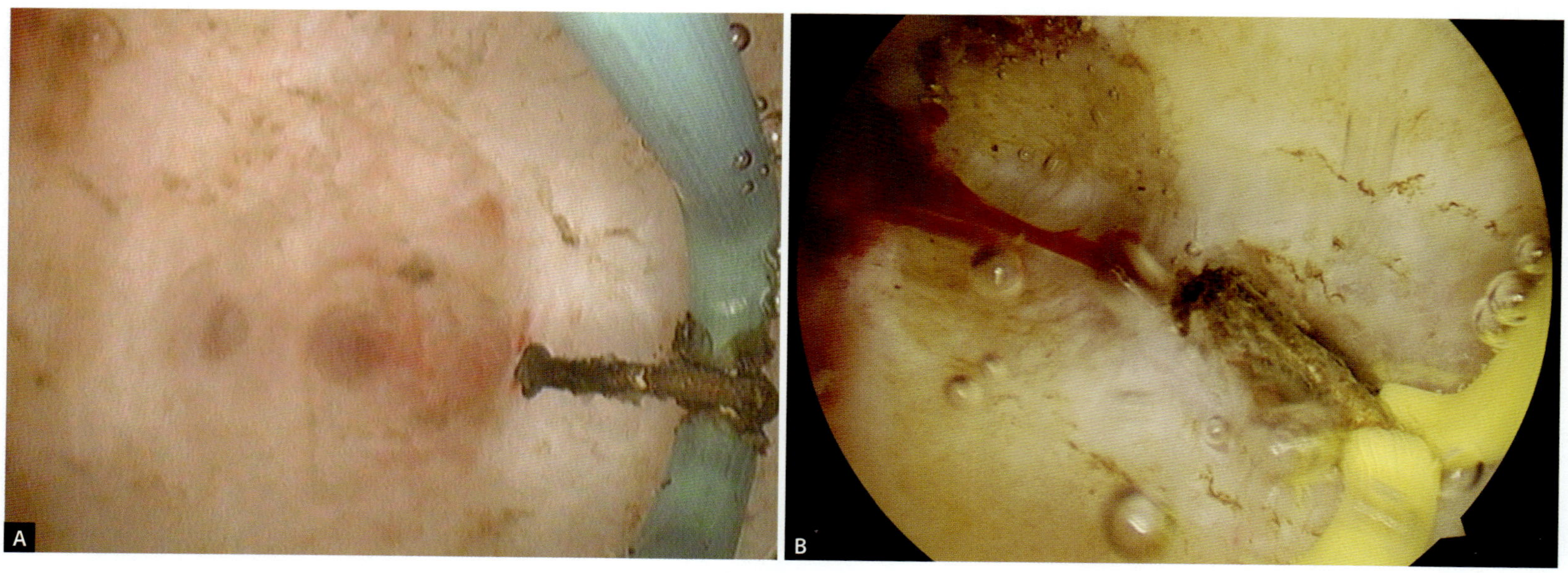

Figs. 6A and B

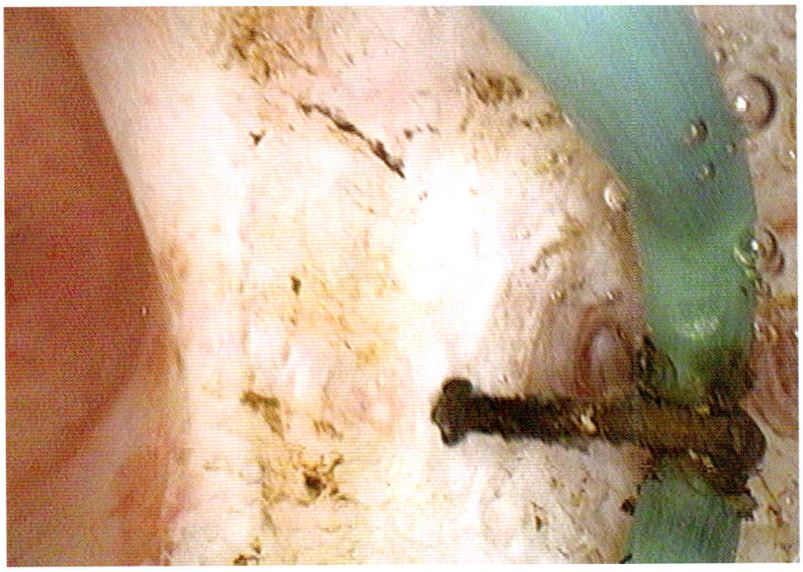

Fig. 6C

Figs. 6A to C: Right side of septum close to right cornua being resected.

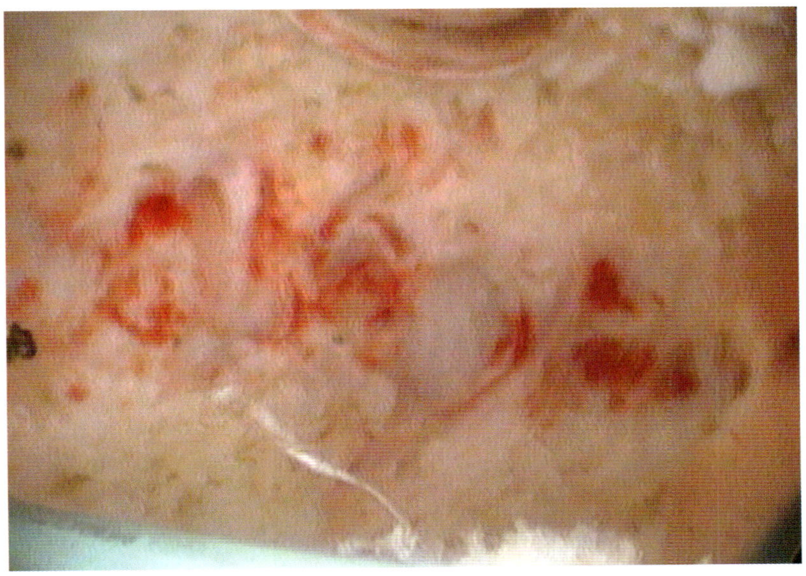

Fig. 7: Bleeding points and myometrial fibers visible at the end of the resection.

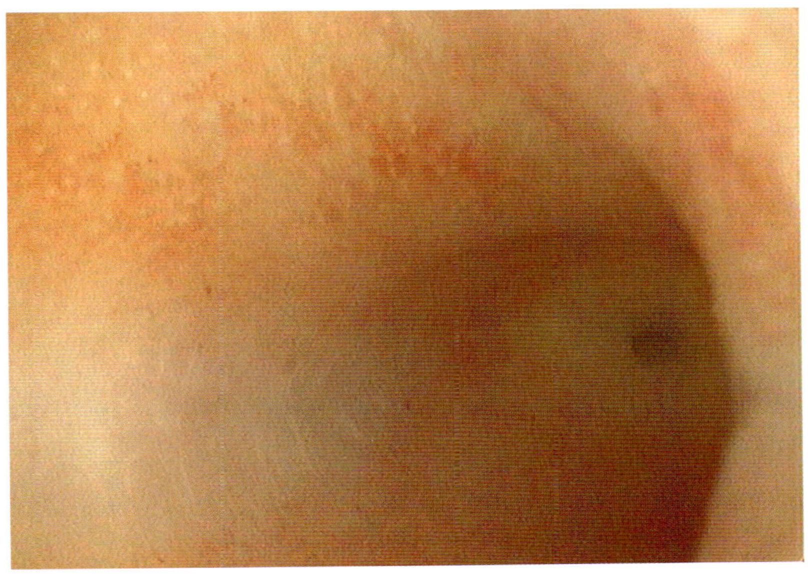

Fig. 8: One side of the septate uterus. Unicornuate cavity mimics like this.

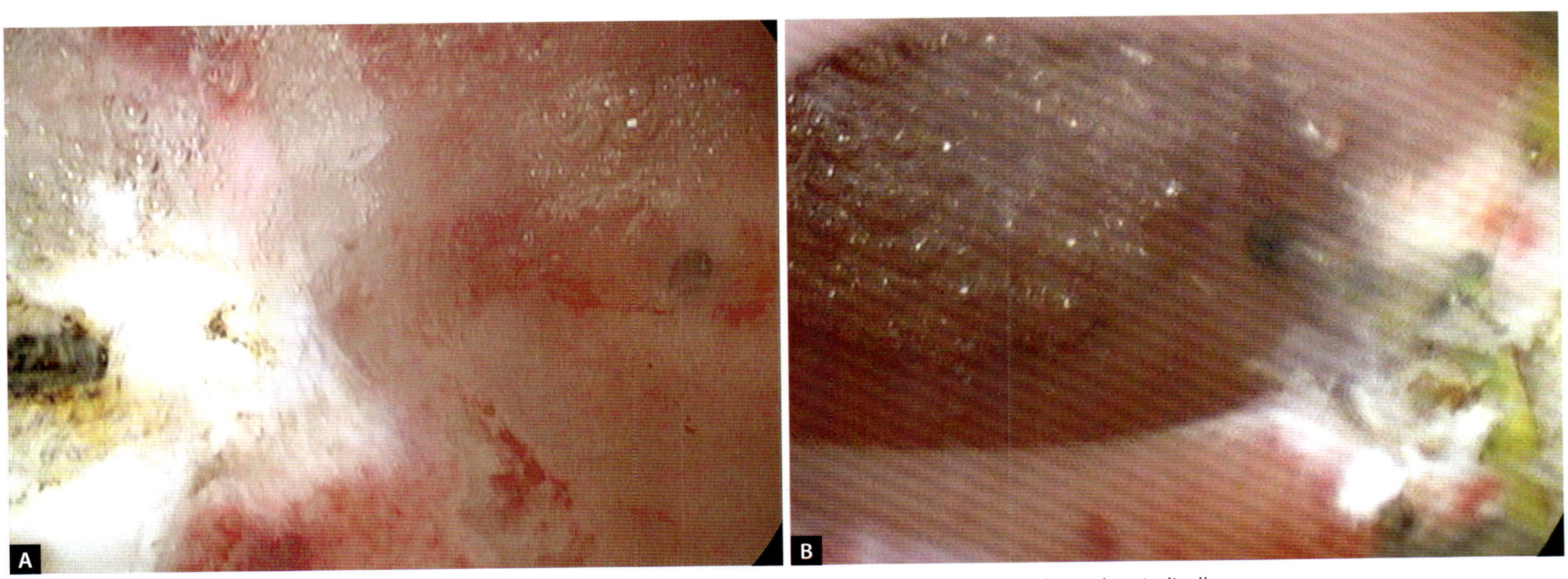

Figs. 9A and B: Fumes and bubbles can disturb the vision which has to be cleaned periodically.

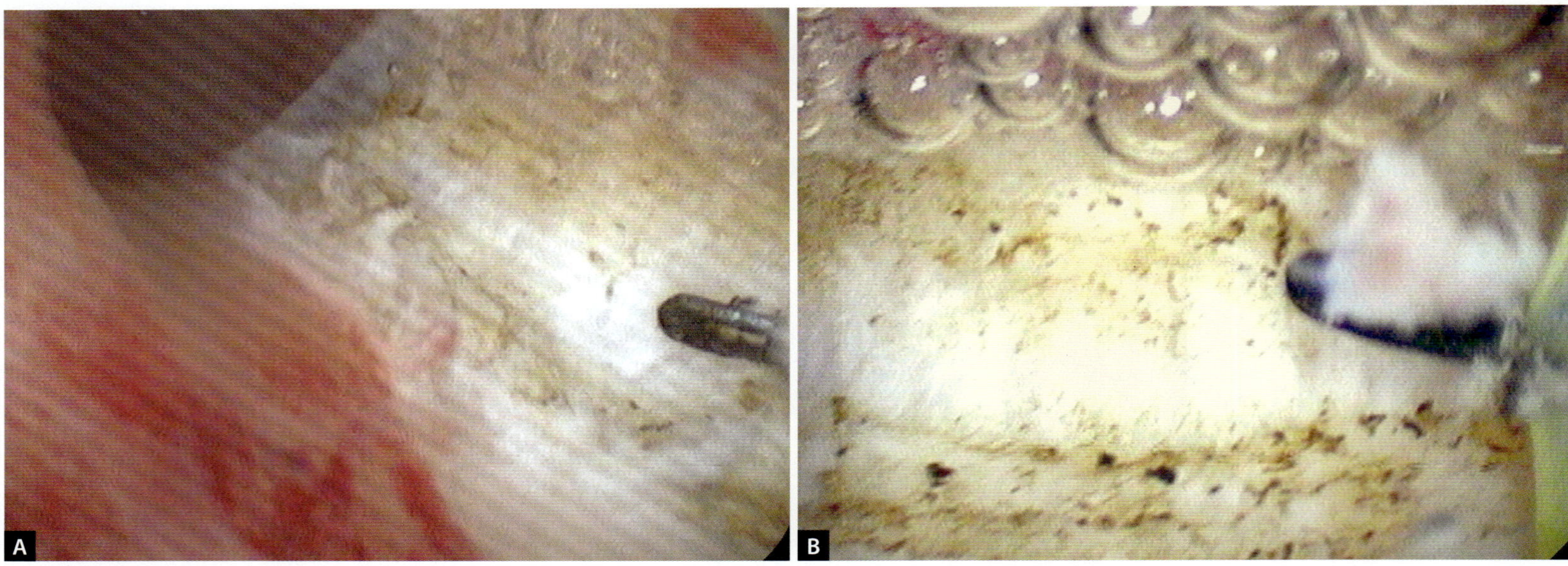

Figs. 10A and B: Posthysteroscopic resection view.

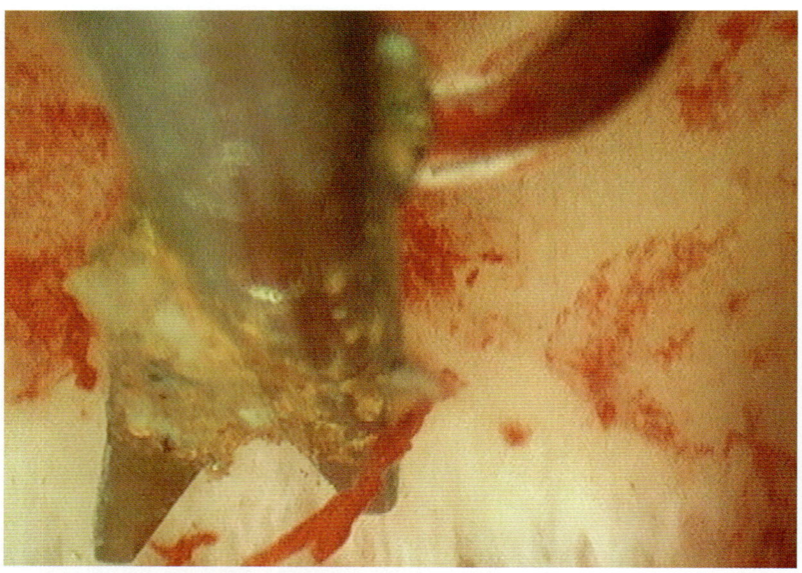

Fig. 11: Septal resection with cold scissors.

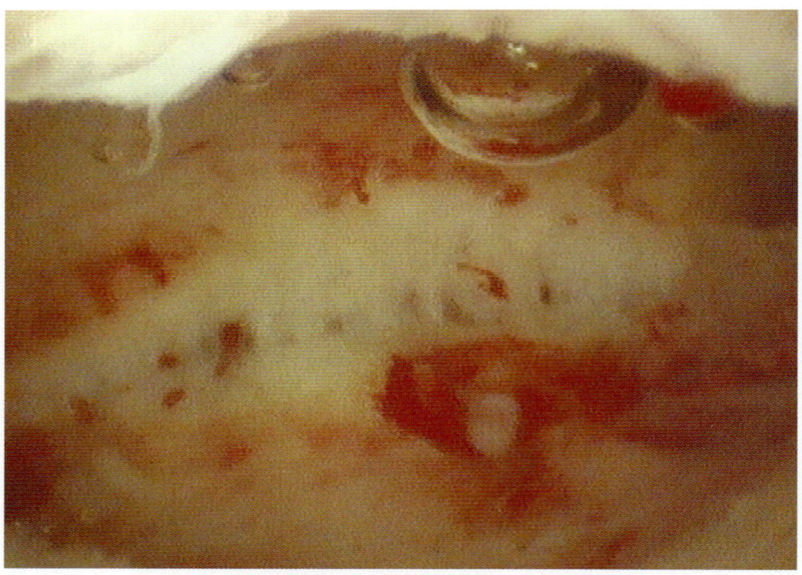

Fig. 12: Postseptal resection uterine cavity.

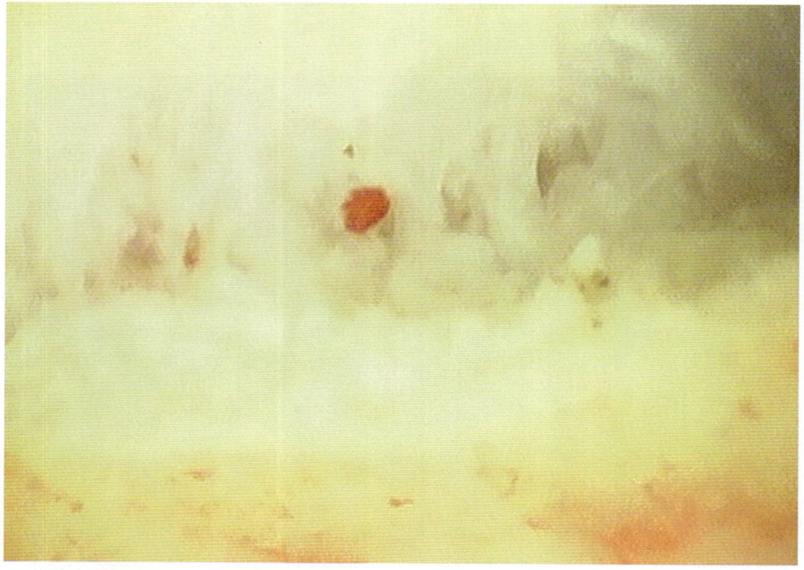

Fig. 13: Postseptal resection (resection done with cold scissors).

SUGGESTED READING

1. Breg A, Sandvik L, Langebrekke A, et al. A randomized trial comparing monopolar electrodes using glycine 1.5% with two different types of bipolar electrodes (TCRis, Versapoint) using saline, in hysteroscopic surgery. Fertil Steril. 2009;91:1273-8.
2. Garuti G, Luerti M. Hysteroscopic bipolar surgery: a valuable progress or a technique under investigation? Curr Opin Obstet Gynecol. 2009;21:329-34.
3. Kothikela S, Bieber EJ, Ying H, et al. Hysteroscopy: evaluation and management of the uterine septum. In: Kavic MS, Nezhat C, Winfield H (Eds). Prevention and Management of Laparoendoscopic Surgical Complications, 3rd edition. New York: Society of Laparoendoscopic Surgeons; 2019. pp. 1-11.
4. Mueller GC, Hussain HK, Smith YR, et al. Müllerian duct anomalies: comparison of MRI diagnosis and clinical diagnosis. AJR Am J Roentgenol. 2007;189:1294-302.
5. Practice Committee of the American Society for Reproductive Medicine. Uterine septum: a guideline. Fertil Steril. 2016;106:530-40.

Accompanying Video: Hysteroscopic septal resection.

CHAPTER

54

Submucosal Leiomyoma

Shubhanjali Sen, G Hemasree, B Ramesh

INTRODUCTION

Uterine leiomyomas are most common tumors of the myometrium with prevalence of 70–80% **(Fig. 1)**. These benign tumors are called myoma, which can be symptomatic or asymptomatic.

INDICATIONS FOR THE HYSTEROSCOPIC REMOVAL OF FIBROID

Submucous fibroid—types 0, 1, and 2 causing:

- Abnormal uterine bleeding
- Infertility
- Recurrent pregnancy loss
- Dysmenorrhea
- Pressure symptoms over the bowel and bladder.

CONTRAINDICATIONS

Hysteroscopic removal of the fibroid is contraindicated in women who have itself contraindication of undergoing hysteroscopic surgery and also fibroids type 2 and intramural fibroid.

Hysteroscopic resection is feasible with the fibroid having an intracavitary component. When the myoma is too large which penetrate the myometrium, it becomes difficult in doing the hysteroscopic resection.

Large fibroids need special skill set in terms of fluid management and even quick removal of the chipped fragments of the myoma.

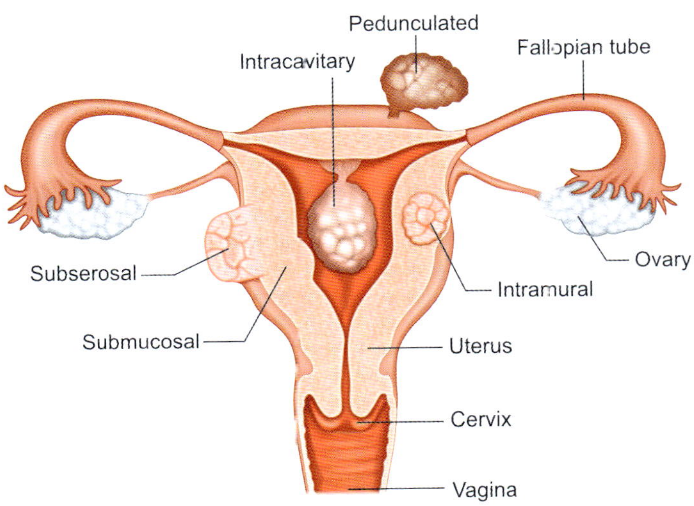

Fig. 1: Myomas of the uterus.

CLASSIFICATION OF THE SUBMUCOUS MYOMA [EUROPEAN SOCIETY FOR GYNECOLOGICAL ENDOSCOPY (ESGE)]

- *Type 0:*
  - Entirely within endometrial cavity
  - No myometrial extension (pedunculated).
- *Type I:*
  - <50% myometrial extension (sessile)
  - <90 angle of myoma surface to uterine wall.
- *Type II:*
  - >50% myometrial extension (sessile)
  - >90 angle of myoma surface to uterine wall.

A recent classification Lasmar classification is perhaps a diagnostic criterion to select the patient for the right approach of the myomectomy **(Fig. 2)**.

EFFECTS ON THE FERTILITY

The pregnancy rate and implantation rate are higher after submucosal myomectomy. The endometrium overlying the submucous myoma shows glandular atrophy, which impairs implantation and nourishment of the embryo and hence, impairs the fertility rate.

DIAGNOSIS OF THE SUBMUCOUS LEIOMYOMA

Transvaginal ultrasonography (TVUS), saline infusion sonography (SIS), magnetic resonance imaging (MRI), and even hysteroscopy are the modalities used for the diagnosis of the submucous fibroid. The goal of the imaging technique is to distinguish between the adenomyosis and leiomyoma.

Three-dimensional (3D) USG is a very calculative diagnostic method which helps in calculating the Lasmar classification. MRI is also superior diagnostic modality as it identifies the proper proportion of the myoma in the endometrial cavity and its relation to the myometrium, which is important during the transcervical resection. Hence, MRI is more sensitive and specific test for the diagnosis.

PREOPERATIVE MANAGEMENT OF THE MYOMA

- Prophylactic antibiotics were administered
- *Progesterone administered:* Depot medroxyprogesterone acetate helps in endometrial atrophy and hence it gives a greater visualization of the endometrium

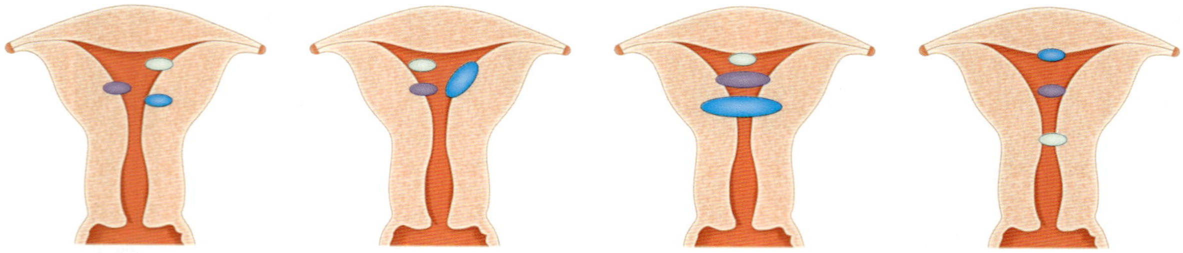

STEP-W classitication

	Size (cm)	Topography	Extension of the base	Penetration	Lateral wall	Total
0	< 2	Low	< 1/3	0	+1	
1	2–5	Middle	1/3 to 2/3	< 50%		
2	> 5	Upper	> 2/3	>50%		

= Score 0

= Score 1

= Score 2

Score	Group	Complexity and therapeutic options
0–4	I	Low complexity hysteroscopic myomectomy
5–6	II	High complexity hysteroscopic myomectomy. Consider GnRH use. Consider two-step hysteroscopic myomectomy
7–9	III	Consider alternative to the hysteroscopic technique

Fig. 2: Lasmar classification.
(GnRH: gonadotropin-releasing hormone)

- *Gonadotropin-releasing hormone (GnRH) agonist:* GnRH analogs decrease the size of the fibroid, but make the dissection of the fibroid from the surrounding difficult. It may lead to vasomotor symptoms and cervical stenosis. In cases of severe bleeding and severe anemia, one dose is sufficient in the view of the cessation of menses and then performing surgery.

MANAGEMENT OF THE SUBMUCOSAL LEIOMYOMA

The most common hysteroscopic technique is transcervical resectoscopic myomectomy (TCRM) which was first reported in 1976.

Other techniques are *dissection, vaporization*, or morcellation, and *excision of submucous myoma*. Leiomyoma up to 4–5 cm can be easily resected with the hysteroscope **(Figs. 3 to 6)**.

Type 0 and 1 will be easily and in one sitting are resected.

Type 2 myoma requires multistage procedure.

TRANSCERVICAL SURGERY FOR LEIOMYOMA

The electrosurgical unit required is monopolar with glycine as the distending media and bipolar with normal saline or Ringer's lactate as distending media.

Principle of the Surgery

Reduction of the leiomyoma volume, creation of amenorrhea to facilitate restoration of hemoglobin and iron stores, and facilitation of the procedure including improved visualization and reduced systemic absorption of distending media.

Cervical Preparation before Transcervical Resectoscopic Myomectomy

Prostaglandins (misoprostol): Prostaglandin E1 (PGE1) 200–400 µg taken orally or vaginally 12–24 hours before surgery facilitates cervical dilatation and minimize the cervical trauma and minimize the trauma.

Technique

Effective performance of hysteroscopic myomectomy requires both appropriate instrumentation and knowledge of the procedure. Small myoma is removed with scissors or hysteroscopic grasping forceps, larger myoma requires a system designed for morcellation, vaporization of the tumor. A proper input output of the fluid is monitored.

Monopolar resectoscope uses cutting current of 80–120 W and the calcified fibroids need 120 W. The wire loop should easily pass through the tissue and if it is not passing through then, the current should be increased.

Resection should be performed from the far end of the fibroid toward the surgeon. The loop should always be visible. It should cut all the way through capsule-to-capsule. The initial incision into the fibroid should be given over the midline and let the edges of the fibroid fall inward leaving behind the panoramic view. The fibroid seems to be firm with whorled appearance while the myometrium seems to be soft and with muscular fascicles.

Pedunculated fibroids that are smaller should be cut from the base. Larger once should be cut into pieces and then detached from the base. The tissue fragments then should be evacuated out with suction or ovum-holding forceps and then sent for histopathological evaluation.

POSTOPERATIVE CARE

- Adequate antibiotics to be given
- Nonsteroidal anti-inflammatory drugs (NSAIDs) to be administered
- Pelvic rest for 4–6 weeks (abstain from swimming, intercourse, and exercises)
- Resume normal daily activities after 3–4 days
- Follow-up after 4–6 weeks.

COMPLICATIONS

The complication rate in dealing small fibroid is 1.4% and for large fibroid it is 6.7%, in total the rate is 1.2–2.6%.

- Uterine perforation
- Intravasation and electrolyte imbalance
- Excessive perioperative bleeding
- Intrauterine adhesions
- Infections
- Glycine toxicity (monopolar cautery).

Postmyomectomy fertility rate is 16.7–76.9% with a mean of 54%.

Steps of Hysteroscopic Myoma Resection (TCRM)

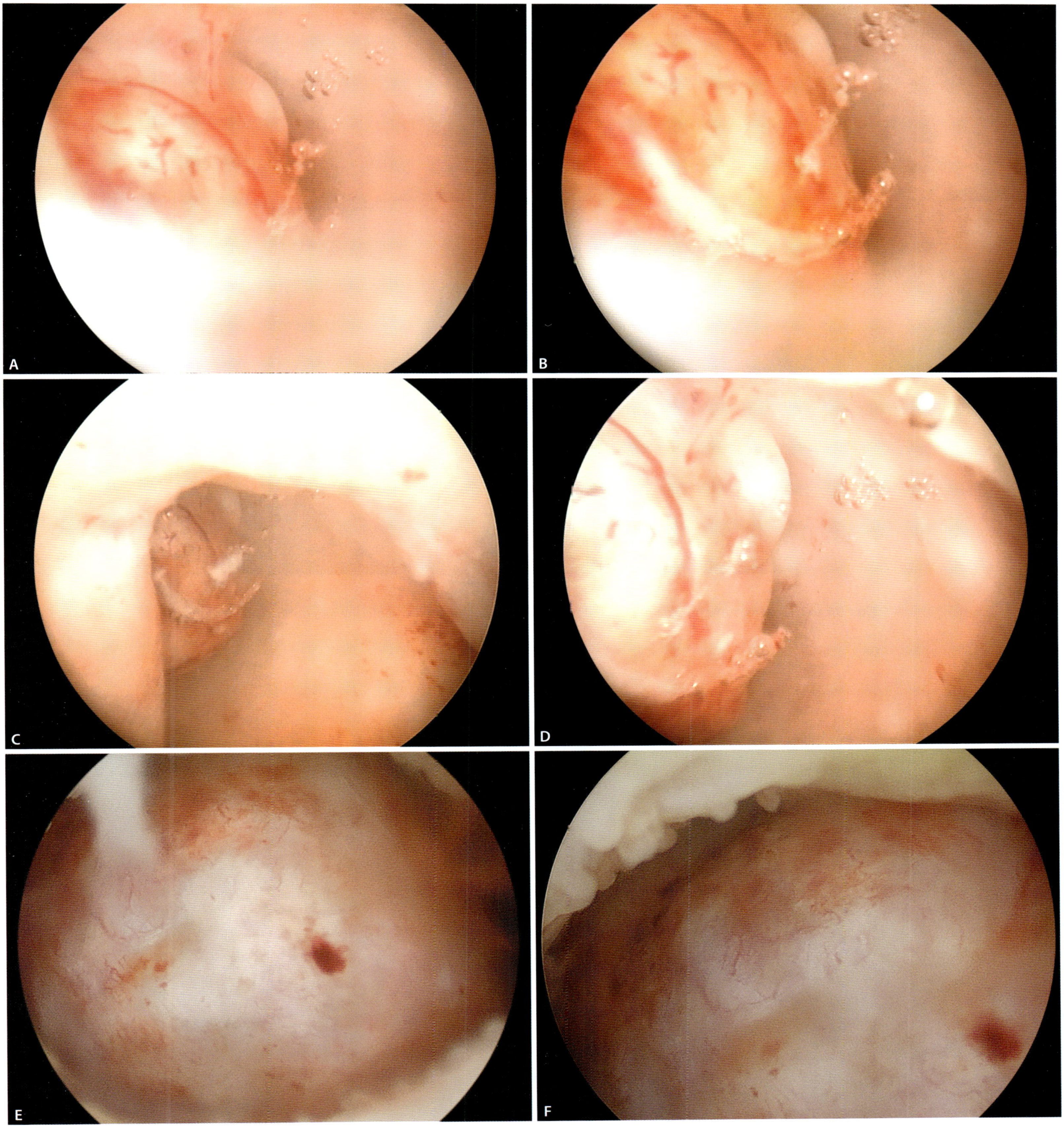

Figs. 3A to F

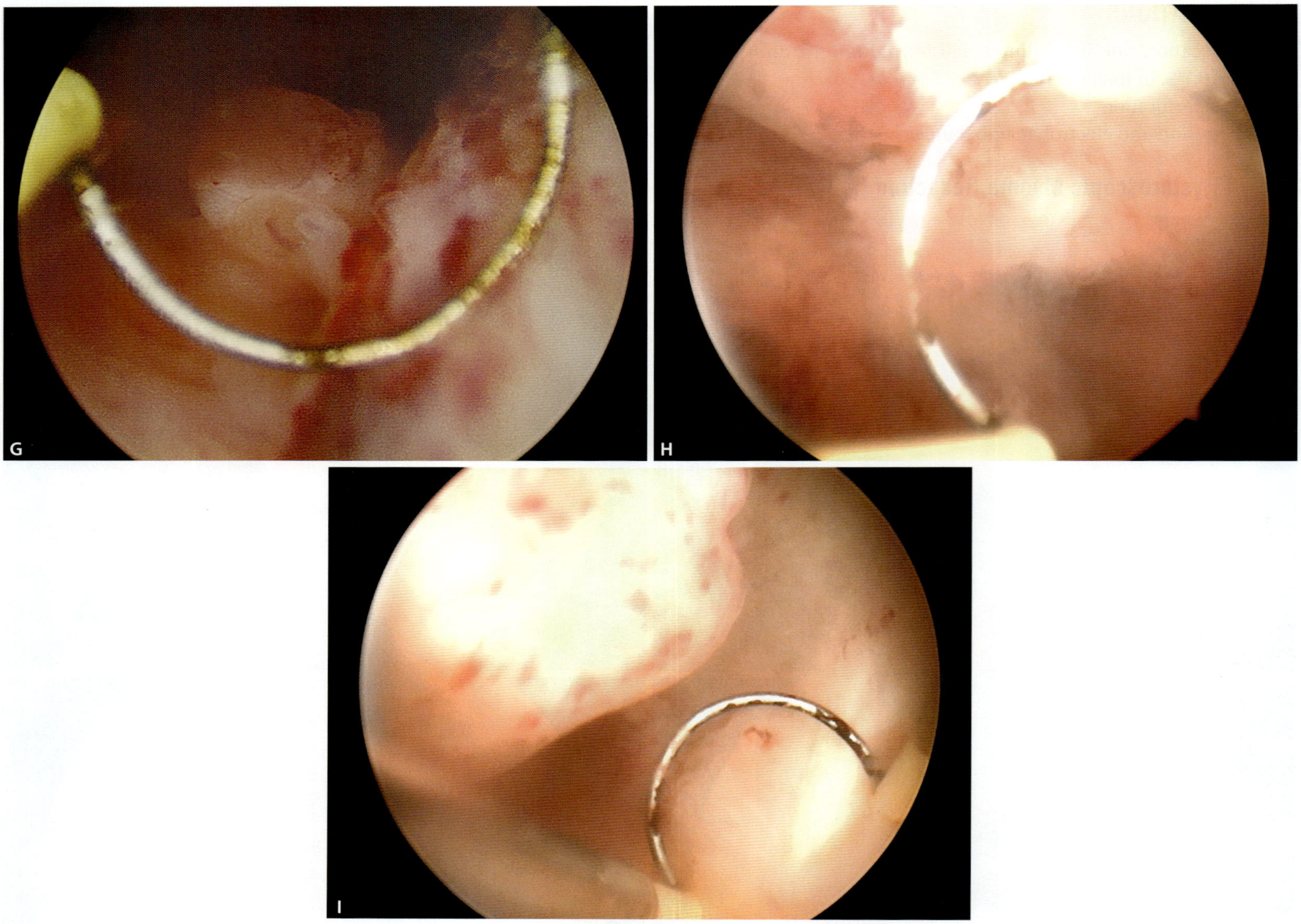

Figs. 3G to I

Figs. 3A to I: Hysteroscopic myoma resection done using monopolar hook and glycine as a distending medium.

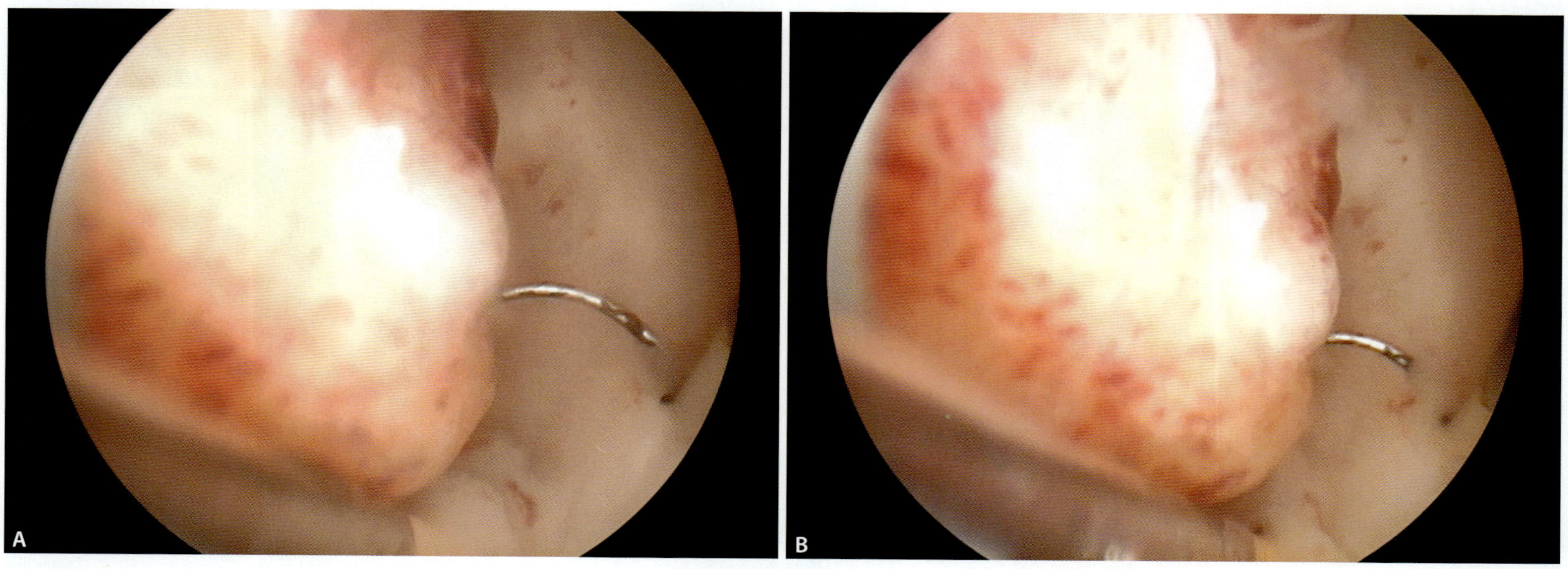

Figs. 4A and B

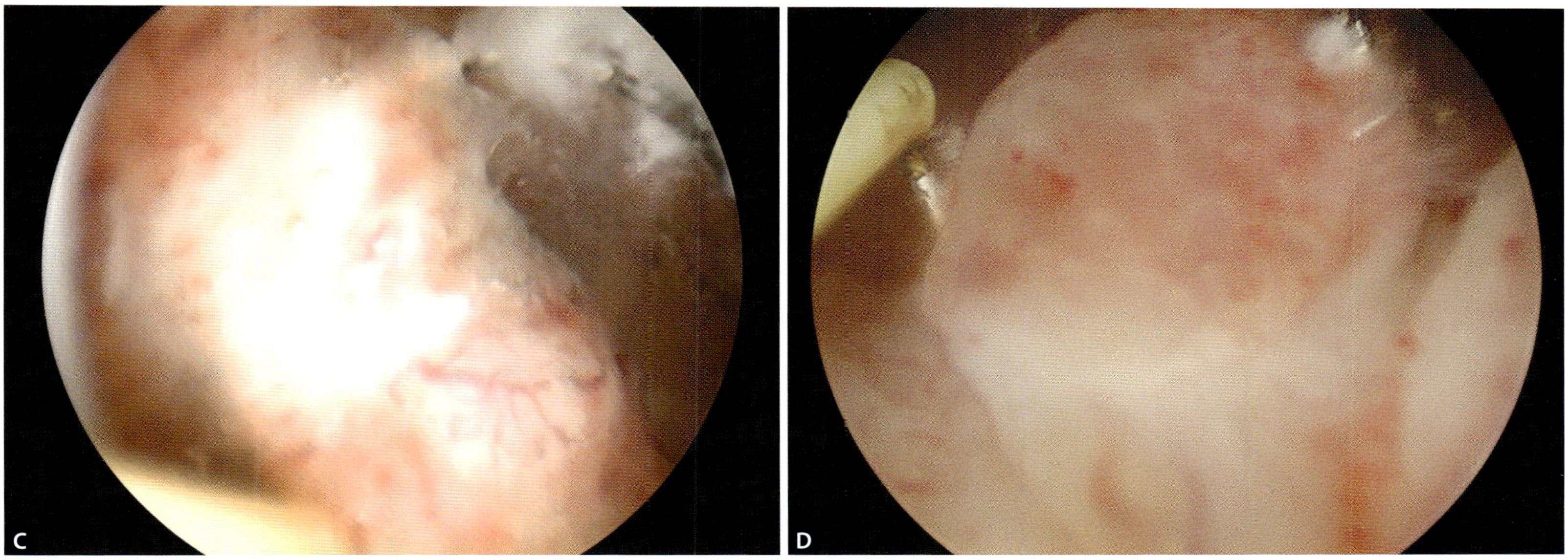

Figs. 4C and D

Figs. 4A to D: The resection should be done from capsule to capsule.

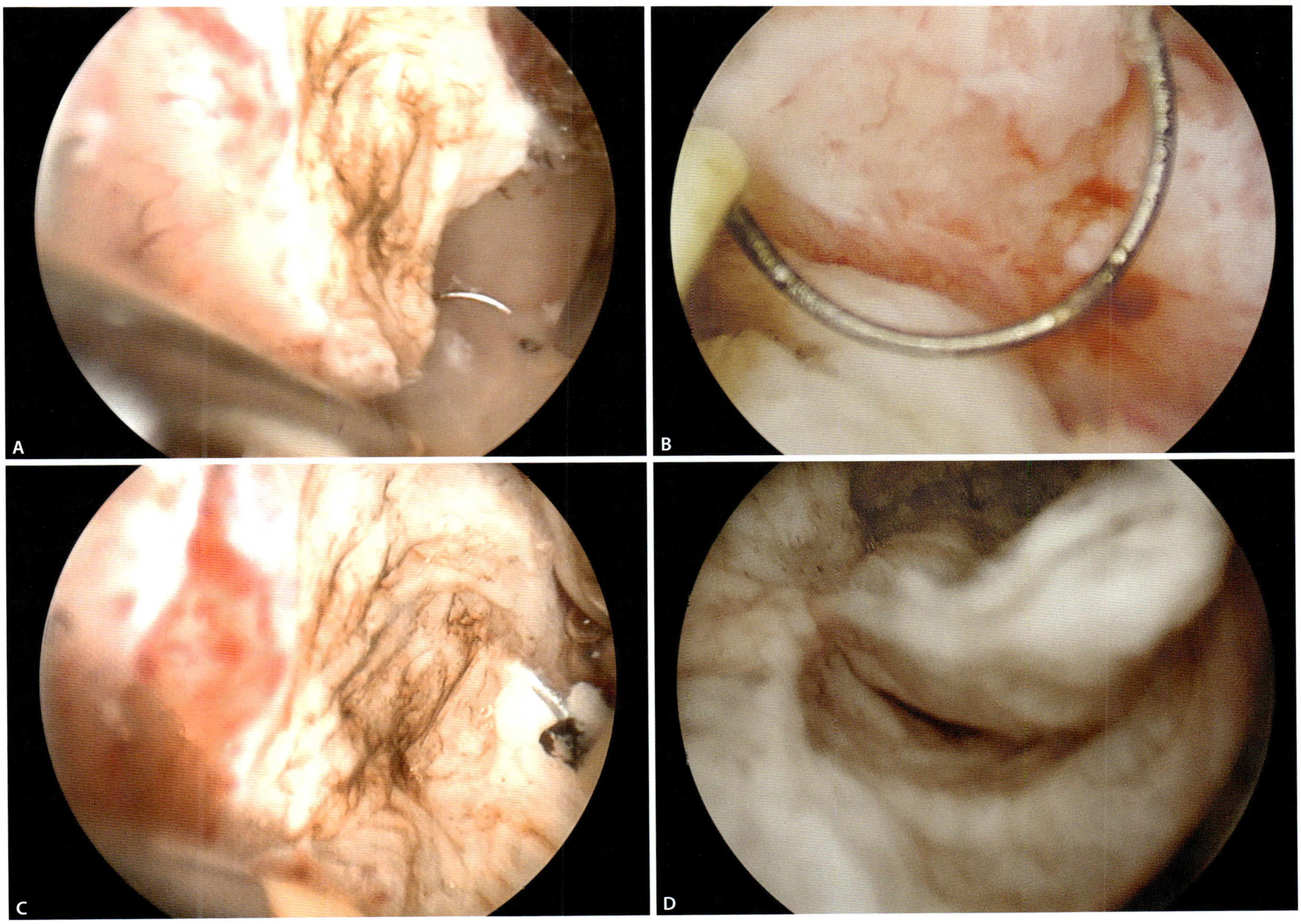

Figs. 5A to D

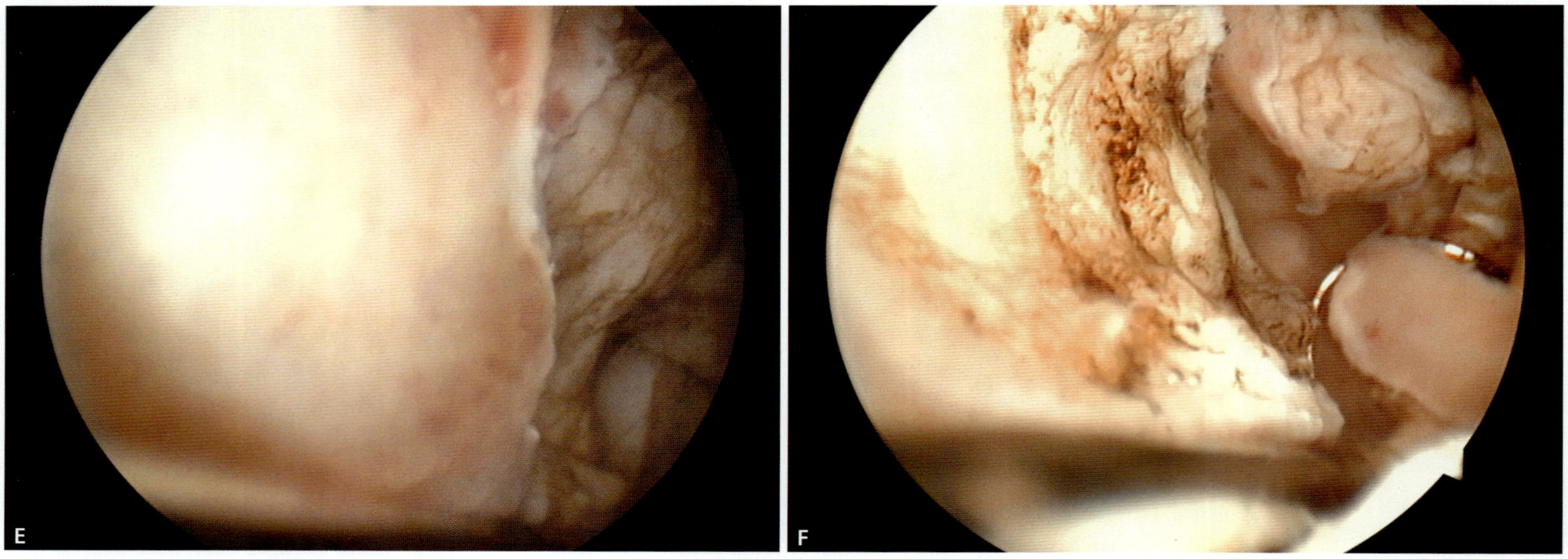

Figs. 5C and F

Figs. 5A to F: The monopolar loop should always be visible.

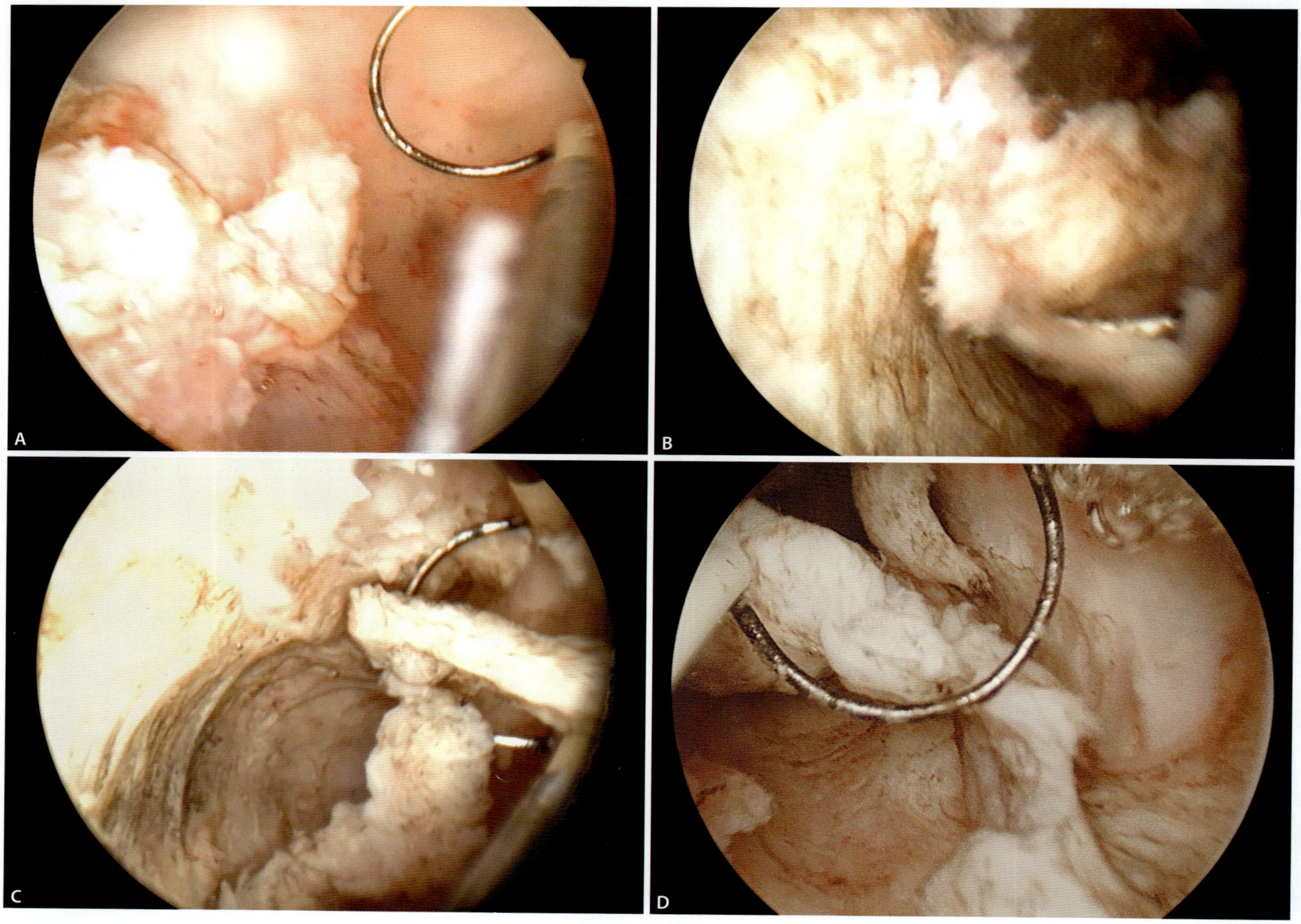

Figs. 6A to D

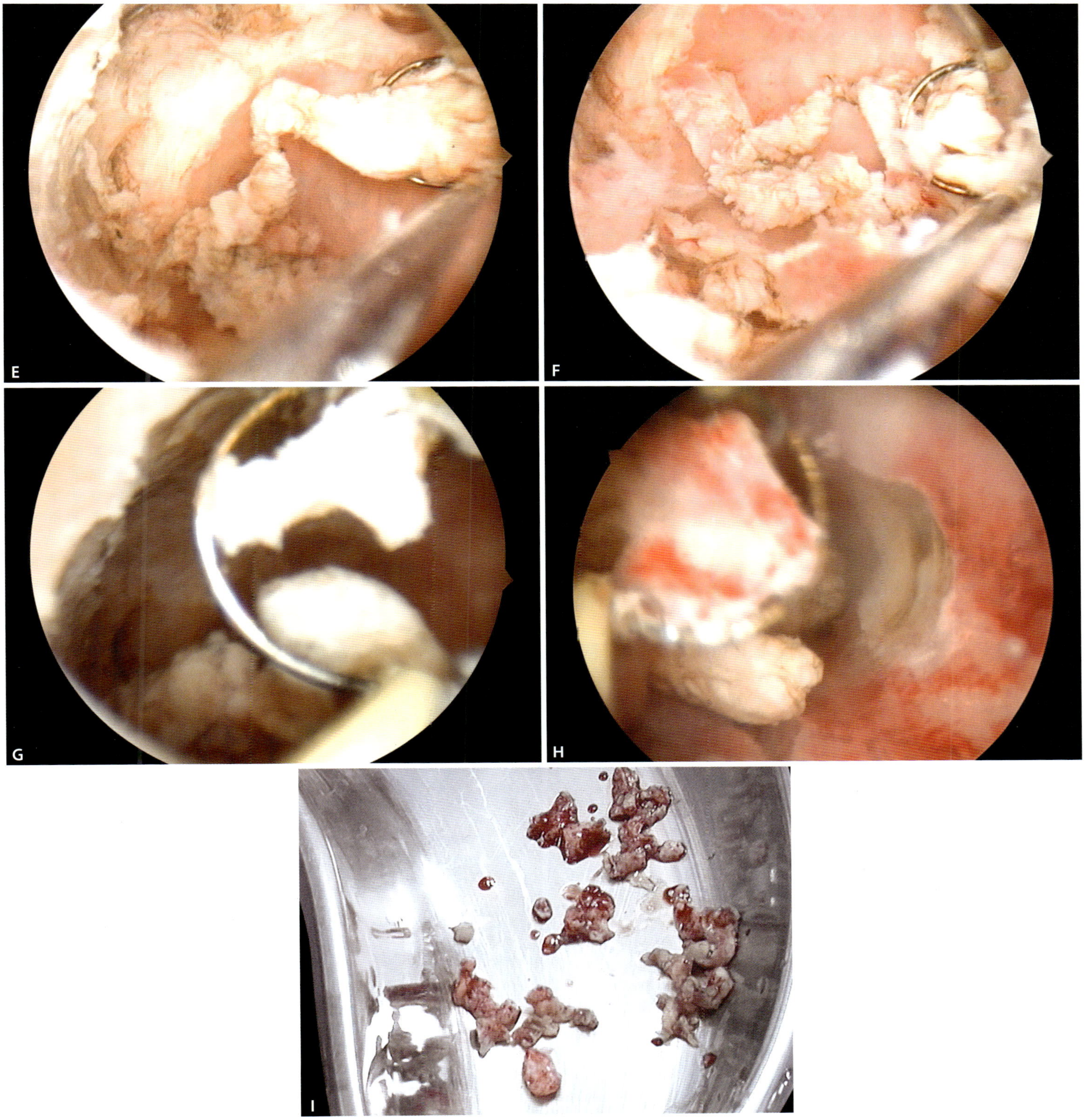

Figs. 6 E to I

Figs. 6A to I: Posthysteroscopic myomectomy, myoma pieces which are sent for histopathological examination (HPE).

SUGGESTED READING

1. American Association of Gynecologic Laparoscopists (AAGL): Advancing Minimally Invasive Gynecology Worldwide. AAGL practice report: practice guidelines for the diagnosis and management of submucous leiomyoma. J Minim Invasive Gynecol. 2012;19:152-71.
2. Botsis D, Papagianni V, Makrakis E, et al. Sonohysterography is superior to transvaginal sonography for the diagnostic approach of irregular uterine bleeding in women of reproductive age. J Clin Ultrasound. 2006; 34:434-9.
3. Camanni M, Bonino L, Tessarolo M, et al. Is it possible to obtain a presurgical Lasmar score for hysteroscopic myomectomy by ultrasound alone? Ultrasound Obstet Gynecol. 2012;40:106-11.
4. Lasmar RB, Dias R, Barrozo PR, et al. Hysteroscopic myomectomy. Braz J Videoendosc Surg. 2008;1:163-70.

Accompanying Video: Hysteroscopic resection of submucous fibroid.

CHAPTER

55

Submucous Fibroid Polypectomy using Bipolar Cautery

Shubhanjali Sen, Minal Kumbhalwar, B Ramesh

INTRODUCTION

When bipolar electrosurgical units are used for the resection of the polyp the advantage is that normal saline is used as the distending media.

PRINCIPLE

In the bipolar set of instruments, both electrodes are introduced into the thermal loop, which are safe. In this way, the current will only have to pass through the tissue with which the thermal loop comes into contact, thus minimizing the danger deriving from the random passage through the corporeal structures. An intrauterine bipolar diathermy allows the use of a normal saline or ringer lactate uterine distension medium. The passage of the electrical energy from the thermal loop to the tissues determines the cutting or coagulation action of the resectoscope.

The bipolar thermal loop for resection is usually smaller than monopolar resectoscope loop.

The advantage of using a bipolar electrosurgical unit is to avoid the complications due to hypotonic, nonconductive and

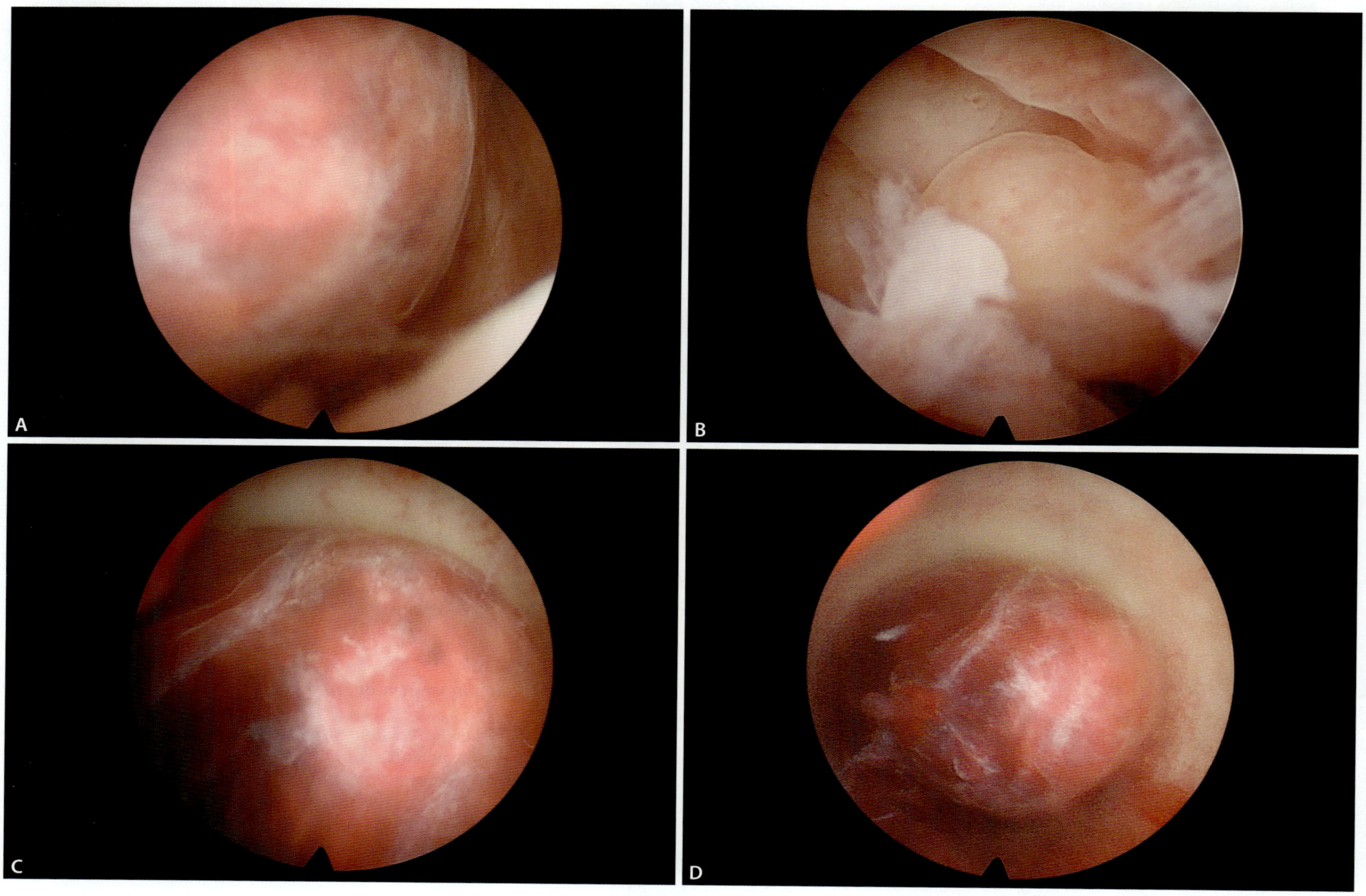

Figs. 1A to D: Bipolar resection.

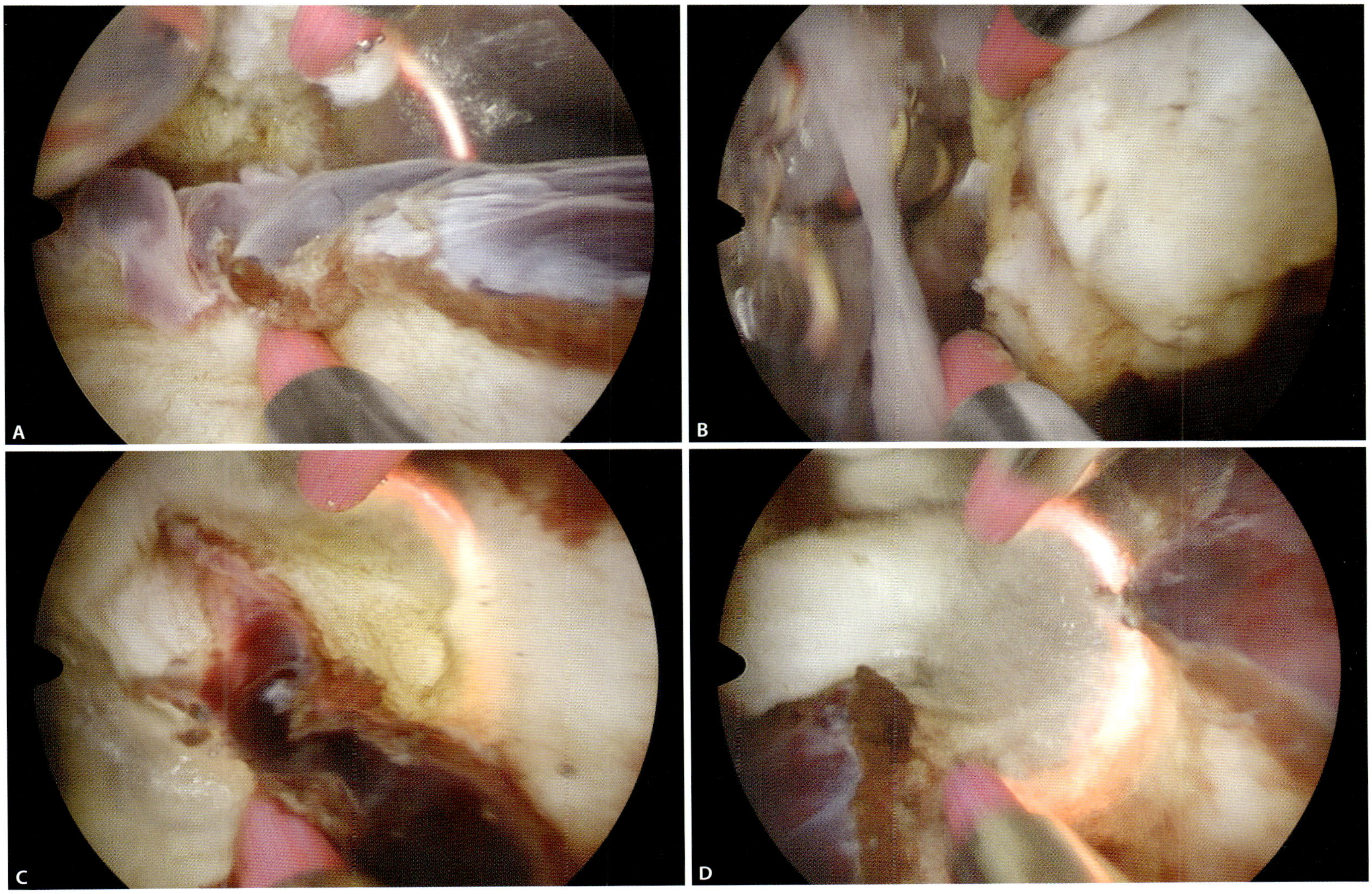

Figs. 2A to D: Bipolar cautery activation gives bright golden sunset arc.

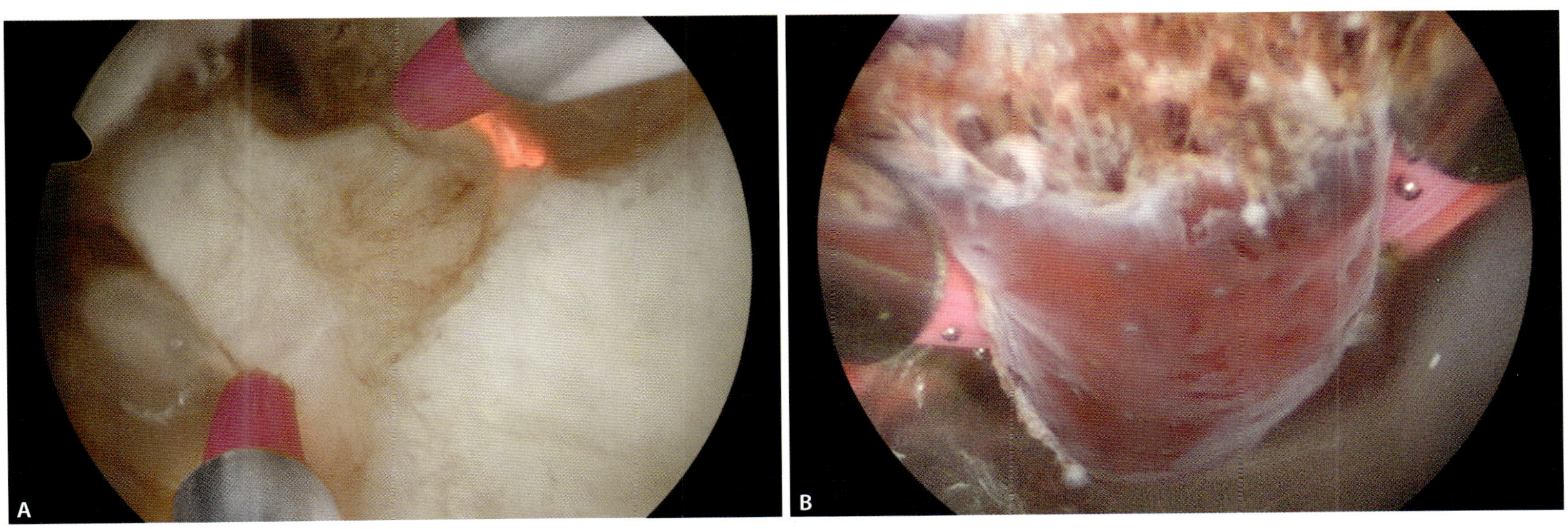

Figs. 3A and B

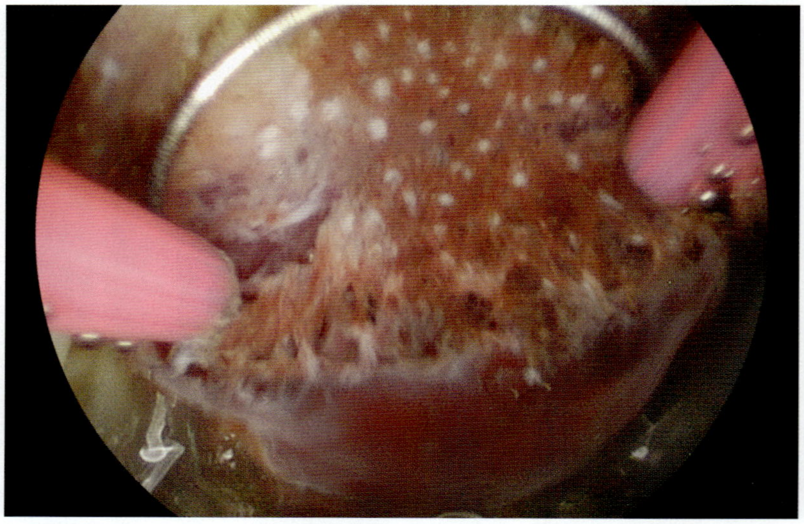

Fig. 3C

Figs. 3A to C: Fibroid resection capsule to capsule.

low viscosity fluid, i.e. glycine. The dreaded disadvantage is hyponatremia, which is caused due to absorption of the fluid through the vasculature. With every 1 liter of fluid deficit 10 mmol/L sodium is decreased. Hyponatremia is due to glycine which, is metabolized, and leads to continuous fall in serum sodium levels. Hyponatremia can lead to bradycardia initially with hypertension, nausea and vomiting and sometimes seizures too. If not corrected on time it may cause pulmonary edema, coma and death.

CHAPTER 56

Laparoscopic Removal of Submucosal Fibroid

Shubhanjali Sen, Isha Rani, B Ramesh

NONHYSTEROSCOPIC METHOD OF SUBMUCOSAL MYOMECTOMY

Abdominal approach may be desirable for the treatment of the submucosal leiomyoma.

INDICATIONS

- When the submucosal fibroid is extending up to the uterine serosa
- With other intramural fibroids or subserosal fibroids to be removed
- Preservation of endometrial surface for the infertile women, as resectoscopic myomectomy may destruct the adjacent endometrium.

Selection of the case for abdominal approach depends on the factors such as size, number, location of the myoma, and presence or absence of coexisting pathology such as adhesions.

Advantage of the laparoscopic approach is to prevent the uterine perforation while doing hysteroscopy.

- Prevention of the uterine rupture
- Protect the endometrial integrity
- Protect from fluid overload complications
- Time required is less
- According to LASMAR classification if the complexity is too high then laparoscopic route should be preferred.

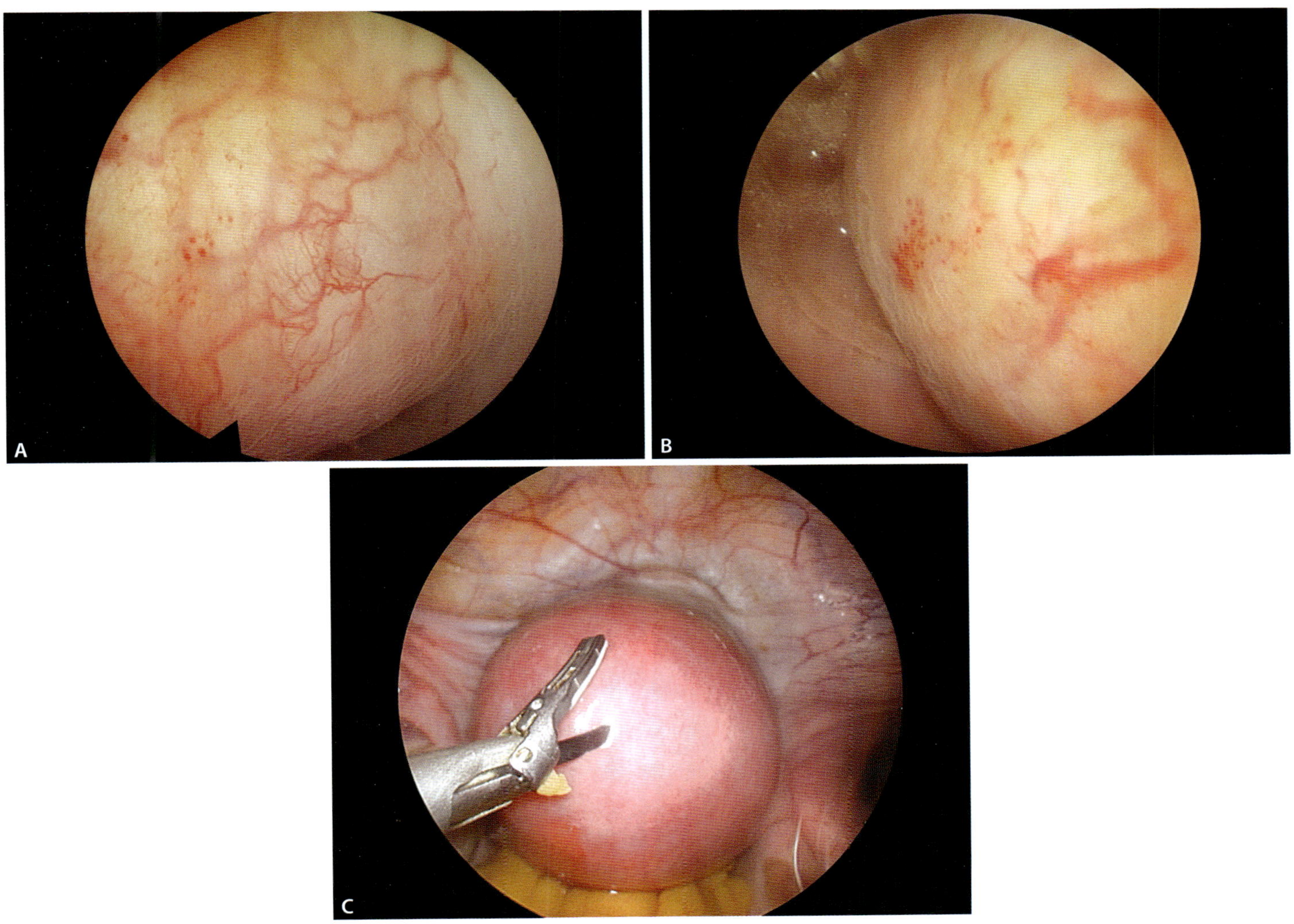

Figs. 1A to C: (A and B) Hysteroscopic view of submucous fibroid; (C) Incision made over uterus using harmonic.

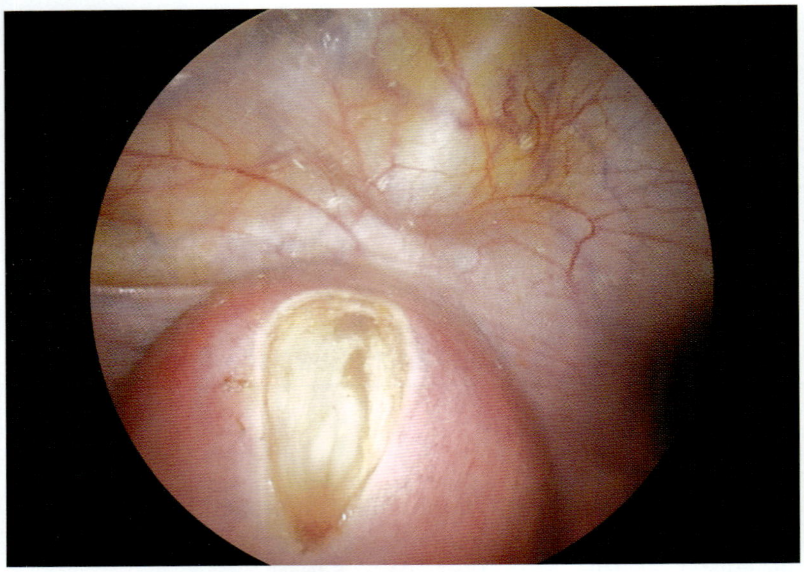

Fig. 2: Myoma exposed.

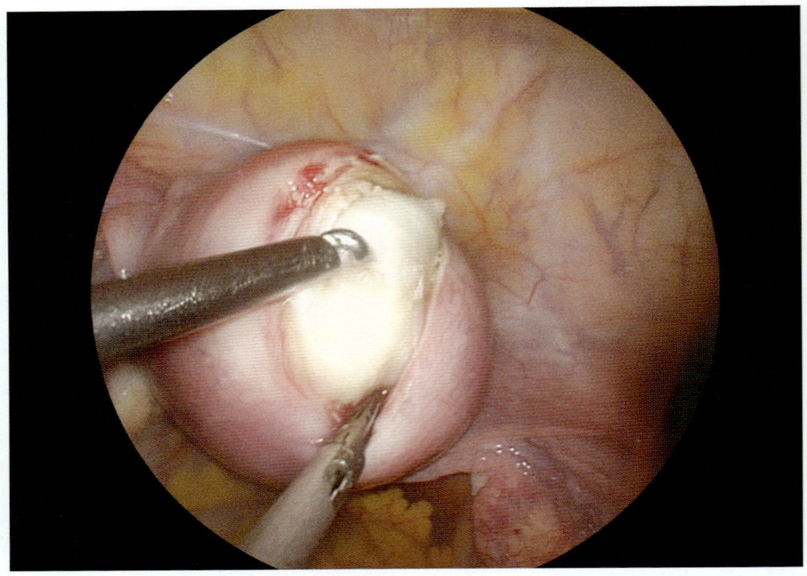

Fig. 3: Myoma screw fixed to submucous fibroid and dissected with harmonic.

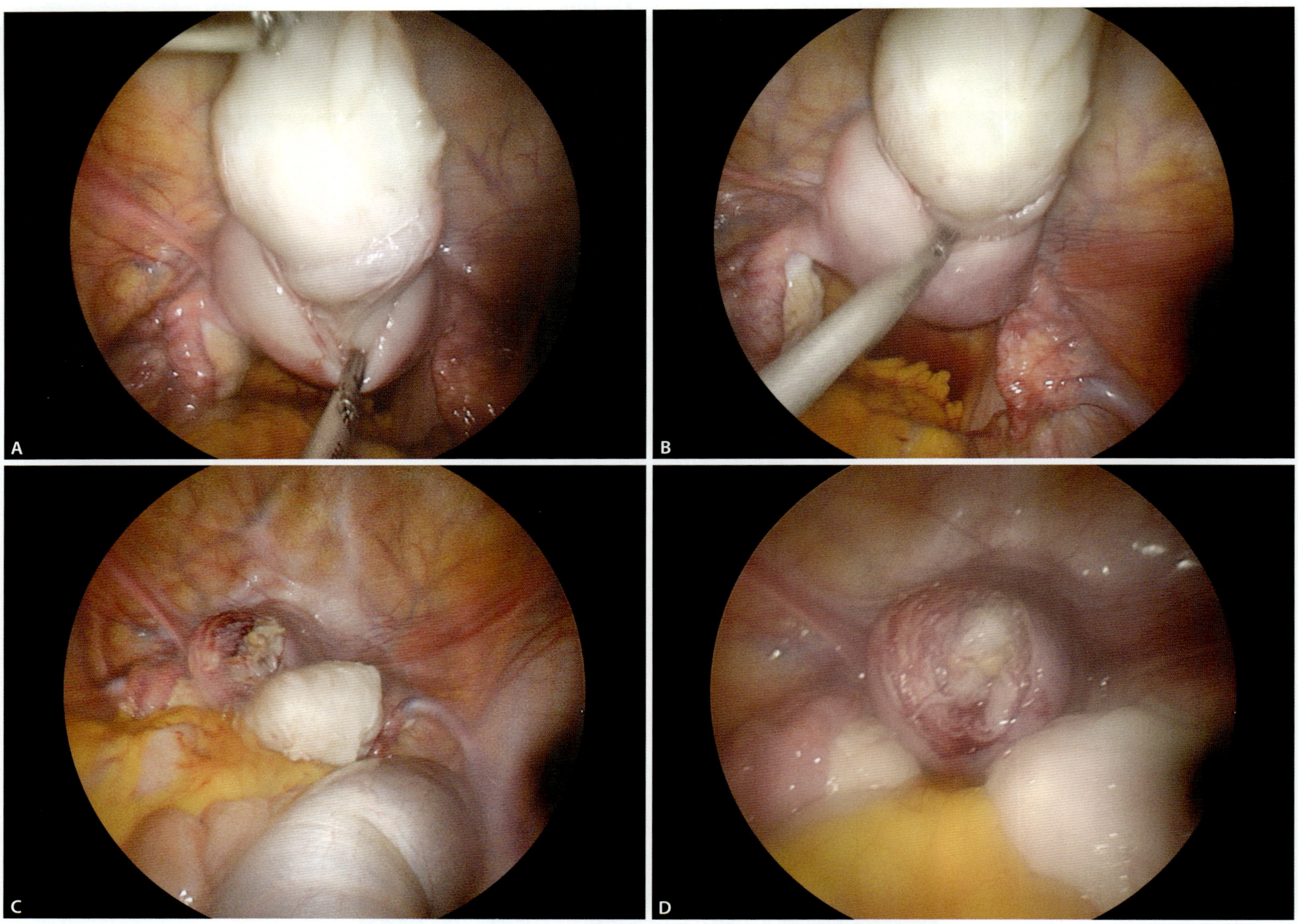

Figs. 4A to D: Myoma enucleated using traction and counter traction.

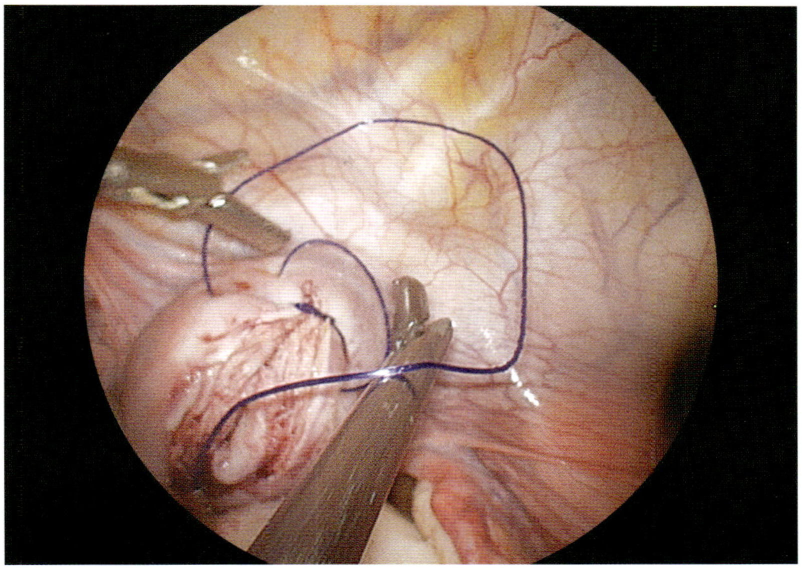

Fig. 4E: Myoma bed sutured with quilled barbed suture taking into consideration that endometrium is everted back into uterine cavity.

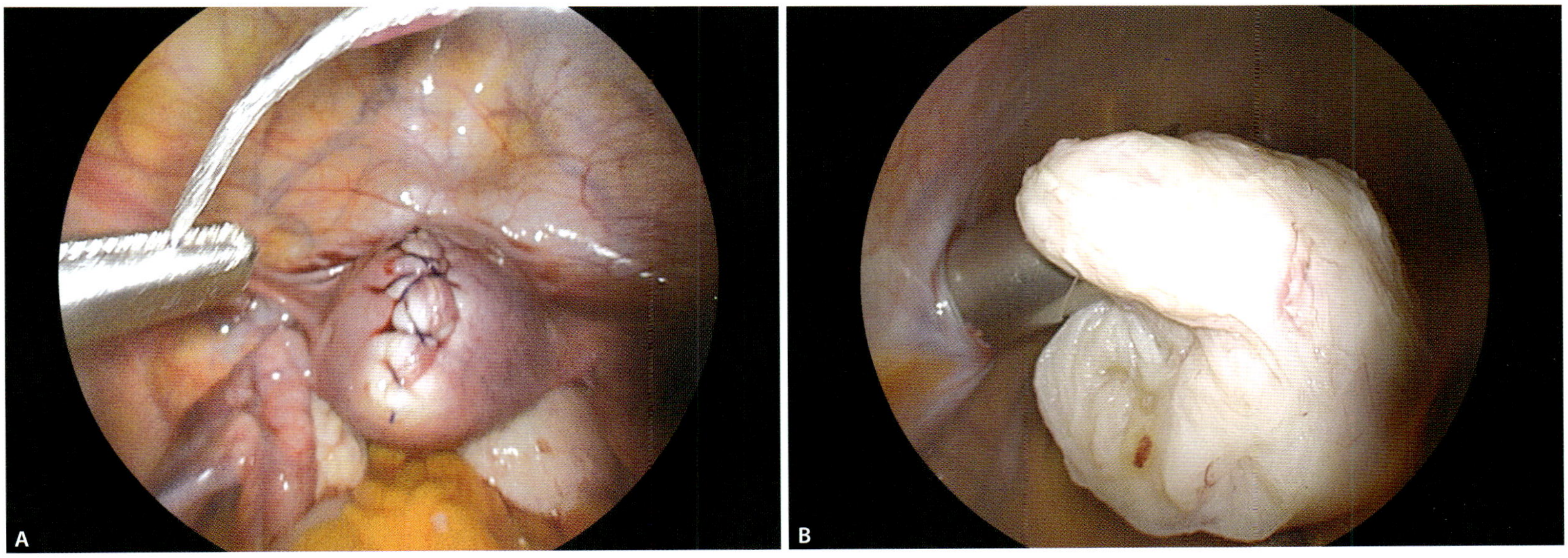

Figs. 5A and B: (A) Hemostasis achieved after suturing; (B) Myoma retrieved with electromechanical morcellation.

Another Big Submucous Fibroid Approached Laparoscopically

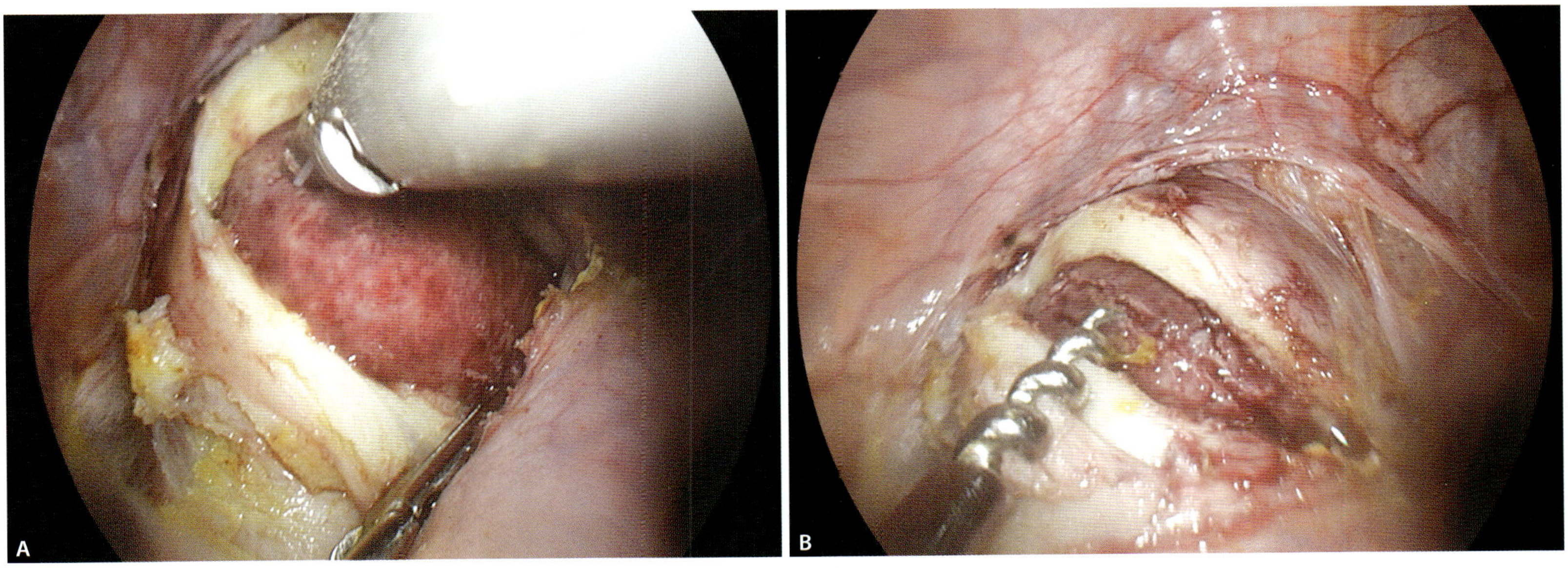

Figs. 6A and B

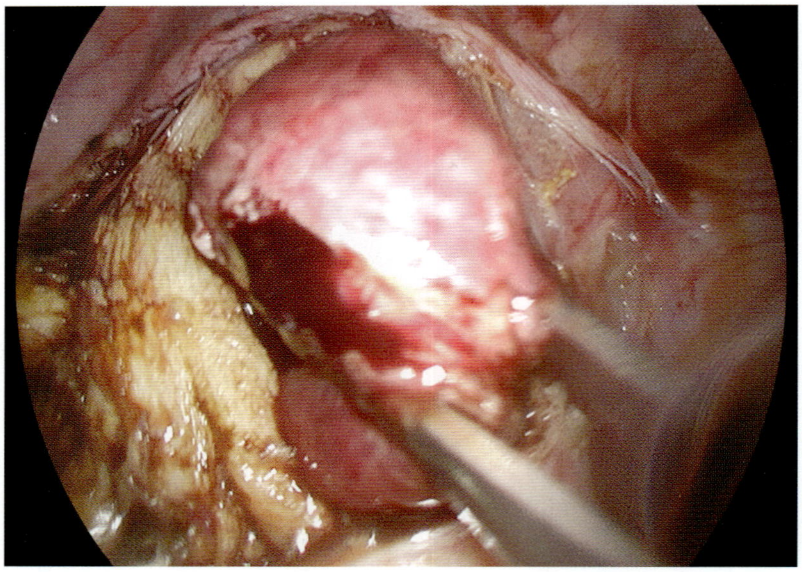

Fig. 6C

Figs. 6A to C: Cavity being opened and myoma grasped.

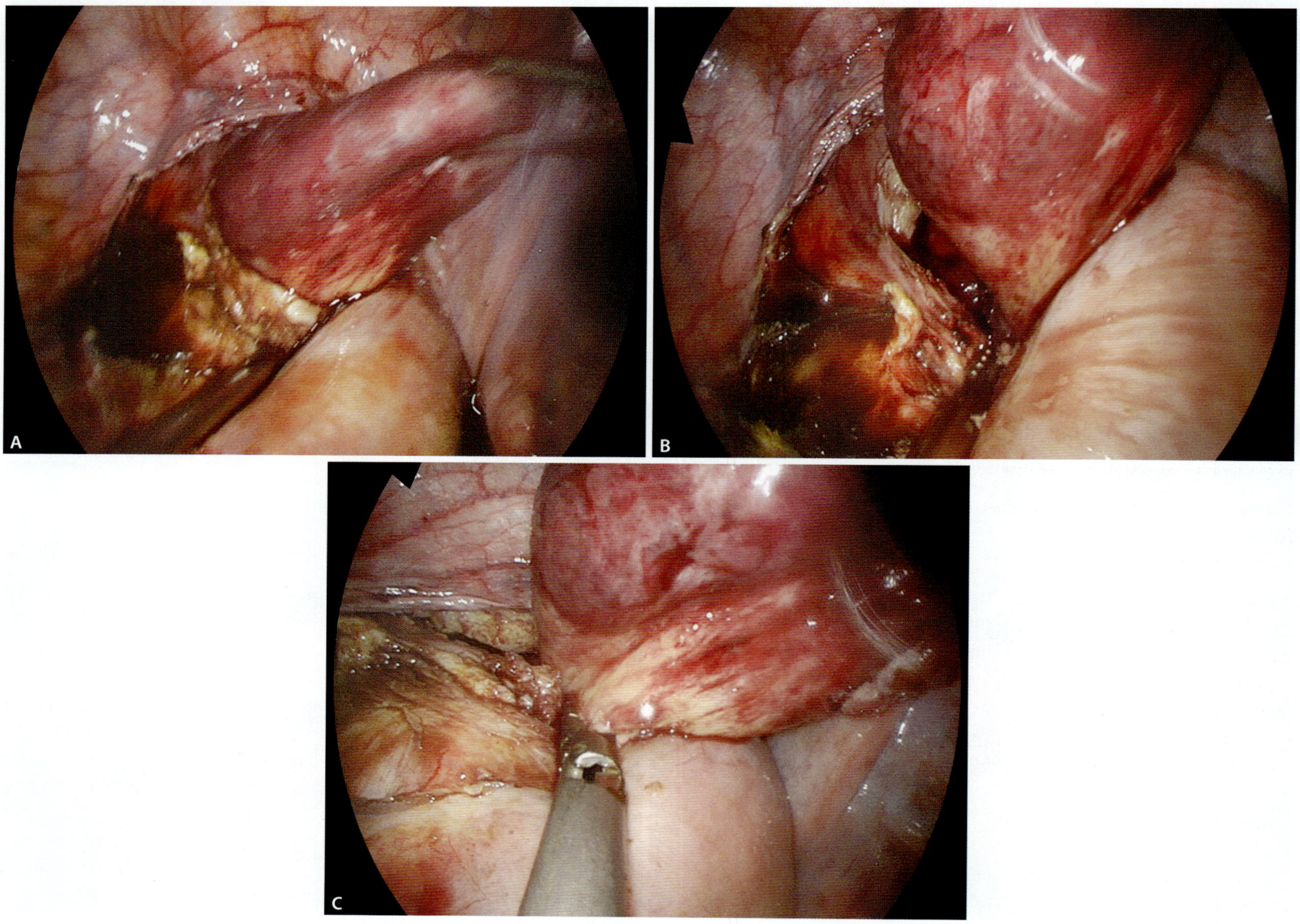

Figs. 7A to C: Base of myoma cauterized for separating myoma from uterus.

CHAPTER

57

Intrauterine Adhesions (Asherman's Syndrome)

Shubhanjali Sen, Isha Rani, B Ramesh

INTRODUCTION

Asherman's syndrome is defined by the presence of intrauterine permanent adhesions, obliterating partially or completely the uterine cavity. Adhesions were first published by Heinrich Fritsch in 1894. After 54 years an Israeli gynecologist Joseph Asherman established the diagnosis in 1948.

SYMPTOMS

Menstrual abnormality (hypomenorrhea, amenorrhea, and hematometra), infertility, dysmenorrhea, subfertility, and recurrent pregnancy loss are indicative for intervention in Asherman's syndrome are commonly encountered problems.

OBJECTIVES OF THE TREATMENT

Primary objective of the intervention is to restore the volume and shape of the uterine cavity to normal and to facilitate communication between the cavity and both the cervical canal and Fallopian tubes.

Secondary objective include treating associated symptoms and preventing recurrence of adhesions.

CLASSIFICATION

Reproductive outcomes correlate with the type of adhesion and the extent of uterine occlusion.

Mild adhesion: Filmy adhesions composed of basalis endometrial tissue producing partial or complete uterine cavity occlusion **(Fig. 1)**.

Moderate adhesions: Fibromuscular adhesions. Thick and covered with endometrium which may bleed on division. They partially or totally occlude the cavity.

Severe adhesions: Adhesions composed of connective tissues only lacks endometrial lining and do not bleed on division. They partially or totally occlude the cavity.

Recently American Society for Reproductive Medicine (ASRM) proposed a scoring system for intrauterine adhesion based on extent of endometrial obliteration, hysteroscopic appearance of the adhesions, and menstrual characteristics of the patient.

Stage 1 (mild): Score 1–4

Stage 2 (moderate): Score 5–8

Stage 3 (severe): Score 9–12

The standardized classification helps in evaluation, reporting, and comparing the results of different modality of treatment and give better outcomes.

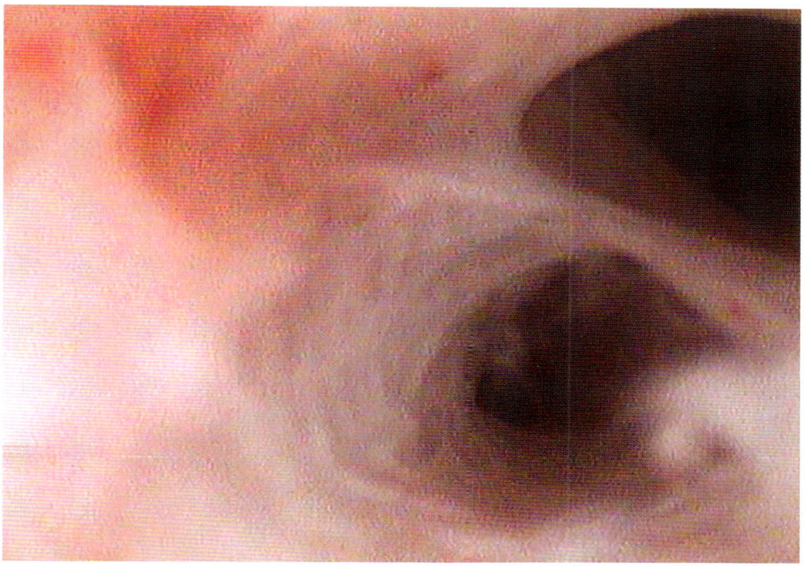

Fig. 1: Adhesions filmy in nature.

MANAGEMENT

Hysteroscopic transcervical division of the adhesions.

TECHNIQUES

1. Nonenergized cold hysteroscopic scissors
2. The resectoscope with monopolar or bipolar radiofrequency energy
3. Fiber optic lasers
4. Mechanical morcellation.

Mild adhesions (stage 1): Simply divided with the tip of hysteroscope.

Moderate (stage 2) and severe (stage 3): Requires scissors, biopsy forceps, electrical energy or mechanical morcellation.

Hysteroscopy

The uterine distention required for hysteroscopy may itself lyse mild adhesions due to distension of the uterine cavity, and blunt dissection may be used using the tip of the hysteroscope. The more lateral the adhesions and greater the density, the more difficult the dissection and greater the risk of perforation. Sometimes it is difficult to diagnose between the adhesions and endometrial lining, so methylene blue is injected to identify the tissue. Monopolar and bipolar electrosurgical instruments are used for adhesiolysis, which creates a precise cutting and good hemostasis **(Figs. 2A to D)**.

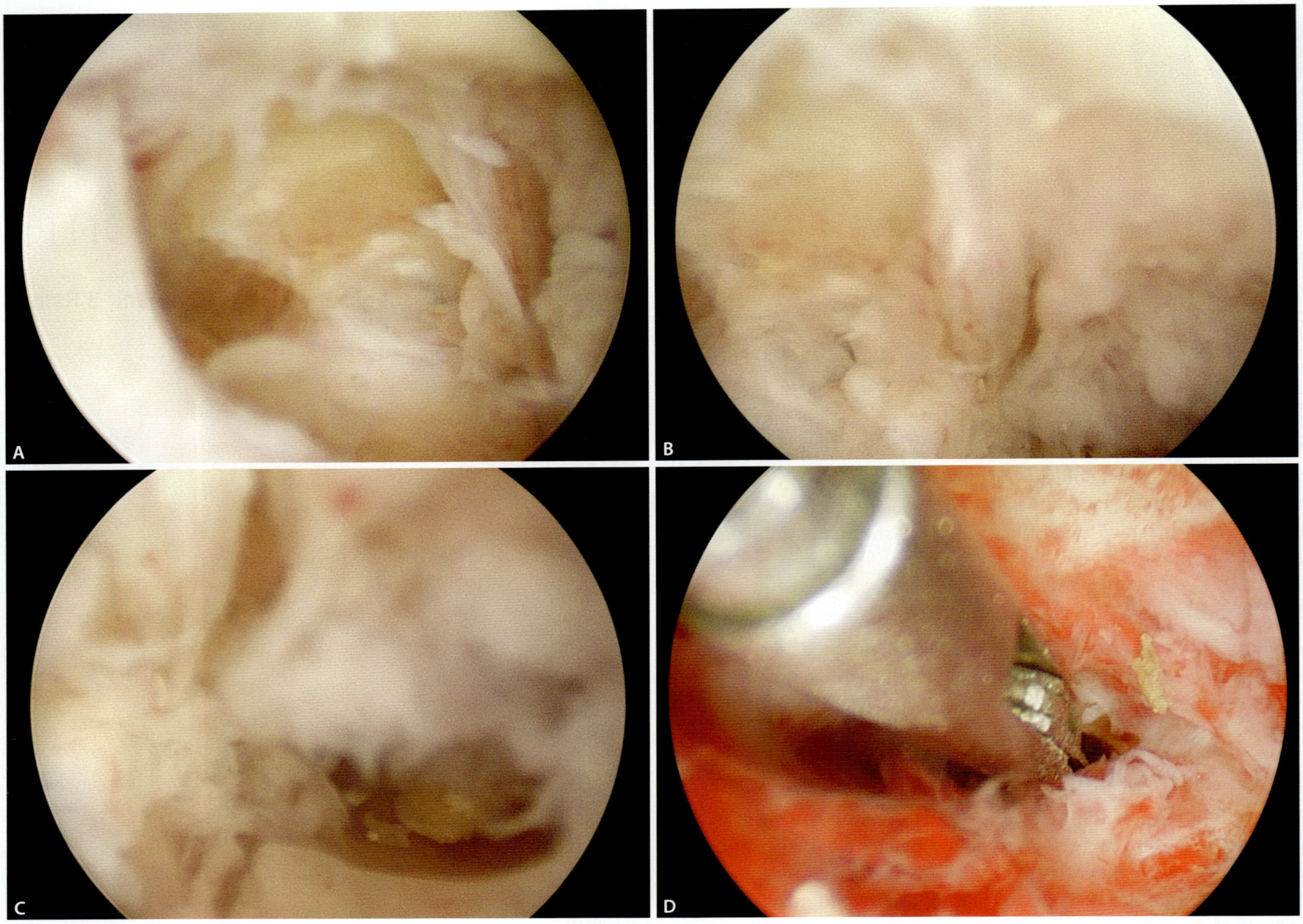

Figs. 2A to D: Adhesiolysis done with scissors.

Adhesiolysis begun inferiorly and was carried out cephalic until a panoramic view of the endometrial cavity was obtained and the tubal ostia are visualized **(Figs. 3 and 4)**. Regeneration of endometrium takes place from the pinkish area to the whitish area **(Fig. 5)**.

Disadvantages: Potential visceral damage, uterine perforation, endometrial damage leading to recurrence of intrauterine adhesions.

Other Hysteroscopic Technique

"Myometrial scoring" 6–8.4 mm deep incision are created in the myometrium using electrosurgery with Collins knife electrode from the fundus to the cervix. These incision enable widening of the uterine cavity. Anatomic success has been reported to be 71%.

Fluoroscopically guided blunt dissection for severe adhesions has been described using hysteroscopically directed Tuohy needle under image intensifier. It is costly and exposes the patient to ionizing radiation.

Ancillary Treatment

Physical Barriers

Insertion of the intrauterine device (IUD) with or without hormonal replacement therapy (estrogen and progesterone) as the treatment does not alter the rates of live births. Copper containing IUD should not be recommended because of its inflammation provoking properties. Hormone therapy alone is itself a good reformation therapy. Foley's catheter was also used but the rate of infertility and amenorrhea is significantly higher **(Figs. 6 to 8)**.

Hormonal Therapy

Postoperative treatment with estrogen therapy (a daily oral of 2.5 mg conjugated equine estrogen with or without opposing progesterone for 2–3 cycles) has been described after surgical treatment of intrauterine adhesions.

Techniques to Increase Vascular Flow to Endometrium

Aspirin, nitroglycerin and sildenafil citrate to increase vascular perfusion to the endometrium and enabling the implantation to happen.

Postoperative Assessment

Evaluation of the uterine cavity after adhesiolysis is very important step for Asherman syndrome (AS). Complete resolution from a single procedure is not possible especially in severe cases where the

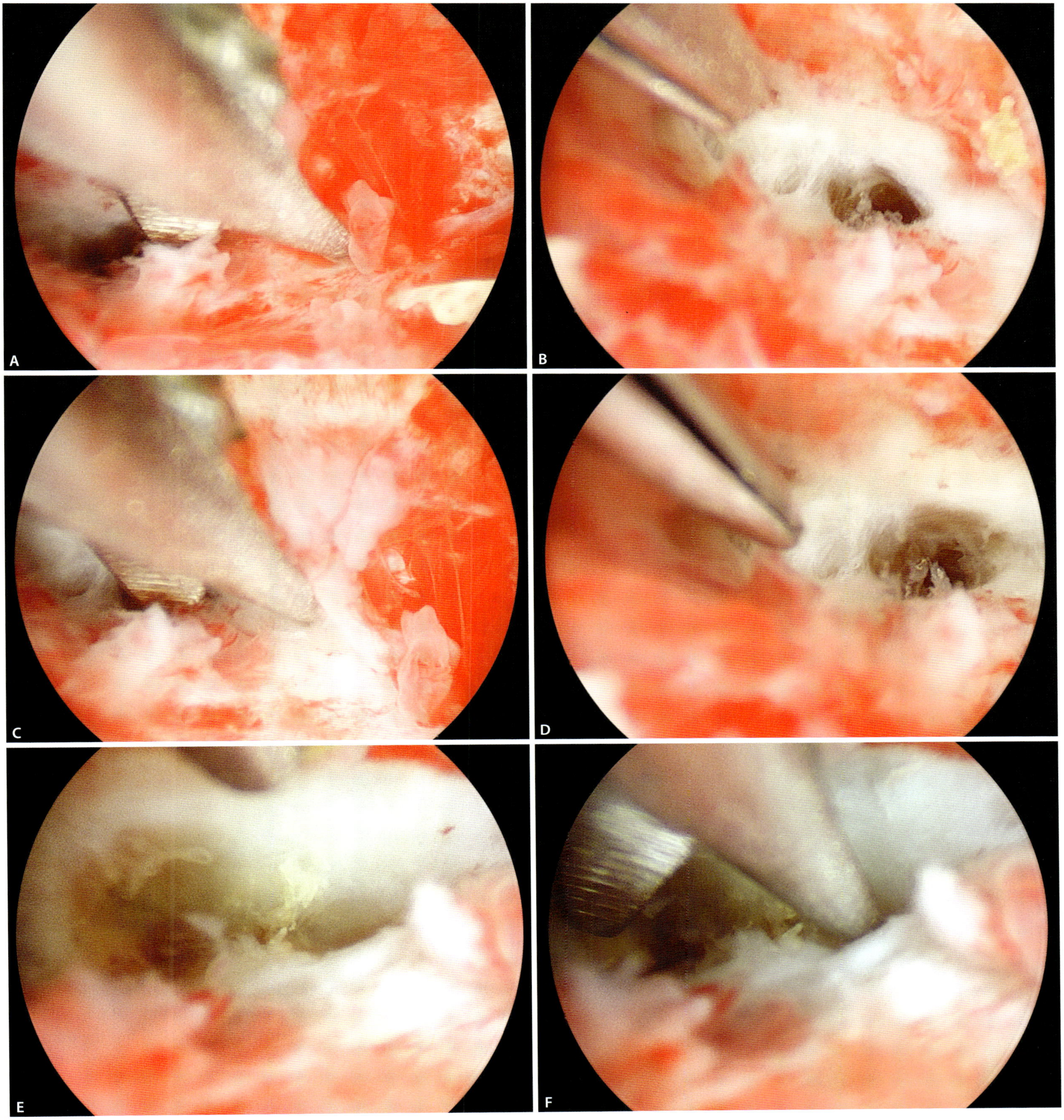

Figs. 3A to F

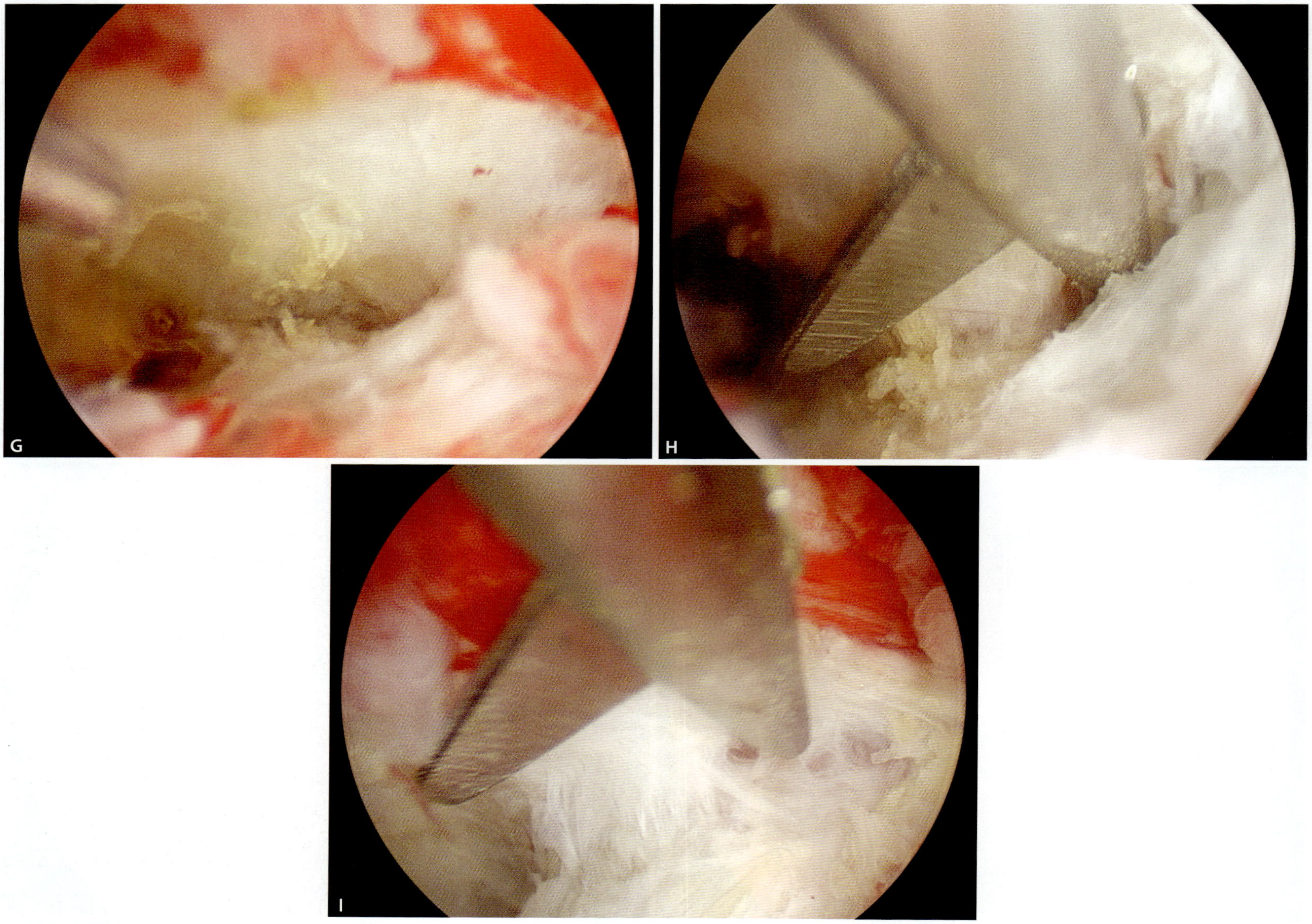

Figs. 3G to I

Figs. 3A to I: Cavity being opened up after initial adhesiolysis.

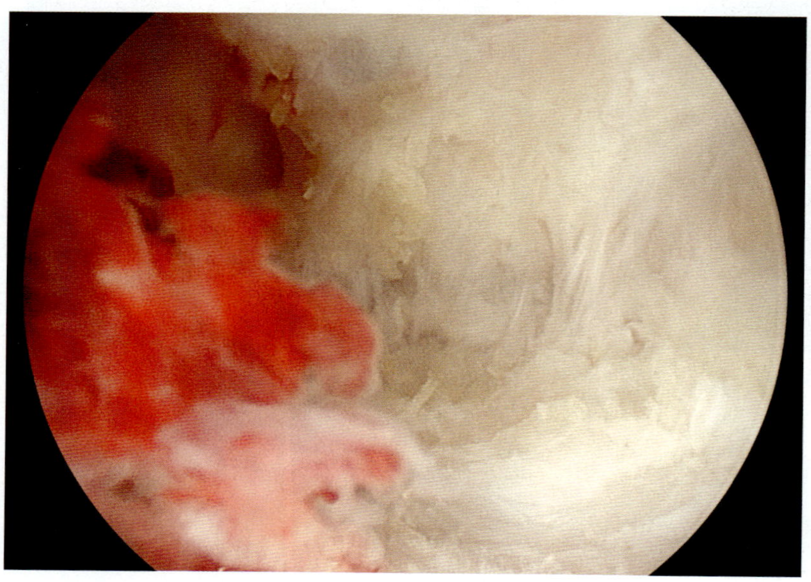

Fig. 4: Cavity is almost formed after adheisolysis.

recurrence rate is very high. The restoration of the menstrual cycle is considered a good marker of success. Most common follow-up modalities are ultrasonography (USG), hysterosalpingography (HSG), and second look hysteroscopy.

Ultrasonography is an accurate and cost-effective tool for measuring the endometrial thickening and for evaluation of normal endometrial development during menstrual cycle. HSG has the advantage to check tubal patency and resolution of thin adhesions from pressure of the liquid contrast medium. HSG is also an investigation of choice because it shows a typical picture of filling defect in the uterine cavity. Hysteroscopy remains the only method which allows an accurate estimation of adhesions recurrence and it is the most commonly used in clinical practice.

Relook hysteroscopy is important for assessment for the formation of the uterine cavity. We may have to repeat 2–3 times and repeated adhesiolysis may be necessary to create the cavity.

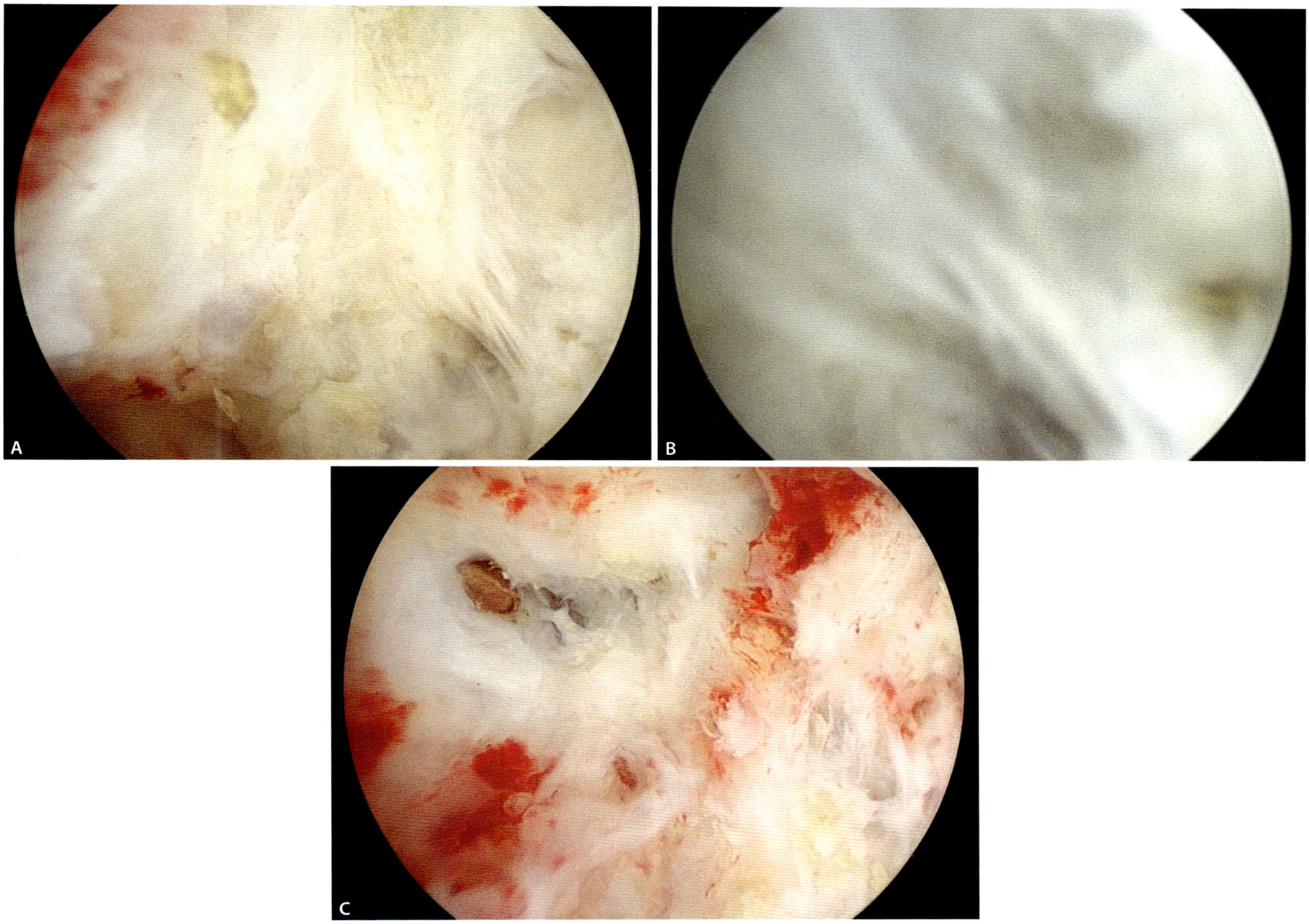

Figs. 5A to C: Final picture of the cavity and the pinkish areas are showing endometrium, the whitish areas are depicting adhesions. Regeneration of the endometrium will take place from the pinkish areas toward whitish areas.

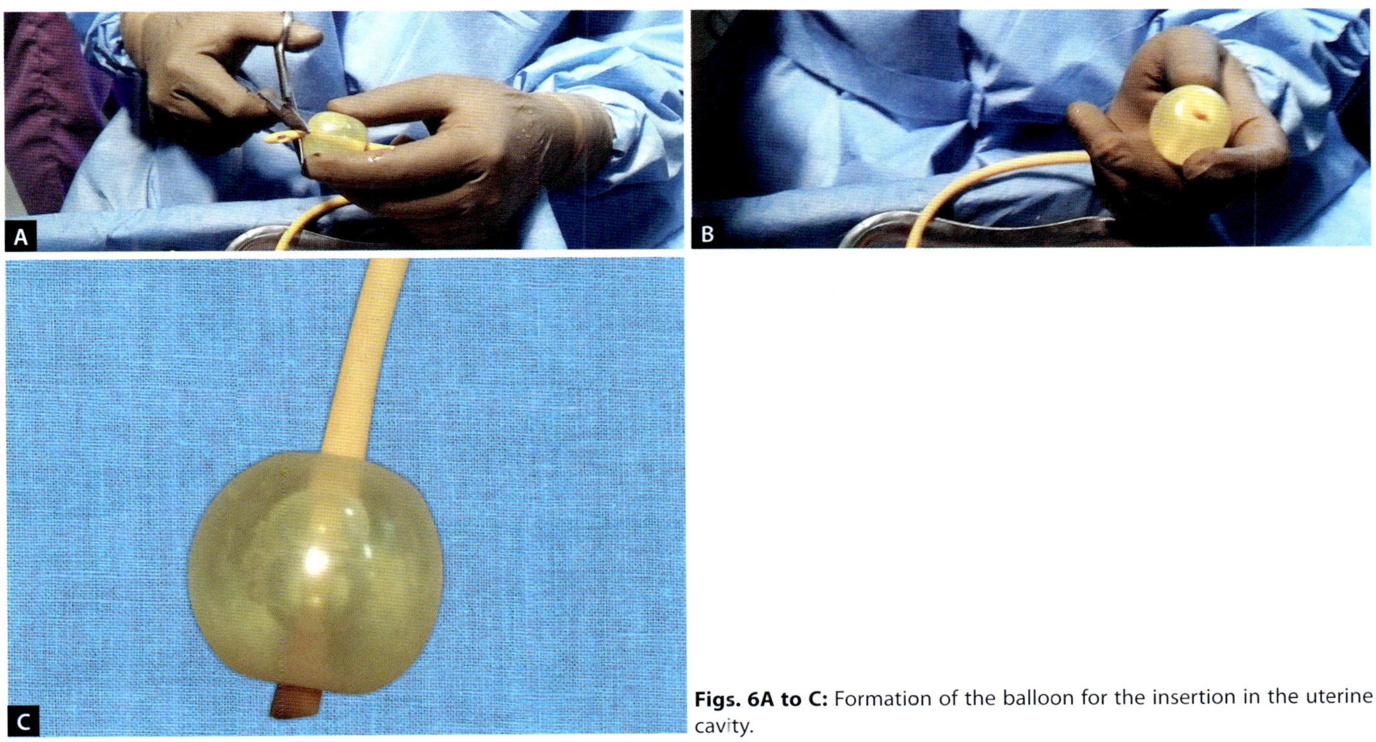

Figs. 6A to C: Formation of the balloon for the insertion in the uterine cavity.

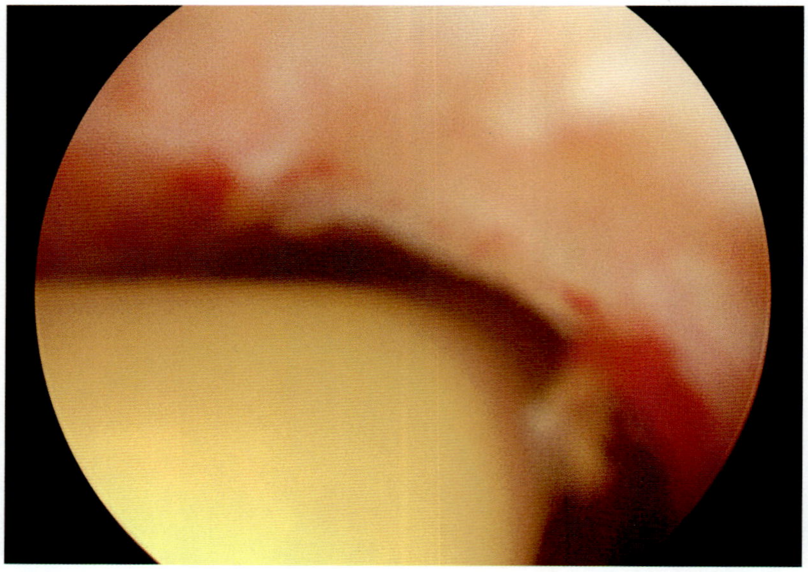

Fig. 7: Foley's catheter inserted into the uterine cavity.

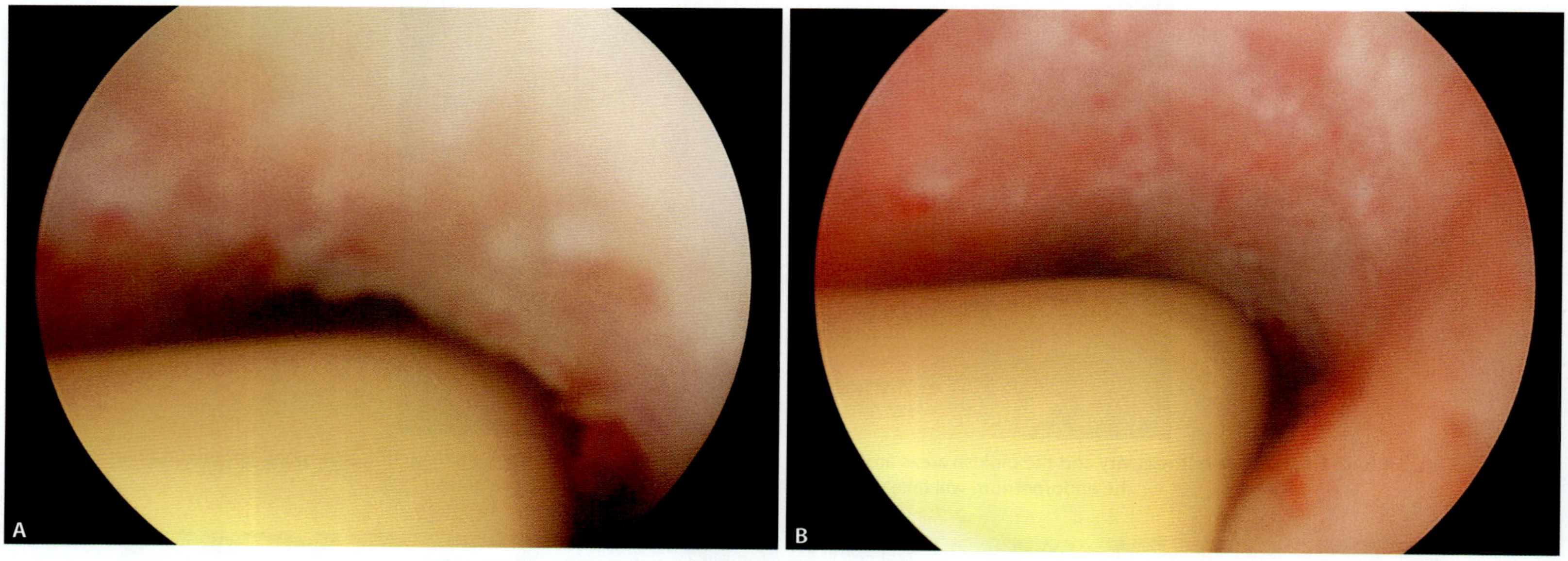

Figs. 8A and B: Confirming the place of the Foley's catheter inside the cavity.

SUGGESTED READING

1. AAGL Advancing Minimally Invasive Gynecology Worldwide. AAGL practice report: practice guidelines for management of intrauterine synechiae. J Minim Invasive Gynecol. 2010;17(1):1-7.
2. Capella-Allouc S, Morsad F, Rongières-Bertrand C, et al. Hysteroscopic treatment of severe Asherman's syndrome and subsequent fertility. Hum Reprod. 1999;14(5):1230-3.
3. Conforti A, Alviggi C, Mollo A, et al. The management of Asherman syndrome: a review of literature. Reprod Biol Endocrinol. 2013;11:118.
4. Yamamoto N, Takeuchi R, Izuchi D, et al. Hysteroscopic adhesiolysis for patient with Asherman's syndrome: menstrual and fertility outcomes. Reprod Med Biol. 2013;12(4):159-66.
5. Zikopoulos KA, Kolibianakis EM, Platteau P, et al. Live delivery rates in subfertile women with Asherman's syndrome after hysteroscopic adhesiolysis using the resectoscope or the Versapoint System. Reprod Biomed Online. 2004;8(6):720-5.

CHAPTER

58

Complications in Hysteroscopy

Shubhanjali Sen, Aditi Rai, B Ramesh

INTRODUCTION

Hysteroscopies are well-established diagnostic and therapeutic procedures with low complication rates. With the advent of fiberoptic light sources and high-resolution lens system. Hysteroscopy has become the most valuable diagnostic and operative tool for the management of the intrauterine pathologies. Adequate distension of the uterine cavity is mandatory for operative and diagnostic hysteroscopy. The most commonly used distension media used are low-viscosity fluids without electrolytes (e.g., 1.5% glycine, dextrose, sorbitol/mannitol and saline) and low-viscosity fluids with electrolytes (Normal saline/ringer lactate).

Complications such as cervical laceration, uterine perforation, intraoperative hemorrhage, vasovagal syndrome, gas embolism, media-related complications and delayed complications like infection and hematometra can occur.[1-3]

MONOPOLAR VERSUS BIPOLAR ELECTROSURGICAL UNIT COMPLICATION

Operative hysteroscopy is usually performed with monopolar electrosurgical unit (ESU) which requires low-viscosity, electrolyte-free hypotonic and isotonic solutions like mannitol (isotonic), sorbitol or 1.5% glycine for distension media. If not taken care about the volume then fluid toxicity and dilutional hyponatremia can occur which results in fatal conditions.

Recently, in view of adverse effects from low-viscosity, electrolyte-free hypotonic solution, bipolar ESU have been introduced in the operative hysteroscopy using 0.9% normal saline as distension media.[4] Targeted biopsies, submucous myomas (type 0 and 1) resection, polypectomy, septum resection, adhesion resection, etc. are common procedures performed hysteroscopically which are time-consuming but rewarding surgeries.[5]

But, if not done in experienced hands, then using monopolar ESU leads to fluid overload in 3–6% of patients[6] causing hypervolemia, laryngeal swelling, hypo-osmolar hyponatremia leading to cerebral edema, hyponatremic hypo-osmolar encephalopathy which lead to permanent brain damage. To avoid fluid overload, skilled surgeon should perform inflow-outflow of intravenous fluid to be meticulously monitored, use of diuretics, correct infusion rates and flow rates and limiting the time for the procedure and if the procedure is taking longer duration then abandon the procedure and shift for second sitting.[7]

If the fluid deficit is 700 mL (glycine), then the patients' vitals, pulse oximetry, urine output and serum sodium should be evaluated intraoperatively.[7] A correction of the hyponatremia is recommended within 24 hours, to prevent cerebral edema,[8] but too rapid correction of the hyponatremia may lead to central pontine myelinolysis (CPM) or osmotic demyelinating syndrome.

Glycine Toxicity

As mentioned earlier, when monopolar resectoscopes are used an low-viscosity electrolyte-free, hypotonic or isotonic, nonconductive fluid like glycine 1.5%, sorbitol 2.7% with mannitol 0.54% mixture, or a mannitol 5%. With glycine, cellular penetration occurs more rapidly than water or dextrose. About 10% of glycine is excreted in urine which results in a brisk osmotic diuresis. Glycine is metabolized in the liver and has a plasma half-life of 85 minutes.

Metabolism leads to increased plasma concentrations of ammonia, serine and oxalate. Hyperammonemia can result in toxic reactions such as visual disturbances and muscle weakness.[9-11] Other side effects associated with the use of glycine include heart failure, hemodilution with hyponatremia, encephalopathy, seizures and gastrointestinal (GI) disturbances such as nausea and vomiting. These occur after a glycine load of 22–35 g (i.e., 1,500–3,500 mL glycine 1.5%).[12] Reports of central nervous system toxicity including hyponatremic encephalopathy and transient blindness from glycine have been reported in the urological and orthopedic literature after prostatectomy and arthroscopy.[9] With glycine, there is a dose-dependent increase of symptoms such as visual disturbance (glycine is an inhibiting neurotransmitter) or excess of ammonia.[13-15]

Sorbitol is metabolized to fructose and glucose. After metabolism, sorbitol and glycine leave free water behind. As they both dilute in the extra- and intracellular compartments, cellular edema and dilutional hyponatremia are the consequences.

Mannitol is inert, distributes only in the extracellular space, and is excreted unchanged by the kidney. Mannitol 3% has the largest sorbitol-mannitol mixture as distension media and glycine 1.5% the smallest plasma dilutional effect.[16,17]

The osmotic diuretic effects of the substances lead to even more sodium loss and thereby worsen hyponatremia.

With a monopolar resectoscope, it seems to be safest to use mannitol or sorbitol/mannitol mixtures because of fewer neurological and cardiovascular compromises.[18]

With a bipolar resectoscope, it is possible to use low-viscosity electrolyte fluids like normal saline and ringer lactate. However, the risk of excessive fluid absorption is still present. An exact determination of the fluid balance is necessary. It is recommended that the procedure is terminated when the fluid absorption reaches 2,000 mL.[18]

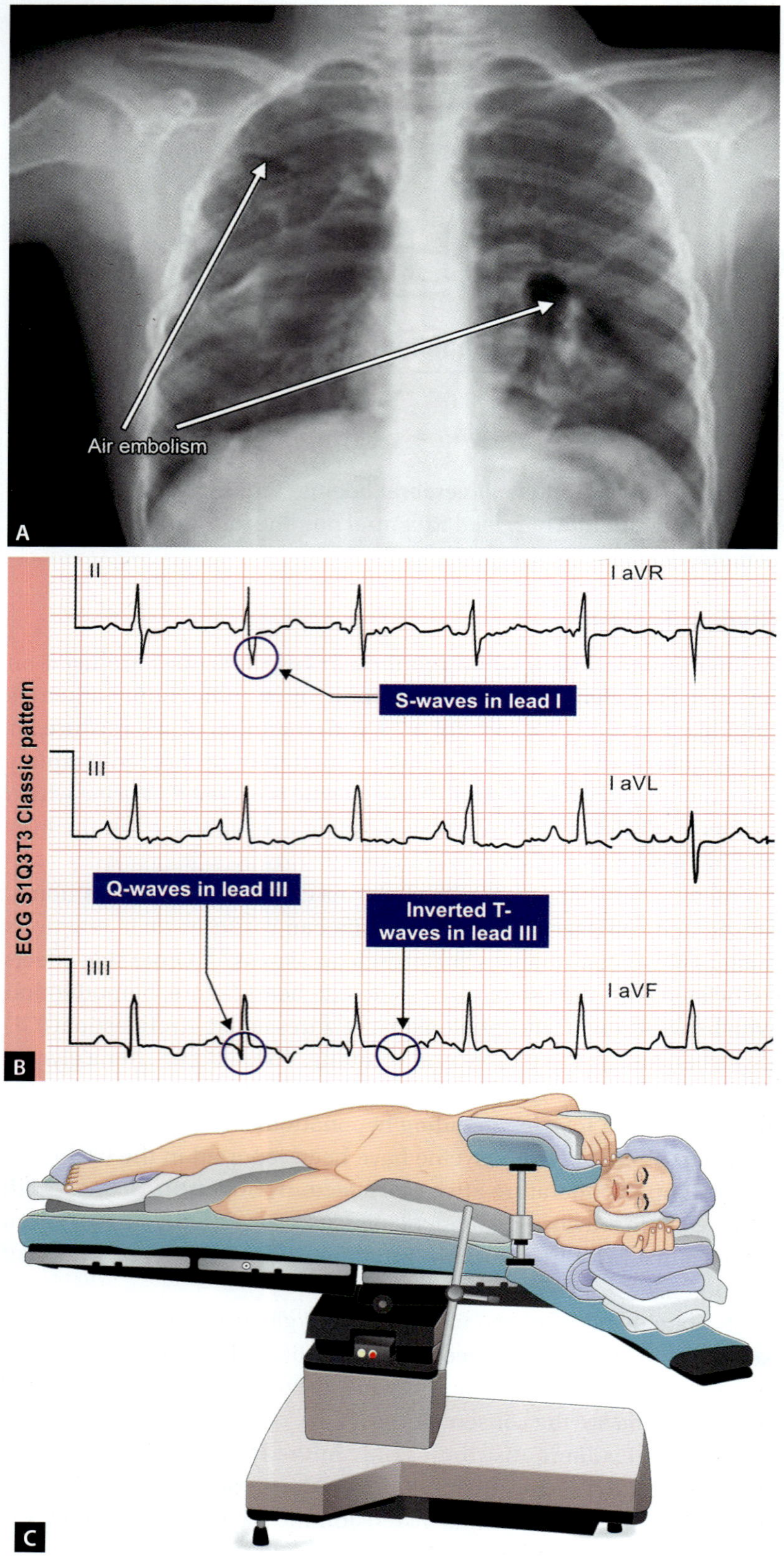

Figs. 1A to C: (A) Air embolism; (B) ECG abnormality; (C) Lateral postion to manage air embolism

Besides, restriction of IV fluids and the use of diuretics during a longer procedure are recommended.[7] The resection time should not exceed 60 minutes[19] although the operation time seems to be less important than the total amounts of fluids used.[20]

The care of the patient suffering from water intoxication involves the removal of excess fluid and correction of the serum sodium level. Because the onset of severe symptoms is often unpredictable, therapy must be undertaken immediately. The rate of correction have been actively debated. Too rapid correction may cause an obscure injury of the brain called CPM.[21,22] The risk of osmotic demyelination appears to be minimal in patients suffering from water overload and acute hyponatremia as a result of operative hysteroscopy. These patients should be treated expeditiously and followed closely. Initially, the serum sodium may be increased by 1–2 mEq/L per hour during the first few hours. There is little reason to attempt to increase the serum sodium by >12 mEq/L in the first 24 hours.

In acute hyponatremia, specific treatment methods are variable but usually include intravenous administration of saline solution and forced diuresis. Both furosemide and mannitol have been advocated to initiate diuresis. Urine output should be accurately measured with an indwelling catheter, and urine sodium concentration should also be evaluated. Adequate intravascular volume is maintained, and sodium is replaced by an infusion of normal saline solution. The rate of infusion will depend on the diuretic response as well as the serum sodium level. Initially, serum electrolytes should be monitored every 4 hours.

GAS EMBOLISM

Gas embolism during operative hysteroscopy is a rare, but well described entity with an incidence ranging from 10 to 50%.[23,24] The true incidence is not known but catastrophic outcomes occur at a rate of 3 in 17,000 procedures.[18] The source of the gas may be ambient air which enters the uterine cavity during the procedure,[18,25,26] or air bubbles within the distension fluid.[18,25,26]

Alternatively, the embolic gas may be carbon dioxide and carbon monoxide, evaporative products of combustion as surgery proceeds.[18,23] Carbon dioxide may be introduced into a large vein via the Veress needle and trapped in the right ventricle, causing right outflow obstruction from the right ventricle into the pulmonary artery.

Indicative features include sudden circulatory collapse, cyanosis, raised jugular venous pressure, a characteristic "millwheel" murmur, a high arterial pCO_2 and a drop in end tidal carbon dioxide concentration. If carbon dioxide insufflation is still ongoing via the Veress needle, it should be stopped immediately and the tubing is disconnected. Escape of blood via the open end of the Veress needle confirms the diagnosis.

How to Recognize?

The earliest sign of carbon dioxide gas embolism is a drop in end tidal carbon dioxide concentration, which is a result of decreased blood flow to the lungs. As all modern anesthetic machines continually record end tidal carbon dioxide concentration, a drop in measurement calls for an immediate halt to further gas being introduced into the peritoneal cavity, followed by investigation to exclude the diagnosis.

How to Manage?

Carbon dioxide insufflation must be stopped immediately, but the Veress needle must not be removed. Cardiopulmonary resuscitation is required. The patient is rolled on to her left side to facilitate expulsion of gas from the ventricle.[27] A central line may also be inserted to aspirate gas from the right ventricle. Alternatively, intracardiac gas aspiration may also be tried.[28]

How to Prevent?

A Veress needle should be inserted with the tap open and without connection to the insufflation machine. If it had been inadvertently

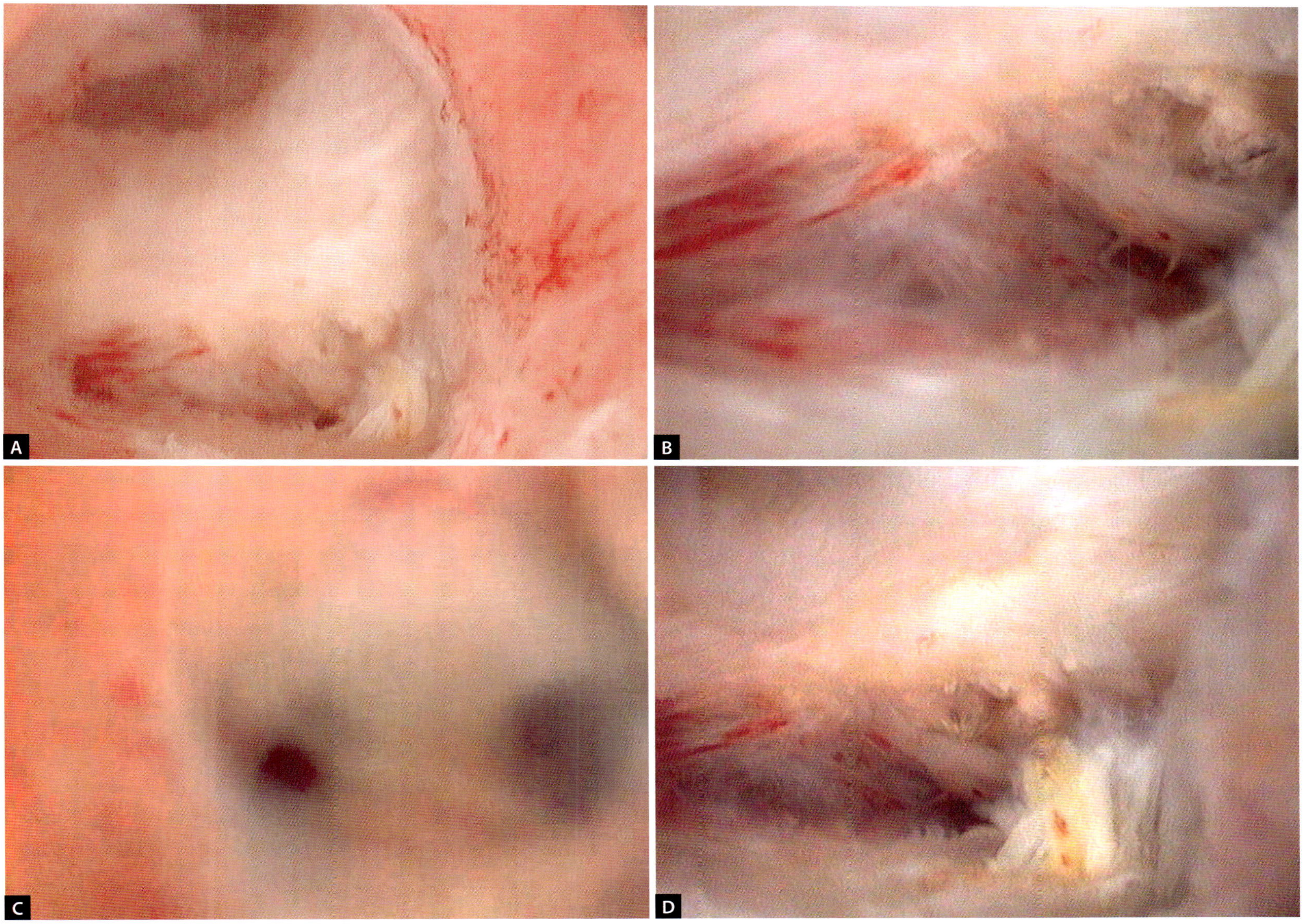

Figs. 2A to D: False passage.

introduced into a large vein, blood would be seen escaping via the open end, as the venous pressure in the vena cava and common iliac vein exceeds that of the atmospheric pressure. As a steep Trendelenburg position decreases venous pressure in the iliac vessels and vena cava, a steep Trendelenburg position should be avoided when creating pneumoperitoneum. Instead, the patient should be in the dorsal position.[29] After pneumoperitoneum has been successfully created, the patient may then be put into the steep Trendelenburg position. Atmospheric air embolism is more dangerous than carbon dioxide embolism because the former is less soluble in blood. For this reason, prior to insufflation, the air in the insufflation tube connected to the carbon dioxide tank should be flushed out. The space in the tube in use in our hospital has been measured to be 25 mL.

UTERINE PERFORATION

Uterine perforation is one possible complication of gynecological procedures including gynecological endoscopic procedures. Recognized risk factors for those undesirable events are: age of the patient, uterine conditions, small uterus, stenotic cervix, prior use of gonadotropin releasing hormone (GnRH) analogs, use of anesthesia or analgesia, patient positioning, extent of the surgery, type of the distending medium, use of thermal energy sources, poor visualization, and lack of uterine distension.[3,30]

Uterine perforation is more common in repeat procedures.[31] Some conditions such as genital tuberculosis have been associated with greater difficulty in carrying out hysteroscopy and hence a higher rate of complications including uterine perforation.[32] Perforations can occur most commonly due to thermal injury, although it can also be caused by use of scissors during resections.[31] Mostly occur in the fundal region or posterior lower segment.[31] Basic preoperative precautions are the first step in avoiding uterine perforation, as with other complications during hysteroscopy, such as inspection of and familiarity with equipment to be used, planning the procedure and briefing the surgical team.[31]

Awareness of contraindications, both in terms of availability of appropriate and familiar equipment and staff and of patient characteristics such as inability to dilate the cervix or distend the uterus is also important.[31] During surgery, the chances of uterine perforation can be minimized by appropriate technique, including always moving the loop toward the operator rather than into the uterus and not activating the power without a clear view of the loop or needle.[33]

In premenstrual women, preoperative self-administration of misoprostol the night before the procedure can assist with cervical ripening and reduce risk of perforation.[33]

"False passage", where the surgeon thinks the hysteroscope is in the uterine cavity can occur, so it is important to be aware of signs

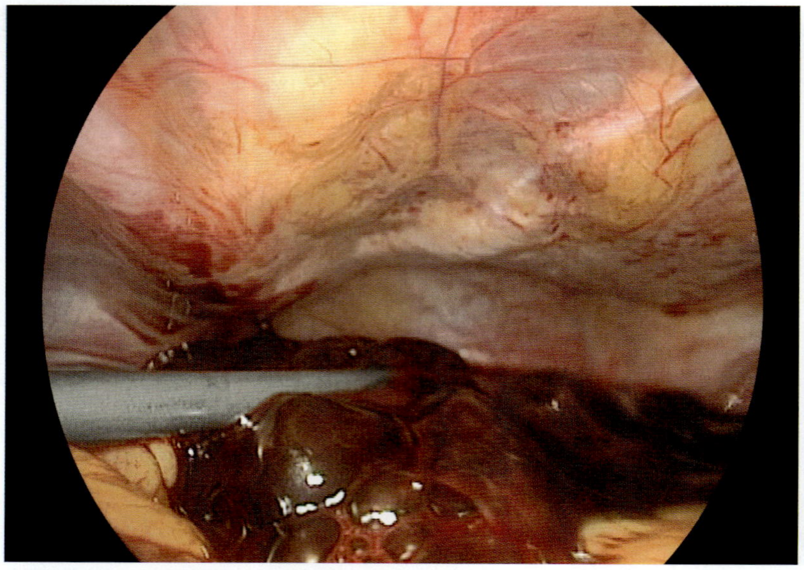

Fig. 3: Hemorrhage posthysteroscopic perforation.

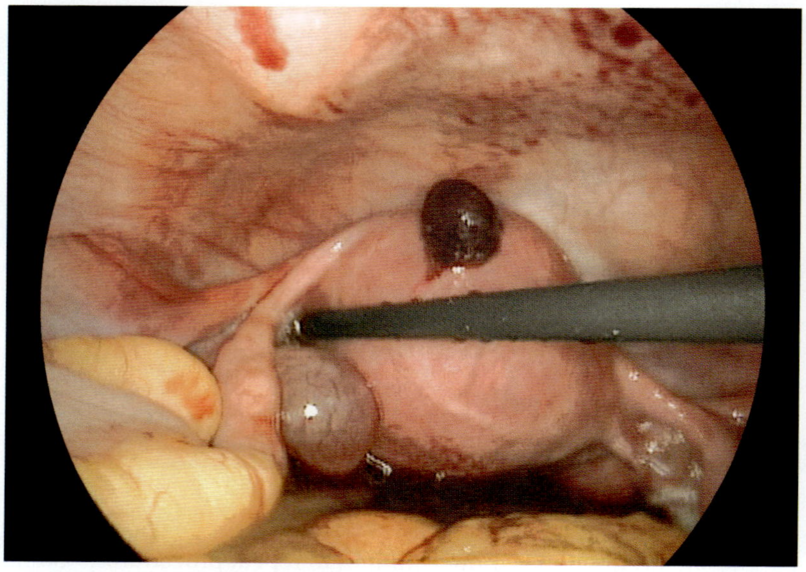

Fig. 4: Hematoma at perforation site.

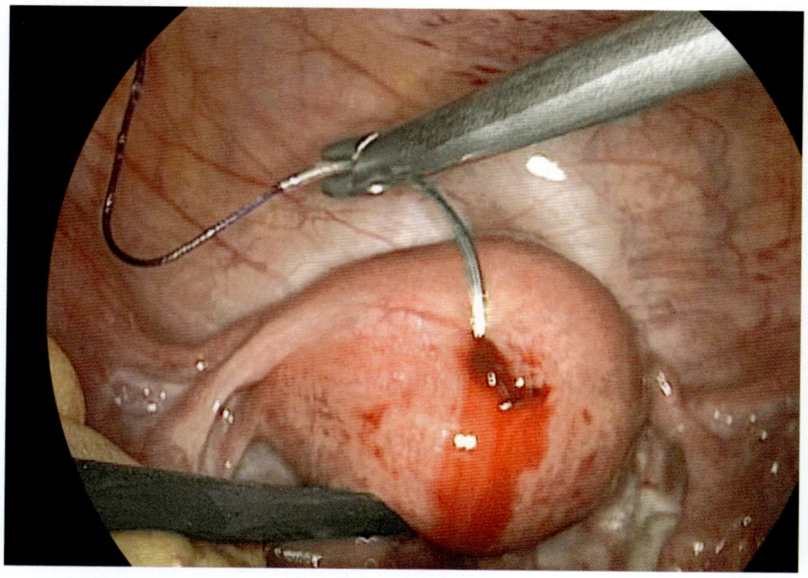

Fig. 5: Perforation site sutured with vicryl no. 1 in interuppted manner.

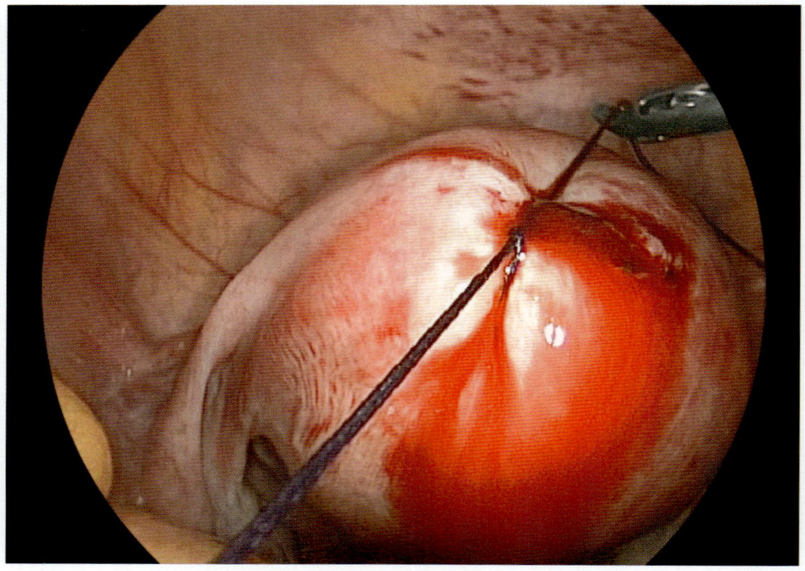

Fig. 6: Perforation site sutured from one angle to other.

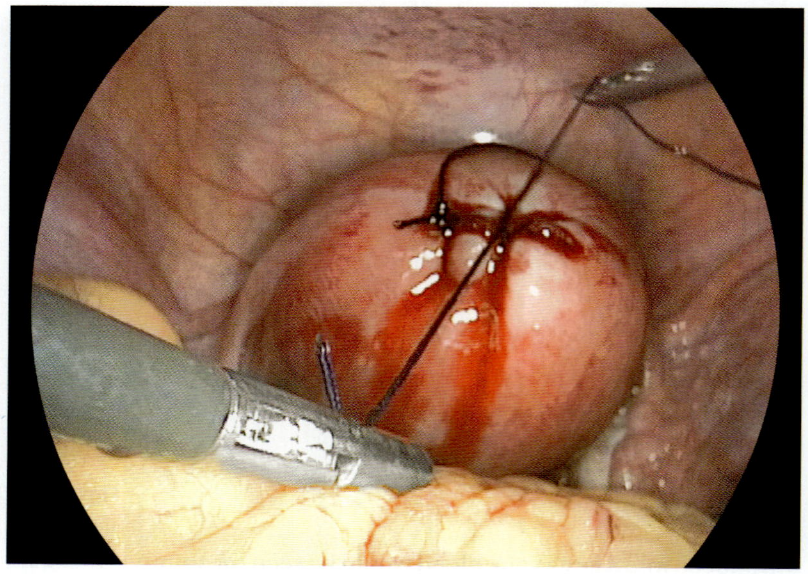

Fig. 7: Complete hemostasis ensured.

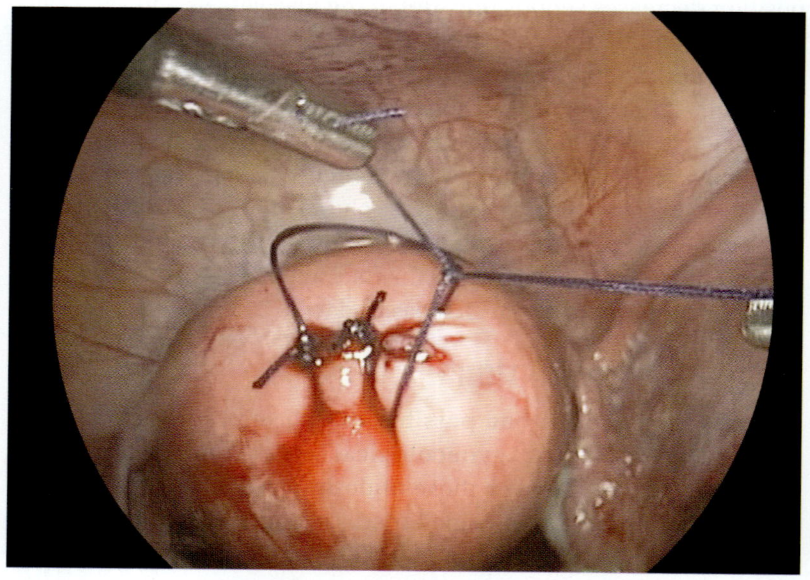

Fig. 8: Mattress interrupted suture placed.

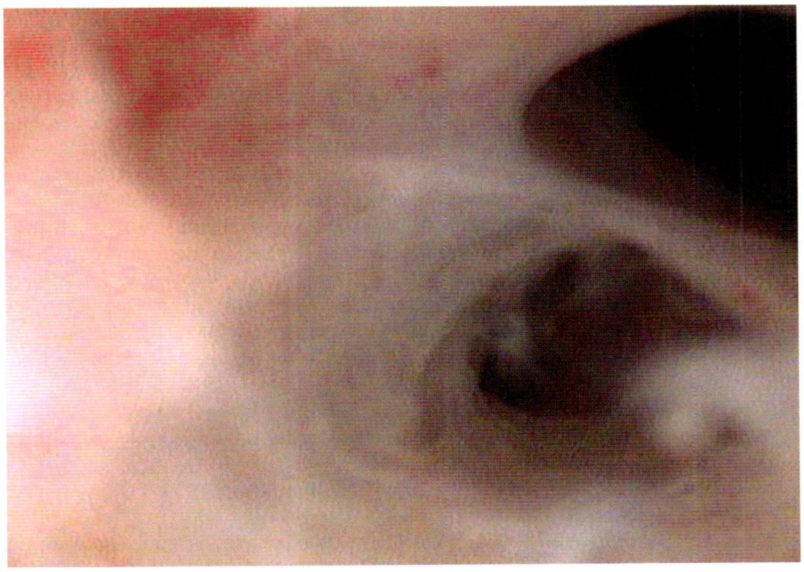

Fig. 9: Adhesions.

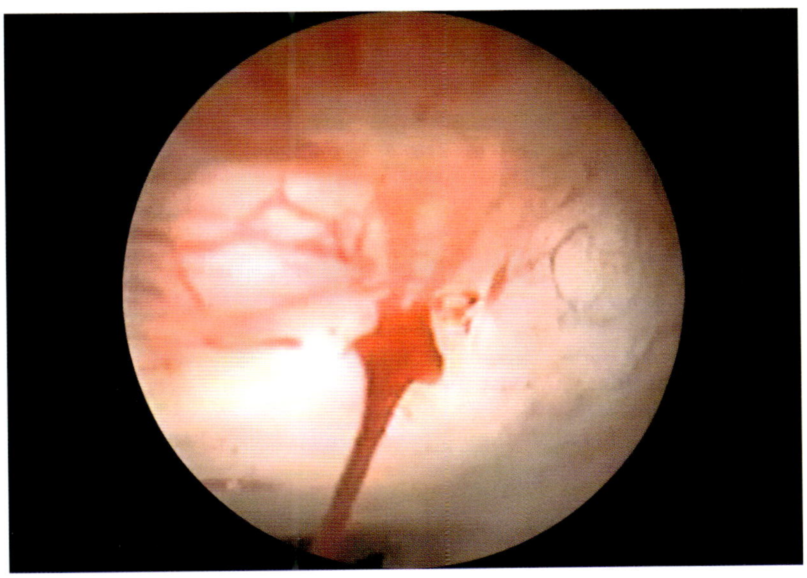

Fig. 10: Bleeding.

of this, including visibility of muscle fibers and tubal ostia, and to stop the procedure even in the absence of detectable perforation as adequate distension could not now be achieved.[31] Risk of false passage can be reduced by cervical dilation with slow, steady pressure, stopping when the internal os opens. If the external but not the internal os is sufficiently dilated, the surgeon should not use force to insert the hysteroscope or resectoscope but use the instrument's inflow to allow dilation of the cervix with fluid pressure.[31] Simultaneous laparoscopy can be helpful in allowing assistants to monitor the serosal surface and guard against perforation.

During myoma removal, excessive traction with the myoma grasper should be avoided. If perforation is imminent, the uterine serosa becomes visible; surgeons should be familiar with this "serosal sign".[31] Generally, uterine perforations do not require treatment but once perforation occurs due to thermal injury, laparoscopy becomes necessary for assessment of overlying organs including the bowel. Any bowel damage detected can then be repaired using mini laparotomy.[31]

Use of intraoperative ultrasound is strongly indicated in endoscopic gynecological surgery, in particular for the reduction and management of uterine perforation in operative hysteroscopy.[34-36]

INTRAUTERINE ADHESIONS

Intrauterine adhesions, in particular, are one of the main long-term complications encountered in operational hysteroscopy.[37-39] While hysteroscopy is used in division of adhesions in hysteroscopic adhesiolysis, recurrence of the adhesions after or as a result of such surgery is a common problem.[39-41] It is critical to address the possibility of development of postoperative adhesions in endoscopically assisted gynecological surgery as the consequences of intrauterine adhesions can include hypomenorrhea, infertility and recurrent pregnancy loss.[38,39] While there are various medications available for the prevention of intraperitoneal adhesions, there are fewer interventions described for prevention of intrauterine adhesions. Possibilities include use of intrauterine balloons, intrauterine contraceptive devices or auto-crosslinked hyaluronan gel such as Hyalobarrier® to prevent adhesions.[38,40] In terms of adhesion formation after surgery, there is evidence to suggest that use of endoscopic techniques with their minimal accessing of the abdominal cavity, less manipulation of sites distal to the surgical site, and gentler and more precise dissection of the relevant structures result in fewer adhesions than open surgery.[42] Methods to minimize adhesions in operative hysteroscopy and combined laparoscopy and hysteroscopic procedures include adherence to basic microsurgery principles, use of extensive irrigation of the abdominal cavity and exploiting the more newly available surgical instruments such as the ultrasonically activated scalpel and monopolar electrocautery.[42] Surgeons should also familiarize themselves with newer surgical techniques which are suggested to reduce adhesion formation, such as temporary ovarian suspension and subserous as opposed to interrupted figure-8 sutures.[42] Use of pharmacological adjuvants can also be considered in management of adhesions, particularly in prevention or minimization, although there is lack of consensus on effectiveness of many suggested agents.[42] Use of preoperative or postoperative GnRH agonists is a promising strategy, as is use of a solid barrier of oxidized regenerated cellulose over traumatized surfaces after hemostasis is complete.[42] There is a need for more randomized control trials on these methods, but surgeons should be mindful of their possibilities in management of adhesion recurrence following endoscopic gynecological surgery.

BLEEDING

Heavy bleeding from the endometrial cavity is uncommon after hysteroscopic surgery in general. If there is continuous bleeding after resection, a Foley catheter can be inserted into the uterine cavity and distended with up to 40 mL of saline until the bleeding settles from a tamponade effect. The balloon can be removed if the bleeding has settled in a few hours. Other pharmacological agents that have been investigated to reduce blood loss at myomectomy include tranexamic acid, prostaglandin E2 analogs (misoprostol and dinoprostone) and ascorbic acid. A more invasive option for controlling bleeding is uterine artery embolization with interventional radiologic techniques if bleeding persists despite above measures.

The advent of the use of ESU (monopolar or bipolar) has reduced the anticipated cases in which bleeding can be a complication.

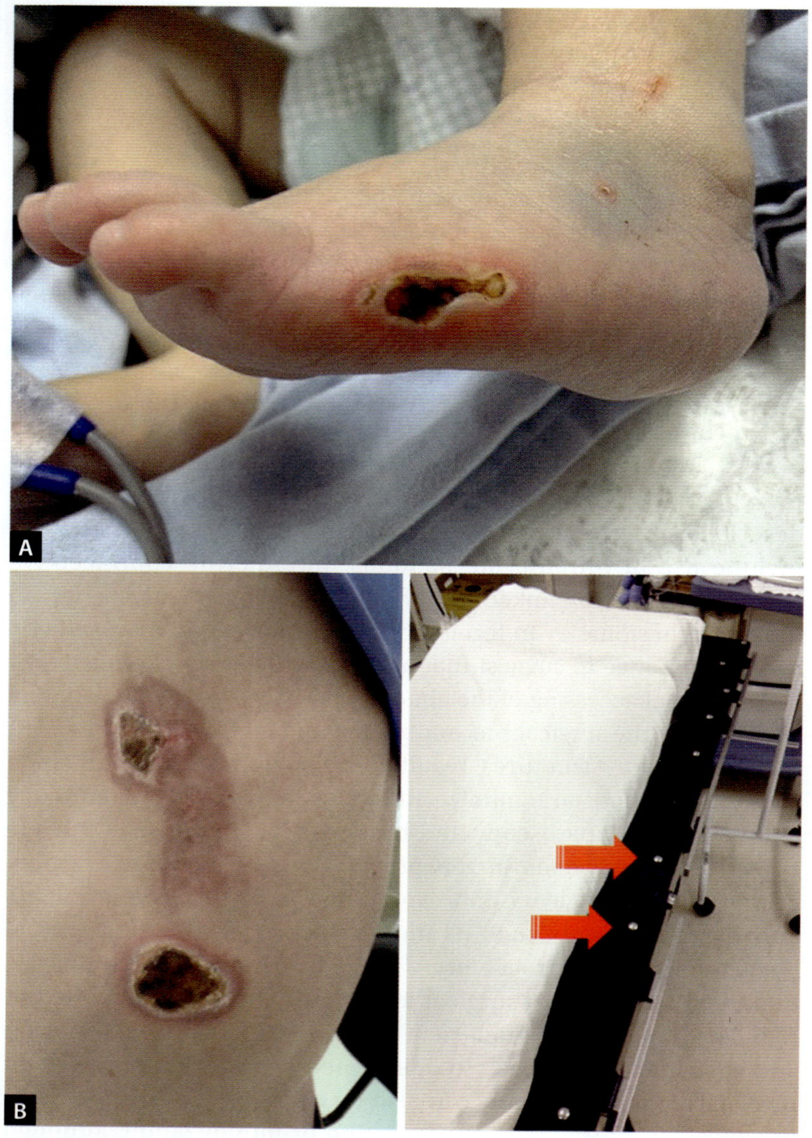

Figs. 11A and B: Thermal burn.

THERMAL BURNS

One must be very careful to avoid unintentional activation of the monopolar or bipolar pedals. If this occurs while the active electrode is resting on the patient, it can cause serious burns to the abdomen, perineum, vagina or vulva. More sinister burns occur when the uterus is perforated by an active electrode causing injury to surrounding structures, most commonly the bowel or blood vessels. This type of injury can be prevented by making sure not to activate the electrode while it is being advanced into the endometrial cavity. It should only be activated when being withdrawn. As discussed before, if a uterine perforation is suspected due to an active electrode, the surgeon must perform an exploratory laparoscopy or laparotomy depending on the extent of perforation.

REFERENCES

1. Bradley LD. Complications in hysteroscopy: Prevention, treatment and legal risk. Curr Opin Obstet Gynecol. 2002;14:409-15.
2. Aydeniz B, Gruber IV, Schauf B, et al. A multicenter survey of complications associated with 21,676 operative hysteroscopies. Eur J Obstet Gynecol Reprod Biol. 2002;104:160-4.
3. Jansen FW, Vredevoogd CB, van Ulzen K, et al. Complications of hysteroscopy: A prospective, multicenter study. Obstet Gynecol. 2000;96:266-70.
4. Kung RC, Vilos GA, Thomas B, et al. A new bipolar system for performing operative hysteroscopy in normal saline. J Am Assoc Gynecol Laparosc. 1999; 6:331-6.
5. Golan A, Zachalka N, Lurie S, et al. Vaginal removal of prolapsed pedunculated submucous myoma: A short, simple, and definitive procedure with minimal morbidity. Arch Gynecol Obstet. 2005;271:11-3.
6. Stotz M, Lampart A, Kochli OR, et al. Intraabdominal bleeding masked by hemodilution after hysteroscopy. Anesthesiology. 2000;93:569-70.
7. Kim AH, Keltz MD, Arici A, et al. Dilutional hyponatremia during hysteroscopic myomectomy with sorbitol-mannitol distention medium. J Am Assoc Gynecol Laparosc. 1995;2(2):237-42.
8. Moritz ML, Ayus JC. The pathophysiology and treatment of hyponatraemic encephalopathy: an update. Nephrol Dial Transplant. 2003;18(12):2486-91.
9. Hahn RG. The transurethral resection syndrome. Acta Anaesthesiol Scand. 1991;35:557-67.
10. Casey WF, Hannon V, Cunningham A, et al. Visual evoked potentials and changes in serum glycine concentration during transurethral resection of the prostate. Br J Anaesth. 1988;60:525-9.
11. Gillett W, Grossman HB, Lee R. Visual disturbances in TUR reaction. Urology. 1985;25:573-5.
12. Ayus JC, Krothapalli RK, Arieff AL. Changing concepts in treatment of severe symptomatic hyponatremia: rapid correction and possible relation to central pontine myelinolysis. Am J Med. 1985;78:897-902.
13. Hahn RG, Sandfeldt L, Nyman CR. Double-blind randomized study of symptoms associated with absorption of glycine 1.5% or mannitol 3% during transurethral resection of the prostate. J Urol. 1998;160(2):397-401.
14. Hahn RG, Shemais H, Essén P. Glycine 1.0% versus glycine 1.5% as irrigating fluid during transurethral resection of the prostate. Br J Urol. 1997; 79(3):394-400.
15. Olsson J, Nilsson A, Hahn RG. Symptoms of the transurethral resection syndrome using glycine as the irrigant. J Urol. 1995;154(1):123-8.
16. Sandfeldt L, Hahn RG. Comparison of urological irrigating fluids containing glycine and mannitol in volunteers. Prostate. 1999;41(2):89-98.
17. Hahn RG, Nilsson A, Ståhle L. Distribution and elimination of the solute and water components of urological irrigating fluids. Scand J Urol Nephrol. 1999;33(1):35-41.
18. Isaacson KB. Complications of hysteroscopy. Obstet Gynecol Clin North Am. 1999;26(1):39-51.
19. Desmond J. Serum osmolality and serum electrolytes in patients who develop dilutional hyponatremia during transurethral resection. Can J Surg. 1970;13(2):116-21.
20. Hahn RG. Fluid absorption in endoscopic surgery. Br J Anaesth. 2006; 96(1):8-20.
21. Ayus JC, Krothapalli RK, Arieff AI. Treatment of symptomatic hyponatremia and its relation to brain damage. N Engl J Med. 1987;5:1190-5.
22. Stern RH. The treatment of hyponatremia: first, do no harm. Am J Med. 1990;88:557-60.
23. Stoloff DR, Isenberg RA, Brill AI. Venous air and gas emboli in operative hysteroscopy. J Am Assoc Gynecol Laparosc. 2001;8:181-92.
24. Brandner P, Neis KJ, Ehmer C. The etiology, frequency, and prevention of gas embolism during CO_2 hysteroscopy. J Am Assoc Gynecol Laparosc. 1999;6:421-8.
25. Spencer MP, Oyama Y. Pulmonary capacity for dissipation of venous gas emboli. Aerospace Med. 1971;42:822-7.
26. Brooks PG. Venous air embolism during operative hysteroscopy. J Am Assoc Gynecol Laparosc. 1997;4:399-402.
27. Yacoub OF, Cardona I, Coveler LA, et al. Carbon dioxide embolism during laparoscopy. Anesthesiology. Anesthesiology. 1982;57(6):533-5.
28. Beck DH, McQuillan PJ. Fatal carbon dioxide embolism and severe haemorrhage during laparoscopic salpingectomy. Br J Anaesth. 1994; 72(2):243-5.
29. Corson SL, Brooks PG, Soderstrom RM. Gynecologic endoscopic gas embolism. Fertil Steril. 1996;65(3):529-33.
30. O'Donovan P, Mc Gurgan P. Complications in hysteroscopy surgery. In: Complications in Gynecological Surgery. London: Springer Science & Business Media BV; 2008. pp. 94-105.
31. Glasser MH. Hysteroscopy: Managing and minimizing operative complications. OBG Manag. 2005;17(2):42-57.
32. Sharma JB, Roy KK, Pushparaj M, et al. Increased difficulties and complications encountered during hysteroscopy in women with genital tuberculosis. J Minim Invasive Gynecol. 2011;18(5):660-5.
33. Istre OI. Managing bleeding, fluid absorption and uterine perforation at hysteroscopy. Best Pract Res Clin Obstet Gynaecol. 2009;23(5):619-29.

34. Kresowik JD, Syrop CH, Van Voorhis, et al. Ultrasound is the optimal choice for guidance in difficult hysteroscopy. Ultrasound Obstet Gynecol. 2012;39(6):715-8.
35. Ma C, Wang Y, Li TC, et al. Trans-abdominal ultrasound guided transvaginal hydrolaparoscopy is associated with reduced complication rate. Eur J Obstet Gynecol Reprod Biol. 2012;160(2):166-9.
36. Criniti A, Lin PC. Applications of intraoperative ultrasound in gynecological surgery. Curr Opin Obstet Gynecol. 2005;17(4):339-42.
37. Alpay Z, Saed GM, Diamond MP. Postoperative adhesions: from formation to prevention. Semin Reprod Med. 2008;26(4):313-21.
38. Mais V, Cirronis MG, Peiretti M, et al. Efficacy of auto-crosslinked hyaluronan gel for adhesion prevention in laparoscopy and hysteroscopy: A systematic review and meta-analysis of randomized controlled trials. Eur J Obstet Gynecol Reprod Biol. 2012;160(1):1-5.
39. Deans R, Abbott J. Review of intrauterine adhesions. J Minim Invasive Gynecol. 2010;17(5):555-69.
40. Lin X, Wei M, Li TC, et al. A comparison of intrauterine balloon, intrauterine contraceptive device and hyaluronic acid gel in the prevention of adhesion reformation following hysteroscopic surgery for Asherman syndrome: a cohort study. Eur J Obstet Gynecol Reprod Biol. 2013;170(2):512-6.
41. Yu D, Wong Y, Cheong Y, et al. Asherman syndrome one century later. Fertil Steril. 2008;89(4):759-79.
42. Nappi C, Di SS, Greco E, et al. Prevention of adhesions in gynaecological endoscopy. Hum Reprod Update. 2007;13(4):379-94.

CHAPTER

59

Transcervical Resection of Endometrium

Shubhanjali Sen, Minal Kumbhalwar, B Ramesh

INTRODUCTION

Transcervical resection of endometrium (TCRE)—this procedure is first-generation endometrial ablation technique. This procedure removes the inner lining of the uterus "endometrium", to grow back. This technique was introduced in 1983. Scottish hysteroscopy audit group study concluded that TCRE has a significant role to play in management of the menorrhagia.

Transcervical resection of endometrium also known as hysteroscopic endometrial resection and hysteroscopic endometrial ablation.

INDICATION

Heavy menstrual bleeding which are not responding to medical management, who has no wish to expand their family (completed family), or who wish to preserve their uterus or contraindicated to hysterectomy.

It can also be performed in:
- Long uterus
- Bicornuate uterus
- Fibroids/polyp
- With 2 or more than 2 previous cesarean section.

Why TCRE is superior to hysterectomy?

This procedure significantly has benefits than hysterectomy.
- Duration of the procedure is significantly short as compared to hysterectomy.
- Postoperative recovery and stay is very short in comparison to hysterectomy.
- Due to better fluid management system, the chances of postoperative fluid overload are negligible now.

PROCEDURE

A daycare procedure, which is of 20–45 minutes done under general anesthesia. Hysteroscope inserted into the cervix and the panoramic view of the uterine cavity is observed, following which resectoscope is used with either loop or roller ball **(Fig. 3C)** for the commencement of the procedure. 1% glycine **(Fig. 8)** is used as the distending medium.

COMPLICATIONS

Intraoperative

- Fluid overload (rarely)
- False passage formation
- Perforation of the uterus.

Postoperative

- Recurrent menorrhagia which is taken up for hysterectomy
- Formation of the hematometra which is usually drained under USG guidance.

POSTOPERATIVE CARE

Patients must be educated about the postoperative bleeding pattern so that psychologically the demands are met in terms of the heavy bleeding.
- Pink to brown discharge can be observed for another 4–5 weeks followed by regular minimal periods or absolute cessation of the periods.
- Dysmenorrhea may or may not be experienced.
- Contraception has to be additionally used as endometrial ablation does not ensure it.
- Normal activities can be resumed from the next day itself.
- Avoid intercourse for 48 hours.

FOLLOW-UP

- Discharged with antibiotics and analgesics
- Weekly basis follow-up and check-up for 3 weeks followed by monthly check-up for 1 year.

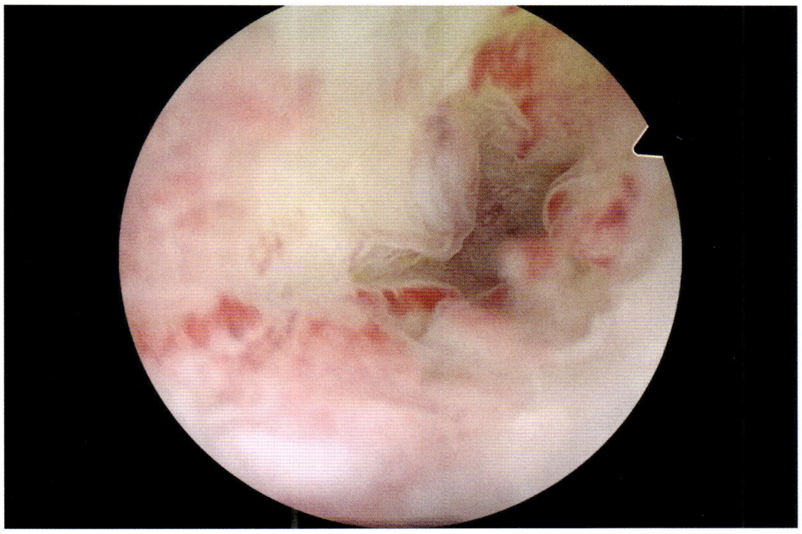

Fig. 1: Endometrial cavity.

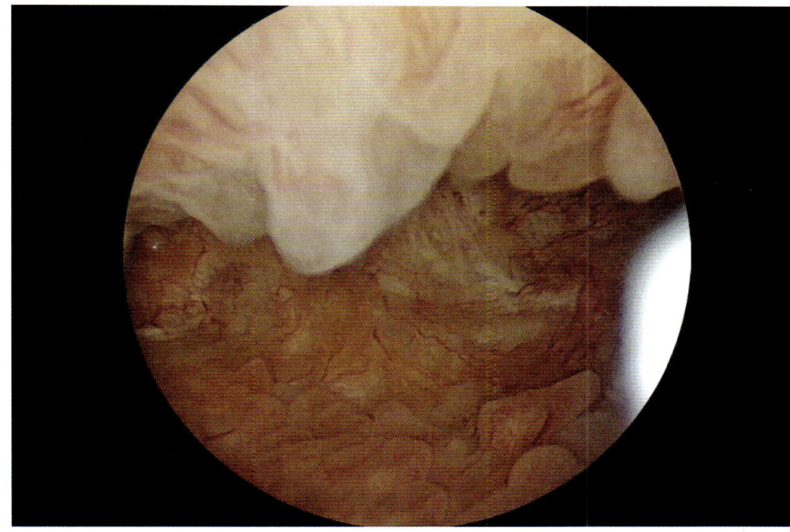

Fig. 2: Endometrial cavity with polypoidal endometrium.

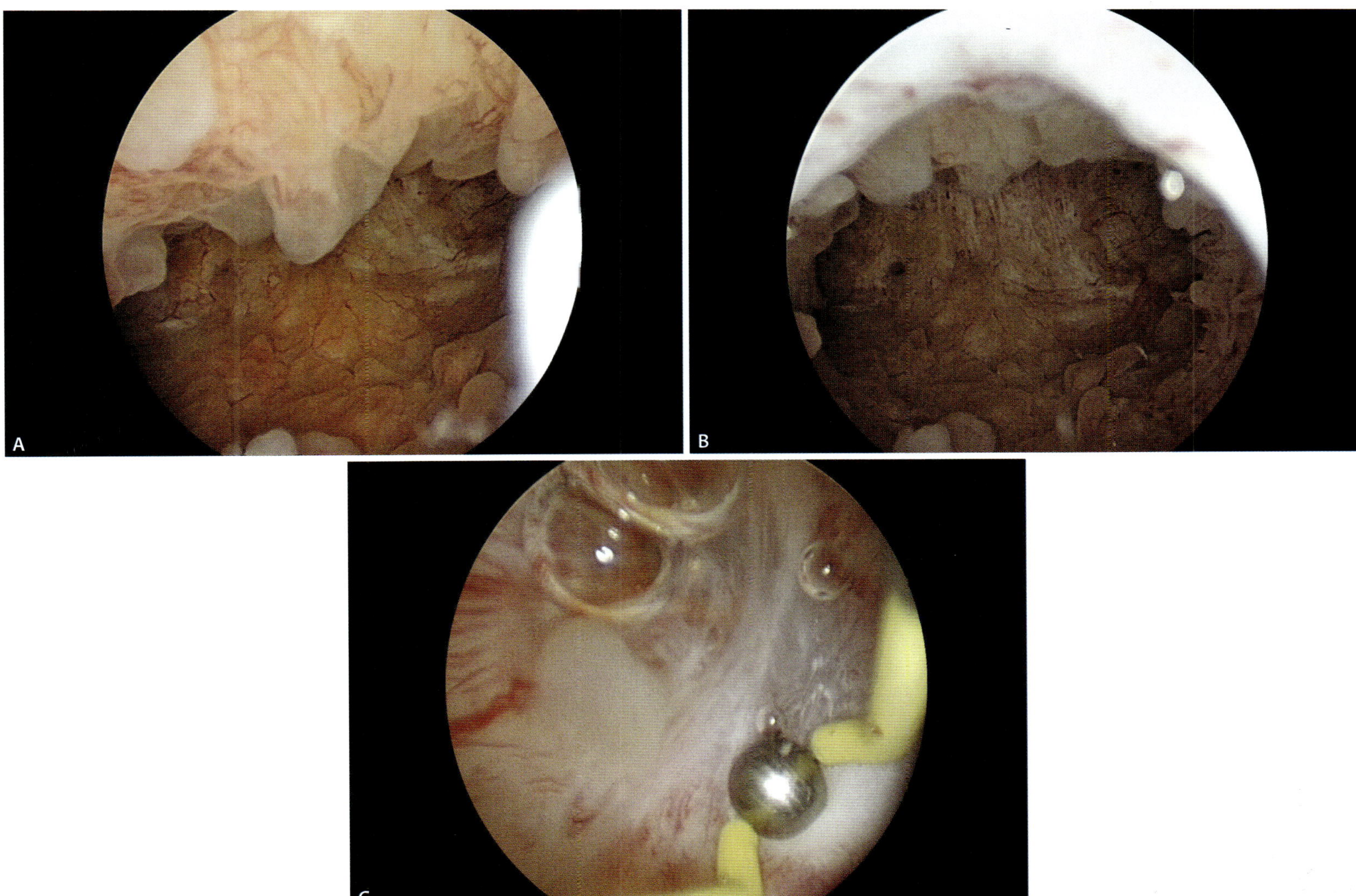

Figs. 3A to C: Roller ball of 26 Fr is used for the ablation of the endometrium with monopolar current and glycine as distention media.

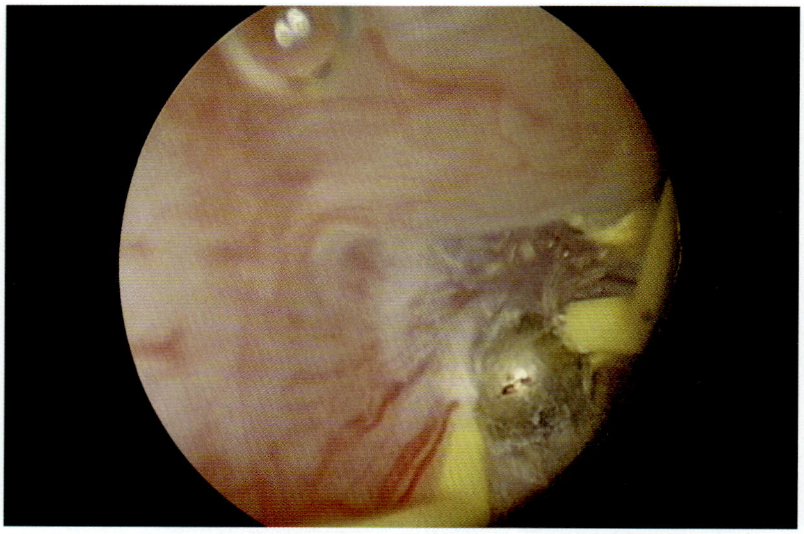

Fig. 4: Roller ball for ablation is used at cornua and fundus.

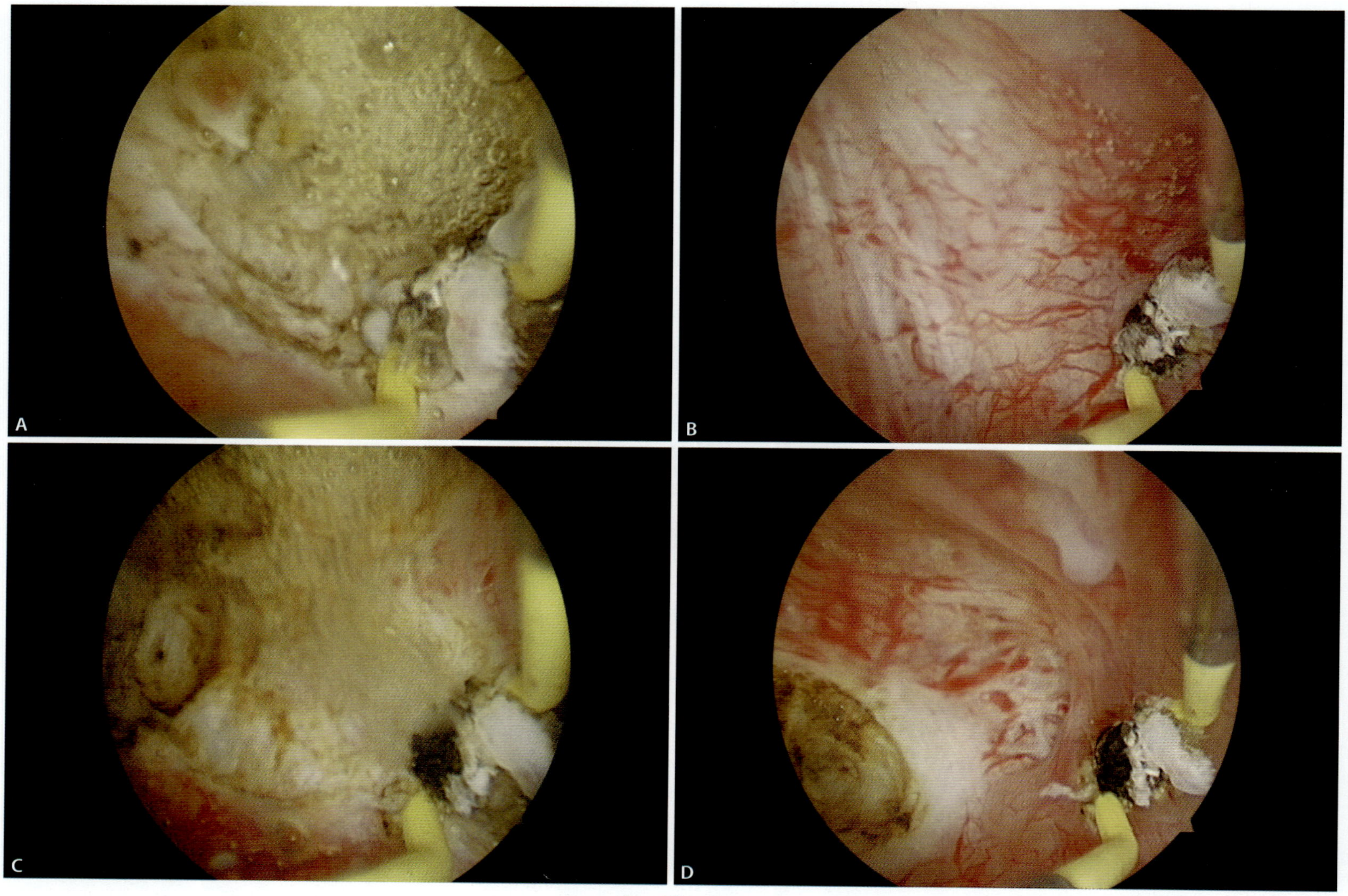

Figs. 5A to D

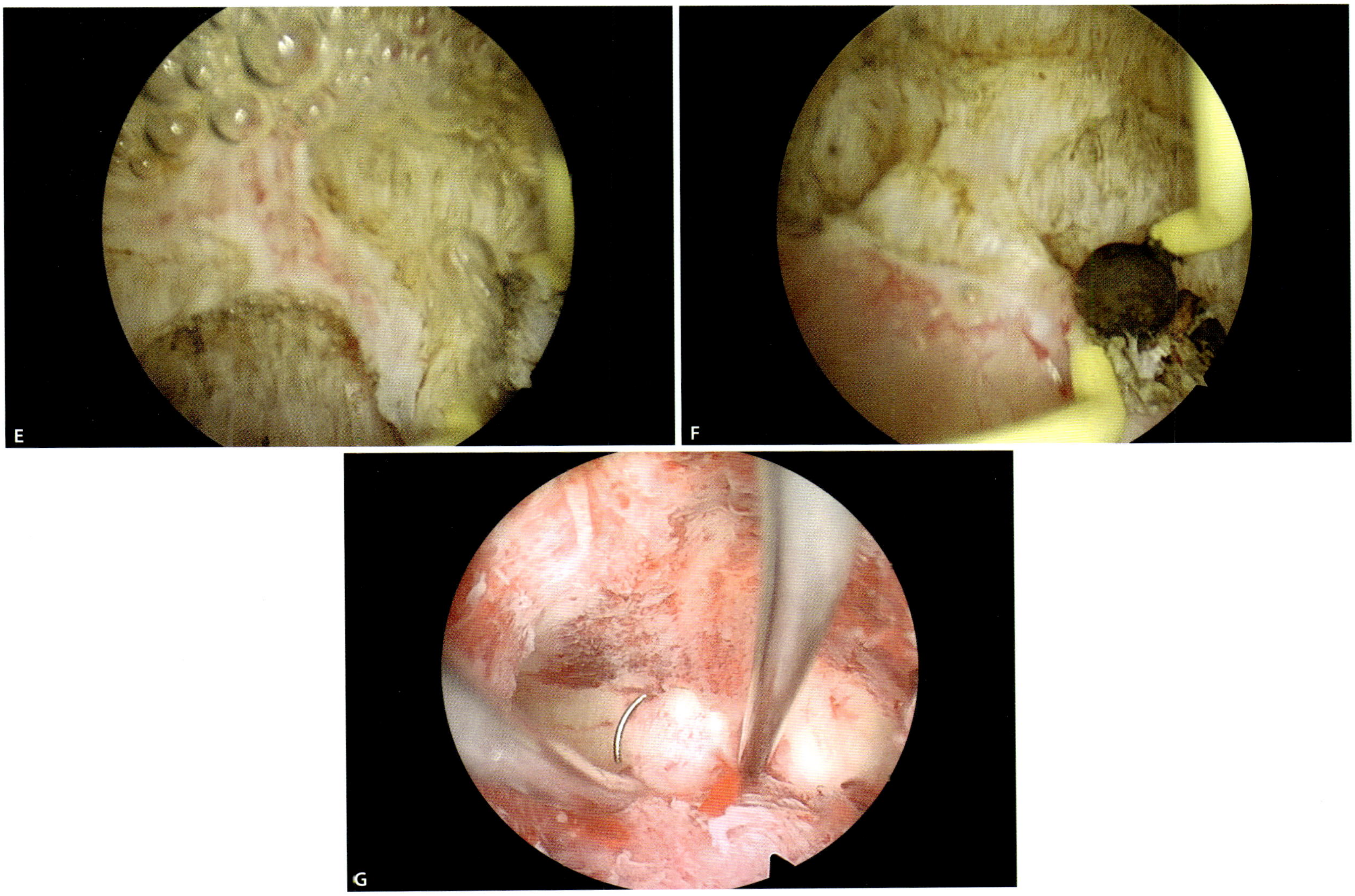

Figs. 5E to G

Figs. 5A to G: Transcervical resection of endometrium is done using a monopolar loop with glycine as a distention medium.

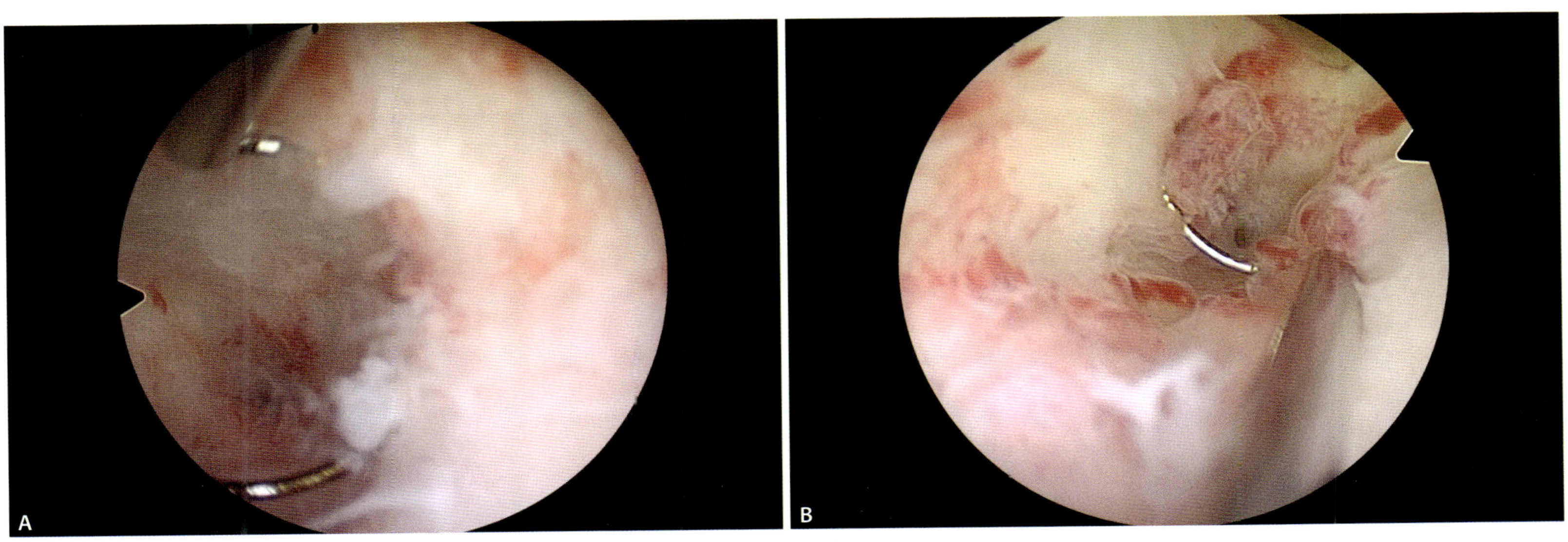

Figs. 6A and B

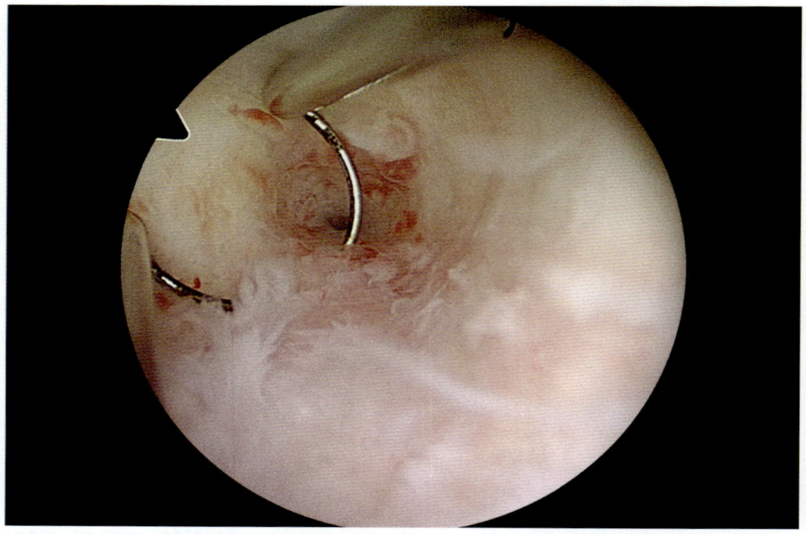

Fig. 6C

Figs. 6A to C: The resection is done as high as possible.

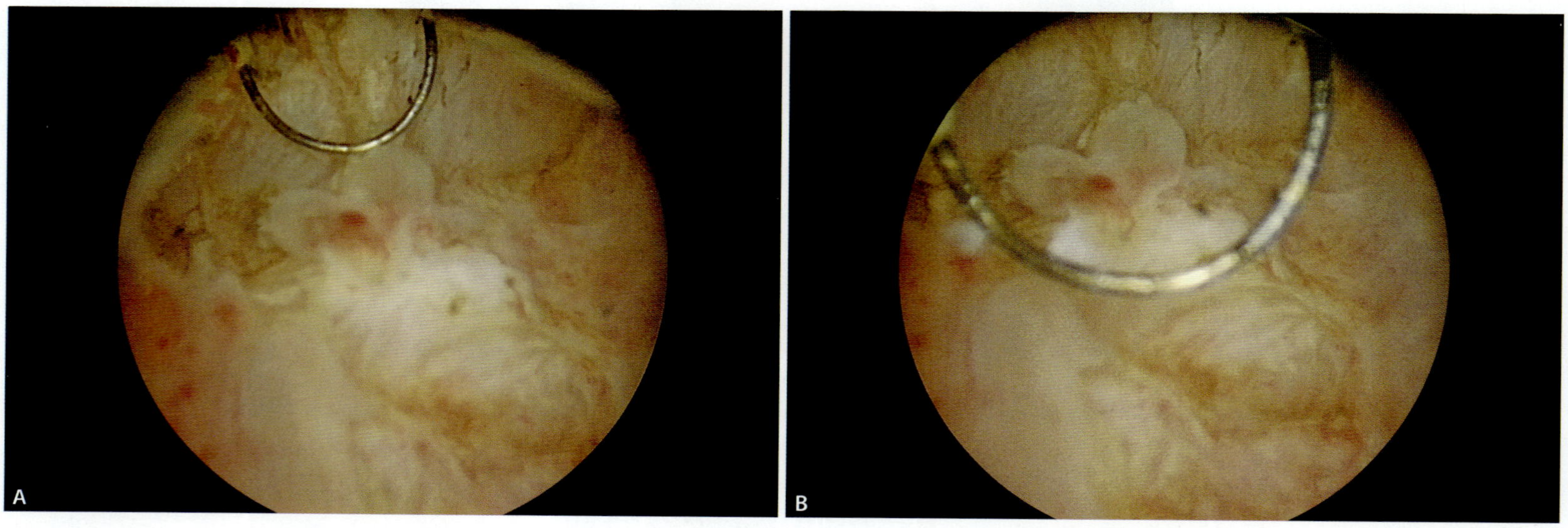

Figs. 7A and B: The resection should not be overdone else the bleeding from the myometrium will start.

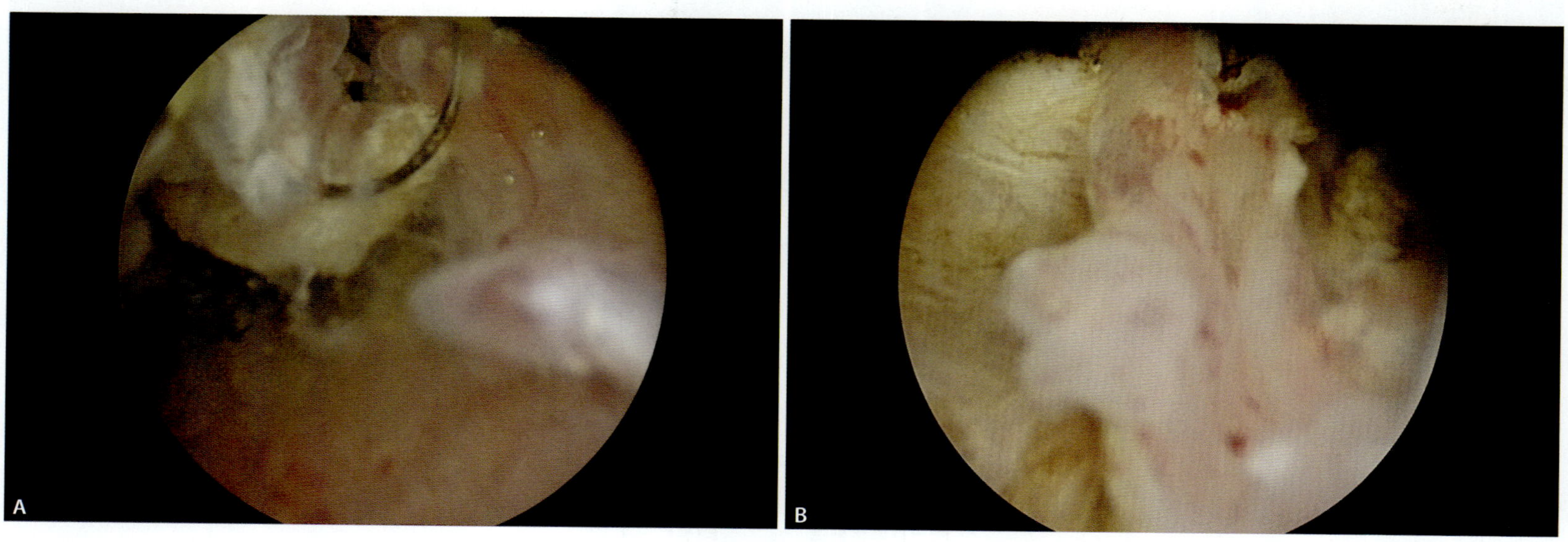

Figs. 8A and B

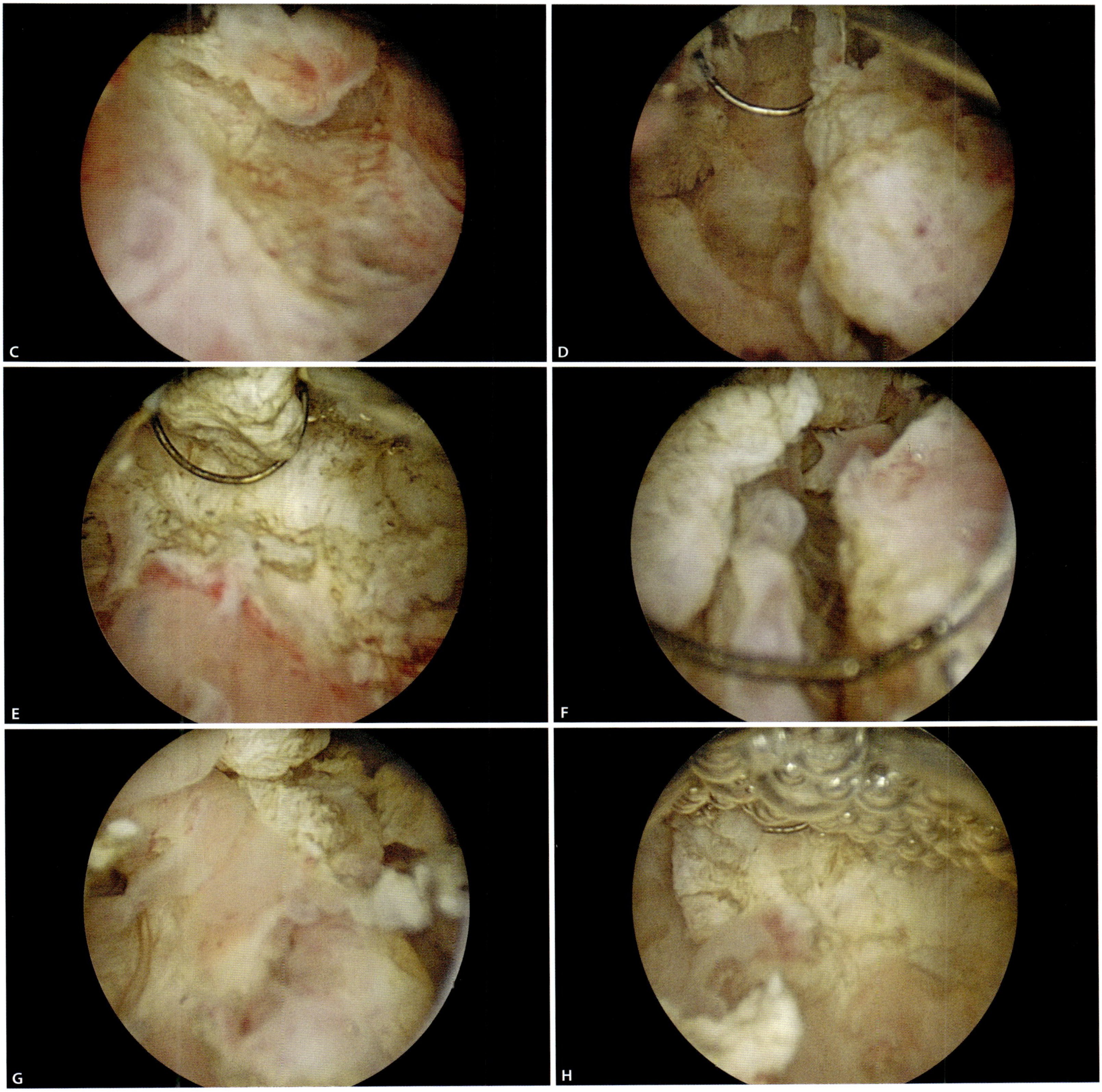

Figs. 8C to H

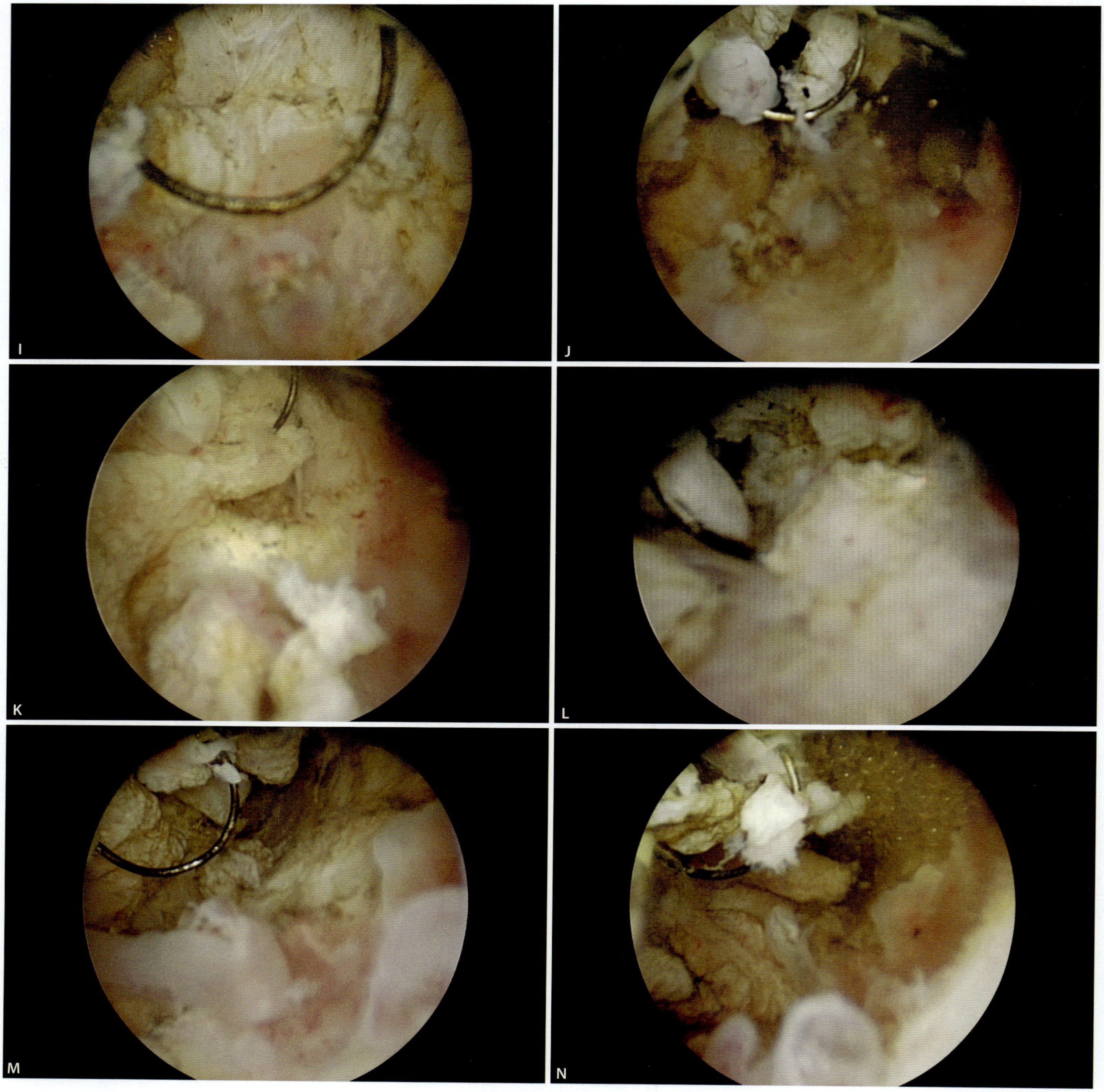

Figs. 8I to N

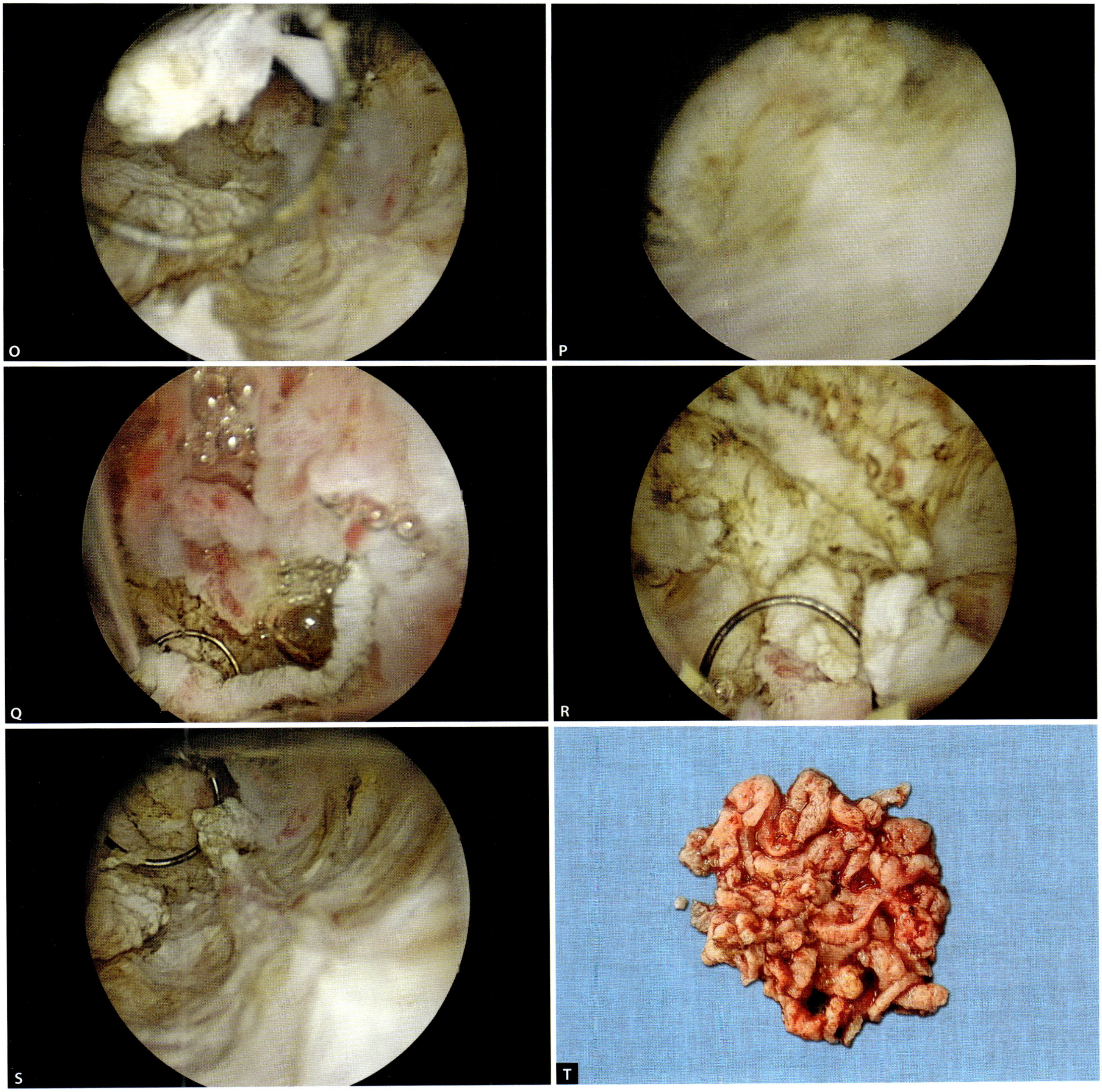

Figs. 8O to T

Figs. 8A to T: After resection, the tissues are retrieved through ovum forceps and sent for histopathology evaluation.

SUGGESTED READING

1. Chandel NP, Bhat VV, Bhat RS, et al. Treatment analysis of transcervical resection of the endometrium in heavy menstrual bleeding. A prospective multicentre therapeutic study in indian scenario. Indian J Obstetr Gynaecol. 2015;2(1):28-35.
2. Fergusson RJ, Lethaby A, Shepperd S, et al. Endometrial resection and ablation versus hysterectomy for heavy menstrual bleeding. Cochrane Database Syst Rev 2013;11:CD000329.
3. Scottish Hysteroscopy Audit Group. A Scottish audit of hysteroscopic surgery for menorrhagia: complications and follow up. Br J ObstetGynaecol. 1995;102:249-54.

Accompanying Video: Transcervical resection of the endometrium (TCRE).

CHAPTER

60

Foreign Body

Shubhanjali Sen, Minal Kumbhalwar, B Ramesh

HYSTEROSCOPIC REMOVAL OF MISPLACED MULTILOAD

Introduction

Lost intrauterine contraceptive device (IUCD) is not uncommon, followed by embedding into the uterine cavity, which cannot be retrieved with curved or straight artery.

Hence, hysteroscopic removal of the lost IUCD is effective treatment of choice.

The extracting instruments used are alligator grasper forceps, hysteroscopic scissors, and cutting loop or Collin's knife. Sometimes laparoscopic grasping forceps are also used.

Superficially embedded IUCD can be very well removed by inserting the grasping forceps through the operating channel and dislodging the IUCD **(Figs. 1 and 2)**.

When the IUCD is free floating with lost threads, partly embedded in the lower segment or completely embedded below the endometrium then a forceful pull is required for its removal. Then laparoscopic grasper is used. The cervix is dilated and laparoscopic grasper is introduced besides the operating channel of the hysteroscope. Cervix to be held with tenaculum or allis to prevent leakage of the distending medium.

Sometimes when the device is completely embedded in the myometrium then Collins knife is required by the experienced surgeons as it might perforate the uterine fundus. Procedure should take care of not damaging the myometrium hence torrential bleeding may start and then bipolar coagulation is required for achieving the hemostasis.

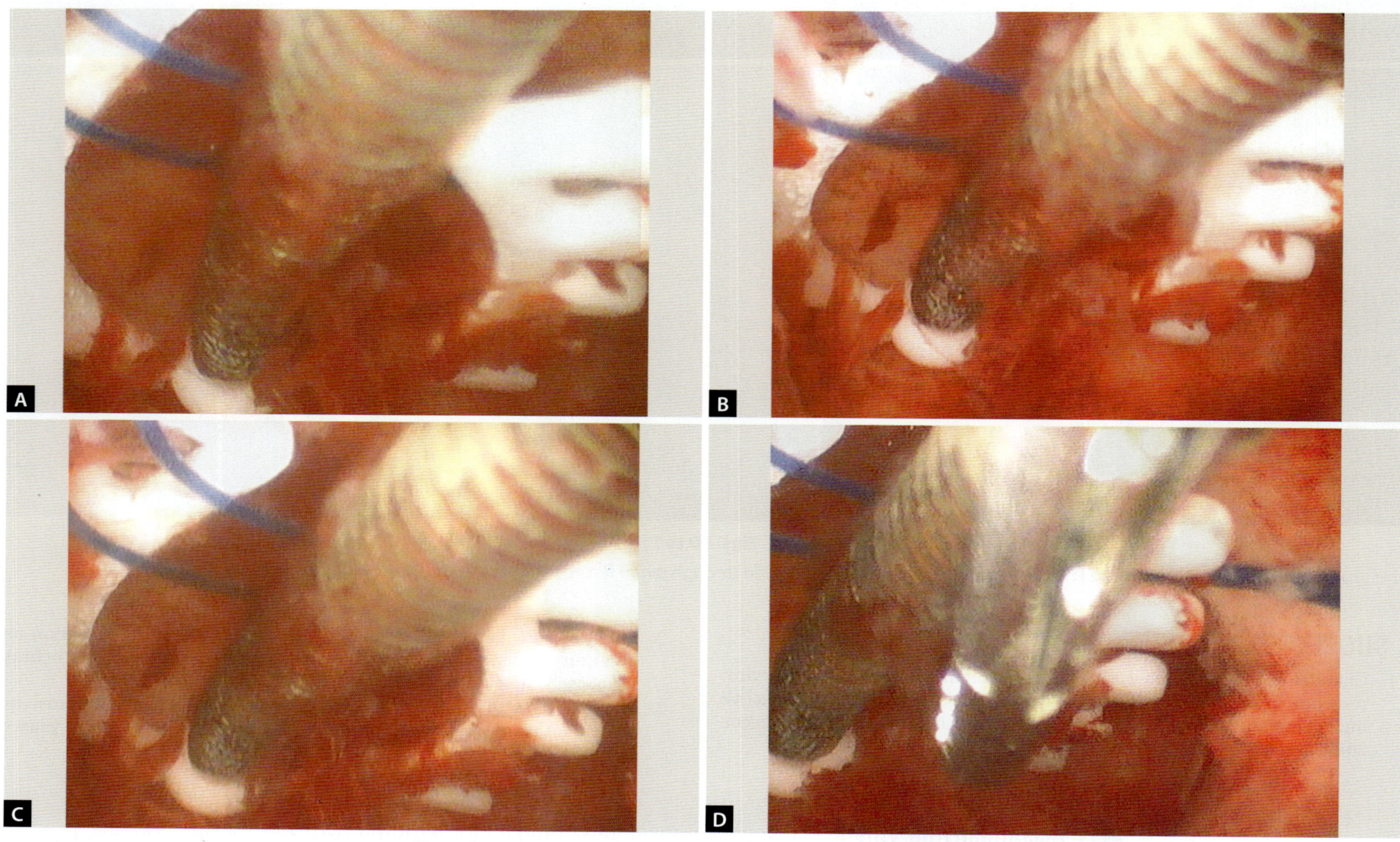

Figs. 1A to D: Hysteroscopic removal of misplaced multiload copper-T.

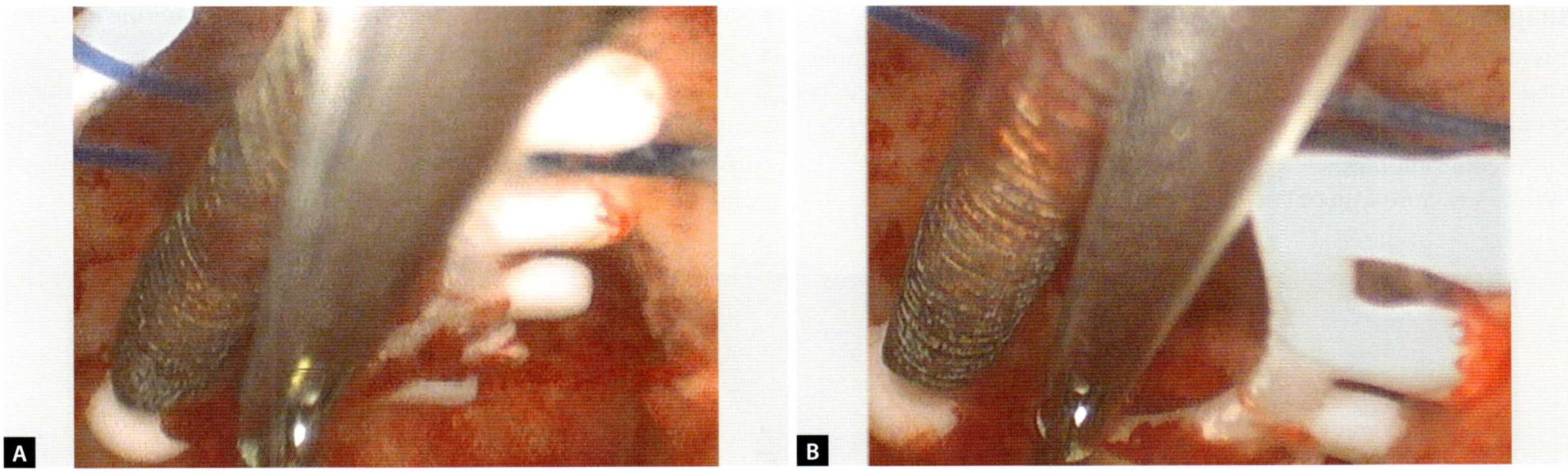

Figs. 2A and B: Using a toothed grasper multiload removed.

Complications

- Nonextraction of the embedded IUCD—ask for an experienced surgeon.
- Check for the IUCD, whether it has perforated the uterus—perform laparoscopy.

Hence, proper planning of the preoperative location of the Cu-T is very important. Keep the ultrasound and laparoscopy handy.

HYSTEROSCOPY DONE FOR RETAINED PRODUCTS OF CONCEPTION

Retained products of conception (RPOC) following the spontaneous abortion, induced abortion, or delivery are common. It leads to abnormal uterine bleeding, abdominal pain, and amenorrhea with fever. Bleeding with infection and fever may be presenting complained.

Diagnosis is done with ultrasonography using a high velocity low-resistance flow with color Doppler.

Treatment

26 Fr cold loop of resectoscope without using any current. Electrical current is only used when bleeding has been encountered or it is a difficult resection **(Figs. 3A and B)**.

The advantage of performing the hysteroscopy during removal of RPOCs is the ability to view the endometrial cavity and repair any abnormality.

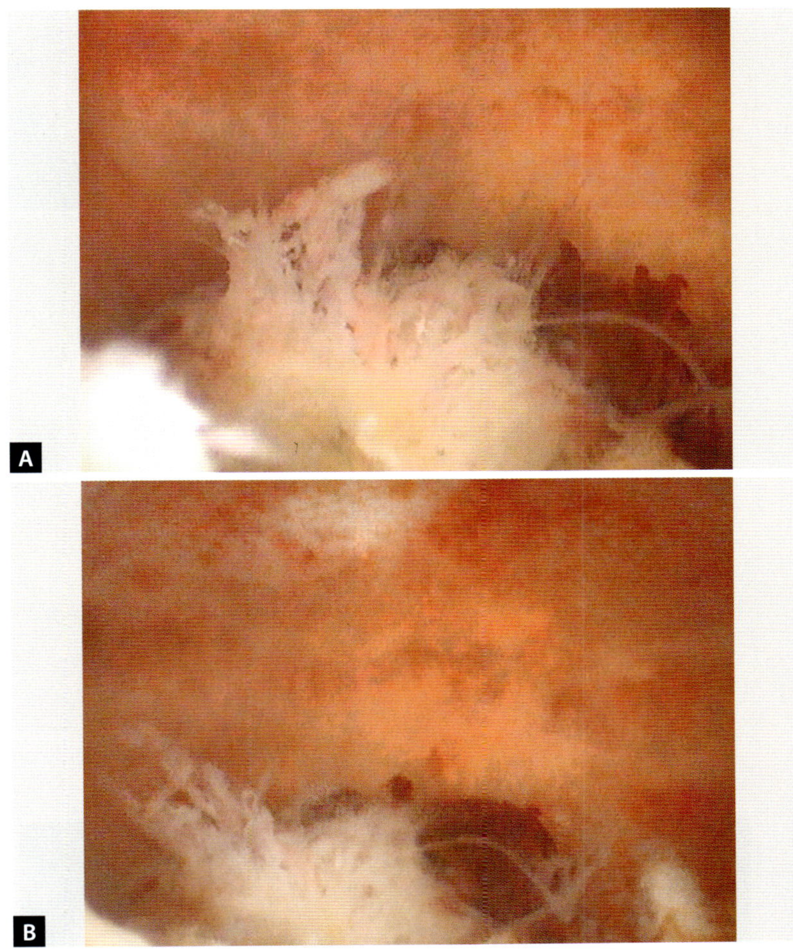

Figs. 3A and B: Hysteroscopy done for retained products of conception.

HYSTEROSCOPIC RETRIEVAL OF OSSEOUS MATERIAL

Introduction

Retained intrauterine fetal bones are one of the factors for infertility and chronic endometritis. It is an uncommon clinical entity with incidence of 0.3 per 10,000 women. There is an increase in the endometrial prostaglandin factor F2 alpha, which prevents the embryo implantation to happen. Prolonged secondary infertility is one of the symptoms, which leads us to the diagnosis.

The suggested theories can be metaplastic transformation of the endometrial stromal cells and implantation of the fetal tissues after abortion.

The retained fragments are an ideal substrate for the bacterial colonization and spread to tubes and cavity thus destroying the functional integrity of the uterine cavity and also potent cause of infertility.

Retained fetal bones are a complication of induced abortion, spontaneous abortion, intrauterine fetal death, and missed abortions.

Symptoms

- Abnormal uterine bleeding
- Dysmenorrhea
- Vaginal discharge
- Pelvic pain
- Acute pelvic pain with purulent vaginal discharge
- Secondary infertility.

Management

Transvaginal ultrasound is the first line of diagnosis modality. Simple ultrasound-based approach to investigate the infertile patient is very effective in making the diagnosis.

Hysteroscopic findings:

- White structure with trabeculated pattern
- White appearing tubular structure embedded in uterine fundus
- Solid bony spicules seen in endometrial cavity.

Hysteroscopy is the successful modality for the removal of the bony fragments, with the help of wire loop resectoscope without current and the fragments are needed to be sent for histopathological evaluation **(Figs. 4 to 9)**.

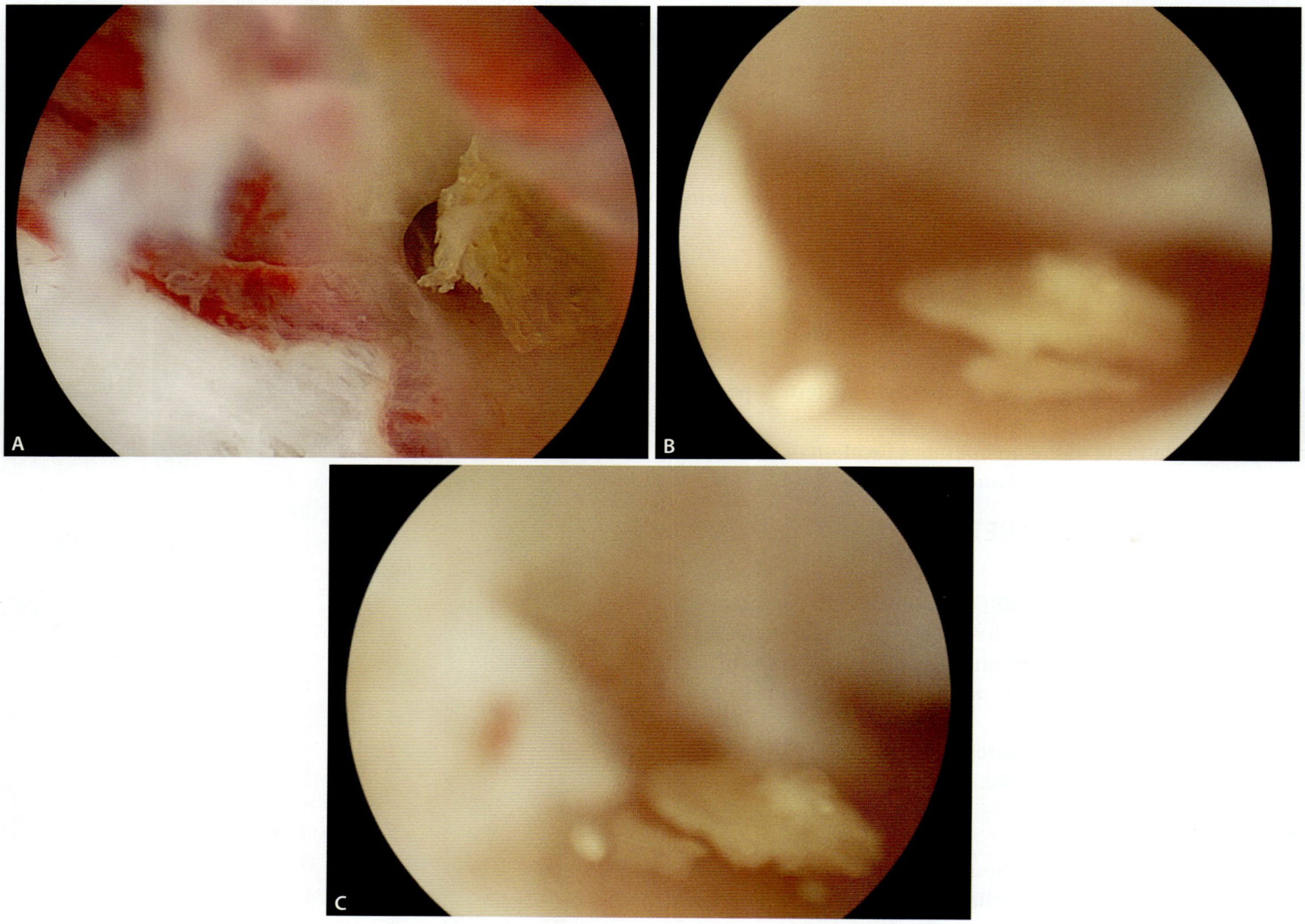

Figs. 4A to C: Hysteroscopic retrieval of osseous material.

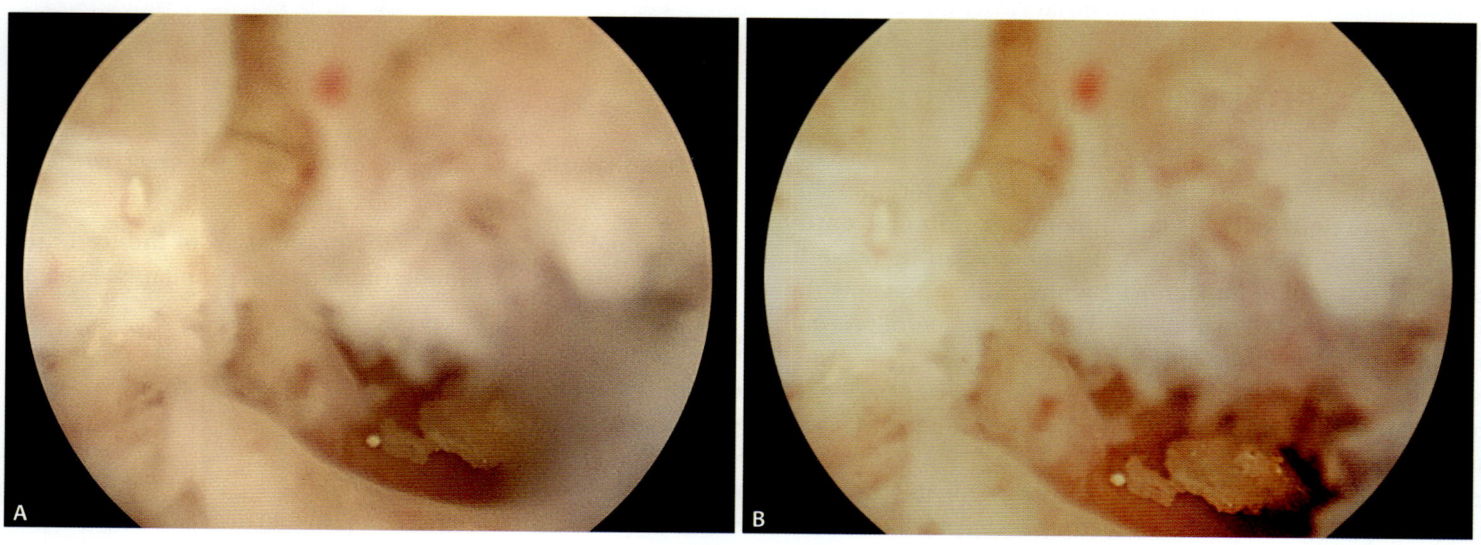

Figs. 5A and B

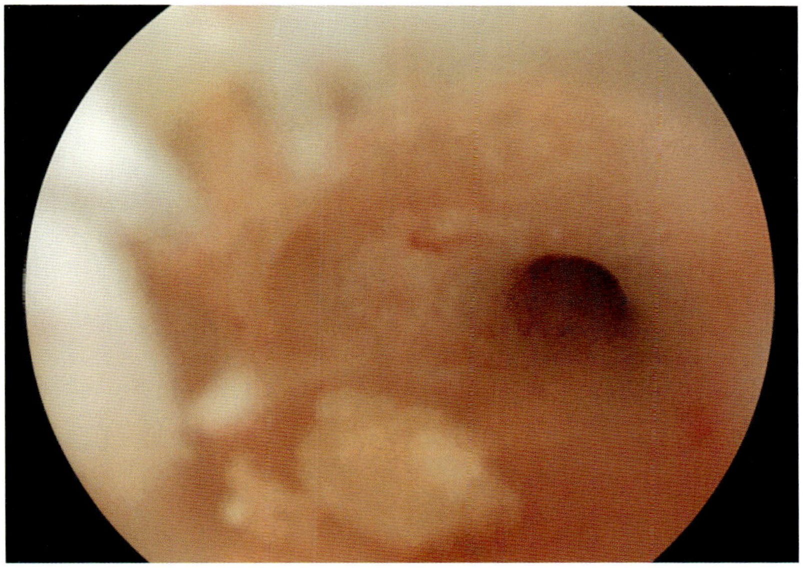

Fig. 5C

Figs. 5A to C: Bits of bone present in the uterine cavity.

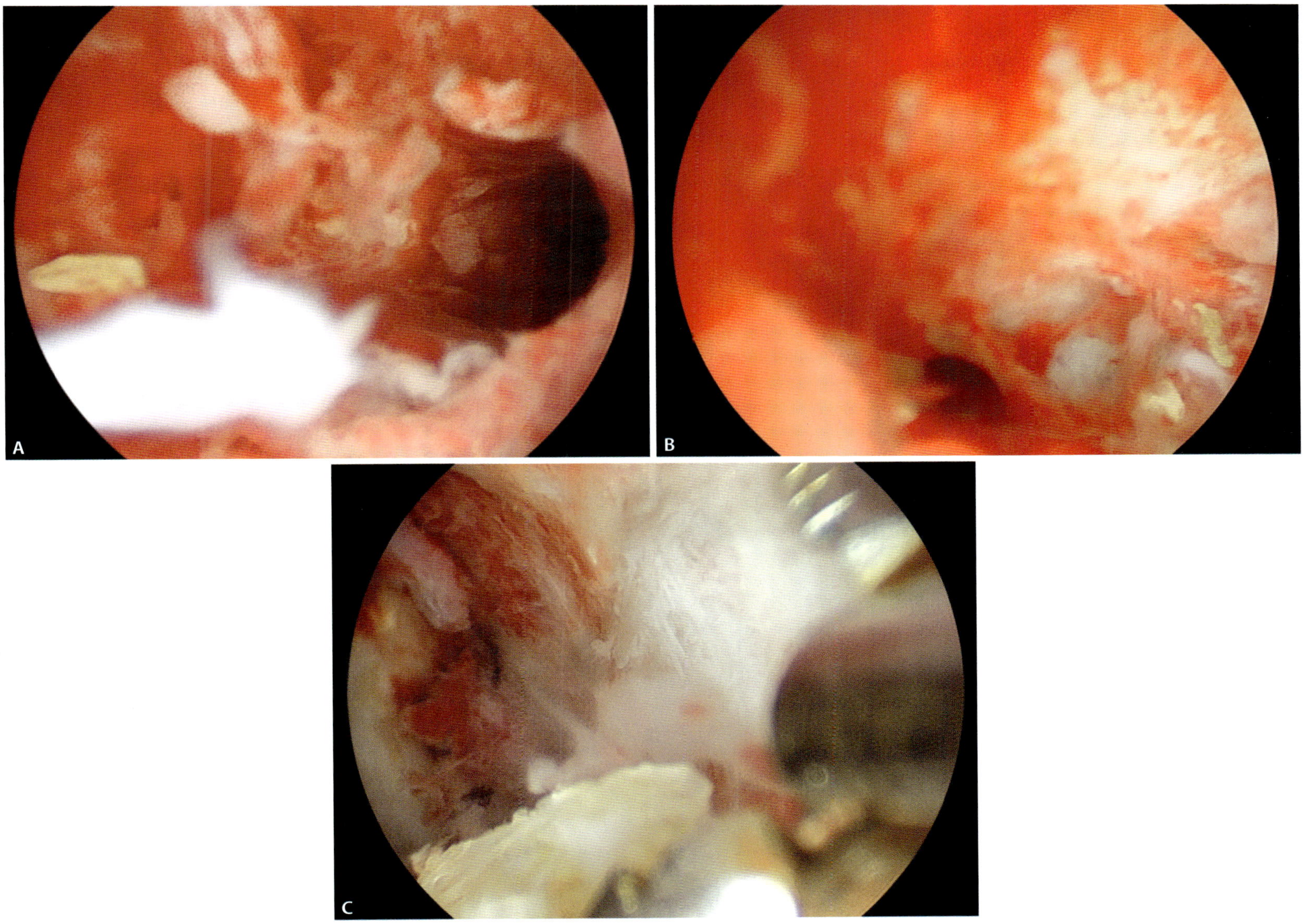

Figs. 6A to C: Bits of bone found near the ostia.

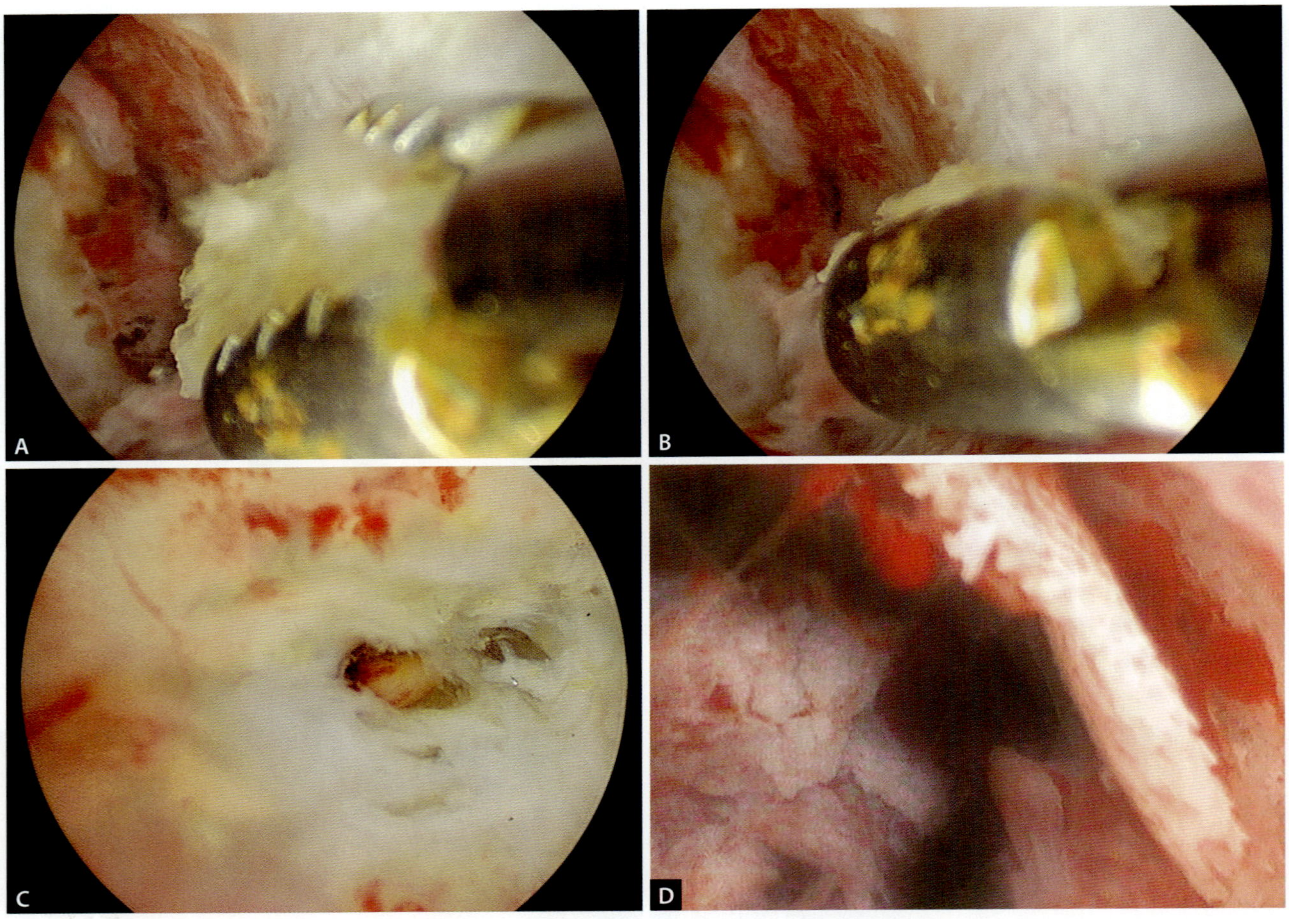

Figs. 7A to D: Bones removed with the help of toothed grasper.

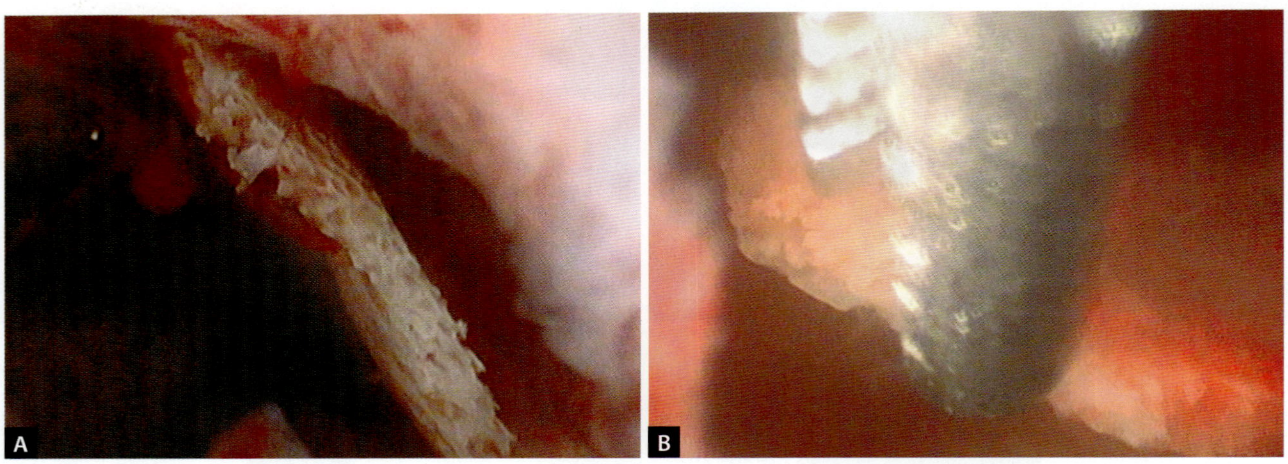

Figs. 8A and B: Old bones present in the endometrial cavity causing infertility to the patient.

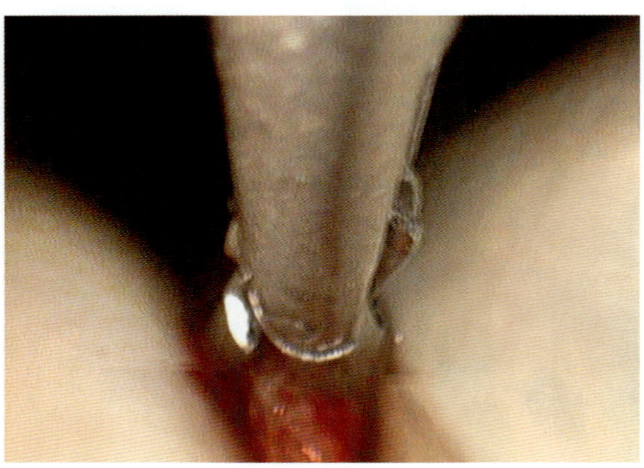

Fig. 9: Removed with the help of toothed grasper.

Transcervical resection of the foreign body (TCRF) is the safe and efficient modality. Simultaneous sonographic visualization of the uterine cavity enhances the confidence of the operating surgeon.

A high spontaneous pregnancy rate may be expected after the removal of the fragments.

CHAPTER

61

Troubleshooting in Hysteroscopy

Shubhanjali Sen, Minal Kumbhalwar, B Ramesh

INTRODUCTION

Hysteroscopy is a combination of coordinated specific actions without any aid or assistance, from managing scope to operating the instruments and making a decision in ultraspeed needs a preprogrammed brain knowledge and experience to mainly troubleshoot your problems in hysteroscopic surgeries.

GENERAL CONSIDERATION TO BE KEPT IN MIND (FIGS. 1 TO 3)

- *Correct position:*
    - Buttocks at the edge of the operating table allowing for the hand to move upward and downward
    - Avoid pressure on prone areas
    - Avoid leaning on the thigh of the patient
- Eyes should always be on screen
- Avoid multiple entries
- Vaginoscopy can be done as it is atraumatic to cervix.

CERVICAL DILATATION

Three landmarks: External cervical orifice, internal cervical orifice, and two tubal ostia.

External cervical os problems: Cervical stenosis, nulliparous external cervical ostium (ECO), and congenital anomaly.

Cervical canal: Adhesions in cervical canal, pathology in cervical canal, congenital anomaly [Diethylstilbestrol (DES) exposure in utero causes T shape uterine anomaly and complete septum].

Internal cervical orifice: Adhesions in internal os, and acutely anteverted and acutely retroverted uterus.

Management of Cervical Stenosis (Figs. 6 to 8)

- Misoprostol 200–400 µg is given one night before vaginally or orally.
- In severe stenosis, misoprostol can be given 2 days prior at bedtime.
- Mechanical dilators should not be used in anticipation of the false passage and cervical laceration.
- *Hysteroscopy:* Using a 2.9 mm hysteroscope and 5 Fr semirigid mechanical instrument, resection of fibrous tissue responsible for stenosis is done. The fibrous ring may be cut at two to three places.
- Nulliparous os will be benefited with modified Bettocchi 1.9 mm hysteroscopy, which does not need any cervical priming.
- If there is congenital vaginal septum, then a good way is to retract the septum nicely to expose the os.
- Laminaria tent can also be used.
- *Mild adhesions:* Under vision, using 5 Fr mechanical scissors can be used for dissection.
- *Moderate and severe adhesions:* Under hysteroscopic vision, using 5 Fr scissors or bipolar electrode.
- *Endocervical polyp:* Base of the polyp identified and transected under vision.

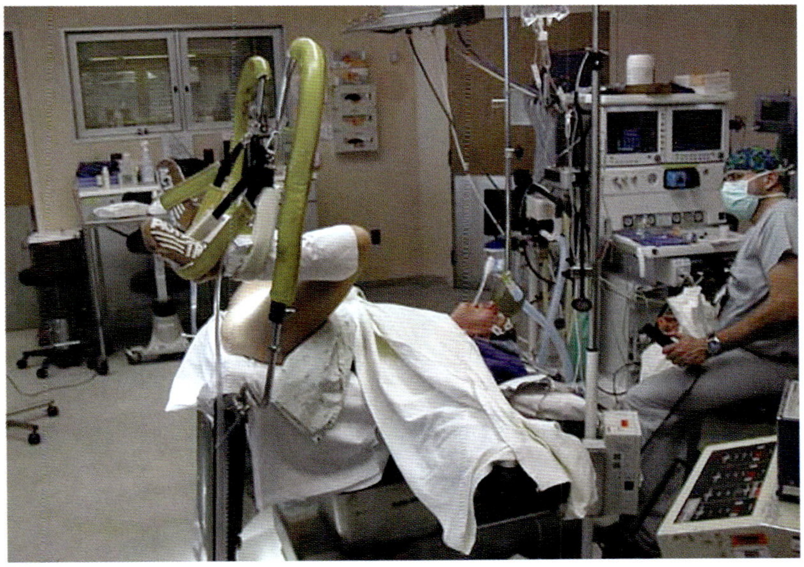

Fig. 1: Operation theater setup.

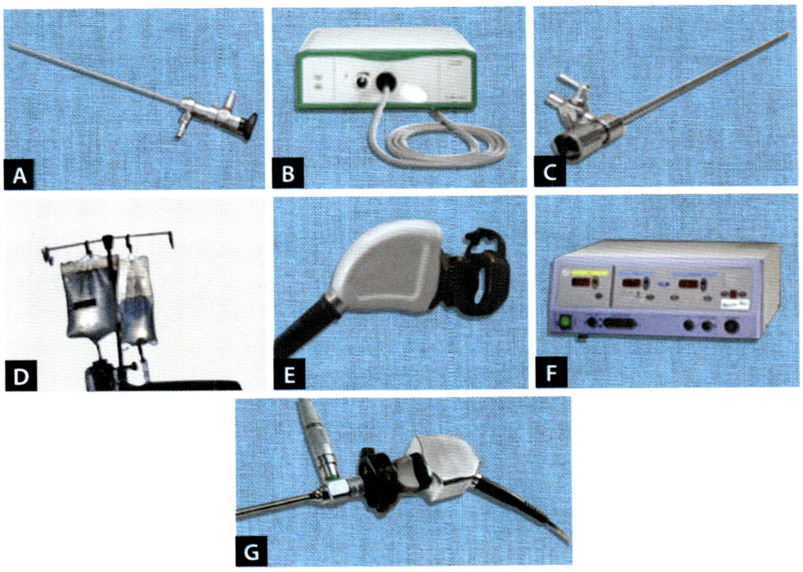

Figs. 2A to G: Assembling the instruments for operative hysteroscopy.

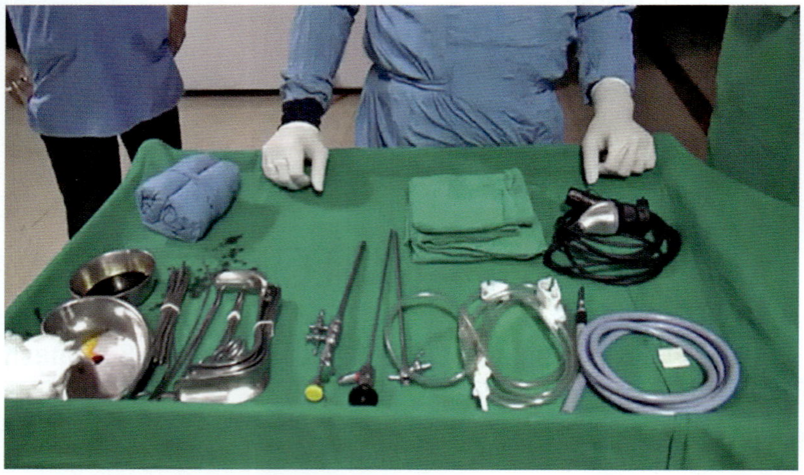

Fig. 3: OT table arrangement for hysteroscopic instruments.

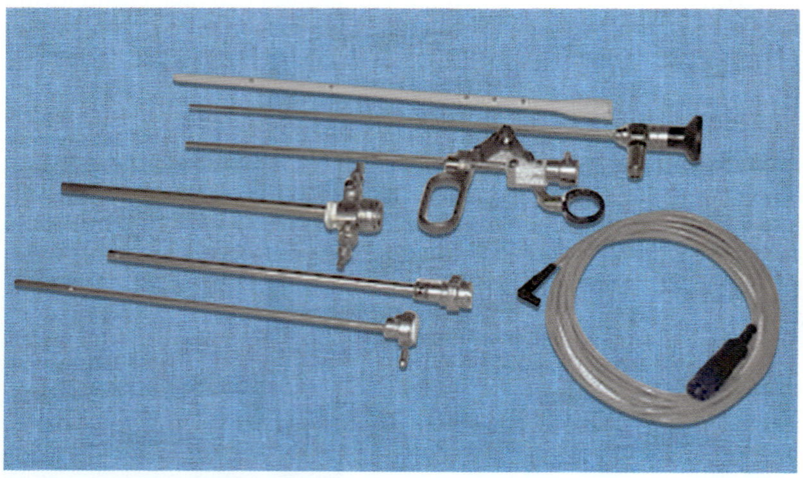

Fig. 4: Resectoscope parts prior to assemble.

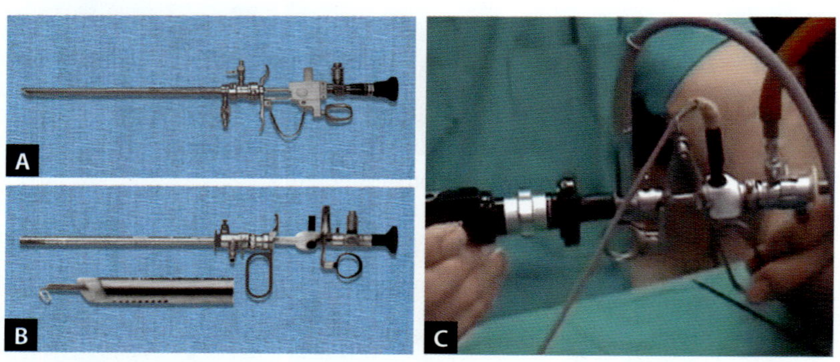

Figs. 5A to C: Assembly of resectoscope with light source, irrigation and electrode.

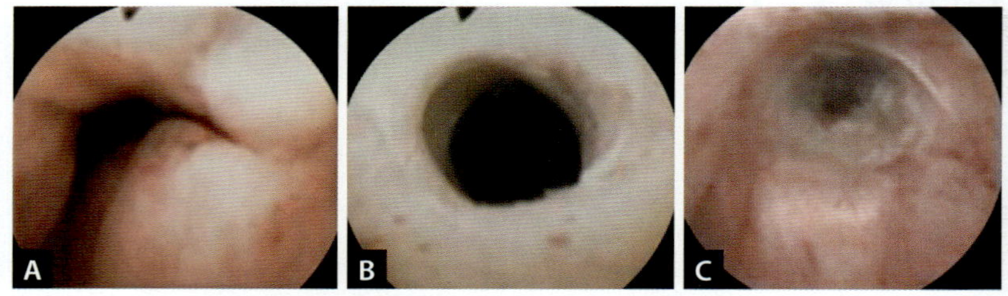

Figs. 6A to C: Stepwise cervical dilatation.

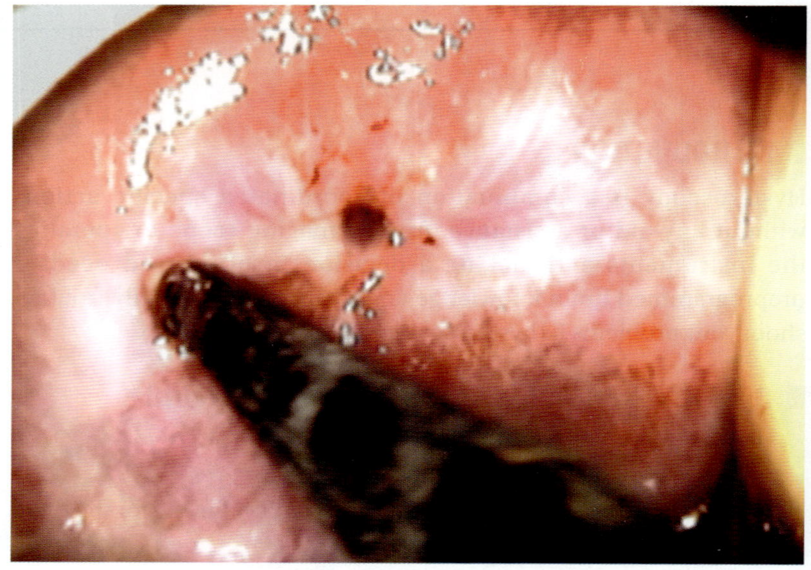

Fig. 7: Stenotic cervical os.

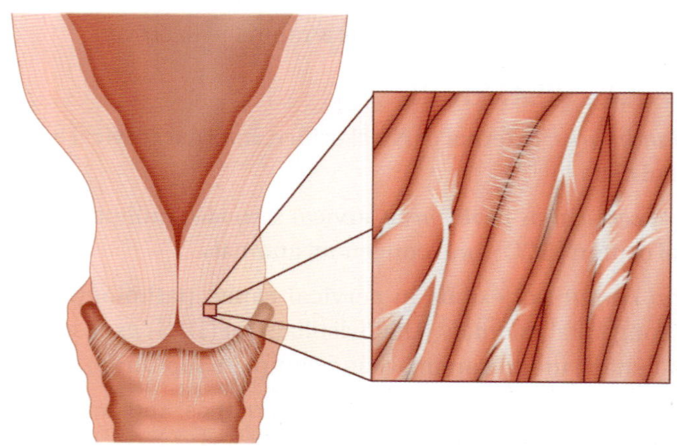

Fig. 8: Muscle fiber arrangement at cervical region.

Acutely anteverted and anteflexed uterus: The os should be in vision and having the hand in downward position in such a way that the camera is below the level of the patient and the scope is directed upward **(Figs. 9 to 11)**.

Retroverted uterus: Keeping the os under the vision, the camera is above the level of the patient and the scope is directed downward.

Lacrimal probes can be used for dilatation in severe stenosis.

Concurrent use of the abdominal ultrasound may help for the better introduction of the dilator preventing the formation of the false passage.

FALSE PASSAGE (FIGS. 13 AND 14)

- To avoid the formation of the false passage, the assembling and the understanding of the direction of the instrument is very important.
- In a 30° telescope, the light cable should be facing downward.
- Keep the os opening in the lower half of the image over the screen.
- Doing this will prevent the hysteroscope to abut into the wall of the cervix and prevent false passage, failed entry, and cervical and uterine perforation.
- *Caution:* Do not redilate the cervix with dilator once the false passage is created as it will invariably lead to uterine perforation.

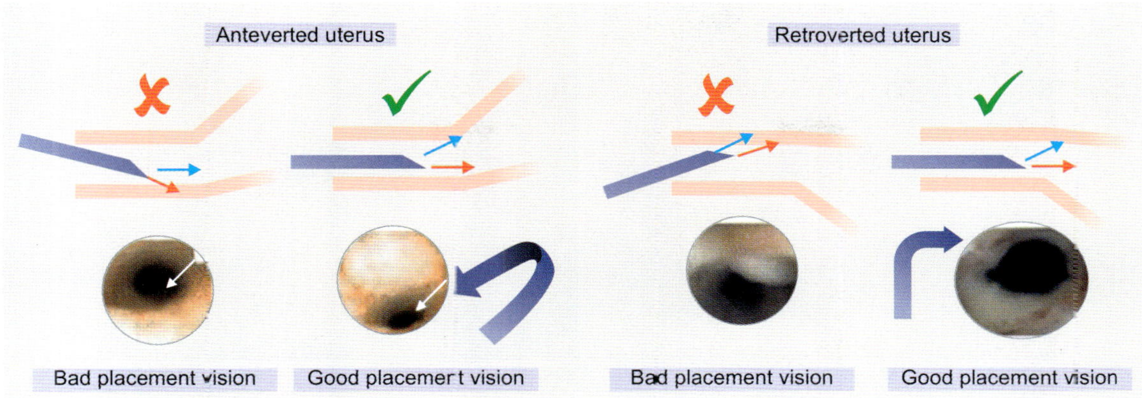

Fig. 9: Demonstration of how to position 30° hysteroscope as per uterine position and the internal cervical os as visualized through scope.

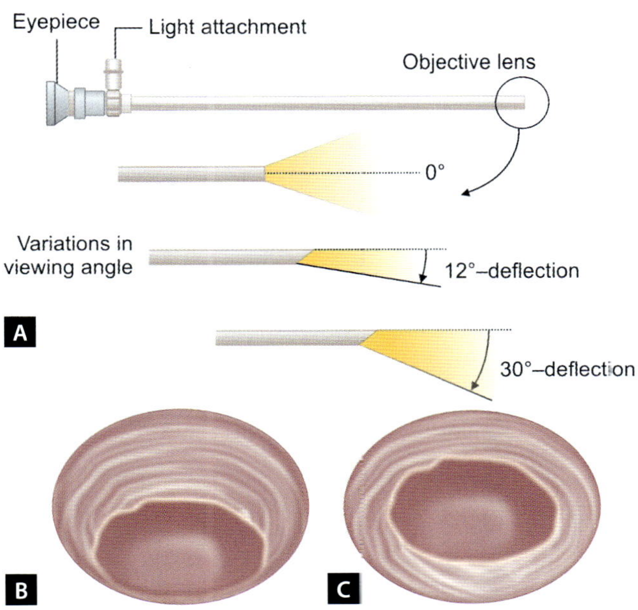

Figs. 10A to C: Different variation in viewing angle.

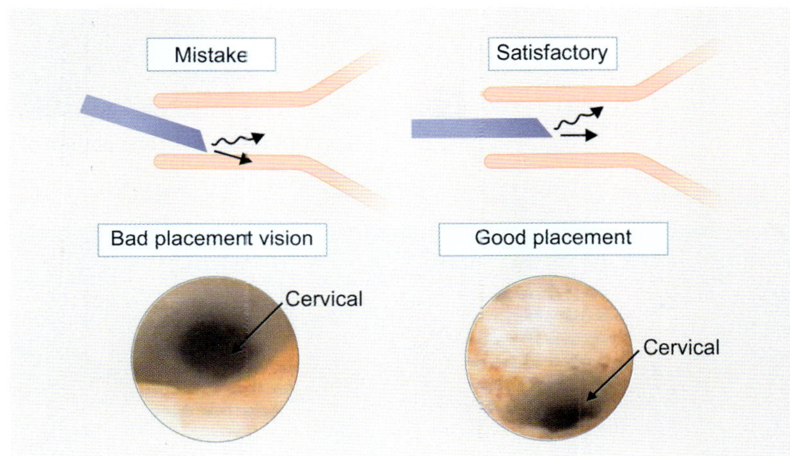

Fig. 11: Defective vision in improper placement of hysteroscope.

- *Causes:* Stenotic cervix, nulliparous cervix, menopausal cervix, and previous surgeries—cervical biopsy, cone biopsy, cryosurgery, acute anteflexion or retroflexion, and prior use of GnRH (gonadotropin-releasing hormone) agonist.

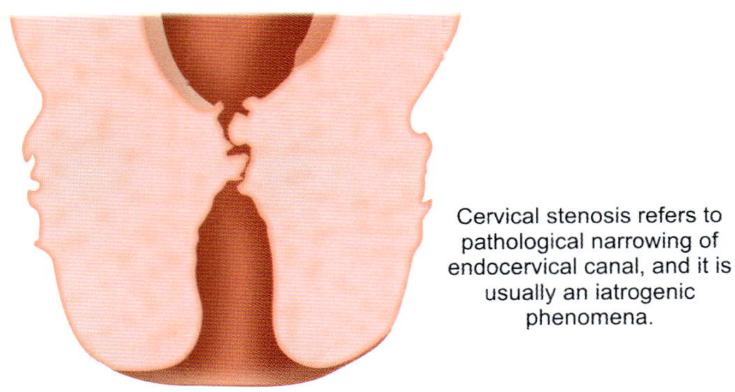

Fig. 12: Cervical stenosis.

Difficulty in Visualizing Cervix

- It happens in menopausal women and prior cervical amputation.
- In such cases, vaginoscopic approach should be adapted for the better visualization of the cervix.
- Using a modified Bettocchi 1.9 mm or standard Bettocchi 2.9 mm scope helps in gradual stretch of the cervix.

Vision and Inadequate Distention

- Adequately dilate the cervix to facilitate overflow.
- Use of continuous flow sheath promoting the lavage of the blood and debris.
- Use of the proper distending media.
- Proper use of the length, diameter, and patency of inflow tubing.
- Adequate pressure infusion device should be used:
    - Using a hysteromat
    - Raising the height of the media bag

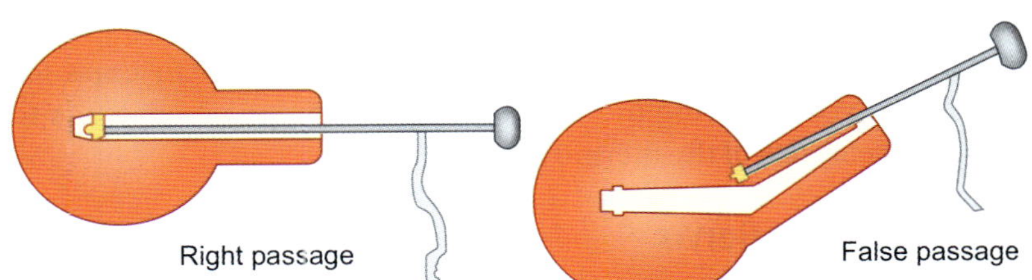

Fig. 13: High chances of false passage depending on version of uterus.

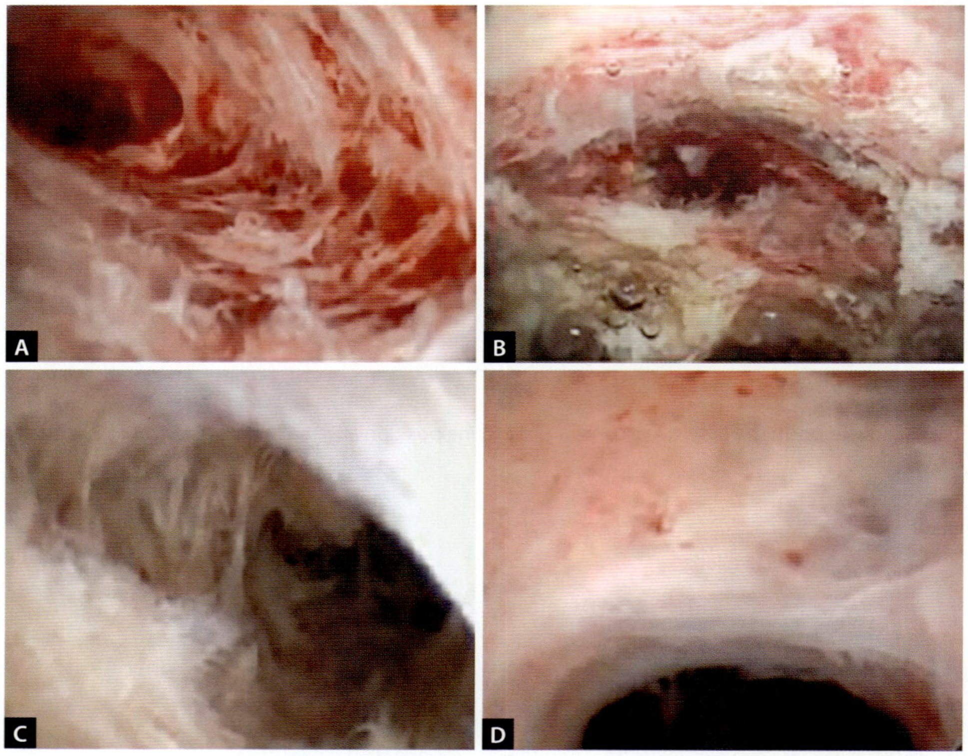

Figs. 14A to D: Criss-cross pattern of the fibers is suggestive of the false passage.

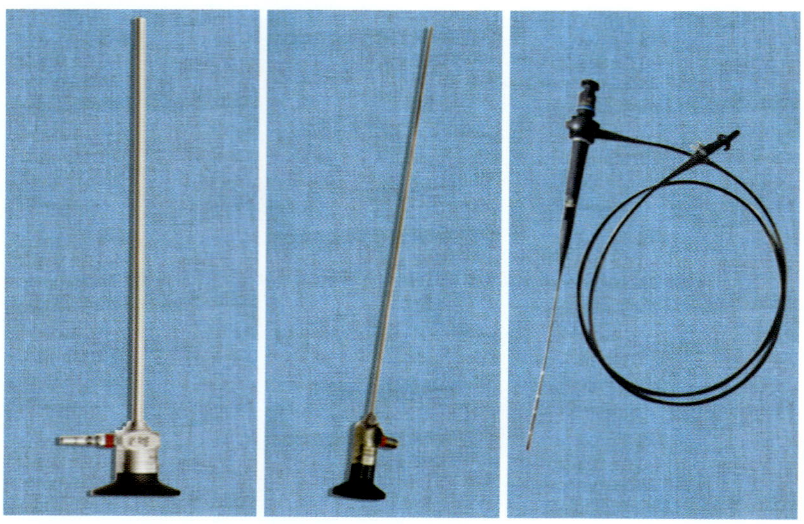

Fig. 15: Hysteroscope.

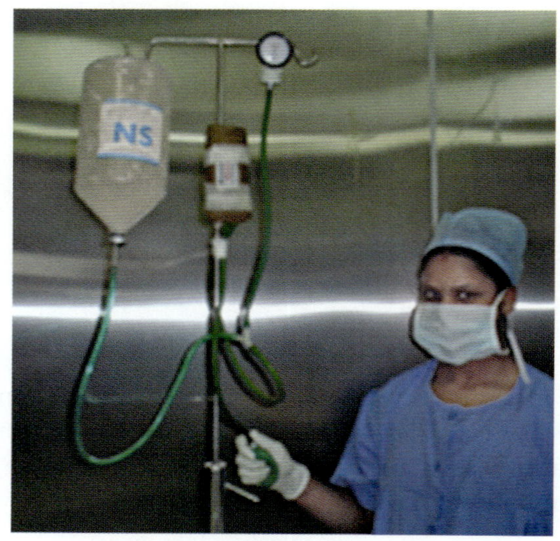

Fig. 16: Irrigation pressure pump.

- Lowering the patient table
- Closing the outflow part
- By applying the tenaculum on either side of an over dilated leaky cervix
- Increasing the pressure of infusion device.

Resection Bleeding/Blocking due to Tissues

Continuous inflow-outflow sheath is used with resectoscope for the proper vision during the operative hysteroscopy which leads to periodic clearance of the uterine cavity.

Leaking around Cervix

If the cervix is overdilated with the dilator, then the cervix will be leaking and the proper visualization of the uterine cavity is not possible.

To prevent this, dilatation should not exceed Hegar's dilator no. 7 to 8.

If the leaking of the cervix occurs, then 1–2 Allis forceps are applied around the cervix.

Uterine Perforation (Figs. 17A to C)

- Occurs when adhesiolysis or any surgical intervention is carried out on the lateral wall or uterine fundus.
- *Two types of perforation:*
  1. *Cold perforation:* Dilator, hysteroscope, and scissors
  2. *Thermal perforation:* Electrosurgical current.
- *Diagnosed:* Sudden loss of the distention despite proper distention medium pressure and flow, intestinal loops/bowel are noted.

Prevention of Glycine Toxicity

- Patient absorbs 20 mL/min of glycine during resection.
- It should not be prolonged for >60 minutes.
- *500 mL deficit:* First alarm
- *750 mL deficit:* Second alarm
    - 20–40 mg Lasix at deficit of 750 mL
    - *Reevaluate serum Na level:*
        - *1.2 L deficit:* Stop surgery preferably
        - *1.5 L deficit:* Never proceed beyond this point.

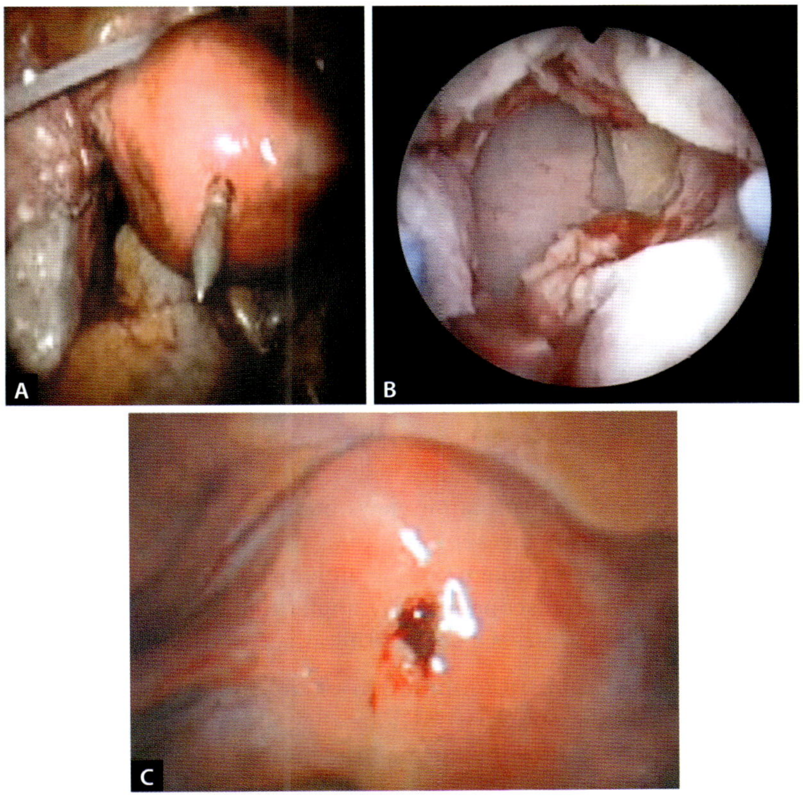

Figs. 17A to C: Perforation site.

- While using bipolar device, fluid deficit permissible is up to 2 L beyond which overload related problems may occur
- Meticulous monitoring of fluid inflow and outflow is the single most important step
- Electronic inflow and outflow monitoring system
- Collection of outflow fluid in a measuring container/suction bottle/commercially available plastic pouch such as drapes.

Intravasation

Contributory factors:

- Length of the surgery
- Partial perforation and false passage, and cervical tears or injury
- Surgery leading to the entry of the myometrium opening larger vascular channel such as myoma resection or division.

Prevention:

- Limit height of the distention bag to 1 m above the patient table
- Use of the electronic machine which can calibrate the flow rate and intrauterine pressure
- Monitoring of input and output of fluid and calculation of the fluid deficit 500–1,000 mL.

Symptomatic Hyponatremia

- Early detection and rapid initiation of treatment
- Early diuresis with furosemide
- Monitoring of input, output, and electrolytes
- Restrict fluid intake
- Supplement oxygen
- Correct sodium levels (<120 mmol/L critical care).

Water Intoxication

- *Excess water absorption:*
    - Hyponatremia
    - Hypokalemia
    - Hypo-osmolality

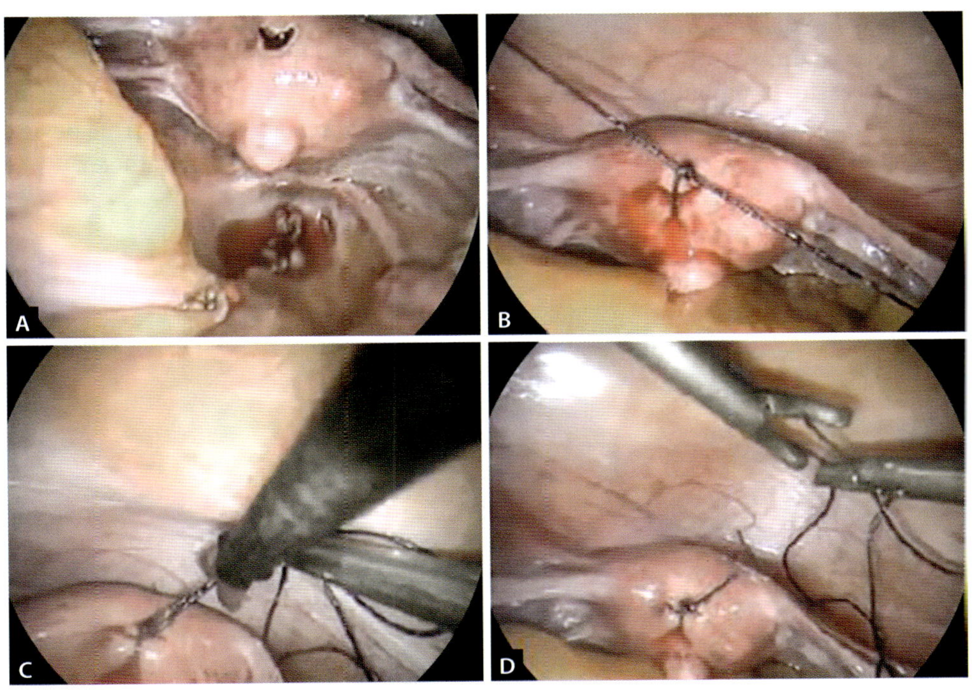

Figs. 18A to D: Suturing of perforation during hysteroscopy.

- Cerebral edema
- Increased ICT
- Cardiac overload.
- *Left heart failure:*
  - Tachypnea
  - Wheezing
  - Frothy edema
  - Arterial hypertension
  - Raised venous pressure
  - Bradycardia
  - Pulmonary edema.

GUIDELINES TO REDUCE COMPLICATIONS WHILE USING ELECTROSURGERY

- Foot pedal to be placed in direct control of the surgeon.
- Dispersive electrode should be securely placed on the thigh. The location should not be scarred or unhealthy.
- *For prevention of the accidental burns:*
  - Advancement of the activated electrode should be under vision
  - The cautery should be checked beforehand
  - Use of electrodes with damaged insulation should be checked
  - Metal speculum should be avoided
- Low-voltage cutting current should be used to avoid current diversion complication.
- Cervix should not be overdilated else it loses the contact between the cervix and sheath leading to current dispersive effect.
- Aggressive increase in power settings should be avoided in case of absence of tissue effect.

PRACTICAL TIPS

- Reducing the size and the diameter of hysteroscope has led to an ambulatory procedure.
- The constant average uterine distention should be <70 mm Hg so that the risk of the passage of the fluid into the abdominal cavity is reduced, thereby making the procedure safe.
- *Vaginoscopic approach:* No touch technique or an atraumatic insertion helps in reducing the pain and discomfort to the patient.
- In virgins or patients with severe vaginal atrophy or stenosis, vaginoscopic approach is very successful in obtaining the desired procedure.
- The pressure to be kept is 30–40 mm Hg.

SPECIAL CONSIDERATIONS

- *Endometrial and endocervical polyps:* 5 Fr scissors used or if the base of the polyp is larger with vascularity, then loop resection is safer.
- *Submucous fibroid:*
  - Difficulty lies in the plane of resection
  - To have a synchronized combined movement of the entire scope and the working element simultaneously.
- *Transcervical resection of the endometrium (TCRE):* The starting point should be a transverse line at the level of the fundus, stop at the level of the white basal layer and shift to the pink endometrial strip until white uterine cavity in not seen. Roller ball electrode should be used to prevent perforation.
  - Two to three layers of resection to be done anteriorly and posteriorly
  - Lateral wall is thin—single superficial layer resection to be done
  - Cornual and fundal region ablated with roller ball electrode as this is only 8 mm and chances of the perforation are high.

To Prevent Hemorrhage

- Do not perform TCRE >3 mm depth of the myometrium.
- Intrauterine pressure (IUP) should not exceed the patient's mean arterial pressure (MAP) as it acts tamponade.
- At the end of the procedure, reduce the IUP and observe the bleeding from the open sinuses.
- *Septal metroplasty:* Panoramic view obtained.
  - At the base of the septum, tubal ostias are visualized and midline traced through septum anteroposterior thickness.
  - Using a resectoscope, slightly angle the Collins knife before assembling the resectoscope to allow access to cornua.

Intrauterine adhesions: Combination of the hysterosalpingogram (HSG) and ultrasonography (USG) are diagnostic of the adhesions. During resection, follow the normal direction of the cavity. Laparoscopic-guided hysteroscopic adhesiolysis is a controlled method of avoiding perforation of the uterus as it transmits the light across the uterine wall and the bulge over the serosal layer which signifies the further hysteroscopic surgery must stop.

Scissors minimizes the risk of destruction of endometrium which are reservoir for future epithelization.

For prevention: Loop intrauterine device (IUD), hormone replacement therapy (HRT), and Foley catheter.

CHAPTER

62

Genital Tuberculosis

Shubhanjali Sen, Isha Rani, B Ramesh

INTRODUCTION

Genital tuberculosis (GTB) is the most common cause of female infertility in developing countries. GTB is found to be 18% of females in India. 5% is responsible to have pelvic inflammatory disease and 10% will have pulmonary tuberculosis.

CLASSICAL HYSTEROSCOPIC FINDINGS ON HYSTEROSCOPY

- Rough dirty looking bizarre pale endometrium with no gland opening **(Figs. 1 and 2)**
- Adhesions **(Figs. 3 and 4)**
- Large whitish tubercles
- Endometrial scarring in endometrium and endocervical area **(Fig. 5)**
- Intraluminal adhesions in interstitial part of Fallopian tube **(Figs. 6A and B)**
- Tubular cavity
- Obliterated cavity
- Ulcers in cavity.

SPECIAL TEST FOR DIAGNOSIS DURING HYSTEROSCOPY

If we perform a vital staining with methylene blue dye. After introduction of the methylene blue dye, the endometrium is seen with hysteroscopy, if the white deposits are still seen, i.e. they have not taken the blue stain then they are the tubercles of the GTB. It appears as starry sky appearance.

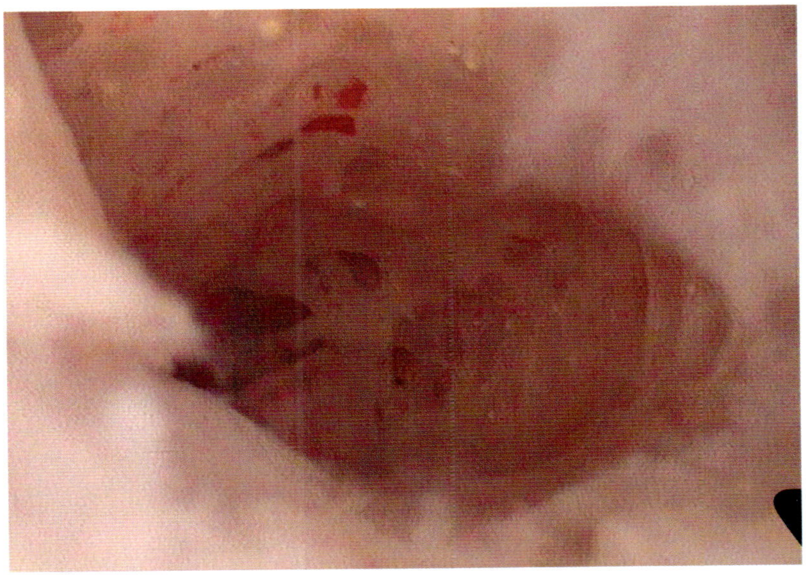

Fig. 1: Whitish small deposits with bizarre pale endometrium.

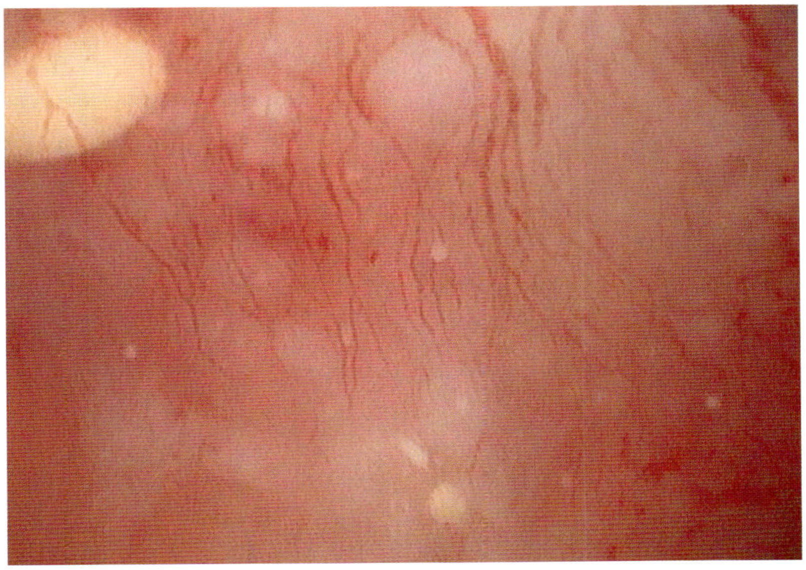

Fig. 2: White tubercles are seen which are pathognomonic of the tuberculosis.

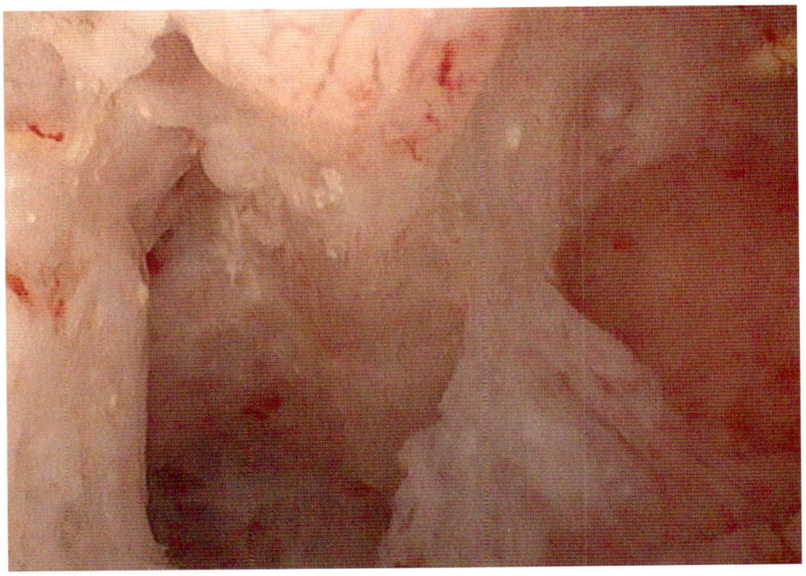

Fig. 3: Endometrial scarring with whitish deposits, tubular obliterated cavity.

EFFECT OF THE DISEASE

Generally, mycobacterium gains access to the body and disseminates into the circulation via the lymphatics. It remains silent throughout

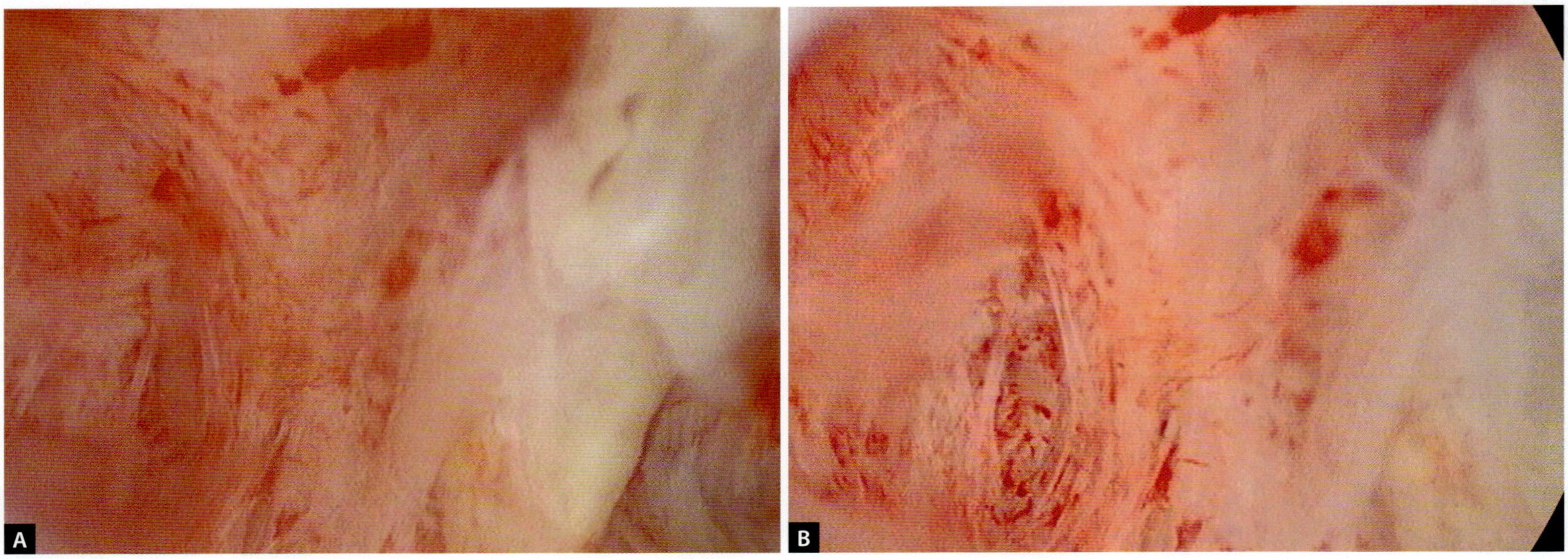

Figs. 4A and B: Adhesions in case of tuberculosis, obliterated cavity.

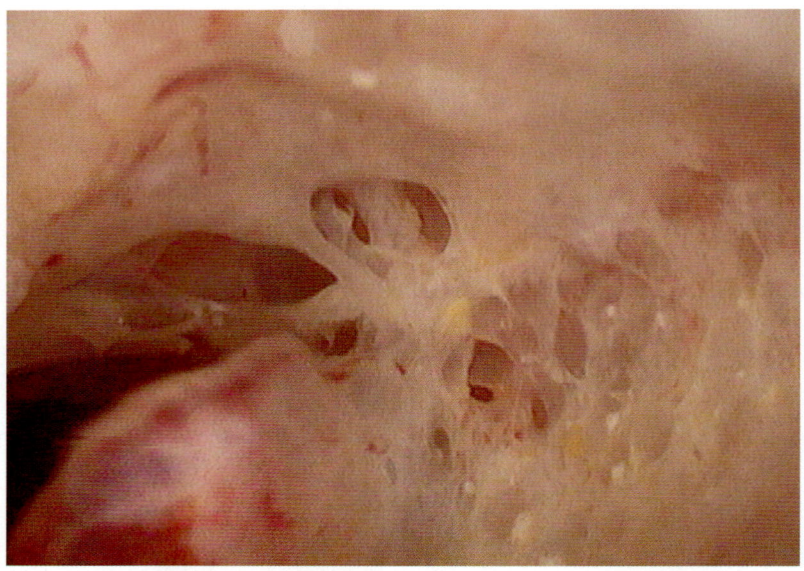

Fig. 5: Endometrial scarring in present, dirty looking endometrium.

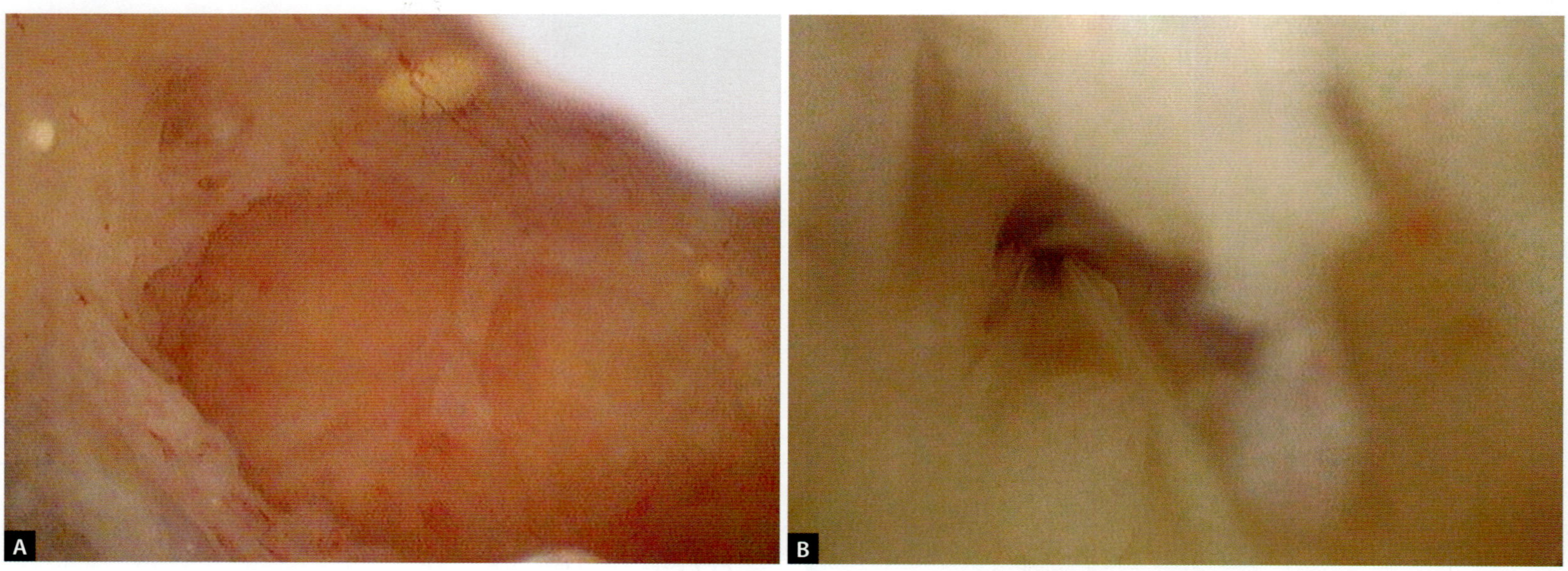

Figs. 6A and B: Cervical stenosis.

life until the immunity is lowered. Increased circulation and hormone dependence of the female genital tract after puberty and sexual activity make its vulnerable for the disease to progress in the genital tract. Tuberculosis of the genitals is usually confined to the endometrium, which is flared up in the fundal area and less in cervical area. Tuberculosis spares the myometrium. The overall involvement of the endometrium is approximately 60–90%.

Tuberculosis causes the endometrial functions abnormal and is associated with tuberculous salpingitis. This leads to severe suppression of the sensitivity of the endometrium to respond to the ovarian hormone and menstrual cycle is disturbed. All these changes will not let the implantation of the embryo to take place.

So, the important idea is to diagnose and treat the tuberculosis early.

MANAGEMENT

Hysteroscopy followed by polymerase chain reaction (PCR) testing for *Mycobacterium tuberculosis* help in early detection of the GTB.

Antitubercular treatment (ATT) consists of four drug regimen, i.e. rifampicin, isoniazid, ethambutol, and pyrazinamide for 2 months, followed by rifampicin and isoniazid for 4 months.

Liver function test (LFT) and renal function test (RFT) with complete blood count (CBC) should be checked every month.

Hysteroscopy to be performed in premenstrual phase.

Side Effects of the Antitubercular Treatment

- Nausea and vomiting managed with domperidone and ranitidine
- Neuralgia and tingling sensation managed with 100 mg pyridoxine/day
- Icterus and abnormal LFT stop the treatment.

TUBERCULOSIS-LAPAROSCOPIC FINDINGS

Adhesions are commonly seen between omentum and anterior abdominal wall **(Figs. 7A to J)**.

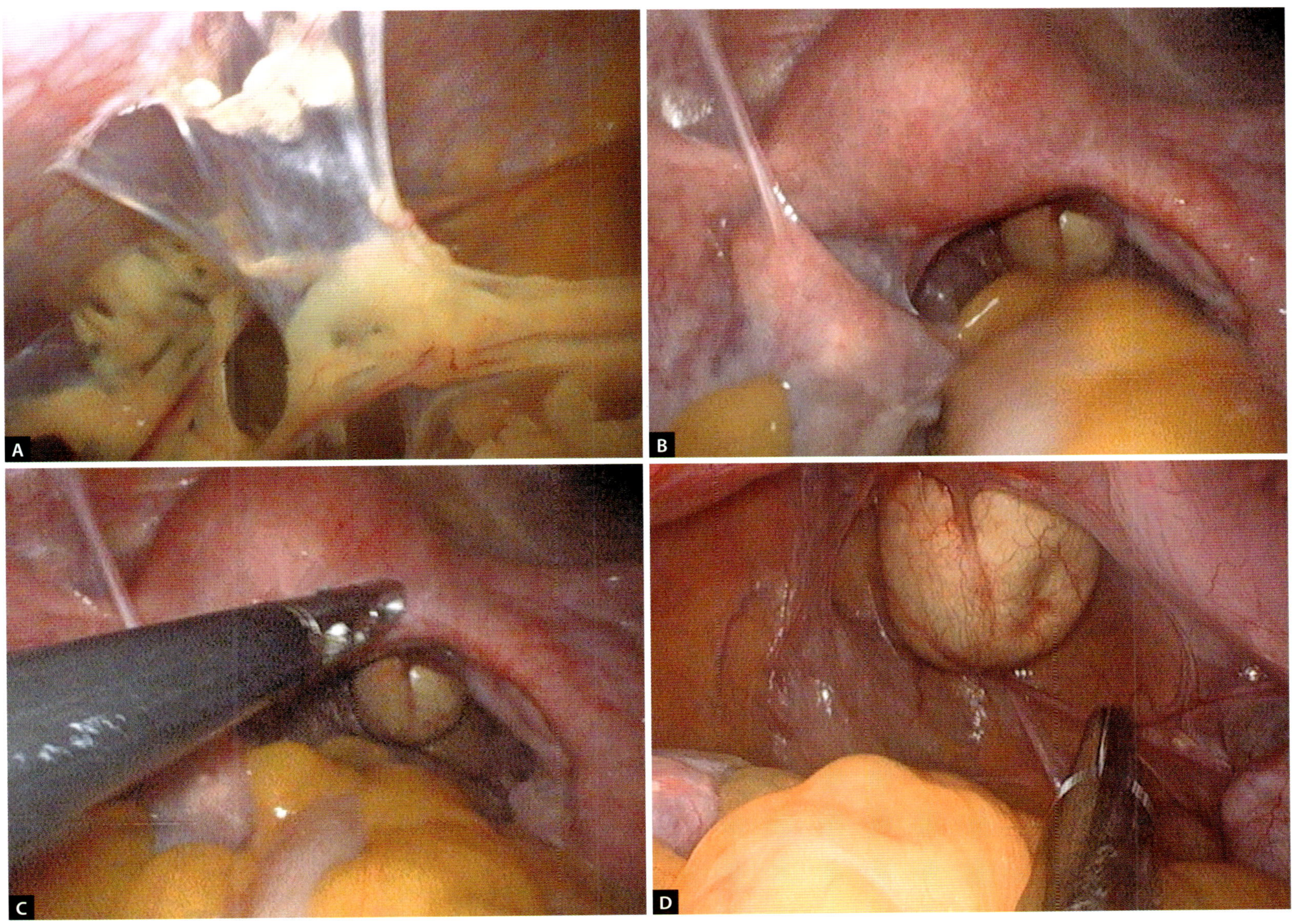

Figs. 7A to D

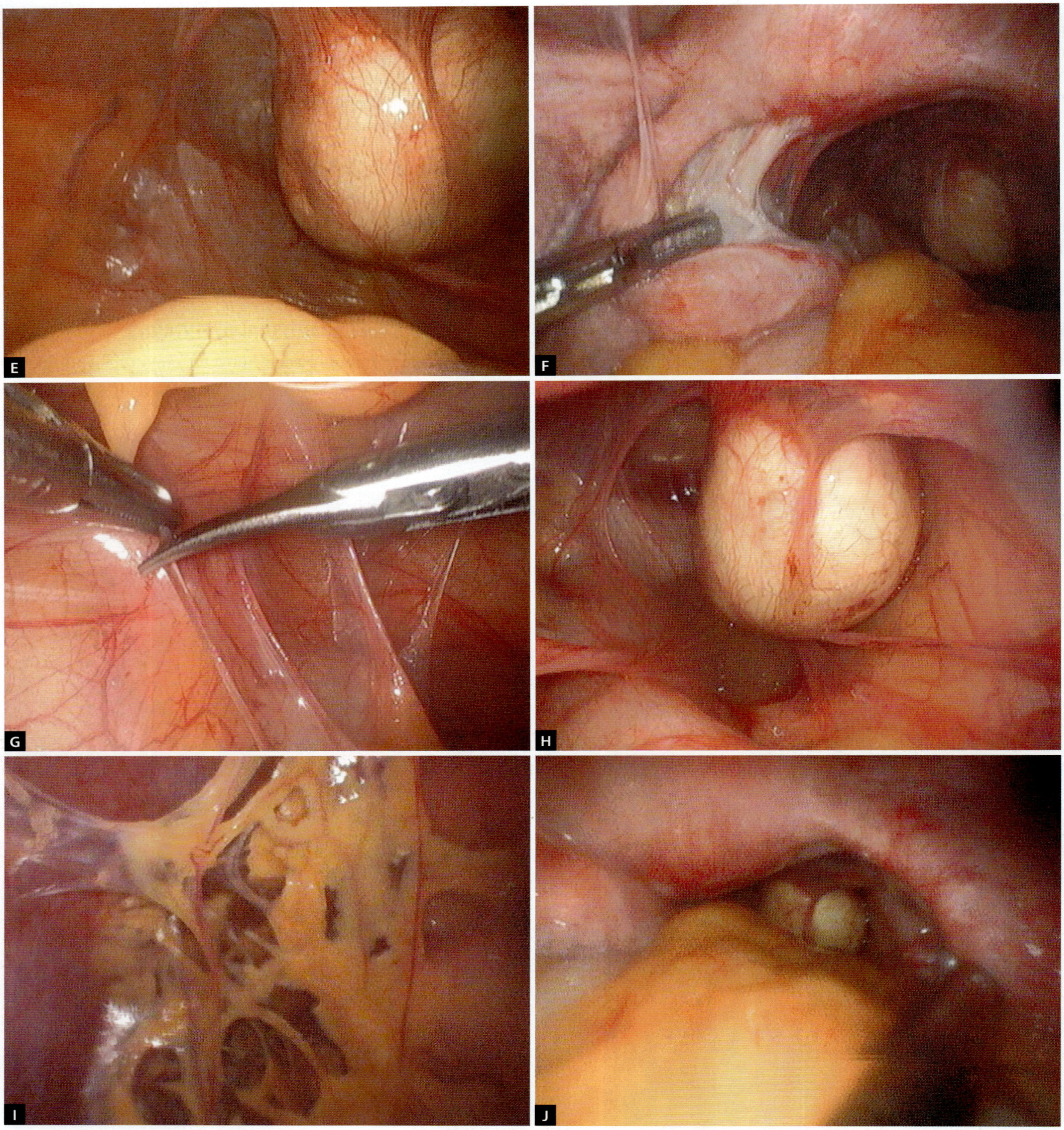

Figs. 7E to J

Figs. 7A to J: Caseous nodule seen, retort-shaped tubes agglutinated to fimbria.

SUGGESTED READING

1. Kumar A, Kumar A. Hysteroscopic marker in endometrial tuberculosis and chronic endomteritis. Mastering the Technique in Hysteroscopy. New Delhi: Jaypee Brothers Medical Publishers; 2017. pp. 603-7.
2. Mohakul SK, Beela VR, Tiru P. Hysteroscopy finding and its correlation with latent endometrium tuberculosis in infertility. Gynecolsurg Springer. 2014;12:31-9.
3. Sharma JB. Current diagnosis and management of female genital tuberculosis. J Obstet Gynaecol India. 2015;65(6):362-71.

CHAPTER

63

Chronic Endometritis

Shubhanjali Sen, Isha Rani, B Ramesh

INTRODUCTION

Chronic endometritis is the subtle inflammatory disease of endometrial mucosa, which is difficult to diagnose. Bacterial pathogens are causative agents like Enterobacteriaceae, *Enterococcus*, *Staphylococcus*, *Mycoplasma*, *Ureaplasma* and *Streptococcus* 17.4% of the patients can be diagnosed hysteroscopically.

SYMPTOMS

- Abnormal uterine bleeding (spotting)
- Pelvic pain
- Infertility
- Leukorrhea
- Failure in implantation of the embryo to endometrium in natural or in vitro fertilization (IVF) pregnancy
- Recurrent pregnancy loss.

ETIOLOGICAL FACTORS

- Medical termination of pregnancy
- Prolonged labor
- Dilatation and curettage
- Intrauterine contraceptive device (IUCD) insertion
- Unsafe sexual intercourse.

HYSTEROSCOPIC FEATURES

- *Strawberry appearance:* Prominent white glandular orifice surrounded by hyperemia localized or scattered.
- Stromal edema **(Fig. 1)**.
- Endometrial thickening (homogeneous or nonhomogeneous).
- Micropolyps <1 mm; strongly suggest chronic endometritis especially smaller one translucent to light **(Fig. 2)**.

  Hysteroscopy to be performed in mid-proliferative period of cycle.

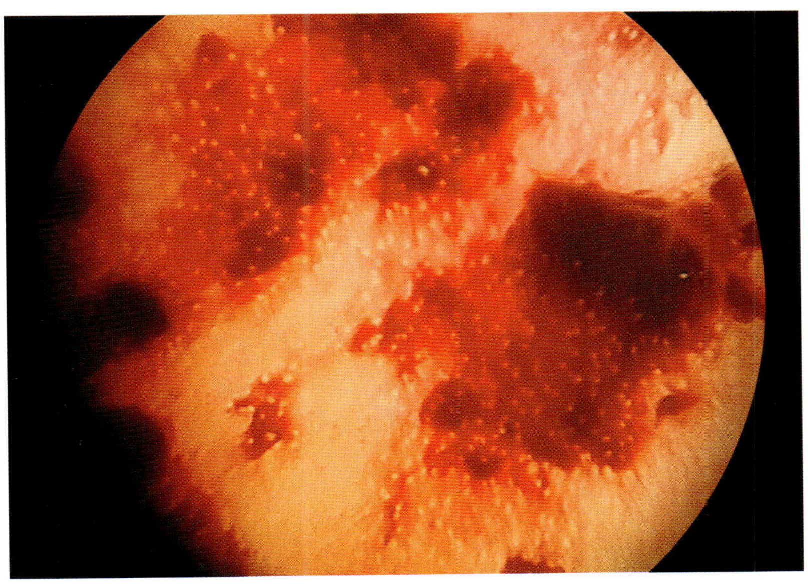

Fig. 1: Strawberry-like appearance.

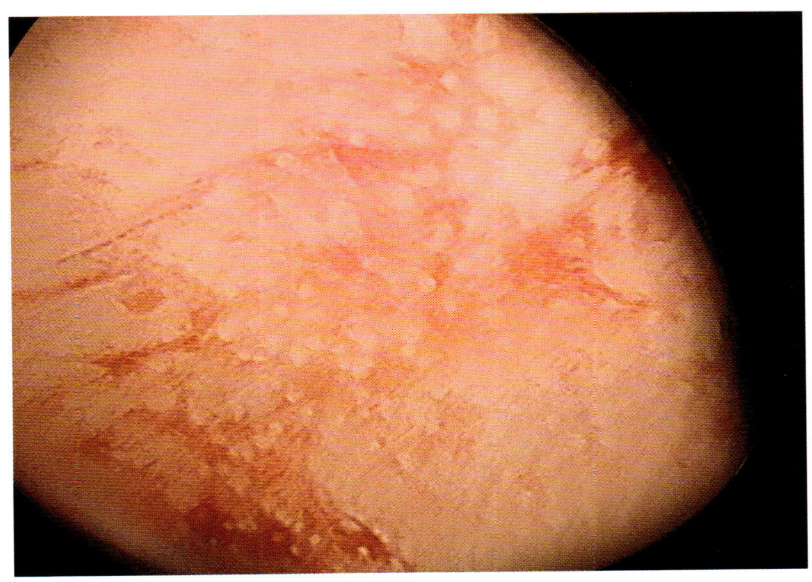

Fig. 2: Micropolyps with stromal edema.

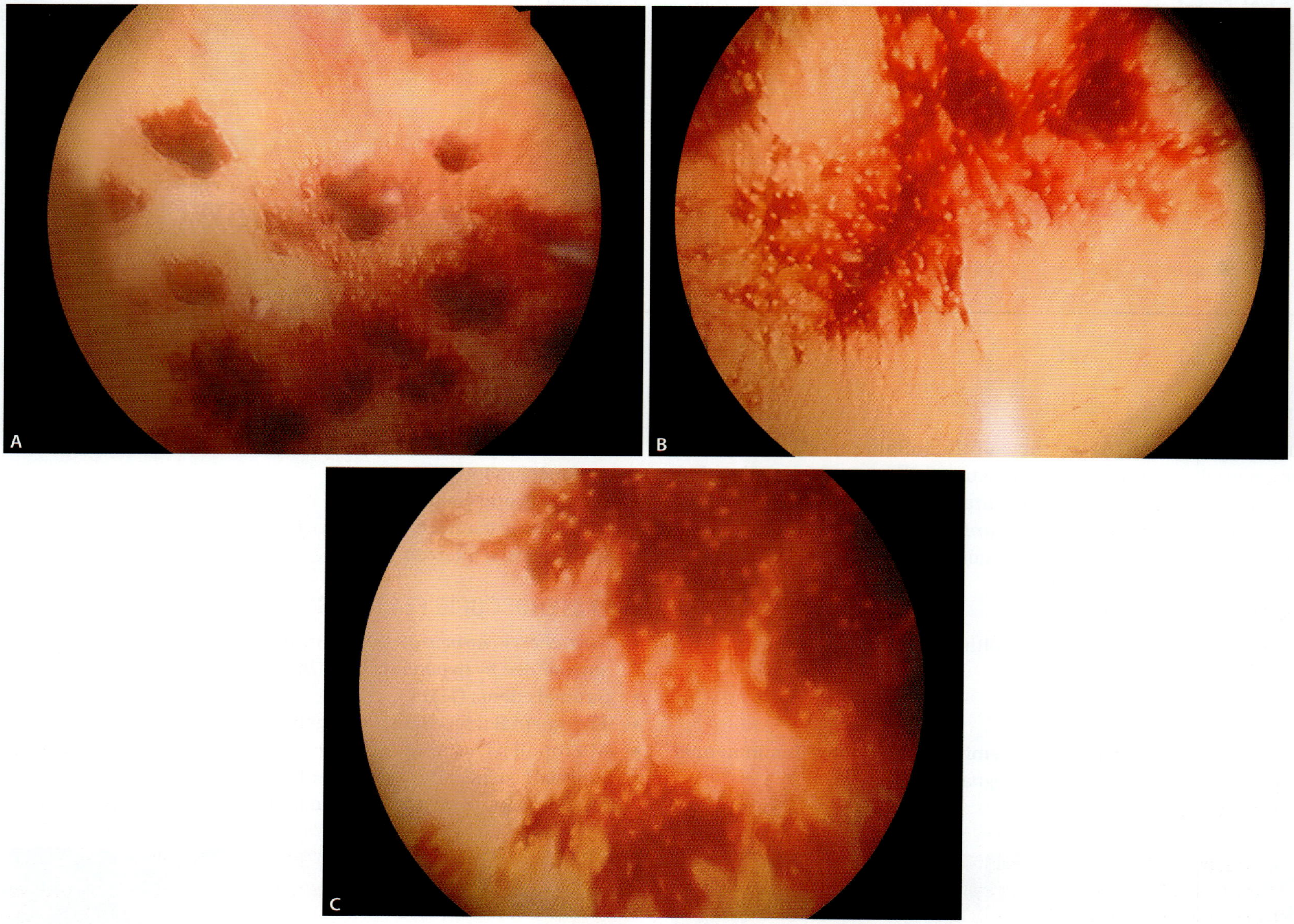

Fig. 3A to C: Various appearance of chronic endometritis.

TREATMENT

Doxycycline 100 mg twice daily for 3 weeks orally taken. Estrogen supplementation 2 mg daily once a day to be taken for 3 months.

SUGGESTED READING

1. Kumar A, Kumar A. Hysteroscopic markers in endometrial tuberculosis and chronic endometritis. In: Shawki O, Deshmukh S, Pacheco LA (Eds). Mastering the Techniques in Hysteroscopy, 1st edition. New Delhi: Jaypee Brothers Medical Publishers (P) Ltd; 2017. pp. 603-7.
2. Moreno I, Cicinelli E, Garcia-Grau I, et al. The diagnosis of chronic endometritis in infertile asymptomatic women: a comparative study of histology, microbial cultures, hysteroscopy, and molecular microbiology. Am J Obstet Gynecol. 2018;218(6):602.e1-602.e16.
3. Song D, Li TC, Zhang Y, et al. Correlation between hysteroscopy findings and chronic endometritis. Fertil Steril. 2019;111(4):772-9.

CHAPTER

64

Vaginoscopy

Shubhanjali Sen, Isha Rani, B Ramesh

VAGINOSCOPIC TECHNIQUE

Hysteroscopy has emerged as the most advanced diagnostic and therapeutic modality in the management of the intrauterine pathology. It is considered as gold standard. It is a safe and most easily performed technique for the definitive diagnosis of intrauterine pathology without the need for any analgesia and anesthesia.

To minimize the pain and discomfort of the patient after procedure, smaller diameter scopes and flexiscopes are developed. Along with this "no touch technique" or "vaginoscopic technique" has come into place so it is atraumatic approach.

Procedure

- After performing bimanual examination in dorsal lithotomy position.
- Parts are cleaned and draped with normal saline and povidone.
- Hysteroscope is introduced into the vagina and labia are closed manually.
- A pressure of 150 mm Hg is normally used for the procedure.
- Normal saline is used as the distending medium.
- Entire vagina and cervix are normally visualized **(Figs. 1 to 4)**.
- External cervical os and internal cervical os are negotiable and we can easily see the uterine cavity with this technique without hampering the cervix **(Figs. 5A and B)**.

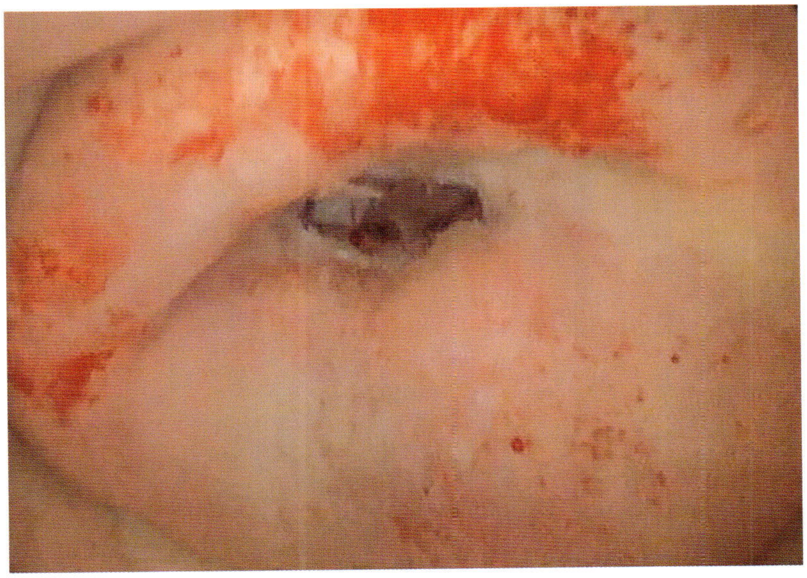

Fig. 1: Cervix with external os.

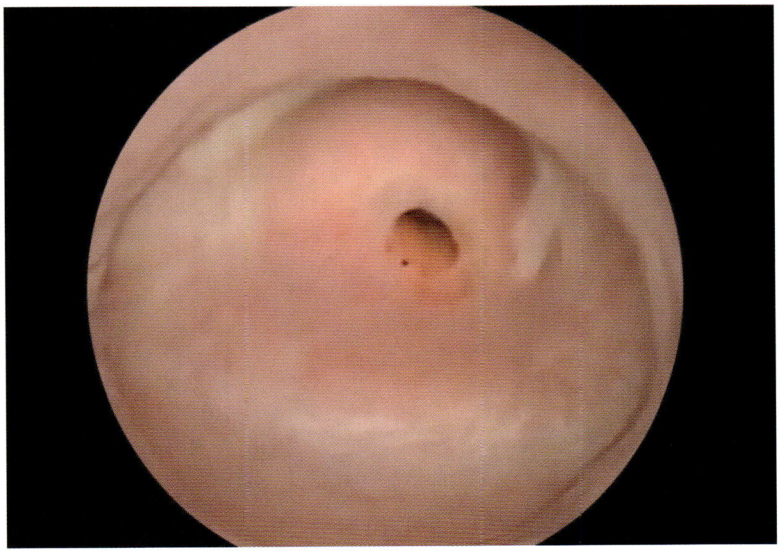

Fig. 2: Vaginal wall visualized after distention.

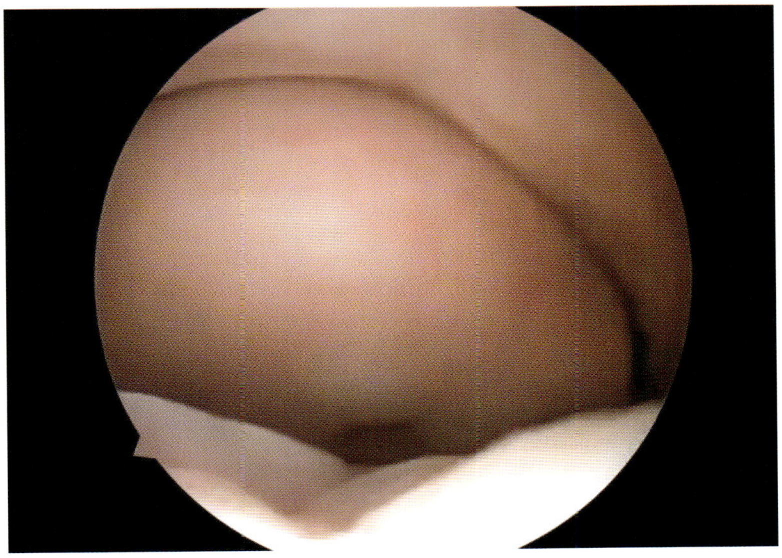

Fig. 3: Vaginal wall collapse in case distention is not well maintained.

Advantages

- No premedication required
- No instrumentation needed like (Sims' speculum, tenaculum like in traditional method)
- Faster procedure than traditional
- Postprocedure compliance of the patient is the same as with traditional method

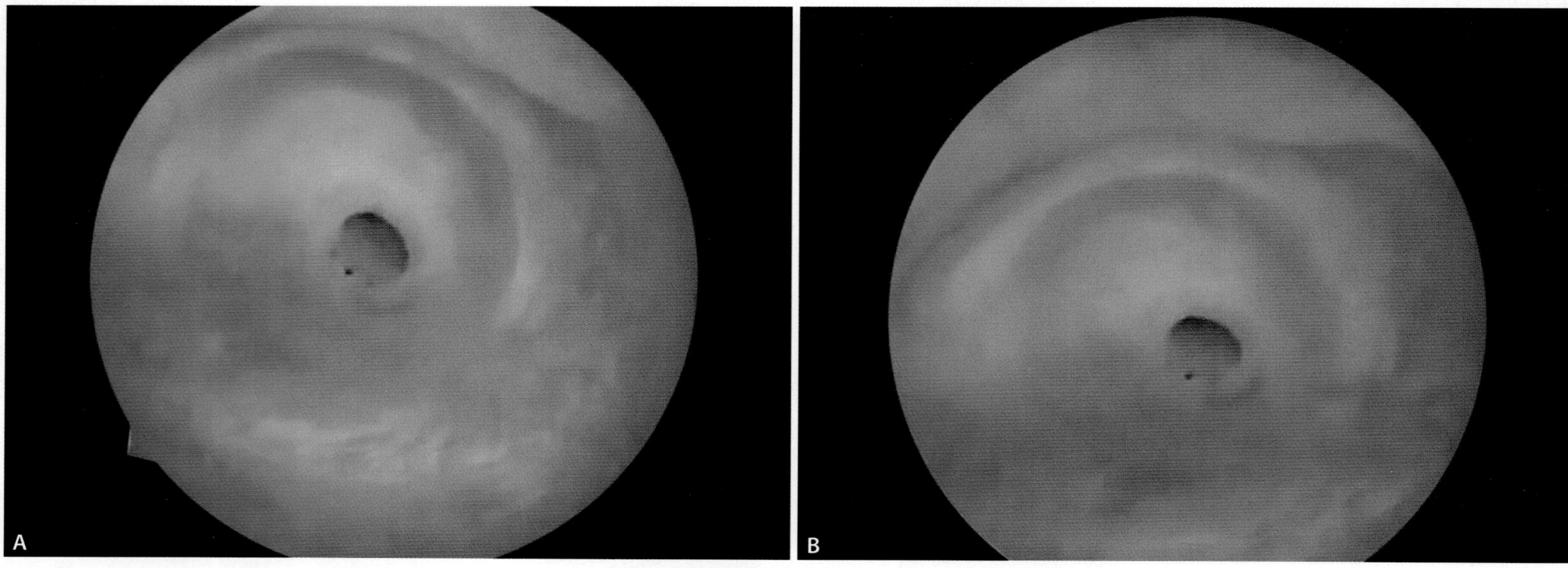

Figs. 4A and B: All vaginal wall visualized.

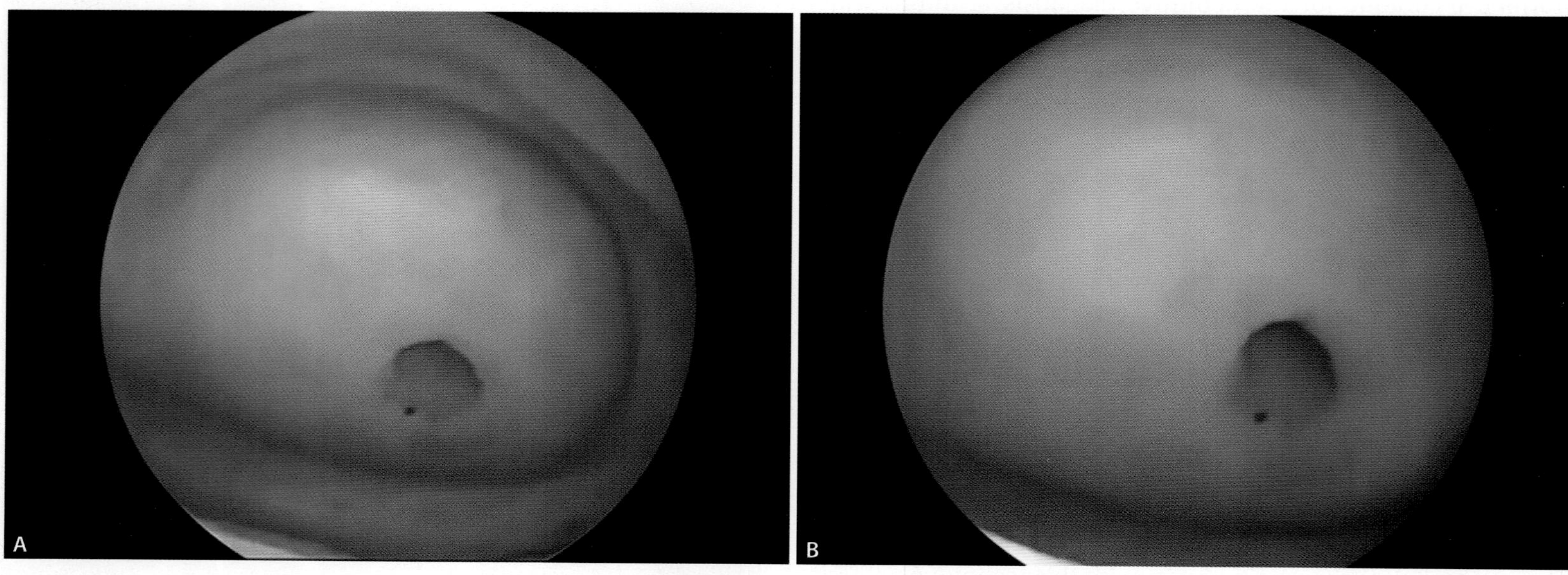

Figs. 5A and B: External os is used as a guide for hysteroscopy.

- For outpatient hysteroscopy
- Well tolerated, feasible, and quick
- Analgesia normally not required after the procedure.

SUGGESTED READING

1. Cooper NA, Smith P, Khan KS, et al. Vaginoscopic approach to outpatient hysteroscopy: a systematic review of the effect on pain. BJOG. 2010;117(5):532-9.
2. Guida M, Di Spiezi Sardo A, Acunzo G, et al. Vaginoscopic versus traditional office hysteroscopy: a randomized controlled study. Hum Reprod. 2006; 21(12):3253-7.
3. Misra R, Sinha M, Mittal S. Vaginohysteroscopy, a patient-friendly technique for outpatient hysteroscopy: experience of the first 100 cases. J Laparoendosc Adv Surg Techniques. 2005;15(3):209-3.
4. Natalia E Desiree GE. Ashley U, et al. Vaginoscopy "no touch" technique: a feasible alternative to paracervical block for in office hysteroscopy [34E]. Obstetr Gynecol. 2019133:60S.

CHAPTER

65

Adenomyosis through Hysteroscope

Shubhanjali Sen, Isha Rani, B Ramesh

ADENOMYOTIC CYST

Refer to **Figures 1 to 3**.

ADENOMYOSIS

Uterine adenomyosis is a common gynecologic disorder of the women with reproductive age group. It is characterized by the presence of ectopic endometrial glands and stroma within myometrium.

Types of Adenomyosis

- *Diffuse type:* Endometrial glands and stroma are extensively intermingled with myometrial muscle fibers with an increase in volume **(Fig. 4)**.
- *Focal:* Single nodular aggregate located in myometrium which may have a histologic spectrum from solid (adenomyoma) to cystic (adenomyotic cyst).

Symptoms

- Dysmenorrhea
- Abnormal uterine bleeding
- Chronic pelvic pain
- Deep dyspareunia.

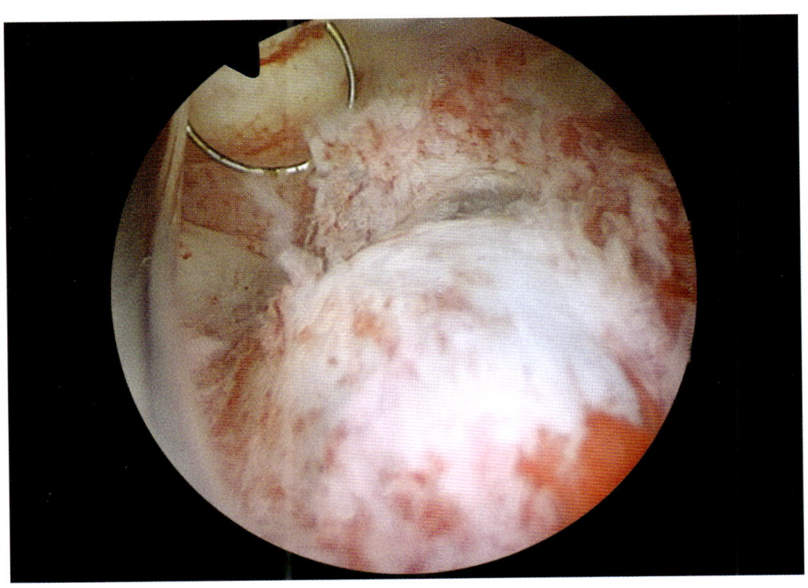

Fig. 1: Adenomyotic cyst seen on posterior wall which was resected with the help of monopolar loop using glycine as the medium.

Diagnosis

- *Transvaginal ultrasound:*
    - *Adenomyomatous nodule:* Oval, hypoechogenic and hyperechogenic nonencapsulated with myometrial thickness with cystic spaces filled with blood >5 mm. Color Doppler revel vascularity which does not circumscribe the lesion and present in orthogonal orientation in relation to the endometrium.

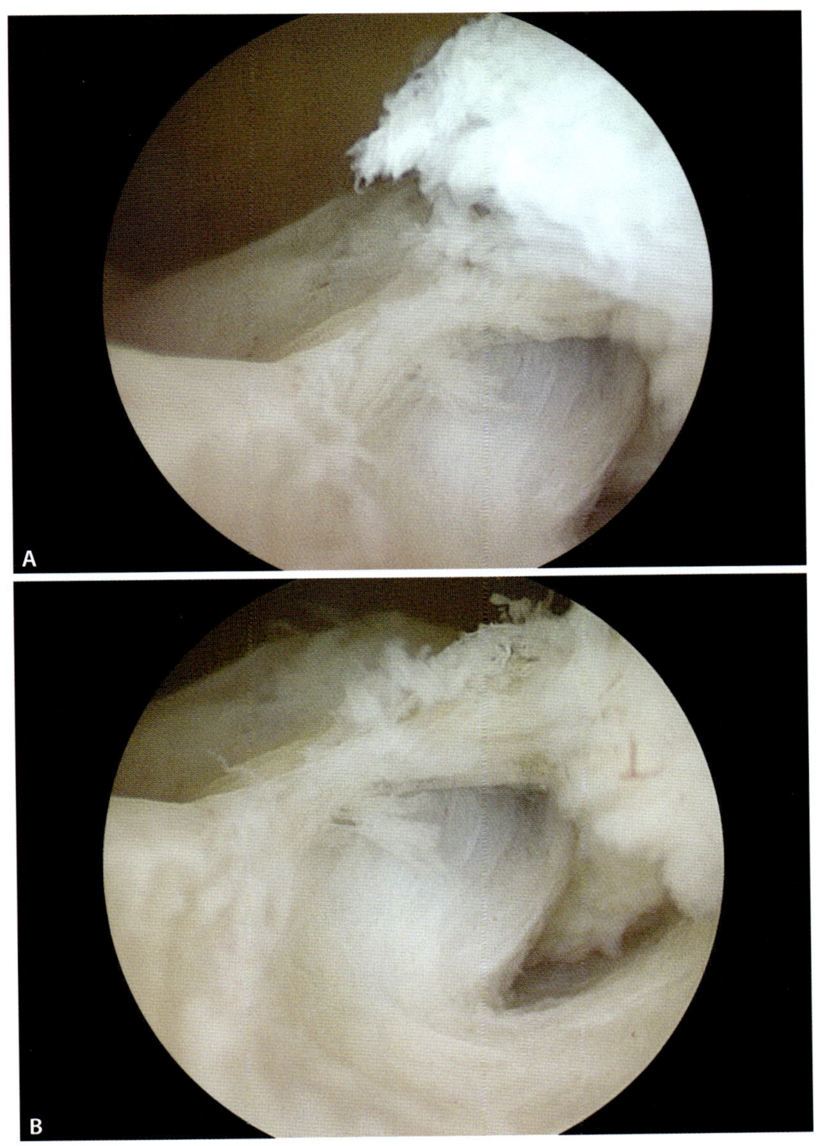

Figs. 2A and B: Adenomyotic cyst.

- *Diffuse:* Uterine fibromyometrium increased volume uterus, asymmetry in thickness of myometrial walls, myometrial linear layers, inhomogeneity, and poorly defined endomyometrial interface.

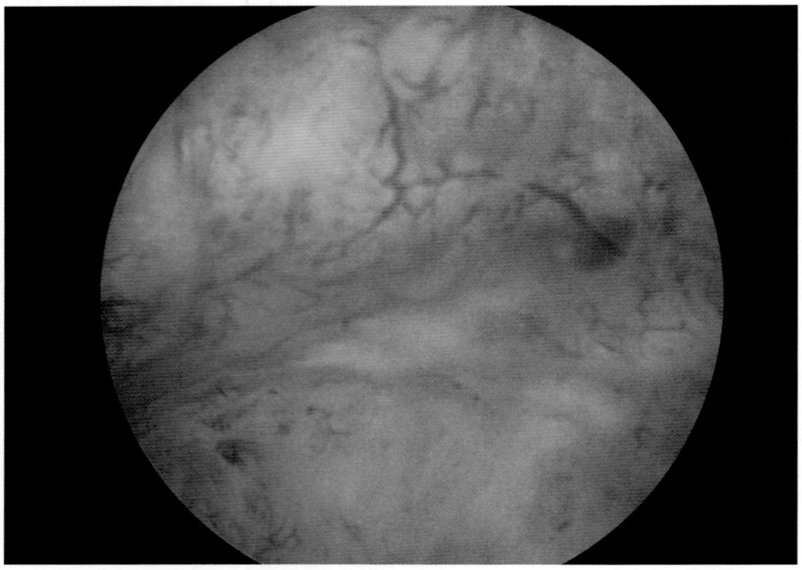

Fig. 3: Hemorrhagic cystic lesion assuming dark blue or chocolate brown appearance.

- *Three-dimensional (3D) transvaginal ultrasound:* Adenomyosis is based on the evaluation of the junctional zone (JZ).
- *MRI:*
    - JZ is easily seen on MRI.
    - JZ depends on thickness, regularity, and interruption.
    - Thickness must be measured at the thickest (JZ maximum) and thinnest (JZ minimum), JZ maximum 15 mm diagnosed with adenomyosis.
- *Hysterosalpingography (HSG):* Lollipop like diverticula (direct sign) is observed. Dilated and prominent spicules are indirect signs.
- *Hysteroscopy:* Direct visualization. Following aspects are indicative of the adenomyosis:
    - Irregular endometrium with tiny openings seen on the endometrial surface
    - Pronounced hypervascularization and endometrial strawberry pattern
    - Fibrous cystic appearance of intrauterine lesions (following three to five episodes of intramyometrial hemorrhage)
    - Hemorrhagic cystic lesions assuming a dark blue or chocolate brown appearance.

Hysteroscopy reveals an irregular endometrial vascular distribution pattern, both during the proliferative and secretory phase.

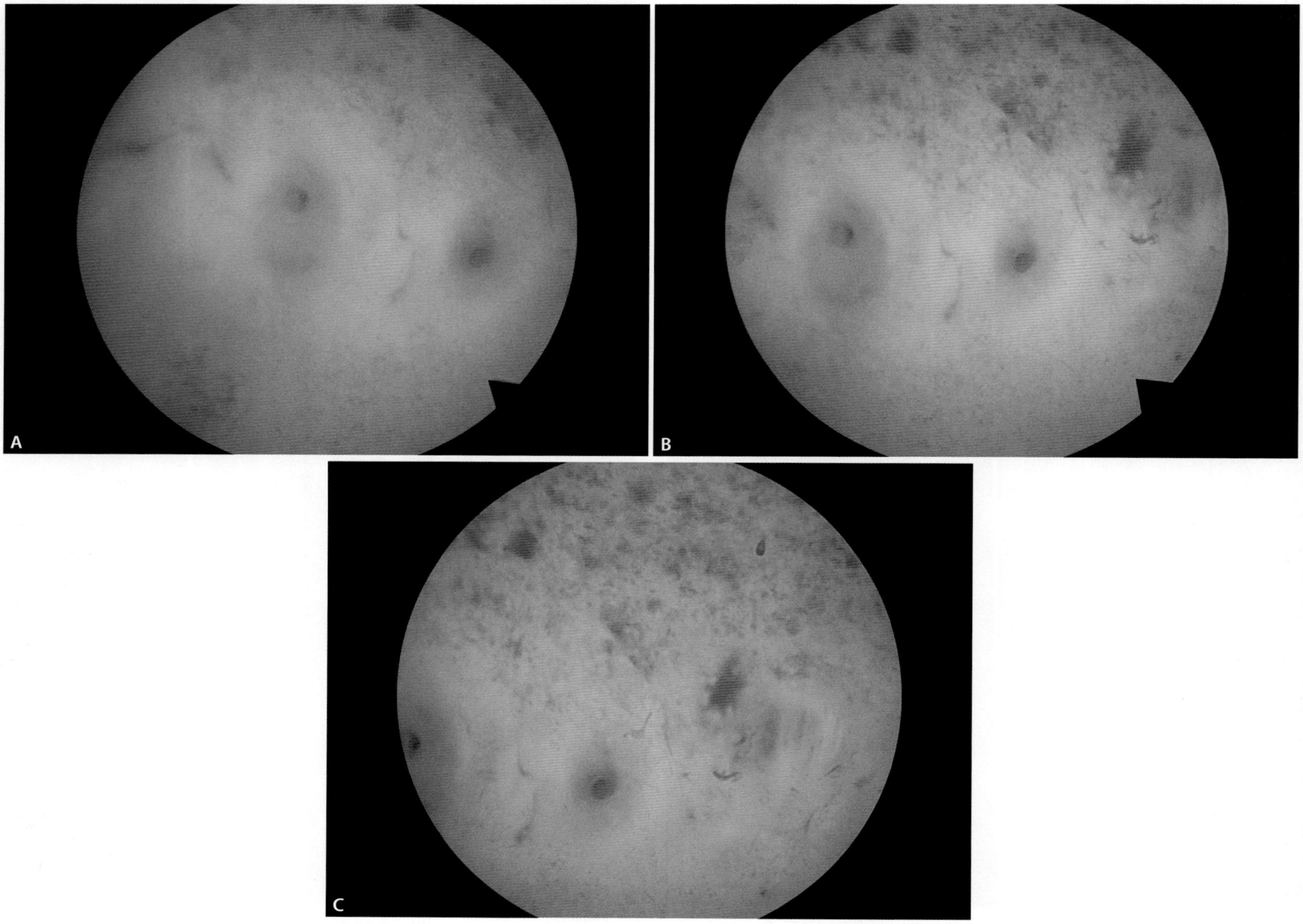

Figs. 4A to C: Irregular endometrium with tiny openings seen, with pronounced hypervascularization.

Hysteroscopic biopsy should be taken from endometrial and myometrial layer and then take a second biopsy deeper which will only include the myometrial tissue.

On resectoscopic biopsy the feature suggestive of adenomyosis are:

- Irregular subendometrial myometrium (spiral/fibrotic)
- Contortion of the normal myoarchitecture
- Presence of the intramural endometrioma.

Recently new gliding system Trophy hysteroscope with 5Fr instrument dissection and coagulation can be done through operative channel.

Management

Several factors like the age and desire for future pregnancy will determine the mode of the treatment.

Medical Approach

Gonadotropin-releasing hormone agonist (GnRHa), levonorgestrel-releasing intrauterine device (LNG-IUD), oral contraceptive pill (OCP), progestogen, and danazol.

The principal limitation of the medical option is that they will induce regression but not eradication of the disease.

Surgical Management

- The uterus to be removed or preserved.
- Hysterectomy (abdominal, vaginal, laparoscopic or robotic) is the final surgical modality of treatment.
- For uterine sparing surgery—fertility enhancing surgery: Adenomyomectomy.
- For uterine sparing surgery not intended for pregnancy: Non-excisional conservative techniques can be done like; laparoscopic electrocoagulation of the myometrium, laparoscopic uterine artery ligation, ablation of the focal adenomyosis with high-frequency ultrasound [high-intensity focused ultrasound (HIFU)], alcohol instillation under ultrasound guidance for the treatment of cystic adenomyosis, radiofrequency ablation of focal adenomyosis and balloon thermoablation for diffuse adenomyosis.

Hysteroscopic Management

Office hysteroscope: Enucleate the superficial focal adenomyoma or to evacuate cystic hemorrhagic lesion less than 1.5 cm with mechanical instrument and bipolar electrode.

Resectoscopic Treatment

- For superficial adenomyotic nodule >1.5 cm and for diffuse superficial adenomyosis; endomyometrectomy who is not requiring to attain pregnancy with endometrial ablation.
- But the technique is different from the transcervical resection of the endometrium (TCRE), as resection of the endometrium as well as myometrium occurs till we see the healthy myometrial tissue. The procedure is accomplished by 3 mm or 5 mm straight loops for the ablation of the fundus and cornual recesses.
- On resecting the focal adenomyoma the receptivity of the endometrium is improved and implantation of the embryo occurs easily.
- Deep diffuse or focal adenomyosis cannot be resected.

SUGGESTED READING

1. Gordts S, Grimbizis G, Campo R. Symptoms and classification of uterine adenomyosis, including the place of hysteroscopy in diagnosis. Fertil Steril. 2018;109(3):380-388.e.1.
2. Spiezio Sardo AD, Calagna G, Santangelo F, et al. The role of hysteroscopy in the diagnosis and treatment of adenomyosis. BioMed Res Int. 2017;2518396:7.
3. Xia W, Zhang D, Zhu Q. Hysteroscopic excision of symptomatic myometrial adenomyosis: feasibility and effectiveness. BJOG. 2017;124:1615-20.
4. Zhang J, Shi W. Treatment of adenomyosis by hysteroscopy. J Minim Invasive Surg. 2015;22;(6):123.

CHAPTER

66

Hysteroscopic Injection of Stem Cell in Infertility Patient with Thin Endometrium

Shubhanjali Sen, G Hemasree, B Ramesh

PROCEDURE

The processed autologous stem cells are loaded in the instilling needle and injected into the subendometrium at multiple sites with the help of hysteroscope.

INDICATIONS

In vitro fertilization (IVF) patients with chronic thin endometrium which do not respond to conservative medical management.

These concentrates in autologous stem cells are taken from the iliac bone of the patient.

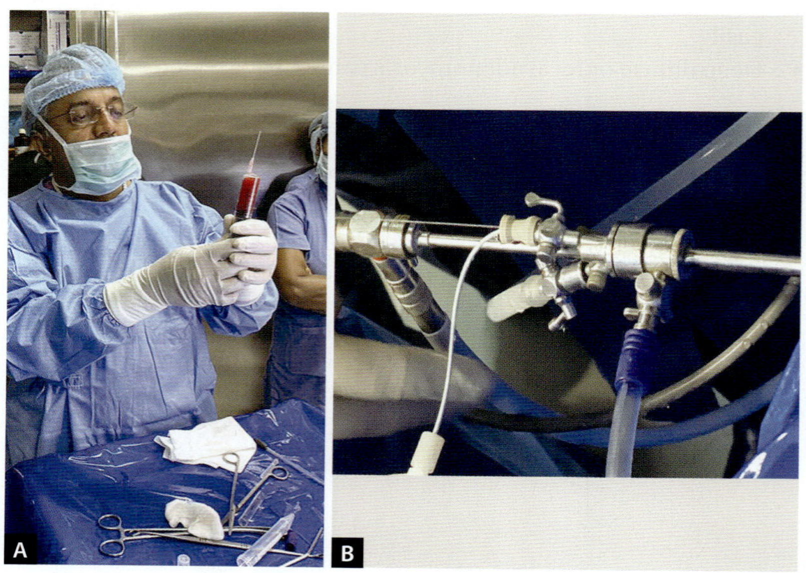

Figs. 1A and B: Loading the processed stem cell.

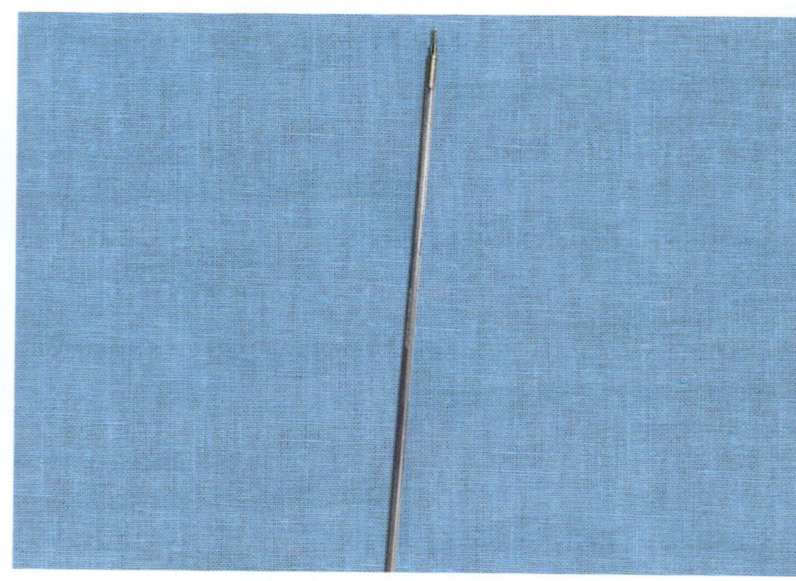

Fig. 2: Stem cell injection needle.

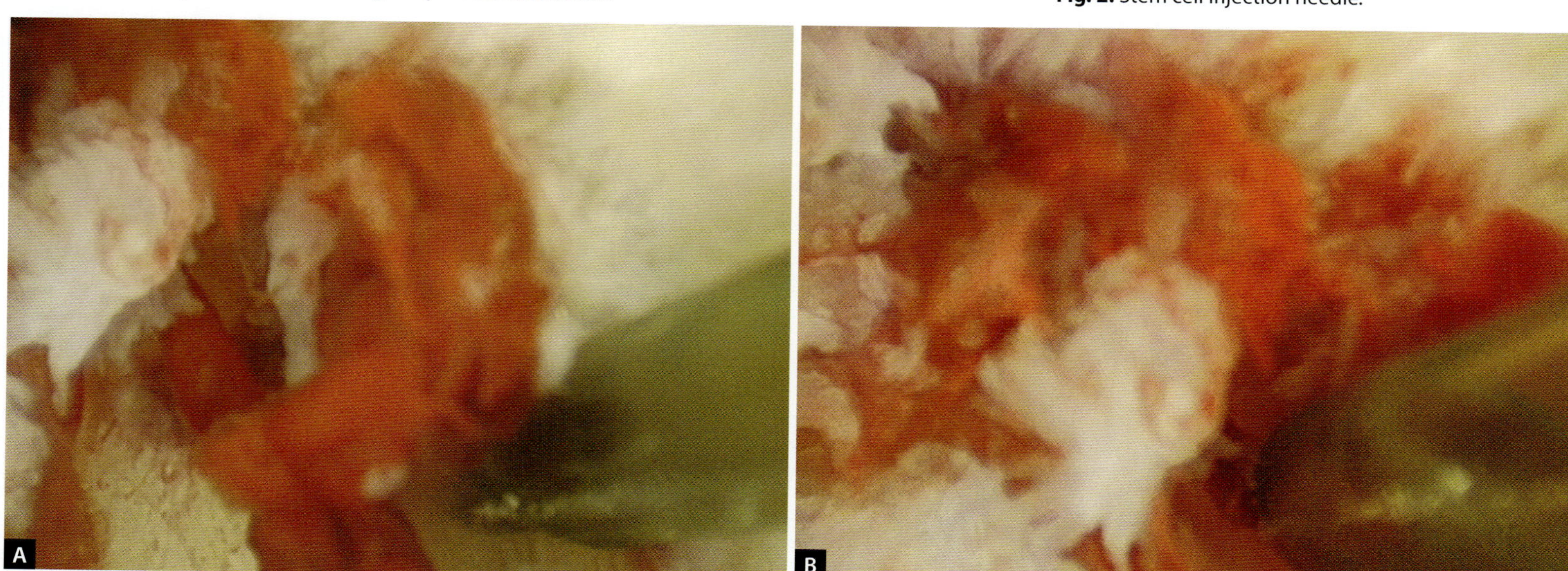

Figs. 3A and B

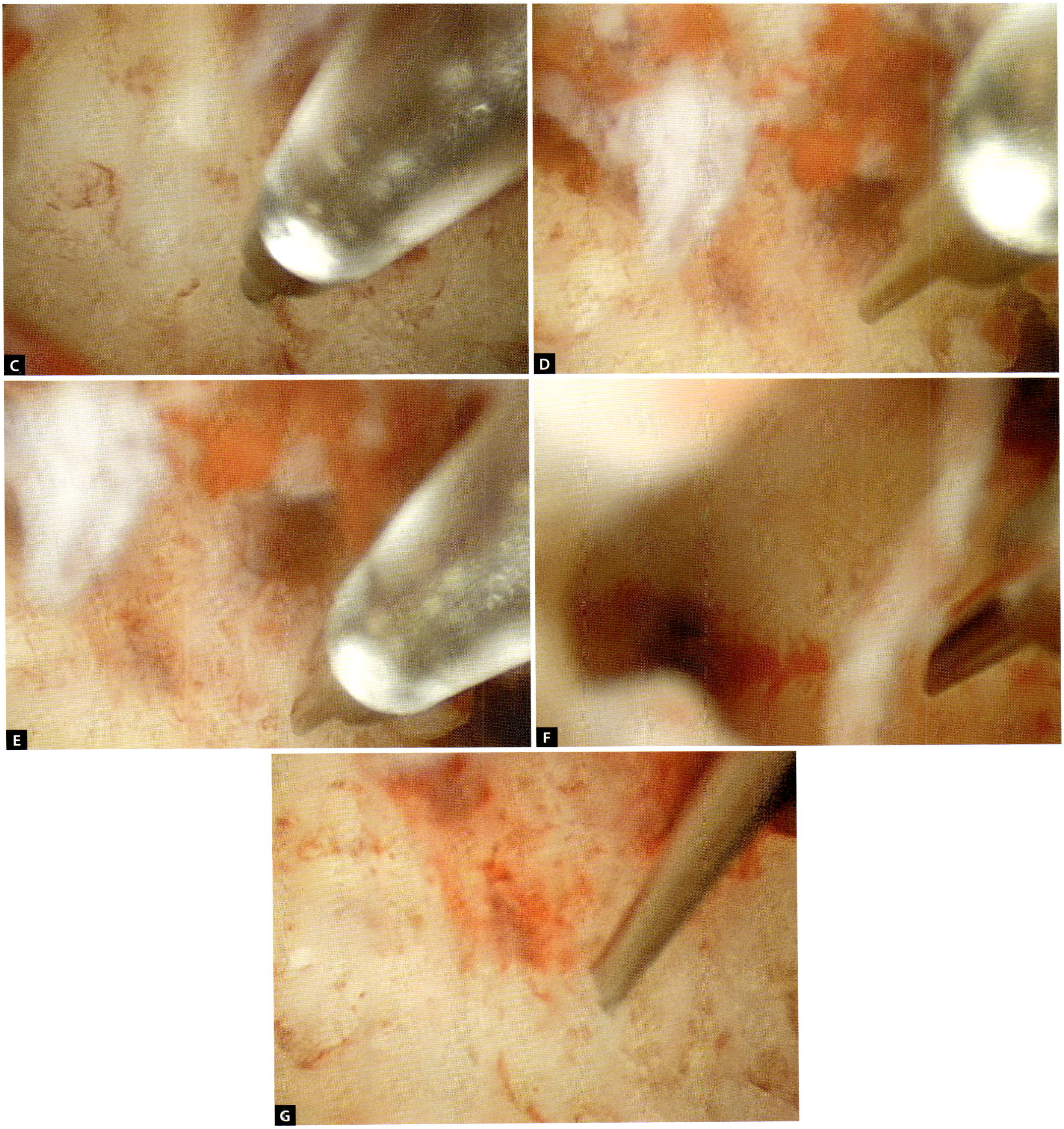

Figs. 3C to G

Figs. 3A to G: Instillation of the processed stem cell into the subendometrium at multiple sites.

3

SECTION

Obstetrics

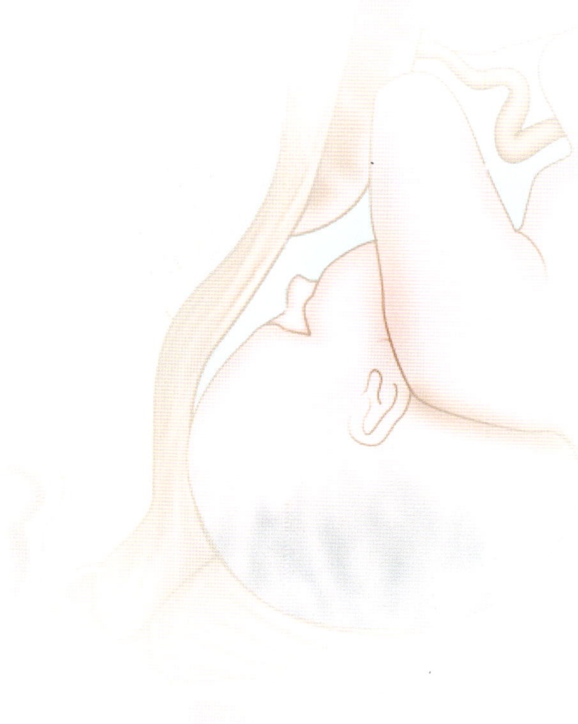

CHAPTER

67

Stages of Labor

Sirisha PSNRS, G Hemasree

INTRODUCTION

Labor is defined as uterine contractions that bring about a demonstrable effacement and dilatation of cervix.

First stage of labor: Onset of true labor pains to the full dilatation of cervix.

Second stage of labor: Full dilation of cervix to delivery of the fetus.

Third stage of labor: Delivery of the fetus to the delivery of the placenta.

FIRST STAGE OF LABOR (FLOWCHART 1)

Flowchart 1: First stage of labor.

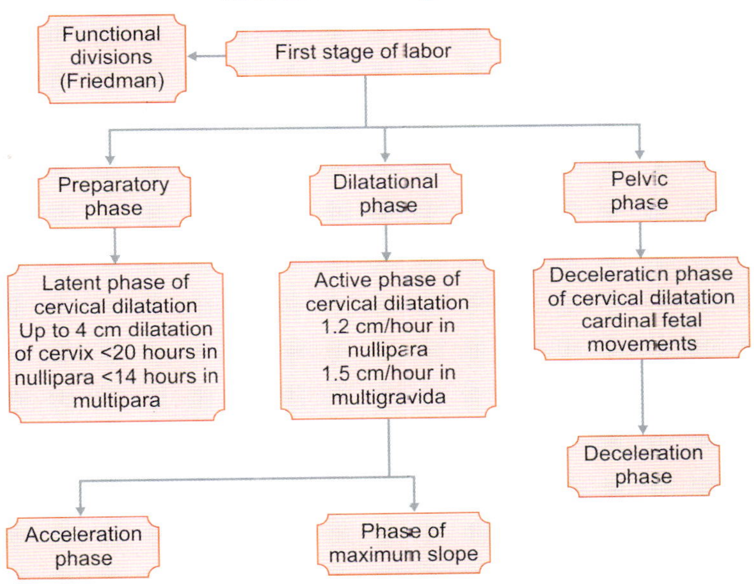

CARDINAL MOVEMENTS OF LABOR

Engagement Descent	First stage
Internal rotation Extension Restitution External rotation	Second stage

SECOND STAGE OF LABOR (FIGS. 1 TO 6)

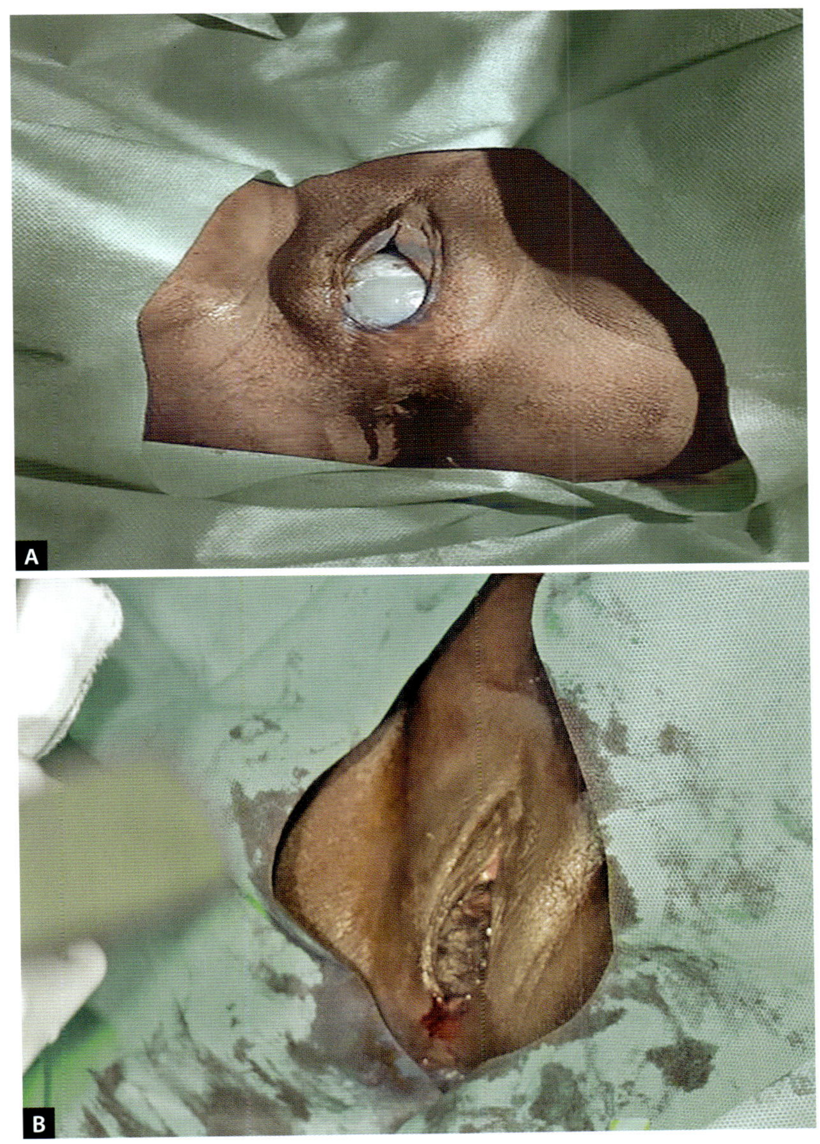

Figs. 1A and B: Crowning: The vulvovaginal opening dilated by fetal head forming a circular opening.

Episiotomy: Incision of the Perineum

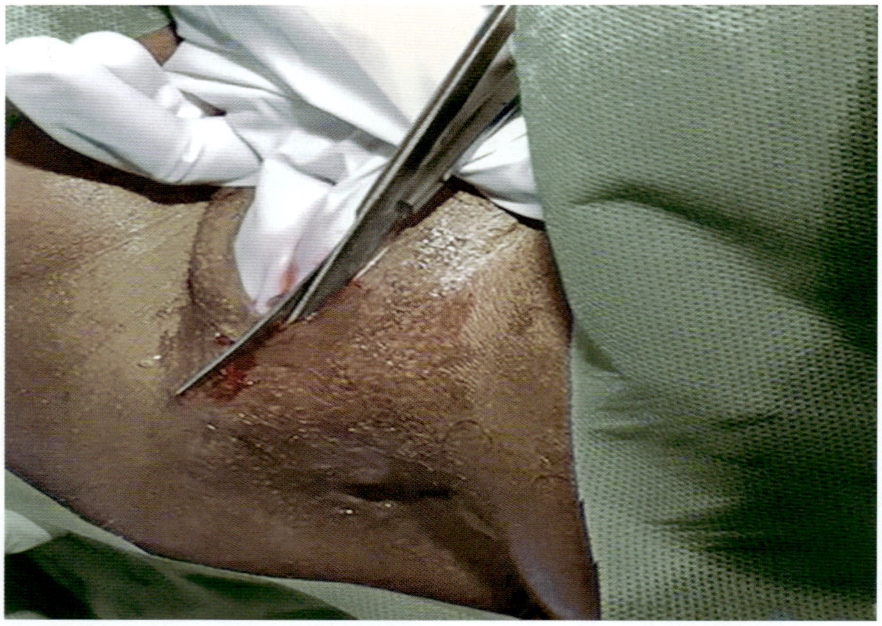

Fig. 2: Episiotomy: Incision of the perineum.
Selective for indications such as shoulder dystocia, breech delivery, instrumental deliveries, occipitoposterior:
- *Timing:* At the time of crowning
- *Type:* Midline, mediolateral.

Delivery of the Fetal Head

Ritgen maneuver: Upward pressure to the fetal chin by the posterior hand while the suboccipital region of the fetal head is held against the symphysis.

Hands poised method: Attendant does not touch the perineum during the delivery of the head.

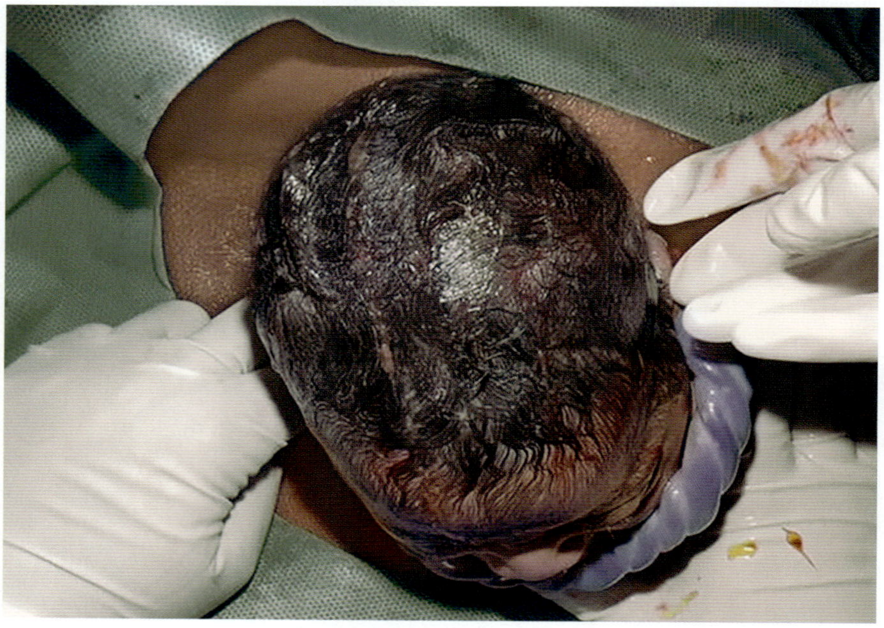

Fig. 3: Delivery of the fetal head.

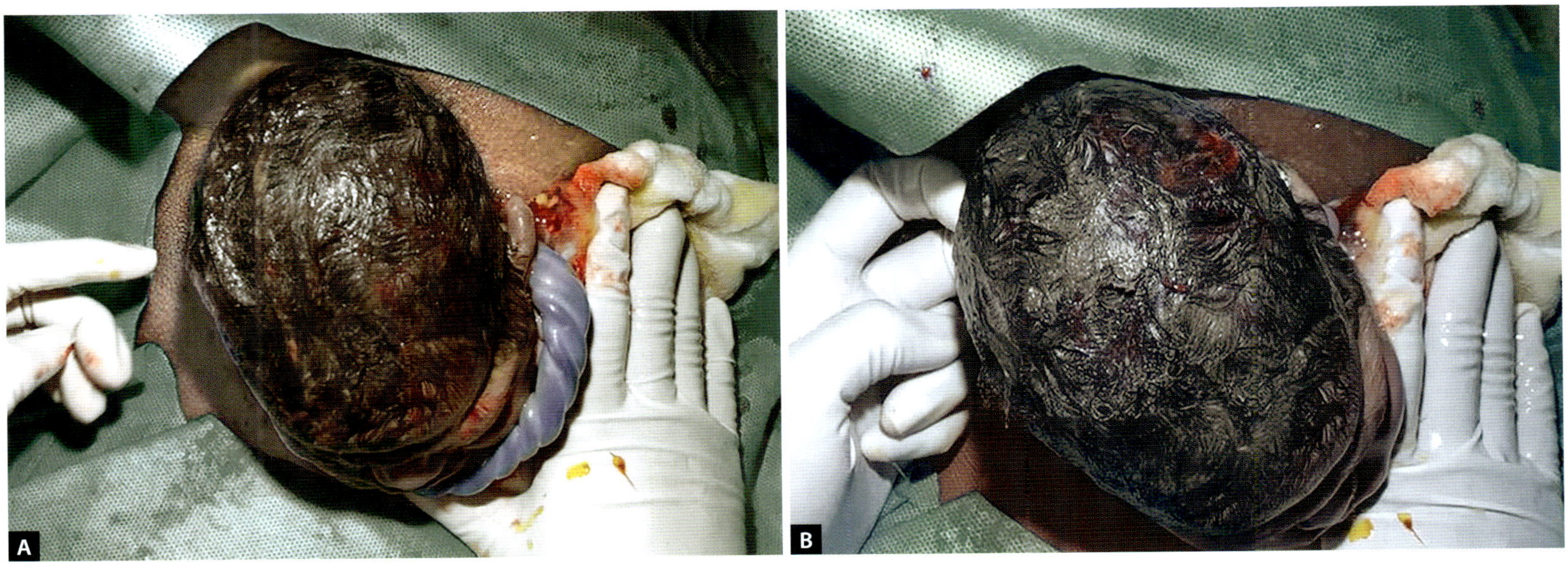

Figs. 4A and B: Restitution: Untwisting of fetal neck.

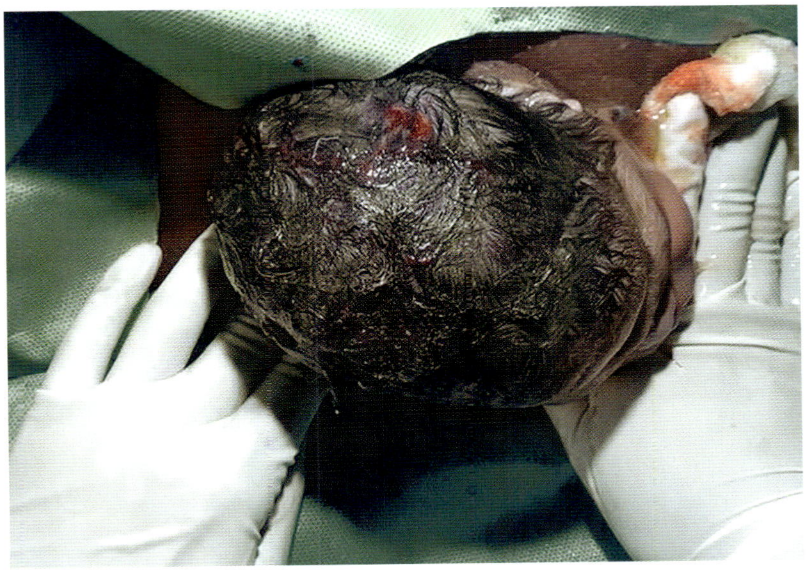

Fig. 5: External rotation: Corresponding to internal rotation of shoulders.

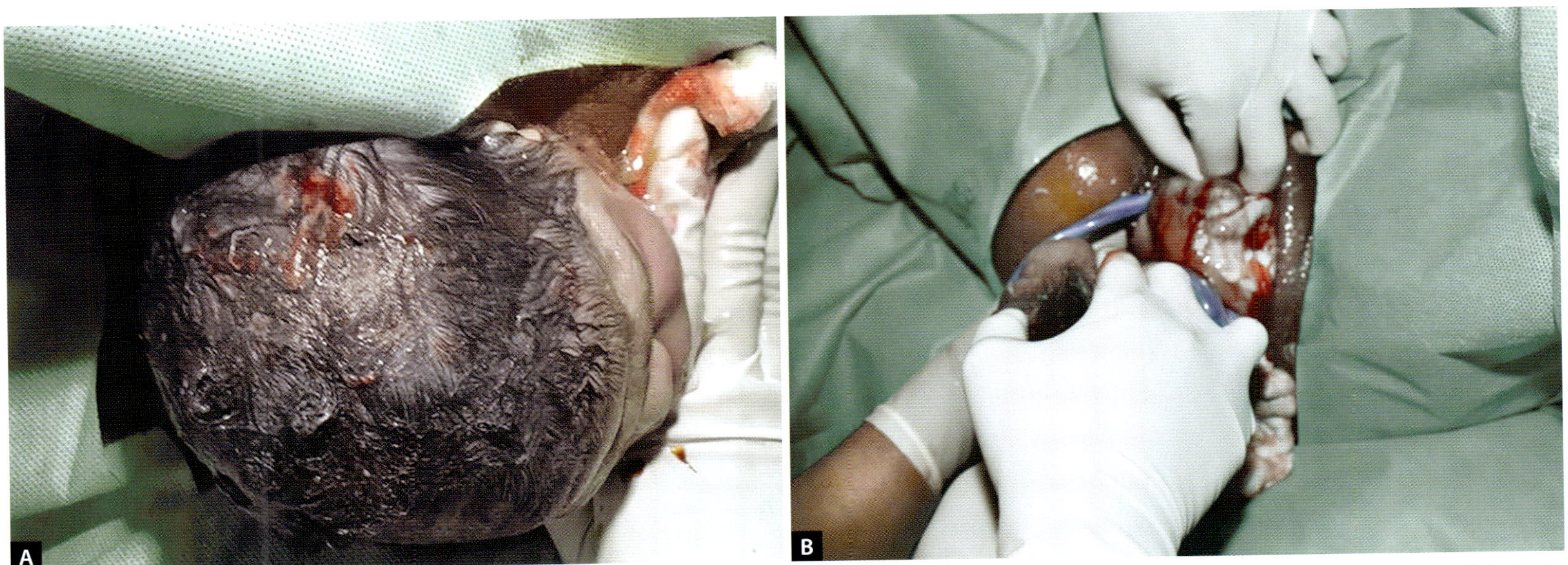

Figs. 6A and B: Delivery of the anterior shoulder by gentle downward traction of the fetal head followed by the delivery of the posterior shoulder and the rest of the body.

THIRD STAGE OF LABOR (FIGS. 7 AND 8)

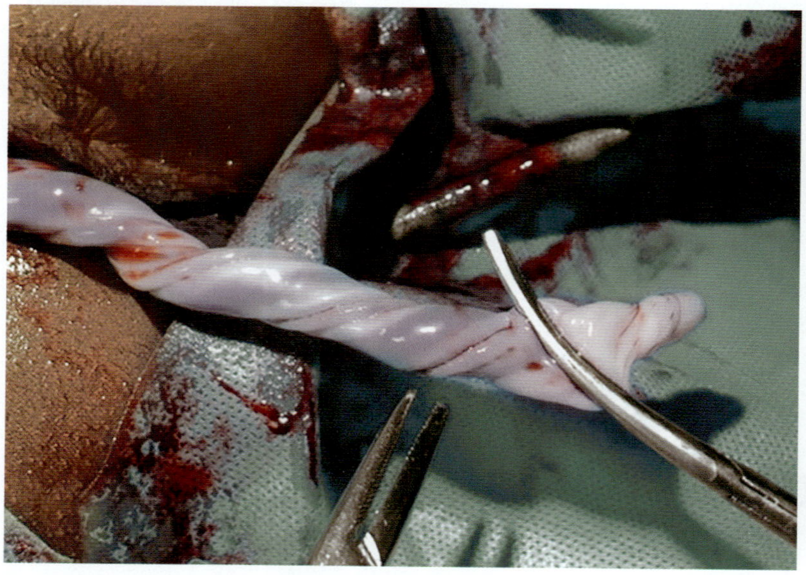

Fig. 7: After the delivery of the baby, cord clamped and cut.
Signs of placental separation: Uterus becomes globular, sudden gush of blood.
Umbilical cord protruding farther out of the vagina.

Active Management of Third Stage of Labor

- Administration of uterotonic
- Cord clamping
- Controlled cord traction for the placental delivery.

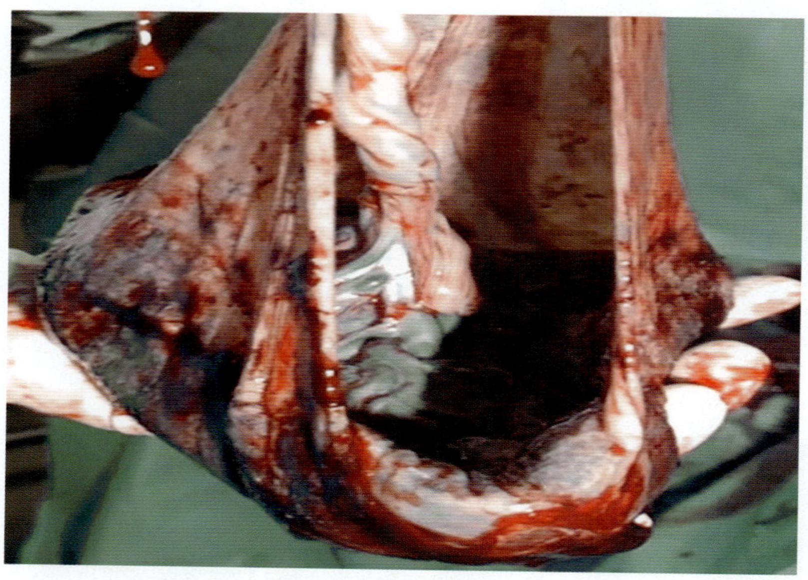

Fig. 8: Active management of third stage of labor.

FOURTH STAGE (TERMED) (FIG. 9)

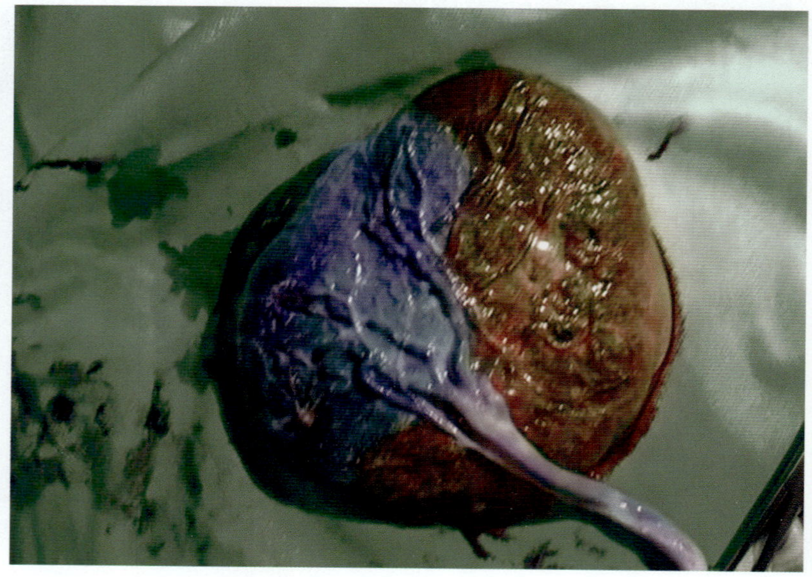

Fig. 9: Fourth stage (termed).
Checking for the completeness of the placenta.
Monitoring for postpartum hemorrhage and vitals for 1 hour.

CHAPTER

68

Vacuum-assisted Vaginal Delivery

Usha Vishwanath, Aditi Rai

It is an operative vaginal delivery with the application of vacuum device with an objective of assisting the laboring woman.

Vacuum extraction is performed for the right indications after fulfilling the necessary criteria which are similar to that of forceps application.

The contraindications for vacuum delivery are as follows:

- Incomplete dilatation of the cervix
- Intact fetal membranes
- Unengaged vertex
- Fetal malpresentation (e.g., breech, transverse lie, brow, and face)
- Suspected cephalopelvic disproportion
- Extreme prematurity

The two types of vacuum cups used are the metal and silastic cups. The cups are available in different sizes, viz., 40 mm, 50 mm, and 60 mm.

Correct placement of the vacuum cup on the fetal scalp is the most important aspect in vacuum delivery. The vacuum cup should be placed symmetrically at the median flexion point which is 2 cm anterior to the posterior fontanelle or 6 cm posterior to the anterior

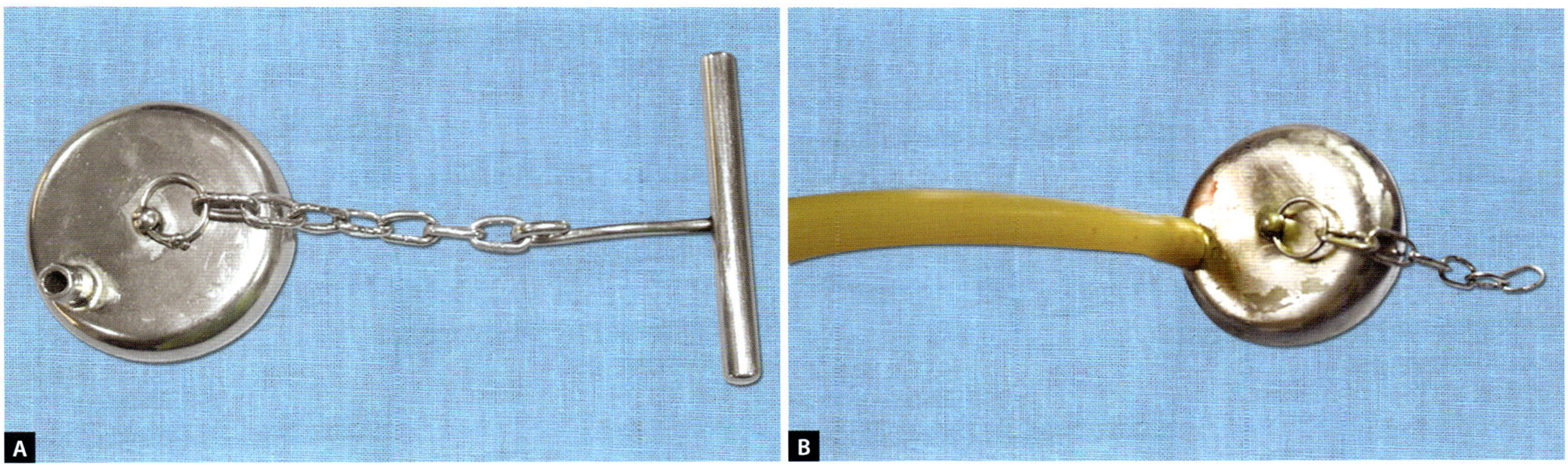

Figs. 1A and B: Vacuum cup, metallic.

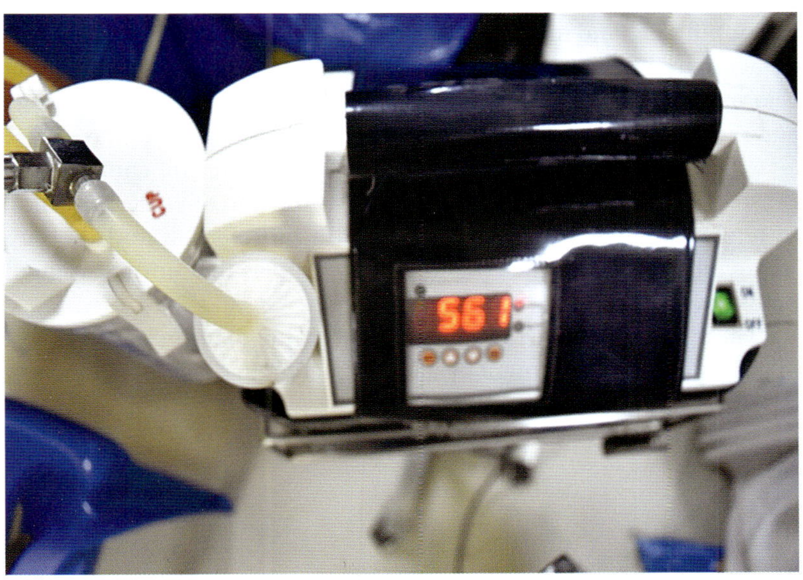

Fig. 2: Suction pump.

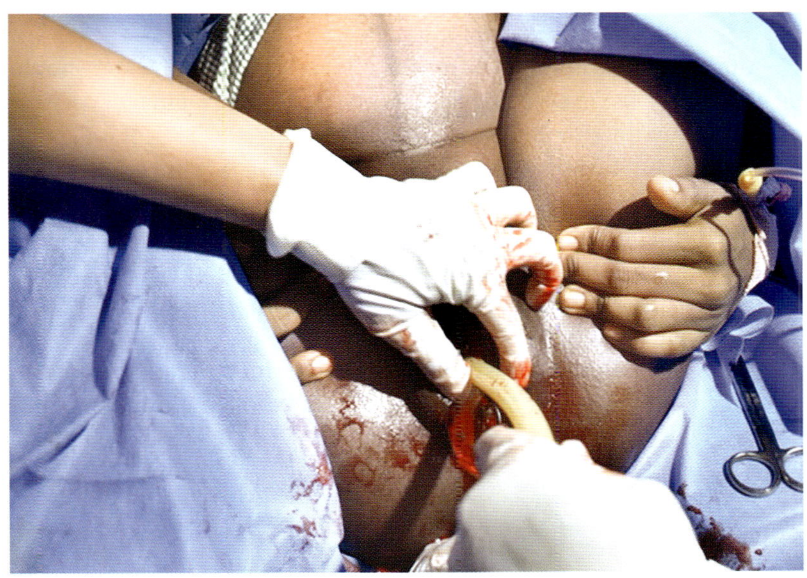

Fig. 3: Cup applied on the fetal head.

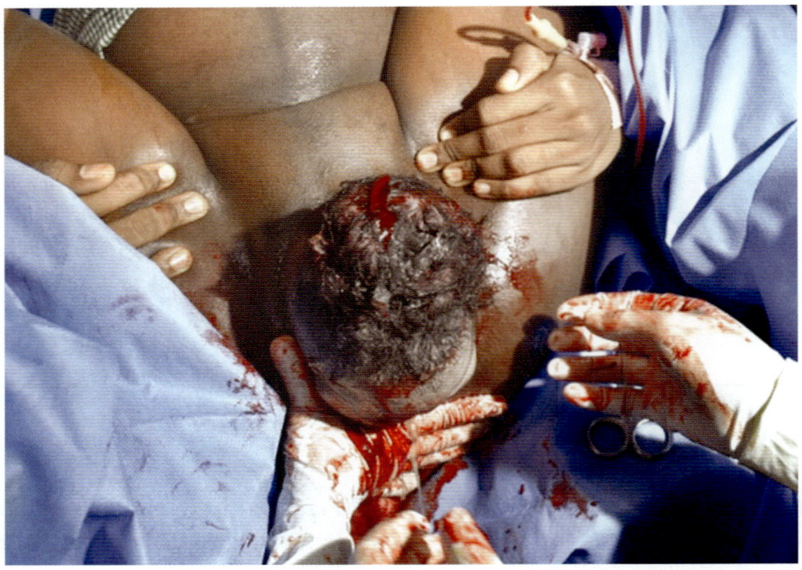

Fig. 4: Delivering the head.

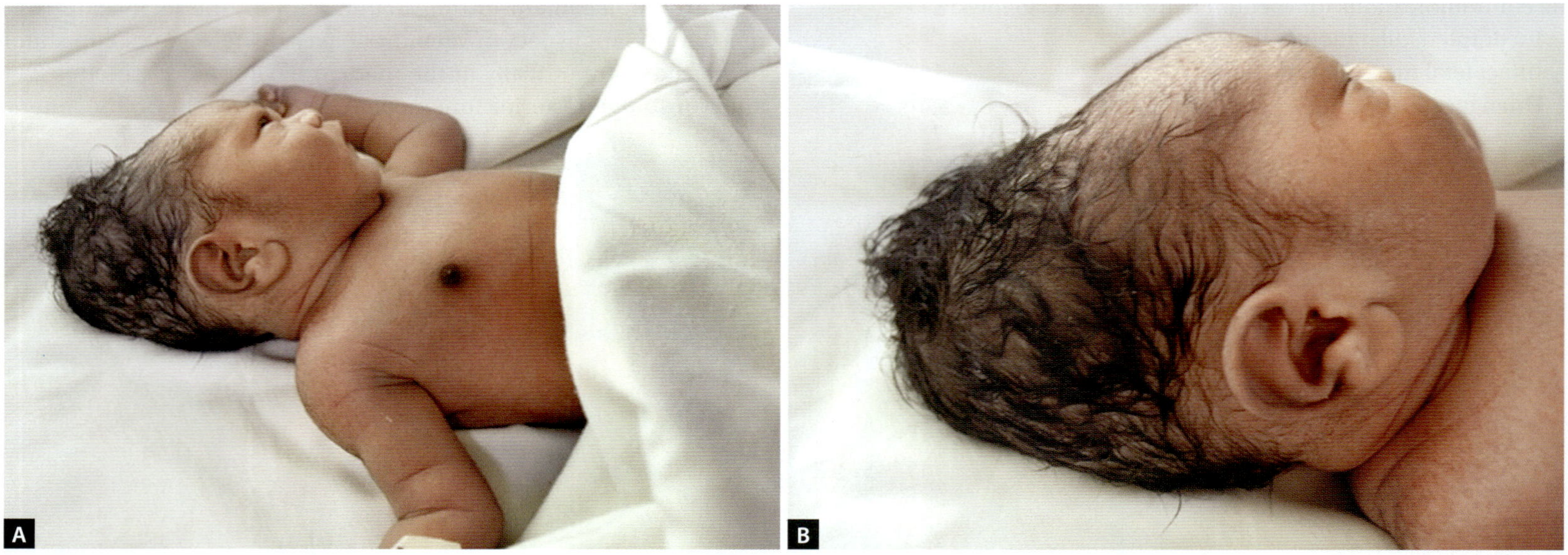

Figs. 5A and B: Caput formation on scalp.

fontanelle. It is essential to remember that the vacuum cup should not be placed on the anterior fontanelle.

After the cup is applied, the entire circumference of the cup should be palpated to make sure that there is no trapping of vaginal or cervical tissues within the vacuum cup.

Previously, it was believed that gradual and slow increase in the vacuum pressure would ensure better attachment of the vacuum cup to the fetal head and thus reduce the chances of failure. A vacuum pressure of 0.6–0.8 kg/cm^2 (500–600 mm Hg) and an artificial caput succedaneum known as chignon can be obtained in less than 2 minutes with a successful outcome.

Once the required pressure has been obtained, it is important to give sustained downward traction should be applied along the pelvic curve using two hands. The dominant hand exerts traction while the nondominant hand monitors the progress of descent and prevents cup detachment by applying counter pressure directly to the vacuum cup. The traction should be applied in concert with uterine contractions and maternal expulsive efforts.

Traction should be discontinued when the uterine contractions cease. The head descends with steady traction and once the crowning of fetal head occurs, the suction should be released and the cup removed. The rest of the baby delivers easily as in a normal vaginal delivery.

There can be failure of vacuum delivery due to improper selection of patients, wrong judgment of station, traction in the wrong direction or faulty application technique.

CHAPTER

69

Pudendal Nerve Block

Sheila K Pillai, Aditi Rai

INTRODUCTION

Pudendal nerve block or saddle block is the type of local anesthesia used commonly in obstetrics.

ANATOMY

Pudendal nerve arises from the sacral plexus in the pelvis. It is derived from the ventral rami of spinal nerves S2-S4. It originates in the pelvis, enters gluteal region through the lower part of the greater sciatic foramen, medial to the internal pudendal vessels. It leaves the gluteal region through lesser sciatic foramen to enter the pudendal canal in the lateral wall of ischioanal fossa. It terminates by dividing into branches. In the posterior part of the pudendal canal, it gives off the inferior rectal nerve and then divides into the two terminal branches, the perineal nerve and the dorsal nerve of clitoris.

The inferior rectal nerve pierces the medial wall of the pudendal canal, crosses the ischioanal fossa from lateral to medial side and supplies the external anal sphincter, skin around the anus, and the lining of the anal canal below the pectineal line.

The perineal nerve which is the larger terminal branch of the pudendal nerve runs forwards below the internal pudendal vessels and terminates by dividing into medial and lateral posterior labial nerves and muscular branches to the urogenital muscles, anterior parts of the external anal sphincter, and the levator ani muscles.

The dorsal nerve of clitoris, which is the smaller terminal branch of the pudendal nerve, runs forwards first in the pudendal canal above the internal pudendal vessels and then in the deep perineal space between these vessels and the pubic arch. Next it passes through the lateral part of the gap between the apex of the perineal membrane and the arcuate pubic ligament, runs on the dorsum of clitoris and supplies the skin of the body of the clitoris and glans.

The pudendal nerve supplies sensory branches to the lower part of vagina and vulva through the inferior rectal and the posterior labial branches. It is the nerve of the perineum. It supplies all the muscles of the perineal space including most of the skin and mucous membrane of perineum.

HISTORY AND TECHNIQUE

The use of pudendal nerve block for vaginal delivery was first reported by King in 1916. It became popular after Klink and Kohl described the modified techniques in 1953 and 1954. Pudendal nerve block is often done in patients not on epidural or spinal anesthesia. The nerve is blocked proximal to its division into the terminal branches. Pudendal nerve block offers satisfactory anesthesia for spontaneous vaginal delivery and outlet forceps delivery. It provides inadequate anesthesia for midforceps delivery, postpartum examination, and repair of upper vagina and cervix. The effectiveness of the procedure depends on the skill of the clinician performing it. The simultaneous infiltration of perineum provides better patient relief.

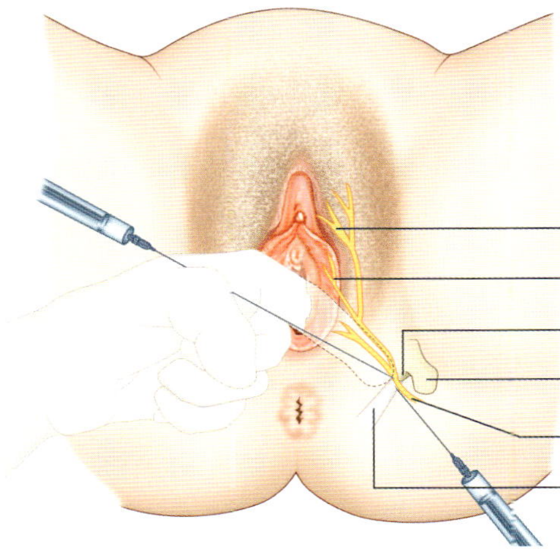

Fig. 1: Pudendal nerve block

The two routes of drug administration are transvaginal and transperineal routes. It can be done immediately prior to delivery or at the beginning of second stage of labor. Pudendal nerve block slightly prolongs the second stage of labor, without increasing the incidence of instrumental deliveries. It does not abolish the urge to bear down completely due to the overlapping innervation of the perineum. For patients not on epidural or spinal analgesia, pudendal nerve block can be performed when the patient complains of vaginal and perineal pain. It has greater efficacy for pain relief of episiotomy and its repair. Pudendal nerve block cannot abolish the pain of uterine contractions. Also as vulva receives sensory innervation from ilioinguinal nerve anteriorly and the perineal branch of the posterior cutaneous nerve of thigh posteriorly the perineal pain will not be completely relieved by pudendal nerve block.

TRANSVAGINAL APPROACH

This approach is commonly used unless the presenting part of the fetus is too low. The patient is put in lithotomy position. The ischial spine is palpated inside the vagina using index finger. The sacrospinous ligament is also palpated and its attachment to the ischial spine is identified. The obstetrician uses a needle guide to prevent injury to vagina or fetus. The needle should protrude about 1–1.5 cm beyond the needle guide to allow adequate penetration to inject the drug. The needle and needle guide are introduced into the vagina with the left hand for the left side of the pelvis and with the right hand for the right side of the pelvis. The needle is introduced through the vaginal mucosa and sacrospinous ligament, just medial and posterior to the ischial spine. The needle passes through the tough sacrospinous ligament and then loss of resistance is felt. As the internal pudendal vessels are very close to the nerve always aspirate for blood before and during the injection of the local anesthetic agent. Typically the needle is steadied and about 7–10 mL of drug is injected on each side. If the procedure is combined with perineal infiltration then care should be taken to note the total dose of the drug given. 2% chloroprocaine or 1% lidocaine can be used. Frequent failure of the procedure is often noted. Sensitivity to the drug used can occur.

TRANSPERINEAL APPROACH

The patient is put in lithotomy position. A skin wheal is made at a point midway between ischial tuberosity and anus. A needle is introduced through the wheal and advanced to reach the ischial spine. After negative aspiration test for blood, 10 mL of the local anesthetic agent is injected. The procedure is repeated on the other side also.

COMPLICATIONS

Complications possible include laceration of vaginal mucosa, systemic toxicity (due to intravascular injection or excessive dose of the drug), vaginal, ischiorectal or retroperitoneal hematoma (due to injury of internal pudendal vessels), and retropsoal or subgluteal abscess. These are very rare. Fetal complications like trauma and inadvertent injection of local anesthetic are rare. Needlestick injury to the obstetricians is also rare but possible complication.

CHAPTER

70

Regular Instruments in Obstetrics and Gynecology

Shwetha Shah, Aditi Rai, B Ramesh

INTRODUCTION

While describing any instrument, it should be held in correct position as it is used in operation theatre. It should be identified correctly, with its complete name, including the name of the person who invented it, describe the parts and mention how it is sterilized, mention how it is introduced, and lastly mention their uses and begin with common indications.

RETRACTORS

Deaver Retractor (Figs. 1A and B)

At its upper end, it has a curved C-shaped blade, attached to a handle and its distal end is curved. It is sterilized by autoclaving.

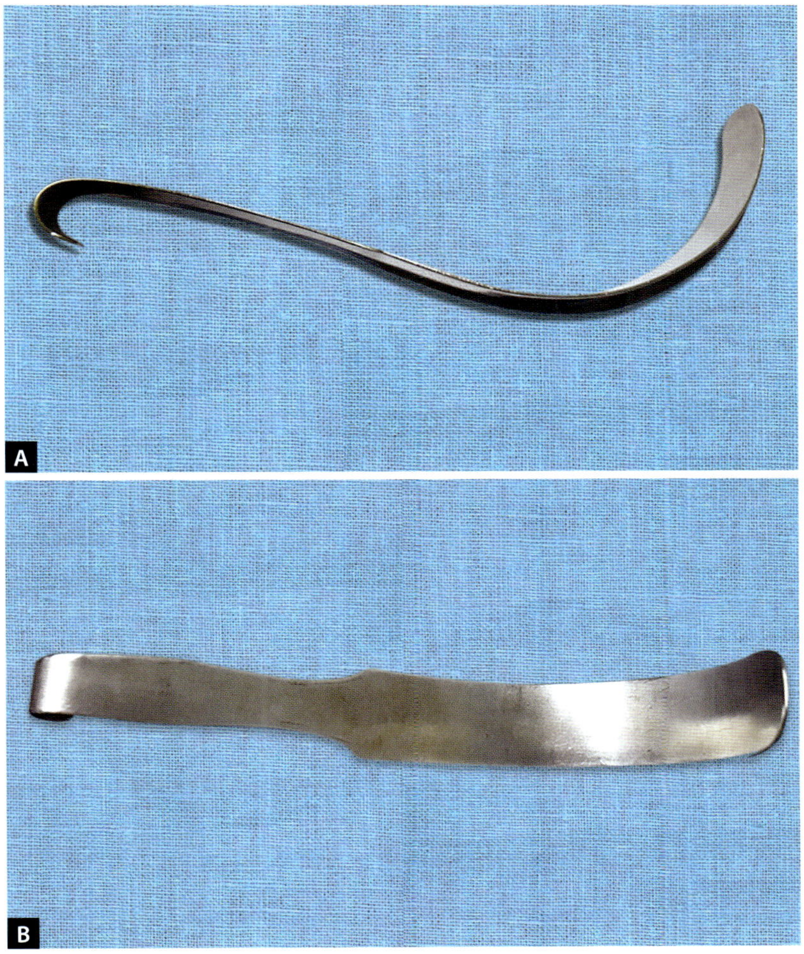

Figs. 1A and B: Deaver retractor.

Uses

To retract intraperitoneal structures like bowel, omentum, bladder and sides of abdominal incision in surgeries like abdominal, vaginal and Wertheim hysterectomy, and exploratory laparotomy.

Method of Insertion

After opening the peritoneal cavity and packing the bowel, it is introduced covered with single mop to keep them retracted from operative field.

Landons Bladder Retractor (Fig. 2)

It is L-shaped retractor having flat blade with a circular opening for finger introduction. It is ideal for vaginal surgeries as the blade is flat and narrow, thus occupying little space in anterior pouch. It is sterilized by autoclaving.

Uses

During vaginal hysterectomy to retract the bladder away from cervix and uterus after the uterovesical (UV) fold has been opened.

Doyen Retractor (Fig. 3)

It is having a broad transverse curved blade at its upper end with a handle. It is sterilized by autoclaving.

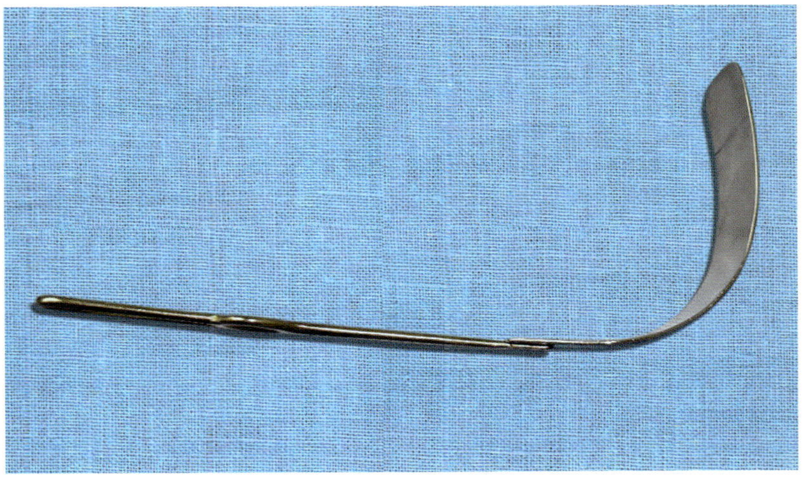

Fig. 2: Landons bladder retractor.

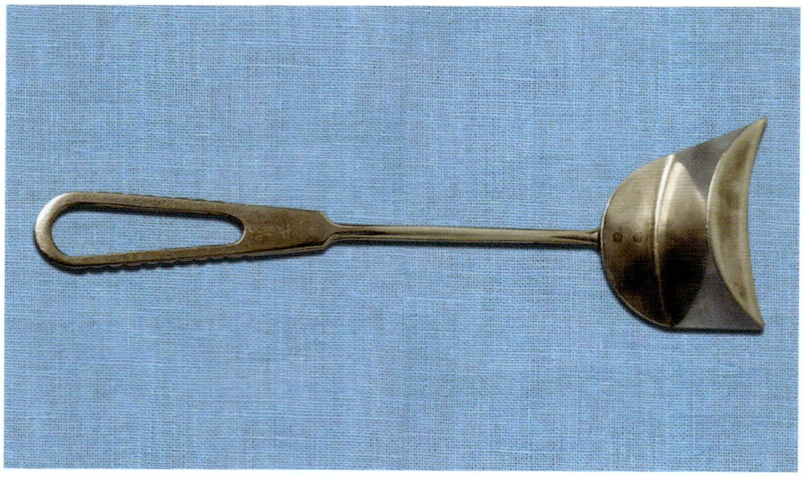

Fig. 3: Doyen retractor.

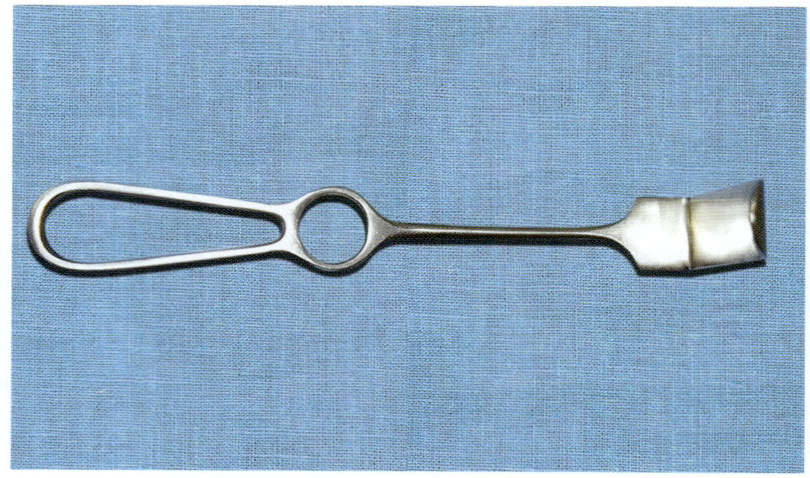

Fig. 4: Right angled retractor.

Uses

- To retract lower angle of abdominal incision.
- *In gynecology:* Abdominal and Wertheim hysterectomy, tuboplasty, exploratory laparotomy, and myomectomy.
- *In obstetrics:* Lower segment cesarean sections and obstetric hysterectomy.

Right Angled Retractor (Fig. 4)

It is used for retraction of sides of skin incision during abdominal and vaginal hysterectomy, tuboplasty, exploratory laparotomy, and during lower segment cesarean section (LSCS).

FORCEPS (FIG. 5)

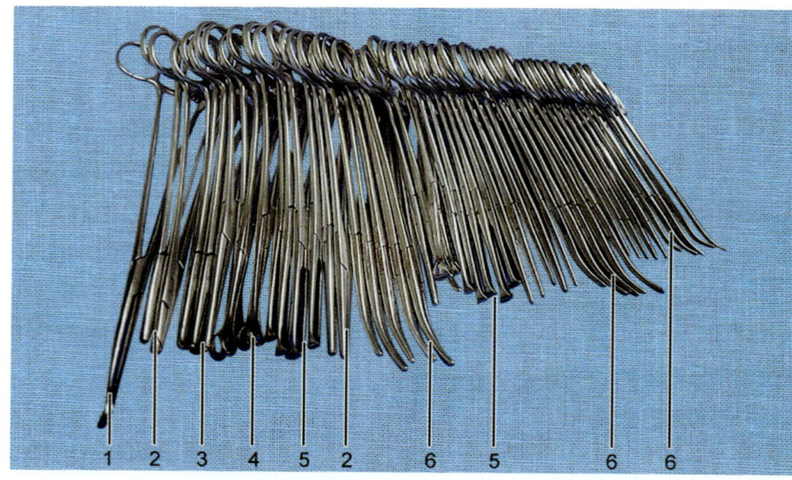

Fig. 5: Different types of forceps.

1. Sponge holding forceps or ring forceps or swab holder

It is a long straight instrument with ring shaped tips which has serrations inside and a handle with two finger rings. It is used for painting and preparing parts preoperatively and to swab out cavities like vagina.

Obstetrics: To hold lips of pregnant cervix during os tightening, for cervical tracing, and to push down the bladder during LSCS.

2. Needle holder

It is used to hold needles while suturing. The tips are blunt and the inner surface of the blade has crisscross serrations with longitudinal groove to secure the needle in place. Long needle holders are used to suture in deep pelvis.

3. Square jaw single-tooth tenaculum or single-tooth vulsellum

It is long curved instrument with its upper end having a single tooth on each blade, with a handle and a ratchet lock. It is used to hold lips of nulliparous cervix. It is used during hysterosalpingography (HSG) and is placed transversely to prevent spillage of dye during chromopertubation.

4. Babcock atraumatic forceps

It is a straight instrument with semicircular fenestrated blades for holding tubular structures and a handle with finger rings and ratchet lock. It is used to hold fallopian tubes in tubal sterilizations, tuboplasty, and in ruptured ectopic pregnancy.

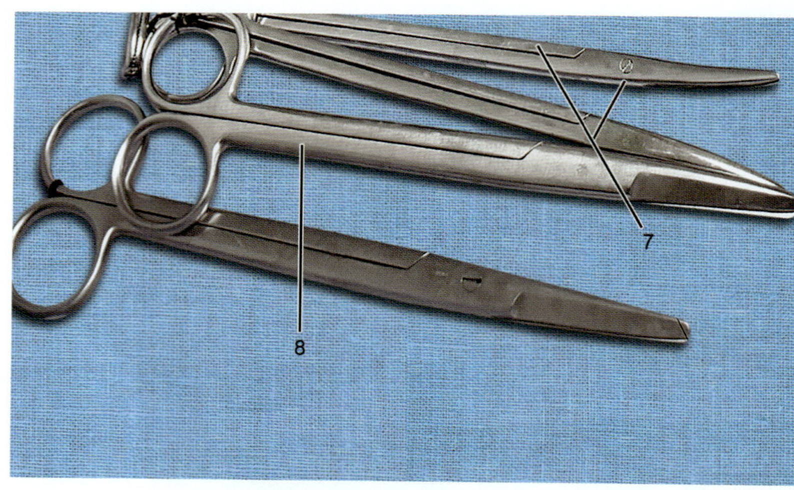

Fig. 6: Metzenbaum and Mayo scissors.

5. Allis tissue holding forceps

Its upper end is curved inwards and has rat teeth which fit into each other, with a handle and a ratchet lock. It is available as long and short. It is used to hold the rectus sheath while opening and closing the abdomen.

In gynecology: To hold edges of vagina in anterior colporrhaphy, colpoperineorrhaphy, during vaginal hysterectomy to open the anterior and posterior pouches.

In obstetrics: During LSCS, to hold the uterine angles, to catch the apex of episiotomy.

6. Hemostatic artery forceps or clamp

It is discovered by Jules-Émile Péan. It is straight or curved available in small, medium, and large sizes. The tip has tapering blades with transverse serrations. It has a handle with three ratchets. The first lock catches the tissue, the second lock clamps the tissue, and third crushes the tissue. Mosquito is a very fine instrument that is used in surgeries like tuboplasty. For holding tissue straight are used and to hold bleeders deep inside pelvis curved are preferred. It is used to secure bleeders, hold peritoneum, to crush the fallopian tube during tubal ligation.

7. Metzenbaum or nelson scissors (Fig. 6)

They are available in various sizes, tips are rounded and sharp, and have longer handle to blade ratio. They are used for cutting delicate tissue and for blunt dissection.

8. Mayo scissors (Fig. 6)

It is heavy duty scissor with narrow but semi blunt edges. It is used to cut fascia and sutures.

CHAPTER

71

Obstetric Forceps

Shwetha Shah, G Hemasree, B Ramesh

DEFINITION

It is a pair of instruments especially designed to assist, the extraction of fetal head or to overcome certain abnormalities either in the power, passage or passenger that interfere in the progress of labor.

In modern obstetrics, the only permissible forceps is an outlet or low forceps and the discussion will be limited to this variety only.

INDICATIONS[1]

Indications of obstetric forceps are given in **Table 1**.

CONTRAINDICATIONS

- Incompletely dilated cervix
- Floating head
- Obstructed labor
- Malpresentations
- Contracted pelvis.

PREREQUISITES FOR FORCEPS APPLICATION[2,3]

Table 2 presents prerequisites for forceps application.

PARTS OF FORCEPS (FIG. 1)

- Blades
- Shank
- Lock
- Handle.

Table 1: Indications of obstetric forceps.

Maternal	*Fetal*
Cut short 2nd stage of labor	Nonreassuring fetal heart
Maternal exhaustion	After coming head of breech
Prolonged 2nd stage	Postmaturity
Conditions where bearing down efforts are to be avoided	

Table 2: prerequisites for forceps application.

Maternal	*Fetal*	*Others*
Fully dilated cervix	Fetal head engaged	Presence of neonatologist
Ruptured membranes	Station exactly known	Informed consent
Pelvis adequate		Experienced obstetrician
Empty bladder, adequate maternal analgesia and anesthesia		Episiotomy Aseptic technique

TECHNIQUE OF FORCEPS APPLICATION (FIGS. 2 TO 11)

- Informed consent obtained.
- Patient is painted and draped.
- Bladder is drained.
- Pelvic examination is done to confirm the required prerequisites for forceps application.

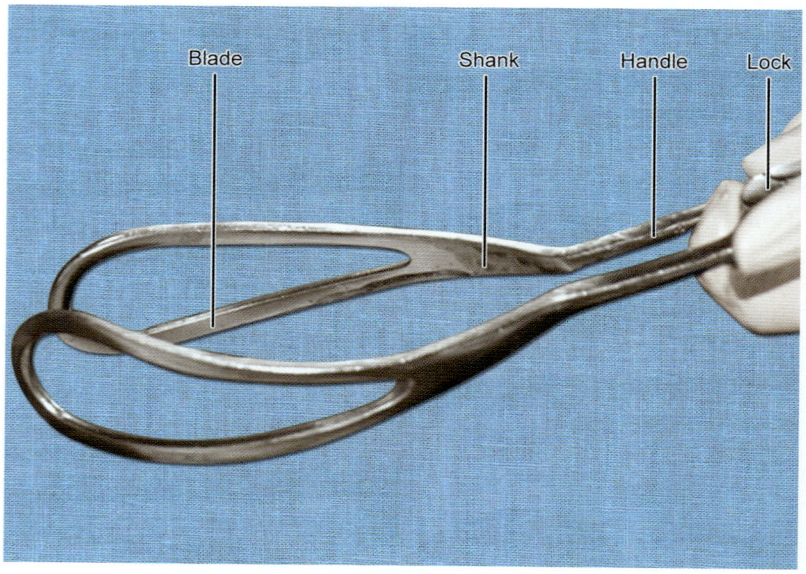

Fig. 1: Parts of forceps.

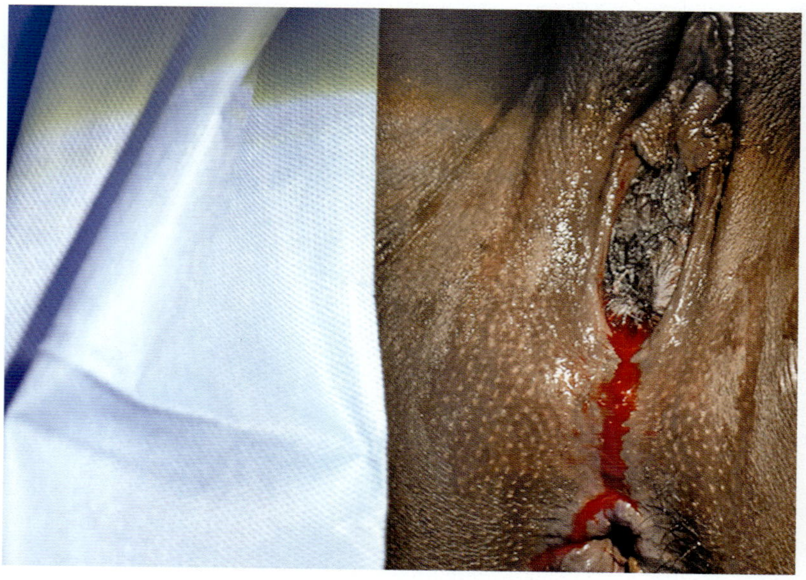

Fig. 2: Fetal head visible at introitus.

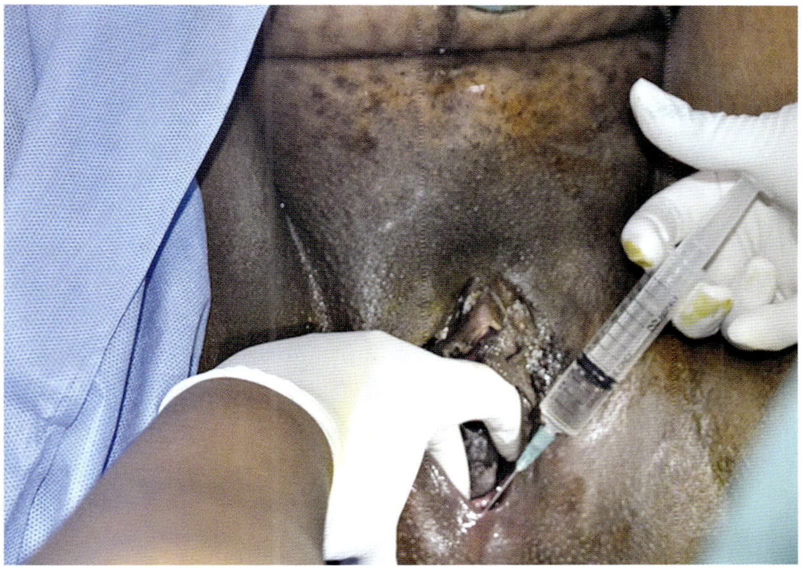

Fig. 3: Adequate local anesthetic infiltrated.

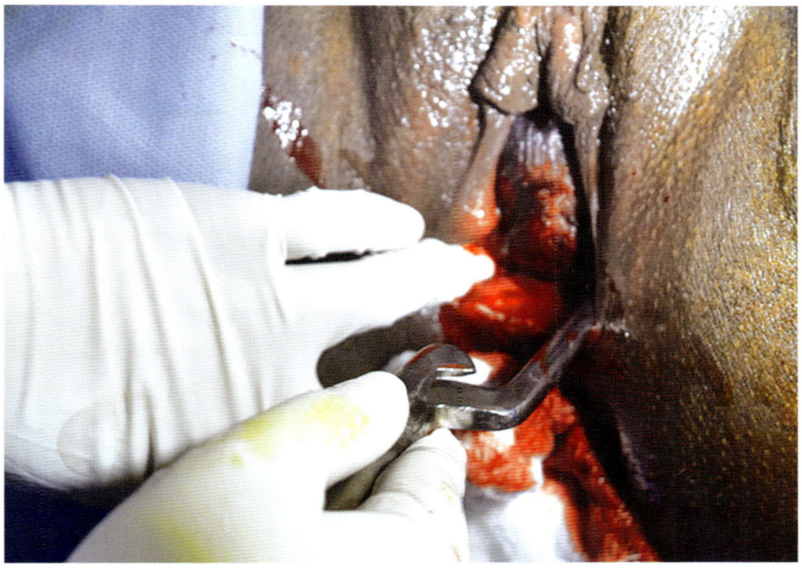

Fig. 6: The blade is rotated so that it lies parallel to the floor.

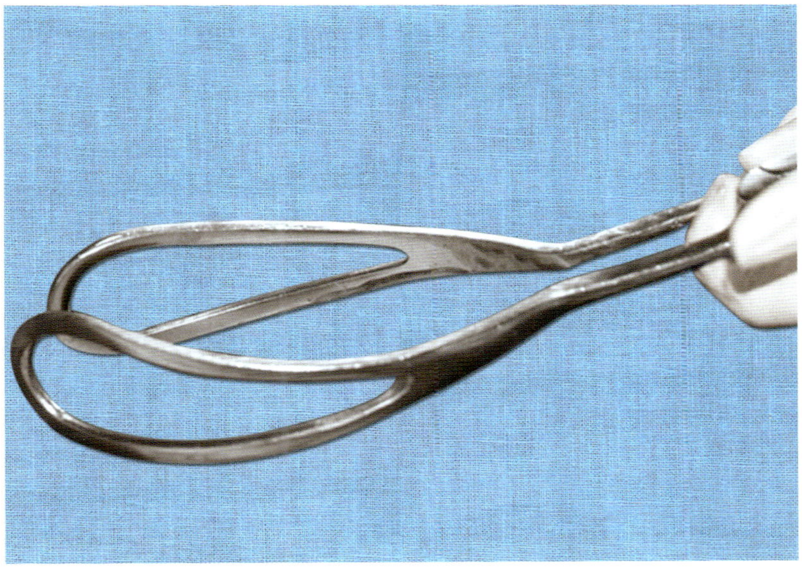

Fig. 4: Articulated forceps before application.

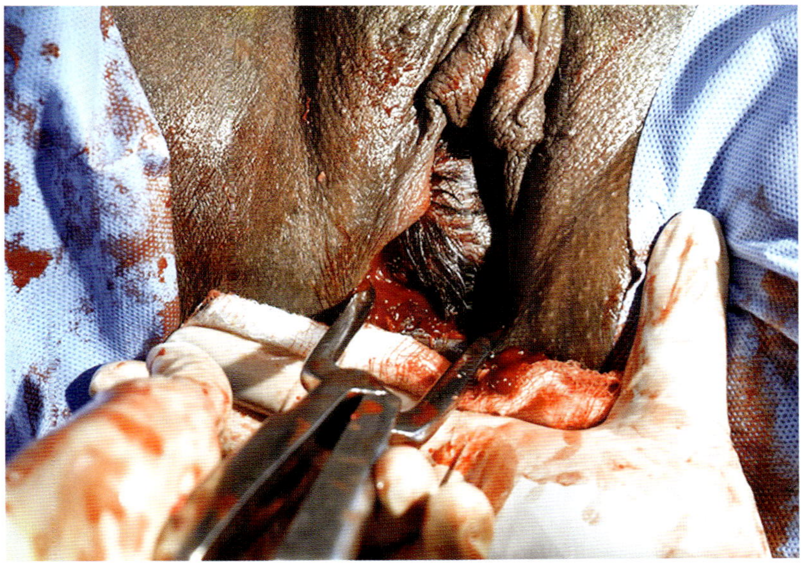

Fig. 7: After the blades of both side are applied correctly they are interlocked.

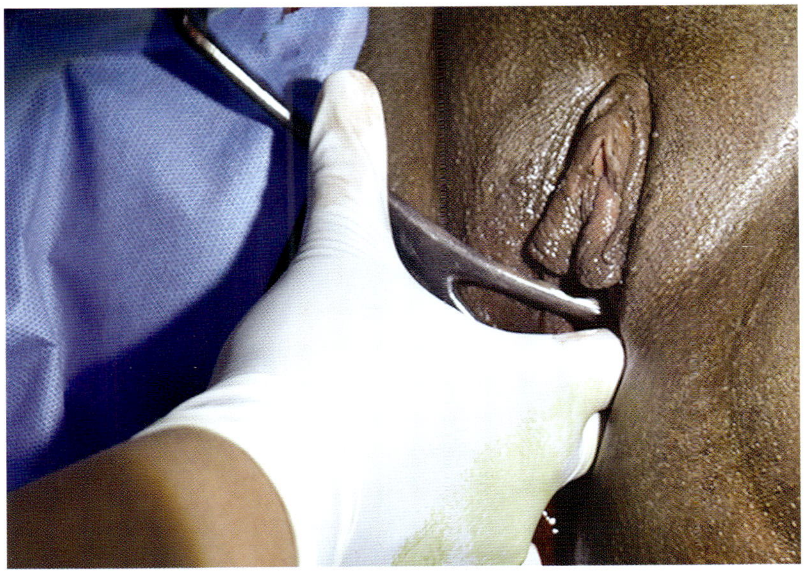

Fig. 5: The left blade is introduced by holding in left hand under guidance of index and middle finger of right hand, kept vaginally and slided till the fenestrum disappears.

COMPLICATIONS[4]

Maternal and fetal complications are presented in **Table 3**.

POSTOPERATIVE CARE

- Prophylactic antibiotics and analgesics should be given
- Routine episiotomy care and perineal hygiene
- Patient should be encouraged to void urine and timing of first voiding should be noted.

FAILED FORCEPS

It is failure of forceps to extract the fetus.

Causes:

- Cannot apply blades
- Blades fail to Interlock
- Blades slip after application
- Failure of blades to rotate.

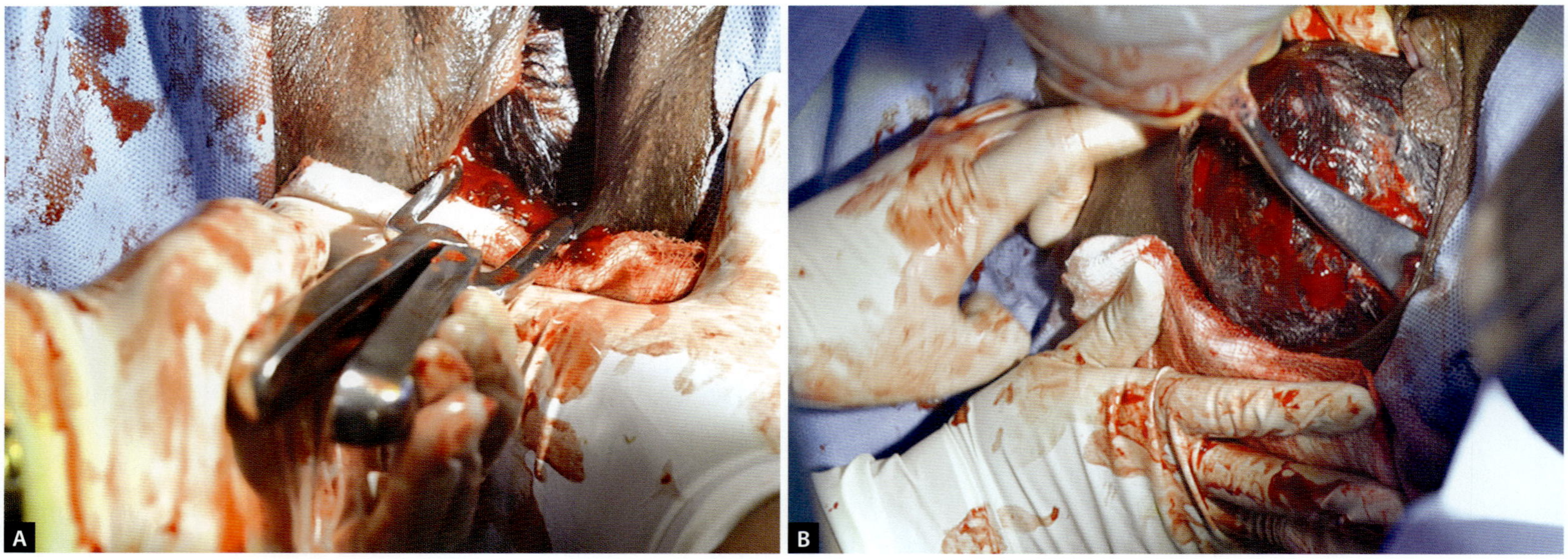

Figs. 8A and B: Traction is first applied in downward direction followed by downward and forward.

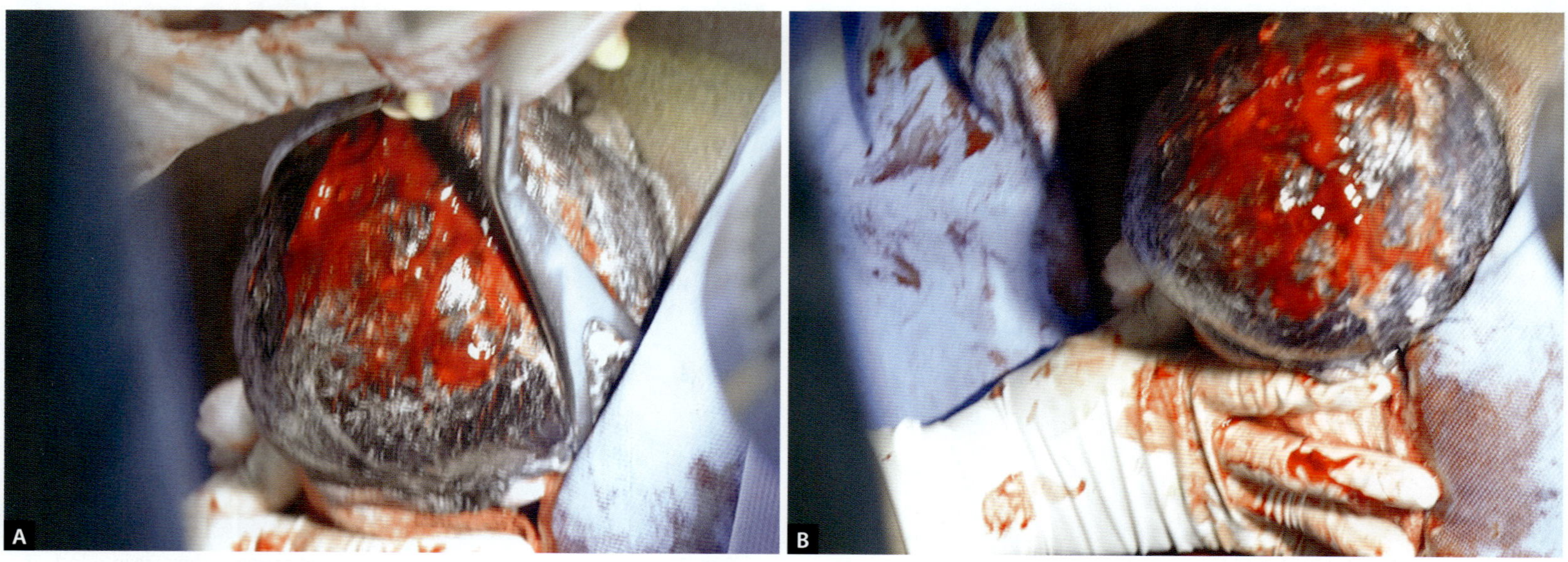

Figs. 9A and B: As soon as the head is delivered the forceps are disengaged and further delivery is aided with help of modified Ritgen maneuver.

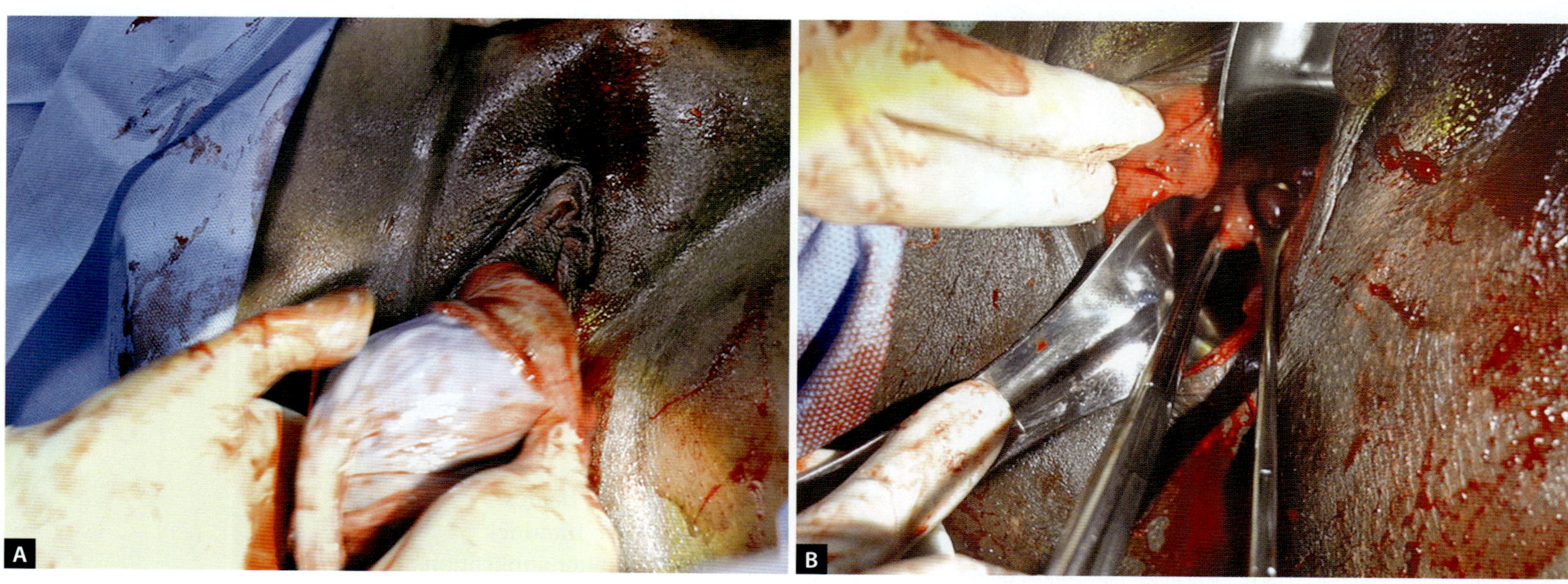

Figs. 10A and B: After placental delivery, cervical tracing is done.

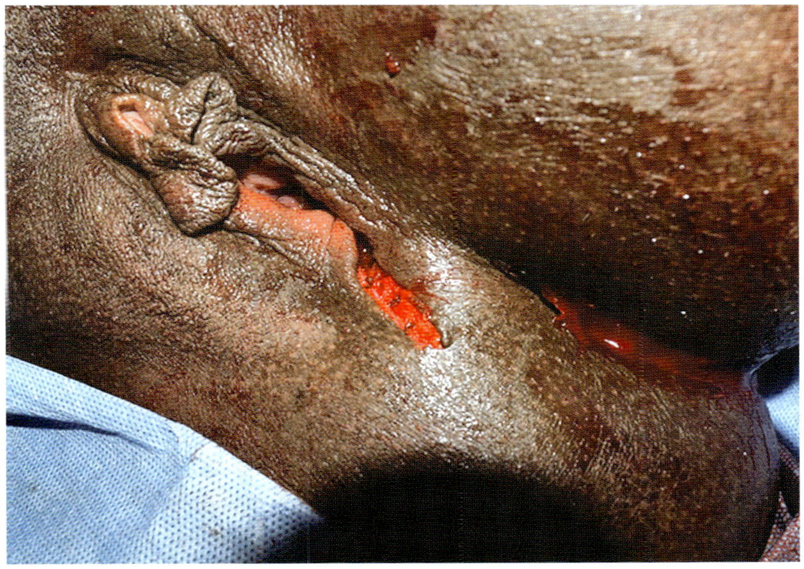

Fig. 11: Episiotomy is sutured in layers.

Table 3: Complications of obstetric forceps.

Maternal		*Fetal*	
Early	*Late*	*Early*	*Late*
Lacerations of cervix, vagina, perineum	Anal sphincter injuries, fecal incontinence	Cephalhematomas, lacerations, bruising	Delayed milestone, cerebral palsy
Extension of episiotomy	Vesicovaginal, rectovaginal fistulas	Depressed skull fractures	Mental retardation
Hematomas	Stress urinary incontinence	Intracranial hemorrhage	Behavioral problems
Postpartum urinary retention	Genital prolapse		

TRIAL OF FORCEPS

Patient is assessed and forceps delivery is attempted, if there is failure of descent of head after two pulls, abandon the application and take patient for lower segment cesarean section (LSCS).

FUTURE OF FORCEPS

It still has place in modern obstetrics provided it is performed judiciously with proper selection of cases and with careful and timely application. It has not only reduced unnecessary cesarean sections, but also maternal and fetal complications due to prolonged labor. Improper training has bought this very important skill to verge of extinction.

REFERENCES

1. British Columbia Reproductive Care Program. Obstetric Guideline 14: Assisted vaginal birth: the use of forceps or vacuum extractor. Vancouver, Canada: BCRCP; 2001.
2. Royal Australian and New Zealand College of Obstetricians and Gynaecologists. College Statement C-Obs 16: instrumental vaginal delivery. Melbourne, Australia: RANZCOG; 2009.
3. Royal Australian and New Zealand College of Obstetricians and Gynaecologists. College Statement C-Obs 13: Guidelines for use of rotational forceps. Melbourne, Australia: RANZCOG; 2009.
4. Dupuis O, Madelenat P, Rudigoz RC. Fecal and urinary incontinence after delivery: risk factors and prevention]. Gynecol Obstet Fertil. 2004;32: 540-8.

CHAPTER

72

Cesarean Section

Sowmya MS, G Hemasree, B Ramesh

INTRODUCTION

A cesarean section is the delivery of a fetus through an abdominal and uterine incision; technically, it is a laparotomy followed by a hysterotomy.[1] This definition considers only the location of the fetus and not whether the fetus is delivered alive or dead.

HISTORY

The first step toward the cesarean operation as it is currently performed was described by Sanger.[2,3] He proposed a procedure that was much less radical and designed to conserve fertility. His operation did not involve hysterectomy and adnexectomy, but instead consisted of removing the peritoneum from a portion of the anterior uterine wall and performing a 2 cm wide wedge resection of the anterior uterine wall. The wedge was cut so that a thick edge of myometrium was adjacent to the peritoneum and a thin edge was adjacent to the endometrial cavity. These modifications allowed the serosal edges to be incorporated into the closure with interrupted silk sutures.[1,4] The technique was further improved on by Garrigues, who did not resect the myometrium but instead simply closed the uterine incision. Other modifications included not dissecting the uterine serosa from the uterus and the introduction of silver wire to approximate the myometrium in addition to the interrupted silk sutures on the serosal surface.[1]

Operative techniques continued to improve during the 18th and 19th centuries. Cesarean section became a safer operation that could be used at an earlier stage in difficult labors, and a number of perioperative and intraoperative modifications emerged. The bladder and the rectum were emptied preoperatively, with catheters and enemas, respectively, to decrease the volume of these organs in the operative field, thereby reducing the risk of injury during the surgical procedure. Preoperative antimicrobial preparation was introduced by Lister in 1876 and included shaving the operative area and applying antiseptic solutions to the operative field. Vaginal douching was also introduced and routinely performed before performing cesarean deliveries.[1]

The technique of laparotomy and site of hysterotomy incision were vigorously debated and modified. Abdominal incisions were made to the right or left of the rectus muscles or in the midline along the linea nigra. The uterine incision was made vertically in the midline, obliquely, transversely through the contractile myometrium, laterally 7.2–10 cm from the fundus, or on the posterior aspect of the uterus.[1]

The first report of uterine closure was not until 1769. A number of suture materials were used to close the uterus, including silver wire, silk, and catgut. Uterine closure was associated with decreased perioperative blood loss. Early surgeons often sutured the uterine incision to the anterior abdominal wall to encourage adhesion formation to reinforce the uterus and allow it to tolerate future gestations.[1]

Closure of the abdominal incision slowly evolved from choosing to leave the wound open and apply only bandages to allow healing by secondary intention to full closure of the abdominal wall. However, the proponents of abdominal closure were in disagreement regarding which layers required reapproximation. Many closed only the skin, whereas others closed all layers. Drainage of the surgical site was also introduced.

Johnson first described a lower segment uterine incision in 1786.[1] In 1908, Selheim suggested that a uterine incision made in the lower uterine segment rather than the contractile segment of the myometrium would decrease blood loss at surgery and decrease blood loss in the event of uterine dehiscence.[1,4]

The development of the modern cesarean operation has not been a recent accomplishment, but instead represents a series of innovations over many centuries of trial and error. Many aspects of the operation as it is commonly performed today are not based on randomized trial or techniques that have been proven to be superior by rigorous study, but instead are the culmination of many years of trial and error.

EPIDEMIOLOGY

There is increasing trend in cesarean section delivery in India. With the increase in institutional deliveries and growing access to gynecological and obstetric care, cesarean section deliveries too have shown an increasing trend. A study by the Indian Council of Medical Research (ICMR) in 33 tertiary care institutions noted that the average cesarean section rate increased from 21.8% in 1993–1994 to 25.4% in 1998–1999.

According to the National Family Health Survey, 1992–1993, two states, Kerala and Goa, have shown the highest percentage of cesarean section deliveries. A rising trend in cesarean section rates, from 11.9% in 1987 to 21.4% in 1996 has been reported from Kerala.

Another study in Jaipur showed that cesarean section rates in a leading private hospital rose from 5% in 1972 to 10% in late 1970s and to 19.7% between 1980 and 1985.

Studies show that in India, the rate of cesarean section delivery is relatively much higher in private hospitals rather than in public health facilities. At the all India level, the rate has increased from 2.9% of the childbirth in 1992–1993 to 7.1% in 1998–1999 and further to 10.2% in 2005–2006.[5]

INDICATIONS

The justification for cesarean section arises from clinical judgment that the interests of mother, fetus or both served by resorting to cesarean delivery in order to avoid the continuation of pregnancy or the onset or the continuation of labor. The conditions that inform this judgment vary widely depending on population served and the clinical skills and facilities are available.[6] The decision to perform an abdominal delivery remains a joint judgment between the physician and patient after carefully weighing the pros and cons of a cesarean delivery versus continued labor and/or operative or spontaneous vaginal delivery.

The indications and proportions of cesarean delivery will vary from country to country and from hospital to hospital. Nonetheless there are four main indications that account for 60–90% of all cesarean section. This includes: repeat cesarean section (35–40%), dystocia (20–35%), breech (10–15%), and fetal distress (10–15%).[7]

PRIMARY CESAREAN SECTION AND REPEAT CESAREAN SECTION

Primary cesarean section is the delivery of the fetus through the maternal abdomen in a gravida who has not previously undergone a cesarean delivery. Repeat cesarean section refers to the gravid who refuses trial of labor or who is not a candidate for vaginal delivery. Common indications for repeat cesarean deliveries include complete placenta previa, breech presentation, fetal lie other than longitudinal after failed external cephalic version, nonreassuring fetal assessment that cannot be further evaluated clinically proven inadequate maternal pelvis, and severe pre-eclampsia hemolysis, elevated liver enzymes, and thrombocytopenia (HELLP) syndrome that is clinically worsening and is remote from delivery, cervical cancer, obstructing fibroid, and acquired immune deficiency. Indications for cesarean delivery can be divided into indications that are of benefit to the mother, the fetus, or both.

Indications for cesarean delivery for maternal benefit include any situation in which it is inadvisable to continue to strive for a vaginal delivery out of concern for maternal outcome. In these situations, the gravida undergoes a major abdominal operation for indications that are likely to decrease her risk for morbidity and/or mortality.

In contrast, when a cesarean section is performed for fetal indications, the mother is undergoing major abdominal surgery when there is no immediate benefit to her but there is potential benefit to the neonate. In these situations, fetal health would be compromised if further efforts toward vaginal delivery are pursued. Indications for abdominal delivery that fall into this classification include delivery of a nonvertex infant or nonreassuring fetal assessment. When counseling the patient before cesarean section regarding the risks and benefits of abdominal delivery, the possibility of morbidity and mortality must be discussed. This point is no less important when counseling for a repeat cesarean delivery.[8]

CLASSIFICATION OF URGENCY

Category 1: Immediate threat to the life of the women or fetus. This will include cesarean section for severe prolonged fetal bradycardia, fetal scalp blood pH < 7.2, cord prolapse, and uterine rupture. These cesareans should occur quickly as possible and certainly within 30 minutes.

Category 2: Maternal or fetal compromise, which is not immediately life-threatening. These include conditions such as antepartum hemorrhage, nonprogressive labor, and labor with maternal or fetal compromise, but not to the degree of category 1. These cases should also be category 1. These cases should also be delivered within 30 minutes if possible, but one has to take into the account the potential risks in meeting this deadline.

Category 3: No maternal or fetal compromise but early delivery required. This will include nonprogressive without maternal or fetal compromise, and women booked for elective cesarean section who are admitted with ruptured membranes or in early labor. It is recommended that these women be delivered within 75 minutes. These are other cases with slowly worsening conditions such as pre-eclampsia and intrauterine growth restriction (IUGR) in which delivery is indicated. If they are preterm and induction of labor is deemed likely to fail an early cesarean delivery is indicated may be necessary.

Category 4: Elective planned cesarean section timed to suit the woman and staff.[9-11]

ANESTHESIA

Regional anesthesia (epidural or spinal) **(Figs. 1 and 2)** should be chosen when possible as it has the least associated maternal and neonatal morbidity **(Figs. 1 and 2)**. General anesthesia may be given if there is need for extreme speed, such as in acute fetal distress, patient preference, and for women in whom regional anesthesia fails (usually less than 5%).

PREOPERATIVE CONSIDERATION

The preoperative assessment should include a full history and physical examination, past medical and surgical history, current medications, drug allergies, and indication for cesarean section.

Unless indicated by other medical complications, a complete blood count, Bispectral Index (BIS), adequate preoperative blood group, and antibody screen are adequate for preoperative blood testing.

To reduce the risk of aspiration pneumonitis women should be offered antacids and drugs (such as H2 receptor antagonists or proton pump inhibitors) to reduce gastric volumes and acidity before cesarean section.

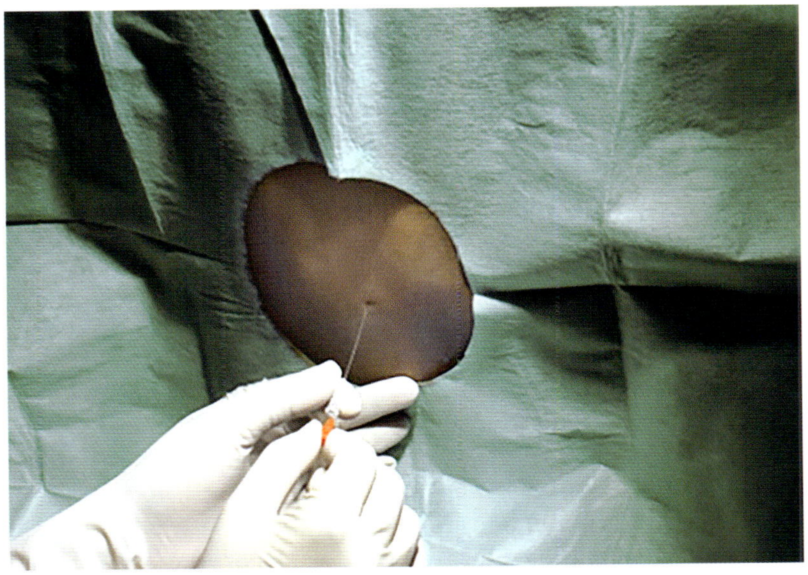

Fig. 1: Regional anesthesia (epidural or spinal).

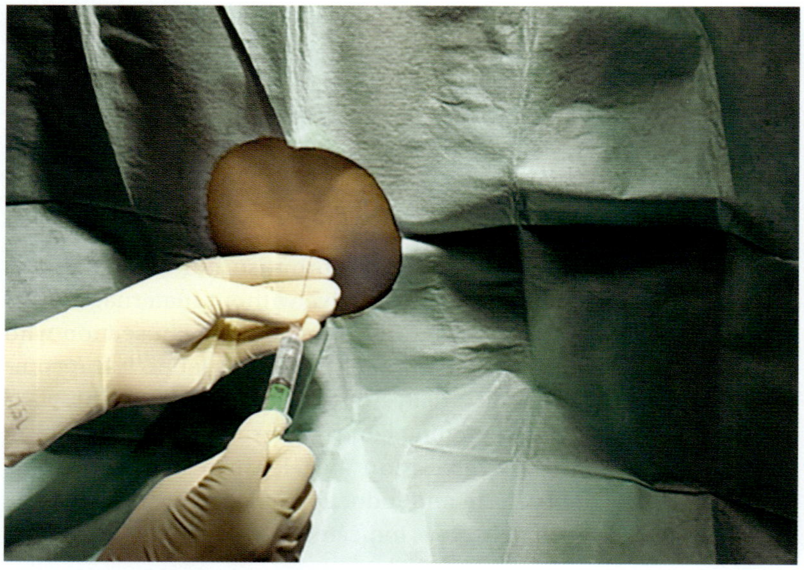

Fig. 2: Regional anesthesia (epidural or spinal).

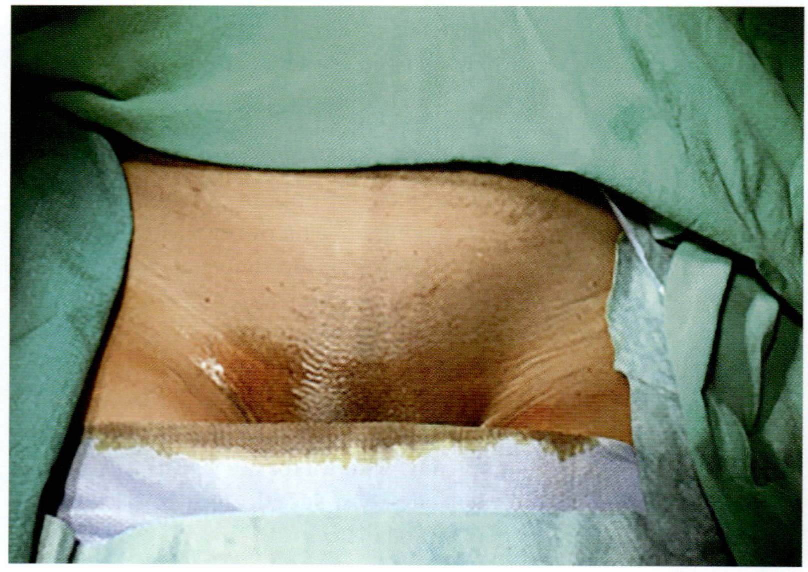

Fig. 3: Draping.

Antiemetics (either pharmacological or acupressure) to reduce nausea and vomiting during cesarean section.

A urinary (Foley) catheter is placed once regional anesthesia is established.

Preoperative shaving of the incision site is not required. If the pubic area over the proposed incision site is thick it can be clipped short, rather than shaved.

Antibiotic prophylaxis should be given both elective and emergency sections and should be administered intravenously after baby is delivered and umbilical cord is clamped. The operating table for cesarean section should have a lateral tilt of 15°, because this reduces maternal hypotension.[6,12]

SURGICAL TECHNIQUES

Skin Incision

A number of skin incisions have been used in abdominal deliveries. The most frequently used type of skin incision is the Pfannenstiel **(Fig. 5)** incision **(Figs. 3 to 5)**.

Other skin incisions used include the Joel-Cohen incision, midline vertical, Maylard, Cherney, right paramedian, and the low transverse. In general, the skin incision should be determined by the physician based on maternal body habitus, clinical situation, time available to deliver the infant, and skill of the surgeon. Midline vertical incisions are generally more hemostatic and require less dissection; therefore, less time from incision to birth than transverse incisions. Transverse incisions fall along the lines of expression of the anterior abdominal wall and therefore should create less pronounced scarring and risk of dehiscence.

Cesarean section should be performed using a transverse abdominal incision because this is associated with less postoperative pain and an improved cosmetic effect compared with a midline incision.[13]

The transverse incision of choice should be the Joel-Cohen incision (a straight skin incision, 3 cm above the symphysis pubis; subsequent tissue layers are opened bluntly and, if necessary, extended with scissors and not a knife), because it is associated with shorter operating times and reduced postoperative febrile morbidity.[13]

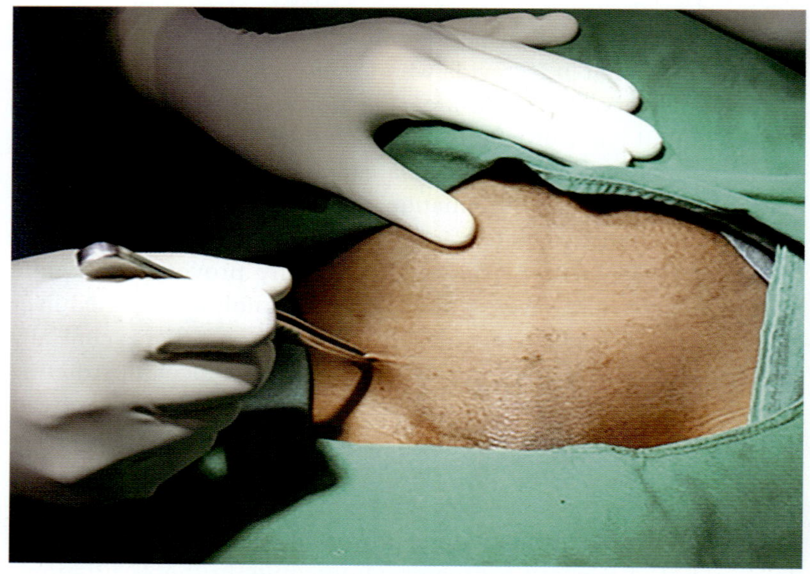

Fig. 4: Checking anesthesia with forceps before giving incision.

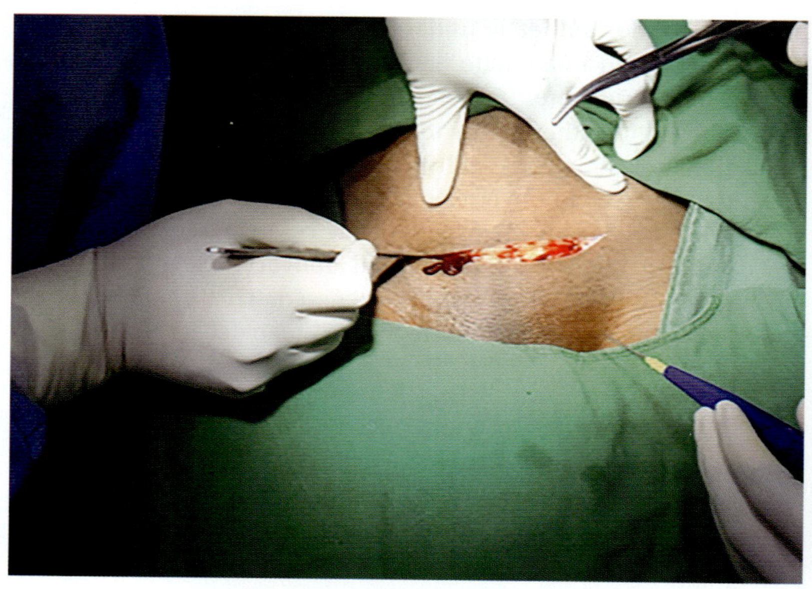

Fig. 5: Skin incision is the Pfannenstiel.

This incision is performed sharply to the level of the anterior rectus fascia **(Fig. 6)**. The anterior rectus fascia is then sharply incised with the scalpel in a transverse manner in the midline to expose the belly of the rectus muscle on either side of the midline. At this time, the incision in the anterior rectus fascia may be extended laterally using either the scalpel or the Mayo scissors.

After the fascia is incised, the anterior rectus fascia can then be dissected from the underlying rectus muscles in both the cephalad and caudad directions. This is accomplished by grasping the cut edges of the fascia with a pair of Allis forceps and using a combination of blunt **(Fig. 7)** and sharp dissection to free the muscle from the overlying fascia **(Figs. 8 and 9)**. This dissection allows the rectus muscles to be retracted laterally without being cut. During this dissection, care must be taken to identify and ligate or electrocoagulate the perforating vessels between the rectus muscles and the anterior fascia; this can be performed at entry, or in the event of an emergency cesarean delivery, at the time of closure. The posterior sheath consists of the fascia of the transversalis muscle and is closely opposed to the peritoneum. These tissues may be incised in either a longitudinal or transverse manner.

Regardless of which manner is chosen, the entry point to open peritoneal cavity should be as high as possible and then extended down under transillumination to avoid injury to the maternal bladder **(Figs. 10 to 12)**.

After opening the peritoneal cavity the uterus is checked for dextrorotation or levorotation the former is more common due to the sigmoid colon. This appraisal of the orientation is important in placing the uterine incision, otherwise it is eccentric and extend into uterine vessels on one side.[7] The loose uterovesical peritoneum is identified **(Fig. 13)**. The attachment of this peritoneum, where it adheres to the surface of uterus, is upper margin of lower uterine segment. The peritoneum should be divided about 2–3 cm below the level of this attachment in the midline and then extended laterally towards each side. The loose areolar tissue between the lower uterine segment and bladder is gently separated with forefinger and doyen or similar retractor placed to move the bladder down and keep it from the line of uterine incision **(Figs. 14 and 15)**.

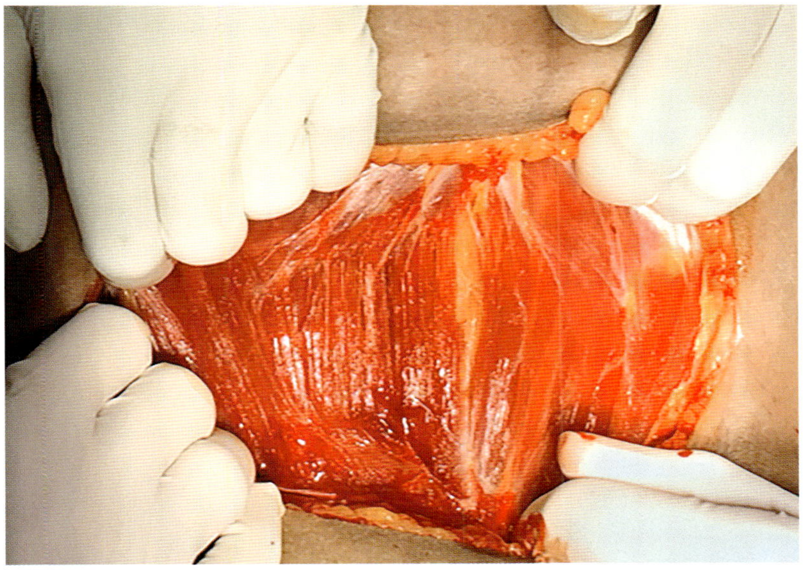

Fig. 7: The anterior rectus fascia can then be dissected from the underlying rectus muscles in both the cephalad and caudad directions.

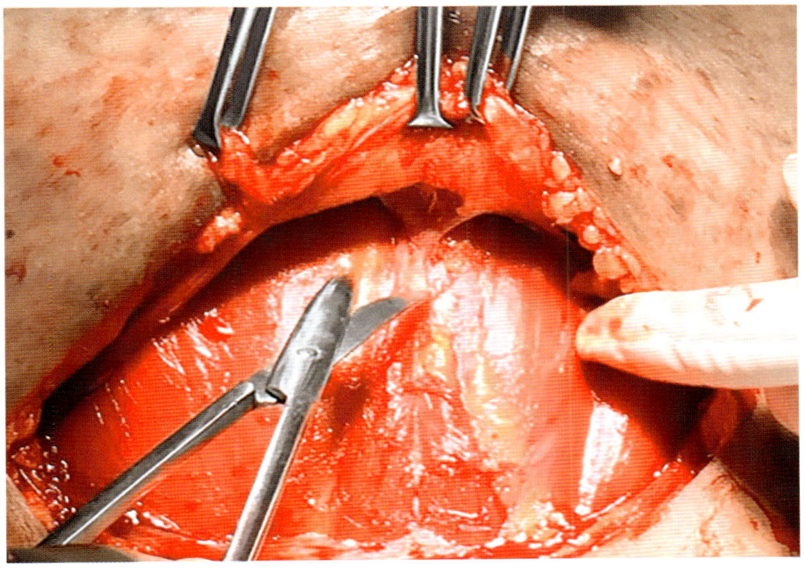

Fig. 8: Sharp dissection to free the muscle from the overlying fascia.

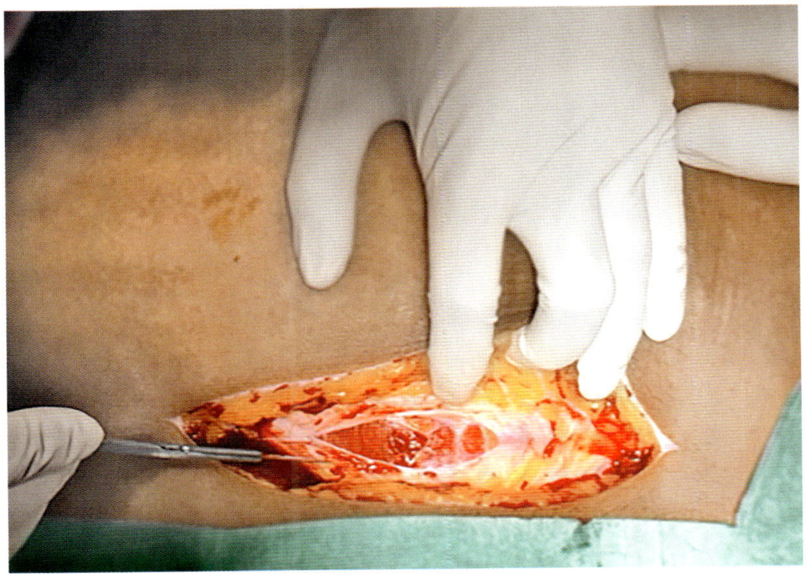

Fig. 6: The anterior rectus fascia is then sharply incised.

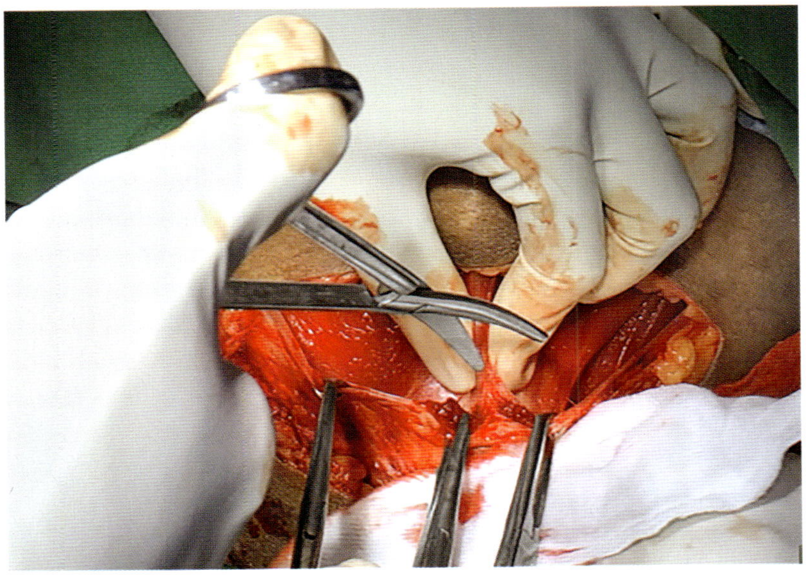

Fig. 9: Sharp dissection to free the muscle from the overlying fascia.

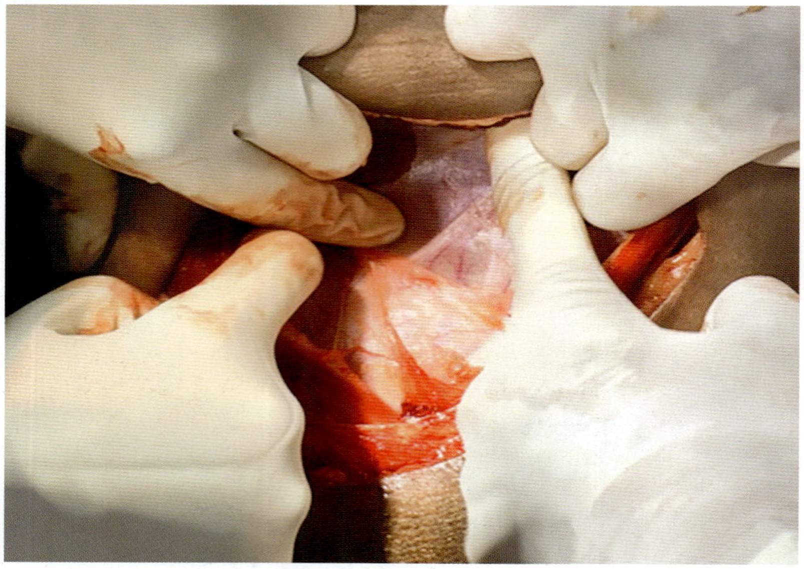

Fig. 10: Separation of peritoneum.

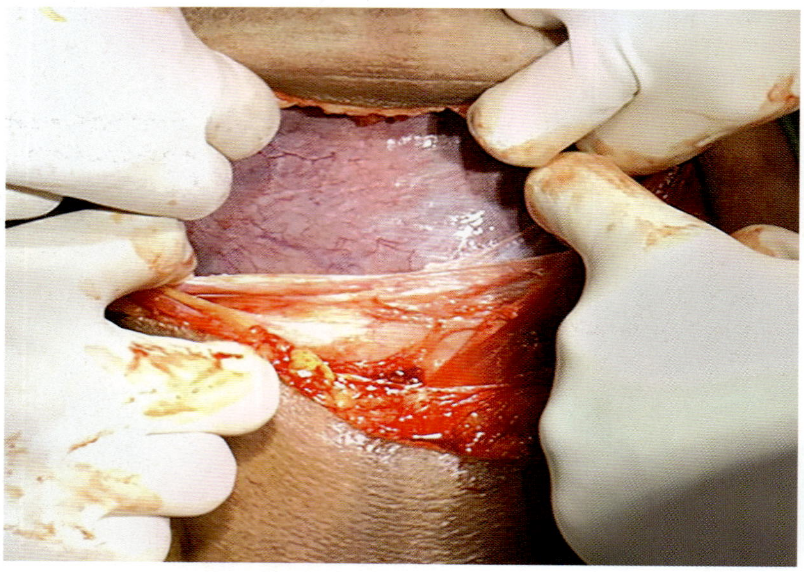

Fig. 11: These tissues may be separated in either a longitudinal or transverse manner.

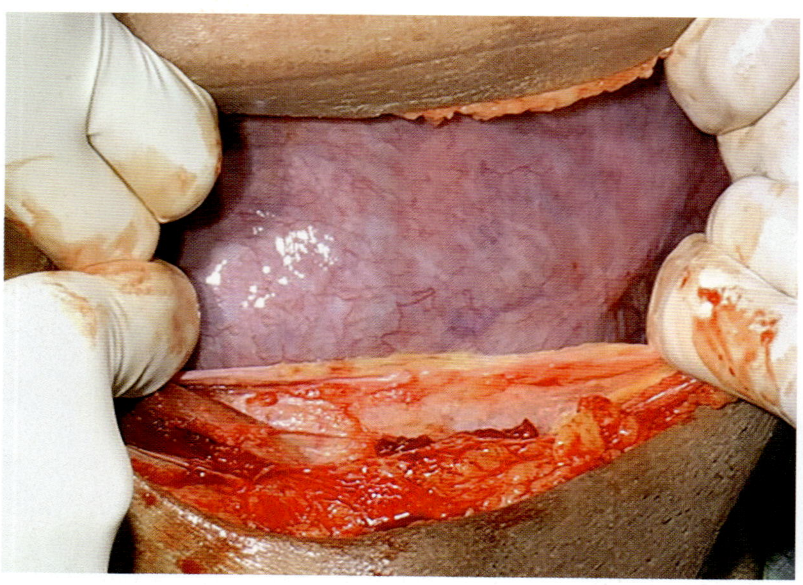

Fig. 12: Peritoneum is opened as high as possible.

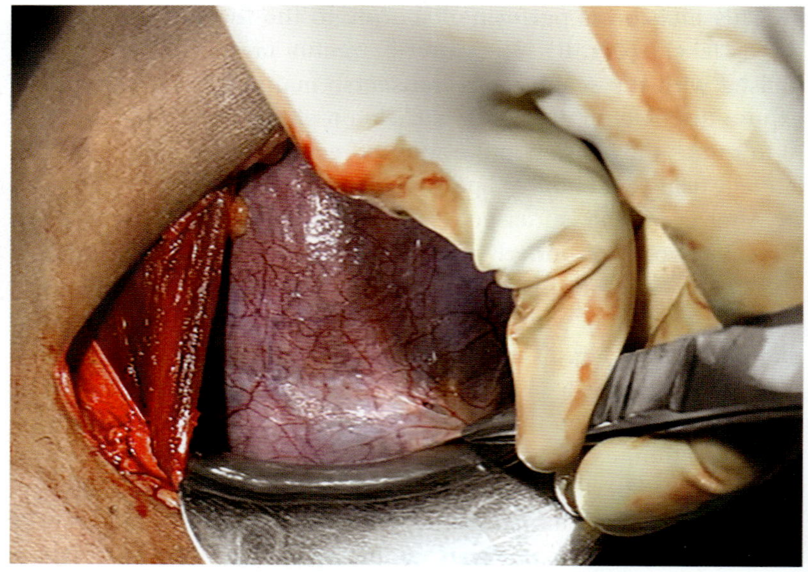

Fig. 13: The loose uterovesical peritoneum is identified.

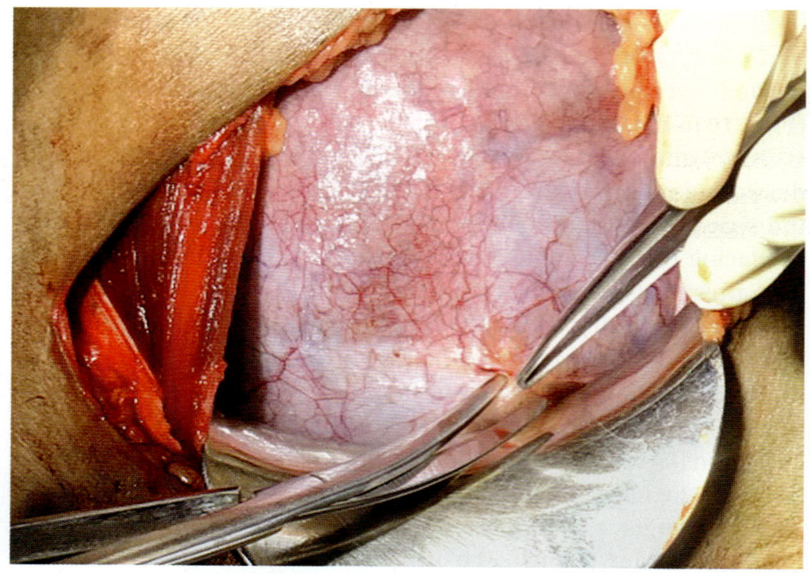

Fig. 14: Bladder is gently separated.

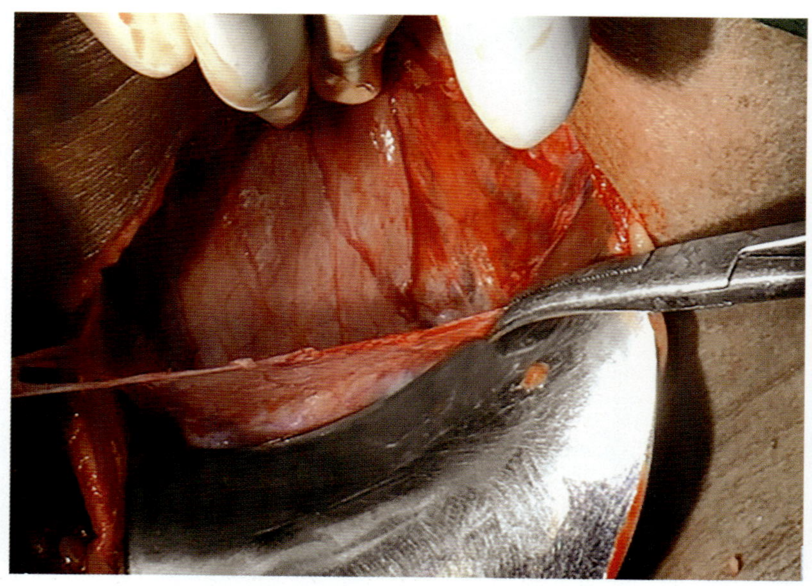

Fig. 15: Retractor placed to move the bladder down.

Identification and placement of incision at uterine wall: Commonly practiced lower segment transverse incision is usually placed about 2–3 cm above the bladder base **(Fig. 16)**. It is very important to remember during cesarean section in advanced labor or in second stage, the lower segment usually is very much stretched and incision is placed relatively higher to avoid the extension laterally and towards vagina. Thick lower segment may pose a problem. There are several alternatives like making J-shaped, J-shaped or T-shaped incision. Occasionally, low midline incision may have to be considered. Using a scalpel and with very gentle strokes make a 2 cm horizontal incision **(Figs. 17 and 18)**. After first stroke and with each succeeding stroke sweep the index finger of opposite hand across the incision so that layers can be clearly seen. When the incision is partially through the muscle, press and release the center of incision with forefinger—if the remaining layer is very thin this will usually raise a "bleb" of membranes which can be incised, almost like a blister, without risk to underlying fetus **(Fig. 19)**. Alternatively, one can use the forefinger or the scalpel handle to, burrow, through the final thin layer. Either way, obsessional attention to the point should almost eliminate the risk of fetal laceration. Intentional extension of the low-transverse incision is necessary in 1–2% of cases.[13] Typically, the extension of the low transverse incision is performed by creating a low vertical incision in the midline, T-ing the uterine incision, or creating a vertical incision at the lateral aspect of the uterine incision, a J-extension. These extensions are commonly performed for malpresentations, poorly developed lower uterine segment, or deep transverse arrest. Incision is then extended laterally using blunt dissection with the fingers. The upward curve of the incision may be created by the surgeons placing their thumbs on the patient's anterior superior iliac spines and index fingers in the uterine incision. By keeping the hand in this position, the incision is pulled open in an arc **(Fig. 20)**.

After the uterine incision has been made, the fetal membranes, if still intact, are ruptured with an Allis clamp. If the fetus is in a noncephalic presentation, leaving the membranes intact until the fetal feet or head can be moved into the uterine incision will increase the ease of delivery. When the fetus is in a cephalic presentation, delivery is performed by the surgeons placing their dominant hand into the uterine cavity and elevating the fetal head into the uterine incision **(Figs. 21 to 23)**. At the same time, an assistant applies firm fundal pressure on breech of infant which facilitates delivery of head.

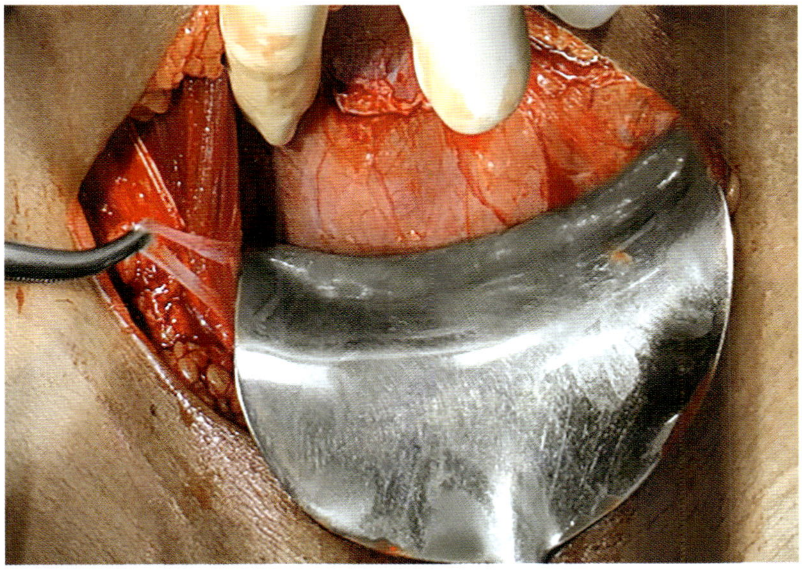

Fig. 16: Lower segment transverse incision is usually placed about 2–3 cm above the bladder base.

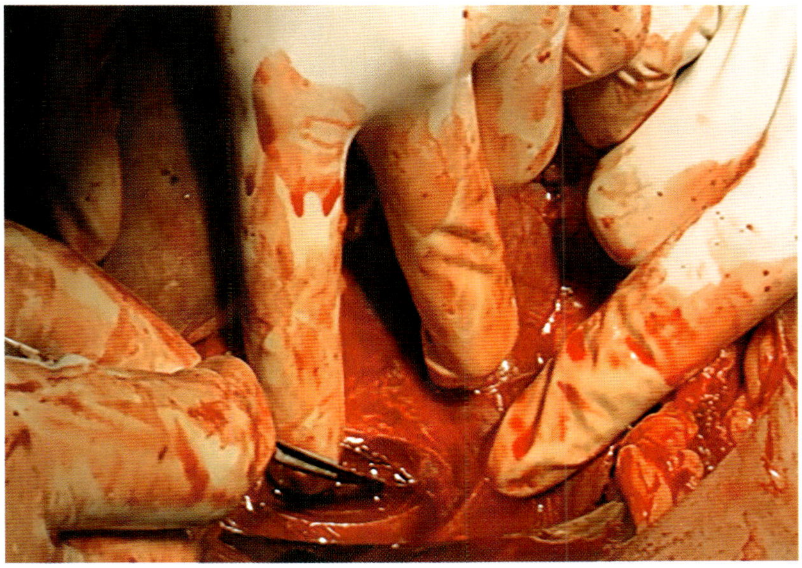

Fig. 18: 2 cm horizontal incision.

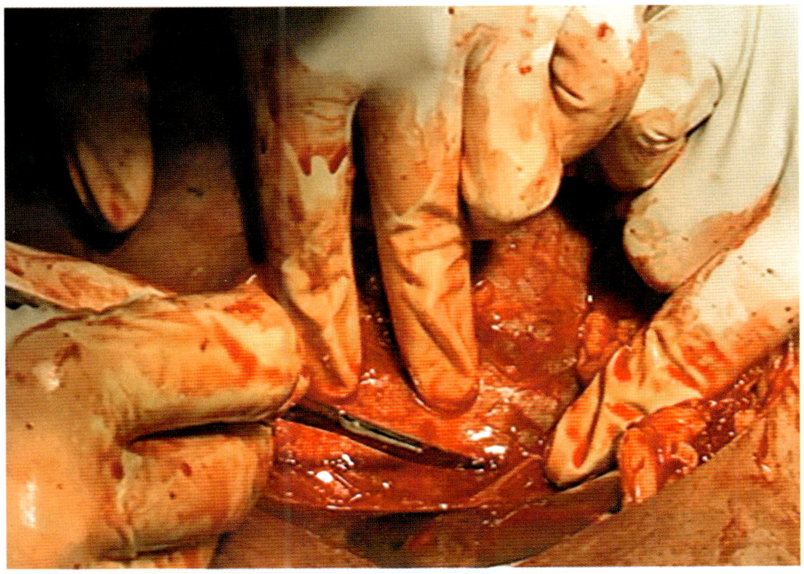

Fig. 17: Lower segment transverse incision.

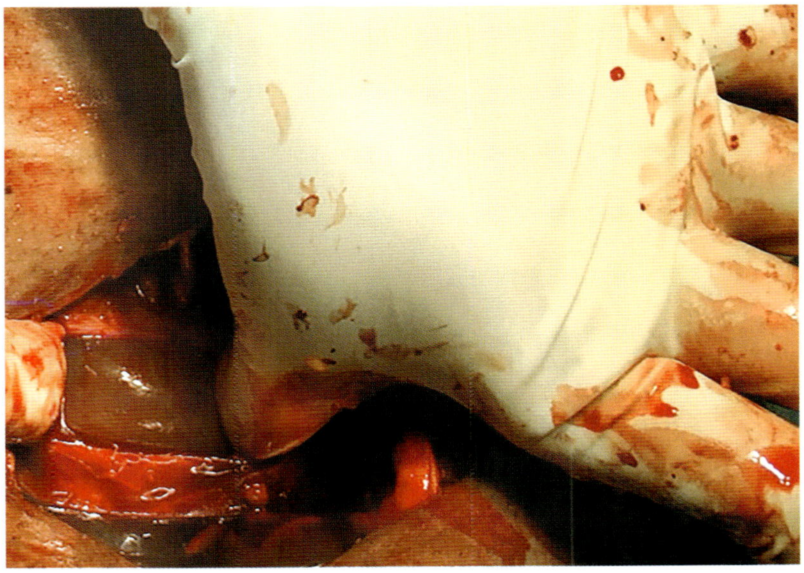

Fig. 19: Lower segment usually is very much stretched.

In elevating the head, the occiput should be identified and the head flexed so that the narrowest diameter passes through the uterine incision. If there is difficulty in delivering the head manually, Simpson's or similar forceps can be used to guide the fetal head through the uterine incision.

Once the head is delivered the oropharynx and nasal passages are cleared, if necessary with gentle suction. At this point, the anesthetist should give 5 units of oxytocin intravenously followed by an oxytocin infusion. Once the infant is completely delivered, it should be rapidly dried and the cord double clamped **(Fig. 24)**. The placenta should be removed by controlled cord traction once signs of separation have occurred **(Figs. 25 and 26)**. Routine manual removal of placenta is discouraged as it increases postoperative blood loss and postoperative sepsis and even acute uterine inversion.[14-16] Once the placenta has been delivered, the uterine cavity should be checked to ensure there are no retained portions of placenta or membranes.

Exteriorization of uterus should not be routinely carried out because it is associated with more pain and does not improve operative outcomes such as hemorrhage and infection[12] **(Figs. 27 and 28)**. On the other hand, if there is an extension of the uterine incision, or the exposure is limited by heavy bleeding, then one should not hesitate to bring the uterus out of the abdominal incision to facilitate hemostasis and repair.

Traditionally, closure of the uterine incision has been in two layers, although increasing numbers of obstetricians have moved to single layer closure. The effectiveness and safety of single layer closure of uterine incision is uncertain. Except within a research context, the uterine incision should be sutured in two layers.[12] The most commonly used sutures are 0 or No. 1 polyglactin (Vicryl) or polyglycolic acid (Dexon). The first layer should include the cut edges of muscle only and not the decidua. It should be a running suture, which avoids the bunching and elevation of tissues seen with continuous locking suture, and facilitates the placement of the second layer which can be either running or locking **(Fig. 29)**. The second layer of sutures should raise a fold of muscle on the upper and lower side to cover the first layer of sutures **(Figs. 30 to 32)**.

Neither the visceral nor the parietal peritoneum should be sutured at cesarean section because this reduces operating time, the need for postoperative analgesia and improves maternal satisfaction.[12] For closure of the abdominal wall some will approximate the medial

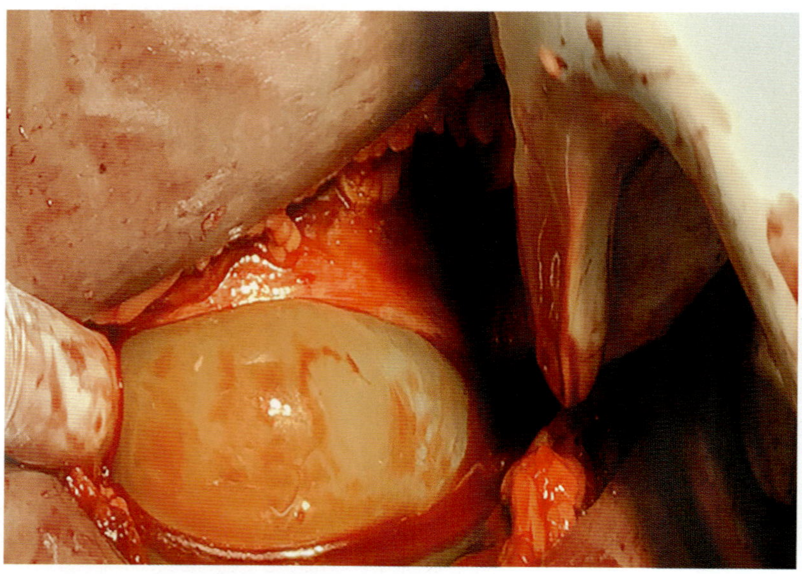

Fig. 20: The fetal membranes, if still intact.

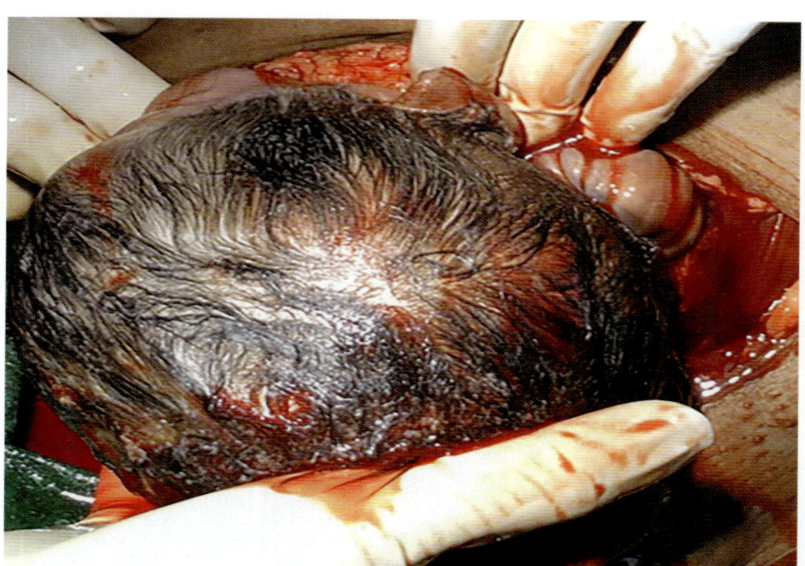

Fig. 21: Delivery of head.

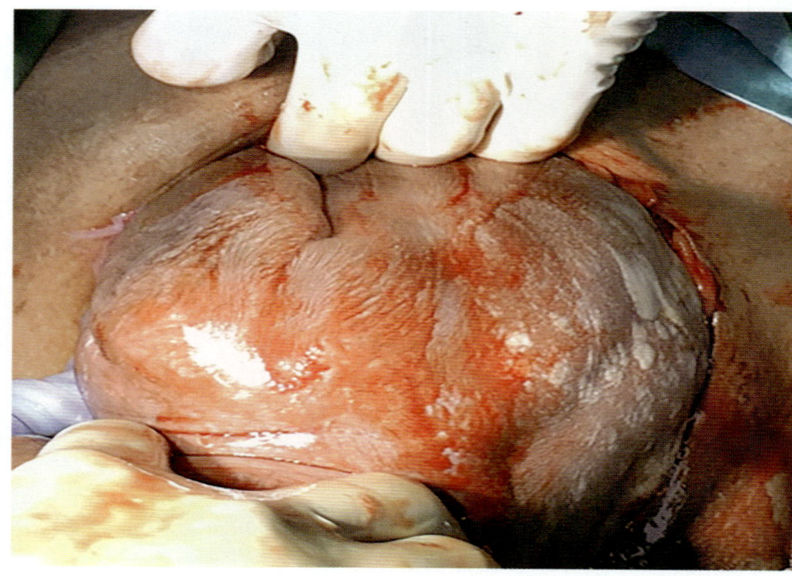

Fig. 22: Guide the fetal head.

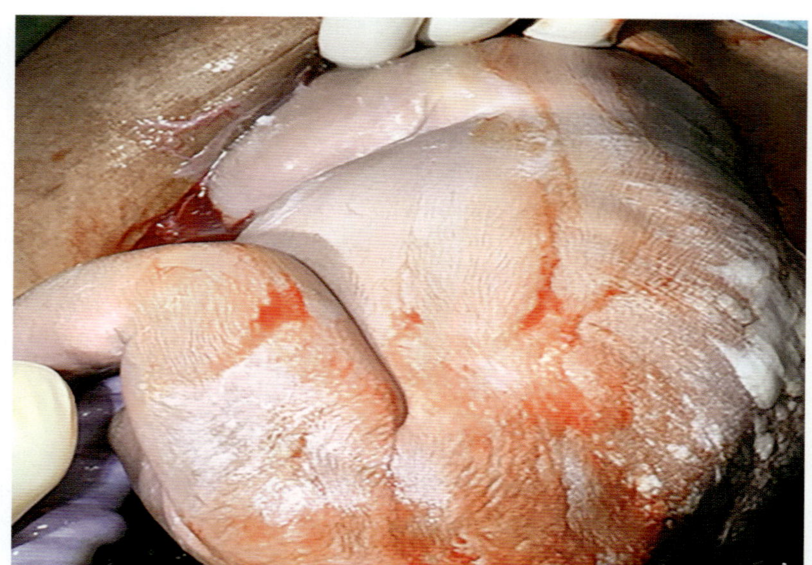

Fig. 23: Infant is completely delivered.

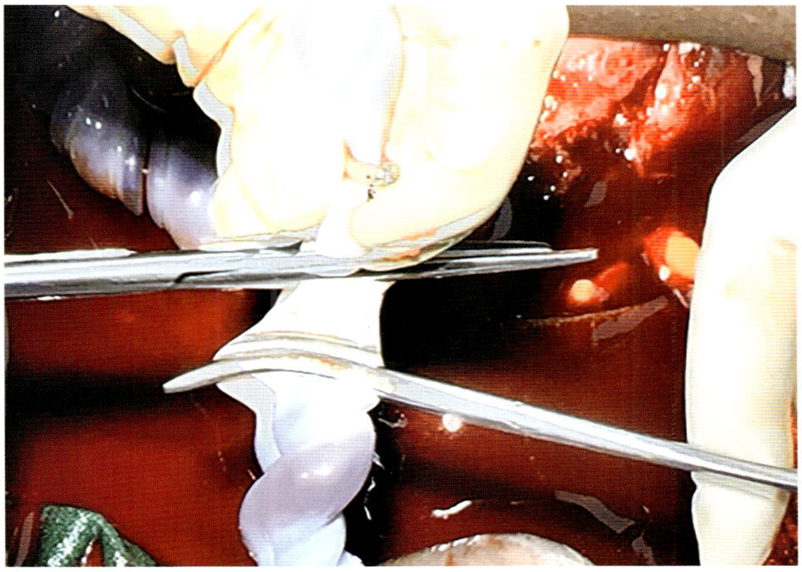

Fig. 24: Cord double clamped.

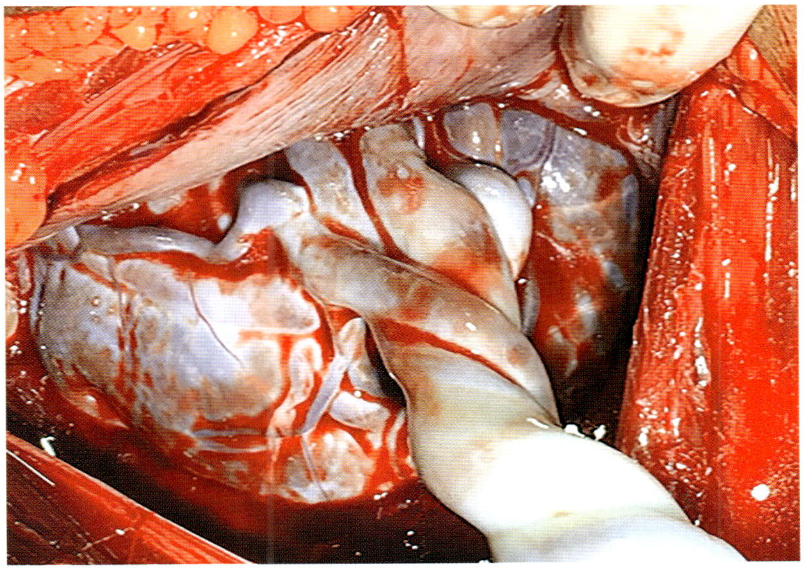

Fig. 25: Placental separation has occurred.

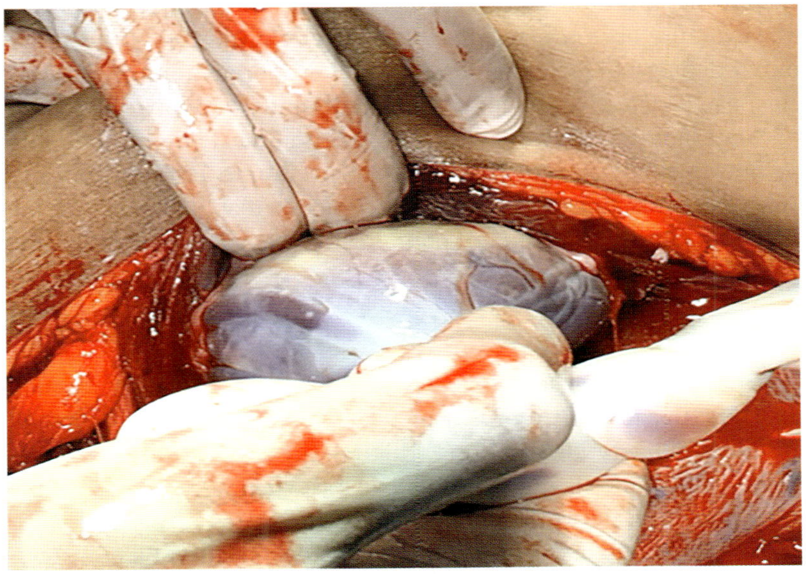

Fig. 26: Removed by controlled cord traction.

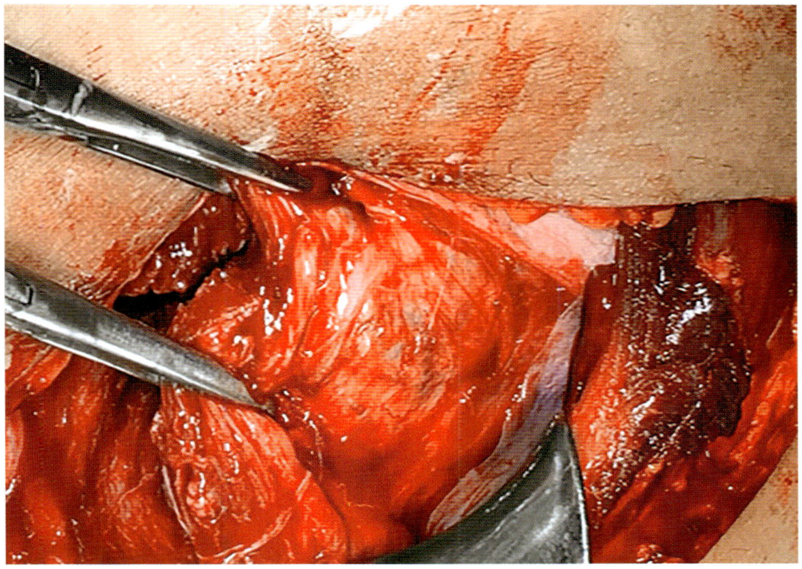

Fig. 27: First layer should include the cut edges.

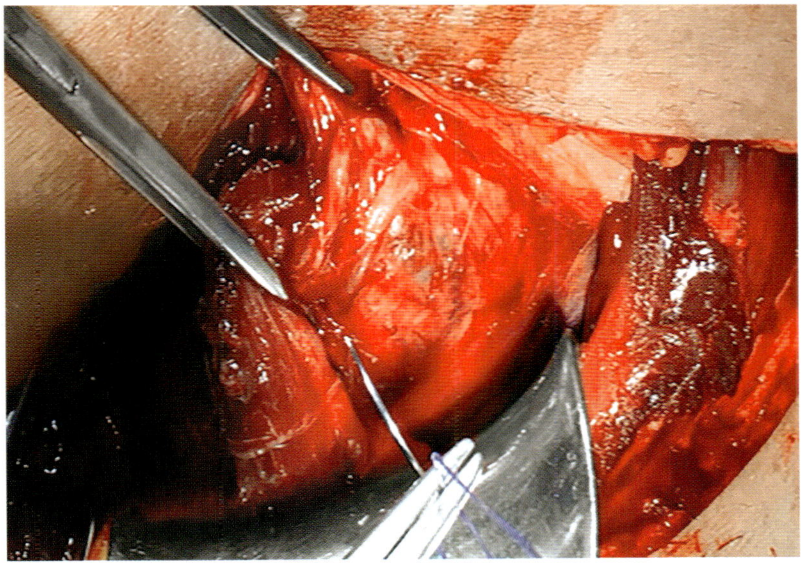

Fig. 28: The first layer should include the cut edges.

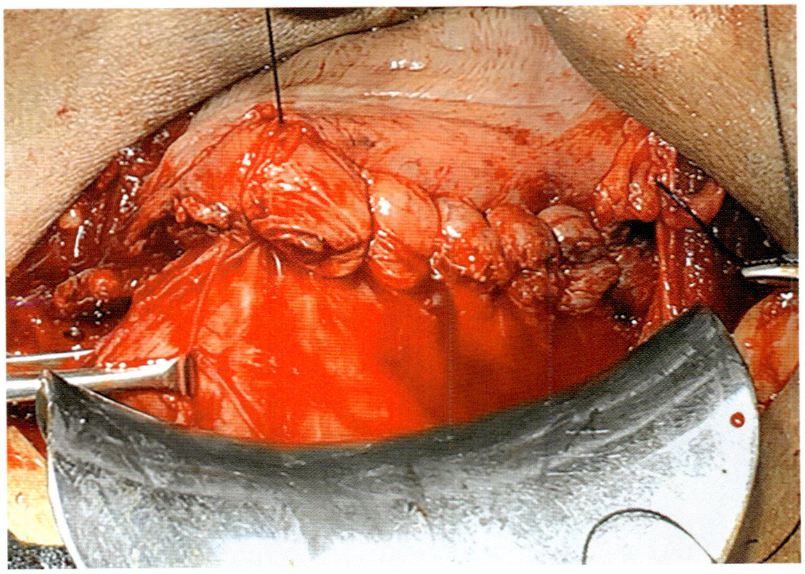

Fig. 29: Continuous running suture.

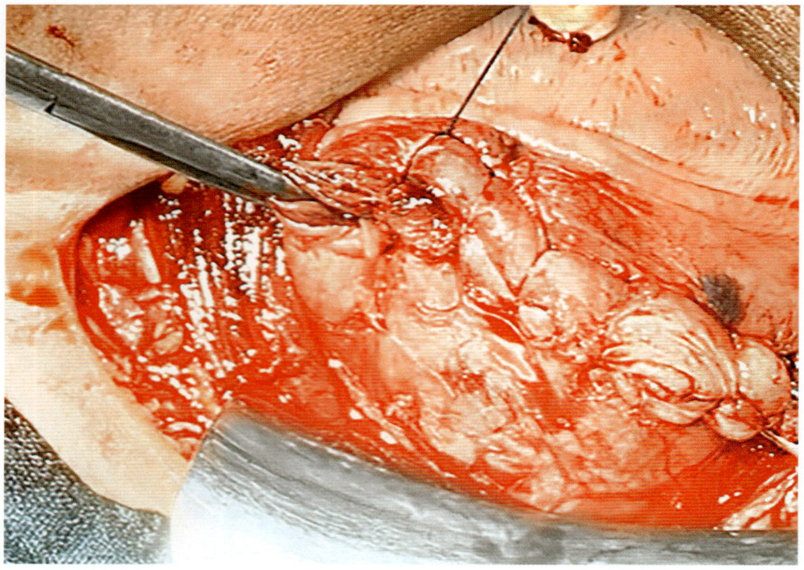

Fig. 30: Uterus closed in 2 layers.

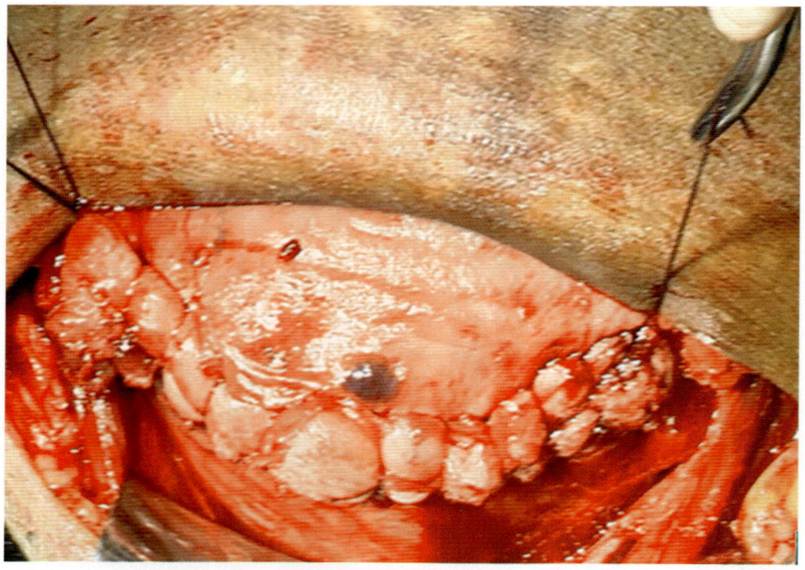

Fig. 31: Uterine angles should be checked.

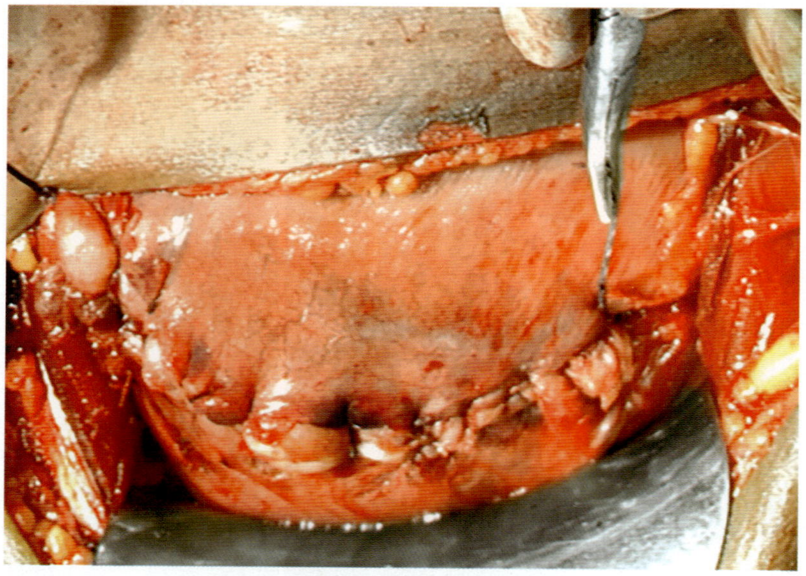

Fig. 32: Homeostasis ensured.

edges of rectus muscle loosely with two or three interrupted and lightly tied sutures, but many omit this step. The rectus sheath is closed with a running suture.

Routine closure of the subcutaneous tissue space should not be used unless the woman has more than 2 cm subcutaneous fat, because it does not reduce the incidence of wound infection. Superficial wound drains should not be used at cesarean section because they do not decrease the incidence of wound infection.[12]

PERIOPERATIVE CARE

- Antibiotic prophylaxis should be given both elective and emergency sections and should be administered intravenously in the form of single dose of a first-generation cephalosporins or ampicillin. In women with prolonged labor and evidence of chorioamnionitis repeat doses of the same antibiotic can be given for the first 48 hours postoperatively.
- Thromboprophylaxis should be offered to woman having cesarean section, because they are at increased risk of venous thromboembolism. The choice of method of prophylaxis (graduated stockings, hydration, early mobilization, and low molecular weight heparin) should take into account risk of thromboembolic disease.
- The Foley catheter can be removed once regional anesthesia has worn off and the woman is ambulant, usually about 12 hours postcesarean.
- Oral fluid and food intake should be administered when the woman feels thirsty or hungry, after confirming bowel peristalsis.
- The wound should be cared for in the standard manner, with occlusive dressings removed on the first postoperative day and the wound examined daily during the hospitalization for evidence of infection, seroma, or hematoma. Skin staples can be removed on the second or third postoperative day with Pfannenstiel incisions.
- The patient may be discharged when she is able to care for herself and her newborn. Many patients are ready to leave the hospital by postoperative day 2 or 3. Discharge instructions should include patient education concerning expectations on activity level, lochia, breastfeeding or milk suppression, contraception, and newborn care.

COMPLICATIONS

Maternal Mortality

As anesthesia and operative techniques have improved, cesarean section has become an increasingly safe and common procedure; however, the obstetrician must always bear in mind that the abdominal delivery of an infant is still a major operative procedure and can be associated with significant mortality and morbidity.

Maternal mortality after cesarean section has been estimated to be between 5.81 and 6.1 per 100,000 procedures. Between 20% and 50% of these deaths are attributable to the cesarean delivery, with the remainder being the result of complications ensured that led to the cesarean section.

Uterine Hemorrhage

Uterine hemorrhage can be caused by atony, lacerations, or retained placenta. Because the uterus usually can be examined at the time of cesarean delivery, determining which of these entities is the cause of the hemorrhage is not as difficult as it is when hemorrhage occurs after a vaginal delivery. Uterine atony continues to be the major cause of hysterectomy at the time of cesarean section. Bleeding can be because of bleeding from the uterine vessels, venous sinus from margins and also from venous sinus of placental beds.

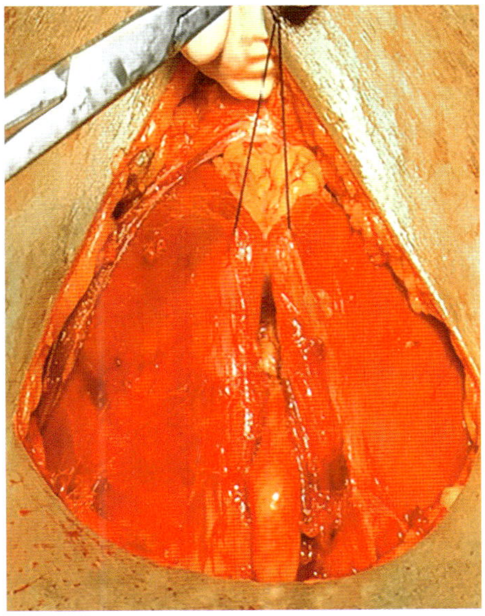

Fig. 33: Muscle approximated.

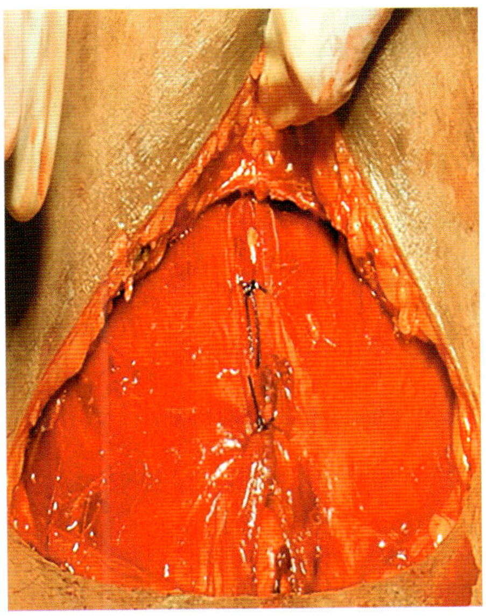

Fig. 34: Muscle c osure done.

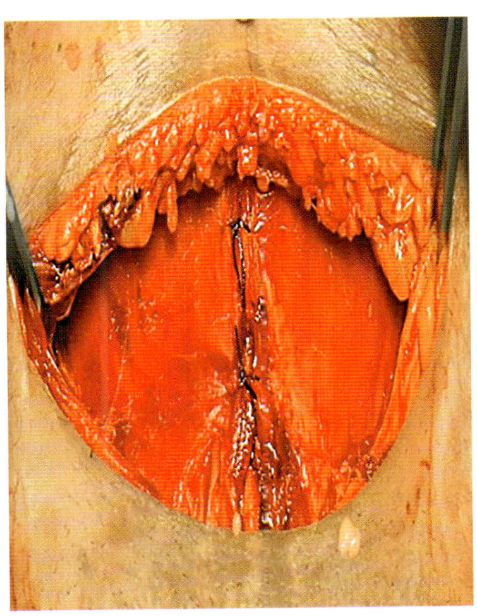

Fig. 35: Angles of rectus sheet is held with Allis forceps.

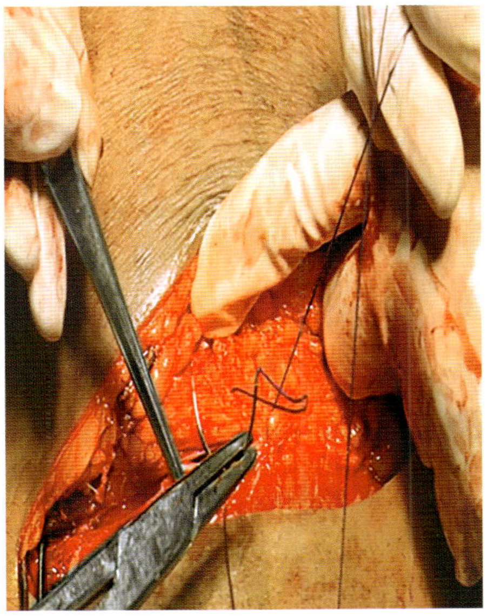

Fig. 36: Rectus sheath closed with PDS1.

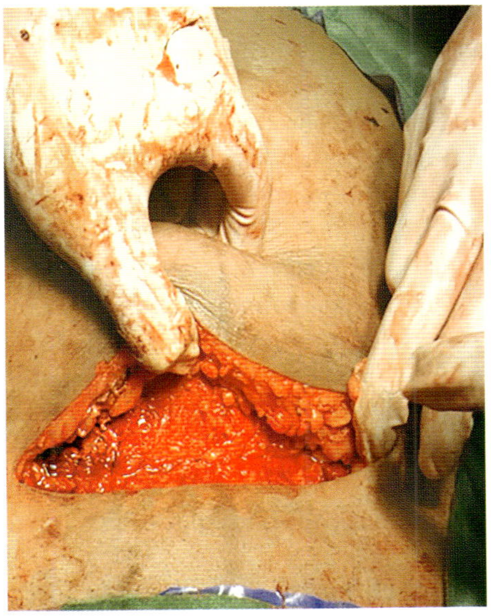

Fig. 37: Rectus sheath closed continuous technique.

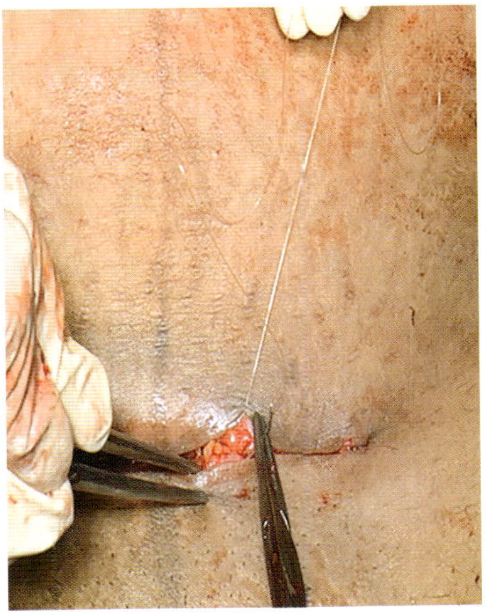

Fig. 38: Skin closed subcutaneous.

Urinary Tract Injury

Injury to the urinary tract is a relatively rare complication of cesarean delivery. The incidences of bladder and ureteral injury are 3% and 1%, respectively.[17] The most common site for bladder injury during cesarean delivery is at the dome of the bladder. Laceration of the bladder should be evaluated by first ensuring that the trigone and ureters are not involved. This may be accomplished by direct visualization of the ureters through a cystotomy incision. If the trigone is not involved and the ureters are functioning, the cystotomy can be closed in two layers. Keeping Foley's catheter for 7–10 days postoperatively is essential. Whenever there is a possibility of inadvertent cystotomy at the time of cesarean section, this can be evaluated by distending the bladder with sterile milk through the Foley catheter and observing the operative field for the appearance of the milk.

Ureteral injury is less common than injury to the bladder. If there is concern during the operative procedure that the ureter has been compromised, the abdomen should not be closed until this possibility has been thoroughly evaluated and excluded or the injury has been identified and corrected. Evaluation of the ureters can be performed by performing a cystotomy in the dome of the bladder and passing an 8-French ureteral stent retrograde through the ureter to the kidney. If ureteral stents are not immediately available, most labor and delivery suites have 8-French pediatric feeding tubes on the neonatal resuscitation cart, and these can be used instead. Another method of evaluating ureteral integrity is to inject 5–10 mL of indigo carmine intravenously and observe for the appearance of the dye at the ureteral orifice. Simply observing the appearance of the dye in the Foley catheter is inadequate to evaluate ureteral patency, because this only guarantees the patency of one ureter. Repair of ureteral injuries is performed as indicated by the level of the injury. Uretero-ureteral anastomosis or ureteral reimplantation with the placement of ureteral stents is the standard. Some minor injuries may be managed by the placement of ureteral catheters alone. Consultation intraoperatively with the appropriate specialist is warranted.

Gastrointestinal Tract Injury

Injury to the bowel at the time of cesarean section is exceedingly rare. An incidence of less than 0.1% has been reported.[17] This low incidence is caused by the displacement of the bowel out of the operative field by the enlarged gravid uterus. The risk of bowel injury is increased in patients with previous abdominal surgery or intra-abdominal adhesions. Injury is usually obvious because of the appearance of bowel contents in the surgical field. These injuries should be quickly identified and isolated to minimize contamination of the peritoneal cavity. Injury to the small bowel can be primarily repaired with a two-layer closure using silk or delayed absorbable suture.[17]

Wound Infections

By definition, any cesarean section is a clean, contaminated operation. Wound infections occur at a rate of approximately 7% after cesarean section when prophylactic antibiotics are not given;[17] this incidence is reduced to 2% with the use of prophylactic antibiotics.[18] Wound infections that occur after cesarean section include endomyometritis, pelvic abscess, incisional abscess, and wound cellulitis. The antibiotic of choice for each infection depends on the location of the infection and the suspected pathogen. Antibiotic therapy should be instituted empirically and adjusted as needed based on culture results. For pelvic abscesses, broad-spectrum antibiotics including anaerobic coverage are required; for superficial wound infections, simply opening the incision and draining the infectious source usually alleviates the problem in patients who do not have signs of systemic infection. Superficial wound cellulitis can usually be treated using penicillinase-resistant penicillin.

Endomyometritis

Endomyometritis complicates up to 80% of cesarean sections performed after the membranes have been ruptured for more than 6 hours in patients who are not administered antibiotic prophylaxis and 30% in patients with intact membranes. The incidence has been shown to be high in patient populations of lower socioeconomic status,[19] in patients that have had six or more vaginal examinations during labor, and in patients with longer duration of rupture of membranes.[20] The rate of uterine infection can be reduced to 5% or less with the use of prophylactic antibiotics given at the time of cord clamp.[21] A single dose of a first-generation cephalosporin is relatively inexpensive and effectively decreases the infection rate.

REFERENCES

1. Gabert HA, Bey M. History and development of cesarean operation. Obstet Gynecol Clin North Am. 1988;15:591-605.
2. Sander M. Speaking before the German Gynecology Association 1885. Am J Obstet Dis Women Child. 1886;19:883.
3. Sanger M. My work in reference to the cesarean operation. Am J Obstet Dis Women Child. 1887;20:593.
4. Boley JP. The history of caesarean section. 1935. CMAJ;1991:145:319-22.
5. Sancheetha G. Increasing trend in Caesarean section delivery in India: role of medicalisation of maternal health. Bangalore: Institute for Social and Economic Change; 2010.
6. Basket TF, Calder AA, Arulkumaran S. Munro Kerr's Operative Obstetrics, 11th edition. Philadelphia: Saunders; 2007.
7. Basket TF, Arulkumaran S. Intrapartum Care. London: RCOG Press; 2001.
8. Lanneau GS, Muffley P, Magann EF. Cesarean birth. Surgical Techniques. Philadelphia: Lippincott Williams & Wilkins; 2004.
9. RCOG. (2004). The National Sentinel Caesarean Section Audit. [online] Available from: https://www.rcog.org.uk/en/guidelines-research-services/audit-quality-improvement/completed-projects/national-sentinel-caesarean-section-audit/. [Last accessed January, 2020].
10. Hoile RW. National Confidential Enquiry in Perioperative Deaths (NCEPOD). Aust Clin Rev. 1993;13(1):11-5.
11. Lukas DN, Yentis SM, Kinsella SM, et al. Urgency of caesarean section: a new classification. J R Soc Med. 2000;93:346-50.
12. NICE. (2011). Caesarean Section (CG132). [online] Available from: https://www.nice.org.uk/guidance/cg132/resources/caesarean-section-pdf-35109507009733. [Last accessed January, 2020].
13. Martin JN Jr, Perry KG Jr, Roberts WE, et al. The case for trial of labor in the patient with a prior low-segment vertical cesarean incision. Am J Obstet Gynecol. 1997;177:144.
14. Hema KR, Johanson R. Techniques for performing caesarean section. Best Pract Res Clin Obstet Gynaecol. 2001;15:17-47.
15. Baska A, Kalan A, Ozkan A, et al. The effect of placental removal method and site of uterine repair on postceasrean endometritis and operative blood loss. Acta Obstet Gynecol Scand. 2005;84:266-9.
16. Bakett TF. Acute uterine inversion: a review of 40 cases. J Obstet Gyneacol Can. 2002;24:953-6.
17. Smith CV, Gallup DG. Management of urinary and gastrointestinal tract injuries. In: Phelan JP, Clark SL (Eds). Cesarean Delivery. New York: Elsevier; 1988.
18. Cunningham FG, Hauth JC, Strong JD, et al. Infectious morbidity following cesarean section: comparison of two treatment regimens. Obstet Gynecol. 1978;52:656-61.
19. Chang PL, Newton ER. Predictors of antibiotic prophylactic failure in post-cesarean endometritis. Obstet Gynecol. 1992;80:117-22.
20. Schwartz WH, Grolle K. The use of prophylactic antibiotics in cesarean section. A review of the literature. J Reprod Med. 1981;26:595-609.
21. Duff P. Prophylactic antibiotics for cesarean delivery: a simple cost-effective strategy for prevention of postoperative morbidity. Am J Obstet Gynecol. 1987;157:794-8.

CHAPTER

73

Cesarean Section in Placenta Previa and Accreta

Usha Rani G, Aditi Rai

INTRODUCTION

Expose the lower segment, incise the uterovesical fold of peritoneum, give a transverse incision on the lower segment about 1.5–2 inches wide. The edges of the uterine incision may be held with Allis forceps to control the bleeding from the veins over the edges of the incision.

The mode of entry into the lower segment should be planned by antenatal placental mapping with ultrasound.

An anterior placenta previa, which is totally covering the lower segment, has to be cut through to facilitate delivery of the baby. Index fingers of both hands are insinuated through the placenta till the membranes are reached. The membranes are ruptured. The uterine incision is extended, either by stretching or by cutting with a pair of scissors. The baby is delivered. The cord should be clamped as soon as the baby has been delivered.

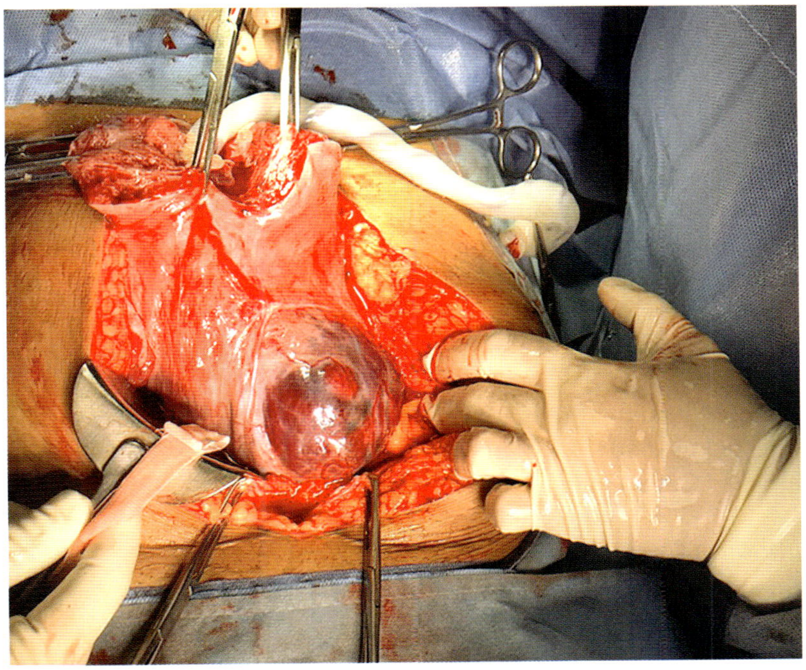

Fig. 1: Placenta accreta.

If the anterior placenta is partly covering the lower segment, the fingers can be passed between the placenta and the uterine wall till it reaches the membranes. The membranes are ruptured and the baby is delivered. The cord should be clamped as soon as the baby has been delivered.

Placental delivery after the delivery of the baby should be individualized. If the placental bed starts to bleed, after the baby's delivery, it should be manually separated and delivered. If the placental bed does not bleed after the delivery of the baby as in the case of posterior placenta previa, wait for spontaneous separation of the placenta.

Postpartum hemorrhage should be anticipated. Uterotonics should be used. Quick ligation of large bleeding vessels at the uterine cut edges should be done before closing the uterine incision.

Bleeding from the placental bed, if excessive can be tackled by:

- Compressing the lower uterine segment using two mops, one placed anteriorly in the uterovesical pouch and the other mop placed posterior to the lower segment.
- By use of vertical or square compression sutures on the lower segment over the areas of bleeding.
- Tamponade of the lower segment with Bakri balloon.

PLACENTA ACCRETA ASSOCIATED WITH PLACENTA PREVIA

When the combination of previa and accreta has been diagnosed antenatally, management should be planned according to the future reproductive needs of the patient.

Incision over the uterus should avoid the placenta. Fundal incision and delivery of the baby can be done. If the placenta is completely adherent, it can be left behind. Preventive surgical or radiological devascularization of the uterus may be beneficial, though not strongly recommended.

In situ hysterectomy in the same sitting as the cesarean section is associated with high morbidity. Placenta can be left behind and hysterectomy can be done after an interval of 6 weeks, if indicated. Placenta accreta is to be managed preferably in a high resource setting.

CHAPTER

74

Cervical Cerclage

Supriya Raina, Isha Rani, B Ramesh

INTRODUCTION

Cervical cerclage (cervical stitch) is a treatment for cervical incompetence. Cervical incompetence refers to intrinsic weakness of cervical tissue that contributes to premature birth not explained by another abnormality.

INDICATIONS FOR CERVICAL CERCLAGE

- Painless cervical dilatation with bulging bag of waters after ruling out overt or subclinical chorioamnionitis
- Women with history of ≥3 second trimester losses
- *Women with high-risk factors:* History of loop electrosurgical excision procedure (LEEP), conization, cervical trauma, and progressive cervical changes by ultrasonography (USG).

CAUSES OF INCOMPETENT CERVIX

- *Congenital:*
  - Müllerian tube defects—bicornuate uterus, septate uterus, and unicornuate uterus
  - Diethylstilbestrol exposure in utero
  - Abnormal collagen tissue—Ehlers-Danlos syndrome, Marfan syndrome
  - Recently, it was suggested that polycystic ovarian syndrome might be associated with cervical insufficiency, especially in women of South Asian or Black origin.[1]
- *Acquired:*
  - Forceful mechanical cervical dilatation
  - Cervical lacerations during labor or delivery.

PATHOPHYSIOLOGY

Cervix is composed of 90% connective tissue and 10% muscular tissue and its ability to retain the products of conception depends on the content and composition of connective tissue. Petersen and Uldbjerg examined cervical collagen in women with cervical insufficiency in nonpregnant state and compared it with women with no cervical insufficiency. They found that they had markedly lower median cervical hydroxyproline concentrations than parous women without cervical insufficiency.[2] Cervical incompetence occurs due to cervical ripening changes remote from term in second trimester itself. Cervix undergoes changes consistent with increased synthesis of collagenases, hyaluronic acid, infiltration by inflammatory cells particularly neutrophils and macrophages. These cause collagen degradation, disruption of collagen structure, increased water content, and increased synthesis of proinflammatory cytokines. As pressure threshold exceeds, cervix starts ripening usually around 18–22 weeks of gestation. In contrast to preterm labor, cervical incompetence does not have preponderance of uterine contractions with it.

CLINICAL FINDINGS

Acute Presentation

Symptoms

Asymptomatic or mild symptoms like pelvic pressure, cramps or backache, and/or a change in the volume, color, or consistency of vaginal discharge. These symptoms begin suddenly in midtrimester (18 and 22 weeks of gestation). Contractions are absent.

Physical Examination

It reveals a soft cervix effaced ≥80% with dilatation of ≥2 cm with bag of waters which might be visible through the external os. Funneling alone should not be considered as a requirement for placement of cervical cerclage. Data do not support the placement of a cerclage on the basis of funneling, but rather on residual cervical length.[3] Active assessment of cervix can be done by various method, transfundal pressure created by applying fundal pressure in the direction of the uterine axis for 15 seconds is more effective than coughing or standing in eliciting cervical changes and signs of progressive second trimester cervical shortening.[4-6]

Tocodynamometry shows no or infrequent contractions at irregular intervals.

A large number of these women with incompetent cervix will be infected as demonstrated by raised white blood cell (WBC) count, elevated C-reactive protein (CRP).

Imaging

Incompetent cervix is characterized by changes depicted in endovaginal USG in second trimester. In these cases, normal T-shaped cervix becomes Y when internal cervical os opens and the amniotic sac starts to herniate into the endocervical canal. Y becomes U with further thinning and opening of cervix. Other important parameter measured is cervical length of unopened portion of cervical canal. Women with <25 mm of cervical length are at greater risk of preterm labor.[3,7-11] Funneling or herniation of membranes into the cervical canal on USG also indicate incompetent os **(Figs. 1A and B)**. Data do not support the placement of a cerclage on the basis of funneling, but rather on residual cervical length.[3]

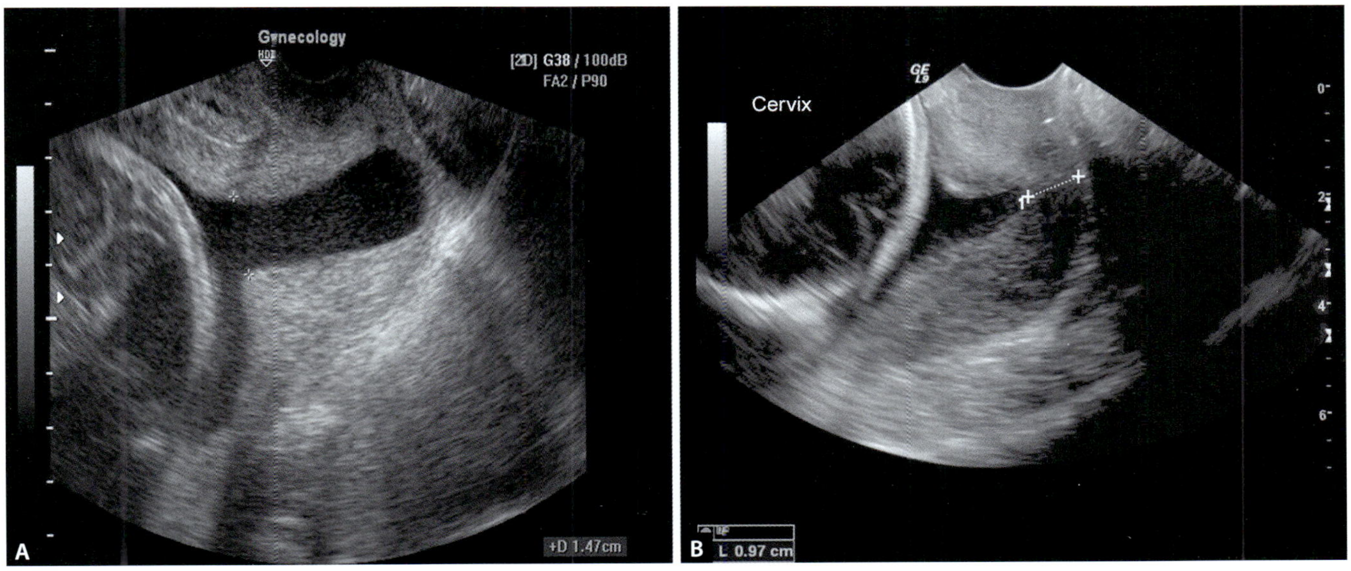

Figs. 1A and B: (A) Funneling and short cervical length seen in incompetent cervix; (B) Short cervical length seen on transvaginal scan.

Cervicovaginal fetal fibronectin (fFN) may be positive, though not confirmatory it has high negative predictive value for onset of preterm labor. In asymptomatic women, the combination of a short (≤25 mm) cervix on ultrasound examination and a positive fFN result is predictive of an increased risk of preterm delivery, though not a marker for cervical incompetence. Two negative tests are reassuring (less than 1% chance of preterm delivery in the next week or two).[12-15]

DIAGNOSIS

The diagnosis of cervical insufficiency is based on either classic historic factors or, preferably, by a combination of historic factors and transvaginal ultrasound (TVU) measurement of cervical length.

- History-based diagnosis of cervical insufficiency—history-based diagnosis of cervical insufficiency in women with ≥2 consecutive prior second-trimester pregnancy losses associated with relatively painless early cervical dilatation *or* ≥3 early (<34 weeks) preterm births in which other causes of pregnancy loss or preterm birth (e.g. infection, placental bleeding, multiple gestation, preterm labor) have been excluded. Risk factors for cervical insufficiency support the diagnosis.
- History, ultrasound, and physical examination-based diagnosis of cervical insufficiency—diagnosis of cervical insufficiency is made in women with one or two prior second-trimester pregnancy losses or preterm births and cervical length ≤25 mm on transvaginal USG examination or advanced cervical changes on physical examination before 24 weeks of gestation.

The diagnosis of cervical insufficiency is usually limited to singleton gestations because the pathogenesis of second-trimester pregnancy loss/preterm delivery in multiple gestations is usually unrelated to a weakened cervix.

APPROACH TO MANAGEMENT

The following approach to management applies to women with singleton pregnancies:

- Candidates for history-indicated cerclage—history-indicated transvaginal cerclage at 12–14 weeks for women with a history-based diagnosis of cervical insufficiency such as three or more second-trimester pregnancy losses associated with painless cervical dilatation.

  In women with recurrent second-trimester losses/preterm births usually with painless cervical dilatation is primarily, and perhaps exclusively, caused by acquired structural weakness of the cervix and can be treated effectively with structural support from a history-indicated cerclage.

  Ideal candidate for cervical cerclage: Either nulliparous or multiparous women at 16–22 weeks of gestation with risk factors for cervical incompetence. History of midtrimester losses, normal CRP, and normal WBC count. Membranes are visible at external os, but not herniating into vagina. Cervical dilatation is less than 3 cm.

  Before admission for cerclage, urinalysis for culture and sensitivity and vaginal cultures for bacterial vaginosis should be taken and any infections if found should be treated.[17-23]

  Some women with history of early preterm births were treated with hydroxyprogesterone caproate weekly from 16 weeks to 36 weeks of gestation.[24-26] Although randomized trials support the benefit of history-indicated cerclage (25% reduction in deliveries <33 weeks) and the benefit of progesterone supplementation[24-26] in this population, no randomized trials have evaluated the efficacy of combination therapy (both history-indicated cerclage and hydroxyprogesterone caproate). One small retrospective study observed that combination therapy (cerclage and hydroxyprogesterone caproate) was more effective than cerclage alone for preventing delivery <24 weeks, but not <28 or 37 weeks.[27] However, the small (n = 33) number of noniatrogenic deliveries <24 weeks precludes a clear conclusion about the efficacy of combined therapy.
- Candidates for ultrasound surveillance and possible ultrasound-indicated cerclage—majority of women with suspected cervical insufficiency do not meet criteria for a history-based diagnosis of cervical insufficiency and, in turn, undergo a history-indicated cerclage. For these women, all with a prior spontaneous preterm birth, administration of hydroxyprogesterone caproate as prophylaxis against preterm delivery is done. Cervical length should be monitored with TVU usually starting at 16 weeks (but sometimes earlier) and apply a cerclage if cervical length is

≤25 mm before 24 weeks.[28] Patients are advised to reduce physical activity, especially those with physical employment, prolonged periods of standing, or frequent and repetitive lifting, although there are no data to confirm or deny the efficacy of bed rest in such cases.[29] The following evidences provide the rationale for this approach of using progesterone and using cervical cerclage:

- In randomized trials, progesterone prophylaxis with hydroxyprogesterone caproate starting at 16 (optimal) to 20 weeks of gestation in women with a history of spontaneous preterm birth and continuing until 36 weeks reduced the risk of recurrent preterm birth
- Women with a short cervix on TVU examination in the second trimester are at increased risk of spontaneous preterm birth
- Placement of a cerclage upon identification of a short cervix (ultrasound-indicated cerclage) is effective in reducing preterm birth.[30] The benefit of ultrasound-indicated cerclage may derive from increasing cervical strength,[31] preventing membranes from being exposed, and retention of the mucus plug.

In a 2011 meta-analysis of randomized trials of women with singleton gestation and prior spontaneous preterm birth and short cervical length ≤25 mm before 24 weeks, placement of an ultrasound-indicated cerclage reduced total neonatal morbidity and mortality by over one-third [15.6% vs. 24.8% without cerclage; relative risk (RR): 0.64; 95% confidence interval (CI): 0.45–0.91], presumably because cerclage reduced the frequency of preterm birth by 30% (delivery <35 weeks; RR: 0.70; 95% CI: 0.55–0.89; 28.4% vs. 41.3% in women without cerclage). Initiate cervical length screening in women with suspected cervical insufficiency at about 14 weeks, but may screen as early as 12 weeks in women with early second-trimester losses, recurrent second-trimester losses, or a prior large cold-knife conization.[32] In women with prior spontaneous preterm birth at 28–36 weeks, initiate screening at 16 weeks. Ultrasound examination is generally repeated every 2 weeks until 24 weeks as long as the cervical length is ≥30 mm and increased to weekly if cervical length is 25–29 mm, with the expectation that preterm cervical changes will precede overt preterm labor or membrane rupture symptoms by 3–6 weeks.

Cerclage stitch is removed at the end of 37 completed weeks of the pregnancy as even when labor starts maturity is confirmed. Approximately 10% of pregnancies end in preterm delivery, i.e. delivery occurring before week 37 of pregnancy. Premature birth is a major concern as there is risk of serious health problems in neonates (newborn babies) including respiratory distress, hypothermia, and infection as a result of preterm delivery more than 85% of long-term disabilities in otherwise healthy babies and 75% of deaths among newborns.

DEMOGRAPHICS: RISK FACTORS FOR PRETERM DELIVERY

- African-American women are at more risk (16–18%) than White women (7–9%)
- Women under 18 years and over 35 years are also at greater risk
- Less educated women are more likely to deliver prematurely
- Smoking during pregnancy is associated with a 20–30% greater risk of delivering prematurely
- Male fetuses are more likely to be born prematurely and have a higher rate of fetal death than female fetuses (a difference of 2.8–9.8%).

PREOPERATIVE PREPARATION

- A complete medical history is taken
- A cervical examination will be necessary to assess the state of the cervix; usually a TVU will be performed
- Nil per oral for a minimum of 6 hours is necessary as the procedure is performed under anesthesia
- The patient should be instructed to avoid sexual intercourse, tampons, and douches for 24 hours before the procedure
- Before the procedure is performed, an intravenous (IV) cannula is placed to administrate fluids and medications
- Elective cervical cerclage is a minor surgical procedure that is generally performed between 12 weeks and 14 weeks of pregnancy (at the beginning of the second trimester) before symptoms of premature labor begin. Emergent cerclages are those placed later in pregnancy when cervical changes have already begun
- The patient will usually receive regional (epidural or spinal) anesthesia during the procedure, although general anesthesia is sometimes used.

TYPES OF CERCLAGE

The cerclage falls into three types:

1. *McDonald stitch:* A purse-string stitch around the cervix to cinch it together. A McDonald cerclage that was described in 1947 is the most commonly performed. It is essentially a purse-string stitch used to close the cervix; the cervix stitching involves a band of suture at the upper part of the cervix while the lower part has already started to efface. This cerclage is usually placed between 16 weeks and 18 weeks of pregnancy. The stitch is removed around the 37th weeks of gestation or earlier if labor starts. This procedure was first described by the Canadian Gynecologist and Obstetrical Pathologist and Surgeon, Ellice McDonald (1876–1955). In McDonald stitch, suture goes through anterior, posterior lips of cervix, lateral aspects of cervix avoiding its arterial supply and purse string is tied either anteriorly or posteriorly **(Figs. 2 to 4)**.
2. *Shirodkar stitch* ***(Figs. 5A to F):*** Shirodkar—a purse-string stitch around the cervix underneath the mucosa of the cervix to help cinch it together. This type of cerclage is less common and

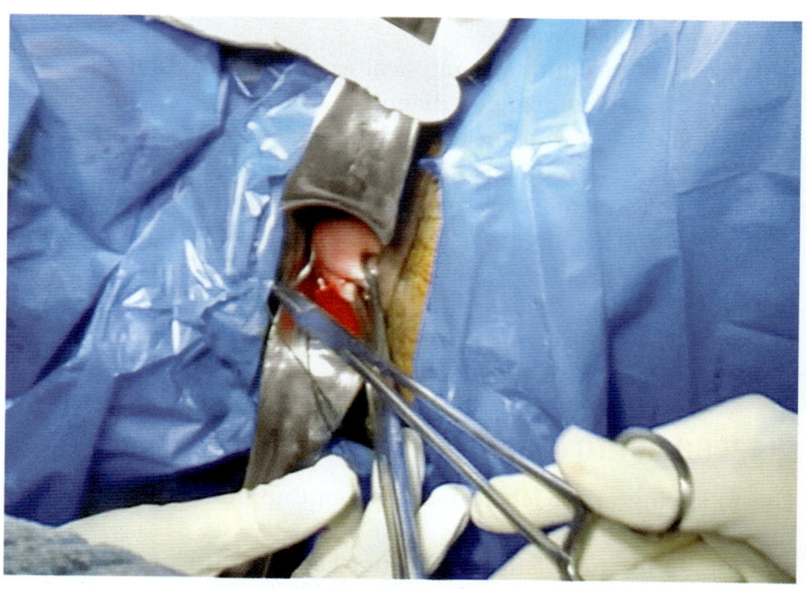

Fig. 2: Anterior lip of cervix is held with sponge holding forceps and suture is passed through it.

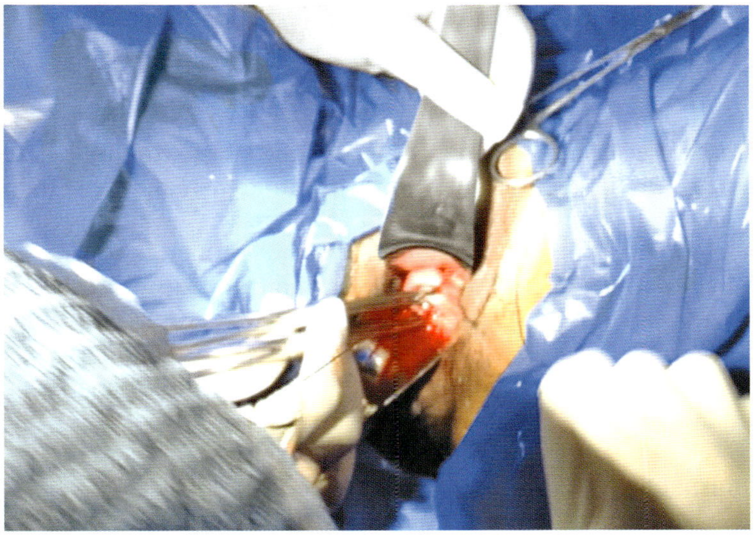

Fig. 3: Suture is passed through lateral and posterior lips of cervix.

technically more difficult than a McDonald. As the stitch is below the mucosal layer and not exposed to the vaginal flora, it is thought (though not proven) to have less risk of infection. The Shirodkar procedure sometimes involves a permanent stitch around the cervix which will not be removed and therefore a cesarean section will be the only way to deliver the baby. The Shirodkar technique was first described by VN Shirodkar in Bombay in 1955. In 1963, Shirodkar traveled to New York City to perform the procedure at the New York Hospital of Special Surgery; the procedure was successful and the baby lived to adulthood. A little incision is made and a special needle is used to tunnel under the mucosa from the incision at 12 o'clock on the cervix to 6 o'clock. Then, the suture is placed back into the 6 o'clock position it just came out of and tunneled under the mucosa back up the other side of the cervix back to 12 o'clock. Finally, the suture is tied tightly and the knots and ends covered over with the mucosa. That buries the suture altogether, possibly reducing the risk of infection (not

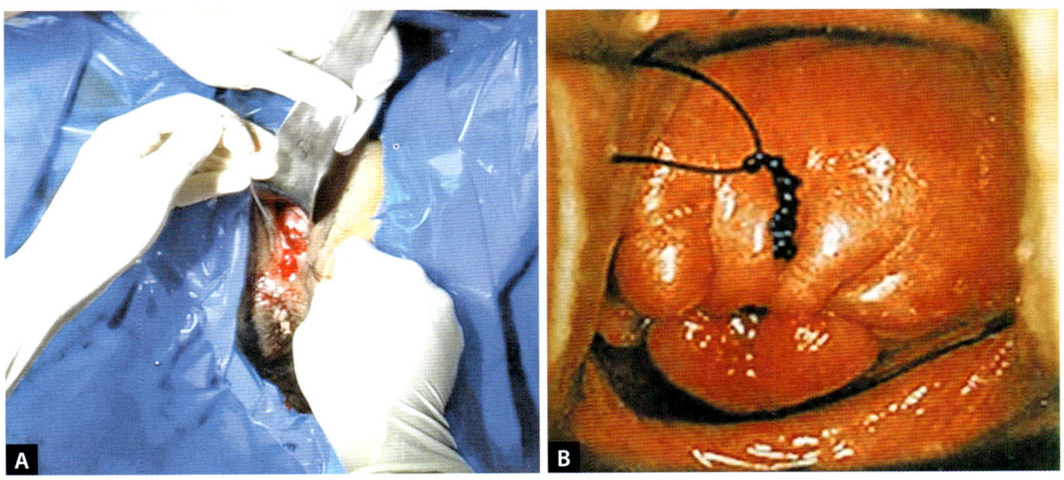

Figs. 4A and B: Stitch being tied anteriorly after taking suture on all four sides of cervix.

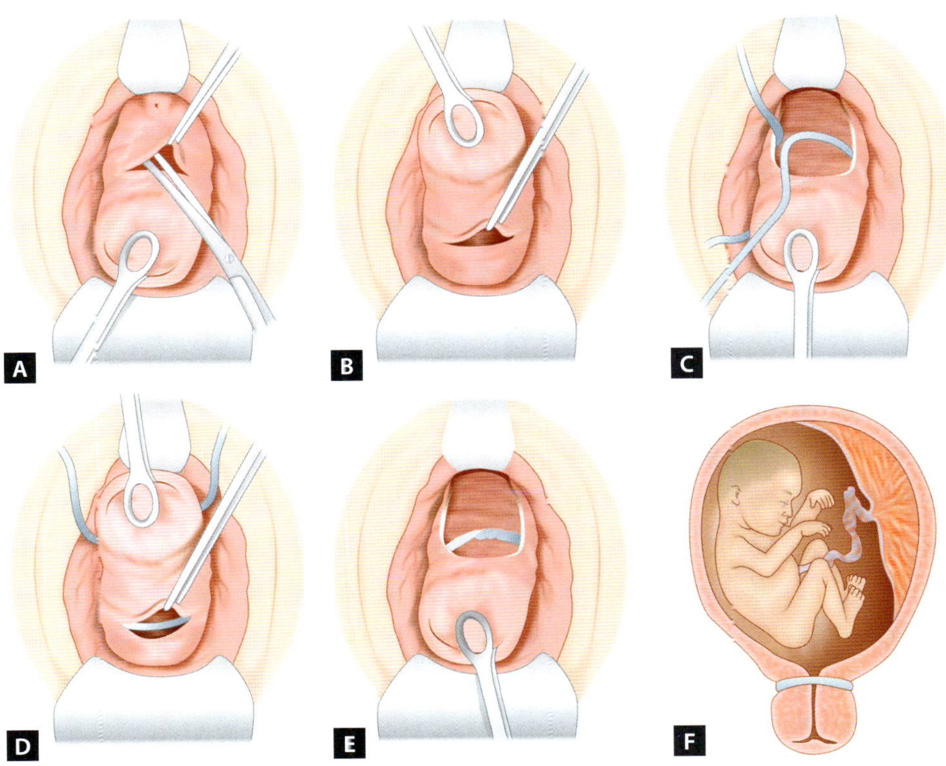

Figs. 5A to F: Shirodkar stitch.

proven) and some feel it is stronger. Both work well, most use McDonald because it is easier.

3. Abdominal cerclage (explained in detail below).

ABDOMINAL CERCLAGE

An abdominal cerclage is a technique of placement of a band at the level of the internal os, as it is not accessible vaginally and requires abdominal placement **(Figs. 6A and B)**. Due to technical difficulty, it is not performed regularly. This is usually performed if the cervix is too short to attempt a standard cerclage, or if a vaginal cerclage has failed or is not possible. However, a few doctors (namely Arthur Haney at the University of Chicago and George Davis at the University of Medicine and Dentistry of New Jersey) are advocating transabdominal cerclage (TAC) to replace vaginal cerclages, due to perceived better outcomes and more pregnancies carried to term.

Procedure

It is performed under anesthesia through a transverse suprapubic incision. The peritoneum overlying the bladder and uterus is divided and the bladder is pushed caudally. The uterine vessels are identified and displaced laterally and a suture is then placed around the cervix at the level of the internal os. The suture is tied posteriorly; this is to allow removal of the suture by posterior colpotomy if necessary, however it is technically more challenging. Some surgeons tie the suture anteriorly.

Until recently, abdominal cerclage required a laparotomy. The uterine vessels have to be dissected from the cervix to allow insertion of the suture medially. The technique is more demanding than that by the vaginal approach and might lead to excessive bleeding from the uterine vessels. Transillumination of the uterine vessels and their branches with a laparoscope and placing the suture through the avascular area of the paracervical tissue medial to the vessels have been proposed. Excessive manipulation of the pregnant uterus could also lead to pregnancy loss. A simpler and less invasive laparoscopic abdominal cerclage would be beneficial.

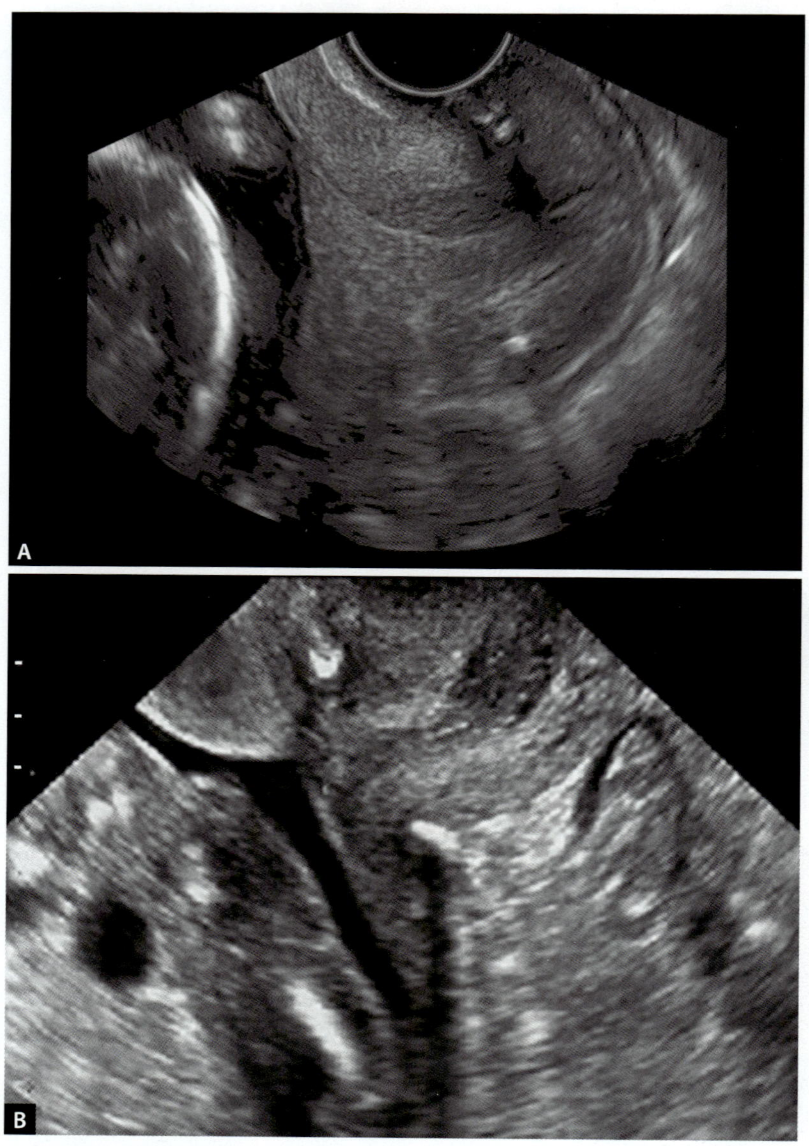

Figs. 6A and B: Ultrasonography (USG) images of an abdominal cerclage in situ.

Laparoscopic Abdominal Cerclage

Advantages

It is less invasive. Advantages of any laparoscopic procedure over laparotomy such as shorter hospitalization, less pain, and faster recovery:

- Minimal uterine manipulation and minimal dissection are required
- Tracking of uterine vessels and creating a window in broad ligament are not necessary; it can be done by piercing broad ligament medial to the uterine vessels. No vessel dissection hence, less risk of bleeding
- The result of laparoscopic abdominal cerclage is equally good as laparotomy. Most cases of abdominal cerclage have been performed during pregnancy, usually after 12 weeks of gestation [after nuchal translucency (NT) scan and dual marker]
- Abdominal cerclage by laparotomy and by laparoscopy has been performed in both pregnant and nonpregnant states. Due to potential risk to the fetus and technically difficulty owing to enlarged uterus, some authors have suggested performing cerclage as an *interval procedure (before pregnancy)*. In patients whose need for abdominal cerclage is clear like patients with documented cervical insufficiency or previous failed vaginal cerclage, performing the procedure in the nonpregnant state has some advantages **(Table 1)**.

Table 1: Difference between interval cerclage and cerclage during pregnancy.

Interval cerclage	*Cerclage during pregnancy*
No fetal risks	Involves fetal risks
Less risks of bleeding for the patient	More maternal risks of bleeding, preterm labor
Easy manipulation with uterine manipulator inserted into the uterus	Difficult manipulation as instrumentation of uterus is not possible in pregnancy
More exposure of anterior surface of uterus as uterus is small	Less exposure of anterior surface of uterus as uterus is difficult to manipulate
Less anesthesia risks in nonpregnant state	More anesthesia risks both to mother and fetus in pregnancy
Mersilene tape can be placed higher without risk of rupturing membranes	Increased chances of rupturing membranes while passing Mersilene tape
Ultrasonography (USG) guidance is not needed in this procedure. Recheck hysteroscopy is done to check proper cerclage placement	Recheck USG is needed to see level of placement of cerclage after surgery and fetal heart both before and after cerclage

LAPAROSCOPIC CERCLAGE IN PREGNANCY (FIGS. 7 TO 14)

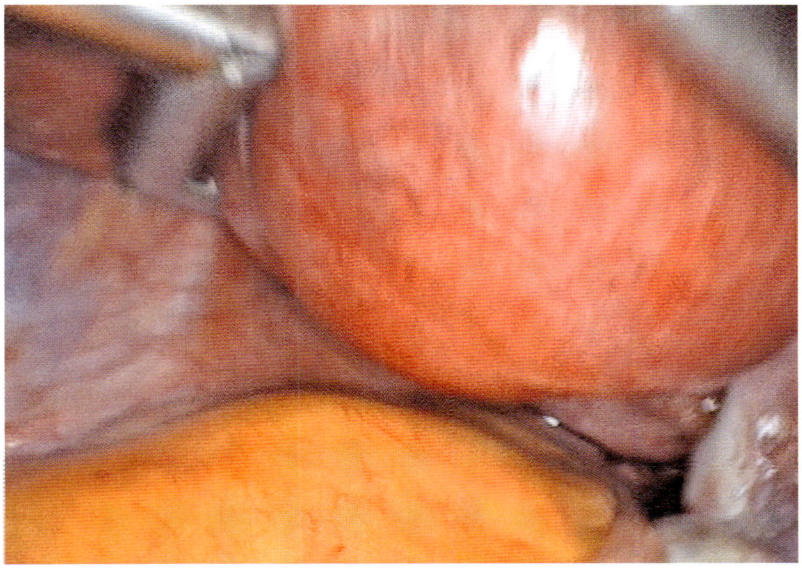

Fig. 7: Bulky uterus in pregnancy is supported with liver retractor.

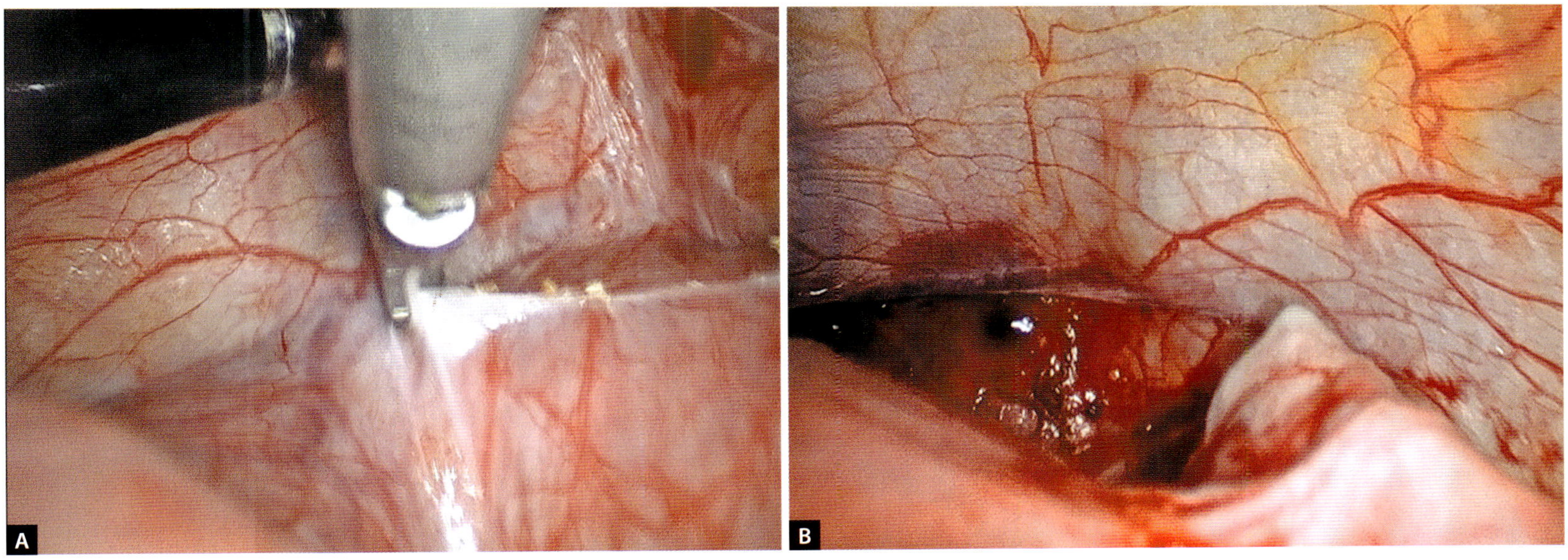

Figs. 8A and B: Bladder is dissected anteriorly.

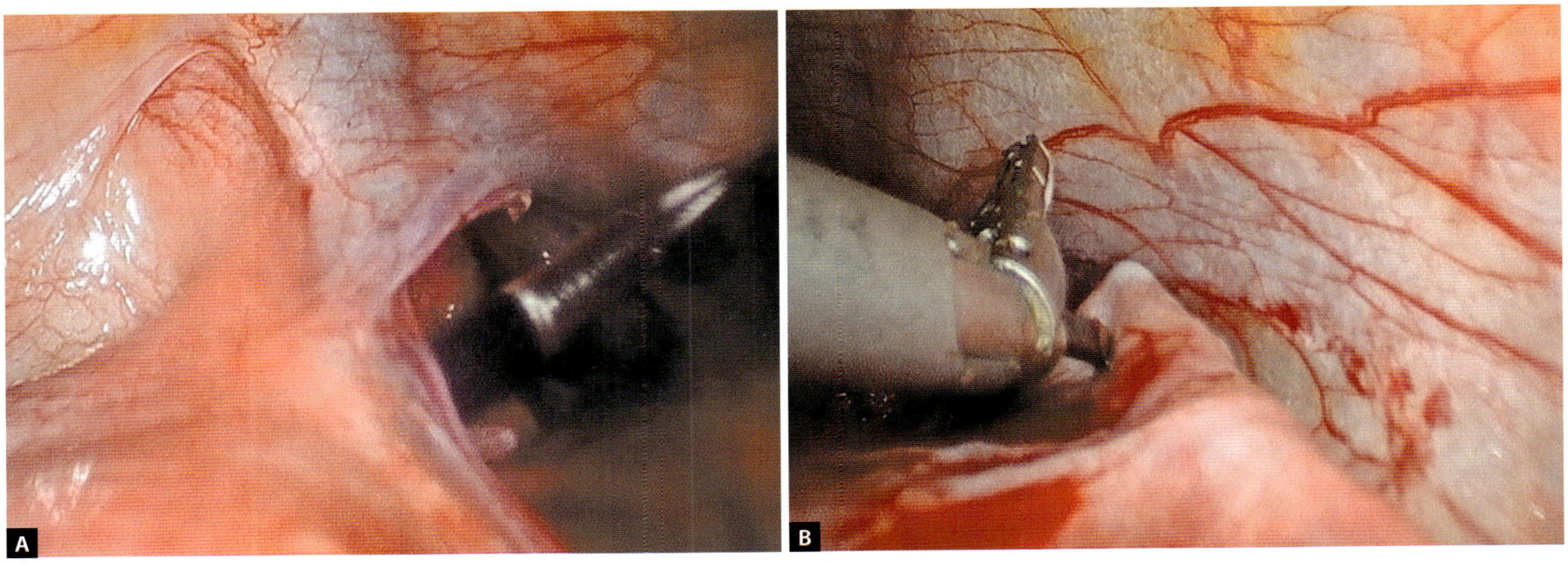

Figs. 9A and B

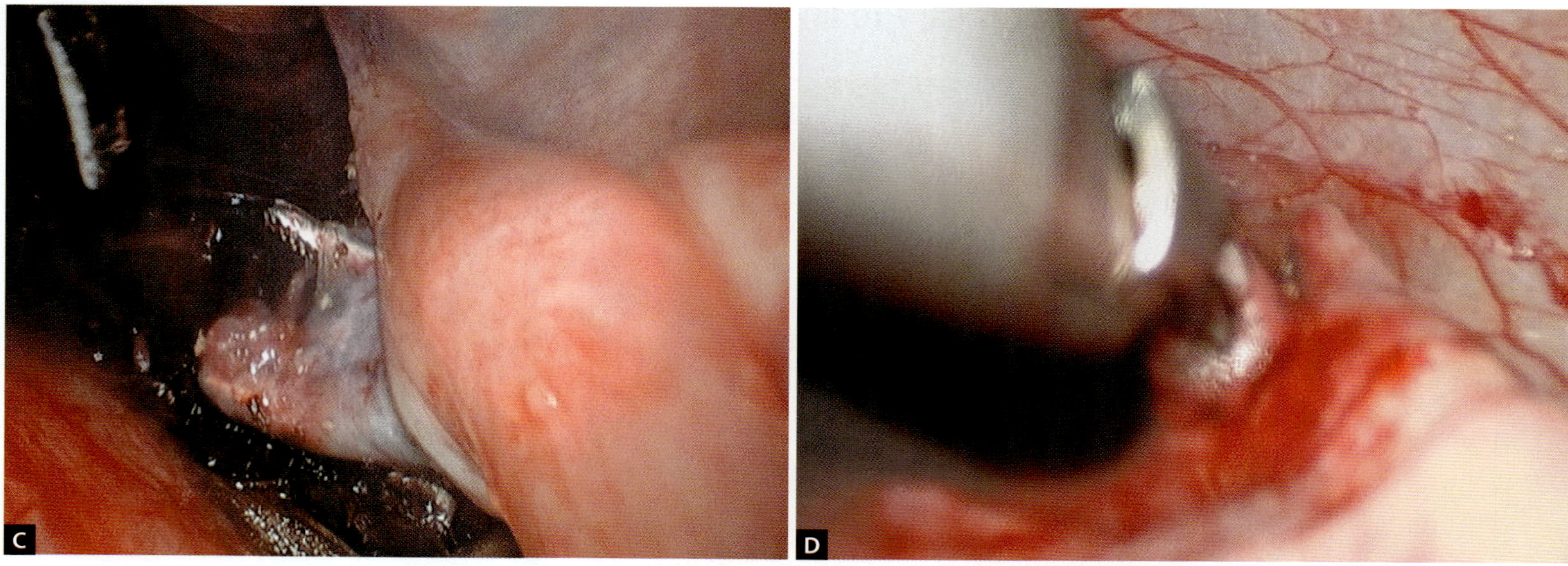

Figs. 9C and D

Figs. 9A to D: Window is made on both sides of broad ligament.

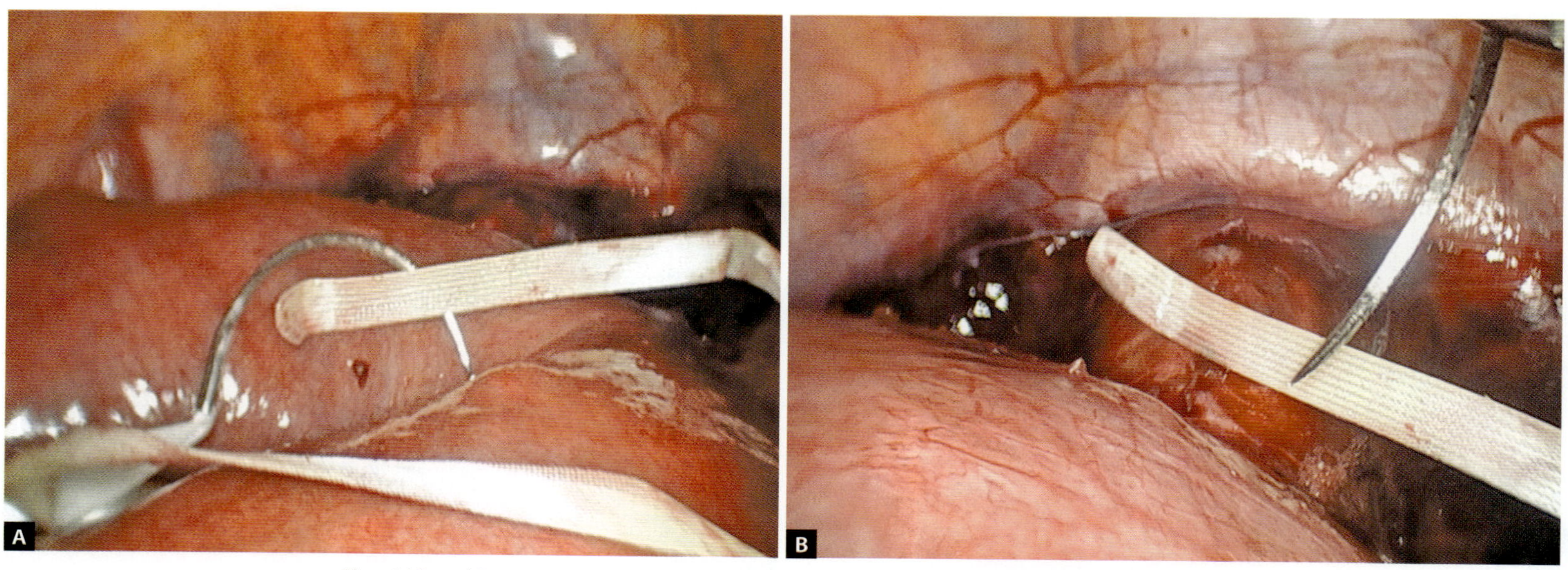

Figs. 10A and B: A 5 mm Mersilene tape is introduced into abdomen through laparoscopic port.

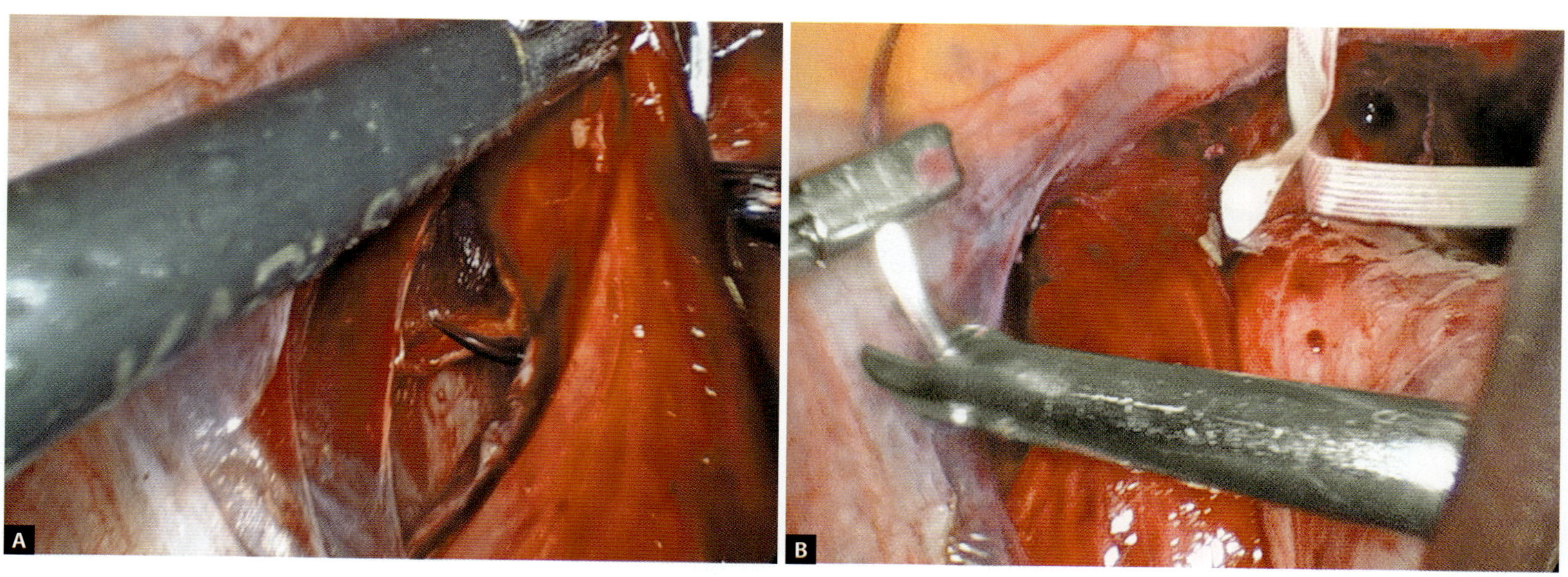

Figs. 11A and B

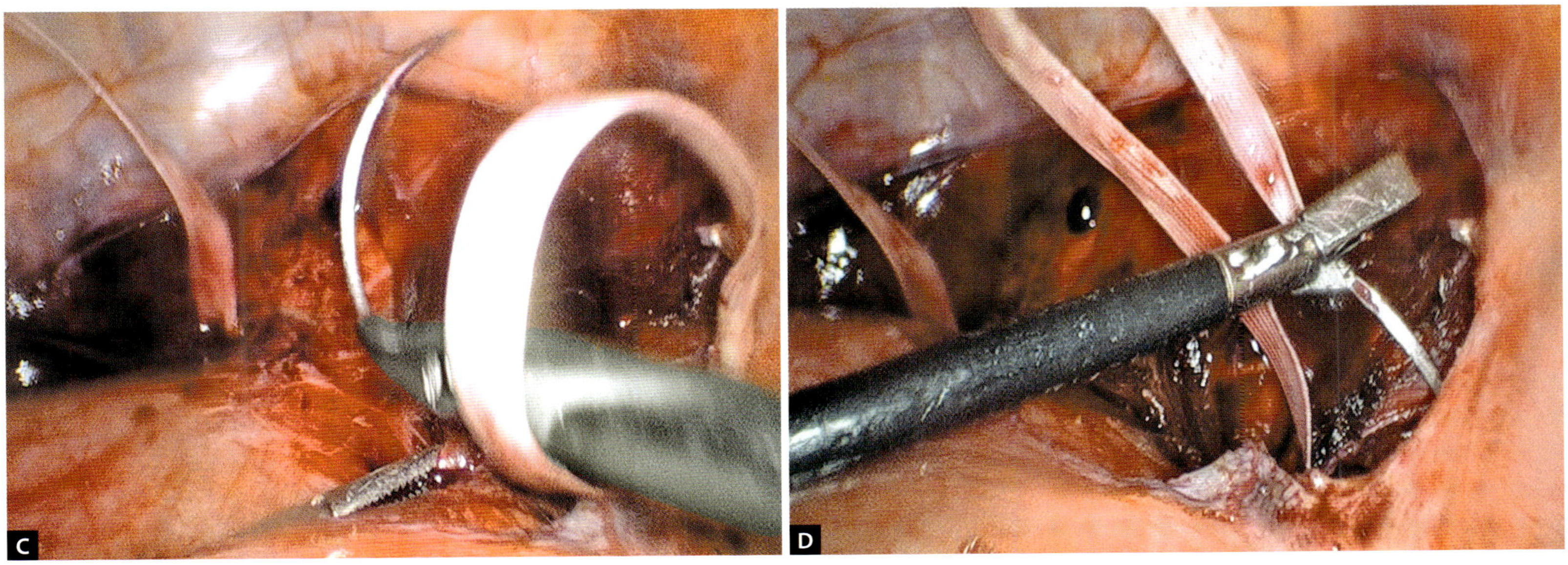

Figs. 11C and D

Figs. 11A to D: Needle of Mersilene tape is introduced on either side of broad ligament.

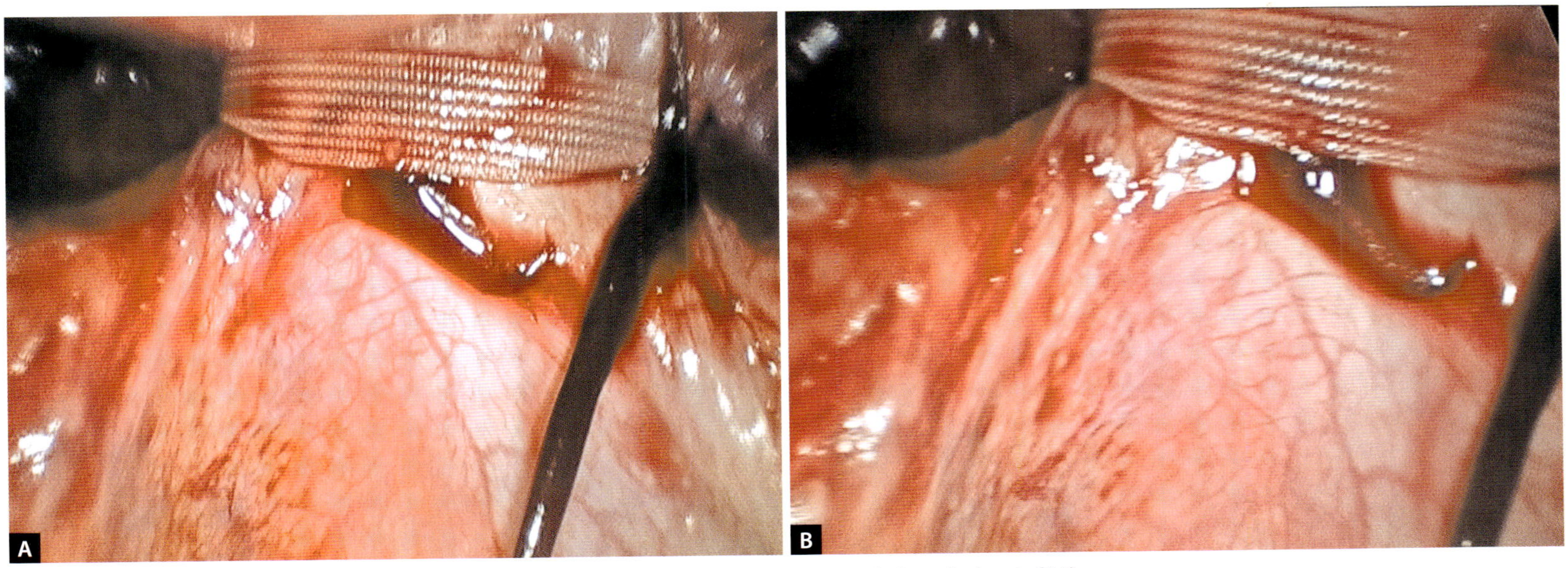

Figs. 12A and B: Mersilene tape is seen posteriorly at the level of isthmus.

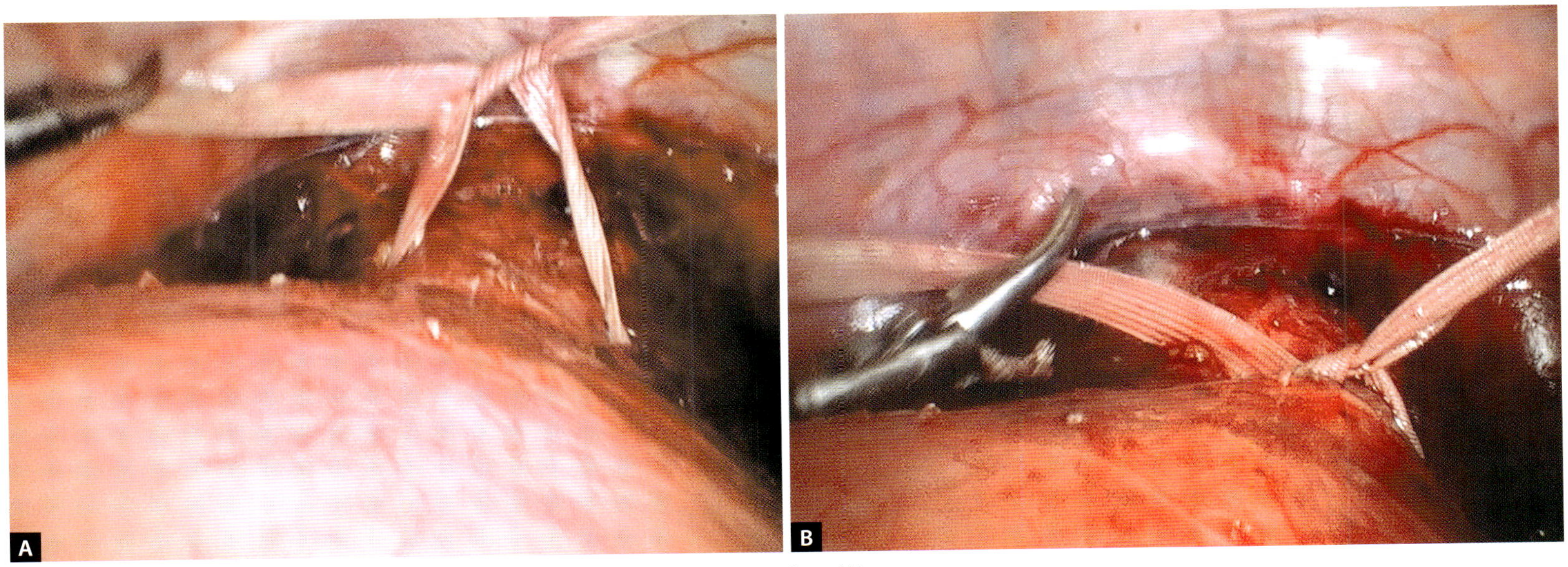

Figs. 13A and B

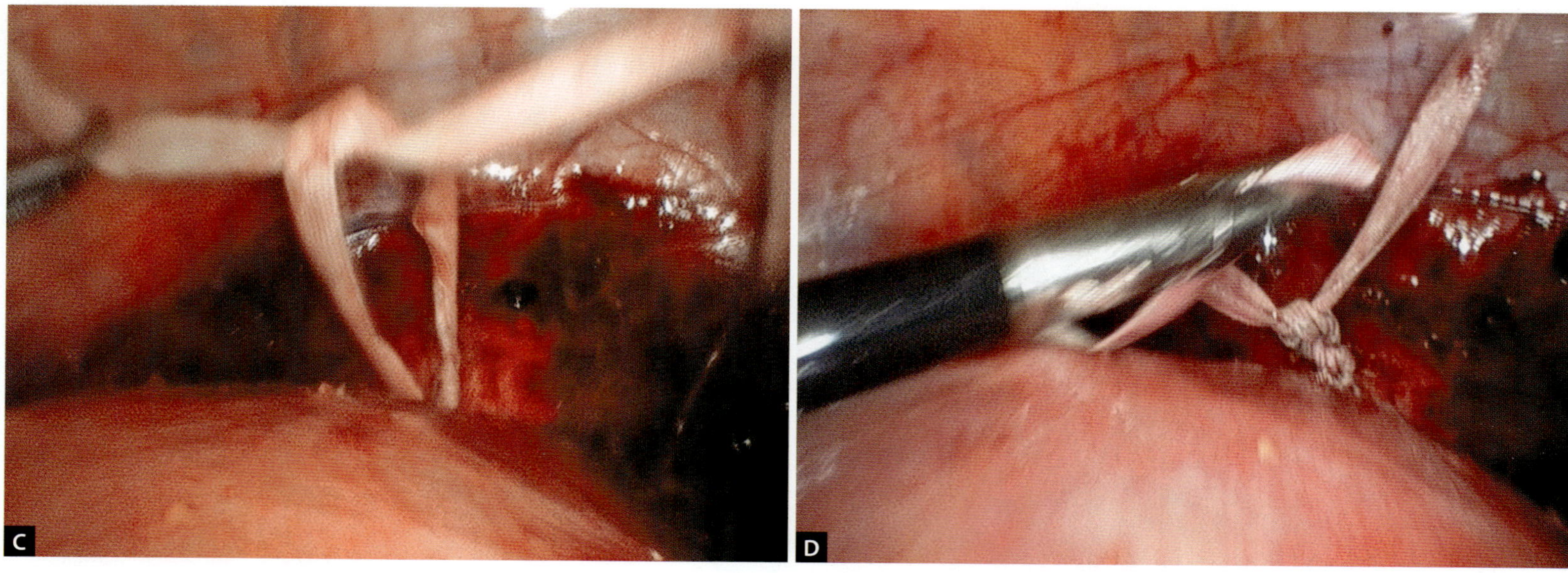

Figs. 13C and D

Figs. 13A to D: Ends of Mersilene tape are tied anteriorly by intracorporeal knotting.

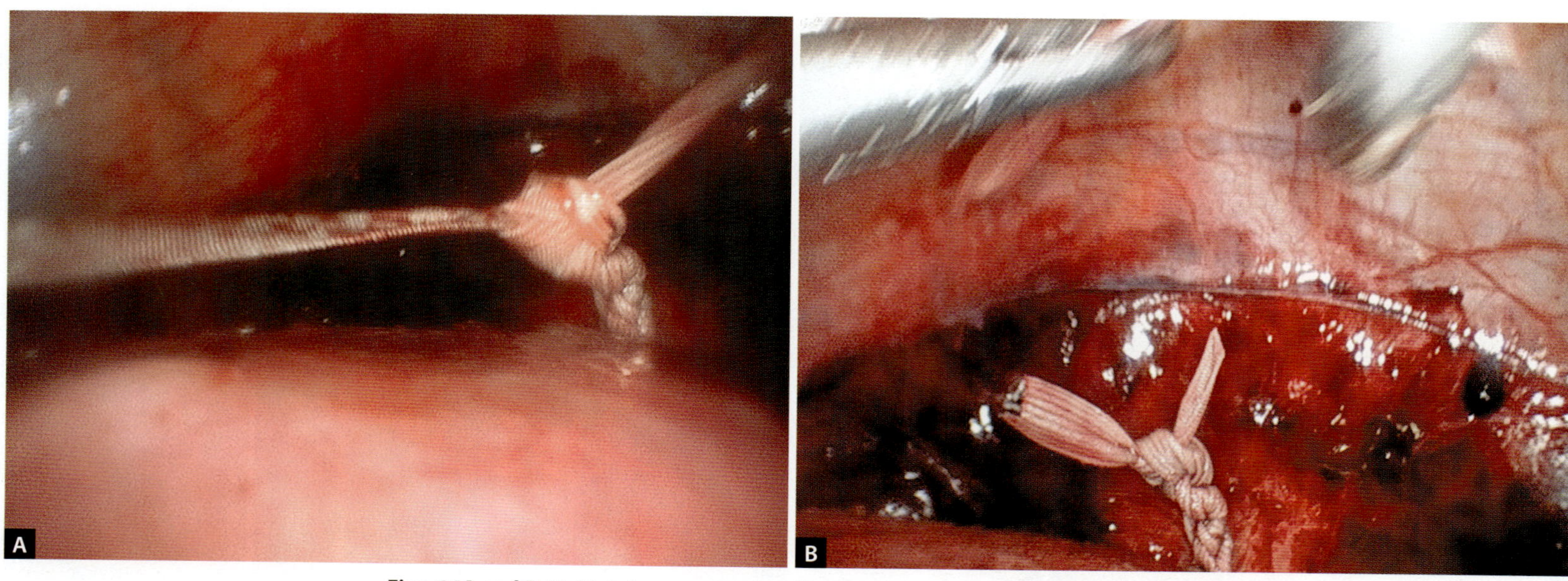

Figs. 14A and B: Multiple knots are fastened in Mersilene tape to avoid knot loosening.

LAPAROSCOPIC INTERVAL CERCLAGE (FIGS. 15 TO 19)

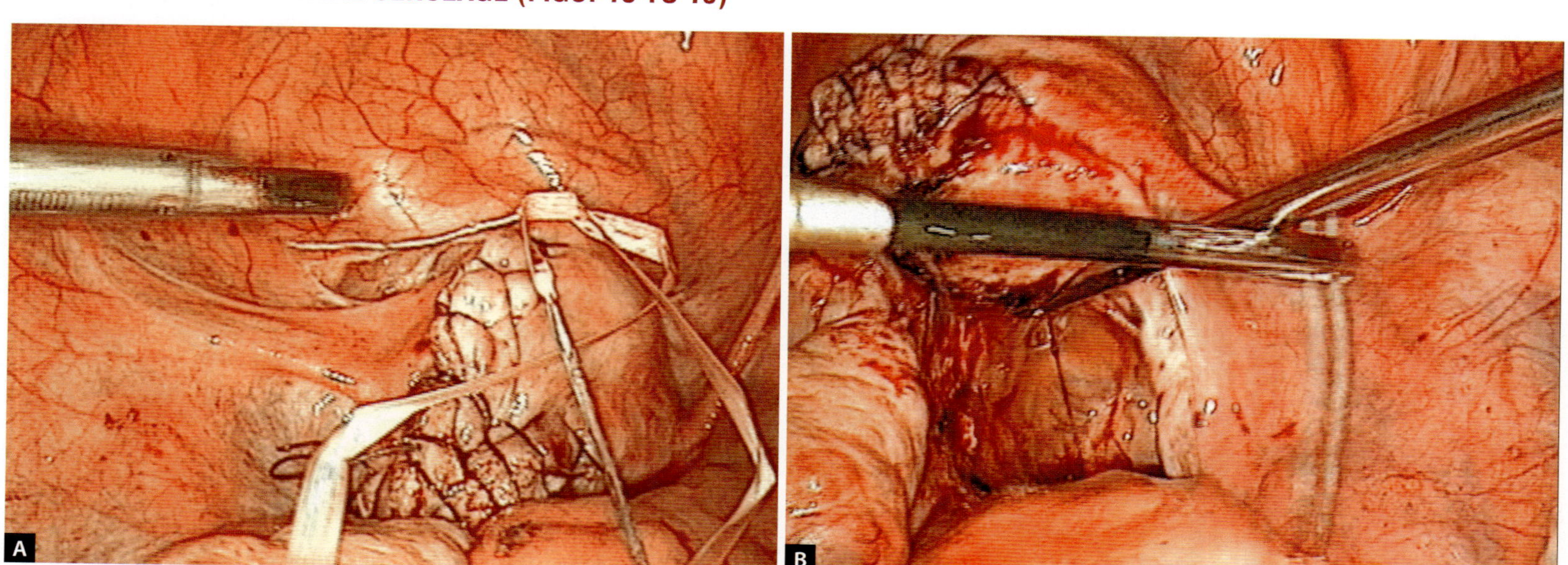

Figs. 15A and B: Mersilene tape is lifted with needle holder and grasper.

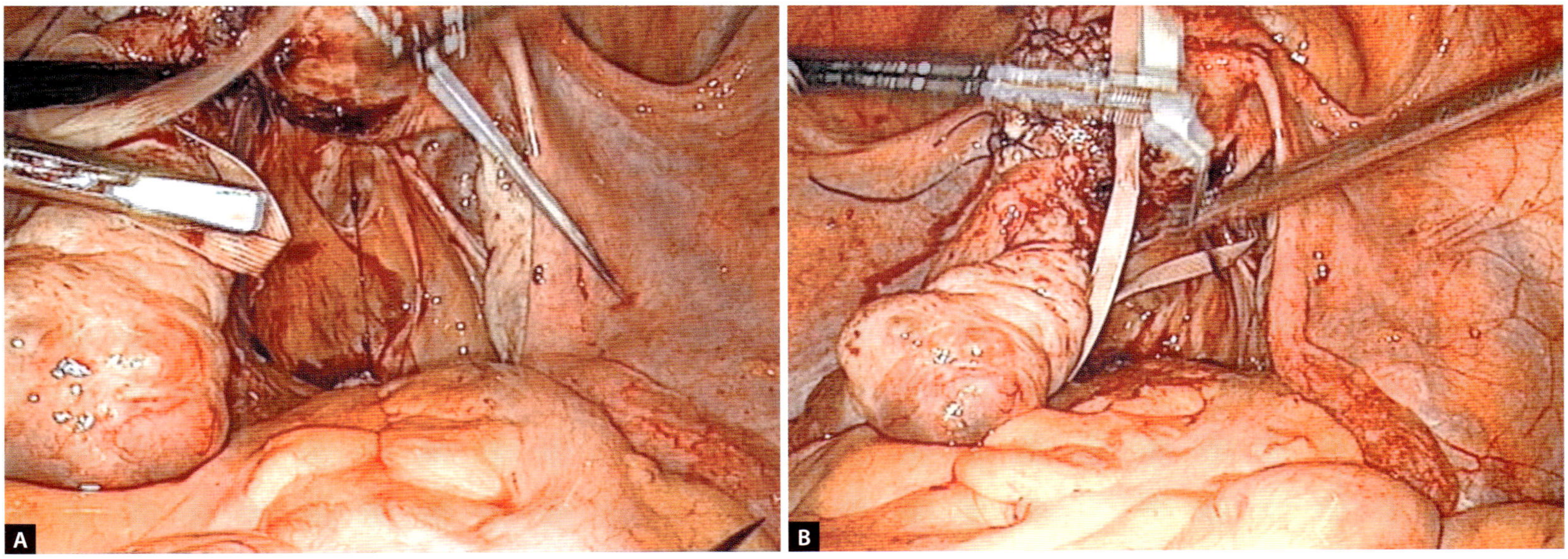

Figs. 16A and B: Needle is being directed to be introduced on one side of cervix at the level of isthmus.

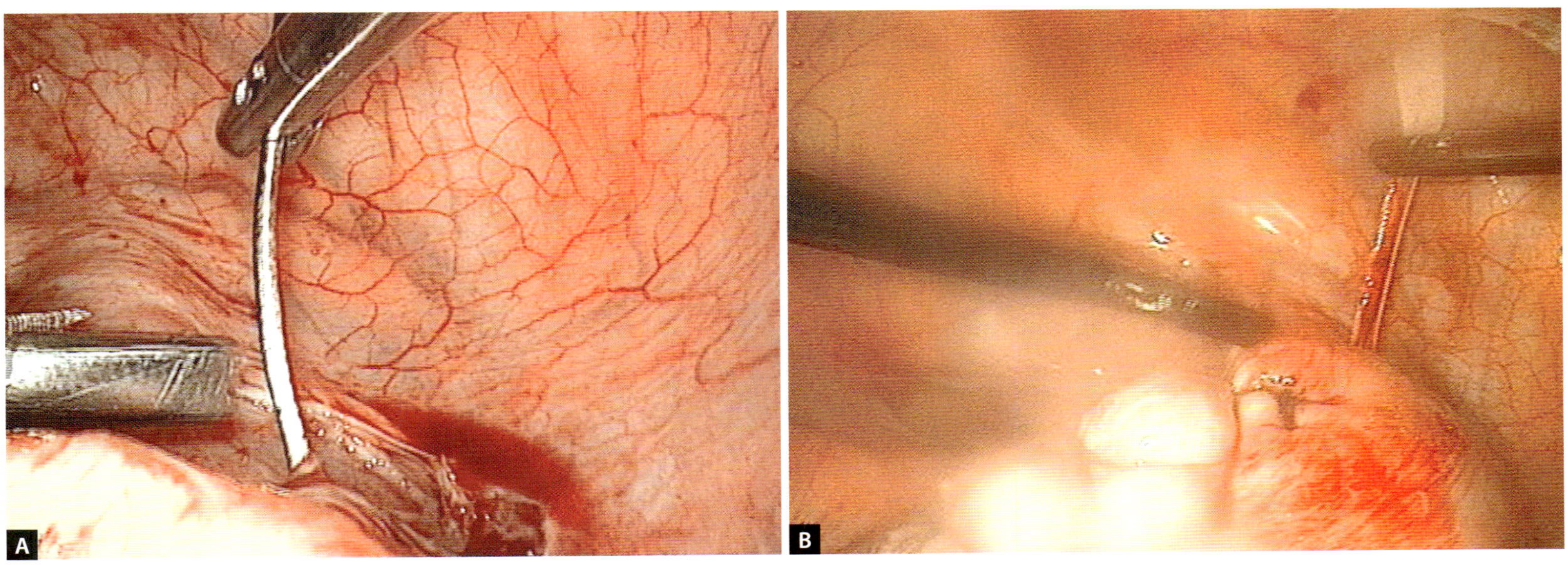

Figs. 17A and B: Mersilene tape is pulled out after passing on one side of uterus.

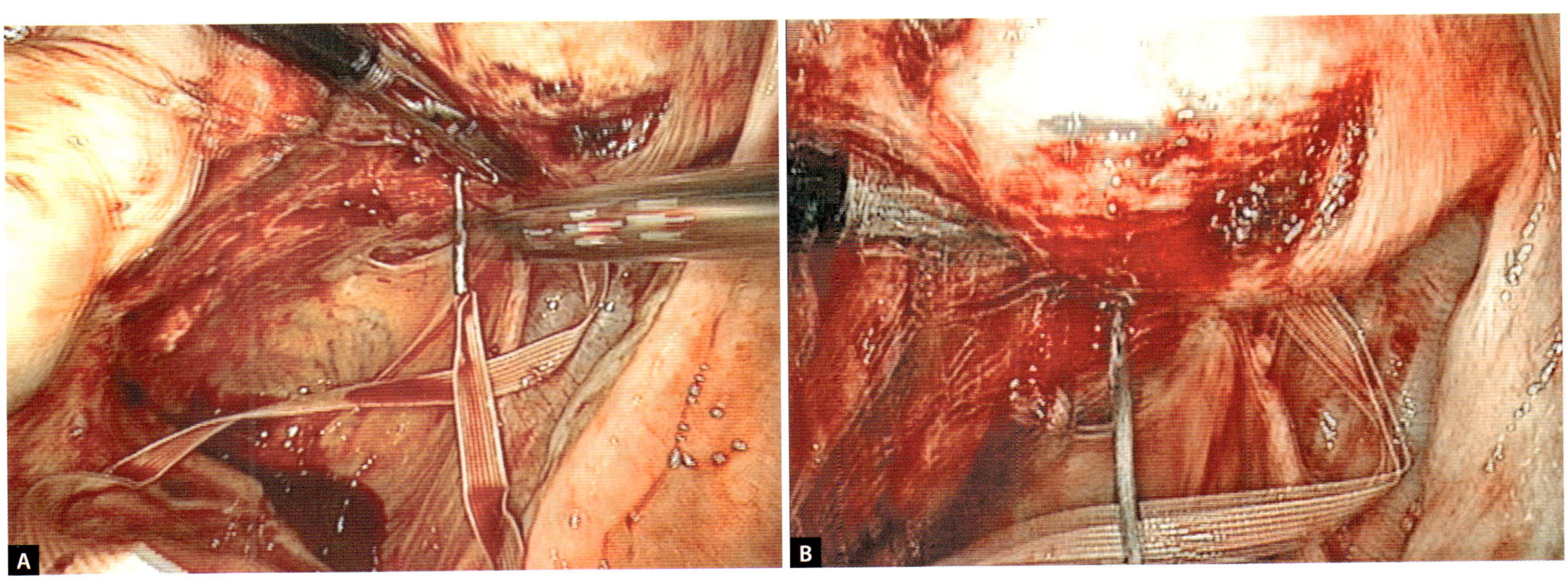

Figs. 18A and B

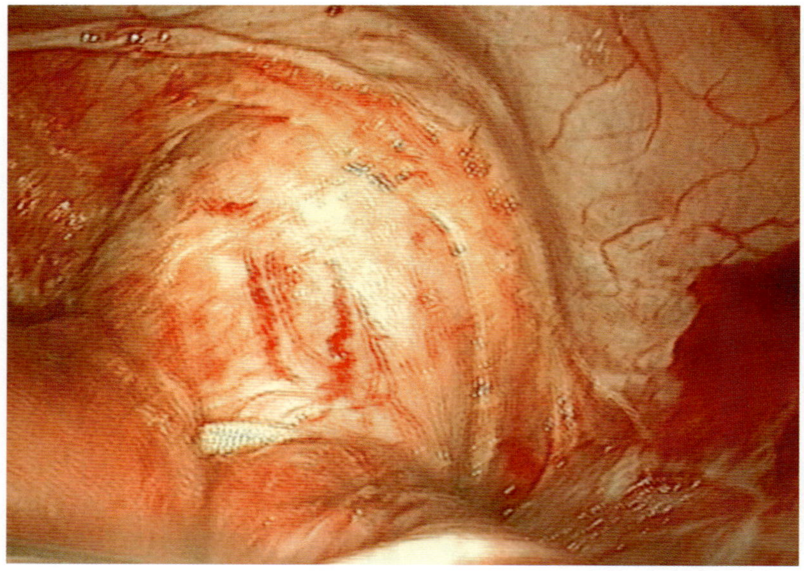

Fig. 18C

Figs. 18A to C: Mersilene tape at the level of isthmus.

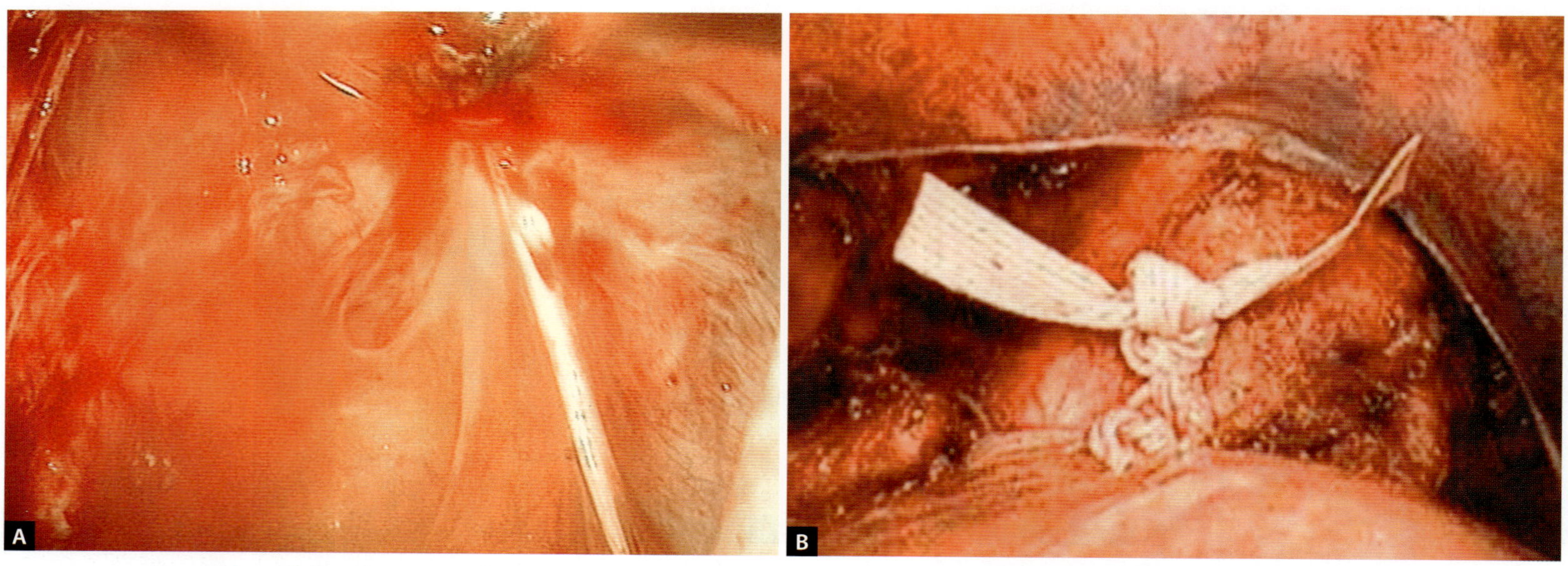

Figs. 19A and B: Mersilene tape with intracorporeal knot (multiple throws) is fastened on anterior aspect of uterus at the level of isthmus.

TECHNIQUE OF LAPAROSCOPIC ABDOMINAL CERCLAGE (FIGS. 7 TO 19)

The procedure is performed under general anesthesia.

The patient is placed in the dorsal lithotomy position followed by insertion of an indwelling catheter. In a nonpregnant state, a uterine manipulator is inserted into the uterine cavity. Laparoscopy is done in the usual fashion, using two secondary trocars at low abdominal quadrants. Depending on the height of the uterus, the secondary trocars are inserted higher than those in the nonpregnant condition and they should be inserted under direct vision. They are placed higher than the level of the uterine fundus.

Cerclage is performed using a 5 mm Mersilene polyester tape. The tape is introduced into the abdominal cavity. The adequate length is about 15 cm. The tape is then passed into the pelvis and positioned behind the uterus. The needle of the tape is held with needle holder and is directed toward the isthmus, medial to the uterine vessel. The cardinal ligament and the cervical body are pierced just above the insertion of the uterosacral ligament and the tip can be seen at the anterior leaf of the broad ligament. The end of the tape is grasped and withdrawn anteriorly. The procedure is then repeated on the opposite side, bringing the other end of the tape anteriorly. The needles on both sides of tape are cut and taken out. Using two laparoscopic needle holders, the two ends of the tape are tied anteriorly with a square knot. It is secured by multiple knots. The excess suture material is trimmed. A C-section is required for women giving birth with a TAC. A TAC can also be placed prepregnancy if a patient has been diagnosed with an incompetent cervix.

Concerns about Abdominal Cerclage in Nonpregnant State

Many concerns have been raised about interval cerclage:

- One such concern is that there might be impaired chance of conception following abdominal cerclage. However, studies showed patients who underwent laparoscopic radical trachelectomy and prophylactic cervical cerclage, 55% of them conceived within 36 months.
- One of the concerns though theoretical relating to cerclage as an interval procedure is when the patient suffers another

miscarriage. However, the cervix can easily be dilated to 8 mm and curettage can be performed in the presence of a cerclage. Alternatively, laparoscopic removal of the cerclage can be performed. A pregnancy of >24 weeks' gestation requires a cesarean delivery or induction can be tried after laparoscopic removal of cerclage.

Advantages of Laparoscopic Abdominal Cerclage Over Vaginal Cerclage

- High placement of the suture
- No risk of slippage of the cerclage
- No foreign body inside the vagina, so no added risk of infection and preterm labor
- The ability to leave the tape in place between pregnancies. To use this technique laparoscopically, the surgeon needs expertise in laparoscopic suturing. A variation on this technique is the robotic-assisted laparoscopic TAC. Decision of performing abdominal cerclage in pregnant or nonpregnant state depends on the treating doctor.

In the pregnant state, the cerclage is usually performed at the end of the first trimester (12–16 weeks) after first trimester aneuploidy screening. In 2004, Groom et al. reported the largest series of 19 prepregnancy TAC with a 100% survival rate and 89% women delivered after 36 weeks. No significant intraoperative, antenatal, intrapartum, and neonatal complications were found.

Some less common methods of cerclage include:

- *Hefner (also known as Wurm) cerclage:* It is a type of rescue cerclage performed when cervical effacement is greater than 80% and cervical dilatation is ≥3 cm. Here after displacing the membranes inside the uterus with Foley's catheter balloon, the lips of cervix are grasped with ring forceps and two U-shaped stitches are placed one vertically from 12 o'clock to 6 o'clock and other horizontal from 3 o'clock to 9 o'clock through the whole thickness of cervix. These are then tied very close to the internal os. Usually, no. 1 Prolene is used.
- *Lash cerclage:* A permanent stitch performed before pregnancy because of trauma to the cervix or an anatomical abnormality.
- *Espinosa Flores operation:* Here, membranes are displaced back into the uterus and two bites into the cervix at 9 and 3 o'clock positions are placed. The suture is inserted first going from anterior to posterior surface and then from posterior to anterior surface. The two ends are tied over the posterior aspect of the cervix. It can be done for both prophylactic and rescue cerclages.

AFTERCARE

After the cerclage has been placed, the patient will be observed for at least several hours (sometimes overnight) to ensure that she does not go into premature labor. Prophylactic tocolytics can be used for a period of 12 hours after the procedure. Patient will then be allowed to return home, but will be instructed to remain in bed or avoid physical activity for 2–3 days. Follow-up appointments will usually take place, so that her doctor can monitor the cervix and stitch and watch for signs of premature labor.

RISKS

Cerclage is generally a safe procedure, but as with any infertility group there are a number of potential complications that may arise during or after surgery. These are given in **Box 1**.

Box 1: Complications of cerclage.

- Risks associated with regional or general anesthesia
- Premature labor
- Premature rupture of membranes
- Cervical dystocia with failure to dilate requiring cesarean section
- Infection of the cervix
- Infection of the amniotic sac (chorioamnionitis)
- Cervical rupture (may occur if the stitch is not removed before onset of labor)
- Injury to the cervix or bladder
- Bleeding.

MORBIDITY AND MORTALITY RATES

About 1–9% of women will experience premature labor after cerclage. The risk of chorioamnionitis is 1–7%, but increases to 30% if cervical dilatation is greater than 1.2 (3 cm). The risks associated with preterm deliveries are far greater. Babies born between 22 weeks and 25 weeks of pregnancy are at significant risk of moderate-to-severe disabilities (46–56%) or death (at 22 weeks, survival is 10–30%, at 24 weeks it is increased to 50%, and at 26 weeks 95%).

RESULTS

Success of cerclage is defined if pregnancy continues till 37 weeks. Success rate for elective cerclage is approximately 80–90% and that for emergency cerclage is 40–60%.

Comparing cerclage with no treatment in women with singleton pregnancy who are at risk of preterm birth, there is obvious reduction in the rate of preterm birth but there is no reduction in death of baby before and after birth. In multiple gestations, there are no significant evidence to suggest that prophylactic cerclage is effective in preventing preterm births and reduction in perinatal deaths and neonatal morbidity.

REFERENCES

1. Feigenbaum SL, Crites Y, Hararah MK, et al. Prevalence of cervical insufficiency in polycystic ovarian syndrome. Hum Reprod. 2012;27:2837-42.
2. Petersen LK, Uldbjerg N. Cervical collagen in non-pregnant women with previous cervical incompetence. Eur J Obstet Gynecol Reprod Biol. 1996;67:41-5.
3. To MS, Skentou C, Liao AW, et al. Cervical length and funneling at 23 weeks of gestation in the prediction of spontaneous early preterm delivery. Ultrasound Obstet Gynecol. 2001;18:200-3.
4. Guzman ER, Pisatowski DM, Vintzileos AM, et al. A comparison of ultrasonographically detected cervical changes in response to transfundal pressure, coughing, and standing in predicting cervical incompetence. Am J Obstet Gynecol. 1997;177:660-5.
5. Guzman ER, Vintzileos AM, McLean DA, et al. The natural history of a positive response to transfundal pressure in women at risk for cervical incompetence. Am J Obstet Gynecol. 1997;176:634-8.
6. Guzman E, Rosenberg J, Houlihan C, et al. A new method using vaginal ultrasound and transfundal pressure to evaluate the asymptomatic incompetent cervix. Obstet Gynecol. 1994;83:248-52.
7. Owen J, Yost N, Berghella V, et al. Mid-trimester endovaginal sonography in women at high risk for spontaneous preterm birth. JAMA. 2001;286:1340-8.
8. Domin CM, Smith EJ, Terplan M. Transvaginal ultrasonographic measurement of cervical length as a predictor of preterm birth: a systematic review with meta-analysis. Ultrasound Q. 2010;26:241-8.
9. Visintine J, Berghella V, Henning D, et al. Cervical length for prediction of preterm birth in women with multiple prior induced abortions. Ultrasound Obstet Gynecol. 2008;31:198-200.
10. Moragianni VA, Aronis KN, Craparo FJ. Biweekly ultrasound assessment of cervical shortening in triplet pregnancies and the effect of cerclage placement. Ultrasound Obstet Gynecol. 2011;37:617-8.
11. Owen J, Yost N, Berghella V, et al. Can shortened midtrimester cervical length predict very early spontaneous preterm birth? Am J Obstet Gynecol. 2004;191:298-303.

12. Goldenberg RL, Iams JD, Mercer BM, et al. The preterm prediction study: the value of new vs standard risk factors in predicting early and all spontaneous preterm births. NICHD MFMU Network. Am J Public Health. 1998;88:233-8.
13. Iams JD, Goldenberg RL, Mercer BM, et al. The preterm prediction study: can low-risk women destined for spontaneous preterm birth be identified? Am J Obstet Gynecol. 2001;184:652-5.
14. Mercer BM, Goldenberg RL, Meis PJ, et al. The Preterm Prediction Study: prediction of preterm premature rupture of membranes through clinical findings and ancillary testing. The National Institute of Child Health and Human Development Maternal-Fetal Medicine Units Network. Am J Obstet Gynecol. 2000;183:738-45.
15. Goldenberg RL, Iams JD, Das A, et al. The Preterm Prediction Study: sequential cervical length and fetal fibronectin testing for the prediction of spontaneous preterm birth. National Institute of Child Health and Human Development Maternal-Fetal Medicine Units Network. Am J Obstet Gynecol. 2000;182:636-43.
16. Lee SE, Romero R, Park CW, et al. The frequency and significance of intraamniotic inflammation in patients with cervical insufficiency. Am J Obstet Gynecol. 2008;198:633.e1-8.
17. Leitich H, Bodner-Adler B, Brunbauer M, et al. Bacterial vaginosis as a risk factor for preterm delivery: a meta-analysis. Am J Obstet Gynecol. 2003;189:139-47.
18. Leitich H, Brunbauer M, Bodner-Adler B, et al. Antibiotic treatment of bacterial vaginosis in pregnancy: a meta-analysis. Am J Obstet Gynecol. 2003;188:752-8.
19. Matijevic R, Grgic O, Knezevic M. Vaginal pH versus cervical length in the mid-trimester as screening predictors of preterm labor in a low-risk population. Int J Gynaecol Obstet. 2010;111:41-4.
20. Ankirskaia AS, Demidova EM, Zemlianaia AA, et al. Genital Mycoplasma as a risk factor of obstetric and perinatal pathology. Vestn Akad Med Nauk SSSR. 1991;6:17-9.
21. Hassan S, Romero R, Hendler I, et al. A sonographic short cervix as the only clinical manifestation of intra-amniotic infection. J Perinat Med. 2006; 34:13-9.
22. Bujold E, Morency AM, Rallu F, et al. Bacteriology of amniotic fluid in women with suspected cervical insufficiency. J Obstet Gynaecol Can. 2008;30:882-7.
23. Oh KJ, Lee SE, Jung H, et al. Detection of ureaplasmas by the polymerase chain reaction in the amniotic fluid of patients with cervical insufficiency. J Perinat Med. 2010;38:261-8.
24. Iams JD, Goldenberg RL, Mercer BM, et al. The Preterm Prediction Study: recurrence risk of spontaneous preterm birth. National Institute of Child Health and Human Development Maternal-Fetal Medicine Units Network. Am J Obstet Gynecol. 1998;178:1035-40.
25. da Fonseca EB, Bittar RE, Carvalho MH, et al. Prophylactic administration of progesterone by vaginal suppository to reduce the incidence of spontaneous preterm birth in women at increased risk: a randomized placebo-controlled double-blind study. Am J Obstet Gynecol. 2003;188:419-24.
26. Meis PJ, Klebanoff M, Thom E, et al. Prevention of recurrent preterm delivery by 17 alpha-hydroxyprogesterone caproate. N Engl J Med. 2003;348:2379-85.
27. Daya S. Efficacy of progesterone support for pregnancy in women with recurrent miscarriage. A meta-analysis of controlled trials. Br J Obstet Gynaecol. 1989;96:275-80.
28. Final report of the Medical Research Council/Royal College of Obstetricians and Gynaecologists multicentre randomised trial of cervical cerclage. MRC/RCOG Working Party on Cervical Cerclage. Br J Obstet Gynaecol. 1993;100:516-23.
29. Sosa C, Althabe F, Belizán J, et al. Bed rest in singleton pregnancies for preventing preterm birth. Cochrane Database Syst Rev. 2004;1:CD003581.
30. Berghella V, Rafael TJ, Szychowski JM, et al. Cerclage for short cervix on ultrasonography in women with singleton gestations and previous preterm birth: a meta-analysis. Obstet Gynecol. 2011;117:663-71.
31. Berghella V, Mackeen AD. Cervical length screening with ultrasound-indicated cerclage compared with history-indicated cerclage for prevention of preterm birth: a meta-analysis. Obstet Gynecol. 2011;118:148-55.
32. Owen J, Hankins G, Iams JD, et al. Multicenter randomized trial of cerclage for preterm birth prevention in high-risk women with shortened midtrimester cervical length. Am J Obstet Gynecol. 2009;201:375.e1-8.

Accompanying Video: Laparoscopic cervical encerclage.

CHAPTER

75

Obstetric Hysterectomy

Jaya V, Aditi Rai

INTRODUCTION

Obstetric hysterectomy is an emergency procedure done to counter intractable bleeding following vaginal delivery or cesarean section. At present, it is being done for abnormal placentation like placenta accreta.

In a retrospective study conducted in Northern India (Chawla et al.) between August 2006 to July 2014, the incidence was 30/100,000 following vaginal delivery and 270/100,000 after cesarean section and overall incidence being 83/100,000. The most common indication is intractable PPH (25%) followed by placenta accreta (21%) and uterine rupture (17.5%). Sepsis and disseminated intravascular coagulation (DIC) account for other causes. Maternal mortality was 17.7% and PNM was 37.5%.

In case of placenta accreta where diagnosis is known earlier, it can be a planned procedure with urologist and interventional radiologist where facilities are available.

The procedure follows the same step as for gynecological hysterectomy. But being an obstetric emergency, as the women may be in shock, subtotal hysterectomy is resorted to. Patient may require postoperative ICU and supportive therapy for DIC and end organ involvement. In case of placenta previa, one has to resort to total hysterectomy as placenta is situated in the LUS and sometimes covering the os. Tubes and ovaries are usually left back as patient is very young. Steps includes clamping the round ligament, corneal structures tubes and ovarian ligament in succession, opening the UV-fold and pushing the bladder down and clamping the uterine artery. The next step is to clamp transversely leaving the cervix. It is easier in case where LSCS has been to clamp transversally at the site of uterine incision and delivering the uterus.

Even when total hysterectomy is attempted, apportion of cervix gets left behind as there is no clear demarcation between cervix and vagina at full dilatation, so screening for Ca cervix is mandatory later on as other women.

The images depict the clamping the corneal structures. It is precautionary to place a drain in conditions like DIC.

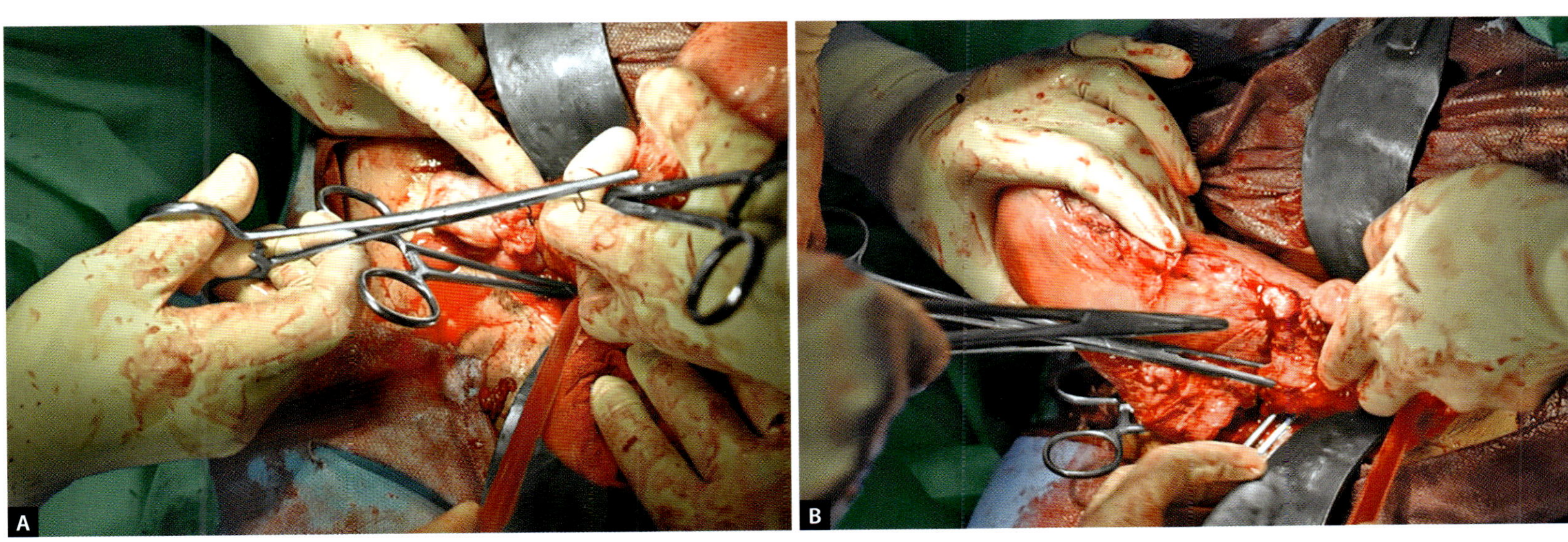

Figs. 1A and B: Uterine arteries exposed.

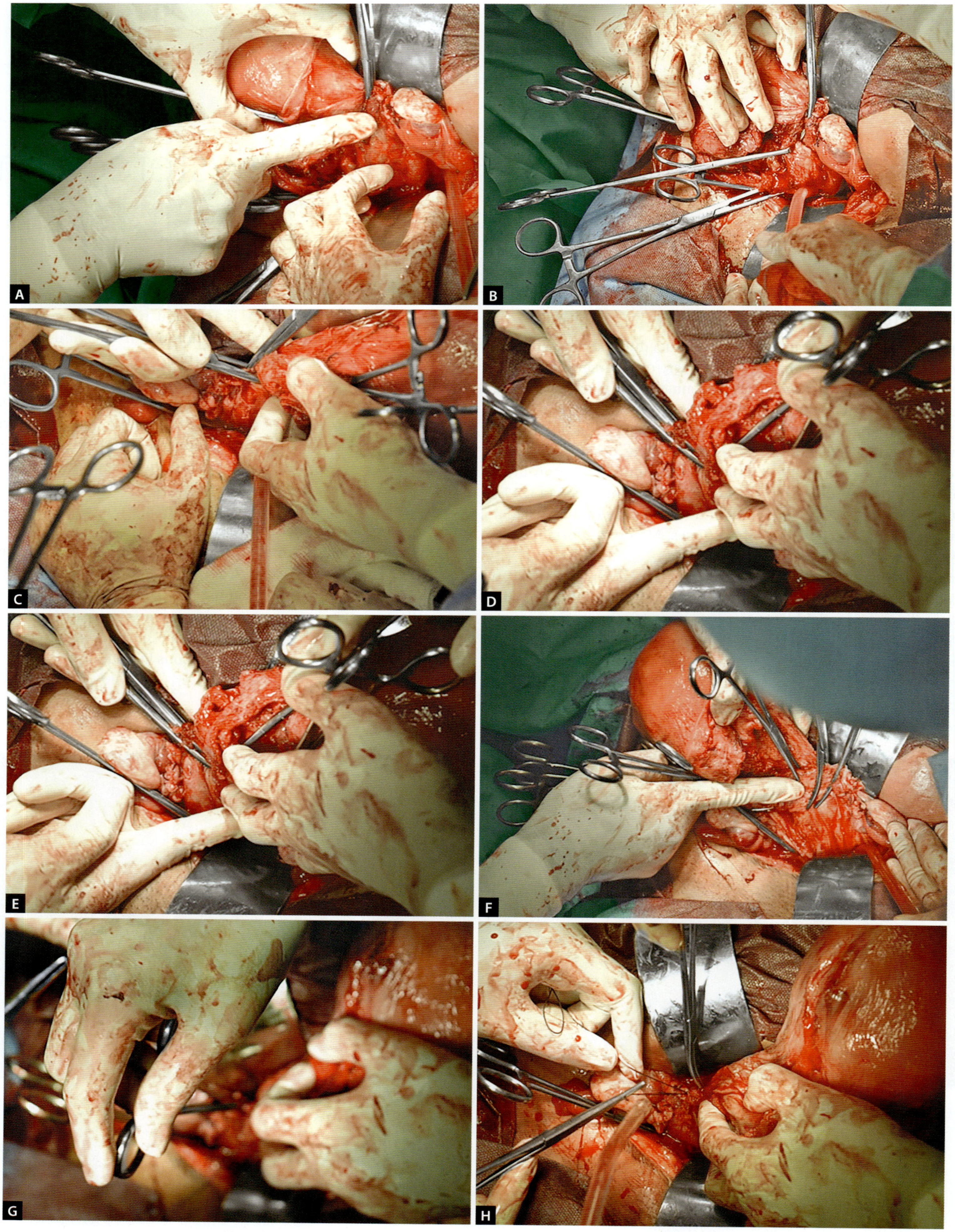

Figs. 2A to H: Bilateral uterine arteries clamped with vicryl no. 1 and cut with scissors.

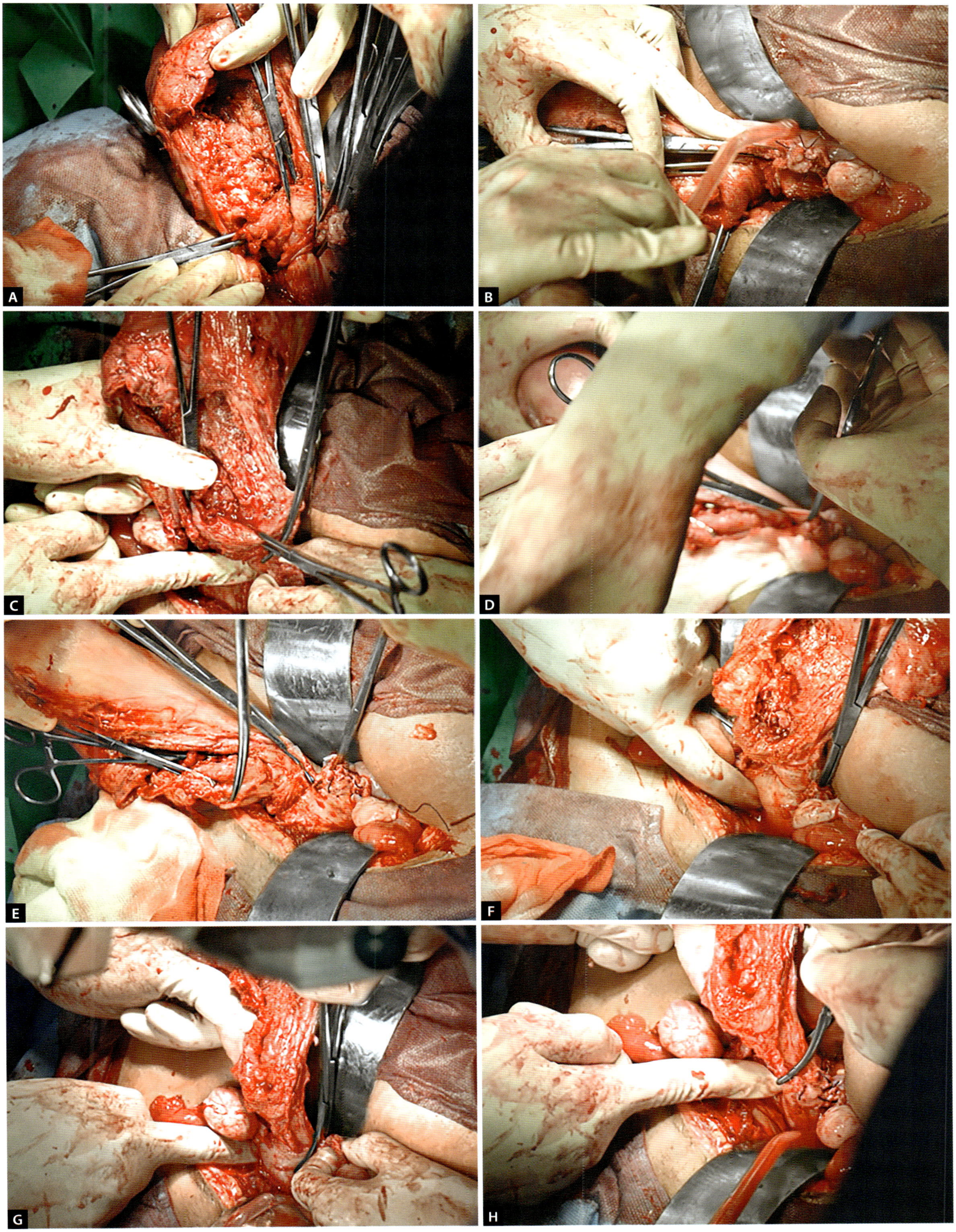

Figs. 3A to H: Bilateral uterosacral and cardinal ligament clamped with vicryl no.1 and cut with scissors.

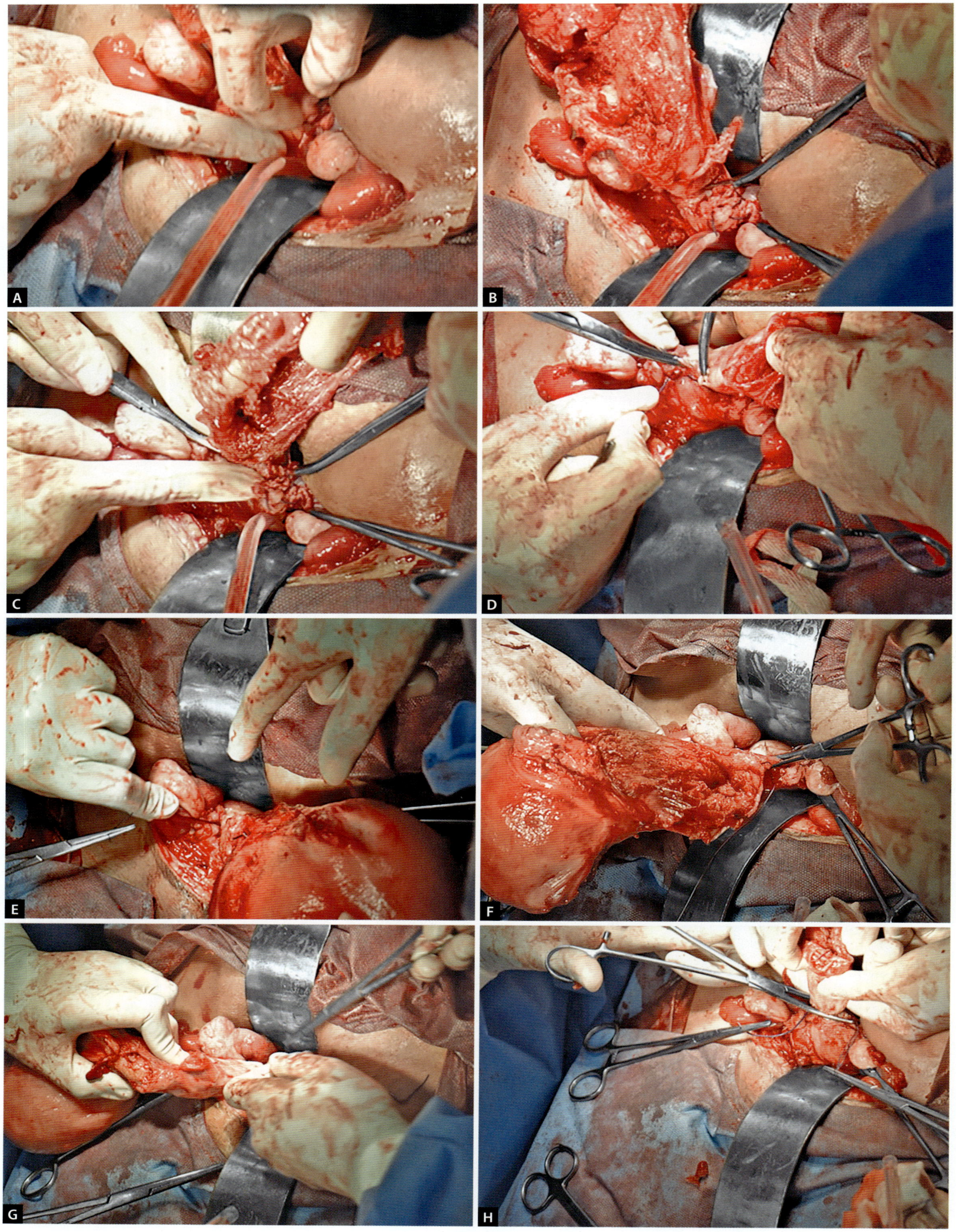

Figs. 4A to H: Supracervical hysterectomy done.

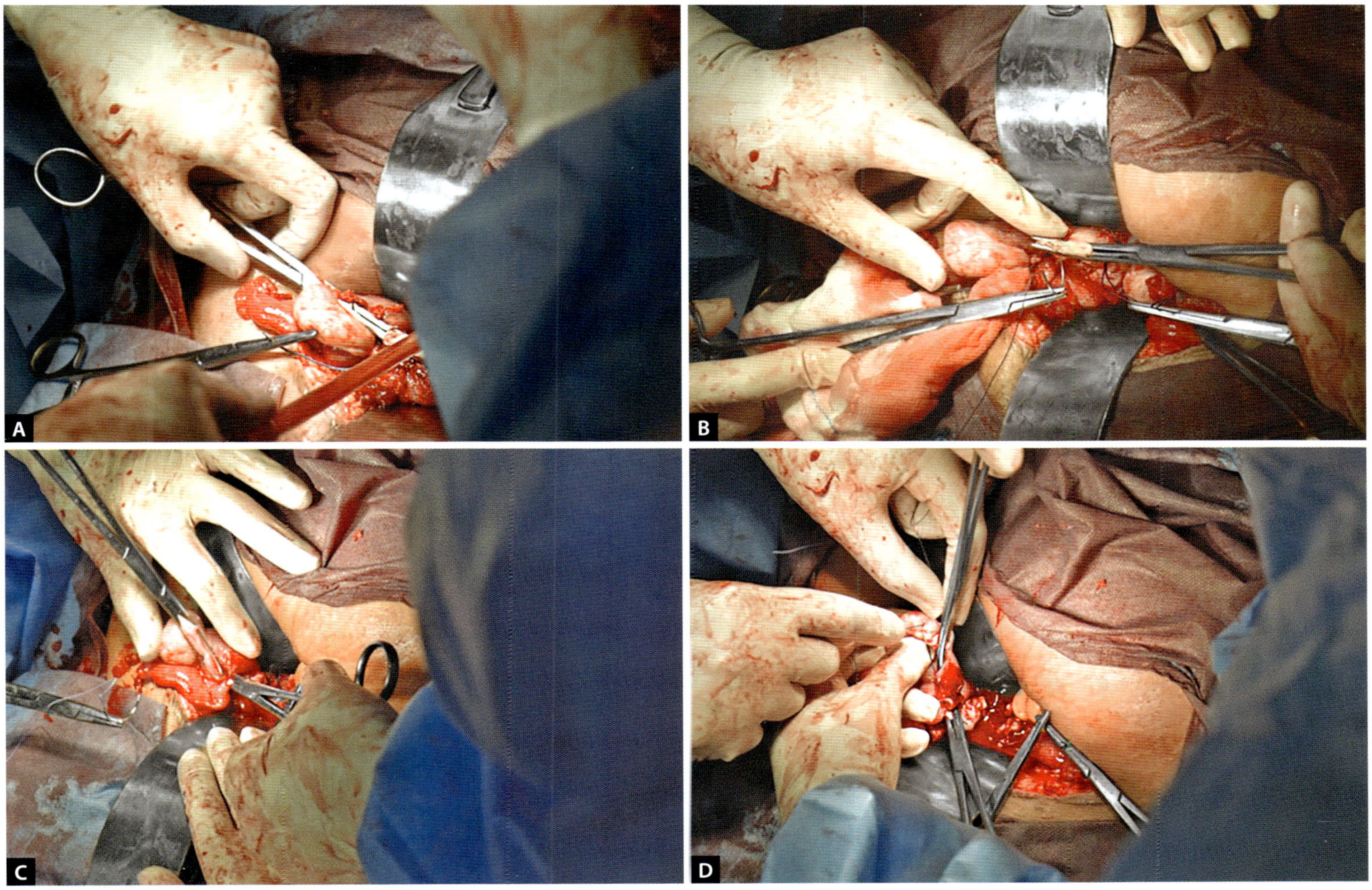

Figs. 5A to D: Vault closed with continous interlocking.

CHAPTER

76

B-Lynch Suture

Bhuvana S, Aditi Rai

INTRODUCTION

Compression sutures are sutures placed externally in various patterns involving the upper and lower uterine segments which function similar to manual compression and facilitates uterine contraction.

B-Lynch described a technique in 1997 to treat uterine atony using a continuous suture to compress the uterus in case of failed medical management for postpartum hemorrhage (PPH) during lower segment cesarean section (LSCS). This technique is being practiced worldwide and was modified by Hayman's in 2002, Cho's suture (square sutures) and horizontal compression sutures have emerged. These are easy to learn and are suitable alternate to obstetric hysterectomy and preserve the fertility potential and save patients' lives.

B-Lynch suture needs a long wide curved needle and a long absorbable suture. After LSCS when we have marked uterine atony, we can have these sutures placed in before closing the uterus.

METHOD

Uterus is exteriorized from the peritoneal cavity. Atraumatic number 1 Vicryl with a long needle is taken and the first bite passes 1.5 cm below and 3 cm lateral on the right end of the incision from outside in and emerges inside out 1.5 cm above and 3.5 cm from the lateral border of the uterus winds around the fundus to pierce the posterior wall and enters outside in to the inner posterior wall 3 cm medial to the lateral border of the uterus and passes horizontally for 3–4 cm and taken inside out at the same corresponding point on the left side inside out. The suture passes over the fundus and taken from back to front and finally emerges through the upper and lower border of the open incision 3 cm from the lateral end and 1.5 cm below the lower edge to meet the suture which is kept long and tied with it. Care should be taken that the assistant compresses the uterus while tying the suture so that vertical compression sutures are tight. Uterine closure is completed in the usual way. Postoperatively oxytocin is continued and can be combined with Bakri balloon tamponade called as sandwich technique. It has an average success rate of 97%.

Hayman's suture is a simple method when uterine incision is already closed. It is quick and easy method to learn. A number 1 atraumatic chromic catgut is passed from below the right lower margin above the reflection of bladder and passes through the anterior and posterior walls to emerge out in the right lower posterior wall which will be held in the fundus and to be tied together after a similar suture is performed on the left side, while the assistant compresses the uterus. It is as efficacious as B-Lynch and has neither future side effects such as uterine synechiae nor does it affect the future fertility. Before closing the abdomen, the surgeon has to ensure that the vaginal bleeding is within normal limits. In our institution, Hayman's suture is practiced widely and has been successful most of the times.

The other sutures are the horizontal compression sutures, Cho's sutures, etc. The square sutures were created by Cho and his colleagues a safer option as the uterine vessels do not cross the anatomy where the stitch is placed.

STEPS OF B-LYNCH SUTURING (FIGS. 1 TO 18)

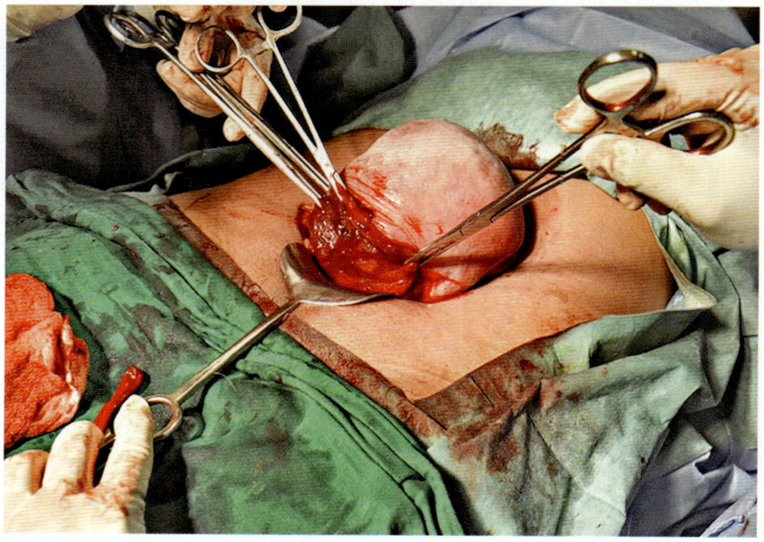

Fig. 1: Step 1.

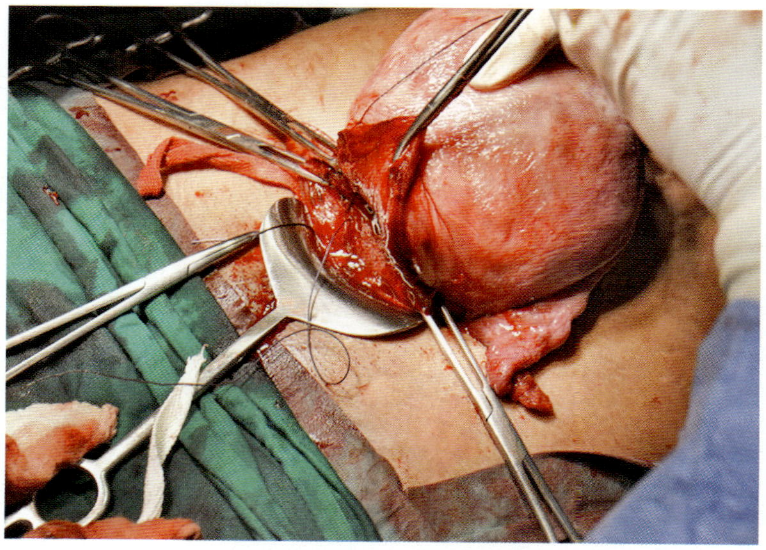

Fig. 2: Step 2—Number 1 Vicryl with a long needle is taken and the first bite passes 1.5 cm below and 3 cm lateral on the right end of the incision from outside in.

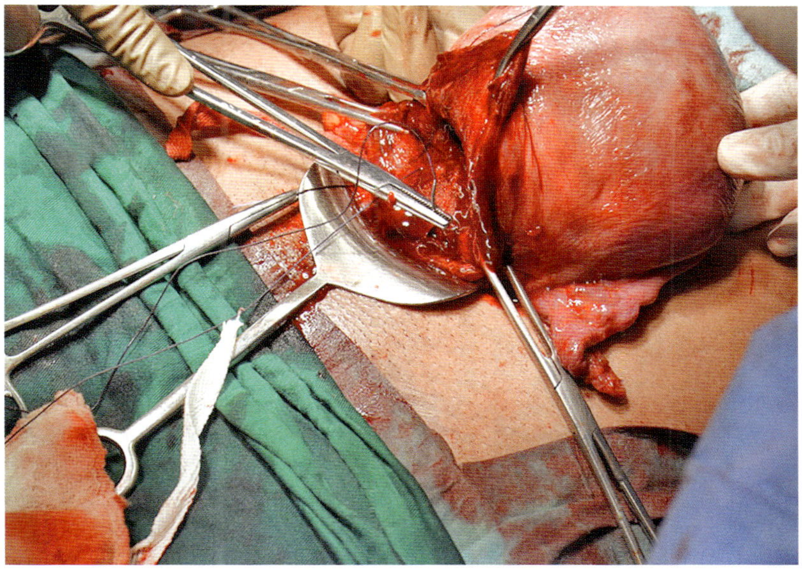

Fig. 3: Step 3.

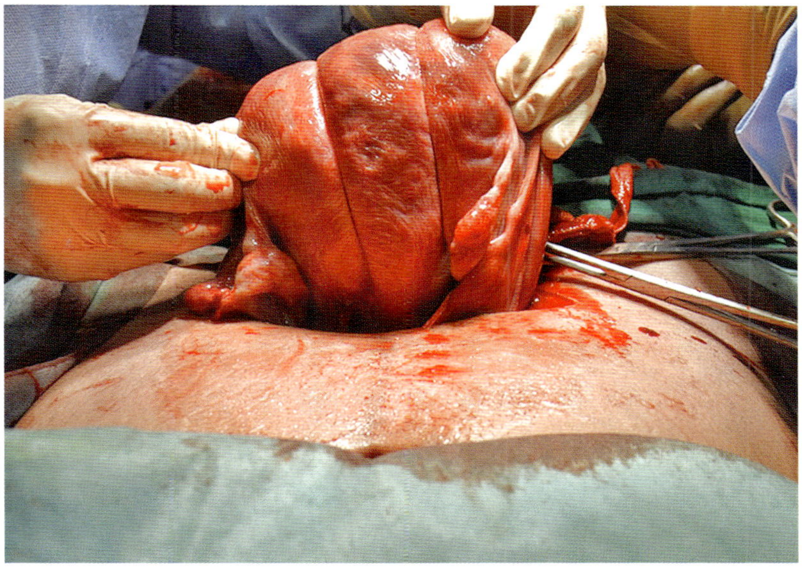

Fig. 6: Step 6—Care should be taken that the assistant compresses the uterus while tying the suture, so that vertical compression sutures are tight.

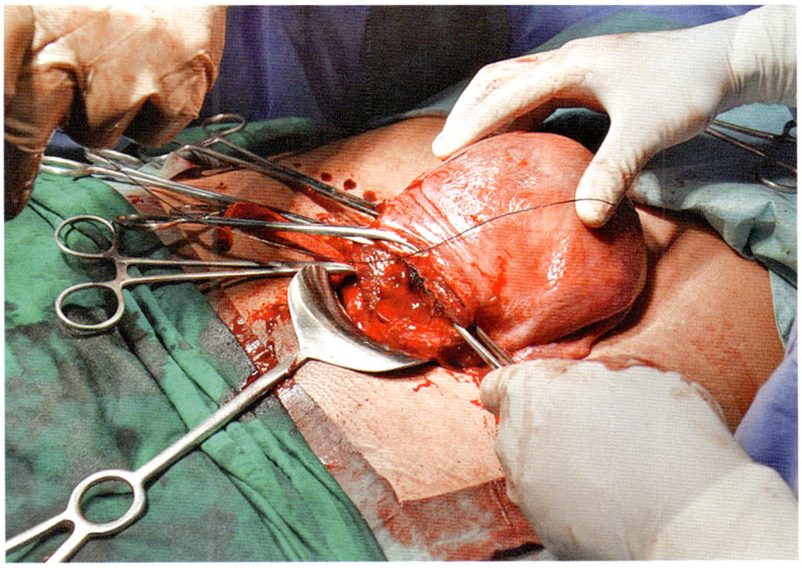

Fig. 4: Step 4—Emerges inside out 1.5 cm above and 3.5 cm from the lateral border of the uterus winds around the fundus to pierce the posterior wall and enters outside in to the inner posterior wall 3 cm medial to the lateral border of the uterus and passes horizontally for 3–4 cm and taken inside out at the same corresponding point on the left side inside out.

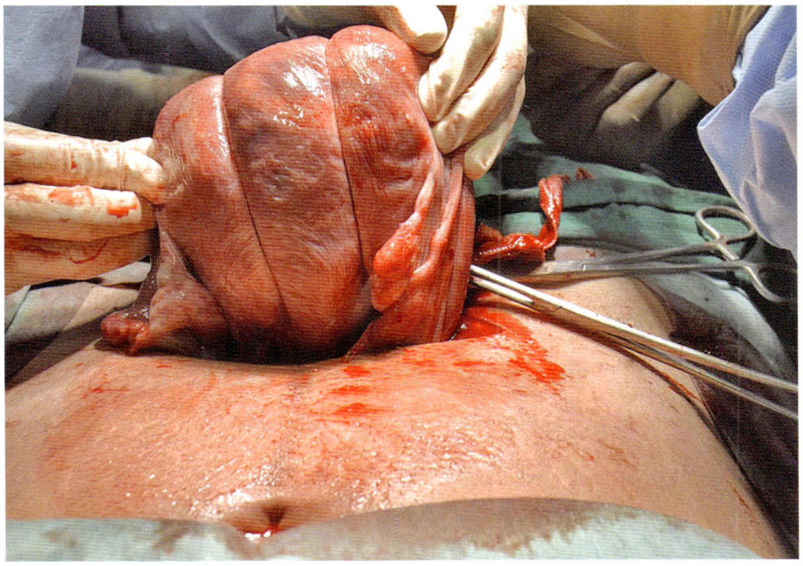

Fig. 7: Step 7—B-Lynch suture in place.

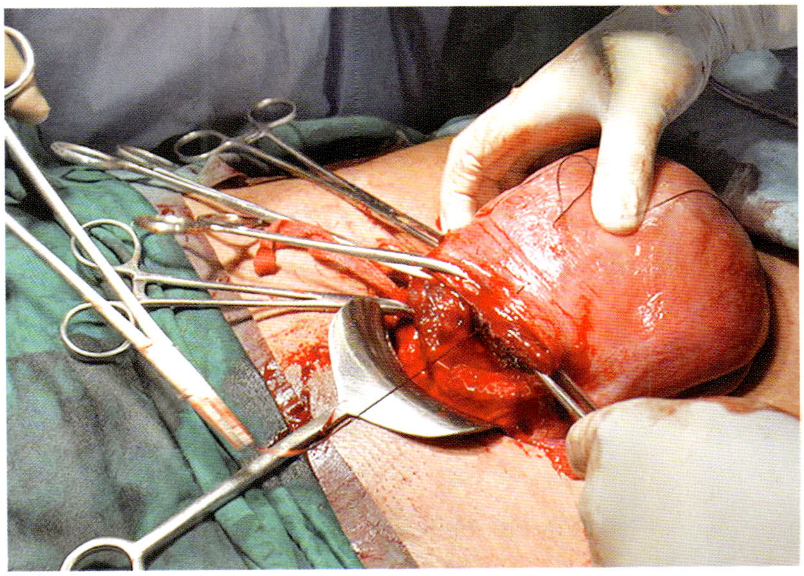

Fig. 5: Step 5—Suture came out through posterior wall of uterus.

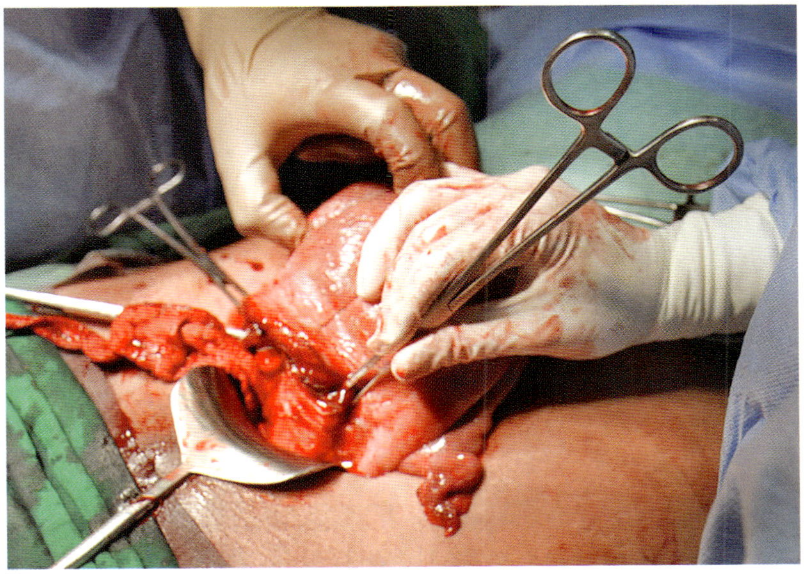

Fig. 3: Step 8.

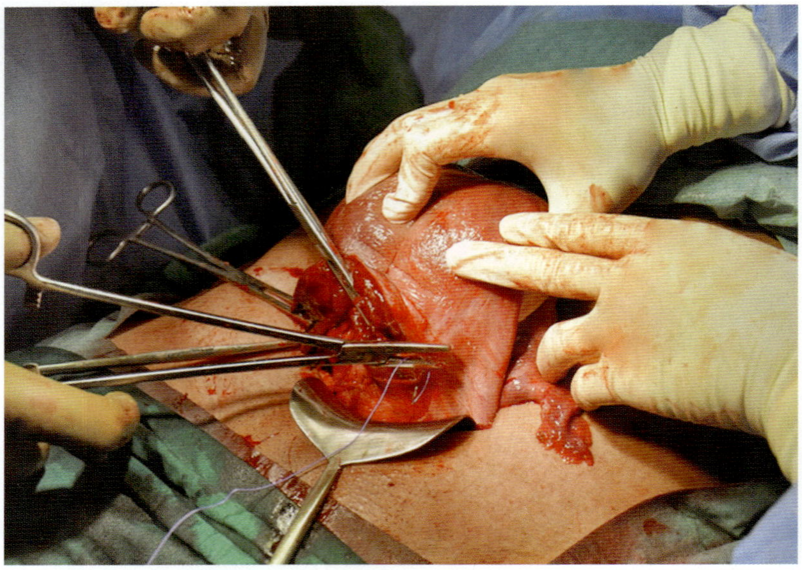

Fig. 9: Step 9—Lower uterine segment closed with vicryl no. 1.

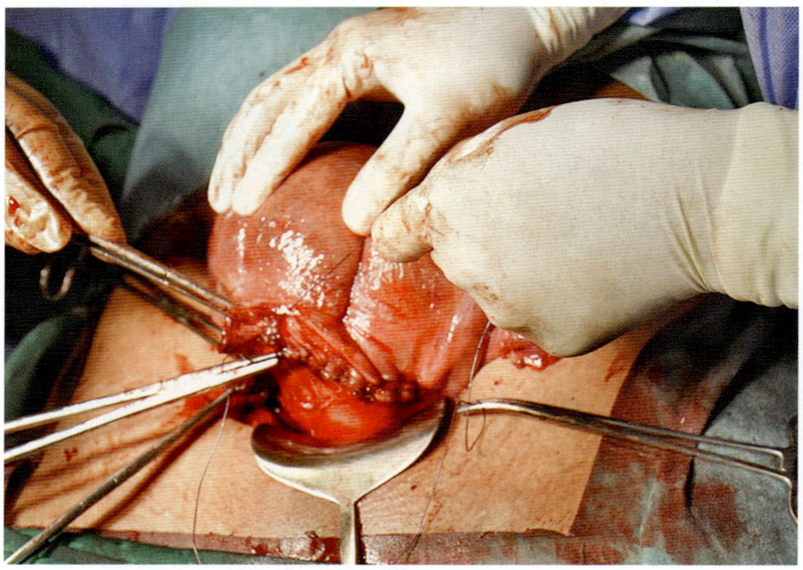

Fig. 10: Step 10.

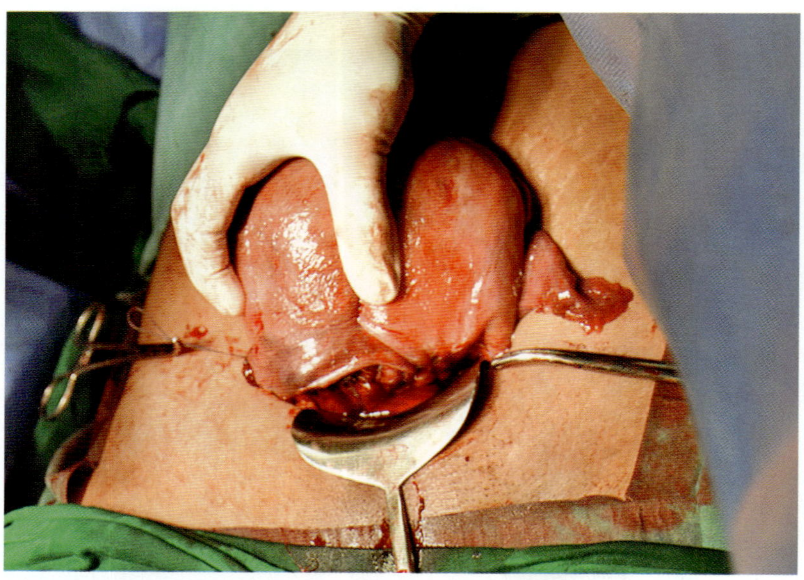

Fig. 11: Step 11.

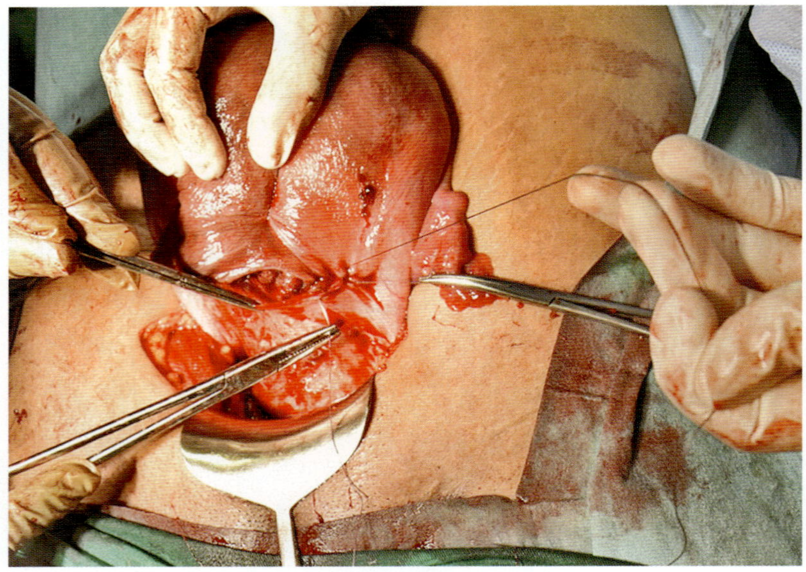

Fig. 12: Step 12.

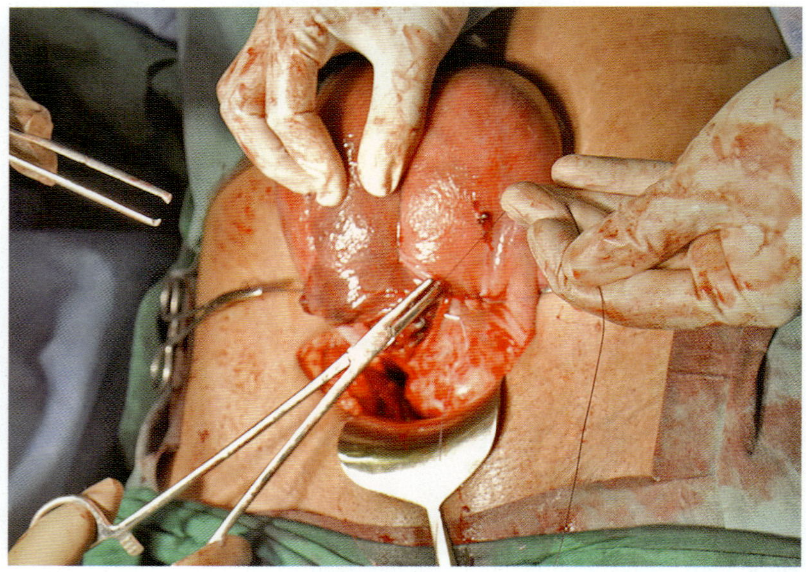

Fig. 13: Step 13.

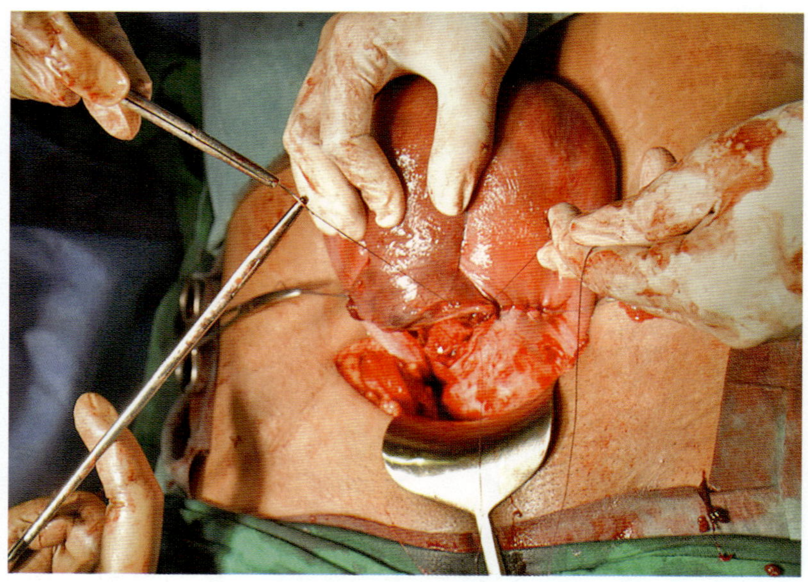

Fig. 14: Step 14.

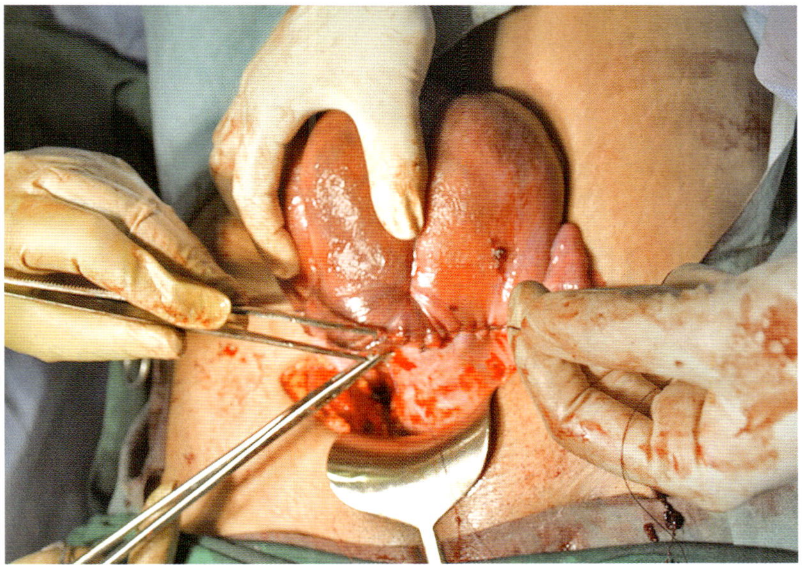

Fig. 15: Step 15.

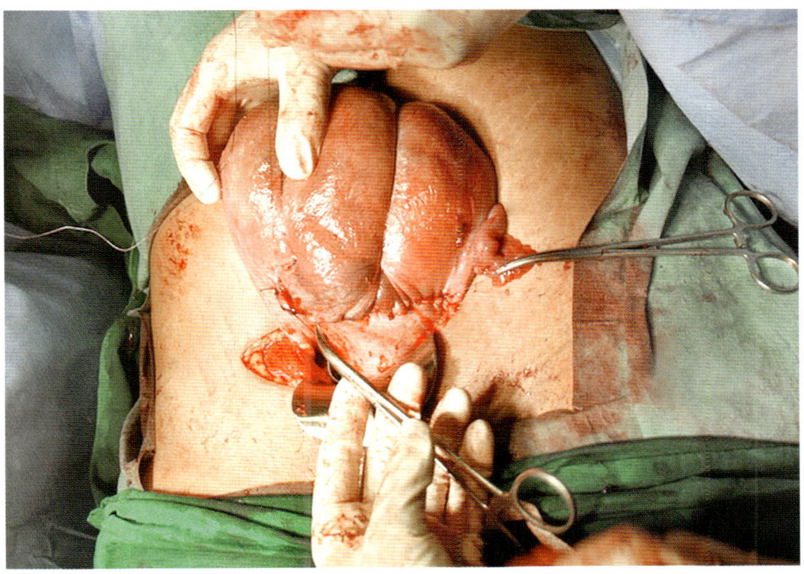

Fig. 16: Step ˊ6.

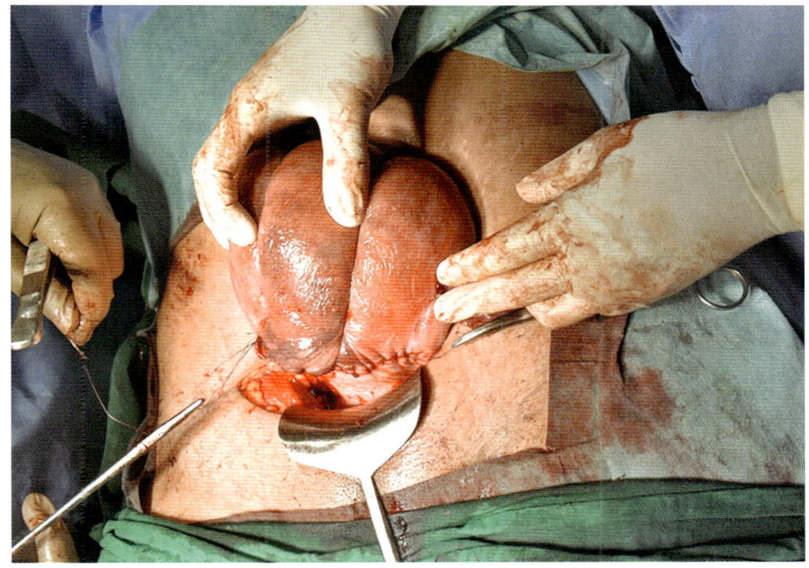

Fig. 17: Step 17.

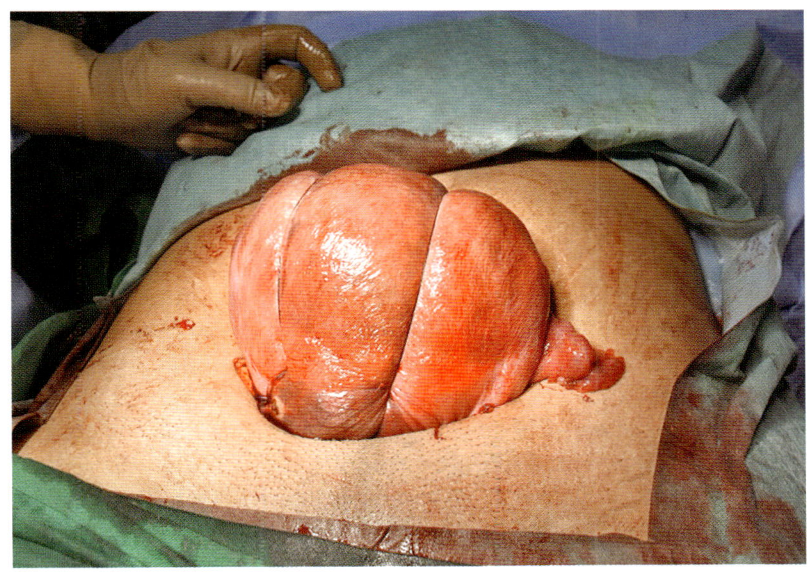

Fig. 18: Step 18—Hemostasis achieved, B-lynch suture in place.

CHAPTER

77

Complete Perineal Tear

Rubina Pandit, Usha Rani G, Isha Rani

BACKGROUND

Perineal Anatomy

The external genitalia of female include mons pubis, labia majora and minora, vestibule, clitoris, and perineal body. Perineal body is a dense connective tissue mass comprising of superficial and deep muscles, including transverse perinei and bulbocavernosus. Inferior to perineal body lies the anal sphincter complex which includes external and internal anal sphincter (IAS). The external anal sphincter (EAS) provides the squeeze pressure to anal canal and is voluntary control. The IAS is responsible for 80% of resting anal canal pressure and is under the control of autonomic nervous system.

INCIDENCE AND DEFINITION

The true incidence of perineal injuries is usually underestimated due to lack of uniformity in definition and failure to correctly diagnose them at the time of delivery. In 2012, the American College of Obstetricians and Gynecologists came up with a standard classification system of perineal lacerations[1] **(Table 1)**. Lacerations extending into or through anal sphincter complex (third and fourth degree) are referred to as obstetric anal sphincter injuries (OASIS). Complete perineal tear (CPT) mainly refers to fourth-degree perineal injury. A button hole injury (where only rectal and vaginal mucosa are involved) if found in isolation should not be classified as third- or fourth-degree perineal tear.

Although the incidence varies depending on patient characteristics, obstetric care provider technique and hospital settings, it is estimated that roughly 53–79% of women will experience some type of lacerations, majority being first and second degree.[2] A recent data from the Nationwide Inpatient Sample has reported an incidence of 3.3% of third-degree perineal tears and 1.1% of fourth-degree perineal lacerations.[3]

Table 1: Classification of perineal lacerations.

Degree	*Definition*
First degree	Injury to perineal skin only
Second degree	Injury to perineum involving perineal muscles but sparing anal sphincter complex
Third degree 3a 3B 3C	Injury to perineum involving anal sphincter complex Less than 50% of external anal sphincter thickness torn More than 50% of external anal sphincter thickness torn Both external and internal anal sphincter torn
Fourth degree	Injury to perineum involving anal sphincter complex and anal epithelium

RISK FACTORS

Maternal Risk Factors

Nulliparity is associated with increased incidence of OASIS, with few authors even reporting a 10-fold higher risk when compared to multiparous females.[4-7] Asian and Indian races also carry a higher risk compared to African American race.[5] Also, increasing fetal weight has also shown an association with increased risk of OASIS, risk being slightly increased with birth weight of over 3,500 g[5] and nearly 2.5-fold increased if birth weight increases beyond 4,000 g.[4] Maternal age, duration of pregnancy, and body mass index were not found to increase the incidence of OASIS.

Labor and Delivery Risk Factors

The strongest risk factors for OASIS include forceps delivery, vacuum-assisted delivery, and midline episiotomy. Majority of studies suggest higher risk with forceps compared with vacuum-assisted deliveries.[8] Other factors associated with increased risk are labor induction, labor augmentation, epidural analgesia, increasing duration of second stage of labor, and vertex malpresentation (primarily occiput posterior).[9] Despite the known risk factors, correctly predicting which patient will suffer from OASIS still remains a challenging task.

DIAGNOSIS

Careful perineal examination including rectum should be performed in all women prior to suturing. Inspection should be performed with proper lighting and adequate analgesia. Palpation is usually carried out with examiner's dominant index finger inserted in anus and ipsilateral thumb placed in vagina and then palpating with a "pin-rolling" movement to assess the thickness.

In case of EAS tear, the ends usually retract and a cavity is palpated along its course. The IAS is a continuation of circular smooth muscle of rectum which is found 6–8 mm cephalad to anal margin and appears pale like a raw white fish. Careful examination of IAS also allows detection of buttonhole injury.[10]

MANAGEMENT

Prevention of Complete Perineal Tear

- *Perineal support:* Whether providing perineal support (person delivering the baby holds perineum with sponge and applies medial pressure) in isolation has any protective effect is still unclear. A Cochrane meta-analysis has failed to show any benefit, although the results were biased by a large randomized controlled trial (RCT) of hands-on versus hands-poised techniques (which included both supporting perineum and slowing the head).[11] According to recent Royal College of Obstetricians and Gynaecologists (RCOG) guideline, warm compression during second stage of labor leads to reductions in OASIS risk.[12]

- *Delivery position:* Majority of studies has not shown any effect on the incidence of CPT on comparing various delivery positions.
- *Episiotomy:* During spontaneous vaginal or instrumental delivery, it is always better to follow the policy of "restricted" episiotomy (only if indicated) than "liberal" use in order to prevent OASIS. Also, when episiotomy is indicated, it is preferable to consider mediolateral episiotomy over a midline incision. The optimal cutting angle should be always more than 45°, ideally around 60°.[10]
- *Instrumental delivery:* When instrumental delivery is performed, vacuum extraction carries comparatively lesser risk of OASIS compared to forceps application. Giving midline episiotomy along with operative vaginal delivery further increases the risk of OASIS and CPT. Certain practices like early forceps removal (after delivery is assured but before largest head diameter is expelled), rotating an occipitoposterior baby to occipitoanterior position, and using minimal maternal efforts during expulsion might assist in limiting the risk of CPT.[13]
- *Others:* Various practices like closed versus open glottis pushing, antepartum perineal massage, delayed pushing, Ritgen's maneuver and water birth have failed to demonstrate any reduction in the incidence of CPT.

Repair of Complete Perineal Tear

Complete perineal tear repair should be performed by an appropriately trained clinician. In case an experienced clinician is not available immediately, repair can be delayed for 8–12 hours with no impact on pelvic floor symptoms or anal incontinence.[14] All CPT repairs should be performed in an operating room with proper lighting under regional or general anesthesia to provide both adequate analgesia and muscle relaxation. The EAS has an inherent tone due to which it has a tendency to retract under its fascial sheath. With adequate muscle relaxation, it is easier to thoroughly evaluate the extent of tear and properly identify the torn sphincter ends.

The patient is placed in dorsal lithotomy position. Perineum and vagina are properly cleaned and draped. A Foley catheter is placed before starting the repair.

Suture Material

Very less studies are available comparing different suture materials for sphincter repair. Both absorbable and delayed absorbable sutures can be used. Use of nonabsorbable sutures may cause stitch abscesses or discomfort feeling mandating their removal.[15]

The suture ends must be cut short. The knots should be covered by overlying superficial perineal muscles to prevent discomfort from suture knot ends. Monofilament sutures are preferred over multifilament due to decreased bacterial adherence and subsequent risk of infection.[16]

Repair of Anal Mucosa

Following a CPT, the anal mucosa can be repaired either by interrupted 3-0 polyglactin (Vicryl) suture with knots tied in anal canal or by submucosal continuous suture using 3-0 polydiaxone (PDS). No studies have demonstrated the superiority of one technique over another with respect to outcomes like recto or anovaginal fistulas. Figure-of-eight technique should be avoided due to risk of ischemia and poor healing of anal mucosa.

Separate Repair of Internal Anal Sphincter (Figs. 1A to C)

Internal anal sphincter damage can cause poor seal with an impaired sampling reflex causing passive incontinence. As compared to EAS, IAS is thin with pale pink appearance, may appear similar to a fascial layer. IAS is best identified by using Allis clamp to grasp retracted EAS fibers and pull towards midline. With traction on EAS edges, IAS can be visualized extending more proximally. When identified, it is advisable to repair IAS separately with interrupted or mattress sutures using 3-0 Vicryl or PDS without any attempt to overlap IAS.[12]

Repair of External Anal Sphincter

There are two primary methods to repair EAS—end-to-end repair and overlapping technique. The EAS torn ends have the tendency to retract due to their inherent tonicity and can be found latero-posteriorly to the tear by palpating the depression downward rather than lateral. The muscle ends are then grasped using Allis clamps **(Figs. 2A and B)**. During repair, it is important to include the fascial sheath in the suture and not just the muscle alone.

End-to-end repair includes direct approximation of torn EAS ends with horizontal mattress sutures using 3-0 PDS or 3-0 Vicryl **(Figs. 3A to D)**. In overlap technique, the EAS torn ends requires more dissection and mobilization. The dissection is done using ischioanal fat present laterally as the landmark. The full length of EAS are then overlapped in a double-breasted manner using interrupted sutures of either 3-0 PDS or 3-0 Vicryl with the goal of overlapping the EAS edges by 1.5–2 cm in the midline. Overlap repair is only possible for 3b or greater OASIS.

Cochrane 2013 meta-analysis has shown better short-term outcomes with less fecal urgency and anal incontinence at 12 months with overlap technique compared to end-to-end repair. However, long-term follow-up till 36 months failed to show superiority of one technique over other.[17] Most of the studies have also showed no difference between the two repair methods. Consequently, the literature does not support the use of a particular repair technique over the other.

Once the anal sphincter is repaired, the rest of the laceration is sutured like a typical second-degree laceration **(Fig. 4)**.

POSTOPERATIVE MANAGEMENT

Antibiotics

In accordance with recent guidelines, prophylactic one dose intravenous antibiotics (second-generation cephalosporin) should be given in order to reduce the risk of perineal wound complications after CPT repair.[1,10]

Bowel Regimen

Stool softeners and oral laxatives like lactulose should be prescribed to women following CPT repair for earlier and less painful bowel motions. Counseling should also include discussing methods to avoid constipation.[1,10]

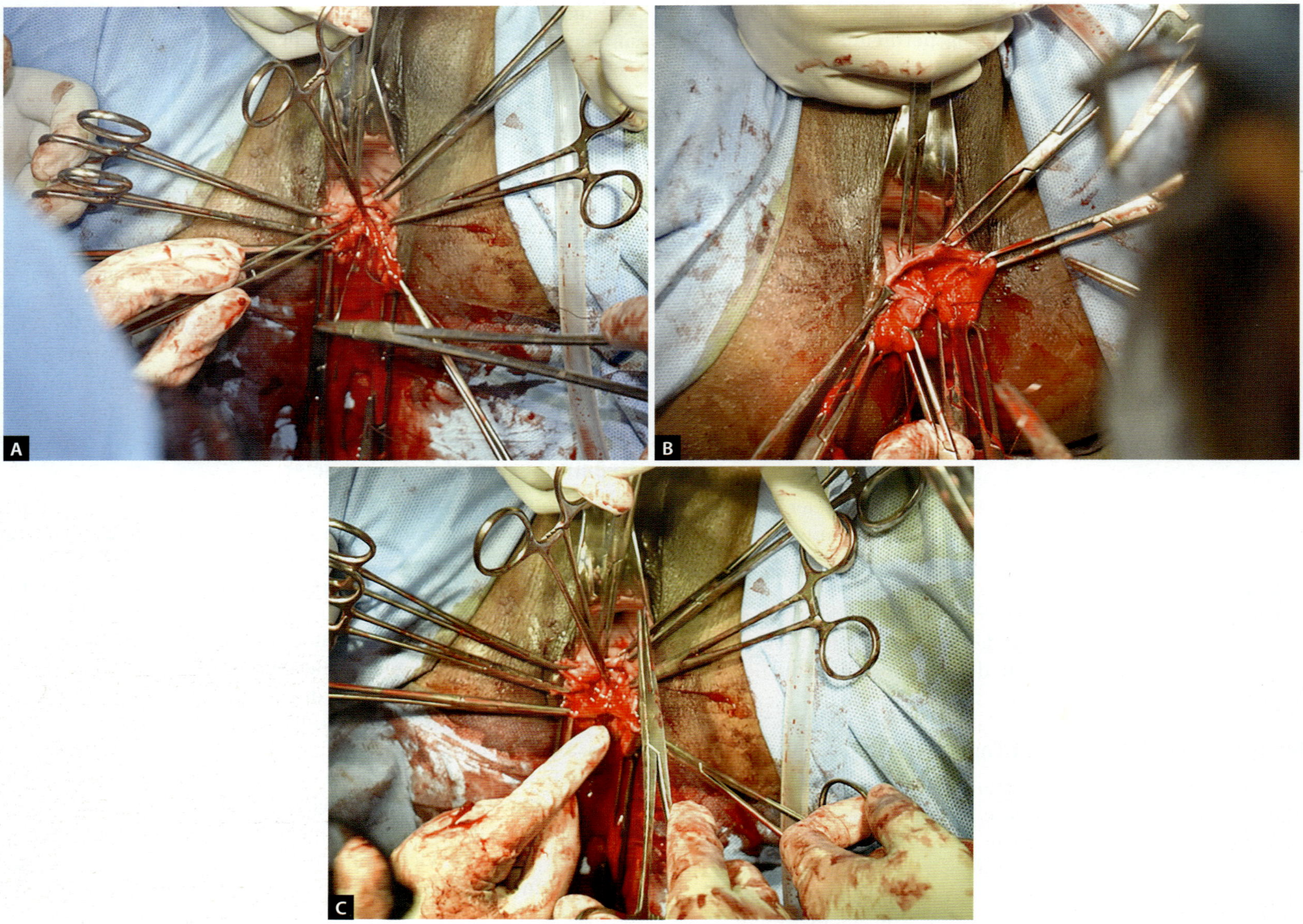

Figs. 1A to C: Internal anal sphincter repair.

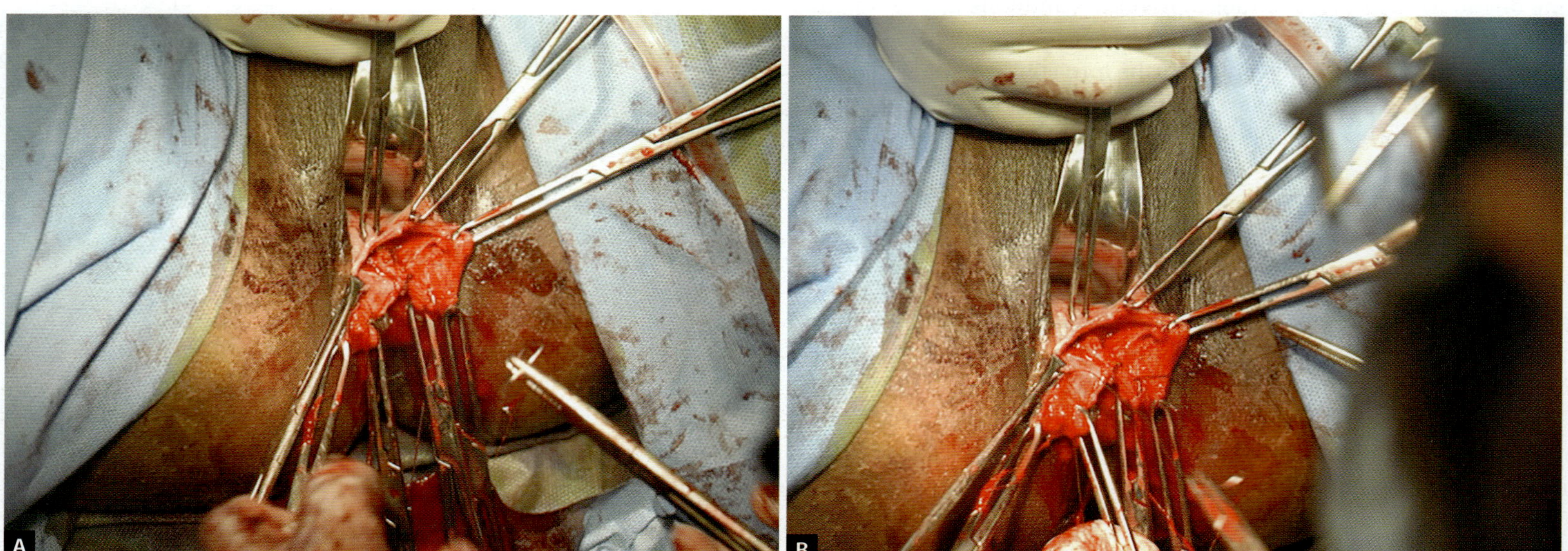

Fig. 2A and B: Torn edges of external anal sphincter held using Allis forceps.

Analgesia

Proper pain control is also an important part of postoperative management following CPT repair. Due to constipating side effect of opioids, nonsteroidal anti-inflammatory drug (NSAID) in conjunction with acetaminophen is preferred as the first line of agent.[10] Opioids, if used, should be combined with stool softeners. There is limited data on

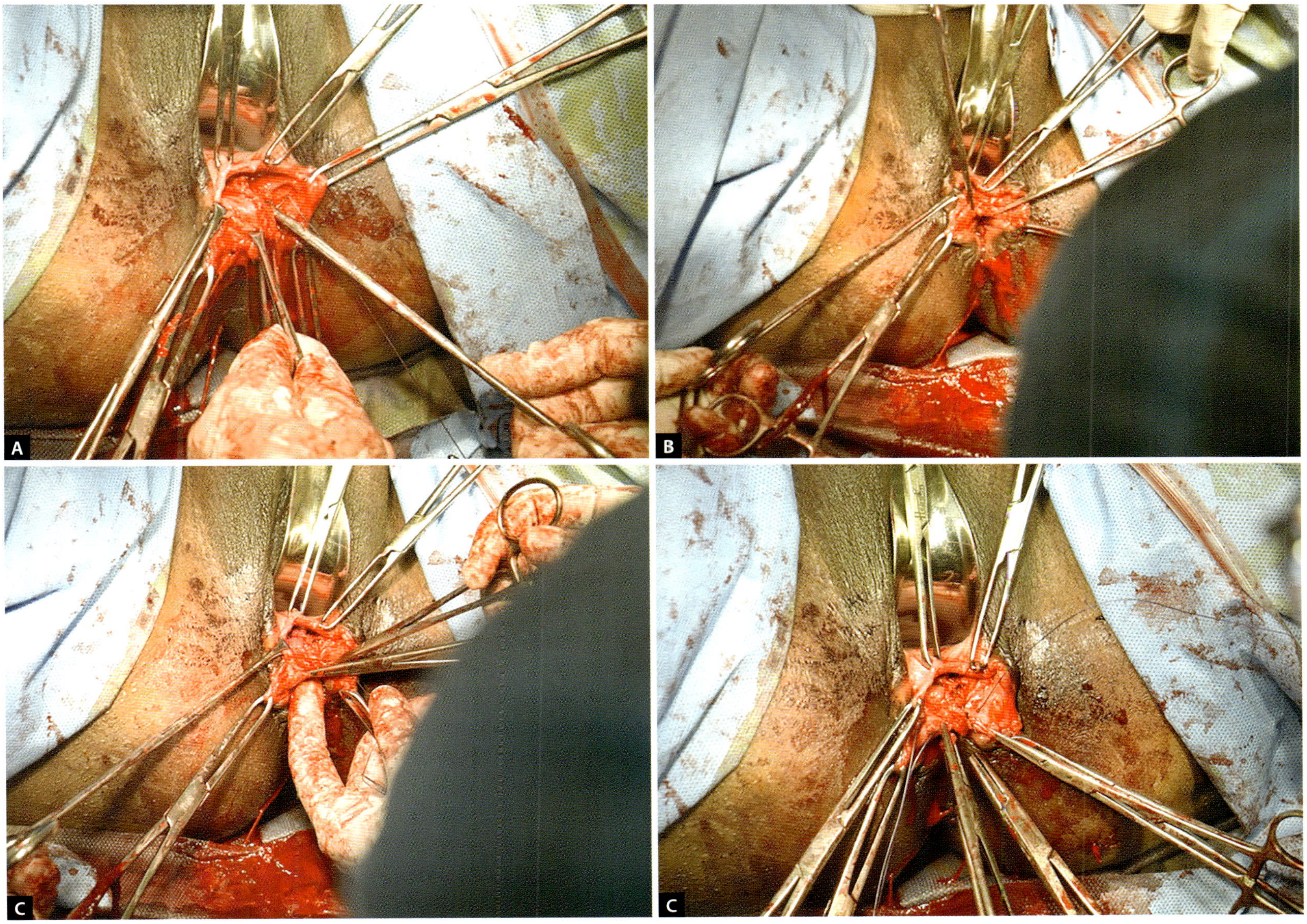

Figs. 3A to D: End-to-end repair of torn external anal sphincter with horizontal mattress sutures.

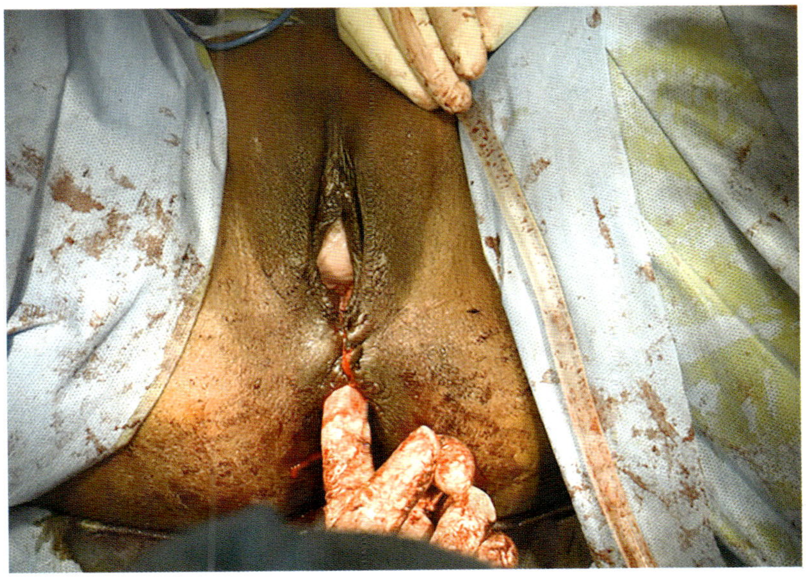

Fig. 4: After complete perineal tear repair.

the effectiveness of local cooling treatments like ice packs, cold bath or cold gel pads applied to perineum. Rectal suppositories should be used with caution in CPT due to theoretical risk of disruption of repair and poor healing of wound.

Follow-up

Patients undergoing CPT repair usually does not require prolong hospitalization. Although standard guidelines for follow-up are lacking, early and consistent follow-up at 2 weekly intervals is recommended for timely and early detection of postoperative complications like wound infection, urinary retention, anal incontinence, etc. Spontaneous voiding needs to be carefully monitored. Any discomfort or inability to pass urine warrants prompt evaluation. Physiotherapy postrepair may be beneficial in postoperative period. Women should be counseled that 60–80% of women are asymptomatic 12 months following CPT repair.[12]

SUBSEQUENT PREGNANCY

Many factors should be taken into account during counseling of women regarding mode of delivery in subsequent pregnancy: the functional status (i.e. short and remote symptoms experienced from index pregnancy), the extent of residual anatomical and/or functional defects, and patient's desire. Although women with a history of OASIS in previous pregnancy have 3.8–5.9-fold greater odds of repeat OASIS in subsequent pregnancy, the absolute risk is still low (3%).[18,19]

After successful CPT repair most women can safely deliver vaginally in next pregnancy. However, RCOG recommend that all women who had sustained OASIS in previous pregnancy and are symptomatic or have abnormal endoanal ultrasonography and/or manometry should have option of elective cesarean birth.[12]

Sustained anal compromise is defined as either:[20]

- External sphincter defect on ultrasound >30° and a maximum squeeze pressure increment of <20 mm Hg on anal manometry
- Defect <30° and a maximum squeeze pressure increment of <20 mm Hg
- No defect and a maximum squeeze pressure increment of <20 mm Hg.

CONCLUSION

Complete perineal tear represent a significant cause of morbidity after vaginal delivery. Careful examination after every delivery is of utmost importance for timely detection and proper management of CPT. Systematic repair of anal sphincter complex should be done by an experienced clinician with close follow-up. Antenatal symptoms evaluation and functional testing can act as a guiding tool in deciding the mode of delivery in future pregnancy.

REFERENCES

1. Committee on Practice Bulletins-Obstetrics. ACOG Practice Bulletin No. 198: Prevention and Management of Obstetric Lacerations at Vaginal Delivery. Obstet Gynecol. 2018;132(3):e87-e102.
2. Smith LA, Price N, Simonite V, et al. Incidence of and risk factors for perineal trauma: a prospective observational study. BMC Pregnancy Childbirth. 2013;13:59.
3. Friedman AM, Ananth CV, Prendergast E, et al. Evaluation of third-degree and fourth-degree laceration rates as quality indicators. Obstet Gynecol. 2015;125:927-37.
4. Richter HE, Brumfield CG, Cliver SP, et al. Risk factors associated with anal sphincter tear: a comparison of primiparous patients, vaginal births after cesarean deliveries, and patients with previous vaginal delivery. Am J Obstet Gynecol. 2002;187(5):1194-8.
5. Meister MR, Cahill AG, Conner SN, et al. Predicting obstetric anal sphincter injuries in a modern obstetric population. Am J Obstet Gynecol. 2016;215(3):310.e1-7.
6. Christianson LM, Bovbjerg VE, McDavitt EC, et al. Risk factors for perineal injury during delivery. Am J Obstet Gynecol. 2003;189(1):255-60.
7. Zetterstrom J, Lopez A, Anzen B, et al. Anal sphincter tears at vaginal delivery: risk factors and clinical outcome of primary repair. Obstet Gynecol. 1999;94(1):21-8.
8. Fitzgerald MP, Weber AM, Howden N, et al. Risk factors for anal sphincter tear during vaginal delivery. Obstet Gynecol. 2007;109(1):29-34.
9. Meister MR, Rosenbloom JI, Lowder JL, et al. Techniques for repair of obstetric anal sphincter injuries. Obstet Gynecol Surv. 2018;73(1): 33-9.
10. Harvey MA, Pierce M, Alter JE, et al. Obstetrical anal sphincter injuries (OASIS): prevention, recognition, and repair. J Obstet Gynaecol Can. 2015;37(12):1131-48.
11. Aasheim V, Nilsen AB, Lukasse M, et al. Perineal techniques during the second stage of labour for reducing perineal trauma. Cochrane Database Syst Rev. 2011;12:CD006672.
12. Royal College of Obstetricians and Gynaecologists. (2015). Third- and fourth-degree perineal tears, Management (Green-top Guideline No. 29). [online] Available from: https://www.rcog.org.uk/en/guidelines-research-services/guidelines/gtg29/. [Last accessed January, 2020].
13. Hirsch E, Haney EI, Gordon TE, et al. Reducing high-order perineal laceration during operative vaginal delivery. Am J Obstet Gynecol. 2008; 198(6):668.e1-5.
14. Nordenstam J, Mellgren A, Altman D, et al. Immediate or delayed repair of obstetric anal sphincter tears—a randomised controlled trial. BJOG. 2008;115:857-65.
15. Duggal N, Mercado C, Daniels K, et al. Antibiotic prophylaxis for prevention of postpartum perineal wound complications: a randomized controlled trial. Obstet Gynecol. 2008;111:1268-73.
16. Katz S, Izhar M, Mirelman D. Bacterial adherence to surgical sutures. A possible factor in suture induced infection. Ann Surg. 1981;194(1): 35-41.
17. Fernando RJ, Sultan AH, Kettle C, et al. Methods of repair for obstetric anal sphincter injury. Cochrane Database Syst Rev. 2013;12:CD002866.
18. Beckmann MM, Garrett AJ. Antenatal perineal massage for reducing perineal trauma. Cochrane Database Syst Rev. 2006;1:CD005123.
19. Altman D, Ragnar I, Ekstrom A, et al. Anal sphincter lacerations and upright delivery postures—a risk analysis from a randomized controlled trial. Int Urogynecol J. 2007;18:141-6.
20. Daly JO, Sultan AH, Van delft KW, et al. Outcome of childbirth after previous obstetric anal sphincter injury. 38th Annual Meeting of the International Urogynecological Association, IUGA. Int Urogynecol J Pelvic Floor Dysfunct. 2013;24(Suppl 1):S69-S70.

SECTION 4

In Vitro Fertilization and Assisted Reproductive Technique

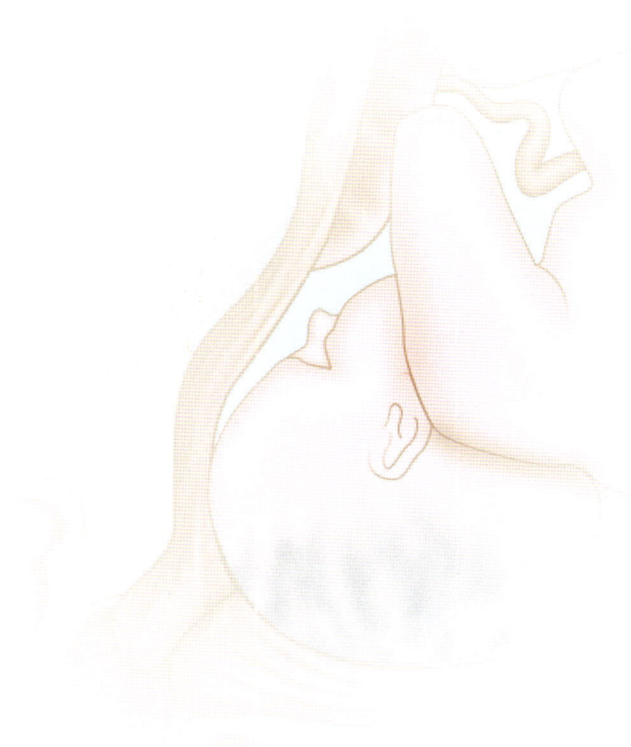

CHAPTER

78 In Vitro Fertilization Techniques: Operation Theater and Laboratory Setup

Ravindranath Nirwani, Shabana Nawaz Ansari, Aditi Rai, B Ramesh

IN VITRO FERTILIZATION OPERATION THEATER

The in vitro fertilization (IVF) operation theater (OT) is a place where all the IVF procedures are carried out in a controlled environment, which includes egg pickup, embryo transfer, and surgical sperm retrieval. Egg pickup is an IVF process in which the eggs are harvested from the patients ovary with the help of ovum pick-up (OPU) needle through ultrasound-guided transvaginal oocyte retrieval technique under general anesthesia **(Figs. 1 and 2)**.

IN VITRO FERTILIZATION LABORATORY (FIGS. 3 TO 8)

The IVF laboratory is a critical part of the IVF process where the eggs that are retrieved from the patient are screened into dishes and are counted and evaluated. IVF is a laboratory procedure from the time eggs are retrieved from a woman until the time the embryo is transferred back into the uterus—a time period of anywhere from 3–5 or 6 days. The laboratory quality and procedures during this time are crucial to the success of IVF. A fertility clinic laboratory is typically run by an embryologist, which is a scientist who is involved in fertility treatment and reproductive research. Embryologists collect eggs, assess, and prepare sperm samples from respective partners, and inject eggs with sperm.

The embryos are handled in the laboratory for several days. After egg retrieval, the embryologist places eggs in an incubator and makes notes on their condition **(Figs. 9 and 10)**. Then, the eggs and sperm are placed together in an incubator to allow fertilization (IVF) or a procedure known as intracytoplasmic sperm injection (ICSI) is performed in which a single sperm is injected into the egg **(Figs. 11 and 12)**.

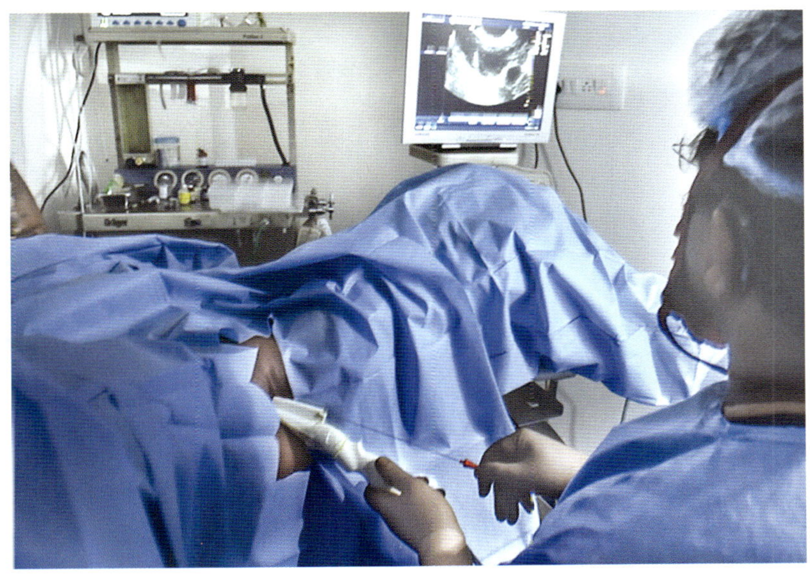

Fig. 2: Egg pickup using ovum pick-up (OPU) needles.

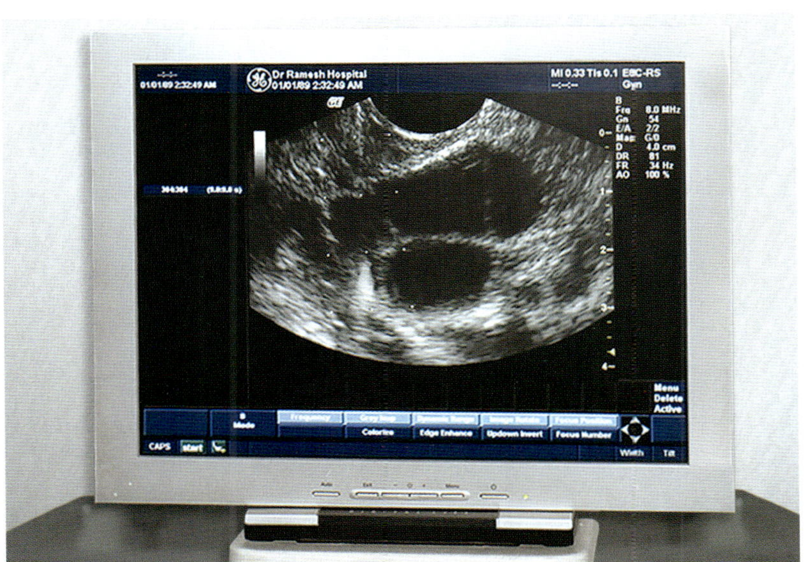

Fig. 1: Ultrasound scan showing matured ovarian follicle, each measuring 18 mm in size.

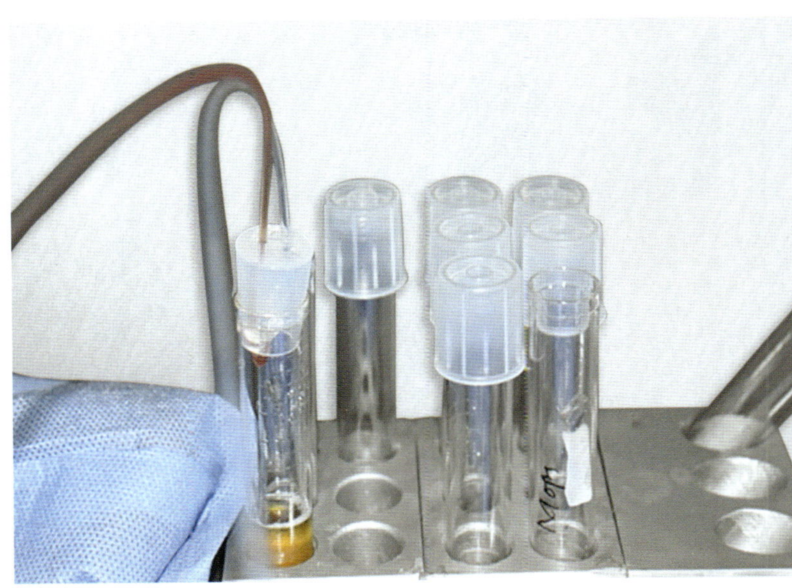

Fig. 3: Aspirated follicles are maintained at 37°C in test tube warmer.

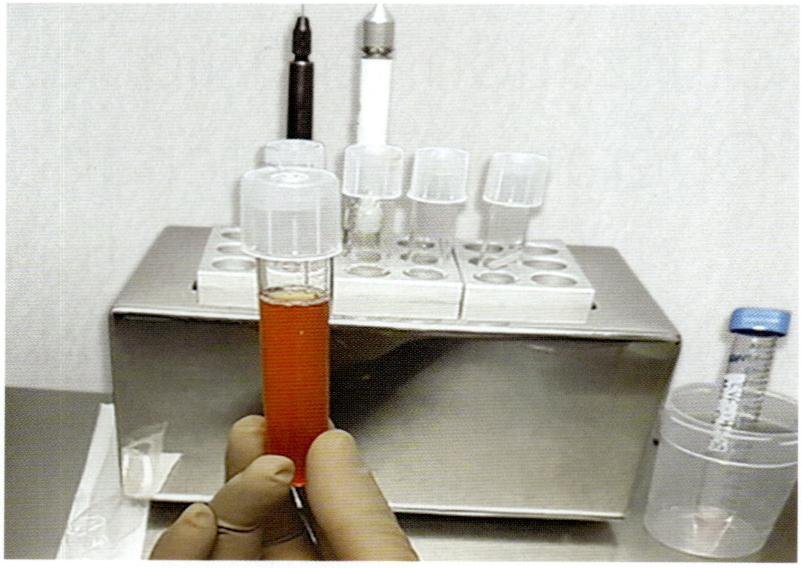

Fig. 4: Test tube showing follicular fluid.

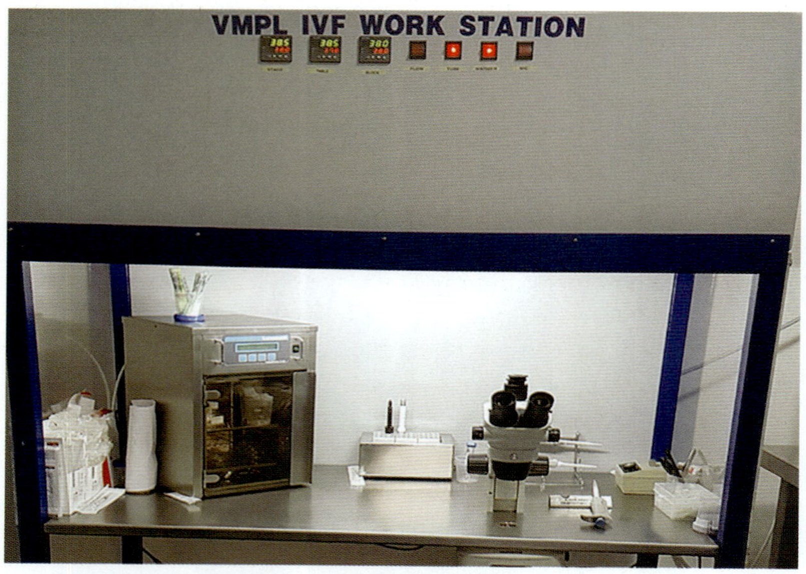

Fig. 5: In vitro fertilization work station having stereozoom microscope and small CO_2 incubator.

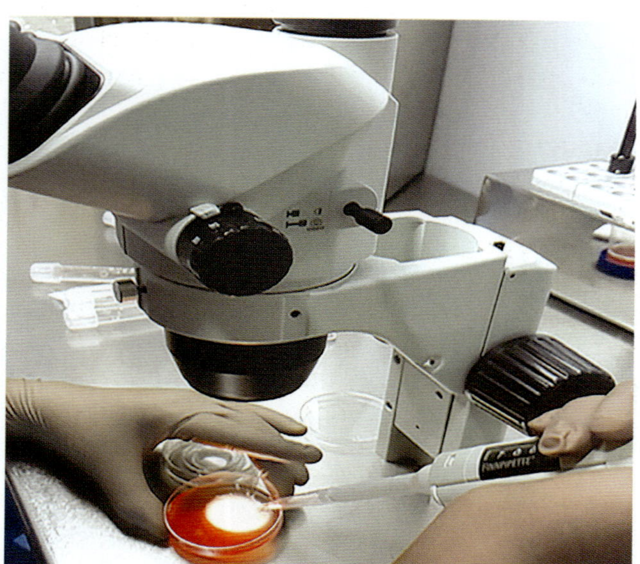

Fig. 6: Aspirated follicular fluid is screened under stereozoom microscope for egg follicles.

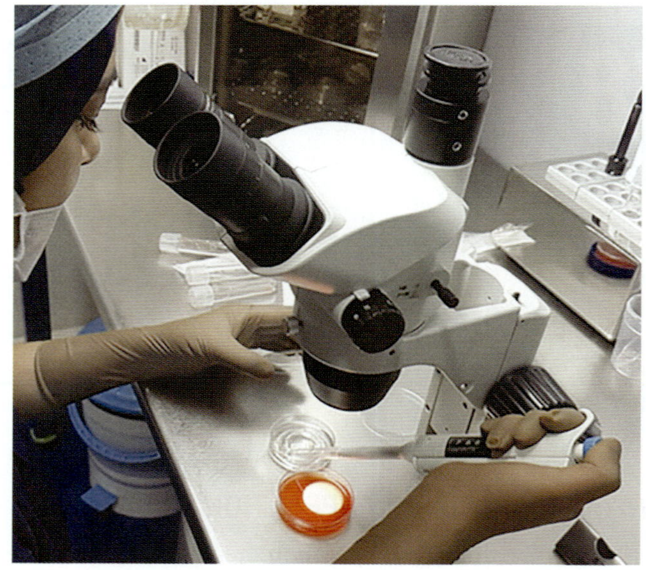

Fig. 7: Screened egg follicles are transferred into center well dish containing flushing medium.

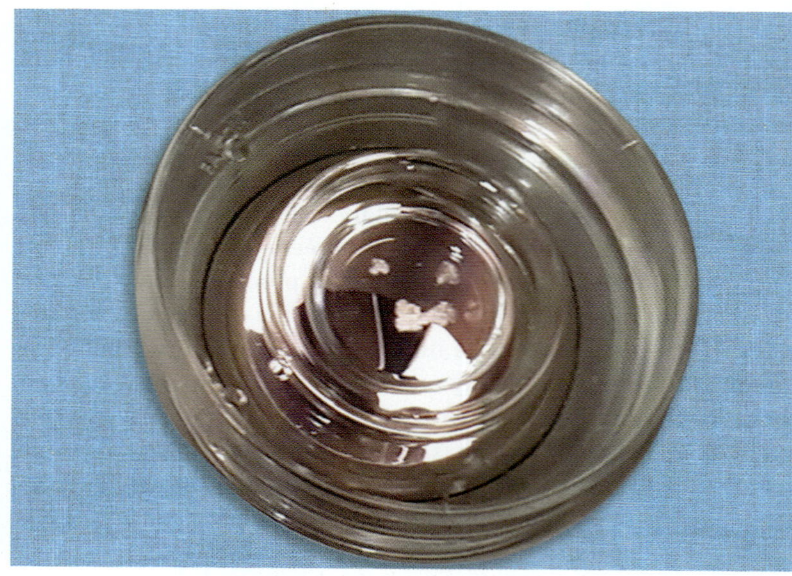

Fig. 8: Egg follicles in dish having fertilization medium.

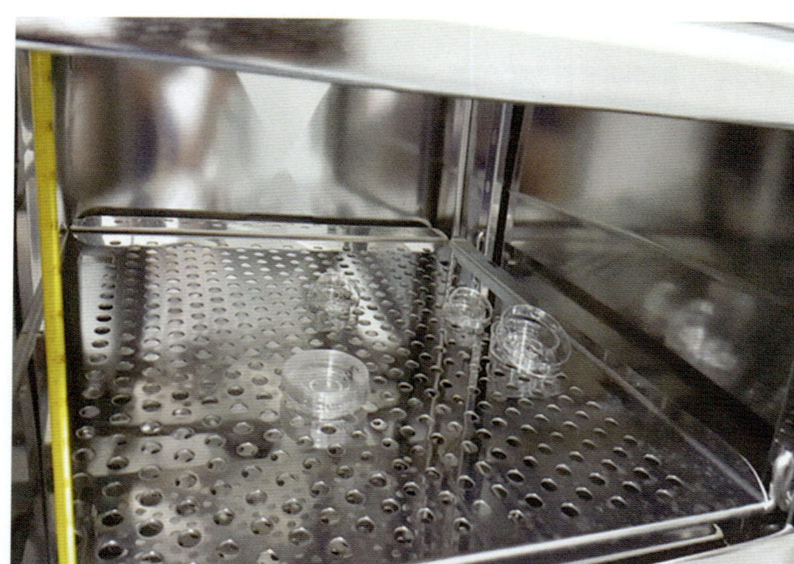

Fig. 9: Dish containing follicles are placed in CO_2 incubator.

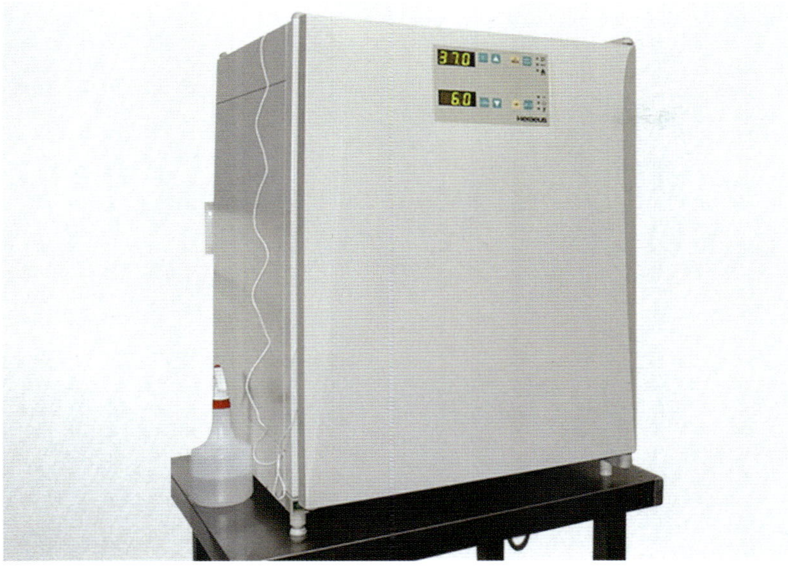

Fig. 10: CO_2 incubator.

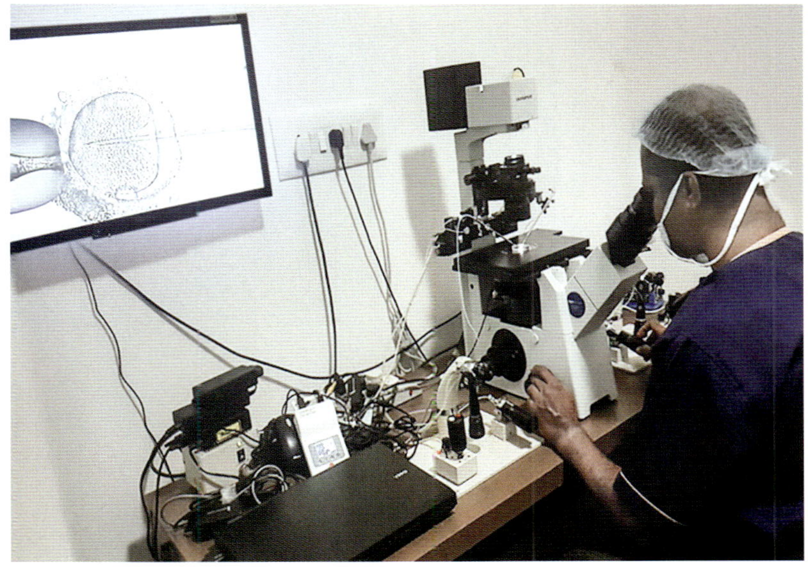

Fig. 12: Performing intracytoplasmic sperm injection.

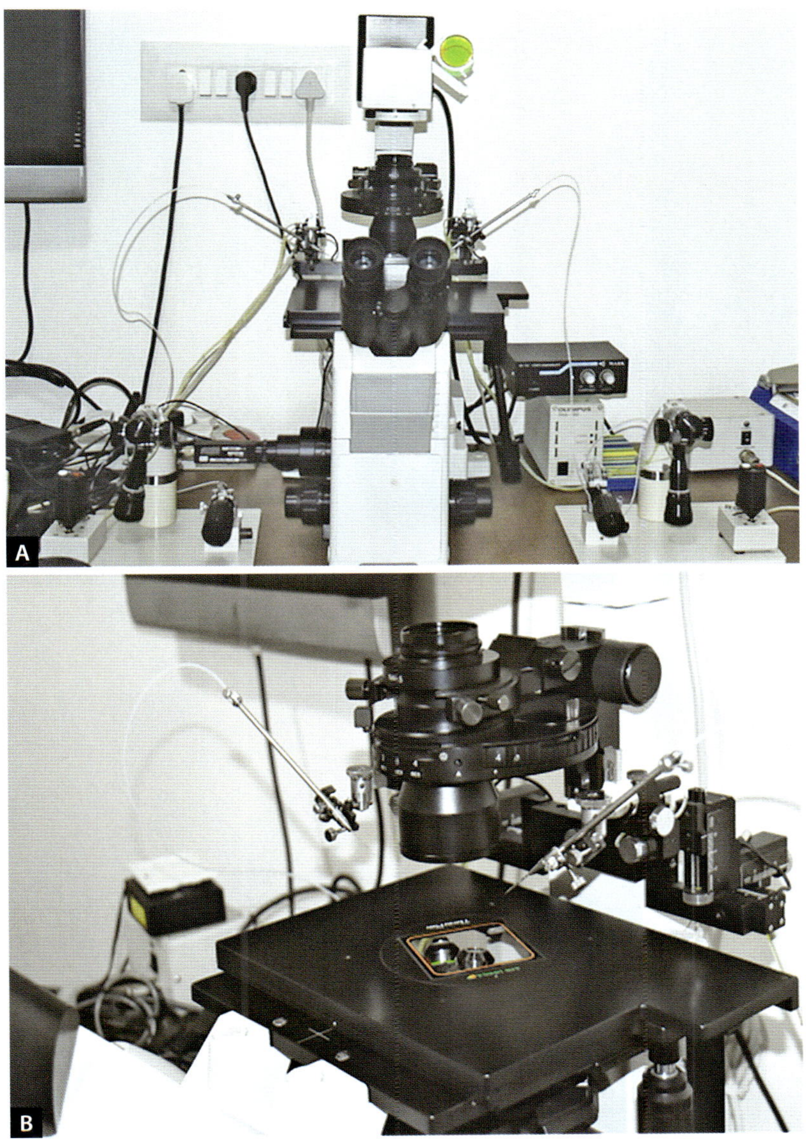

Figs. 11A and B: Intracytoplasmic sperm injection machine.

The day after retrieval is called day 1, and the embryos, which at this point are single-celled zygotes with two pronuclei are assessed. On day 2, the embryo typically divides into a four-cell embryo, and on day 3 it typically becomes a six- to eight-cell embryo. Embryos are assessed on Days 2 and 3 for transfer or placement into a blastocyst media until day 5 or 6. Days 4–5, the embryo is a morula. Days 5–7, the embryos are blastocysts.

DIFFERENT STAGES OF EMBRYOS STARTING FROM DAY 0 TO DAY 5 (FIGS. 13 TO 17)

Embryos are typically transferred on day 3 or day 5. The embryologist assesses the embryos carefully to see which day it would be better to transfer. Before the embryos are transferred, the embryologist evaluates them for their morphological appearance and grades them on a scale of one to four. The embryos that have the best characteristics and are dividing normally are thought to be more likely to successfully implant.

LASER-ASSISTED HATCHING (FIGS. 18 TO 21)

The unfertilized egg is surrounded by a shell called zona pellucida. The zona pellucida ensures that only one sperm cell enters and thus fertilizes the egg. After fertilization of the egg, zona pellucida keeps the cells of the embryo together. During the cleavage stages and in vitro culture of the human embryo, zona pellucida gets harder, possibly due to the culture conditions. Laser-assisted hatching (LAH) with the LYKOS® or ZILOS-tk® uses a highly focused infrared laser beam to remove the zona pellucida in very precise increments. Indications of LAH are presented in **Table 1**.

The problem of a harder zona pellucida is that the embryo may not hatch or use excessive energy for getting out. LAH is one out of several methods to help the fertilized egg to hatch out and attach to the uterus. Other methods are acid or mechanical hatching of one part of zona pellucida. Recent meta-research (comparison of different relevant researches) showed that women who have undergone repeated IVF treatments without results, double their chances of a pregnancy by use of assisted laser hatching.

EMBRYO BIOPSY FOR PREIMPLANTATION GENETIC SCREENING

One of the most powerful tools available in reproductive medicine is preimplantation genetic diagnosis (PGD). Through PGD, doctors and

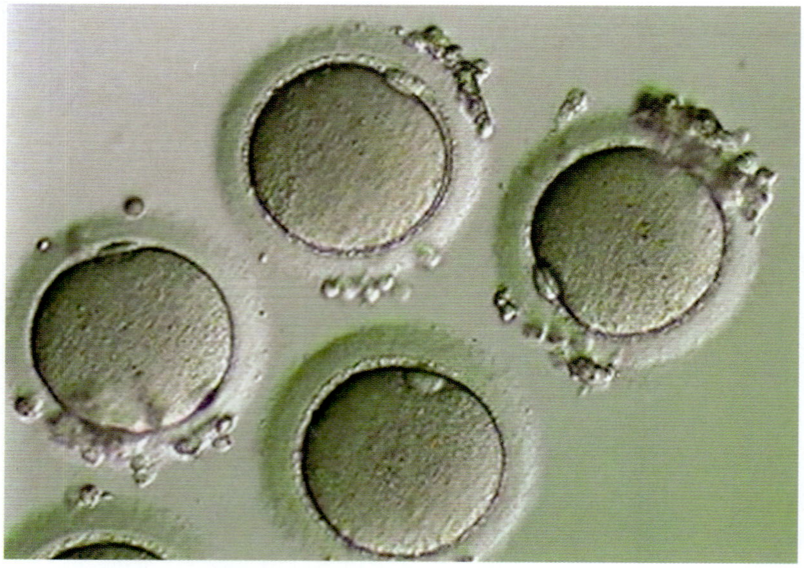

Fig. 13: Day 0, oocytes after denudation.

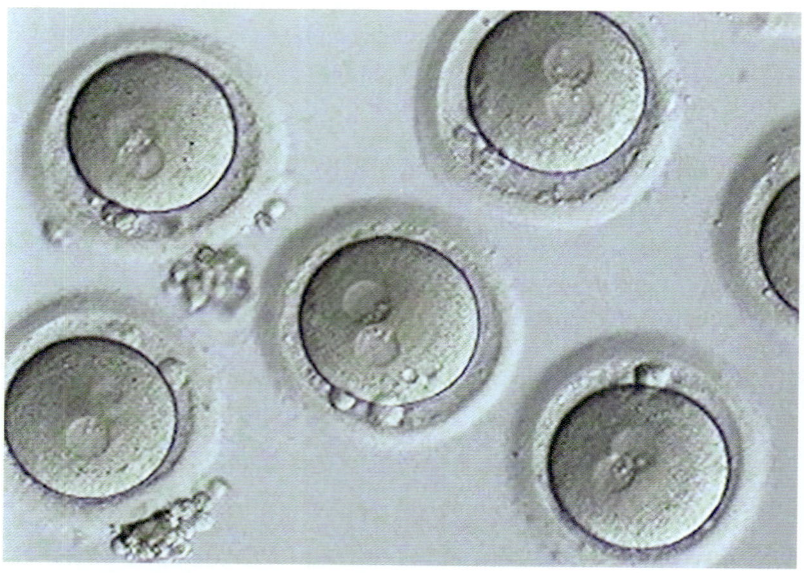

Fig. 14: Day 1, fertilized zygote showing two pronuclei (2PN) stage.

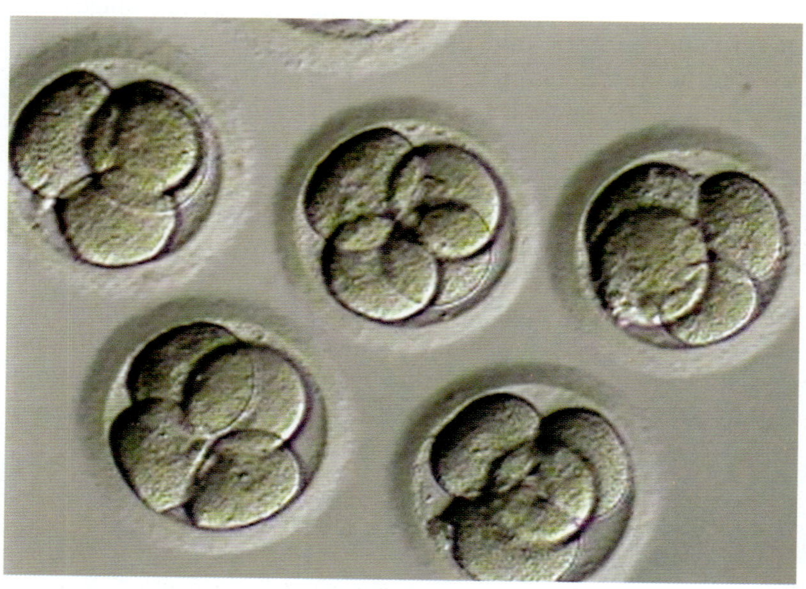

Fig. 15: Day 2, embryos showing four-cell stage.

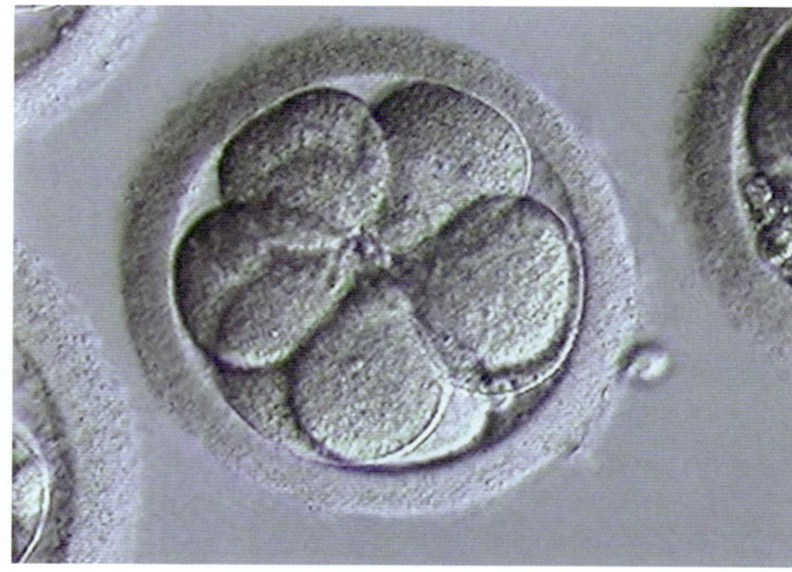

Fig. 16: Day 3, embryo showing eight-cell stage.

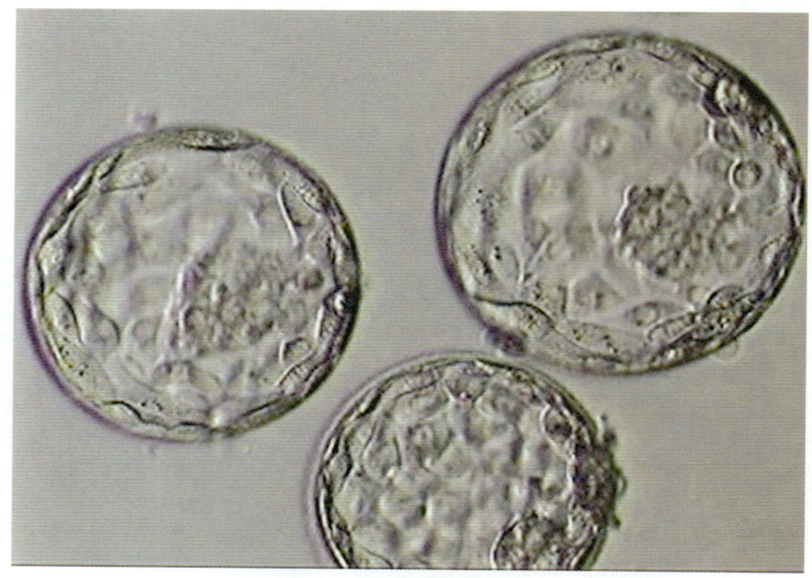

Fig. 17: Day 5, showing blastocyst stage.

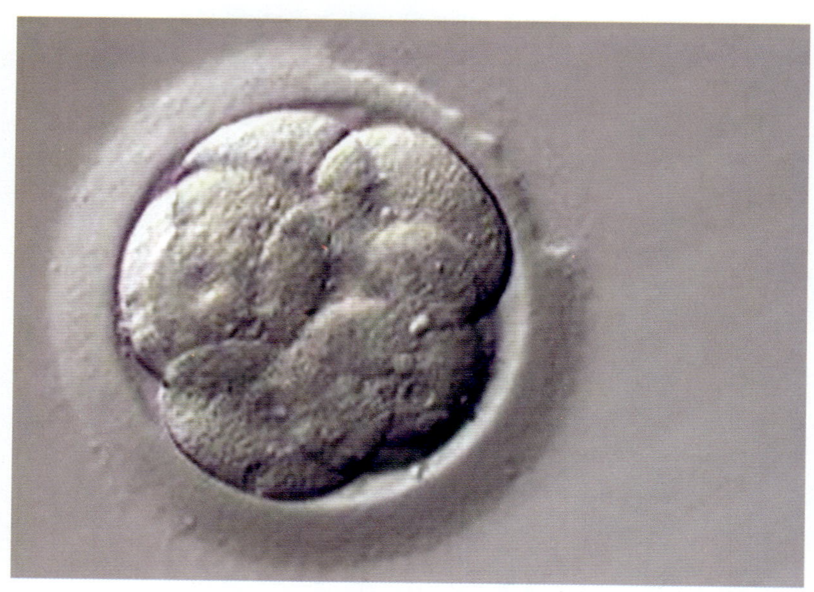

Fig. 18: Laser-assisted hatching of day 3, embryo having harder zona after thawing procedure.

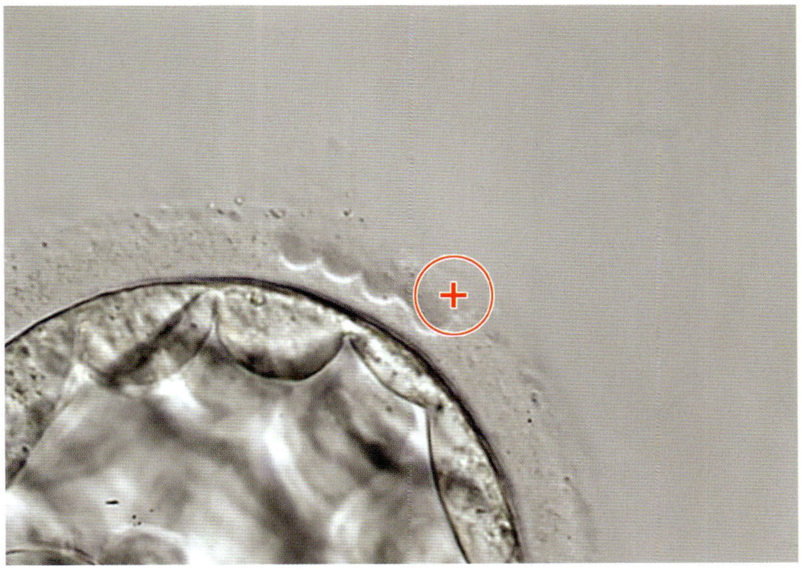

Fig. 19: Laser-assisted hatching of day 5, blastocyst having thick zona.

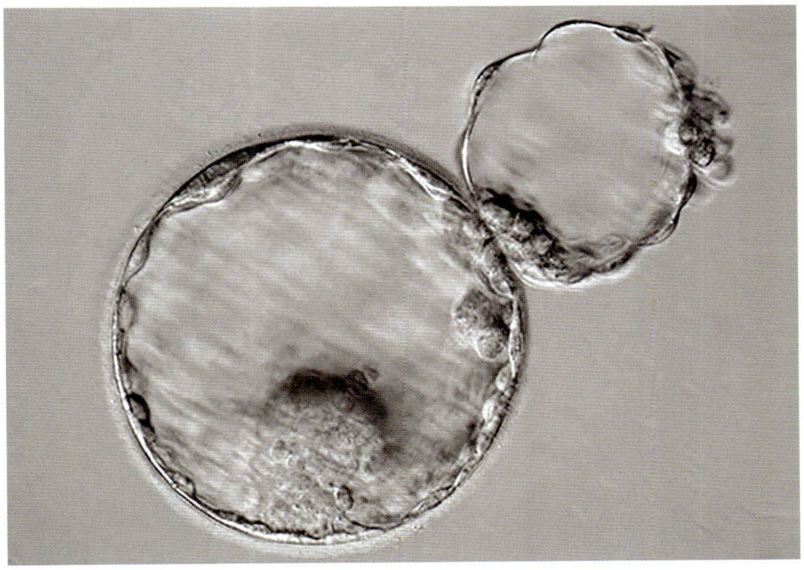

Fig. 20: Hatching out of trophectoderm cells after laser-assisted hatching.

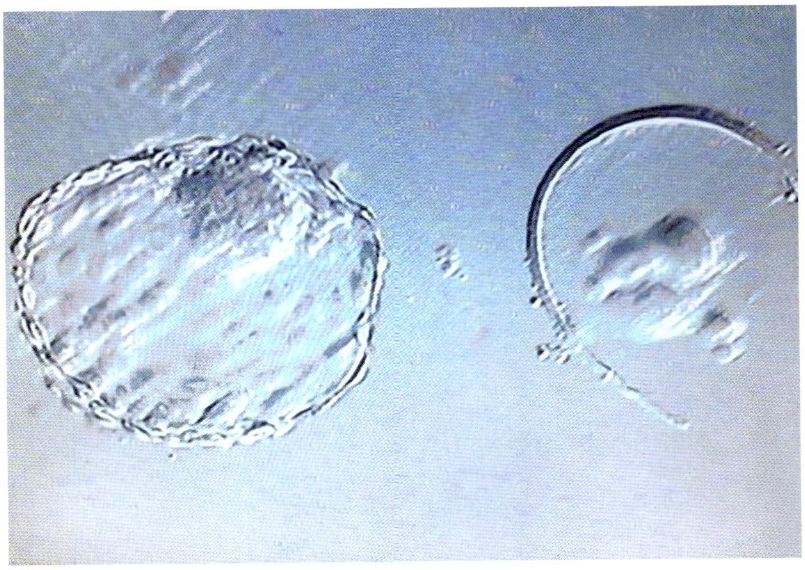

Fig. 21: Completely hatched out blastocyst after laser-assisted hatching.

Table 1: Indications for LAH.

Age	*Women over 37 years old*
Hormonal status	Women with an elevated baseline level of follicular stimulating hormone (FSH)
Embryo quality	Women with poor prognosis embryos, including conditions such as a thick zona pellucida, slow cell division rate, or high cell fragmentation
IVF attempts	Women who have failed one or more IVF cycles
Frozen embryos	Women using frozen/thawed embryos, which may have hardened zona pellucida

(IVF: in vitro fertilization; LAH: laser-assisted hatching)

patients can learn about the genetic content of an embryo before it is implanted into the uterus. This information includes the number of chromosomes an embryo contains (normal is 46), the gender of the embryo and in some cases, if the embryo is affected by a specific genetic disease (like cystic fibrosis). Ultimately, PGD can both help prevent genetic disease and improve success rates for IVF.

To perform PGD, several general steps are required, which are as follows:

- Embryos are created through IVF
- The embryos grow in the IVF laboratory for 3–5 days
- A precise biopsy procedure is used to remove a/some cell(s) from the embryo
- The removed cells are transported to a deoxyribonucleic acid (DNA) laboratory for analysis
- The results of the DNA analysis are sent back to our IVF laboratory
- Genetically healthy embryos are transferred into the uterus.

The PGD biopsy can be performed anytime from the 3rd to the 5th day after an embryo is formed. The decision of which day to biopsy depends on several factors. Both day 3 and day 5 biopsy have their own advantages and disadvantages.

Day 3 Biopsy (Figs. 22 to 25)

On the 3rd day after embryo formation, most embryos will be comprised of eight cells (each cell is called a blastomere). A biopsy at this point, removes one of the eight cells for analysis.

Advantages

- It involves fresh embryo transfer, does not require freezing—less expensive.
- Can be transferred within the same cycle, no need to wait for next cycle.

Disadvantages

- Only one cell can be biopsied, less genetic material—more chances of getting inaccurate results.
- Day 3 biopsy is more traumatic or damaging to the embryo than a day 5 biopsy.

Day 5 Biopsy (Figs. 26 to 29)

On the 5th day after embryo formation, most embryos are comprised of more than 100 cells. A biopsy at this point includes the removal of 10–15 cells.

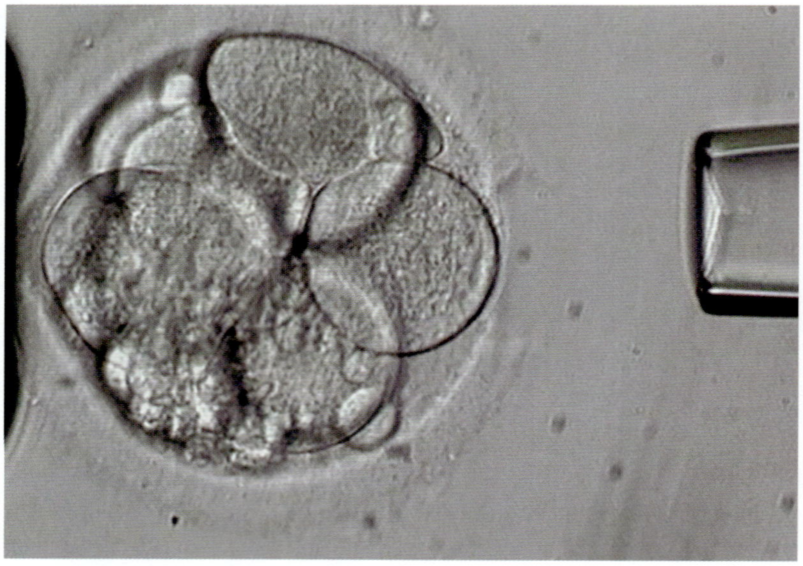

Fig. 22: Seven-cell embryo, on day 3 after in vitro fertilization held in place on a micromanipulator with a holding pipette, laser is used to create a hole through the shell of embryo.

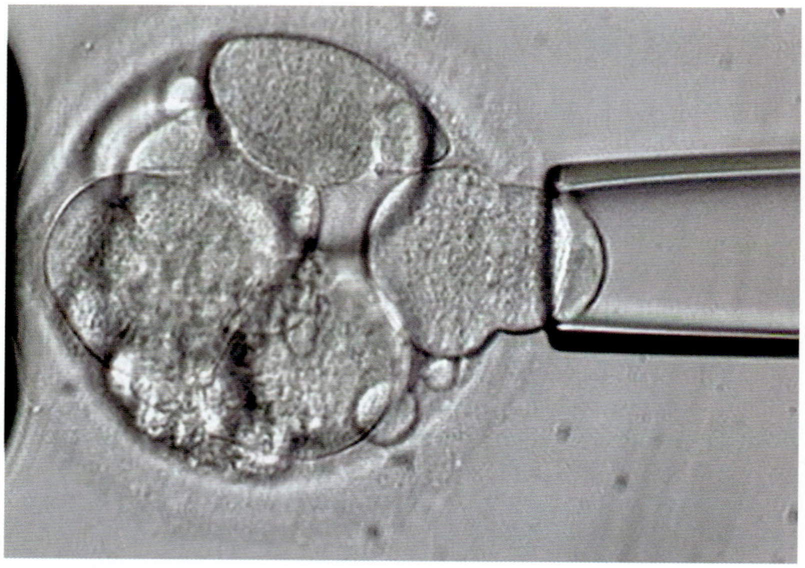

Fig. 23: A single blastomere is dislodged from embryo.

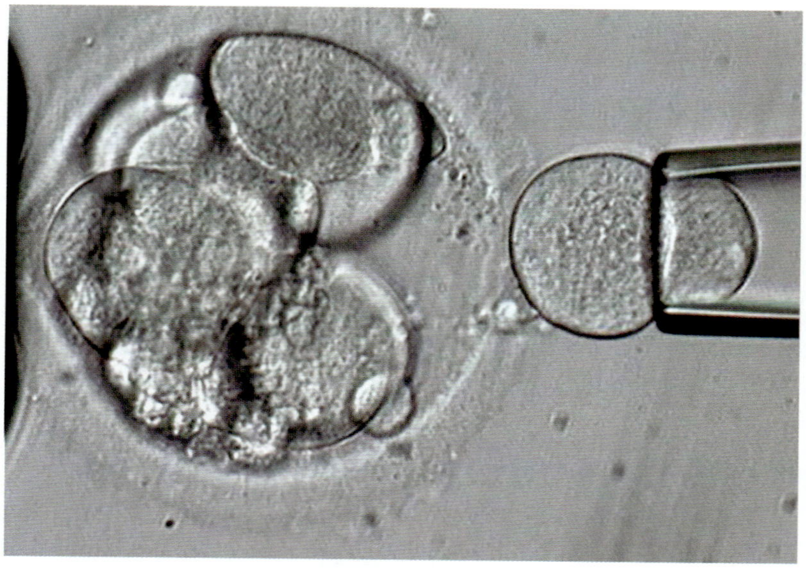

Fig. 24: The blastomere is being removed.

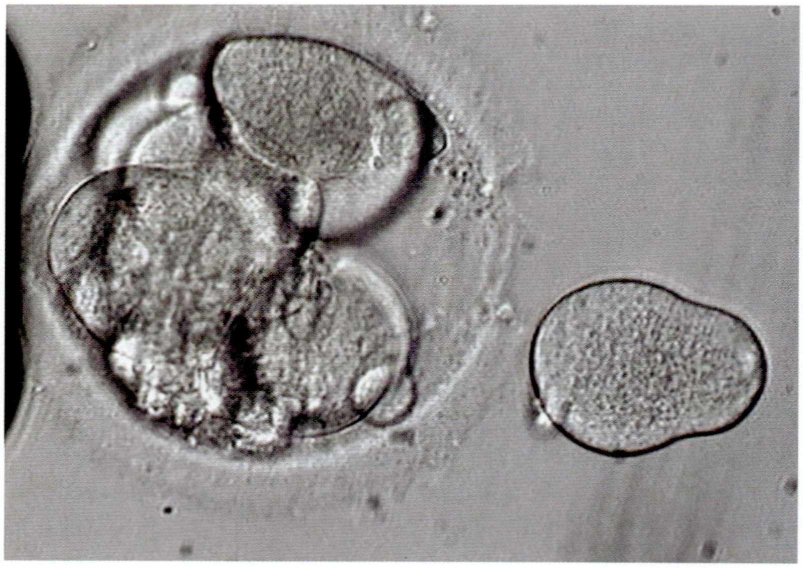

Fig. 25: The embryo biopsy has been completed successfully as the biopsied embryo is intact after the biopsy.

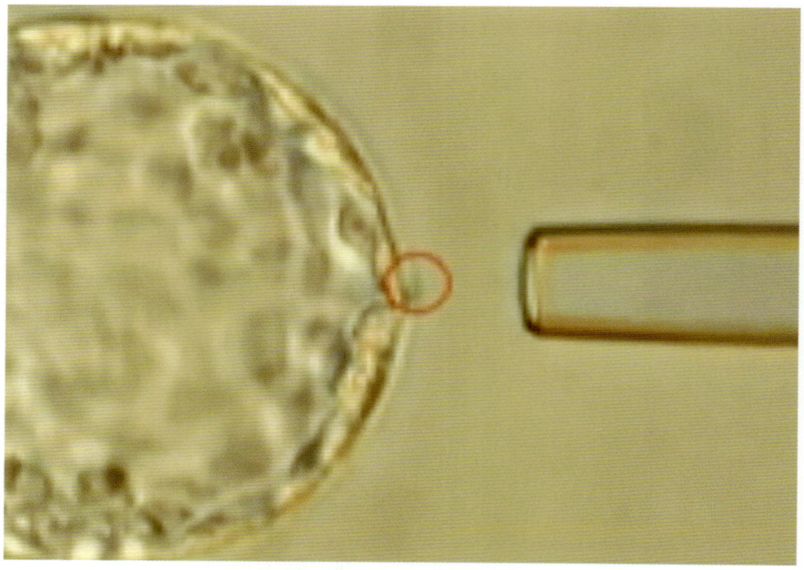

Fig. 26: Blastocyst is held in position with holding pipette. Laser is used to create hole.

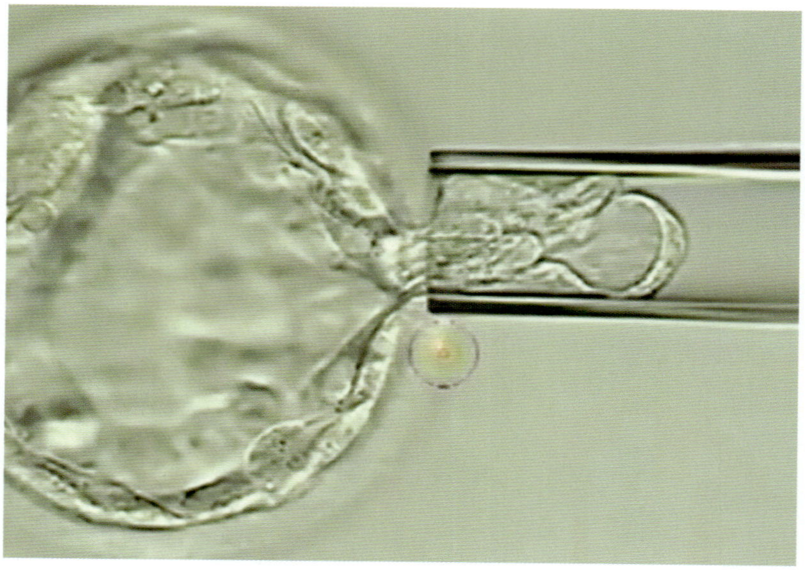

Fig. 27: Gentle suction is applied on trophectoderm cells.

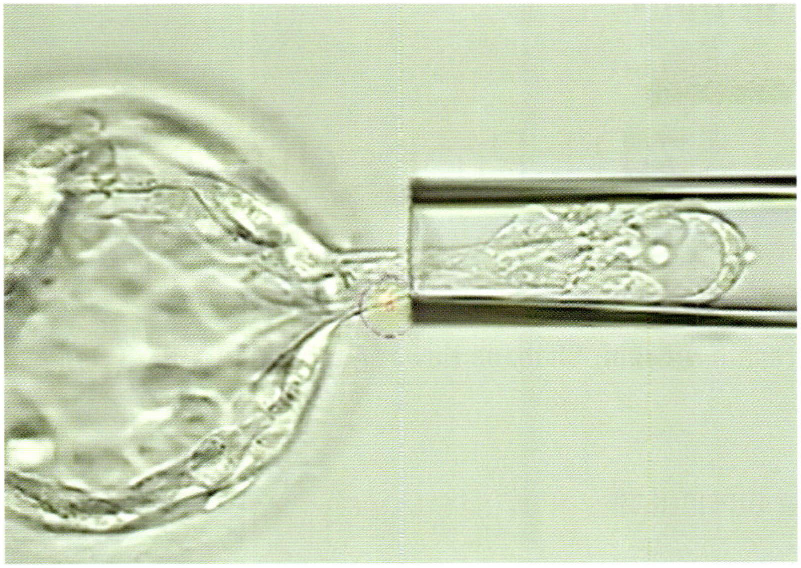

Fig. 28: Trophectoderm cells pulled out little and laser is applied to cleave the cells.

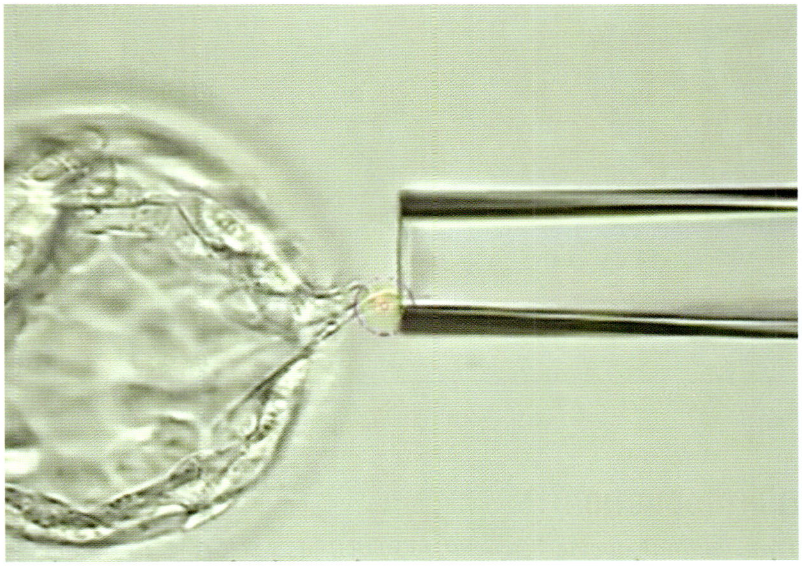

Fig. 29: Trophectoderm biopsy has been successfully completed.

Advantages

- More genetic material (from 10–15 cells), there is less theoretical chance for inaccurate or incomplete results when the DNA is analyzed.
- A second advantage is that the day 5 embryo is potentially more resilient to the biopsy than a day 3 embryo.

Disadvantage

The biggest disadvantage of a day 5 biopsy is that it requires that the embryos are frozen.

CHAPTER

79

ART Procedures and Oocyte Retrieval

Ravindranath Nirwani, Shabana Nawaz Ansari, Aditi Rai, B Ramesh

INTRODUCTION

Transvaginal oocyte retrieval (TVOR), also referred to as *oocyte retrieval (OCR)*, is a technique used in *in vitro fertilization* (IVF) in order to remove *oocytes* from the *ovary* of a woman, enabling *fertilization outside the body*. TVOR is more properly referred to as *transvaginal ovum retrieval* when the oocytes have matured into *ova*, as is normally the case in IVF. TVOR is currently performed with a *transvaginal ultrasound* transducer with an attached needle under general anesthesia. OCR is typically performed 35–36 hours after human chorionic gonadotropin (hCG) administration by a transvaginal sonography-guided technique.

TECHNIQUE

Patient put in lithotomy position. External genitalia cleansed with normal saline and vagina flushed. Vaginal ultrasound probe introduced and the target ovary focused and fixed in the center of the biopsy line. Using the aspiration needle **(Figs. 1A and B)**, the follicle entered with sharp jab at its maximum width. Suction vacuum **(Fig. 2)** applied and follicle aspirated until it is fully collapsed. The aspirated fluid is then collected in the test tube and handed over to the embryologist to check for the oocyte cumulus complex **(Figs. 3A and B)**. The process is continued till all the follicles are completely aspirated from both the ovaries. After completion, the needle is withdrawn, and *hemostasis* is achieved. The procedure usually lasts 20–60 minutes. Postprocedure vagina and cervix examined for bleeding.

DIFFICULTIES IN OVUM PICKUP

- Stuck ovary
- Endometriomas
- Bleeding from ovarian vessels
- Hydrosalpinx
- Empty follicle syndrome.

COMPLICATIONS

- *Vaginal bleeding:* 1.4–18.4%
- Intraperitoneal bleeding
- *Infections:* 0.2–0.55%.

EMBRYO TRANSFER

Embryo transfer refers to a step in the process of assisted reproduction in which *embryos* are placed into the *uterus* of a female with the intent to establish a *pregnancy*.

- Fresh ET
- Frozen ET

The outcome from using cryopreserved embryos has uniformly been positive, pregnancy rates are increased following FET, and perinatal outcomes are less affected, compared to ET in the same cycle as ovarian hyperstimulation was performed.

In a stimulated or a cycle where a "frozen" embryo is transferred, the recipient woman could be given first estrogen preparations (about 2 weeks), then a combination of estrogen and progesterone so

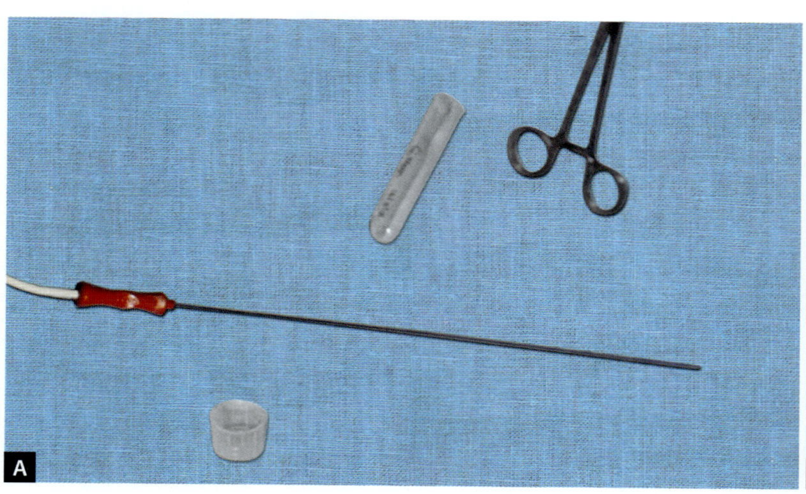

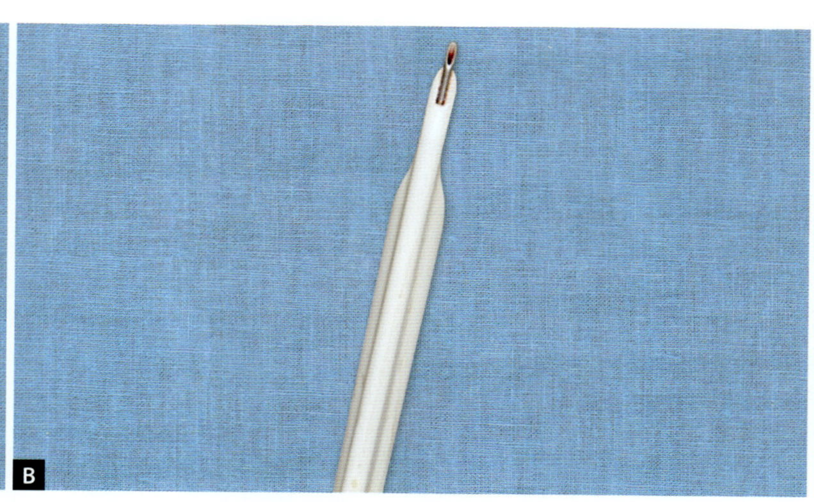

Figs. 1A and B: (A) Oocyte pickup needle (OPU needle); (B) Needle guider.

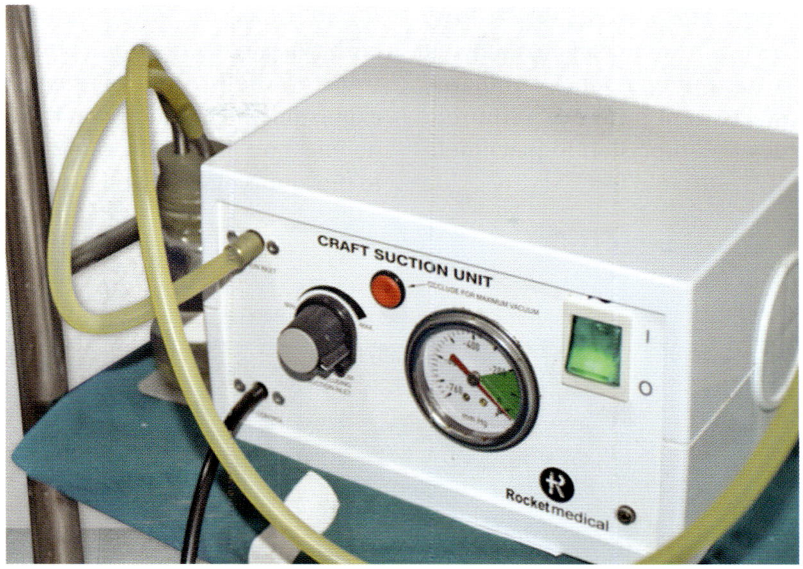

Fig. 2: Suction pump.

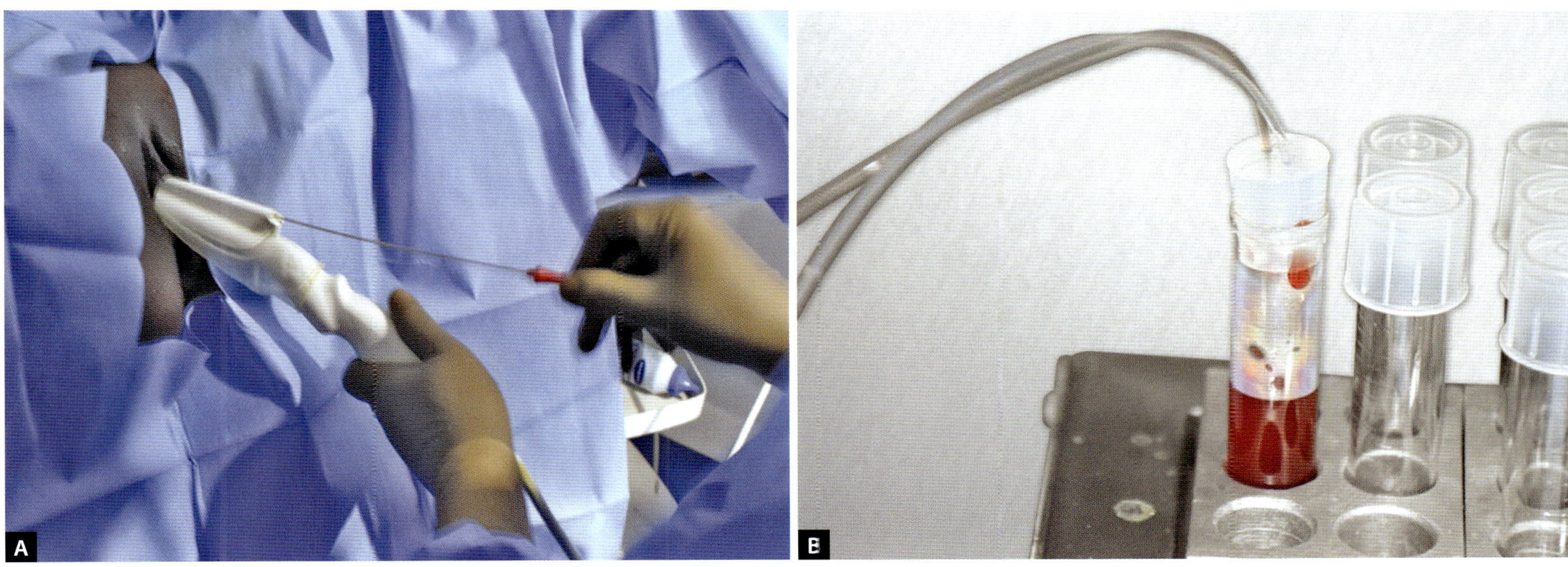

Figs. 3A and B: (A) Oocyte aspiration using OPU needle; (B) Aspirated oocytes maintained at 37°C in test tube warmer.

that the lining becomes receptive for the embryo. The time of receptivity is the implantation window.

Timing

Embryo transfer can be performed after various durations of embryo culture, conferring different stages in embryogenesis. The main stages at which ET is performed are cleavage stage (day 2–4 after coincubation) or the blastocyst stage (day 5 or 6 after coincubation). Laboratories have developed grading methods to judge oocyte and embryo quality, in order to optimize pregnancy rates. Time-lapse microscopy system for IVF was approved for clinical use, since 2009 **(Fig. 4)**.

Procedure

A speculum is placed in the vagina to visualize the cervix, which is cleansed with saline solution or culture media **(Figs. 6A to G)**. The catheter is inserted through the cervical canal and advanced into the uterine cavity. A soft transfer catheter is loaded with the embryos and handed to the clinician after confirmation of the patient's identity.

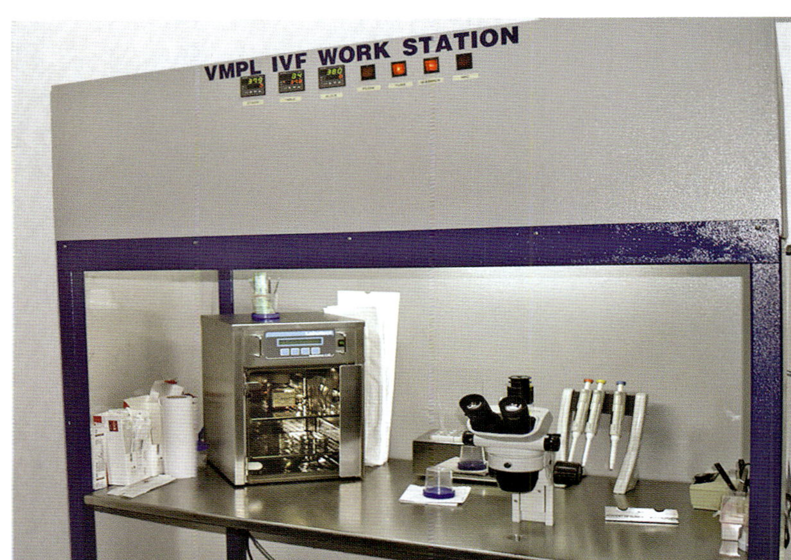

Fig. 4: In vitro fertilization workstation.

Under ultrasound guidance, embryos are placed 1–2 cm from the uterine fundus **(Figs. 5 and 7)**. There is evidence of a significant increase in clinical pregnancy using ultrasound guidance compared with only "clinical touch". Anesthesia is generally not required. Single ETs in particular require accuracy and precision in placement within the uterine cavity.

After insertion of the catheter, the contents are expelled and the embryos are deposited. Limited evidence supports making trial transfers before performing the procedure with embryos. After expulsion, the duration that the catheter remains inside the uterus has no effect on pregnancy rates. After withdrawal, the catheter is handed to the embryologist, who inspects it for retained embryos **(Table 1)**.

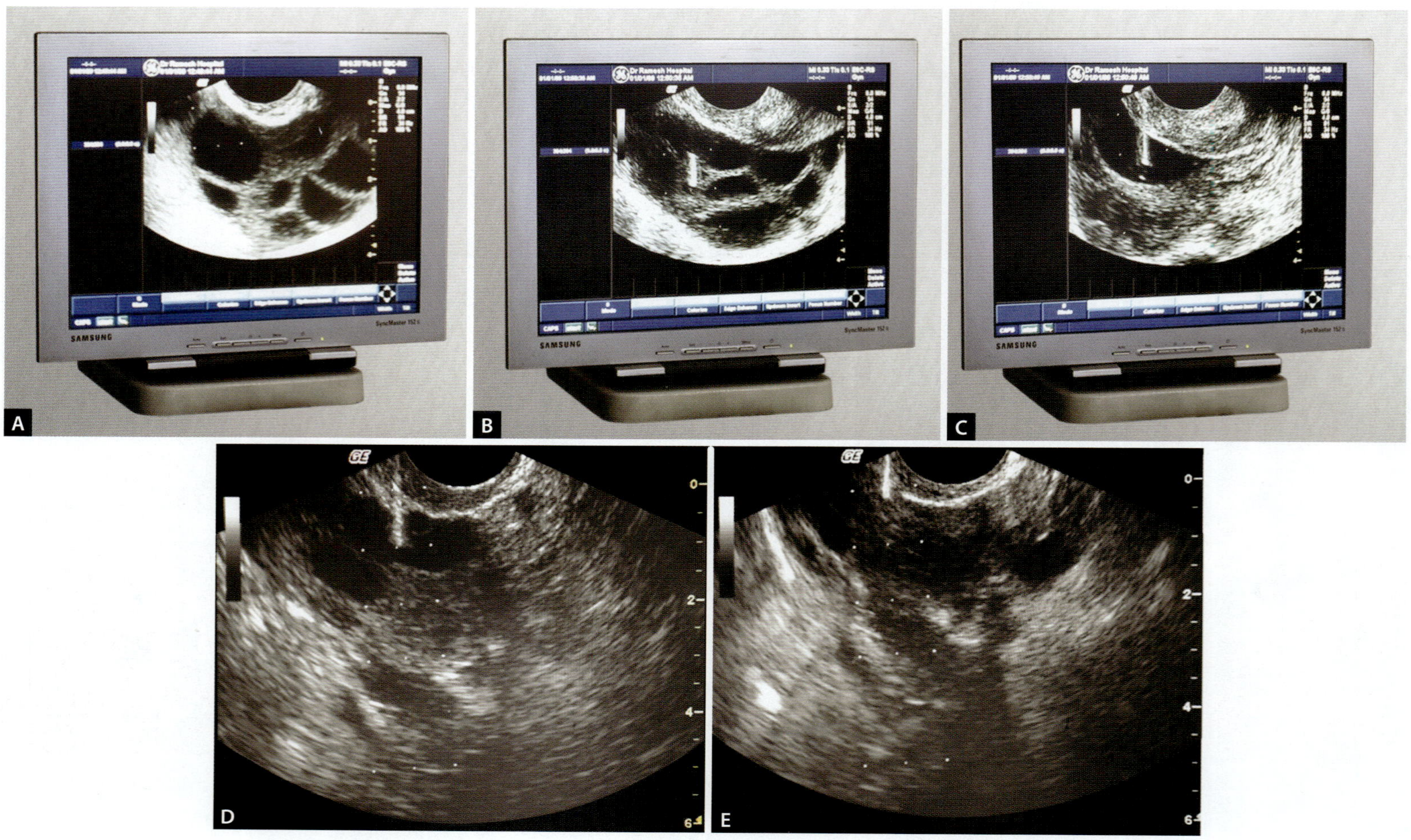

Figs. 5A to E: (A) US Scan showing matured follicle; (B) US scan showing matured follicle (16–18 Gauze) from the ovaries; (C and D) Gentle suction pressure (80–120 mm Hg) is applied to aspirate the follicles; (E) Follicle is aspirated completely.

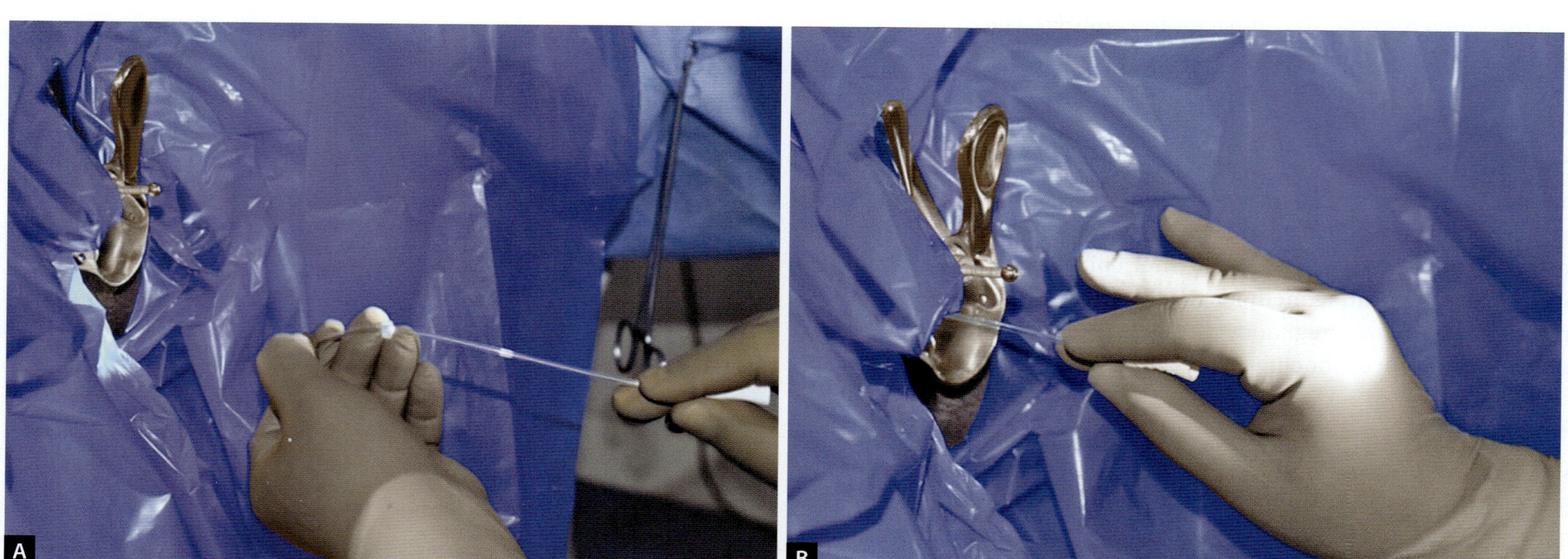

Figs. 6A and B

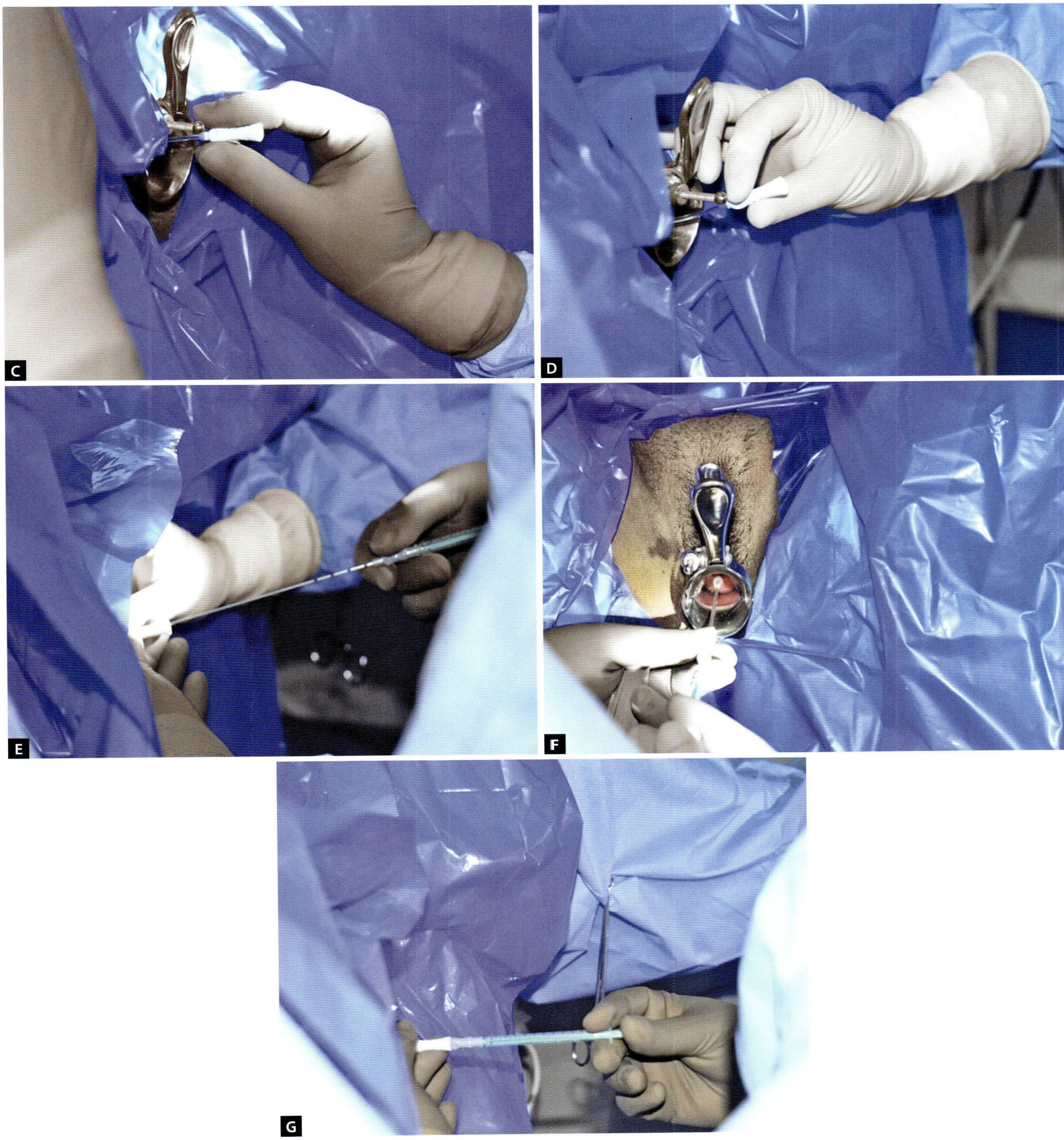

Figs. 6C to G

Figs. 6A to G: (A and B) A speculum is placed in the vagina to visualize the cervix; (C to D) An outer sheath catheter is inserted through cervix into the uterine cavity; (E and F) An embryo loaded soft catheter is inserted through outer sheath catheter into the uterine cavity; (G) Loaded embryo is completely pushed into the uterus.

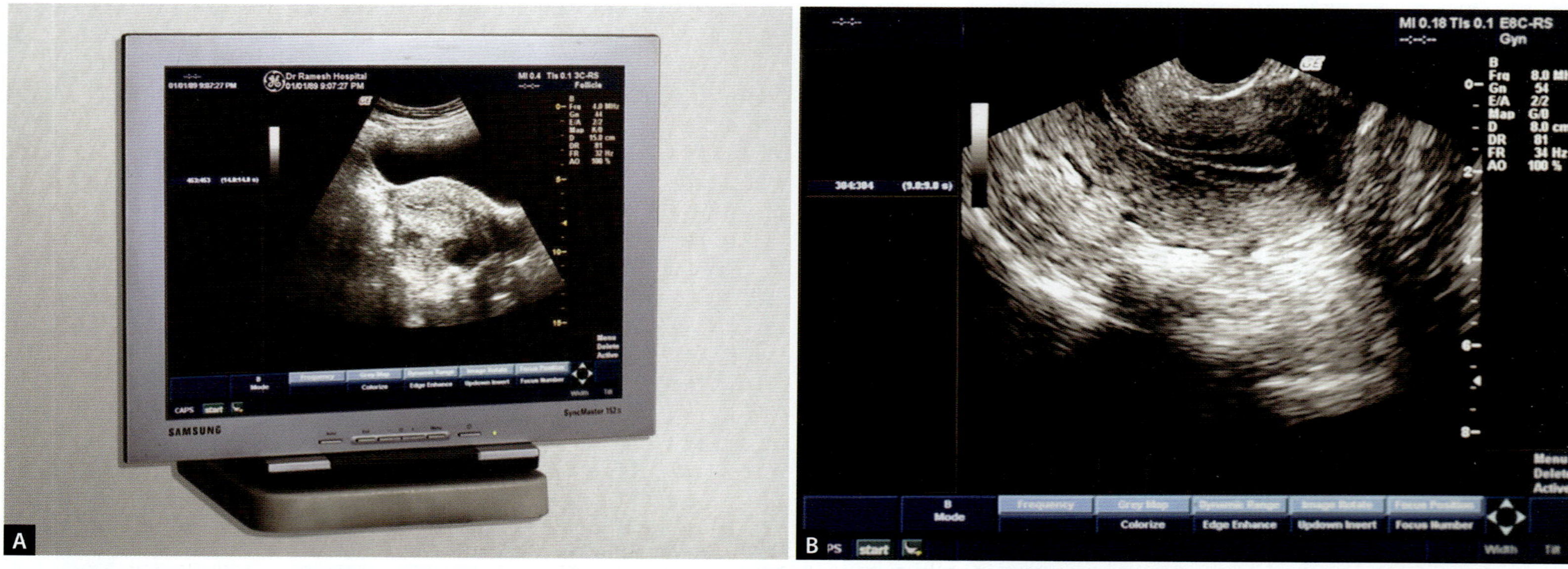

Figs. 7A and B: Ultrasound-guided embryo transfer.

Table 1: Recommendation for the limit to the number of embryo to transfer.

Age	*Attempt no.*	*Embryos transferred*
<37 years	1st	1
	2nd	1 if top-quality
	3rd	No more than 2
37–39 years	1st and 2nd	1 if top-quality
		2 if no top-quality
	3rd	No more than 2
40–42 years		2

TESTICULAR SPERM EXTRACTION

Testicular sperm extraction (TESE) is a surgical sperm retrieval procedure used in fertility treatment for men who have no sperm in their ejaculate. TESE is used for men with both obstructive and nonobstructive azoospermia. These men have no sperm in their ejaculate because either there is a blockage in the route between the site of sperm production (the testes) and ejaculation or because there is a partial or complete failure in sperm production in the testes.

Testicular sperm extraction is a minor theater procedure carried out on an outpatient basis under local anesthesia. Sperm are retrieved from the testes and can be used to achieve fertilization of eggs in the laboratory. However, because the numbers of sperm that retrieved is often very low, it is necessary to combine TESE with intracytoplasmic sperm injection (ICSI). The consultant may advise that TESE is carried out in advance of any fertility treatment to confirm that sperm production is occurring. If suitable numbers of sperm are identified on this occasion, it is sometimes possible to freeze the testicular extract and to thaw and use this sample for subsequent treatment. More commonly, however, once it has been confirmed that sperm production is occurring, the TESE procedure is repeated on the day of the egg retrieval and the fresh sample used for ICSI. Again, providing that there are suitable numbers of sperm present, the sample can sometimes be frozen for use in future treatment cycles **(Figs. 8 and 9)**.

Sperm Retrieval Techniques

There are a few different types of sperm retrieval procedures that can be used depending on your individual situation. Each of these extraction techniques has certain benefits and drawbacks.

Percutaneous Epididymal Sperm Aspiration

Percutaneous epididymal sperm aspiration (PESA) is typically the first choice for sperm retrieval, and is done by inserting a needle through the scrotum into the epididymis to collect a small amount of sperm.

Microscopic Epididymal Sperm Aspiration

Microscopic epididymal sperm aspiration is slightly more invasive technique than PESA and uses microsurgical techniques to collect sperm from the epididymis.

Testicular Sperm Extraction and Microscopic Testicular Sperm Extraction

Testicular sperm extraction is done either using a needle or a small incision to collect a small sample of the testis tissue for extraction of sperm. In cases of very *low sperm production*, a technique known as microscopic TESE (MicroTESE) is used to collect sperm from the testis.

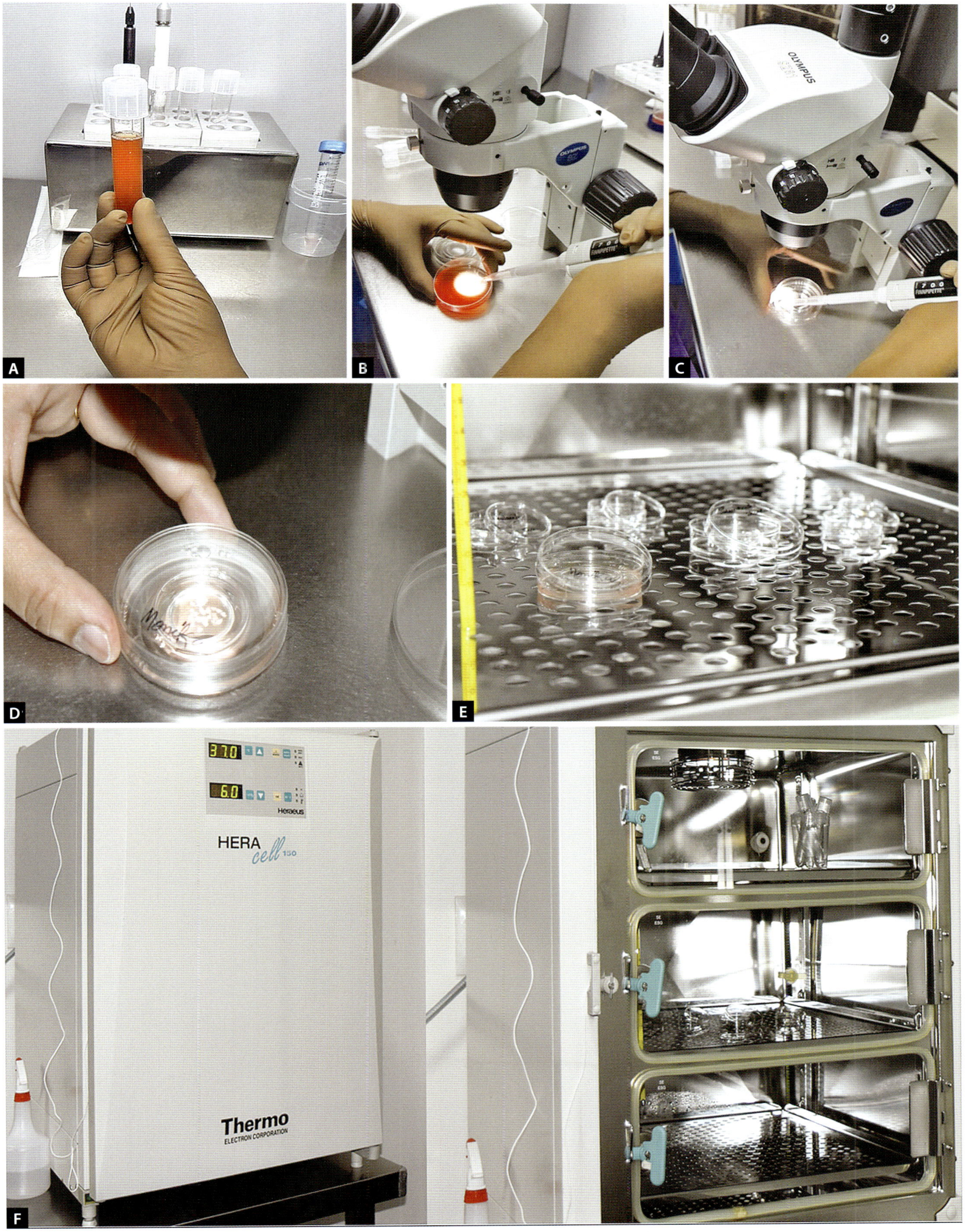

Figs. 8A to F: (A) Test tube showing follicular fluid; (B) Screening of follicular fluid under stereozoom; (C) Washing and transferring the follicles into flushing medium; (D) Follicles are resuspended into fertilization medium; (E) Dish containing follicles are placed into CO_2 Incubator At 37°C; (F) CO_2 incubator (inside and outside view).

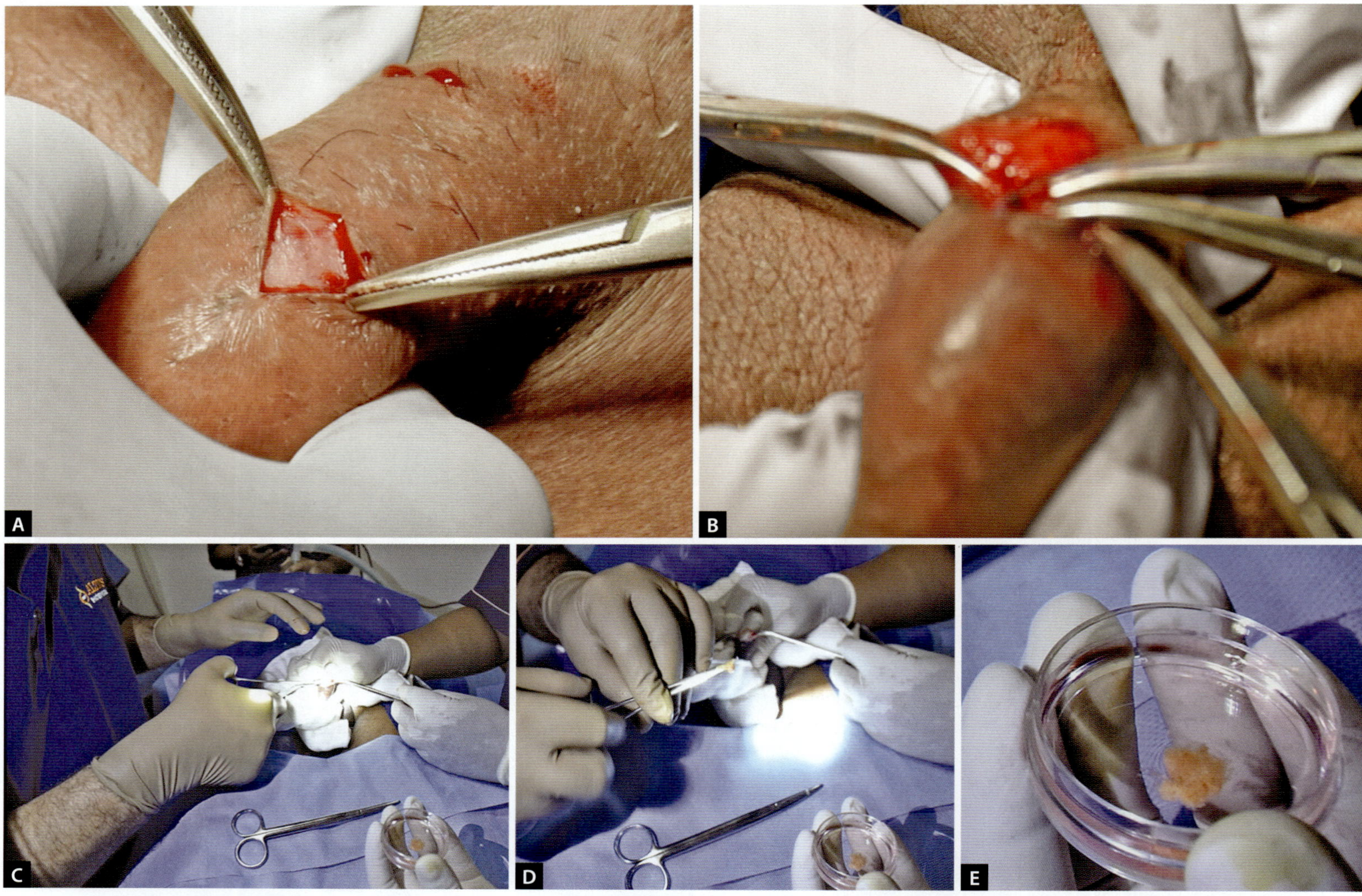

Figs. 9A to E: (A) TESE incision; (B) Deep incision; (C and D) Collection of seminiferous tubules; (E) Freshly collected seminiferous tubules.

5

SECTION

Single-port Surgeries in Gynecology

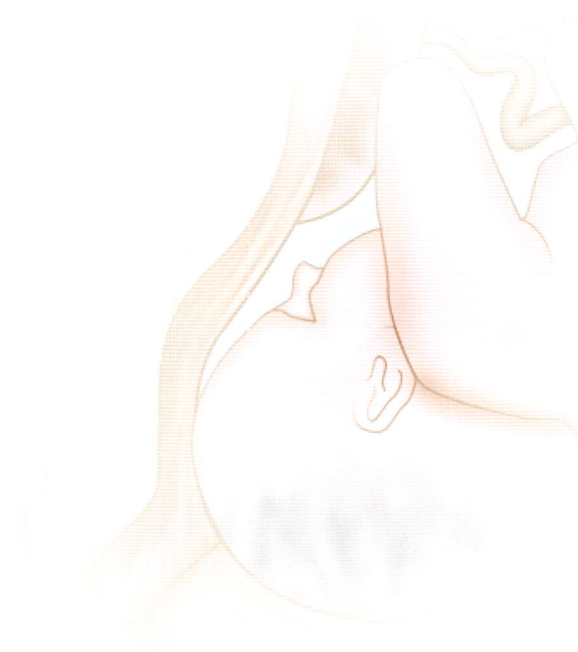

CHAPTER

80

Abdominal Access in LESS

B Ramesh, Aditi Rai

INTRODUCTION

Access through a single incision differentiates laparoendoscopic single-site (LESS) surgery from traditional multiport surgery. It is an important facet of LESS, as it should not only allow the telescope and various hand instruments through a single small incision, but also facilitate the movement of instruments for effective performance of surgery.

UMBILICUS: THE SITE OF ENTRY

Umbilicus is the site of choice as both pelvis and abdomen is accessible through it. Good cosmesis is another advantage as umbilicus being a natural cicatrix, conceals the scar if proper reconstruction is done. Entry into the peritoneal cavity can be obtained through a vertical umbilical skin incision or an inverted omega circumumbilical incision.

There are three approaches to performing laparoscopic surgery via a single incision:[1]

1. *Operative laparoscope:* This approach has been widely used by gynecologists to perform tubal sterilization. The operative laparoscope (Laprocator) has a side channel along the shaft of the instrument, which allows passage of a ring applicator to perform banding, or instrument for coagulation of the Fallopian tubes.
2. *Single skin incision with multiple fascial incision:* With this approach, multiple 5–10 mm trocars are inserted next to each other for access to the abdominal cavity. Small bridges are cut between the fascial incisions to enable organ retrieval.[2,3]
3. *Specialized access ports:* These are commercially available devices with multiple channels to access the abdominal cavity. The ports have been described in Chapter 81.

Use of Operative Laparoscope in Single-port Laparoscopy (Figs.1A and B)

Similar to single-port surgery, other techniques have been developed to reduce the invasiveness of laparoscopic surgeries and increase the cosmetic appeal like the two-port surgery and NOTES (natural orifice transluminal endoscopic surgery). The two port and laparoscopic assisted techniques utilize an operative laparoscope through one port while an accessory port assists in retraction and dissection of tissues and helps in triangulation.[4] The use of single-port laparoscopy to detort the ovary and treat ovarian cysts, while sparing the ovarian tissue itself, has been described in the literature.[5-7] These methods have been shown to be feasible, safe, effective and provide minimal postoperative pain and bleeding with improved cosmesis. Limitations of this technique are common to other procedures involving the operative laparoscope. Depth perception is a challenge when using the original "operating laparoscopes" because the laparoscope and the operating instrument are aligned in the same plane.[8] There are fewer degrees of freedom between the instruments, inside and outside the abdominal cavity, which limits the surgeon's movements. These problems of the operating laparoscope can be alleviated to some extent by use of intrauterine manipulator to change the position of the uterus, use of a 30° angled laparoscope to allow better visualization and to perform surgery with a combination of standard and long instruments.[7] Last but not least, the operating laparoscope has only one side channel for instrumentation which limits the type of procedures that can be performed by this method. In comparison, the specialized multiple access ports available for single-port laparoscopic surgery contain three to four 5-mm channels, which make more complex procedures feasible.

Single-incision but Multiport Technique (Curcillo and King Technique) (Figs. 2A to F)

The transumbilical technique for cholecystectomy, without additional incisions, was described first by Navarra et al. in 1997 and later Piskun et al. in 1999,[9,10] but failed to gain popularity due to lack of proper instrumentation. This was further refined and popularized by Curcillo and King in 2007 and published subsequently with their original technique of entry.[11,12] In their technique, a skin incision at the umbilicus, allows a flap of the umbilicus to be raised, allowing for 3–4 separate sheath incisions at distances of 2–3 cm from each other in the "Mickey Mouse" configuration. This makes it possible to insert three or even four low profile trocars, which can permit one optic and two working instruments and the possibility of an additional grasping instrument as well. Low profile and short trocars further reduce the clashing of the instruments close to the abdominal wall.[13] These fascial defects are placed at a short distance from each other. If angulation is used to enter these fascial defects, better maneuverability and maintenance of pneumoperitoneum is ensured. The disadvantage with this method is loss of pneumoperitoneum and that the defects left behind (Swiss cheese appearance) may not allow proper approximation and may lead to fascial weakening.

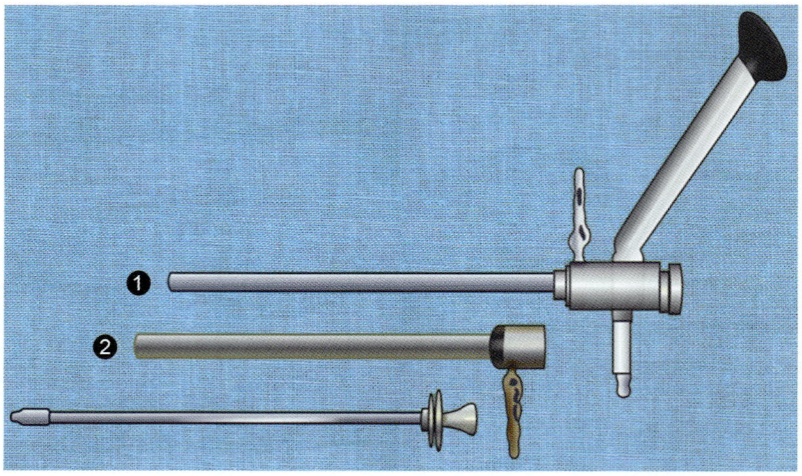

Fig. 1A: Operative laparoscope: The Frazee operative laparoscope (KARL STORZ, Tuttlingen, Germany) is an 8-mm straight-viewing Hopkins laparoscope, 30-cm length, with a 5-mm working channel.

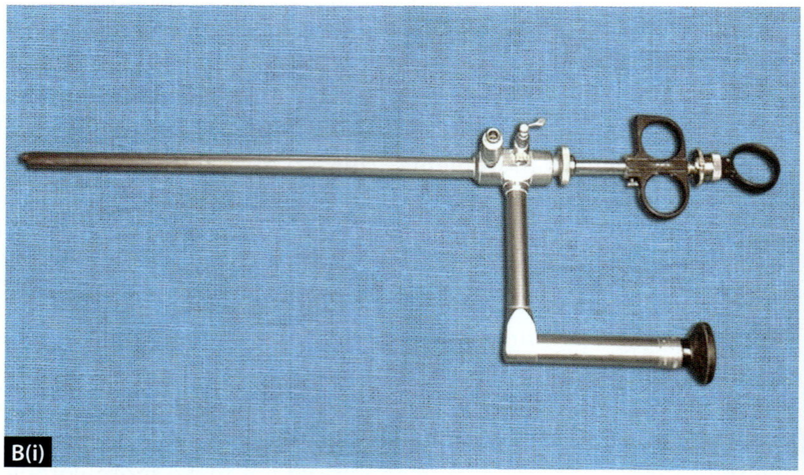

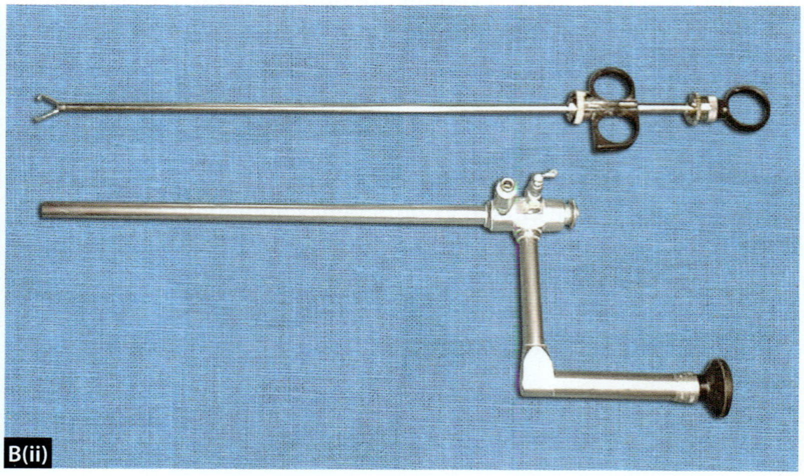

Figs. 1B(i and ii): Laparocator (for laproscopic tubal ligation with Fallope rings): (i) Laprocator channel (operative laparoscope) with offset eyepiece and operating channel. The ring applicator for application of Fallope channel rings is seen with prongs at the distal end; (ii) The ring applicator has been inserted through the operating channel. *Courtesy:* Dr Sharda Patra, Assoc Prof (Department of Obstetrics & Gynecology, Lady Hardinge Medical College, New Delhi).

Use of a Specialized Multichannel Access Device

The third and widely used technique is use of specially designed multichannel devices. These are commercially available devices, which can be inserted through a single opening in the umbilicus. These ports have 3–4 openings, which permit the placement of 3 or 4 instruments. One of the earliest multichannel devices was the R-Port (Advanced Surgical Concepts, Wicklow, United Kingdom). It was just a single-gel interphase that could be perforated many times to get the instruments in. But there was a problem of loss of pneumoperitoneum with this. Now a wide variety of access devices is available. These new access devices permitted the surgeon to insert more than two instruments and an optic, with trocars as in the GelPort and the SILS™ port and without as in the R-Port™, through the same port.[14-17] The articulating or angulated instruments can be inserted through these devices along with an optic to overcome problems of loss of triangulation **(Fig. 3)**.[13,18] The access device is inserted through an incision between 20 mm and 25 mm depending on the port and the organ to be accessed.[19] For details of various access ports, refer chapter 81.

OPERATIVE PROCEDURE: ACCESS IN LESS

Entry (Figs. 4A to N)

After administrating anesthesia and routine preparation of the patient, the right-handed surgeon stands on left side of the patient. The umbilicus is cleaned with Betadine solution.

Preventive local anesthesia: A dilute 10–20 mL solution of local anesthetic (0.5% bupivacaine with epinephrine) is administered topically in the peritoneum before skin incision is made. It is known as preemptive anesthesia. It is known to reduce postoperative pain intensity and requirement of analgesic in patients treated with local anesthetic before surgery as compared to local anesthetic administered postoperatively.[20,21] Transmission of pain signals evoked by tissue damage leads to sensitization of the peripheral and central pain pathways. Preemptive analgesia reduces this sensitization. Owing to this "protective" effect on the nociceptive system, preemptive analgesia is more effective than a similar analgesic treatment initiated after surgery.[22] Hence, it is preferable to prevent or "preempt" the neurophysiological and biochemical consequences

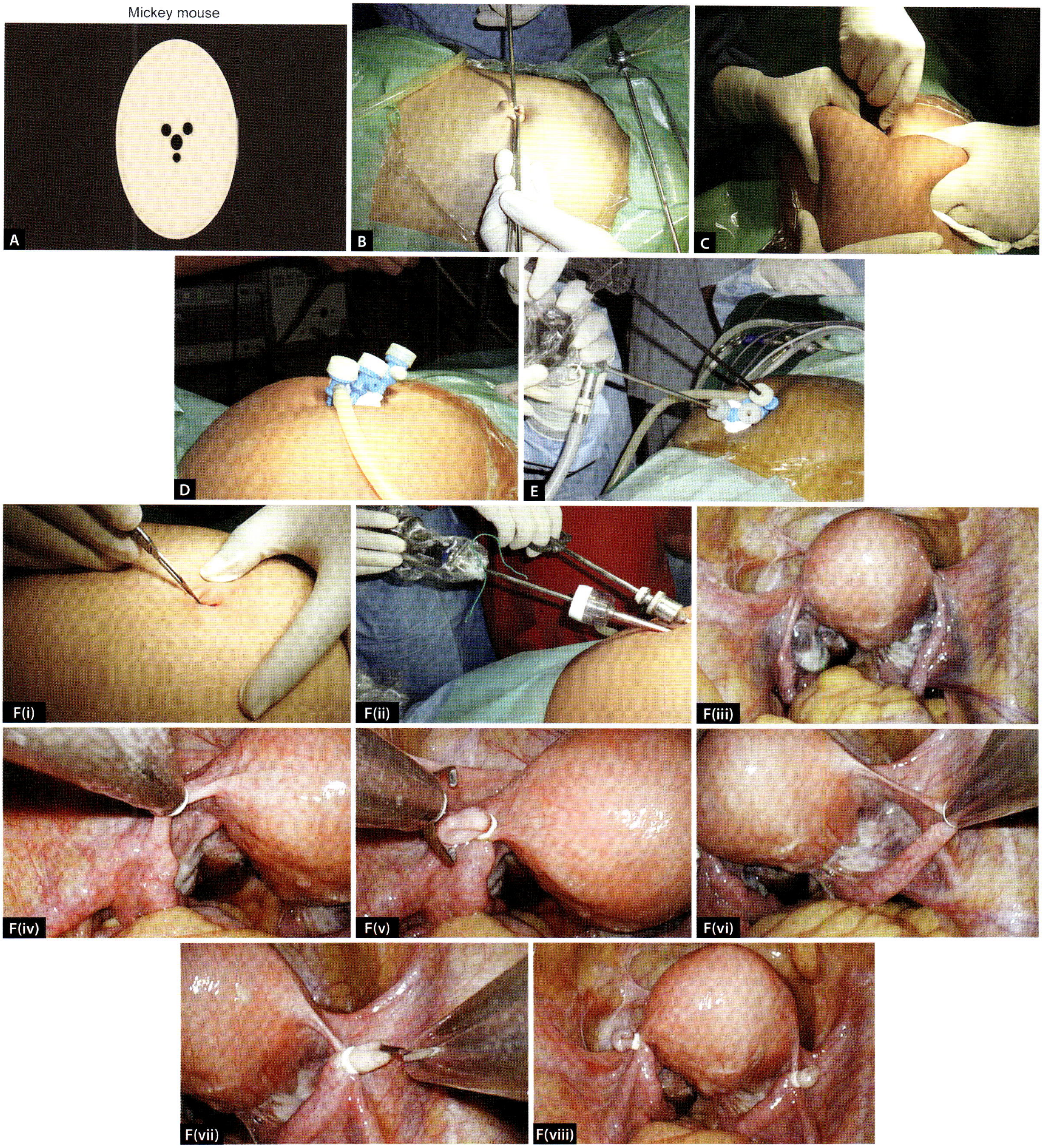

Figs. 2A to F: Curcillo and King method. Single skin with multiple fascial incisions: (A) Diagrammatic representation; (B) Incision is planned at the umbilicus; (C) First 5-mm trocar inserted through the fascia; (D) Three 5-mm trocars through different fascial but single skin incision; (E) Salpingectomy being performed. 5-mm telescope and grasper inserted through two trocars; (F) Laparoscopic tubal ligation with Fallope rings. Two trocars have been inserted through a single skin incision in the umbilicus with two fascial incisions: (i) Incision for access; (ii) Endoeye and ring applicator seen through two trocars in the same incision; (iii to viii) Laparoscopic view of tubal ligation with Fallope rings using ring applicator.

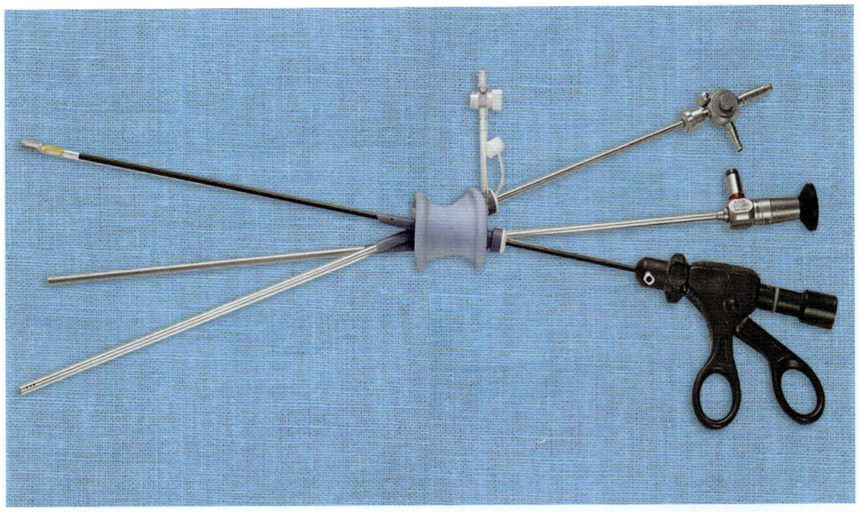

Fig. 3: Instruments and telescope (5 mm 30° long) through Covidien SILS port.

of a noxious input to the central nervous system (CNS) rather than to begin treatment when these consequences are already established.[23]

The abdominal entry through the umbilicus is made with open Hasson technique. It should be remembered that the size of the skin incision is independent of the fascial incisions. Since cosmesis postoperatively is an important factor for consideration, all efforts should be made to avoid the disfigurement of the umbilicus. Especially for female patients, as in gynecological procedures, it is expected that any disfigurement of the umbilicus will negate all benefits of single access surgery and can lead to patient dissatisfaction.

Important Considerations

- Proper preoperative preparation of the umbilicus. Patients are instructed to clean the umbilicus thoroughly before reporting to the hospital. Preoperative prepping by ward nurse includes cleaning with soap solution and Betadine.
- Skin incision should mimic natural creases—either a curved infraumbilical incision also known as "Omega"-type incision or a "J"-shaped or "hockey stick incision" can be given.[24] The shape of the incision will depend on the size and configuration of the umbilical crater.
- No part of the incision should lie outside the umbilical crater.[24]
- Umbilical stalk should not be cut; instead the fascia can be entered at the base where the stalk is attached.[24]

Use of the circumumbilical inverted omega incision allows for placement of multiple trocars through separate fascial incisions through umbilicus or multichannel access ports, provides a site for specimen removal, and potentially enhances cosmesis in this patient population. The choice to use a vertical or an inverted omega incision rests with the surgeon. After making the incision, the dissection is done up to the rectus sheath by using blunt dissection. The rectus sheath is held with artery forceps and lifted and a small nick is given with scissors. Once the fascial defect is created, it can be extended by using a blunt artery forceps and stretching it both horizontally and vertically. It is a good practice to hold the rectus sheath with stay sutures before putting in the access port. This helps as a guide to the sheath when the fascial closure is done. The stay sutures are removed when the fascia is being closed. The access port is then inserted into the incision.

Closure (Figs. 5A to C)

At the conclusion of each case, the fascia and underlying peritoneum are isolated and closed with delayed absorbable suture in a running fashion with 0-Vicryl suture (Ethicon, Somerville, NJ). If the umbilical stalk is cut, it is identified and reattached to the fascia with an anchoring stitch by use of 0-Vicryl suture, and the skin is closed with subcuticular absorbable sutures with 3-0 Monocryl. The fascia can also be closed with interrupted, "Figure-of-8" delayed absorbable sutures.[25] In a retrospective study conducted by Kevin Stepp et al., there were no significant differences in intraoperative or postoperative complications, wound complications, postoperative antibiotic use, or 6 week patient satisfaction between the two incision types.[26]

Review of literature: The method for access was described by Rivas et al. in their case series on single incision laparoscopic cholecystectomy.[27] The umbilicus was everted by pulling the deepest point of the umbilical scar (inner ring) out of its inward position. A 1.5–2 cm transumbilical incision then was performed in a vertical fashion without extension of this incision beyond the outer limits of the umbilical folds. By incising the rectus sheath, direct access into the abdomen was obtained. Through this opening, a low-profile, 5-mm trocar was placed under direct vision without the need for an introducer or previous pneumoperitoneum. Only for cases in which the entry site into the abdomen is not readily identified after the stalk had been incised, is pneumoperitoneum obtained with the use of a Veress needle.[25]

In Curcillo and King method,[11,12] after adequate pneumoperitoneum has been obtained, a second 5-mm port is placed through the same skin incision, but approximately 5 mm above the first port. Only if needed is an additional 5-mm trocar placed inferiorly or laterally through the same skin incision but at a different fascial site. The use of three different fascial incisions could lead to loss of pneumoperitoneum, which can be avoided by not making such openings too near each other (should be at least 2 mm apart).

Therefore, abdominal access through a single incision in the umbilicus defines laparoendoscopic single-site surgery (LESS). The type of incision and ports depends on the procedure, skill, and comfort of the patient. The surgeon should be careful about maintaining the integrity of the umbilicus during access and closure. If these principles are followed, excellent cosmetic benefit and satisfaction can be provided to the patient without compromising on the operative procedure.

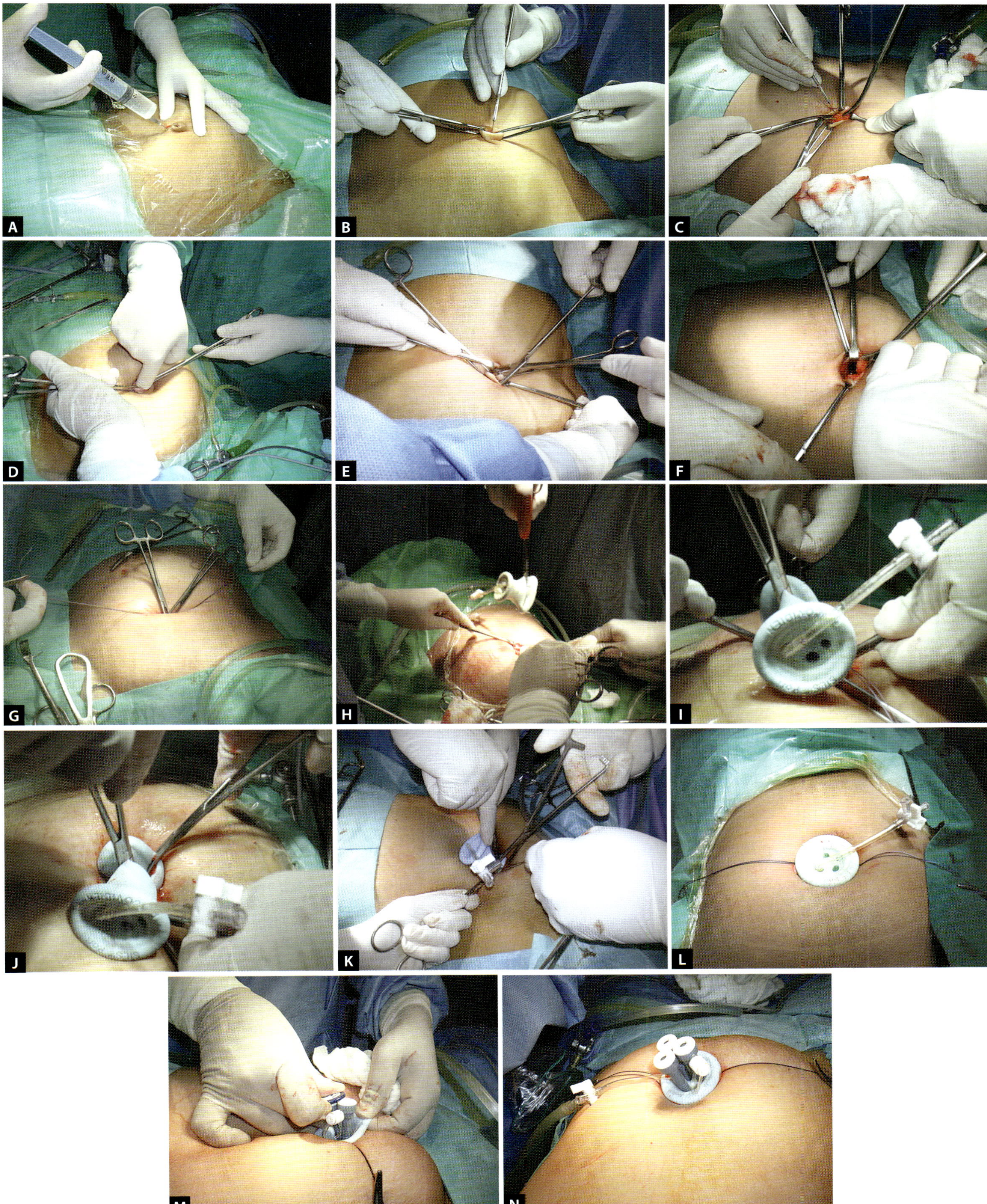

Figs. 4A to N: Procedure for single incision access using SILS port (Covidien). (A) Local anesthetic instillation; (B) Making vertical incision. The margins of the umbilicus are held with Allis forceps; (C) Subcutaneous sharp dissection; (D) Blunt dissection and palpation of rectus sheath; (E) Extension of the fascial incision with a long artery forceps; (F) Access has been obtained into the peritoneal cavity; (G) Stay sutures at the margins of the rectus sheath; (H) SILS port (Covidien) being held with artery forceps for insertion; (I to K) Steps on insertion of Covidien port into the incision; (L) Access port fully inserted; (M) Insertion of 5-mm trocars; (N) SILS port with three 5-mm trocars.

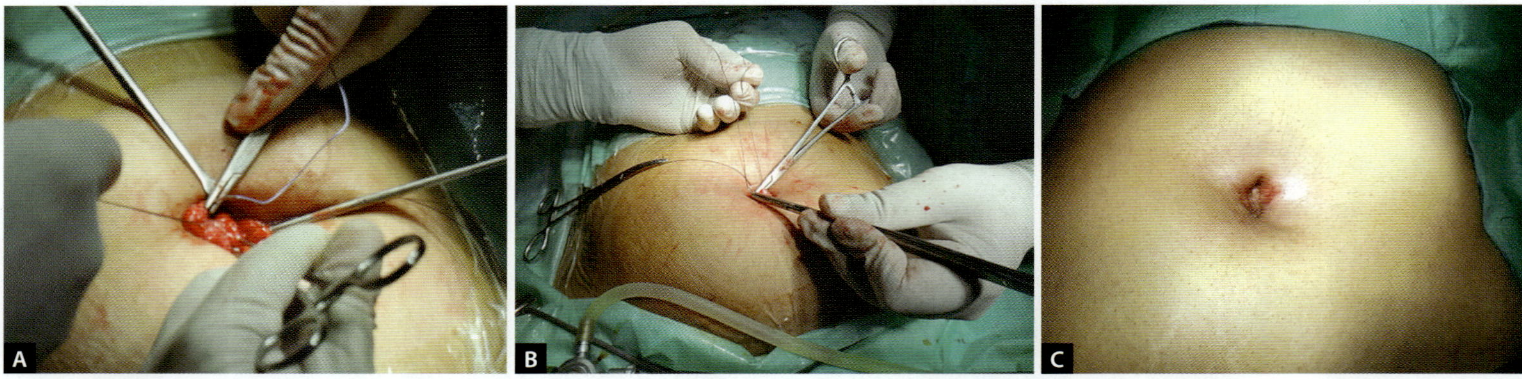

Figs. 5A to C: Closure. (A and B) Closure of the incision; (C) Scar after closure.

KEY POINTS

- Access though a single incision defines laparoendoscopic single-site surgery
- Site of access is the umbilicus
- Anatomical configuration of the umbilicus should be maintained during incision and closure
- Type of incision depends on shape and size of umbilicus and surgeon's preference
- Local infiltration of anesthetic preoperatively provides enhanced postoperative pain relief.

REFERENCES

1. Uppal S, Frumovitz M, Escobar P, et al. Laparoendoscopic single-site surgery in gynecology: review of literature and available technology. J Minim Invasive Gynecol. 2011;18:12-23.
2. Podolsky ER, Curcillo PG 2nd. Single port access (SPA) surgery—a 24-month experience. J Gastrointest Surg. 2010;14:759-67.
3. Tacchino R, Greco F, Matera D. Single-incision laparoscopic cholecystectomy: surgery without a visible scar. Surg Endosc. 2009;23:896-99.
4. Khosla A, Ponsky TA. Use of operative laparoscopes in single-port surgery. A forgotten tool. J Minim Access Surg. 2011;7(1):116-20.
5. Li YT, Kuon LC, Lee PN, et al. Laparoscopic detorsion of twisted ovary. J Chin Med Assoc. 2005;68(12):595-8.
6. Kosumi T, Kubota A, Usui N, et al. Laparoscopic ovarian cystectomy using a single umbilical puncture method. Surg Laparosc Endosc Percutan Tech. 2001;11(1):63-57.
7. Fagotti A, Fanfani F, Marocco F, et al. Laparoendoscopic single-site surgery (LESS) for ovarian cyst enucleation: report of first 3 cases. Fertil Steril. 2009;92:1168;e13-6.
8. Bedaiwy MA, Escobar PF, Pinkerton J, et al. Laparoendoscopic single-site salpingectomy in isthmic and ampullary ectopic pregnancy: preliminary report and technique. J Minim Invasive Gynecol. 2011;18:230-3.
9. Navarra G, Pozza E, Occhionorelli S, et al. One-wound laparoscopic cholecystectomy. Br J Surg. 1997;84:695.
10. Piskun G, Rajpal S. Transumbilical laparoscopic cholecystectomy utilizes no incisions outside the umbilicus. J Laparoendosc Adv Surg Tech A. 1999;9:361-4.
11. Castellucci SA, Curcillo PG, Ginsberg PC, et al. Single port access adrenalectomy. J Endourol. 2008;22:1573-6.
12. Podolsky ER, Rottman SJ, Poblete H, et al. Single-port access (SPA) cholecystectomy: a completely transumbilical approach. J Laparoendosc Adv Surg Tech A. 2009;19:219-22.
13. Raman JD, Bensalah K, Bagrodia A, et al. Laboratory and clinical development of single keyhole umbilical nephrectomy. Urology. 2007;70:1039-42.
14. Rane A, Kommu S, Eddy B, et al. Clinical evaluation of a novel laparoscopic port (R-Port) and evolution of the single laparoscopic port procedure (SLiPP). J Endourol. 2007;21:A22-3.
15. Rane A, Rao P. Single-port-access nephrectomy and other laparoscopic urologic procedures using a novel laparoscopic port (R-port). Urology. 2008;72:260-63.
16. Rao PP, Bhagwat SM, Rane A. The feasibility of single-port laparoscopic cholecystectomy: a pilot study of 20 cases. HPB (Oxford). 2008;10: 336-40.
17. Kaouk JH, Haber GP, Goel RK, et al Single-port laparoscopic surgery in urology: initial experience. Urology. 2008;71:3-63.
18. Raman JD, Cadeddu JA, Rao P, et al. Single-incision laparoscopic surgery: initial urological experience and comparison with natural-orifice transluminal endoscopic surgery. BJU Int. 2008;101:1493-6.
19. Rao PP, Rao PP, Bhagwat S. Single-incision laparoscopic surgery—current status and controversies. J Minim Access Surg. 2011;7(1):6-16.
20. Pasqualucci A, de Angelis V, Contardo R, et al. Preemptive analgesia: intraperitoneal local anesthetic in laparoscopic cholecystectomy. A randomized, double blind, placebo-controlled study. Anesthesiology. 1996;85(1):11-20.
21. Ke RW, Portera SG, Bagous W, et al. A randomized, double-blinded trial of preemptive analgesia in laparoscopy. Obstet Gynecol. 1998;92(6): 972-75.
22. Dahl JB, Møiniche S. Pre-emptive analgesia. Br Med Bull. 2004;71:13-27.
23. Woolf CJ, Chong MS. Preemptive analgesia—treating postoperative pain by preventing the establishment of central sensitization. Anesth Analg. 1993;77:362-79.
24. Sobolewski C, Yeung PP Jr, Hart S. Laparoendoscopic single-site surgery in gynaecology. Obstet Gynecol Clin North Am. 2011;38:741-5.
25. Gunderson CC, Knight J, Ybanez-Morano J, et al. The risk of umbilical hernia and other complications with laparoendoscopic single-site surgery. J Minim Invasive Gynecol. 2012;19:40-5.
26. Kane S, Stepp KJ. Circumumbilical (Omega) incision use in laparoendoscopic single-site (LESS) gynecologic surgery. J Minim Invasive Gynecol. 2011;18:S148.
27. Rivas H, Varela E, Scott D. Single-incision laparoscopic cholecystectomy: initial evaluation of a large series of patients. Surg Endosc. 2010;24: 1403-12.

CHAPTER

81

Instruments and Ports

B Ramesh, Aditi Rai

INTRODUCTION

Laparoendoscopic single-site surgery (LESS) requires surgery to be completely performed through a single access point, i.e. through the umbilicus. There are three approaches to obtain access, through an operating laparoscope, multiple fascial incisions through a single skin incision and commercially available specialized access ports.[1] The inherent difficulties of LESS like instrument manipulation through a crowded operating space and potential for collision can be mitigated to some extent by specialized instruments. The various access techniques in LESS have been described in Chapter 80. In this chapter we will describe commercially available multichannel access ports and instruments specifically designed for single-port surgeries.

ACCESS PORTS[1-3]

TRIPORT AND QUADPORT ACCESS SYSTEM

(Olympus America, Inc, Center Valley. A)[1,2] **(Fig. 1)**.

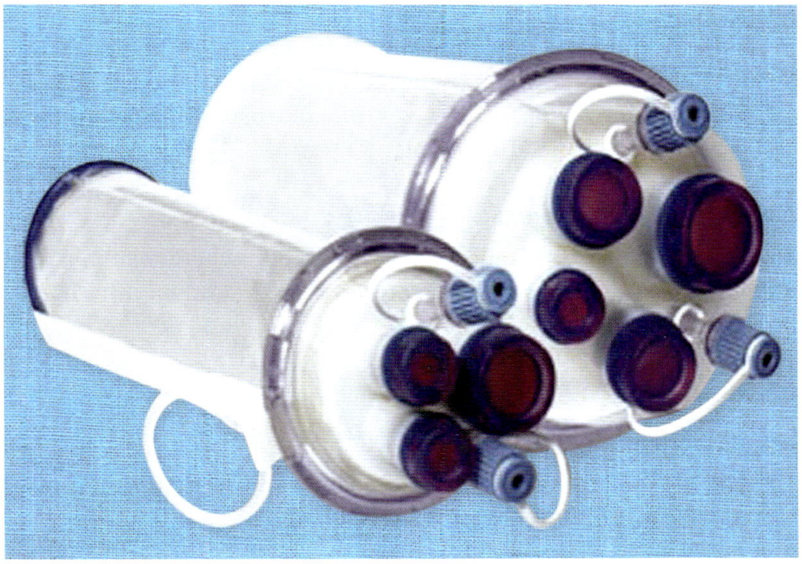

Fig. 1: TriPort and Quadport.
Courtesy: Olympus website.

Component Parts

The TriPort initially introduced as the R-Port and QuadPort have two components:

1. An outer multichannel valve and
2. A fascial retractor with an inner and outer ring connected by a retractable sleeve.

The TriPort has two 5 mm channels, one 12 mm channel, with insufflation line. It requires incisions ranging from 12 to 25 mm and allows the passage of three instruments. The QuadPort has 4 legs: one 5 mm, two 10 mm, and one 15 mm in diameter. The device can be used with fascial incisions ranging from 25 to 65 mm. Each port is covered with a simple valve of thermoplastic elastomer that maintains pneumoperitoneum. To minimize friction between instruments and the port, some amount of lubrication is essential.[2]

Deployment

For insertion, a skin and fascial incision is made and the distal ring is loaded into an introducer. The introducer is used to bluntly pierce the abdominal wall and push the distal ring into the abdominal cavity. The inner ring expands once it is pushed out of the introducer. Then the introducer is removed, the retracting sleeve is grasped at the proximal end and the outer ring is passed downward over it to create a tight seal with the abdominal wall. The excess sleeve is then cut away. Once in place, the multi-instrument access port accommodates up to three (TriPort) or four (QuadPort) instruments to be used simultaneously.

Advantages[1,2]

- Multiple instruments can be placed and removed without loss of pneumoperitoneum.
- The TriPort can be safely introduced through controlled deployment.
- It can also be easily removed and replaced as in the case of specimen removal as the current formation of this device allows the entire diaphragm that contains the channels to be removed and replaced.
- It has the ability to adapt to abdominal walls of various thicknesses up to 10 cm.
- Plastic valves and a low profile allow passage of curved instruments and provide a wider field of view once the laparoscope is inserted through one of the valves. Similarly, the short channels afford greater angle of distraction compared with standard rigid trocars, increasing the achievable triangulation between the instruments.
- The angle of the different ports helps to reduce instrument crowding.

Drawbacks of Triport and QuadPort Devices[1]

- The main drawback of the TriPort design is the gel valves. They have been known to come apart when excessive manipulation of instruments take place.
- Lubrication of instruments is necessary to prevent valve damage. With each instrument passage, lubricant needs to be applied.
- Once the valve is removed, reinsertion is easy, but seal maintenance remains inconsistent.
- The sleeve may get damaged resulting in loss of pneumoperitoneum.
- Maximum depth of 10 cm limits use of the system in obese patients.

QuadPort

The larger QuadPort is commercially available with one 5 mm port, two 10 mm ports, and one 15 mm port, allowing up to four instruments to be used through a single incision between 2.5 cm and 6.5 cm in length. Flexible ports enhance access to the surgical site and accommodate different types and sizes of laparoscopic instruments; conventional, bent and articulating.

Advantage of QuadPort over TriPort

The QuadPort has an advantage over the TriPort when organ retrieval would necessitate a fascial incision between 25 and 65 mm. Also it provides four ports.

X-CONE

(KARL STORZ, Tuttlingen, Germany)[1,3] **(Figs. 2 and 3)**.

The X-cone consists of two metal halves that once within the peritoneal cavity are joined together by a silicone cap. Within the cap, there are three access channels that can accommodate instruments up to 12 mm in diameter. It is inserted through a 2–2.5-cm incision. The ENDOCONE requires a 3.5-cm incision, but permits the passage of more instruments than any other access device. It contains channels for six 5 mm instruments and two 12 mm instruments. These devices when used together with curved instruments enhance the triangulation in single-port surgery.

Deployment (Fig. 3)

After making an incision at the umbilicus, stay sutures are taken on the rectus sheath. The stay sutures are held firmly and uniformly and first half of the X-cone placed inside. The second half of the X-cone is now inserted under visualization. The inner part of the access system is now closed. After correct positioning, the tension on the fascial sutures is relieved and outer working access of the port system is closed together. The X-cone must be placed with the insufflation stopcock at 12 noon. The silicone cap or seal is then placed on the access channel.

GELPORT AND GELPOINT SYSTEM

The GelPort and GelPoint system **(Fig. 4)** (Applied Medical Resources Corp, Rancho Santa Margarita, California)

The GelPort system is an innovative sealing device that permits abdominal access and frequent instrument exchange during surgery, while preserving the pneumoperitoneum.[4] The GelPort system has previously been used for hand-assisted laparoscopy.

Component Parts

- A GelSeal cap.
- Alexis wound retractor with a flexible inner ring connected to an outer ring with a clear sheath. The outer ring has a diameter of approximately 10 cm. A GelSeal cap fits over the outer ring.
- Four self-retaining low profile trocars with an obturator: for easier insertion of laparoscopic instruments through the gel interface.

GelSeal Cap

Offers a pseudoabdomen platform for triangulation of standard laparoscopic instrumentation and provides a flexible fulcrum for improved instrument articulation. It maintains pneumoperitoneum for continuous access and visualization.

Alexis Wound Retractor

It retracts the abdominal wall in an atraumatic manner. It facilitates specimen retrieval and protects the incision site.

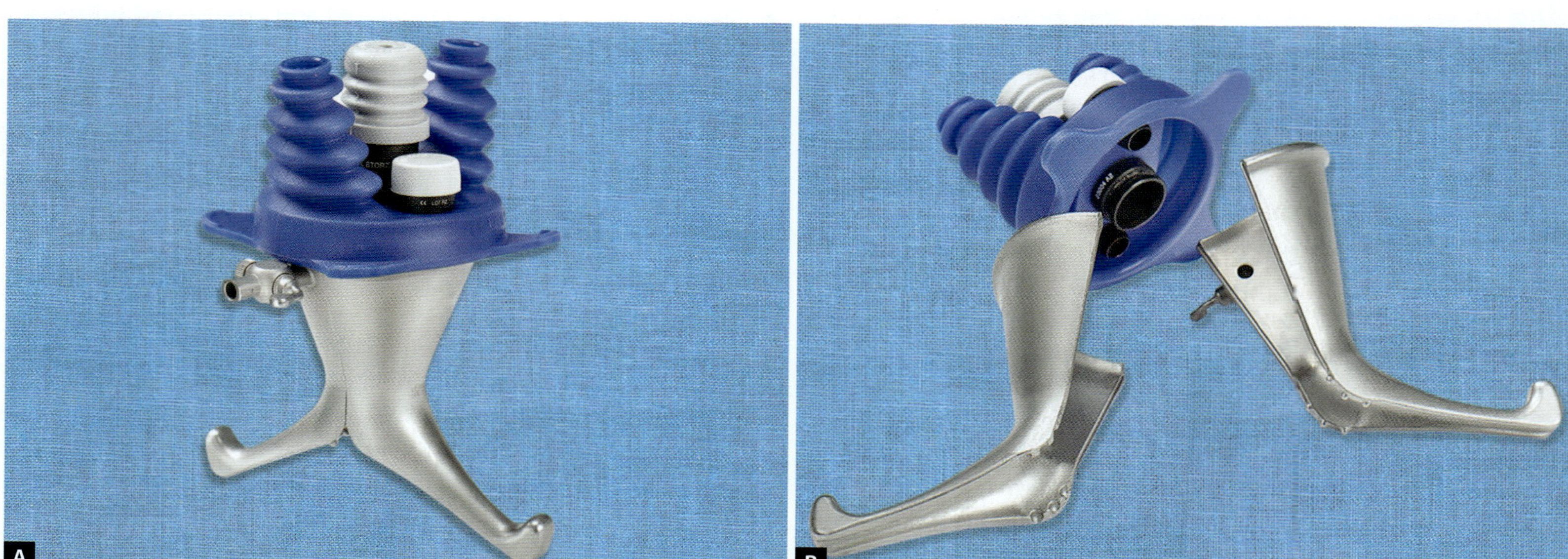

Figs. 2A and B: X-cone access device from KARL STORZ.

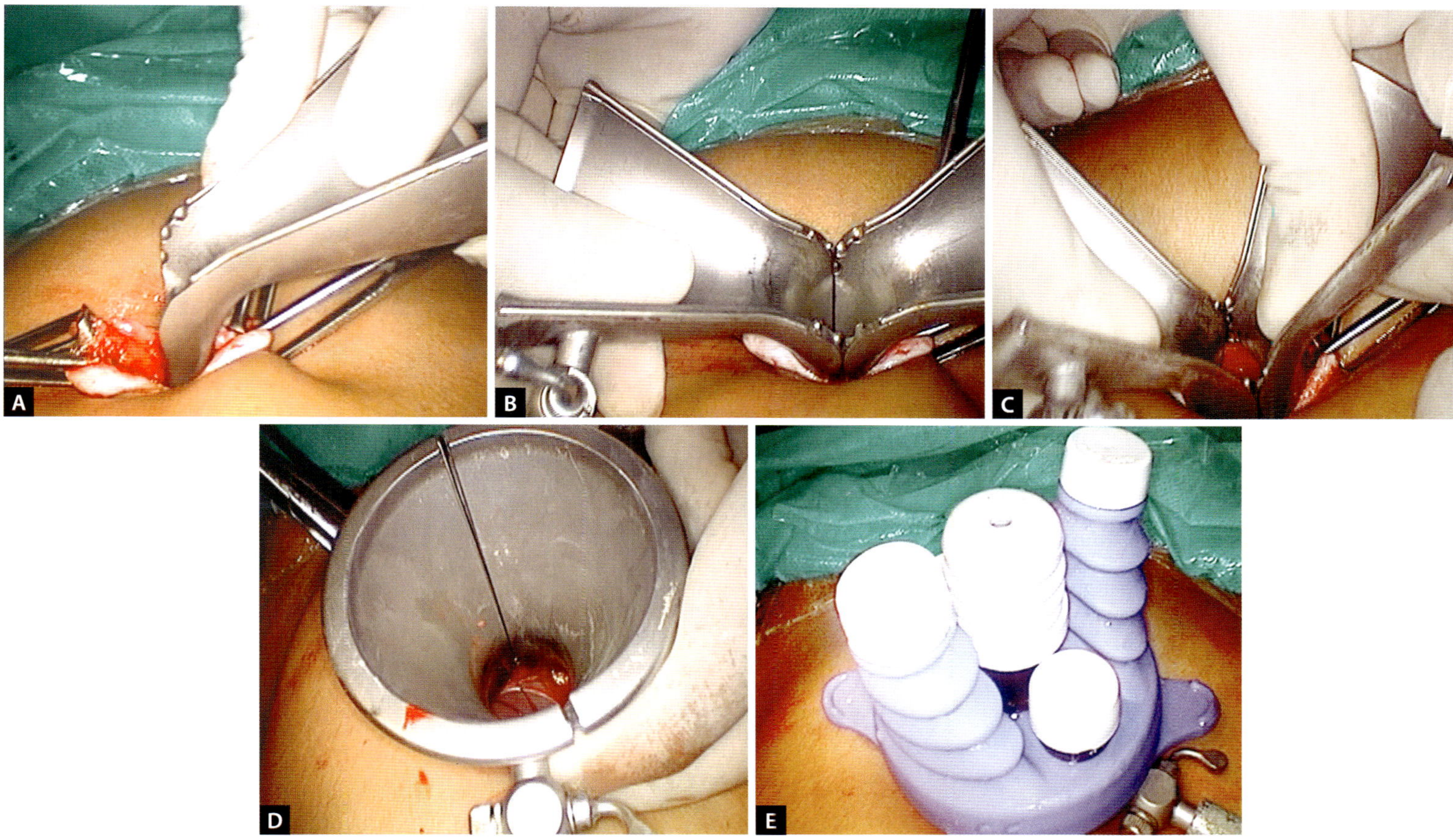

Figs. 3A to E: Deployment of X-cone through the umbilicus.

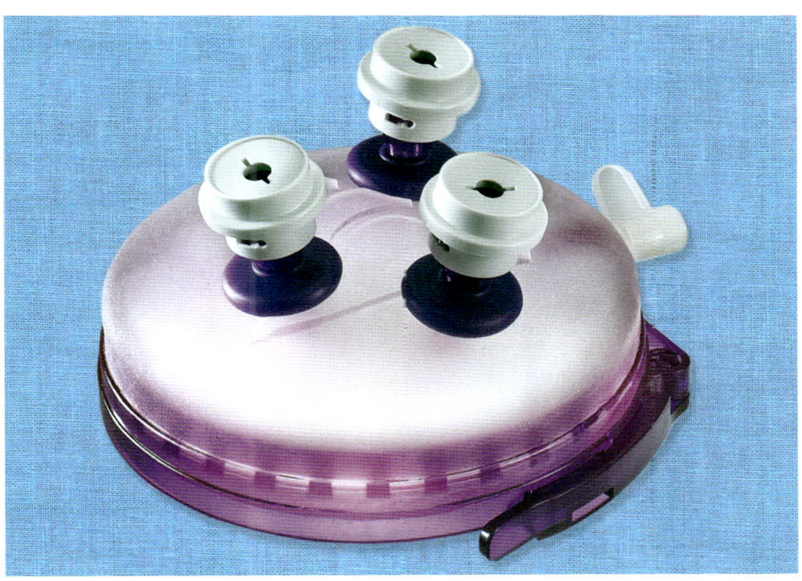

Fig. 4: GelSeal cap with self-retaining ports.

Self-retaining Ports

- Float above incision, e.g. above abdominal wall to maximize internal working diameter.
- Accommodates both 5 mm and 10 mm instrumentation.
- Low profile design offers freedom of movement.

Deployment

Before making an incision, the GelPort is prepared by placing transparent, adhesive film over the central gel opening. A 2–3-cm curvilinear subumbilical skin incision is made and the fascia is then identified. The fascia is elevated, a 2-cm transverse or vertical incision is made and the peritoneal cavity is entered. The GelPort's flexible intra-abdominal ring is tagged with a suture before collapsing it and then the ring is inserted into the abdominal cavity. The GelPort cap is attached to the extraperitoneal ring without rolling the ring and "tightening" it to the abdominal wall. A 5 or 10 mm laparoscopic trocar is inserted through the GelPort and under direct observation and the abdomen is insufflated with CO_2. Because the extraperitoneal GelPort ring is not "rolled" tightly against the abdominal wall, a CO_2-filled space (e.g. pseudoabdomen) is produced. The pseudoabdomen provides for greater versatility, enhancing mobility, flexibility, and surgical access. The trocars are inserted through the gel, but not into the abdominal cavity.[4]

The *advantages* of the GelPort system for LESS surgery include:

- The versatility of the GelSeal cap enables placement of instruments of different shapes and sizes, the GelSeal cap creates a pseudoabdomen that floats above the fascial incision.[3]
- The 10 cm diameter of the outer ring reduces instrument crowding.
- Fader and Escobar et al.[5] used the GelPort system for robotic-assisted LESS surgery in gynecology and reported that the larger outside dimension of the GelSeal cap reduces crowding of the robotic arms. A retrospective review of the GelPort system in pelvic surgery concluded that this system is favorable for single-port surgery, because the device provides circumferential access and retraction.[4]
- The major advantage is that it provides a "flexible fulcrum" for the manipulation of the laparoscope and instruments, even without trocars. When used without trocars, extracorporeal instrument crowding is minimized.[2]

One *disadvantage* of the GelPort system is the large slit in the GelSeal, which can sometimes leak gas. The addition of the GelSeal cap in the GelPoint platform has alleviated this problem. Moreover, in obese patients, use of the GelPort system can be complicated given the increased distance between the skin and the fascia.[1] These have been overcome in GelPoint by using 10 cm outer ring, which reduces instrument crowding and provides circumferential access and retraction.[4]

SILS PORT

The SILS port (Covidien Inc, Norwalk, cT, USA)[1,3] **(Figs. 5A to C)** is a single use multiple instrument access device for single-port laparoscopic surgery made with an elastic polymer in a dumbbell shape. The port fits a 2.5-cm incision and allows for three custom-made trocars of up to 12 mm in size with one three-way stopcock for the purpose of insufflation or smoke evacuation. The elastic material allows the port to conform to the shape of the abdominal wall to maintain pneumoperitoneum as well as access of multiple cannulas of different sizes.

The SILS™ port is comprised of the following components:

- 5 mm and 5 mm to 12 mm cannulae.
- 5 mm and 12 mm blunt-tipped obturators.
- Multiple instrument access port.
- Insufflation/smoke evacuation tubing and stopcock.

Deployment: A 2-cm skin incision is made in the umbilicus by open method to facilitate the insertion of the SILS Port. Blunt dissection through the fascia and peritoneum by standard Hasson technique is recommended. Manipulation of the access port into the incision may be carried out digitally, or with the help of an artery forceps applied obliquely over the SILS port. Continuous rotation and pushing of the obturator/cannula assembly when inserting will ensure a smooth entry into the access port into the abdominal cavity (refer Chapter 80 **Figs. 4A to N**).

Advantages

- The port is durable and withstands significant manipulation.
- Easy placement.

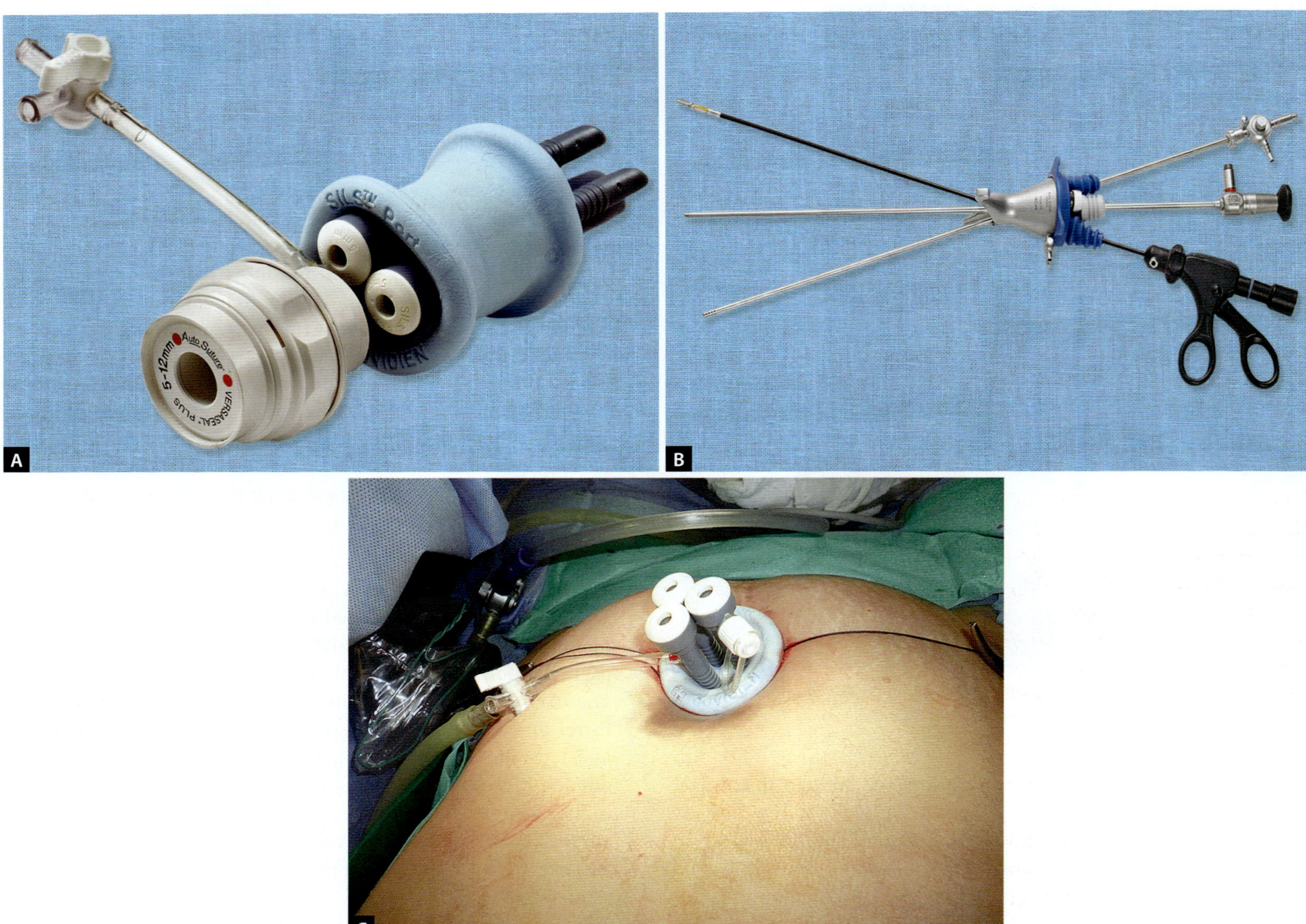

Figs. 5A to C: SILS port. (A) 5 mm and 12 mm cannulas though access port; (B) Multiple instrument access port with instruments; (C) SILS port placed through the umbilicus for hysterectomy procedure.

- Availability of the dedicated SILS kit with multiple compatible instruments and open entry into the peritoneal cavity.
- The removable caps on the cannulas make small specimen retrieval easier.
- Individual ports use a traditional laparoscopic seal, which helps to minimize gas leak.

Drawbacks

- It is a single use access device and adds to the cost of the surgical procedure.
- The SILS port has only one length and therefore has a limited range of abdominal wall thickness that it will accommodate.
- Removal and reinsertion is challenging and has a steeper learning curve than some of the other port choices.
- Larger specimen retrieval requires removal of the entire access port.

SSL PORT[1,3]

The *SSL access system (Ethicon Endo-surgery, Inc, Cincinnati, OH, USA)* is a newly developed low-profile access system with detachable seal cap with separate wound retractors.

Seal cap assembly containing two 5 mm ports and one 15 mm port is attached to the flexible access retractor.

The seal cap rotates 360° independent of the access retractor.

Component Parts

The device consists of a retractor and a seal cap. The two sizes of the retractors enable proper placement, depending on the depth of abdominal wall:

- The smaller 2 cm retractor for walls up to 4 cm deep.
- The larger 4 cm retractor for abdominal walls up to 7 cm deep.

Deployment

A single 1.5–3.5 cm incision is required for insertion of this port. An insertion tool is provided to facilitate placement of fixed length retractors.

Advantages

- Unique to the device is the 360° rotation of the seal cap independent of the retractor to change orientation intraoperatively without losing pneumoperitoneum, which enables quick reorientation of instruments during procedures and reduces the need for instrument exchanges.
- The removable cap allows for easier retrieval of specimen without removing the wound retractor while the rigid body provides a fulcrum for instrumentation.

TRANSENTERIX SPIDER

TransEnterix's Inc (TransEnterix, Durham, NC) approach in single-port surgery is a flexible catheter technology borrowed or adapted from interventional medicine. This approach "hybrid cross-platform technology" promises to make this system unique both in clinical reach and procedural capability.[6] This device was developed by a cardiologist who transferred the technology of directable catheters from endovascular procedures to a port with directable channels.

Component Parts

It houses two rigid and two flexible ports. The rigid ports are for the insertion of rigid laparoscopic instruments and transenteric flexible catheter-based instruments are inserted through the flexible ports for the purpose of grasping, dissecting, ligating or coagulating tissue. The flexible instruments provide high level of dexterity.

WOUND RETRACTOR AND GLOVE

This is an inexpensive homemade port. It has two parts **(Fig. 6)**:

1. *Wound retractor (Alexis; Applied Medical, Rancho Santa Margarita, CA):* The wound retractor is composed of a distal ring, a proximal ring and a cylindrical connecting sleeve.
2. *Surgical glove:* Trocar sheaths are inserted into three fingers of the glove. Then glove is draped around the rim of the wound retractor.

Deployment

A 2-cm incision is created in the umbilicus with the open Hasson technique. A small wound retractor is inserted into the wound opening transumbilically. Once it is fixed in the umbilical opening, it retracts the wound edges laterally. This makes a small vertical incision a wider and rounder opening. The glove with trocar sheaths is draped around the rim of the wound retractor and insufflation is done **(Figs. 7A to E)**.

Advantages[7,8]

- Elastic nature of the glove enables it to have a good purchase on the ring and potentially achieves an airtight seal.
- Multiple fingers of the glove functions as multiple channels for instruments.
- Elastic nature of glove allows greater manipulation of instruments.
- Specimen extraction can be done easily through the wound retractor without much difficulty as it retracts and stretches the incision. The glove can be easily detached from the wound retractor to extract the tissue.

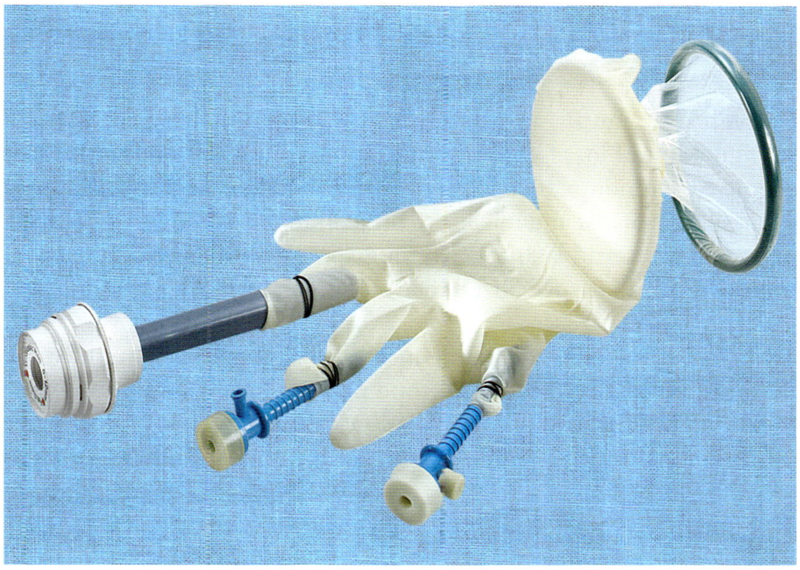

Fig. 6: Alexis wound retractor with the glove inserted over the rim of the retractor. Fingers of the glove function as multiple channels for instruments.

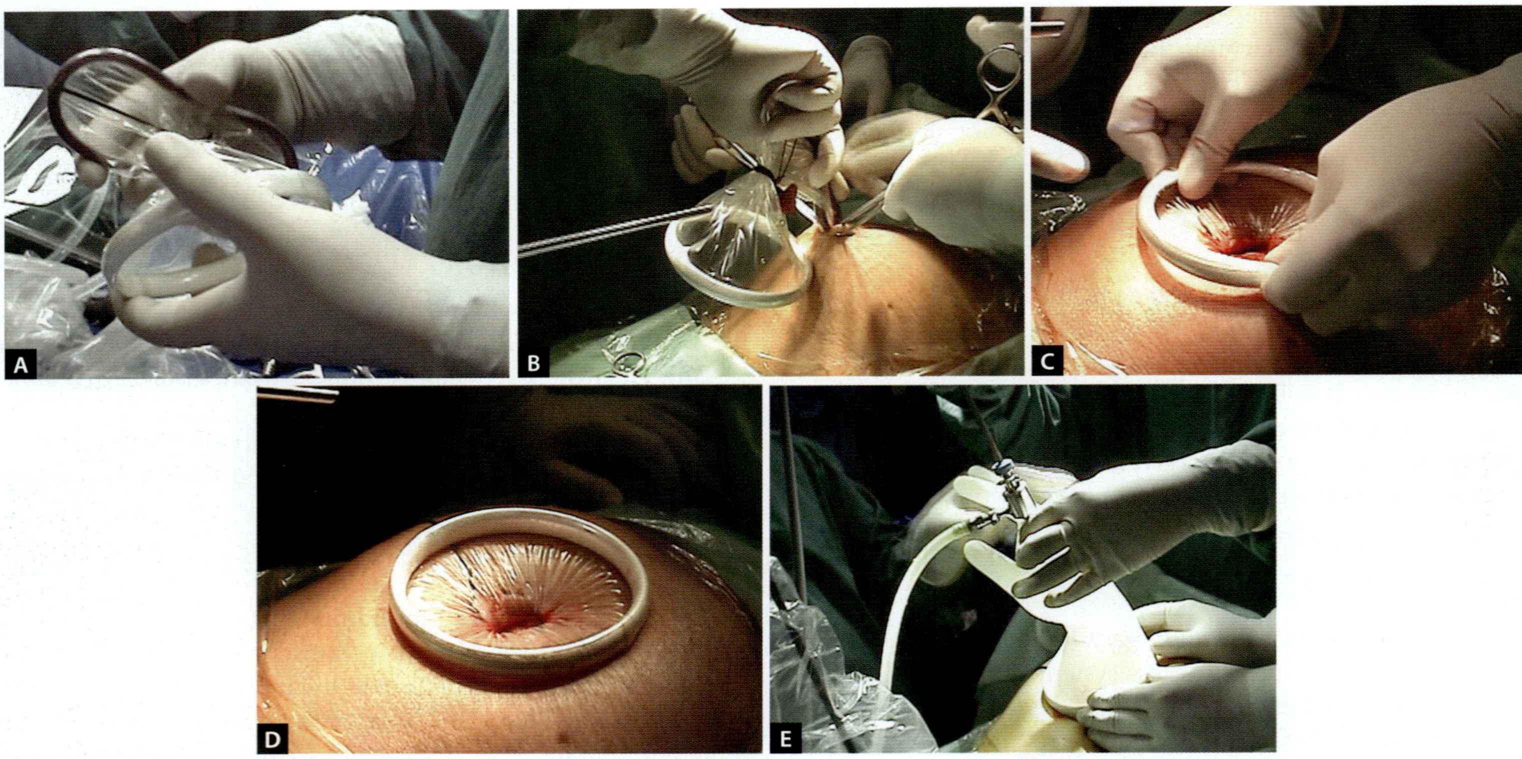

Figs. 7A to E: Placement of Alexis wound retractor into the peritoneal cavity through an umbilical incision. A glove forms airtight seal with the fingers of the glove accommodating the trocars.

- It may decrease port-site infection, bleeding and subcutaneous emphysema because of the tamponade effect of the wound retractor. Many studies in LESS have demonstrated the feasibility of this access port.[7-9]
- Relatively cheap as compared to commercial devices.

Disadvantages[1]

- *Cumbersome setup:* Though the glove forms an airtight seal with the wound retractor there is a potential loss of pneumoperitoneum with glove leak.
- Excessive manipulation at the port site may lead to slippage of glove leading to loss of pneumoperitoneum.

INSTRUMENTS

Conventional multiport laparoscopy utilizes the principle of triangulation of forces from two different points. If standard laparoscopic instruments are inserted from the single-port, the effect of triangulation is lost and it leads to difficult manipulation and collision of instruments and reduced working space for the surgeon. Hence, there is a need for specialized instruments to improve ergonomics of LESS procedure.

Use of curved or articulating instruments can partially reduce the inherent problems of LESS. Despite parallel insertion of the instruments, an internal type of triangulation is created.[3] This approximates the tips of instruments taking handles away from each other.

USE OF VARIOUS INSTRUMENTS IN LESS

Standard (Straight) Laparoscopic Instruments

All conventional laparoscopic instruments can be used for LESS surgery. Use of the standard instruments provides reasonable exposure and does not add extra cost to the surgery. It also reduces the extended time associated with the learning curve with new instruments. As new techniques develop, their versatility is important.[10] The standard instruments, however may be appropriate only for simple procedures; complex surgeries will require specialized instrumentation. Long length straight instruments are better suited to LESS **(Figs. 8 to 10)**.

Use of 1.9 mm Needle Instruments

Needle instruments have been used to retract gallbladder in LESS cholecystectomy. But use in LESS is controversial. To increase the surgeon's confidence and thereby patient safety, LESCAR endorses the discretionary adjunctive use of 1.9 mm needle instruments during LESS surgery. These 1.9 mm instruments have three potential advantages due to facilitation of instrument triangulation, tissue retraction and intracorporeal suturing and knot tying along the lines of standard multiport laparoscopy (refer Chapter 86, **Figs. 2A and B**).

- Enhanced patient safety.
- Increased intraoperative dexterity.
- An expanded clinical repertoire of LESS surgery with immediate effect.

But, to be accepted in LESS reliability, tensile strength, design and variety need to be improved.[11]

Curved Instruments (Figs. 11 to 13)

- The "S-PORTAL" instruments (KARL STORZ and Co Tuttlingen, Germany) has four curves, which results in the instrument tip and the handle coming in the same line and this gives the surgeon the feeling of using virtual trocars with triangulation without crossing hands. Apart from this, S-PORTAL® has curved instruments specifically aims at solving the problems of triangulation and ergonomics in LESS surgery.[12]

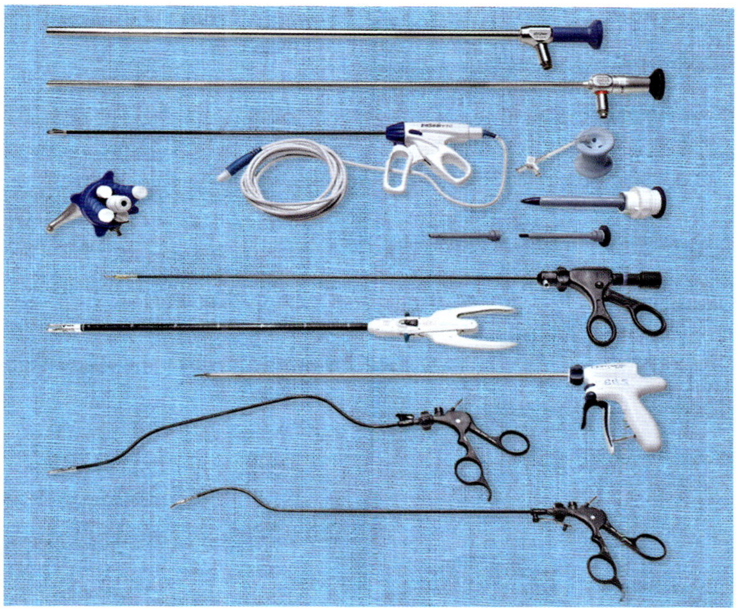

Fig. 8: Various access ports and instruments used in LESS.

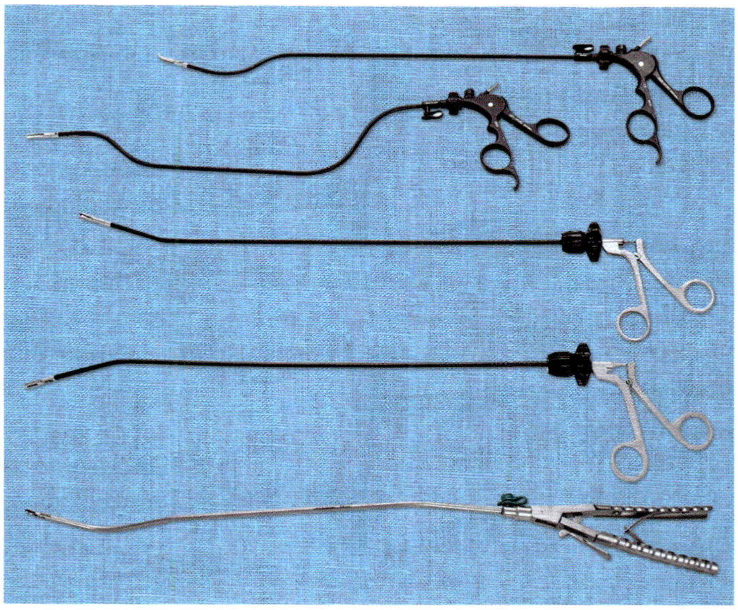

Fig. 11: Curved instruments for LESS.

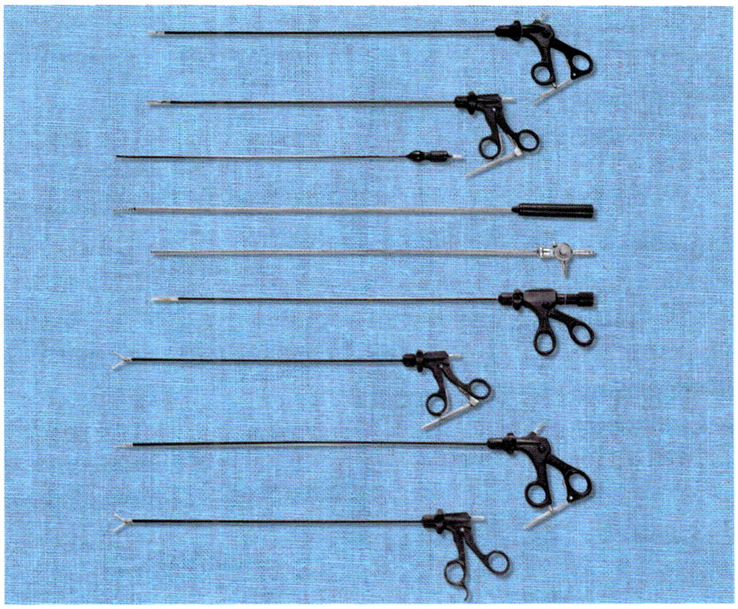

Fig. 9: Straight instruments used in LESS.

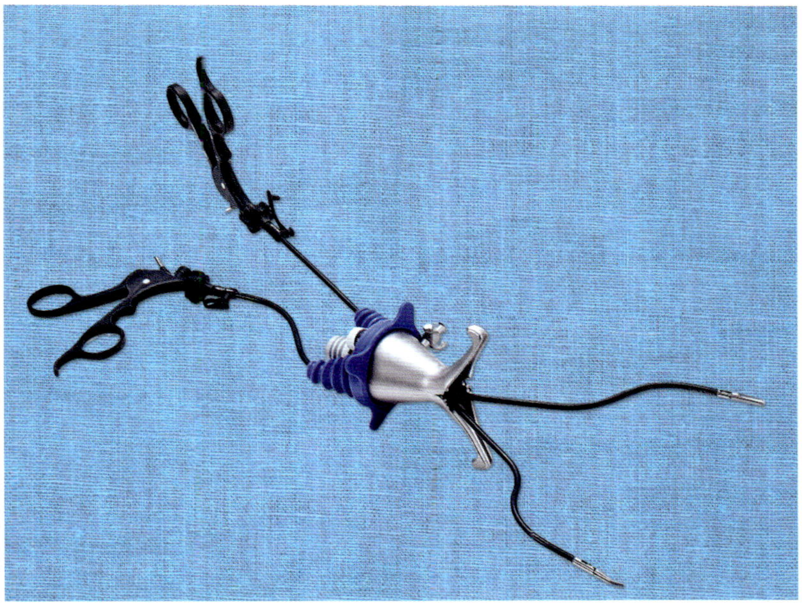

Fig. 12: Triangulation effect due to two curved instruments through access port (X-cone).

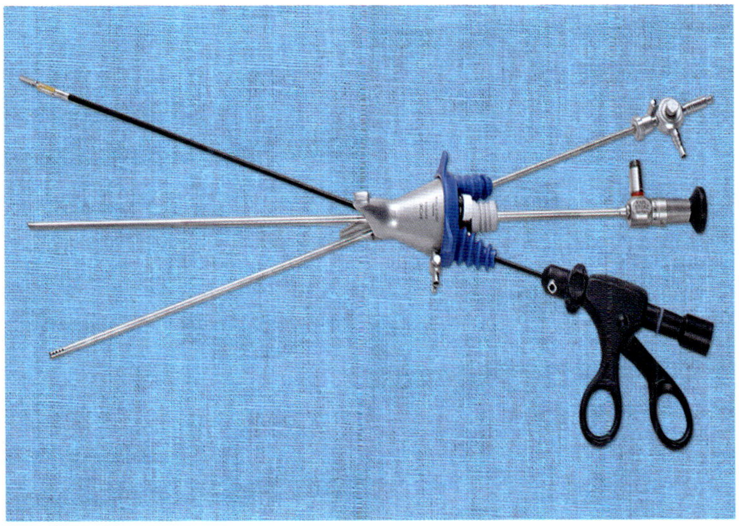

Fig. 10: Optics (5 mm long scope) and instruments through single-access port.

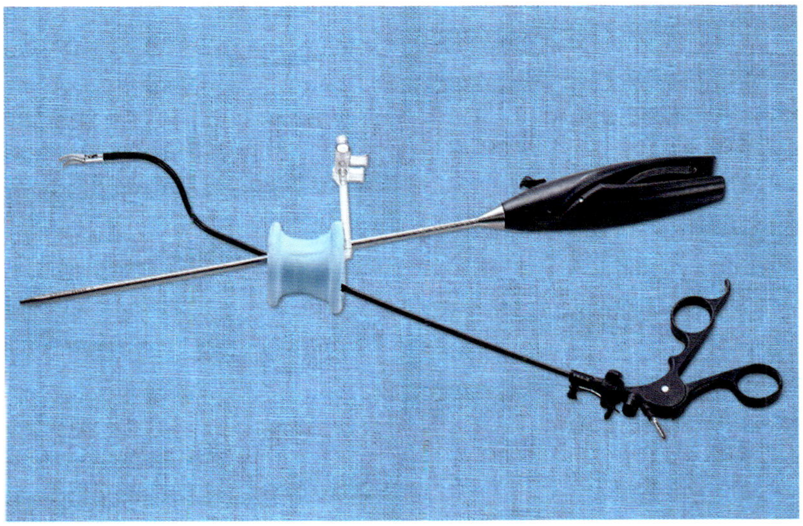

Fig. 13: Use of one straight needle holder and curved grasper facilitates suturing.

- Olympus (Orangeburg, NY, USA) offers HiQ™ LS curved 5 mm H hand instruments. These are reusable rigid instruments with angulated distal and proximal ends and rotator action.[12]
- Surgiquest™ (Orange, CT, USA) has a range of curved instruments that are designed specifically for LESS surgery.[12]

In an extensively ergonomic study performed by Manukyan and colleagues, the curved instrument was significantly more efficient with respect to economy of motions and quality of performance in the experimental setup of laparoscopic rectosigmoid resection.[13] Stolzenberg et al. concluded that prebent instruments were less time consuming and had a better maneuverability in comparison to flexible instruments in LESS surgery.[14]

Wristed Instruments (Articulated)

Many articulated instruments are available in the market, which claim to offer added advantages of maneuverability at the tip.

RealHand Instruments[1,15]

RealHand high-dexterity instruments (Novare Surgical Systems, Inc., Cupertino, California) are designed to mirror the surgeon's hand direction with the added benefit of tactile feedback. They are 5 mm instruments in which the handle is connected to the tip by several cables, this enables 360° articulation that mimics the movement of the surgeon's hand and therefore, provides 7° of freedom of movement.

- A major advantage of these instruments is the dexterity they allow the surgeon, enabling him or her to overcome limited triangulation. Currently, 11 different RealHand instrument tips are available including the ThermaSeal tip, which uses thermal energy to denature protein structures and create high-integrity seals and clean divisions. Standard graspers, scissors and needle holders with added range of movement are also available.
- The potential disadvantages of these instruments include a long learning curve and relatively high cost.

The initial experience in using these instruments in gynecology was reported by Rettenmaier et al. in the setting of traditional three-point laparoscopy.[16]

Autonomy Laparo-Angle Instruments[1,15]

Like the RealHand instruments, Autonomy Laparo-Angle instruments (Cambridge Endoscopic Devices, Inc., Framingham, Massachusetts) provide a 360° articulating head that mimics the surgeon's movements. Unlike the RealHand instruments, the Autonomy Laparo-Angle instruments include a mechanism to rotate the instrument head after locking at any angle and a finger socket to open and close the distal jaws. There is a proximal bending section that translates the movements of the surgeon's wrist to the tip of the instrument. There is also an "angle" locking mechanism to lock the distal tip at any angle to facilitate a better working angle on the outside.

SILS Kit with Roticulator Instruments[1]

The SILS kit for LESS surgery (Covidien) is made to accompany the SILS port. The SILS kit includes roticulator instruments with distal ends with limited range of movement of 0–80°. As the distal end is pushed out from its outer sheath, the angle of the extended bent portion increases.

The handle also enables the surgeon to rotate the distal instrument 360°, similar to what is possible with traditional laparoscopic instruments. The instrument tips include dissectors, scissors and graspers. Several of the roticulator instruments have monopolar cautery attachments. *The major advantages* of these instruments include their availability as an SILS kit, which minimizes compatibility issues and these instruments are less costly than RealHand or Laparo-Angle instruments.

The disadvantages include limited movement of the instrument tip, which does not allow translation of the surgeons' hand movements, as is possible with RealHand or Laparo-Angle instruments.

Roticulating instruments: Intracorporeal suturing during SILS will be greatly facilitated with the introduction of 5 mm handheld surgical manipulators with 6° of freedom. These enable graded flexion of the distal segment of the instrument and through the incorporation of an internal wrist enabling rotation of the tip and jaws, greatly facilitate both continuous and interrupted suturing.[17]

Dutta published the first cases of LESS splenectomies and LESS cholecystectomies performed in the pediatric age group using RealHand® HD instruments (Novare Surgical Systems) and a thermal ligation device (Thermaseal®; Novare Surgical Systems, Cupertino, CA, USA).[18]

A significant learning curve was demonstrated when the first-generation novel articulating needle driver (Cambridge Endo, Framingham, MA, USA) was compared with a conventional laparoscopic needle driver (KARL STORZ and Co. KG) by evaluating the completion of standardized laparoscopic suturing task by novices. This may be secondary due to the complexity of physical maneuvers required for their use.[19]

Instruments for Hemostasis (Fig. 14)

LigaSure™ tissue fusion technology, including LigaSure Advance™ and Valleylab™ mode (Covidien Norwalk, CT, USA), are integral part and can become an ideal hemostatic tool for MISS surgery. Sure and rapid means of establishing hemostasis with thermal energy delivery systems, staples, clips and sutures equivalent in efficiency to that of standard multiport laparoscopy are essential. Ultrasonic energy is another option for hemostasis and devices like Harmonic™ (Ethicon Endo-Surgery Inc., Cincinnati, OH, USA), AutoSonix™ (Autosuture; CovidienNorwalk, CT, USA), and SonosurgX™ (Olympus, Hamburg, Germany) have been well established in conventional laparoscopy. These instruments are routinely used in LESS surgery.[12] The longer version of Harmonic and Enseal (Ethicon Endo-Surgery) is more suitable for LESS.

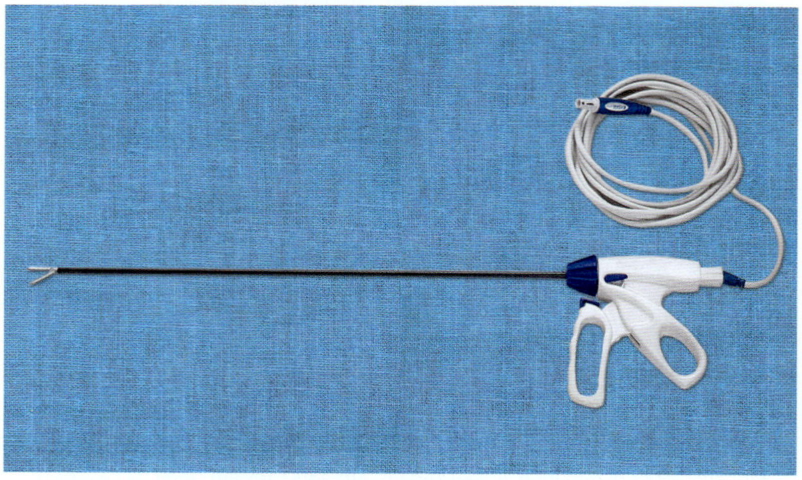

Fig. 14: Longer version of Enseal (Ethicon Endo-Surgery Inc., Cincinnati, OH, USA).

KEY POINTS

Use of instruments in LESS:

- Use of long instruments reduces crowding in LESS surgeries
- Use of combination of curved and straight instruments to create triangulation internally
- Use of vessel sealing devices for hemostasis
- Avoid lateral movements. They are difficult due to reduced operating space and can lead to collisions. The movements in LESS are more in upward-downward direction
- Keep the instruments in different horizontal planes above the level of the patient externally. It keeps the instrument handles away and prevents collisions.[3]

FUTURE TRENDS: "SMART INSTRUMENTS"

A prototype of modular surgical instrument with artificial intelligence was made, which needs further refinement and validation.[20]

There have been reports regarding the laparoscopic use of the Radius® surgical system (Tuebingen Scientific, Tübingen, Germany), mechanical manipulators (MM) with 6° of freedom, with ergonomic hand-arm movements and interchangeable endo-effectors.[21,22] Such instruments represent an intermediate stage in the field of minimally invasive surgery between traditional laparoscopic and electromechanic robotical systems. These may change the face of laparoscopic surgery in times to come.

REFERENCES

1. Uppal S, Frumovitz M, Escobar P, et al Laparoendoscopic single-site surgery in gynecology: review of literature and available technology. J Minim Invasive Gynecol. 2010;18:12-23.
2. Tsai AY, Selzer DJ. Single-port laparoscopic surgery. Adv. Surg. 2010;44:1-27.
3. Sobolewski C, Yeung PP Jr, Hart S. Laparoendoscopic single-site surgery in gynecology. Obstet Gynecol Clin North Am. 2011;38(4):741-55.
4. Rettenmaier MA, Abaid LN, Erwin MR, et al. A retrospective review of the GelPort system in single-port access pelvic surgery. J Minim Invasive Gynecol. 2009;16:743-7.
5. Escobar PF, Fader AN, Paraiso MF, et al. Robotic assisted laparoendoscopic single-site surgery in gynecology: initial report and technique. J Minim Invasive Gynecol. 2009;16:589-91.
6. Escobar PF, Starks D, Fader AN, et al. Laparoendoscopic single-site and natural orifice surgery in gynecology. Fertil Steril. 2010;94:2497-502.
7. Kim TJ, Lee YY, Kim MJ, et al. Single port access laparoscopic adnexal surgery. J Minim Invasive Gynecol. 2009;16:612-5.
8. Kim YW, Park BJ, Ro DY, et al. Single-port laparoscopic myomectomy using a new single-port transumbilical morcellation system: initial clinical study. J Minim Invasive Gynecol. 2010;17:587-92.
9. Kim YB, Lee JR, Moon JM, et al. Clinical application of single-port laparoscopic surgery for various indications. J Minim Invasive Gynecol. 2010;17: S128-S151.
10. Podolsky ER, Curcillo PG 2nd. Single port access (SPA) surgery—a 24-month experience. J Gastrointest Surg. 2010;14:759-67.
11. Gill IS, Advincula AP, Aron M, et al. Consensus statement of the consortium for laparoendoscopic single-site surgery. Surg Endosc. 2010;24:762-8.
12. Dhumane PW, Diana M, Leroy J, et al. Minimally invasive single-site surgery for the digestive system: a technological review. J Minim Access Surg. 2011;7(1):40-51.
13. Manukyan GA, Waseda M, Inaki N, et al. Ergonomics with the use of curved versus straight laparoscopic graspers during rectosigmoid resection: results of a multiprofile comparative study. Surg Endosc. 2007;21:1079-89.
14. Stolzenburg JU, Kallidonis P, Oh MA et al. Comparative assessment of laparoscopic single-site surgery instruments to conventional laparoscopic in laboratory setting. J Endourol. 2010;24:239-45.
15. McDonald ER, Brownlee E, Ahmed I. New tools for a new job—single-port laparoscopic surgery equipment. Med Equip Insights. 2009:2:1-7.
16. Rettenmaier MA, Lopez K, Graham CL, et al. RealHand high dexterity instruments for the treatment of stage I uterine malignancy. JSLS. 2009; 13:27-31.
17. Cuschieri A. Single-incision laparoscopic surgery. J Minim Access Surg. 2011;7(1):3-5.
18. Dutta S. Early experience with single-incision laparoscopic surgery: eliminating the scar from abdominal operations. J Pediatr Surg. 2009;44: 1741-5.
19. Tuncel A, Lucas S, Bensalah K, et al. A randomized comparison of conventional vs articulating laparoscopic needle-drivers for performing standardized suturing tasks by laparoscopy-naive subjects. BJU Int. 2008; 101:727-30.
20. Miller DJ, Nelson CA, Oleynikov D. Shortened OR time and decreased patient risk through use of a modular surgical instrument with artificial intelligence. Surg Endosc. 2009;23:1099-105.
21. Coscarella G, Di Lorenzo N, Gacek I. The radius surgical system: preliminary experience with new laparoscopic device. Minim Invasive Ther Allied Technol. 2005;14:332-3.
22. Di Lorenzo N, Camperchioli I, Gaspari AL. Radius surgical system and conventional laparoscopic instruments in abdominal surgery: application, learning curve and ergonomy. Surg Oncol. 2007;16:S69-72.

CHAPTER

82

LESS Concomitant Procedures

B Ramesh, Pooja Sharma, Isha Rani

INTRODUCTION

Laparoendoscopic single-site (LESS) surgery is widely getting accepted in various surgical modalities like general surgery, urology, and gynecology. LESS provides the surgeon the opportunity to perform more complex surgical procedures through a single entry site. Single-port surgery has various advantages of improved cosmesis, LESS pain and reduction of other port site complications.[1-5] Feasibility of LESS in various gynecologic procedures like hysterectomy, myomectomy and adnexal procedures like ovarian cystectomy and management of ectopic pregnancy has also been reported.[6-11] The universal nature of umbilicus as the single laparoscopic port among various surgical specialties enables the performance of concomitant surgeries via this single incision. This is because the umbilicus is a standard site for initial port placement used to perform multiple general surgery, urologic, and gynecologic procedures **(Figs. 1A and B)**.[12]

Various gynecological and surgical procedures can be combined in LESS surgeries. The commonly performed surgical procedures like cholecystectomy and appendectomy can be performed with gynecologic procedures like hysterectomy and adnexal surgery. The advantages of concurrent procedures are single hospitalization, LESS anesthesia exposure, LESS morbidity and reduced operative time as compared to two operative procedures done separately.[13] If concomitant surgeries are performed by traditional multiport laparoscopy, it would involve separate multiple trocar entries for gynecologic and surgical procedures. More the skin incisions, more the chances of bleeding, pain, wound infection, hematoma, trocar-site hernia, and adhesion formation. These problems could be minimized using access through the single-port. Recent advances have further minimized morbidity and improved cosmesis in laparoscopic surgery. This advantage is more pronounced in obese individuals who are prone to wound related complications. In procedures like cholecystectomy with hysterectomy, tissue retrieval becomes easier through the colpotomy wound. The feasibility of single-port surgery in cholecystectomy has been described.[14,15] Various gynecologic procedures like tubal ligation, salpingectomy, removal of adnexal tumors, hysterectomy and pelvic and para-aortic node dissection have been performed by single-port laparoscopy.[8,16] If traditional multiport laparoscopy is used for concomitant procedures, the number of ports will increase considerably increasing risk of port complications since the same port sites cannot be used for gynecologic and surgical procedures. LESS can be performed for concomitant procedures overcoming these disadvantages. Before performing concomitant LESS procedures, the patients are informed about the operative strategy of having a single incision in the abdomen with a possibility of several more incisions or a conversion to an open technique.

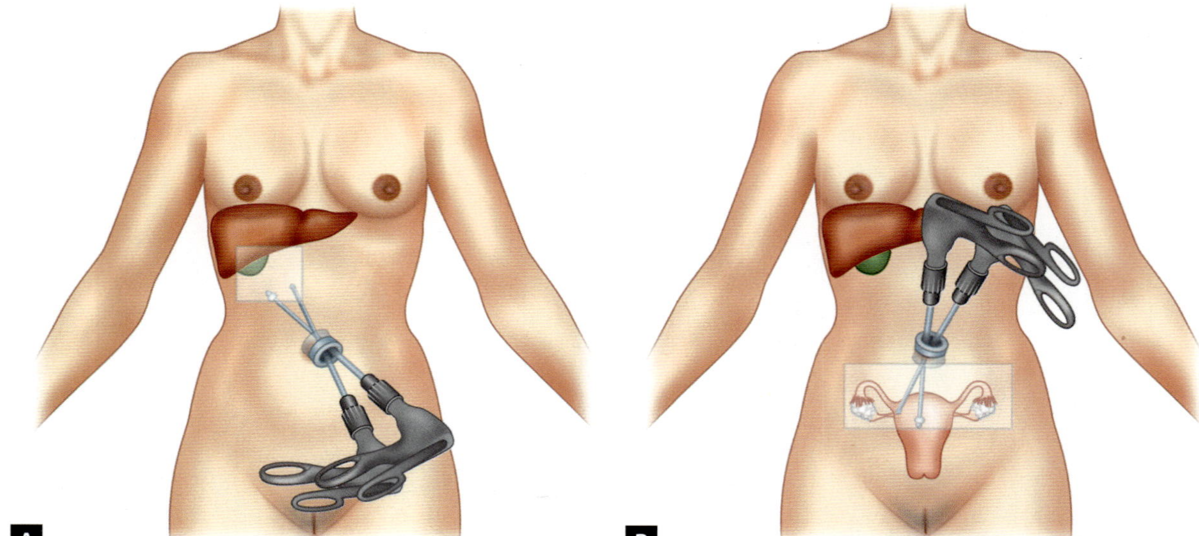

A B

Figs. 1A and B: Umbilicus can be used as approach for both upper abdomen and pelvic procedures.

Concomitant gynecological and surgical procedures:

- Total laparoscopic hysterectomy with cholecystectomy/appendectomy
- Adnexal procedures with appendectomy/cholecystectomy
- Pelvic adhesiolysis with appendectomy/cholecystectomy
- Laparoscopic mesh hernia repair with gynecologic procedures
- Operative laparoscopy for endometriosis with surgical procedures
- Open umbilical hernia repair with LESS procedure.

LIMITATIONS

The performance of concomitant procedures in LESS is limited by extensive pathology. For example, in combined hysterectomy and cholecystectomy, the performance of LESS is limited by the size of the uterus. Any extensive pathology like extensive adhesions and extensive endometriosis would limit the successful performance of single-port surgery. Also, the performance of concurrent LESS procedures will require both laparoscopic surgeon and gynecologic endoscopist skilled in single-port surgery.

REVIEW OF LITERATURE

The first case of LESS concomitant hysterectomy and cholecystectomy was described by Hart et al. and its feasibility demonstrated. The patient was a parous lady with menorrhagia and dysmenorrhea with fibroid uterus and concurrent cholecystitis with cholelithiasis. A concurrent LESS cholecystectomy and hysterectomy was performed. The procedure was completed in 3 hours without any intraoperative or postoperative complications.[12] Inclusion criteria for cholecystectomy would be patients in overall good health without complex biliary disease (including choledocolithiasis) or extensive previous abdominal surgery. Criteria for hysterectomy will exclude very large uteri and those with extensive adhesions or endometriosis. Both general laparoscopic surgeon and gynecologic laparoscopic surgeon skilled in LESS are essential for the procedure. Ultimately the difficulty of procedure that can be performed will depend on skill and ability of the surgeon(s).

The age group of women undergoing hysterectomy for menorrhagia and cholelithiasis is similar. The exact incidence of women requiring concurrent cholecystectomy and hysterectomy is unknown. Patsner et al.[17] found that of 950 major abdominal operations performed over 66 months because of known or suspected gynecologic malignant lesions, 35 patients (3.6%) also underwent concomitant cholecystectomy because of cholelithiasis. Wadhwa et al.[13] reported performing 145 combined endoscopic surgical procedures from January 1999 to December 2002, of which seven were combined laparoscopic cholecystectomy and open hysterectomy procedures. Malfetano et al.[18] described performance of 46 incidental cholecystectomy procedures during surgery for gynecologic malignant lesions from October 1985 to September 1989. Twenty-three patients (50%) had a preoperative diagnosis of cholelithiasis and in the remaining 23 patients, substantial gallbladder disease was diagnosed intraoperatively.

To perform conventional laparoscopic cholecystectomy, general surgeons place the primary trocar through the umbilicus and two 5-mm trocars in a right and left subcostal position and one 10-mm trocar in the epigastrium, respectively, to enable retraction of the gallbladder, preparation of the Calot triangle and dissection of the cystic duct and artery. In contrast, two 5-mm accessory ports are inserted lateral to the inferior epigastric vessels bilaterally and one 5- or 10-mm port suprapubically by the gynecologic endoscopist. It signifies that for a concomitant procedure to be performed, an increased number of ports (up to 6) will be required for the successful completion of the surgery **(Figs. 2 to 4)**. It is evident than, if both the surgeries can be performed through a single incision in the umbilicus, it will be of great benefit to the patient. Since a large number of cholecystectomies and hysterectomies are being performed annually, and the paradigm shift toward minimally invasive approach, concomitant LESS procedures will become order of the day.

Daniela Surico et al.[19] reported a case of single-port simultaneous ovarian cystectomy and cholecystectomy which was successfully completed without the need of extraumbilical skin incision or conversion to standard laparoscopy. Histologic evaluation confirmed the presence of cholelithiasis and an ovarian endometrioid cyst. Operative time was 132 minutes, estimated blood loss was 35 mL and no intraoperative complications occurred. Postoperative recovery was uneventful and patient was discharged 24 hours after surgery. At 1 month follow-up excellent cosmesis was obtained and patient was satisfied with the end result. In 2009, O'Hanlan[6] reported the first two cases of patients who underwent LESS total laparoscopic hysterectomy, bilateral salpingo-oophorectomy and concomitant appendectomy.

Another important possibility is combination of open umbilical hernia repair and LESS procedure. We performed this case of umbilical hernia repair with LESS hysterectomy. The patient presented with complaints of hernia at the umbilicus with fibroid induced menorrhagia. Skin incision was given. Hernial sac was dissected and contents of the sac were reduced. The opening was then utilized to place the single-incision laparoscopic surgery (SILS) Covidien port and then LESS hysterectomy was carried out **(Figs. 5A to J)**. After completion of the hysterectomy, the hernial repair was carried out. Therefore, presence of small umbilical hernia is not an absolute contraindication to LESS. In fact, it may be the preferred route of surgery in these types of cases.

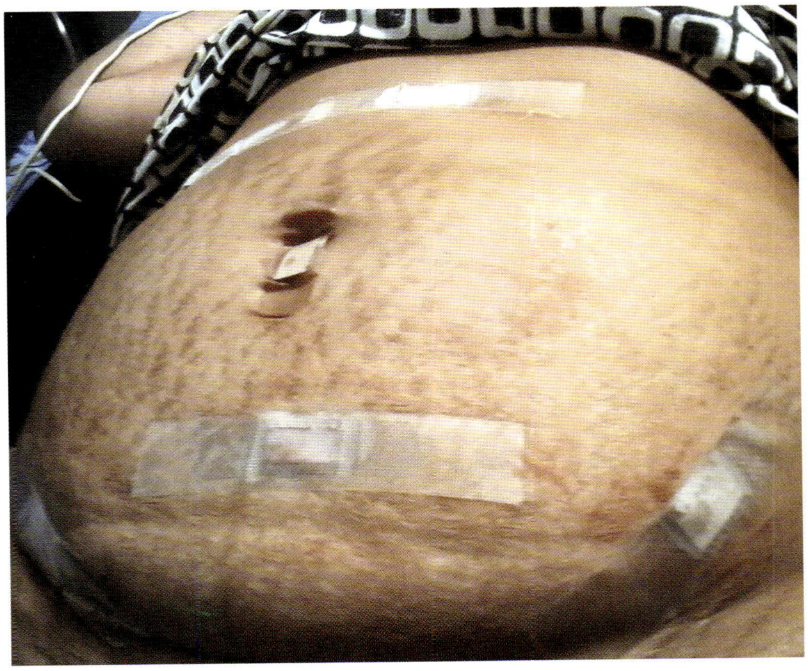

Fig. 2A: Abdominal incisions in a patient who underwent combined cholecystectomy and hysterectomy by multiport laparoscopy. First postoperative day.

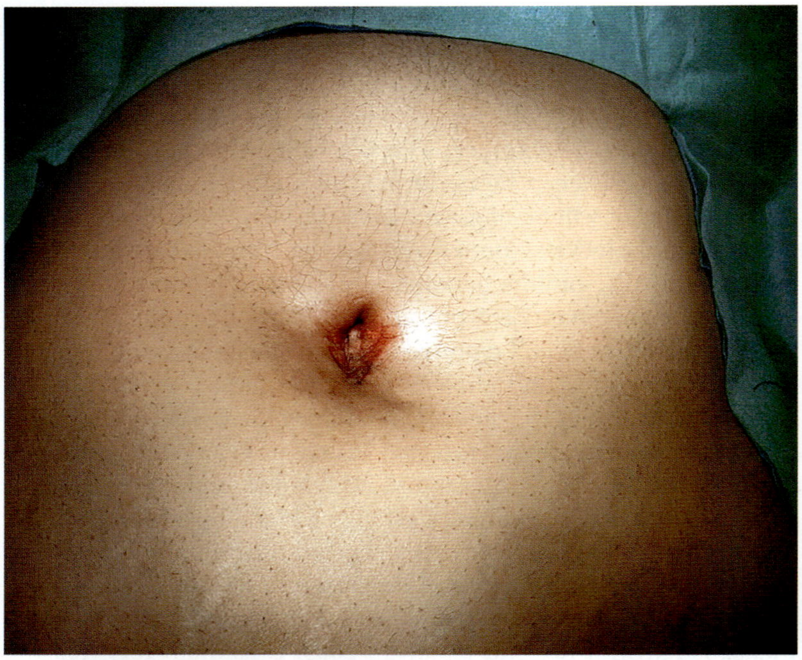

Fig. 2B: Abdominal wound of a patient after single-incision laparoscopic surgery. Immediate postoperative picture.

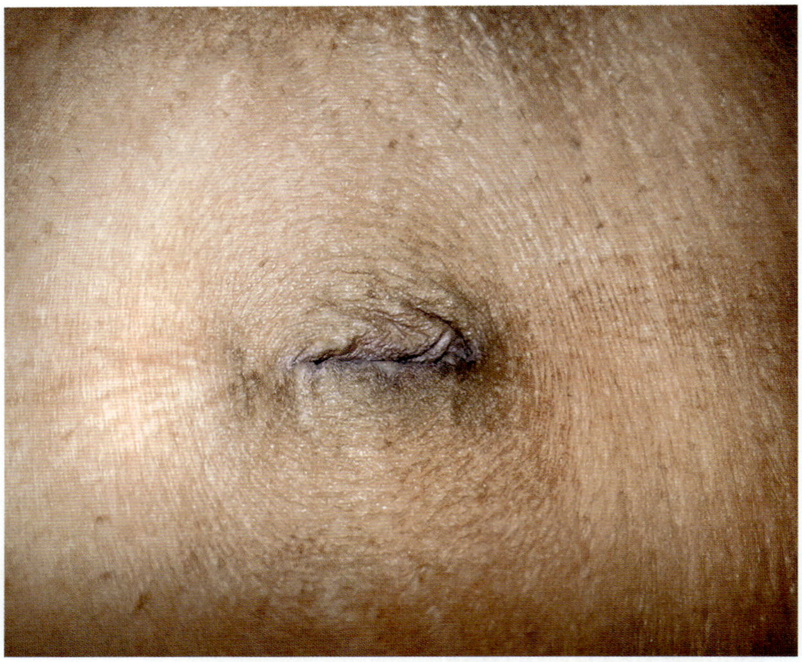

Fig. 2C: Follow-up picture of laparoendoscopic single-site (LESS) scar in a patient who underwent LESS combined cholecystectomy and hysterectomy (1½ years postsurgery).

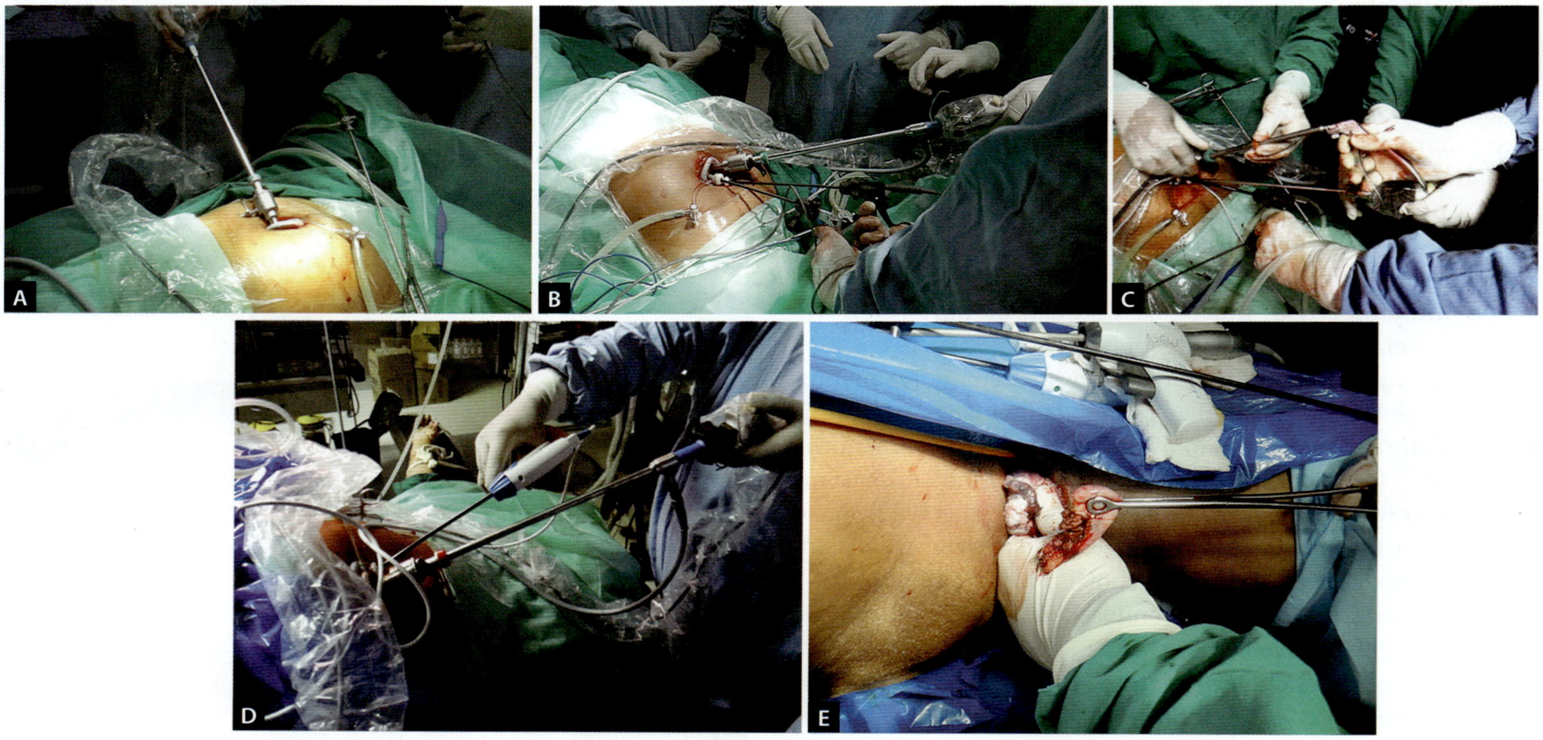

Figs. 3A to E: Concurrent laparoendoscopic single-site (LESS) cholecystectomy and hysterectomy: External view. (A) Visualization of the gallbladder; (B) Dissection of the gallbladder. Note the head up position during cholecystectomy; (C) Vascular clips being applied; (D) Hysterectomy being performed in the same patient. The position has been changed to Trendelenburg or head low position. Enseal (vessel sealing device) is being used to coagulate uterine vessels; (E) Specimen retrieval. Gallbladder and uterus with tube and ovaries being removed through the colpotomy.

The performance of concomitant procedures using LESS is feasible and safe. This may be relevant particularly in surgery for benign conditions like cholecystectomy, appendectomy with gynecologic procedures. The contraindications for concomitant procedures will be extensive or malignant disease like suspected ovarian malignancy, dense adhesions or extensive endometriosis, but the main determinant of feasibility is the skill of the surgeon. It can be facilitated with use of flexible endoscopes like Endoeye and specialized instruments like Roticulator instruments. Also the endoscopic surgeons need to increase and reinvent their surgical skills and techniques. It requires a multidisciplinary approach and cooperation involving endoscopic surgeons from the specialties of gynecology and general surgery.

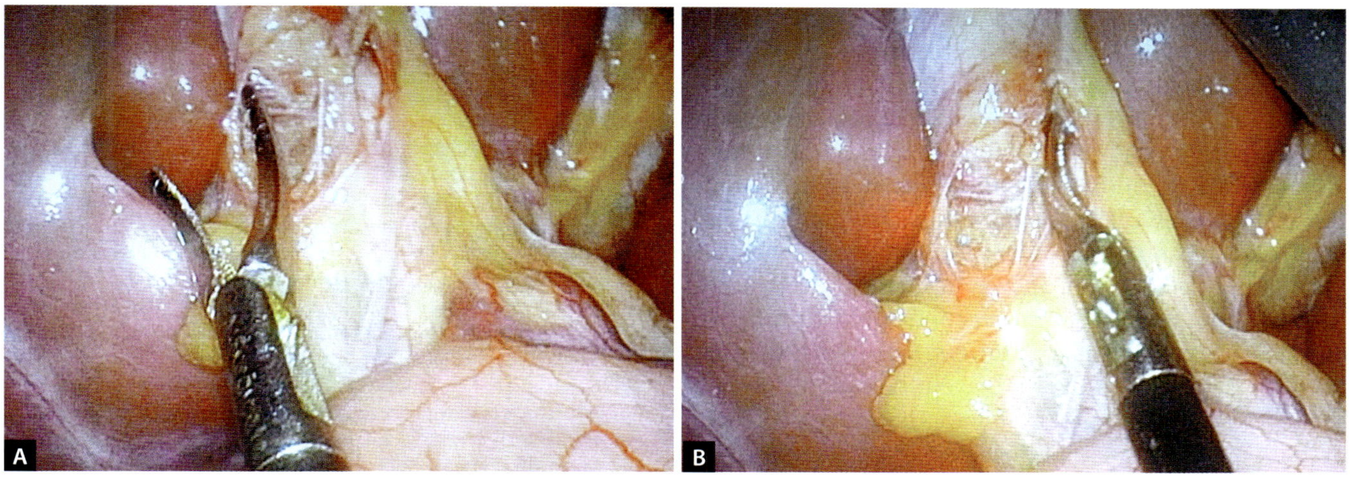

Figs. 4A and B: Dissection of gallbladder in laparoendoscopic single-site (LESS) concurrent cholecystectomy and hysterectomy: Laparoscopic view.

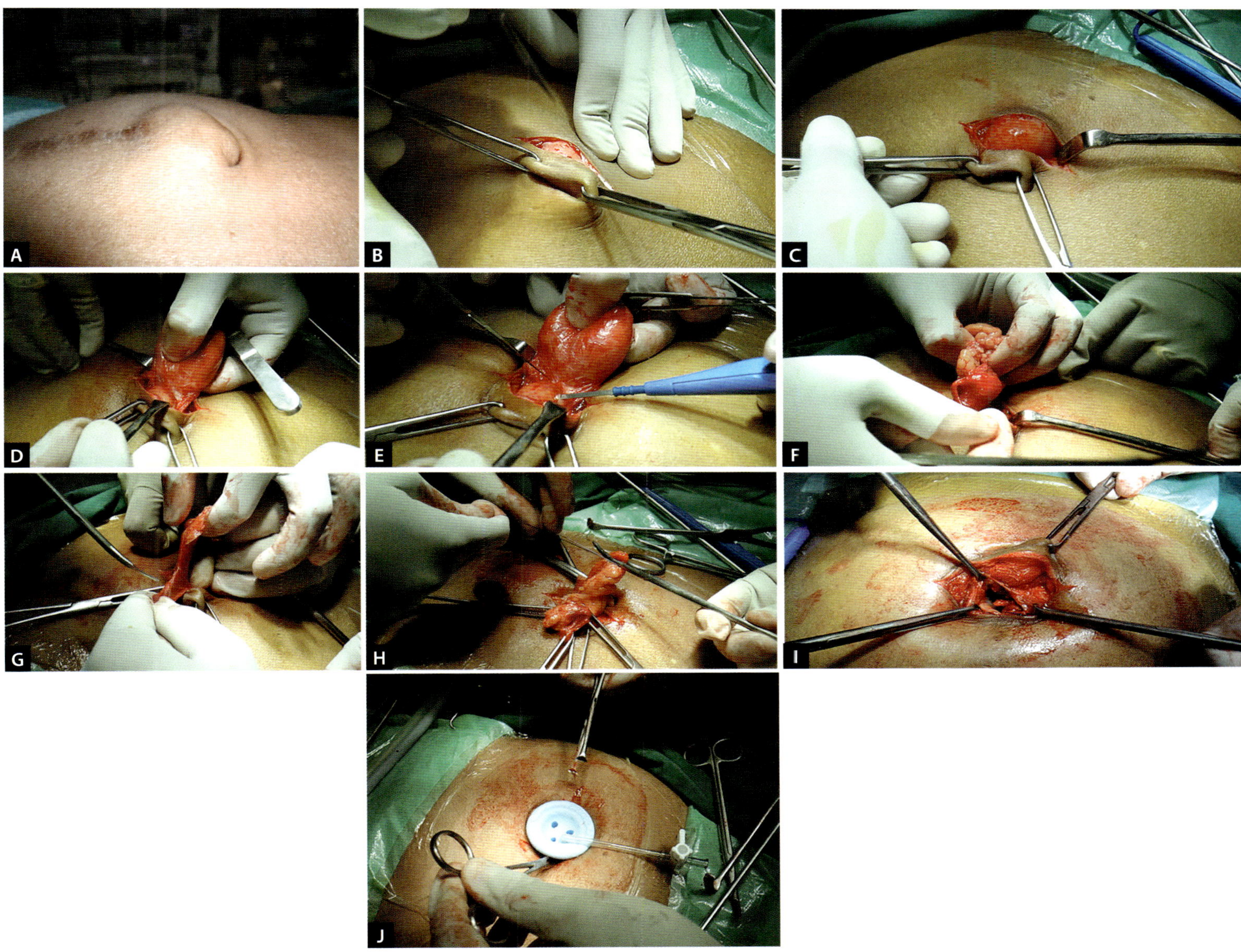

Figs. 5A to J: Concurrent umbilical hernia repair and LESS hysterectomy. (A) Umbilical hernia; (B) Skin incision being given; (C) Skin incision retracted; bulge can be appreciated; (D and E) hernial sac being dissected; (F) Omentum can be visualized in the hernial sac; (G) Omentum separated from the hernial sac; (H) Bleeding vessel in the omentum is being tied; (I) Hernial contents have been reduced and the peritoneal cavity can be seen; and (J) Covidien SILS port has been inserted through the incision. LESS hysterectomy was then carried out.

FUTURE OF CONCURRENT SURGERY IN LESS

As more and more procedures in various surgical specialties are being performed by single-port, we can expect many more concurrent procedures to be performed in the future. A recent case series has reported on patients undergoing laparoscopic bariatric surgery who desired gynecologic surgeries at the same time.[20] Four patients had bilateral tubal ligation and one patient had a total laparoscopic hysterectomy with bilateral salpingo-oophorectomy at the time of laparoscopic bariatric surgery. None of the cases had an increase in estimated blood loss. In those cases who underwent concurrent tubal ligation, there was no significant increase in operative time. There was no additional morbidity or complications in this group of patients. The authors concluded that there is clearly a correlation between morbid obesity and gynecologic issues, such menstrual dysfunction, fibroids, PCOS, subfertility, endometrial hyperplasia and cancer, urinary and fecal incontinence and pelvic prolapse. In these patients, there is merit in combining two surgeries imparting maximal benefit to the patient. In this series, multiport laparoscopy was used. Since LESS is being used for both bariatric and gynecologic procedures, in future a combination of these surgeries by single-port approach is a valid and advantageous option. These may include combination of fertility enhancing surgeries like ovarian drilling in PCOS with bariatric procedures like gastric banding, sleeve gastrectomy and gastric bypass procedures.

As the technology and surgical skill improves, more and more abdominal and pelvic surgeries will come under the purview of LESS surgery and in future any combination of abdominal and pelvic surgery will be possible through single-port. It gives an entirely new perspective to the concept of minimally invasive surgery.

CONCLUSION

Many gynecologic and surgical procedures can be performed concurrently through single incision by LESS. Concurrent procedures can provide enhanced benefit to the patient like signle hospitalization and improved cosmesis. Both surgeon and gynecologic endoscopist should be well versed with single port surgery.

REFERENCES

1. Pelosi MA, Pelosi MA III. Laparoscopic hysterectomy with bilateral salpingo-oophorectomy using a single umbilical puncture. N J Med.1991; 88:721-6.
2. Pelosi MA, Pelosi MA III. Laparoscopic supracervical hysterectomy using a single-umbilical puncture. J Reprod Med. 1992;37:777-84.
3. Hernandez JM, Morton CA, Ross S, et al. Laparoendoscopic single site cholecystectomy: the first 100 patients. Am Surg. 2009;75:1030.
4. Chow A, Purkayastha S, Paraskeva P. Appendicectomy and cholecystectomy using single-incision laparoscopic surgery (SILS): the first UK experience. Surg Innov. 2009;16:211-7.
5. Desai MM, Berger AK, Brandina R, et al. Laparoendoscopic single-site surgery: initial hundred patients. Urology. 2009;74:805-12.
6. O'Hanlan KA. First single-incision type 7 total laparoscopic hysterectomy, adnexectomy and appendectomy. Gynecol Surg. 2010;7:379-82.
7. Kim TJ, Lee YY, Kim MJ, et al. Single-port access laparoscopic adnexal surgery. J Minim Invasive Gynecol. 2009;16:612-5.
8. Fader AN, Escobar P. Laparoendoscopic single-site surgery (LESS) in gynecologic oncology: technique and initial report. Gynecol Oncol. 2009; 114:157-61.
9. Savaris RF, Cavazzola LT. Ectopic pregnancy: laparoendoscopic single-site surgery: laparoscopic surgery through a single cutaneous incision. Fertil Steril. 2009;92:1170.e5-e7.
10. Yoon BS, Park H, Seong SJ, et al. Single-port laparoscopic salpingectomy for the surgical treatment of ectopic pregnancy. J Minim Invasive Gynecol. 2010;17:26-9.
11. Fagotti A, Fanfani F, Marocco F, et al. Laparoendoscopic single-site surgery (LESS) for ovarian cyst enucleation: report of first 3 cases. Fertil Steril. 2009;92:1168.e13-6.
12. Hart S, Ross S, Rosemurgy A. Laparoendoscopic single-site combined cholecystectomy and hysterectomy. J Minim Invasive Gynecol. 2010;17: 798-801.
13. Wadhwa A, Chowbey P, Sharma A, et al. Combined procedures in laparoscopic surgery. Surg Laparosc Endosc Percutan Tech. 2003;13:382-6.
14. Romanelli JR, Earle DB. Single-port laparoscopic surgery: an overview. Surg Endosc. 2009;23:1419-27.
15. Langwieler TE, Nimmesgern T, Back M. Single-port access in laparoscopic cholecystectomy. Surg Endosc. 2009;23:1138-41.
16. Rettenmeier MA, Abaid LN, Erwin MR, et al. A retrospective review of the GelPort system in single-port access pelvic surgery. J Minim Invasive Gynecol. 2009;16:743-7.
17. Patsner B, Mann W, Arato M, et al. Cholecystectomy accompanying major abdominal surgery for gynecologic cancer. Gynecol Oncol. 1989;32: 46-8.
18. Malfetano JH, MacDowell RT, O'Hare MM. Incidental cholecystectomy in the treatment of gynecologic malignancy. J Gynecol Surg. 1990;6:195-8.
19. Surico D, Gentilli S, Vigone A, et al. Laparoendoscopic single-site surgery for treatment of concomitant ovarian cystectomy and cholecystectomy J Minim Invasive Gynecol. 2010;17:656-9.
20. Scheib SA, Curlin H, Thomassee M, et al. Combining gynecologic surgery at time of laparoscopic bariatric surgery. J Minim Invasive Gynecol. 2012; 19:S151-S178.

CHAPTER

83

LESS: Our Experience—Tips and Tricks for Beginners

B Ramesh, Aditi Rai

"Experience is not what happens to a man; it is what a man does with what happens to him."

—Aldous Huxley

INTRODUCTION

In the following pages, we describe our experience with laparo-endoscopic single-site (LESS) surgery. It includes the difficulties faced and how they were overcome. This chapter includes certain key points, which we understood with performance of different kinds of LESS surgeries; which can be a guide to laparoscopic surgeons with keen interest in single-port surgeries. Last, but not the least, the learning curve has to be followed and gradual progress from simpler to complex procedures is the way forward. The reader should understand that only the name is "LESS"; a great effort and dedication is required by the surgeon to become accomplished in this approach. Also, only those who are fairly accomplished in multiport laparoscopy should embark into the field of single-port surgery. It is very important to understand the basic principle, access, specific instrumentation and difference or modification in technique from multiport laparoscopy. And as experience increases, one can improvise and innovate to overcome the limitations and increase the efficacy of surgery. Last but not least, the surgeon should remember that the most important fact is the outcome of surgery; and irrespective of the approach, the principle and safety of the surgery should never be compromised. As we started single-port surgeries, we faced a lot of difficulties. As we did more and more surgeries, we modified our technique; new instrumentation also contributed to overcoming these difficulties.

One can read through this chapter to understand what one might face during the learning phase of LESS and incorporate this knowledge in the performance of surgery.

ACCESS: THE INCISION IN THE UMBILICUS

The first difficulty we faced was in inserting the access port itself. The port placement in LESS is similar to open laparoscopy; gynecologic laparoscopic surgeons usually are not used to the open approach. Initially, we used to enter through and through the umbilicus cutting through all layers. We realized that this created a problem in wound healing, wound infection thereby affecting cosmesis. Later, we switched to starting the incision at the center of umbilicus and slightly extending beyond inferior margin. With this modification, healing is better and the configuration of the umbilicus is maintained. We do not prefer the infraumbilical-curved incision.

Tips and Tricks

- *Preoperative cleaning of the umbilicus is very essential:*
  - Patient should be asked to clean the umbilicus before reporting for surgery.
  - In the preoperative ward, the importance of preparation of umbilicus with soap solution and Betadine should be emphasized upon the nursing staff.
  - Finally, during cleaning and draping on the operating table, special attention has to be paid to the umbilicus.
  - It should be remembered postoperative wound infection at the umbilicus can defeat the purpose of single incision access surgery.
- *Plan the incision:*
  - Incision type and length depends on the type of the umbilicus and the comfort of the surgeon.
  - Cosmesis is important from the patient's perspective.
- *Maintain umbilical integrity:*
  - Avoid cutting the umbilical stalk.

ACCESS: INSERTION OF THE ACCESS PORT

Insertion of the access port through the incision also was difficult in the initial stages. X-cone (Karl Storz) is slightly easier to insert since it has two metallic halves, which can be inserted separately and reassembled inside. X-cone, for the same reason has the advantage of easy insertion of needle and suture material and also in tissue retrieval as the silicon cap can be removed and then reattached. When using the Covidien SILS port, though it is flexible we found the insertion slightly difficult in the early cases. We found that taking two stay sutures in the rectus fascia with Vicryl no 1 may be helpful. The advantage of stay suture is that it helps in lifting the abdominal wall during insertion of the port. Also it helps in identification of the rectus fascia during closure. The stay sutures are removed after suturing of the rectus sheath. We hold the Covidien port obliquely with an artery forceps and retract the edges of the skin and rectus sheath with right-angled retractors. This facilitates insertion of the port. The steps of insertion are shown in the chapter on abdominal access.

Tips and Tricks

- Retract skin and fascial edges before insertion.
- Stay sutures on rectus fascia to facilitate both insertion of port and closure of incision.

CHOICE OF ACCESS PORT

Gas leakage through the access port is a common and frustrating problem in single-port laparoscopic surgeries. We have used wound retractor with surgical glove and various commercially available access ports in our LESS procedures.

Homemade Port-wound Retractor and Surgical Glove

It is a cheaper alternative to the commercially available access ports. The material of the glove is stretchable and provides great space for the manipulation of the instruments. The insertion of materials like mesh and suture material is easy, as only the glove portion has to be removed. Similarly, tissue retrieval becomes easier. The first disadvantage is that the assembly of the port may sometimes be difficult. The proper fitting of the glove on the retractor is not maintained as the glove has the tendency to slip. Also, sometimes on manipulation, the glove can pop out leading to sudden loss of pneumoperitoneum.

X-cone (Karl Storz)

It is a reusable device. Insertion is easier as described earlier. One of the problems that we faced with X-cone was that with manipulation the cap disengages from the metal halves leading to loss of pneumoperitoneum. Insertion of suture material and tissue retrieval is easier.

SILS Covidien Port

We are using the SILS port for most of our LESS procedures. After the initial difficulty we faced, the insertion is easy because of the flexible nature of the port. We only need an incision of 2 cm length to insert this port. We have not faced the problem of gas leakage with this port. The insertion of needle and suture is slightly difficult in SILS port. Also, for tissue retrieval, the whole port has to be removed.

In Gelport, the range of movement is better. We found the insertion of Triport cumbersome.

Tips and Tricks

- Weigh the pros and cons of each access port.
- Choice of access port lies with the surgeon.
- Fascial incision should be optimum—should allow easy insertion as well as prevent loss of pneumoperitoneum.

CLOSURE OF THE INCISION

The closure of the umbilical incision is very important to achieve the benefits of better cosmetic effect. As emphasized earlier, stay sutures should be placed at the margins of the rectus sheath after access is obtained. During closure, the margins can be lifted up to be identified and exposed properly and facilitate closure. The sheath is closed with Vicryl no 1. If required, a second layer of sutures can strengthen closure. If the umbilical stalk has been cut, it has to be reattached to the fascia to restore the normal anatomy of the umbilicus. The dead space in the subcutaneous tissue has to be completely obliterated to prevent hematoma or seroma formation. Wound infection, if it occurs, can lead to fascial weakening and umbilical hernia in the future. Also, it negates all the cosmetic benefits of the single incision. For proper umbilical reconstruction, we took the advice of a plastic surgeon in the initial cases. The cosmetic results and patient satisfaction has been very good.

Tips and Tricks

- Proper closure of the fascial incision by identifying margins of the rectus sheath essential.
- No dead space should be left during closure.
- Proper umbilical reconstruction is mandatory.

VISION AND OPTICS

One of the major problem one faces during performance of an LESS procedure as compared to conventional multiport laparoscopic surgery is reduced vision. When we started doing single-port laparoscopic surgeries, we used standard length rigid 5 mm 0° laparoscope. The vision was restricted and surgery was difficult. To overcome this problem we tried using 10 mm 0° laparoscope. The marginal improvement in visualization was offset by restriction in manipulation and collision of instruments because of the increase in size.

To overcome instrument collision, we shifted to 10 mm long (52 cm) bariatric scope. It reduced instrument clashing but still occupied more space. Now we use a 5 mm 30° long rigid bariatric scope. Because of the long length, it keeps the camera away from the access port, 30° angle improves the area of visualization and it occupies less space than 10 mm laparoscope.

Recently, we have started using flexible tip 5 mm laparoscope (ENDOEYE). The deflectable distal tip provides a 100° field of view in all directions. The light cable is parallel to the laparoscope and not at right angle to the other scope. This does not obstruct the hand movements of the surgeon. The Endoeye has greatly improved vision and facilitated instrument manipulation. We feel the flexible tip endoscopes are ideal for performance of LESS procedures, but cost may be a constraining factor. If flexible tip endoscope is not available, long bariatric 5 mm 30° scope is an acceptable alternative.

Another point to consider is holding of the camera. Earlier in our single-port procedures, the assistant used to hold the camera and surgeon used to operate with one hand. The problem, which occurs with this in single-port laparoscopy, is that sometimes the assistant is not able to correctly anticipate the movements of the surgeon. In LESS, because the vision and operating space is already reduced, lack of proper coordination between the camera and instruments increases the operative difficulty. So, we feel the surgeon operating from the left side of the patient can hold the camera in the right hand and the instrument in the left hand if only one instrument is being used with the camera assistant on standby. This also reduces hand collision extracorporeally. We feel there is a learning curve for the camera assistant also in single-port laparoscopy.

Tips and Tricks

- Reduced vision is an important limiting factor in LESS.
- Flexible tip endoscopes are ideal.
- Long bariatric 5 mm 30° laparoscope is an acceptable alternative.

INSTRUMENT MANIPULATION AND TRIANGULATION

Inherent problems of LESS are reduced working space, lack of triangulation seen in multiport laparoscopy and clashing of instruments. Certain points should be kept in mind to minimize these problems. To reduce collision, a combination of long and short instruments can be used. These instruments will be at different planes, leading to effective manipulation. It is important that the instruments are introduced in parallel and should not cross each other. To create triangulation in the operating space, we have found the use of articulating instruments to be useful. In addition, we find use of one articulating and one straight instrument to be very useful in tissue manipulation without instrument collision. In our experience, we have found the combination of straight and articulating instruments to be ergonomically better than two articulating instruments.

There are two kinds of curved instruments, which are available—single curve and double curve. We find both the insertion through the access port and intracorporeal manipulation of double curve instruments very cumbersome. We routinely use only single-curve instruments.

Tips and Tricks

- Restricted instrument manipulation and loss of triangulation specific problems of LESS procedures.
- Use of articulating and curved instruments can offset these problems to some extent.
- Use of long instruments and combination of straight and curved instruments is ideal.
- Use of flexible trocars facilitates insertion and manipulation of curved instruments.

SUTURING

Suturing is the most difficult aspect of any kind of laparoscopic surgery and this is true for single-port laparoscopic surgery. Intracorporeal suturing and knot tying in LESS requires skill and technique of the highest order. Suturing and knot tying using two straight instruments is a very difficult task. Use of articulating instruments is useful in this. We have found the use of one curved instrument and straight needle holder makes suturing more efficient. Even holding the needle is difficult in LESS. Use of self-righting needle driver facilitates this action. The other techniques that we use are single handed suturing with barbed suture in myoma bed closure in LESS myomectomy and vault closure in LESS hysterectomy. Barbed suture is very useful in LESS procedures as knotting is not essential. Another method of suturing is the Endostitch. SILS stitch is a modification, which has been developed for single-port surgeries. It is a longer instrument and has a deflectable tip. The problem with these devices is that in deep myomas, suturing is not feasible.

Tips and Tricks

- Combination of one straight and one curved instrument is ideal.
- Self-righting needle holder and devices like Endostitch may be useful.
- Barbed suture is advantageous as knotting is not required.

HEMOSTASIS

Control of bleeding in LESS can be achieved with bipolar coagulation and vessel sealing devices. Longer version of these such as Enseal is available which can be used in LESS. We believe that LESS surgeries have almost zero-tolerance for bleeding. Once significant bleeding occurs, vision is further reduced and it is difficult to manage. One should always take utmost care to prevent unnecessary bleeding.

Tips and Tricks

Prevent bleeding. One should not hesitate to place an extra port to control hemorrhage.

TISSUE RETRIEVAL

Tissue retrieval is easier in LESS because of 2–2.5 cm umbilical incision. In multiport laparoscopy, the lateral port incision has to be extended in case of removal of adnexal masses and morcellation of fibroids. This extension of lateral incision increases the trocar site complications like nerve injuries, vessel injuries, wound complication, and hernias.

Morcellation of fibroids can be done by umbilical morcellation (3–4 cm fibroids) or transvaginal morcellation (4–8 cm fibroids). It must be remembered that in umbilical morcellation, only the side of morcellator is seen and the end on view is not obtained. So one has to be very careful in this step of LESS myomectomy.

SPECIFIC SITUATIONS

LESS Total Laparoscopic Hysterectomy

- Combination of Ultrasonic Shears (HARMONIC SCALPEL) and bipolar device or vessel sealer is ideal. The ultrasonic device can be used for bladder dissection and bipolar or vessel sealer for coagulating the infundibulopelvic and uterine pedicles. The vessel sealing devices like Enseal are better as both coagulating and cutting can be performed by the same device and repeated instrument changes are not required.
- During bladder dissection, the instrument movement is an anterior posterior movement rather than lateral movement in LESS. This is because lateral movement can cause instrument collisions.
- The vessel sealer or the bipolar forceps is applied obliquely to the uterine pedicle in LESS as compared to perpendicular application in multiport laparoscopic hysterectomy.

LESS Myomectomy

- *Myoma screw:* For enucleation of myoma, we use a combination of long myoma screw and scissors. This step of traction and countertraction is more difficult in single-port myomectomy. The direction of traction has to change multiple times to facilitate enucleation.
- As described in hysterectomy, movements are anterior-posterior and above–downward rather than lateral movements.

LEARNING CURVE

As in multiport laparoscopic surgery, LESS also has a learning curve. It is advised that only endoscopic surgeons competent in multiport laparoscopy should embark on single-port laparoscopic surgeries. Initially, one can start with simpler procedures like salpingectomy, oophorectomy that involve coagulation and cutting. Once one is fairly familiar with these surgeries one can proceed to simple hysterectomy with vaginal vault closure. The next level of difficulty is in procedures with movements of traction and countertraction. Then one can start with simpler myomectomies and intracorporeal suturing. One should always proceed from simpler to complicated procedures. In case of intraoperative difficulty, one must not hesitate to convert to multiport laparoscopy.

Ours is a dedicated gynecologic endoscopy tertiary level hospital and infertility center. We get all kind of complicated cases as referrals from all over Karnataka and neighboring states. **Tables 1 to 6** shows the analysis of the LESS surgeries performed at our center.

COMPLICATIONS

The incidence of complications in our cases is very low because of the careful selection of cases. The complications were:

- *Placement of extra lateral port:* This happened in three cases of LESS hysterectomy. In the first case, it was because of heavy bleeding. One lateral side port was placed and the bleeding vessel was coagulated. In the second case, there was technical difficulty due to dense adhesions. And the third a case of a large 20-week size uterus with fibroids. The manipulation and visualization was difficult in this case.
- *Wound infection:* We had about 5 cases of wound infection. This was during initial part of the learning curve. Four cases responded to conservative treatment; the fifth patient had to undergo debridement and resuturing. With the proper preoperative cleaning of umbilicus and proper patient follow-up, the incidence of wound infection has decreased.
- *Umbilical hernia:* One patient developed umbilical hernia. She had undergone combined cholecystectomy and hysterectomy and was diabetic. Umbilical hernia repair was done for her.
- During our course of LESS, there were no visceral injuries.

Table 1: Distribution of laparoendoscopic single-site (LESS) gynecologic surgeries performed (from 2007 till Jan2013).

	Type of surgery	*No. of cases performed*
1.	LESS hysterectomy	108
2.	LESS myomectomy	25
3.	LESS for ectopic pregnancy	9
4.	LESS oophorectomy	7
5.	LESS ovarian/paraovarian cystectomy	22
6.	LESS cholecystectomy	4
7.	LESS hysterectomy with cholecystectomy	8
8.	LESS hysterectomy with appendicectomy	5
9.	NOTES appendicectomy	4
10.	NOTES cholecystectomy	1
	Total number of cases	*193*

NOTE: All cholecystectomies and appendicectomies were performed by general laparoscopic surgeon well-versed in LESS. See pie chart below.

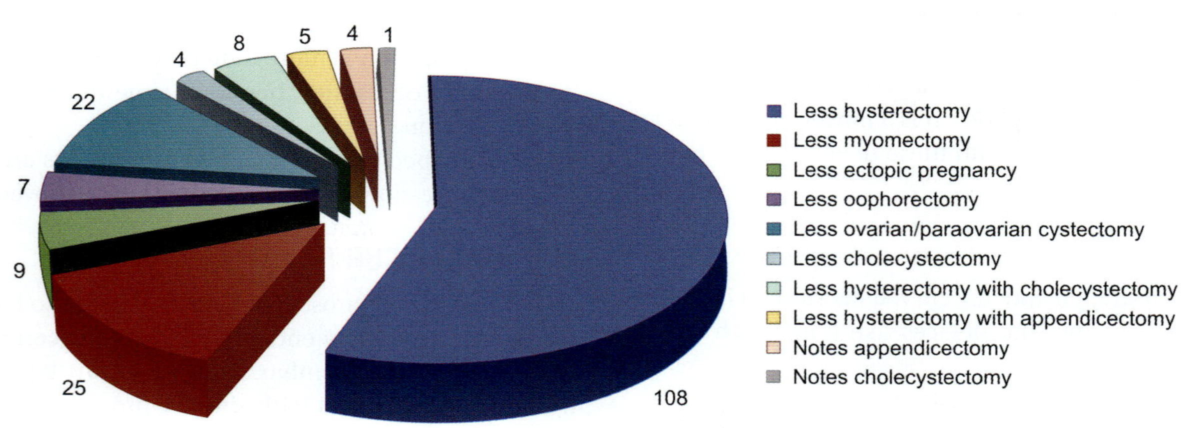

Table 2: Access ports used.	
1.	Single skin/multiple fascial incisions method—4
2.	Access ports used
	Covidien SILS port—112
	X-cone—42
	Gelport—3
	Wound retractor and glove—30
	Triport—2
LESS hysterectomy (this number is exclusive of the concurrent procedures). See the bar graph below.	

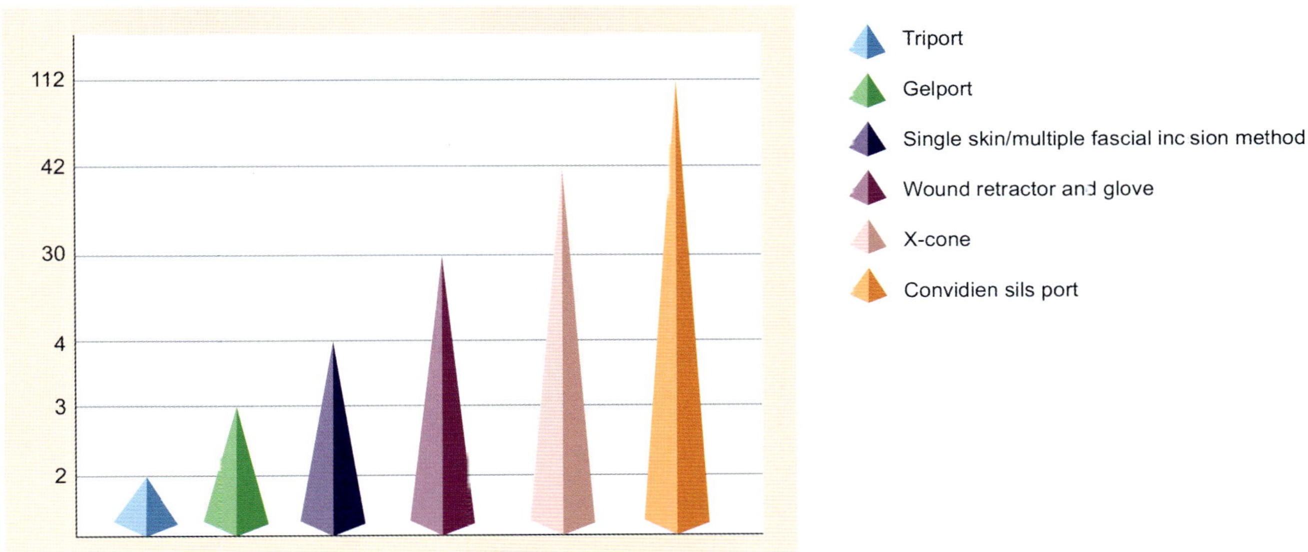

Table 3: Type of hysterectomy.
Total laparoscopic hysterectomy—106
Laparoscopic-assisted vaginal hysterectomy—2

Table 4: Indications of laparoendoscopic single-site (LESS) hysterectomy.
Abnormal uterine bleeding—53
Fibroid uterus—41
Adenomyosis—12
Chronic pelvic pain—2
The maximum size of uterus removed by LESS approach was 16–18 weeks

Table 5: Laparoendoscopic single-site (LESS) myomectomy: location of fibroid.
Post wall—11
Anterior wall—9
Fundal—4
Lower body posterior wall—1
Maximum size of myoma removed was 10 cm

Table 6: Tissue retrieval in fibroids.
Umbilical mechanical morcellation-2
Umbilical electromechanical morcellation-10
Transvaginal colpotomy-1
Transvaginal electromechanical morcellation-12

CONCLUSION

The above chapter describes the authors' experience of LESS surgery. The above points are meant to highlight the challenges one might face in the process of developing this skill and their probable solutions. The surgeon has to go through his or her learning curve to become proficient in the art of single-port laparoscopic surgeries.

"People never learn anything by being told, they have to find out for themselves."

—Paulo Coelho

Accompanying Video: Single port hysterectomy (SILS).

CHAPTER

84

Optics for Laparoendoscopic Single-site Surgery

B Ramesh, Aditi Rai

INTRODUCTION

The insertion of the scope and instruments together in parallel through a single access port in laparoendoscopic single-site surgery (LESS) makes visualization of the operative field restricted and difficult. Everyone would agree that vision is an essential component of laparoscopy. Improper visualization can decrease operative efficiency and increase risk of complications. In single-port laparoscopy, due to close proximity of instruments and the scope, these problems are compounded. This chapter will discuss the optical options available for LESS that can overcome this limitation to some extent.

LAPAROSCOPE

The commonly used laparoscopes can be straight diagnostic and angled operative. Endoscopes can be rigid or flexible. In rigid scopes, all components are aligned together. And most rigid scopes are focused with a camera coupler. The components of the endoscope are objective lens, eyepiece and transmission system. The Hopkins rod lens system, the shaft of the laparoscope contains quartz rods that provide clear vision.[1] In flexible scopes, fiber-optic bundles are present. The newer version of laparoscopes is "chip on the tip" in which camera and scope are incorporated together. The laparoscopes may have different viewing angles such as 0°, 30°, and 90°. The degree of angulation depends on a prism in the objective lens. A schematic representation of a telescope is shown in **Figure 1**.

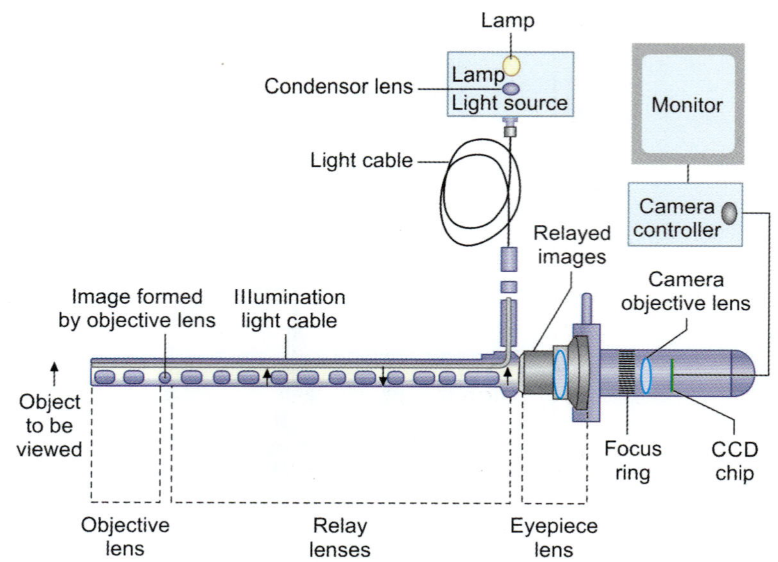

Fig. 1: Schematic diagrammatic representation of a 0-degree telescope. The fiber optics directs the light to the tip. The image of the tissue is formed by the objective lens and transmitted through the rod lens system. This is then perceived by the surgeon at the eyepiece. In videolaparoscopy, the image is transmitted to the monitor via the camera.

Rod lenses and reversal system: The reversal system consists of a series of rod lenses made of glass. They serve to transmit the image within the endoscope, i.e. they relay the image captured by the objective lens to the eyepiece lens. They provide a clearly higher light transmission efficiency compared to conventional lenses where the area filled with air between the lenses is relatively large. Advantages of rods lens system over conventional laparoscopes, is that, the glass rods in the Hopkins telescope provides a larger image, greater light transmission and improved clarity of vision.

Camera head: Camera head houses the adapter and charged coupled device (CCD). The CCD captures light and converts it to digital data that is recorded by the camera and relayed to the monitor.

Fiber-optic endoscope: Rigid endoscopes have superior image quality compared to flexible endoscopes as the rod-lens relay system gives better light transmission than a fiber bundle.

Design of a chip-on-the-tip endoscope: The camera and scope is incorporated together. The camera chip is taken out of the camera head and placed at the distal end of the scope, i.e. the endoscope tip itself contains a camera sensor or the CCD. This technology does away with the optical lenses an image passes through when chip is in the camera head. This requires less light than do standard cameras because the light is not lost in the light cord and rod lenses. The image generated in the objective lens is guided onto to the video chip. The latter converts the optical signals into electrical signals and transmits them to the camera controller. The image suffers minimal loss, interference and distortion compared to standard scopes. These laparoscopes have four ways deflection for greater flexibility and all round viewing angles.

The various advantages of chip on the tip design **(Fig. 2)** (*Courtesy*: OLYMPUS) are:

- The optics are designed to maximize the performance of the CCD.
- Since fewer lenses are required, higher contrast imaging is facilitated by the reduction in the reflected noise that occurs at the lens surface.
- It allows a wider field of view and better spatial orientation **(Fig. 2A)**.
- The system has fewer lenses; this reduces light absorption occurring inside the lens. This allows bright, natural color imaging, and better depth perception.

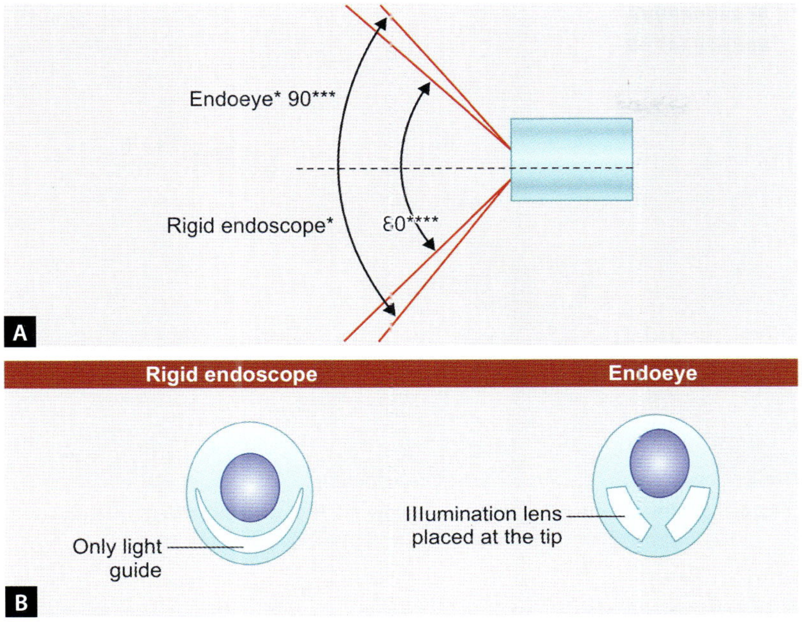

Figs. 2A and B: (A) Endoeye allows wider field of view and better spatial orientation; (B) Appropriate light distribution is facilitated by illumination lenses placed at the tip.

- The illumination lenses are placed at the tip allowing appropriate light distribution **(Fig. 2B)**.
- Inside the scope only cables are housed except at the tip. So there is very little deterioration of image quality.

OPTICS OPTIONS FOR LESS

Traditional 5 and 10 mm cameras can be used for LESS surgery. The use of traditional laparoscopy cameras increases instrument crowding. There are *four ways in which to reduce the crowding* and provide a stable image during the procedure.[2]

- Use of bariatric-length, rigid, 5 mm scopes to offset the instrument length during the surgery and reduce crowding.
- Use of 30° scopes to enhance the viewing angle.
- Use of a laparoscopic camera-scope combination with an in-line light cord and a low-profile camera head to reduce the tangling of light source coming in at a 90° angle with a traditional laparoscopic camera.
- Use of specialized laparoscopic camera for single-port surgery with a deflectable tip.

Conventional Laparoscopes

Thirty-degree endoscope (5 mm and 10 mm) is the most common endoscope used for LESS surgery today. High-fidelity vision is necessary for intraoperative visualization of anatomic regions and structures. The surgeon should be able to visualize structures from differing perspectives, preferably offline from the axis of the instruments.

Modified Laparoscopes (Fig. 3)

- Long telescopes; Both Karl Storz endoscopy (Tuttlingen, Germany) and Stryker endoscopy (San Jose, CA, USA) have modified their existing endoscopes to develop 5 mm, 30° telescopes that are 50 cm long. The extra length removes the camera head and light cord from the operative field. But, the added length reduces the brightness of the scope and visualization can be poor in larger patients.

EndoCAMeleon™ is a 10 mm rigid scope with adjusting knob for selection of viewing direction angle from a range of 0° to 120° EndoCAMeleon (Karl Storz) has a rotating camera chip within the tip.

- Operating laparoscopes with 45° or 90° angled eyepieces with an operating channel (5.5–7 mm) for instruments. They can be of value in LESS surgery to put the endoscope away and increase working space for the instruments.
- A laparoscopic camera-scope combination with an in-line light cord and a low-profile camera head.

Endoeye (Figs. 4 to 7)

The deflectable-tip Endoeye video laparoscope (Olympus America, Center Valley, Pennsylvania) was approved by the US Food and Drug Administration in 2005 and has been commercially available since then, long before single-port surgery became mainstream. This laparoscope has an outer diameter of 5 mm for a standard video resolution camera and 10 mm for the high-definition video resolution camera. The distal tip is flexible and hosts the camera, enabling enhanced angulation range.[3]

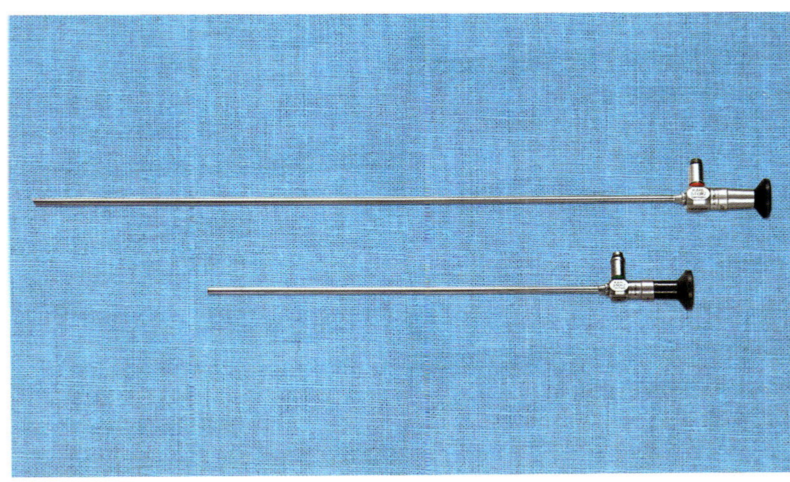

Fig. 3: 5 mm 30° long telescope 0° and 0° 5 mm small telescope.

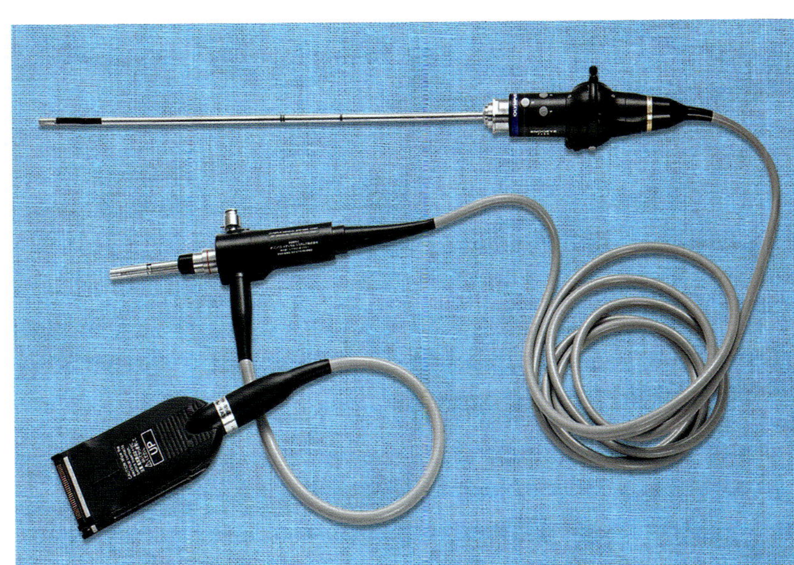

Fig. 4: One-piece design that integrates the light cable and camera system into the laparoscope allows easy intraoperative maneuvering.

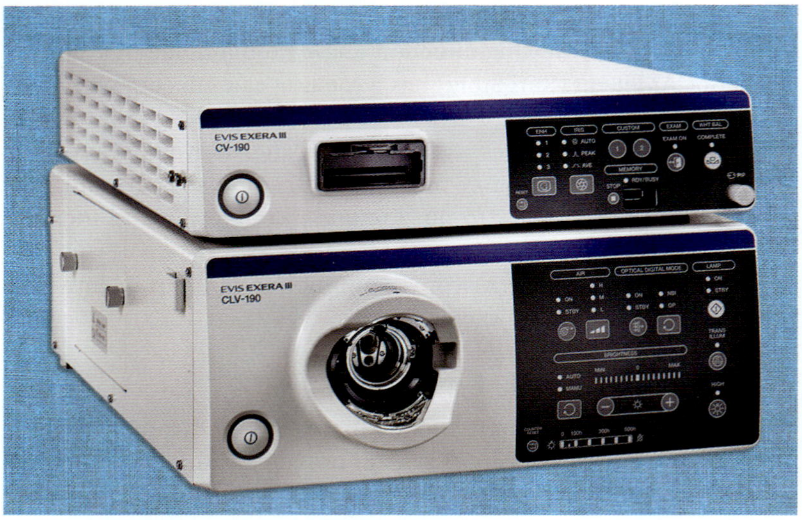

Fig. 5: Xenon light source and the camera unit for the Endoeye.

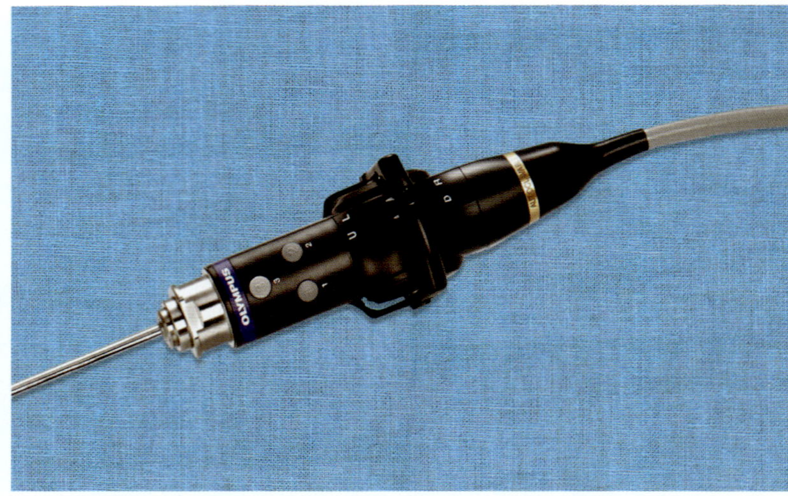

Fig. 6: Switches can be programmed to allow the remote control of frequently used functions such as image capturing and zoom.

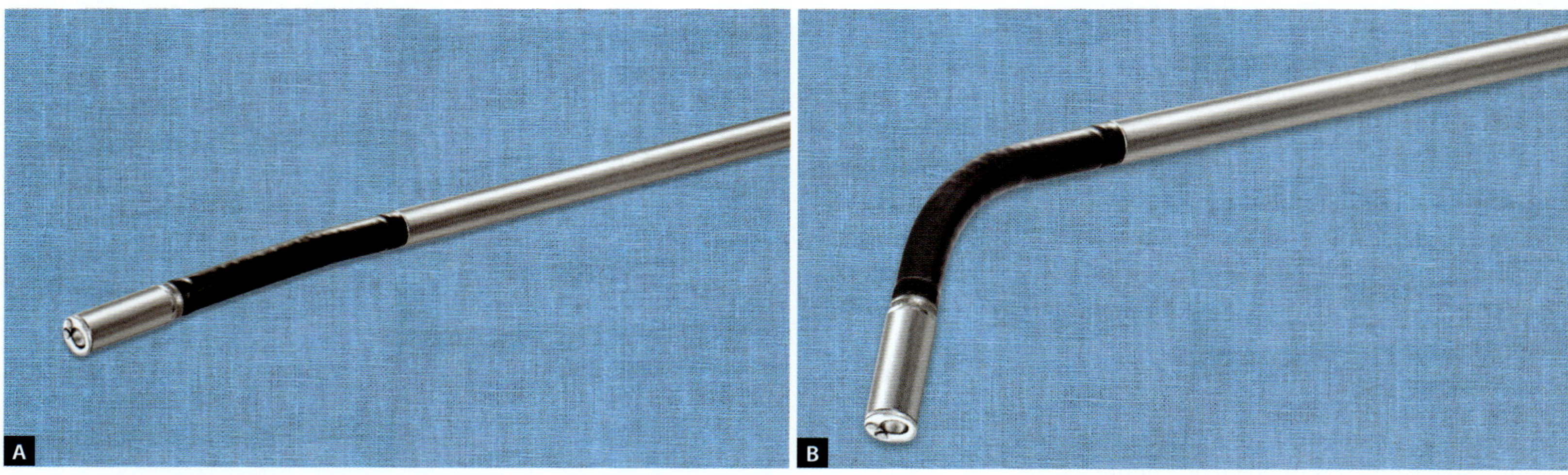

Figs. 7A and 8B: Angulation in four directions and shorter bending section allows for easier orientation even in narrow cavities.

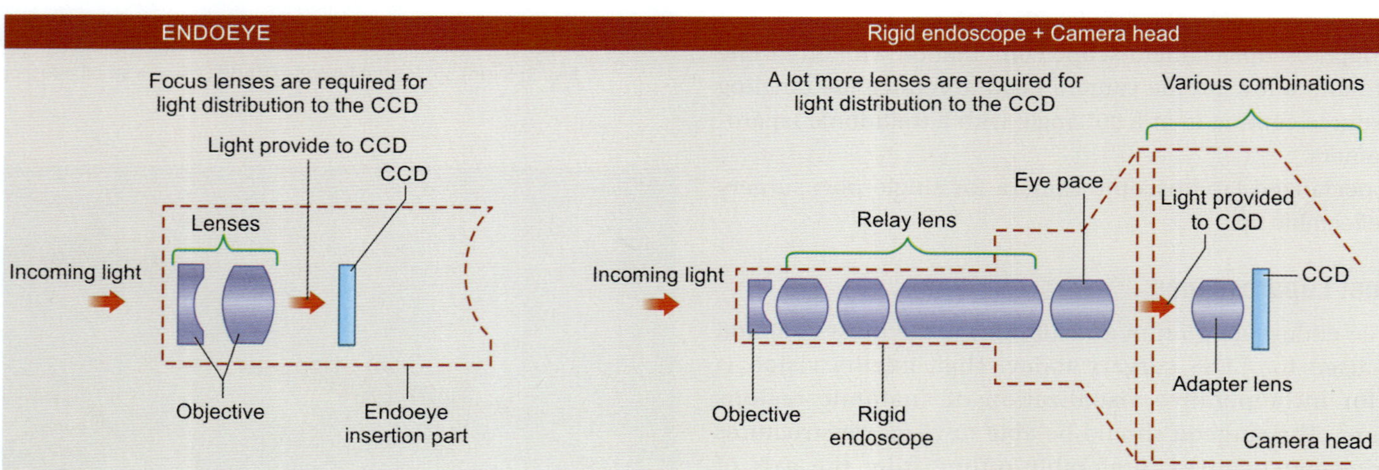

Fig. 8: Fewer focus lenses required for light distribution to charged coupled device (CCD) as compared to rigid endoscope where an array of relay lenses are required.

The 5 mm autoclavable, endoscope with integrated camera and light cable with a deflectable tip is tailor made for LESS surgeries.

Endoeye technology: Conventional flexible endoscopes use optical fibers to carry images from the scope tip to the eyepiece, generating images. The Endoeye uses a distally mounted CCD for providing brighter images, color reproduction, greater depth of field and focus free operation. The innovative distal chip design, by placing the CCD at the scope tip, has eliminated the need for a separate camera head and provides the convenience of automatic focus and light intensity regulation **(Figs. 8 and 9)**. The deflectable tip provides a complete 100° field of view to visually capture the desired location. Angulation control allows smooth deflection in four directions. The Olympus LTF-VP is

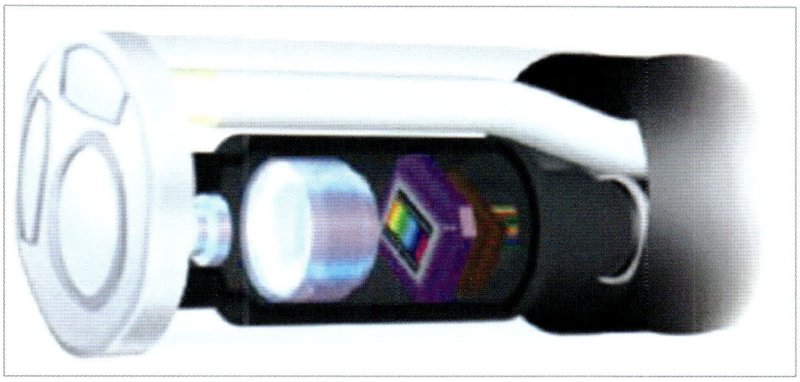

Fig. 9: The distally mounted charged coupled device (CCD) delivers a brighter image, color reproduction, larger depth of field, and focus-free operation.

a 5.4-mm diameter flexible videoscope. This helps make endoscopic surgery less invasive. The small diameter allows entry through 5 mm ports and its flexible tip allows observation from angles not possible with a rigid 10 mm diameter scope. LTF-VH HD Endoeye is a 10-mm flexible video laparoscope.

The major advantage of the deflectable-tip Endoeye in single-port surgery is that less movement is necessary at the port site to move the camera, which reduces collision with other instruments in the limited space. The major disadvantage of this scope is incompatibility with other video platforms, necessitating an entire new setup and, hence, relatively high cost.[3]

Stryker-Ideal Eyes-HD-articulating Laparoscope

It is a 10 mm laparoscope with an integrated cable. It allows over 100° flexion in all directions.

CONCLUSION

Good vision and clarity is one of the most important aspects of laparoscopy. Visualization of details of the anatomy is quintessential to the efficiency and outcome of surgery. The surgeon should be able to visualize the tissues from various angles and offline from the axis of instruments. This becomes more relevant in the performance of complex procedures.

Slender, angled view scopes and now the "chip on the tip design" endoscopes can improve the visibility for the surgeon and make LESS procedures feasible.

REFERENCES

1. Ocampo J, Nutis M, Nezhat C, et al. Equipment. In: Nezhat C, Nezhat F, Nezhat C (Eds). Nezhat's Operative Gynecologic Laparoscopy and Hysteroscopy, 3rd edition. New York: Cambridge University Press; 2008. pp. 9-35.
2. Uppal S, Frumovitz M, Escobar P, et al. Laparoendoscopic single-site surgery in gynecology: review of literature and available technology. J Minim Invasive Gynecol. 2010;18:12-23.
3. Kikuchi I, Kumakiri J, Kuroda K, et al. A novel modification of traditional 2-port laparoscopic surgery using a 5-mm flexible Scope. J Minim Invasive Gynecol. 2009;16:734-8.
4. Hackethal A, Ionesi-Pasacica J, Eskef K, et al. Transvaginal NOTES with semi-rigid and rigid endoscopes that allow adjustable viewing angles. Arch Gynecol Obstet. 2010.

CHAPTER

85

Specimen Retrieval

B Ramesh, Aditi Rai

INTRODUCTION

In the past decade or so, minimally invasive surgery has advanced by leaps and bounds to a level unimaginable years ago. More and more procedures are being attempted laparoscopically, imparting benefits of smaller, cosmetic incisions with less morbidity and faster recovery to the patient. Single-port laparoscopy or laparoendoscopic single site (LESS) is a step forward in that direction. Tissue retrieval can be described as the sine qua non of minimally invasive surgery. Sometimes, it can be a daunting task as the organ or tissue has to be brought out through a small incision. This chapter covers this aspect in various types of single-port surgeries.

The various methods of tissue retrieval in LESS are **(Table 1)**:

- Use of 10 mm claw forceps through umbilical access port
- Colpotomy
- Use of endobag
- Transumbilical mechanical morcellation
- Electromechanical morcellation with a power morcellator
  - Umbilical
  - Vaginal
  - Transcervical (in supracervical hysterectomy).

Table 1: Methods of tissue retrieval in laparoendoscopic single site (LESS).

Surgery	*Specimen*	*Method(s) of retrieval*
Myomectomy	Fibroid	Transumbilical mechanical
		Transumbilical electromechanical
		Transvaginal electromechanical
		Colpotomy
Ectopic pregnancy-salpingostomy/salpingectomy	Products of conception/Fallopian tube	Through 10 mm port with claw forceps
Oophorectomy	Ovary/tubo-ovarian mass	Endobag through umbilicus/colpotomy
Ovarian/paraovarian cystectomy	Cyst lining	Through 10 mm port with claw forceps
		Colpotomy
		Endobag through umbilicus/colpotomy
Appendicectomy	Appendix	Through 10 mm port with claw forceps/Endobag
Cholecystectomy	Gallbladder	Endobag through umbilicus
Hysterectomy	Uterus	Through vaginal vault by mechanical morcellation with knife/abdominal electromechanical morcellation
Supracervical hysterectomy	Uterus	Transcervical morcellation

THROUGH THE UMBILICAL ACCESS PORT USING CLAW FORCEPS

Small specimens like cyst lining of ovarian or paraovarian cysts, ectopic pregnancy, Fallopian tube and appendix can be removed through a 10-mm claw forceps. At the end of the surgical procedure, a 10-mm trocar is inserted through the umbilical access port through one of the channels **(Fig. 1A)**. A 10-mm standard claw forceps is inserted through this trocar and tissue can be grasped **(Figs. 1B and C)**. Sometimes if the grasping of the tissue is difficult a toothed grasper can be introduced through another channel and help to feed the grasper to the claw forceps. Tissue can then be removed. If some difficulty is faced during removal, radial cuts are made to reduce its bulk and easy withdrawal.

COLPOTOMY

An incision can be made through the pouch of Douglas (POD) for tissue retrieval. This method can be used for larger or thicker cyst linings or small fibroids. An incision is made in the POD either vaginally or laparoscopically. A sponge on holder or with a colposcopy center (CCL) extractor delineates vagina. It has a ball-shaped head that delineates the vagina and helps the surgeon to make the incision laparoscopically. An incision is made between the uterosacral ligaments using a monopolar hook or ultrasonic shears. Alternatively, the surgeon goes to the vaginal end and makes an incision in the posterior fornix. A claw forceps (10 mm) is inserted though an opening in the ball of CCL extractor and can be used to grasp the specimen or endobag **(Figs. 2A and B)**. This can then be pulled out. Incision is then sutured vaginally or laparoscopically.

Advantages of Colpotomy

It is a relatively cheap and easy method.

Disadvantages of Colpotomy

- Not feasible in
  - Obliteration of POD with endometriosis and adhesions
  - Patients who are not sexually active.
- Loss of pneumoperitoneum—this problem can be overcome using a CCL extractor.

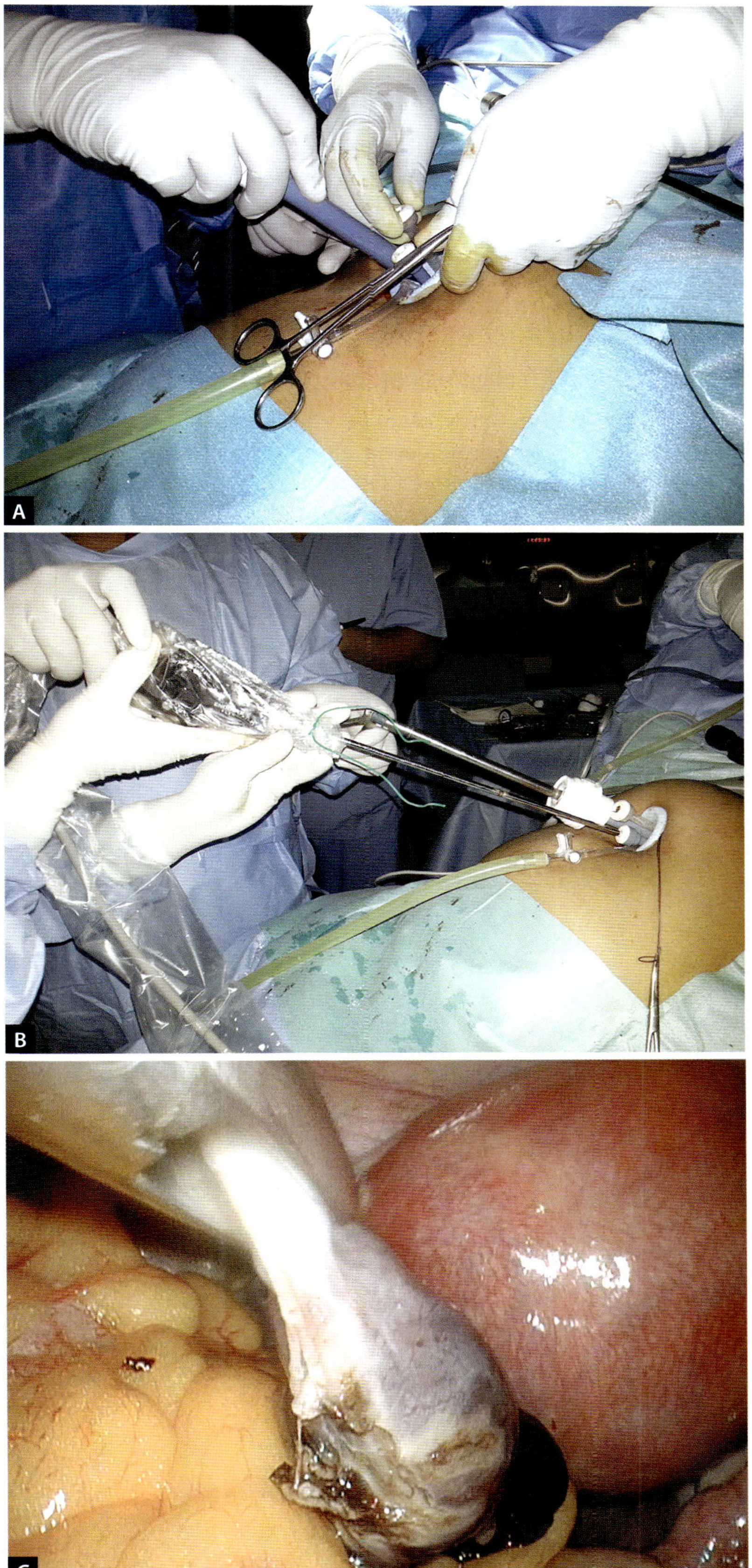

Figs. 1A to C: (A) Inserting 10 mm trocar through Covidien SILS port; (B) 10 mm trocar through the SILS port with 10 mm claw forceps. Flexible scope Endoeye is inserted through 5 mm trocar; (C) 10 mm claw forceps holding salpingectomy specimen. Laparoscopic view.

- Scarring of vagina leading to dyspareunia.
- Injury to surrounding structures like rectum.
- Postoperative adhesions in the pouch of Douglas.

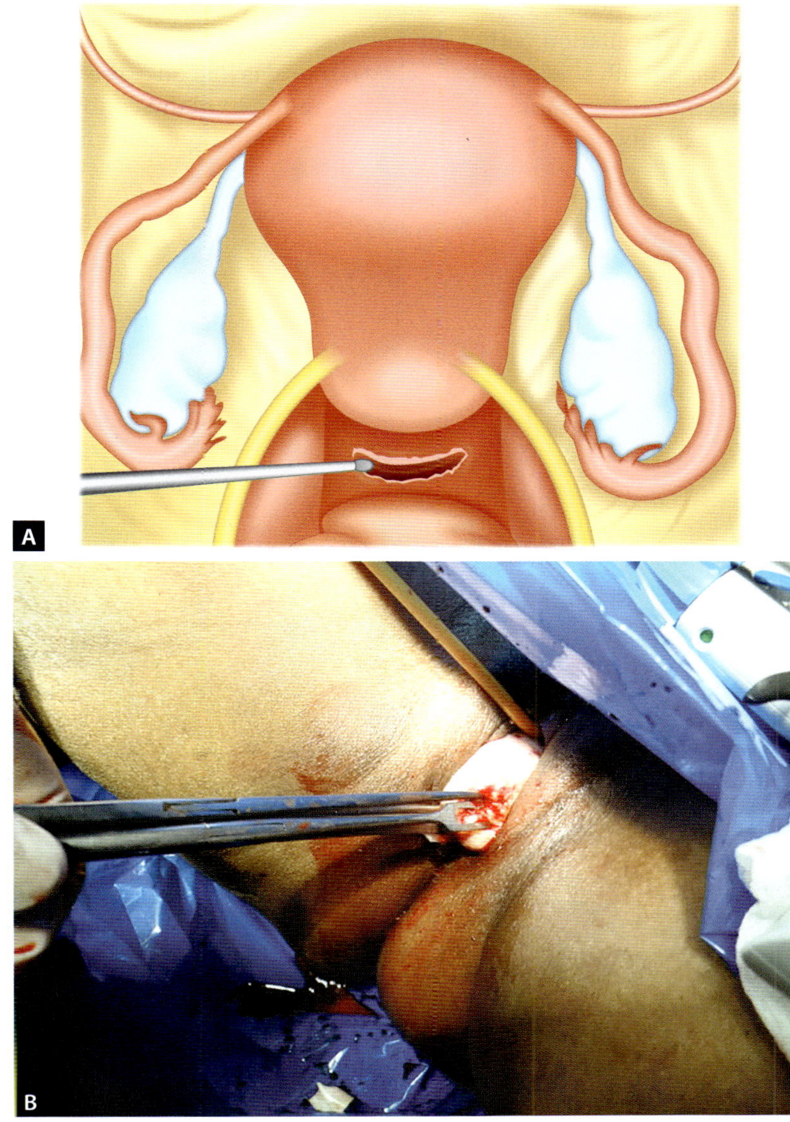

Figs. 2A and B: (A) Colpotomy incision given between two uterosacral ligaments; (B) Fibroid being removed through colpotomy site in a case of LESS myomectomy.

ENDOBAG

In case of specimens in which spillage has to be avoided, like ovarian cysts, the removal should be done in an endobag. The ideal endobag should be easy to see and manipulate within the abdomen, strong, and impermeable to infectious and malignant tissue.[1] There are various commercially available endobags like Endo Catch Gold (Autosuture, Inc., Norwalk, CT, USA), Endopouch Retriever (Ethicon Endo-surgery, Cincinnati, OH, USA), and Espiner E-Sacs (Espiner Medical Products, Clevedon, UK). A low cost endobag can be made with sterile surgical gloves **(Fig. 3)**. Silk 1 suture can be tied around the glove excluding the fingers part and cutting that end. Endobags are generally used for ovarian cysts like endometriotic and dermoid cysts. It is recommended that in this kind of cysts the enucleation should be done inside the endobag to prevent spillage. The contents of the cyst can be suctioned inside the bag. The endobag with cyst wall is brought toward the umbilical opening, holding it with a claw forceps. The access port is then removed and the endobag is pulled into the opening. The margins of the endobag are brought out through the incision and it is gradually pulled out **(Figs. 4A to H)**. If the cyst is big, it can be decompressed or mechanically morcellated at the umbilicus within the bag and then delivered through the incision. Care must be taken to avoid rupture of the endobag. In case mechanical morcellation is difficult, electrical morcellation within the endobag may be undertaken. The disadvantage with single-port endobag retrieval is that once the access port is removed, we cannot visualize the inner part of the endobag as the telescope is removed. When glove and wound retractor is used as the access port, the retrieval becomes easier because of the space provided by the wound retractor.[2]

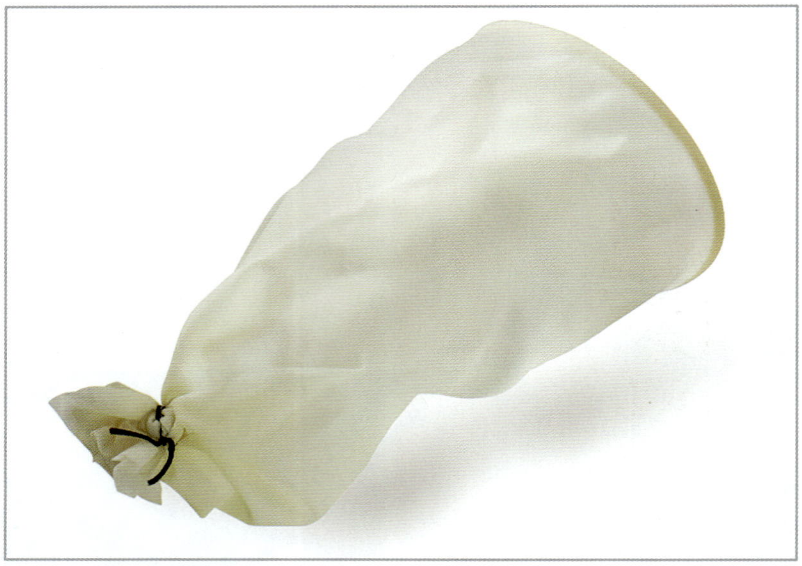

Fig. 3: Homemade endobag.

TRANSUMBILICAL MECHANICAL MORCELLATION

The myoma is brought up to the incision using the tenaculum after removing the port. Then the myoma is pulled further in the incision and carefully morcellated at the level of the incision using a knife. The fascia is closed with 0-Vicryl suture **(Figs. 5A to E)**.

ELECTROMECHANICAL MORCELLATION WITH A POWER MORCELLATOR

Transumbilical Electromechanical (Figs. 6A to F)

Retrieval of myoma may also be done by electromechanical morcellation through umbilicus or alternatively through the pouch of Douglas. In umbilical morcellation, 10 or 15 mm morcellator is inserted through one opening in the port and a toothed grasper through another. The morcellator is directly inserted after removing one of the trocars through one of the channels. The flexibility of SILS Covidien port allows 15 mm morcellator to be inserted without difficulty. The toothed grasper is used to feed the myoma, which is held in claw forceps introduced through the morcellator. The claw forceps is then drawn into the morcellator and morcellation is done. The main disadvantage of transumbilical morcellation is that panoramic view of morcellation

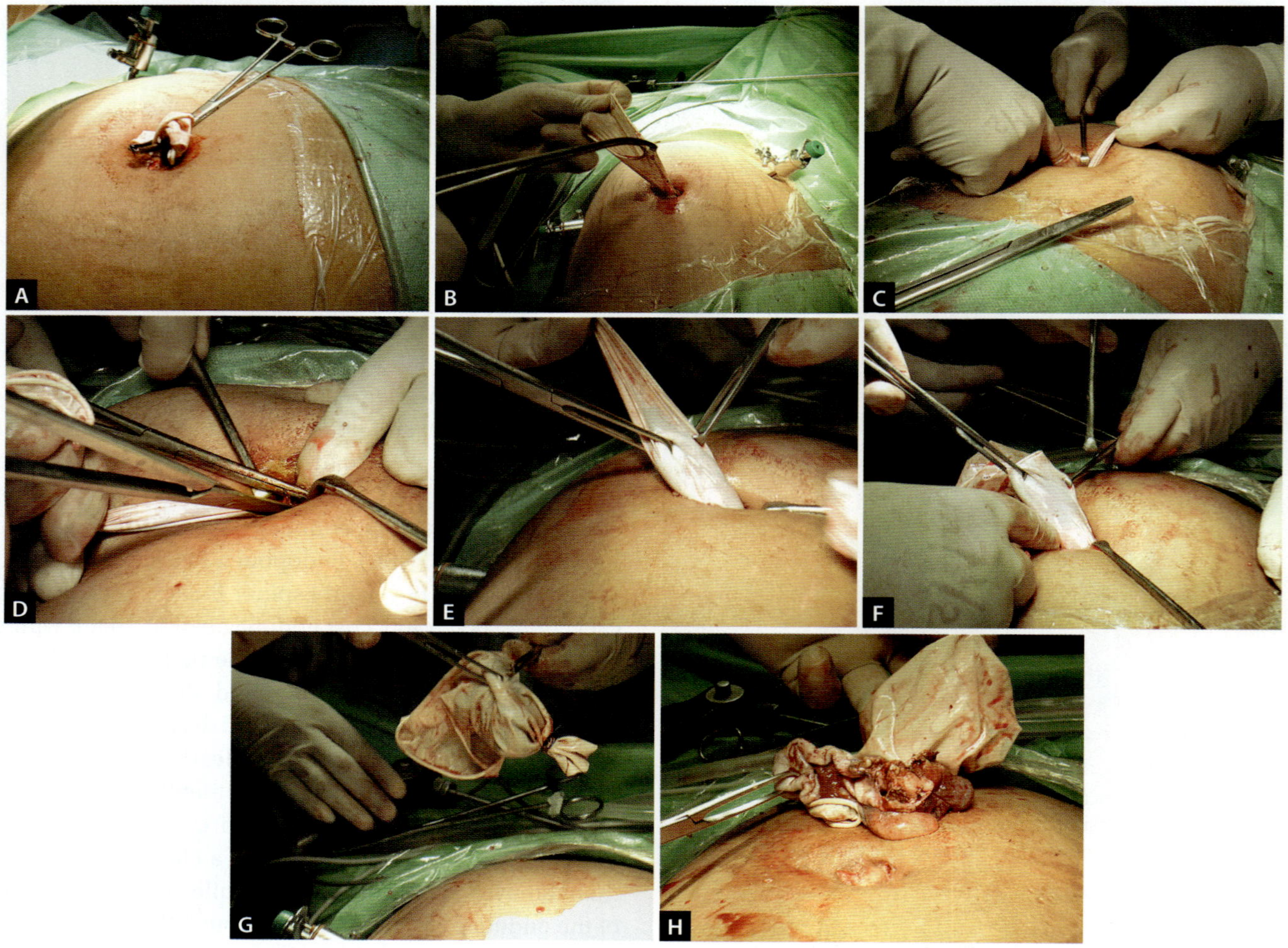

Figs. 4A to H: Tissue retrieval (ovarian cyst lining) through umbilical port site. (A) Endobag with tissue is brought out to the umbilicus. The access port has been removed; (B) Margins of the endobag are held by long artery forceps; (C and D) The endobag is held while the skin incision is retracted with right angled retractor to increase space; (E and F) The endobag is gradually delivered out; (G) The endobag with the cyst is completely out of the incision; (H) Cyst lining out of the endobag.

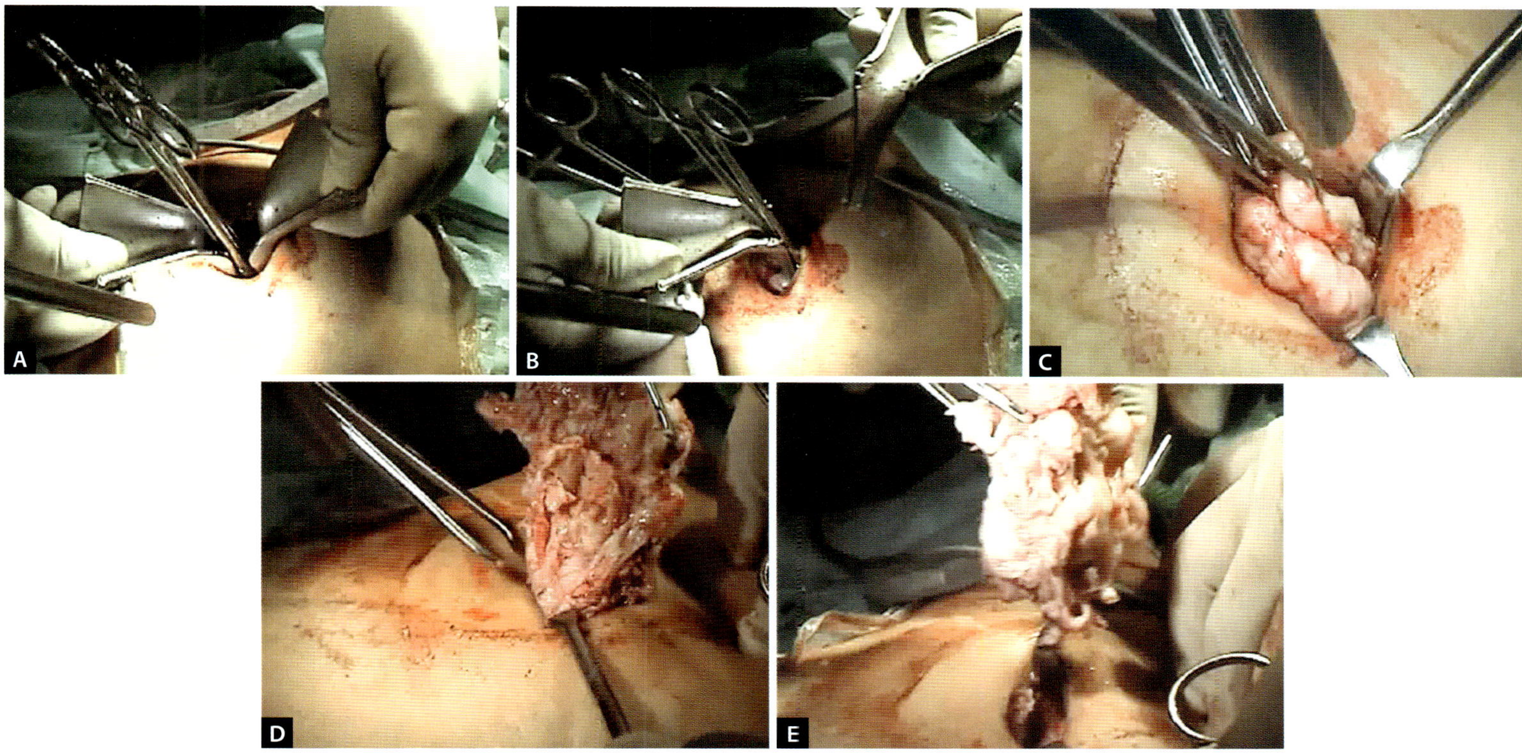

Figs. 5A to E: Transumbilical mechanical morcellation. (A and E) X-cone access port being taken out of the incision. The fibroid specimen is held by Allis forceps; (C) After the port is removed, the fibroid is brought out into the incision; (D) The fibroid is being mechanically morcellated and pulled out; (E) The fibroid is completely out of the incision.

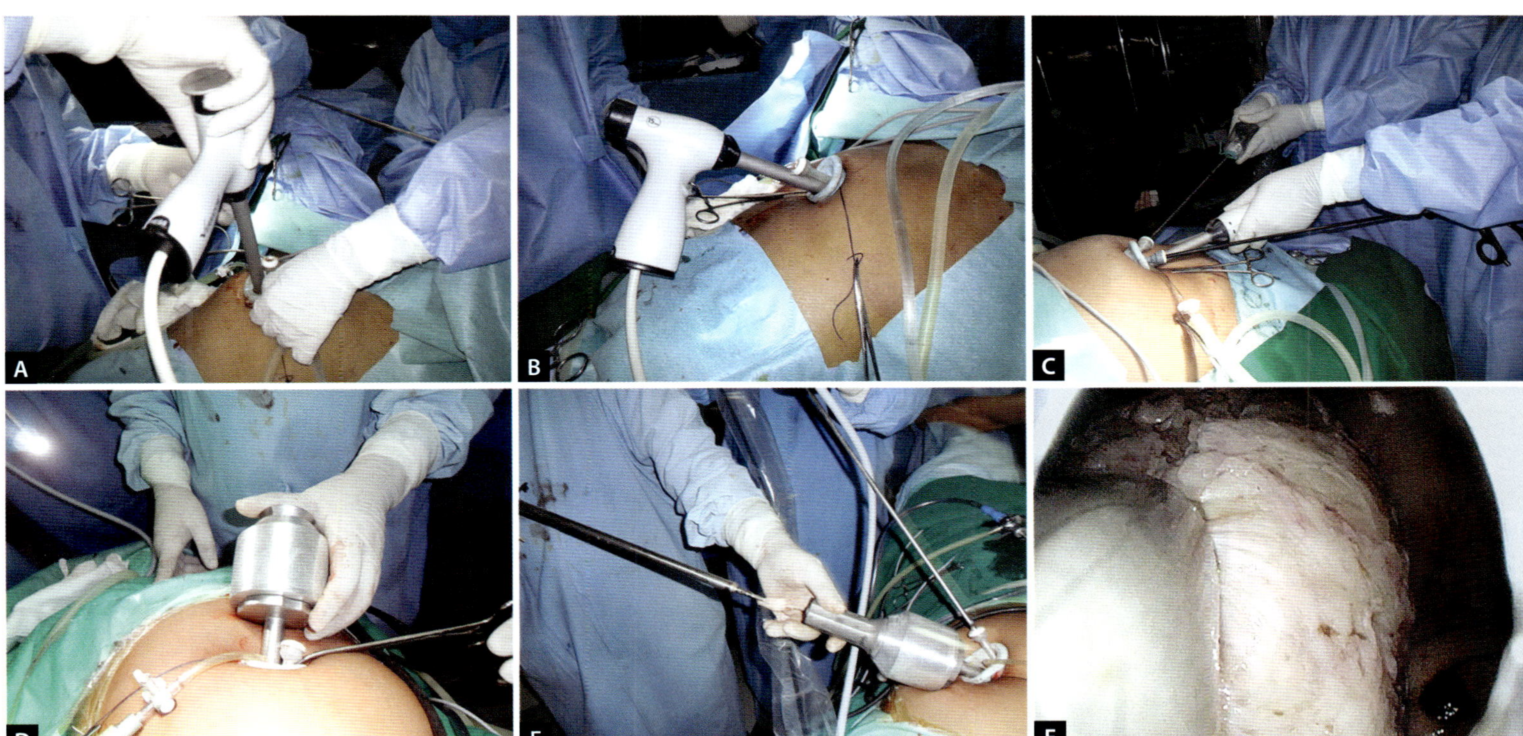

Figs. 6A to F: Transumbilical electromechanical morcellation. (A) Insertion of morcellator (Versator) through channel in SILS port. Note that the morcellator is inserted without a trocar; (B) Position of inserted morcellator; (C) Transumbilical morcellation being performed in a case of LESS myomectomy. The Endoeye (5 mm flexible telescope) and long toothed grasper are seen entering the abdomen through 5 mm trocars; (D) Rotocut G1 morcellator (Karl Storz, Tuttlingen, Germany). Rotocut G1 morcellator inserted through SILS port; (E) Morcellated fibroid specimen being removed with 15 mm claw forceps. In this case, 5 mm rigid 30° telescope is being used; (F) Umbilical morcellation: Laparoscopic view.

is not seen and the view of blade is very limited. The transumbilical morcellation with morcellator was described by Kim et al.[3] in cases of single-port myomectomy with glove and wound retractor as access port. The authors felt that use of surgical glove enables the transit of a 15-mm morcellator through a small umbilical incision. For extraction of the cut tissue, glove can be detached from the wound retractor. Also, the use of wound retractor increases the space available to remove the tissue this method may be also be used for ovarian cysts.

Transvaginal Electromechanical (Figs. 7A to I)

The surgeon inspects the vaginal side after completion of the myomectomy. The posterior lip of the cervix is held by an Allis forceps and retracted anteriorly and the vaginal surface is visualized. A sponge on holder is used to push the posterior vaginal fornix and the location is visualized laparoscopically to ensure the correct position between the two uterosacral ligaments and away from rectum. A 1.5-cm transverse superficial incision is made vaginally to facilitate the introduction of the morcellator under continuous laparoscopic vision. The morcellators with long blade like SAWALHE (Karl Storz GmbH & co. KG, Tuttlingen Germany) or GYNECARE X-TRACT (Ethicon Inc, Somerville, NJ) are preferred for vaginal morcellation. During morcellation, pneumoperitoneum is increased to 20 mm Hg to ensure good visualization and panoramic view. A 10-mm claw forceps was used to guide the myoma into the morcellator and morcellation was done carefully. The morcellator is removed under vision and the adjacent structures were carefully inspected. The vaginal incision is left unsutured. The author has used this method of morcellation through the POD in both multiport and single-port myomectomy with good results.

Precautions during Electromechanical Morcellation

- The intra-abdominal pressure should be raised to 20 mm Hg before starting morcellation.
- The morcellator blade should be visualized at all times.
- Only the person handling the morcellator should activate the control.
- Immediately after finishing the morcellation, it should be switched off to prevent inadvertent activation.
- All small bits of fibroid should be removed meticulously after exploring the abdominal cavity. If myoma bits are left behind, they may attach to a vascular structure, develop blood supply, and grow as *iatrogenic* parasitic fibroids.
- Vaginal morcellation through the pouch of Douglas
    - The patient should be brought beyond the edge of the table
    - Long blade morcellator should be preferred
    - The blade should extend beyond the uterus to prevent injury
    - Should not be attempted in cases where the pouch is obliterated by some pathology like endometriosis and adhesions.

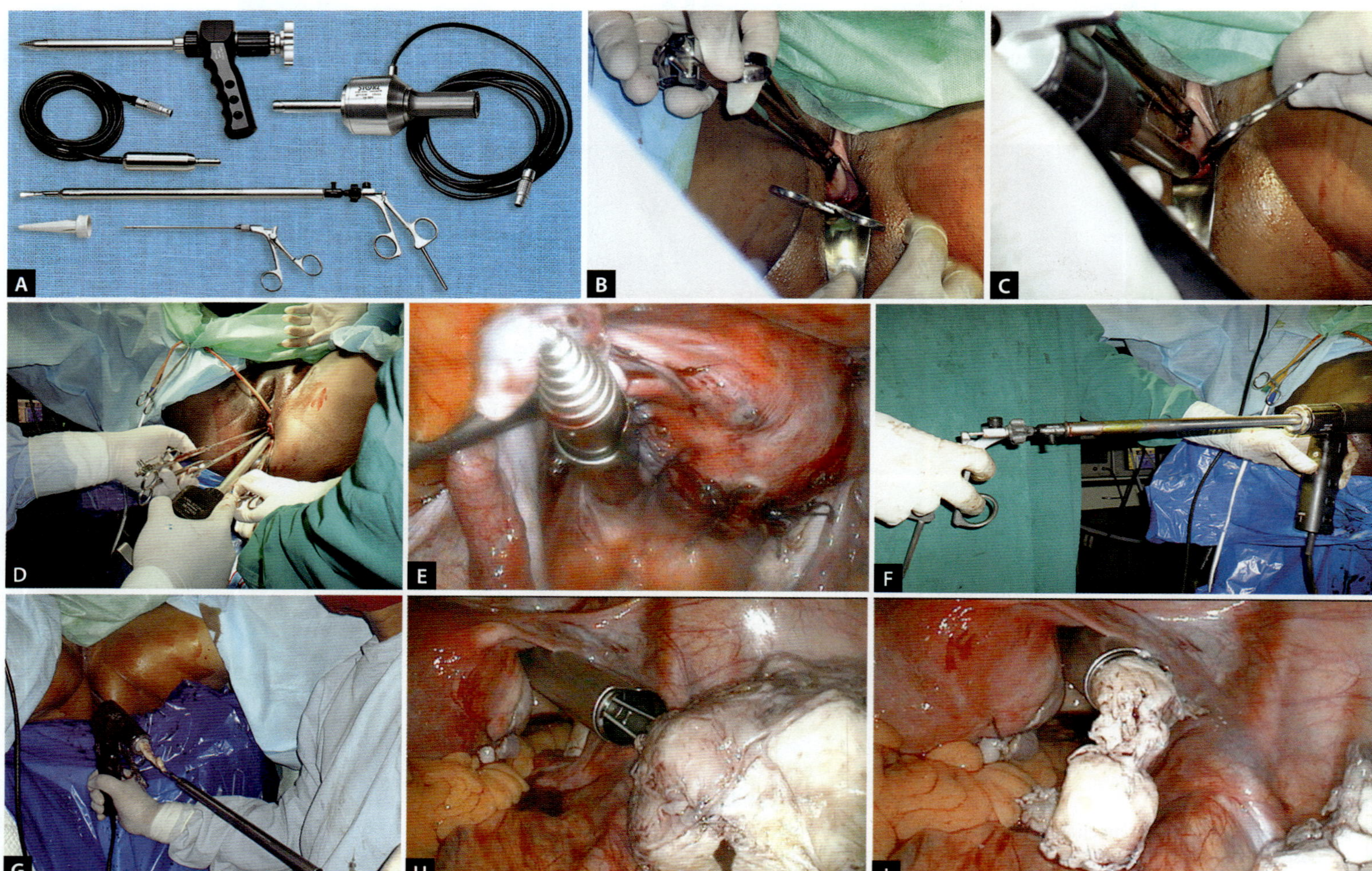

Figs. 7A to I: Transvaginal electromechanical morcellation. (A) Sawalhe (Karl Storz) (left) and Rotocut G1 (Karl Storz) (right) morcellators. Morcellators with long blade like Sawalhe is more suited to vaginal morcellation; (B) Incision made in the posterior fornix; (C) Insertion of Sawalhe morcellator; (D) Morcellator inserted through the pouch of Douglas under laparoscopic guidance. Note the uterine manipulator used to antevert the uterus during insertion and morcellation; (E) Sawalhe morcellator inserted through the pouch of Douglas: laparoscopic view; (F and G) 15 mm claw forceps is used to grasp and pull out morcellated myoma strips; (H and I) Myoma being morcellated through the pouch of Douglas: laparoscopic view.

Advantages of Transvaginal Morcellation over Transumbilical Morcellation in Less Myomectomy

- Visualization is better in vaginal route as scope is inserted through the umbilicus and whole length of blade can be seen whereas in transumbilical route since the telescope and morcellator are both inserted through the umbilicus, vision is compromised.
- In vaginal route, the morcellator is inserted through the vagina whereas the toothed grasper which is used to feed the fibroid into the morcellator goes through the umbilical port. Hence collision is reduced. In transumbilical method, the toothed grasper and the morcellator both enter through the umbilical access port, hence leading to collision.

Transcervical Morcellation (of Uterus in Supracervical Hysterectomy)

Rosenblatt et al. described a newer technique of transcervical morcellation of uterus in cases of supracervical hysterectomy in 2010.[4] It was described in multiport supracervical hysterectomy to avoid the enlargement of lateral side port incision for the morcellator, which is a site of considerable pain for the patient. Avoiding the lateral extension the incidence of pain, injury, wound infection, and trocar site hernia can be reduced. In these cases laparoscopic supracervical hysterectomy was performed in the usual fashion. After complete transection of the uterine fundus from the cervical stump, the uterine manipulator was removed. The coring of cervix was done by a 10-mm flat myoma screw (Karl Storz GmbH & Co., Tuttlingen, Germany) or 15 mm classic intrafascial supracervical hysterectomy (CISH) instrument set (Wisap GmbH, Munich, Germany) after sounding the cervix to determine the axis of the cervical canal. Regardless of instrumentation, the entire coring procedure is performed with direct laparoscopic visualization of the pelvis to ensure no injury to internal organs. When coring of the endocervix is complete, the serrated blade is removed and the morcellator is advanced into the pelvic cavity for removal of the uterus. Morcellation is performed using a 10-mm tenaculum placed through the morcellator. The laparoscopic assistant orients the specimen for the tenaculum in such a manner as to maintain the morcellator blade on the outer surface of the uterine corpus. Using the "core-guard" lip on the morcellator also facilitates this process. When the specimen has been completely removed, the defect in the cervix is closed to prevent herniation of bowel or adnexa through the cervix. When the specimen has been completely removed, the defect in the cervix is closed to prevent herniation of bowel or adnexa through the cervix. Yoon et al.[5] used the technique of transcervical morcellation in cases of LESS subtotal hysterectomy. Supracervical hysterectomy was performed using Harmonic Ace and Roticulator instruments. The cervix was dilated via the vaginal approach up to No. 15 Hegar dilator. Then, the Semm morcellator (15-mm serrated blade; Wisap, Sauerlach-München, Germany) was inserted through the dilated cervical os and the uterus was removed using the transcervical morcellator with the assistance of the endoscopic grasper to hold the removed uterus. After the uterus was completely removed hemostasis was ensured using bipolar coagulation. Reperitonization of cervical stump was done.

Transumbilical morcellation is done with electromechanical morcellator through access port. Through the access port, movement is restricted because the morcellator (15 mm), telescope and laparoscopic grasper are inserted together into a small opening. However, if cervical canal is used as another port, it enables morcellation without limiting the range of motion. Also the morcellating blade is visualized in its entire length as against umbilical morcellation where vision is restricted. In case of single-port subtotal hysterectomy transcervical morcellation can be a source of infection. In single incision access procedures, the transcervical route can reduce crowding around the umbilical wound. In addition, the transumbilical morcellator with the serrated entrance could damage the glove during insertion into the umbilical wound, which the after is could result in air leakage if glove and wound retractor is used as access device. Therefore, transcervical morcellation is the preferable technique in LESS subtotal hysterectomy.[5]

KEY POINTS

- Tissue retrieval in LESS requires techniques similar to multiport laparoscopy with slight modification.
- Morcellation in LESS myomectomy may be done transumbilically or transvaginally.
- Transvaginal route has advantages over transumbilical route.
- Transcervical morcellation for LESS subtotal hysterectomy.

REFERENCES

1. Heinberg E, Pasic R. Tissue retrieval in endoscopic surgery. In: Pasic RP, Levine RL (Eds). A Practical Manual of Laparoscopy and Minimally Invasive Surgery: A Clinical Cookbook, 2nd edition. United Kingdom: Informa UK Limited; 2007. pp. 239-49.
2. Kim TJ, Lee YY, Kim MJ, et al. Single-port access laparoscopic adnexal surgery. J Minim Invasive Gynecol. 2009;16:612-5.
3. Kim YW, Park BJ, Ro DY, et al. Single-port laparoscopic myomectomy using a new single-port transumbilical morcellation system: initial clinical study. J Minim Invasive Gynecol. 2010;17:587-92.
4. Rosenblatt P, Makai G, DiSciullo A. Laparoscopic supracervical hysterectomy with transcervical morcellation: initial experience. J Minim Invasive Gynecol. 2010;17:331-6.
5. Yoon G1, Kim TJ, Lee YY, et al. Single-port access subtotal hysterectomy with transcervical morcellation: a pilot study. J Minim Invasive Gynecol. 2010;17:78-81.

CHAPTER

86

Suturing Techniques in LESS

B Ramesh, Madhuri V, Aditi Rai

INTRODUCTION

Minimal access surgery has evolved from small multiple incisions (conventional laparoscopy) to single incision [laparoendoscopic single-site (LESS)] to no incision (NOTES). Now almost all abdominal surgical procedures are feasible through laparoscopic approach. Intracorporeal suturing and knot tying is the most challenging and daunting task of laparoscopic surgery which requires a lot of diligence and patience to master. For performance of advanced laparoscopy, intracorporeal suturing is an absolutely essential rate-limiting step with a long learning curve.[1,2]

In laparoendoscopic single-site surgery, the approach to the abdominal cavity is made through a single incision in the umbilicus. The inherent difficulties of loss of triangulation, limited vision and reduced operating space makes intracorporeal suturing a task of herculean proportions for a laparoscopic surgeon venturing into LESS. In this chapter, we will discuss the difficulties, techniques and methods of suturing in LESS.

TECHNICAL COMPLEXITY OF SUTURING IN LESS

Despite the advances in the fields of optics, imaging and instrumentation, laparoscopic suturing and knot tying, entail patience and experience, and are difficult, time consuming, and frustrating[3] more so in LESS.

Reasons for the technical complexity in LESS:

- Restriction of surgeon's vision
- Difficult instrument handling and manipulation
- Lack of tactile perception
- Limited working space
- Need for excellent hand-eye coordination and manual dexterity.[4]
- When the angle between the working instruments is narrow and the working area is limited, ligation and suturing are substantially difficult to perform.
- Inadequate control of the instrument compromising a surgeon's ability to tighten the knot in LESS.

In conventional laparoscopy, position of entry of the optic and other instruments can be appropriately selected according to the type of the surgical procedure to allow comfortable suturing. On the other hand, in LESS the optic and hand instruments enter through the same port in the same plane in parallel. This configuration complicates the surgical procedure and renders suturing difficult.

PRINCIPLES OF LAPAROSCOPIC SUTURING

For effective endosuturing, triadic relationships of port sites are very important, with the optical port in the center and suturing ports on either side. Suturing in traditional laparoscopic surgery is accomplished using two contralateral or ipsilateral ports using needle holders/needle holder and grasping forceps. The port placement in traditional laparoscopic surgery allows for a perfect triangulation, which facilitates laparoscopic suturing **(Fig. 1)**.

Since all instruments in LESS pass through a single incision in the umbilicus, there is lack of triangulation, inline viewing, and instrument crowding at port site. The ideal port position is difficult to achieve in the operating room in all cases in LESS. In fact wide spread acceptance of LESS may be hindered due to these difficulties. It is particularly challenging to form a loop around the hand instrument when there is limited working space and instruments are parallel to each other. The narrow space, and parallel positioning of instruments and the laparoscope permits only to and fro motion in the longitudinal plane of the instruments (inline movement) **(Figs. 2A and B)**.

Some of these problems can be mitigated with articulating instruments. They create internal triangulation in spite of parallel insertion and facilitate loop formation for suturing. Hence, suturing can be performed in spite of these limitations in LESS. Many new instruments and methods have been developed to overcome these difficulties in conventional laparoscopic surgery **(Fig. 2C)**. In this chapter, the techniques which can be adapted in LESS with considerable ease are described.

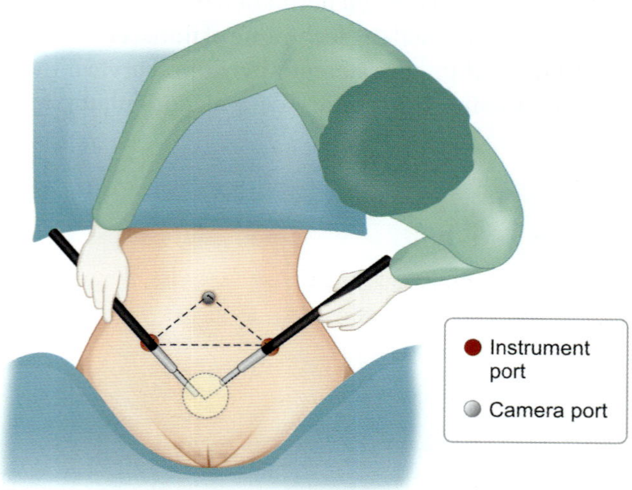

Fig. 1: Port positioning for suturing in multiport laparoscopy.

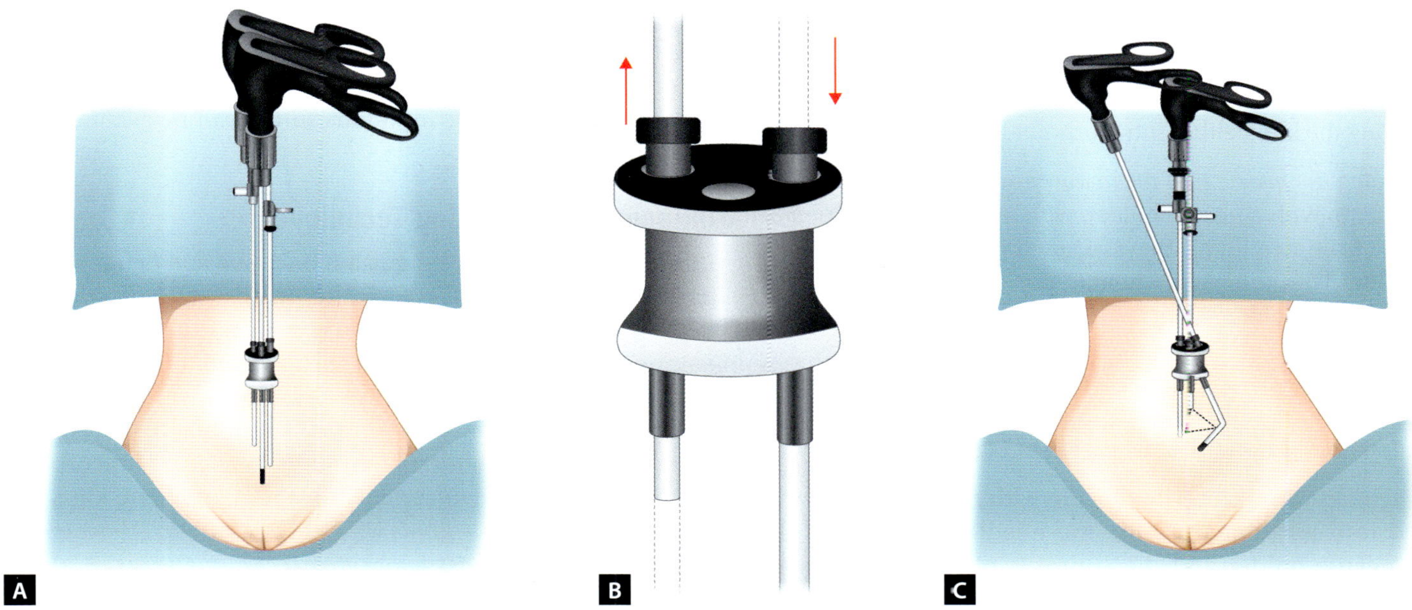

Figs. 2A to C: Instruments through the LESS port for suturing. (A) Showing the narrow angle between instruments in single-port; (B) Showing forward and backward movement of instruments in one plane; and (C) Articulating instrument facilitates triangulation.

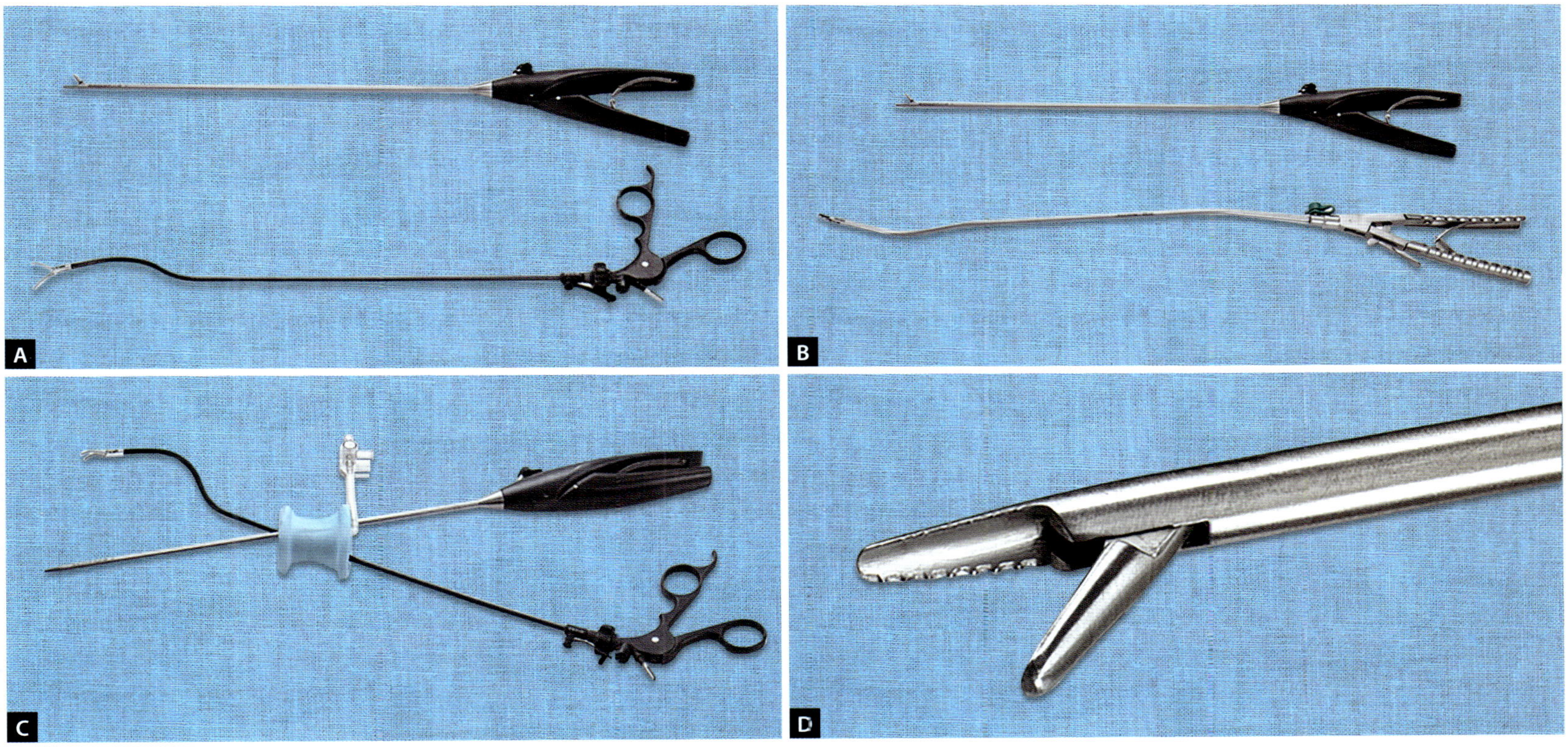

Figs. 3A to D: (A to C) Needle holders for suturing in LESS; (D) Self-righting needle holder from Aesculap, B Braun.

INSTRUMENTATION FOR SUTURING

Apart from the straight graspers and needle holders, specially designed instruments for laparoendoscopic single-site surgery LESS are available, which facilitate suturing.

Articulating instruments: Refer Chapter 81 "Instruments and Ports".

Needle holders ***(Figs. 3A to D):*** An important principle in suturing in the abdomen is that the surgeon should be in control of the needle at all times. In laparotomy, the needle holder can hold a needle securely during suturing. In laparoscopy, it has been difficult to reproduce this great grasping force. The needle tends to angulate and rotate in the laparoscopic needle holder. In the abdomen the needle requires positioning in the needle holder with the aid of another instrument before suturing.[5]

The initial difficulty that the surgeon faces in suturing is to hold the needle in the correct position. As the movement of instruments is only inline, lateral movement or movement independent of the other instrument is difficult. The reusable self-righting needle holders automatically orients the needle vertically, providing both needle and suture manipulation in the same instrument.

STEPS OF SUTURING

The three important steps in endoscopic suturing are introduction of the needle and suture into the abdominal cavity, placing the suture ligature, and tying the knot, either intracorporeally or extracorporeally.

Step 1: Introducing the needle into the abdominal cavity: The needle is held close to the tip with a needle holder, with the curve of the needle along the axis of the needle holder as shown in **Figures 4A and B**. The needle holder with the needle held in position is driven into the 12 mm trocar of the Covidien port or 10 mm trocar if Curcillo and King method is used.

The needle can also be introduced into the peritoneal cavity by holding the suture material 3–4 cm away from the needle hub and driving them into the 10 mm trocar as shown in **Figures 4C to E**.

Step 2: Placing the suture: Once the needle with the suture material is introduced into peritoneal cavity, the needle is held with the self-righting needle holder and the suture is placed in the tissue to be approximated with the help of a grasper in the other hand. An articulating grasper in the other hand is preferred.

Step 3: Knot-tying: The suturing in LESS can be performed as a continuous suturing technique or an interrupted technique. The initial knot of a continuous suture can be accomplished in several ways:[3,6]

- Performing an intracorporeal knot with a needle holder and an assistant needle holder.
- Extracorporeal knot tying by the following methods:
  - Creating a slipknot or a preformed loop on the distal end of the suture (having pierced the tissues with a needle, this one is pulled through the preformed loop, which, after having been tied, functions as a lock).
  - Sliding the knot using Clarke's knot pusher.
- Using special threads furnished with reabsorbable clips.
- Barbed suture with one end knotted before introducing or V-Loc, which is available with a preformed loop.
- Endostitch Autosuture or SILS Stitch device with first knot placed by passing the needle through a preformed loop extracorporeally or knot performed intraperitoneally.

The ideal length of a suture for the intracorporeal performance of a separate stitch is 10 cm, a length that makes the knot-tying maneuvers easier. In the performance of a continuous suture, the thread should be 15 cm long, thus allowing the surgeon a way to accomplish the final knot.[7]

The final knot of a continuous suture can be accomplished using Aberdeen or twist knot.

Intracorporeal Knotting Technique

Intracorporeal knots avoid tension on tissue and hence are most often used to fix tissue and less often for hemostasis since they cannot be tied with the same strength as extracorporeal knots. They are also used for anchoring a running suture, such as used for vaginal vault closure following total laparoscopic hysterectomy, myoma bed closure after myomectomy, peritoneal closure, repair of bladder lacerations, or on tissue that is likely to tear if tension is applied.[3] Intracorporeal knots can be accomplished in various methods like square knot, mayoknot, ligature knot or double knots which are described elsewhere.[8]

Intracorporeal twist knot-tying technique **(Figs. 5 and 6)** is an intracorporeal knotting technique that can be adapted to use in single-port laparoscopic suturing as this technique requires forward and backward hand movements in one plane in other words in line movements of the suturing instruments and can be accomplished with instruments lying parallel to each other as in LESS.

Technique of twist knotting: After passing the needle through the tissue, the needle end of the suture is grasped with the needle holder and rotated around its axis three times, thus forming three loops. After the loops are formed, the suture is released and grasped with the grasper while the needle holder that has the loops around its shaft, grasps the short tail of the suture, pulling it back through the formed loops thus forming a surgeon's knot. Applying tension on both ends of the suture sets the knot that is resistant to slippage and can be secured with an additional square knot.

The intracorporeal knotting can be accomplished in LESS by yet another simple technique similar to the twist knot. This technique consists in holding the needle with its concavity bent downward or, toward the operating surgeon. The curved and rigid structure of the needle allows the needle holder to act on it and makes it possible to perform quickly and simply the execution of the spyres around the needle holder **(Figs. 7 and 8)**.[9,10]

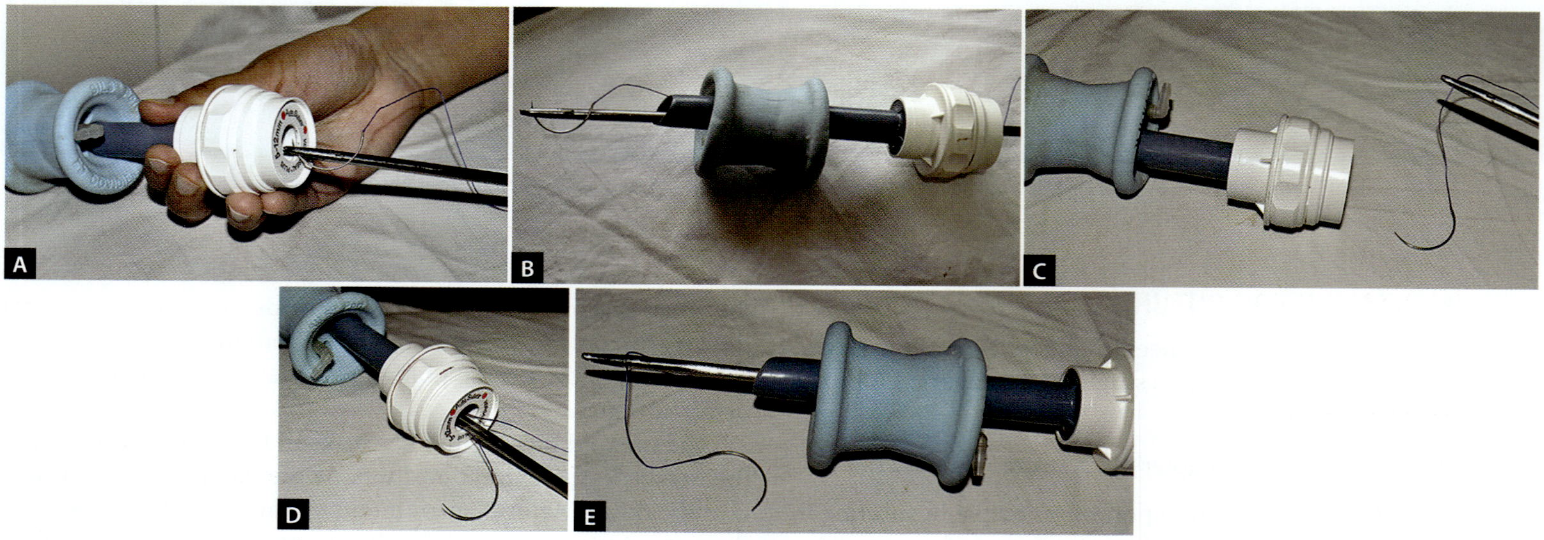

Figs. 4A to E: Needle introduction techniques in LESS. Single-port laparoscopic surgery in gynecology.

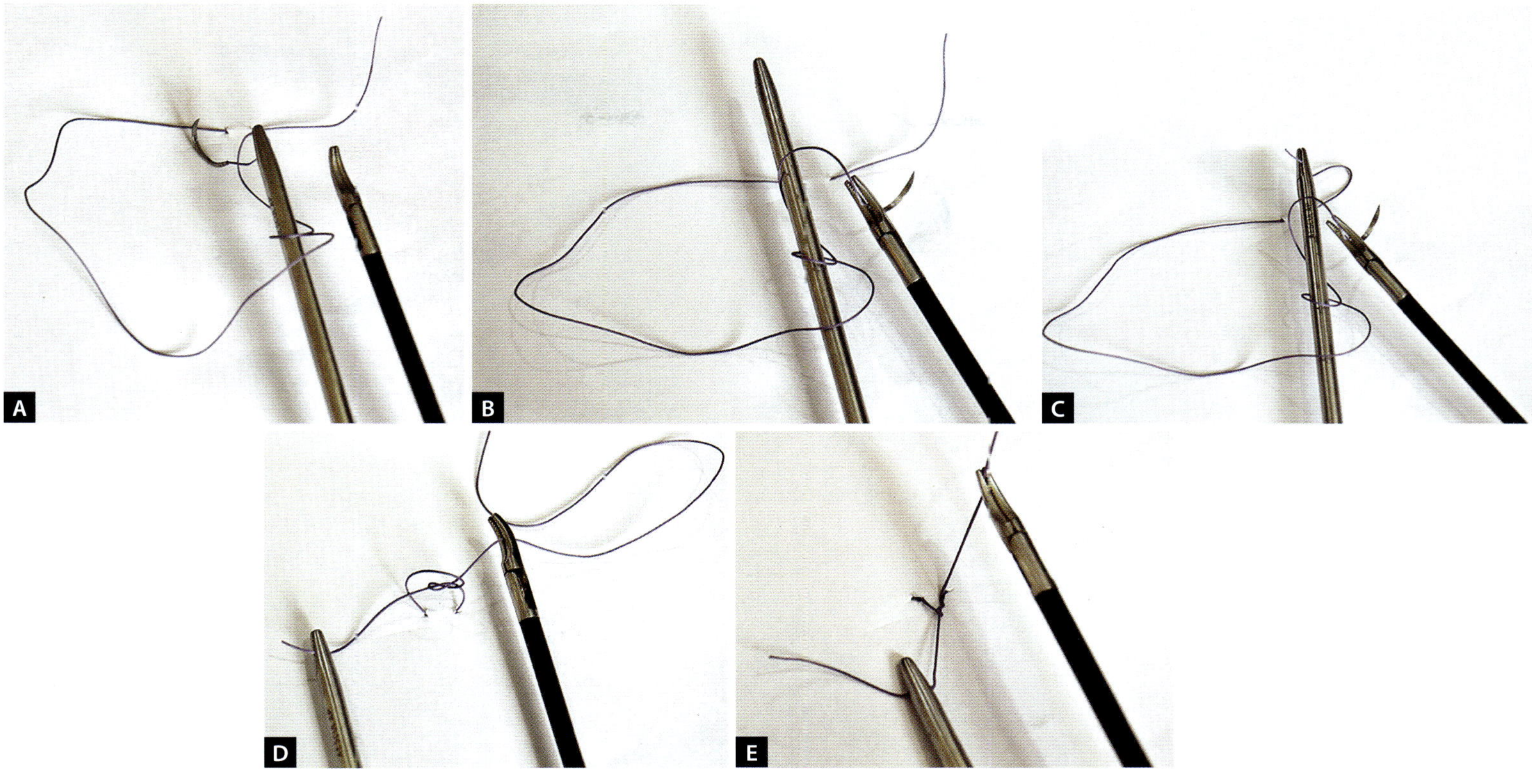

Figs. 5A to E: (A) The long tail of the suture is held with the needle driver 3–4 cm from the hub and a counterclockwise C loop is formed around the needle driver; (B) The suture is released by the needle driver and grasped by the grasper; (C) The suture tail is now held with needle holder and pulled back through the loop; (D) The knot is tied by pulling both ends in opposite directions; (E) The first knot formed. A second clockwise loop is made and the knot is tied in the same fashion.

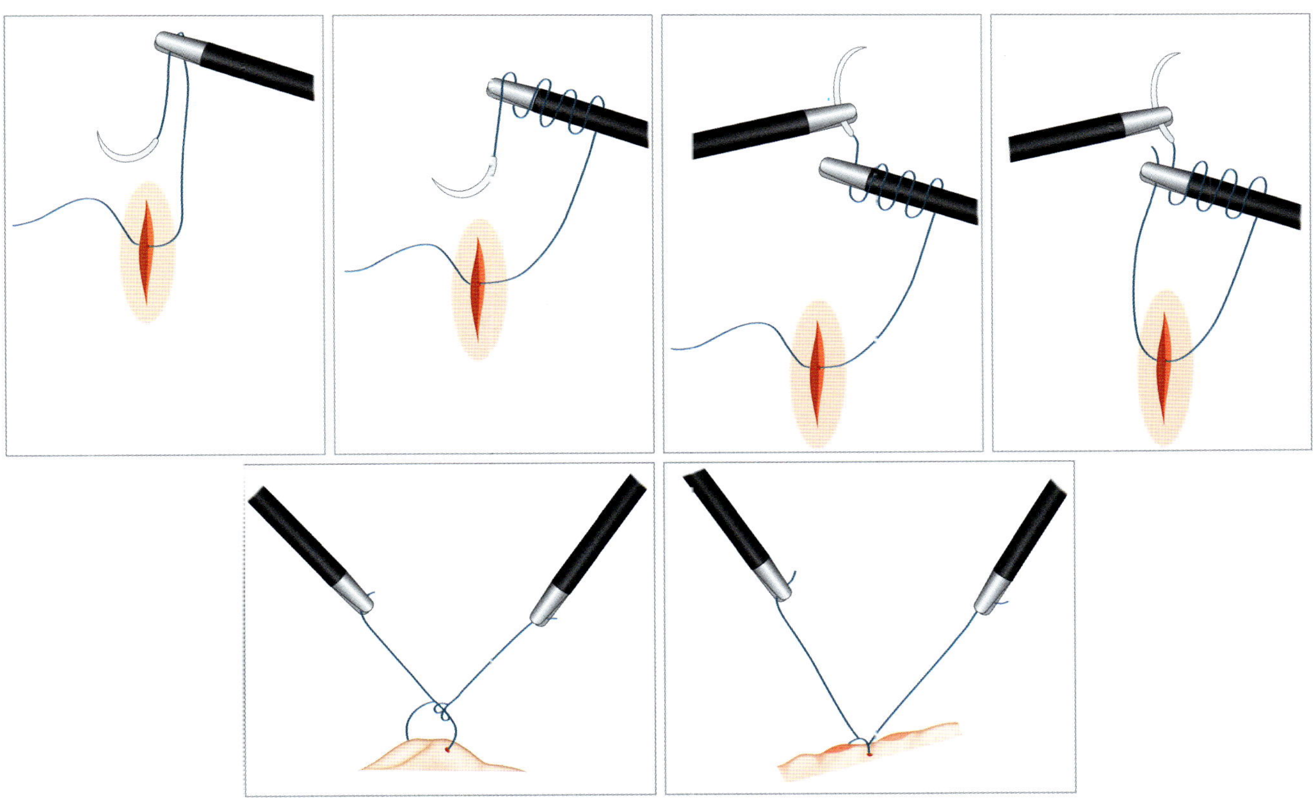

Fig. 6: Internal square knot.

Extracorporeal Knotting Technique for LESS

Extracorporeal knotting technique for LESS: Extracorporeal knot tying by either a preformed loop on the distal end of the suture or sliding the knot using Clarke's knot pusher can be used in LESS surgeries.[3,8]

- Sliding the knot using Clarke's knot pusher is used in LESS in a similar way as described elsewhere.[8]
- A simple method to create a preformed loop is described here. Form a complete loop, be it simple or double, introduce the

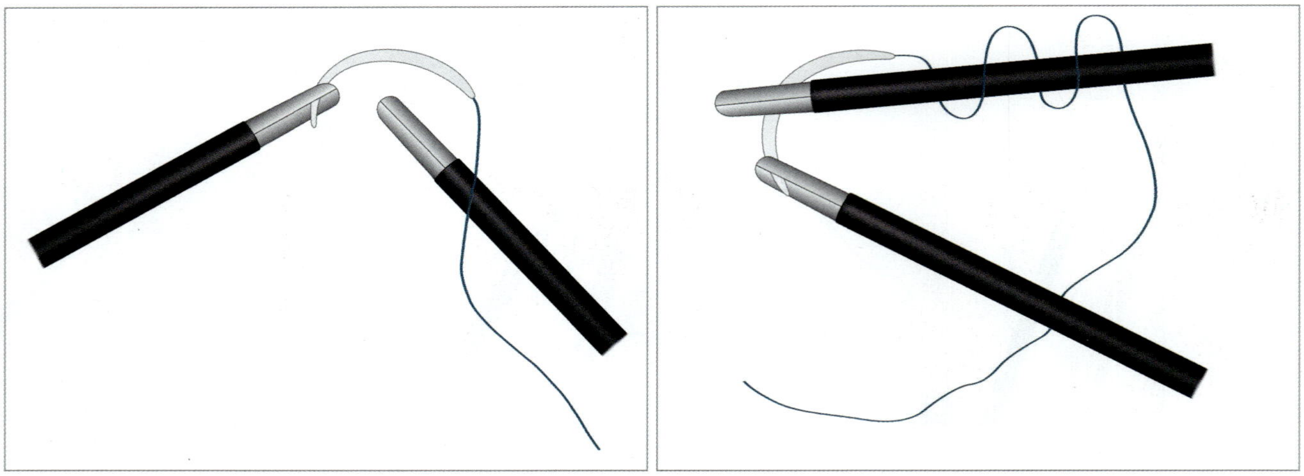

Fig. 7: A simple intracorporeal knotting technique.

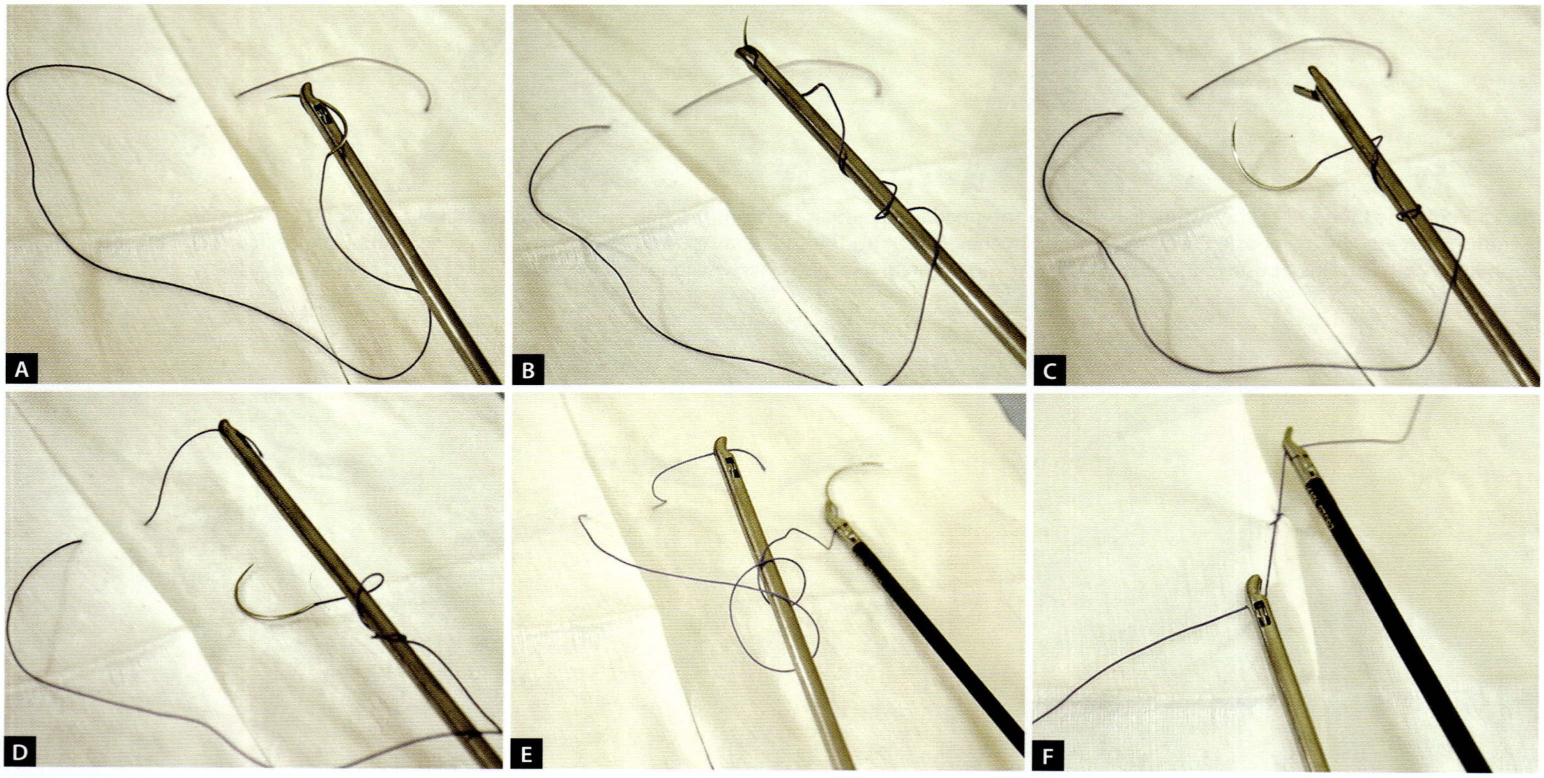

Figs. 8A and F: (A) Hold the needle with its concavity bent downward; (B) Rotate the axis of the needle holder holding the needle in the jaws; (C) Drop the needle held by the jaws of the needle holder; (D and E) The needle holder grasps the tail end and the grasper grasps the suture close to the needle; (F) Knot is formed by applying tension on both ends of suture. Repeat this to perform the second knot.

site b inside the loop in order to generate a new loop inside the already existing one and then the ends of the thread a and c are retracted, keeping in countertraction the end b, which will form the height of the extracorporeally formed preformed loop **(Figs. 9A and B)**. Slide the loop over the needle holder to introduce into the peritoneal cavity for suturing.

REVIEW OF LITERATURE

Toshiaki Endo et al.[11] have devised a remarkably simple knot-tying technique that can be applied during LESS with an access port with a Roticulator and a straight-type needle driver. They determined that, after transfixing the needle, the long tail of the thread should be grasped at around 90° relative to the long axis of tip of the Roticulator, which is articulated at 80°. This automatically forms an ideal C-loop because of gravitation. The authors suggest the needle attached to the long tail should face the distal side from the tip of Roticulator (from the surgeon's perspective) and the apex of the C-loop is then toward the proximal side from the tip of the Roticulator (from the perspective of the surgeon). This thread position facilitates knot-tying. The upper arm of the C-loop should then be entwined by applying a series of axial spinning movements to the rod of the needle driver, during which time the jaws of the needle driver should be kept open so the thread does not slip off of the rod. This technique does not require any special skills and any surgeon able to perform intracorporeal suturing should also be able to easily perform this knotting technique in SILS **(Fig. 10)**.

The "side winding" intracorporeal knot tying technique was described by, Baki Ekci which can be used, even when the surgeon has only a limited view of the scope and instruments. To conduct this

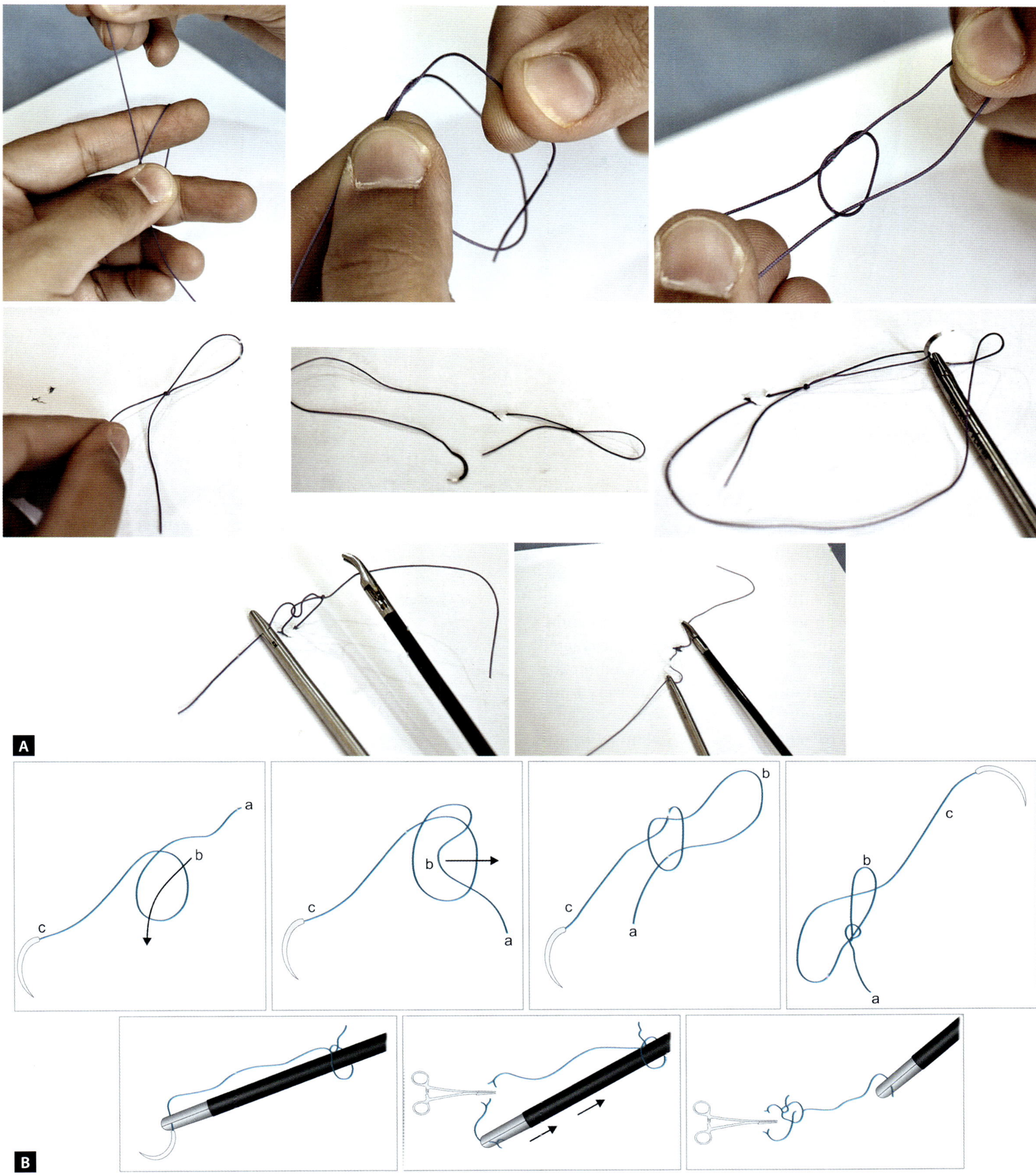

Figs. 9A and B: Technique of accomplishing a preformed loop and its introduction into peritoneal cavity by sliding the loop over the needle driver.

technique the author uses a flexible grasping forceps (Roticulator Endo Grasp) to hold up the tissue and the stitch, and a needle holder. In the first step, the Roticulator Endo Grasp is opened in the knotting area, and the suture is wound around twice. The suture is grasped with the Roticulator instrument at a point a few centimeters distal to the exit of the suture from the tissue. The reef knot is converted into a slip knot by applying distracting forces on the suture material at the two opposite points. After the first knot has been tightened, the instrument is removed, and the procedure is repeated until the desired number of knots has been made.[12]

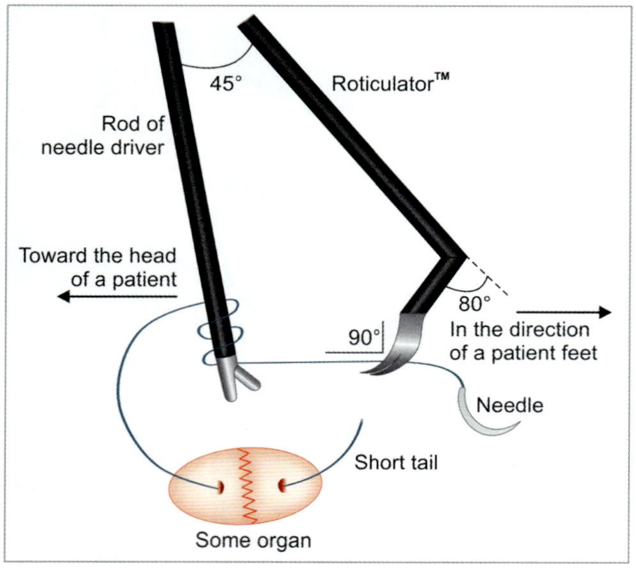

Fig. 10: Roticulator andograsp and suture technique.

CONTINUOUS SUTURING WITH BARBED SUTURE

Most surgeons find the suture technique of interrupted sutures as used in total laparoscopic hysterectomy vaginal vault closure or myoma base closure difficult through a single-port. An alternative suture material called barbed suture has been used to facilitate continuous suturing providing the strength of "continuous interrupted" suture without knots. Bidirectional barbed sutures are created by cutting barbs into the suture with the barbs facing in a direction opposite that of the needle. Barbed suture self-anchors at every 1 mm of tissue, yielding more consistent wound apposition. Because bidirectional barbed sutures self-anchor and are balanced by the countervailing barbs, no knots are required.[13,14] We have used single-handed suturing while using barbed sutures as the sutures are held by the barbs and does not require knotting.

ENDOSTITCH DEVICE/SILS STITCH DEVICE (FIGS. 11 AND 12)[15,16]

Endostitch device/SILS stitch device (US Surgical Corp., Norwalk, Ct 2008) serviced by Covidien is a l0-mm disposable, automatic, and endoscopic suturing device that has been designed to make laparoscopic suturing less frustrating and more user friendly. It is used for both intracorporeal and extracorporeal knot tying using one hand (one handed device). EndoStitch™ single-use suturing device has two jaws and consists of four main parts: a handle, a toggle lever, a needle holder secured inside the jaws and a needle. It is 38 cm long. SILS stitch has a 43-cm shaft length and can be used with ease in LESS surgeries for suturing.[6]

EndoStitch (Fig. 8A)

Needle loader: The suturing needle is loaded from the disposable loading unit.

The needle: The needle is straight, about 9 mm long, has two pointed ends, and the suture attachment is in the middle. It is held in one jaw and can be passed to the other jaw by closing the handle and flipping the toggle levers located on the handle.

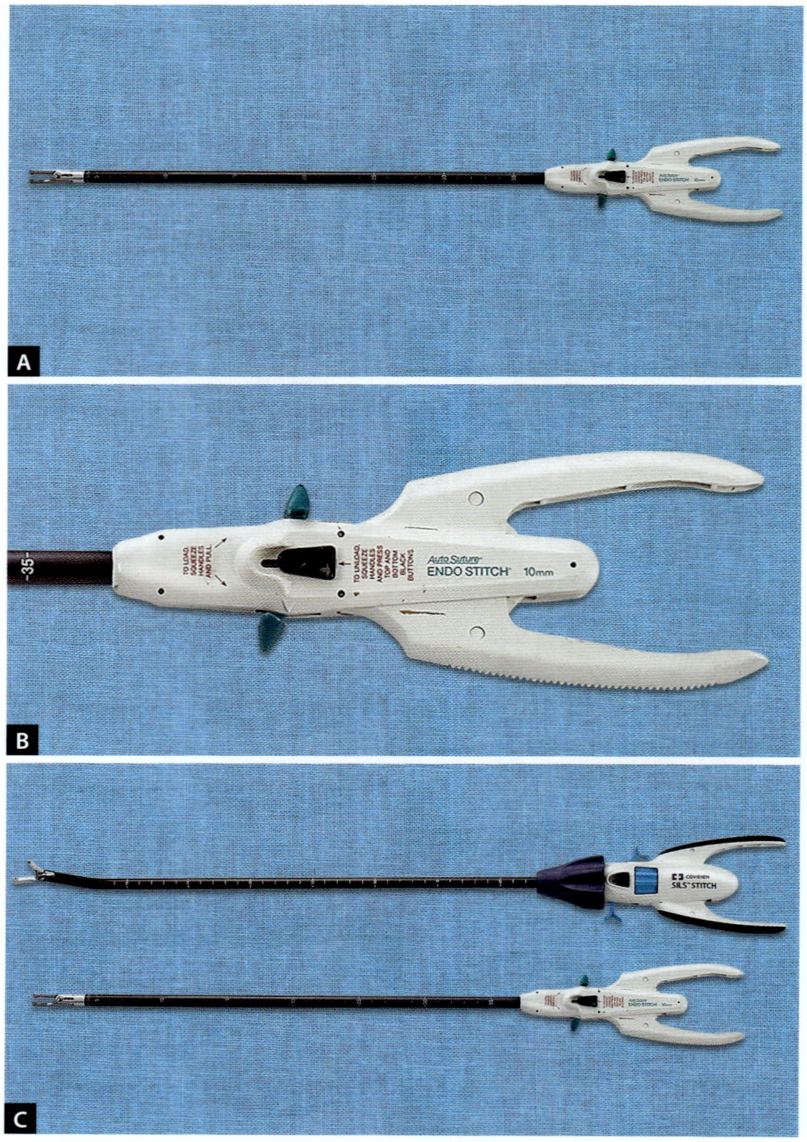

Figs. 11A to C: (A) SILS stitch and Endostitch. The handle (top) and jaws (bottom) of the Endo Stitch laparoscopic suturing instrument. There are two toggle levers on the handle and the upper needle on the jaws, which contains a suture; (B) The handle of endostitch: Note the two toggle levers, two black unloading buttons (one on the front and one on the back) and two handles; (C) SILS stitch and endostitch: Note the articulation possible at the tip of the SILS stitch instrument and the difference in the length of the instruments.

The jaws: The jaws of the EndoStitch instrument are 4 mm wide. To further assist in placing the needle as close to the tissue as possible, the needle is offset to one side of the jaws.

The handle ***(Fig. 8B)****:* The handle section consists of two toggle levers, two black unloading buttons (one on the front and one on the back) and two handles.

The shaft: The shaft of the EndoStitch 10 mm instrument is 36 cm in length to provide enhanced access to the tissue site.

Technique of suturing with EndoStitch/SILS stitch: The Endo stitch may be used to place running or interrupted stitches, intracorporeal or extracorporeal in soft tissue during laparoscopic surgery. The tissue to be sutured is positioned inside the EndoStitch jaws. By pressing the handles, the jaws are closed, driving the needle through the tissue, and flipping the toggle lever, the needle is passed to the opposite jaw.

Releasing the handle opens the jaws and pulls the suture through the tissue, leaving the tail. This device makes suturing easy and fast, and it can be used in a number of ways for knot tying. Aside from cost,

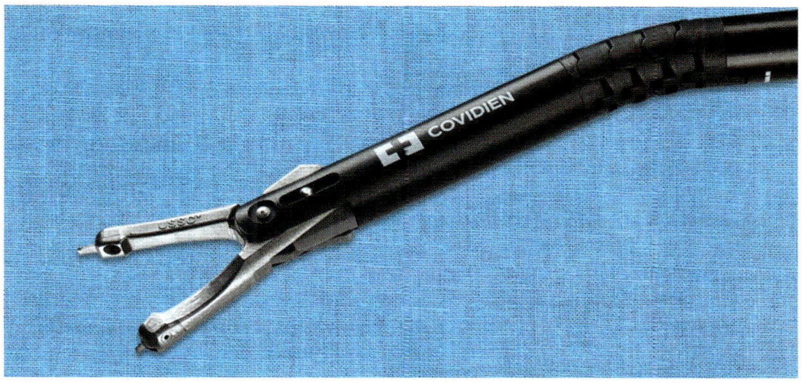

Fig. 12: Jaws of the SILS stitch similar to the jaws of EndoStitch.

a disadvantage of this instrument is difficulty placing the stitch through large pedicles.[17]

The EndoStitch can be effectively used to place extracorporeal knots using the 48 cm polysorb material suture available. The needle is loaded on to the jaws of the endostitch device and the loaded device is introduced into the 10 mm trocar. The free end of the suture is held with the nondominant hand or by an assistant. After placing the suture in the tissue to be approximated, the EndoStitch device is brought out of the trocar and an extracorporeal knot is performed and is slid down using the closed jaws of the EndoStitch.

SILS STITCH ARTICULATING SUTURING DEVICE

The SILS™ Stitch (Covidien, Mansfield, MA) is based on the same technology as the EndoStitch with the added advantage of articulation up to 75° and rotation up to 360°. This enables surgeons to operate in tight spaces during advanced laparoscopic procedures, and to reach

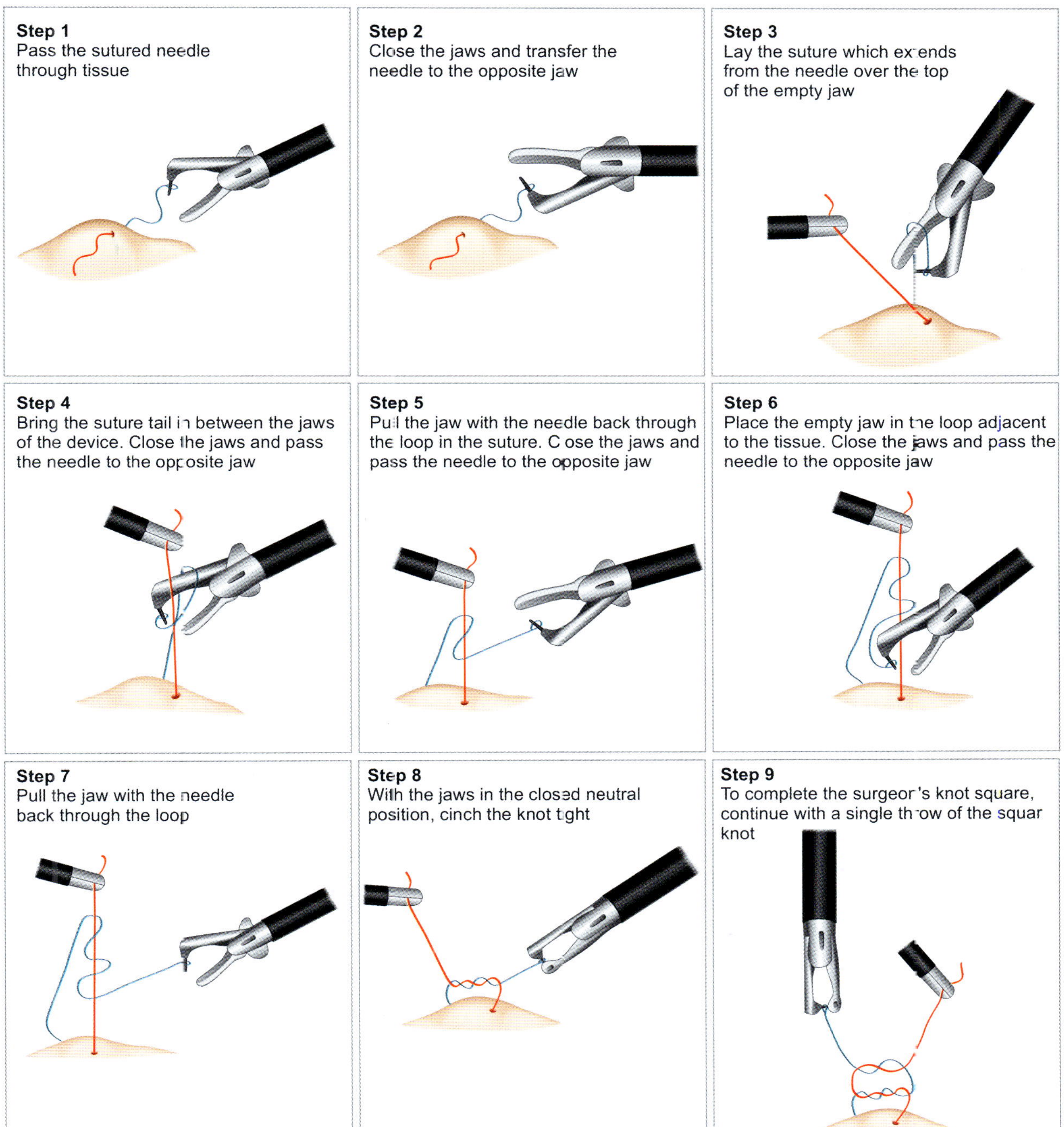

Fig. 13: Intracorporeal knotting technique using Endostitch.

tissues in their natural anatomical position rather than pulling or manipulating tissue into the suturing device.[14]

The longer shaft **(Fig. 8D)** and greater maneuverability enables LESS surgeries. The SILS™ Stitch instrument was designed to be compatible with the current Endo Stitch™ reloads or single-use loading units (SULUs), which include Surgidac™, Polysorb™, Sofsilk™, and Bralon™ sutures. Loading and unloading of the new instrument is almost identical to the loading and unloading of the current Endo Stitch™ device **(Fig. 13)**.

CONCLUSION

Suturing is one of the most trying aspects of conventional laparoscopy requiring a lot of skill, practice and patience. It is to be expected that the same is true of LESS, and to a greater degree. In LESS, suturing can be facilitated by flexible tip endoscopes, articulating instruments, self-righting needle holders, and specialized suturing devices. Also, few of the techniques used for suturing and knot tying in conventional laparoscopy can be modified and incorporated in LESS along with specialized techniques like single-handed suturing. Still, there is great scope for improvement in this area and we believe innovations will simplify the art of suturing further. This will definitely escalate the adoption of LESS by many more laparoscopic surgeons.

KEY POINTS

- Suturing in LESS requires a great degree of skill and manual dexterity.
- Specialized instruments and optics facilitate suturing.
- Automated suturing devices can enable easier suturing in LESS.

REFERENCES

1. Kawano T, Nishikage T. Open-jaw technique in laparoscopic knot tying. Surg Endosc. 2008;22:269-70.
2. Croce E, Olmi S. Intracorporeal knot-tying and suturing techniques in laparoscopic surgery: technical details. JSLS. 2000;4:17-22.
3. Meilahn JE. The need for improving laparoscopic suturing and knot tying. J Laparoendosc Surg. 1992;2:267.
4. Ekci B. A simple technique for knot tying in single incision laparoscopic surgery (SILS). Clinics (Sao Paulo). 2010;65:1055-7.
5. Henry Clarke suturing and ligating history of operative laparoscopy: The first thirty years: © January 15, 2000.
6. Sanfilippo JS, Solnik, MJ. Operative laparoscopy. Glob Libr Women's Med. 2008; DOI 10.3843/GLOWM.10088.
7. Croce E, Olmi S, Azzola M, et al. Knot-tying and suturing technique in laparoscopic surgery. Eur J Coelio Surg. 1997;3:35-40.
8. Khullar R.. Endo suturing and tissue approximation in laparoscopic surgery, www.iages.org.in/media/files/c_57_64. pdf [Last accessed January, 2020].
9. Ko ST, Airan MC. Therapeutic laparoscopic suturing techniques. Surg Endosc. 1992;6:41-6.
10. Pennings JL, Kenyon T, Swanstrom L. The knit stitch. An improved method of laparoscopic knot tying. Surg Endosc. 1995;9:537-40.
11. Endo T, Nagasawa K, Umemura K, et al. A remarkably easy knot-tying technique for single-incision laparoscopic surgery with the SILS port for gynecologic diseases. J Minim Invasive Gynecol. 2011;18:500-2.
12. Ekçi B. A simple technique for knot tying in single incision laparoscopic surgery (SILS), Clinics (Sao Paulo). 2010;65:1055-7.
13. Einarsson JI, Chavan NR, Suzuki Y, et al. Use of bidirectional barbed suture in laparoscopic myomectomy: evaluation of perioperative outcomes, safety, and efficacy. J Minim Invasive Gynecol. 2011;18:92-5.
14. Langebrekke A, Qvigstad E. Total laparoscopic hysterectomy with single-port access without vaginal surgery. J Minim Invasive Gynecol. 2009;16:609-11.
15. Hart S. The benefits of automated suturing devices in gynecologic endoscopic surgeries: the Endo Stitch and SILS Stitch. Surg Technol Int. 2012;22:159-64.
16. Endostitch product manual. www.autosuture.com.
17. Pasic R, Levine RL. Laparoscopic suturing and ligation techniques. J Am Assoc Gynecol Laparosc. 1995;3:67-79.

CHAPTER

87

Vaginal Route Single-site Surgery (Transvaginal NOTES)

B Ramesh, Aditi Rai

INTRODUCTION

Minimally invasive surgery has moved from the concept of decreasing the size of incision to almost scarless surgery. Laparoendoscopic single-site (LESS) is a step in this direction as the configuration of the umbilicus hides the single incision scar. Natural orifice transluminal endoscopic surgery (NOTES) is an emerging technique of surgery that completely eliminates abdominal incisions and incision related complications such as wound infections, incisional hernia, postoperative pain, and adhesions.[1]

The concept of natural orifice surgery refers to access through a natural opening in the body to perform intra-abdominal surgery. While the NOTES working group includes transgastric peritoneal access, NESA (New European Surgical Academy), the first European-based NOS working group has explored the transdouglas route. The difference between the terms "NOS" and "NOTES" is not accidental. "T" in NOTES stands for transluminal. NOS includes NOTES because it refers to all surgical procedures performed through all body openings.[2,3] The most commonly used approaches for NOTES are:

- *Transgastric approach:* The abdominal surgeries are performed though the lumen of the stomach. A double channel endoscope is used and procedures are performed after making a gastrostomy. Procedures like appendectomy, cholecystectomy, and tubal occlusion have been tried with this approach. The problem with this approach is difficulty in closure of the gastrostomy due to improper visualization. A detailed description of transgastric NOTES is beyond the scope of this chapter.
- *Transvaginal approach:* Single-port approach for intra-abdominal procedures though the pouch of Douglas **(Fig. 1)**.

Note: Transumbilical single incision surgery (also known as E-NOTES) is now classified as laparoendoscopic single-site surgery or LESS. In this chapter we will briefly discuss the current status of transvaginal NOTES procedures.

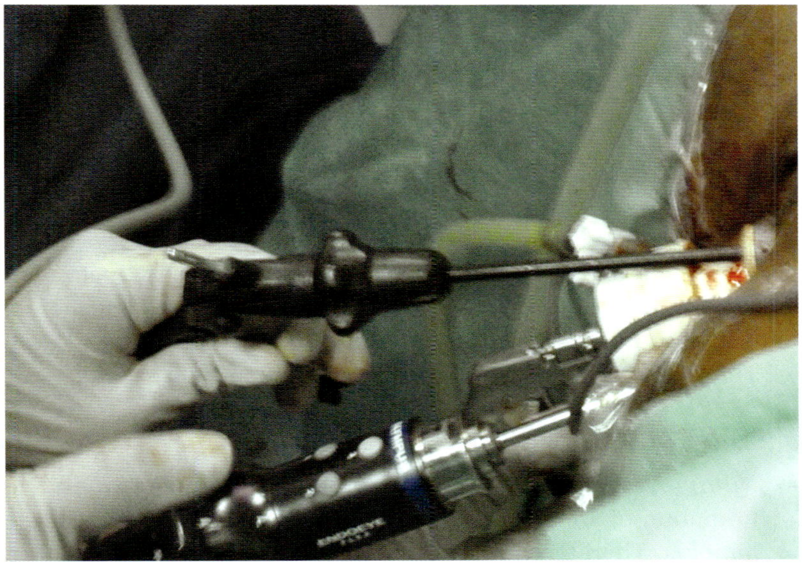

Fig. 1: Transvaginal natural orifice transluminal endoscopic surgery (NOTES).

ADVANTAGES OF VAGINAL ROUTE

- *Simple entry:* The incision into the vagina through the posterior fornix is easy, can be performed with available instruments, and is under vision. Many procedures have been performed through the vaginal route by gynecologists over the years. The transgastric route in comparison is complex and requires endoscopic guidance for entry through the mouth, esophagus, and stomach.
- *Adequate working space:* The dimensions of the pouch of Douglas have been measured toward its routine use in surgical procedures. The physiological diameter of the pouch of Douglas was found to range between 20 and 34 mm[4] which is suited to operative intervention.
- *Flexibility of vaginal wall and ligaments:* As the sacrouterine ligaments have a lateral sway, instruments with a wider diameter can be introduced into the peritoneal cavity without causing any mechanical damage to the posterior wall of the vaginal wall and its attached structures.[5] The vaginal walls allow easy maneuverability of the instruments.
- *Straight view:* For upper abdominal procedures like cholecystectomy, the transvaginal access provides a direct end on view through the endoscope and orientation is easier. But, because of the same reason, procedures in the pelvis become more difficult.
- *Easy closure:* The vaginal walls generally heal without scarring. The vagina can be closed from outside with simple suturing under vision without the need of expensive devices.
- *Less risk of vascular injury:* The introduction of the instruments is done under vision and parallel to the major blood vessels, thus minimizing the risk of injury.[2]
- *Lower insufflation pressure:* Because the traditional 14 mm Hg CO_2 pressure is not needed for the introduction of the device, the working pressure in vaginal NOTES is less, not exceeding 8–9 mm Hg. This will enable procedures to be performed with epidural anesthesia.[2] In future, gasless laparoscopy is a possibility if abdomen can be lifted with an effective device.

- *Surgeon's comfort:* As any other vaginal procedure, the surgeon can sit and perform the procedure, increasing surgeon's comfort.[2]
- *Easier disinfection:* The risk of contamination of peritoneal cavity in this route is less than the transgastric route as vagina can be cleaned and disinfected more easily than mouth, esophagus, and stomach.[2]

DISADVANTAGES OF VAGINAL ROUTE

- Though entry through the pouch of Douglas is simple and routinely practiced by gynecologists for vaginal procedures like hysterectomy, there is inherent risk of injury to any structure like bowel adherent adjacent to the site. To overcome this, a mini laparoscope at the umbilicus to guide entry can be used (Hybrid NOTES). This allows the scope and instruments to be introduced under vision.
- There is concern about scarring and formation of adhesions in the vagina following the procedure. This can lead to dyspareunia or may interfere with fertility. This may preclude its use in nulliparous patients.
- In multipara, the laxity of the vaginal wall may interfere with the maintenance of pneumoperitoneum because of persistent leakage of gas.
- For performance of gynecological procedures, the view is not direct. The endoscope has to be retroflexed to obtain proper visualization of the operative field. This requires proper training and one there is a long learning curve.
- This route cannot be used in all patients and in male patients.

CONTRAINDICATIONS

- *Nulliparous patients:* There is concern about postoperative formation of adhesions leading to iatrogenic infertility in these patients. Therefore, transvaginal NOTES should be avoided in patients desiring future fertility.
- *Severe endometriosis:* In cases of severe endometriosis with obliteration of the pouch of Douglas, entry through vaginal route carries risk of injury to adjacent structures and should be avoided.
- *Adhesions in the pouch of Douglas:* A history of previous pelvic inflammatory disease or previous surgery for pelvic disease should be considered as a contraindication for this route.
- *Active vaginal infection:* Vaginitis or vaginal discharge should be actively treated aggressively with local treatment and oral antibiotics to clear the infection before surgery. If entry is performed in presence of infection, it can spread to the peritoneal cavity leading to peritonitis.
- *Complex surgical procedures:* Single incision access surgeries have an inherent problem of lack of triangulation. In cases of transvaginal NOTES, the view is retroflected. These factors preclude the performance of complicated surgeries by this route.[6]
- *Suspected adnexal lesions:* In suspicious adnexal masses, full surgical staging is mandatory irrespective of the route employed. Transvaginal NOTES may not allow optimal surgical staging and rupture of the mass with spillage of tumor cells is a distinct possibility.[6]

TECHNICAL DIFFICULTIES

As NOTES involves the use of operating instruments in line with the light source and endoscope, difficulties associated with poor visibility, maintenance of spatial orientation, maneuverability, and grasping are evident.[2] These technical difficulties are well demonstrated in the literature for the transvaginal NOTES.[7-9]

- There is limited control of instruments during surgery.
- The instruments are inserted through the two working channels of the flexible endoscopes, arriving in parallel into the peritoneal cavity. There is lack of triangulation, which restricts movements and manipulation.
- The endoscope does not stabilize intra-abdominally; leads to repeated loss of view of the operative field. This reduces the efficiency of the surgeon and increases operative time.
- Though in upper abdominal surgeries such as cholecystectomy end on view is obtained in transvaginal NOTES, the performance of pelvic procedures becomes difficult because of the same reason. In pelvic procedures a Retroflected view is obtained, which is an upside down and reversed image. It is difficult of the surgeon to visually analyze the movement of the instruments and the endoscope. And sometimes only a lateral view of the target tissue is possible. Thereby, upper abdominal procedures may be easier to perform than pelvic procedures with this technique.

PROCEDURE

For transvaginal NOTES, patient is put in lithotomy position. Any infection of the vagina has to be ruled out. Vagina is cleaned with povidone-iodine solution. The posterior wall of the vagina is retracted with a Sims speculum and anterior wall with an anterior vaginal wall retractor. The posterior lip of the cervix is held by Allis forceps and is retracted anteriorly. This exposes the posterior fornix. Vaginal mucosa in the posterior fornix is opened by a 2-cm incision in the pouch of Douglas region at the junction of the cervix and vagina. The peritoneum of the pouch of Douglas is identified by sharp dissection and opened. The access port is then inserted and peritoneal cavity is insufflated with CO_2. The transvaginal access can also be performed under laparoscopic guidance to rule out any adhesion or obliteration of the pouch of Douglas.

TRANSDOUGLAS ENDOSCOPIC DEVICE[2,5]

Because of the difficulties and technical challenges in performance of NOTES with available instrumentation, a new device known as the Transdouglas Endoscopic Device (TED) has been developed. The investigators believe that the performance of NOTES transvaginally requires instruments that are configured according to pelvic anatomy.

This device has a diameter of 35 mm and it consists of working channels in sizes from 3 mm to 5 mm in diameter, integrated with insufflation and a control system. The device has two moveable joints which enables the TED to form an "S" or a "U" shape. The "S" shape is designed for procedures in the upper abdomen and the "U" form for operations in the pelvis. Flexibility and wide optic vision are the two important features of this device. Still work is being done to determine the surgical methodology, choice of procedures and patient and feasibility of this device.

The expected disadvantages of the transdouglas approach using the TED:[2,5]

1. For morcellation, a second abdominal entry is required as it will not be possible to introduce it through the pouch of Douglas with its limited dimensions.
2. As no other instrument can be introduced simultaneously, all necessary components have to be incorporated in the device to be able to perform procedures.

APPLICATION OF NOTES IN GYNECOLOGY

The transvaginal NOTES approach utilized by surgeons and urologists to perform cholecystectomy, appendectomy and nephrectomy;[10,11] this approach has not become popular in gynecology because of the greater technical difficulty in performing surgery in the pelvis. The technique of transvaginal hydrolaparoscopy uses specially designed instruments applied via the posterior vaginal fornix using fluid medium has been used for diagnostic procedures in infertility cases.[12,13] There is no report of it being used for more complex procedures.

Recently two reports of transvaginal NOTES in adnexal procedures have been published. Ahn et al.[14] used transvaginal NOTES to perform adnexal procedures in 10 patients. They concluded that surgery for benign adnexal pathology was feasible through this approach and comparable to LESS and multiport surgery in terms of postoperative pain and hospital stay. The authors suggested that performance of transvaginal NOTES can be performed by a surgeon well versed with transumbilical single-port laparoscopy in properly selected patients. They suggested that care must be taken to prevent inadvertent laceration of the rectum, blood vessels or the ureter by excessive force. The authors also suggested that Trendelenburg position is preferred to prevent rectal injury.

Lee et al.[15] published a study on transvaginal NOTES for adnexal procedures using surgical glove and wound retractor. Their preliminary results showed that transvaginal NOTES is feasible in selected patients.

CONCLUSION

Transvaginal NOTES is still in the process of evolution. It use in gynecologic procedures is still in the initial stages. This is because of restricted view and technical difficulties in operations in the pelvis with NOTES approach. It may be feasible in carefully selected patients; but more studies are required to evaluate its true place in minimally invasive surgery.

REFERENCES

1. McGee MF, Rosen MJ, Marks J, et al. A primer on natural orifice transluminal endoscopic surgery: building a new paradigm. Surg Inn. 2006;13:86-93.
2. Stark M, Benhidjeb T. Natural orifice surgery: transdouglas surgery—a new concept. JSLS. 2008;12:295-8.
3. Stark M, Benhidjeb T. Natural Orifice Surgery working group [letter to the editor]. Gastrointest Endosc. 2007;66:208-10.
4. Harlaar JJ, Kleinrensink GJ, Hop WC, et al. The anatomical limits of the posterior vaginal vault toward its use as route for intra-abdominal procedures. Surg Endosc. 2008;22:1910-2.
5. Stark M, Di Renzo GC, Benhidjeb T. Natural orifice surgery (NOS)—toward a single-port transdouglas approach for intra-abdominal procedures. Eur J Obstet Gynecol Reprod Biol. 2010;148:114-7.
6. Kondo W, Branco AW, Branco Filho AJ, et al. Transvaginal Natural Orifice Transluminal Endoscopic Surgery (Notes): Surgical Technique and Results. Adv Gynecol Endosc. 2011.
7. Branco AW, Branco Filho AJ, Kondo W, et al. Hybrid transvaginal nephrectomy. Eur Urol. 2008;53:1290-4.
8. Branco Filho AJ, Noda RW, Kondo W, et al. Initial experience with hybrid transvaginal cholecystectomy. Gastrointest Endosc. 2007;66:1245-8.
9. Kondo W, Noda RW, Branco AW, et al. Transvaginal endoscopic tubal sterilization. J Laparoendosc Adv Surg Tech A. 2009;19:59-61.
10. Horgan S, Cullen JP, Talamini MA, et al Natural orifice surgery: initial clinical experience. Surg Endosc. 2009;23:1512-8.
11. Kaouk JH, White WM, Goel RK, et al. NOTES transvaginal nephrectomy: first human experience. Urology. 2009;74:5-8.
12. Darai E, Dessolle L, Lecuru F, et al. Transvaginal hydrolaparoscopy compared with laparoscopy for the evaluation of infertile women: a prospective comparative blind study. Hum Reprod. 2000;15:2379-82.
13. Moore ML, Cohen M, Liu GY. Experience with 109 cases of transvaginal hydrolaparoscopy. J Am Assoc Gynecol Laparosc. 2003;10:282-5.
14. Ahn KH, Song JY, Kim SH, et al. Transvaginal single-port natural orifice transluminal endoscopic surgery for benign uterine adnexal pathologies. J Minim Invasive Gynecol. 2012;19:631-5.
15. Chyi-Long Lee, Kai-Yun Wu, Hsuan Su, et al. Transvaginal natural-orifice transluminal endoscopic surgery (NOTES) in adnexal procedures. J Minim Invasive Gynecol. 2012;19:509-13.

Index

Page numbers followed by *b* refer to box, *f* refer to figure, *fc* refer to flowchart, and *t* refer to table

C

G

H

M

N

Q

R

S